Clinical Medicine

Clinical Medicine

A textbook for medical students and doctors

Second Edition

Edited by

Parveen J Kumar BSc, MD, FRCP

*Senior Lecturer, Medical College of St Bartholomew's Hospital, London, and
Honorary Consultant Physician, St Bartholomew's and Homerton Hospitals, London*

and

Michael L Clark MD, FRCP

*Senior Lecturer, Medical College of St Bartholomew's Hospital, London and
Consultant Physician, St Bartholomew's Hospital, London*

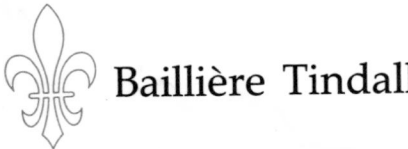 Baillière Tindall

This book is printed on acid free paper.

Baillière Tindall 24–28 Oval Road
W.B. Saunders London NW1 7DX

The Curtis Center
Independence Square West
Philadelphia, PA 19106–3399

55 Horner Avenue
Toronto, Ontario M8Z 4X6, Canada

Harcourt Brace Jovanovich (Australia) Pty Ltd,
30–52 Smidmore St
Marrickville, NSW 2204, Australia

Harcourt Brace Jovanovich Japan Inc.
Ichibancho Central Building, 22–1 Ichibancho
Chiyoda-ku, Tokyo 102, Japan

First Edition published 1987

Second Edition 1990

Typeset by Columns Type Design and Production Services, Reading
Printed in Great Britain by Cambus Litho, East Kilbride, Scotland

British Library Cataloguing in Publication Data

Clinical Medicine. 2nd Edn.
  1. Pathology   2. Medicine
  I. Kumar, PJ   II. Clark, ML
  616   RB111

ISBN 0–7020–1391–9

Contents

List of Contributors

LRI Baker MA, MD, FRCP,
Consultant Physician,
Department of Nephrology,
St Bartholomew's Hospital,
London
Renal disease

A John Camm BSc, MD, FRCP, FACC,
Professor of Clinical Cardiology,
St George's Hospital Medical School,
London
Cardiovascular disease

WR Cattell MD, FRCP, FRCP(E),
Physician and Senior Consultant Nephrologist,
St Bartholomew's Hospital,
London
Renal disease; Water, electrolyte and acid-base homeostasis

AW Clare MD, FRCPsych, FRCPI,
Professor of Clinical Psychiatry,
Trinity College Dublin;
Medical Director,
St Patrick's Hospital,
Dublin
Psychological medicine

Michael L Clark MD, FRCP,
Senior Lecturer,
Medical College of St Bartholomew's Hospital;
Consultant Physician,
Department of Gastroenterology,
St Bartholomew's Hospital,
London
Nutrition; Gastroenterology; Liver, biliary tract and pancreatic diseases; Environmental disorders

Charles RA Clarke MB, BChir, FRCP,
Consultant Neurologist,
St Bartholomew's Hospital and Whipps Cross Hospital,
London
Environmental disorders; Neurology and muscle disease

Diana Cundell BSc,
Research Assistant,
Academic Department of Respiratory Medicine,
Medical College of St Bartholomew's Hospital,
London
Immunology

Robert J Davies MA, MD, FRCP,
Reader in Respiratory Medicine,
Academic Department of Respiratory Medicine,
Medical College of St Bartholomew's Hospital,
London
Immunology; Respiratory disease

Paul L Drury MA, MRCP,
Consultant Physician,
Diabetic Unit,
King's College Hospital and Greenwich District Hospital
London
Endocrinology

MJG Farthing MD, FRCP,
Wellcome Senior Lecturer and Honorary Consultant Physician,
Department of Gastroenterology,
Medical College of St Bartholomew's Hospital,
London
Infectious diseases and tropical medicine

EAM Gale MA, MB, FRCP,
Senior Lecturer and Consultant Physician,
Director, Department of Diabetes and Immunogenetics,
Medical College of St Bartholomew's Hospital,
London
Diabetes and other disorders of metabolism

RN Greenwood BSc(Eng), ACGI, MSc, MBChB, MRCP,
Consultant Nephrologist,
Lister Hospital,
Stevenage
Renal disease

CJ Hinds FRCP, FFARCS,
Consultant and Senior Lecturer,
Department of Anaesthesia and Intensive Care,
St Bartholomew's Hospital,
London
Intensive care

EC Huskisson, MD, FRCP,
Senior Lecturer and Consultant Physician,
Department of Rheumatology,
St Bartholomew's Hospital,
London
Rheumatology and bone disease

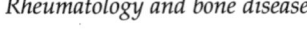

JDT Kirby FRCP,
Consultant Physician,
Department of Dermatology,
St Bartholomew's Hospital,
London
Dermatology

Parveen J Kumar BSc, MD, FRCP,
Senior Lecturer,
Medical College of St Bartholomew's Hospital;
Honorary Consultant Physician,
Department of Gastroenterology,
St Bartholomew's and Homerton Hospitals
London
Genetics and molecular biology; Gastroenterology;
Liver, biliary tract and pancreatic diseases

David A Levison MD, FRCPath,
Professor of Clinical Histopathology,
UMDS Guy's Hospital
London
Histopathology

JS Malpas DPhil, FRCP, FRCR,
Professor of Medical Oncology and
Director, Imperial Cancer Research Fund,
Department of Medical Oncology,
Medical College of St Bartholomew's Hospital,
London
Diseases of the blood; Medical oncology

MF Murphy MD, MRCP, MRCPath,
Senior Lecturer and Honorary Consultant in
Haematology,
Department of Haematology,
Medical College of St Bartholomew's Hospital,
London
Diseases of the blood

RM Pearson MA, MB, MRCP,
Consultant Physician (Clinical Pharmacology),
Harold Wood Hospital;
Senior Lecturer,
Department of Clinical Pharmacology,
Medical College of St Bartholomew's Hospital,
London
Poisoning

DDK Rolston MD, MNAMS, DM,
Associate Professor of Gastroenterology,
Department of Gastroenterology and
Wellcome Research Unit,
Christian Medical College Hospital,
Vellore, India
Infectious diseases and tropical medicine

P Turner MD, FRCP,
Professor of Clinical Pharmacology,
Medical College of St Bartholomew's Hospital,
London
Adverse drug reactions

WF Jackson MA, MB, BChir, FRCP,
Medical Producer, British Medical Television;
Executive Producer, Royal Society of Medicine Television Producer;
Formerly Honorary Consultant; Department of Medicine,
Guy's Hospital, London;
Formerly Editorial Director, Medicine International, Oxford

Editorial Consultant to the First Edition

Preface to the First Edition

There must be a good reason to write a new textbook of medicine when there are already a number on the market. It seemed to us that none of those currently available adequately conveyed the detail and background needed for medical practice in the late 1980s and 1990s. We have tried to strike a balance between exciting new developments in medical research and the vast quantity of established fact that needs to be absorbed by today's student. For this reason each chapter attempts to link scientific advances with clinical practice so that the management of disease can be based on sound physiological concepts.

This book is designed for both medical students and practising doctors and we have tried to produce a detailed but comprehensible text that bridges the gap between the purely introductory and the larger reference works. Tropical diseases have been included, and because the book will have a worldwide distribution we have discussed the presentation of disease as seen in developing countries. Disorders seen only in childhood have been excluded as these are well covered in other texts and would make this book too large. However, there are chapters on intensive care, nutrition, adverse drug reactions, poisoning and environmental medicine, which are often neglected yet play an important role in modern medical practice. There is inevitably an enormous chapter on infectious diseases but we felt that a description of all infectious agents should be included for quick reference; this chapter also contains basic information on antibiotic chemotherapy and a section on epidemiology and host resistance. A short chapter on genetics, molecular biology and immunology provides the basic principles of these subjects. Today's clinical students will have covered much of this in their preclinical course, but we hope that established practitioners will find it a useful introduction. Specific genetic and immunological disorders are covered in appropriate chapters.

We have concentrated on the management of disease but, within the text, have highlighted details of practical procedures and emergency therapy so that this book will be an invaluable companion in clinical practice. The practising clinician can use the book for reference or as a quick and easy guide to the management of an individual patient. Each chapter contains many tables and figures as an aid to learning. There are many cross-references, so that it is easy to move through different parts of the book to pursue different aspects of a particular topic and repetition has been minimized.

The contributors are all actively engaged in both clinical and research work, so the text has been written by clinicians who are not only in the forefront of medical advance but who also do ward rounds and outpatient clinics. At the time of writing all the contributors were working at St Bartholomew's Hospital, London, and thus combine a unified teaching approach with high academic standards.

We would like to thank all our colleagues for their hard work and cooperation and also our families and the many friends who have supported us during the preparation of this book.

Parveen Kumar
Michael Clark

Preface to the Second Edition

This edition has become necessary because of the rapid acceleration in medical knowledge that has taken place over the last three years. The book has become a 'standard' text in many medical colleges throughout the world and we have therefore had the benefit of considerable feedback on the first innovative edition. We have also conducted our own survey amongst students, junior medical staff, consultants and general practitioners. As a result of this consultation we have kept the basic format intact but each chapter has been carefully scrutinized to remove redundant material and to insert new advances. For example, Chapter 1 has had some rare infective disorders removed, but the whole section on HIV infection (AIDS) has been expanded.

We have tried to keep the book the same length, but inevitably there has been some increase in pages, due to more figures, X-rays and scans, as well as to new sections on cell biology, care of the dying and an increased emphasis on molecular biology throughout the book. The authors remain essentially the same, even though a number have moved to other hospitals and medical schools. Their commitment to the book is evident by the careful way in which each of the chapters has been updated and revised as necessary.

We have once again retained the extensive cross referencing in order to reduce repetition and to integrate the whole subject of clinical medicine. We have therefore not felt it necessary to have separate chapters for example, on epidemiology and the diseases of the elderly, as these are integral parts of each chapter. We have retained the Appendices as these have proved extremely popular. This book's success has partly depended on its clear style and format. We have tried to make this new edition even more 'user friendly' and therefore added colour.

Finally we would like to thank all our colleagues and friends, and especially our families for their continuing support.

Parveen Kumar
Michael Clark

Acknowledgements

We would like to thank all our colleagues and medical students who have helped us in the preparation of both the first and now the second edition. In particular for this edition we would like to thank Dr Graeme Alexander, Dr Robert Allan, Dr Pierre Bouloux, Dr Elizabeth Fagan, Dr Richard Greenwood, Dr David Leaver, Professor Andrew Lister, Dr Alison Maclean, Dr Anthony Nathan, Dr Ray Powles, Dr Anthony Raine, Dr Ama Rohatiner, Dr Simon Roselaar, Dr David Westaby and Dr Peter White.

Seán Duggan and Carol Parr from Baillière Tindall have given valuable help and advice. Dr William Jackson helped with the original format of the book which has contributed much to its success and this contribution is acknowledged again.

Every effort has been made to check the drug dosages given in this book. However, as it is possible that some errors have been missed or that dosage schedules have been revised the reader is strongly urged to consult the drug companies' literature before administering any of the drugs listed.

1

Infectious Diseases and Tropical Medicine

and schistosomiasis. New infective agents continue to be identified and include *Helicobacter pylori* and the new hepatitis virus C. Human immunodeficiency virus (HIV) infection continues to increase. There is an increasing problem of infections in the immunosuppressed, not only in those with HIV but also in organ transplant recipients and those receiving anticancer chemotherapy.

The control of infectious diseases world-wide has been vastly improved by the use of effective vaccines and antimicrobial agents. Technological advances in molecular biology have also improved diagnosis, treatment and the development of new vaccines.

Table 1.1 League table of infectious diseases world-wide.

Disease	Esimated morbidity (No. of cases in thousands per year)	Estimated mortality (No. of deaths in thousands per year)
Diarrhoeal disease	3 000 000– 5 000 000	10 000
Respiratory infection	?	5 000
Malaria	150 000	1 500
Measles	80 000	1 000
Schistosomiasis	20 000	1 000
Whooping cough	20 000	400
Neonatal tetanus	?	150

Introduction

Global impact

Infectious diseases are the commonest afflictions of mankind and are a major source of morbidity and mortality in both developed and developing countries. Table 1.1 shows estimated morbidity and mortality figures for the common infectious diseases.

Increase in world travel in the past 30–40 years has brought Westerners into contact with a number of diseases unusual in the West, such as malaria

Epidemiology

The prevalence of infectious diseases varies markedly throughout the world and depends on climatic conditions, sanitation, the quality of the water supply, and to some extent the specific disease resistance of the indigenous population at risk. The continuance of infectious diseases in a human population requires:

● Reservoirs of infection
● Effective modes of transmission

Reservoirs

Human reservoirs are necessary for the agents of those diseases that (under natural conditions) exclusively afflict humans. Specific examples of such diseases are hepatitis A and B, cholera and shigellosis. Many sites in the body act as permanent reservoirs for microorganisms:

- Skin, e.g. *Staphylococcus epidermidis*
- Nasopharynx, e.g. meningococci
- Intestinal tract, e.g. *Giardia, Entamoeba histolytica*—both can continue to colonize after clinical recovery

Viruses may remain in the body for many months or years, notable examples being hepatitis B virus and the neurotropic herpesviruses.

Helminths may remain in the circulation (e.g. schistosomes in the portal vein) or lymphatic system (e.g. filarial worms) for many years, the former constantly producing millions of ova, a high proportion of which are deposited back into the environment.

Animal reservoirs of human disease are also important both in the Western and Third Worlds. The following are common examples of zoonoses (infections that can be transmitted from animals, except arthropods, to man):

- From battery-farmed chickens—*Salmonella* or *Campylobacter jejuni* infection
- From domestic cats—*Toxoplasma gondii* infection
- From domestic and wild animals—*Giardia* infection
- From cattle—*Cryptosporidium parvum* infection

Diseases that rely on arthropods for their transmission include malaria, yellow fever, Dengue fever and rickettsial infections.

Environment reservoirs may also act as a temporary lodging place for some bacteria, viruses and parasites.

Water contaminated with enteropathogens is a constant cause of concern in the tropics; water may also be a reservoir of hepatitis A virus. Cysts of some protozoa, notably *Giardia*, may remain viable despite apparently effective water-purification procedures.

Soil is also a source of the agents of human disease, particularly spore-forming bacteria such as *Clostridium* spp. and *Bacillus anthracis*, whose spores can remain viable under suitable climatic conditions for many months.

Transmission

Airborne spread. Some viruses, bacteria and bacterial spores can be carried directly by the wind. Some are generally spread by droplets in the air, e.g. influenza viruses, and other microorganisms such as *Legionella* are spread by aerosol, characteristically from air-conditioning units.

Spread by direct contact. This includes:

- Person-to-person spread, e.g. skin infections (impetigo, ringworm and scabies) and sexually transmitted diseases
- Faecal–oral spread, particularly amongst children in residential institutions, e.g. shigellosis, giardiasis and hepatitis A
- Inoculation of infection, e.g. transfusion of blood or blood products containing hepatitis B, C or HIV or by contaminated needles (drug abusers, medical and paramedical personnel)
- Insect bites, e.g. mosquitoes (malaria), sandfly (leishmaniasis), ticks (babesiosis) and bugs (Chagas' disease)
- Entry through the skin, which occurs with the larval forms of some helminths that can survive in soil or water, e.g. *Schistosoma, Strongyloides* and hookworm

Spread by food and water. Contaminated food and water is the usual mode of transmission of enteropathogens. Some bacteria, such as *Shigella*, require as few as 102 organisms to initiate infection, whereas others like *Vibrio cholerae* require approximately 10^8 organisms. Cysts of parasites such as *Giardia* and *Entamoeba histolytica* can survive in water for many months and are relatively resistant to water-treatment procedures.

Spread by fomites. Transmission of infection can occur between persons via an inanimate object, e.g. bed linen, books.

Principles and basic mechanisms

Figure 1.1 summarizes the important steps that occur during the pathogenesis of infection.

Specificity

Some infectious agents are strictly species selective. Amoebiasis, for example, only naturally affects humans. Even within a species, relative resistance is apparent, such as the decreased susceptibility of Duffy blood group negative individuals to *Plasmodium vivax* malaria.

Microorganisms are also highly specific with respect to the organ or tissue that they infect. This predilection for specific sites in the body relates partly to the *milieu exterieur*, i.e. the immediate environment in which the organism finds itself; for

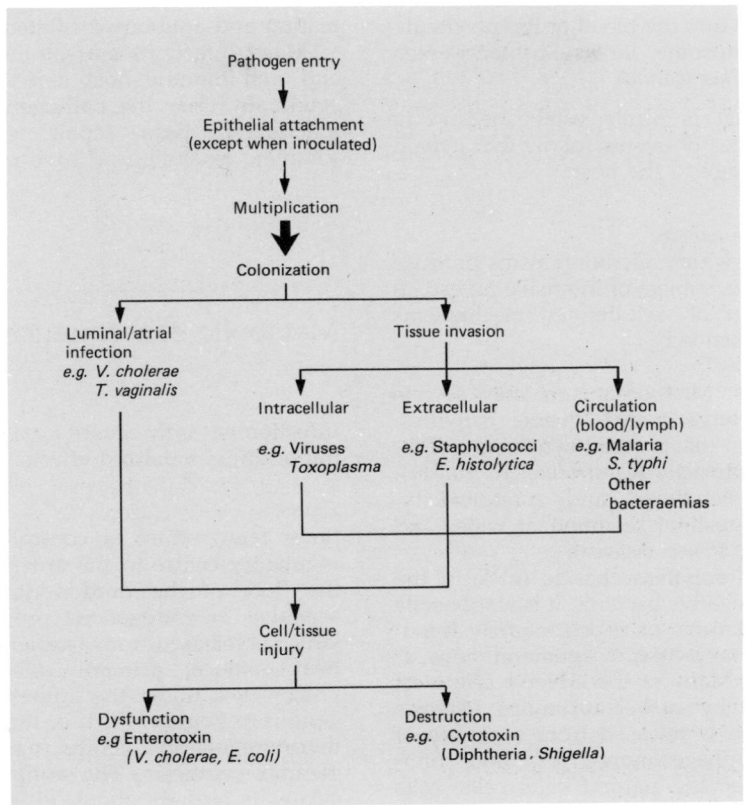

Fig. 1.1 The pathogenesis of infection.

example, anaerobic organisms colonize the highly anaerobic colon, whereas aerobic organisms are generally found in the mouth, pharynx and proximal intestinal tract. Other organisms that clearly show selectivity are:

- *Streptococcus pneumoniae* (respiratory tract)
- *Escherichia coli* (urinary and alimentary tract)

Even within a species of bacterium such as *Escherichia coli*, different strains will show selectivity towards a particular organ, e.g. the enterotoxigenic *E. coli* causes acute diarrhoeal disease, whereas the uropathogenic *E. coli* is responsible for urinary tract infection.

Even within an organ a pathogen may show selectivity for a particular cell type. In the intestine, for example, rotavirus predominantly invades and destroys intestinal epithelial cells on the upper portion of the villus, whereas reovirus selectively enters the body through the specialized epithelial cells, known as M cells, that cover the Peyer's patches.

Epithelial attachment
Many bacteria attach to the epithelial substratum by specific organelles called pili (or fimbriae) that contain a surface lectin(s): a protein or glycoprotein that recognizes specific sugar residues on the host cell. Such is the specificity of this attachment mechanism that it limits enterotoxigenic *Escherichia coli* infection, for example, to certain species. Some viruses and protozoa (*Plasmodium*, *Entamoeba histolytica*) also interact with their target-cell surface membrane by a similar mechanism. Other parasites such as hookworm have specific attachment organelles (buccal plates) that firmly grip the intestinal epithelium.

Multiplication and colonization
These follow epithelial attachment. Pathogens may then either remain within the lumen of the organ that they have colonized or may invade the tissues.

Invasion
Invasion may result in:

- An intracellular location for the pathogen (e.g. viruses, *Toxoplasma*, *Leishmania*, *Plasmodium*)
- An extracellular location for the pathogen (e.g. mycobacteria, staphylococci and *E. histolytica*)

- Invasion directly into the blood or lymph circulation (e.g. schistosome larvae, trypanosomes, *Leishmania* and *Plasmodium*)

Once the pathogen is firmly established in its target tissue, a series of events follow that usually culminates in damage to the host.

Tissue dysfunction or damage
The mechanism by which microorganisms produce disease has been the subject of intensive investigation and a number of well-defined mechanisms have now been described.

Exo- and endotoxins. Microorganisms may secrete exotoxins. These have many diverse activities, including inhibition of protein synthesis (diphtheria toxin), neurotoxicity (*Clostridium perfringens*, *C. tetani* and *C. botulinum*) and enterotoxicity, which results in intestinal secretion of water and electrolytes (*E. coli*, *Vibrio cholerae*).

Endotoxin is a lipopolysaccharide (LPS) in the cell wall of Gram-negative bacteria. It is responsible for many of the features of shock, namely hypotension, fever, intravascular coagulation and, at high doses, death. Many of the adverse effects of LPS are mediated by cachectin/tumour necrosis factor (TNF), which is released from a variety of phagocytic (macrophages/monocytes) and non-phagocytic (lymphocytes, natural killer cells) cells in response to infections and inflammatory stimuli (Table 1.2). TNF itself then stimulates the release of a cascade of other mediators involved in inflammation and tissue remodelling, e.g. Interleukins 1 and 6, prostaglandins, leukotrienes, corticotrophin.

Table 1.2 Factors that trigger TNF biosynthesis.

Bacterial endotoxin (LPS)
Toxic shock syndrome toxin—1(TSST-1)
Mycobacterial cord factor
Virus
Complement component, C5a
Interleukin-1 (IL-1)
Fungal and protozoal antigens

Tissue invasion. *Staphylococcus aureus* has tissue-invasive qualities, e.g. abscess formation and bacteraemia, as well as producing toxins causing diarrhoea and a toxin responsible for a widespread erythema (staphylococcal scalded skin syndrome). Similarly, some pathogenic *E. coli* can produce tissue invasion without production of a specific toxin.

Secondary immunological phenomena. All organisms can initiate secondary immunological mechanisms, e.g. complement activation, immune complex formation and antibody-mediated cytolysis of cells.

Many infections are self-limiting, and immune and non-immune host defence mechanisms will eventually clear the pathogens. This is generally followed by tissue repair, which may result in complete resolution or leave residual damage.

Metabolic consequences

Infection not only causes local damage but also has important generalized effects.

Fever
Body temperature is controlled by the thermoregulatory centre in the anterior hypothalamus in the floor of the third ventricle. This centre is sensitive to endogenous pyrogen (interleukin 1) which is released from a variety of cells involved in host defence, primarily blood monocytes and phagocytes, under the influence of microbial exogenous pyrogens. IL-1 is thought to act on the thermoregulatory centre by increasing prostaglandin synthesis. The antipyretic effect of salicylates is brought about, at least in part, through its inhibitory effects on prostaglandin synthetase.

Fever production is thought to have a positive effect on the course of infection. However, for every 1°C rise in temperature, there is a 13% increase in basal metabolic rate and oxygen consumption. Fever therefore leads to increased energy requirements at a time when anorexia leads to decreased food intake. The normal compensatory mechanisms in starvation, e.g. mobilization of fat stores, are inhibited in acute infections. This leads to an increase in skeletal muscle breakdown, releasing amino acids, which, via gluconeogenesis, are used to provide energy.

In chronic infection there is time for adaptation and the body is able to utilize fat stores more effectively and thus weight loss is much slower.

Protein metabolism
During acute infection major changes occur in protein metabolism:

- There is a diversion of synthesis away from somatic and circulating proteins such as albumin towards acute-phase proteins such as C-reactive protein, haptoglobin, alpha-1-antitrypsin, caeruloplasmin and fibrinogen.
- Protein synthesis is also directed towards immunoglobulin production and there is production of lymphocytes, neutrophils and other phagocytic cells.

- There is a marked increase in nitrogen losses, which may reach 10–15 g per day.

Mineral metabolism and acid–base balance
Mineral metabolism and acid–base balance are disturbed during acute infection. In general, sodium and water are retained, principally owing to the effects of increased levels of aldosterone and inappropriate secretion of antidiuretic hormone. During the convalescent period after acute infection, a diuresis may occur. Acid–base balance disturbance is common, and includes respiratory alkalosis following tachypnoea related to fever, respiratory acidosis and hypoxaemia associated with pneumonia, and metabolic acidosis associated with septicaemia.

In acute infection these changes are mild and resolve promptly without specific intervention. However, in situations where infections are prolonged and resolution is slow, supportive care may be necessary, particularly with respect to managing nutritional deficits and electrolyte and acid–base disturbances.

Host defence (see also Chapter 2)

The human body has natural resistance to infection as well as the ability to develop acquired resistance to specific pathogens when necessary.

Natural resistance (see p. 125)

Body surface
The epithelial barriers of skin and mucous membranes are the primary lines of defence. In the bronchial tree, retrograde beating of cilia and intermittent coughing and expectoration provide a simple mechanism for keeping the upper airways free of invading pathogens. In the intestine, villus movement and peristalsis are usually antegrade, and tend to expel pathogens through the anus.

Chemical factors such as gastric acid are particularly active against certain enteropathogens, namely *Salmonella* sp., *Shigella* sp. and *Vibrio cholerae*, while the low pH of the urine inhibits the growth of many urinary pathogens.

The gel-forming properties of mucus form a sticky trap both for normal flora and for pathogens, and constant secretion of mucus results in a continuous shedding of organisms from a variety of body sites.

The normal microbial flora play a vital role in impeding the growth of certain pathogens; for example, certain non-pathogenic *E. coli* produce colicins that are lethal to *Salmonella* and *Shigella*.

Surface immunoglobulins are found on all mucous membranes and are active during the early phase of colonization. Secretory IgA is particularly important since it is resistant to the action of proteolytic enzymes. However, gonococci, meningococci and some streptococci produce IgA proteases able to cleave secretory IgA (which accounts for approximately 40% of the IgA secreted).

Extracellular fluids
Natural antibodies are present in these fluids, some of which neutralize toxins, others act as opsonins and promote phagocytosis, while others activate complement, resulting in bacteriolysis. Beta lysin is released from platelets in inflammatory exudates and has the ability to kill Gram-positive bacteria. C-reactive protein is also involved in complement activation. In the presence of viruses, some cells produce substances called interferons. These have broad-spectrum antiviral activity that is not limited to the invading virus.

Phagocytic cells
Organisms may be carried by lymphatics and trapped in lymph nodes, where they become a target for phagocytosis by macrophages. Failing this they will ultimately enter the circulation and be ingested by circulating neutrophils or by phagocytic cells in the liver (Kupffer's cells), spleen, bone marrow, pituitary or adrenal gland.

Acquired resistance

Antibodies
The presence of foreign antigens leads to the transformation of B lymphocytes into plasma cells that produce immunoglobulin (Ig). The primary response is the production of IgM. IgM is an active cell agglutinin and also activates complement via the classical pathway. It is, however, a large molecule and does not cross the placenta. Within 10–14 days the IgG response begins, and IgG becomes the predominant antibody in the circulation. IgG antibodies can act:

- As opsonins by forming a bridge between the pathogen (Fab portion) and the phagocytic neutrophil (Fc portion)
- As antitoxins
- As complement activators
- By taking part in antibody-dependent cell-mediated cytotoxicity
- By blocking attachment of microbial pathogens to the substratum or preventing entry into the cell (e.g. blocking entry of the malarial parasite into the red cell)

Secretory immunity to specific organisms occurs in many luminal and atrial (e.g. vaginal) infections, and often involves blocking of the attachment of microorganisms (e.g. *Vibrio cholerae*, influenza virus

—see p. 65) to the epithelium. Not all antibody production during infection is useful, as many antibodies have no protective function whatsoever, although they may be useful for serodiagnosis.

Cell-mediated immunity
T lymphocytes are particularly important in those diseases in which immunity is not acquired by circulating antibodies. Cell-mediated immunity is important in fungal and viral infections, in some bacterial infections (leprosy, brucellosis, tuberculosis and syphilis) and in some parasitic infections (leishmaniasis and schistosomiasis). Some T lymphocytes are cytotoxic, recognizing and destroying cells that bear a foreign antigen (virus-infected cells). In addition, sensitized T lymphocytes produce lymphokines that activate and attract macrophages to the site of infection.

T lymphocytes survive for long periods and therefore provide lasting protection against infection.

The immunological response to infection generally involves both humoral and cellular mechanisms; for example, specific antibodies may limit the spread of a virus, but sensitized T lymphocytes are required for its elimination.

Host susceptibility

Many factors are known to influence an individual's susceptibility to infection. Individuals at the extremes of life are more susceptible to infection. The infant has a relatively immature immune

Table 1.3 Opportunistic infections.

Predisposing factors	Infectious agents
Primary immunodeficiency	
Antibody defects (hypo- or agammaglobinaemia, selective IgA deficiency)	Bacteria (respiratory, intestinal and urinary)
Cell-mediated defects (Swiss, Wiskott–Aldrich or DiGeorge's syndrome)	
Combined defects (severe combined immunodeficiency)	Viruses, bacteria and fungi (e.g. *Candida*)
Malignant disorders, e.g. leukaemia, lymphoma	
Diminished cell-mediated immunity, neutropenia	Viruses (CMV, VZV, HSV), Gram-negative organisms (causing bacteraemia), fungi
Infection with HIV	
Diminished cell-mediated immunity	Viruses (CMV) *Pneumocystis, Cryptosporidium* atypical mycobacteria
Allograft recipients (renal, bone marrow, heart)	
Diminished cell-mediated immunity	Enterobacteriaceae, *Pseudomonas* or Gram-negative bacteria (all causing bacteraemia), herpesviruses, fungi
Bone marrow failure	
Neutropenia	Enterobacteriaceae, *Pseudomonas, Candida* (causing bacteraemia or disseminated infection), herpesvirus
Defective clearance of pathogens	
Splenectomy	
Cystic fibrosis disease	Pneumococcal and other bacterial pathogens
Gut motility disorders	
Endotracheal tube	Gut aerobes and anaerobes, *Pseudomonas, Klebsiella,* Enterobacteriaceae
Liver disease	
Tissue, vessel and organ implants	
Prosthetic heart valve	
CSF shunt	Bacteria and *Candida*. Often organisms of low pathogenic potential, e.g. *Staphylococcus epidermidis*
Peritoneal dialysis catheter	
Central venous catheter	

system and in the early neonatal period relies heavily on transplacental passage of immunoglobulin (IgG) from its mother and of secretory immunoglobulin (sIgA) in colostrum and breast milk. Immune function in the elderly is less effective than in the younger adult and may be further modified by impaired nutrition. There are also some genetic determinants of susceptibility to infection, a good example being the relative resistance of individuals carrying the HbS gene (sickle-cell trait) to malaria. HLA haplotypes may also play a part in determining the host response to infection, possibly through linkage with immune response genes.

Diabetics have increased numbers of infections, particularly pyogenic infections, as do patients with both primary and secondary immunodeficiency.

Opportunistic infection

Opportunistic infection occurs in individuals with compromised host defence mechanisms. Sometimes the infecting agent is not a normal pathogen. The clinical presentation is often atypical, leading to diagnostic difficulty. The failure of local defence mechanisms leads to an absence of signs of infection, such as fever and pus.

Opportunistic infections are noted for their chronicity and for their resistance to conventional antimicrobial chemotherapy. Table 1.3 summarizes the important situations in which opportunistic infection may arise and the infectious agents commonly associated with these diseases.

Interaction between nutrition and infection

Undernutrition impairs host defence (Fig. 1.2). Natural resistance to infection is lowered by alterations in the integrity of body surfaces, the reduced ability to repair epithelia, and the reduction in gastric acid production. In addition, immunological abnormalities are found:

- Tissue and circulating macrophage function is impaired
- T lymphocyte function is depressed
- The total lymphocyte count is below 1×10^9 cells per litre, which is indicative of a relatively immunocompromised host
- Cell-mediated immunity is in a state of anergy, i.e. the body fails to respond to a recall antigen such as the Mantoux test
- Antibody production is less sensitive to undernutrition, but in severe malnutrition depression in both circulating and secretory immunity are detectable. This is of importance clinically in that vaccination (e.g. against polio) may have to be more aggressive in malnutrition before protective immunity is achieved
- Complement levels fall rapidly in severe acute malnutrition and remain low during long periods of established suboptimal nutritional status. Complement levels have been used as a biochemical marker of nutritional status

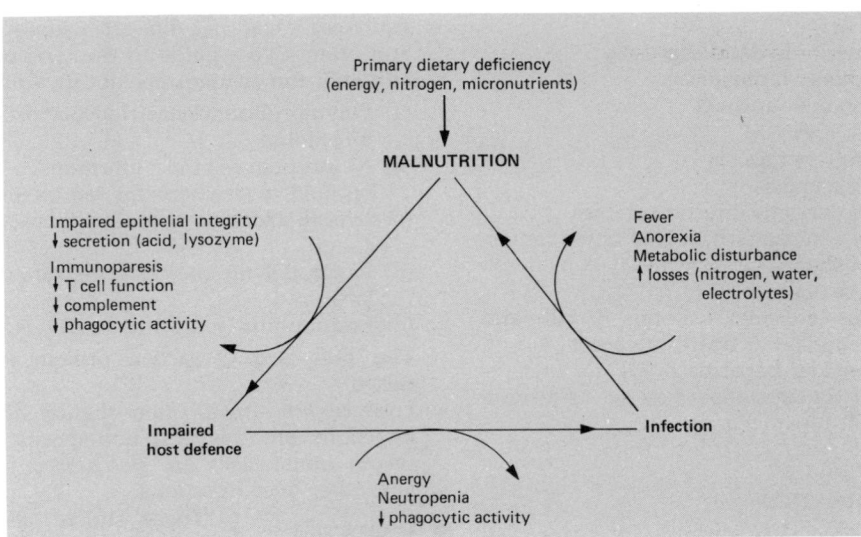

Fig. 1.2 Nutrition–infection–host defence: a complex interaction.

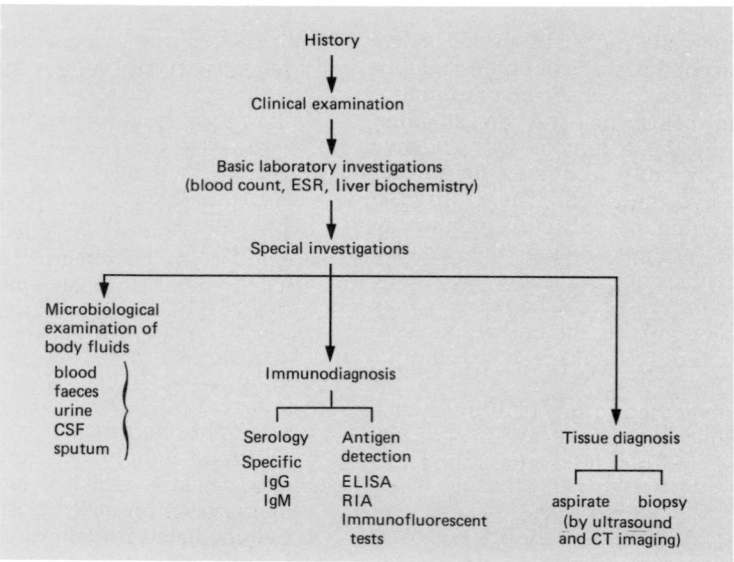

Fig. 1.3 An approach to the diagnosis of infectious diseases.

Diagnosis (Fig. 1.3)

HISTORY

Particular attention should be paid to the following:

- Foreign travel—remembering that certain diseases can exist both in the tropics and Europe, e.g. leishmaniasis, giardiasis
- Immigrants—country of origin
- Food and water—food poisoning is extremely common
- Occupation, e.g.
    sheep farmers—hydatid disease
    sewer workers—leptospirosis
    leather workers—anthrax
- Domestic pets, e.g.
    budgerigars—psittacosis
    cats—toxoplasmosis
    dogs—*Toxicara canis* infection, rabies
- Sexual activity—hepatitis B, mixed enteric infections and HIV should be particularly considered in male homosexuals
- Drug addiction—consider hepatitis B, HIV and pyogenic infections, e.g. staphylococcal
- Tattooing—consider hepatitis B, HIV
- Injections and transfusions—may act as a route of transmission for infections

CLINICAL EXAMINATION

A general examination should be performed with particular attention to skin rashes, lymphadeno-pathy and hepatosplenomegaly. In cases of sexually transmitted diseases the perineum, rectum and vagina should be inspected. The presence of a fever is helpful, but less emphasis is now placed on fever patterns because of improved laboratory diagnosis. High swinging fevers are characteristically seen with localized pus.

INVESTIGATION

Tests should be performed as appropriate. If the diagnosis is obvious, e.g. a measles rash is present, no tests are necessary. The list below gives examples of situations in which tests are useful.

- *Full blood count and film* are usually performed and often give a guide to the type of infection, although the changes are not invariable:
    (a) Polymorphonuclear leucocytosis—bacterial infections
    (b) Neutropenia—viral infections, brucellosis, typhoid, overwhelming septicaemia
    (c) Lymphocytosis—viral infections, whooping cough
    (d) Atypical lymphocytes—infectious mononucleosis
    (e) Eosinophilia—parasitic infections, helminths
    The ESR and C-reactive protein are usually raised
- *Liver biochemistry* is often slightly abnormal in infections but this is a non-specific sign. The serum transferases are also raised in hepatitis and other liver infections
- *Urine analysis*
- *Chest X-ray*
  These should also be performed, even in the absence of symptoms and signs

Further investigations are often required to make the specific diagnosis:

- Blood culture
- Microscopic examination and culture of appropriate body fluids, e.g. urine, faeces, CSF, sputum
- Viruses can be identified in the above body fluids by:
  (a) Electron microscopy
  (b) Tissue culture (cytomegalovirus)
  (c) Immunological antigen capture techniques (rotavirus)
- Immunodiagnosis—immunological techniques are now available for the identification of:
  (a) *Pathogen-specific antigens* using polyvalent antisera or monoclonal antibodies
  (b) *Specific serological responses* to infection using immunodiffusion, complement fixation, indirect haemagglutination, indirect immunofluorescence or enzyme-linked immunosorbent assay (ELISA)

A high titre of IgM specific to a pathogen (e.g. hepatitis A or B virus, cytomegalovirus) is diagnostic of a recent infection. In infection a single raised IgG is unhelpful as this only indicates a previous rather than a current infection. However, a rising titre can confirm the diagnosis (e.g. in brucellosis or mycoplasma infection).

These immunological techniques are particularly useful in the identification of pathogens that are difficult to culture by standard microbiological techniques or intracellular pathogens that require tissue culture

- Tissue diagnosis—biopsy/aspiration with isolation of pathogen:
  (a) Bone marrow/liver biopsy for generalized infections such as tuberculosis, leishmaniasis
  (b) Rarely, if the above technique is negative, splenic aspiration for leishmaniasis
  (c) Transbronchial biopsy for *Pneumocystis carinii* infection
- Imaging procedures—ultrasound and CT scan (with needle aspiration) for abscesses in liver, lung, brain or abdomen

Pyrexia of unknown origin (PUO)

A major diagnostic problem is the patient who has a pyrexia, either intermittent or continuous, that lasts for 3 weeks or more and in whom routine investigations have failed to reveal a cause. PUO may merely be an unusual presentation of a common disease. Table 1.4 shows some of the common causes of PUO.

Age is an important pointer, since cancer and the connective tissue diseases are more common in the elderly.

Immunocompromised individuals are at particu-

Table 1.4 Common causes of pyrexia of unknown origin (PUO).

Infection (40%)
Pyogenic abscess, e.g. liver
Tuberculosis
Urinary infection
Biliary infection
Subacute infective endocarditis
EBV infection
CMV infection
Q fever
Toxoplasmosis
Brucellosis
Cancer (30%)
Lymphomas
Leukaemia
Solid tumours, e.g.
renal carcinoma
hepatocellular carcinoma
pancreatic carcinoma
Immunogenic (20%)
Drugs
Connective tissue and autoimmune diseases, e.g.
rheumatoid disease
systemic lupus erythematosus
polyarteritis nodosa
polymyalgia/cranial arteritis
Sarcoidosis
Factitious (1–5%)
Switching thermometers
Injection of pyrogenic material
Remain unknown (5–9%)

lar risk of infectious disease and often present with a particularly unusual spectrum of infections (see p. 6).

An aggressive approach to the diagnosis of PUO is justified since there is a good chance that determination of a specific diagnosis will influence management and result in curative treatment. It is always worth repeating the history and examination since new signs may have evolved since the patient's initial admission to hospital. All drug therapy should be reassessed and, if possible, stopped.

INVESTIGATION

First-line investigations such as a full blood count, blood culture, urinalysis, routine blood chemistry and chest X-ray should be repeated.

Other investigations

- CT and ultrasound scanning are particularly

valuable in revealing primary and secondary neoplastic diseases and also for showing occult abscesses. MRI is occasionally useful.

- Aspiration or needle biopsy under imaging control provides a histological diagnosis.
- Laparoscopy may be required to confirm a gynaecological cause, e.g. pelvic inflammatory disease, multiple peritoneal metastases or tuberculous peritonitis.
- Needle biopsy of the liver (histology and culture) may be required to confirm granulomatous hepatitis, tuberculosis or metastatic cancer
- Scanning with gallium-59, which is taken up by polymorphs, or indium-111 labelled leucocytes, can localize an abscess.

Laparotomy is rarely performed since the advent of more sophisticated imaging and guided-biopsy techniques.

Septicaemia

The term *bacteraemia* refers to the transient presence of organisms in the blood (generally without causing symptoms) as a result of local infection or penetrating injury.

The term *septicaemia*, on the other hand, is usually reserved for when bacteria or fungi are actually multiplying in the blood, usually with the production of severe systemic symptoms such as fever and hypotension.

Pyaemia describes the serious situation when, in a septicaemia, organisms and neutrophil polymorphs embolize to many sites in the body causing abscesses, notably in the lungs, liver and brain.

Septicaemia has an extremely high mortality and demands immediate attention.

CAUSES

The term *primary septicaemia* is used to describe the situation when the focus of infection is not apparent. Such patients are generally elderly, undernourished or suffering from chronic disease, particularly alcoholic cirrhosis and diabetes.

The common sites of infection and infective

Table 1.5 Septicaemia in a previously healthy adult.

Site of origin	Usual pathogen(s)
Skin	*Staphylococcus aureus* and other Gram-positive cocci
Urinary tract	*Escherichia coli* and other aerobic Gram-negative rods
Respiratory tract	*Streptococcus pneumoniae*
Gallbladder or bowel	*Streptococcus faecalis*, *E. coli* and other Gram-negative rods *Bacteroides fragilis*
Pelvic organs	*Neisseria gonorrhoeae*, anaerobes

agents responsible for *secondary septicaemia* are shown in Tables 1.5 and 1.6. Pneumococcus and *Haemophilus influenzae* are common causes of septicaemia in children, whereas in neonates Gram-negative rods and group B streptococci are the most likely aetiological agents. *Neisseria gonorrhoeae* is a common cause of septicaemia in young adults, but it is usually mild without serious effects. Intravenous drug abusers frequently suffer bacteraemia and septicaemia often caused by *Staphylococcus aureus*, *Pseudomonas* and *Serratia*.

CLINICAL FEATURES

Fever, rigors and hypotension are the cardinal features of severe septicaemia. However, the illness may be preceded by less specific symptoms such as headache, lethargy, apprehension and subtle changes in conscious level. Other clinical features and their pathogenesis are shown in Table 1.7.

INVESTIGATION

Septicaemia is almost always treated initially on the basis of a clinical diagnosis after appropriate specimens have been sent to the laboratory. Probable origins of infection and likely pathogens must be sought on the basis of a careful history and examination. The type of infection will clearly differ in hospitalized and otherwise previously healthy adults (see Tables 1.5 and 1.6). Body fluids or other specimens (blood, urine, CSF, tissue or abscess aspirates) should be submitted to full microbiological examination. Imaging investigations such as ultrasonography and CT scan may be required.

Table 1.6 Septicaemia in hospitalized patients.

Clinical problem	Usual pathogen(s)
Urinary catheter	*Escherichia coli*, *Klebsiella*, *Proteus*, *Serratia*, *Pseudomonas*
Intravenous catheter	*Staphylococcus aureus* and *S. epidermidis*, *Klebsiella*, *Pseudomonas*, *Candida albicans*
Peritoneal catheter	*S. epidermidis*
Post-surgery:	
Wound infection	*Staphylococcus aureus*, *Escherichia coli*, anaerobes (depending on site)
Deep infection	Depends on anatomical location
Burns	Gram-positive cocci, *Pseudomonas*, *Candida albicans*
Immunocompromised patients	Any of the above

Table 1.7 Special clinical features of septicaemia.

Clinical feature	Cause and effect
Hypotension ('endotoxic shock')	Liberation of bacterial endotoxin (cell-wall lipopolysaccharide) that reduces vascular tone and increases permeability
Pulmonary oedema and adult respiratory distress syndrome (ARDS)	Increased permeability of the alveolar capillary endothelium, impaired gas exchange and hypoxia
Disseminated intravascular coagulation (DIC)	Activation of blood coagulation by endothelial damage, endotoxins and immune complexes

Catheters or cannulae, which might be sources of infection, should be removed and sent for culture.

TREATMENT

Antibiotic therapy should be commenced immediately. If the organism and its antibiotic sensitivities are unknown, a combination of drugs should be chosen to cover the likely pathogens. If there is an obvious site of skin sepsis, drugs such as flucloxacillin (1 g 6-hourly i.v.) and an aminoglycoside to cover *Staphylococcus aureus* should be used. If bowel sepsis is suspected, then a broader-spectrum drug of the cephalosporin group (e.g. cefoxitin 1–2 g every 6–8 h i.m. or i.v.) would be advisable. In the absence of any helpful clinical guidelines, a combination of a penicillin drug that is active against *Pseudomonas* (carbenicillin 5 g every 4–6 h by slow i.v. injection, or ticarcillin 15–20 g in divided doses) with an aminoglycoside such as tobramycin (3–5 mg·kg^{-1} daily in divided doses every 8 h) should be given. Metronidazole (1 g every 8 h by rectum) is often added to provide additional cover against anaerobic organisms. Steroids should not be used for the treatment of septicaemia or septicaemic shock.

Antimicrobial chemotherapy

Widespread and often inappropriate use of antibiotics has led to increasing numbers of organisms with multiple drug resistance. Antibiotics are not required for minor infections.

Although the majority of antibiotics are relatively safe drugs, important toxic effects do occur when used in the incorrect dosage and in the presence of other disease states, notably renal disease. In addition, antibacterial therapy may result in secondary yeast or fungal infection or may facilitate the growth of a second bacterial pathogen, such as *Clostridium difficile*, an important cause of antibiotic-associated colitis.

Choice of drug
Blind therapy. Antimicrobial therapy is often begun before the organism is identified and its antibiotic sensitivities known. The choice of drug(s) is therefore dependent on a clinical diagnosis and a knowledge of the organisms likely to be involved in a given situation. Before beginning 'blind' therapy it is essential to obtain appropriate body fluids or other specimens for microbiological examination. Adjustments to the antibiotic regimen can then be made, if necessary, when antibiotic sensitivities are available.

Spectrum of activity. The spectrum of antibacterial activity of the drug chosen should ideally be as narrow as possible, as it will then have fewer detrimental effects on the normal bacterial flora of the host. 'Blind' therapy, however, by necessity generally covers a broader spectrum than required.

Bactericidal vs. bacteriostatic. In the majority of infections there is no firm evidence that bactericidal drugs (penicillins, cephalosporins, aminoglycosides) are more effective than bacteriostatic drugs, but it is generally considered important to use the former in the treatment of bacterial endocarditis and in patients in whom host defence mechanisms are compromised.

Patient factors. In addition to age and pregnancy, the following factors should be considered.

- *The site of infection.* The chosen drug must be able to gain access to the part of the body involved. The brain, eye, biliary tract, prostate and loculated abscesses are inaccessible to many drugs.
- *Renal and hepatic function.* Impaired renal or hepatic function necessitates a major modification of the dose regimen or even complete avoidance of certain drugs. Care should be taken when using aminoglycosides, carbenicillin, ticarcillin, flucytosine and some antitubercular agents in patients with renal impairment. Other drugs, such as nalidixic acid, tetracycline and vancomycin, should be avoided altogether.

Dose
This is influenced by the type of infection to be treated and the age of the patient. Bacterial endocarditis and deep-seated abscesses (e.g. in brain or lung) generally require high-dose therapy for several weeks.

Route of administration
Some drugs (e.g. some of the cephalosporins) are only available as intravenous preparations, but many antibiotics are well-absorbed by the oral route and generally there is no advantage to the patient for therapy to be administered by the more expensive parenteral route. Patient compliance must, however, be taken into account.

Duration of therapy
With more potent drugs, only short courses or even single doses may be required.

Monitoring
In serious infections (e.g. subacute infective endocarditis), monitoring of circulating drug concentra-
tions is important for assessing efficacy of treatment. Drug concentrations can be measured directly in serum, but the efficacy of therapy is best determined by serum bactericidal assay just before and at a standard time after administration of antibiotics. The highest dilution of serum that completely kills the causative organism can then be determined.

Monitoring for toxicity is particularly important with the aminoglycoside antibiotics. Concentrations are determined immediately before ('trough' levels) and usually 15–30 min after intravenous administration of the drug. High 'trough' levels of $> 2~\mu g \cdot ml^{-1}$ are considered to be the most important factor in causing the oto- and nephrotoxicity commonly seen with these agents.

Table 1.8 Antibiotic chemoprophylaxis.

Clinical problem	Aim	Drug regimen
Rheumatic fever	To prevent recurrence and further cardiac damage	Phenoxymethylpenicillin 500 mg or erythromycin 250 mg twice daily if penicillin-sensitive
Infective endocarditis	To prevent infection on abnormal, prosthetic or homograft heart valves following potentially bacteraemic procedures	*Dental/oropharyngeal procedures* Oral amoxycillin 3 g 1 h before (erythromycin for penicillin-sensitive individuals—1.5 g 1 h before and 500 mg 6 h after). *For 'high-risk' patients and genitourinary instrumentation* i.m. amoxycillin 1 g + i.m. gentamicin 1.5 mg·kg⁻¹ before and oral amoxycillin 500 mg 6 h after procedure *Gastrointestinal procedures (for prosthetic valves only)* Amoxycillin 1 g i.m. plus gentamicin i.m. 1.5 mg·kg⁻¹ before and oral amoxycillin 500 mg 6 h after procedure
Meningitis: Due to meningo-cocci	To prevent infection in close contacts	Rifampicin 600 mg twice daily for 2 days
Due to *Haemophilus influenzae*	To reduce nasopharyngeal carriage	Rifampicin 10–20 mg·kg⁻¹ daily for 4 days
Tuberculosis	To prevent infection in exposed (close contacts) tuberculin-negative individuals, infants of infected mothers and immunosuppressed patients	Oral isoniazid 5 mg·kg⁻¹ daily for 6–12 months
Malaria	To prevent infection	Oral chloroquine 400–500 mg as a single dose each week, 2 weeks before and for 6 weeks after leaving endemic area. Where chloroquine resistance occurs (get advice and see p. 88)

Combination antibiotic therapy
Combinations of antibiotics are commonly used in the empirical treatment of many serious infections such as septicaemia, meningitis, tuberculosis and endocarditis, but some care must be taken in the choice of drugs within such combinations. There is still some concern that a combination of a bactericidal and a bacteriostatic antibiotic may impair their therapeutic efficacy. However, this concept is by no means universally applicable, since the bacteriostatic drug tetracycline and the bactericidal drug rifampicin are thought to be synergistic. Generally, combinations of bactericidal drugs are at least additive and in some situations are synergistic, whereas combinations of bacteriostatic drugs are generally only additive.

Antibiotic chemoprophylaxis
This is required in certain disease states (see Table 1.8).

Mechanisms of resistance to antimicrobial agents

The development or acquisition of resistance to an antibiotic by bacteria invariably involves a mutation at a single point in a gene or transfer of genetic material from another organism (see Fig. 1.4). Single-point mutations occur in *E. coli*, for example, at the rate of approximately 1 per 10^5–10^7 cell divisions. A mutation resulting in antibiotic resistance by this mechanism would involve alteration of a single nucleotide base.

Larger fragments of DNA may be introduced into a bacterium either by transfer of 'naked' DNA or via a bacteriophage (a virus) DNA vector. Both the former (transformation) and the latter (transduction) are dependent on integration of this new DNA into the recipient chromosomal DNA. This requires a high degree of homology between the donor and recipient chromosomal DNA.

Finally, antibiotic resistance can be transferred from one bacterium to another by conjugation, when extra chromosomal DNA (a plasmid) containing the resistance factor (R factor) is passed from one cell into another during direct contact. Transfer of such R factor plasmids can occur between unrelated bacterial strains and involve large amounts of DNA.

Transformation is probably the least clinically important mechanism, whereas transduction and R factor transfer are probably the most important for the sudden emergence of multiple antibiotic resistance in a single bacterium.

ANTIBACTERIAL DRUGS

Naturally occurring compounds

Penicillins
Structure. Penicillins, like cephalosporins, have a beta-lactam ring fused to a thiazolidine ring (see Fig. 1.5).

Relatively minor changes to the side-chain of benzyl penicillin render the phenoxymethyl derivative acid resistant and allow it to be absorbed well when given orally. The presence of an amino group in the phenyl radical of benzyl penicillin increases the antimicrobial spectrum of the native penicillin and makes it active against both Gram-negative and Gram-positive organisms. More extensive modification of the side-chain (e.g. as in cloxacillin) renders the drug insensitive to bacterial penicillinase, a major advance in treating infections caused by penicillinase (beta-lactamase)-producing staphylococci.

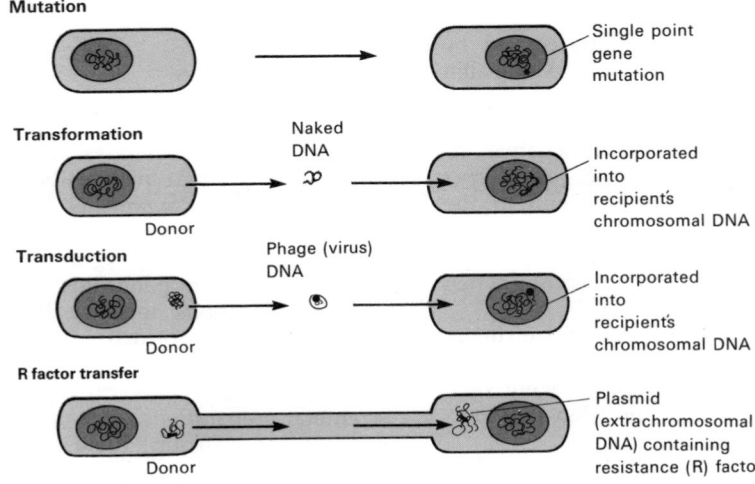

Fig. 1.4 Mechanisms of resistance to antimicrobial drugs.

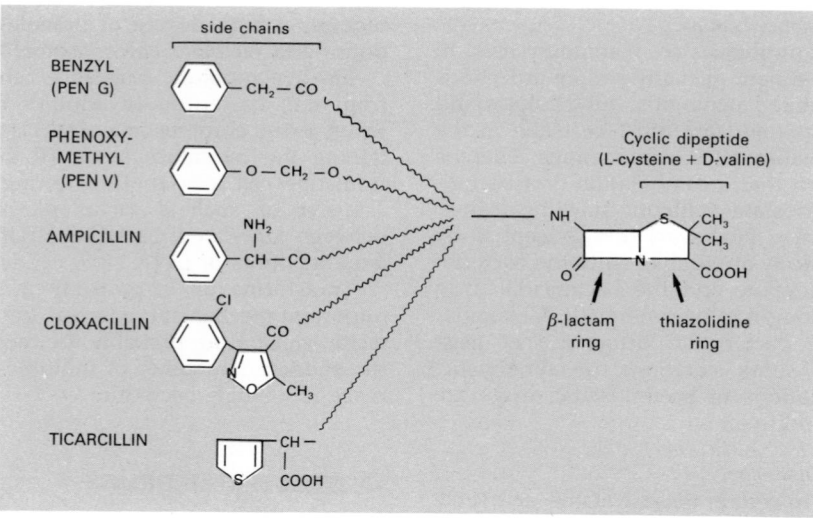

Fig. 1.5 The structure of penicillins.

Mechanisms of action. Penicillins block the terminal cross-linking reaction (between alanine and glycine) of bacterial cell-wall mucopeptide formation. Penicillins and other beta-lactam antibiotics bind to and inactivate specific penicillin-binding proteins (PBPs) which are peptidases involved in the final stages of cell wall assembly and remodelling during growth and division.

Indications for use. Benzyl penicillin can only be given parenterally and is the drug of choice for serious infections, notably infective endocarditis, pneumococcal, meningococcal, streptococcal and gonococcal infections, clostridial infections (tetanus, gas gangrene), actinomycosis, anthrax, and spirochaetal infections (syphilis, yaws).

Phenoxymethylpenicillin (penicillin V) is an oral preparation that is chiefly used as maintenance therapy for rheumatic fever prophylaxis.

Flucloxacillin is used in infections caused by penicillinase-producing staphylococci. Methicillin is also effective but must be given by injection.

Ampicillin is susceptible to penicillinase, but its antimicrobial activity includes Gram-negative organisms such as *Salmonella*, *Shigella*, *E. coli*, *Haemophilus influenzae* and *Proteus*. It is useful in the treatment of urinary tract and upper respiratory tract infections. Amoxycillin has a similar sphere of activity to ampicillin, but is better absorbed when given by mouth.

Clavulanic acid is a powerful inhibitor of many bacterial beta-lactamases and when given in combination with an otherwise susceptible agent such as amoxycillin or ticarcillin can broaden the spectrum of activity of the drug.

The extended-spectrum penicillins, carbenicillin and ticarcillin are active against *Pseudomonas* infection and the acylureidopenicillin derivatives (azlocillin, mezlocillin, piperacillin) have increased activity against Gram-negative organisms, including *Pseudomonas*, compared with other penicillins. However, they are susceptible to staphylococcal beta-lactamases and are therefore not reliable for treating staphylococcal disease.

Resistance. Bacteria producing penicillinase are resistant to some penicillins.

Interactions. Penicillins inactivate aminoglycosides when mixed in the same solution.

Toxicity. Hypersensitivity (skin rash, urticaria, anaphylaxis), encephalopathy and tubulo-interstitial nephritis can occur. Ampicillin also produces a hypersensitivity rash in approximately 90% of patients with infectious mononucleosis who receive this drug. Generally, the penicillins are very safe.

Cephalosporins

The cephalosporins have major advantages over the penicillins in that they are innately resistant to staphylococcal penicillinases and have a broader range of activity that includes both Gram-negative and Gram-positive organisms. Like the penicillins they have a beta-lactam ring, but this is associated with a dihydrothiazine ring in place of the thiazolidine ring found in penicillins (see Fig. 1.6). Side-chain modifications increase their potency and range of activity. Structural modifications have produced orally active drugs such as cephalexin and cephradine and a variety of highly potent parenteral preparations such as cefuroxime, cephamandole and cefoxitin (Table 1.9).

Mechanism of action. Like penicillins, cephalosporins inhibit bacterial cell-wall synthesis.

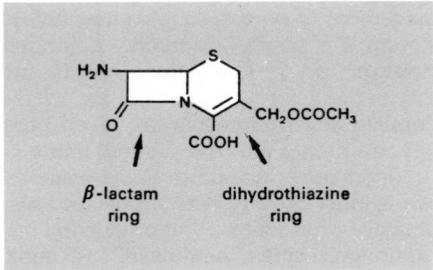

Fig. 1.6 The structure of a cephalosporin.

Indications for use. These potent broad-spectrum antibiotics are useful for the treatment of serious systemic infections, particularly when the precise nature of the infection is unknown. They are commonly used for serious post-operative sepsis and in immunocompromised patients, particularly during treatment of leukaemia and other malignancies.

Resistance. Cephalosporins generally resist the action of beta-lactamase-producing bacteria.

Interactions. Increased nephrotoxicity is seen when cephalosporins are used in conjunction with other nephrotoxic antibiotics such as aminoglycosides and some diuretics.

Toxicity. This is as for penicillin; some patients are allergic to both groups of drugs. The early cephalosporins caused proximal tubule damage, although the newer derivatives have less nephrotoxic effects.

Monobactams
Aztreonam is the only member of this class currently available.

Structure. Aztreonam is a synthetic analogue of an

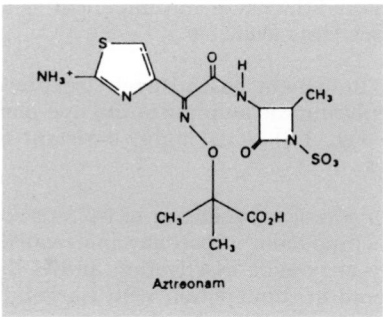

Fig. 1.7 The structure of monobactams.

antibiotic found in soil bacteria (see Fig. 1.7), with a novel structure containing beta-lactam ring in core configuration.

Mechanism of action is inhibition of bacterial cell wall synthesis. It is resistant to most beta-lactamases and does not induce beta-lactamase production.

Indications for use. Aztreonam's spectrum of activity is limited to aerobic Gram-negative bacilli, thus resembling aminoglycosides. With the exception of urinary tract infections, aztreonam should be used in combination with metronidazole (for anaerobes) and an agent active against Gram-positive cocci (a

Table 1.9 Cephalosporins—some examples.

	Activity	Use
First generation Cephazolin Cephalothin Cephalexin (oral)	Gram-positive cocci	Surgical prophylaxis Penicillin allergy
Second generation Cefuroxime Cephamandole Cefoxitin Cefaclor (oral) Cephradine (oral)	Extended spectrum and more effective than first generation against *E. coli, Klebsiella* spp. and *Pr. mirabilis*	Resistant *H. influenzae*, mixed aerobic–anaerobic infections (combined with aminoglycoside)
Third generation Cefotaxime[a] Ceftazidime Latamoxef disodium[b]	Broad spectrum; more potent against aerobic Gram-negative bacteria than first or second generation	Especially Enterobacteriaceae, *Ps. aeruginosa, B. fragilis* and *N. gonorrhoeae*

[a] Penetrates CSF.
[b] Not a true cephalosporin (has an oxygen instead of a sulphur molecule in the dihydrothiazine ring).

penicillin or erythromycin). It may eventually replace aminoglycosides in combination therapy.

Toxicity is as for beta-lactam antibiotics.

Carbapenems
N-formimidoyl thienamycin (Imipenem) is the only drug of this class available.

Structure. Imipenem has a novel structure with a carbon replacing the sulphur in the five-membered ring (see Fig. 1.8). It is highly resistant to beta-lactamases.

Mechanism of action. Inhibition of bacterial cell wall synthesis. Imipenem is partially inactivated in the kidney by enzymatic inactivation and is therefore administered in combination with cilastatin.

Indications for use. Imipenem has the broadest spectrum of activity of all known antibiotics. It is active against Gram-positive cocci (similar potency to penicillins), Gram-negative organisms and anaerobes (similar potency to metronidazole and clindamycin). It should only rarely be used for community-acquired infection, its main indications being nosocomial infections when multiple resistant Gram-negative bacilli or mixed aerobe and anaerobe infections are suspected.

Toxicity is similar to that of other beta-lactam antibiotics. Nausea, vomiting and diarrhoea occur in less than 5%. There is no evidence of nephrotoxicity or coagulation abnormalities.

Aminoglycosides
Structure. These antibiotics are derived from *Streptomyces* species and are polycationic compounds of amino sugars (Fig. 1.9).

Mechanisms of action. Aminoglycosides interrupt bacterial protein synthesis by inhibiting ribosomal function (messenger and transfer RNA).

Indications for use. Streptomycin is bactericidal for susceptible organisms. Neomycin is only used for the topical treatment of eye and skin infections and orally for preoperative 'bowel sterilization' and in

the management of portosystemic encephalopathy. Even though it is poorly absorbed, prolonged oral administration can produce toxic effects such as ototoxicity.

Gentamicin and tobramycin are given parenterally. They are highly effective against many Gram-negative organisms including *Pseudomonas*. They are active against *Streptococcus faecalis* and also the beta-lactamase-producing staphylococci. The newer aminoglycosides, netilmicin and amikacin, have a similar spectrum of antibacterial activity and are generally resistant to the aminoglycoside-inactivating enzymes produced by some bacteria. Their use should be restricted to gentamicin-resistant organisms.

Resistance. Some bacteria produce phosphorylating, adenylating or acetylating enzymes that inactivate aminoglycoside antibiotics. These enzymes are coded for and transferred by R factors (extra-chromosomal DNA).

Interactions. Enhanced nephrotoxicity occurs with other nephrotoxic drugs, ototoxicity with some diuretics, and neuromuscular blockade with curari-form drugs.

Toxicity. Aminoglycosides are nephrotoxic and ototoxic (vestibular and auditory), particularly in the elderly. Blood levels must be checked (p. 12).

Tetracyclines
Structure. These are bacteriostatic drugs possessing a four-ring hydronaphthacene nucleus (see Fig. 1.10). Variation of the native compound is obtained by different substitutions to give, for example, oxy- and chlortetracycline, or doxycycline.

Mechanism of action. Tetracyclines inhibit bacterial protein synthesis by interrupting ribosomal function (transfer RNA).

Indications for use. Tetracyclines are active against Gram-positive and Gram-negative bacteria but their use is now limited. Tetracycline is used for the treatment of acne and rosacea. Tetracyclines are also active against *Vibrio cholerae, Rickettsia,*

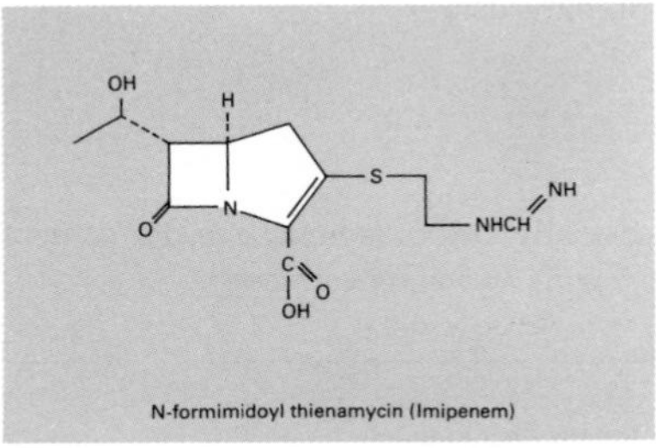

N-formimidoyl thienamycin (Imipenem)

Fig. 1.8 The structure of imipenem.

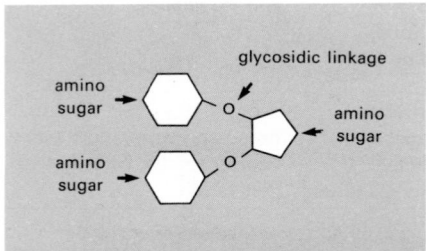

glycosidic linkage

amino sugar

amino sugar

amino sugar

Fig. 1.9 The structure of an aminoglycoside.

Mycoplasma, Coxiella burnetii, Chlamydia and *Brucella.*

Resistance. Some bacteria possess reduced bacterial cell permeability to tetracycline, which is coded for by an R factor. Resistance is particularly important in infections with pneumococci and *Haemophilus influenzae.*

Interactions. The efficacy of tetracyclines is reduced by antacids, barbiturates and oral iron-replacement therapy.

Toxicity. Tetracyclines are generally safe drugs, but they may enhance established or incipient renal failure, although doxycycline is safer than others in this group. They cause brown discoloration of growing teeth, and thus these drugs are not given to children or pregnant women. Photosensitivity can occur.

Erythromycin
Structure. Erythromycin consists of a lactone ring with unusual sugar side-chains.

Mechanism of action. Erythromycin inhibits protein synthesis by interrupting ribosomal function.

Indications for use. Erythromycin has a similar antibacterial spectrum to penicillin and is useful in individuals with penicillin sensitivity. It can be given orally or parenterally. It is included in the treatment regimen of all pneumonias as many are due to *Mycoplasma.* It is effective in the treatment of infections due to *Bordetella pertussis* (whooping cough), *Legionella, Campylobacter, Chlamydia, Coxiella* and *Listeria.*

Toxicity. Erythromycin estolate may produce cholestatic jaundice after prolonged treatment.

Chloramphenicol
Structure. Chloramphenicol is the only naturally occurring antibiotic containing nitrobenzene (see Fig. 1.11). This structure is probably important for

its toxicity in humans and for its activity against bacteria.

Mechanism of action. Chloramphenicol is structurally similar to uridine-5-phosphate and competes with messenger RNA for ribosomal binding. It also inhibits peptidyl transferase.

Indications for use. Despite its toxicity, chloramphenicol is indicated for the treatment of severe infection due to *Salmonella typhi* and *paratyphi* (enteric fevers) and severe infections due to *Haemophilus influenzae* (meningitis and acute epiglottitis). It is also active against *Yersinia pestis* (plague) and is used topically for purulent conjunctivitis.

Resistance. Bacterial R factors code for acetylating enzymes that can inactivate chloramphenicol and also reduce bacterial cell permeability to this agent.

Interactions. Chloramphenicol enhances the activity of anticoagulants, phenytoin and oral hypoglycaemic agents.

Toxicity. Severe irreversible bone marrow suppression is rare but nevertheless restricts the usage of this drug to the indications above and for ill patients. Chloramphenicol should not be given to premature infants or neonates because of their inability to conjugate and excrete this drug; high blood levels lead to circulatory collapse and the often fatal 'grey baby syndrome'.

Fusidic acid
Structure. Fusidic acid has a structure resembling that of bile salts.

Mechanism of action. It is a potent inhibitor of bacterial protein synthesis. Its entry into cells is facilitated by the detergent properties inherent in its structure.

Indications for use. Fusidic acid is mainly used for penicillinase-producing *Staphylococcus aureus* infections such as osteomyelitis or endocarditis, and for

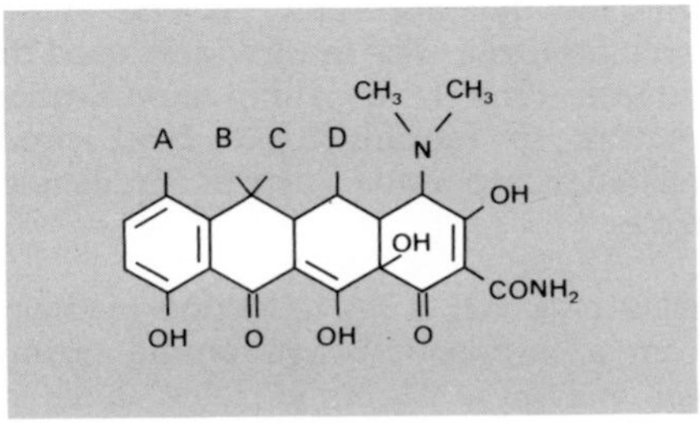

Fig. 1.10 The structure of tetracycline. Substitution of CH_3, OH or H at positions A to D produces variants of tetracycline.

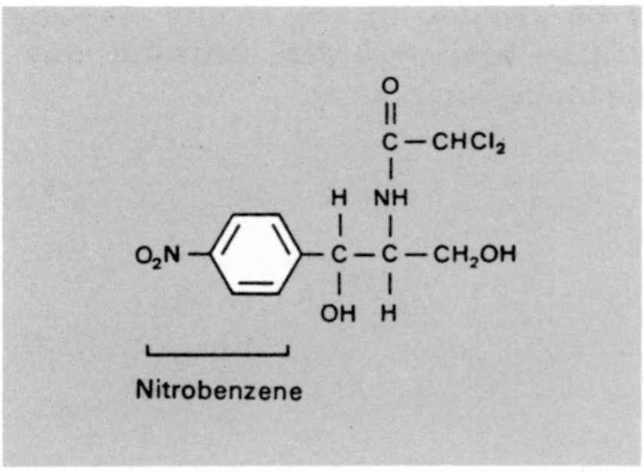

Fig. 1.11 The structure of chloramphenicol.

other staphylococcal infections associated with bacteraemia or septicaemia. The drug is well absorbed orally but is relatively expensive. It is well concentrated in bone.

Resistance may occur rapidly and is the reason why fusidic acid is given in combination with another antibiotic.

Toxicity. Fusidic acid may occasionally be hepatotoxic but is generally a safe drug and if necessary can be given during pregnancy.

Synthetic compounds

Sulphonamides
Structure. The sulphonamides are all derivatives of the prototype sulphanilamide (see Fig. 1.12).

Mechanism of action. Sulphonamides block thymidine and purine synthesis by inhibiting microbial folic acid synthesis. Trimethoprim also inhibits folic acid synthesis.

Indications for use. Sulphamethoxazole is mainly used in combination with trimethoprim co-trimoxazole for treatment of *Pneumocystis carinii* infection. Trimethoprim alone is now used for other infections such as urinary tract infections and acute-on-chronic bronchitis. Sulphapyridine in combination with 5-aminosalicylic acid (i.e. sulphasalazine) is used in inflammatory bowel disease.

Resistance. Bacteria may become resistant to sulphonamides by production of sulphonamide-resistant dihydropteroate synthetase and by altering bacterial cell permeability to these agents.

Interactions. Sulphonamides potentiate oral anticoagulants and hypoglycaemic agents.

Toxicity. Sulphonamides cause thrombocytopenia, folate deficiency and megaloblastic anaemia and haemolysis in individuals with glucose-6-phosphate dehydrogenase deficiency, and therefore should not be used in such people. Co-trimoxazole should be avoided in the elderly if possible, as deaths have been recorded, probably due to the sulphonamide component.

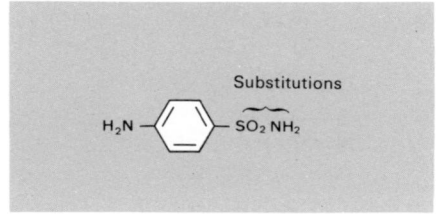

Substitutions

H_2N —⬡— $SO_2\,NH_2$

Fig. 1.12 The structure of a sulphonamide.

Quinolones
The new quinolone antibiotics, such as ciprofloxacin, are useful oral broad-spectrum antibiotics, related structurally to nalidixic acid. The latter achieves only low serum concentrations after oral administration and its use has been limited to the urinary tract where it is concentrated.

Structure—see Fig. 1.13.

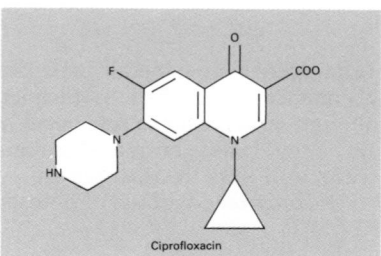

Ciprofloxacin

Fig. 1.13 The structure of a quinolone.

Mechanism of action. This group of bactericidal drugs inhibit bacterial DNA synthesis by inhibiting DNA gyrase, the enzyme responsible for maintaining the superhelical twists in DNA.

Indications for use. Ciprofloxacin should be reserved for infections caused by organisms resistant to standard drugs at the moment. The extended spectrum quinolones such as ciprofloxacin have activity against Gram-negative and some Gram-positive bacteria. Useful in Gram-negative septicaemia, skin and bone infections, gastrointestinal, urinary and respiratory tract infections, meningococcal carriage and in some sexually transmitted diseases such as gonorrhoea and NSU due to *Chlamydia trachomatis*.

Toxicity. Gastrointestinal disturbances, photosensitive rashes and occasional neurotoxicity can occur.

Nitroimidazoles
Structure. These agents are active against anaerobic organisms, notably anaerobic bacteria and some pathogenic protozoa. The most widely used drug is metronidazole (Fig. 1.14). Minor modifications in the structure of nitroimidazole have produced other related compounds such as tinidazole and nimorazole.

Mechanisms of action. After reduction of their nitro group to a nitrosohydroxyl amino group by microbial enzymes, nitroimidazoles cause strand breaks in microbial DNA.

Indications for use. Metronidazole is of major importance in the treatment of anaerobic bacterial

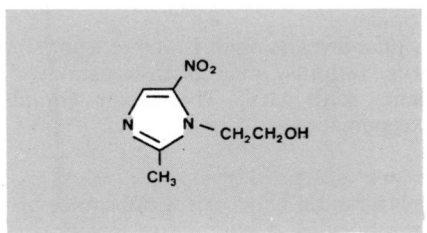

Fig. 1.14 The structure of metronidazole, a nitro-imidazole.

infection, particularly that due to *Bacteroides*. It is also used prophylactically in colonic surgery. It may be given orally, by suppository (entirely satisfactory blood levels can be obtained by this route) or intravenously (very expensive). It is also the treatment of choice for amoebiasis, giardiasis and infection with *Trichomonas vaginalis*.

Interactions. Nitroimidazoles can produce a disulphuram-like reaction with ethanol.

Toxicity. Nitroimidazoles are tumorigenic in animals and mutagenic for bacteria, although carcinogenicity has not been described in humans. They cause a metallic taste, and peripheral neuro-pathy with prolonged use. They should be avoided in pregnancy.

Vancomycin
Vancomycin is produced by *Streptomyces orientalis*.

Structure. Vancomycin is a complex and unusual glycopeptide primarily active against Gram-positive bacteria.

Mechanism of action. Vancomycin inhibits cell-wall synthesis and is bactericidal.

Indications for use. Vancomycin is given orally for *Clostridium difficile*-related pseudomembranous enterocolitis and intravenously in methicillin-resistant *Staphylococcus aureus* (MRSA) infections. It is expensive and its use should be restricted to these two conditions.

Toxicity. Vancomycin can cause ototoxicity and nephrotoxicity. Care must be taken to avoid extravasation at the injection site as this causes necrosis and thrombophlebitis.

ANTIFUNGAL DRUGS

Naturally occurring compounds

Polyenes
The most potent of these is amphotericin B, which

is used intravenously in severe systemic fungal infections. Nephrotoxicity is a major problem and dosage levels must take into account background renal function. Nystatin is not absorbed through mucous membranes and is therefore useful for the treatment of oral and enteric candidiasis and for vaginal infection. It can only be given orally or as pessaries. Polyenes react with the sterols in fungal membranes, increasing permeability and thus damaging the organism.

Griseofulvin
This naturally occurring antifungal is concentrated in keratin and is therefore useful for chronic fungal infection of nails, although treatment may be required for many months. It is also widely used for the treatment of ringworm.

Synthetic drugs

Imidazoles such as miconazole (Fig. 1.15), keto-conazole and clotrimazole are all active against strictly aerobic organisms:

- Clotrimazole is used topically for the treatment of ringworm.
- Miconazole is a potent systemic antifungal that may be used with amphotericin B in severe systemic fungal infection and is active both orally and parenterally.
- Ketoconazole is active orally but can produce liver damage. It is effective in deep mycoses including invasive aspergillosis, cryptococcosis, histoplasmosis and blastomycosis.
- Fluconazole is noted for its ability to enter cerebrospinal fluid (CSF) and is used for treatment of central nervous system (CNS) infection with *Cryptococcus neoformans*.
- Itraconazole fails to penetrate CSF. It is used for vulvovaginal candidiasis. Toxicity is mild.

The fluorinated pyridine derivative, flucytosine, is usually used in combination with amphotericin B for systemic fungal infection. Side-effects are uncommon, although it may cause bone marrow suppression. It is active when given both orally and parenterally.

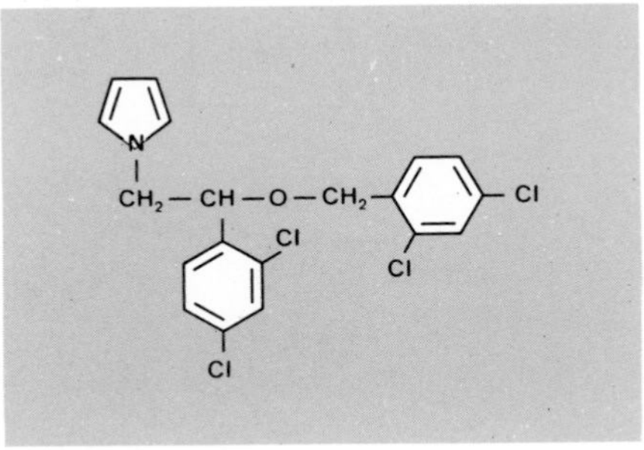

Fig. 1.15 The structure of miconazole, an imidazole.

ANTIVIRAL DRUGS

Idoxuridine

This agent is active against herpes simplex virus (HSV) as a 5% solution with dimethyl sulphoxide (DMSO), but to be effective it must be applied to the skin before the appearance of vesicles. It is also effective as a 0.1% solution when instilled into the eye for HSV keratitis. Similar topical use in herpes zoster probably alters the clinical course of the illness if given early.

Vidarabine (adenine arabinoside)

This agent may be given intravenously and is active against HSV and varicella zoster virus (VZV). It is also used in severe varicella infection (chickenpox). Its major effects include bone marrow suppression and renal impairment.

Acyclovir

This agent is relatively free from side-effects and is effective against many herpes virus infections. Oral and topical preparations are available for the treatment of HSV infections. An intravenous preparation can be used for the treatment of systemic virus infection in the immunocompromised host, particularly VZV infections, and also for primary HSV infection e.g. encephalitis.

Ribavirin (Tribarvirin)

Given during the first week of lassa fever this drug reduces mortality from about 50% to 5%. Oral prophylaxis for 10 days is indicated for contacts.

Azidodeoxythymidine (AZT)

AZT (zidovudine) (Fig. 1.16), a thymidine analogue inhibits HIV reverse transcriptase and thereby impairs viral replication. It is strongly recommended for HIV patients in Group IV (see p. 71), particularly those with opportunistic infection and neurological disease. Bone marrow toxicity is frequent (ca. 30%) and serious. Polymyositis and an encephalitis-like syndrome may also occur.

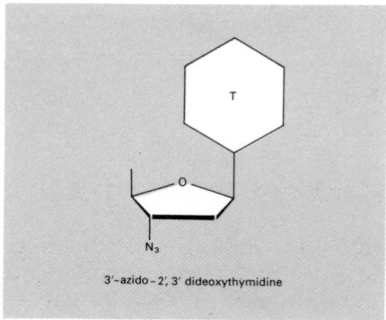

3'-azido-2', 3' dideoxythymidine

Fig. 1.16 The structure of AZT.

Ganciclovir

This guanine analogue is active against cytomegalovirus retinitis and gastrointestinal disease in patients with HIV. The major complication is neutropenia.

Interferon (see p. 137)

This is a naturally occurring substance produced by T lymphocytes during virus infection. Interferon production occurs in response to many different viruses and production stimulated by one virus may confer protection against a second viral invader. Recombinant DNA technology has enabled this substance to be produced commercially and it is currently being evaluated as a treatment for acute and chronic hepatitis and herpesvirus infections.

Prevention

Although effective antimicrobial chemotherapy is available for many diseases, the ultimate aim of any infectious disease control programme is to prevent infection occurring. This may be achieved either by:

- Eliminating the source or mode of transmission of an infection
- Reducing host susceptibility to environmental pathogens

Control of sources and transmission

Water and food supplies constitute a major reservoir of infection and careful surveillance of supplies reduces the incidence of many diseases e.g. acute diarrhoeal disease, bovine TB.

Screening of blood donors has proved essential to control the spread of hepatitis and HIV. Definition of high-risk carrier populations, such as male homosexuals and immigrants from endemic areas of infectious disease is also important.

Reduction of host susceptibility

Immunization has changed the course and natural history of many infectious diseases. Passive immunization by administering preformed antibody, either in the form of immune serum or purified gamma globulin, provides short-term immunity and has been effective in both the prevention and treatment of a number of bacterial and viral diseases (Table 1.10). Long-lasting immunity is,

Table 1.10 Examples of passive immunization available.

Infection	Antibody	Indication	Efficacy
Bacterial			
Tetanus	Human tetanus immune globulin	Prevention and treatment	+
Diphtheria	Horse serum	Prevention and treatment	±
Botulism	Horse serum	Treatment	±
Viral			
Hepatitis A			
Measles	Human normal immune globulin	Prevention	+
Rubella			
Hepatitis B	Human hepatitis B immune globulin	Prevention	+
Varicella zoster	Human varicella zoster immune globulin	Prevention	+
Rabies	Human rabies immune globulin	Prevention	+

however, only achieved by active immunization with a live attenuated organism, a dead organism or an antigen preparation of part of an organism, ideally produced by recombinant DNA technology. Active immunization may also be performed with microbial toxin (either native or modified), in which case the immunogen is called a toxoid. Important preparations available for active immunization are shown in Table 1.11. The active immunization schedule currently recommended in the UK is summarized in Table 1.12.

Table 1.11 Preparations available for active immunization.

Live vaccines
Oral polio (Sabin)
Measles
Mumps
Rubella
Yellow fever
BCG

Dead organisms, crude or purified extracts
HBV
Pertussis
Typhoid
Polio (Salk)
Influenza
Cholera
Meningococci (group A and C)
Rabies
Pneumococcal

Toxoids
Diphtheria
Tetanus

Recombinant vaccines
HBV

Table 1.12 Immunization schedule recommended in the UK.

Year of life	Vaccines	Dose schedule
1	DTP plus OPV *or* DT (if P contraindicated)	At 3, 5 and 9–12 months
1–2	MMR	Single dose[a]
School entry	Booster DT plus OPV	Single dose
10–14 (females)	Rubella	Single dose
10–14	BCG (tuberculin-negative individuals)	Single dose[b]
15–18	T plus OPV	Single dose

DTP = diphtheria (D)/tetanus (T)/pertussis (P) (triple vaccine); OPV = oral polio vaccine; MMR = measles, mumps and rubella (single antigen measles vaccine still available if MMR refused); BCG = bacille Calmette–Guérin.
[a] Can be given at any age > 1 year.
[b] Interval of 3 weeks between rubella and BCG.

Bacterial infections

Gram-positive cocci

STAPHYLOCOCCAL INFECTIONS

Staphylococci are aerobic, facultatively anaerobic, Gram-positive cocci. They contain a number of cellular antigens and produce enzymes such as coagulase as well as toxins such as enterotoxin. Their pathogenicity correlates most closely with the production of the coagulase enzymes. Three patho-

Table 1.13 Host factors that increase susceptibility to staphylococcal infections (predominantly *Staphylococcus aureus*).

Injury to skin or mucous membranes, e.g.
    abrasions
    trauma (accidental or surgical)
    burns
    insect bites

Metabolic abnormalities, e.g.
    diabetes mellitus
    uraemia

Foreign bodies[a], e.g.
    intravenous and other indwelling catheters
    cardiac and orthopaedic prostheses
    tracheostomies

Abnormal leucocyte function, e.g.
    Job's syndrome
    Chédiak-Higashi syndrome
    steroid therapy
    drug-induced leucopenia

Post-viral infections, e.g.
    influenza

Miscellaneous conditions, e.g.
    excess alcohol consumption
    malnutrition
    malignancies
    old age

---

[a] Often *Staphylococcus epidermidis*.

genic species are recognized. *Staphylococcus aureus* is coagulase positive and *S. epidermidis* and *S. saprophyticus* are coagulase negative. Staphylococci are part of the normal microflora of the human skin, the upper respiratory tract, especially the nasopharynx, and the intestinal tract. Twenty-five per cent of the population are permanent carriers of *S. aureus*.

Approximately 20% of all human staphylococcal infections are autogenous. Transmission is most frequently by direct contact with an infected individual but may be airborne or via fomites. Several predisposing host factors have been identified (Table 1.13).

The organism can cause a wide clinical spectrum of diseases. These are usually localized, but infection may spread, resulting in bacteraemia or metastatic infection. Table 1.14 shows a list of conditions due to *S. aureus*; a few of these will be considered below.

Skin infections

These are discussed on p. 1021.

Osteomyelitis

Acute osteomyelitis is almost always due to staphylococcal infection. It occurs predominantly in males between the ages of 3 and 12 years, usually affecting the lower limbs. A history of trauma is often present. The diaphysis is initially involved, with subsequent spread of the infection to the periosteum and the subcutaneous tissues. Signs of inflammation are present. The child is usually irritable and febrile. There is leucocytosis and blood cultures are positive in about 75% of patients.

Osteomyelitis involving the vertebrae occurs in adults over 50 years of age. The onset is insidious, with pain; often there are no other features of infection.

Radiographs are usually normal in the first week after onset in both varieties of osteomyelitis.

Food poisoning (see Table 1.21)

This results from ingestion of food contaminated with pre-formed heat-stable enterotoxin. *S. aureus*

Table 1.14 Clinical conditions produced by *Staphylococcus aureus*.

Due to invasion

Skin:
    Furuncles
    Cellulitis
    Impetigo
    Carbuncles

Lungs:
    Pneumonia
    Lung abscesses

Heart:
    Endocarditis
    Pericarditis

Central nervous system:
    Meningitis
    Brain abscesses

Bones and joints:
    Osteomyelitis

Miscellaneous:
    Parotitis
    Pyomyositis
    Septicaemia
    Enterocolitis

Due to toxin

Staphylococcal food poisoning

Scalded-skin syndrome:
    Generalized erythema
    Bullous impetigo
    Staphylococcal scarlet fever

Toxic shock syndrome

---

accounts for approximately 5% of all food poisoning in the UK. Contamination is usually from an infected individual.

Foods such as canned foods, processed meats, milk and cheese favour the growth of *S. aureus*. The illness is manifest within 6 h of ingestion of contaminated foods and affects close to 100% of individuals who have eaten such foods. In contrast to food poisoning due to other organisms, staphylococcal food poisoning is characterized by the presence of persistent vomiting. Fever, when present, is usually below 38°C. Abdominal discomfort, diarrhoea or dysentery may be present. No specific treatment is necessary as the illness is short-lived (12–24 h); however, supportive treatment with fluids and electrolytes is occasionally indicated.

Acute staphylococcal enterocolitis
This presents as a more severe fulminant clinical syndrome, typically following broad spectrum antibiotics. Pseudomembranes may be seen at sigmoidoscopy.

Toxic shock syndrome (TSS)

Staphylococci that produce the toxic shock syndrome toxin-1 (TSST-1) are responsible for this syndrome. TSS is seen most frequently in menstruating women below the age of 30 years who use Mg^{2+}-chelating tampons. However, it can occur in other situations and men and children are not exempt. It is characterized by the abrupt onset of fever, a diffuse macular erythema, vomiting, diarrhoea, severe myalgia and shock. Blood cultures are negative and anti-TSST-1 antibodies are present in low concentrations in serum. Treatment is supportive. Antibiotics are usually given, although the syndrome is produced by the exotoxin. Mortality is about 10%.

Scalded skin syndrome (SSS)

Scalded skin syndrome is caused by staphylococci which elaborate the toxin exfoliatin. It is seen in children under 5 years of age and is characterized by a painful macular skin rash followed by bullae and generalized shedding of the epidermis.

TREATMENT

Any local lesion, e.g. an abscess, should be drained. Systemic infection is treated with antibiotics. Hospital-acquired infections are usually penicillin-resistant and therefore treatment is with flucloxacillin or nafcillin, usually together with fusidic acid. Seventy per cent of infections acquired outside the hospital are penicillin-sensitive and a penicillin is the drug of choice. Increasing antibiotic resistance is still a problem and most hospitals have restrictions on the use of single antibiotics. The control of staphylococcal cross-infection as discussed below is important.

Methicillin-resistant *Staphylococcus aureus* (MRSA) were detected in 1961 soon after methicillin was introduced. Such strains were only resistant to beta-lactam antibiotics and never caused serious problems. The MRSA strains that emerged first in Australia in the late 1970s and have spread worldwide are resistant to many other antibiotics, including aminoglycosides. These are now referred to as MARSA (methicillin-aminoglycoside-resistant *S. aureus*). There have been many outbreaks of infection, particularly in patients in tertiary referral centres, in the seriously ill and in those with surgical wounds and venous access sites. Origin of infection is often 'another hospital' or from healthy staff carriers. Control is essential and involves:

- Close and constant microbiological surveillance both before and during attacks
- Immediate isolation of infected individuals
- Appropriate management of the carrier state

Although topical antibiotics have been used to eradicate nasal colonization their efficacy is now in doubt. Careful handwashing with chlorhexidine solution is still widely recommended. MARSA can now be treated with vancomycin but teichoplanin and the quinolones are likely to be effective.

STREPTOCOCCAL INFECTIONS

Streptococci are round or ovoid Gram-positive, bacteria. Virulence is attributed to the cell-wall M protein and the production by some streptococci of hyaluronidase, DNAses or streptokinase. The spread of streptococci is mediated by direct contact, fomites or airborne droplet infection. Group A beta-haemolytic streptococci (*Streptococcus pyogenes*) are responsible for over 95% of human infections (Table 1.15). Group B streptococci frequently produce neonatal sepsis and meningitis, and group C, F and G organisms occasionally cause pharyngitis and group D endocarditis and septicaemia. Alpha-haemolytic streptococci (known collectively as *S. viridans*) found commonly in the mouth, e.g. *S. sanguis* and *S. mitior* as well as *S. mutans*, a non-haemolytic streptococcus, cause three-quarters of all streptococcal endocarditis.

S. pneumoniae is the commonest cause of pneumonia (see p. 672).

Scarlet fever

Scarlet fever occurs when the infectious organism (usually a group A streptococcus) produces erythrogenic toxin in an individual who does not possess neutralizing antitoxin antibodies.

Table 1.15 Diseases caused by streptococci.

Suppurative

Skin:
  Impetigo
  Pyoderma
  Erysipelas
  Cellulitis

Pharyngeal:
  Pharyngitis
  Tonsillitis
  Peritonsillar abscess

Infections confined to women:
  Puerperal sepsis
  Endometritis

Pulmonary:
  Pneumonia
  Empyema

Others:
  Osteomyelitis
  Infective endocarditis
  Meningitis
  Peritonitis
  Lymphangitis
  Bacteraemia

Non-suppurative
Rheumatic fever
Glomerulonephritis
Scarlet fever

CLINICAL FEATURES

The incubation period of this relatively mild disease of childhood is 2–4 days following a streptococcal infection, usually in the pharynx. Regional lymphadenopathy, fever, rigors, headache and vomiting are present. The rash, which usually appears on the second day of illness, initially occurs on the neck but rapidly becomes punctate, erythematous and generalized. It is typically absent from the face, palms and soles, and is prominent in the flexures. The rash usually lasts about 5 days and is followed by extensive desquamation of the skin. The face is flushed with characteristic circumoral pallor. Early in the disease the tongue has a white coating through which prominent bright red papillae can be seen ('strawberry tongue'). Later the white coating disappears, leaving a raw-looking, bright red colour ('raspberry tongue').

Scarlet fever may be complicated by the development of peritonsillar or retropharyngeal abscesses and otitis media.

DIAGNOSIS

The diagnosis is established by the typical clinical features and culture of throat swabs, where the organisms are usually found in abundance or more rapidly by latex agglutination of throat swab extracts. Elevated anti-streptolysin O and anti-DNAse B levels in the serum are indicative of streptococcal infection.

TREATMENT

Treatment is directed at preventing the non-suppurative complications of streptococcal infections (see Table 1.15).

Penicillin is the drug of choice and may be given orally as phenoxymethylpenicillin 125 mg four times daily for 10 days or as a single intramuscular injection of benzathine penicillin 916 mg in adults. Individuals allergic to penicillin can be treated effectively with erythromycin 250 mg four times daily for 10 days.

The role of tonsillectomy in preventing further attacks of pharyngitis remains controversial.

PREVENTION

Chemoprophylaxis with penicillin or erythromycin should be given in epidemics.

Erysipelas

Erysipelas is an acute, rapidly progressive infection of the skin that is almost always due to group A streptococci. It usually occurs in the very young, the elderly, the debilitated or the immunosuppressed. The onset is abrupt; fever, headache and vomiting are common. The erythematous skin lesion, which is usually on the face, enlarges rapidly and has a sharply demarcated raised edge. Vesicles and bullae appear within this lesion, which then rupture, leaving crusts on the surface. Regional lymphadenopathy is common. Bacteraemia, when present, is associated with a high mortality rate. Treatment with penicillin is rapidly effective.

Rheumatic fever

This is discussed on p. 583.

Acute glomerulonephritis

This is discussed on p. 435.

Gram-negative cocci

NEISSERIAL INFECTIONS

Neisseria are Gram-negative diplococci. *N. meningitidis* and *N. gonorrhoeae* are the only two bacteria in this group that are commonly pathogenic to humans.

Meningococcal infection

Meningococci (*N. meningitidis*) are ubiquitous. However, group A is commonly found in Africa and group B on the European and American continents. The incidence of groups C, Y and W135 infections is steadily rising world-wide. Group A is responsible for epidemics of meningitis and group B and C for sporadic infections. Its virulence is attributed to the polysaccharide capsule (which resists phagocytosis) and the lipopolysaccharide-endotoxin complex (which is responsible for its clinical toxicity). Transmission is by droplet infection or direct contact. Humans are the only known reservoirs. Following transmission, *N. meningitides* colonize the nasopharynx preferentially because of the humidity, increased carbon dioxide tension and specific receptor substances synthesized by the nasopharynx to which they adhere. Invasiveness of the organism appears to be almost solely dependent on the amount of specific antimeningococcal bactericidal antibody in the host. A history of a recent viral respiratory infection is common.

CLINICAL FEATURES

Four major clinical syndromes due to meningococci are recognized:

- *Meningococcaemia* may occur alone or in association with meningitis. It is characterized by the presence of headache, fever, malaise and myalgia. The patient looks toxic, and has tachycardia and tachypnoea. Skin manifestations occur early and consist of a purpuric rash and/or petechiae that also affect the conjunctivae.
- *Fulminant meningococcaemia* (Waterhouse–Friederichsen syndrome) occurs in about 10% of patients. It is characterized by an extremely rapid downhill clinical course, with extensive haemorrhage into the skin, hypotension, shock, confusion, coma and death within a few hours of the onset of symptoms. Disseminated intravascular coagulation (DIC), due to activation of the complement system, may further complicate the clinical picture. Haemorrhage into the adrenal glands may or may not be present. Without prompt treatment, the mortality rate approaches 100%.
- *Meningococcal meningitis* presents with fever, nausea, vomiting, headache, photophobia, altered consciousness and neck rigidity. The clinical presentation is indistinguishable from other acute bacterial meningitides (see p. 930).
- *Chronic meningococcaemia* is rare. It is characterized by intermittent fever, a maculopapular rash, arthralgia and splenomegaly. Blood cultures are positive during bacteraemic episodes.

N. meningitidis may also rarely result in polyarthritis, pericarditis and nephritis.

DIAGNOSIS

This is established by demonstrating meningococci in body fluids such as blood, CSF, petechial or joint aspirates. The CSF is turbid with an increase in neutrophils and protein. Counterimmunoelectrophoresis and latex agglutination to the polysaccharide antigen of group A, C, D and Y have recently been found useful.

TREATMENT

Benzylpenicillin is the treatment of choice, the dose being 1.2–2.4 g i.v. 4-hourly for adults. Ampicillin is equally effective. Chloramphenicol (75–100 mg·kg^{-1}) is the drug of choice in individuals allergic to penicillin. Treatment for shock (p. 716) and DIC (p. 343) should be instituted. Steroids should not be used in meningococcal meningitis.

PREVENTION AND CONTROL

Penicillin does not affect the carrier state. Family contacts of patients are protected effectively by rifampicin 600 mg two times daily for two days. Immunoprophylaxis with a quadrivalent vaccine against group A, C, Y and W135 organisms is effective.

Gonorrhoea

Gonorrhoea is caused by *N. gonorrhoeae*. It is discussed further on p. 48.

Gram-positive bacilli

CORYNEBACTERIA INFECTION

Corynebacterium diphtheriae is a Gram-positive, club-shaped bacillus. Three morphological varieties are recognized—*mitis*, *intermedius* and *gravis*. Of these, *mitis* is generally associated with mild infections. Only corynebacteria exposed to the bacteriophage beta, which carries the *tox*$^+$ gene are capable of toxin production. The toxin has two subunits, A and B. Subunit A is responsible for clinical toxicity. Subunit B serves only to transport the toxin component to specific receptors, present chiefly on the myocardium and in the peripheral nervous system. Humans are the only natural hosts.

Diphtheria

Diphtheria caused by *C. diphtheriae* occurs worldwide. Its incidence in the West has fallen dramatically following widespread active immunization.

Transmission is mainly through airborne droplet infection and rarely through fomites.

CLINICAL FEATURES

The incubation period varies from 2 to 7 days. Diphtheria is essentially a disease of childhood. The manifestations may be regarded as local (due to the membrane) or systemic (due to exotoxin). The presence of a membrane, however, is not essential to the diagnosis. The illness is insidious in onset and is associated with tachycardia and low-grade fever. If complicated by infection with other bacteria such as *Streptococcus pyogenes*, fever is high and spiking.

Nasal diphtheria is characterized by the presence of a unilateral, serosanguinous nasal discharge that crusts around the external nares.

Pharyngeal diphtheria is associated with the greatest toxicity and is characterized by marked tonsillar and pharyngeal inflammation and the presence of a membrane. This tough greyish-white membrane is formed by fibrin, bacteria, epithelial cells, mononuclear cells and polymorphs, and is firmly adherent to the underlying tissue. Regional lymphadenopathy is prominent and produces the so-called 'bull-neck'.

Laryngeal diphtheria is usually a result of extension of the membrane from the pharynx. A husky voice, a brassy cough, and later dyspnoea and cyanosis due to respiratory obstruction are common features.

Clinically evident myocarditis occurs, often weeks later, in patients with pharyngeal or laryngeal diphtheria. Acute circulatory failure due to myocarditis may occur in convalescent individuals around the 10th day of illness and is usually fatal. Neurological manifestations may occur either early in the disease (palatal and pharyngeal wall paralysis) or several weeks after its onset (cranial nerve palsies, paraesthesias, peripheral neuropathy or, rarely, encephalitis).

Cutaneous diphtheria is increasingly being seen in association with burns and in individuals with poor personal hygiene. Typically the ulcer is punched-out with undermined edges and is covered with a greyish-white to brownish adherent membrane. Constitutional symptoms are uncommon.

DIAGNOSIS

This must be made on clinical grounds since therapy is usually urgent and bacteriological results of culture studies and toxin production cannot be awaited.

TREATMENT

The patient should be isolated and bed rest advised. Antitoxin therapy is the only specific treatment. It must be instituted rapidly to prevent further fixation of toxin to tissue receptors, since fixed toxin is not neutralized by antitoxin. Depending on the severity, 20 000 to 120 000 units of horse-serum antitoxin should be administered intravenously after an initial test dose to exclude any allergic reaction. There is a risk of anaphylaxis immediately after antitoxin administration and of serum sickness 2–3 weeks later. Antibiotics should be administered concurrently to eliminate the organisms and thereby remove the source of toxin production. Procaine penicillin, 1.2 g i.m., once daily for 7 days is usually effective.

The cardiac and neurological complications need intensive therapy, as described on p. 705.

PREVENTION

Diphtheria can be effectively prevented by active immunization in childhood (see p. 21).

All contacts of the patient should have throat swabs sent for culture; those with a positive result should be treated with penicillin or erythromycin and active immunization or a booster dose of toxoid given.

LISTERIAL INFECTION

Listeria monocytogenes is a non-spore-forming, facultatively anaerobic bacillus that is motile at 20–25°C. It grows optimally at 30–37°C but can multiply at 4°C and survive heating to 60°C. It is found worldwide and is widely disseminated in the environment. Listeriosis predominantly occurs perinatally but may occasionally occur in immunocompromised adults. It causes abortions, septicaemia and meningitis. The mortality rate is high. Recent concern has arisen because of the increasing number of food-borne outbreaks in the past 10 years. Foods most commonly implicated are raw vegetables, coleslaw, milk, soft cheeses, chicken and paté. Cook–chill catering has come under scrutiny, the implication being that the organism can survive if reheating is inadequate.

Diagnosis is established by blood or CSF culture. Treatment is with ampicillin and gentamicin. Erythromycin, co-trimoxazole or rifampicin are alternatives.

CLOSTRIDIAL INFECTIONS

Clostridium is a Gram-positive, spore-forming, obligatory anaerobic bacillus. Some species, such as *C. botulinum* and *C. tetani*, produce potent neurotoxins, whereas *C. perfringens* produces numerous enzymes and only occasionally an enterotoxin (see Table 1.21). All clostridia that are pathogenic to humans produce exotoxins and require a low redox potential for growth. They are normal commensals of human and animal gastrointestinal tracts, and are widely distributed in soil, where, as spores, they may survive for many years in adverse conditions.

Tetanus

Tetanus occurs when a wound is contaminated by *C. tetani* in unimmunized individuals. The wound may be trivial and disregarded by the patient. The clinical manifestations of the disease are due to the potent neurotoxin, tetanospasmin. Tetanospasmin acts on both the alpha and gamma motor systems at synapses, resulting in disinhibition. It also produces neuromuscular blockade and skeletal muscle spasm, and acts on the sympathetic nervous system. The end result is marked flexor muscle spasm and autonomic dysfunction. The organism is not invasive.

CLINICAL FEATURES

The incubation period varies from a few days to several weeks. Four clinical varieties are recognized.

Generalized tetanus is the commonest form. Initially the patient complains of feeling unwell. This is followed by trismus (lock-jaw) due to masseter muscle spasm. Spasm of the facial muscles produces the characteristic grinning expression known as risus sardonicus. If the disease is severe, painful reflex spasms develop, usually within 24–72 h of the initial symptoms. The interval between the first symptom and the first spasm is referred to as the 'onset time'. The spasms may occur spontaneously but are easily precipitated by noise, handling of the patient or by light. The frequency of spasms usually increases and respiration becomes impaired due to laryngeal spasm. Oesophageal and urethral spasm lead to dysphagia and urinary retention, respectively. Arching of the neck and back muscles (opisthotonus) occurs. Autonomic dysfunction is evidenced by tachycardia, a labile blood pressure, sweating and cardiac arrhythmias. Patients with tetanus are mentally alert.

Death results from aspiration, hypoxia, respiratory failure, cardiac arrest or exhaustion. Mild cases with rigidity usually recover. Poor prognostic indicators are:

- Short incubation period
- Short onset time
- Cephalic tetanus
- Extremes of age
- 'Skin poppers' (narcotic addicts who inject drugs subcutaneously)

Localized tetanus. Pain and stiffness is confined to the site of the wound. The tone of the surrounding muscles is increased. Recovery usually occurs.

Cephalic tetanus an uncommon form and invariably fatal. It usually occurs when the portal of entry of *C. tetani* is the middle ear. Cranial nerve abnormalities, particularly of the seventh nerve, are usual. Generalized tetanus may or may not develop.

Tetanus neonatorum occurs in neonates owing to infection of the umbilical stump. Failure to thrive, poor sucking, grimacing and irritability are followed by rapid development of intense rigidity and spasms. Mortality approaches 100%.

DIAGNOSIS

Few diseases resemble tetanus in its fully developed form. The diagnosis is therefore a clinical one. Rarely, *C. tetani* may be isolated from wounds.

Phenothiazine overdosage, strychnine poisoning, meningitis and tetany can mimic tetanus.

TREATMENT

Nursing care. Improvement in nursing-care techniques has contributed more than any other single measure to the decrease in the mortality rate from 60% to nearer 20%. Patients are nursed in a quiet, isolated, well-ventilated, darkened room. Intragastric feeds may be necessary; bladder and bowel care are also important.

Wound debridement should be carried out where indicated.

Antibiotics and antitoxin. Both antibiotics and antitoxin should be administered, even in the absence of an obvious wound. Intravenous penicillin is the drug of choice. Human antitetanus immunoglobulin 2000–3000 units i.m. should be given to neutralize any circulating toxin; it has no effect on fixed toxin. If human antitetanus immunoglobulin is not available, immune equine tetanus immunoglobulin 10 000–20 000 units i.m. should be given, after excluding allergy to this product.

Antitoxin administrations

Most antitoxins are heterologous and therefore dangerous hypersensitivity reactions are common.

Prior to treatment:
- Question patient about:
  (a) Allergic conditions, e.g. asthma, hayfever
  (b) Previous antitoxin administration.
- Read instructions on antitoxin package carefully.
- Always give a subcutaneous test dose.

Control of spasms. Diazepam is the drug of choice. Up to 120 mg per 24 h may be required to control spasm and rigidity in adults. Beta-blocking drugs may be useful to control autonomic dysfunction.

The role of corticosteroids is controversial. Curarization and artificial respiratory support is best left to specialist units. The judicious use of a tracheostomy may be helpful in averting death.

Active immunization. Once recovery has occurred, active immunization should be instituted, as immunity following tetanus is incomplete.

PREVENTION

Tetanus is an eminently preventable disease and all persons should be immunized regardless of age. Those who work in a contaminated environment, such as farmers, are particularly at risk. Active immunization with either plain toxoid or the alum-adsorbed toxoid can be given. Of these, the latter is superior. Initially two doses of 0.5 ml of the toxoid are given intramuscularly at 8-week intervals. The third dose is given 6–12 months later as a booster. Subsequent boosters are required at 5-year intervals. Infant immunization schedules in the UK include tetanus (see Table 1.12).

Protection by passive immunization with either the equine or human antitetanus toxin is short-lived, lasting only about 2 weeks.

Botulism

Botulism is caused by *C. botulinum*. This organism is found in the soil and food is easily contaminated with the spores, which can survive heating to 100°C. The organisms proliferate in preserved canned foods and produce toxins. Only three types of neurotoxin—A, B and E—have been shown consistently to produce disease in humans. The toxins, which are the most potent known to man, result in marked neuromuscular blockade. They are heat-labile and are inactivated by heating at 80°C for 30 min or at 100°C for 10 min.

Three clinical forms are recognized:

- Foodborne: ingestion of pre-formed toxin usually in home canned or bottled food
- Infant botulism: Toxin production *in vivo*
- Wound botulism

CLINICAL FEATURES

Nausea, vomiting and diarrhoea are early symptoms and usually occur 18–20 h after ingesting contaminated food. Neurological symptoms dominate the clinical picture and include blurred vision and diplopia. Laryngeal and pharyngeal paralysis occur, and later generalized paralysis; consciousness is not altered. Respiratory insufficiency may occur. The marked cholinergic blockade results in urinary retention and constipation. Fever is unusual.

A strabismus occurs due to lateral rectus weakness and the pupil is fixed mid position or dilated and unresponsive to light or accommodation.

DIAGNOSIS

The presence of toxin in faeces, serum or suspected food items is demonstrated by injecting the material into mice. The differential diagnosis includes the Guillain–Barré syndrome and myasthenia gravis.

TREATMENT

Treatment is supportive and should be directed at maintaining adequate respiration, with assisted ventilation if necessary. Intravenous administration of 20 ml of antitoxin is followed by 10 ml 2–4 h later and then every 12–24 h as necessary. The role of antibiotics has not been adequately evaluated. Guanidine hydrochloride in doses of 15–40 mg·kg^{-1} improves botulism-induced paralysis by reversing the intramuscular blockage.

PROGNOSIS

The overall mortality rate for botulism is high (50–70%) but patients who survive the acute paralysis can recover completely.

Gas gangrene

Gas gangrene (clostridial myonecrosis) is commonly caused by *C. perfringens*. *C. novyi* and *C. septicum* are less frequently implicated. Gas gangrene occurs in lacerated wounds associated with fractures or retained foreign bodies. It is characterized by the onset of inordinately severe pain, with thickened induration and oedema at the injury site. When gas gangrene occurs in a limb, the part distal to the injury becomes cold and pulseless. Blebs occur and discharge a watery fluid, which later becomes haemorrhagic. The involved muscles at first appear pale and oedematous, but later they become beefy-red in colour and then brownish-black and frankly gangrenous. The characteristic crepitus of gas gangrene is a late feature. Systemic signs of toxicity are prominent. The patient is febrile, tachypnoeic and has a marked tachycardia. Hypotension, renal failure and hepatic failure develop as terminal events. Consciousness remains unaltered.

TREATMENT

Treatment consists of adequate surgical debridement, with parenteral penicillin or chloramphenicol combined with another antibiotic to cover aerobic and anaerobic organisms that are frequent wound contaminants. The role of anti-gas gangrene toxin and hyperbaric oxygen is controversial.

Pseudomembranous colitis

Pseudomembranous colitis is caused by the A and B toxins produced by *C. difficile*. It usually occurs a few days after institution of antibiotic therapy, although it has been known to occur even a month after discontinuing antibiotics. Clindamycin has been most frequently implicated, but ampicillin, tetracycline, lincomycin and the cephalosporins have also been causally related to some cases. Fever, diarrhoea (rarely with blood) and abdominal cramps are usual. Sigmoidoscopic examination may reveal a markedly erythematous, ulcerated mucosa covered by a membrane-like material although in about 20% of patients only the ascending colon is involved. A normal sigmoidoscopy therefore does not exclude infection. The presence of this membrane is not essential to the diagnosis.

DIAGNOSIS

Identification of the toxin (by observing its cytopathic effect on cells in tissue culture) in stool specimens is usually diagnostic but the test can be unreliable. Culture of the organism alone is insufficient as 5% of healthy adults carry *C. difficile*. Both the organism and its toxin are commonly found in healthy neonates in whom it has no pathological significance.

TREATMENT

All suspected antibiotics should be discontinued. Vancomycin 125 mg orally, four times daily, for 10 days, has until recently been the drug of choice. Metronidazole and bacitracin are also effective and considerably less expensive.

BACILLUS INFECTIONS

Anthrax

Anthrax, is caused by *Bacillus anthracis*. Its spores are extremely hardy and withstand extremes of temperature and humidity. The organism is capable of toxin production and this property correlates most closely with its virulence. The disease occurs world-wide. Epidemics have been reported in the Gambia, in both North and South America and in southern Europe. Transmission is through direct contact with an infected animal and is seen in farmers, butchers and dealers in wool and animal hides. Spores can also be ingested or inhaled.

CLINICAL FEATURES

The incubation period varies from 1 to 5 days.
The *cutaneous* form is the commonest mode of presentation and is seen most frequently in the tropics. It is self-limiting in the majority of patients. Typically, a small erythematous, maculopapular lesion is present that subsequently vesiculates and undergoes ulceration, with formation of a central black eschar. Occasionally the perivesicular oedema is marked and toxaemia may be present.

Respiratory involvement (woolsorter's disease) due to inhalation of spores results in a nonproductive cough, fever and retrosternal discomfort. Pleural effusions are common. In some patients there is apparent clinical improvement followed by the abrupt onset of dyspnoea, marked cyanosis and death.

Gastrointestinal anthrax presents as severe gastroenteritis. Haematemesis and bloody diarrhoea may occur.

DIAGNOSIS

Diagnosis is established by demonstrating the organism in smears or by culture. Detection of a fourfold increase in antibodies measured by indirect microhaemagglutination or enzyme-linked immunoabsorbent assay (ELISA) in paired sera (i.e. acute and convalescent samples) is diagnostic.

TREATMENT

Penicillin is the drug of choice. In mild cutaneous infections, phenoxymethylpenicillin 500 mg four times daily for 2 weeks is adequate. In more severe infections, e.g. when septicaemia is present, up to 24 g of intravenous penicillin is required daily. Sulphonamides, chloramphenicol and tetracycline have also been used successfully. The role of steroids in fulminant anthrax infections is questionable.

Any infected animal that dies should be burned and the area in which it was housed disinfected. Where animal husbandry is poor, mass vaccination of animals may prevent widespread contamination.

Vaccination of exposed workers is effective.

Bacillus cereus infection

This Gram-positive, aerobic, spore-forming bacillus can cause food poisoning and wound sepsis.

OTHER ORGANISMS

Cat-scratch disease

Seven to 14 days after a scratch or bite, a small red papule appears at the site associated with regional lymph-node enlargement. Lymphadenopathy may persist for several weeks and suppurate in up to 40%. The disease may progress systemically with encephalitis, neuroretinitis, arthritis, hepatitis, osteolytic bone lesions and pleurisy. Recently a cell-wall-defective Gram-positive bacilli has been identified as the cause. The organism is sensitive to some cephalosporins (cefoxitin, cefotaxime) and aminoglycosides (gentamicin, tobramycin).

Gram-negative bacilli

BRUCELLOSIS (Malta fever, undulant fever)

Brucella is a Gram-negative coccobacillus. Three species are recognized—*abortus*, *melitensis* and *suis*. Brucellosis is a zoonosis and has a world-wide distribution (Table 1.16), although it has been virtually eliminated from cattle in the UK. The organism does not withstand pasteurization. The brucella endotoxin (a cell-wall lipopolysaccharide) is responsible for systemic symptoms and host hypersensitivity accounts for formation of granulomas. The organisms usually gain entry into the human body via the mouth, though less frequently they may enter via the respiratory tract, genital tract or abraded skin. The bacilli travel in the lymphatics and infect lymph nodes. This is followed by haematogenous spread with ultimate localization of the bacilli in the reticuloendothelial system. Spread is largely by the ingestion of raw milk from infected cattle. The disease often occurs in workers in close contact with animals or carcasses.

CLINICAL FEATURES

The incubation period varies from 1 to 3 weeks. The onset of *acute brucellosis* is insidious, with malaise, headache, weakness, generalized myalgia and night sweats. The fever pattern is classically undulant, although continuous and intermittent patterns are frequent. Lymphadenopathy, hepatomegaly and spinal tenderness may also be present. The presence of splenomegaly is indicative of severe infection. Arthritis, spondylitis, bursitis, osteomyelitis, orchitis, epididymitis, meningoencephalitis and endocarditis have all been described, especially in infections with *B. melitensis* or *B. suis*.

Chronic brucellosis is characterized by easy fatiguability, myalgia, occasional bouts of fever and depression, which may persist for several months. Splenomegaly is present. It needs to be distinguished from other causes of prolonged fever (p. 9).

Localized brucellosis is uncommon. Bones and joints, spleen, endocardium, lungs, urinary tract and nervous system may be involved. Systemic symptoms occur in less than one-third. Antibody titres are low. Diagnosis is established by culturing the organisms from the involved site.

DIAGNOSIS

Blood cultures are positive during the acute phase of illness in 50% of patients. Serological tests are of greater value. The *Brucella* agglutination test, which demonstrates a fourfold or greater rise in titre over a 4-week period, is highly suggestive of brucellosis. A single titre greater than 1 in 60 is also suggestive of brucellosis in the appropriate clinical setting. An elevated serum IgG level detected by extraction with 2-mercaptoethanol (2-ME) is evidence of current or recent infection. A negative 2-ME test excludes chronic brucellosis. Specific *Brucella* immunoglobulins can be detected by the ELISA technique.

TREATMENT

Tetracycline 500 mg orally four times daily is given combined with rifampicin 800 mg once daily for 6 weeks, but relapses occur. Alternatively, tetracycline can be combined with streptomycin, which is usually only given for the first 2 weeks of treatment. Co-trimoxazole 960 mg two times daily is also effective.

PREVENTION AND CONTROL

Prevention and control involves careful attention to hygiene when handling infected animals, eradication of infection in infected animals, and pasteurization of milk. No vaccine is available for use in humans.

Table 1.16 Main geographical distribution and natural hosts of the *Brucella* species.

Organism	Geographical distribution	Natural host
B. abortus	World-wide, except northern Europe, Japan, Yugoslavia	Cattle
B. melitensis	Mediterranean region (especially Malta), Middle East	Goats and sheep
B. suis	Far East, USA	Pigs
B. canis[a]		Beagles

[a] Rarely causes disease in humans.

BORDETELLA INFECTIONS

Bordetella is a Gram-negative coccobacillus. B. pertussis causes pertussis (whooping cough). B. parapertussis and B. bronchiseptica produce milder infections.

Pertussis

Pertussis occurs world-wide. Humans are both the natural hosts and reservoirs of infection. Pertussis is highly contagious and is spread by droplet infection. In its early stages it is indistinguishable from other types of upper respiratory tract infection and hence spread occurs easily. Epidemics are common and have increased in the UK since the safety of the whooping cough vaccine was questioned.

CLINICAL FEATURES

The incubation period varies from 7 to 14 days. It is a disease of childhood, with 90% of cases occurring below 5 years of age. However, no age is exempt. During the catarrhal stage the patient is highly infectious, and cultures from respiratory secretions are positive in over 90% of patients. Malaise, anorexia, mucoid rhinorrhoea and conjunctivitis are present. The paroxysmal stage, so called because of the characteristic paroxysms of coughing, begins about a week later. Paroxysms with the classic inspiratory whoop are seen only in younger individuals in whom the lumen of the respiratory tract is compromised by mucus secretion and mucosal oedema. The whoop results from air being forcefully drawn through the narrowed tract. These paroxysms usually terminate in vomiting. Conjunctival suffusion and petechiae and ulceration of the frenulum of the tongue are usual. Lymphocytosis due to the elaboration of lymphocyte-promoting factor by B. pertussis is characteristic; lymphocytes may account for over 90% of the total white blood cell count. This stage lasts approximately two weeks and may be associated with several complications, including bronchitis, lobar pneumonia, atelectasis, rectal prolapse and inguinal hernia. Cerebral anoxia may occur, especially in younger children, resulting in convulsions. Bronchiectasis is a late sequel.

DIAGNOSIS

The diagnosis is suggested clinically by the characteristic whoop and a history of contact with an infected individual. It is confirmed by growing the organism in culture. Cultures of swabs of nasopharyngeal secretions result in a higher positive yield than cultures of 'cough plates'.

TREATMENT

If the disease is recognized in the catarrhal stage, erythromycin will abort or decrease the severity of the infection. In the paroxysmal stage antibiotics have little role to play in altering the course of the illness.

PREVENTION AND CONTROL

Affected individuals should be isolated to prevent contact with others. This is particularly important in hostels and boarding schools. Pertussis is an easily preventable disease and effective active immunization is available (see Table 1.11). A Japanese vaccine that is less reactogenic than the currently used whole-cell vaccine is being evaluated.

HAEMOPHILUS INFECTIONS

Haemophilus is a Gram-negative pleomorphic, coccobacillus. Those pathogenic to humans include H. influenzae, H. ducreyi and H. parainfluenzae. In general, non-encapsulated forms produce luminal infections, e.g. bronchitis, and encapsulated organisms produce invasive disease, e.g. meningitis. Haemophilus is a normal commensal of the upper respiratory tract and is found in about 80% of healthy individuals.

Of the six antigenic types of H. influenzae identified, type b is the most important in humans and demonstrates the greatest pathogenicity, especially in children below 5 years of age. It can produce disease in several human organs (Table 1.17). Infection is generally autogenous and hence sporadic cases are common.

Table 1.17 Major clinical syndromes associated with *Haemophilus influenzae*.

Respiratory system
Sinusitis
Bronchitis
Pneumonia

Central nervous system
Meningitis
Brain abscess

Cardiac system
Endocarditis
Pericarditis

Miscellaneous
Septic arthritis
Cellulitis
Epiglottitis
Otitis media

High risk factors include:

- Children, 6–48 months
- Sickle cell disease
- Splenectomy
- Hypogammaglobulinaemia
- Treated Hodgkin's disease
- Alcohol abuse

There is evidence of increasing immunity to *Haemophilus* with age. This is related to the presence of anticapsular and specific bactericidal antibodies. Cross-reacting antibodies to other Gram-negative bacteria can also contribute to immunity. Adults with impaired host defence mechanisms, e.g. alcoholics, appear to have an increased risk of infection. A history suggestive of an antecedent viral fever is usual.

Infections with *Haemophilus influenzae*

H. influenzae infections have a world-wide distribution.

Meningitis
H. influenzae is the commonest cause of meningitis in the second year of life. The clinical features are described on p. 930.
  Generally the response to treatment is slow. About 25% of children have permanent residual neurological deficits such as deafness.

Epiglottitis
This is characterized by a dramatically rapid course and fatal outcome in children if appropriate treatment is not instituted. The onset is acute with high fever, pooling of oropharyngeal secretions, dysphagia and marked respiratory distress. Examination reveals a markedly swollen and inflamed epiglottis.

Pneumonia
H. influenzae type b accounts for about 30% of all childhood bacterial pneumonias and 3–6% of pneumonias in adults.

DIAGNOSIS

This is made by isolation and culture of the organism. Counterimmunoelectrophoresis can be used to detect type b capsular antigen in 75% of patients.

TREATMENT

Treatment is urgent, as delay may result in a high mortality, especially in patients with meningitis and epiglottitis. In these conditions the drug of choice is chloramphenicol 50–100 mg·kg^{-1} per day i.v. for children and 4 g per day i.v. for 7–10 days for adults. Ampicillin can be used for less severe cases, but resistance to this drug is increasing.

PREVENTION

Children in close contact with an infected individual are at an increased risk of developing the disease. Rifampicin 20 mg·kg^{-1} for 4 days is helpful. Recently, a purified capsular antigen vaccine has been tried with variable success.

CHOLERA

Cholera is caused by the curved, actively motile, flagellated Gram-negative bacillus, *Vibrio cholerae*. The organism is killed by temperatures of 100°C in a few seconds but can survive in ice for up to 6 weeks. The El Tor biotype has replaced the classical biotype as the major cause of cholera. This is because the El Tor *V. cholerae* is a hardier organism. Infection with the El Tor biotype is frequently unrecognized because it produces milder clinical symptoms; a chronic gall-bladder carrier state can result in about 3% of all infected adults. All three strains (Inaba, Ogawa and Hikojima) are pathogenic. The fertile, humid Gangetic plains of West Bengal have traditionally been regarded as 'the home of cholera'. However, the seventh and most recent pandemic of cholera, which was caused by the El Tor biotype, affected large areas of Asia, North Africa and Southern Europe. Humans are the only known natural hosts. Transmission is by the faecal–oral route. Contaminated water plays a major role in the dissemination of cholera, although contaminated foods and contact carriers may be instrumental in the spread during epidemics.

Achlorhydria or hypochlorhydria facilitates passage of the cholera bacilli into the small intestine, where they proliferate and elaborate an exotoxin with A and B subunits. The B subunit binds to specific GM1 ganglioside receptors and the A subunit activates the intracellular enzyme adenylate cyclase. This produces elevation of 3'5'-cyclic AMP, which in turn produces massive secretion of isotonic fluid into the intestinal lumen (see p. 222). The toxin is bound irreversibly to the receptor site where it exerts its effect for 24–48 h. The clinical effects are produced by the toxin and the organism is not invasive.

CLINICAL FEATURES

The incubation period varies from a few hours to 6 days. The majority of patients with cholera have a mild illness that cannot be distinguished clinically from diarrhoea due to other infective causes. Classically, however, three phases are recognized in the untreated disease. The *evacuation phase* is characterized by the abrupt onset of painless, profuse, watery diarrhoea, associated with vomiting in the severe forms. 'Rice water' stools, so called because of mucus flecks floating in the watery stools, are characteristic of this stage. If appropriate supportive treatment is not given, the patient passes on to the *collapse phase*. This is characterized by features of circulatory shock (cold clammy skin, tachycardia, hypotension and peripheral cyanosis) and dehydration (sunken eyes, hollow cheeks and a diminished urine output). The patient, though apathetic, is usually lucid. Muscle cramps may be severe. Children may, in addition, present with convulsions due to hypoglycaemia. At this stage renal failure and aspiration of vomitus present major problems. Should the patient survive this stage, he then enters into the *recovery phase*, with a gradual return to normal of clinical and biochemical parameters in 1–3 days.

Cholera sicca is an uncommon but severe form of cholera. It presents with massive outpouring of fluid and electrolytes into dilated intestinal loops. Diarrhoea and vomiting do not occur and hence the disease is frequently not recognized. The mortality rate is high.

DIAGNOSIS

Diagnosis is largely clinical. Examination of freshly passed stools may demonstrate rapidly motile organisms. This is not diagnostic, as *Campylobacter jejuni* may also give a similar appearance. However, demonstration of the rapidly motile vibrios by dark-field illumination and subsequent inhibition of their movement with type-specific antisera is diagnostic.

Stool and rectal swabs should be taken for culture.

TREATMENT

With appropriate and effective rehydration therapy, mortality has decreased to less than 1%. Rehydration is mainly oral, but intravenous therapy is occasionally required.

- **Oral rehydration**, for maintenance therapy or for correction of mild to moderate dehydration, is best carried out by giving a glucose–electrolyte solution. The World Health Organisation (WHO) ORS and numerous commercial preparations of varying composition are available (Table 1.18). Mildly dehydrated individuals should be given ORS 50 ml·kg^{-1} in the first 4 h followed by a maintenance solution of a 100 ml·kg^{-1} daily until the diarrhoea stops. For moderate dehydration, ORS 100 ml·kg^{-1} is given within the first 4 h followed by 10–15 ml·kg^{-1} per hour. Recently rice- and wheat-based electrolyte solutions have been found to be effective and actually reduce stool volume as well as rehydrating.

- **Intravenous rehydration** is required only for severely dehydrated individuals with features of collapse. Intravenous solutions recommended by WHO include Ringer's lactate solution and the 'Diarrhoea Treatment Solution' (sodium chloride 4.0 g, sodium acetate 6.5 g, potassium chloride 1.0 g, and glucose 9.0 g, per litre). Several litres of intravenous fluid are usually required to overcome the features of shock. Maintenance of hydration is effectively carried out by oral rehydration solutions.

Antibiotics such as tetracycline 250 mg four times daily for 3 days or doxycycline help to eradicate the infection, decrease stool output and shorten the duration of the illness dramatically. Drug resistance is becoming an increasing problem.

Table 1.18 Oral rehydration solutions (ORS) available in the UK.

	Sodium (mmol·L^{-1})	Potassium (mmol·L^{-1})	Chloride (mmol·L^{-1})	Bicarbonate (mmol·L^{-1})	Glucose (mmol·L^{-1})	Citrate (mmol·L^{-1})
WHO/UNICEF	or 90	20	80	30	111	—
	90	20	80	—	111	10
Sodium chloride and oral glucose powder compound	35	20	37	18	200	—
Dioralyte	35	20	37	18	200	—
Rehidrat[a]	50	20	50	20	91	9
Dextrolyte[b]	35	13.4	30.5	—	200	—
Electrolade	50	20	40	—	111	10
Pedialyte MS[c]	45	20	35	—	139	10
RS[c]	75	20	65	—	139	10

[a] Plus fructose 2 mmol·L^{-1} and sucrose 94 mmol·L^{-1}.
[b] Plus lactate 7.7 mmol·L^{-1}.
[c] MS, maintenance solution; RS, rehydration solution.

Table 1.19 Patterns of gut infection.

	Non-inflammatory	Inflammatory	Penetrating
Major location:	Jejunum	Colon	Ileum
Clinical presentation:	Watery diarrhoea	Dysentery	Enteric fever
Common pathogens:	*Vibrio cholerae* Enterotoxigenic *Escherichia coli*	*Shigella* sp. Enteroinvasive *Escherichia coli* *Salmonella* sp. *Clostridium difficile* *Campylobacter jejuni* *Entamoeba histolytica* (see p. 88)	*Salmonella typhi* *Yersinia enterocolitica*
Pathogenetic mechanisms:	Enterotoxin (CT, LT, ST) production causing intestinal secretion of water and electrolytes	Invasion of gut epithelium ± cytotoxin release	Invasion and bacteraemia

CT = cholera toxin; LT and ST = *E. coli* heat-labile and heat-stable toxins.

PREVENTION AND CONTROL

Immunization with currently available vaccines results in poor immunity and is no longer recommended. Attenuated live cholera vaccines are under intensive evaluation. Chemoprophylaxis with tetracycline 500 mg two times daily for 3 days for adults and 125 mg daily for children is effective. The most effective preventive measures, however, are good hygiene and sanitary living conditions.

Table 1.19 compares the pattern of infection caused by *Vibrio cholerae* with the patterns of infection caused by other gut organisms.

ENTEROBACTERIACEAE INFECTIONS

The Enterobacteriaceae is a diverse group of aerobic Gram-negative organisms. Included in this category are *Escherichia coli*, *Salmonella* and *Shigella*.

Escherichia coli infection

Escherichia coli is commonly responsible for urinary tract infections, bacteraemia, neonatal meningitis, and peritoneal and biliary infections. Such infections are indistinguishable from similar clinical conditions caused by other bacteria.

E. coli responsible for enteric disease have different serotype characteristics from those that cause disease elsewhere in the body. Four main categories of *E. coli* capable of producing human diarrhoeal disease are recognized.

Enterotoxigenic E. coli (ETEC) produces a diarrhoeal illness that is mediated through a heat-labile toxin (LT) and/or a heat-stable toxin (ST). Toxin production is genetically encoded by transferable DNA plasmids. LT resembles cholera toxin in its mode of action since it also acts via cyclic AMP and is associated with massive secretion of water and electrolytes into the intestinal lumen. ST activates guanylate cyclase with elevation of cyclic GMP levels and subsequent secretion of water and electrolytes (see Fig. 4.27a, p. 222). Clinically ETEC produces three syndromes:

- An illness indistinguishable from severe cholera
- 'Traveller's diarrhoea', a milder disease (other causes are shown in Table 1.20)
- Diarrhoea of varying severity in children, especially in developing countries.

Enteroinvasive E. coli (ETEC) produces an illness similar to that produced by *Shigella* (see below).

Enteropathogenic E. coli (EPEC) attaches to and damages intestinal epithelium, producing diarrhoea, primarily in children below 2 years of age. Toxins are thought to be involved in the production of diarrhoea. Epidemics are common, especially in nurseries.

Table 1.20 Causes of traveller's diarrhoea.

Pathogen	Proportion of cases (%)
Enterotoxigenic *Escherichia coli*	40–75
Shigella sp.	0–15
Salmonella sp.	0–10
Rotavirus, Norwalk family of viruses	0–10
Giardia lamblia, *Entamoeba histolytica*	0–3
Unknown	22–25

Enterohaemorrhagic E. coli (EHEC) produce a shiga-like cytotoxin that causes bloody diarrhoea and colitis. Fever is unusual. Outbreaks have been linked with contaminated food, particularly hamburgers.

TREATMENT

Oral administration of fluids and electrolytes is the mainstay of therapy. Many *E. coli* gut infections are self-limiting and require no specific antimicrobial therapy. For severe infection, particularly with colitis and a systemic illness, ampicillin 2 g daily or co-trimoxazole 960 mg twice daily can be given. Gentamicin 2–5 mg·kg^{-1} daily or tobramycin 3–5 mg·kg^{-1} daily in divided 8-hourly doses are effective alternatives in severe illness with septicaemia.

Trimethoprim 200 mg once daily is effective prophylaxis against traveller's diarrhoea due to ETEC, and early treatment with the standard therapeutic dose of 200 mg two times daily for 3–5 days will shorten the duration of the illness.

Salmonellosis

Salmonella is a Gram-negative, generally motile bacillus. Biochemically three species are recognized —*S. typhi* and *S. paratyphi*, *S. choleraesuis* and *S. enteritidis*. Their thermal death point is 60°C but they can withstand freezing and dry conditions for prolonged periods of time. Although salmonellae have a world-wide distribution, they usually result in disease only where there is poor hygiene and overcrowding. Transmission occurs by ingestion of contaminated foods (particularly eggs and poultry products) or water. In the past few years there has been a dramatic increase in *S. enteritidis* phage type 4 illnesses owing to widespread contamination of battery chickens. The organism is found in the alimentary tract, the oviducts and within the egg itself. In the UK, spread is often by carriers, usually food handlers, who contaminate the food. Following ingestion, the salmonellae colonize the small intestine and proliferate in Peyer's patches. They are then carried through the lymphatics, enter the bloodstream, and are thereby transported to the reticuloendothelial system.

A spectrum of clinical syndromes due to *Salmonella* is recognized:

- Enteric fever (typhoid or paratyphoid fever)
- Enterocolitis
- Extra-intestinal focal infections, e.g. osteomyelitis
- Food poisoning
- Carriers

Typhoid fever

This is caused by *S. typhi*. Humans are the only known reservoirs. The incubation period is usually 10–14 days. The onset is insidious, with headache being a prominent symptom. The fever is remittent and gradually increases in severity in a step-ladder fashion over 3–4 days. Cough, sore throat and altered behaviour may also be present. Constipation is usually present initially and diarrhoea only occurs late in the disease. Physical examination during the first week reveals a toxic individual with a relative bradycardia. During the second week several physical signs can be elicited. An erythematous maculopapular rash that blanches on pressure and is referred to as 'rose spots' appears, chiefly on the upper abdomen and thorax, and lasts for only 2–3 days. These spots are not easily visible on dark-skinned patients. A soft splenomegaly occurs in about 75% of patients. Cervical lymphadenopathy (present in about 30% of patients), hepatomegaly (present in about 30% of patients) and right iliac fossa tenderness are other physical signs that may be present. The third week of illness, aptly referred to as 'the week of complications', is the time when the majority of complications occur. These include lobar pneumonia, haemolytic anaemia, meningitis, peripheral neuropathy, acute cholecystitis, urinary tract infection and osteomyelitis. Intestinal perforation occurs in 2–3% and intestinal haemorrhage in 2–8%. The fourth week of illness ('the week of convalescence') is characterized by a gradual return to health.

DIAGNOSIS

Leucopenia is present. Blood cultures are positive in about 80% during the first week and 30% in the third week. Urine cultures are helpful during the second week and stool cultures during the second to fourth week. Marrow cultures are occasionally helpful. Of the serological tests the Widal test, which measures serum agglutinins against the O and H antigens, is most helpful; a fourfold increase in titre in sequential blood samples is suggestive of *Salmonella* infection.

CARRIERS

Carriers can be divided into chronic carriers, defined as individuals who excrete *Salmonella* for at least 1 year, and convalescent carriers. The presence of Vi agglutinin in the serum in a dilution greater than 1 : 10 is suggestive of a carrier state. Since the gall-bladder is frequently the focus of infection, duodenal aspirates for culture of the bile-containing duodenal juice may yield useful information.

TREATMENT

Chloramphenicol (75 mg·kg^{-1} daily in four divided doses) remains the drug of choice, despite increasing resistance. It is 4–6 days before the temperature shows signs of diminishing, although subjective improvement is noted earlier. Treatment should be continued for 2 weeks. Co-trimoxazole 960 mg daily is also effective; again therapy should be continued for 2 weeks. Ampicillin 6 g daily is a useful alternative. Complications such as intestinal perforation or haemorrhage may occur despite adequate treatment. These complications can often be managed conservatively.

Eradication of a carrier state can be difficult, but ampicillin 4–6 g daily with probenicid 2 g daily for 6 weeks may be effective. Chemotherapy does not effect a cure in about 40%. In such individuals cholecystectomy remains the only mode of treatment.

PREVENTION AND CONTROL

This includes provision of safe drinking water, sanitary disposal of excreta and proper attention to hygiene by those who handle food. The parenteral monovalent typhoid vaccine is used as it is less likely to produce local and systemic reactions, but protection is incomplete and relatively short-lived (1 year). An attenuated strain of S. typhi (Ty 21a) is being evaluated as a live oral vaccine and appears to confer moderately good protection for 3 years.

Paratyphoid fever
Paratyphoid fever is due to S. paratyphi A, B or C. They result in an illness clinically indistinguishable from typhoid fever. However, paratyphoid fever is a milder illness. Treatment is with co-trimoxazole 960 mg daily for two weeks.

Enterocolitis
This is an acute, short-lived infection, and is usually due to S. enteritidis serotype typhimurium. It is generally mild, lasting 2–3 days, and presents with fever, malaise, cramping abdominal pain, bloody diarrhoea and vomiting. Occasionally a cholera-like picture may be present. Treatment is symptomatic. This Salmonella is an important cause of food poisoning; other organisms responsible are shown in Table 1.21.

As with typhoid fever, a chronic carrier state may develop. Treatment is as described for S. typhi carriers.

Shigellosis (bacillary dysentery)

Shigellosis is an acute self-limiting intestinal infection caused by one of four species of Gram-negative non-spore-forming bacilli. These include *Shigella dysenteriae, S. flexneri, S. boydii* and *S. sonnei*. While all of them are enteroinvasive, S. dysenteriae type 1 and some strains of S. flexneri and S. sonnei have been demonstrated to elaborate a toxin that is enterotoxic, neurotoxic and cytotoxic. Like salmonellosis, shigellosis is found world-wide and is more prevalent in areas with poor hygiene and overcrowding. Transmission is by the faecal–oral route.

Table 1.21 Bacterial causes of food poisoning.

Organism	Source	Incubation period	Symptoms	Diagnosis	Recovery
Staphylococcus aureus	Contaminated food, usually by humans	2–6 h	Diarrhoea, vomiting and dehydration	Culture organism in vomitus or remaining food	Rapid (few hours)
Bacillus cereus	Spores in food survive boiling	1–6 h	Diarrhoea, vomiting and dehydration	Culture organism in faeces and food	Rapid
Clostridium perfringens	Spores in food survive boiling	8–22 h	Watery diarrhoea and cramping pain	Culture organism in faeces and food	2–3 days
Clostridium botulinum	Spores survive cooking but only germinate in anaerobic conditions, e.g. canned or bottled foods	18–36 h	Brief diarrhoea and paralysis due to neuromuscular blockade	Demonstrate toxin in food or faeces	10–14 days
Salmonella enteritidis[a]	Bowels of animals, especially fowl	12–24 h	Abrupt diarrhoea, fever and vomiting	Culture organism in stool	Usually 2–5 days, but may be up to 2 weeks
Campylobacter jejuni	Bowels of animals, especially fowl; also in milk	48–96 h	Diarrhoea ± blood, fever, malaise and abdominal pain	Culture organism in stool	3–5 days

Non-microbial toxins such as dinoflagellate plankton toxin in shellfish ('red tide'), scrombotoxin from some varieties of spoiled fish (see p. 753) and red kidney bean toxin (haemagglutinin) from partially cooked beans also cause acute diarrhoea.
[a] Many strains, including S. typhimurium.

CLINICAL FEATURES

The incubation period is short, usually being 2 days. The onset is acute, with fever, malaise, abdominal pain and watery diarrhoea. As the disease increases in intensity, bloody diarrhoea with mucus, tenesmus, faecal urgency and severe cramping abdominal pain becomes prominent. Nausea, vomiting, headache and convulsions (in children) may occur and have been attributed to the neurotoxin. When the disease is due to *S. dysenteriae*, which is responsible for the more fulminant forms of shigellosis, a cholera-like picture is occasionally seen. Sigmoidoscopy shows the presence of a markedly hyperaemic and inflamed mucosa, with transversely distributed ulcers with rugged undermined edges. The appearances are often indistinguishable from other dysenteric infections and from non-specific inflammatory bowel disease. Complications may be mild (arthritis, conjunctivitis, morbilliform rash) or life-threatening, such as colonic perforation, septicaemia and the haemolytic uraemic syndrome.

DIAGNOSIS

The diagnosis is made on the basis of a stool culture.

TREATMENT

Treatment is symptomatic. In severe illness, ampicillin 50–100 mg·kg^{-1} daily in children and 2 g daily in adults or nalidixic acid 1 g four times daily may decrease the severity of illness.

Public health measures, particularly the disposal of excreta and the provision of potable water, prevent infection. Outbreaks in schools can only be controlled by good hygiene.

CAMPYLOBACTER INFECTION

Campylobacter jejuni is a Gram-negative, motile, curved spiral rod that is microaerophilic and thus fails to multiply under aerobic or strict anaerobic conditions. *Campylobacter jejuni* causes acute diarrhoea, sometimes with blood, and is now one of the most common causes of acute gastroenteritis in the UK.

CLINICAL FEATURES

Symptoms begin 2–5 days after eating infected material (usually chicken or milk), the commonest being fever, headache and malaise. These are followed rapidly by diarrhoea, often with blood and quite severe cramping abdominal pain. The patient generally appears unwell. Sigmoidoscopy can show the changes of acute colitis, which may be indistinguishable from those of ulcerative colitis.

DIAGNOSIS

Direct phase microscopy of a wet mount of stool may reveal the motile curved rods resembling 'flying birds'. The organism may be cultured on special media within 48 h. In severe infections the organism may be cultured from the blood.

TREATMENT

In the majority of cases, *Campylobacter* enteritis is a self-limiting illness, resolving in 5–7 days. Although the organism is sensitive to erythromycin, there is no evidence that treatment with this antibiotic alters the natural history of the infection. However, if systemic symptoms continue in association with persistent bacteraemia, antibiotics are usually administered.

HELICOBACTER (previously known as a campylobacter) (see p. 188)

H. pylori, a curved Gram-negative organism, colonizes the gastric epithelium beneath the mucus layer and in areas of gastric metaplasia such as occur in the duodenum and oesophagus. *H. pylori* is noted for its ability to produce urease, which is thought to be involved in the pathogenesis of disease.

YERSINIA INFECTIONS

The only three major human pathogens are *Yersinia pestis*, which causes plague, and *Y. pseudotuberculosis* and *Y. enterocolitica*, which cause mesenteric lymphadenitis and enterocolitis, respectively.

Y. enterocolitica and *Y. pseudotuberculosis* infections

These result in a number of clinical syndromes depending on the host's age and immune status. Patients may present with enterocolitis, acute mesenteric lymphadenitis or terminal ileitis. Enterocolitis is characterized by the presence of fever, diarrhoea and severe abdominal pain, which may lead to a mistaken diagnosis of appendicitis. Arthritis (sometimes with Reiter's syndrome—see p. 403) and erythema nodosum are seen and are immunologically mediated.

This is usually a self-limiting disease and no treatment is required. In very severe cases, tetracycline 1 g daily may be given.

Plague

Plague is caused by *Y. pestis*, a Gram-negative, pleomorphic bacterium. Nowadays it is mainly limited to animals, but sporadic cases of plague, as well as occasional epidemics, occur world-wide in humans. The major reservoirs are woodland rodents, which transmit infection to domestic rats (*Rattus rattus*). The vector is the rat flea, *Xenopsylla cheopis*. These fleas bite humans when there is a sudden decline in the rat population. Occasionally, spread of the organisms may be through infected faeces being rubbed into skin wounds or through inhalation of droplets.

Virulence is attributed to the presence of the endotoxin, exotoxin and fraction I (a soluble protein that prevents phagocytosis of the organism). Clinical manifestations are attributed to the lipopolysaccharide endotoxin.

CLINICAL FEATURES

Four clinical forms are recognized—bubonic, pneumonic, septicaemic and cutaneous plague.

Bubonic plague is the commonest form and occurs in about 90% of infected individuals. The incubation period is about a week. The onset of illness is acute, with high fever, chills, headache, myalgia, nausea, vomiting and, when severe, prostration. This is rapidly followed by the development of lymphadenopathy, most commonly involving the inguinal lymph nodes (buboes). Characteristically these are matted and tender, and suppurate in 1–2 weeks. Petechiae, ecchymoses and bleeding from the gastrointestinal tract, the respiratory tract and the genitourinary tract may occur. Mental confusion follows the development of toxaemia.

Pneumonic plague is characterized by the abrupt onset of features of a fulminant pneumonia with bloody sputum, marked respiratory distress, cyanosis and death in almost all affected patients.

Septicaemic plague presents as an acute fulminant infection with evidence of shock and disseminated intravascular coagulation. If left untreated, death usually occurs in 2–5 days. Lymphadenopathy is unusual.

Cutaneous plague presents either as a pustule, eschar or papule or an extensive purpura, which can become necrotic and gangrenous.

DIAGNOSIS

The diagnosis is easily established by demonstrating the organism in lymph node aspirates, in blood cultures or on examination of sputum.

TREATMENT

Treatment is urgent and should be instituted before the results of culture studies are available. Several antimicrobial drugs are effective, including streptomycin 0.5 g i.m. every 4 h for 48 h followed by 0.5 g every 6 h for 5 days, or tetracycline 2–3 g daily for 14 days.

PREVENTION AND CONTROL

Prevention of plague is largely dependent on the control of the flea population and the use of potent antiflea agents such as 2% aldrin. Outhouses, or huts, should be sprayed with insecticides that are effective against the local flea. Rodents should not be killed until the fleas are under control as the fleas will leave dead rodents to bite humans. Tetracycline 500 mg four times daily or sulphonamides 2–4 g daily for 7 days are effective chemoprophylactic agents. Patients themselves can be infective when the buboes break down; patients with pneumonic plague can spread the organism by droplet spread. A partially effective formalin-killed vaccine is available for use by travellers to plague-endemic areas.

TULARAEMIA

Tularaemia is due to infection by *Francisella tularensis*, a Gram-negative organism. It is primarily a zoonosis, affecting mainly rodents, including rabbits and squirrels. Vectors are ticks, flies and mosquitoes. Humans are infected by handling infected animals or from vector bites. The micro-organisms enter through the skin or through minor abrasions in the mouth or conjunctivae. Occasionally infection occurs from contaminated water or from eating uncooked meat. The disease occurs world-wide and is frequently seen in the USA, particularly in hunters and butchers.

CLINICAL FEATURES

The incubation period of 2–7 days is followed by a generalized illness. A number of clinical syndromes can be seen:

- The ulceroglandular form is the commonest. A papule occurs at the site of inoculation. This ulcerates and is followed by tender, suppurative lymphadenopathy. Infected material entering the eye is followed by a purulent conjunctivitis with periauricular lymphadenopathy.
- Pneumonic forms present with cough, chest pain and eventually a pneumonia, sometimes accompanied by a pericarditis.
- The septicaemic form presents with the sudden onset of a fever, myalgia, headache and shock.

DIAGNOSIS

Diagnosis is by culture of the organism or by a rising titre seen on a bacterial agglutination test.

TREATMENT

Treatment is with streptomycin or more usually gentamicin. The patient should be isolated.

PREVENTION

In endemic areas all wild animals should be handled using gloves. Infected meat and water should be adequately cooked. A vaccine is available for laboratory staff handling possibly infected animals.

GLANDERS

Glanders is caused by a Gram-negative bacillus, *Pseudomonas mallei*. It affects mainly horses but can be transmitted to man, mainly horse handlers. The disease is acquired by inhalation or inoculation of infected material. In the acute state, the patient is toxic with a high fever and delirium. There is an ulceration of the upper respiratory tract with eventual pneumonia, empyema and lung abscess. Septicaemia develops, which was fatal prior to antibiotics becoming available. Treatment is with sulphonamides.

MELIOIDOSIS

Melioidosis is due to the Gram-negative bacillus, *Pseudomonas pseudomallei*, which is a soil saprophyte. It infects humans (particularly diabetics or traumatized patients) by penetrating through skin abrasions, occasionally by inhalation, or via ingestion of contaminated water. It is found world-wide, but occurs mainly in South-East Asia.

Septicaemia with abscesses in the lung, kidney, liver and spleen may occur. The central nervous system may be involved. The prognosis is poor. A chronic form, usually presenting with an unresolved pneumonia, also occurs.

Diagnosis is by culture of the organism. An indirect haemagglutination test is positive after 1 week.

TREATMENT

The patient should be barrier-nursed and treated with ceftazidime.

PASTEURELLOSIS

Pasteurelloses are infections primarily of animals. Three species are known to infect man, the commonest being *Pasteurella multocida*, which is also the most virulent. All these organisms are commensal in the nasopharynx and gastrointestinal tract of a number of domestic and wild mammals. Transmission to humans may occur through a bite or scratch.

CLINICAL FEATURES

Focal soft tissue infection with marked erythema, severe tenderness and regional lymphadenopathy may be present. These organisms are also responsible for chronic respiratory infections, bacteraemia, and brain and renal abscesses.

TREATMENT

Penicillin is the drug of choice and should be given parenterally as benzylpenicillin 1–2 g every 4 h.

LEGIONNAIRES' DISEASE

This is caused by the fastidious *Legionella pneumophila*, a weakly Gram-negative, catalase-positive bacillus. It is described on p. 674.

BACTEROIDES INFECTION

Bacteroides is an obligatory anaerobic, Gram-negative bacillus. *B. fragilis* is the most important anaerobic human pathogen and is a normal commensal in the human large gut. It does not produce an endotoxin and because of its polysaccharide capsule it resists phagocytosis. *B. fragilis* also produces heparinase, which may be involved in the development of thrombophlebitis, and beta-lactamases, which inhibit the action of penicillin. It is not a highly invasive organism and grows best in necrotic tissues.

CLINICAL FEATURES

Seventy-five per cent of all intra-abdominal infections, particularly postoperative infections, are caused by anaerobes. *Bacteroides* is a frequent cause of hepatic, subhepatic, pelvic and splenic abscesses. The pus has a characteristic putrid smell. *Bacteroides* also causes pelvic infections and may result in endometritis, Bartholin's abscess and pelvic peritonitis. Bacteraemia and Fournier's gangrene are also caused by *B. fragilis*.

DIAGNOSIS

This depends on strict anaerobic culture with special media. Recently gas–liquid chromatography has been used to detect the volatile fatty acids produced by anaerobic bacteria.

TREATMENT

Surgery is usually required as well as chemotherapy. Metronidazole (1–2 g daily by mouth or 1 g 8-hourly by rectum) is the drug of choice; it is also used prophylactically in colorectal surgery, with a dramatic reduction in postoperative infections.

Actinomycetes

Actinomycetes are Gram-positive, branching higher bacteria (not fungi) and include *Actinomyces israelii*, *Nocardia asteroides* and *N. brasiliensis*.

Actinomyces is a normal mouth and intestine commensal, but *Nocardia* is a soil saprophyte. *Actinomyces* produces an illness characterized by chronicity and poor infectivity. It has a world-wide distribution. Disease due to *N. asteroides* is frequently seen in the USA and Europe, whereas *N. brasiliensis* gives rise to disease more commonly in southern Asia.

Actinomycosis

In actinomycosis, characteristic clusters of organisms referred to as 'sulphur granules' are formed. *Actinomyces* is a rare cause of disease in the Western World. Three clinical forms of disease are recognized:

- The *cervicofacial variety* usually occurs following dental extraction. It is often indolent and slowly progressive, associated with little pain, and results in induration and localized swelling of the lower part of the mandible ('lumpy jaw'). Lymphadenopathy is uncommon. Occasionally acute inflammation occurs.
- The *thoracic variety* follows inhalation of these organisms into a previously damaged lung. The clinical picture is not distinctive and is often mistaken for malignancy or tuberculosis. Symptoms such as fever, malaise, chest pain and haemoptysis are present. Empyema occurs in 25% of patients and local extension produces chest-wall sinuses with discharge of sulphur granules.
- *Abdominal actinomycosis* most frequently affects the caecum. Characteristically, a hard indurated mass is felt in the right iliac fossa. Later, sinuses develop. The differential diagnosis includes malignancy, tuberculosis, Crohn's disease and amoeboma. Pelvic actinomycosis appears to be increasing with wider use of intrauterine contraceptive devices.

TREATMENT

Treatment involves surgery, and penicillin is the drug of choice. High-dose i.v. penicillin is given for 4–6 weeks followed by oral penicillin for some weeks after clinical resolution. Tetracyclines are also effective.

Nocardiosis

CLINICAL FEATURES

Nocardia gives rise to two distinct clinical entities:

- *Pulmonary disease* presents with cough, fever, and haemoptysis. Pleural involvement and empyema may occur.
- *Mycetoma* is the result of local invasion by *Nocardia* and presents as a painless swelling, usually on the sole of the foot (Madura foot). The swelling of the affected part of the body continues inexorably. Nodules gradually appear from which purulent fluid containing characteristic 'grains' of the organisms are discharged. Systemic symptoms and regional lymphadenopathy are distinctly uncommon. Sinuses may occur several years after the onset of the first symptom.

Mycetoma may also be produced by several other members of actinomycetes, including *Actinomadura* and *Streptomyces*. It is then referred to as an actinomycetoma. When caused by true fungi belonging to Eumycetes, e.g. *Madurella mycetomi* or *Petriellidium boydii*, it is referred to as eumycetoma. The clinical presentation, with the exception of differently coloured 'grains', is similar to that of mycetoma.

DIAGNOSIS

This is often difficult to establish, as *Nocardia* is not easily detected in sputum cultures or on histological section.

TREATMENT

Treatment consists of adequate surgical drainage of the pus combined with prolonged chemotherapy. The drug of choice is sulphadiazine in doses of up to 9 g daily. Co-trimoxazole may also be used.

Mycobacteria

Mycobacteria are acid-fast, aerobic bacilli that grow extremely slowly. The cell wall contains complex lipids and glycolipids, one of which—the cord factor—is responsible for producing granulomas. No extracellular enzyme or toxins have been identified. The capacity of mycobacteria to produce disease is therefore attributed to their ability to multiply within phagocytic cells and to withstand intracellular enzymatic digestion.

A clinical classification of mycobacteria is shown in Table 1.22.

Table 1.22 Classification of *Mycobacterium* species based on their capacity to produce disease.

Species	Disease produced
Obligate intracellular bacteria:	
M. leprae	Leprosy
Facultative intracellular bacteria:	
M. tuberculosis	Most cases of human tuberculosis
M. bovis	Cattle and rarely human tuberculosis
Rare forms:	
M. avium–intracellulare	Fowl and human tuberculosis particularly in HIV infection
M. paratuberculosis	Johne's disease (chronic granulomatous enteritis) in cattle
M. scrofulaceum	Lymph node infection
M. kansasii	Human tuberculosis

Tuberculosis

Tuberculosis is largely due to *Mycobacterium tuberculosis*.

EPIDEMIOLOGY

Tuberculosis is present world-wide with an extremely high prevalence in Asian countries, where 60–80% of children below the age of 14 years are infected. Tuberculosis is spread predominantly by droplet infection.

The prevalence of tuberculosis increases with poor social conditions, inadequate nutrition and overcrowding.

PATHOLOGY

The characteristic lesion is a granuloma with central caseation and Langhans' giant cells.

The primary infection usually involves the lungs, but can involve other areas such as the ileocaecal region of the gastrointestinal tract. It is almost always accompanied by lymph node involvement.

In most people the primary infection heals leaving some surviving tubercle bacilli. With a lowering of host resistance these are reactivated producing local spread as well as haematogenous spread to all organs of the body, including the lungs, bones and kidneys. This particularly occurs in the elderly, in alcoholics, in patients with diabetes mellitus, lung disease, or after gastrectomy, as well as in patients who are on corticosteroids or are immunosuppressed.

Occasionally the primary infection progresses locally to a more widespread lesion; haematogenous spread can also occur.

Tuberculosis in the adult is therefore usually the result of reactivation of old disease, occasionally a primary infection or, more rarely, re-infection.

CLINICAL FEATURES

Pulmonary tuberculosis is the commonest form; this is described on p. 678, along with the chemotherapeutic regimens.

Tuberculosis also affects other organs, including:

- The gastrointestinal tract—mainly the ileocaecal area, but occasionally the peritoneum is affected, producing ascites (see p. 209)
- The genitourinary system—the kidney is mainly involved, but tuberculosis is also the cause of painless, craggy swellings in the epididymis and salpingitis, tubal abscesses and infertility in females
- The central nervous system—tuberculous meningitis and tuberculomas
- The skeletal system—arthritis and osteomyelitis with cold abscess formation can occur
- The skin—inducing lupus vulgaris
- The eye—producing choroiditis, iridocyclitis or phylctenular keratoconjunctivitis
- The pericardium—producing constrictive pericarditis
- The adrenal glands—causing destruction and producing Addison's disease
- The lymph nodes—this is a common mode of presentation, especially in young adults and children. Any group of lymph nodes may be involved but hilar and paratracheal lymph nodes are the commonest. Initially the nodes are firm and discrete but later they become matted and can suppurate and form sinuses.

Scrofula is the term used to describe massive cervical lymph node enlargement. It is most often due to *M. tuberculosis*, and rarely due to *M. scrofulaceum* or *M. kansasii*. Signs of acute inflammation are absent.

Leprosy (Hansen's disease)

The causative organism is the acid-fast bacillus *M. leprae*. Unlike other mycobacteria, it does not grow in artificial media or even in tissue culture. While inability to culture the organism obtained from lesions and secretions is suggestive of *M. leprae*, it is not diagnostic. The following additional properties have recently been found to be useful in its identification:

- Loss of acid fastness following pyridine extraction.

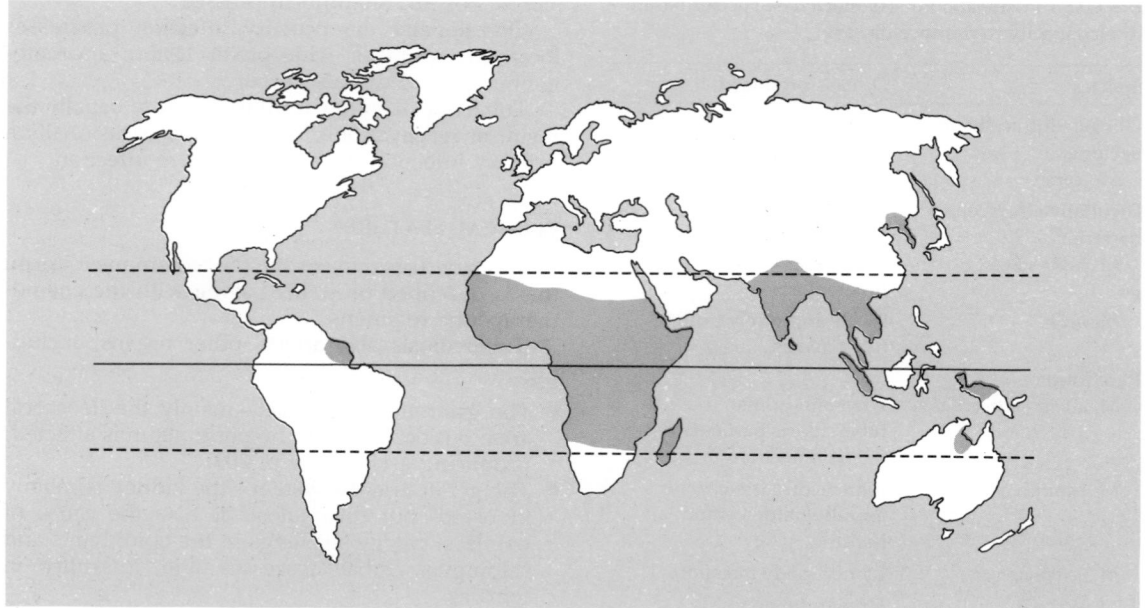

Fig. 1.17 The geographical distribution of leprosy, showing areas where the prevalence is 5 in 1000 or greater.

- The ability of the organism to grow slowly in the foot-pad of mice. Other mycobacteria also grow in the foot-pad of mice, but these produce distinct histological changes.
- The ability of *M. leprae* to oxidize 3,4-dihydroxy-phenylalanine to pigmented products.
- The ability of this organism to invade peripheral nerves, a property not demonstrated by other mycobacteria.

Leprosy is found primarily in Asia and Africa (Fig. 1.17). Endemic foci are still present in the USSR and parts of the USA. Of the 15 million people with leprosy world-wide, about two-thirds are in Asia. The precise mode of transmission is unknown; it is likely that nasal secretions play an important role.

Once an individual has been infected, subsequent progression to clinical disease appears to be dependent on several factors:

- Sex—males appear to be more susceptible than females. In India, the ratio of affected males to females is 2 : 1.
- Genetic susceptibility—studies in twins have shown a concordance in identical but not in non-identical twins.
- The immunological response of the individual to the bacillus.

CLASSIFICATION

Two polar types of leprosy are recognized:

- *Tuberculoid leprosy*—a localized disease that occurs in individuals who exhibit a marked immunological resistance to the organism.
- *Lepromatous leprosy*—a generalized disease that occurs in individuals with impaired cell-mediated immunity.

Two subdivisions of lepromatous leprosy are included in the classification. The patient is said to have the 'subpolar' lepromatous (LL$_s$) form when he has passed through a borderline phase before becoming lepromatous, and the polar lepromatous (LL$_p$) form when the patient is lepromatous throughout.

The following types are also recognized:

- *Borderline leprosy* has features of both the polar varieties and is subdivided into borderline-tuberculoid (BT), borderline (BB) and borderline-lepromatous (BL). Borderline leprosy is an unstable state characterized by increasing numbers of *M. leprae* bacilli and decreasing numbers of lymphocytes.
- *Indeterminate leprosy* is characterized by one or more hypopigmented, sometimes erythematous, ill-defined macules of variable size. Sensation, sweating and hair growth over the macules are usually normal.
- *Neuritic leprosy* is not associated with skin lesions. The affected nerve is enlarged and firm and sensory loss in the area of the nerve's distribution is present.

Two indices are currently in use to evaluate the

response to treatment of patients in whom the skin-smear test for acid-fast bacilli is positive:

- *Bacteriological index* (BI). This index is an objective way of evaluating the response to treatment. The skin-smear is graded from 1+ to 6+ depending upon the number of bacilli present per high-power field. The BI is calculated by taking the mean result of four slide examinations. For example, a decrease in BI from 6 to 3.5 on therapy indicates a good response to treatment.
- Morphological index (MI). This is the percentage of solid staining acid-fast bacilli on smears (solid bacilli represent viable bacteria). A patient with an MI of 0% is not infectious.

CLINICAL FEATURES

The incubation period varies from 2 to 6 years, although it may be as short as a few months or as long as 20 years. Leprosy should be considered in any individual who presents with hypopigmented skin patches associated with loss of sensation, especially to touch or temperature, and evidence of nerve involvement (thickening or tenderness), in whom non-cultivable acid-fast bacilli have been identified in skin smears.

The onset of leprosy is generally insidious. However, acute onset is known to occur and patients may present with a transient rash, with features of an acute febrile illness, with evidence of nerve involvement, or with any combination of these.

CLINICAL SPECTRUM

Tuberculoid leprosy (TT)

In tuberculoid leprosy the infection is localized because the patient has unimpaired cell-mediated immunity. The characteristic usually single skin lesion is a hypopigmented, anaesthetic patch with thickened, clearly demarcated edges, central healing and atrophy. The face, gluteal region and extremities are most commonly affected. Frequently the nerve leading to this hypopigmented patch and the regional nerve trunk are thickened and tender. Unlike other parts of the body, a tuberculoid patch on the face is not anaesthetic. Nerve involvement leads to marked muscle atrophy. Tuberculoid lesions are known to heal spontaneously.

Borderline-tuberculoid (BT) leprosy

Resembles TT but skin lesions are usually more numerous, smaller and may be present as small 'stellite' lesions around larger ones. Peripheral but not cutaneous nerves are thickened, leading to deformity of hands and feet.

Borderline (BB) leprosy

Skin lesions are numerous varying in size and form (macules, papules, plaques). The annular, rimmed lesion with punched out, hypopigmented anaesthetic centre is characteristic. There is widespread nerve involvement and limb deformity.

Borderline-lepromatous (BL) leprosy

There are a large number of florid asymmetrical skin lesions of variable form, which are strongly positive for acid-fast bacilli. Skin between the lesions is normal and often negative for bacilli.

Lepromatous leprosy (LL)

Although practically every organ can be involved, the changes in the skin are the earliest and most obvious manifestation. Peripheral oedema and rhinitis are the earliest symptoms. The skin lesions predominantly occur on the face, the gluteal region and the upper and lower limbs. They may be macules, papules, nodules or plaques. Of these, the macule is the earliest lesion. Infiltration is most noticeable in the ear lobes. Thinning of the lateral margins of the eyebrows is characteristic. The mucous membranes are frequently involved, resulting in nasal stuffiness, laryngitis and hoarseness of the voice. Nasal septal perforation with collapse of the nasal cartilages produces a saddle-nose deformity. With progression of the disease, the typical leonine facies due to infiltration of the skin becomes apparent. Glove and stocking anaesthesia, gynaecomastia, testicular atrophy, icthyosis and nerve palsies (facial, ulnar, median and radial) develop late in the disease. Neurotrophic atrophy affecting the phalanges leads to the gradual disappearance of fingers. Nerve involvement is less pronounced than in tuberculoid leprosy.

Lucio's phenomenon is seen only in Mexico and Central America, where lepromatous leprosy is associated with an endarteritis which results in skin ulceration. The ulcers are large, with undermined edges and markedly necrotic bases. Smears from the base generally reveal numerous acid-fast bacilli. Healing is by scar formation. Treatment is wide surgical excision with skin grafts. Chemotherapy alone is ineffective in healing ulcers.

The lepromin test

This is a measure of host resistance to leprosy and not a test for detecting leprosy. 0.1 ml of a suspension of dead bacilli (either Mitsuda lepromin or the Dharmendra lepromin) is injected intradermally. Two reactions are observed:

- The early Fernandez reaction becomes positive in 48 h and reflects the *sensitivity* of the tissue to the leprosy bacilli protein.
- The late (Mitsuda) reaction develops in 4–5 weeks and reflects the resistance of the host to

the bacteria. This reaction is strongly positive in tuberculoid leprosy and is negative in lepromatous leprosy.

Lepra reactions

Lepra reactions are immunologically mediated acute reactions that occur in patients with the borderline or lepromatous spectrum of disease. Two forms are recognized.

Erythema nodosum leprosum (ENL; type II lepra reaction) is a humoral antibody response to an antigen–antibody complex (i.e. a type III hypersensitivity reaction). It is seen in 50% of patients with treated LL. It is characterized by fever, arthralgia and crops of painful, subcutaneous erythematous nodules. It may last from a few days to several weeks.

The *borderline reaction* (type I lepra reaction) is seen following treatment of patients with borderline disease; it is a type IV delayed hypersensitivity reaction. Both upgrading or reversal reactions (i.e. a clinical change towards a more tuberculoid form) and downgrading reactions (i.e. a change towards the lepromatous form) can occur. The borderline reaction is characterized by acute inflammation of pre-existing borderline lesions. Neurological deficits such as an ulnar nerve palsy may occur abruptly.

DIAGNOSIS

The diagnosis of leprosy is essentially clinical. Patients should be examined in adequate natural light. The demonstration of acid-fast bacilli in smears from the skin or nasal mucosa is highly suggestive. Occasionally nerve biopsies are helpful. The definitive diagnosis is established by cultivating the organisms in the foot-pads of mice.

TREATMENT

Leprosy should be treated in specialist centres with adequate physiotherapy and occupational therapy support. Multi-drug therapy is now essential because of developing drug resistance (up to 20% of cases are resistant to dapsone).

Dapsone (DDS), a folate synthetase inhibitor, is bacteriostatic. It has the advantage of being cheap and well tolerated. Side-effects are few and include haemolytic anaemia and sulphaemoglobinaemia. In 1982 the World Health Organization recommended that for multi-bacillary forms of leprosy (BB, BL and LL types) it should be taken on a daily basis (100 mg) along with rifampicin 600 mg once monthly and clofazimine 50 mg daily with an extra dose of 300 mg monthly. The monthly doses are given under supervision. This triple therapy should be given for a minimum of 2 years or continued until a patient's skin smears become negative for acid-fast bacilli. However, in paucibacillary forms (TT or BT) 6 months' therapy with DDS 100 mg daily and rifampicin 600 mg monthly is recommended.

The major disadvantage with clofazimine is that it is a dye and causes a generalized reddish-brown pigmentation in light-skinned individuals and a slate grey pigmentation in dark-skinned individuals. Ethionamide is a suitable alternative. Acedapsone (DADDS), a depot sulphone, has been used with some success.

Surgery and physiotherapy play an important role in the management of trophic ulcers and deformities of the hands, feet and face.

Treatment of lepra reactions

Treatment of lepra reactions is urgent, as irreversible eye and nerve damage can occur with amazing rapidity. Anti-leprosy therapy must be continued. Type II lepra reactions (ENL) are effectively treated with analgesics, chloroquine, clofazimine and antipyretics. Thalidomide, a drug known for its potent teratogenic effects, is by far the most effective in the ENL reaction, but must be used with caution. Prednisolone 30–40 mg daily for a few weeks is effective in type I reactions.

PREVENTION AND CONTROL

This depends on rapid treatment of infected patients, particularly those with LL and BL, to decrease the bacterial reservoir. It is spread by close contact, but only a small proportion of contacts—approximately 1%—develop the disease. Anti-leprosy vaccines are under clinical trial; the efficacy of the BCG vaccine against leprosy is debatable. Mass chemoprophylaxis is impracticable and its efficacy in household contacts has not been established.

Mycobacterial ulcer

Also known as Buruli ulcer, after the Buruli region in Uganda, this condition occurs in tropical, rural areas near rivers, e.g. in Zaire, Nigeria and Malaysia. It is caused by *M. ulcerans*. The disease is contracted by swimming in infected water. Initially a small subcutaneous nodule develops. This undergoes ulceration that involves the subcutaneous tissue, muscle and fascial planes. The ulcers are usually large, with undermined edges and markedly necrotic bases. Smears taken from necrotic tissue generally reveal numerous acid-fast bacilli. Treatment is wide surgical excision with skin grafts. Antituberculous therapy is ineffective.

Mycoplasma

Mycoplasma is a small free-living, motile bacterium that lacks a cell wall. *Mycoplasma pneumoniae* is found world-wide and may cause up to 20% of pneumonias. Infection is endemic but epidemics also occur, the infection being spread by airborne droplets between close contacts. *M. pneumoniae* infection is found most commonly in childhood, adolescence and early adulthood.

The oropharynx, trachea and bronchi are commonly involved, but there is frequently infiltration into the lung, causing pneumonia.

The clinical features and treatment are described on p. 672.

M. hominis and *Ureaplasma urealyticum* cause non-specific urethritis and cervicitis.

Sexually transmitted diseases (STDs)

The incidence of many sexually transmitted diseases has increased substantially during the last 30 years. Even syphilis, which had shown a gradual decline in the first half of this century, has increased in the last two decades, largely in the male homosexual population. The rising rates of gonorrhoea, non-specific urethritis and herpes simplex virus infection are largely due to the increased numbers of sexual contacts (homosexual and heterosexual) that many individuals make during adolescence and early adulthood. Other factors that contribute to increased transmission rates relate to the fact that women and homosexual men may carry STDs without symptoms, and that venerophobia is less pronounced since the advent of effective treatment for many sexually transmitted diseases. However, the most recent figures suggest that these diseases are again declining, largely due to the threat of HIV infection and the increased use of condoms.

The organisms responsible for specific STDs are summarized in Table 1.23. Full clinical features of the illnesses they cause are given elsewhere.

HISTORY

In addition to the general medical history it is important to take a detailed history of sexual contacts (heterosexual and homosexual), with particular emphasis on whether these were regular or casual and the specific nature of the sexual activity, namely, genital, orogenital, oroanal or anogenital. It is also important to know whether there is a past

Table 1.23 Sexually transmitted diseases and their causative organisms.

Sexually transmitted diseases	Causative organism
Bacterial	
Syphilis (see p. 46)	*Treponema pallidum*
Gonorrhoea (see p. 48), ophthalmia neonatorum	*Neisseria gonorrhoeae*
Non-specific vaginitis	*Gardnerella vaginalis*
Granuloma inguinale (p. 49)	*Calymmatobacterium granulomatis*
Chancroid (p. 49)	*Haemophilus ducreyi*
Non-specific urethritis, proctitis, cervicitis (p. 49)	*Chlamydia trachomatis*
	Ureaplasma urealyticum
Pelvic inflammatory disease	*Mycoplasma hominis*
Lymphogranuloma venereum (p. 49)	*Chlamydia trachomatis* (L 1,2,3 serotype)
Viral	
Genital herpes, cervical cancer	Herpes simplex virus (HSV 2 and 1)
AIDS (p. 68)	HIV-1, ? HIV-2
Genital warts (p. 1026)	Papillomavirus
Molluscum contagiosium	Pox virus
Hepatitis (p. 251)	HBV, HCV, CMV
Fungal	
Vaginal 'thrush', balanitis (p. 1027)	*Candida albicans*
Protozoal	
Vaginitis, urethritis, balanoposthitis (p. 91)	*Trichomonas vaginalis*
Arthropods	
Genital scabies	*Sarcoptes scabei*
Pediculosis pubis	*Phthisus pubis*

history of STD and whether any specific antimicrobial therapy has been received recently.

EXAMINATION

General examination should include a search for neurological or cardiovascular evidence of advanced syphilis, and for lymphadenopathy, Kaposi's sarcoma and opportunistic infection in patients suspected of acquired immunodeficiency syndrome (AIDS). In men with urethral discharge, a Gram-stain for leucocytes and organisms should be made and a wet preparation should be examined for *Trichomonas vaginalis*. Material should also be dried on a slide for examination by an immuno-fluorescent technique for *Chlamydia*. Many laboratories are now able to culture *Chlamydia* in tissue culture cell lines. Microbiological culture for gonococci and, if possible, *Ureaplasma* should be performed. Smears from the urethral meatus of women should also be examined by Gram-stain and cultured for gonococci. Smears should also be taken from the lateral and posterior fornix of the vagina and from the cervical os for examination by Gram-stain and culture.

In men with balanitis and balanoposthitis (inflammation of the glans penis and prepuce), smears should be taken for Gram-staining and for microbiological culture of *Candida* and aerobic and anaerobic bacteria, including *Haemophilus ducreyi*. Careful examination should be made for the vesicles of HSV; if in doubt, material should be sent in transport medium for virus culture.

When anorectal infection is suspected, proctoscopy should be performed and rectal smears examined by Gram-stain and cultured, particularly for gonococci. Similarly, throat swabs should be performed when there has been orogenital contact. Blood should be taken for syphilis serology (VDRL test and TPHA), for hepatitis B and C markers, particularly in high-risk individuals (male homosexuals, bisexuals, intravenous drug abusers) and also for antibody to HIV in individuals suspected of AIDS (after counselling).

TREATMENT, PREVENTION AND CONTROL

Treatments for individual sexually transmitted diseases are given elsewhere.

Prevention of STD must be tackled on many fronts, including health education at school and through the media, the use of protective measures, particularly condoms, avoidance of sexual contact with individuals known to have STD or in high-risk groups, and ultimately by vaccine development, which will probably be particularly important for the control of AIDS.

Historically, contact tracing has been an important community-based approach to the control of STD, but the rising incidence rates would suggest that this method is failing, largely because of the increased numbers of casual sexual contacts that now commonly occur. Many individuals, particularly male homosexuals, regularly present themselves to STD clinics for regular check-ups, since it is now widely known that asymptomatic carriage of infection, particularly in the rectum, is common.

Many diseases not classically regarded as STDs are transmitted by sexual contact in male homosexuals (Table 1.24). These should be searched for in patients presenting at an STD clinic, particularly individuals with diarrhoea or other bowel symptoms, and those with weight loss, intermittent fever and malaise.

Table 1.24 Additional organisms that are sexually transmitted in male homosexuals.

Viruses:
   Human immunodeficiency virus (HIV)
   Hepatitis B virus and D (delta virus)
   Hepatitis A virus
   Hepatitis C virus (rare)
   Cytomegalovirus

Bacteria:
   Salmonella spp.
   Shigella spp.
   Campylobacter jejuni

Protozoa:
   Giardia lamblia
   Entamoeba histolytica
   Cryptosporidium spp.
   Microsporidium spp.
   Isospora belli
   Sarcocystis spp.

Helminths:
   Strongyloides stercoralis
   Trichuris trichiura
   Enterobius vermicularis

'Gay bowel disease' is the term used to describe diarrhoea occurring in homosexuals. Diarrhoea may be related to a variety of infecting organisms, which are often multiple. Protozoa as well as bacteria can be found. *Giardia* and *Cryptosporidium* can involve both the small and large bowel.

Syphilis

Treponema pallidum is a motile spirochaete that is generally acquired by close sexual contact, the organism entering the new host through breaches in squamous or columnar epithelium. Primary infection of non-genital sites may occasionally occur in medical personnel. A fetus can acquire the infection by transplacental passage of the organism from an infected mother during the later stages of pregnancy, giving rise to congenital syphilis.

Both congenital and acquired syphilis have early and late stages, each of which has classical clinical features (Table 1.25).

Primary

Two to four weeks after exposure to the pathogen a papule develops, usually on a genital site (penis, labia or cervix), that soon ulcerates to become the painless, hard chancre. This is associated with painless, regional lymphadenopathy. One of the commonest sites to see a chancre nowadays is in the anus of homosexual men. The primary chancre heals, usually within a few weeks.

Table 1.25 Classification and clinical features of syphilis.

	Clinical features
	Acquired
Early stages	
Primary	Hard chancre
	Painless, regional lymphadenopathy
Secondary	*General:* Fever, malaise, arthralgia, sore throat and generalized lymphadenopathy
	Skin: Red/brown maculopapular non-itchy, sometimes scaly rash; condylomata lata
	Mucous membrane: Mucous patches, 'snail-track' ulcers in oropharynx and on genitalia
Late stages	
Tertiary	*Late benign:* Gummas (bone and viscera)
	Cardiovascular: Aortitis and aortic regurgitation
	Neurosyphilis: Meningovascular involvement, general paralysis of the insane (GPI) and tabes dorsalis
	Congenital
Early stages	Stillbirth or failure to thrive
	'Snuffles' (nasal infection with discharge)
	Skin and mucous membrane lesions as in secondary syphilis
Late stages	'Stigmata': Hutchinson's teeth, 'sabre' tibia and abnormalities of long bones
	Keratitis, uveitis, facial gummas and CNS disease

Secondary

Two or three months after the chancre has healed, variable combinations of fever, sore throat, malaise and arthralgia occur. Signs include:

- Generalized lymphadenopathy
- Generalized skin rashes involving the whole body with the exception of the face, but including the palms and soles of the feet—common
- Condylomata lata—warty, plaque-like lesions found in the perianal area and other moist body sites
- Superficial confluent ulcers—found in the mouth and on the external genitalia

After a few months the features of secondary syphilis abate, but in up to 20% of individuals may recur during a period known as early latency. After one year the period of late latency is entered; this may continue for many years before the late stages of syphilis become apparent.

Tertiary

Late benign syphilis generally involves the skin and the bones. Gummas (granulomatous, sometimes ulcerating, lesions) can occur anywhere in the skin, frequently at sites of trauma. They are commonly found in the skull, tibia, fibula and clavicle, although any bone may be involved. Visceral gummas occur mainly in the liver (hepar lobatum) and the testes. Cardiovascular and neurosyphilis are discussed in detail elsewhere (see p. 624 and p. 933).

Congenital syphilis

Congenital syphilis usually becomes apparent between the second and sixth week after birth, early signs being nasal discharge, skin and mucous membrane lesions, and failure to thrive. Signs of late syphilis generally do not appear until after 2 years of age and take the form of 'stigmata' relating to early damage to developing structures, particularly teeth and long bones. Other late manifestations parallel those of adult tertiary syphilis (see Table 1.25).

DIAGNOSIS

Treponemes may be identified by dark-ground illumination microscopy and are present in chancres and in the mucosal patches of secondary infection. Individuals with either primary or secondary disease are highly infectious.

Serological tests are helpful in the diagnosis of syphilis. The Wassermann reaction (WR) has now been superseded. The VDRL (Venereal Disease Research Laboratory) cardiolipin antigen test is a useful screening test and is positive within 3–4 weeks after the primary infection. It generally becomes negative by 6 months after treatment. However, this test also becomes negative in untreated patients (50% of patients with late stage syphilis).

False-positive results may occur in other infectious diseases, particularly:

- Infectious mononucleosis
- Hepatitis
- Mycoplasma infections
- Some protozoal infections

They may also occur in some patients with:

- Cirrhosis
- Malignancy
- Autoimmune disease

The *T. pallidum* immobilization (TPI) test is the

most specific test but is now rarely used except in reference centres. It remains positive for years after successful treatment. However, it is an expensive test and is now becoming replaced by the *T. pallidum* haemagglutination assay (TPHA) and fluorescent treponema antibodies absorbed (FTA-ABS) test, both of which are highly specific. The FTA-ABS test is positive in more than 90% of patients with primary infection and in all patients with latent and late syphilis. It remains positive for life, even after treatment. Activity on the VDRL test correlates most closely with active infection.

Examination of the CSF for evidence of neurosyphilis (p. 933) and a chest X-ray to determine the extent of cardiovascular disease should also be performed.

TREATMENT

Early syphilis (primary or secondary) should be treated with long-acting procaine penicillin 1.2 g daily by intramuscular injection for 10 days. When compliance is in doubt, a single injection of benzathine penicillin 2.4 g will maintain adequate levels of drug for approximately 2 weeks. For late stage syphilis, particularly when there is cardiovascular or neurological involvement, the treatment course should be extended to between 2 and 3 weeks. For patients sensitive to penicillin, tetracycline or erythromycin, 500 mg four times daily for 2 weeks is effective.

The Jarisch–Herxheimer reaction is due to release of endotoxin when large numbers of organisms are killed by antibiotics, and is seen in 50% of patients with primary syphilis. It occurs about 8 h after the first injection and usually consists of mild fever, malaise and headache lasting a few hours. In secondary syphilis, 90% of patients are affected. In tertiary syphilis a severe reaction, although rare, can occur so that prednisolone is often given 24 h before the antibiotic treatment. Penicillin should not be withheld because of the Jarisch–Herxheimer reaction; since it is not a dose-related phenomenon, there is no value in giving a smaller dose.

Gonorrhoea

Gonorrhoea, which is caused by *Neisseria gonorrhoeae*, occurs world-wide but has reached epidemic proportions in the USA. Transmission is commonly through sexual contact, although nonsexual transmission is possible; for example, an infected mother may pass on the infection to a newborn child, usually resulting in gonococcal conjunctivitis.

CLINICAL FEATURES

A small percentage of males and 30–40% of females with gonorrhoea are asymptomatic. Symp-tomatic males usually present within 3–5 days with urethritis characterized by a purulent urethral discharge, meatal oedema, dysuria and frequency of micturition. Local complications are rare, but periurethral abscesses and epididymitis can occur. In symptomatic females, gonorrhoea results in a purulent vaginal discharge, frequency of micturition and anorectal discomfort; bartholinitis may occur. Male homosexuals are often asymptomatic but anal and pharyngeal involvement is not uncommon. Disseminated gonococcal infection produces fever, malaise, myalgia and a diffuse pustular and erythematous rash. Joint involvement with an asymmetrical tenosynovitis and arthritis, meningitis and perihepatitis (Fitz–Hugh–Curtis syndrome) have also been reported.

Pelvic inflammatory disease is the commonest complication of gonorrhoea in women. There is ascending infection leading to endometritis and salpingitis. This presents acutely with lower abdominal pain, tenderness and fever. Treatment should be started quickly to avoid the late complication of infertility. In men, sterility following epididymo-orchitis and urethral stricture are the main complications.

DIAGNOSIS

Though the clinical presentation is suggestive, definitive diagnosis can only be made by identifying the organisms in smears or by culturing them in special media (Thayer–Martin or New York City medium) from discharge, blood or joint fluid. No serological tests have been found useful. Other sexually transmitted diseases such as syphilis should be looked for and treated appropriately.

TREATMENT

Procaine penicillin (2.4 g in men, 4.8 g in women i.m.) with 1 g of probenicid orally as a single dose, ampicillin 2 g as a single oral dose with 1 g probenicid orally (repeated for women), or tetracycline 0.5 g by mouth four times daily for 7 days is usually effective. The procaine penicillin/ probenicid regimen has the advantage of being effective against syphilis, but has no effect on *Chlamydia trachomatis* infections. Tetracycline, however, effectively eradicates *Chlamydia trachomatis* infection but not syphilis. Anorectal gonorrhoea should be treated only with a procaine penicillin/ probenicid combination. Spectinomycin (2 g in men, 4 g in women, as a single intramuscular dose) and cefotaxime are useful for treating penicillinase-producing *N. gonorrhoeae* and in patients who are allergic to penicillin.

Post-gonococcal urethritis should be treated with tetracycline. Contacts should be traced and treated appropriately.

Lymphogranuloma venereum (LGV)

Chlamydia trachomatis types 1, 2 and 3 (p. 55) is responsible for this sexually transmitted infection. It is endemic in the tropics, with the highest incidences in Africa, India and South-East Asia.

CLINICAL FEATURES

The primary lesion is a painless ulcerating papule on the genitalia and only occurs in one-quarter of the patients. A few days after this heals, regional lymphadenopathy develops. The lymph nodes are painful and fixed and the overlying skin develops a dusky erythematous appearance. Finally, nodes may become fluctuant (buboes) and may rupture. Acute LGV may present as proctitis with perirectal abscesses, the appearances sometimes resembling anorectal Crohn's disease.

DIAGNOSIS

The diagnosis is made on the basis of:

- The characteristic clinical picture
- Isolation of an LGV strain of *C. trachomatis* (only possible in specialized laboratories)
- Immunofluorescence using specific monoclonal antibodies for identifying organisms in pus from a bubo
- A rising titre in a complement-fixation test

The intradermal Frei test is non-specific and unreliable. Great care must be taken to exclude syphilis and genital herpes.

TREATMENT

Early treatment with oxytetracycline 500 mg four times daily for at least 2 weeks is generally necessary. Chronic infection may result in extensive scarring and abscess and sinus formation and surgical drainage may be required. Sexual partners should also be treated.

Urethritis and cervicitis

Chlamydia trachomatis is an important cause of urethritis (non-gonococcal or non-specific urethritis, NSU). Symptoms of burning pain on micturition and urethral discharge begin a variable time after exposure. Chronic infection can lead to urethral stricture. The same organism may also infect the uterine cervix but in many cases causes no symptoms. The organism is also associated with pelvic inflammatory disease in women, which may result in infertility. It is also a cause of proctitis in homosexuals.

Treatment with oxytetracycline 250 mg four times daily for 2–3 weeks is best given to both partners, followed by a 2-week course of erythromycin if symptoms recur.

Chancroid

Chancroid (soft chancre) is an acute sexually transmitted disease caused by *Haemophilus ducreyi*. It occurs chiefly in tropical countries, with occasional outbreaks in the USA and Europe.

CLINICAL FEATURES

The incubation period is 3–7 days. Initially a papule forms, which then ulcerates and in about 3 days results in an irregular, variably sized, tender ulcer with undermined edges and a necrotic base. It is not unusual for multiple ulcers to coalesce to form a giant ulcer. Lesions are generally on the penis in men and on any part of the perineum in women. Regional lymphadenopathy is usual and may, if left untreated, result in abscess formation and suppuration. A feeling of being unwell and mild fever are common.

DIAGNOSIS

Clinical differentiation of chancroid from other sexually transmitted diseases such as syphilis, herpes simplex and lymphogranuloma venereum is difficult. The diagnosis is confirmed only when the organism is isolated in culture from the ulcer or from enlarged lymph nodes, but not all clinical cases are culture-positive.

TREATMENT

H. ducreyi is sensitive to tetracycline (500 mg four times daily for 1–3 weeks) and sulphonamides. Other useful drugs include co-trimoxazole, erythromycin, streptomycin and kanamycin.

Granuloma inguinale

Granuloma inguinale is the least common of all sexually transmitted diseases in North America and Europe, but is endemic in the tropics and subtropics, particularly the Caribbean, South-East Asia and South India. Infection is caused by *Calymmatobacterium granulomatis*, a short, encapsulated Gram-negative bacillus. The infection was also known as Donovanosis, the organism originally being known as Donovan's body. Although sexual contact appears to be the most important mode of transmission, the infection rates are low, even between sexual partners of many years' standing.

CLINICAL FEATURES

In the vast majority of patients, the characteristic, heaped-up ulcerating lesion with prolific red granulation tissue appears on the external genitalia, perianal skin or the inguinal region within

1–4 weeks of exposure. However, almost any cutaneous or mucous membrane sites can be involved, including the mouth and anorectal regions. Extension of the primary infection from the external genitalia to the inguinal regions produces the characteristic lesion, the 'pseudo-bubo'.

DIAGNOSIS

The clinical appearance usually strongly suggests the diagnosis but *C. granulomatis* (Donovan bodies) may be identified intracellularly in scrapings or biopsies of an ulcer. Culture or serological methods of diagnosis are not available.

TREATMENT

Antibiotic treatment should be given for at least 10–14 days. Tetracycline 500 mg four times daily, streptomycin 1 g twice daily i.m. or ampicillin 500 mg four times daily are the three most commonly used drugs. Alternatives include erythromycin and chloramphenicol.

Spirochaetes

Important spirochaetal infections include those due to *Treponema* (syphilis, bejel, yaws and pinta) and *Borrelia* (the relapsing fevers, tropical ulcer and cancrum oris) (Table 1.26).

Table 1.26 Spirochaetal infections.

Disease	Organism
Syphilis	*Treponema pallidum*
Bejel (endemic non-venereal syphilis)	*Treponema pallidum* variant
Yaws	*Treponema pertenue*
Pinta	*Treponema carateum*
Leptospirosis (Weil's disease)	*Leptospira icterohaemorrhagiae*
Canicola fever	*Leptospira canicola*
Louse-borne relapsing fever	*Borrelia recurrentis*
Tick-borne relapsing fever	*Borrelia duttonii*
Cancrum oris	*Borrelia vincenti*
Lyme disease	*Borrelia burgdorferi*
Rate-bite fever	*Spirillum minus* *Streptobacillus moniliformis*

Syphilis

This is described on p. 46.

Bejel (endemic non-venereal syphilis) yaws and pinta

These diseases are endemic throughout the tropical and subtropical regions of the world (see Fig. 1.18).

Bejel
A variant strain of *Treponema pallidum*, sometimes referred to as *T. pallidum endemicum*, is responsible for this infection and is spread by non-venereal routes in situations where hygiene is poor. The organism enters through abrasions in the skin. The disease is found in children and differs from venereal syphilis in that a primary lesion is not commonly seen, although the late stages are indistinguishable from syphilis. Specific treponemal serology tests cannot differentiate these conditions and treatment is the same as for syphilis.

Yaws
Apart from syphilis, yaws is the most widespread of the treponemal diseases. It is spread by direct contact, usually in children, the organism again entering through damaged skin. After an incubation period of weeks or months, a primary inflammatory reaction occurs at the inoculation site, from which organisms can be isolated. Dissemination of the organism leads to multiple papular lesions containing treponemes; these skin lesions usually involve the palms and soles. There may also be bone involvement, particularly the long bones and those of the hand.

In late yaws bony lesions may progress to cause gross destruction and disfigurement, particularly of the skull and facial bones, the interphalangeal joints and the long bones. Plantar hyperkeratosis is characteristic. Like syphilis, there may be a latent period between the early and late phases of the disease, but visceral, neurological and cardiovascular problems do not occur. Serological tests for syphilis are positive. Treatment is with long-acting penicillin which, together with improved hygiene, has substantially reduced the prevalence of this disease.

Pinta
Pinta is restricted mainly to Central and South America but otherwise closely resembles endemic syphilis. The primary lesion is a pruritic red papule, usually on the hand or foot. It may become scaly but never ulcerates and is generally associated with regional lymphadenopathy. In the later stages similar lesions can continue to crop for up to 1 year associated with generalized lymphadenopathy. Eventually the lesions heal, leaving hyper-

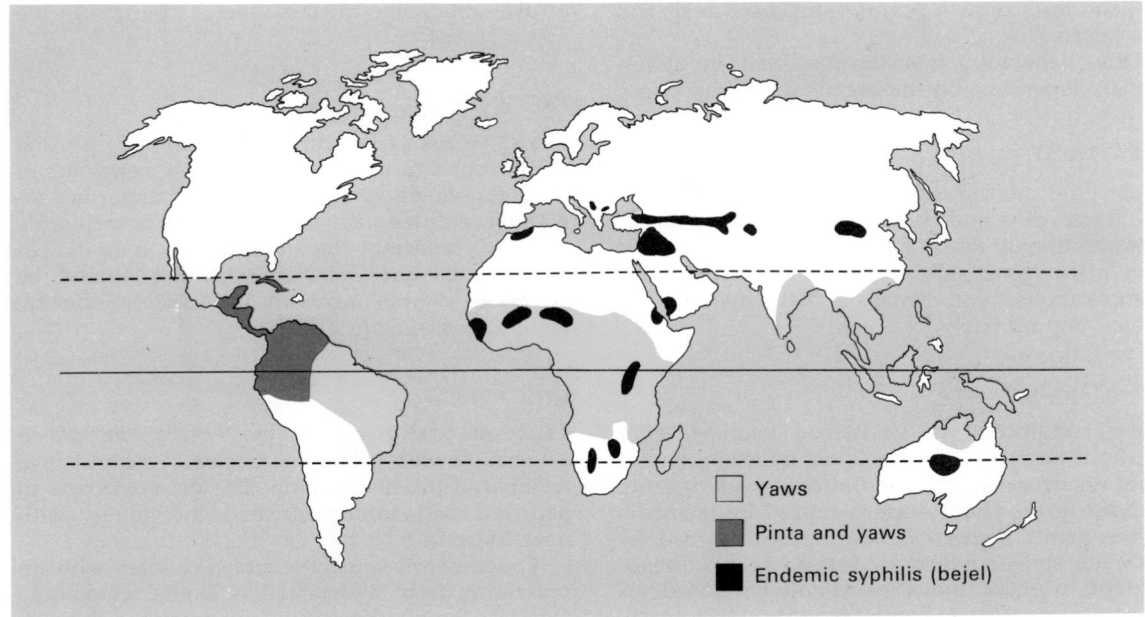

Fig. 1.18 The geographical distribution of bejel, yaws and pinta.

pigmented or depigmented patches. Syphilis serology is positive and treatment is as for other treponemal infections by long-acting penicillin.

Leptospirosis

This zoonosis is most commonly caused by *Leptospira icterohaemorrhagiae* (from rodents), when infection is known as Weil's disease, or *L. canicola* (from dogs and pigs). Leptospires are excreted in the animal urine, to which humans may then be exposed. Certain occupational groups are particularly at risk, namely veterinarians, those involved in animal husbandry, abattoir workers and, in the past, miners and sewer workers. Pet owners and those who take part in water sports in inland waters are also exposed to the infection. Weil described a disease that consisted of jaundice, haemorrhage and renal impairment due to *L. icterohaemorrhagiae* but, fortunately, only 10–15% of patients suffer such a severe illness, the majority escaping with a benign self-limiting illness without jaundice.

CLINICAL FEATURES

The incubation period is usually 10 days (range 2–26 days). Leptospirosis has two phases: a leptospiraemic phase lasting up to a week, followed by an immune phase, which is generally separated from the former phase by an asymptomatic period of 1–3 days.

The leptospiraemic phase is similar to many acute systemic infections, and is characterized by severe headache, fever, malaise, anorexia and myalgia. The majority of patients have suffusion of the conjunctivae. Infrequently there is hepatosplenomegaly, lymphadenopathy and various skin rashes.

During the immune phase of the illness 50% of patients have meningism, about one third of whom have CSF lymphocytosis and a modest elevation of CSF protein concentration. The majority recover uneventfully at this stage. However, a small proportion go on to develop tender hepatomegaly, jaundice, haemolytic anaemia, oliguric renal failure with microscopic haematuria, and occasionally cardiac involvement characterized by atrial and ventricular dysrhythmias and congestive cardiac failure. The mortality of Weil's disease is still unacceptably high at between 5–20%.

DIAGNOSIS

Although diagnosis is most often made clinically:

- Leptospires can be cultured from blood or CSF during the first week of the illness. A minority of patients excrete the organism in the urine during the second week of the illness and may continue to do so for a further 2–4 weeks.
- Specific IgM leptospiral antibodies appear by the end of the first week and are useful diagnostically.

- Blood tests show a polymorpholeucocytosis and a raised ESR.
- Other laboratory investigations may be abnormal, depending on the organs involved.

TREATMENT

Leptospires are sensitive to penicillins, erythromycin, tetracycline and chloramphenicol. Penicillin is most commonly used (2.4 g daily for 1 week) and should be given at any stage of the illness. Complications, e.g. renal or liver failure, are treated appropriately.

The relapsing fevers

These conditions are so named because, after apparent recovery from the initial infection, one or more recurrences may occur after a week or more without fever. The disease is caused by members of the genus *Borrelia*. *B. recurrentis* is spread by body lice and *B. duttonii* by soft ticks. The disease is found in Africa, India, the Middle East, Mediterranean Europe and South America. The louse-borne variety occurs in epidemics when humans live in close contact in impoverished conditions and the tick-borne disease is found in areas where traditional mud huts are the form of shelter for both humans and the tick.

CLINICAL FEATURES

Symptoms begin 7–10 days after infection and consist of a high fever of abrupt onset with rigors, generalized myalgia and headache. A petechial or ecchymotic rash may be seen. The general condition then deteriorates, with delirium, hepatosplenomegaly, jaundice, haemorrhagic problems and circulatory collapse. Although complete recovery may occur at this time, the majority experience one or more relapses of diminishing severity approximately 1 week after the initial illness. Without specific treatment, approximately one third of patients will die.

Louse and tick-borne relapsing fevers are clinically similar, although louse-borne fever tends to have a shorter initial illness with more frequent relapses.

DIAGNOSIS

Spirochaetes can be demonstrated microscopically in the blood during febrile episodes.

TREATMENT

Penicillin or tetracycline çan be used, although both give rise to a severe Jarisch–Herxheimer reaction (see p. 48). Some strains of *Borrelia duttonii* are resistant to penicillin, so it is advisable to use tetracycline for this type of infection in the first instance.

PREVENTION

Ticks live for years and remain infected, passing the infection to their progeny. These reservoirs of infection should be controlled by spraying houses with insecticides such as 2% benzene hexachloride and by reducing the number of rodents. In contrast, patients infested with lice should be deloused by washing with 1% Lysol or dusting with 10% dicophane (DDT).

Cancrum oris

Cancrum oris is caused by *Borrelia vincentii* in association with anaerobic bacteria, commonly a member of the fusobacteria. The disease occurs in deprived and undernourished individuals with poor hygiene.

Cancrum oris usually occurs in children who are recovering from a debilitating illness, commonly measles. Rapidly progressive gangrenous destruction of the inner aspect of the mouth and cheek occurs, which may continue to progress even after treatment with penicillin. The mortality is high, probably reflecting the underlying poor physical state of the patient.

Lyme disease

This disease was first recognized in 1975 and the causative agent, *Borellia burgdorferi*, was finally identified in 1983. The disease is transmitted by *Ixodes dammini* or related ixodid ticks. It was originally described in Lyme, Connecticut, but is now known to occur in many parts of the USA, in Europe and in Australia.

CLINICAL FEATURES

The first stage of the illness consists of the unique and characteristic skin lesion—erythema chronicum migrans, often accompanied by headache, fever, malaise, myalgia, arthralgia and lymphadenopathy. The second stage follows weeks or months later, when some patients develop neurological (meningoencephalitis, cranial or peripheral neuropathies) or cardiac (myocarditis) problems. Finally, the third stage of the disease consists of arthritis, which recurs in attacks for several years, often with associated erosion of cartilage and bone. Arthritis has not been seen in patients in the UK.

DIAGNOSIS

The clinical features and epidemiological considerations are usually strongly suggestive of infection with this spirochaete, but the diagnosis can be

Table 1.27 Rickettsial infections.

Disease	Organism	Vector
Typhus fevers:		
Epidemic typhus	Rickettsia prowazekii	Human lice
Endemic (murine) typhus	Rickettsia typhi (R. mooseri)	Rat flea
Rocky Mountain spotted fever	Rickettsia ricketsii	Tick
Scrub typhus	Rickettsia tsutsugamushi	Larval mite
Rickettsial pox	Rickettsia akari	Mite
Trench fever	Rochalimaea quintana	Human lice
Q fever	Coxiella burnetii	None

confirmed by isolation of the organisms from blood, skin lesions or CSF. The yield is low by this technique; however, serological testing, particularly for specific IgM antibodies, is highly effective.

TREATMENT

Penicillin or tetracycline given early in the course of the disease shortens the duration of the illness in approximately 50% of patients. High-dose parenteral penicillin (benzathine penicillin, 2.4 g weekly for 3 weeks) or intravenous benzyl penicillin (2 g daily for 10 days) should be given.

Rat bite fevers

Two spirochaetes, *Spirillum minus* and *Streptobacillus moniliformis*, produce similar febrile illnesses following rat bites. Although the wound initially heals, 1–3 weeks later a local inflammatory response occurs that may be associated with swelling and ulceration. Systemic sequelae of generalized infection are then evident and periodic fevers may continue for several weeks. *Spirillum minus* causes a milder illness with a shorter incubation period and less-prolonged sequelae.

DIAGNOSIS

Spirochaetes can be identified in aspirates from the inflammatory site, from a regional lymph node (*Spirillum minus*), or from the blood (*Streptobacillus moniliformis*). Serological tests are available and may be helpful in diagnosis.

TREATMENT

Both organisms are sensitive to penicillin and tetracycline.

Rickettsiae and similar organisms

Rickettsiae are small bacteria that are spread to humans by arthropod vectors, namely, human body lice, fleas, ticks and larval mites. Rickettsiae inhabit the alimentary tract of these arthropods and the disease is spread to the human host by inoculation of their faeces through human skin, generally by irritation and scratching. Rickettsiae multiply intracellularly and can enter most mammalian cells, although the main lesion produced is a vasculitis due to invasion of endothelial cells of small blood vessels. Thus multi-system involvement is usual. The causative organisms and arthropod vectors for rickettsial infections are shown in Table 1.27.

CLINICAL FEATURES

Epidemic typhus
This is the most important rickettsial infection. Major outbreaks of typhus fever have occurred, mainly during famines and wars. It is found in Africa, Mexico, South America and Asia.

The incubation period is 1–3 weeks followed by an abrupt febrile illness associated with profound malaise and generalized myalgia. After 2 or 3 days the fever remains constant at around 40°C. Headache is severe and there may be conjunctivitis with orbital pain. A measles-like eruption appears around the fifth day, the macules increasing in size and eventually becoming purpuric in character. At the end of the first week, signs of meningoencephalitis are evident and CNS involvement may progress to stupor or coma, sometimes with extrapyramidal involvement. At the height of the illness, splenomegaly, pneumonia, myocarditis and gangrene at the peripheries may be evident. Oliguric renal failure occurs in fulminating disease, which is usually fatal. Recovery begins in the third week but is generally slow.

The disease may recur many years after the initial attack owing to rickettsiae that lie dormant in lymph nodes. The recrudescence is known as Brill–Zinsser disease. The factors that precipitate recurrence are not clearly defined, although other infections may be important.

Endemic (murine) typhus

This is a rat infection that is inadvertently spread to man by a rickettsiae-carrying rat flea. The disease closely resembles epidemic typhus but is much milder and rarely fatal.

Rocky Mountain spotted fever

Infected hard ticks transmit this infection to humans, the same arthropod vector being responsible for other tick-borne typhus fevers in Africa, India and the Mediterranean (Rickettsia conorii), in Central Asia and the Far East (Rickettsia siberica), and in Australia (Rickettsia australis).

Rocky Mountain spotted fever is limited to North and South America. As in other tick-borne typhus fevers, many patients will be able to give an account of tick bites or exposure to ticks. Clinical features closely resemble those of epidemic typhus, although the incubation period may be shorter and an eschar (crusted necrotic papule) may develop at the site of the bite in association with regional lymphadenopathy. The typical, generalized maculopapular rash occurs, which includes the palms and soles of the feet. The rash eventually becomes petechial. Neurological, haematological and cardiovascular complications occur as in epidemic typhus.

Scrub typhus

Found throughout Asia and the Western Pacific, this disease is spread by larval trombiculid mites (chiggers). Like tick-borne typhus, an eschar can often be found. Again the clinical illness resembles that of epidemic typhus, with an abrupt onset febrile illness, rash and severe toxaemia. Bronchitis and interstitial pneumonia occur commonly but physical findings in the chest are minimal. The infection may recur despite treatment with antibiotics.

Rickettsial pox and trench fever

Rickettsial pox is an urban disease described initially in New York City in 1946. A rodent mite was responsible for the spread of the infection to humans, the epidemic being related to massive expansion of the mouse community in large apartment buildings. The disease is mild, but similar in character to other rickettsial infections. Trench fever is also a relatively mild illness but multiple relapses are common. Although the causative agent of both these diseases, Rochalimaea

Table 1.28 Weil–Felix reaction[a] in rickettsial infections.

Rickettsial infection	Proteus strain[b]	
	OX19	OXK
Typhus fevers:		
Epidemic typhus	+	−
Endemic typhus	+	−
Rocky Mountain spotted fever	+	−
Scrub typhus	−	+
Rickettsial pox	−	−
Trench fever	−	−
Q fever	−	−

[a] Agglutination of Proteus strains by patients' serum.
[b] + = positive result (i.e. agglutination occurs);
− = negative result.

quintana, was originally classified with the rickettsiae, it is now known that the organism does not demand an intracellular existence and may be cultured on bacteriological media. Both of these diseases are now rare and rickettsial pox may have disappeared completely.

DIAGNOSIS

The diagnosis is generally made on the basis of the history and clinical course of the illness. Although the causative organisms can be isolated by inoculation of infected blood into laboratory animals, this is laborious and may take several weeks.

Serodiagnosis using the Weil–Felix Proteus agglutination test, which relies on the fact that Rickettsia and Proteus OX strains have common antigens, has been used for more than 50 years. Typical results of this test in different rickettsial infections are shown in Table 1.28. The Weil–Felix test is now being replaced by a complement-fixation test.

TREATMENT

Chloramphenicol 50 mg·kg^{-1} is given as an initial dose, followed by the same total dose given daily in three or four divided doses. Improvement generally occurs in 48 h; treatment should continue for at least 24 h after the fever has abated. Alternatively, tetracycline 2 g daily may be given. Corticosteroids are also used in severely ill patients.

CONTROL

This is achieved by control of vectors, namely lice, fleas, mites and ticks. Lice and fleas can be eradicated from clothing by insecticides (0.5% malathion or dicophane [DDT]). Chemical repellants are also useful. Control of rodents is vital.

Bites from ticks and mites should be avoided by wearing protective clothing on exposed areas of the body, especially in high-risk regions. Mites can also be destroyed by chemical spraying from the air.

Q fever

Q fever is a zoonosis due to the rickettsia-like organism *Coxiella burnetii*. This organism is smaller than true rickettsiae, more resistant to physical and chemical injury and has a negative Weil–Felix reaction, since it does not share common antigens with *Proteus*. Clinically, Q fever differs from rickettsial illnesses as the rash is not a major feature and transmission of the disease to humans is independent of an arthropod vector. Important modes of spread to man are thought to be dust, aerosols and milk from infected cows. *Coxiella burnetii* is widespread in domestic and farm animals. It is spread between them by ticks, which constitute an important arthropod reservoir of the disease.

CLINICAL FEATURES

Fever begins insidiously, together with other symptoms of an influenza-like illness, 1–2 weeks after exposure. The acute illness may resolve spontaneously without treatment, but with persisting infection, symptoms and signs of pneumonia may develop, followed by endocarditis. A petechial rash may be apparent at this stage. Occasionally epididymo-orchitis, uveitis and osteomyelitis may be present. Untreated chronic infection is usually fatal.

DIAGNOSIS

Serodiagnosis by complement fixation tests is important since *C. burnetii* is an obligate intracellular organism and does not grow on standard microbiological culture media. The organism possesses two classes of antigens, phase I and phase II. Antibodies to the phase I antigens appear later in the illness than antibodies to the phase II antigens; high titres are diagnostic in endocarditis. Persistently high titres of both antibodies confirm chronic infection.

TREATMENT

Tetracycline is the treatment of choice for acute infection. For endocarditis a prolonged course of treatment is required, clindamycin often being given in association with tetracycline. Co-trimoxazole and rifampicin may also be useful.

Chlamydiae

Although chlamydiae were once thought to be large viruses, it is now clear that they are true intracellular bacteria with a cell wall and both DNA and RNA, and are susceptible to a range of antibiotics. They are ubiquitous and found in almost every avian and mammalian species and it has been estimated that up to 20% of the human population is infected with this organism. They are highly infectious, but rarely kill their host. There are two species—*Chlamydia trachomatis* and *C. psittaci*; Table 1.29 shows the diseases produced.

Table 1.29 *Chlamydia* infections.

Disease	Organism
Trachoma	C. trachomatis
Lymphogranuloma venereum	C. trachomatis (Serotypes L 1, 2 and 3)
Urethritis, cervicitis, proctitis	C. trachomatis
Psittacosis	C. psittaci

Trachoma

This is the commonest cause of blindness in the world and is found in the tropics and the Middle East. It is entirely preventable. It commonly occurs in children and is probably spread by direct transmission or possibly by flies.

Infection is bilateral and begins in the conjunctiva, with marked inflammation and scarring. Scarring of the upper eyelid causes entropion, leaving the cornea exposed to further damage. The corneal scarring that eventually occurs leads to blindness. The changes in the eye are sometimes accompanied by an upper respiratory tract infection.

Trachoma may also occur as an acute ophthalmic infection in the neonate.

DIAGNOSIS

The diagnosis is generally established by:

- The typical clinical picture
- The presence of intracytoplasmic inclusion bodies in conjunctival cells

TREATMENT

Tetracycline ointment applied locally each day for 2–3 months is effective, as is systemic therapy with oral tetracycline or sulphonamide. Once infection has been controlled, surgery may be required for eyelid reconstruction and for treatment of corneal opacities. Community health education with respect to hygiene and earlier case reporting could make a substantial impact on disease prevalence.

Genital infections

Lymphogranuloma venereum (LGV) is caused by *C. trachomatis* serotypes L 1, 2 and 3 and is described on p. 49.

Genital infections are also caused by other strains of *C. trachomatis* (see p. 49).

Psittacosis (ornithosis)

Although originally thought to be limited to the psittacine birds (parrots, parakeets and macaws), it is now known that the disease is widely spread amongst many species of birds, including pigeons, turkeys, ducks and chickens, hence the broader term 'ornithosis'. Human infection is related to exposure to infected birds and is therefore a true zoonosis. The causative organism, *C. psittaci*, is excreted in avian secretions; it can be isolated for prolonged periods from birds who have apparently recovered from infection. The organism gains entry to the human host by inhalation.

CLINICAL FEATURES AND TREATMENT

These are discussed on p. 674.

Viral infections

Viruses are much smaller than other microorganisms and contain either DNA or RNA. Since they are metabolically inert, they must live intracellularly, using the host cell for synthesis of viral proteins and nucleic acid. Viruses have a central nucleic acid core surrounded by a protein coat that is antigenically unique for a particular virus. The protein coat (capsid) imparts a helical or icosahedral structure to the virus. Some viruses also possess an envelope consisting of lipid and protein (Fig. 1.19).

Hepatitis viruses are discussed on p. 252.

DNA viruses

Details of the structure, size and classification of DNA viruses are shown in Table 1.30.

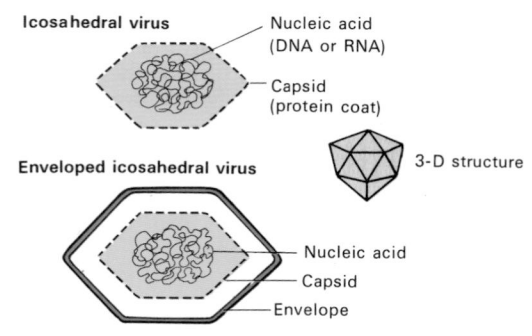

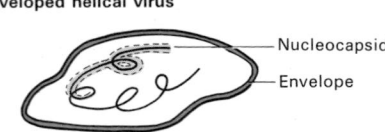

Fig. 1.19 The basic structure of viruses.

ADENOVIRUSES

Adenovirus infection commonly presents as an acute pharyngitis. By school age the majority of children show serological evidence of previous infection. Certain subtypes produce an acute conjunctivitis associated with pharyngitis. In adults, adenovirus causes acute follicular conjunctivitis and rarely pneumonia that is clinically similar to that produced by *Mycoplasma* (see p. 672). Adenovirus has also been implicated as a cause of gastroenteritis (p. 62) without respiratory disease and may be responsible for acute mesenteric lymphadenitis in children and young adults.

HERPESVIRUSES

Herpes simplex virus (HSV) infection

Two types of HSV have been identified: HSV-1 is the major cause of herpetic stomatitis, herpes labialis ('cold sore'), keratoconjunctivitis and encephalitis, whereas HSV-2 causes genital herpes and may also be responsible for systemic infection in the immunocompromised host. These divisions, however, are not rigid, for HSV-1 can give rise to genital herpes.

Primary inoculation of the infection is via skin or mucous membrane. The initial infection may go unnoticed or may produce a severe inflammatory reaction. The virus then remains latent, most commonly in the trigeminal nerve, but may be reactivated by trauma, febrile illnesses and ultraviolet radiation, producing the recurrent form of

Table 1.30 Human DNA viruses.[a]

| Structure | | Approximate | | |
Symmetry	Envelope	size	Group	Viruses
Icosahedral	−	80 nm	Adenovirus	Adenoviruses
Icosahedral	+	100 nm	Herpesvirus	Herpes simplex virus types 1 and 2
				Varicella zoster virus
				Cytomegalovirus
				Epstein–Barr virus
Icosahedral	−	50 nm	Papovavirus	Human papillomavirus
				Polyomavirus
Icosahedral	−	?38 nm	Parvovirus	Parvovirus B19
Complex	+	300 nm	Poxvirus	Variola virus
				Vaccinia virus

[a] For hepatitis viruses see p. 252.

the disease known as herpes labialis ('cold sore'). Recurrent infections occur in one third of patients.

In genital herpes the primary infection is usually more severe and recurrences are inevitable. The virus remains latent in the sacral ganglia and during recurrence can produce a radiculomyelopathy, with pain in the groin, buttocks and upper thighs. Primary anorectal herpes infection is now common in male homosexuals.

Immunocompromised patients such as those receiving intensive cancer chemotherapy or those with the acquired immunodeficiency syndrome (AIDS) may develop disseminated HSV infection involving many of the viscera. In severe cases death may result from severe hepatitis and encephalitis.

Neonates may develop primary HSV infection following vaginal delivery in the presence of active genital HSV infection in the mother. Caesarean section should therefore be performed in the presence of active genital HSV infection.

Humoral antibody levels increase following primary infection, but mononuclear cell responses are probably more important in preventing dissemination of disease.

The clinical picture, diagnosis and treatment are described on p. 1024.

Varicella zoster virus (VZV) infection

VZV produces two distinct diseases—varicella (chickenpox) and herpes zoster (shingles). The primary infection is chickenpox. It usually occurs in childhood, the virus entering through the mucosa of the upper respiratory tract. The primary infection almost never occurs twice in the same individual. The virus then remains latent in sensory and motor nerve cells for many years. It may recur as localized disease limited to a dermatome innervated by a single spinal or cranial sensory ganglion (shingles) and/or may affect a motor nerve such as the facial nerve, causing facial palsy. Shingles is never the result of a primary infection. Patients with chickenpox or shingles are infective, the virus being spread from fresh skin lesions by direct contact or airborne transmission.

CLINICAL FEATURES

Fourteen to twenty-one days after exposure to VZV, a brief prodromal illness of fever, headache and malaise heralds the eruption of chickenpox, characterized by the rapid progression of macules to papules to vesicles to pustules in a matter of hours. In young children the prodromal illness may be very mild or absent. The illness tends to be more severe in older children and can be debilitating in adults. The lesions occur on the face, scalp and trunk, and to a much lesser extent on the extremities. It is characteristic to see skin lesions at all stages of development on the same area of skin. Fever subsides as soon as new lesions cease to appear. Eventually the pustules crust and heal without scarring.

Important complications of chickenpox include pneumonia, which generally begins 1–6 days after the skin eruption. Pulmonary symptoms are usually more striking than the physical findings, although a chest radiograph usually shows diffuse changes throughout both lung fields. Central nervous system involvement occurs in about 1 per 1000 and most commonly presents as an acute truncal cerebellar ataxia. The immunocompromised are susceptible to disseminated infection with multi-organ involvement.

Shingles (p. 1025) occurs in adults, particularly the elderly, producing an identical skin lesion to chickenpox, although restricted to a sensory nerve distribution.

TREATMENT

Chickenpox requires no treatment in healthy children and infection results in life-long immunity. However, the disease may be fatal in the immunodeficient or the immunosuppressed, when it is reasonable to use passive immunization with varicella zoster immunoglobulin (VZIg). In the immunocompromised host it is also reasonable to give acyclovir (500 mg·m^2 three times daily i.v. for 7 days) or vidarabine (10 mg·kg^{-1} daily i.v. for 7 days).

Cytomegalovirus (CMV) infection

Infection with CMV is found world-wide and has its most profound effects as an opportunistic infection in the immunocompromised, particularly in recipients of bone-marrow and solid organ transplants and in patients with AIDS. Ninety per cent of patients with AIDS are infected with CMV and 95% of this population have disseminated CMV at autopsy. A large proportion of the adult population has serological evidence of previous exposure to the virus, although infection is generally symptomless.

CLINICAL FEATURES

In healthy adults CMV causes an illness similar to infectious mononucleosis, with fever, lymphocytosis with atypical lymphocytes, and hepatitis. Infection may be spread by blood transfusion. Disseminated fatal infection with widespread visceral involvement occurs in the immunocompromised including encephalitis, retinitis, pneumonitis and diffuse involvement of the gastrointestinal tract.

Intrauterine infection may have serious consequences on the fetus; there is generally CNS involvement causing microcephaly and motor disorders, often associated with jaundice, hepatosplenomegaly, thrombocytopenia and haemolytic anaemia. In older children CMV infection presents as hepatitis with or without jaundice.

DIAGNOSIS

Serological tests can identify past (IgG) or current (IgM) infection. The virus can also be identified in tissue culture by the presence of characteristic intranuclear 'owl's eye' inclusions.

TREATMENT

In the immunocompetent, infection is usually self-limiting and no specific treatment is required. In the immunosuppressed, ganciclovir (2.5 mg·kg^{-1} three times daily for 14–21 days) reduces retinitis and gastrointestinal damage and can eliminate CMV from blood, urine and respiratory secretions. It is less effective against pneumonitis and encephalitis. Drug resistance has been reported.

Epstein-Barr virus (EBV) infection

This virus causes an acute febrile illness known as infectious mononucleosis (glandular fever), which occurs world-wide in adolescents and young adults. EBV is probably transmitted in saliva and by aerosol.

CLINICAL FEATURES

The predominant symptoms are fever, headache, malaise and sore throat. Palatal petechiae and a transient macular rash are common, the latter occurring in 90% of patients who have received ampicillin for the sore throat. Cervical lymphadenopathy, particularly of the posterior cervical nodes, and splenomegaly are characteristic. Mild hepatitis is common, but other complications such as myocarditis, meningitis, mesenteric adenitis and splenic rupture are rare. Although some young adults remain debilitated and depressed for some months after infection, the evidence for the occurrence of latency and reactivation of the virus in healthy individuals is controversial, although these are thought to occur in immunocompromised patients.

DIAGNOSIS

EBV infection should be strongly suspected if atypical mononuclear cells (glandular fever cells) are found in the peripheral blood. It can be confirmed during the second week of infection by a positive Paul–Bunnell reaction, which detects heterophile antibodies (IgM) that agglutinate sheep erythrocytes. False positives can occur in other conditions such as hepatitis, Hodgkin's disease and acute leukaemia. Specific EBV IgM antibodies indicate recent infection by the virus. The Mono-spot test is a sensitive and easily performed screening test. Clinically similar illnesses are produced by CMV and toxoplasmosis but these can be distinguished serologically.

TREATMENT

The majority of cases require no specific treatment and recovery is rapid. Corticosteroid therapy is advised when there is neurological involvement, e.g. encephalitis, meningitis, Guillain–Barré syndrome or when there is marked thrombocytopenia or haemolysis. Corticosteroid therapy has also been used when malaise and intermittent fever are prolonged but this is not recommended.

EBV is also considered to be the aetiological agent responsible for Burkitt's lymphoma and nasopharyngeal carcinoma.

PAPOVAVIRUSES

These small viruses tend to produce chronic infections, often with evidence of latency. They are capable of inducing neoplasia in some animal species and were among the first viruses to be implicated in tumorigenesis. Human papilloma-virus is responsible for the common wart and has recently been implicated as a cause of carcinoma of the anal canal. The human BK virus, polyoma-virus, is the only other human virus of importance in this group. It is generally found in immuno-suppressed individuals and may be detected in the urine of between 15 and 40% of renal transplant patients, in patients receiving cytotoxic chemo-therapy and in those with immunodeficiency states, notably the Wiskott–Aldrich syndrome.

For genital warts see p. 1026.

PARVOVIRUSES

Human parvovirus B19 produces:

- Erythema infectiosum (fifth disease) a common infection in schoolchildren. The rash is typically on the face (slapped-cheek appearance). The patient is well and the rash can recur over weeks or months.
- Asymptomatic infection occurs in 20% of children.
- Moderately severe self-limiting arthropathy.
- Aplastic crises in patients with chronic haemoly-sis, e.g. sickle cell disease.
- Chronic infection with anaemia in immunocom-promised subjects.

POXVIRUSES

Smallpox (variola)

This disease has now been eradicated following an aggressive vaccination policy and careful detection of new cases. All remaining viruses in laboratories have been destroyed.

Vaccinia virus

This is a laboratory virus and does not occur in nature in either man or animals. Its origins are uncertain but it is thought to be a derivative of the variola or cowpox virus used by Jenner for vaccination against smallpox. Vaccination is now not recommended except for laboratory personnel handling the virus for experimental purposes. Should the disease reappear, herd immunity would be very low and widespread dissemination of the disease might result.

RNA viruses (Table 1.31)

PICORNAVIRUSES

Poliovirus infection (poliomyelitis)

Poliomyelitis occurs when a susceptible individual is infected with poliovirus type I, II or III. These viruses have a marked propensity for the nervous system, especially the anterior horn cells of the spinal cord and cranial nerve motor nuclei. Polio-myelitis is found world-wide but its incidence has decreased dramatically following improvements in sanitation, hygiene and the widespread use of polio vaccines. Spread is usually via the faecal–oral route, as the virus is excreted in the faeces.

CLINICAL FEATURES

The incubation period varies from 10 to 14 days. Although polio is essentially a disease of child-hood, no age is exempt. The clinical manifestations vary considerably:

- *Inapparent infection* is common and occurs in 95% of infected individuals.
- *Abortive poliomyelitis* occurs in approximately 4–5% and is characterized by the presence of fever, sore throat and myalgia. The illness is self-limiting and of short duration.
- *Non-paralytic poliomyelitis* has features of abortive poliomyelitis as well as signs of meningeal irritation, but recovery is complete.
- *Paralytic poliomyelitis* occurs in approximately 0.1% of all infected individuals. Several factors predispose to the development of paralysis:
    male sex
    exercise early in the illness
    trauma, surgery or intramuscular injection which localize the paralysis
    recent tonsillectomy (bulbar poliomyelitis)
    HLA 3 and 7

This form of the disease is characterized initially by features simulating abortive poliomyelitis. Symptoms subside for 4–5 days, only to recur in greater severity with signs of meningeal irrita-tion and muscle pain, which is most prominent in the neck and lumbar region. These symptoms persist for a few days and are followed by the onset of asymmetric paralysis without sensory involvement. The paralysis is usually confined to the lower limbs in children under 5 years of age

Table 1.31 Human RNA viruses.

Structure		Approximate size	Group	Viruses	
Symmetry	Envelope				
Icosahedral	−	30 nm	Picornavirus	Poliovirus Coxsackievirus Echovirus Enterovirus Rhinovirus	} Enteroviruses
Icosahedral	−	80 nm	Reovirus	Reovirus Rotavirus	
Icosahedral	+	50–80 nm	Togavirus	Rubella virus Alphaviruses Flaviviruses	} Arbovirus
Helical	+	80–120 nm	Orthomyxovirus	Influenza viruses A, B and C	
Helical	+	100–300 nm	Paramyxovirus	Measles virus Mumps virus Respiratory syncytial virus	
Helical	+	60–175 nm	Rhabdovirus	Rabies virus Vesicular stomatitis virus	
Helical	+	100 nm	Retrovirus	Human immunodeficiency virus (HIV)	
Helical	+	100–300 nm	Arenavirus	Lassa virus Lymphocytic choriomeningitis virus	
Pleomorphic	+	Filaments or circular forms; 100 × 130–2600 nm	—	Marburg virus Ebola virus	

and the upper limbs in older children, whereas in adults it manifests as paraplegia or quadriplegia.

- Bulbar poliomyelitis occurs in 5–30% and is characterized by the presence of cranial nerve involvement. Soft palate, pharyngeal and laryngeal muscle palsies are common.

Aspiration pneumonia, myocarditis, paralytic ileus and urinary calculi are late complications of all types of poliomyelitis.

Post-polio syndrome refers to an increase in the degree of muscle atrophy of an affected limb many years after the primary attack.

DIAGNOSIS

The diagnosis is a clinical one. Distinction from the Guillain–Barré syndrome is easily made by the absence of sensory involvement and the asymmetrical nature of the paralysis in poliomyelitis.

TREATMENT

Treatment is symptomatic. Bedrest is essential during the early course of the illness. Respiratory support with intermittent positive pressure respiration is required if the muscles of respiration are involved. Once the acute phase of the illness has subsided, occupational therapy, physiotherapy and occasionally surgery play an important role in patient rehabilitation.

PREVENTION AND CONTROL

Immunization has dramatically decreased the prevalence of this disease world-wide. Trivalent oral poliovaccine (OPV) (active virus) is used (see Table 1.12); occasionally, inactivated poliovirus vaccine is used intramuscularly.

Coxsackie-, echo- and enterovirus infection

These viruses are spread by the faecal–oral route. They each have a number of different types and are responsible for a broad spectrum of disease involving the skin and mucous membranes, muscles, nerves, the heart (see Table 1.32), and rarely other organs, such as the liver and pancreas.

Table 1.32 Picornavirus infections (excluding poliovirus and rhinovirus).

Disease	Coxsackievirus A (types A_1–A_{22}, A_{24})	Coxsackievirus B (types B_1–B_6)	Echovirus (types 1–9, 11–27, 29–33)	Enterovirus (types 68–71)
Cutaneous and oropharyngeal				
Herpangina	+++	+	+	
Hand, foot and mouth	+++	+		+
Erythematous rashes	+	+	+++	
Neurological				
Paralytic	+		±	+
Meningitis	++	++	+++	+
Encephalitis	++	++	±	+
Cardiac				
Myo- and pericarditis	+	+++	+	
Muscle				
Myositis (Bornholm disease)	+	+++	+	

Skin and oropharyngeal disease
There is a vesicular eruption on the fauces, palate and uvula (herpangina). The lesions eventually evolve into aphthous ulcers. The illness is usually associated with fever and headache but is short-lived, recovery occurring within a few days.

Hand, foot and mouth disease
Oral lesions are similar to those seen in herpangina but may be more extensive in the oropharynx. However, vesicles and a maculopapular eruption also appear on the palms of the hands and the soles of the feet. This infection commonly affects children; recovery occurs within a week.

Neurological disease
Other enteroviruses in addition to poliovirus can cause a broad range of neurological disease, including meningitis, encephalitis, and a paralytic disease characteristic of poliomyelitis.

Heart and muscle disease
Viruses are an important cause of acute myocarditis and pericarditis, from which, in general, there is complete recovery. However, these viruses can also cause chronic congestive cardiomyopathy and, rarely, constrictive pericarditis.

Skeletal muscle involvement, particularly of the intercostal muscles, is an important feature of Bornholm disease, a febrile illness usually due to Coxsackievirus B. The infection affects both children and adults and may be complicated by meningitis or cardiac involvement.

Rhinovirus infection

Rhinovirus is responsible for the common cold (p. 649); peak incidence rates occur in the colder months, especially spring and autumn. There are multiple rhinovirus immunotypes, which makes vaccine control impracticable.

REOVIRUS

Reovirus infection

Reovirus infection occurs mainly in children, causing mild respiratory symptoms and diarrhoea. A few deaths have been reported following disseminated infection of brain, liver, heart and lungs.

Rotavirus infection
Rotavirus (Latin *rota* = wheel) is so named because of its characteristic circular outline with radiating spokes. It is responsible world-wide for both sporadic cases and epidemics of diarrhoea, and is presently one of the most important causes of childhood diarrhoea. The prevalence is higher during the winter months.

Other viruses associated with gastroenteritis are shown in Table 1.33.

Clinically the illness is characterized by vomiting, fever, diarrhoea, and the metabolic consequences of water and electrolyte loss. Histology of the jejunal mucosa in children shows shortening of the villi, with crypt hyperplasia and mononuclear cell infiltration of the lamina propria. Diagnosis can be established by ELISA for the detection of rotavirus antigen in faeces but this is rarely

Table 1.33 Viruses associated with gastroenteritis.

Rotavirus (Groups A, B, C, D and E)

Enteric adenovirus (types 40 and 41)

Norwalk and related viruses

Calicivirus

Astrovirus

Parvovirus

Other small round viruses

indicated clinically, since infection is self-limiting and there is no specific treatment.

Treatment is directed at overcoming the effects of water and electrolyte imbalance with adequate oral rehydration therapy and, when indicated, intravenous fluids. Antibiotics should not be prescribed.

Adults may become infected with rotavirus but symptoms are mild or absent.

Rotavirus vaccines are under evaluation. Live, attenuated, oral bovine rotavirus vaccines (RIT 4237 and WC3) are moderately effective in the industrialized world but less so in the developing world. Reabsortant rotaviruses are being constructed by recombinant DNA technology that have an attenuated animal rotavirus 'backbone' but contain RNA inserts from human rotavirus in an attempt to improve immunogenicity.

TOGAVIRUSES

These can be divided into the rubella virus and the arboviruses.

Rubella

Rubella ('German measles') is caused by a spherical, enveloped fragile RNA virus that is easily killed by heat and ultraviolet light. While the disease can occur sporadically, epidemics are not uncommon. It has a world-wide distribution. Spread of the virus is via droplets; maximum infectivity occurs during the time the rash is present.

CLINICAL FEATURES

The incubation period varies from 14 to 21 days, averaging 18 days. The clinical features are largely age-determined, with symptoms being mild or even absent in children under 5 years of age. The peak incidence of the disease is at 15 years.

During the prodrome the patient complains of malaise and fever. Mild conjunctivitis and lymphadenopathy may be present. The distribution of the lymphadenopathy is characteristic and involves the suboccipital, post-auricular and posterior cervical groups of lymph nodes. Small petechial lesions on the soft palate (Forchheimer spots) are suggestive but not diagnostic. Splenomegaly may be present.

The eruptive or exanthematous phase usually occurs within the first 7 days of the initial symptoms. The rash first appears on the forehead and then spreads to involve the trunk and the limbs. It is pinkish-red, macular and discrete, although some of these lesions may coalesce. It usually fades by the second day and rarely persists beyond the third day after its appearance.

COMPLICATIONS

Complications are rare; they include superadded pulmonary bacterial infection, arthralgia, haemorrhagic manifestations due to thrombocytopenia, encephalitis and the *congenital rubella syndrome*. Rubella affects the fetuses of 50–70% of all women who contract the infection during the first trimester of pregnancy. The incidence of congenital abnormalities diminishes in the second and third trimesters. Congenital rubella syndrome is characterized by the presence of fetal cardiac malformations, especially patent ductus arteriosus and ventricular septal defect, eye lesions, especially cataracts, microcephaly, mental retardation and deafness. The *expanded rubella syndrome* consists of the manifestations of the congenital rubella syndrome plus hepatosplenomegaly, myocarditis, interstitial pneumonia and metaphyseal bone lesions.

DIAGNOSIS

This is usually clinical. It can be confirmed by culturing the virus from throat swabs or urine or by demonstrating an increased antibody titre (measured using the sensitive haemagglutination inhibition test) in the second of two successive blood samples taken 14 days apart.

TREATMENT

Treatment is symptomatic.

PREVENTION

Prevention of rubella is important. Human immunoglobulin can decrease the symptoms of this already mild illness, but does not prevent the teratogenic effects. Several live attenuated rubella vaccines have been used with great success in preventing this illness and these have been successfully combined with the measles and mumps vaccine. The side-effects of vaccination have been dramatically decreased by using vaccines prepared in human embryonic fibroblast cultures (RA 27/3 vaccine). Use of the vaccine is contraindicated during pregnancy or if there is a likelihood of pregnancy within 3 months of immunization. Complication of immunization during pregnancy is less than 2%.

Arbovirus (arthropod-borne) infection

Arboviruses are zoonotic viruses, with the possible exception of the O'nyong-nyong fever virus of which humans are the only known vertebrate hosts. They are transmitted through the bites of insects, especially mosquitoes and ticks, although infection can result from the ingestion of contaminated foods or inhalation of these organisms. Over 385 viruses are classified as arboviruses. *Culex*, *Aedes* and *Anopheles* mosquitoes account for the transmission of the majority of these.

Although the majority of arbovirus diseases are generally mild, epidemics are frequent and when these occur the mortality is high. In general, the incubation period is less than 10 days. The illness tends to be biphasic and, as in other viral fevers, pyrexia, conjunctival suffusion, a rash, retro-orbital pain, myalgia and arthralgia are common. Lymphadenopathy is seen in dengue. Lifelong immunity after an infection is usual. In some of these viral fevers, haemorrhage is a feature (Table 1.34), although its pathogenesis is speculative. Increased vascular permeability, capillary fragility and disseminated intravascular coagulation have been implicated. Encephalitis may be prominent in some fevers.

Alphaviruses
The 24 viruses of this group are all transmitted by

Table 1.34 Viral infections associated with haemorrhagic manifestations.

Arbovirus
Mosquito-borne:
  Yellow fever (urban and sylvan)
  Dengue haemorrhagic fever
  Chikungunya
  Rift Valley fever
Tick-borne:
  Congo and Crimean haemorrhagic fevers
  Kyasanur Forest disease
  Omsk haemorrhagic fever

Arenavirus
Argentinian haemorrhagic fever
Bolivian haemorrhagic fever
Lassa fever
Epidemic haemorrhagic fever

Picornavirus
Acute haemorrhagic conjunctivitis

Paramyxovirus
Atypical measles

mosquitoes; eight result in human disease. These viruses are globally distributed and tend to acquire their names from the location where they were first isolated (such as Ross River, Eastern Venezuelan, and Western encephalitis viruses) or by the local expression for a major symptom caused by the virus (such as chikungunya meaning 'chronic bleeding'). Infection is characterized by fever, skin rash, arthralgia, myalgia and sometimes encephalitis.

Flaviviruses
There are 60 viruses in this group, some of which are transmitted by ticks and others by mosquitoes.

Yellow fever

Yellow fever, caused by a flavivirus, results in an illness of widely varying severity. It is a disease confined to Africa and South America between latitudes 15° north and 15° south of the equator. For poorly understood reasons, yellow fever has not been reported from Asia, despite the fact that climatic conditions are suitable and the vector, *Aedes aegypti*, is common. The infection is transmitted in the wild by *A. africanus* in Africa and the *Haemagogus* species in South and Central America. These mosquitoes are responsible for maintaining infection in monkeys, which form the sylvan reservoir. *A. aegypti* and the *Haemagogus* species are responsible for transmission of this disease from monkeys to humans in Africa and South and Central America, respectively. Once infected, a mosquito remains so for its whole life.

CLINICAL FEATURES

The incubation period varies from 3 to 6 days. When the infection is mild, the disease is indistinguishable from other viral fevers such as influenza or dengue. Classically, however, jaundice, proteinuria and haemorrhage occur.

Three phases in the illness are recognized. Initially the patient presents with a high fever of acute onset, usually 39–40°C, which then returns to normal in 4–5 days. During this time, headache is prominent. Retrobulbar pain, myalgia, arthralgia, a flushed face and suffused conjunctivae are common. Epigastric discomfort and vomiting are present when the illness is severe. Relative bradycardia (Faget's sign) is present from the second day of illness. The patient then makes an apparent recovery and feels well for several days. Following this 'phase of calm' the patient again develops increasing fever, deepening jaundice and hepatomegaly. Ecchymosis, bleeding from the gums, haematemesis and melaena may occur. Coma, which is usually a result of uraemia or haemorrhagic shock, occurs for a few hours preceding death. The mortality rate is up to 40% in severe cases.

DIAGNOSIS

The diagnosis is established by isolating the virus (when possible) from blood during the first three days of illness, by demonstrating increasing neutralizing antibody titres, or by finding the typical histological lesions on liver biopsy. These include mid-zone necrosis, fatty degeneration and intracellular hyaline necrosis (Councilman bodies).

TREATMENT

Treatment is supportive. Bed rest, analgesics, and maintenance of fluid and electrolyte balance are important.

PREVENTION AND CONTROL

Yellow fever is an internationally notifiable disease. It is easily prevented using either the 17-day chick embryo vaccine, which is more popular, or the Dakar vaccine. Eradication of the breeding places of the vectors will help in decreasing the prevalence of the disease.

Dengue

Dengue is a viral disease found mainly in Asia and Africa, although it has been reported from the USA as well. Four different antigenic varieties of the dengue virus are recognized and all are transmitted by the daytime-biting *Aedes aegypti*. Humans are infective during the first three days of the illness (viraemic stage). Mosquitoes become infective about 2 weeks after feeding on an infected individual, and remain so for the rest of their lives. The disease is usually endemic, but epidemics have been recorded. Immunity after the illness is partial.

CLINICAL FEATURES

The incubation period varies from 5 to 6 days. Two clinical forms are recognized.

Classic dengue fever is characterized by the abrupt onset of fever, malaise, headache, retrobulbar pain which worsens on eye movements, conjunctival suffusion and severe backache, which is a prominent symptom. Lymphadenopathy, petechiae on the soft palate and skin rashes may also occur. The rash is transient and morbilliform. It appears on the limbs and then spreads to involve the trunk. Desquamation occurs subsequently. Cough is uncommon. The fever subsides after 3–4 days, the temperature remains normal for a couple of days, and then the fever returns, together with the features already mentioned, but is milder. This biphasic or saddleback pattern is considered characteristic. Severe fatigue, a feeling of being unwell and depression are common for several weeks after the fever has subsided.

Dengue haemorrhagic fever is a severe form of dengue fever and is believed to be the result of two sequential infections with different dengue serotypes. It is a disease of children and has been described almost exclusively in South-East Asia. The disease has a mild start, often with symptoms of an upper respiratory tract infection. This is then followed by the abrupt onset of shock and haemorrhage into the skin and ear, epistaxis, haematemesis and melaena known as the dengue shock syndrome. Serum complement levels are depressed and there is laboratory evidence of a consumptive coagulopathy.

DIAGNOSIS

Isolation of the dengue virus by tissue culture in sera obtained during the first few days of illness is diagnostic. Demonstration of rising antibody titres by neutralization (most specific), haemagglutination inhibition or complement-fixing antibodies in sequential serum samples is presumptive evidence of dengue virus infection.

TREATMENT

Treatment is symptomatic.

Rift Valley fever

Rift Valley fever is primarily an acute febrile illness of livestock, sheep, goats and camels. It is found in southern and eastern Africa. The vector in east Africa is *Culex pipiens* and in south Africa, *Aedes caballus*. Following an incubation period of 3–6 days, the patient has an acute febrile illness that is difficult to distinguish clinically from other viral fevers. The temperature pattern is usually biphasic. The initial febrile illness lasts 2–4 days and is followed by a remission and a second febrile episode. Complications are indicative of severe infection and include retinopathy, meningoencephalitis, haemorrhagic manifestations and hepatic necrosis. Mortality approaches 50% in severe forms of the illness. Treatment is symptomatic.

Japanese encephalitis

Japanese encephalitis is a mosquito-borne encephalitis caused by a flavivirus. It has been reported most frequently from the rice-growing countries of South-East Asia and the Far East. *Culex tritaeniorhynchus* is the most important vector and feeds mainly on pigs as well as birds such as herons and sparrows. Humans are accidental hosts.

As with other viral infections, the clinical manifestations are variable. The onset is heralded by severe rigors. Fever, headache and malaise last from 1 to 6 days. Weight loss is prominent. In the acute encephalitic stage the fever is high (38–41°C), neck rigidity occurs and neurological signs such as altered consciousness, hemiparesis and convulsions develop. Mental deterioration occurs over a period of 3–4 days and culminates in coma. Mortality varies from 7% to 40% and is higher in children. Residual neurological defects such as deafness, emotional lability and hemiparesis occur in about 70% of patients who have had CNS involvement. Convalescence is prolonged. Antibody detection in serum and CSF by IgM capture ELISA is a useful rapid diagnostic test. An inactivated mouse brain vaccine is effective and available. Treatment is symptomatic.

ORTHOMYXOVIRUSES

Influenza

Three types of influenza virus are recognized—A, B and C. The influenza A virus is a spherical or filamentous enveloped virus. Haemagglutinin, a surface glycopeptide, aids attachment of the virus to the wall of susceptible host cells at specific receptor sites. Cell penetration, probably by pinocytosis, and release of replicated viruses from the cell surface is effected by budding through the cell membrane or by the action of viral neuraminidase.

- *Influenza A* is generally responsible for pandemics and epidemics.
- *Influenza B* often causes smaller or localized and milder outbreaks, e.g. in camps or schools.
- *Influenza C* rarely produces disease in humans.

Antigenic shift (major antigenic change within an influenza subtype) usually heralds the onset of a pandemic.

Sporadic cases of influenza and outbreaks among groups of people living in a confined environment are frequent. The incidence increases during the winter months, when crowding is common. Spread is mainly by droplet infection but fomites and direct contact have also been implicated.

The clinical features, diagnosis, treatment and prophylaxis of influenza are discussed on p. 653.

PARAMYXOVIRUSES

These are a heterogeneous group of enveloped viruses of varying size that are responsible for parainfluenza, mumps, measles and respiratory infection.

Parainfluenza

Parainfluenza is caused by the parainfluenza viruses types I to IV, which have a world-wide distribution. Type IV has been identified only in the USA.

Parainfluenza is essentially a disease of children and presents with features similar to the common cold. When severe, a brassy cough with inspiratory stridor and features of laryngotracheobronchitis (croup) are present. Treatment is symptomatic. The role of steroids is controversial.

Measles (rubeola)

Measles is a highly communicable disease that occurs world-wide. With the introduction of aggressive immunizaticn policies, the incidence of measles has fallen dramatically in the West, but it still remains one of the commonest childhood infections in developing countries, where it is associated with a high morbidity and mortality. It is spread by droplet infection.

CLINICAL FEATURES

The incubation period varies from 8 to 14 days. Two distinct phases of the disease can be recognized.

Typical measles

- *The infectious pre-eruptive and catarrhal stage.* This is the stage of viraemia and viral dissemination. Malaise, fever, rhinorrhoea, cough, conjunctival suffusion and the pathognomonic Koplik's spots are present during this stage. Koplik's spots are small, greyish, irregular lesions surrounded by an erythematous base and are found in greatest numbers on the mucous membrane opposite the second molar tooth. They occur a day or two before the onset of the rash.
- *The non-infectious eruptive or exanthematous stage.* This is characterized by the presence of a maculopapular rash (Table 1.35) that initially occurs on the face, chiefly the forehead, and then spreads rapidly to involve the rest of the body. At first the rash is discrete but later it may become confluent and patchy, especially on the face and neck. It fades in about a week and leaves behind a brownish discoloration with desquamation.

Although measles is a relatively mild disease in the healthy child, it carries a high mortality in the malnourished and in those who have other diseases. Complications are common in such individuals and include bacterial pneumonia, bronchitis, otitis media and gastroenteritis. Less commonly, myocarditis, hepatitis and encephalomyelitis may occur. The virus has also been implicated in the rare condition subacute sclerosing panencephalitis.

Maternal measles, unlike rubella, does not cause congenital fetal abnormalities. It is, however,

Table 1.35 Some viral infections associated with a maculopapular rash.

Adenovirus infection

Arbovirus infection

Measles

Cytomegalovirus infection

Enterovirus infection

Hepatitis B virus

Infectious mononucleosis

Rubella

Rubeola

associated with spontaneous abortions and premature delivery.

Atypical measles is a severe illness that usually occurs in individuals who have previously received the inactivated vaccine and are exposed to wild measles virus. The high fever (> 40°C), myalgia, abdominal pain and cough are followed by vesicles, petechiae and purpura. Skin lesions may be mistaken for scarlet fever, meningococcaemia or varicella. Pneumonia invariably occurs and the pulmonary infiltrates may persist for years.

DIAGNOSIS

The clinical features are distinctive and hence serological tests, such as the haemagglutination inhibition test, are rarely used to confirm the diagnosis. The measles virus is difficult to culture.

TREATMENT

Treatment is symptomatic. Antibiotics are indicated only if secondary bacterial infection occurs.

PREVENTION

A previous attack of measles confers a high degree of immunity and second attacks are uncommon.

Human immunoglobulin 0.25 ml·kg^{-1} given within 5 days of exposure effectively aborts an attack of measles. It is indicated for previously unimmunized children below 3 years of age, during pregnancy, and in those with debilitating disease.

Active immunization involves a single dose of 0.5 ml live attenuated measles vaccine given subcutaneously. The measles vaccine has recently been adapted for administration as an aerosol.

Mumps

Mumps is the result of infection with an intermediate-sized paramyxovirus. It is spread by droplet infection, by direct contact or through fomites. Humans are the only known natural hosts. The peak period of infectivity is 2–3 days before the onset of the parotitis and for 3 days afterwards.

CLINICAL FEATURES

The incubation period averages 18 days. Although no age is exempt, it is primarily a disease of school-aged children and young adults; it is uncommon before the age of 2 years. The prodromal symptoms are non-specific and include fever, malaise, headache and anorexia. This is usually followed by severe pain over the parotid glands, with either unilateral or bilateral parotid swelling. The enlarged parotid glands obscure the angle of the mandible and may elevate the ear lobe, which does not occur in cervical lymph-node enlargement. Trismus due to pain is common at this stage. Submandibular gland involvement occurs less frequently.

COMPLICATIONS

Central nervous system involvement is the commonest extra-salivary-gland manifestation of mumps. Clinical meningitis occurs in 5% of all infected patients, and 30% of patients with CNS involvement have no evidence of parotid gland involvement.

Epididymo-orchitis develops in about one-third of patients who develop mumps after puberty. Bilateral testicular involvement results in sterility in only a small percentage of these patients.

Pancreatitis, oophoritis, myocarditis, mastitis, hepatitis and polyarthritis may also occur.

DIAGNOSIS

The diagnosis of mumps is on the basis of the clinical features. In doubtful cases, serological demonstration of a fourfold rise in antibodies detected by complement fixation or indirect haemagglutination or neutralization tests on acute and convalescent sera is diagnostic.

TREATMENT

Treatment is symptomatic. Attention should be given to adequate nutrition and mouth care. Analgesics should be used to relieve pain. The role of steroids in the treatment of mumps orchitis is controversial.

PREVENTION

Live attenuated mumps virus vaccine given as a single 0.5 ml intramuscular dose can prevent the disease in children over the age of 1 year. This vaccine should not be used in children below this age as it interferes with transplacentally acquired maternal antibodies. Vaccination is contraindicated in immunosuppressed individuals, during pregnancy, or in those with severe febrile illnesses, because the live attenuated vaccine may cause disease.

Respiratory syncytial virus infection

Respiratory syncytial virus is a paramyxovirus that causes many respiratory infections. It is a common cause of bronchiolitis in infants, which is complicated by pneumonia in approximately 10% of cases.

RHABDOVIRUSES

Rabies

Rabies is a major problem in some countries and carries a high mortality.

The rabies virus is bullet-shaped and has spike-like structures arising from its surface containing glycoproteins that cause the host to produce neutralizing, haemagglutination-inhibiting antibodies. The virus has a marked affinity for nervous tissue and the salivary glands. It exists in two major epidemiological settings:

- *Urban rabies*, which is most frequently transmitted to humans through rabid dogs and, less frequently, cats.
- *Sylvan (wild) rabies*, which is maintained in the wild by a host of animal reservoirs such as foxes, skunks, jackals, mongooses and bats

With the exception of Australia, New Zealand and the Antarctic, human rabies has been reported from all continents. Transmission is through the bite of an infected animal. However, only 50% of rabid bites result in clinical disease. Human-to-human transmission is rare. Rabid animals can also transmit the disease by licking abraded skin or mucosa. Rarely, airborne droplet infection occurs.

Having entered the human body, the viruses replicate in the muscle cells near the entry wound. They penetrate the nerve endings and travel in the axoplasm to the spinal cord and brain. In the central nervous system the viruses again proliferate before they spread to the salivary glands, lungs, kidneys and other organs via the autonomic nerves.

CLINICAL FEATURES

The incubation period is variable and may range from a few weeks to several years; on average it is 1–3 months. In general, bites on the head, face and neck have a shorter incubation period than those elsewhere. In humans, two distinct clinical varieties of rabies are recognized:

- 'Furious rabies'—the classical variety
- 'Dumb rabies'—the paralytic variety

Furious rabies
The only characteristic feature in the prodromal period is the presence of pain and tingling at the site of the initial wound. Fever, malaise and headache are also present. About 10 days later, marked anxiety and agitation or depressive features develop. Hallucinations, bizarre behaviour and paralysis may also occur. Hyperexcitability, the hallmark of this form of rabies, is precipitated by auditory or visual stimuli. Hydrophobia (fear of water) is present in 50% of patients and is due to severe pharyngeal spasms on attempting to eat or drink. Aerophobia (fear of air) is considered pathognomonic of rabies. Examination reveals hyper-reflexia, spasticity, and evidence of sympathetic overactivity indicated by pupillary dilatation and diaphoresis.

The patient goes on to develop convulsions, respiratory paralysis and cardiac arrhythmias. Death usually occurs in 10–14 days.

Dumb rabies
Dumb rabies, or paralytic rabies, presents with a symmetrical ascending paralysis resembling the Guillain–Barré syndrome. This variety of rabies commonly occurs after bites from rabid bats.

It is unusual for patients to survive an attack of rabies; only a few cures have been documented.

DIAGNOSIS

The diagnosis of rabies is generally made clinically. Recently, fluorescent antibody has been used to detect rabies antigen in corneal impressions or in salivary secretions; this is a useful test. The classical Negri bodies are detected at post mortem in 90% of all patients with rabies; these are eosinophilic, ovoid bodies, 2–10 nm in diameter, seen in greatest numbers in the cells of the hippocampus and the cerebellum.

TREATMENT

Once the disease is established, therapy is symptomatic. The patient should be nursed in a quiet, darkened room. Nutritional, respiratory and cardiovascular support may be necessary.

Drugs such as morphine, diazepam and chlorpromazine should be used liberally in patients who are excitable.

The wound should be carefully cleaned, adequately debrided and left open. Cauterization of the wound with one of the quaternary ammonium compounds such as cetrimide or 1% benzalkonium chloride should then be performed. Antirabies serum injected locally around the site of the wound can be helpful.

PREVENTION

The vaccine of choice is the human diploid cell strain vaccine (HDCSV).

Post-exposure prophylaxis

Five 1.0 ml doses of HDCSV should be given intramuscularly: the first dose is given on day 0 and is followed by injections on days 3, 7, 14 and 28. Duck embryo vaccine (DEV), a killed virus vaccine, is another safe alternative. Reactions to these vaccines are uncommon.

Pre-exposure prophylaxis

This is given to individuals with a high risk of contracting rabies, e.g. laboratory workers, animal handlers and veterinarians. HDCSV 1.0 ml intramuscularly on days 0, 7 and 21 should provide effective immunity. If DEV is used, two 1.0 ml subcutaneous injections 1 month apart, followed by a third dose at 6 months also offers adequate protection. Vaccines of nervous-tissue origin are still used in some parts of the world. These, however, are associated with significant side-effects and are best avoided if HDCSV or DEV is available.

Vesicular stomatitis

Vesicular stomatitis is a viral disease of animals. In humans the virus produces a severe influenza-like infection. Sore throat and cervical or submandibular lymphadenopathy are usual. Raised vesicular lesions on the buccal mucosa are characteristic. Occasionally these vesicles may be seen on the fingers. The disease is self-limiting and rarely lasts more than 5 days.

RETROVIRUSES

Infection with human immunodeficiency virus (HIV)

HIV is the virus responsible for the acquired immunodeficiency syndrome (AIDS), which probably first became apparent in 1979 but was not fully appraised by clinicians and scientists until 1981. The syndrome is characterized by a profound defect in cell-mediated immunity resulting in opportunistic infections, particularly *Pneumocystis carinii* pneumonia, and otherwise uncommon malignancies such as Kaposi's sarcoma.

The virus

HIV belongs to a family of retroviruses (Table 1.36) distinguished from other RNA viruses by their

Table 1.36 Human lymphotropic retroviruses.

Subfamily	Virus	Disease
Lentivirus	HIV-1	AIDS
	HIV-2	AIDS?
Oncovirus	HTLV-1[a]	Adult T cell leukaemic-lymphoma
		Tropical spastic paraparesis
	HTLV-2	T-cell hairy leukaemia

[a] HTLV = human T-cell leukaemia virus.

ability to replicate through a DNA intermediate using an enzyme, reverse transcriptase (Fig. 1.20). HIV-1 and the related virus HIV-2 are further classified as lentiviruses ('slow' viruses) because of their slowly progressive clinical effects.

The virus has an envelope containing a glycoprotein (gp) of 120 kD molecular weight that binds to the CD4 receptor of CD4 lymphocytes (Figs 1.20, 1.21). The virus replicates by making a DNA copy (provirus) of its diploid RNA (using reverse transcriptase), which then becomes inserted into the host cell chromosomal DNA. This then provides RNA genomes for a progeny of new viruses.

HIV probably destroys CD4 cells by several mechanisms:

- Budding of new virions from infected cells damages cell membranes (Fig. 1.21).
- Expression of gp120 on the surface of infected CD4 cells allows other non-infected CD4 cells to bind to them via CD4 receptors producing a 'raft' of cells known as a syncytium (Fig. 1.22a).
- Immune-mediated cell death via cytotoxic T cells or natural killer cells directed to gp120 on the surface either of infected cells (Fig. 1.22b) or following binding of free gp120 to CD4 receptors (Fig. 1.22c).

EPIDEMIOLOGY

AIDS is transmitted by sexual contact and blood products. These limited modes of transmission have resulted in the emergence of well-defined risk groups (Table 1.37).

The origins of HIV are unknown, although HIV-1 was present in Africa in 1959. It is thought either that the virus was transmitted to humans from primates (a Simian immunodeficiency virus, $S1V_{MAC}$ was first identified from a Rhesus monkey in 1985) or that HIV evolved in man from a non-pathogenic human ancestor lentivirus.

Three epidemiological patterns of HIV infection and AIDS have emerged:

- N. America, Western Europe, Australia
  - homosexual and bisexual men
  - slow emergence of heterosexual transmission
  - i.v. drug abuse

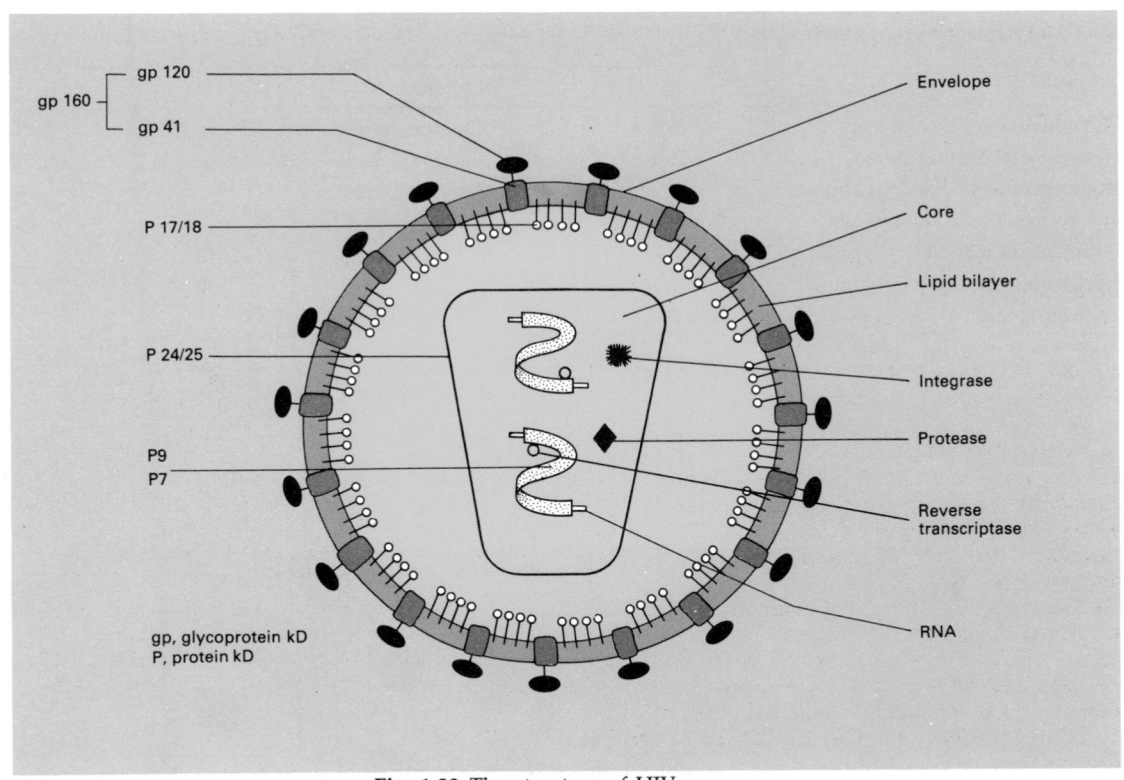

Fig. 1.20 The structure of HIV.

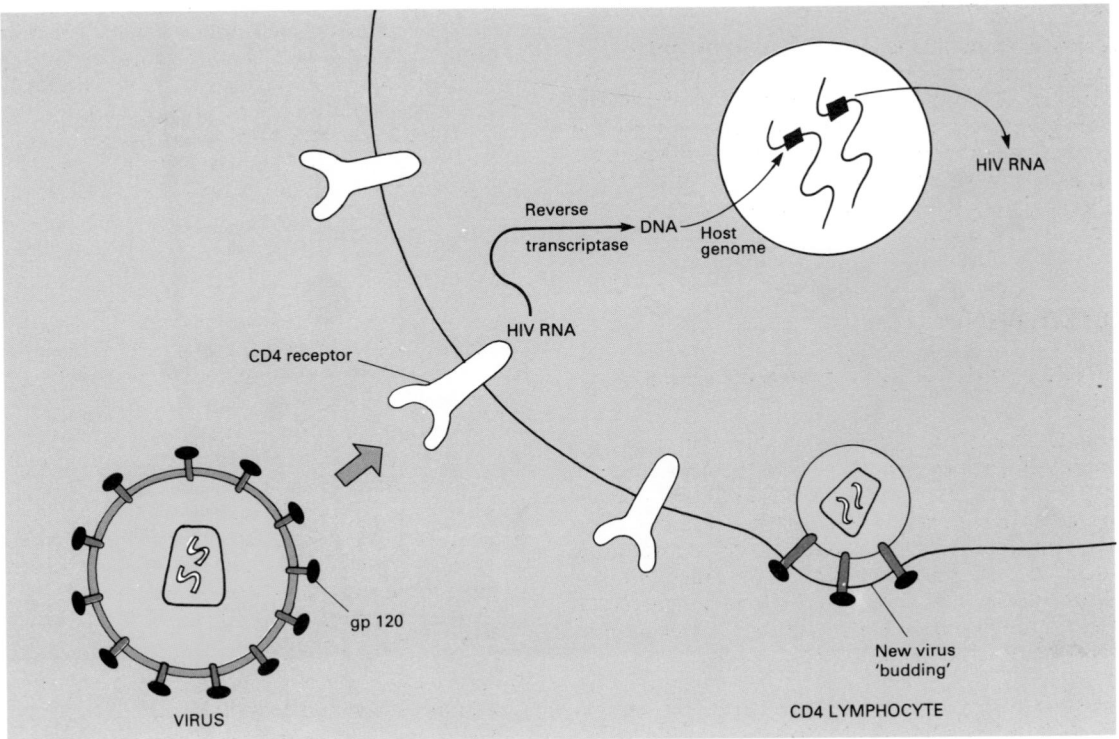

Fig. 1.21 HIV entry and replication in CD4 T lymphocytes (see text).

Table 1.37 Population groups with AIDS.

Adults		Children	
Homosexual or bisexual men	63%	Children whose mothers have AIDS	78%
Heterosexual drug abusers	19%	Recipients of blood/blood products	13%
Homosexual/bisexual drug abusers	7%	Haemophiliacs	6%
Heterosexual men and women	4%	Undetermined	3%
Recipients of blood/blood products	3%		
Haemophiliacs	1%		
Undetermined	3%		

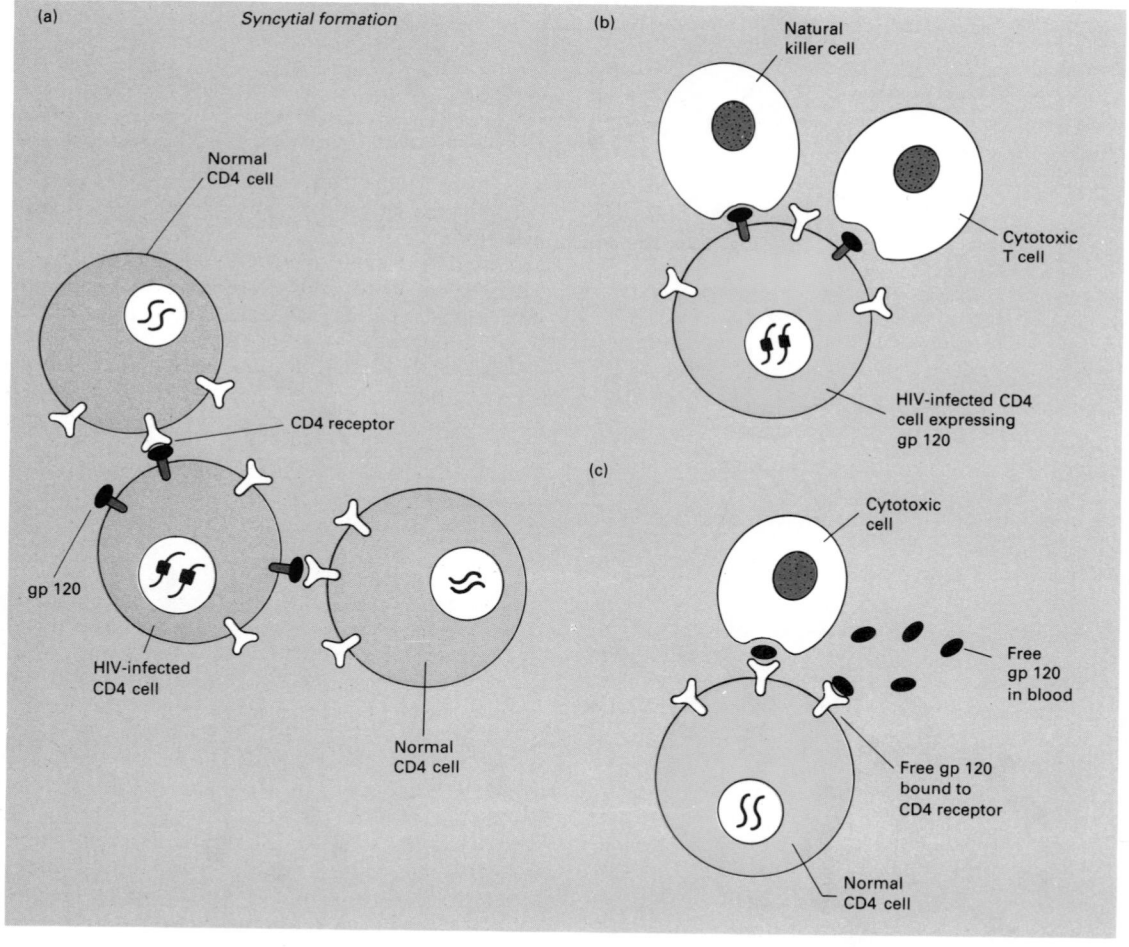

Fig. 1.22 The mechanism of CD4 lymphocyte destruction by HIV (see text).

Table 1.38 Summary of classification system for HIV infections.

Group I	Acute infection (transient symptoms with seroconversion)
Group II	Asymptomatic infection
Group III	Persistent generalized lymphadenopathy
Group IV	Other manifestations:
	(a) Chronic constitutional disease, e.g. lassitude, fever (> 1 month), weight loss (> 10%), diarrhoea (> 1 month)
	(b) Neurological disease, e.g. dementia (subacute encephalitis), peripheral neuropathy, atypical aseptic meningitis
	(c) Specified secondary infections (see Table 1.39)
	(d) Specified secondary cancers, e.g. Kaposi's sarcoma, primary brain lymphoma, squamous carcinomas (anal canal, tongue), Burkitt's lymphoma
	(e) Other conditions, e.g. diarrhoea

- Sub-Saharan Africa, Latin America
  - heterosexuals, prostitutes
  - blood transfusion (in areas where not tested)
  - perinatal (some cities 5–15% pregnant women infected)
- North Africa, Middle East, Eastern Europe, Asia, Pacific
  - HIV arrived mid 1980s
  - accounts for only 1% of reported cases
  - contacts from above groups

The incubation period appears to depend on the mode of transmission, varying from approximately 1 year following sexual contact to up to 9 years after transfusion of contaminated blood. Infants born to women with AIDS may develop the disease within a few months, with 30% affected by the age of 18 months.

The total number of reported cases of HIV infections is now well in excess of 150 000, with a current mortality rate of over 40%. The mortality for the full syndrome would appear to be almost 100%. It has been estimated that 100 million will be infected by 1991.

CLINICAL FEATURES

A broad spectrum of disease is caused by HIV (Table 1.38). Immediately after infection the virus commonly causes an acute febrile illness that might be mistaken for influenza or infectious mononucleosis. The individual may then remain symptom-free for months or several years, and then present with progressive weight loss, intermittent fever, generalized lymphadenopathy,

Table 1.39 Organisms causing opportunistic infections in AIDS.

Bacteria
Mycobacterium avium-intracellulare[a]
M. kansasii[a]
M. tuberculosis[a]
Viruses
Cytomegalovirus[a]
Herpes simplex virus[a]
Herpes zoster (multidermatomal)[a]
Fungi
Candida sp.[a]
Histoplasma spp.
Cryptococcus neoformans
Parasites
Pneumocystis carinii
Cryptosporidium sp.
Isospora belli
Strongyloides stercoralis[a]
Toxoplasma gondii
Sarcocystis spp.

[a] Often with disseminated infection.

chronic diarrhoea, one or more opportunistic infections (see Table 1.39), widespread Kaposi's sarcoma, and even a progressive encephalopathy. The Walter Reed (WR) classification relates progression of HIV infection to AIDS with the CD4 blood count (see Fig. 1.23).

Most individuals infected with HIV will eventually go on to develop the complete syndrome of AIDS (group IV, Table 1.38) with 50–70% developing symptomatic disease in 10 years.

The details of systematic involvement are discussed in the appropriate chapters.

DIAGNOSIS

The diagnosis should be suspected in individuals from a high-risk group with all or some of the clinical features of AIDS. These patients should have no other obvious cause for immunodeficiency with or without opportunistic infection. The presence of the virus can now be confirmed by detecting the presence of antibody to HIV by ELISA. Before the test is performed, patients should be carefully counselled on the implications of a positive test. There are multiple immunological abnormalities in AIDS, the characteristic pattern being lymphopenia, with a quantitative and qualitative defect in the CD4 inducer/helper subset of T cells resulting in a marked defect in cell-mediated immunity. In addition there are B cell abnormalities, with polyclonal activation of B cells and increased immunoglobulin secretion, causing hypergammaglobulinaemia.

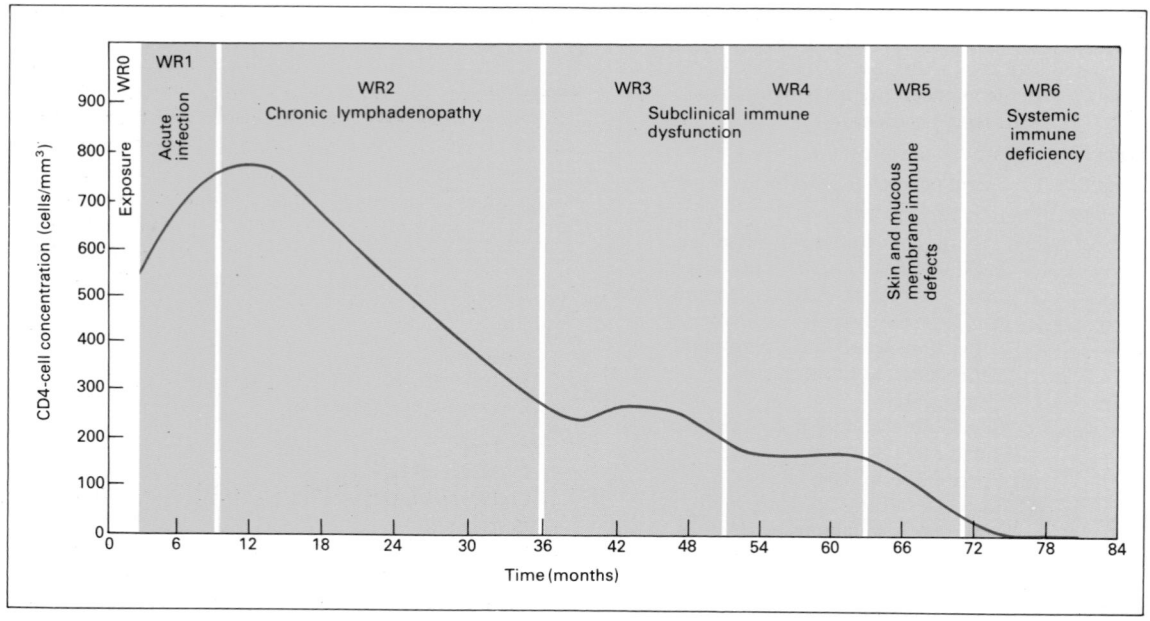

Fig. 1.23 Walter Reed (WR) classification of HIV infection.

TREATMENT

Although there is no cure for AIDS, certain drugs, particularly azidothymidine (AZT, zidovudine) can reduce the progression of early symptomatic disease to AIDS. It is unclear how early the drug should be given in the course of the illness, although trials are underway to answer this question. Toxicity of AZT includes bone marrow suppression, myopathy and encephalopathy. Other potentially useful drugs include 2′,3′-dideoxycytidine (ddC) and phosphonoformate.

Treatment and supportive management of opportunistic infections remains a critical part of the care of AIDS patients (see Table 1.39).

PREVENTION

To contain the present HIV pandemic, changes in sexual practices ('safe sex', use of condoms) and screening of all blood products for HIV are essential. Vaccine development is underway using a variety of strategies:

● Killed whole virus
● HIV subunit (gp 160, gp 120)
● HIV subunit in virus vector (e.g. HIV/vaccinia recombinant)
● Anti-idiotype (antibody against CD$_4$)

ARENAVIRUSES

Arenaviruses are pleomorphic, round or oval viruses with diameters ranging from 50 to 300 nm. The virion surface has club-shaped projections, and the virus itself contains a variable number of characteristic electron-dense granules that represent host ribosomes. Infection with the prototype virus of this group produces lymphocytic choriomeningitis. Arenaviruses are also responsible for Argentinian and Bolivian haemorrhagic fevers and Lassa fever.

Lassa fever

This illness was first documented in the town of Lassa, Nigeria, in 1969 and is confined to sub-Saharan West Africa (Nigeria, Liberia and Sierra Leone). The multimammate rat, *Mastomys natalensis*, is known to be a reservoir. Humans are infected by ingesting foods contaminated by rat urine or saliva containing the virus. Direct inoculation and inhalation of this virus are also common modes of spread of this disease.

CLINICAL FEATURES

The incubation period varies from 1 to 24 days. The disease is insidious in onset and is characterized by fever, myalgia, severe backache, malaise and headache. A transient maculopapular rash may be present. Sore throat and lymphadenopathy occur in over 50% of patients. In severe cases epistaxis and gastrointestinal bleeding may occur, hence the classification of Lassa fever as a viral haemorrhagic fever. The fever usually lasts from 1 to 3 weeks and recovery within a month of the onset of illness is usual. However, death occurs in 15–20% of hospitalized patients, usually from irreversible hypovolaemic shock.

DIAGNOSIS

The diagnosis is established by serial serological tests (including the Lassa-specific IgM titre) or by culturing the virus from the throat, serum or urine.

TREATMENT

Treatment is supportive. Human convalescent serum has produced some clinical improvement but its value has been questioned. Ribavirin, an antiviral drug, has been useful in preventing haemorrhagic manifestations in rhesus monkeys and dramatically reduces mortality in human infection.

In non-endemic countries, strict isolation procedures should be used, the patient ideally being nursed in a flexible-film isolator or by medical and nursing staff wearing full protective clothing, including respirators or ventilated hoods. Prevention of spread of the virus is best achieved by treating patients in the endemic area where they contracted the disease, since a high proportion of the local population will be immune.

Lymphocytic choriomeningitis (LCM)

This infection is a zoonosis, the natural reservoir of the LCM virus being the house mouse. Infection is characterized by either:

- Non-nervous-system illness, with fever, malaise, myalgia, headache, arthralgia and vomiting.
- A typical aseptic meningitis-type illness, with signs of meningism in addition to the above symptoms. Occasionally, a more severe form occurs, with encephalitis leading to disturbance of consciousness.

This illness is generally self-limiting and requires no specific treatment.

MARBURG VIRUS DISEASE AND EBOLA VIRUS DISEASE

These severe, haemorrhagic, febrile illnesses are discussed together because their clinical manifestations are similar. These diseases are named after Marburg in Germany and the Ebola river region in the Sudan and Zaire where these viruses were first isolated. The natural reservoir for these viruses has not been identified and the precise mode of spread from one individual to another has not been elucidated.

The illness is characterized by the acute onset of severe headache, severe myalgia and high fever, followed by prostration. On about the fifth day of illness a non-pruritic maculopapular rash develops on the face and then spreads to the rest of the body. Diarrhoea is profuse and is associated with abdominal cramps and vomiting. Haematemesis, melaena or haemoptysis may occur between the seventh and sixteenth day. Hepatosplenomegaly and facial oedema are usually present. In Ebola virus disease, chest pain and a dry cough are prominent symptoms.

Treatment is symptomatic. Convalescent human serum appears to decrease the severity of the attack.

POST-VIRAL/CHRONIC FATIGUE SYNDROME
(see p. 972)
Viral illnesses have been implicated aetiologically, including those due to EBV, Coxsackie B viruses, ECHO viruses, CMV and hepatitis A virus. Non-viral causes such as allergy to *Candida* spp. have also been proposed.

The proportion of patients with 'organic' diagnoses remains uncertain. Recent studies suggest that two-thirds of patients with a symptom duration of more than 6 months have an underlying psychiatric disorder.

Fungal infections

Morphologically, fungi can be grouped into two major categories:

- Yeasts, which reproduce by budding
- Moulds, which grow by branching and longitudinal extensions of hyphae

Dimorphic fungi are those that behave as yeasts in the host but as moulds *in vitro*, e.g. *Histoplasma* and *Sporothrix*. Despite the fact that fungi are ubiquitous, fungal infections are uncommon. Fungal infections are transmitted by inhalation of spores or by contact with the skin.

Diseases are usually divided into:

- Systemic
- Subcutaneous
- Superficial

Systemic mycoses are unusual, but opportunistic mycoses can cause disease in immunocompromised patients. Fungi do not produce endotoxin, but exotoxin, e.g. aflatoxin, production has been documented *in vitro*. Fungi may also produce allergic pulmonary disease (see p. 687).

In general, human fungal infections are indolent and respond poorly to treatment. Some fungi such as *Candida albicans* are human commensals.

Systemic fungal infections

Histoplasmosis

Histoplasmosis is caused by *Histoplasma capsulatum*, a non-encapsulated, dimorphic fungus. Spores can survive in moist soil for several years, particularly when it is enriched by bird and bat droppings. Histoplasmosis occurs world-wide and is commonly seen in Ohio and the Mississippi river valley. Transmission is mainly by inhalation of the spores.

CLINICAL FEATURES

Figure 1.24 summarizes the pathogenesis, main clinical forms and sequelae of *Histoplasma* infection.

Primary pulmonary histoplasmosis is usually asymptomatic. The only evidence of infection is conversion of a histoplasmin skin test from negative to positive, and radiological features similar to those seen with the Ghon primary complex of tuberculosis (see p. 678). Calcification in the lungs, spleen and liver occurs in patients from areas of high endemicity. When symptomatic, primary pulmonary histoplasmosis generally presents as a mild influenza-like illness, with fever, chills, myalgia and cough. The systemic symptoms are pronounced in severe disease.

Complications such as atelectasis, secondary bacterial pneumonia, pleural effusions, erythema nodosum and erythema multiforme may also occur.

Chronic pulmonary histoplasmosis is clinically indistinguishable from pulmonary tuberculosis (see p. 679). It is usually seen in white males over the age of 50 years. Radiologically, pulmonary cavities, infiltrates and characteristic fibrous streaking from the periphery towards the hilum are seen.

Disseminated histoplasmosis resembles disseminated tuberculosis clinically. Fever, lymphadenopathy, hepatosplenomegaly, weight loss, leucopenia and thrombocytopenia are common. Rarely, features of meningitis, hepatitis, Addison's disease, endocarditis and peritonitis may dominate the clinical picture.

DIAGNOSIS

Definitive diagnosis is possible only by culturing the fungi or by demonstrating them on histological sections. The histoplasmin skin test is usually positive.

Antibodies usually develop within 3 weeks of the onset of illness and are best detected by the complement-fixation test. Titres above 1 : 32 are suggestive of *Histoplasma* infection. Agar gel diffusion and latex agglutination antibody tests may also be helpful.

TREATMENT

Only severe acute pulmonary histoplasmosis, chronic histoplasmosis and acute disseminated histoplasmosis require therapy. Intravenous amphotericin 0.5–0.6 mg·kg^{-1} daily or 1.0–1.2 mg·kg^{-1} on alternate days for 10 weeks is the mainstay of therapy. The less-toxic antifungal

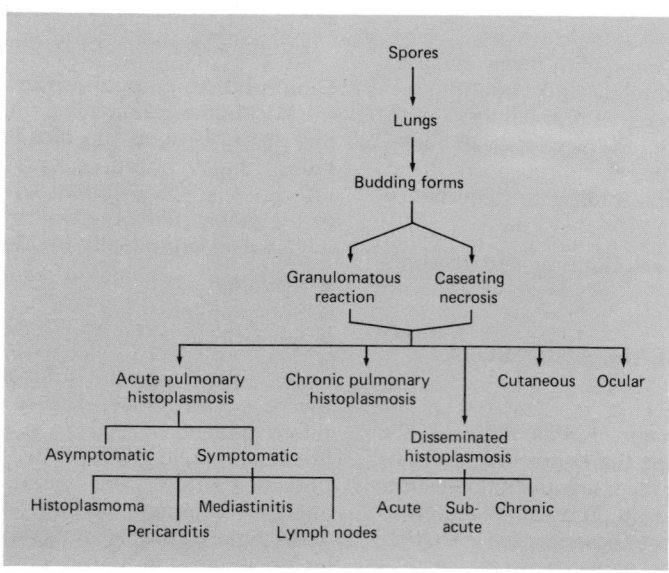

Fig. 1.24 A summary of the pathogenesis, main clinical forms and sequelae of *Histoplasma* infection.

agent ketoconazole is effective, as are the newer agents itraconazole and fluconazole. Surgical excision of histoplasmomas (pulmonary granuloma due to *H. capsulatum*) or chronic cavitatory lung lesions and release of adhesions following mediastinitis is often required.

African histoplasmosis

African histoplasmosis is caused by *Histoplasma duboisii*, the spores of which are larger than that of *H. capsulatum*. Skin lesions, e.g. abscesses, nodules, lymph node involvement and lytic bone lesions are prominent. Pulmonary lesions do not occur. Treatment is similar to that for *H. capsulatum* infection.

Aspergillosis

Aspergillosis is caused by several dimorphic fungi of the Aspergillus species. Of these, *Aspergillus fumigatus* is the commonest cause of disease in humans, although *A. flavus* and *A. niger* have also been implicated as pathogens. These fungi are ubiquitous in the environment and are commonly found on decaying leaves and trees. Humans are infected by inhalation of the spores. Disease manifestation depends on the dose of the spores inhaled as well as the immune response of the host. Three major forms of the disease are recognized:

- *Bronchopulmonary allergic aspergillosis* (p. 687), with symptoms suggestive of bronchial asthma.
- *Aspergilloma* (p. 689), sometimes referred to as a pulmonary mycetoma.
- *Fulminant disease*, which occurs in immunosuppressed patients, presenting as acute pneumonia, meningitis or an intracerebral abscess, lytic bone lesions, and granulomatous lesions in the liver; less commonly endocarditis, paranasal *Aspergillus* granuloma or keratitis may occur. Urgent treatment with intravenous amphotericin is required.

The diagnosis and treatment are described in more detail on p. 688.

Cryptococcosis

Cryptococcosis is caused by the yeast-like fungus, *Cryptococcus neoformans*. It has a world-wide distribution and appears to be spread by birds, especially pigeons, in their droppings. The spores gain entry into the body through the respiratory tract, where they elicit a granulomatous reaction. Pulmonary symptoms are, however, uncommon and meningitis, which is clinically indistinguishable from bacterial meningitis, is the usual mode of presentation.

Lung cavitation, hilar lymphadenopathy, pleural effusions and occasionally pulmonary fibrosis occur. Less commonly, the skin and bones are involved.

DIAGNOSIS

This is established by demonstrating the organisms in appropriately stained tissue sections. A positive latex cryptococcal agglutinin test performed on the CSF is diagnostic of cryptococcosis.

TREATMENT

Amphotericin (0.3–0.5 mg·kg^{-1} daily i.v.) alone or in combination with flucytosine (100–200 mg·kg^{-1} daily) has reduced the mortality of this once always fatal condition. Therapy should be continued for 3 months if meningitis is present. Fluconazole has greater CSF penetration and is likely to become the treatment of choice.

Coccidioidomycosis

Coccidioidomycosis is caused by the non-budding spherical form (spherule) of *Coccidioides immitis*. This is a soil saprophyte and is found in the southern United States, Central America and parts of South America.

Humans are infected by inhalation of the thick-walled barrel-shaped spores called arthrospores. Occasionally epidemics of coccidioidomycosis have been documented following dust storms.

CLINICAL FEATURES

The majority of patients are asymptomatic. Infection is detected by the conversion of a skin test using either coccidioidin (extract from a culture of mycelial growth of *C. immitis*) or spherulin (the soluble fraction from a culture of *C. immitis* spherules) from negative to positive.

Acute pulmonary coccidioidomycosis presents, after an incubation period of about 10 days, with fever, malaise, cough and expectoration. Erythema nodosum, erythema multiforme, phlyctenular conjunctivitis and, less commonly, pleural effusions may occur. Complete recovery is usual. Pulmonary cavitation with haemoptysis, pulmonary fibrosis, meningitis, lytic bone lesions, hepatosplenomegaly, and skin ulcers and abscesses may occur in severe disease.

DIAGNOSIS

Because of the high infectivity of this fungus, and consequent risk to laboratory personnel, serological tests (rather than culture of the organism) are widely used for diagnosis. These include the highly specific latex agglutination and precipitin tests. A positive complement-fixation test performed on the CSF is diagnostic of coccidioido-mycosis meningitis.

TREATMENT

Mild pulmonary infections are self-limiting and require no treatment, but progressive and disseminated disease requires urgent therapy. Amphotericin is the drug of choice. Surgical excision of cavitatory pulmonary lesions or localized bone lesions may be necessary. For meningitis, intrathecal amphotericin may be required; the role of steroids remains controversial. Ketoconazole or miconazole can be of value.

Blastomycosis

Blastomycosis is a systemic infection caused by the biphasic fungus *Blastomyces dermatitidis*. Although initially believed to be confined to certain parts of North America, it has recently been reported in Canada, Africa, Israel, Eastern Europe and Saudi Arabia.

CLINICAL FEATURES

Blastomycosis primarily involves the skin, where it presents as non-itchy papular lesions that later develop into ulcers with red verrucous margins. The ulcers are initially confined to the exposed parts of the body but later involve the unexposed parts as well. Atrophy and scarring may occur. Pulmonary involvement presents as a solitary lesion resembling a malignancy or gives rise to radiological features similar to the primary complex of tuberculosis. Systemic symptoms such as fever, malaise, cough and weight loss are usually present. Bone lesions are common and present as painful swellings.

DIAGNOSIS

The diagnosis is confirmed by demonstrating the organism in histological sections or by culture. Serology is not useful because of the marked cross-reactivity of antibodies to *Blastomyces* with *Histoplasma*.

TREATMENT

The drug of choice is amphotericin.

Invasive zygomycosis

Invasive zygomycosis, mucormycosis, is rare and is caused by several fungi, including *Mucor*, *Rhizopus* and *Absidia*. It occurs in ill patients. The hallmark of the disease is vascular invasion with marked haemorrhagic necrosis.

Rhinocerebral mucormycosis is the commonest form. Nasal stuffiness, facial pain and oedema, and necrotic, black nasal turbinates are characteristic. It is rare and is mainly seen in diabetics with ketoacidosis. Other forms include pulmonary and disseminated infection (immunosuppressed), gastrointestinal infection (in malnutrition) and cutaneous involvement (in burns). Treatment is with amphotericin. This condition is invariably fatal if left untreated.

Candidiasis

Candidiasis is the most common fungal infection in humans and is caused by *Candida albicans*. *Candida* are small asexual fungi. All the species that are pathogenic to humans are normal oropharyngeal and gastrointestinal commensals. Candidiasis is found world-wide.

CLINICAL FEATURES

Practically any organ in the body can be invaded by *Candida*, but oral thrush (p. 179) is the commonest form. This is seen in the very young, in the elderly, following antibiotic therapy and in those who are immunosuppressed. Candidal oesophagitis may present with painful dysphagia.

Cutaneous candidiasis (p. 1027) typically occurs in intertriginous areas. It is also an important cause of paronychia, balanitis and vaginitis.

Chronic mucocutaneous candidiasis is a rare manifestation, usually occurring in children, and is associated with a T-cell defect. It presents with hyperkeratotic plaque-like lesions on the skin, especially the face, and on the finger nails. It is associated with several endocrinopathies, including hypothyroidism and hypoparathyroidism. Less commonly dissemination of candidiasis may lead to a haematogenous spread, with meningitis, pulmonary involvement, endocarditis or osteomyelitis.

DIAGNOSIS

The fungi can be demonstrated in scrapings from infected lesions or in tissue secretions.

TREATMENT

This varies depending on the site and severity of infection. Oral lesions respond to nystatin, oral amphotericin or miconazole. For more severe systemic infections, parenteral therapy with amphotericin or ketoconazole, or oral therapy with flucytosine 50–75 mg·kg^{-1} daily for 2–3 weeks may be required.

Pneumocystis carinii infection

Pneumocystis carinii is an important cause of interstitial pneumonia in the immunocompromised host. The taxonomy of *P. carinii* remains controversial but recent studies suggest that it is a fungus; some authorities regard it as a protozoan whilst others prefer to leave it unclassified. The organism exists as a trophozoite, which is probably motile and reproduces by binary fission. After the trophozoite invades the lung parenchyma, its wall thickens and forms a cyst. On maturation, further division takes place to yield eight merozoites which, after cyst wall rupture, develop into trophozoites.

CLINICAL FEATURES

Infection is probably common in infancy but most infections in otherwise healthy infants remain undetected. Outbreaks in infant nurseries have been reported but are now less common. Infection in adults is associated with a major defect in cell-mediated immune mechanisms. Thus, infection with *P. carinii* is one of the most common opportunistic infections in AIDS (affecting 80%) and an important cause of death in these patients. The illness presents as a severe pneumonia with progressive respiratory distress, a non-productive cough, tachypnoea, hypoxia and fever. Physical signs in the chest are minimal or absent. Chest radiographs generally show bilateral diffuse granular opacities spreading from the hilar region and initially sparing the periphery. These radiographic changes may develop late; they may be absent for 1 or 2 days even in a patient with severe dyspnoea.

DIAGNOSIS

Demonstration of the organism in lung tissue is essential to make a confident diagnosis of *Pneumocystis* infection. The organism cannot easily be isolated from sputum or aspirated pulmonary secretions. The currently favoured way to detect the organism is in lung tissue obtained by transbronchial biopsy during fibre-optic bronchoscopy or open lung biopsy. Needle aspiration of lung parenchyma has been used in the past but has a high complication rate (pneumothorax or haemorrhage) and is no longer in general use.

TREATMENT

High-dose co-trimoxazole (640 mg trimethoprim, 3.2 g sulphamethoxazole) 12-hourly, usually intravenously initially, is given for 2–4 weeks. Co-trimoxazole is useful in protecting high-risk patients from *P. carinii* infection. Other drugs used to treat this infection include pentamidine, and a combination of pyrimethamine and sulfadoxine

appears to be an effective prophylactic preparation. Monthly inhaled pentamidine aerosol is also useful for prophylaxis after infection.

Local fungal infections

Dermatophytosis

Dermatophytoses are chronic fungal infections of keratinous structures such as the skin, hair or nails (see p. 1028). *Trichophyton*, *Microsporum* and *Epidermophyton* are traditionally referred to as dermatophytes, although other fungi such as *Candida* can also infect keratinous structures.

Sporotrichosis

Sporotrichosis is due to the saprophytic fungus *Sporothrix schenckii*, which is found world-wide. Infection usually follows cutaneous inoculation, at the site of which a reddish, non-tender, maculopapular lesion, referred to as 'plaque sporotrichosis' develops. Pulmonary involvement and disseminated disease rarely occur.

TREATMENT

Treatment with saturated potassium iodide (10–12 ml daily orally for adults) is curative in the cutaneous form. Amphotericin or miconazole is required for systemic infection.

Subcutaneous zygomycosis

Subcutaneous zygomycosis is caused by several filamentous fungi of the *Basidio bolus* genus. The disease usually remains confined to the subcutaneous tissues and muscle fascia. It presents as a brawny, woody infiltration involving the limbs, neck and trunk. Less commonly, the pharyngeal and orbital regions may be affected.

Treatment is with saturated potassium iodide solution given orally.

Chromomycosis

Chromomycosis (chromoblastomycosis) is caused by fungi of the genus *Philalophora* and *Cladosporium carrionii*. It presents initially as a small papule, usually at the site of a previous injury. This persists for several months before ulcerating. The lesion later becomes warty and encrusted and gradually spreads. Satellite lesions may be present. Itching is frequent. The drug of choice is flucytosine in combination with amphotericin in small doses.

Rhinosporidiosis

Rhinosporidiosis is caused by *Rhinosporidium seeberi*. This organism has not been cultured. Although recognized world-wide, it is seen mainly in South India and Sri Lanka. Mucosal lesions present as polyps that are friable and vascular; the nose, nasopharynx and soft palate are most frequently involved. Haematogenous dissemination may occur. Treatment is surgical excision and cautery.

Protozoal infections

Blood and tissue infections

LEISHMANIASIS

Three clinical entities caused by *Leishmania* have been described:

- Visceral leishmaniasis (kala-azar)
- Cutaneous leishmaniasis of the New World
- Cutaneous leishmaniasis of the Old World

The geographical distribution is shown in Fig. 1.25.

The life-cycle of the parasite involves two stages:

1 The *amastigote* (Leishman–Donovan body) occurs in vertebrate hosts such as humans, dogs or rodents. The parasites infect macrophages and reticuloendothelial cells and multiply until the cells rupture, releasing the organisms into the circulation. When the female sandfly (*Phlebotomus* or *Lutzomyia*) bites an infected host, it draws blood containing the amastigotes.
2 In the sandfly the parasites develop into the infective *promastigotes*, which move to the salivary glands in about 10 days.

The cycle is completed by the sandfly's biting another vertebrate.

The presentation in humans is dependent on the patient's cellular immunity as well as the parasite species.

In the *kala-azar syndrome* there is little or no immune response and the reticuloendothelial system is laden with amastigote-laden histiocytes. In subjects with an increased immune response, hepatic and lymph node granulomas are found and either there are no clinical symptoms or a localized lesion is seen.

Inapparent infection is common in endemic areas and is recognized by the high incidence of leishmanin-positive skin tests. There is usually no previous history of skin ulceration or systemic disease. Infection is eradicated by the immune system and the subject is left with permanent immunity to that species of *Leishmania*.

Visceral leishmaniasis (kala-azar)

Visceral leishmaniasis is caused by *L. donovani* and occurs in Asia, the Mediterranean, South America and Africa. Dogs, foxes, jackals and wild rodents can be reservoirs, but in India humans are the only known reservoir. Primary skin lesions (leishmaniomas) are usually small, but can be found at the site of the sandfly bite.

The disease usually affects young people. The incubation period may be months or years. The onset is abrupt or insidious. The patient feels remarkably well despite many symptoms and signs. Fever occurs and may exhibit a characteristic biphasic pattern. Cough is frequent and diarrhoea may occur. The skin is dry and rough and with time becomes pigmented. Splenic enlargement may be massive and hypersplenism is chiefly responsible for the pancytopenia seen. Epistaxis may occur due to thrombocytopenia. Hepatomegaly is less prominent than the splenomegaly. In African kala-azar, warty skin eruptions and lymphadenopathy also occur. If left untreated, death occurs within three years in the majority of patients and is due to pulmonary or gastrointestinal superinfection, to which these patients are predisposed.

Infantile kala-azar is seen chiefly in the Mediterranean region and is a disease of children below the age of 5 years.

Post-kala-azar dermal leishmaniasis (PKDL) occurs 1–2 years after successful treatment for visceral leishmaniasis in a small proportion of patients in India and less often in Africa. It is characterized by macular, erythematous lesions and pale pink nodules on the face.

INVESTIGATION AND DIAGNOSIS

- The characteristic Leishman–Donovan bodies may be demonstrated in buffy coat preparations of blood or in bone-marrow smears or lymphnode, liver or spleen aspirates.
- The organism can be cultured in the Nicolle–Novy–MacNeal culture medium.
- Complement-fixing antibodies may be detected by indirect immunofluorescence, ELISA and haemagglutination.
- Formol gel test is positive owing to hyperglobulinaemia.

An intradermal leishmanin skin test (a test of delayed hypersensitivity) is of no value in diagnosis since it is negative early in the course of the disease.

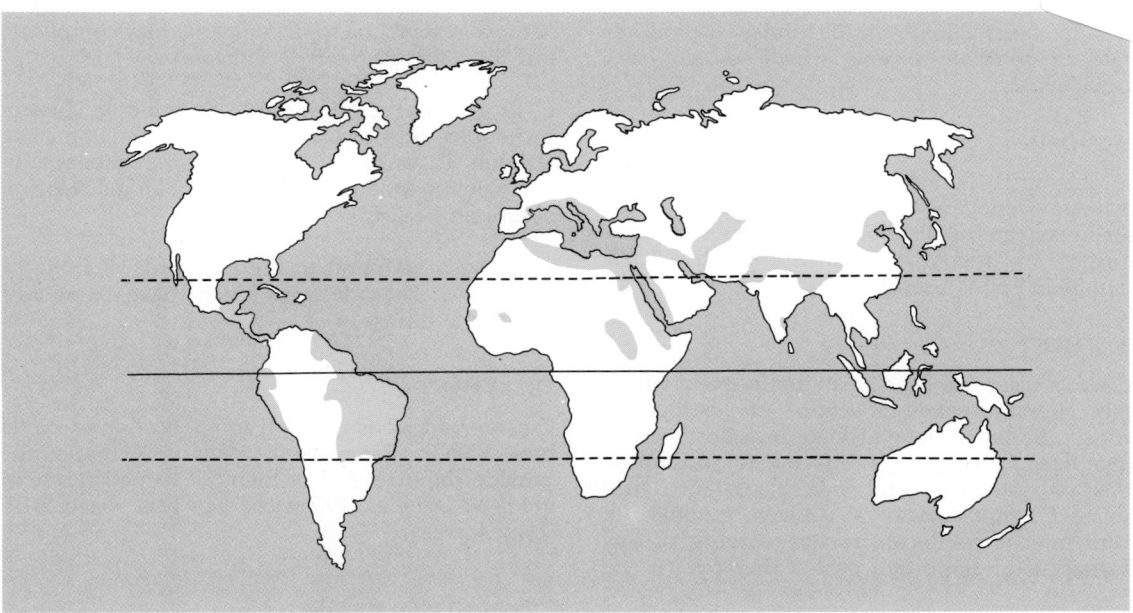

Fig. 1.25 The geographical distribution of leishmaniasis.

TREATMENT

Response to therapy varies. African kala-azar is relatively resistant to treatment and the duration of therapy is necessarily longer. Pentavalent antimony compounds are the drugs of choice. Sodium stibogluconate 30 mg·kg^{-1} in adults should be continued for at least 40 days. Meglumine antimonate 50 mg·kg^{-1} daily for 10–30 days is a useful alternative.

Intercurrent pulmonary infections should be treated with appropriate antibiotics. Blood transfusions are rarely required.

Intravenous amphotericin or pentamidine (up to four courses of 3 mg·kg^{-1} daily for 10 days) may be required for patients whose initial response to therapy is poor. Pentamidine is ineffective in the treatment of PKDL.

PREVENTION

In endemic areas control of vectors plays an important part. Spraying with an effective insecticide should be carried out at regular intervals. There should also be an attempt to decrease the reservoir of infection by destroying infected animals and treating infected humans early.

Cutaneous leishmaniasis of the New World (American cutaneous leishmaniasis)

Four forms are recognized:

Chiclero's ulcer

This is caused by *L. mexicana* and is found in Mexico, Guatemala, Brazil, Venezuela and Panama. It occurs on the exposed parts of the body, and runs a benign course with spontaneous healing within 6 months. However, infection of the pinna (chiclero's ear) results in gross destruction of the external ear. A lesion at this site may persist for over 20 years.

Espundia (mucocutaneous leishmaniasis)

This is caused by *L. braziliensis* and is found in Brazil, Ecuador, Bolivia, Uruguay and northern Argentina. Initially painful, itchy nodules appear on the lower limbs, and then ulcerate. Lymphangitis is usual. Healing occurs spontaneously in 6 months.

Several years later, secondary lesions develop at mucocutaneous junctions such as the nasopharynx. There is evidence of nasal obstruction, ulceration, septal perforation and destruction of the nasal cartilages. Death usually occurs from secondary bacterial infection or aspiration.

Diffuse cutaneous leishmaniasis

This is caused by *L. amazonensis* and is characterized by diffuse infiltration of the skin by Leishman–Donovan bodies. Visceral lesions are absent. Clinically this chronic condition resembles lepromatous leprosy, although it does not involve the nasal septum.

Uta

Uta is a similar disease to diffuse cutaneous leishmaniasis and is caused by *L. peruviana*. It occurs in cooler climates in the Andes. It produces single or multiple ulcers, which usually heal spontaneously.

DIAGNOSIS

The diagnosis is established by demonstrating Leishman–Donovan bodies in spleen or bone-marrow smears or histological sections of tissues. Parasites are scanty and hence a positive leishmanin skin test is useful.

TREATMENT

Chiclero's ulcer has been treated effectively with a single intramuscular injection of cycloguanil pamoate. Sodium stibogluconate in a dose similar to that used for kala-azar is effective for most other forms of cutaneous and mucocutaneous leishmaniasis. Amphotericin is usually required for severe infections. Reconstructive surgery of any deformity is an important part of therapy.

Cutaneous leishmaniasis of the Old World

This is a mild form of leishmaniasis caused by *L. tropica* or *L. aethiopica*. *L. tropica* is found in urban areas of the Mediterranean, USSR and India.

L. tropica minor causes a red pruritic papule that ulcerates (oriental sore) and heals by scarring. Leishmaniasis recidiva, which is characterized by features resembling lupus vulgaris, may complicate this form of cutaneous leishmaniasis.

L. tropica major usually results in multiple clusters of nodules that ulcerate. A marked inflammatory reaction is present. Regional lymphadenopathy and satellite lesions are common. Marked scarring occurs on healing.

L. aethiopica is found in the highlands of Ethiopia and Kenya. The cutaneous lesions have a tendency to become diffuse.

TREATMENT

Cutaneous lesions respond to application of direct heat (40°C). Pentavalent antimony compounds provide the mainstay of therapy. In patients with indolent lesions, levamisole has been used with some success.

TRYPANOSOMIASIS

Trypanosomes are protozoa that at some stage of their life-cycle have a flagellum. The development of the trypanosomes consists of several stages. They usually exist as trypomastigotes in vertebrate hosts such as humans, although some may also exist as amastigotes, e.g. *Trypanosoma cruzi*. Two main types of development of the parasite in its

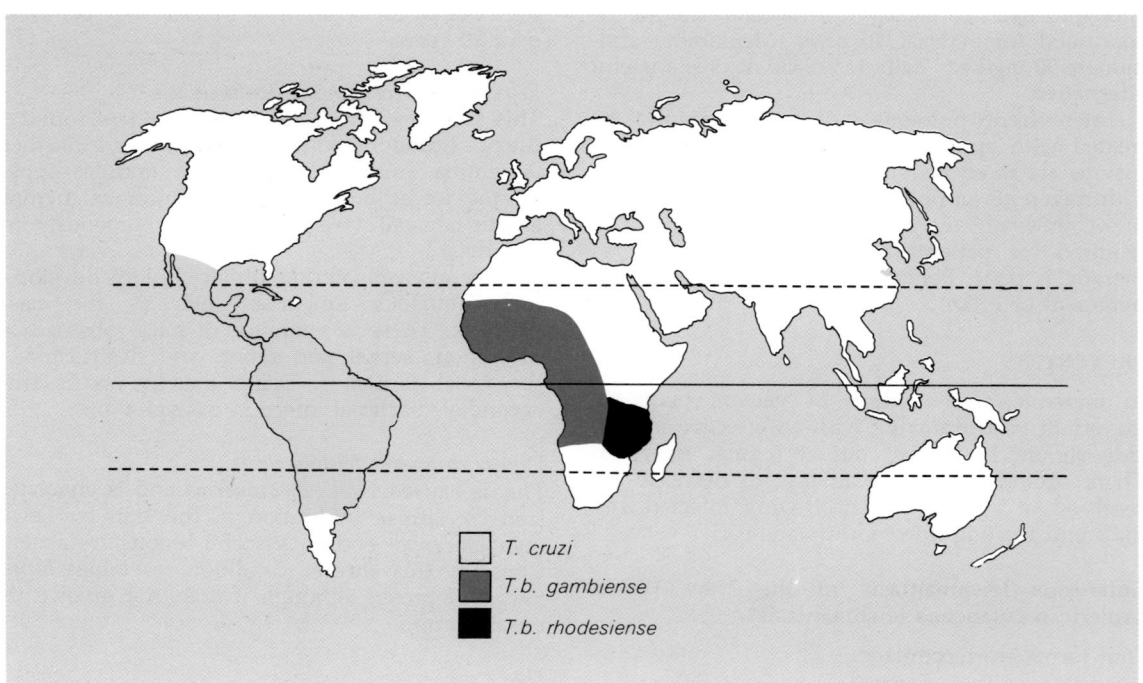

Fig. 1.26 The geographical distribution of trypanosomiasis.

vector are recognized:

- *Anterior station development* (salivaria), where the organism is transmitted through the bite of the insect (e.g. *T. brucei*)
- *Posterior station development* (stercoraria), where transmission occurs by rubbing faecal matter from the insect into the bite wound or conjunctiva (e.g. *T. cruzi*)

African trypanosomiasis

African trypanosomiasis (sleeping sickness) follows the bite of the tsetse fly and is caused by *T. brucei*, which develops by anterior station. *T. brucei* is found in west and central Africa between the 20° north and 20° south parallels of latitude (Fig. 1.26). Two clinical forms are recognized (Table 1.40):

- *Gambian sleeping sickness* is found mainly in West Africa, but also in southern Sudan and Uganda
- *Rhodesian sleeping sickness*, which is found from Ethiopia in the north to Botswana in the south

Gambian sleeping sickness is caused by *T. b. gambiense* and transmitted to humans by the tsetse fly species *Glossina palpalis* and *G. tachinoides*. Humans are the only important reservoirs.

   T. b. rhodesiense, the causative agent of Rhodesian sleeping sickness, is a zoonosis and is transmitted by *Glossina pallidipes*, *G. morsitans*, *G. swynnertoni*, and *G. palpalis*. Pigs are possible reservoirs of *T. b. rhodesiense*.

   Tsetse flies are daylight biting and both males and females can be infected. Following the bite of a tsetse fly, metacyclic forms (the infective forms of trypomastigotes) are deposited into the subcutaneous tissue, where a marked perivascular reaction occurs. Lymphatics are then invaded, followed by spread to the lymph nodes. Invasion of the bloodstream occurs in 2 or 3 weeks, at which time the organisms reach all parts of the body, especially the CNS. In the CNS they elicit a marked perivascular mononuclear infiltration that results in leptomeningitis or encephalomyelitis. The presence of a toxin, although postulated, has not been demonstrated.

CLINICAL FEATURES

The incubation period is about 3 weeks. The clinical manifestations of Gambian and Rhodesian sleeping sickness are similar. Gambian sleeping sickness is a chronic illness with symptom-free periods, while Rhodesian sleeping sickness is an acute, more severe form, and death usually occurs within a year, often due to myocarditis. Features of CNS involvement are therefore less prominent in the Rhodesian form (Table 1.40).

   Following a bite by an infected tsetse fly, a

Table 1.40 Comparison between Gambian and Rhodesian sleeping sickness.

	Gambian	Rhodesian
Causative agent:	*Trypanosoma brucei gambiense*	*Trypanosoma brucei rhodesiense*
Main insect vector:	*Glossina palpalis*	*Glossina morsitans*
Transmission:	Anterior station	Anterior station
Reservoir:	Humans (pigs, goats, cattle, ? dogs)	Humans, wild animals (antelopes and hogs), cattle
Geographical distribution:	West Africa (Gambia to Congo), central Africa, scattered areas in east Africa	East Africa
Clincal features		
Duration:	Chronic	Acute
Severity:	Mild	Severe
Trypanosoma chancre:	Uncommon	Common
Fever:	Insidious and low grade	Acute and with large variations
Lymphadenopathy:	Prominent, especially posterior cervical group (Winterbottom's sign)	Less prominent
Hepatosplenomegaly:	Present	Present
CNS abnormalities:	Marked	Less marked
Other organs involved	Uncommon	Common
Treatment with melarsoprol:	Effective	Ineffective
Chemoprophylaxis:	Effective	Less effective

nodule appears at the site of the bite. This is referred to as a trypanosoma chancre and is seen more commonly in Rhodesian sleeping sickness and in Caucasians. Tachycardia and persistent headache are common. Spontaneous healing of the chancre is followed by haematogenous dissemination.

The lymph glands are discrete, non-tender and have a peculiar rubbery consistency. Splenomegaly and hepatomegaly may also occur. After a variable period of time, there is evidence of central nervous system involvement and features of a chronic meningoencephalomyelitis with behavioural changes. The patient loses interest in his surroundings, becomes apathetic, has a mask-like facies, and a tendency to fall asleep during the day and inability to sleep at night. The eyelids tend to droop, there is facial puffiness, the lower lips are swollen and hang loosely and the patient's attention span decreases. Later, tremor of the hands, areas of hyperaesthesia, especially over the ulnar nerve (Kerandel's sign), choreiform movements, seizures and finally coma develop. Myocarditis, hepatitis, petechiae and pleural effusions may occur, particularly in Rhodesian sleeping sickness.

Unusual manifestations
An erythematous, patchy, annular rash that fades in a week may be seen in the early stages of infection in Caucasians. Facial oedema, paraesthesiae, periosteitis, especially of the tibia resulting in hyperaesthesia, iridocyclitis and choroiditis may occur. Endocrine dysfunction may develop, manifesting as amenorrhoea or impotence.

DIAGNOSIS

The definitive diagnosis depends on demonstrating trypomastigotes in the peripheral blood, lymph node aspirates or CSF. If the organism is not easily demonstrated, concentration techniques should be utilized. IgM levels in the serum and CSF are markedly elevated.

TREATMENT

Therapy is usually effective if commenced before CNS symptoms develop.

Suramin, a polysulphated compound, is given intravenously; initially 0.1 g is given as a test dose to exclude an idiosyncratic reaction, followed by 1.0 g i.v. on the 1st, 3rd, 7th, 14th and 21st days. If proteinuria or haematuria develop, therapy should be discontinued. Pentamidine 3–4 mg·kg^{-1} intramuscularly on alternate days for 10 injections is an effective alternative. Rapid intravenous injection of pentamidine results in hypotension.

Although suramin and pentamidine have been found to be effective and should be used initially to control the fever, they do not cross the blood–brain barrier. It is currently believed that relapse or failure to respond to therapy will occur when CNS involvement occurs early in the disease. Hence drugs that penetrate the blood–brain barrier are being recommended as part of the initial treatment of trypanosomiasis. Melarsoprol, a trivalent arsenic, is used most widely for this purpose. Three to four consecutive injections of 2.0–3.6 mg·kg^{-1} body weight (up to a maximum of 250 mg per injection) are given intravenously. The course is usually repeated after an interval of 2 weeks. Major side-effects include an acute encephalitis-like condition and skin rashes.

A water-soluble analogue of melarsoprol, melarsonyl potassium, has also been found effective in Gambian but not in Rhodesian sleeping sickness.

Nitrofurazone 10 mg·kg^{-1} in divided doses three times daily for 10 days has also been found to be useful in cerebral trypanosomiasis. Peripheral neuropathy and haemolytic anaemia may be troublesome side-effects in patients with glucose-6-phosphate dehydrogenase deficiency.

PREVENTION AND CONTROL

Elimination of the vector—the tsetse fly—by insecticides or by making environmental conditions unsuitable for its inhabitation would effectively eradicate trypanosomiasis. Both these approaches require formidable mobilization of manpower and money. Insect repellents should be used when visiting endemic areas.

A single intramuscular prophylactic injection of pentamidine 4 mg·kg^{-1} body weight (up to a maximum dose of 300 mg) gives effective protection against Gambian sleeping sickness, but is less effective against Rhodesian sleeping sickness.

African trypanosomiasis in children

In children the early manifestations and CNS symptoms overlap. Lymphadenopathy and neurological abnormalities may occur together. Seizures and choreiform movements are not uncommon. Treatment is as for the adult form.

American trypanosomiasis (Chagas' disease)

This is a zoonotic disease caused by *T. cruzi* that is transmitted by various reduviid insects. The principal vectors are *Triatoma infestans*, and *Rhodnius prolixus* (Latin America) and *Panstrongylus megistus* (Venezuela). Once infected, these insects remain infective for at least 2 years. Humans constitute the main reservoir, although domesticated and wild animals are also important reservoirs. Humans are infected when a bite is contaminated by the faeces of an infected insect or when infected faeces are rubbed into an abrasion or mucosal surface such as the conjunctiva. Less commonly the infection may spread via blood transfusions or transplacentally.

Chagas' disease is confined to South and Central America. Occasional cases have also been reported from southern Texas.

CLINICAL FEATURES

The incubation period varies from 1 to 3 weeks. Two clinically distinct presentations are recognized:

Acute Chagas' disease
Acute Chagas' disease predominantly affects children. An erythematous, indurated papule (chagoma) develops at the site of bite, and is associated with regional lymphadenopathy. This resolves spontaneously. If the portal of entry is the conjunctiva, unilateral periorbital and palpebral oedema (Romana's sign), conjunctivitis and preauricular lymphadenopathy develop. Systemic findings such as fever, a transient morbilliform or urticarial rash, a peculiar gelatinous oedema of the face and trunk, tender lymphadenopathy and hepatosplenomegaly may be present. Death may occur in a small proportion of patients owing to myocarditis or meningoencephalitis. More commonly the patient recovers completely in a few weeks.

Chronic Chagas' disease
Chronic Chagas' disease occurs in previously asymptomatic individuals. It is due to an autoimmune reaction mediated by cytotoxic T cells and antibodies against the endocardium, vascular tissue and striated muscle, together with myenteric plexus damage by amastigotes. The heart is invariably involved. The patient may complain of chest pain, dyspnoea or syncope. Cardiac abnormalities and arrhythmias are usual. Signs of right-sided cardiac failure may be present. Thromboembolic phenomena may occur.

With gastrointestinal involvement, mega-oesophagus, leading to dysphagia and aspiration pneumonia, and megacolon, giving constipation and progressive abdominal distension, may occur. Dilatation of the biliary tree and of the bronchi have also been documented.

DIAGNOSIS

In acute Chagas' disease trypomastigotes may be demonstrated in peripheral blood. If parasites are not demonstrated in the blood, xenodiagnosis may be used: a parasite-free laboratory-reared vector feeds on a patient suspected to have the disease and 2–3 weeks later the intestinal contents of the vector are examined for parasites.

In chronic Chagas' disease complement fixation (Machado–Guerreiro reaction), indirect fluorescent antibody or haemagglutination tests may be used.

Radiological assessment of gastrointestinal abnormalities is helpful.

TREATMENT

Nifurtimox, a nitrofurazone derivative, has been found to be useful in acute disease. The dose is $20 \text{ mg} \cdot \text{kg}^{-1}$ daily for children below the age of 2 and $8–10 \text{ mg} \cdot \text{kg}^{-1}$ daily for 3–4 months in older children and adults. Side-effects are few and include transient leucopenia, vomiting, sleeplessness and paraesthesiae. Benzimidazole is a useful alternative drug.

Over 80% of patients with the acute form of the disease and slightly more with the chronic form are cured of the infection.

PREVENTION AND CONTROL

No vaccine or chemoprophylactic agent is available. Prevention therefore involves the regular spraying of houses with benzene hexachloride in order to decrease the vector population.

TOXOPLASMOSIS

Toxoplasmosis is caused by *Toxoplasma gondii*, an intracellular protozoon, which requires for completion of its life-cycle a definitive host, e.g. a cat, sheep or pig, and an intermediate host, e.g. a human. Infection of humans occurs either congenitally or by ingestion of foodstuffs contaminated by infected cat faeces or lamb or pork contaminated with *T. gondii* cysts. Toxoplasmosis is rare in the UK.

CLINICAL FEATURES

Five major clinical forms of toxoplasmosis are recognized:

1 *Asymptomatic lymphadenopathy*, the commonest mode of presentation.
2 *Lymphadenopathy*, usually involving the cervical lymph nodes and associated with a febrile illness. This may clinically be indistinguishable from infectious mononucleosis but the Paul–Bunnell test is negative.
3 *Neurological abnormalities*, which include neck stiffness and headache, associated with sore throat and maculopapular rashes. The CSF is under pressure and the level of protein is elevated.
4 An *acute febrile illness*, with a maculopapular rash, hepatosplenomegaly and reactive lymphocytes in the peripheral blood. Uveitis, chorioretinitis, myocarditis and hepatitis may occur.

In the immunocompromised host, features present in the acute febrile and neurological forms are prominent.

5 *Congenital toxoplasmosis*, in which the symptoms and signs are indicative of CNS involvement. The characteristic 'syndrome of Savin', which comprises internal hydrocephalus, chorioretinitis, convulsions and cerebral calcification, may be seen. Tremors, nystagmus, micro-ophthalmia and pneumonitis are also present. The prognosis is usually poor, the survivors generally exhibiting mental retardation, epilepsy and spastic paraplegia.

DIAGNOSIS

Serological tests are the mainstay of diagnosis of acquired infection. The Sabin–Feldman dye test, a measure of IgG antibodies, has been widely used. Antibodies can also be detected by indirect fluorescence or indirect haemagglutination. Raised antibody levels are common in the general population and only a rising antibody titre is highly suggestive of toxoplasmosis. The IgM–immunofluorescent antibody (IgM–IFA) test is particularly useful for detecting acute infection since titres rise early and fall rapidly.

T. gondii can be isolated by injecting the peritoneum of mice with tissue extracts, e.g. bone marrow, body fluids or CSF when available, and examining the peritoneal fluid 6–10 days later for the organism.

TREATMENT

Most patients require no therapy as the disease is mild. Pyrimethamine (25–50 mg three times daily) and sulphadiazine (4–5 g daily) are used in combination for severe disease since they are synergistic. Therapy should be continued for at least 1 month. Since pyrimethamine is teratogenic, spiramycin is a useful alternative during pregnancy. Steroids are probably useful in ocular toxoplasmosis.

PREVENTION

Domestic cats that kill mice and birds are the chief source of infection and care should be taken in handling their faeces.

BABESIOSIS

This is a tick-borne disease, found chiefly in North America and Europe, and is occasionally transmitted to humans, especially those who are immunosuppressed. The causative organism is the plasmodium-like *Babesia microti*. The incubation period averages 10 days. In patients with normal splenic function, the symptoms are mild and usually comprise fever, nausea, myalgia, chills, vomiting and abdominal pain. Hepatosplenomeg-aly and mild to moderate haemolytic anaemia may also be present. In splenectomized individuals, systemic symptoms are more pronounced and haemolysis is associated with haemoglobinuria, jaundice and renal failure. Examination of a peripheral blood smear may reveal the characteristic plasmodium-like organisms.

TREATMENT

Treatment is mainly symptomatic. In severe cases pentamidine may be used but is effective only in reducing the numbers of but not eradicating the parasite. Chloroquine is reasonably effective.

MALARIA

Malaria affects more than 100 million people each year and has a mortality rate of 1%.

Endemic and epidemic malaria are found in all countries between the 30° south and 40° north lines of latitude (Fig. 1.27). Malaria is primarily a disease of hot, humid countries at altitudes less than 2200 metres above mean sea level, where conditions are ideal for prolific breeding of the mosquito vector, *Anopheles*. It is endemic in India, in parts of Africa and parts of South and Central America. Malaria may also be transmitted by blood transfusion and by importation of infected mosquitoes by air, so-called airport malaria.

In humans, malaria is caused by four species of *Plasmodium*:

- *P. vivax* and *P. ovale* cause tertian malaria.
- *P. falciparum* causes malignant tertian malaria.
- *P. malariae* causes quartan malaria.

The four species are distinguishable from each other on examination of peripheral blood smears.

P. ovale has been reported predominantly from East and West Africa. *P. vivax* is the major species in temperate zones, whereas in the tropics all forms of malaria are seen. With present-day ease and speed of travel, sporadic cases of malaria are being increasingly recognized. Unfortunately, the initial impact of the WHO eradication programme lost its impetus in several countries in the early 1970s and malaria has once more become a major cause of morbidity and mortality in tropical and subtropical countries.

Humans, the intermediate hosts, are infected following the bite of an infected female *Anopheles* mosquito, the definitive host. The parasite can also be transmitted by blood transfusion, transplacentally, and, increasingly, between drug addicts who use improperly cleaned syringes.

The introduction of sporozoites, the infective form of the parasite, through the skin by the *Anopheles* mosquito heralds the commencement of

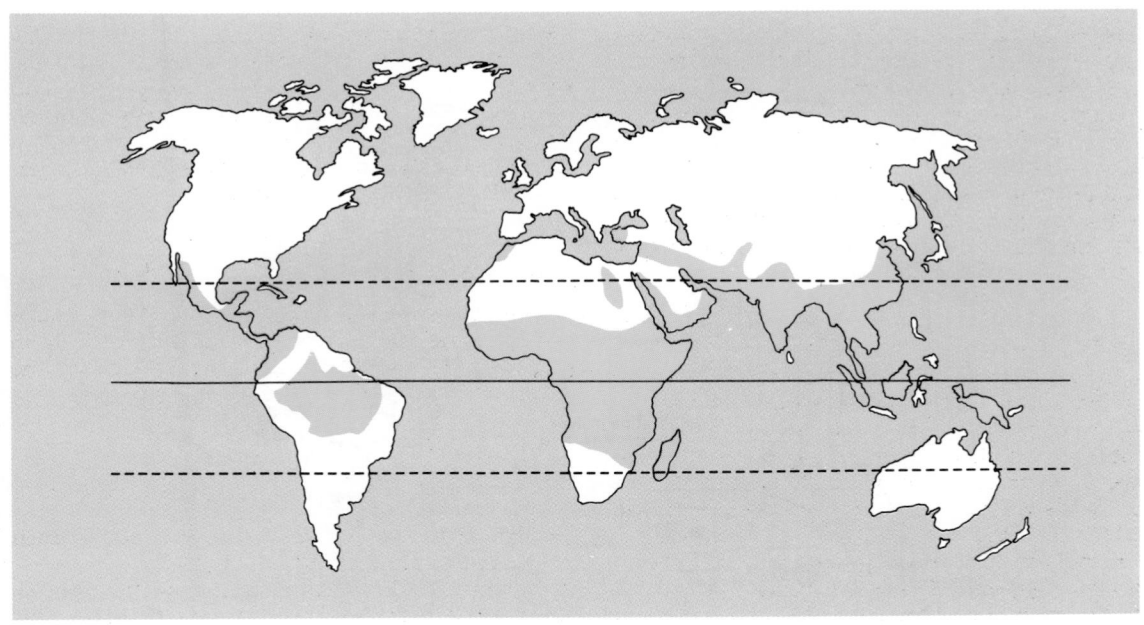

Fig. 1.27 The geographical distribution of malaria.

the human cycle (Fig. 1.28). The following stages occur.

Pre-erythrocytic schizogony
During this phase clinical symptoms are absent and humans are not infective. Those sporozoites that are not removed by the body's defence mechanisms undergo development within the liver. A variable number of days later, micromerozoites are liberated (primary attack). Other sporozoites (*P. vivax* and probably *P. ovale*) remain in a latent form in the liver as hypnozoites.

Erythrocytic schizogony
This is the phase when red blood cells (RBCs) become infected by the micromerozoites. In the RBCs they pass through several stages of development, namely trophozoites, schizonts and finally merozoites. These asexual parasitic forms are found in peripheral blood about 12 days after inoculation of the sporozoites in *P. vivax* infection and 9 days in *P. falciparum* infection. The different *Plasmodium* species differ in their ability to invade RBCs. *P. falciparum* is capable of invading all RBCs, especially young RBCs. It therefore has the potential to produce the most severe form of malaria. *P. vivax* and *P. ovale* preferentially invade reticulocytes and young RBCs, whereas *P. malariae* invades senescent RBCs. Each cycle in the red cells terminates with rupture of the cell and release of merozoites into the circulation. This occurs every 48 h in *P. falciparum* infection, every 48–72 h in *P.*

vivax and *P. ovale* infection, and approximately every 72 h in *P. malariae*.

Gametogony
The erythrocytic phase may continue for a considerable period of time before the stage of gametogony occurs. In this stage a few merozoites develop into the sexual form of the parasites known as gametocytes. Of these only the mature forms are found in peripheral blood. At this stage the patient is infective.

Exoerythrocytic schizogony
This fourth stage, which occurs in the liver, is found only with *P. vivax*, probably *P. ovale* and possibly *P. malariae* infections. It does not occur with *P. falciparum* infection and is believed to be responsible for the relapses in *P. vivax* and *P. ovale* infections. The parasites in this phase are referred to as hypnozoites.

When an *Anopheles* mosquito ingests human blood containing gametocytes it marks the commencement of the sexual cycle in the mosquito. The external incubation period varies from 7 to 20 days.

IMMUNITY

This may be natural or acquired. Natural immunity is present in individuals of West African extraction who are blood group Duffy-negative (FyFy) and therefore lack the specific receptor on the RBC

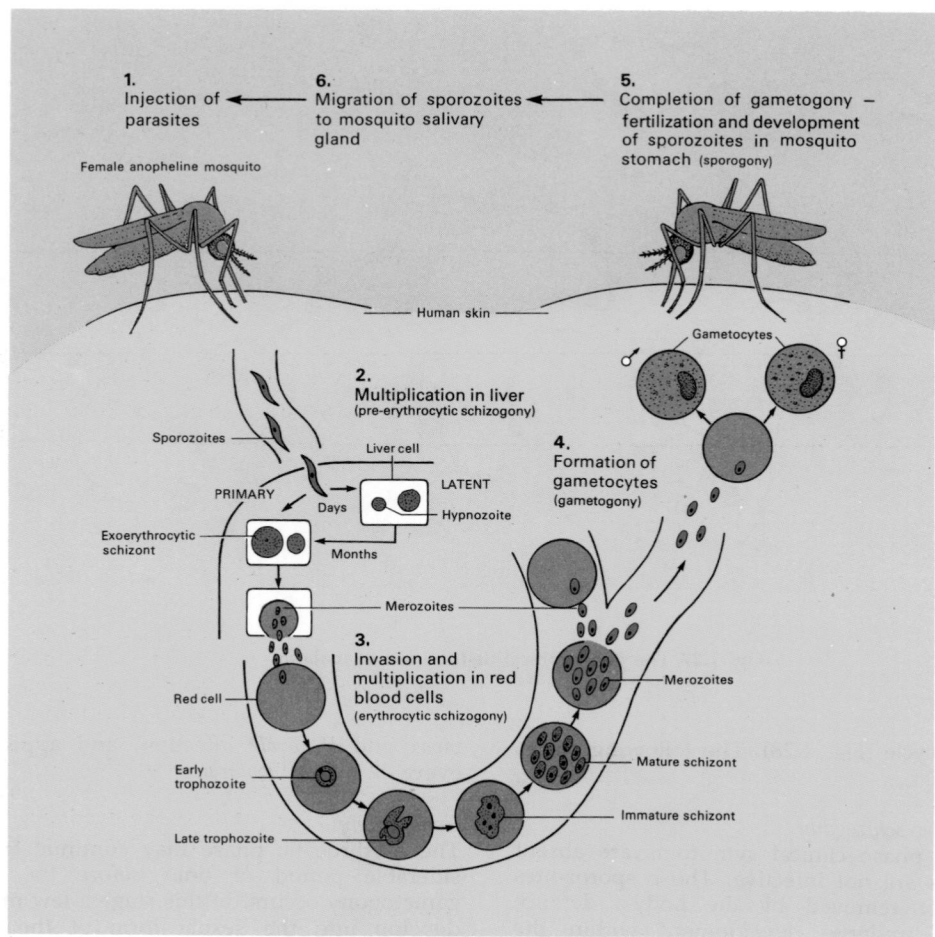

Fig. 1.28 A schematic life-cycle of *Plasmodium vivax*.

surface to which the merozoites attach. They cannot develop *P. vivax* malaria. The presence of haemoglobin S, glucose-6-phosphate dehydrogenase deficiency, thalassaemia and pyruvate kinase deficiency also offer resistance against *P. falciparum*. The presence of abnormal haemoglobins or altered red cell metabolism retards *P. falciparum* maturation and reduces the severity of the disease.

The spleen plays an important role in natural immunity, since splenectomized individuals are highly susceptible to the malarial parasite.

Infants are protected by the transfer of maternal IgG antibodies across the placenta.

Partial immunity may be acquired following an attack of malaria, and is attributed to macrophage stimulation by T cells.

CLINICAL FEATURES

The incubation period varies, being:

- 10–14 days in *P. vivax*, *P. ovale* and *P. falciparum*
- 18 days–6 weeks in *P. malariae* infection

Although individual variations in clinical presentation are noted, febrile paroxysms, anaemia, splenomegaly and hepatomegaly are usually present. Malarial febrile paroxysms typically have three stages:

1 The *'cold stage'* is characterized by marked vasoconstriction and lasts from 30 min to 1 h. The patient feels intensely cold and uncomfortable. There is marked shivering. The temperature rises rapidly, often to as high as 41°C.
2 The *'hot stage'* abruptly follows and lasts for 2–6 h. The patient feels intensely hot and uncomfortable. Delirium may be present.
3 The *'sweating stage'* then occurs, during which the bedclothes are drenched. The patient feels fatigued and exhausted but otherwise well and often sleeps. The fever is due to schizont rupture

and the release of pyrogens.

Herpes labialis frequently occurs in established malaria. Anaemia is usually present and is largely a result of haemolysis.

P. vivax and P. ovale

The fever occurs every other day when established. These species of *Plasmodium* give rise to a clinically mild infection. The presence of an exoerythrocytic stage is responsible for relapses and makes eradication of the organisms difficult.

P. malariae

This is usually a mild disease with a fever, but tends to run a more chronic course. The nephrotic syndrome can complicate this type of malaria and may be fatal between the ages of 4 and 5 years. Because of its chronicity, the patient develops a sallow complexion, marked muscle wasting, mild icterus and massive splenomegaly. Growth retardation may occur in children.

P. falciparum

This is potentially the most severe form of malaria (pernicious malaria), with high levels of parasitaemia. Infected RBCs develop peculiar knob-like surface projections that facilitate adhesion of these RBCs to the endothelium of blood vessels. The consequent vascular occlusion causes severe organ damage, chiefly in the kidneys, liver, brain and gastrointestinal tract. The prodrome tends to be severe. The fever follows no particular pattern. Splenomegaly tends to occur late and the characteristic cold, hot and sweating stages are not prominent. The following clinical forms of falciparum malaria are recognized and are likely to occur when more than 5% of RBCs are parasitized:

- *Cerebral malaria* is characterized by a marked elevation in body temperature, a rapid deterioration in consciousness, convulsions, coma and death.
- *Algid malaria* is characterized by the presence of severe vomiting, diarrhoea and peripheral circulatory collapse.
- *Septicaemic malaria* results in a high, continuous fever, vomiting and signs and symptoms mimicking typhoid fever. Pulmonary circulatory insufficiency may be present, with cough, haemoptysis and features of shock lung. The hepatorenal syndrome and spontaneous splenic rupture may also occur.
- *Blackwater fever*, so called because of the production of dark brown-black urine owing to intravascular haemolysis, is seen only in falciparum malaria. It can be precipitated by very small amounts of quinine in quinine-sensitive cases.

This is a rapidly progressive illness characterized by the abrupt onset of fever, marked haemolysis, haemoglobinuria, hyperbilirubinaemia, vomiting, circulatory collapse and acute renal failure. Malarial parasites cannot usually be detected in peripheral blood smears after the onset of intravascular haemolysis.

Tropical splenomegaly syndrome

Tropical splenomegaly syndrome is seen in areas where malaria is hyperendemic. It is uncommon before 10 years of age. Characteristic features are massive splenomegaly, marked elevation in serum IgM levels, and IgM aggregates (detected by immunofluorescence) in Kupffer's cells in the liver. The splenomegaly responds to antimalarial therapy. However, malarial parasites are not detected in the spleen or peripheral blood smears.

PREVALENCE

The following indices are used to measure the prevalence of malaria:

- The *spleen rate*, defined as the percentage of children between 2 and 10 years of age with splenomegaly, is used as a measure of the endemicity of malaria in a community.
- The *infant parasite rate*, defined as the percentage of infants below 1 year of age in whom malarial parasites are demonstrable in peripheral blood smears, is regarded as the most sensitive index of transmission of malaria to a locality.

DIAGNOSIS

The parasite can be demonstrated in either thin or thick peripheral blood smears stained with Giemsa, Wright or Leishman stains. Two to three blood smears taken each day for 3 or 4 days and found to be negative are necessary before a patient is declared malaria-free.

Serological methods are not widely used but include indirect immunofluorescence, indirect haemagglutination and gel diffusion techniques.

Enzyme-linked immunosorbent assays (ELISA) for antigen detection and probes for parasite DNA are currently being evaluated.

TREATMENT

General
Analgesics and antipyretics such as aspirin and paracetamol are given as necessary. Intravenous fluids may be required to combat dehydration and shock.

Treatment of an acute attack
The 4-aminoquinolines are the drugs of choice. Chloroquine-sensitive malaria is treated with

chloroquine 600 mg of the base followed by 300 mg in 6 h and then 150 mg twice daily for 3 days, or amodiaquine hydrochloride 600 mg of the base followed by 400–600 mg daily for 2 days up to a total maximum dose of 2400 mg.

Chloroquine-resistant malaria is treated with quinine sulphate 650 mg three times daily for 5 days given in combination with pyrimethamine 25 mg twice daily for 3 days and sulphadiazine 500 mg twice daily for 5 days. Alternatively, quinine sulphate may be followed by a single dose of sulfadoxine 1.5 g combined with pyrimethamine 75 mg (available as Fansidar). Unfortunately, widespread resistance to this drug is developing. Mefloquine is a recently synthesized quinolone, is useful in chloroquine and some quinine-resistant cases; again resistance to this is developing. Halofantrine, an amino alochol, is a promising drug for resistant cases. Both these last two drugs are too expensive for widespread use.

Drug side-effects. These drugs are potentially toxic. With quinine, tinnitus, haemolytic anaemia and drug fever may occur. Chloroquine may cause vomiting, abdominal pain, agranulocytosis or convulsions.

Eradication
P. falciparum. Chloroquine alone or in combination with either pyrimethamine 25 mg or primaquine 45 mg as a single dose effects a radical cure because there is no exoerythrocytic stage in falciparum malaria.

P. vivax, P. malariae and *P. ovale.* Primaquine, an 8-aminoquinoline, is essential for eliminating the exoerythrocytic cycle and effecting a radical cure. A course of one of the 4-aminoquinolines should be followed by primaquine 7.5 mg daily for 14 days. Alternatively, 300 mg chloroquine combined with 45 mg primaquine once a week for 8 weeks is also effective.

Treatment of severe malaria (more than 1% of RBCs infected) or any of the pernicious forms of falciparum malaria constitutes a medical emergency. Therapy is initially with intravenous chloroquine 5 mg·kg^{-1} or quinine hydrochloride 10 mg·kg^{-1}, with the dose being repeated every 8 h until oral therapy can be tolerated.

PREVENTION AND CONTROL

Owing to changing patterns of resistance, advice about chemoprophylaxis should be sought prior to leaving for a malaria-endemic area. Chemoprophylaxis is essential for those visiting endemic areas; generally chloroquine 400–500 mg once a week in areas where there is no chloroquine resistance, but where there is resistance it should be combined

with proguanil 200 mg daily or in South-East Asia or Papua New Guinea dapsone/pyrimethamine (malaprim) one tablet (100 mg and 125 mg respectively) each week as above. Prophylaxis should be continued for 6 weeks after leaving a high-risk area.

On the basis of the 1979 WHO Expert Committee report on malaria, the following preventive measures have been suggested. Measures to be applied to the community include prevention of man–vector contact, destruction of adult mosquitoes and mosquito larvae, and active elimination of human infection by presumptive treatment (i.e. treatment of all fevers in endemic areas with antimalarials) and radical treatment. Measures to be applied to individuals include use of mosquito repellents, chemoprophylaxis and chemotherapy where indicated.

Intestinal and genital infections

Amoebiasis

The most important human disease due to amoebae is amoebiasis, which is caused by *Entamoeba histolytica*. This intestinal pathogen can be differentiated from other enteric amoebae such as *Entamoeba hartmani*, *Entamoeba coli* and *Endolimax nana*, since *E. histolytica* is the only amoeba found in the intestine that phagocytoses red blood cells. It occurs world-wide, although much higher incidence rates are found in the tropics and subtropics. It can be found in active male homosexuals who carry the pathogen (usually strains of low virulence) and between whom it is spread by sexual contact.

LIFE-CYCLE AND PATHOGENESIS

The organism exists both as a motile trophozoite and as a cyst that can survive outside the body. Cysts are transmitted chiefly by ingestion of contaminated food or water or spread directly by person-to-person contact. Trophozoites emerge from the cyst in the small intestine and then pass on to the colon, where they multiply (Fig. 1.29). Many individuals can carry the pathogen without obvious evidence of clinical disease (asymptomatic cyst passers). However, under certain conditions, *E. histolytica* trophozoites invade the colonic epithelium, probably with the aid of their own cytotoxins and proteolytic enzymes. The parasites continue to multiply and finally frank ulceration of the mucosa occurs. If penetration continues trophozoites may enter the portal vein, via which

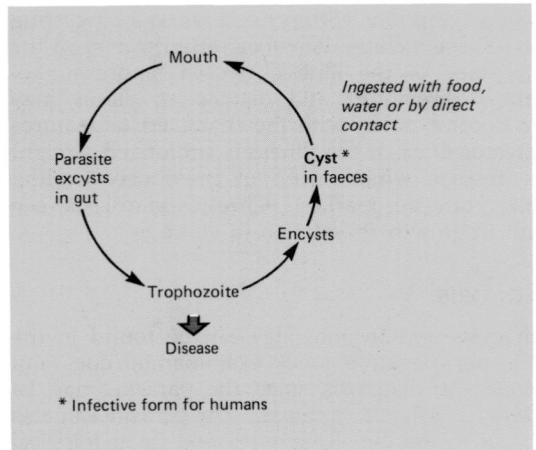

Fig. 1.29 A schematic life-cycle of intestinal protozoa.

they reach the liver and cause hepatitis and intrahepatic abscesses. This invasive form of the disease is particularly serious and unless treated promptly is often fatal.

CLINICAL FEATURES

The incubation period is highly variable and may be as short as a few days or as long as several months or even a year. The presentation of amoebic colitis may be:

- Gradual onset with mild intermittent diarrhoea and abdominal discomfort, usually progressing to bloody diarrhoea with mucus. Systemic manifestations such as headache, nausea and anorexia are often present.
- Severe acute (amoebic) dysentery, closely resembling that due to *Shigella* (bacillary dysentery).
- A fulminating colitis.

Typically, patients with amoebic colitis appear less unwell than those with bacillary dysentery, fever is low-grade or absent, and dehydration is unusual.

COMPLICATIONS

Complications are unusual, but include:

- Progression of fulminant colitis to toxic dilatation of the colon with perforation and peritonitis.
- Chronic infection leading to stricture formation.
- Severe haemorrhage.
- Development of a mass of fibrotic granulation tissue (amoeboma), most commonly in the caecum or rectosigmoid region. Amoebomas occur in 10% of patients and may bleed, cause obstruction, intussuscept and are sometimes

mistaken for a carcinoma.
- Amoebic liver abscess, which often develops in the absence of a recent episode of colitis. Tender hepatomegaly, a high swinging fever and profound malaise are characteristic, although early in the course of the disease both symptoms and signs may be minimal. The clinical features are described in more detail on p. 276.

DIAGNOSIS

Serodiagnosis

The amoebic fluorescent antibody titre (FAT) is positive in at least 90% of patients with liver abscess and 75% with active colitis. Seropositivity is low in asymptomatic cyst passers.

Colonic disease

Direct examination of colonic exudate obtained at sigmoidoscopy or of freshly passed stool as a saline-wet mount is the most rapid and least expensive way of confirming amoebic infection. *E. histolytica* trophozoites must be distinguished from non-pathogenic amoebae and from polymorphonuclear leucocytes, with which they are sometimes confused. Cysts may also be present in the stool. Sigmoidoscopy and barium enema examination may show colonic ulceration but are rarely diagnostic.

Liver disease

Liver abscess should be suspected if the serum alkaline phosphatase is elevated, even when clinical signs are absent. Hepatic ultrasound scan should confirm the presence of an abscess, which may be either single or multiple. Pus from an amoebic abscess has a classic 'anchovy sauce' appearance and may contain trophozoites.

TREATMENT

Metronidazole 800 mg three times daily for 5 days is given in amoebic colitis and a more prolonged course for 10–14 days in liver abscess or other extra-intestinal spread.

An alternative drug is the newer nitroimidazole derivative, tinidazole. Dehydroemetine is used when nitroimidazoles fail (rarely). Diloxanide furoate is a luminal amoebicide and may be a helpful adjunct in clearing cysts.

Large, tense abscesses in the liver may require percutaneous drainage, using an ultrasound scan to localize accurately the abscess and to position the drainage needle.

CONTROL AND PREVENTION

This disease will be difficult to eradicate because of the substantial human reservoir of asymptomatic cases. There is no immediate hope of vaccine development, particularly as the same individual may experience several episodes of amoebic infection, indicating that only partial protective immunity develops after exposure to the pathogen. Improved standards of personal hygiene and water quality are important. Cysts are destroyed by boiling water for at least 10 minutes, but the effects of chlorination are variable.

Balantidiasis

Balantidium coli is the only ciliate that produces clinically significant infection in humans. It is found throughout the tropics, particularly in Central and South America, Iran, Papua New Guinea and the Philippines. It is usually carried by pigs and infection is most common in those communities that live in close association with swine. Its life-cycle is identical to that of *Entamoeba histolytica*.

B. coli produces a dysenteric illness owing to invasion of the distal ileal and colonic mucosa. The colitis may be acute and fulminant and if untreated may be fatal. Trophozoites rather than cysts are found in the stool. Treatment is with tetracycline, ampicillin or metronidazole.

Giardiasis

Giardia lamblia is a flagellate that is found worldwide. It causes small-intestinal disease, with diarrhoea and malabsorption. Prevalence is high throughout the tropics. It is an important cause of traveller's diarrhoea world-wide. In certain parts of Europe, the USSR, and in some rural and mountainous areas of North America, large waterborne epidemics have been reported. Person-to-person spread is common in day nurseries and residential institutions and between male homosexuals. Like *Entamoeba histolytica*, the organism exists both as a trophozoite and a cyst, the latter being the form in which the protozoon is transmitted.

The organism colonizes and multiplies within the small intestine and may remain there without causing detriment to the host. Severe malabsorption may occur and is thought to be related to morphological damage to the small intestine; changes in villus architecture vary from mild partial villus atrophy to rarely subtotal villus atrophy. The mechanism by which *Giardia* causes alteration in mucosal architecture and produces diarrhoea and intestinal malabsorption is unknown. There is evidence that the morphological damage may be immune-mediated. Bacterial overgrowth has also been found in association with giardiasis and may contribute to fat malabsorption.

CLINICAL FEATURES

Many individuals excreting *Giardia* cysts have no symptoms and are therefore carriers. Others develop symptoms within 1 or 2 weeks of ingesting cysts. These include diarrhoea, often watery in the early stage of the illness, nausea, anorexia, abdominal discomfort and distension. Stools may then become paler, with the characteristic features of steatorrhoea. If the illness is prolonged, weight loss ensues, which, even in previously healthy adults, can be marked. Chronic giardiasis can result in growth retardation in children.

DIAGNOSIS

Both cysts and trophozoites can be found in the stool, but negative stool examination does not exclude the diagnosis since the parasite may be excreted at irregular intervals. The parasite can also be seen in duodenal aspirates and in histological sections of jejunal mucosa. Raised specific anti-*Giardia* IgG and, in acute infections, IgM antibodies are found.

TREATMENT

Metronidazole 2 g as a single dose on three successive days will cure the majority of infections, although sometimes a second or third course is necessary. Preventive measures are similar to those outlined for *E. histolytica*.

Cryptosporidium

This organism is found world-wide. It produces a devastating diarrhoeal illness in patients with immunodeficiency, particularly those with AIDS. It has recently become a recognized cause of gastroenteritis, particularly in children.

The parasite is able to reproduce both sexually and asexually and has a life-cycle in the intestine very similar to that of *Plasmodium*. The disease is spread by oocysts excreted in the faeces.

CLINICAL FEATURES

In healthy individuals cryptosporidiosis is a self-limiting illness lasting for 7–10 days. Acute watery diarrhoea is associated with fever and general malaise, but otherwise the disease follows a benign course. In the immunocompromised patient diarrhoea is followed by severe weight loss and general debility, contributing significantly to the downhill course of AIDS. Occasionally toxic dilatation of the colon can occur. A syndrome of right upper quadrant abdominal pain, raised alkaline phosphatase and the typical bile duct abnormalities of sclerosing cholangitis is seen in AIDS patients.

DIAGNOSIS

The parasite can be detected in intestinal biopsies but is now most commonly found in faeces (as oocysts) using concentration techniques and a modified Ziehl-Neelsen stain.

TREATMENT

As yet there is no effective treatment for this infection, although spiramycin, erythromycin and clindamycin can reduce diarrhoea. AZT can clear infection temporarily in AIDS.

Trichomoniasis

Trichomonas vaginalis is a flagellate that causes vaginitis and urethritis. The resulting vaginal discharge is profuse, greenish and malodorous and associated with vulval irritation. The organism also colonizes the male urethra, where it may produce little or no effect or may alternatively cause frank urethritis. Infection is transmitted sexually. Motile trichomonads can be readily seen in wet preparations or urethral or vaginal discharge. Infection responds to metronidazole (2 g as a single oral dose) and it is advisable to also treat the patient's sexual partner.

Helminthic infections

Nematode (roundworm) infections

FILARIASIS

Several nematodes belonging to the superfamily Filarioidea are responsible for filariasis (Table 1.41). The adult worms are thread-like. Females are larger than males. The viviparous females give birth to larvae known as microfilariae. The microfilariae of various species can be easily differen-tiated from each other by the presence or absence of a sheath and the pattern of nuclear distribution in the tail. These nematodes require two hosts to complete their life-cycle.

Bancroftian and Malayan filariasis

Wuchereria bancrofti is found mainly in the tropics and subtropics, in northern Australia, Pacific Islands, West and Central Africa, South America and India. *Brugia malayi* infection is less wide-spread than Bancroftian filariasis and is found in India, southern China, Malaysia, Indonesia and Borneo (Fig. 1.30). Humans are the definitive hosts and mosquitoes of various types are the inter-mediate hosts. Humans are the only known reservoirs of Bancroftian filariasis, whereas, in addition to humans, animals such as cats are reservoirs of Malayan filariasis. *Cutex fatigans* is the main vector of Bancroftian filariasis. *Aedes* and *Anopheles* species have also been implicated. The major vector for Malayan filariasis is *Mansonia annulifera*.

Following the bite of an infected mosquito, the larvae penetrate the skin, enter the lymphatics and are carried to the regional lymph nodes. Here they grow and mature for up to 18 months. After fertilization the microfilariae produced are carried from the lymphatics into the blood; they do not produce any symptoms or signs. Adult worms produce lymphangitis, which is believed to be a hypersensitivity reaction. The lymphangitis is fol-lowed by fibrosis, a granulomatous reaction and later irreversible lymphatic blockade. Secondary bacterial infection may add considerably to the inflammatory response and resultant fibrosis.

CLINICAL FEATURES

Following an incubation period that averages 10–12 months, the patient presents with fever ranging from 39 to 41°C accompanied by lymphangitis, both of which usually subside in 3–5 days.

Table 1.41 Habitat, vectors and major clinical manifestations of some nematodes of the superfamily Filarioidea.

Organism	Habitat of adult worms in humans	Vector	Clinical manifestations
Wuchereria bancrofti	Lymphatics, lymph nodes	*Culex, Aedes, Anopheles*	Fever, lymphangitis, elephantiasis of limbs, breasts and scrotum
Brugia malayi	Lymphatics	*Mansonia*	Fever, lymphangitis, elephantiasis (scrotal involvement is uncommon)
Loa loa	Subcutaneous tissue, subconjunctiva	*Chrysops*	'Calabar swellings', urticaria
Onchocerca volvulus	Subcutaneous tissue	*Simulium*	Subcutaneous nodules, elephantiasis, ocular lesions
Dipetalonema	Body cavities	*Culicoides*	Occasionally dermatitis

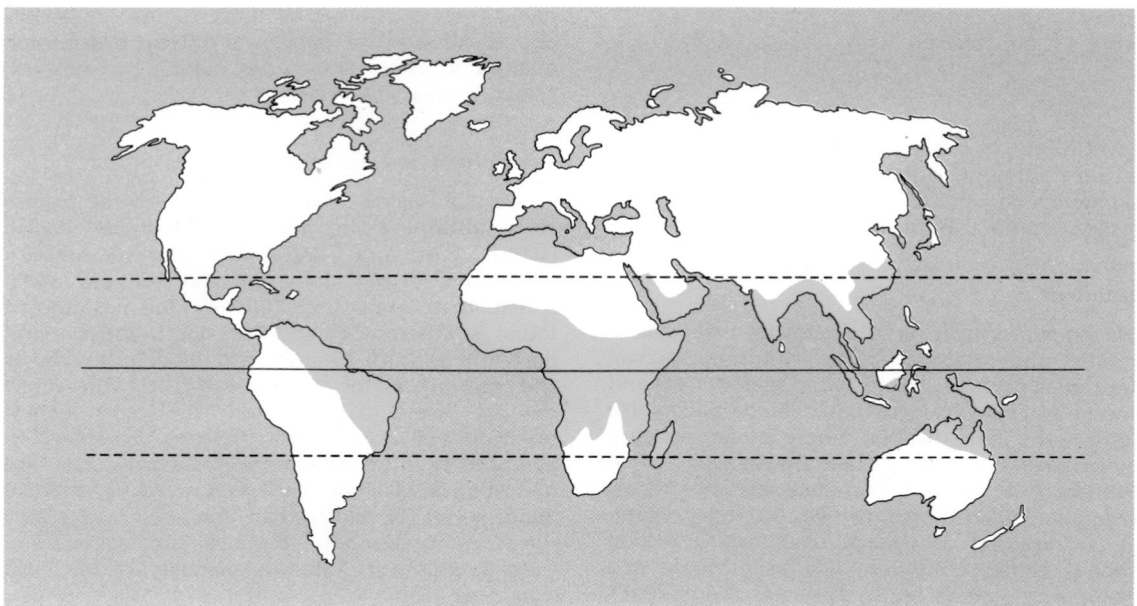

Fig. 1.30 The geographical distribution of filariasis.

Lymphangitis typically involves the lymphatics of the lower or upper limbs or of the abdomen. Involvement of the lymphatics of the epididymis, testis and spermatic cord occurs almost exclusively in Bancroftian filariasis. The involved superficial lymphatics appears as red streaks on the skin, and are tender and cord-like. The inflammation may subside either with treatment or spontaneously but there is a tendency for recurrences. The inflammatory phase is usually followed by the obstructive phase, which is characterized by features of lymphatic blockade. Many sites may be affected, but lower limb and scrotal oedema occur frequently. Long-standing obstruction produces thick, rough skin, which occasionally ulcerates. Less frequently chyluria, chylous ascites and pleural effusions occur. The obstructive phase may be punctuated by episodes of acute lymphangitis.

DIAGNOSIS

The clinical presentation is characteristic. Eosinophilia and the presence of microfilariae in thin or thick peripheral blood smears is diagnostic. Since *W. bancrofti* and *B. malayi* are released into the peripheral circulation at night, blood for examination should be taken between 9 p.m. and 1 a.m. If, despite repeated examination, microfilariae cannot be demonstrated in thick or thin blood smears, diethylcarbamazine 100 mg given as a single dose followed by blood removal 30 min later for examination may give a positive yield. Various parasite-concentration techniques such as Knott's concentration or membrane filtration techniques have resulted in a higher positive yield. Serological tests are not specific.

TREATMENT

Diethylcarbamazine (DEC) 2–6 mg·kg^{-1} daily in three divided doses for 2–3 weeks is recommended. A second course after 6 weeks increases the cure rate. The WHO Expert Committee has recommended that a total of 72 mg·kg^{-1} be given for eradication of Bancroftian filariasis and 30–40 mg·kg^{-1} for Malayan filariasis. DEC is filaricidal. Following initiation of therapy, marked allergic reactions can occur and require concomitant administration of antihistamines or steroids.

Associated bacterial infections should be appropriately treated. Reconstructive surgery plays an important role in removing unsightly tissue.

PREVENTION AND CONTROL

Mass chemotherapy with DEC has been effective in decreasing the *microfilariae rate* (the percentage of individuals who have microfilariae in a unit volume of their blood in a given population) and the *microfilariae density* (the number of microfilariae per unit volume of blood in individual patients). Primary prophylaxis should be aimed at vector control and protection of humans from mosquitoes.

Tropical eosinophilia

Tropical eosinophilia has been attributed to microfilariae such as *Dirofilaria* and more recently to *W. bancrofti* and *B. malayi*. Two forms are recognized, one characterized by lymphadenopathy and splenomegaly, and the other by cough, bronchospasm and an asthma-like picture (see p. 689).

Loiasis

Loiasis is caused by *Loa loa*. As in Bancroftian and Malayan filariasis, the microfilariae of *L. loa* do not produce any symptoms. Unlike in Bancroftian filariasis, the microfilariae are found in the peripheral circulation mainly during the day. The disease is confined to the hot, humid, swampy areas of West and Central Africa, in which environment the deerfly vectors *Chrysops silacea* and *Chrysops dimidiata* thrive. Following the bite of a female *Chrysops*, the microfilariae are introduced into the skin of the human host and tend to migrate in the subcutaneous tissues. They have a predilection for subconjunctival and periorbital tissues.

CLINICAL FEATURES

The main feature of loiasis is *Calabar swellings*, which are painless, localized, transient, hot, soft-tissue swellings, often near joints. They persist for periods varying from a few hours to several weeks. They occur more commonly during the hotter months and may be preceded by numbness and tingling. They are produced by toxin released from the adult worm.

Urticaria, pruritus, lymphoedema, arthritis and chorioretinitis may occur.

A picture resembling meningoencephalitis that occurs only during treatment is thought to be an allergic reaction.

DIAGNOSIS

The worm can be seen in subcutaneous tissues or crossing the conjunctivae.

The characteristic microfilariae may be demonstrable in peripheral blood smears. Serological tests such as the complement-fixation test are also useful.

TREATMENT

Diethylcarbamazine (DEC) 2–6 mg·kg^{-1} is effective against both adult worms and microfilariae. Treatment should be continued for 2–3 weeks.

PREVENTION AND CONTROL

Prevention is best effected by adequate personal protection. In addition, houses should be sprayed with dieldrin. Mass treatment of all the inhabitants of villages with DEC 2 mg·kg^{-1} daily for 3 days has reduced the incidence of this disease.

Onchocerciasis

Onchocerciasis is produced by the filarial worm *Onchocerca volvulus*. The gravid female has a life-expectancy of 15 years. The microfilariae are found in the skin and subcutaneous tissue. Man is the only known definitive host and the day-biting female blackfly of genus *Simulium* is the vector; the species involved are *S. damnosum* and *S. naevi* in Africa and *S. metallicum* in Venezuela. The disease is confined to west, central and east Africa, Central and South America, and southern parts of Saudi Arabia.

CLINICAL FEATURES

The incubation period averages 1 year. Initially a papular, reddish, itchy rash develops. With repeated infections, characteristic subcutaneous nodules of various sizes appear. Usually they number fewer than 10 and are unevenly distributed over the body. In chronic disease, lichenification, xeroderma, pseudoichthyosis and atrophy of the skin occur. The nodules may be associated with the development of genital elephantiasis, hydrocele and the so-called 'hanging groin', in which large folds of wrinkled and thickened skin develop in the groin.

Ocular lesions represent the most serious manifestation of this disease and are the cause of up to 15% of the blindness in some areas. Initially the patient complains of lacrimation, photophobia and a foreign-body sensation in the eye. Conjunctivitis, iridocyclitis, chorioretinitis, secondary glaucoma and optic atrophy may occur. The eye lesions have been attributed to toxin production by the microfilariae and adult worms, mechanical irritation and hypersensitivity.

DIAGNOSIS

This is established by demonstrating microfilariae in snips of bloodless tissue obtained from the nodules and kept in saline for 30 min to 1 h before microscopic examination. The organism may also be identified in the anterior chamber of the eye by slit-lamp examination. Mazzotti's test is suggestive of the diagnosis and is positive if pruritus and a rash develop within a few hours of taking 50–100 mg of diethylcarbamazine (DEC) orally. Serological tests are not helpful in the indigenous population as the positivity rate is high. Eosinophilia occurs.

TREATMENT

In endemic areas not all people require treatment. The major indications for treatment are:

- The threat of eye damage
- Severe pruritus

Ivermectin, a new broad-spectrum antiparasitic drug is effective in filariasis and is now the drug of choice. A single dose of 150 µg·kg^{-1} orally produces a prolonged reduction in microfilarial levels. Annual re-treatment must be given until the adult worms die.

PREVENTION AND CONTROL

Prevention and control are confined to personal protection and attempts at destroying the vector. Chemoprophylaxis has not been found to be practical or effective.

DRACUNCULIASIS

Dracunculiasis (guinea worm infection) results from infection with *Dracunculus medinensis*. It is found sporadically throughout the tropics but is common in certain parts of India, central, east and west Africa, Pakistan, the Middle East, parts of South America and the eastern regions of the USSR.

Humans are the definitive host and are infected by ingestion of water containing infected *Cyclops*. The larvae are liberated in the human stomach by the action of acid. These penetrate the intestinal wall, where the male dies after fertilizing the female. The gravid female than wanders in connective tissue for several months before emerging through the skin. On reaching the skin, it elicits an allergic reaction with blister formation and later protrusion of the worm associated with the discharge of motile larvae. The larvae are then taken up by *Cyclops*, which once again are infective to man.

CLINICAL FEATURES

A generalized reaction can occur that is associated with nausea, vomiting, generalized urticaria and diarrhoea. These symptoms abate with rupture of the blister. Secondary bacterial infection, especially with streptococci, is common and results in cellulitis and abscess formation. In Nigeria, tetanus is a frequent complication. If attempts at extraction of the worm result in damage to it, intense cellulitis may occur. Arthritis, synovitis, ankylosis of joints and epididymitis are rare sequelae.

DIAGNOSIS

Keeping the appropriate part of the body immersed in water may induce the worm to wriggle out. Fluorescent antibody tests are useful. Radiography may reveal the presence of the worm.

TREATMENT

Gradual physical extraction of the worm by winding it carefully around a stick is the treatment of choice. It may take several days before the entire worm is extruded. Niridazole and thiabendazole are of questionable value in facilitating worm extrusion.

PREVENTION AND CONTROL

Prevention of this parasitosis is easily effected by chemically treating infected sources of water.

ANIMAL NEMATODES

Toxocariasis

Toxocariasis (visceral larva migrans) occurs worldwide and is caused by *Toxocara canis* or *T. cati*. The adult worm is found in the intestine of dogs and cats. The infective ova are passed in animal faeces and may be accidentally ingested by humans. The liberated larvae penetrate the intestinal wall and reach the liver and lung via the circulation. Epidemiologically, puppies are the most important natural hosts and the infection is most commonly seen in children between 1 and 4 years of age. Several viscera may be involved (visceral larva migrans) and the clinical manifestations are dependent on the organ involved and the intensity of infection. Eosinophilia is common. Urticaria and dermatitis may occur. With pulmonary involvement the presentation is that of bronchial asthma. Chest radiographs may reveal transient pulmonary infiltrates. Splenomegaly and hepatomegaly may occur. Rarely involvement of the myocardium and central nervous system may result in death. Eye involvement (ocular larva migrans) produces a retinoblastoma-like picture; other organs are usually spared.

DIAGNOSIS

The presence of marked eosinophilia, hepatomegaly, and elevated plasma IgG, IgM and IgE is suggestive, as is the identification of foreign-body eosinophilic granulomas in histological sections. Recently detection of specific antibodies by ELISA has been found to be useful.

TREATMENT

Treatment is difficult to evaluate in view of the mild nature of the illness and the tendency for spontaneous cure. Diethyl-carbamazine 2–6 mg·kg^{-1} daily in divided doses for 3 weeks or thiabendazole 25 mg·kg^{-1} twice daily for 5 days is probably effective.

Cutaneous larva migrans

Cutaneous larve migrans (creeping eruption) is a disease of the hot, humid areas of tropical and subtropical countries. It is caused by the dog and cat hookworms. *Ancylostoma braziliense* and *A. caninum* and, occasionally, the human parasites *A. duodenale*, *Necator americanus* and *Strongyloides stercoralis*, the adult forms of which are found in the intestine of the host (see p. 96). The filariform larve emerges from the ova passed in the faeces and penetrates intact human skin. An itchy papule develops at the site of larval entry. Two to three days later a markedly itchy, erythematous, serpiginous skin lesion develops. This is due to the larva, which migrates slowly at 1–2 mm per day. The skin over the lesion may vesiculate. Healing occurs by crusting. Although the lesions are more frequent on the lower limbs, any part of the body may be affected. Secondary bacterial infection may result in a mistaken diagnosis of pyoderma. The only systemic manifestations are transient pulmonary infiltrates and occasional breathlessness. Eosinophilia is seen.

TREATMENT

Thiabendazole applied locally as a 10% solution or given systemically (25 mg·kg^{-1} for 5 days) is effective.

Anisakiasis

Anisakiasis (herring worm disease) is caused by the larval stage of several species of *Anisakis*, and possibly of the related nematode *Phocanema*, which are found in abundance in herring, and dolphins, whales and other large sea mammals. The disease is prevalent in Japan and northern Europe, where raw herring and other raw fish are considered a delicacy. In Japan the illness is characterized by an acute gastric syndrome that presents as epigastric pain, nausea and vomiting. Upper gastrointestinal endoscopy may reveal the presence of larvae in the gastric mucosa. In contrast, in Europe the small intestine is predominantly involved and the patient presents with colicky, generalized abdominal pain and fever. Eosinophilia is unusual.

Trichinosis

This is caused by the intestinal nematode, *Trichi-nella spiralis*. The larval form is found in rats, hares, pigs, dogs and cats. Although cases of trichinosis have been reported from all parts of the world, it is found predominantly in the USA and Europe. It is uncommon in India. Transmission to humans occurs when improperly cooked meats, contaminated with infective larvae, are eaten.

CLINICAL FEATURES

Vomiting, diarrhoea, abdominal pain and headache occur 24–72 h after ingestion of contaminated meat. The severity of the clinical manifestations depends on the number of infecting larvae.

The larvae mature into the adult form in the intestine, where they reproduce and discharge larvae into the circulation. When these larvae migrate into the bloodstream and striated muscles (a stage that lasts 10–21 days), periorbital oedema, conjunctivitis, photophobia, fever with chills, and muscle pain and spasm occur. An urticarial rash, diarrhoea, dyspnoea and pleurisy may also occur. Myocardial and central nervous system involvement is unusual and, if it occurs, may result in death. In the next stage of development, larvae encyst in striated muscle. During encystment symptoms gradually subside, although weakness, muscle pain and cramps may persist for several months.

DIAGNOSIS

A firm diagnosis can be made on the clinical presentation, marked eosinophilia, and positive serology using ELISA. If necessary the diagnosis can be established by biopsying the deltoid or gastrocnemius muscle 3 weeks after the onset of illness and demonstrating the presence of the larvae.

TREATMENT

Analgesics, sedatives and bed rest are the mainstays of treatment. Steroids are indicated only in the presence of myocarditis, central nervous system involvement or marked allergic phenomena. Thiabendazole 25 mg·kg^{-1} body weight twice daily for 7 days is effective against intestinal worms and larvae.

INTESTINAL NEMATODE INFECTION (Table 1.42)

Some adult nematodes live within the intestinal lumen. The disease is spread to man (Fig. 1.31):

- Passively by ingesting infective eggs, as occurs with *Ascaris lumbricoides* ('roundworm'), *Trichuris trichiura* (whipworm) and *Enterobius vermicularis* (threadworm)

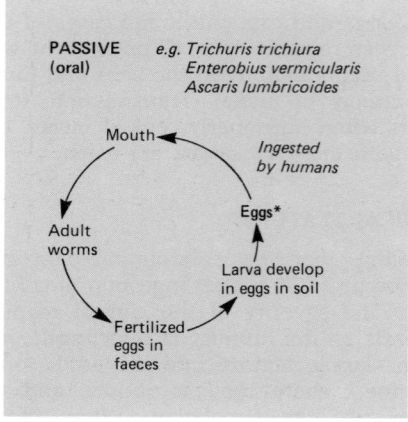
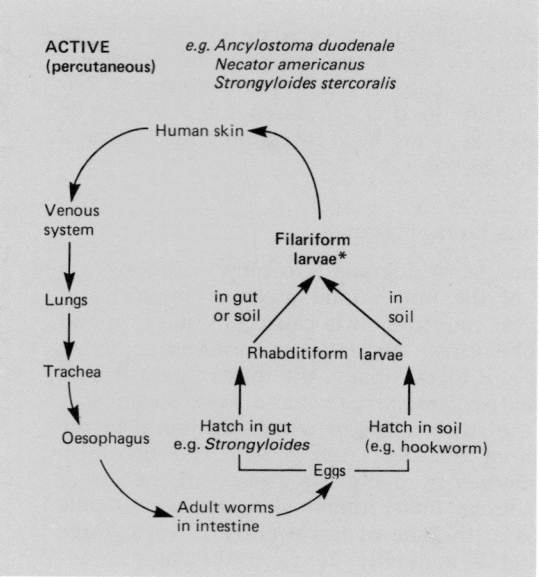

Fig. 1.31 Schematic life-cycles of intestinal nematodes.

● Actively by percutaneous spread of filariform larvae that penetrate the skin (hookworm and *Strongyloides*)

Ascaris deviates from the simplified life-cycle shown in Fig. 1.31 in that it invades the duodenum and enters the venous system, via which it reaches the lungs. The worm is eventually expectorated and swallowed, entering the intestine where it completes its maturation. *Strongyloides* is the only nematode that is able to complete its life-cycle in man; its rhabditiform larvae, which hatch in the intestine, are able to re-infect the host by penetrating the intestinal wall and entering the venous system.

Strongyloidiasis

Strongyloides stercoralis is found world-wide but is particularly common in warm, wet regions such as

parts of Central America and south-east Asia. Infection can persist for decades and is still being discovered in war veterans, particularly prisoners of war who worked on the Burma–Thailand railway and veterans from Vietnam. Adult worms inhabit the crypts of the small intestine, causing little damage, but in heavy infection worms are embedded in the mucosa, and cause an inflammatory response with mucosal injury. The worms are passed in the stools and autoinfection is common.

CLINICAL FEATURES

After penetration of the skin by the filariform larvae, a local reaction occurs characterized by itching, erythema, oedema and urticaria. This subsides within 2 days. A week later, migration of the adolescent worms causes irritation of the upper airways, producing cough and occasionally more

Table 1.42 Intestinal nematode (roundworm) infections.

Organism	Site	Clinical manifestations
Strongyloides stercoralis	Small intestine	Malabsorption
Hookworm: *Ancylostoma duodenale* and *Necator americanus*	Small intestine	Iron-deficiency anaemia
Capillaria philippinensis	Small intestine	Malabsorption
Ascaris lumbricoides ('roundworm')	Small intestine	? Undernutrition, intestinal obstruction
Trichuris trichiura (whipworm)	Large intestine	Usually nil, colitis, rectal prolapse
Enterobius vermicularis (threadworm)	Large intestine	Usually nil, pruritus ani

severe respiratory symptoms. After about 3 weeks, intestinal colonization occurs, often leading to abdominal discomfort, intermittent diarrhoea and constipation. These symptoms can be mild and may pass unnoticed. However, in some individuals, heavy infection may lead to persistent diarrhoea, nausea, anorexia and evidence of intestinal malabsorption, notably steatorrhoea. Hypoalbuminaemia and weight loss also occur. Disseminated strongyloidiasis is a very serious and often fatal condition and has been described in patients receiving corticosteroid or other immunosuppressive therapy or in those who are immunocompromised for other reasons.

DIAGNOSIS

Motile rhabditiform larvae can be detected in fresh stool or in duodenal aspirate. Eosinophilia is common. In heavy infection, anaemia and biochemical evidence of malabsorption are found.

TREATMENT

Treatment consists of thiabendazole 1.5 g twice daily for 2 days. Therapy should be given for at least 5 days (often longer) in the hyperinfected patient with disseminated disease. Albendazole is also effective. As the mortality is high in this group owing to an accompanying Gram-negative septicaemia, treatment should include i.v. broad-spectrum antibiotics.

Hookworm infection

Hookworm is seen world-wide and affects approximately 25% of the world's population. *Ancylostoma duodenale* is found in Europe, the Middle East and North Africa, whereas *Necator americanus* is found in the Western Hemisphere, sub-Saharan Africa, south-east Asia and the Far East.

Adult worms inhabit the small intestine and attach firmly to the intestinal mucosa by the teeth or cutting plates in their large buccal capsule. Blood loss is approximately 0.2 ml per day in *A. duodenale* infection (5- to 10-fold less with *N. americanus*); in heavy infection it has been estimated that up to 100 ml of blood is lost daily.

CLINICAL FEATURES

Local irritation at the site of larval entry in the skin is known as 'ground itch', but this rapidly disappears to be followed some 2 weeks later by mild and transitory pulmonary symptoms. Most patients are asymptomatic once the larvae have reached the small intestine. Some patients experience ulcer-like symptoms and those with heavy chronic infection eventually develop symptoms and signs of anaemia. Hookworm infection is the commonest cause of iron-deficiency anaemia world-wide.

DIAGNOSIS

Hookworm ova appear in the stool, the number of eggs present giving a guide to the severity of the infection. Early in the infection, eosinophilia may be found in the peripheral blood. This is followed later by the appearance of iron-deficiency anaemia.

TREATMENT

Mebendazole 100 mg twice daily for 3 days is effective in both types of hookworm, although the infection may not be cleared with a single course of treatment.

Ascaris lumbricoides ('roundworm') infection

Ascaris lumbricoides is a large worm that is found world-wide but is particularly common in poor rural communities where there is heavy faecal contamination of the immediate environment. Infection may be entirely asymptomatic, although heavy infections are associated with nausea, vomiting, abdominal discomfort and anorexia. Worms may obstruct the small intestine, the commonest site being at the ileocaecal valve. Worms occasionally invade the appendix, causing acute appendicitis, or the bile duct, resulting in biliary obstruction and suppurative cholangitis. The nutritional impact of *Ascaris* infection in children is controversial, although it is likely that heavy infection in malnourished children certainly compounds the situation, largely by competition for host nutrients.

DIAGNOSIS

Ascaris eggs may be identified in the stool and occasionally adult worms emerge from the mouth or the anus.

TREATMENT

Mebendazole 100 mg twice daily for 3 days or a single dose of piperazine (100 mg·kg^{-1}) or pyrantel pamoate (10 mg·kg^{-1}) are effective. Surgical intervention may be required for intestinal or biliary obstruction.

Trichuris trichiura (whipworm) infection

Trichuris trichiura is a common parasite and is found world-wide. Prevalence varies from 1% to 90%, being highest in poor communities with inadequate sanitation. Adult worms are most commonly found in the distal ileum and caecum, although in heavy infection no part of the colon is spared. The adult worm embeds its cephalic region into the intestinal mucosa, leaving the distal tail free within the lumen. Such invasion damages the intestinal mucosa and in heavy infection overt colonic and rectal ulceration may result, leading to significant blood and protein loss.

CLINICAL FEATURES

Most infections are asymptomatic and haematological or biochemical deficits do not occur provided nutritional intake is adequate. Heavy infection is associated with diarrhoea with blood and mucus, often associated with abdominal discomfort, tenesmus, anorexia and weight loss. Involvement of the appendix can cause appendicitis, and rectal prolapse has been reported in children.

DIAGNOSIS

Stool examination confirms the presence of typical barrel-shaped eggs. Proctosigmoidoscopy may reveal adult worms firmly attached to the rectal mucosa.

TREATMENT

Mebendazole (100 mg twice daily for 3 days) or a single dose of pyrantel pamoate (10 mg·kg^{-1}) are effective therapies.

Enterobius vermicularis (threadworm) infection

This parasite occurs world-wide but is more prevalent in temperate and cold climates. Children are most commonly infected, but it may affect whole families, inhabitants of residential institutions, and any group of people living in overcrowded circumstances. Adult worms reside largely in the colon, the female migrating to the anus to deposit embryonated eggs on the perianal and perineal areas. Superficial damage to the colonic mucosa occurs during heavy infection and secondary bacterial infection of these lesions may rarely result in submucosal abscesses.

CLINICAL FEATURES

Intense pruritus ani is usually the only symptom of threadworm infection. This is usually nocturnal and related to egg-laying in the perianal region by the female worms. Scratching results in dissemination of eggs and autoinfection. Infection has little significance while the parasite remains within the intestinal lumen, although on occasions migration occurs to the peritoneum and the viscera may be involved.

DIAGNOSIS

Diagnosis is best achieved by applying a piece of clear adhesive tape to the perianal region; this tape may then be examined microscopically for the presence of adherent eggs. Adult worms may be observed leaving the anus by the child's parents.

TREATMENT

A single dose of mebendazole 100 mg followed by a second dose 2 weeks later is usually effective. Alternatives include pyrantel pamoate or piperazine. Family members should also be treated.

Trematode (fluke) infections (Table 1.43)

BLOOD INFECTIONS

Schistosomiasis (bilharzia)

Three major species of schistosomes produce human disease. These have marked differences in geographical distribution (Fig. 1.32). Prevalence is dependent on the presence of a susceptible intermediate snail host and faecal contamination of water supplies. The size of snail populations varies with the season and availability of freshwater

Table 1.43 Trematode (fluke) infection.

Organism	Location	Major disease site(s)
Schistosoma mansoni	Mesenteric veins	Liver, colon
Schistosoma japonicum	Mesenteric veins	Liver, colon, small intestine
Schistosoma haematobium	Pelvic veins, vesical plexus	Bladder, distal colon, rectum
Fasciola hepatica	Bile ducts	Bile ducts, liver
Clonorchis sinensis	Bile ducts	Bile ducts, liver
Fasciolopis buski	Small intestine	Small intestine
Paragonimus westermani	Lung	Lung

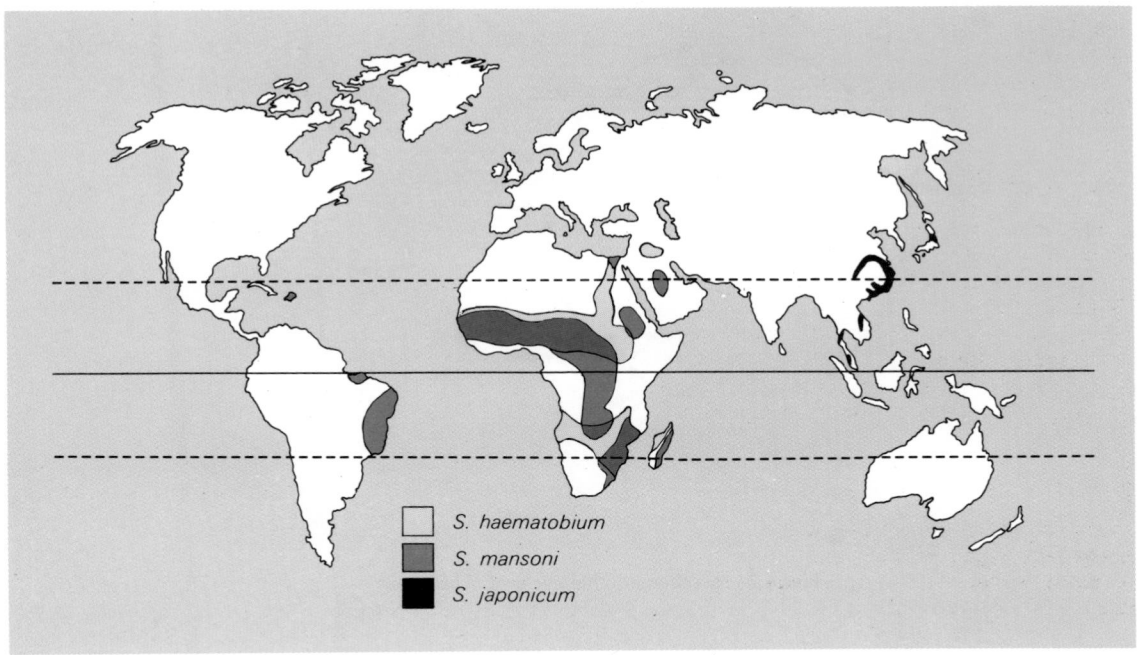

Fig. 1.32 The geographical distribution of *Schistosoma*.

breeding grounds. An increase in the world prevalence of schistosomiasis is partly due to dam construction and irrigation programmes.

LIFE-CYCLE AND PATHOGENESIS

Human infection occurs after penetration of the skin or mucous membranes by cercariae, the infective form of the parasite that is liberated into fresh water by the specific intermediate snail host (Fig. 1.33). Cercariae penetrate unbroken skin and migrate as schistosomules through the venous circulation to the liver, where the adult worms mature. Eventually pairs of male and female worms migrate upstream along the portal vein to the mesenteric venules, until the calibre of the vessels halts their progress. They remain in this location for many years copulating continuously and producing enormous numbers of eggs. To complete the life-cycle, eggs must leave the body, either by penetrating the intestinal wall (*Schistosoma mansoni* and *S. japonicum*) or the bladder wall (*S. haematobium*) and returning to the environment via faeces or urine, respectively. The larvae (miracidia) develop inside the eggs but do not hatch until they arrive in fresh water, when they search actively for the specific snail host to invade. Once inside the snail, multiplication occurs, a single miracidium producing up to a 100 000 cercariae released at the rate of 5000 per day.

Eggs retained in host tissues, particularly the liver, urinary bladder and intestine, are responsible for the clinical manifestations of schistosomiasis. Egg antigens initiate both immediate and delayed-type hypersensitivity reactions with granuloma formation. Humoral substances such as lymphokines, macrophage migration inhibitory factor and fibroblast stimulating factors are found at the site of these granulomas and presumably support the cellular inflammatory response. Healing eventually occurs by fibrosis.

CLINICAL FEATURES

The first clinical sign of an acute infection is a local inflammatory response at the site of the invading cercariae known as 'swimmer's itch'. Within a week or more there is a generalized allergic response characterized by fever, urticaria, eosinophilia, myalgia and malaise. Nausea, vomiting and profuse diarrhoea are common, as are respiratory symptoms, particularly cough. Clinical findings at this time include generalized lymphadenopathy, hepatosplenomegaly and signs of patchy pneumonia. In Asia the acute disease is called Katayama fever. It is most pronounced in infection with *S. japonicum* and *S. mansoni*.

Chronic schistosomiasis varies in its clinical presentation depending on the type of schistosome involved.

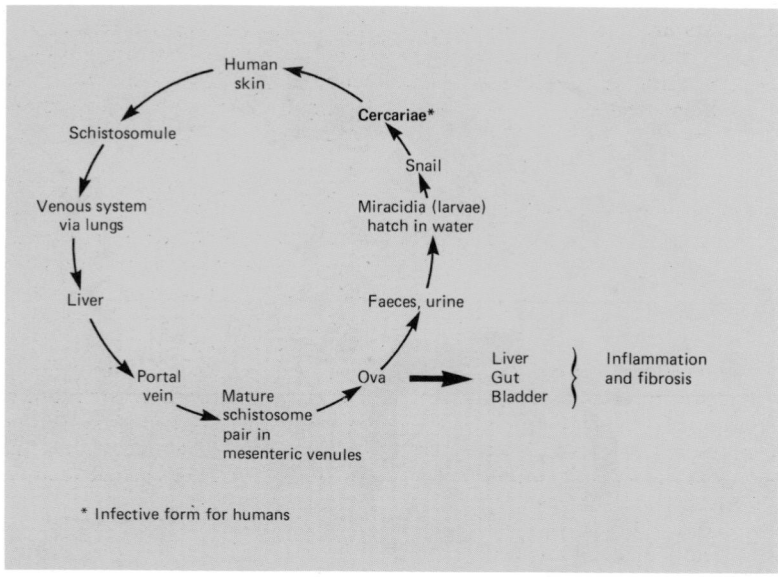

Fig. 1.33 A schematic life-cycle of *Schistosoma*.

S. mansoni and S. japonicum

S. mansoni is found predominantly in Africa, South America and the West Indies, whereas *S. japonicum* is common in China and other specific sites in South-East Asia.

S. mansoni predominantly affects the colon, where the presence of ova produces macroscopic lesions such as mucosal granularity, erythema and superficial ulceration. However, a particularly severe form of colonic disease is seen in Egyptians, with gross ulceration and polyp formation, particularly in the rectosigmoid; extensive polyposis results in significant blood and protein loss from the colon. Progressive fibrosis in the intestinal wall leads to rigidity and stricture formation, although intestinal obstruction is rare. A localized granulomatous reaction in the intestine (pseudotumour or bilharzioma) may be mistaken for a colonic cancer.

The development of granulomatous hepatitis, followed by progressive periportal fibrosis and portal hypertension, is signified by marked hepatosplenomegaly, often associated with oesophageal varices. In advanced cases death is due to the complications of portal hypertension, as hepatocellular function remains remarkably good.

S. japonicum affects the small intestine and proximal colon in addition to causing fibrotic liver disease. *S. japonicum* produces larger numbers of eggs than *S. mansoni*, which accounts for the more extensive pattern of disease and the frequency of ectopic deposition of ova, particularly in the lungs, spinal cord and brain. The latter may result in fits or hemiplegia.

Epithelial dysplasia in the colon has been reported in patients with chronic *S. japonicum* colitis, and it is now clear that this condition has premalignant potential in endemic areas.

S. haematobium

This is predominantly a urinary tract schistosome found predominantly in Egypt, east Africa and the Middle East. Chronic inflammation is found in the bladder, ureters and urethra, causing urinary frequency, dysuria and haematuria. Chronic infection leads to obstructive uropathy, chronic pyelonephritis and renal failure, and contraction of the bladder. Epidemiological studies confirm an association between bladder carcinoma and this infection. The internal genitalia may be involved and rectal inflammation and ulceration may be found in up to 70% of patients.

DIAGNOSIS

In endemic areas a confident diagnosis can often be obtained on clinical grounds. Confirmation is achieved by detecting the characteristic eggs in the stools, the urine or in a rectal biopsy. Different species of *Schistosoma* can be distinguished not only by the clinical pattern but also by egg morphology.

A plain abdominal radiograph may reveal intramural calcification in the wall of the bladder or the colon. Barium contrast studies of the colon show spiculating mucosal ulceration, polyposis, strictures, and possibly a mass lesion that could either be a bilharzioma or, in the case of *S. japonicum* infection, a carcinoma.

Intravenous urography may confirm an obstructive uropathy and demonstrate bladder contraction.

Immunodiagnostic tests are available, the most sensitive of which detect antibodies against a gut-associated polysaccharide antigen by either ELISA or by indirect immunofluorescence.

TREATMENT

The two major objectives of treatment of schisto-somiasis are:

- Reduction in egg production
- Prevention or reduction of tissue damage by eggs already *in situ*

In endemic and hyperendemic areas, curative therapy is usually inappropriate, since reinfection occurs rapidly, whereas infected individuals who are no longer exposed to the parasite can be effectively treated. Suppressive non-curative chemotherapeutic approaches have been used in mass treatment programmes in Egypt with good clinical improvement following a reduction in the 'worm burden'. All antischistosomal drugs have the same effect: they cause worms to leave the mesenteric and vesical veins and to enter the liver and lungs where they are eventually destroyed by host tissue responses.

Praziquantel is active against all species of schistosome and is probably the drug of choice as it is well tolerated and relatively free from serious side-effects. A single dose ($40 \text{ mg} \cdot \text{kg}^{-1}$) cures more than 90% of patients with *S. haematobium*, with slightly lower rates against *S. mansoni*. *S. japonicum* is best treated with a total dose of $60 \text{ mg} \cdot \text{kg}^{-1}$ given in divided doses over 1 or 2 days.

Oxamniquine is active against *S. mansoni* and metriphonate against *S. haematobium*. Niridazole has been superseded.

Colonoscopic polypectomy can control the number of colonic polyps, but surgery may be required to relieve obstructive uropathy and for inflammatory masses in the central nervous system.

LIVER AND BILIARY TRACT INFECTIONS

Fascioliasis

Fasciola hepatica infects sheep, goats and cattle, in which it produces liver disease, and is only accidentally transmitted to man via consumption of wild watercress grown on the grazing land of infected animals. The disease is found world-wide, including the United Kingdom. Animals excrete eggs in their faeces, from which ciliated miracidia emerge. These enter the freshwater snail (the intermediate host) in which larval development takes place. Eventually cercaria are released and these encyst on aquatic or surface vegetation.

After ingestion by a mammalian host, the parasites excyst, migrate through the intestinal wall and penetrate the liver capsule after traversing the peritoneal cavity. Immature flukes reach the bile duct by passing through liver parenchyma and after maturation begin to produce eggs. Adult flukes remain within the biliary tract for many years.

CLINICAL FEATURES

Early symptoms of intermittent fever, malaise, weight loss, right upper quadrant pain and urticaria relate to migration of flukes through the liver and generally occur 2–3 months after infection.

A second phase of the illness relates to the presence of flukes in the biliary tract, where they can cause obstruction with jaundice and cholangitis, although infection may remain asymptomatic. Flukes have been found in many ectopic sites, including lung, brain and skin.

DIAGNOSIS

Eosinophilia is common in the early phase of the illness and is often associated with liver biochemical abnormalities and a positive complement fixation test. Ova are not found in the stool until the second phase of the illness when the mature flukes are established in the biliary tract. However, in up to 30% of cases, stools remain negative; the diagnosis can then be confirmed either by identifying ova in duodenal aspirate or by serological tests. Treatment is with bithionol $30–50 \text{ mg} \cdot \text{kg}^{-1}$ for 10–15 doses given either daily or on alternate days.

Clonorchiasis

Clonorchis sinensis is a common fluke of the dog, cat and pig that affects millions of animals in the Far East, particularly Indochina, Japan, Korea, Hong Kong and Vietnam. A related fluke, *Opisthorchis felineus*, also affects foxes and is found predominantly in India, the Philippines, Korea and Japan. The life-cycles of both these flukes are similar to that of *Fasciola hepatica*, except that freshwater fish become infected by the cercaria and thereby function as a second intermediate host. Human infection occurs by ingestion of infected raw fish.

CLINICAL FEATURES

Infected individuals may remain symptom-free, although prolonged exposure with heavy infection results in recurrent cholestatic jaundice, suppurative cholangitis, liver abscess and cholangiocarcinoma.

DIAGNOSIS

The diagnosis is made on microscopic examination of faeces or duodenal aspirate.

TREATMENT

Praziquantel 25 mg·kg^{-1} as a single dose is the treatment of choice.

INTESTINAL INFECTIONS

Fasciolopsiasis

Fasciolopsis buski causes intestinal infection in man and pigs. There are two intermediate hosts— freshwater snails and water plants. Human infection is initiated by oral contact with contaminated water plants. These large flukes, which are several centimetres in length, are common in China, Vietnam, Thailand and Taiwan.

Mucosal ulceration and inflammation are apparent at the site of attachment in the intestine; abscess formation, haemorrhage and occasionally bowel obstruction may result. The symptoms are usually non-specific. Heavy infection in children may simulate or precipitate protein–energy malnutrition. Anaemia and eosinophilia are common.

DIAGNOSIS

The diagnosis may be simple if the patient is vomiting or passing flukes per rectum, but may be confirmed by identifying ova in the stools.

TREATMENT

Treatment is with tetrachloroethylene 0.12 ml·kg^{-1} as a single dose (maximum dose of 5 ml) or dichlorophen 100 mg·kg^{-1} as a single dose (which may be repeated 1 week later).

Cestode (tapeworm) infections

Tapeworms belong to the subclass Cestoda. These are flat worms measuring from a few millimetres (*Echinococcus granulosus*) to several metres in length (*Taenia saginata*). Structurally they consist of a head that is adorned with suckers and hooks (*Taenia solium*) or suckers alone (*T. saginata*). The head is attached via a short slender neck to several segments or proglottids that form a chain-like structure or strobila. The terminal proglottid is the most mature. The entire worm is covered with a continuous elastic cuticle. Tapeworms are devoid of a gastrointestinal tract or vascular system; nutrients are absorbed directly through the cuticle. They are hermaphrodites and cross-fertilization between proglottids is frequent.

Adults live in the intestinal tract of vertebrates, whereas the larvae (oncospheres) exist in the

tissues of vertebrates and invertebrates. Infection is transmitted to humans by ingestion of meats infected with larval forms. Four tapeworms commonly infect humans: *T. saginata*, *T. solium*, *Diphyllobothrium latum* and *Hymenolepis nana*.

Taenia saginata (beef tapeworm) infection

T. saginata measures up to 10 m in length, inhabits the upper jejunum, and is prevalent in humans in all beef-eating countries. The majority of patients are asymptomatic. Symptoms are mild, with vague epigastric and abdominal pain, and occasional diarrhoea and vomiting. Weight loss is unusual. Rarely, appendicitis and pancreatitis due to obstruction of the appendix and pancreatic ducts, respectively, by the adult worms may occur. The commonest symptom is the presence of proglottids in the faeces, bed or underclothing.

DIAGNOSIS

The presence of proglottids, which are visible macroscopically, or the eggs, which are seen microscopically, in the faeces or perianal region is diagnostic. A higher positive yield is obtained by examining perianal clear adhesive tape swabs for ova, in which case the scolex (the head) or proglottids are required to establish the species.

TREATMENT

Praziquantal 10 mg·kg^{-1} as a single dose is probably the treatment of choice. Niclosamide 2 g as a single chewed dose is also effective.

PREVENTION

Prevention is easily effected by careful inspection of beef for cysticerci (encysted larval forms). Refrigeration of beef at $-10°C$ for 5 days or cooking it at $57°C$ for a few minutes destroys the cysticerci.

Taenia solium infection and cysticercosis

Taenia solium (the pork tapeworm) measures up to 6 m in length. It has a world-wide distribution but is seen most frequently in eastern Europe, South-East Asia and Africa. In the adult form it lives in the human upper jejunum. The clinical features are similar to those caused by *T. saginata*.

Treatment is similar to that for *T. saginata*. However, because release of ova can occur during treatment and, theoretically, these could be carried back into the stomach, releasing the intermediate larval stage, treatment for *T. solium* should be followed by a saline purge.

Human cysticercosis
Cysticercosis occurs after autoinfection or hetero-infection by eggs of *T. solium* and invasion of

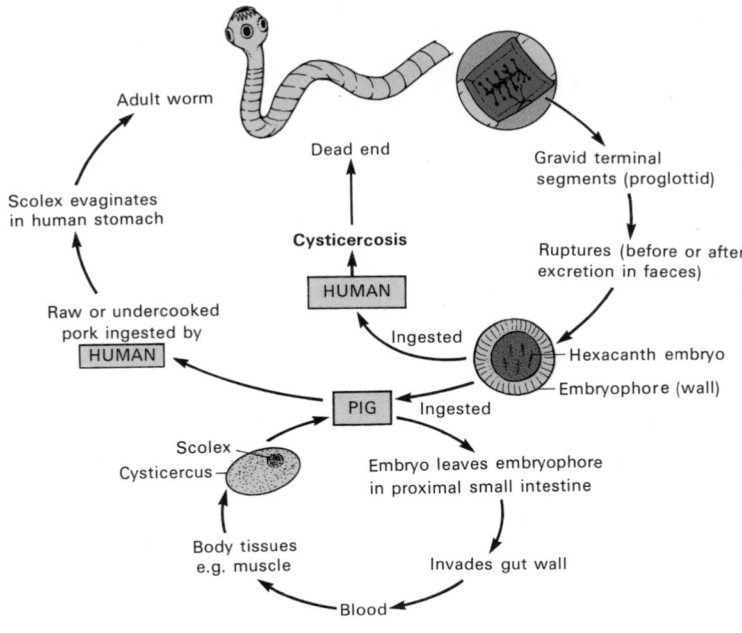

Fig. 1.34 A schematic life-cycle of *Taenia solium*.

tissues by the intermediate larval form *Cysticercus cellulosae* (Fig. 1.34). Cysticercosis is most commonly seen in parts of Asia, Africa and South America. Cysticerci may develop in any tissue in the body. Most commonly, however, three clinical forms are recognized:

- *Cerebral cysticercosis* may present as various forms of epilepsy, as a space-occupying lesion or as focal neurological deficits including hemiplegia and behavioural changes.
- *Ocular cysticercosis* may present as retinitis, uveitis, conjunctivitis or choroidal atrophy. Blindness may ensue.
- *Subcutaneous cysticercosis* presents as small, pea-sized, hard nodules in the subcutaneous tissue.

The diagnosis is established by biopsying a subcutaneous nodule and demonstrating the characteristic translucent membrane. Radiography may demonstrate calcified degenerating cysticerci. CT brain scan should be performed when subcutaneous cysticercosis has been diagnosed. Indirect haemagglutination tests are useful.

Treatment involves surgical excision of the cysticerci. Praziquantel is the drug of choice for cysticercosis.

Diphyllobothrium latum infection

Diphyllobothriasis is particularly prevalent in Scandinavian countries, the Baltic region, Japan and the lake region of Switzerland. Infection in humans, the definitive host, results from ingestion of fish that contain the infective plerocercoid form. The adult tapeworm measures several metres in length. The proglottids differ from those of *Taenia* in that they are more wide than long. The adult worm usually attaches itself to the jejunum.

The clinical features are usually mild and consist of vague abdominal discomfort, anorexia, nausea and vomiting. Megaloblastic anaemia, due to competitive utilization of ingested vitamin B_{12} by the parasite, may occur in a small percentage of patients. Rarely, intestinal obstruction occurs.

Treatment is similar to that described for *T. saginata*.

Hydatid disease

Hydatid disease occurs when humans ingest the hexacanth embryos of the dog tapeworm, *Echinococcus granulosus* or of *E. multilocularis*.

Human infection with *E. granulosus* frequently occurs in early childhood by direct contact with infected dogs, or by eating uncooked, improperly washed vegetables contaminated with infected canine faeces. In the duodenum the hexacanth embryos hatch, penetrate the intestinal wall, enter the portal system and are then carried to the liver. Further dissemination of embryos to the lung and

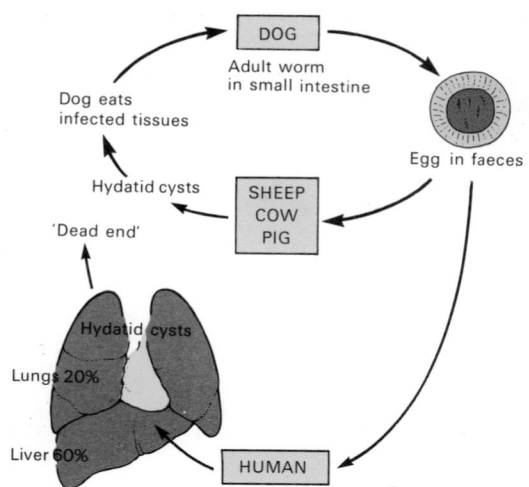

Fig. 1.35 A schematic life-cycle of *Echinococcus granulosus*.

to almost every organ in the body may occur, where they form hydatid cysts (Fig. 1.35). The disease is seen in all parts of the world, particularly in those countries where sheep and cattle-raising constitutes an important means of livelihood. These animals perpetuate the life-cycle of the parasite.

Symptoms largely depend upon the site of the unilocular hydatid cyst. The liver is the commonest site for cyst formation (60%), followed by the lung (20%), kidneys (3%) and brain (1%). In the liver the majority of cysts are situated in the right lobe. The symptoms are those of a slowly growing benign tumour. Pressure on the bile ducts may cause jaundice. Rupture into the abdominal cavity, pleural cavity or biliary tree may occur. In the latter instance, intermittent jaundice, abdominal pain

and fever associated with eosinophilia result. A cyst rupturing into a bronchus may result in its expectoration and spontaneous cure, but if secondary infection supervenes a chronic pulmonary abscess will form. Haemoptysis, dyspnoea and chest pain may lead to a mistaken diagnosis of malignancy. Focal seizures may occur if cysts are present in the brain. Renal involvement produces lumbar pain and haematuria. Calcification of the cyst occurs in about 40% of cases.

The alveolar hydatid cyst caused by *E. multilocularis* results from its larval stage. *E. multilocularis* is seen in parts of Canada, the USSR, and Alaska. Foxes and small rodents constitute the intermediate hosts; humans are accidental hosts. The majority of the lesions are in the liver and metastasis may occur.

The diagnosis and treatment of hydatid disease are described on p. 276.

Further reading

Bannister B (1983) *Infectious Diseases*. London: Baillière Tindall.

Braude AI (1985) *Infectious Diseases and Medical Microbiology*, 2nd edn. Philadelphia: WB Saunders.

Farthing MJG & Keusch GT (1989) *Enteric Infection: Mechanisms, Manifestations and Management*. London: Chapman and Hall.

Mandel GL, Douglas RG & Bennett JE (1985) *Principles and Practice of Infectious Diseases*, 2nd edn. New York: John Wiley.

Manson-Bahr PEC & Bell D (1987) *Manson's Tropical Diseases*, 19th edn. London: Baillière Tindall.

Youmans, GP, Paterson PY & Sommers HM (eds) (1985) *The Biologic and Clinical Basis of Infectious Diseases*, 3rd edn. Philadelphia: WB Saunders.

2

The Basics of Genetics, Molecular and Cell Biology and Immunology

Before these disorders are considered the basic mechanisms will first be described.

A glossary of terms commonly used in genetics can be found on p. 148.

Molecular basis of genetics

Genetic information is stored in the form of double-stranded DNA. Each strand of DNA is made up of a deoxyribose phosphate backbone and a series of purine [adenine (A) and guanine (G)] and pyrimidine [thymine (T) and cytosine (C)] bases. The two strands of DNA are held together by hydrogen bonds between the bases. As T always pairs with A, and G with C, there are only four possible pairs of nucleotides—TA, AT, GC and CG. The nucleus of each diploid cell contains 6×10^9 base pairs worth of DNA and of this 5×10^6 are likely to be transcriptionally active. DNA in a cell is coiled around histone proteins to form nucleosomes and further condensed into chromosomes that are seen at metaphase.

Three adjacent nucleotides (a codon) code for a particular amino acid—e.g. AGA for arginine, TTC for phenylalanine. There are only 20 common amino acids but 64 possible codon combinations that make up the genetic code. This means that some amino acids are coded by more than one triplet; other codons are used as signals for 'initiating' or 'terminating' polypeptide-chain synthesis, while others read as 'nonsense' and no amino acid is produced.

GENES

A gene is a portion of DNA that codes for a single polypeptide sequence (called a cistron). There are two main types:

- *Structural genes*, which are responsible for syn-

This chapter serves as an introduction and describes the essential facts required for an understanding of genetics, molecular biology and immunology.

Only the broad mechanisms of pathogenesis of diseases are discussed here but *details of the abnormalities found within each disease state are discussed with the clinical findings elsewhere in this book.*

Genetics, molecular and cell biology

Introduction

Genetic disorders are assuming a greater importance since our increased understanding of molecular biology. Very few genetic disorders can be treated effectively and the emphasis is towards prenatal diagnosis and genetic counselling.

Human diseases can be due to entirely genetic or environmental causes (unifactorial) or to a combination of both factors (multifactorial).

Genetic disorders can be divided into:

- *Unifactorial* genetic disorders—usually due to single gene defects. These disorders are numerous, although each individual disorder is rare. There is a clear pattern of inheritance with a high risk to relatives.
- *Multifactorial*. These are common, have no clear pattern of inheritance and there is a low risk to relatives.
- *Chromosomal* defects are rare and have no clear pattern of inheritance. There is a low risk to relatives.

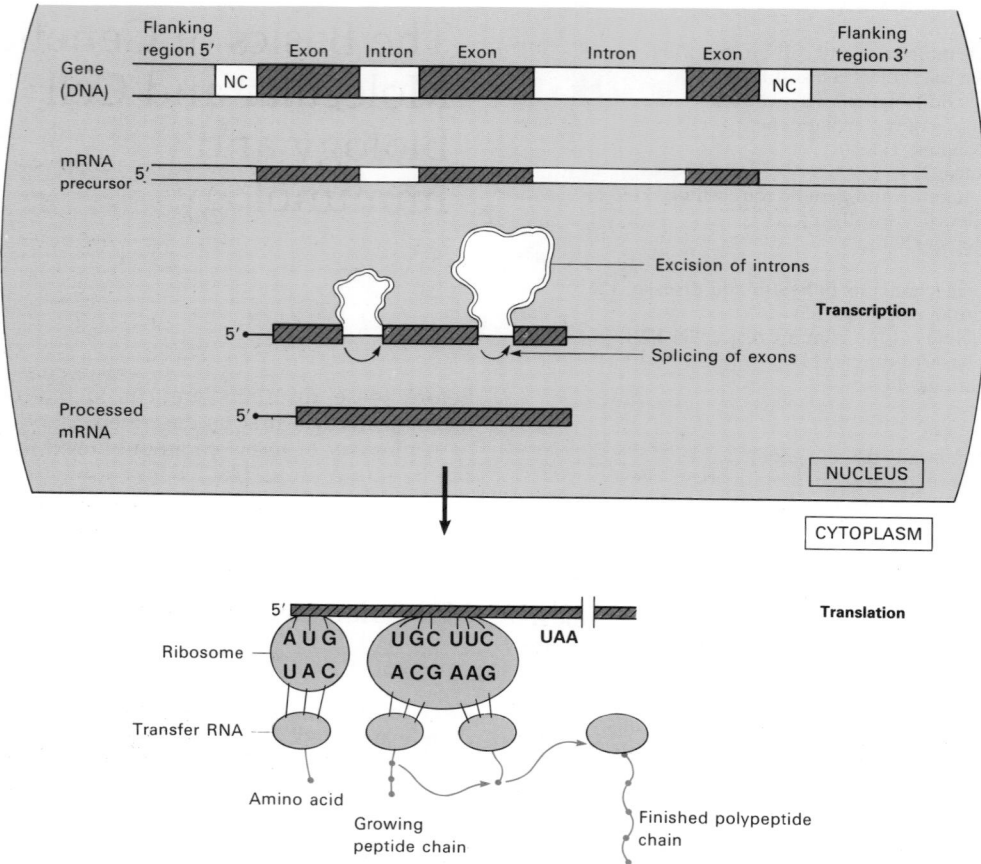

Fig. 2.1 Genetic control of protein synthesis. NC = non-coding; mRNA = messenger RNA; AUG = 'start' coding sequence; UAA = 'stop' coding sequence.

thesis of specific proteins, e.g. enzymes, haemoglobin and collagen
- *Control genes*, which are thought to modify the action of structural genes

Genes consist of lengths of DNA that contain sufficient nucleotide triplets to code for the appropriate number of amino acids in the polypeptide chains of a particular protein. However, these coding sequences (called exons) are interrupted by intervening sequences (IVS) that are non-coding (called introns) at various positions (see below).

TRANSCRIPTION AND TRANSLATION (Fig. 2.1)

Genetic information is carried from the nucleus to the cytoplasm by messenger RNA (mRNA), which acts as a template for protein synthesis. RNA is found mainly in the nucleolus and cytoplasm and is similar in structure to DNA except that thymine is replaced by uracil (U).

Each base in the mRNA molecule is lined up opposite to the corresponding base in the DNA—C to G, G to C, T to A and A to U (instead of T).

This initial mRNA is a complete transcription of one strand of DNA and therefore contains both introns and exons. Before leaving the nucleus, the introns are excised and the exons are spliced together. The mRNA migrates out of the nucleus into the cytoplasm. Polysomes (groups of ribosomes) become attached to the mRNA; these will carry the growing peptide chain. This definitive mRNA now has the exact coding sequence for the order of amino acids in a polypeptide chain. It also contains specific 'start' (e.g. AUG) and 'stop' (e.g. UAA) codons, which determine the points of initiation and termination of peptide-chain synthesis.

In the cytoplasm each molecule of transfer RNA (tRNA) is specific for one amino acid and has three unpaired nucleotide bases (the anti-codon) that correspond to the appropriate codons of the mRNA.

The mRNA therefore can act as a template—a particular codon in the mRNA is related through the tRNA to specific amino acids. The ribosome moves along the mRNA like a 'zipper', linking the assembled amino acids to form a polypeptide chain (protein synthesis).

The regulation of protein synthesis is extremely complex and not entirely understood. The rates of transcription and protein production are thought to be regulated by sequences in the 'flanking' regions at each end of the genes. The NC (non-coding) region directs the production of mRNA regions that are not translated into a protein product.

CHANGES IN DNA (MUTATIONS)

Changes in DNA are random and can be inherited. Many different types are recognized e.g. point mutations, insertions, deletions, rearrangements, duplications, gene fusion and gene invasion.

Substitution

This is the simplest type of change and involves the substitution of one base or one triplet for another. For example, the triplet AAA, which codes for phenylalanine, may become AGA, which codes for serine.

Whether a substitution produces a clinical disorder or not depends on whether it results in a change in a critical part of the protein molecule produced. Fortunately, many substitutions have no effect on the function or stability of the proteins produced as several triplets code for the same amino acid. However, in others the effects may be severe; for example, in sickle cell disease a change in the DNA results in the substitution of valine for glutamic acid and the production of HbS rather than HbA. Over 300 variants of haemoglobin have been described, as single amino-acid changes can alter the electrophoretic mobility of the haemoglobin molecule. Many others, however, remain undetected, as some substitutions do not alter the protein sufficiently to change the electrophoretic mobility.

Other examples include glucose-6-phosphate deficiency in Africans, which is known to result from the production of an enzyme variant with a single amino-acid mutation. DNA substitution is also seen in a rare form of diabetes in which a change in a single amino acid prevents the normal cleavage of pro-insulin to insulin.

Insertion or deletion

Insertion or deletion of one or more bases is a more serious change, as it results in the alteration of the rest of the following sequence (frame-shift). For example, if the original code was:

TAA GGA GAG TTT

and the third nucleotide (A) is deleted, the sequence becomes:

TAG GAG AGT TT . . .

Deletions of part or all of the structural gene cause changes in amino-acid sequences. This type of change is responsible for some forms of thalassaemia and deletion in the dystrophin gene results in Duchenne muscular dystrophy.

Normal chain termination occurs when the ribosomes on the mRNA reach one of the chain termination codons (e.g. UAA, UAG or UGA). Mutations can involve these termination codons as well. For example, premature termination may occur when a coding sequence for 'termination' of a polypeptide chain is produced by a mutation. Alternatively, a chain may not terminate correctly when instead of the sequence reading 'stop' it allows the insertion of another amino acid. Haemoglobin Constant Spring—a haemoglobin variant—is formed when, instead of the 'stop' sequence, there is a single base change allowing the insertion of an extra amino acid.

Analysis and isolation of genes

TECHNIQUES OF DNA ANALYSIS

Applications

DNA analysis is mainly carried out for:

- Prenatal diagnosis of Mendelian disorders
- Detecting carriers of X-linked recessive disorders
- The pre-symptomatic diagnosis of autosomal dominant disorders

It may clarify the diagnosis in genetic disorders associated with specific mutations or gene deletions. Index cases are usually diagnosed by conventional methods, e.g. haemoglobin electrophoresis for thalassaemia or a muscle biopsy for Duchenne muscular dystrophy.

Techniques for DNA analysis include both biochemical and bacteriological steps and involve:

- The isolation of a human gene from cells
- Its incorporation into a vector, e.g. a plasmid, bacteriophage or cosmid (recombinant step)
- The introduction of the vector into an organism, e.g. a bacterium
- The production of multiple 'copies' of the gene (cloning)
- Subsequent selection and harvesting

Amino-acid sequencing techniques for DNA permit positive identification of the gene under study.

DNA extraction. DNA can be extracted from any nucleated cell and can be stored indefinitely (particulary useful for family studies) as it is stable. In practice 10–20 ml of whole blood (white cells) or chorionic villus material are used.

DNA fragmentation and electrophoresis. Genomic DNA can be cut into a number of fragments by *restriction enzymes* obtained from bacteria. These restriction endonucleases are bacterial enzymes that recognize their own individually specific DNA sequence and cleave double-stranded DNA at these sites. For example, the DNA of the micro-organism *Escherichia coli* RY 13 is cleaved by the restriction enzyme Eco RI at the points indicated below:

$$5' \text{ G} \downarrow \text{AATTC } 3'$$
$$3' \text{ CTTAA} \uparrow \text{G } 5'$$

These fragments can be separated by electrophoresis, with smaller fragments migrating faster down the agarose gel. The gel denatures DNA into single strands. Fragment size can be determined by using known markers on the gel.

Southern blotting (Fig. 2.2). The above DNA fragments are transferred on to a nitrocellulose filter (placed on top of the gel) by fluid rising through the gel. DNA sticks very firmly to the filter. DNA fragments can be analysed by mixing with a DNA probe (see below) in a hybridization reaction.

Molecular hybridization. A fundamental property of

strands of DNA is that when two strands are separated, e.g. by heating, they will always re-associate and stick together again because of their complementary base sequences. The presence or position of a particular gene can therefore be identified using a gene 'probe' consisting of DNA with a base sequence that is complementary to that of the gene.

Gene probes and gene cloning. A probe is a piece of single-stranded DNA, radiolabelled with [32]P. Complementary DNA (cDNA) probes can be synthesized from the messenger RNA of the gene under study using reverse transcriptase. They can be cloned by incorporating the DNA fragment (not whole genes) into vector DNA such as a bacterial plasmid (Fig. 2.3). *Plasmids* are extremely simple organelles that live and replicate in the cytoplasm of bacteria. They consist of a circular ring of DNA that can be cleaved by a specific restriction endonuclease to produce a linear structure.

The DNA for insertion into a vector is broken up by using restriction enzymes and is mixed with the plasmids and joined by a ligase. Some plasmids in the mixture now incorporate the foreign DNA and re-form into circular structures (see Fig. 2.3). These re-formed plasmids and some suitable bacteria are then mixed together and a small proportion of the plasmids will enter the bacterial cytoplasm. These bacteria can be selected out by different techniques; for example, the plasmid may confer antibiotic resistance to the bacteria and this

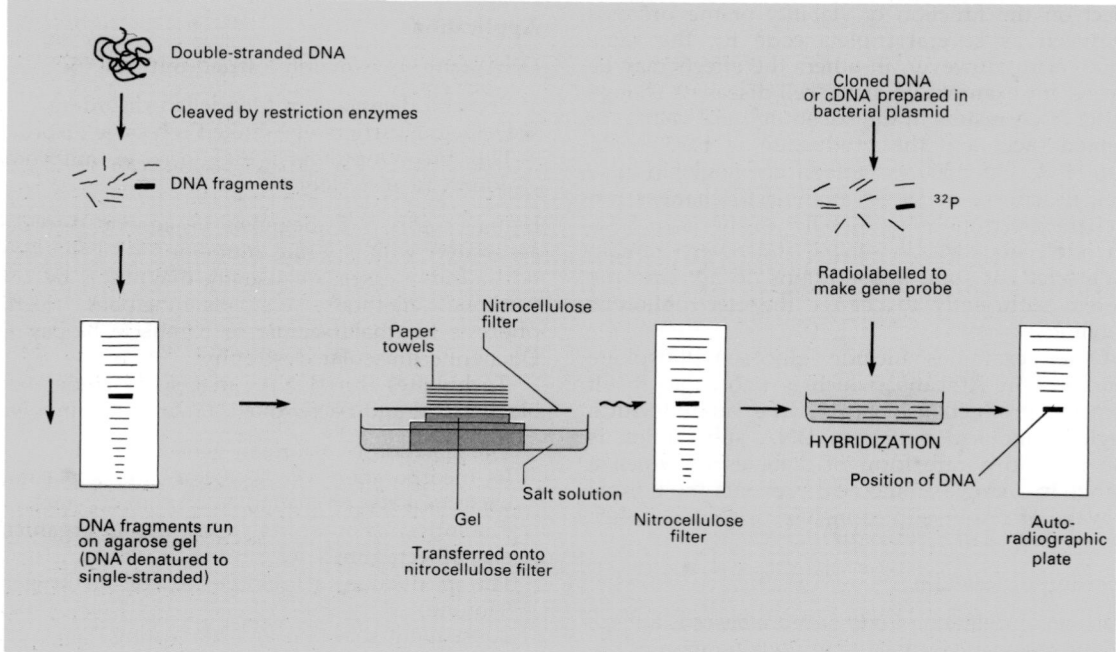

Fig. 2.2 Techniques of Southern blotting, showing detection of a specific DNA gene using a specific radiolabelled DNA probe.

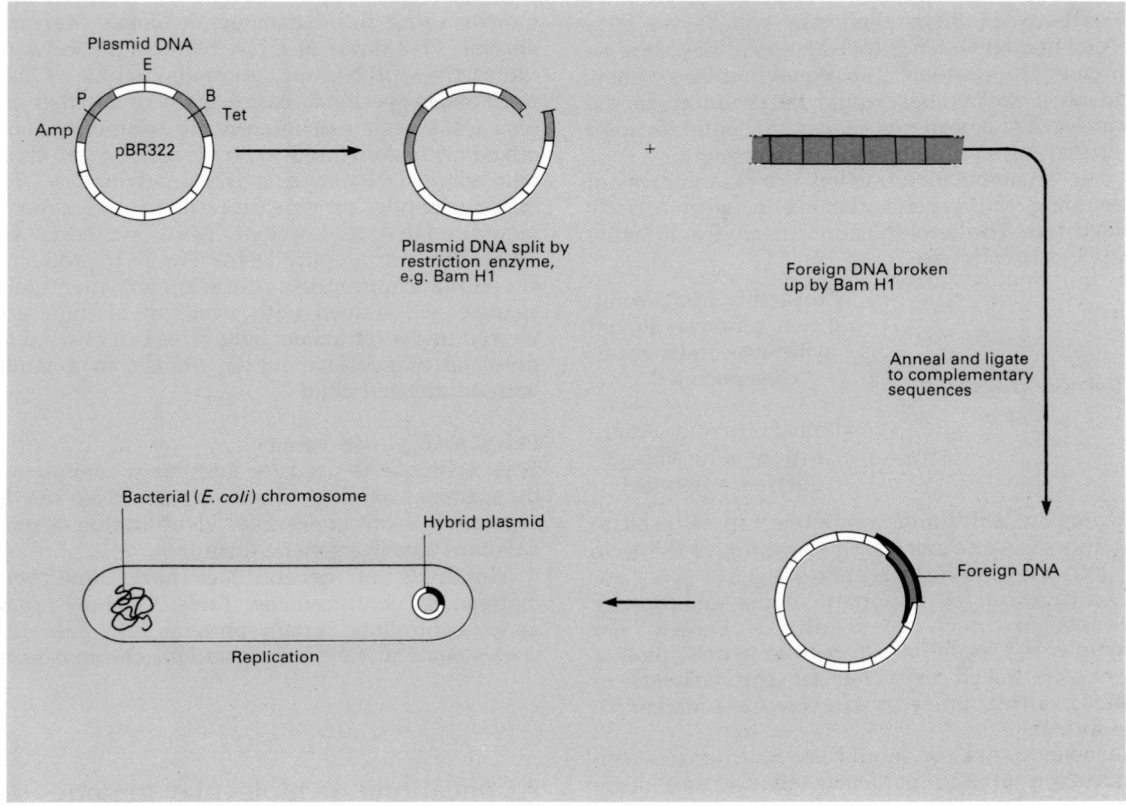

Fig. 2.3 Recombinant DNA technique, showing incorporation of foreign DNA into a plasmid. Amp, ampicillin resistance; Tet, tetracycline resistance. Restriction enzyme sites: B = Bam H1; E = Eco R1; P = Pst 1.

can be detected on culture. Using the technique of hybridization, bacterial colonies can be screened to search for the particular clone that contains the inserted DNA. If one is found it can be grown in large quantities to produce the required DNA.

DNA probe hybridization (gene mapping)
The manufactured radiolabelled probe is added to the solution for hybridization with the nitrocellular filter blotted with the patient's DNA. The probe will bind to a matching DNA sequence and this can be identified by using autoradiography. By using different enzymes for cleavage it is possible to build up restriction enzyme maps of appropriate areas of the genome.

A similar technique using RNA fragments is known as 'Northern blotting', and one using virus polypeptides that can be reacted with specific antibody is called 'Western blotting'.

Gene libraries
There are now gene libraries and banks of cloned DNA fragments with known sequences growing in suitable hosts such as *E. coli*. This allows easy identification of individual genes for given amino-

acid sequences and the manufacture of probes for gene mapping.

Gene sequencing
The structure of individual genes can be determined by rapid methods for sequencing the base pairs. In principle, [^{32}P] DNA is divided into aliquots, each of which is treated with a different chemical to produce a different purine or pyrimidine or combinations of these, e.g. G, A + G, C + T, C. These are then separated electrophoretically and the sequence is read off on a radiograph of the gel. This method has been used for the identification of many single-gene disorders.

Genetic linkage and analysis
Loci on the same chromosomes are said to be syntenic. If the loci occupied by two genes are very close together then it is less likely that they will be separated during the crossing-over process during meiosis and will therefore be transmitted together, i.e. closely linked. Crossing-over is random along the chromosome and may take place at different points in successive meiosis. If the loci are far enough apart always to have one or more cross-

overs between them, then they will have a 50% recombination which is the same as if they were on different chromosomes, i.e. equal numbers of new and old combinations would be produced in the gametes. Thus, syntenic genes sufficiently far apart will also have an independent assortment.

The 'recombination fraction' is a practical way of describing the genetic distance between closely linked loci. The recombination fraction in a family can be calculated as:

$$\text{Relative probability (linkage)} = \frac{\text{Probability of a sibship if two genes are linked with a recombination frequency } \theta}{\text{Probability of a sibship if there is no linkage between two loci}}$$

Calculation tables and computers can be used to produce, for convenience, a logarithm of the ratio or 'lod' score (from logarithm odds).

Linkage can be important in the detection of diseases in which no marker is known. For example, if a locus for a particular genetic disease is closely linked to a normal chromosomal or genetic variant, the latter can serve as a marker for the former.

However, linkage should not be confused with association of two particular diseases, as some genes have considerable protein polymorphisms.

Linkage disequilibrium is described under HLA histocompatibility antigens on p. 119.

Restriction fragment length polymorphisms (RFLPs)
DNA is composed of coding and non-coding sequences, and variations (point mutations) are common in the latter regions. When these variations in the non-coding regions affect the restriction enzyme cleavage sites, digestion will produce DNA fragments of *different* sizes (restriction fragment length polymorphisms). RFLPs are common and if they occur in or near a known gene they can be used as markers for a particular genetic disorder. If a person is heterozygous for an RFLP, there will be two different band patterns for each of a pair of chromosomes. Thus, a single chromosome region can be tracked through a family. Before this can be done, however, a family must have DNA analysis performed to see whether there is indeed a variation in the fragment size detected by a specific probe; the particular fragment must then be identified and looked for in relatives or in a pregnancy. For example, RFLPs can be used in Huntington's chorea, where the gene on chromosome 4 has not yet been cloned and the DNA polymorphism is close to the disease gene.

Polymerase chain reaction (PCR)
Small amounts of DNA can be amplified enor-

mously using this technique. It allows the rapid analysis (1–2 days) of DNA without the need for radioactive probes or autoradiography. Oligonucleotides specific to base sequences at either end of a DNA region of interest are synthesized and mixed with denatured genomic DNA (e.g. chorionic villus DNA) and a DNA polymerase. The oligonucleotide primers anneal to the complementary DNA and initiate DNA synthesis and replication and amplify DNA. The PCR product is cut with the appropriate restriction enzyme, run on agarose gel, stained with ethidium bromide and viewed under ultraviolet light. This can be used for pre-natal diagnosis of cystic fibrosis in a family with an affected child.

Pulsed field gel electrophoresis
This technique is used for long-range mapping of the genome as large fragments of DNA can be separated. It can be used for identification of gene deletions causing genetic disorders.

Hundreds of genetic loci have now been mapped on chromosomes. Table 2.1 shows some genes controlling certain proteins and Table 2.2 shows some disease loci on various chromosomes.

Applications of molecular genetics

The use of molecular biological techniques in genetics will undoubtedly have a large impact on the investigation, diagnosis, treatment and control

Table 2.1 Chromosomal localization of genes controlling certain proteins.

Chromosome	
1	Rhesus blood group
	Duffy blood group
5	Haemopoietic growth factors (some)
6	Major histocompatibility complex
	HLA-A, B, C, D
	Properdin factor B
	Complement 4
7	Erythropoietin
9	ABO blood groups
11	β, γ and δ globin chains of haemoglobin
	Insulin
14	α-1-Antitrypsin
16	Haptoglobin
	α-Globin chain of Hb
19	Complement C3

Table 2.2 Examples of some disorders with known chromosomal localization.

Chromosome	
1	Elliptocytosis Gaucher's disease types I, II and III
4	Huntington's chorea
5	Familial adenomatous polyposis
6	Haemochromatosis 21-Hydroxylase deficiency
7	Cystic fibrosis
9	Friedreich's ataxia Tuberose sclerosis
11	Sickle cell anaemia β-Thalassaemias Acute intermittent porphyria Diabetes mellitus (rare forms)
12	Phenylketonuria von Willebrand's disease
13	Wilson's disease Retinoblastoma
14	α-1-Antitrypsin deficiency Variegate porphyria
16	Polycystic kidney (adult type) α-Thalassaemias
17	Pompé disease
18	Familial amyloidosis Non-Hodgkin's lymphoma (some)
19	Dystrophia myotonica Familial hypercholesterolaemia
21	Familial Alzheimer's disease Homocystinuria
22	Di George syndrome
X-linked	Haemophilia A and B Duchenne muscular dystrophy G-6PD deficiency Fragile X mental retardation Hunter's syndrome Lesch Nyhan syndrome Retinitis pigmentosa

of genetic disorders. Some of the applications include:

- The investigation of gene structure, function and mapping, e.g. immunoglobulin genes, globin genes
- The control of genetic disease, e.g. prenatal diagnosis, carrier detection
- The diagnosis of genetic disorders, e.g. sickle cell disease, Huntington's chorea
- The biosynthesis of substances, e.g. insulin, growth hormone, vaccines
- The future treatment of genetic disease by the insertion of cloned normal genes and deletion of abnormal genes

Very careful control and supervision of gene manipulation will, however, be necessary because of its potential hazards and ethical implications.

Chromosomes

Every nucleated cell in the body, excepting the gametes, has 46 chromosomes. Each chromosome contains one molecule of double-stranded DNA. There are two *sex* and 44 *autosomal* chromosomes. Chromosomes are numbered from the largest (No. 1) to the smallest (No. 22).

During division, a chromosome consists of two identical chromatids joined together at a centromere (Fig. 2.4). The centromere can be at three

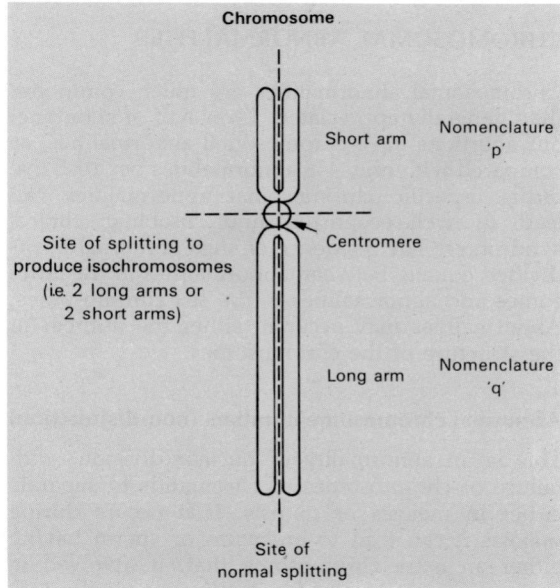

Fig. 2.4 A schematic diagram showing the structure of a chromosome with the sites at which it can split. The nomenclature for describing loci on chromosomes is as follows:

Number of chromosome or X or Y + short arm (p) or long arm (q)

The region or subregion is defined by transverse light and dark bands stained with quinacrine or giemsa and numbered from the centromere outwards.

Chromosome constitution	= chromosome number + sex chromosome + abnormality
Example 46 XX	= normal female
47 XX + 21	= trisomy 21 (Down's syndrome)
46 XYt (2; 19) (p21; p12)	= translocation between chromosome 2 and 19 with breaking at band p21 and p12 on the short arm.

locations: viz. central (metacentric), nearer one end than the other (submetacentric) or at one extreme end (acrocentric).

The two members of each pair of autosomes (one derived from each parent) resemble one another (they are homologous). However, the sex chromosomes differ—in the female the sex chromosomes are homologous (XX) but in the male pair they are not (XY).

During cell division (*mitosis*), each chromosome divides into two so that each daughter nucleus has the same number of chromosomes as its parent cell. During gametogenesis, however, the number of chromosomes is halved by *meiosis* so that after conception the number of chromosomes remains the same and is not doubled. In the female, each ovum contains one or other X chromosome but, in the male, the sperm bears either an X or a Y chromosome.

CHROMOSOMAL ABNORMALITIES

Chromosomal abnormalities are much commoner than generally appreciated. Over half of spontaneous abortions have chromosomal abnormalities, as compared with only 4–6 abnormalities per 1000 live births. Specific chromosomal abnormalities can lead to well-recognized and disabling clinical syndromes. The incidence of such abnormalities is divided equally between abnormalities in the autosomes and abnormalities in the sex chromosomes. Abnormalities may occur in either the number or the structure of the chromosomes.

Abnormal chromosome numbers (non-disjunction)

This is an abnormality of nuclear division, with failure of chromosomes or chromatids to separate either in meiosis or mitosis. If it occurs during meiosis it can lead to an ovum or sperm having either an extra chromosome that, if involved in conception, produces a fetus with an extra chromosome (i.e. three instead of two of a given type—called trisomy) or only one (monosomy). Fetuses with the latter defect are usually non-viable. Non-disjunction can occur with autosomes or sex chromosomes.

Occasionally, non-disjunction can occur during mitosis shortly after two gametes have united. It will then result in the formation of two cell lines, each with a different chromosome complement. This occurs more often with the sex chromosome, and is called 'mosaicism'.

Abnormal chromosome structure

Common chromosomal abnormalities include:

● *Translocation* (t):
  Reciprocal. This occurs when any two homo-

logous chromosomes lying together break simultaneously and a portion of one joins up with a portion of the other. Here the cell still has 46 chromosomes, but the structure of two of them has been rearranged. The carrier of this balanced reciprocal translocation is healthy but, if at meiosis the homologous pair separate and a child gets one normal and one abnormal chromosome, i.e. an unbalanced translocation, development can be disturbed.

Robertsonian translocation is clinically more important and occurs when two acrocentric chromosomes join and the short arm is lost leaving only 45 chromosomes. This translocation is again balanced as no genetic material is lost and the individual is healthy. The offspring, however, have a risk of an unbalanced arrangement and the risk depends on which acrocentric chromosome is involved. Clinically important is the 14/21 translocation and a woman with this karyotype has a 1 : 8 risk of a Down's baby (a male carrier has a 1 : 50 risk). However, they have a 50% risk of producing a carrier like themselves, hence the importance of genetic family studies. Relatives should be alerted about the risk of a Down's offspring and should have their chromosomes checked.

● *Deletion* (del). This is a loss of a section of chromosome together with the genes contained in it; for example, in the *cri du chat* syndrome there is a deletion of the short arm of chromosome 5 and in the Prader–Willi syndrome, a deletion of chromosome 15 (del (15) (q 11–13)).
● *Inversion* (inv). This is an end-to-end reversal of a segment within a chromosome, e.g. abcdefgh becomes abcdhgfe.
● *Fragile sites* (fra). In this a particular chromosome site is fragile and has a tendency to break, e.g. the fragile site near the end of the X chromosome in Fragile X syndrome.
● *Duplication*. This is where part of the chromosome is duplicated, e.g. abcdef becomes abcabcdef.

Abnormalities of chromosome number or structure can be seen in both autosomes and sex chromosomes; some of the resulting syndromes are shown in Table 2.3. Many individuals have an extra sex chromosome that remains unrecognized. However, since this abnormality is associated with an increased incidence of mental retardation and psychiatric problems, a disproportionate number of such individuals are seen in psychiatric and mental institutions.

Mitochondrial chromosome

Mitochondria are unique and contain their own genetic material—2–10 copies of double-stranded circular DNA in the cytoplasm. This DNA is

Table 2.3 Chromosomal abnormalities—examples of a few syndromes.

Syndrome	Chromosome karyotype	Incidence and risks	Clinical features	Mortality
AUTOSOMAL ABNORMALITIES				
Down's syndrome	47, + 21 (95%) Mosaicism Translocation } (5%)	1 : 650 (Risk with 20–29 year old mother = 1 : 1000; > 45 year old mother = 1 : 30)	Flat facies, slanting eyes, epicanthic folds, small ears, simian crease, short stubby fingers, hypotonia, variable mental retardation, congenital heart disease (up to 50%)	High in first year, but some survive to adulthood
Patau's syndrome	47, + 13	1 : 5000	Low-set ears, cleft lip and palate, polydactyly, micro-ophthalmia, mental retardation	Rarely survive for more than a few weeks
Edwards' syndrome	47, + 18	1 : 3000	Low-set ears, micrognathia, rocker-bottom feet, mental retardation	Rarely survive for more than a few weeks
SEX CHROMOSOME ABNORMALITIES				
Fragile X syndrome	46, XX, fra (X) 46, XY, fra (X)	1 : 2000	Mental retardation predominantly in males. Macroorchidism	
Female Turner's syndrome	45, XO	1 : 2500	Infantilism, primary amenorrhoea, short stature, webbed neck, cubitus valgus, normal IQ	
Triple X syndrome	47, XXX	1 : 1000	No distinctive somatic features, mental retardation	
Others	48, XXXX 49, XXXXX	Rare	Amenorrhoea, infertility, mental retardation	
Male Klinefelter's syndrome	47, XXY (or XXYY)	1 : 1000 (more in sons of older mothers)	Decreased crown–pubis: pubis–heel ratio, eunuchoid, testicular atrophy, infertility, gynaecomastia, mental retardation (20%; related to number of X chromosomes)	
Double Y syndrome	47, XYY	1 : 800	Tall, fertile, minor mental and psychiatric illness, high incidence in tall criminals	
Others	48, XXXY 49, XXXXY		Mental retardation, testicular atrophy	

different from nuclear DNA: it is transmitted only by mothers and has few introns and a slightly different genetic code, e.g. UGA codon is read as 'tryptophan' and not 'stop'. Thirteen proteins are coded for and all are components of the mitochondrial respiratory chain and oxidative phosphorylation. Deletion defects in DNA produce mitochondrial myopathies and encephalopathies. Skeletal muscle biopsies show 'ragged red fibres'. Many syndromes have been described, e.g. mitochondrial encephalomyopathy, lactic acidosis and stroke-like episodes (MELAS).

Chromosome examination

Chromosomes can only be seen in actively dividing cells. Lymphocytes from the peripheral blood are therefore stimulated by phytohaemogglutanin for these studies. Amniotic fluid, placental cells from chorionic villus sampling, bone marrow and other tissues (e.g. skin) can also be used. Culture and preparation takes about three days for lymphocytes but now computer-assisted image analysis and fluorescence-activated cell sorters are being developed. On staining, for example with the Giemsa stain, the chromosomes show a distinctive pattern of light and dark bands, enabling each chromosome to be identified.

Inheritance

UNIFACTORIAL INHERITANCE

Monogenetic disorders can be inherited as dominant, recessive or sex-linked characteristics. As chromosomes are present in duplicate, nearly all the genes are represented twice.

A harmful mutation of one allele (i.e. heterozygous) will usually cause no harm if the other is normal. However, if both alleles are affected (i.e. homozygous), the mutation will be expressed as disease. The conditions produced are known as *recessive* disorders.

Alternatively, at the same loci, a single normal gene may not be adequate for the normal functioning of the individual. In this situation a single harmful mutation in one allele will manifest itself as disease; this is known as a *dominant* disorder.

Tables 2.4 and 2.5 give a list of inherited diseases. Some diseases show a racial or geographical prevalence. Thalassaemia is seen mainly in Greeks, south-east Asians and Italians, porphyria variegata occurs more frequently in the South African white population, and Tay–Sachs disease particularly occurs in Ashkenazi Jews.

Inheritance occurs according to simple Mendel-

Indications for chromosomal analysis

Chromosome studies may be performed for various reasons at the following times:

- *Antenatal*
  (a) Sexing of fetus in X-linked disorders
  (b) Diagnosis of autosomal trisomy
  (c) Pregnancies in women over 35 y
- *In the neonate*
  (a) Congenital malformations
  (b) Suspicion of trisomy
  (c) Ambiguous genitalia
- *In the adolescent*
  (a) Primary amenorrhoea or failure of pubertal development
  (b) Growth retardation
- *In the adult*
  (a) Screening of patients with a child with a chromosomal abnormality for further genetic counselling
  (b) Infertility or recurrent miscarriages
  (c) Mental handicap
  (d) Certain malignant disorders e.g. leukaemias

---

ian laws, making predictions of disease in offspring and therefore genetic counselling more straightforward. Disorders are usually due to defects of a single gene.

Autosomal dominant disorders (see Fig. 2.5a, Table 2.4)

A dominant gene can be manifested in the heterozygous form and is transmitted by an affected person to half his offspring (whether male or female). These disorders have a greater variability than recessive disorders and can often be traced through many generations of the family.

Estimation of risk for counselling families can, however, be difficult because:

- Incomplete penetrance may occur if patients have a dominant gene but it does not manifest itself clinically in them. This gives the appearance of the gene having 'skipped' a generation.
- The age of onset may be variable. Presymptomatic detection of patients with the 'mutant' gene should be carried out particularly in families with dystrophia myotonica or Huntington's chorea.
- Dominant traits are extremely variable in severity (*variable expression*) and a mildly affected parent may have a severely affected child.
- New cases in a previously unaffected family are usually the result of a new mutation, illegitimacy or one parent being minimally affected and therefore undiagnosed. If it is a mutation, the risk of a further affected child is negligible. Most cases of achondroplasia are due to new mutations.

Table 2.4 Autosomal dominant disorders—examples.

Achondroplasia
Acute intermittent porphyria
Adult polycystic disease
Alzheimer's disease (familial)
α-1-Antitrypsin deficiency
C_1 esterase inhibitor deficiency
Crigler–Najjar syndrome type II
Epidermolysis bullosa (some forms)
Familial adenomatous polyposis
Familial hypercholesterolaemia
Facio-scapulohumeral dystrophy
Hereditary angio-oedema
Hereditary elliptocytosis
Hereditary haemorrhagic telangiectasia
Hereditary spherocytosis
Huntington's chorea
Marfan's syndrome
Dystrophia myotonica
Neurofibromatosis
Osteogenesis imperfecta (some forms)
Peutz–Jegher's syndrome
Rotor syndrome
Tuberose sclerosis
von Willebrand's disease

Table 2.5 Autosomal recessive disorders—examples.

Albinism (occulocutaneous)
Ataxia telangiectasia
Crigler–Najjar syndrome type I
Congenital adrenal hyperplasia
Cystic fibrosis
Deafness (some forms)
Dubin–Johnson syndrome
Epidermolysis bullosa (some forms)
Fanconi syndrome
Friedreich's ataxia
Galactosaemia
Gaucher's disease
Glycogen storage disease
Haemochromatosis
Homocystinuria
Hurler's syndrome (mucopolysaccharidosis I)
Infantile polycystic kidney disease
Laurence–Moon–Biedl syndrome
Phenylketonuria
Sickle cell disease
Tay–Sachs disease
β-Thalassaemia
Wilson's disease

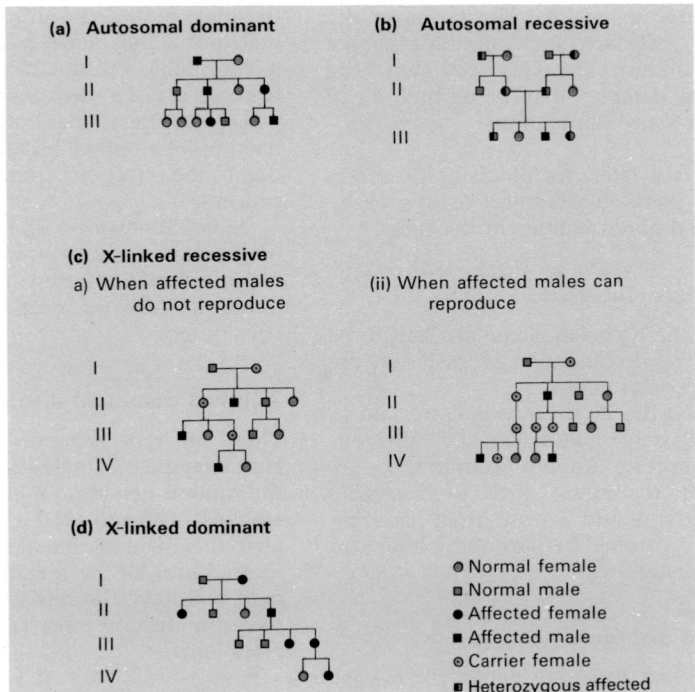

Fig. 2.5 Different modes of inheritance. (a) Autosomal dominant. (b) Autosomal recessive. (c) X-linked recessive. (d) X-linked dominant.

The overall incidence of autosomal dominant disorders is 7 per 1000 live births.

Autosomal recessive disorders (see Fig. 2.5b; Table 2.5)

These disorders only occur when an individual is homozygous for that gene; the parents will be unaffected healthy carriers (heterozygous for the gene). There is usually no family history, although the defective gene is passed from generation to generation. The offspring of an affected person will be healthy heterozygotes unless the affected person had married a carrier. If carriers marry, the offspring have a 1 : 4 chance of being homozygous and affected; a 1 : 2 chance of being a carrier; and a 1 : 4 chance of being genetically normal. Consanguinity increases the risk of a recessive disorder. A first-cousin marriage has an increased risk of 3% (above the risk in the general population) of having an abnormal child.

The clinical features of autosomal recessive disorders are usually severe; patients often present in the first few years of life and have a high mortality.

Many inborn errors of metabolism are recessive diseases. The commonest recessive disease in the UK is cystic fibrosis, with 1 in 22 of the population being a carrier. Cystic fibrosis affects 1 in every 2000 live births.

The overall incidence of autosomal recessive disorders is about 2.5 per 1000 live births in the UK. World-wide, diseases such as thalassaemia and sickle cell disease are very common; the frequency of these diseases may be as high as 20 per 1000 births in some populations.

Prenatal diagnosis (see later) for recessive disorders may be possible using biochemical assays or by detecting structural abnormalities in the fetus.

Sex-linked disorders (Table 2.6)

Genes carried on the X chromosome are said to be X-linked and can be dominant or recessive in the same way as autosomal genes.

Genes carried on the Y chromosome are said to be Y-linked and only males can be affected. However, there are no known examples of Y-linked single-gene disorders, with the possible exception of hairy ears and azoospermia (spermatogenesis may be controlled by part of the long arm of the Y chromosome).

X-linked recessive disorders (see Fig. 2.5c)

In the male, X-linked recessive genes are always manifested as there is no normal gene on an additional X chromosome (as there is in the female) to oppose the action of the abnormal gene. In the

Table 2.6 X-linked disorders—examples.

Recessive

Albinism (ocular)
Becker's muscular dystrophy
Christmas disease
Colour blindness
Duchenne muscular dystrophy
Fabry's disease
Glucose-6-phosphate dehydrogenase deficiency
Haemophilia A, B
Hunter's syndrome (mucopolysaccharidosis II)
Lesch–Nyhan syndrome
Menkes syndrome
Mental retardation (with or without fragile site)
Nephrogenic diabetes insipidus
Wiskott–Aldrich syndrome

Dominant

Vitamin D-resistant rickets

female, X-linked recessive genes are only manifested when the gene is homozygous. These conditions therefore usually affect males. They are transmitted by healthy female carriers or affected males if they survive to reproduce.

The best known example of an X-linked recessive disorder is haemophilia. Half the female offspring of a carrier female (married to a normal man) will be carriers and half will be normal; half the male offspring will have haemophilia and half will not. The male offspring of a male with haemophilia will not have the disease as long as his wife is not a carrier, but all the female offspring will be carriers. Very rarely a female will have haemophilia, either because she is homozygous or due to the effect of Lyonization, which is a random process.

A family history is not always positive, since new mutations are common. However, if a family history shows affected males in different generations, a Y-linked recessive disorder should be considered.

X-linked dominant disorders (see Fig. 2.5d)

These are rare. Vitamin D-resistant rickets is the best example. Females who are heterozygous for the mutant gene and males with the gene on their single X chromosome will manifest the disease. Half the male or female offspring of an affected mother and all the female offspring of an affected man will have the disease. Affected males tend to have the disease more severely than the heterozygous female.

Sex-limited inheritance

Occasionally a gene can be carried on an autosome

but manifests itself only in one sex. For example, frontal baldness is an autosomal dominant disorder in males but behaves as a recessive disorder in females.

MULTIFACTORIAL INHERITANCE

Characteristics resulting from a combination of genetic and environmental factors are said to be multifactorial; those involving multiple genes can also be said to be polygenic. Measurements of most biological factors, e.g. height, show a variation between individuals in a population and a uni-modal, symmetrical (Gaussian) frequency distribution curve can be drawn. This variability is due to variation in the genetic factors, the environmental factors or both. Environmental factors may play an important part in determining some characteristics, such as weight, whilst other characteristics such as intelligence or height may be largely genetically determined. The genetic component is thought to be due to the additive effects of a number of alleles at a number of loci (polygenic), many of which can be individually identified using molecular biological techniques. One such condition that has been studied is congenital pyloric stenosis. This is commoner in boys but if it occurs in girls the latter have a larger number of affected relatives. This difference suggests that a larger number of the relevant genes are required to produce the disease in girls than in boys.

Other conditions that may have a polygenic inheritance are shown in Table 2.7.

POPULATION GENETICS

The genetic constitution of a population depends on many factors. The Hardy–Weinberg equilibrium is a concept, based on a mathematical equation, that describes the outcome of random mating within populations. It states that 'in the absence of mutation, non-random mating, selection and genetic drift, the genetic constitution of the population remains the same from one generation to the next'.

This genetic principle has clinical significance in terms of the number of abnormal genes in the total gene pool of a population. The Hardy–Weinberg equation states that:

$$p^2 + 2pq + q^2 = 1$$

where p is the frequency of the normal gene in the population, q is the frequency of the abnormal gene, p^2 is the frequency of the normal homozygote, q^2 is the frequency of the affected abnormal homozygote, $2pq$ is the carrier frequency, and $p + q = 1$.

This equation can be used, for example, to find

Table 2.7 Some conditions that may have a polygenic inheritance.

Hypertension
Peptic ulceration
Rheumatoid arthritis
Diabetes mellitus
Epilepsy
Ischaemic heart disease
Congenital dislocation of the hip
Cleft palate
Pyloric stenosis
Congenital heart disease
Neural tube defects

the frequency of heterozygous carriers in cystic fibrosis: The incidence of cystic fibrosis is 1 in 2000 live births. Thus,

$$q^2 = 1/2000$$
$$q = \sqrt{(1/2000)} = 1/44$$
and $p = 1 - q = 43/44$

The carrier frequency is represented by $2pq$, i.e. $2 \times (43/44) \times (1/44) = 1/22$.

Thus, 1 in every 22 persons in the population is a heterozygous carrier for cystic fibrosis.

Clinical genetics and genetic counselling

Genetic disorders pose considerable health and economic problems because often there is no effective therapy. The prevalence of these disorders is shown in Table 2.8. In any pregnancy the risk of a serious developmental abnormality is approximately 1 in 30 pregnancies; approximately 15% of paediatric in-patients have a multifactorial disorder with a predominantly genetic element. The emphasis must therefore be on prevention.

People with a history of a congenital abnormality in a member of their family often seek advice as to why it happened and about the risks of producing a further abnormal offspring. Interviews must be conducted with great sensitivity and psychological insight, as parents may feel a sense of guilt and blame themselves for the abnormality in their child.

The *aims* of genetic counselling should include:

- Establishing an accurate diagnosis
- Information on prognosis and follow-up
- Estimation of the risk in future pregnancy of

developing or transmitting a disorder
- Genetic screening—prenatal diagnosis, carrier detection, genetic registers
- Continued support and follow-up

Counselling should be non-directive, with the couple making their own decisions on the basis of an accurate presentation of the facts and risks in a way that they can understand.

- *History.* A full and careful history should be taken. The pregnancy history, drug, alcohol ingestion during pregnancy and maternal illnesses, e.g. diabetes, should be detailed.
- *Examination* of the child may help in diagnosing a genetically abnormal child with characteristic features, e.g. trisomy 21, or whether a genetically normal fetus was damaged *in utero*.
- *Drawing a family tree* is essential. Questions should be asked about abortions, stillbirths, deaths, marriages, consanguinity and medical history of family members. Diagnoses may need verification from other hospital reports.
- *Estimation of risk* should be based on the pattern of inheritance. Mendelian disorders (see earlier) carry a high risk; chromosomal abnormalities a low risk. Empirical risks may be obtained from population or family studies.
- *Carrier detection* is offered in autosomal recessive disorders for conditions that are relatively common, e.g. screening for β-thalassaemia (Asian and Mediterranean populations), sickle cell disease (African origin) and Tay–Sachs disease (Ashkenazi Jews).
- *Pre-natal diagnosis.* For families at risk of genetic disease an intrauterine diagnosis is important either to reassure parents if the fetus is unaffected or to allow termination of the pregnancy. It should be carried out if there is a high genetic risk of a severe disorder (particularly if the prenatal test is reliable) and if no treatment is available for the particular disorder.

Table 2.8 Prevalence of genetic disease.[a]

Type	Prevalence per 1000 population (estimated)
Single gene	
Autosomal dominant	2–10
Autosomal recessive	2
X-linked recessive	1–2
Chromosomal abnormalities	6–7
Common disorders with appreciable genetic component	7–10
Congenital malformation	20
Total	38–51

[a] From Kingston H (1989) Clinical genetic services, *British Medical Journal* **298**: 306–307, with permission.

The techniques available and their uses are shown in Table 2.9. Amniocentesis (see box) and ultrasonography are widely available. High-resolution ultrasonography has replaced amniocentesis in some centres for the diagnosis of neural-tube defects. Chorionic villus sampling (transcervical or transabdominal under ultrasound guidance) can be performed at an earlier time (8–12 weeks' gestation) and has the advantage of earlier and easier termination if necessary. Embryo biopsy is now technically feasible; after *in vitro* fertilization and embryo culture, biopsy and DNA analysis of one or two embryonal cells at 8–16 cell stage is undertaken.

- *Screening of maternal serum* has limited uses apart from measuring α-fetoprotein. High concentrations are seen in fetuses with open neural-tube defects (80%), and some other fetal abnormalities.
- *Genetic registers*, held on computers, allow the tracing and follow-up of family members, and are particularly useful for disorders amenable to DNA analysis e.g. Huntington's chorea, familial adenomatous polyposis, myotonia dystrophica and Duchenne muscular dystrophy.
- *Ethical issues* may arise on the basis of religious beliefs or on whether an abortion should be carried out for minor defects. Presymptomatic testing for Huntington's chorea is also a problem as some young family members may wish to know the risk (with appropriate counselling of its implications) whilst others do not want to

Amniocentesis

- This is performed at 14–17 weeks' gestation as an out-patient
- Ultrasound is used to localize placenta and to detect the presence of twins
- Sterile precautions are used during aspiration of approximately 20 ml of amniotic fluid via the transabdominal route
- The specimen is centrifuged and:
  (a) The *supernatant* is used for chemical analysis to detect defects such as the adrenogenital syndrome (17-hydroxyprogesterone) or mucopolysaccharidases (glycosaminoglycosis), α-fetoprotein and acetylcholinesterase are raised in neural tube defects, anterior abdominal wall defects, congenital nephrosis. Alkaline phosphatase and γ-glutamyltranspeptidase for cystic fibrosis. The fluid is normally clear. Blood suggests puncture of placenta. Discoloration may suggest impending fetal death.
  (b) The *cell deposit* can be cultured and used for cytogenetics (or chromosomal anomalies), enzyme studies for the detection of inborn errors of metabolism such as Tay–Sachs disease, single gene defects by DNA analysis, fetal sexing for X-linked disorders.

Table 2.9 Methods available for prenatal diagnosis.

Technique	Risk and trimester for performing test	Comment
Ultrasonography	Safe 2nd trimester	Structural abnormalities e.g. neural tube defects, skeletal abnormalities Also used as part of the techniques below
Amniocentesis	Risk < 1% 2nd trimester	Chromosomal analysis. Measurement of α fetoprotein or acetyl cholinesterase Biochemical analysis Widely available
Fetoscopy	Risk 3% 2nd trimester	Direct examination Fetal sampling Highly specialized
Chorionic villus sampling	Risk 2% 1st trimester	Chromosomal and DNA analysis Biochemical analysis Highly specialized

know. Cousin marriages in ethnic minorities may also pose a problem.

In many common conditions only an empirical assessment of the risk can be given. This should be carefully explained to the individuals seeking advice and the risks should be put in perspective. Unless the type of inheritance is straightforward, it is advisable to send couples to the nearest genetic clinic.

TREATMENT OF GENETIC DISORDERS

- *Conventional* therapy consists of controlling rather than curing the genetic effect. Examples include anticonvulsant therapy in tuberose sclerosis, dietary phenylalanine restriction in phenylketonuria, avoidance of fava bean in G-6PD deficiency, avoiding drugs that precipitate porphyria, e.g. barbiturates, oestrogens, and Factor VIII replacement in haemophilia A.

Other conditions (e.g. muscular dystrophy) will require physiotherapy, orthopaedic therapy, treatment of infections, home modifications, help with schooling and family support. Lay organizations may provide extra help.

- *Gene product replacement.* Production of insulin and growth hormone by recombinant DNA techniques.
- *Gene therapy.* In theory this involves manipulation of the genome directly to repair a defect which could cure a genetic disorder. In future it may be possible to remove bone marrow cells from a patient with β-thalassaemia, culture the cells *in vitro* and infect them with a retrovirus carrying an insertion of a human β-globin gene; cells with normal β-globin would then be selected and replaced into the patient's bone marrow. There are ethical problems and also the possibility of an increased risk of neoplasia.

Human leucocyte antigens (HLA)

The HLA system consists of a series of closely linked genetic loci situated in the major histocompatibility complex (MHC) on the short arm of chromosome 6. Figure 2.6 shows the classification of these antigens. The class 1, or A, B and C, series of genes are expressed on all nucleated cells, whereas the class II series of genes are expressed predominantly on B lymphocytes. A feature of these loci is that they are highly polymorphic, i.e. a large number of different alleles occur; more than 20 HLA-A, 40 HLA-B, 10 HLA-C, 15 HLA-DR, 3 HLA-DQ and 6 HLA-DP antigens have been identified so far. The class III series of genes express complement.

GENETIC LINKAGE

The genes at a given locus are inherited as codominants, so that each individual expresses both alleles, one transmitted from the mother and the other from the father. Because of the close linkage between the loci, all the genes in the MHC tend to be inherited together. The term 'haplotype' is used to indicate the particular set of HLA genes an individual carries on each chromosome 6.

'Crossing over' can occur within the HLA region. However, certain alleles occur more frequently in the same haplotype than expected by chance and this is known as linkage disequilibrium; for example, the haplotype A1,B8 occurs more frequently than would be expected from the individual gene frequencies of A1 or B8.

There is a wide inter-racial variation in HLA antigens; for example, the HLA haplotype A1, B8 is found mainly in Caucasians, while the antigen B42 is seen only in Blacks.

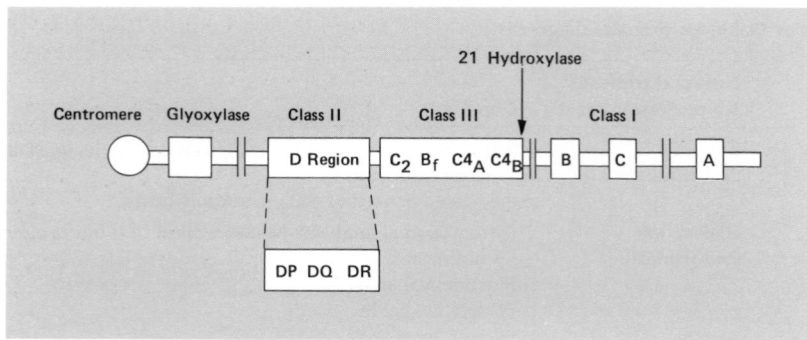

Fig. 2.6 Human leucocyte antigens (HLA). A schematic diagram of the short arm of chromosome 6, showing the position of different HLA antigen classes.

Products of the HLA genes

The HLA genes code for cell-surface glycoproteins that extend from the plasma membrane to the cytoplasm and are known as class I and class II molecules. These glycoproteins consist of two chains of unequal size (alpha and beta chains), and are antigenic.

Class I molecules (Fig. 2.7)

Class I antigens are expressed on all cell types except erythrocytes and trophoblasts. Striated muscle cells and liver parenchymal cells are normally negative but become strongly positive in inflammatory reactions.

HLA-A, -B and -C antigens can be distinguished

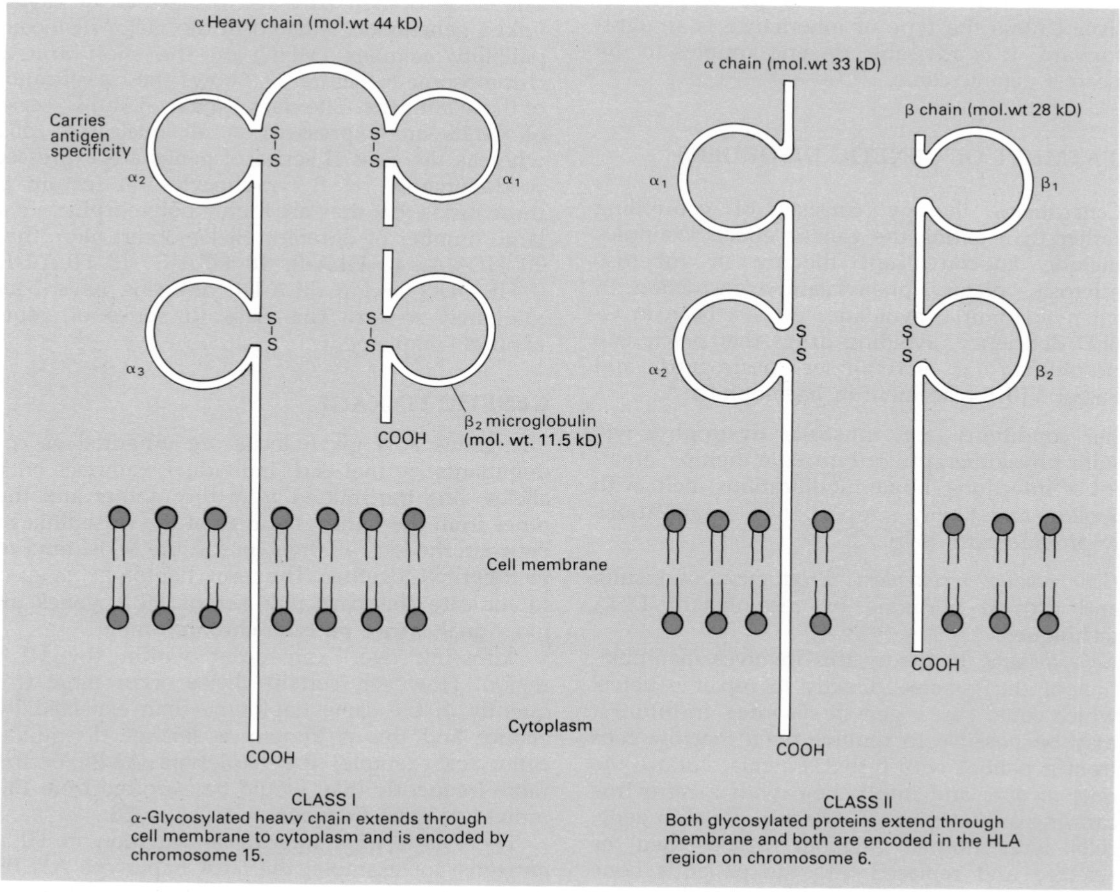

CLASS I
α-Glycosylated heavy chain extends through cell membrane to cytoplasm and is encoded by chromosome 15.

CLASS II
Both glycosylated proteins extend through membrane and both are encoded in the HLA region on chromosome 6.

Fig. 2.7 Histocompatibility antigens—class I and class II.

serologically by the microlymphocytotoxic test. Lymphocytes from the peripheral blood are incubated with a range of antibodies of known specificity (obtained from parous women or immunized individuals) in the presence of complement and trypan blue dye (which penetrates and stains cells with a damaged cell membrane). If the antibody does not react with the antigen, the lymphocytes survive and exclude the dye; in a positive reaction the dye enters the dead cells, indicating the presence of the specific antigen on that cell.

Class II molecules (Fig. 2.7)

Class II antigens are expressed on B cells, monocytes, dendritic cells and activated T cells. Inflammation causes aberrant class II expression in many other tissues. They are important in presenting antigens to certain subpopulations of T cells.

HLA-D antigens are recognized by the mixed lymphocyte culture (MLC) technique, which requires a panel of different HLA-D homozygous standard typing cells. The homozygous typing cell (HTC) is treated with mitomycin or irradiation to prevent it dividing when it is cultured with the test responder lymphocytes. The latter will not proliferate (measured by incorporation of tritiated thymidine) if it possesses the same D antigen as the HTC, but it will proliferate if it lacks this antigen. The DR (D-related) antigens are very closely related to D antigens and are also detected on B cells (B cell alloantigens) using a cytotoxic antibody test. These antigens are probably the counterpart of the 'immune-associated' (Ia) antigens on the surface of B cells and macrophages in the mouse.

Immunoregulatory function of HLA molecules

In the mouse, the *Ir* gene controls the magnitude of the immune response by helping T cell recognition of the macrophage-bound antigen. Thus, T cells use HLA antigens as recognition molecules (Fig. 2.8). Helper T (T_H) cells (identified by monoclonal antibody CD4) usually use class II antigens, whilst cytotoxic T cells (identified with monoclonal antibody CD8) generally use class I antigens. Thus:

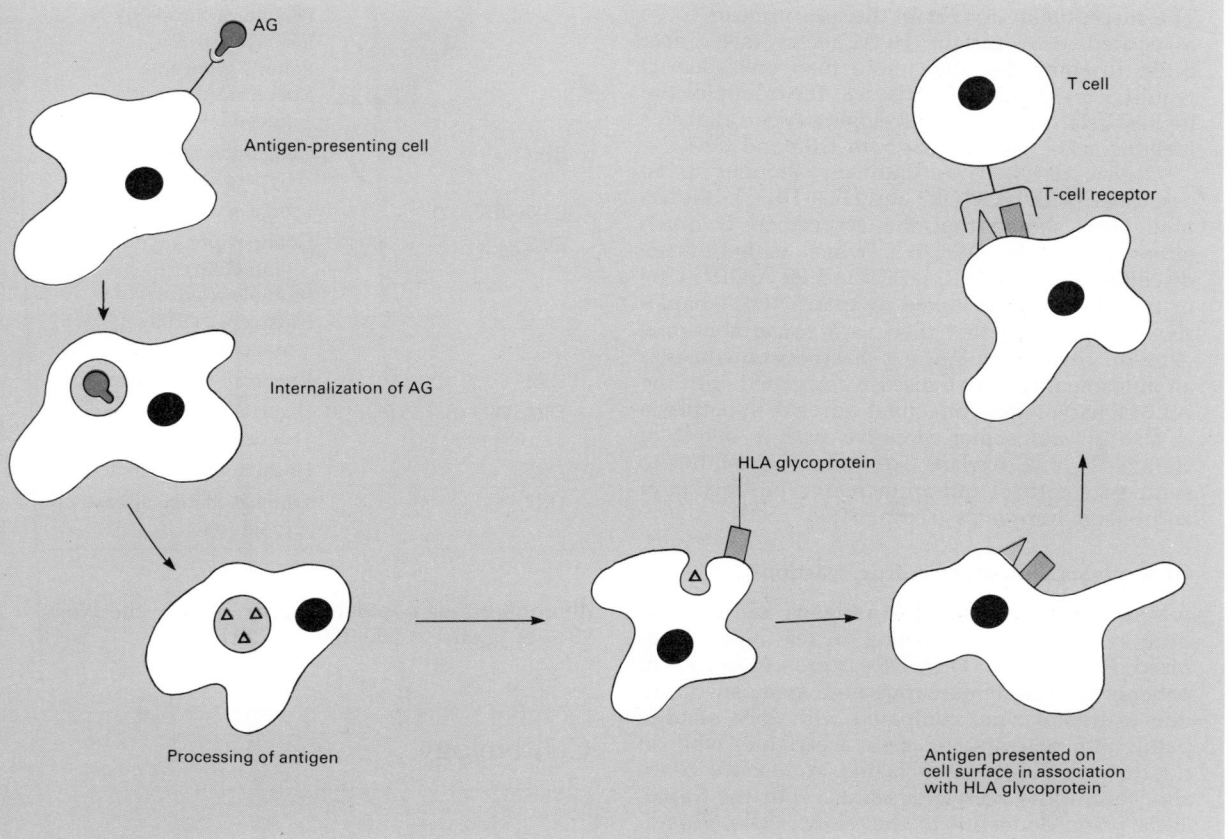

Fig. 2.8 Processing of antigen by macrophage (antigen-presenting cell) followed by T-cell recognition of macrophage-bound antigen via the HLA glycoprotein.

- T$_H$ cells only cooperate with B cells if they share the same Ia (HLA-DR) antigens.
- Macrophages presenting an antigen to a T$_H$ cell must also share the same Ia (DR) antigen in order to stimulate it.
- Cytotoxic T cells also require the same class I HLA molecules to be present on the target cell for cytotoxicity. For example, cytotoxic lymphocytes lyse target cells that have been infected with the specific virus and carry one or more of the same class I antigens, but do not lyse target cells infected with a different virus and/or which do not share the same class I antigens.

Transplantation requirements

Tissue typing for organ grafting requires HLA typing for A, B, C and DR antigens. The match should be as close as possible, as this increases graft survival. Requirements for matching in bone-marrow transplantation are much more stringent, as the rejection process can be either host-versus-graft or graft-versus-host (see p. 362).

Genetic markers and disease associations

The susceptibility to certain diseases appears to be associated with certain HLA alleles (see Table 2.10). In some disorders more than one allele is required to produce the disease; for example, the highest relative risk for developing type I diabetes mellitus is the presence of both DR3 and DR4.

Coeliac disease was originally thought to be associated with HLA-DR3 and HLA-DR7, but it has now been shown that the association is much stronger with HLA-DQW2, which is in linkage disequilibrium with HLA-DR3 and HLA-DR7. One or two diseases are linked to specific HLA haplotypes, suggesting that there is a single abnormal gene on chromosome 6, e.g. haemochromatosis is an autosomal recessive disease associated with the A3,B14 haplotype; congenital adrenal hyperplasia is also an autosomal recessive with a defect of steroid 21 hydroxylase, resulting in failure to synthesize cortisol and an increased production of androgenic hormones (see p. 816).

HLA alleles and adverse drug reactions

Associations between HLA antigens and adverse drug reactions are becoming increasingly recognized. For example, HLA-DR4 is present in 75% of patients with systemic lupus erythematosus (SLE) due to hydralazine, compared with 25% of idiopathic SLE patients and slow acetylators who do not develop SLE on hydralazine. Autosomal genes also control the acetylator status, with the 'rapid' allele being dominant to the 'slow' allele. Homozygotes for the 'slow' allele have reduced levels of N-acetyltransferase in the liver. Acetylation is the controlling factor for the rate of drug metabolism. The percentage of rapid acetylators varies in different ethnic populations, viz. 50% in the West, 90% of Japanese and 100% in Eskimos.

Table 2.10 HLA-associated diseases.

A3, B14	Haemochromatosis
A28	Schizophrenia
B5	Behçet's syndrome
	Polycystic kidney disease
	Ulcerative colitis
B8	Tuberculoid leprosy (Asians)
B8, DR3	Chronic active hepatitis (autoimmune)
	Dermatitis herpetiformis
	Graves's disease
	Idiopathic membranous glomerulonephritis
	Myasthenia gravis (without thymoma)
	Addison's disease
	Sjögren's syndrome
	Systemic lupus erythematosus
B8, DR3, DR7, DQW2	Coeliac disease
B27	Acute anterior uveitis
	Ankylosing spondylitis
	Psoriatic arthropathy
	Reactive arthritis
	Reiter's syndrome
	Rheumatoid arthritis (juvenile)
BW47	Congenital adrenal hyperplasia
CW6 (B13, 17)	Psoriasis vulgaris
DR2	Goodpasture's syndrome (anti-GBM)
	Multiple sclerosis
	Narcolepsy (100% association)
DR4	Rheumatoid arthritis
DR4, DR3 (B8, 15 [62] 18)	Diabetes mellitus (insulin-dependent)
DR5	Hashimoto's thyroiditis
DR7	Minimal change disease (nephrotic)

Cell biology

Each eukaryotic cell has a cell membrane (plasmalemma) that separates it from the environment and compartmentalizes many highly specialized organelles.

Cell membrane
This consists of a bilayer of non-polar or amphipathic lipid molecules with phospholipids, cholesterol and glycolipids with proteins and carbohydrates inserted into it. It is a dynamic fluid compartment and acts as a barrier for water and hydrophilic solutes. The viscosity of this bilayer is controlled by modifying the fatty acyls of its phospholipid.

The cell membrane has several functions:

● Proteins present in the lipid bilayer act as channels for various ions, 'pumps' for selective transport of ions, e.g. sodium, specific carriers for metabolites, e.g. amino acids.
● Specific receptor molecules present on the outer surface of the membrane of target cells interact with physiological ligands, e.g. hormones, lipoproteins, immunoglobulins, peptide hormones, neurotransmitters (first messengers). The activated receptor then interacts with an enzyme system that produces a second messenger, usually cyclic adenosine monophosphate (cAMP). This in turn triggers a chain of intracellular reactions that eventually leads to the usual response of the cell to its physiological ligand (see Fig. 11.2, p. 513). Receptors, e.g. insulin receptor, have now been isolated and consist of large glycoproteins. Defective or damaged receptors can lead to disease states, e.g. acetylcholine receptor in myasthenia gravis, lipoprotein (LDL) receptor in familial hypercholesterolaemia.
● Cell : cell recognition and communication. At certain points the cell membrane is fused to its neighbouring cell and intercellular channels allow diffusion of ions or small molecules.
● Differentiated domains. Certain areas of the cell membrane are structurally different. For example, the low-density-lipoprotein (LDL) receptor lies in an invagination or a 'pit'. This pit is coated with heavy and light chains of *clathrin*. These coated pits become detached and form coated vesicles. Absorptive cells have a characteristic brush border with microvilli containing enzymes for food digestion.

Nucleus
This contains the cell's genome, consisting of DNA and all the apparatus for replication and transcription into RNA (see p. 106). When the cell is not dividing, the nuclear envelope—consisting of an outer and inner membrane—separates it from the cytoplasm. The outer membrane is continuous with the endoplasmic reticulum. During cell division, chromosomes becomes visible. The *cell cycle* starts with an active phase :G_1 (G = gap), during which the cell synthesizes RNA, proteins, lipids and polysaccharides. G_1 is followed by S (synthesis), during which the genome (DNA) is replicated. A short inactive phase (G_2) is followed by mitosis (see Fig. 7.6, p. 354).

Cytoplasm
This contains many specialized organelles that serve different functions. These include storage of substances, e.g. glycogen and lipids, the synthesis of essential substances, e.g. amino acids, fatty acids, monosaccharides, the metabolism of these substances, and protein synthesis and translation. Microtubules are cylindrical structures formed from the protein tubulin; they help to maintain the structure of the cells and form channels for communication between the subcellular organelles. These organelles are:

● *Endoplasmic reticulum*. This is a network of channels throughout the cytoplasm from the nucleus to the cell membrane. It is divided into:
  The *nuclear membrane* surrounding the nucleus and controlling traffic in and out of the nucleus
  The *rough endoplasmic reticulum* (RER), which is lined by ribosomes that synthesize proteins
  The *smooth endoplasmic reticulum* (SER), consisting of tubules and vesicles containing microsomes
  ER is involved in the processing of secretory proteins. Some contain enzyme systems (e.g. mixed-function oxygenases, including cytochrome P450) that hydroxylate hydrophobic compounds, making them more soluble and therefore easier to metabolize (e.g. vitamin D) or eliminate (e.g. drugs).
● *Golgi apparatus*. This consists of channels or vesicles. Functions include modification and packaging of secretory proteins, transport of lysosomal enzymes to lysosomes and storage. The Golgi apparatus acts as a focal point for the complex intracellular traffic that takes place between all of the subcellular components.
● *Mitochondria*. These consist of double membranes with an extensively infolded inner membrane forming cristae. It contains enzymes responsible for oxidative phosphorylation, the citric acid cycle, the electron-transport chain and ATP synthesis.
● *Lysosomes*. These contain digestive enzymes, mostly acid hydrolases, capable of digesting most constituents of cells and tissues. The substrates can enter the lysosome directly or via the Golgi apparatus.

Cell traffic
It is apparent from the above that traffic through the cell is continuous and many of the subcellular organelles play a part in processing an individual substance. The signals that control this trafficking are unclear. An example of cellular and intracellular movement is given in Fig. 2.9.

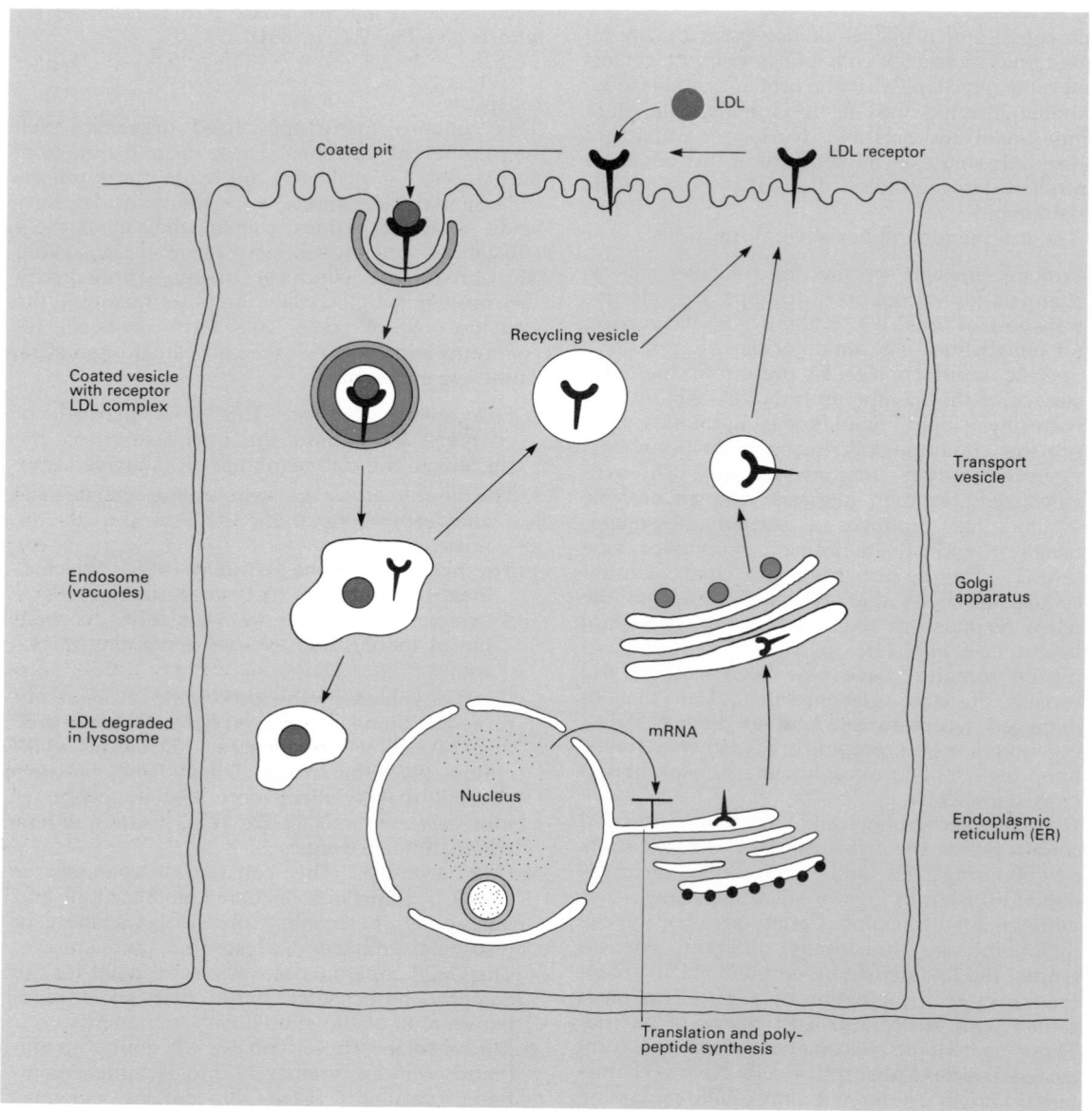

Fig. 2.9 Receptor-mediated endocytosis. LDL receptors are formed in the ER and transported via the Golgi apparatus to the cell surface. LDLs bind to these receptors, are internalized and taken up by the endosome. The receptor is recycled back to the surface, while the LDL is broken down by the lysosomes, freeing cholesterol needed for membrane synthesis.

Immune mechanisms in health and disease

INTRODUCTION

Functionally, immunological competence can be divided into that resulting from the genetic consti-

tution of the host (natural or innate immunity) and that resulting from stimulation with a foreign substance (acquired immunity). Natural immunity is the first line of defence, whereas acquired immunity produces a specific response to an antigen and retains its 'memory' for future contact with that particular antigen. Exposure of an individual to a foreign antigen thus elicits an immune response which results in:

- Elimination of the foreign material
- Protection against future contact with that antigen

Natural immunity

Natural immunity is dependent on the make-up of the host. Protection is afforded by mechanical barriers and secretions, by extracellular fluids and by phagocytic cells.

Mechanical barriers and secretions
- Intact skin provides a physical barrier. Shedding of desquamated skin removes microorganisms.
- Mucosal surfaces trap bacteria and other foreign material in an adhesive blanket of mucus. Cilia in the respiratory tract sweep the mucus and microorganisms towards the mouth where they are eliminated by coughing or swallowing.
- Body fluids e.g. tears, sweat, contain bacteriostatic substances, such as lactic acid. The flow of these fluids sweeps away organisms.
- Mucous membranes also secrete antimicrobial factors, e.g. lysozyme, lactoferrin and secretory IgA. Some organisms, e.g. gonococci, meningococci and some streptococci, produce IgA proteases that are able to cleave secretory IgA.
- Normal microbial flora play a vital role in impeding the growth of bacteria, e.g. certain non-pathogenic *E. coli* produce colicins that are lethal to *Salmonella* and *Shigella*.

Extracellular fluids
Natural antibodies are present in these fluids. Some neutralize toxins, some act as opsonins and promote phagocytosis, and some activate complement resulting in bacteriolysis.

- Beta-lysin is released from platelets and acts against Gram-positive bacteria.
- C-reactive protein (CRP) is involved in complement activation.
- Interferons are produced by some cells and these have a broad spectrum antiviral activity.
- Gastric acid is antimicrobial.
- Basic proteins derived from damaged cells in an inflammatory response have antimicrobial activity e.g. protamine, spermine, spermidine.
- Human milk contains a lipase.
- Lysozyme, a mucolytic enzyme found in neutrophils, acts on the cell wall of Gram-positive bacteria, resulting in lysis.

Phagocytic cells
Macrophages and neutrophils, phagocytose organisms in the circulation, lymph nodes, liver, spleen, bone marrow, pituitary or adrenal glands.

Acquired immunity

Acquired immunity is the immunological response to infection and involves:

- Humoral immunity involving antibody production and complement
- Cell-mediated immunity

These will be described below.

Immune responses conferring protection against disease can be induced by direct infection or by artificial exposure of the individual to inactive forms of the infectious organism, i.e. immunization.

A glossary of terms commonly used in immunology can be found on p. 149.

Lymphoid tissue

Lymphoid organs appear early in gestation. The thymus appears first, producing cells at 8 weeks that become immunocompetent by 11 weeks. The total population of the lymphoid tissue is completed by 16 weeks of gestation.

Lymphocytes are distributed in all organs, tissues and interstitial fluids except the brain. Many lymphocytes constitute a 'circulating pool' and are constantly entering and leaving the blood and lymph. Other lymphocytes are concentrated in certain areas and constitute lymphoid organs. Lymphoid tissues in man are the bone marrow, spleen, thymus, lymph nodes and mucosally associated lymphoid tissue (MALT). MALT is present in the gut, pharynx, bronchi, breast, genitourinary system and the salivary and lacrimal glands.

The resting lymphoid tissue consists of three areas:

- The cortex, which contains B lymphocytes
- The paracortex, which contains T lymphocytes
- The medulla, which contains connective tissue

Following antigenic stimulation the following changes result:

- The cortex contains actively dividing cells.
- The paracortex contains blast-like cells and 'germinal centres' containing actively dividing cells.
- The medulla is packed with plasma cells secreting antibodies; each plasma cell lives for a few days.

The immune response

The immune response has two limbs:

- The *afferent limb* is concerned with the recognition of the antigen, the processing of this antigen, and the induction of the immune response.

- The *efferent limb*, activated by contact with the antigen, sets in motion a series of cellular and humoral mechanisms against the antigen.

This series of events involves cooperation between lymphocytes and phagocytic cells and the release of many soluble factors termed cytokines (see below).

Cells participating in the immune response

All cells involved in the immune response are derived from a common stem cell in the marrow (see p. 295). This gives rise to the lymphoid progenitor cells, which then produce lymphocytes, or the myeloid progenitor, which then produces macrophages, monocytes, eosinophils, neutrophils and mast cells.

Lymphocytes

Lymphocytes account for up to 45% of the circulating blood leucocytes. They are divided into:

- T lymphocytes (70% of total lymphocytes)
- B lymphocytes (20% of total)
- 'Null' cells (10% of total)

T and B cells (Fig. 2.10) communicate either by

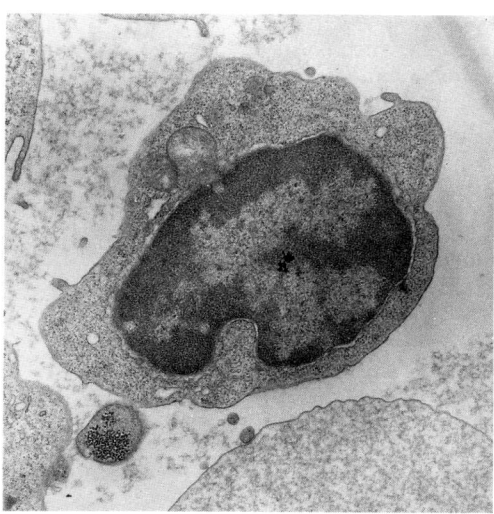

Fig. 2.10 Electron micrograph of B and T lymphocytes.

direct contact or by soluble factors. Immunological memory is carried by long-living T and B cells.

T lymphocytes
These cells migrate from the bone marrow to the thymus where they are processed by the thymic epithelial cell hormone, which transforms them into immunocompetent cells. During maturation there is a progressive expression of selected cell-surface markers (Table 2.11a) and activation of genes that will eventually encode for the α and β chains that will make up the T cell receptor. T cells are activated to form 'blast' cells by specific antigens as well as non-specific mitogens such as phytohaemagglutinin (PHA); the latter can be demonstrated *in vitro*. This activation involves macrophages, which process and present the antigen to the lymphocytes (see Fig. 2.8).

T lymphocytes are divided into subsets depending on their role in the immune response, either regulating antibody production or taking part in delayed hypersensitivity reactions:

- T helper (T_H)
- T suppressor (T_S)
- T cytotoxic (T_C)
- T delayed hypersensitivity (T_D)

Surface phenotypes divide them into CD4$^+$ (T_H, T_S) and CD8$^+$ (T_S and T_C). CD4$^+$ T cells recognize antigens when they are presented to them by antigen-presenting cells in association with MHC class II molecules; CD8$^+$ T cells recognize antigen with MHC class I molecules. T cells can be further divided into subsets by the use of monoclonal antibodies that react with surface molecules on the T cells (Table 2.11a).

T cell receptor (TR)
This consists of α and β chains, similar to the immunoglobulin light chains, with variable *N*-terminal ends. The β chain contains two constant regions. There are several hypervariable regions and if the molecule were arranged like an antibody it would form an antigen-binding site. The T cell receptor for helper and cytotoxic cells is very similar.

The following factors are important in T cell function:

- T_H and B cell interaction is essential for an optimal humoral response to most antigens.
- T-cell-mediated immunity can be transferred by giving T cells to a genetically compatible individual.
- T-cell interaction with antigen releases non-specific factors called *lymphokines* (cytokines) that amplify the immunological response (see p. 136).
- T lymphocytes live for months or years.

Table 2.11a T cells—monoclonal antibodies and surface antigens.

Monoclonal antibodies/ synonyms	Antigen	Antigen Mol.wt (kD)	Distribution	Comments
PAN-T cell				
Anti-T$_1$ Leu 1	CD5	69	All mature T cells Few B cells	? Monokine receptor
Anti-T$_3$ } Leu 4	CD3	19–26	All mature T cells	Anti-CD3 activates T cells Receptor ? calcium channel
Anti-T$_{11}$ Leu 5 E rosette receptor	CD2	55	T cells All thymocytes Some NK cells	Greatest density on T$_S$ cells and thymocytes E associated protein
T cell subset				
Anti-T$_4$ Leu 3	CD4	62	50–60% periph. T cells Most thymocytes	T helper cells Class II MHC restricted Receptor for HTLV-3
Anti-T8 Leu 2	CD8	33, 76	25–35% periph. T cells Most thymocytes	Cytotoxic and suppressor T cells Class I MHC restricted
Anti-T$_6$ Leu 6	CD1	49, 12	80% thymocytes	Specific for cortical thymocytes Related to class I
Inducible activation marker				
Anti-TAC IL-2r	CD25	55	Activated T cells	Recognizes IL-2 receptor Blocks IL-2 binding Blocks proliferation Inducible by antigen and mitogen
Anti-T$_9$	None	44	Majority of activated T cells. Few thymocytes	Transferrin receptor

Table 2.11b Receptors and surface antigens present on T and B lymphocytes.

	Lymphocytes		Comments
	T	B	
Receptors			
Complement	−	+	
C3b	−	+	
C4b			
Immunoglobulin	−	+	Receptors mainly for IgM but also for IgA, IgG and IgE Most are of low affinity, but 10% have high affinity receptors for IgG. It has been suggested these are 'null' cells
Sheep erythrocyte (E receptor)	+	−	Present on 60–65% of all circulating T lymphocytes
Surface antigens/markers			
1a	+	−	Present on circulating lymphocytes and involved in cell–cell cooperation
Immunoglobulin	−	+	

B lymphocytes

These are derived from the bone marrow, are thought to be processed in the fetal liver and spleen and the adult bone marrow (in mammals), and live for days or weeks. They are transformed into antibody-producing plasma cells. Antibody synthesis is inhibited by T_S cells.

T and B lymphocytes also differ in their surface receptors and markers (Table 2.11b).

'Null cells'

These lymphocytes do not possess the phenotype markers of either T or B cells but are characterized by the possession of Fc receptors for IgG. They originate in the bone marrow. Some may be identical to 'killer' (K) cells, which have cytotoxic properties against target cells coated with antibody, and some may be 'natural killer' (NK) cells, which are thought to lyse certain tumour cells.

Mononuclear phagocytes (p. 333)

These are present as tissue macrophages and blood monocytes. Mononuclear phagocytes bear surface receptors for IgG and the complement components C3 and C5 and low-affinity receptors for IgE. They are also thought to possess receptors for cytokines such as γ-interferon and migration inhibitory factor (MIF), although these have not yet been characterized.

The primary activities of mononuclear phagocytes are:

- The engulfment and digestion of cell debris and foreign material. This is important in non-specific immunity.
- The presentation of partially degraded antigen–antibody complexes or free antigen to T and B cells. This is important in humoral immunity.

Neutrophils (p. 331)

Polymorphonuclear granulocytes (neutrophils) live for 6–20 h and constitute approximately 60% of the total number of leucocytes. They bear surface receptors for IgA, IgG and complement components.

Neutrophils are the characteristic cells of acute inflammation and play a primary role in non-specific immunity by engulfing and digesting microorganisms; their absence usually proves fatal.

Mast cells and basophils

Mast cells are present in the skin and mucosal surfaces and basophils circulate in the blood. Although direct proof of a common origin is lacking for these cells, they are commonly linked together owing to their similar mediator content and mechanisms of activation.

Both mast cells and basophils are involved in immediate hypersensitivity reactions, when they release mediators following allergen binding to their surface (see Fig. 12.32). They bear receptors for the complement components C3 and C5 and high-affinity receptors for IgE.

The numbers of circulating basophils in non-allergic individuals is small but shows an increase in patients with allergic disease. They are also seen in the secretions of patients with allergic rhinitis.

Mast cells consist of at least two distinct populations, which are distinguished by their enzymic content. The T mast cells contain trypsin alone and were formerly termed mucosal mast cells owing to their location near mucosal surfaces. The TC mast cells contain both trypsin and chymotrypsin and were formerly described as connective tissue mast cells, owing to their location. Some of the properties of T and TC mast cells are outlined in Table 2.12.

Eosinophils (see p. 332)

These are seen in the circulation in allergic diseases and helminth infections and in the secretions of patients with allergic rhinitis. Eosinophils live for between 6 and 20 h. They bear receptors for IgG

Table 2.12 Mast cells—properties of T and TC cells.[a]

	T mast cells	TC mast cells
Location	Mucosal surfaces	Connective tissue
Major proteoglycan	Chondroitin sulphate	Heparin
Cytoplasmic IgE	+	−
Histamine content	+	++
Histamine release following stimulation with basic amines	−	+
Major arachidonic acid metabolite $LTC_4 : PGD_2$	25 : 1	1 : 40
Staining after formaldehyde fixation	−	+

[a] T = trypsin; C = chymotrypsin.

and the complement components C3 and C5 and also possess low-affinity receptors for IgE.

The primary activities of eosinophils are:

- The engulfment and/or digestion of antigen–antibody complexes. This is important in the immune response against helminth infestation (see Cellular Immunity, p. 135).
- The release of enzymes that are able to inactivate biologically active substances such as histamine. This is important in Type 1 hypersensitivity reactions.
- The release of granule proteins that damage helminths during parasitic infections and disrupt respiratory epithelium, mimicking the pathological changes observed in bronchial asthma (see Type 1 hypersensitivity reactions below).

Four eosinophil granular components are involved in mediating damage:

- *Major basic protein (MBP)*. MBP is the major protein component of eosinophil granules and directly damages helminths, producing ballooning and detachment of the tegumental membrane. Exposure of respiratory epithelium to MBP results in desquamation and disruption of the cells.
- *Eosinophil cationic protein (ECP)*. ECP is present in the matrix of eosinophil granules and its deposition has been seen in the kidneys of patients with renal disease, certain types of myocardial infarction and allergic gastroenteritis. It is highly toxic to parasites, being 8–10 times more active than MBP, producing complete fragmentation and disruption of the organisms. ECP is a potent neurotoxin.
- *Eosinophil-derived neurotoxin (EDN)*. EDN is released from the matrix of eosinophil granules and can damage myelinated neurons in experimental animals.
- *Eosinophil peroxidase (EPO)*. EPO is localized in the granule matrix of the eosinophil and in combination with a halide and H_2O_2 can kill bacteria, helminths and tumour cells; it inactivates leukotrienes C_4 and D_4 and causes mast-cell degranulation.

Antigen-presenting cells

- Cells of the monocytic/macrophage series carry HLA class II antigens and present antigens to T_H cells. Dendritic cells express HLA class II antigens on their surface and activate T_H cells. They are found in many organs, particularly in T cell areas of lymph nodes.
- Other dendritic cells (class II negative) have immunoglobulin Fc receptors and receptors for C3b for the capture of immune complexes. They are localized to B cell areas.

TYPES OF IMMUNE RESPONSE

The ability of a substance to induce an immune response is termed its antigenicity and is determined by the size, foreignness and complexity of the material. The type of immune response will depend on the antigen and the immunological maturity of the immune system. It can take the form of humoral antibody production, immune tolerance or a cell-mediated response.

HUMORAL RESPONSE

Antigens

Antigens are defined as substances that elicit immune responses in vertebrate animals. Microorganisms, even simple ones, bear a number of different antigens on their surfaces and are therefore too complex to allow the generation of an antibody against the entire organism. Instead, antibodies are directed against specific areas of the surface antigens, termed *epitopes*. Each antigen consists of a number of epitopes, which may be a repeated single unit or several structures. Antisera produced against microorganisms consist of a number of different antibodies, each being specific for the epitope against which it has been raised.

Antibody–antigen reactions

Antibody affinity
For an antibody to bind to an antigen, the two moieties must be sufficiently complementary in structure to allow them to fit closely enough for non-covalent bonding to occur, termed 'goodness of fit'. The non-covalent forces between antibody and antigen are mediated by hydrogen bonding and hydrostatic, Van der Waals' and hydrophobic binding forces. Of these, hydrophobic forces may account for up to 50% of the total strength of the antibody–antigen bond.

Antibody specificity
Although each antibody is specific for a particular epitope on an antigen, epitopes may themselves be present on more than one antigen. If this occurs, then some of the antibodies raised against one antigen will react with the corresponding epitope(s) in another that contains the same epitope. This phenomenon is termed 'cross-reactivity' and explains why antisera raised against certain organisms will react with those of others.

Antibody production
Lymphocytes and cells of the monocyte–macrophage series play a central role in antibody production:

- Macrophages, present on mucosal surfaces and

in tissues, trap the antigen and partially degrade it.

- This degraded antigen is carried on the surface of the macrophage as small, highly immunogenic peptides in association with cell antigens and presented to T and B lymphocytes.
- Receptive T and B lymphocytes undergo 'blast formation' producing a clone (family of cells).

Prior to antigen exposure, a few antigen–specific lymphocytes arise by random mutation. Initial exposure to antigen results in the appearance of circulating antibodies within 3 days and maximal antibody production by 7–10 days. This primary response is chiefly mounted by antibodies of the IgM class and also results in the generation of 'memory' T and B cells that can rapidly proliferate on re-exposure to antigen. Subsequent exposure to the same antigen results in the generation of IgG antibodies. During the secondary antigenic challenge, antibodies appear more quickly and reach a higher titre.

Proliferation of T and B cells produces:

- Plasma cells from B lymphocytes, which synthesize antibody
- T helper cells (T_H cells), which cooperate with plasma cells in the synthesis of certain antibodies
- T suppressor cells (T_S cells), which regulate antibody synthesis

The synthesis of antibody can be stimulated in two ways (Fig. 2.11):

T-independent antigens

T-independent antigens are believed to be able to directly stimulate B cells to synthesize antibody and two mechanisms of activation by these antigens have been suggested:

- T-independent antigens are polymeric (consisting of single repeated units) and this could allow them to cross-link the B cells' antigen receptors triggering antibody production.
- T-independent antigens are mitogenic, so that the second signal for antibody production may be delivered via the B cell mitogen receptor.

This is the method by which antibody production against antigens such as *Escherichia coli* and pneumococcal polysaccharides is stimulated.

T-dependent antigens

T-dependent antigens require cooperation between T and B cells to synthesize antibodies. Antigen binds to T cells via their TR receptors and to B cells via their immunoglobulin (Ig) receptors and help is then delivered directly to the B cell. This is the method by which antibody production against antigens such as serum proteins and erythrocytes is stimulated.

Various soluble factors are also generated by the actions of antigen on T cells and macrophages that stimulate the proliferation and activation of T and B cells; these are summarized in Table 2.13.

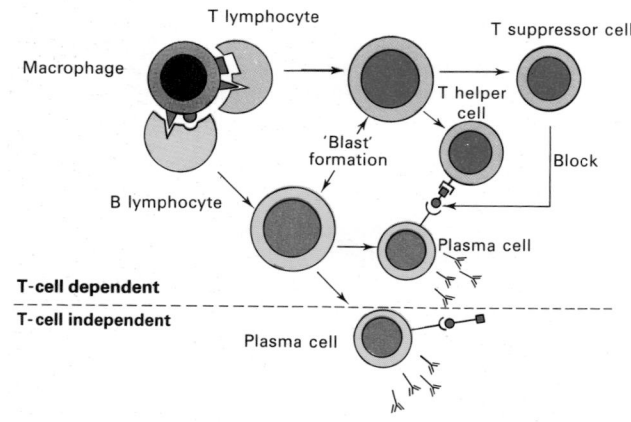

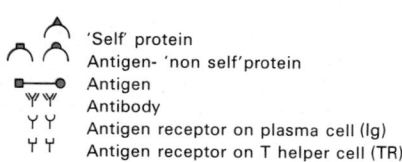

	'Self' protein
	Antigen- 'non self' protein
	Antigen
	Antibody
	Antigen receptor on plasma cell (Ig)
	Antigen receptor on T helper cell (TR)

Fig. 2.11 T-cell dependent and independent antibody production. The macrophage presents an antigen to the T or B lymphocytes, which undergo blast formation. Further differentiation leads to the formation of T helper and suppressor cells and plasma cells. Further cooperation between T helper cells and plasma cells leads to the production of antibodies, except with certain antigens (see text), when T-cell cooperation is not required.

Table 2.13 Some soluble T cell and macrophage factors involved in antibody synthesis (see also p. 137).

Factor	Antigen specific/ non-specific	Source	Target	Effect
Genetically restricted factor (GRF)	Specific	Macrophages	T cells	Induces T_H cells
Helper factor	Specific	T_H cells	B cells/macrophages	Induces B cells
Suppressor factor	Specific	T_S cells	T cells	Suppresses T cells
Interleukin-1 (IL-1)	Non-specific	Macrophages Other cells	T and B cells	Promotes multiplication and activation
Interleukin-2 (IL-2)	Non-specific	T_H cells in presence of macrophages	T and B cells	T cell proliferation and activation B-cell differentiation
Interleukin-4 (IL-4)	Non-specific	T_H cells in presence of macrophages	B cells	Synergy with IL-1 in B-cell activation
Interleukin-6 (IL-6)	Non-specific	Macrophages Fibroblasts	B cells	B-cell differentiation

The interactions between macrophages, T lymphocytes and B lymphocytes (as shown in Fig. 2.11) occur primarily within lymphoid tissue.

Immunoglobulins

These are a group of glycoproteins present in the serum and in tissue fluids whose production is induced on exposure to antigen. Immunoglobulins (Ig) consist of four polypeptide chains (two identical heavy chains and two identical light chains) that are linked together by disulphide bonds to form the basic subunit structure as represented in Figs 2.12 and 2.13. The genes for immunoglobulins are encoded on three chromosomes: chromosome 2 for κ light chains, 22 for λ light chains and 14 for the heavy chain.

There are five types of heavy chain: alpha (α), delta (δ), epsilon (ε), gamma (γ) and mu (μ), and two types of light chain, kappa (κ) and lambda (λ).

Immunoglobulin molecules are divided into five distinct classes on the basis of the heavy chain (that forms the immunoglobulin molecule). These classes are IgA (α chain), IgD (δ chain), IgE (ε chain), IgG (γ chain) and IgM (μ chain).

Papain splits immunoglobulins into two regions:

- A fragment with which antibody combines (Fab). This is divided into a variable (V) and constant homology (CH1) region or domain. The V region, or paratope, is unique for each antibody.
- A constant region fragment (Fc) that determines the class of immunoglobulin. It contains two CH domains (CH2 and CH3) in IgA, IgD and IgG and an additional one (CH4) in IgM and IgE, as these have larger heavy chains.

The constant region determines the cytophilic activities of the immunoglobulin e.g. in the case of IgG:

- *CH1*: Binding of the C4b fragment of complement
- *CH2*: Control of C1q complement fixation and the catabolic rate of the whole molecule

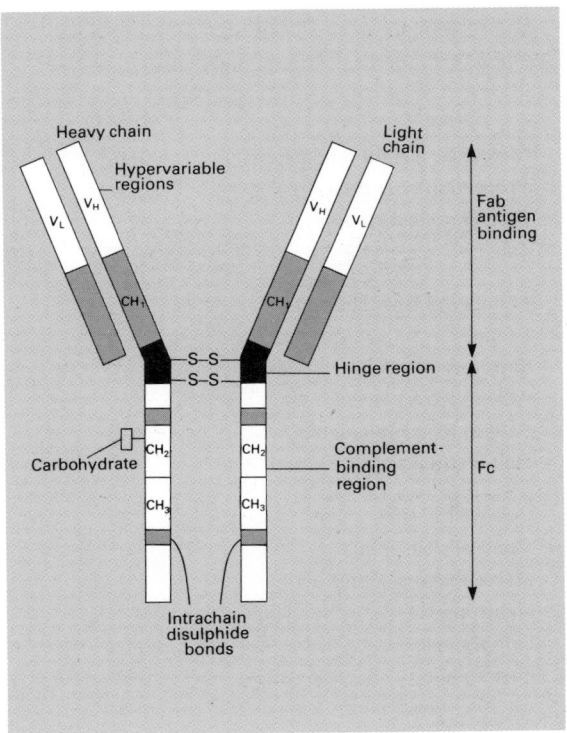

Fig. 2.12 Basic subunit structure of immunoglobulins.

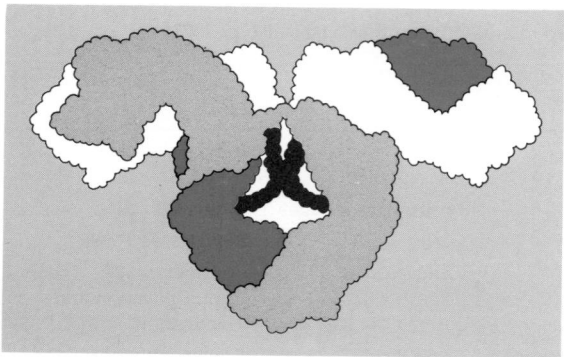

Fig. 2.13 Computer-generated model of IgG. Redrawn from *New Scientist* (1989), No. 1661.

- Interaction between CH2 and CH3. Binding to staphylococcal protein A and the Fc receptors of neutrophils and NK cells
- *CH3*: Binding to the Fc receptor of macrophages and monocytes

Immunoglobulin heterogeneity is also determined by three types of genetic variation as illustrated in Fig. 2.14:

- *Isotypic variation*. This refers to the genetic variation within the heavy and light chain CH regions that results in the formation of various heavy- and light-chain classes and subclasses, e.g. four IgG heavy-chain isotypes, IgG_1, IgG_2, IgG_3, IgG_4. The variants produced are present in

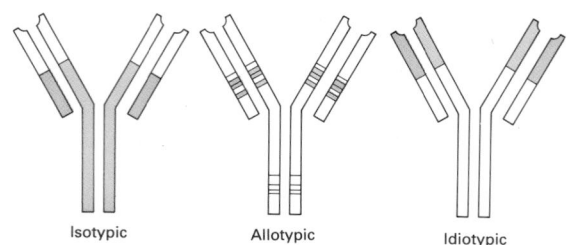

Fig. 2.14 Isotypic, allotypic and idiotypic variations of immunoglobulins.

all healthy members of a particular species.
- *Allotypic variation*. This refers to genetic variants of CH domains of the heavy and light chains that are not present in all members of a particular species. There are three groups, viz. Gm specifications found only on IgG; Km on k light chains of immunoglobulins and determined by a single amino-acid substitution at position 153 or 191 of k chain; and allotypes restricted to IgA and IgM.
- *Idiotypic variation*. This refers to variation in the V regions of the heavy and light chains, which are specific to each antibody molecule's combin-

Table 2.14 Properties of immunoglobulins (Ig).

	IgA	sIgA[a]	IgD	IgE	IgG	IgM
Molecular weight (kilodaltons)	160	400	185	200	150	900
Proportion of Ig pool	15%	—	1%	Trace	70–75%	10%
Number of subclasses	2 (IgA_1, IgA_2)	2 (IgA_1, IgA_2)	1	1	4 (IgG_1, IgG_2, IgG_3, IgG_4)	2 IgM_1, IgM_2
Number of basic subunits	1	2	1	1	1	5
J chain[b]	—	+	—	—	—	+
Secretory piece[c]	—	+	—	—	—	—[d]
Able to cross placenta	—	—	—	—	+	—
Able to fix complement	±	+	—	—	+	+
Half-life (days)	6	—	3	> 30	23	5
Cytophilic binding						
Mast cells/basophils	—	—	—	+	—	—
Macrophages/monocytes	—	—	—	+	+	—
Neutrophils	+	+	—	—	+	—
Lymphocytes	+	+	—	+	+	+
Eosinophils	—	—	—	+	+	—

[a] Secretory IgA.
[b] Joining chain—links immunoglobulin subunits together.
[c] Allows immunoglobulins to resist proteolysis; molecular weight = 60 kD.
[d] Present on secretory IgM.

ing site. These have been subdivided into α idiotopes, which are out of reach of the antigen binding site; β idiotopes, which are close to the antigen binding site; and γ idiotopes, which are those formed by the antigen binding site itself.

The different classes vary both in their structure and their physicochemical properties (Table 2.14).

- *Immunoglobulin A*. IgA represents 15–20% of the human serum immunoglobulin pool and is the predominant immunoglobulin in secretions, e.g. gut. Secretory IgA (sIgA) is chiefly dimeric, with the two subunits joined together by a joining or J chain, and is protected from proteolysis by combining with a protein termed the secretory component. It plays a primary role in mucosal immunity through the fixation of complement via the alternative pathway and by preventing the adherence of microorganisms at mucosal surfaces. Some organisms e.g. *Neisseria meningitidis* can overcome this by producing an IgA protease.
- *Immunoglobulin D*. IgD accounts for less than 1% of the total plasma immunoglobulin but is present on circulating lymphocytes. Its role is, as yet, unknown although it is believed to be involved in lymphocyte differentiation.
- *Immunoglobulin E*. IgE is present in trace amounts and is a serum monomeric protein that is present on the membranes of basophils and mast cells. It plays a primary role in the defence against helminthic infection and in allergic disease IgE can fix complement via the alternative pathway.
- *Immunoglobulin G*. IgG is a monomeric protein accounting for 70–75% of serum immunoglobulin. The majority of antibody production during secondary immune responses is of this class, as are antitoxin antibodies. IgG (except IgG$_4$) can fix complement via the classical pathway.
- *Immunoglobulin M*. IgM represents 10% of the total serum pool. This pentameric molecule joined together by five J chains is also found in secretions where, like sIgA, it possesses a secretory piece to prevent proteolysis. The majority of antibodies synthesized during primary immune responses are of this class. IgM can fix complement via the classical pathway.

COMPLEMENT

Complement is a series of nine plasma proteins that become bound to antigen–antibody complexes in a specific sequence (cascade) and contribute to humoral immunity in two main ways:

- *Opsonization and phagocytosis*. The binding of complement and/or antibody to the surface of a

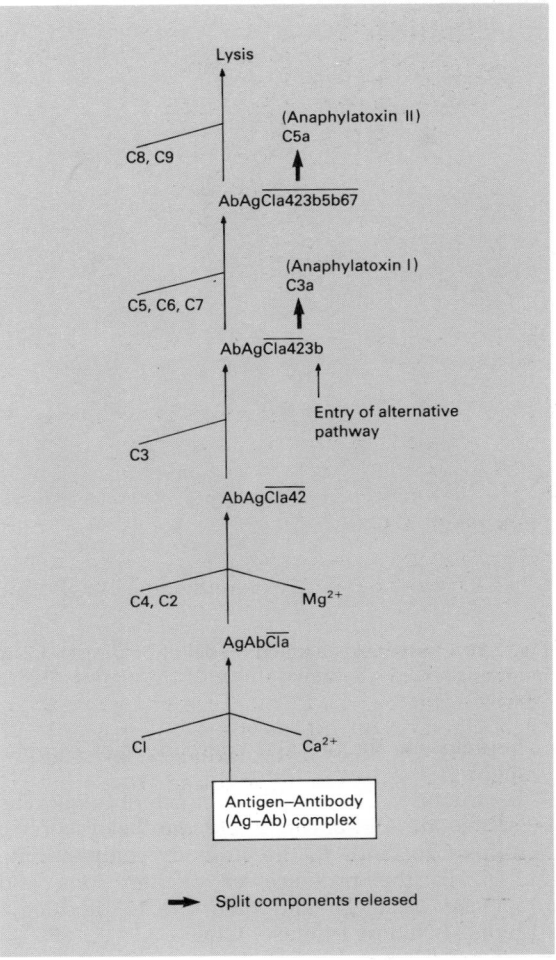

Fig. 2.15 The classical pathway of complement activation.

microorganism attracts phagocytes towards it and facilitates the phagocytosis and elimination of the organism.
- *Complement fixation*. The fixation of complement to the surface of a microorganism results in both its opsonization and, if the complement cascade is completed, lysis of the organism

Binding, or fixation, of complement results in either the lysis or engulfment by phagocytes of the antigen, and can occur by two major routes—the classical and the alternative pathways.

The classical pathway

The classical pathway is triggered either by two IgG antibodies or by one IgM being bound to antigenic material as summarized in Fig. 2.15.

- The Fc sites of the antibody/antibodies produce a

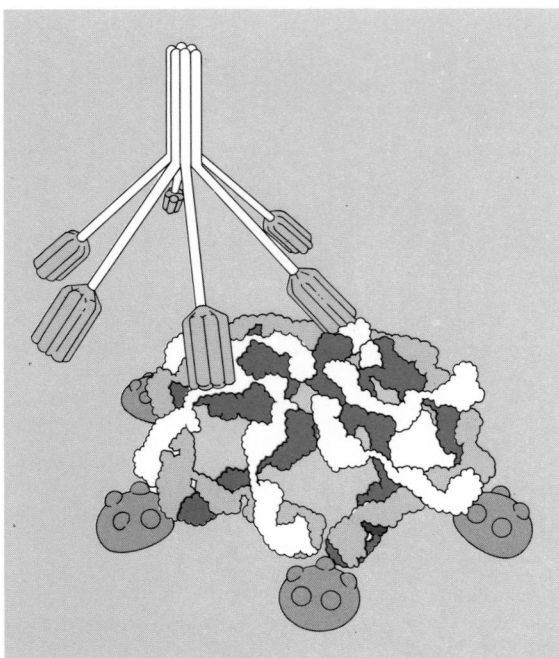

Fig. 2.16 Computer-generated model of binding of C1 to immunoglobulin. Redrawn from *New Scientist* (1989), No. 1661.

binding site for the first component of complement—C1.

- In structure, C1 resembles a bunch of tulips. The 'stems' are C1s and C1r and the 'heads' of the tulips C1q binds to the antibody complex (Fig. 2.16) in the presence of calcium ions and activates first C1r and then C1s to produce a serine–histidine esterase, C1a.
- C4 and C2 next bind to the complex. C1a splits off a 6000-dalton protein from C4 and the remaining C4b fragment complexes with C2 in the presence of magnesium ions. Following the loss of a 30 000-dalton fragment from C2, C4b2b binds to the complex. C1a activates the C42 complex to form C3 convertase.
- The binding of C3 to the complex causes the particles that are being coated to agglutinate (immune adherence). C3 convertase cleaves a 9000-dalton protein from C3 (C3a) and the remaining larger fragment is bound to the complex.
- C5, C6 and C7 bind to the complex with the liberation of a 15 000-dalton protein from C5 (C5a). The C567 complex tends to polymerize and form micelles in free solution. In this state it is highly reactive and will attach itself to any nearby cell's lipid bilayer. This produces a phenomenon known as 'bystander lysis' in which non-target cells are also destroyed.
- C8 causes cells to become 'leaky' and C9 lyses the antigenic material.

Several biologically active molecules are generated during the complement cascade:

- C3a (anaphylatoxin I) is chemotactic for neutrophils and liberates histamine from mast cells. It also produces smooth-muscle contraction and erythema and oedema in the skin. Receptors for this complement component are present on monocytes, neutrophils, mast cells, basophils and eosinophils.
- C3b enhances adherence to and engulfment of antigenic particles by phagocytes. Receptors for this complement component are present on neutrophils, eosinophils, macrophages and monocytes.
- C4b is similar to C3b but less effective.
- C5a (anaphylatoxin II) is chemotactic for neutrophils and activates them to produce leukotrienes, especially leukotriene B_4. Like C3a, C5a also produces mast-cell degranulation and smooth-muscle contraction. Receptors for this complement component are present on monocytes, neutrophils, mast cells, basophils and eosinophils.
- C567 is chemotactic for neutrophils.

Modulation of the classical complement cascade is achieved by:

- C1a esterase inhibitor
- Anaphylatoxin inactivator (attacks C3a and C5a)

The alternative pathway

The alternative pathway can be triggered by IgA, IgE, cobra venom and bacterial endotoxins and is summarized in Fig. 2.17. It is initiated by particle-bound C3b that is thought to be continuously formed in small amounts by the actions of proteolytic enzymes present in body fluids.

- Factor B is bound to C3b in the presence of magnesium ions. The binding of this 80 000-dalton protein is controlled by the presence of another factor, termed Factor H, which competes with Factor B for the C3b-binding site. Which of the two factors is bound depends on the surface to which the C3b is attached.
- The C3bB complex is susceptible to enzymatic cleavage by Factor D. This results in the loss of a 33 000-dalton Ba protein and the formation of a C3bBb complex, which is stabilized by the binding of properdin. C3bBb is the alternative pathway equivalent to C3 convertase and the binding of another molecule of C3b results in the formation of C5 convertase.
- C3 convertase also produces a positive feedback loop that enhances the rate at which complement is fixed.
- C5, C6, C7, C8 and C9 bind as in the classical pathway with the liberation of C5a.

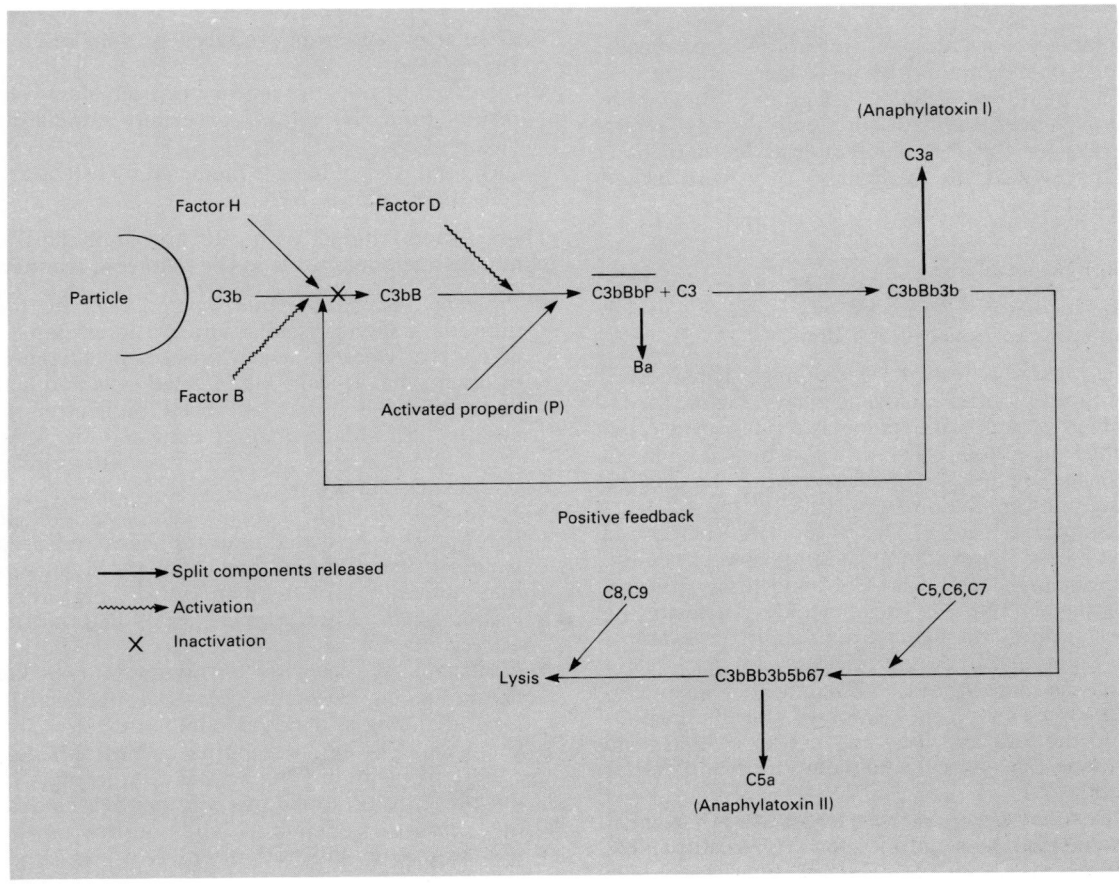

Fig. 2.17 The alternative pathway of complement activation.

Modulation of the alternative complement cascade is achieved by:

- Factor H
- C3b inactivator (C3 INH)

CELLULAR IMMUNITY

Cellular immune responses primarily involve the activation of T cells by antigen-presenting cells and are those in which antibody plays a subordinate role. They are involved in immunity against intracellular viruses, parasites and bacteria resistant to phagocytosis.

Antigen presentation

Antigen presentation by macrophages to T cells results in these cells releasing a factor that induces the antigen-presenting cell to generate interleukin 1 (IL-1). IL-1 production activates the T cell to produce IL-2, which drives the antigenically activated cells to proliferate.

Cell-mediated cytotoxicity

Lysis of cells by specific T_C cells and by NK cells results from the close binding of these cells to their targets. Binding results from:

- Antigen-specific receptors on the T_C cells. No antibody is required to elicit this binding and the T cells generally survive following lysing of the target cell, often to kill more targets. This form of cellular toxicity is important in eliminating virally-infected cells.
- Determinants recognized by NK cells. NK cells bind to their targets and, in the presence of calcium, 'modify' the target so that it then lyses independently of the NK cell. These cells also release a cytotoxic factor with similar activities.
- Antibody or Fc receptors on K cells. This form of cell-mediated cytotoxicity involves the recognition by K cells of the Fc portion of antibody bound to the target cell and the subsequent lysing of the cell. This may be important in the elimination of tumour-infected cells.

Cytokines

Cytokines are a group of proteins released chiefly by activated lymphocytes and macrophages and which modulate cellular immunity. They have generally been divided into lymphokines, which are released by activated lymphocytes, and interleukins, which are a 'family' of seven related proteins.

Lymphokines

These mediators, generated by activated T and B lymphocytes have several actions:

- *Macrophage activation.* Macrophage activation is induced by macrophage activation factor (MAF), which increases the killing and phagocytic capacities of these cells. Once activated, macrophages are prevented from leaving the area by migration-inhibition factor (MIF).
- *Eosinophil activation.* This is mediated by several cytokines including granulocyte colony-stimulating factor (GM-CSF) and tumour necrosis factor (TNF β). These cytokines activate the eosinophils and increase their ability for example to kill antibody coated *Schistosoma*.
- *Leucocyte chemotaxis.* Chemotactic cytokines attract eosinophils, basophils and neutrophils into the area and they are then prevented from leaving by leucocyte migration-inhibitory factor (LIF).
- *Destruction of non-leucocyte target cells* is mediated by the cytokines lymphotoxin (TNFα) and TNFβ. TNF α and β increase the killing of susceptible

cells by NK cells.

- Cellular exudation is produced by skin reactive factor (SRF).
- Increased turnover of leucocytes from stem cells results from the release of colony-stimulating factors (CSF).
- Increased lysis of bone is mediated by osteoclast-activating factor (OAF).

These factors interact with cells and antibodies to eliminate microorganisms in the following manner:

- *Prevention of viral spread* (Fig. 2.18). In the immune response against viruses, interferons α and γ are released, which prevent proliferation of organisms. T_C cells kill infected cells and halt viral spread if it has not been transferred to another cell. Macrophages, activated by MAF from sensitized T cells, break intracellular bridges, preventing viral spread.
- *Elimination of bacteria and protozoa resistant to phagocytosis.* Activated macrophages released from sensitized T cells can eliminate organisms that normally survive phagocytosis, e.g. *Toxoplasma gondii*, *Mycobacterium leprae* and *Listeria monocytogenes*.
- *Elimination of helminths.* Antibodies can kill helminths, e.g. *Schistosoma mansonii*, by mechanisms involving antibody-dependent cytotoxicity. Cytotoxic cells, e.g. eosinophils or macrophages, adhere to helminths via Fc and C3 receptors in the presence of antibodies. Eosinophils bind to the opsonized helminth and destroy it by releasing eosinophil cationic protein and major basic protein.

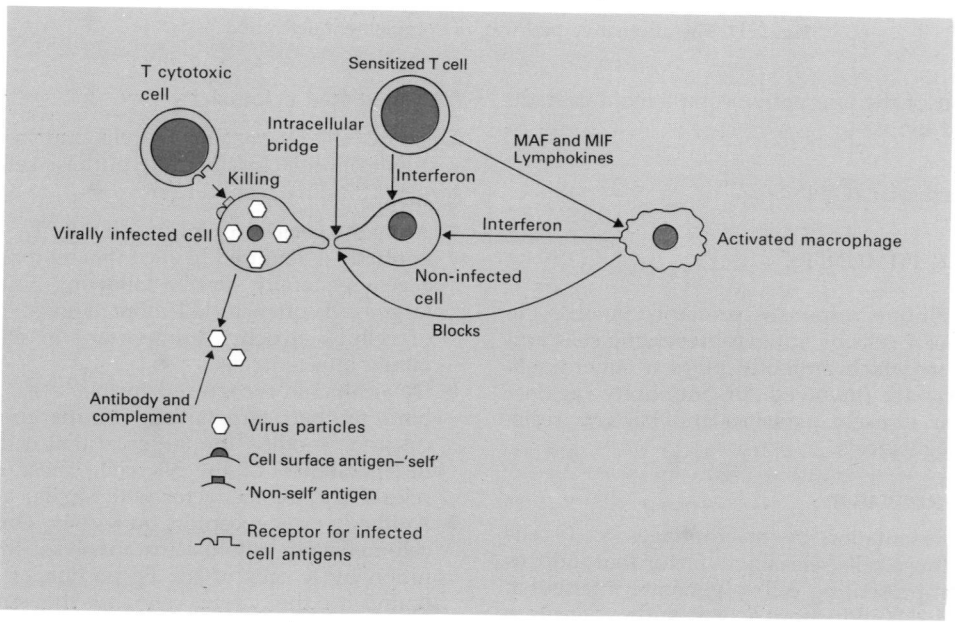

Fig. 2.18 Cell-mediated immunity against viruses (see text). MAF = macrophage-activation factor, MIF = macrophage-inhibition factor.

Interleukins

The interleukins are a group of proteins that pass signals between cells of the immune system. They are generated by a wide variety of cell types including T cells, macrophages and epithelial cells and interact to control the cellular immune response. They are also involved in haemopoiesis.

- *Interleukin 1 (IL-1)*. IL-1 (leucocyte activating factor LAF) is released from macrophages, fibroblasts, endothelial and epithelial cells. It stimulates the proliferation of T and B cells, increases bone resorption and induces prostaglandin synthesis. In its membrane-bound form on macrophages it also stimulates lymphocyte activation and differentiation.
- *Interleukin 2 (IL-2)*. IL-2 (T-cell replacing factor, TRF and T-cell growth factor) is released by activated T cells and is a co-factor for the growth and differentiation of T and B cells. It also increases the cytotoxic activity of monocytes, T cells and NK cells. IL-2 receptors appear on T cells after polyclonal activation of the T-cell receptor. They are of high affinity and have two distinct polypeptide chains, each of which contains an IL-2 binding site.
- *Interleukin 3 (IL-3)*. IL-3 (multicolony-stimulating factor, multi-CSF) is also released by activated T cells and stimulates the growth of haemopoietic stem and progenitor cells. It has also been shown, at least in mice, to support mast cell growth.
- *Interleukin 4 (IL-4)*. IL-4 (B-cell growth factor, BCGF and B-cell stimulating factor, BSF-1) is released by T cells and is a growth factor for B cells, some T cells, myeloid and erythroid precursors, all of which have an IL-4 receptor. IL-4 is important for immunoglobulin isotype regulation.
- *Interleukin 5 (IL-5)*. IL-5 is released by activated T cells and induces eosinophil differentiation (CFU-EO), activated B-cell proliferation and IgA synthesis.
- *Interleukin 6 (IL-6)*. IL-6 is released by fibroblasts and macrophages and induces B-cell differentiation and expression of acute phase reactants on hepatocytes. IL-6 receptors are present on various cell types. IL-6 may be involved in the pathogenesis of certain autoimmune diseases.
- *Interleukin 7 (IL-7)*. IL-7 (lymphopoietin 1) is released by bone-marrow cells and serves as a growth factor for the early lymphoid precursors of both B and T cells.

Interferons

Interferons (IFN) are regulatory proteins produced by virus-infected cells and interfere with virus replication. There are three main types of interferons:

- IFN-α, encoded by over 20 genes on chromosome 9 for over 15 functionally different alphas
- IFN-β, encoded by a single gene near α on chromosome 9
- IFN-γ, encoded by a single gene on chromosome 12

Each contains 165–187 amino acids and has a molecular weight in the range 17–25 kD.

IFNs can be induced by:

- Viruses, bacteria, double-stranded RNA (IFN-α and -β)
- Mitogens and antigens (IFN-γ)
- Other protein regulators e.g. cytokines (TNF, IL-1, IL-2), colony-stimulating factors

IFN-α is mainly produced in peripheral blood mononuclear cells; IFN-β in fibroblasts and epithelial cells. IFNs are also produced constitutively in other sites of the body e.g. peritoneum.

IFN cell receptors

Two different cell-surface receptors are widely distributed in the body, viz. IFN-α and IFN-β share a 110–130 kD receptor encoded by chromosome 21; IFN-γ receptor is probably a product of a single mRNA and has a molecular weight of 54 kD and is encoded by chromosome 6.

Actions and uses (see Table 2.15)
IFNs control cellular actions by binding to cell-surface receptors and transiently and rapidly inhibiting translation of viral mRNA by stimulating protein kinase and a ribonuclease that destroys viral mRNA.

Table 2.15 Some actions of interferons.[a]

Action	IFN-α	IFN-β	IFN-γ
B cells			
Activation	—	—	Yes
Proliferation	No	—	—
Differentiation	—	—	Yes
T cells			
Stimulate growth	—	—	Yes
Cytotoxic	Yes	—	Yes
Cytostatic	Yes	Yes	Yes
Induction of anti-viral			
state	Yes	Yes	Yes
class I MHC	Yes	Yes	Yes
class II MHC	No	No	Yes
Antitumour activity	Yes	Yes	Yes
Induce fever	Yes	Yes	Yes
Vaccine adjuvant			
properties	—	—	Yes

[a] Data from Balkwill F (1989) Lancet i, pp. 1060–1062, (with permission).

Interferons confer resistance to infection by many RNA and DNA viruses. They can:

- control immune responses by, for example, inducing MHC class I and II genes or inducing cell-surface receptors for Fc portion of IgG or for other cytokines, e.g. TNF. IFN-γ appears to have a more central role in immune regulation; it is a macrophage-activating factor, enhancing cytotoxic activity of NK cells.
- control cell growth and differentiation. IFN-α and IFN-β are potent inhibitors of normal and malignant cell growth; some cells are arrested at G1 phase, the proto-oncogene *c-myc* is inhibited.
- be used in anticancer therapy, e.g. IFN-α used in hairy cell leukaemia, chronic myelocytic leukaemia, multiple myeloma, essential thrombocythaemia, lymphoma, solid tumours (AIDS-related Kaposi's tumour).
- be used in infectious diseases e.g. chronic hepatitis B, leprosy.

IMMUNE TOLERANCE AND AUTOIMMUNITY

When cells from the immune system of an animal that has not reached immunological maturity are exposed to antigenic material they are unable to produce antibodies against it. This state of specific unreactivity which can also be acquired in adults is termed 'immunological tolerance'.

B-cell tolerance

Tolerance can be induced in B cells in four ways:

- *Clonal abortion.* When immature B cells encounter low concentrations of antigen, this may cause the immature clone to abort.
- *Clonal exhaustion.* Repeated antigenic challenge can result in removal of all mature functional B-cell clones leading to clonal exhaustion.
- *Functional deletion.* Absence of specific T-cell help, required for antibody synthesis, and presence of specific T_S results in an inability of the B cells to function properly.
- Antibody forming cell blockade. Large doses of antigen can lead to effective tolerization as the antigen is recognized as 'self'.

T-cell tolerance

Tolerance can be induced in T cells in three ways:

- *Clonal abortion.* Immature T cells may abort when they encounter antigen in a similar way to B cells.
- *Functional deletion.* Subsets of mature T cells, e.g.

T_C, T_H, may be deleted.
- *T suppression.* Specific T suppressor cells may be generated that inhibit the activities of other T or B cells.

Forbidden clones

Immunological tolerance to the body's own tissue is thought to be acquired during fetal life, and therefore the body does not mount significant antibodies against its own tissues. Nevertheless, some clones of cells that can produce 'autoantibody' ('forbidden clones') are thought to be produced throughout life and are either:

- Suppressed by large amounts of 'self' antigen
- Suppressed by antigen-specific T_S cells

Autoimmunity is the loss of tolerance to 'self'-antigens. Autoantibodies are produced to a wide variety of antigens. These autoantibodies may be organ-specific (e.g. intrinsic factor antibodies in pernicious anaemia, thyroid antibodies in Hashimoto's disease) or non-organ specific (e.g. antinuclear factor in systemic lupus erythematosus).

Three mechanisms are involved in the pathogenesis:

- Immune complex disease, in which complexes formed between autoantibodies and antigens deposit in various tissues, e.g. glomeruli.
- Circulating autoantibodies react with antigens on surfaces of cells, stimulating release of inflammatory mediators or complement or activating cytotoxic cells. The latter two will lead to cell lysis.
- Cell-mediated immunity. Sensitized T cells may injure cells directly or indirectly by releasing lymphokines.

In some diseases, more than one of the mechanisms above may be involved, e.g. in SLE. In other conditions, autoantibodies may bind to the cell-surface receptors and interfere with their function, e.g. autoantibodies to acetylcholine receptors on the motor end-plate in myasthenia gravis. In a similar way, antibodies to hormone receptors may alter their function, e.g. autoantibodies to the thyrotrophin receptor (long-acting thyroid stimulator, LATS) causes excess hormone secretion in Graves's disease. Experimentally, a foreign antigen that resembles a self-antigen can induce an autoimmune reaction (molecular mimicry), e.g. experimental allergic encephalitis. In humans this mechanism may apply in the encephalitis seen following rabies vaccination with inactivated rabies virus grown in neural tissue of animals.

Abnormalities of the immune response

IMMUNODEFICIENCY DISEASES

Some individuals are unable to produce an immune response to antigenic material and are termed immunodeficient. Immunodeficiency may be inherited or may occur as a result of infection or drug therapy. It includes defects in antibody production, complement fixation, and lymphocyte and phagocyte functioning.

Antibody deficiency syndromes
Table 2.16 shows syndromes associated with defective antibody production.

Complement deficiencies
Deficiencies of the following can occur:

- C1 esterase inhibitor, causing hereditary angioedema (see p. 1015) (the deficiency is inherited in an autosomal dominant manner)
- C1q, leading to persistent skin lesions (discoid lupus erythematosus)
- C1q, C1r, C4 or C2, causing an increased tendency to immune complex vasculitis
- C3 or C3b inhibitor, leading to exhaustion of the alternative pathway and associated with Klinefelter's syndrome
- C5, C6, C7 or C8, caused by a genetic defect and leading to recurrent infections with *Neisseria*

Immunodeficiency disease involving defective T lymphocyte functions

In these diseases, cell-mediated immunity is impaired in all cases. They include:

- *Thymic aplasia*, either with hypoparathyroidism (DiGeorge's syndrome) or with normal parathyroids (Nezelof syndrome). Antibody production is normal but patients usually die in infancy. Fungal infections are common (see p. 76).
- *Purine nucleoside phosphorylase deficiency.* Antibody production is normal but some patients also have abnormal red blood cells.
- *Ataxia telangiectasia.* This is inherited as an autosomal recessive and is associated with selective IgA deficiency, cerebellar ataxia and oculocutaneous telangiectasia. Onset is early and children die in the second decade owing to infections.
- *Wiskott–Aldrich syndrome.* This is an X-linked recessive defect thought to involve faulty presentation of antigen by macrophages. Males present with thrombocytopenia, eczema and

recurrent infections. The immunoglobulins are normal but no antibody is produced against polysaccharide antigens.

- *Bloom's syndrome.* Immunoglobulin levels are reduced, with sometimes only IgA being affected. Lymphomas are seen.
- *Severe combined immunodeficiency* (SCID). This presents in the first few months of life and has a variable inheritance. No specific antibodies are produced and low numbers of T and B lymphocytes are seen. Death is usual before the age of 2 years. It can occur in association with other diseases, e.g. short-limbed dwarfism.

Immunodeficiency disease involving defective phagocyte functions

Patients suffer from repeated infections, mainly involving the skin. Diseases include:

- *Job's syndrome.* High levels of serum IgE and defective neutrophil chemotaxis are seen.
- *Chronic granulomatous disease* (CGD). This is a sex-linked disease in which chemotaxis is normal but intracellular killing of catalase-positive organisms in polymorphonuclear leucocytes and macrophages is impaired.
- *Chédiak–Higashi syndrome.* Neutrophil lysosomal formation is affected, leading to impaired killing. It is associated with oculocutaneous albinism, and staphylococcal and candidal infections are common.
- *Myeloperoxidase deficiency.* This is an autosomally recessive-linked disease producing reduced levels of myeloperoxidase enzyme in neutrophils and monocytes. Systemic candidiasis is common.

HYPERSENSITIVITY REACTIONS

Immunological priming can lead, on further exposure to antigen, to either secondary boosting of the immune response or an excessive damaging reaction termed hypersensitivity. Six types of hypersensitivity have been described (Fig. 2.19, Table 2.17): types I, II, III and V are mediated by antibody and types IV and VI by cellular mechanisms. In practice, these reactions may not necessarily occur singly. For example, types II–VI may be involved in producing autoimmune diseases.

Type I reaction (reaginic/anaphylactic/immediate hypersensitivity reaction)

This is an allergic reaction produced within 30 min of exposure to a specific allergen. Allergens, e.g. house dust, pollens, animal danders or moulds, only elicit reactions in certain genetically predis-

Table 2.16 Immunodeficiency syndromes associated with defective antibody production.

Syndrome	Antibodies/immunoglobulins	Circulating B lymphocytes	Circulating T lymphocytes	Comments
X-linked 'agammaglobulinaemia'	Small amounts of IgG and IgM	Absent	Immature	Familial. Sometimes only male offspring and siblings affected
Transient hypogammaglobulinaemia in childhood	Produced against potent antigens, e.g. tetanus toxoid, only	Normal	Low numbers of T helper cells	Recurrent infections
Late onset primary hypogammaglobulinaemia	Low levels, especially of IgA	Normal, produce mainly IgM	Fail to differentiate. Some patients have increased numbers of T suppressor cells	Recurrent respiratory tract infections, especially *H. influenzae*. Also gut infections, haematological abnormalities and arthritis
Functional antibody deficiency	Impaired response to antigens such as tetanus toxoid	Normal	Normal	Mechanisms unknown. May follow chronic infection or smoking
Thymoma and hypogammaglobulinaemia	Low IgA. Moderate hypogammaglobulinaemia	Absent (also precursors)	Normal	Patients usually 40–70 years of age at presentation
Low IgG and IgA with hyper-IgM	Low levels of IgG and IgA, high levels of IgM			
IgA deficiency	IgG and IgM normal, IgM and IgD found in secretions	Normal	Normal	
IgG subclass deficiencies	IgM and IgA normal. Sometimes IgG normal, except for one subclass			Sometimes familial
IgM deficiency	Normal	Normal	T helper cell defect	Rare. Usually other immunoglobulins involved

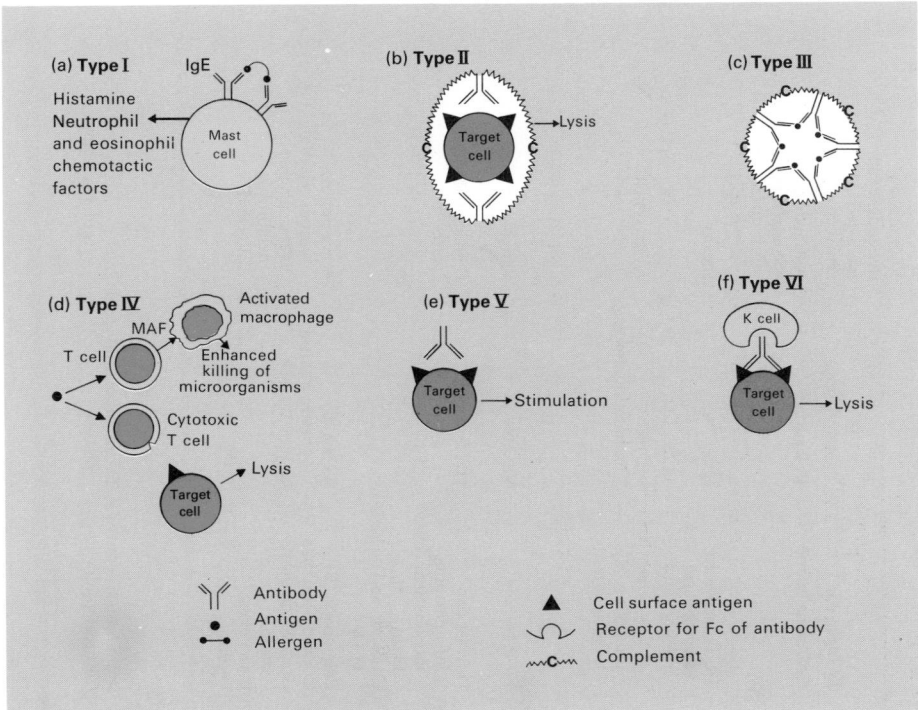

Fig. 2.19 Hypersensitivity reactions. (a) Type I: immediate anaphylactic hypersensitivity. (b) Type II: membrane damage/cytolytic hypersensitivity. (c) Type III: immune complex hypersensitivity. (d) Type IV: delayed hypersensitivity. (e) Type V: stimulatory hypersensitivity. (f) Type VI: antibody-dependent cell-mediated cytotoxicity (ADCC). MAF = macrophage-activating factor.

posed individuals, who are said to be atopic (see p. 664). Atopy is diagnosed on skin prick testing (see Fig. 12.18, p. 648) when a reaction is elicited by sensitizing allergens. Type I reactions can be passively transferred by injection of serum containing IgE antibody into the skin (passive cutaneous anaphylaxis). The antibody will remain fixed to the mast cells in the skin for up to 4–5 days and an injection of the antigen will produce a wheal and flare reaction (Prausnitz–Küstner reaction).

Type I reactions are mediated via allergen-specific antibodies of the IgE class and occur as follows.

- Allergen inhalation or ingestion results in local generation of specific IgE via the interaction of macrophages and receptive B and T_H cells.
- Locally produced allergen-specific IgE then binds to the Fc receptors of mast cells and, to a lesser extent, eosinophils and macrophages sensitizing them. IgE also enters the circulation, where it sensitizes basophils.
- Subsequent exposure to allergen results in the cross-linking of the IgE antibodies on the sensitized cells and to mediator release (see Fig. 2.19).

Binding of allergen to sensitized cells results in the *de novo* synthesis and/or release of several inflammatory mediators:

- *Histamine.* Present as a preformed mediator in sensitized mast cells and basophils, histamine produces vasodilatation and bronchial smooth-muscle constriction.
- *Arachidonic acid metabolites.* Arachidonic acid is generated in sensitized cells from membrane lipids following the binding of specific allergen. It is subsequently metabolized to produce prostaglandins (cyclo-oxygenase pathway), leukotrienes (lipo-oxygenase pathway) or platelet-activating factor (PAF acetylation), depending on which cell type is being activated (see Fig. 12.30). Leukotrienes and prostaglandins are together termed *eicosanoids*.

The arachidonic acid metabolites involved in Type I hypersensitivity reactions are PAF, leukotrienes (LT) B_4, C_4, D_4 and E_4 and prostaglandins (PG) D_2, E_2 and $F_{2\alpha}$. They have four main actions:

- *Inflammatory cell mucosal infiltration.* This is mediated by LTB_4 and PAF, which attract and activate neutrophils, eosinophils and monocytes/macrophages. LTB_4 is released by activated mast cells and macrophages and PAF is released by mast cells, neutrophils and eosinophils.
- *Bronchoconstriction.* This is mediated by several metabolites including PAF, LTC_4, LTD_4 and LTE_4 and PGD_2 and $PGF_{2\alpha}$. LTC_4 and PGD_2 are

Table 2.17 Summary of hypersensitivity reactions.

	I (immediate)	II (cytotoxic)	III (immune complex)	IV (delayed)	V (stimulating)	VI (antibody-dependent cell-mediated cytoxocity)[a]
Antigens	Pollens, moulds, mites, drugs, food and parasites	Cell surface or tissue bound	Exogenous (bacteria, fungi, parasites) Autoantigens	Cell/tissue bound	Cell surface	Antibody complexed on cell surface of target cells
Mediators	IgE and mast cells	IgG, IgM and complement	IgG, IgM, IgA and complement	T_D, T_C activated macrophages and lymphokines	IgG	K cells
Diagnostic tests	Skin prick tests—wheal and flare RAST	Coombs' test Indirect immunofluorescence (antibodies) Red cell agglutination Precipitating antibodies	Skin test—oedema, erythema (Arthus reaction) Immune complexes	Skin test—erythema induration (e.g. tuberculin test)	Indirect immunofluorescence	As for type II
Time taken for reaction to develop	15–30 min	Rapid	4–12 h	12–48 h	Variable	Variable
Histology	Oedema, vasodilatation, mast cell degranulation, eosinophils	Damage to target cells	Acute inflammatory reaction, neutrophils, vasculitis	Perivascular inflammation, mononuclear cells, fibrin Caseation and necrosis in TB	Hypertrophy	Damage to target cells
Diseases and conditions produced	Asthma (extrinsic) Eczema (atopic) Urticaria Allergic rhinitis Anaphylaxis	Autoimmune haemolytic anaemia Transfusion reactions Haemolytic disease of newborn Goodpasture's syndrome Addisonian pernicious anaemia Myasthenia gravis	Autoimmune e.g. SLE, glomerulonephritis, rheumatoid arthritis Low-grade persistent infections, e.g. viral hepatitis Disease caused by environmental antigens, e.g. farmer's lung	Pulmonary TB Contact dermatitis Graft-versus-host disease Insect bites Leprosy	Neonatal hyperthyroidism Graves' disease	Autoimmune tumour rejection Defence against helminthic infection
Treatment	Antigen avoidance Antihistamines Corticosteroids (usually topical) Sodium cromoglycate	Exchange transfusion Plasmapheresis	Corticosteroids Immunosuppressives Plasmapheresis	Immunosuppressives Corticosteroids	Treatment of individual disease	Treat symptomatically

[a] Type VI hypersensitivity may also be classified with type II reactions.

the major arachidonic acid metabolites released by mast cells. The remaining eicosanoids are generated by human lung tissue and/or alveolar macrophages.

- Bronchial mucosal oedema is mediated by LTC_4 and LTD_4 and PGE_2. PGE_2 is released from alveolar macrophages and human lung tissue.
- Mucus hypersecretion is mediated by LTC_4 and LTD_4.

— IgG Ab reacting with cell surface Ag

Type II reactions (cytotoxic/membrane reactions)

— IgG Ab reacting with cell surface (r) → signalling

In this type of reaction, antibodies of the IgG or IgM class are directed against cell-surface or tissue antigens. These antibodies interact via their Fc regions and fix complement. Antibodies are produced against epitopes on the patient's own cells and can lead to the development of autoimmune diseases, e.g. autoimmune haemolytic anaemia.

Antibodies can also 'block' a receptor site, preventing its normal function: for example, in insulin-resistant diabetes antibodies react with the insulin receptors. In this particular type of reaction, complement is not involved.

In certain conditions, IgG autoantibodies are present but it is not clear whether they are involved in the pathogenesis of the disease, e.g. intrinsic factor antibodies are found in pernicious anaemia.

Type III reactions (immune-complex-mediated hypersensitivity reactions)

Antibodies (IgG or IgM) can complex with antigen to form immune complexes. These are usually removed by the reticuloendothelial system, but a hypersensitivity reaction can sometimes occur when these complexes are deposited in the tissues. Complement is activated and this results in an inflammatory reaction leading to cellular damage.

Immune complexes can be:

- *Soluble.* These are formed when the antigen is in excess and can be produced, for example, by injecting large amounts of xenogeneic serum into the circulation, leading to 'serum sickness'.
- *Insoluble.* These precipitates are formed when the concentrations of antibody and antigen are equivalent or when there is an excess of antibody. The size of the complexes determines the site at which they are deposited. An intradermal injection of antigen in a patient with a high circulating level of antibody will produce a red, oedematous area at the site of the injection within 4–12 h. This is called the 'Arthus reaction'. Examples of conditions in which insoluble complexes are formed include pulmonary aspergillosis (when the complexes are deposited in bronchial walls) and erythema nodosum (when the complexes are deposited in the vessels).

Tissue damage occurs as follows.

- Complement fixation leads to generation of C3a and C5a.
- C3a and C5a have chemotactic properties and cause release of vasoactive amines from mast cells and basophils.
- Vascular permeability is thus increased and polymorphonuclear leucocytes are sequestered.
- Lysosomal enzymes are released and cause tissue damage.
- Complexes also interact with platelets through their Fc receptors, causing them to aggregate and microthrombi to form.

The diseases produced by immune complex deposition can be divided according to the type of antigen.

- Autoimmune diseases, e.g. systemic lupus erythematosus, are caused by the production of an antibody to a *self-antigen*, which leads to immune complex formation and deposition.
- Low-grade persistent infection with a *microbial antigen* with a weak antibody response leads to chronic immune complex formation, e.g. in viral hepatitis B or staphylococcal infective endocarditis.
- Repeated inhalation of an *environmental antigen*—moulds or an animal antigen—can produce an extrinsic allergic alveolitis, e.g. farmer's lung disease. The antibodies are IgG rather than IgE.

IVa1 = Ag presented to Th1 cells eg RhA
IVa2 = Ag " to Th2 cells eg Asthma
IVb = CD8+ cytotoxic recognise Ag on surface of target cells

Type IV reactions (cell-mediated/delayed hypersensitivity reactions)

eg IDDM.

These reactions take more than 12 h to develop and can be produced in several ways. Type IV reactions can be transferred from one animal to another by certain types of lymphocytes but not by serum.

The reaction is mediated by:

- T delayed hypersensitivity cells (T_D) that have become sensitized to a particular antigen previously: these release lymphokines and interleukins (see Cellular Immunity, p. 135).
- T cytotoxic cells (T_C), which directly damage infected target cells, e.g. virus-infected cells, allogeneic cells or host cells in graft-versus-host disease.

Cell recruitment in type IV reactions is initially neutrophil in nature (within a few hours) and is followed by lymphocyte and macrophage infiltration (24–48 h).

Type IV reactions are seen in association with viral infections, tuberculosis and brucellosis. They have also been implicated in autoimmune diseases such as Hashimoto's thyroiditis and homograft rejection.

Type V reaction (stimulating antibody reaction)

Antibodies of the IgG class directed against cell-surface antigens can 'stimulate' some cells instead of killing them. They may be important in the pathogenesis of neonatal hyperthyroidism, as IgG stimulating antibodies directed against thyroid cells would be capable of crossing the placenta.

Type VI reaction (antibody-dependent cell-mediated cytotoxicity; ADCC)

Killer lymphocytes (K cells) can lyse target cells coated with antibody. They are 'activated' by antigen–antibody complexes. The K cells interact with the Fc region of cell-bound antibody, and destroy the target cells by the release of proteolytic enzymes.

Type VI reactions are involved in autoimmune diseases, tumour rejection and defence against helminthic parasites.

Genetic basis of cancer

Although some patients may have an inherited predisposition to cancer, e.g. familial adenomatous polyposis, most neoplastic transformation involves genetic alterations within cells. Oncogenes are genes that are present in normal cells but which, in cancer cells, become altered in their structure or expression. They share some homology with genes of oncogenic retroviruses, from which they derive their names: e.g. c-myc from v-myc—a gene found in avian myelocytomatosis virus; c-abl from v-abl—a gene found in Abelson murine leukaemia virus. The human genome contains between 20 and 100 genes and these are divided into proto-oncogenes (precursors) or cellular oncogenes (part of a normal cell). Very few of these genes have been completely sequenced but it is thought they are extremely heterogeneous (molecular weight 20 000 to 150 000) and may be membrane bound, soluble in the cell cytoplasm or bound to cellular DNA.

Oncogenes can be activated by:

● *Viral stimulation.* Retroviruses causing cancer in animals can activate oncogenes when they infect a cell. The viral RNA is transcribed by reverse transcriptase into viral DNA, which enters the host nucleus and is incorporated into cellular DNA (chromosomes). This may activate a proto-oncogene and alter the function of the cell. Alternatively, the virus itself may pick up the cellular proto-oncogene, incorporate it into its own viral genome and possibly infect another host cell, e.g. Rous sarcoma virus in chickens.

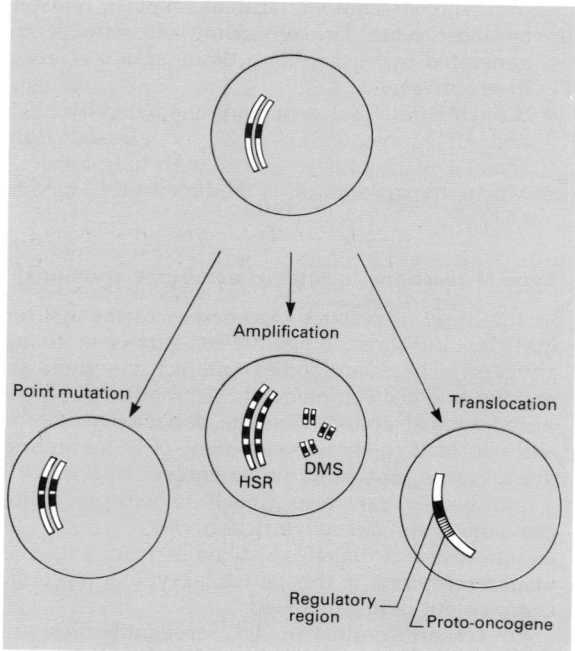

Fig. 2.20 Activation of cellular oncogenes (see text). HSR = homogeneous staining region; DMs = double minutes.

● *Non-viral stimulation* (Fig. 2.20). Proto-oncogenes, like other genes, contain structural and control regions and changes in either region can produce an active oncogene. Structural point mutations can be induced by carcinogens throughout the proto-oncogenes but oncogenic activation will only occur if they are at certain critical points, e.g. the bcr-abl hybrid protein in the Philadelphia chromosome in CML (p. 363). Alternatively, if a mutation affects the amount, rather than the structure of an encoded protein, the regulation of the encoded protein will be affected. For example, regulatory changes can be produced by translocation or amplification of a segment of chromosome containing a proto-oncogene. In Burkitt's lymphoma, by *trans-location*, the regulatory segment of the *myc* proto-oncogene is replaced by a regulatory segment of an unrelated immunoglobulin. This *myc* trans-location restructures a gene that encodes normal protein but that is, now, not appropriately regulated.

Amplification can also affect the *myc* gene; here, instead of the normal two copies of genes on autosomal chromosomes, multiple copies of the gene appear either within the chromosomes (homogeneously staining regions, HSRs) or as extra-chromosomal particles (double minutes), e.g.

amplification of N-*myc* in neuroblastomas or N-*myc* or L-*myc* in some small-cell carcinomas.

Other mutational changes may occur at the karyotypic level—either activating oncogenes or inactivating tumour-suppressing genes.

- *Genetic susceptibility.* Activated oncogenes cannot be transmitted and therefore cannot account for hereditary factors. However, genetic sequences that are distinct from oncogenes have been found and predispose to certain types of cancer. The mode of action of these cancer-susceptibility genes is not clearly understood but these may act in many ways, e.g. affecting the ability of the immune system to recognize tumour cells, the rate at which carcinogens act at target organs or the ability of cells to repair DNA.

Cancer susceptibility genes are thought to play a part in the familial predisposition to retinoblastomas, Wilms' tumour or familial adenomatous polyposis. These genes may act in *normal* tissues by suppressing growth and proliferation (anti-oncogenes) but if inactivated, e.g. by a random somatic mutation, will trigger growth. Normal tissue in these patients will probably contain a normal allele of the gene and an abnormal inactive allele from the affected parent. Thus, if the normal allele is inactivated, tumour growth will result.

ONCOGENE PRODUCTS AND GROWTH REGULATION

Proto-oncogenes encode proteins that are known to participate in the regulation of normal cellular proliferation (Fig. 2.21). For example:

- The product of *c-sis* has the same amino-acid structure as a platelet-derived growth factor (PDGF), a protein known to increase cellular activity.
- The product of *c-erb B* has the same structure as the epidermal growth factor receptor. This factor activates protein kinases within cells, increasing their growth.
- The product of *c-myc* is involved in cell cycle control.

Alteration in the structure or control of these genes could be important in the control of cell growth and the development of malignant potential. Monoclonal antibodies to oncogenic proteins are being developed so that assays of oncogenes in normal and abnormal cells can be made. DNA hybridization techniques have already shown vast increases of certain genes in tumour tissues, e.g. N-*myc* in neuroblastoma.

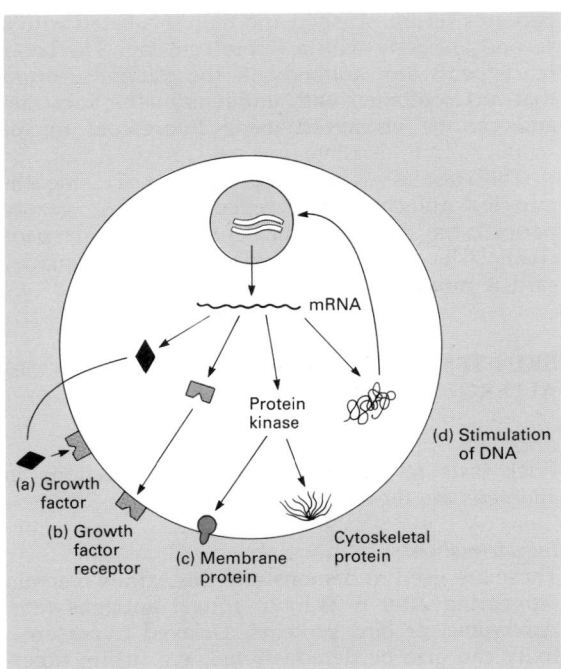

Fig. 2.21 Effect of oncogene products on cellular function. (a) *c-sis* affecting platelet-derived growth factor. (b) *c-erb B* increasing epidermal growth factor receptor. (c) *c-abl* increasing protein kinases, which alter cellular structure. (d) *c-myc* stimulation of DNA.

Investigations

MEASUREMENT OF IMMUNOGLOBULINS AND OTHER PROTEINS

Immunoprecipitation
Immune precipitates are formed when antigen and antibody are combined in proportions of near to equivalence. This technique is used for estimation of the concentration of many proteins.

In the single radial immunodiffusion test, an antiserum specific for the heavy chain of the immunoglobulin to be measured is mixed with melted agar and poured on to a plate. When it is set, holes are cut and the patient's serum as well as a series of control immunoglobulins to form a standard curve are placed in the wells. The diameter of precipitate produced is measured and read off the standard curve to give the actual concentration.

Immunoelectrophoresis

This involves separation of antigens present in, for example, serum by placing an electric charge across it on an agar plate. Positively charged proteins move to the negative electrode and vice versa. A longitudinal trough is then cut in the agar parallel to the direction of the current and filled with antibody. The antibody diffuses into the agar, and arcs of precipitates form where antigen and antibody meet. The plates can then be stained. Serum protein electrophoresis will screen for paraproteins (monoclonal bands).

In counter-current electrophoresis the pH of the gel is chosen so that the antibody is positively charged and the antigen is negatively charged. On passing a current, the antigen and antibody move towards each other and precipitate; this increases the sensitivity of the test. In rocket electrophoresis, antigens are electrophoresed into an antibody-containing gel.

For the measurement of cryoglobulin (i.e. immunoglobulins that form precipitates in the cold), a fresh specimen of blood should be taken in a warm syringe and allowed to clot at 37°C. The serum should then be left at 4°C for 48 h to precipitate the cryoglobulin. The precipitate redissolves on warming back to 37°C, at which temperature the tests are then performed.

Bence Jones proteins (free monoclonal light chains) are detected in concentrated urine on cellulose acetate electrophoresis, when an M band is seen. The presence of monoclonal free $\varkappa$ or λ light chains can be confirmed using immunoelectrophoresis.

Radioimmunoassay (RIA), enzyme-linked immunoabsorbent assay (ELISA) and the radioallergosorbent test (RAST)

These are extremely sensitive methods of detecting antigens and antibodies in low concentrations.

RIA. This is described on p. 768.

ELISA. This method is like RIA but the ligand used not only detects the antibody but is also coupled to an enzyme (e.g. peroxidase), which can be visualized by adding chromogen. Chromogen is colourless but becomes coloured when the enzyme portion of the ligand acts on it. The coloured end-product, i.e. the amount of antibody, is measured by optical density scanning of the plate.

RAST. This test measures IgE to a specific antigen. It is like RIA but the allergen (antigen) is bound to a tiny cellulose disc rather than a large plastic plate, thus increasing the ability of the test to detect tiny amounts of IgE in the serum. The ligand used is labelled anti-IgE antibody.

Antibodies that can be detected include intrinsic factor antibody, double-stranded DNA antibody, glomerular basement membrane antibody, acetylcholine receptor antibody and platelet antibody. Specific IgE antibodies to inhalants or food can also be measured.

Autoantibodies

These can be detected by haemagglutination, indirect immunofluorescence or counter-current immunoelectrophoresis.

Haemagglutination. This depends on the ability of the antibody to cross-link surface antigens on red blood cells. The antibody is serially diluted in wells with saline; positive and negative controls are also used. A red-cell suspension is added to each well. If no antibody is present the cells settle to form a pellet; if antibody is present, it agglutinates the red cells to form a hazy red appearance.

This test is used to detect rheumatoid factor, thyroglobulin antibody, thyroid microsomal antibody and erythrocyte autoantibodies (Coombs' test; see p. 321).

Indirect immunofluorescence. This detects autoantibodies and antibodies to tissues and cellular antigens. Sections of frozen animal tissues (e.g. liver, kidney, stomach or thyroid) are cut at −20°C on a cryostat. The sections are incubated with the patient's serum, washed and then incubated with a second antibody with a fluorescein tag. The latter reacts with any antibody in the patient's serum that has combined with antigens in the substrate and can be visualized using fluorescent microscopy.

This test is used to detect nuclear, smooth-muscle, mitochondrial, reticulin, DNA, gastric parietal cell, thyroid microsomal, adrenal, pancreatic islet cell, salivary gland, skeletal muscle, cardiac muscle and skin antibodies.

SKIN TESTS FOR ANTIGENS AND ALLERGENS

Prick tests

Prick tests for type I IgE-mediated reactions to allergens are described on p. 648.

Intradermal tests

These are used to demonstrate the Arthus reaction (appearing after 6–24 h) to fungal antigens (e.g. *Aspergillus*) or bird proteins. Delayed hypersensitivity can also be demonstrated, e.g. using tuberculin in the Mantoux test (p. 681). Immune deficiency can be assessed by testing with a panel of common antigens such as *Candida albicans*, streptokinase–streptodornase or mumps virus. Ninety-five per cent of normal adults respond to at least one of these antigens. Children not exposed to these antigens can be tested by sensitization followed by a challenge with dinitrochlorobenzene (DNCB).

Patch tests (see p. 1006)

These demonstrate delayed hypersensitivity to a variety of sensitizing antigens in contact dermatitis, e.g. ointments, rubber extracts or metallic ions.

DETECTION OF IMMUNE COMPLEXES

Immune complexes can be detected by looking for evidence of complex deposition in tissues using direct immunofluorescence or by measuring complexes in the blood or in body fluids. There are many methods based on either the physical properties (e.g. morphology and size) or biological properties of the immune complexes. The latter include complement binding (e.g. the C1q binding assay) or cell binding either to Fc receptors (e.g. platelet aggregation) or to Fc and C3b receptors (e.g. Raji cell assay).

All methods detect aggregated immunoglobulin and therefore immune complexes are sometimes difficult to distinguish from non-specifically aggregated immunoglobulins. These tests are not routinely performed and are not essential for the diagnosis of diseases thought to be mediated by immune complexes.

LYMPHOCYTE SEPARATION

Lymphocytes can be separated from other blood constituents by using their different densities. Diluted defibrinated whole blood is layered on top of Ficoll Isopaque and centrifuged. The lymphocytes settle at the plasma–Ficoll interface, whilst other blood constituents fall to the bottom.

Human T lymphocytes have receptors for sheep red cells and form rosettes when mixed together. They can be separated from non-rosetting B cells by using Ficoll gradients as above.

Lymphocyte subpopulations can also be separated on antibody-sensitized plates, when antigen-positive cells bind to the plate and antigen-negative cells are washed off. Thus, T cells can be separated from B cells by using anti-Ig that binds B cells or T_H from T_S by using the appropriate antibody.

Monoclonal antisera can distinguish and quantitate helper T cells, which stain with horseradish peroxidase linked CD4, from suppressor-cytotoxic T cells, which stain with linked CD8 (OKT8).

B lymphocytes have surface immunoglobulins that can be identified by direct immunofluorescence using fluorescein-conjugated antisera to human immunoglobulin. They can then be counted with a fluorescent microscope or by using a fluorescence-activated cell sorter (FACS).

IN VITRO TESTS OF CELL-MEDIATED IMMUNITY

Lymphocyte transformation test

When sensitized lymphocytes are cultured with the appropriate antigen they undergo blast transformation and DNA is synthesized. This can be measured by adding tritiated thymidine 16 h before the cells are harvested. Thymidine is taken up by the cells and incorporated into DNA. The radioactivity of the cells is measured; a high count indicates lymphocyte transformation and thus sensitivity to the antigen.

Macrophage-migration inhibition test

Lymphocytes produce lymphokines when exposed to a sensitizing antigen. One of these lymphokines is the macrophage-migration inhibition factor (MIF). Macrophages and lymphocytes are packed into capillary tubes and cultured in media with and without antigen. If migration of the cells out of the

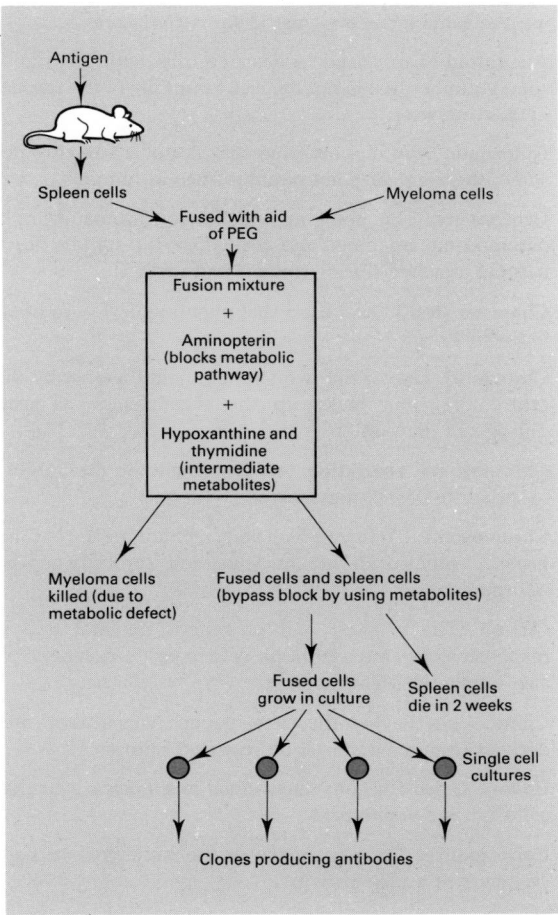

Fig. 2.22 Monoclonal antibody production. PEG = polyethylene glycol.

capillary tubes is inhibited, it suggests that the lymphocytes are sensitive to the antigen and are producing MIF.

MONOCLONAL ANTIBODY PRODUCTION

This involves the production of a cell that can generate a single specific antibody (Fig. 2.22).

Glossary

TERMS COMMONLY USED IN GENETICS

Acrocentric. Term used to describe a chromosome in which the centromere lies close to one end, producing one long and one short arm.

Allele (allelomorph). Alternative form of a gene occupying the same locus on a particular chromosome.

Aneuploid. Term used to describe cells with a chromosomal number that is not the exact multiple of the normal haploid number.

Autosome. Any chromosome that is not a sex chromosome; there are 22 pairs of autosomes in humans.

Centromere. The point at which two chromatids of a chromosome are joined and also where the spindle fibres become attached during mitosis and meiosis.

Character (trait). An observable phenotypic feature of an individual.

Chromatid. One of the two strands, held together by the centromere, that make up the chromosome as seen during cell division.

Chromosomal aberration. An abnormality in the number or structure of a chromosome.

Chromosome. A thread-like body containing DNA and protein, situated in the nucleus, and carrying genetic information.

Cistron. The smallest unit of genetic material that is responsible for the synthesis of a specific polypeptide; also known as a gene.

Clone. Cells having the same genetic constitution and derived from a single cell by repeated mitoses.

Codon. Three adjacent nucleotides in a nucleic acid that code for one amino acid.

Concordance. The occurrence of the same trait in both members of a pair of twins.

Cytokines. Groups of proteins that modulate cellular immunity and are released mainly by activated lymphocytes and macrophages.

Deletion. Loss of a part of a chromosome.

Diploid. Term used to describe cells containing two sets of chromosomes.

Dominant. Term used to describe a trait expressed in individuals who are heterozygous for a particular gene.

Exon. A segment of a gene that is represented in the mRNA product (coding sequence).

Expressivity. The degree to which the effect of a gene is expressed.

Gene. Part of a DNA molecule that directs the synthesis of a specific polypeptide chain; it consists of many codons.

3′ The end of a gene at which transcription ceases.
5′ The end of a gene at which transcription begins.

Gene pool. The total genetic information contained in all the genes in a breeding population at a given time.

Genetic marker. A genetically controlled phenotypic feature used in inheritance studies.

Genetics. The science of heredity and variation.

Genome. The total amount of genetic material in the cell.

Genotype. The genetic constitution of an individual.

Haploid. Term used to describe the cells containing one set of chromosomes.

Heterozygote. An individual possessing two different alleles at the corresponding loci on a pair of homologous chromosomes.

Homozygote. An individual possessing identical alleles at the corresponding loci on a pair of homologous chromosomes.

Hybrid. The progeny of a cross between two genetically different organisms.

Hybridization. The pairing of complementary DNA or RNA strands to give DNA–DNA or DNA–RNA strands; for example, it is used to search for particular DNA fragments after Southern blotting.

Intron. A segment of a gene not represented in the RNA product because it has been removed through splicing together of exons on either side of it.

Karyotype. The number, size and shape of the chromosomes in a cell.

Linkage disequilibrium. The association of particular alleles at two linked loci more frequently than expected by chance.

Locus. The site of a gene on a chromosome.

Monosomy. Loss of one chromosome of a homologous pair, resulting in 45 chromosomes.

Non-disjunction. Failure of a chromosome pair to separate during cell division, resulting in both chromosomes passing to the same daughter cell.

Nucleotide. The basic unit of nucleic acids, which is made up of a pyrimidine or purine base, a pentose sugar and a phosphate group.

Mosaics. Patients with two different cell lines in their constitution.

Oncogenes. Genes present in normal cells but which, in cancer cells, become altered in their structure or expression.

Penetrance. The proportion of individuals with a particular genotype who also have the corresponding phenotype. Full penetrance occurs when a dominant trait is always seen in an individual with one such allele, or when a recessive trait is seen in all individuals possessing two such alleles.

Phenotype. The appearance of an individual, resulting from the effects of both environment and genes.

Ploidy. Term that describes the number of chromosome sets, viz. 23 = haploid (1 set), 46 = diploid (2 sets).

Proto-oncogene. A normal gene with the potential to become activated into an oncogene.

Polymerase chain reaction (PCR). Technique for rapid analysis of DNA. Oligonucleotide primers corresponding to each end of DNA of interest are synthesized and amplified in genomic DNA.

Pulsed field gel electrophoresis. Technique for separation of large fragments of DNA.

Recessive. Term used to describe a trait expressed in individuals who are homozygous for a particular gene but not seen in the heterozygote.

Restriction-fragment length polymorphisms (RFLPs). When variations in non-coding DNA sequences affect restriction-enzyme cleavage sites, DNA fragments of different sizes (RFLPs) will result from enzyme digestion.

Sex linkage. Genes carried on the sex chromosomes.

'Somy'. Term referring to the number of copies of an individual chromosome per cell, e.g. 'trisomy' = 3 copies.

Synteny. Term used to describe genes on the same chromosome.

Transcription. The process by which genetic information is transmitted from the DNA in the chromosomes to messenger RNA.

Translation. The process by which genetic information from messenger RNA is 'translated' into protein synthesis.

Translocation. The transfer of a piece of one chromosome to another non-homologous chromosome.

Trisomy. Representation of a chromosome three times rather than twice, giving a total of 47 chromosomes.

TERMS COMMONLY USED IN IMMUNOLOGY

Allergen. An antigen provoking an allergic response. The term is usually restricted to antigens such as grass pollen involved in type I hypersensitivity.

Allergy. *See* Immune response.

Allotype. Genetically determined epitopes that vary between different members of the same species, e.g. blood group antigens.

Antibody. An immunoglobulin capable of binding to an antigen via specific areas of the protein termed combining sites.

Antigen. A substance that produces an immune response when introduced into a vertebrate animal.

Atopy. Genetically determined tendency to develop immediate hypersensitivity/allergic reactions to common allergens involving the production of immunoglobulin E.

Complement. A serum enzyme cascade usually activated by antibody–antigen complexes; the enzymes released are capable of lysing red cells, nucleated cells and bacteria to which antibody is attached.

Cell cooperation. Cell interaction that is either between T and B lymphocytes, which leads to antibody production, or between T lymphocytes, which regulates humoral immunity.

Cell-mediated immunity. Specific immunity that is dependent on T lymphocytes.

Epitope. An antigenic determinant of known molecular structure present on complex antigens.

Graft-versus-host reaction. The response of a graft containing immunologically functional cells against its non-identical host or recipient.

Idiotype. The unique determinant present in the antigen combining site of an antibody.

Immune response. The development of a state of altered reactivity following exposure to an antigen. It may be cell-mediated, humoral or both.

Immunoglobulin. A glycoprotein composed of heavy and light polypeptide chains; the class to which an immunoglobulin belongs is determined by the type of heavy chain.

Immunological tolerance. The development of a specific unresponsiveness to a particular antigen that, in other circumstances, is capable of inducing an immune reaction.

Interleukins. A group of molecules that are involved in signalling between cells of the immune system. They are released by several cell types, including lymphocytes.

Isotypes. Antigenic variation common to all members of the same species, e.g. differences in the immunoglobulin chains and classes.

Lymphokine. A generic term used for substances other than antibodies that are released from sensitized lymphocytes and are intracellular mediators of the immune response.

Monoclonal antibody. An antibody produced by a single clone (family) of cells.

Opsonization. The coating of, for example, microorganisms with either antibody or antibody and complement. Opsonization facilitates phagocytosis of the particles.

Paratope. The part of an antibody that combines with the epitope of an antigen.

Phagocytosis. The process of engulfment of particles, e.g. microorganisms, by cells.

Syngeneic (isogeneic). Term used to describe cells or tissues transferred between genetically identical individuals (e.g. identical twins).

Vaccine. Material containing antigens. May be:
- *Inactivated* (containing organisms incapable of replication, e.g. whooping cough vaccines)
- *Live* (actual pathogen given by unusual route, e.g.contagious bovine pleuropneumonia vaccine)
- *Attenuated* (live vaccine containing organisms treated to lose their virulence, e.g. polio and BCG vaccines)
- *Heterologous* (protecting against organisms not present in the vaccine by cross-reaction, e.g. cowpox vaccine protects against smallpox)

Xenogeneic (heterogeneic). Used to describe cells or tissues transferred between different species.

Further reading

Emery AEH & Mueller RF (1988) *Elements of Medical Genetics*, 7th edn. Edinburgh: Churchill Livingstone.

Fraser Roberts JA & Pembury ME (1985) *An Introduction to Medical Genetics*, 8th edn. Oxford: Oxford University Press.

Galton DJ (1985) *Molecular Genetics of Common Metabolic Disease*. London: Edward Arnold.

Harper PS (1984) *Practical Genetic Counselling*, 2nd edn. Bristol: John Wright.

Kingston Helen M (1989) *ABC of Clinical Genetics*. London: British Medical Journal.

Male D, Champion B & Cooke A (1987) *Advanced Immunology*. London: Gower Medical/Churchill Livingstone.

McKusick VA (1983) *Mendelian Inheritance in Man*, 6th edn. Baltimore: Johns Hopkins University Press.

McKusick VA (1988) *The Human Gene Map*. Baltimore: Johns Hopkins University Press.

Roitt I, Brostoff J & Male D (1988) *Immunology*. London: Gower Medical/Churchill Livingstone.

Strober W & James SP (1988) The interleukins. *Paediatric Research* **24**: 111–119.

Weatherall DJ (1986) *The New Genetics in Clinical Practice*, 2nd edn. Oxford: Oxford University Press.

3

Nutrition

to help him avoid any 'food faddism' that can easily develop as a result of extensive advertising based on commercial interests rather than concerns about health.

Water and electrolyte balance

Water and electrolyte balance is dealt with fully in Chapter 10. Approximately 1 litre of water per day is required in the diet to balance insensible losses, but much more is usually drunk, the kidneys being able to excrete large quantities.

Dietary sodium is variable in the range of 4–12 g a day. It has been recommended that this should be decreased by 3 g a day in view of a possible link between dietary sodium and hypertension (p. 615).

Introduction

In developed countries, excess food is available and the commonest nutritional problem is obesity. in the developing countries, lack of food and poor usage of the available food results in protein–energy malnutrion.

Diet and disease are interrelated in many ways. First, diet is a causative factor in the development of certain diseases. Excess energy intake, particularly when high in animal (saturated) fat content, is thought to be responsible for a number of diseases, including ischaemic heart disease and diabetes. The importance of the relationship between nutrition and cancer has been realized in recent years, largely owing to epidemiological studies. There is evidence that vitamin A deficiency may be associated with certain tumours and a high fat intake is also thought to be of importance in producing cancer. Numerous carcinogens, either intentionally added to food (e.g. nitrates for preserving foods) or accidental contaminants (e.g. moulds producing aflatoxin and fungi) may also be involved in the development of cancer.

Second, special diets are necessary to control certain disease states, e.g. a low-sodium diet can be used in renal and liver disease and a gluten-free diet in coeliac disease.

Finally, the proportion of processed foods eaten may affect the development of disease. A number of processed convenience foods have a high sugar and high fat content and therefore predispose to obesity and dental caries. They also have a low fibre content, and dietary fibre is possibly important in the prevention of a number of diseases (see p. 153).

A link between diet and disease is also present when industrial pollution of food supplies occurs, e.g. with insecticides, herbicides or preservatives.

The overall role of the doctor is not only to advise the patient to take a balanced diet but also

Energy balance

Food is necessary to provide the body with energy (Fig. 3.1). The oxidation of carbohydrate, fat and protein eventually leads to the generation of high-energy bonds in adenotriphosphate (ATP), which is then used for all energy requirements. In addition to providing energy, some of these oxidative products are utilized to generate the carbohydrates, fats and proteins of which the body is composed (Table 3.1).

The normal energy requirements for man are variable and depend on:

- Body size: more food is usually required by a 70 kg than a 40 kg man.
- Age: with increasing age there is a reduction in physical activity and metabolically active tissues in the body. The basal metabolic rate (BMR)

Table 3.1 Normal composition of a 70 kg man.

	kg	Per cent of body weight
Water	42	60
Fat	13	18
Protein	11	16
Carbohydrate	0.5	0.7
Minerals	3.5	5.2

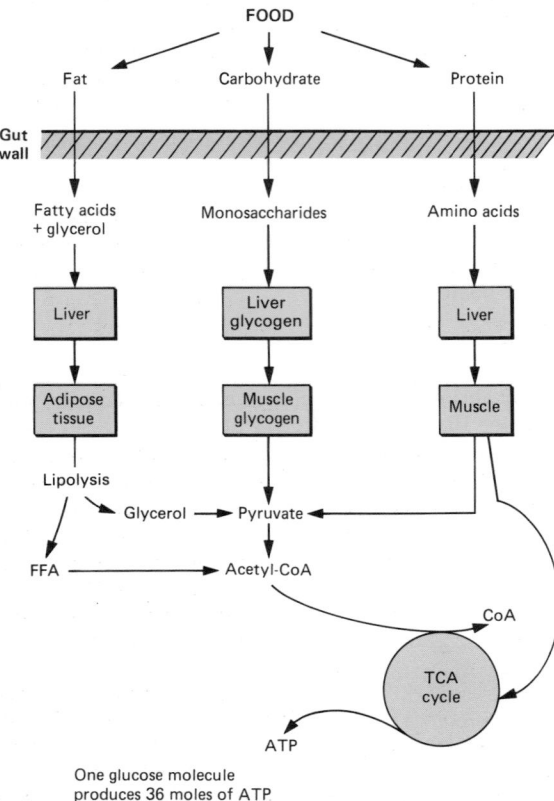

One glucose molecule
produces 36 moles of ATP

Fig. 3.1 The production of energy from food.

Table 3.2 Approximate energy expenditure of a normal adult per day.

	kcal	kJ
Male		
Rest	500	2100
Light work	1000	4200
Heavy work	2500	10500
Female		
Rest	420	1760
Light work	840	3250
Heavy work	1500	6300

decreases by up to 10% per decade.
- Environment: activity falls in extreme hot and cold climates and the BMR also decreases in heat.
- Physical activity: Table 3.2 shows the approximate energy expenditure of normal adults at rest and during different work activities.

Energy requirements also increase during the growing period, with pregnancy and lactation, and following infection or trauma.

In the basal state, energy demands for muscle are 30% of the total energy required, abdominal organs 25%, brain 20% and heart 10%. The increase in muscle energy requirements during exercise is 10-fold.

Energy is derived from various stores. The fat content of the body is extremely variable; it may be increased twofold in an obese subject. One-third of protein (e.g. in bone) is unavailable as an energy source, muscle being the main available protein source. Muscle contains three times its own weight of water and protein breakdown provides only 4 kcal (17 kJ) of energy per gram. Adipose tissue is therefore an efficient way of storing energy and is the only major source of fuel available, apart from muscle protein, in the long-term fasting state. Fat is broken down into free fatty acids and ketone bodies, and protein into amino acids, prior to oxidation to provide energy. Carbohydrate stores are small, consisting of glycogen in the liver and a small amount of circulating glucose.

The average daily energy intake in developed countries of a 70 kg man is 2700 kcal (approximately 12 000 kJ). These calories are normally provided as approximately.

- 320 kcal (1360 kJ) of protein (80 g)
- 1200 kcal (4800 kJ) of carbohydrate (300 g)
- 1125 kcal (4625 kJ) of fat (125 g)

Recommendations from the Health Education Council in the UK suggest a decrease in the fat content of the diet and an increase in complex carbohydrates, with the protein content remaining much the same.

Body weight depends on energy balance, which in turn depends on the balance between intake and expenditure. Intake depends partly on food availability but also on a number of complex interrelationships that include the stimulus of good food, the role of hunger, metabolic changes, e.g. hypoglycaemia, and the pleasure and habit of eating. Some people are able to keep their body weight constant within a few kilograms for many years but most gradually increase their weight owing to a small but continuous increase of intake over expenditure.

Protein

The recommended daily intake of protein is 0.8 g·kg^{-1} per day, with protein representing at least 10% of the total energy intake. Most affluent people eat more than this, consuming 80–100 g of protein per day. The total amount of nitrogen excreted in the urine represents the balance between protein breakdown and synthesis. In order to maintain nitrogen balance, at least 40–50 g of protein are needed. The amount of protein required to maintain nitrogen balance in a particular individual can be calculated from the amount of nitrogen excreted in the urine using the following equation:

Urinary nitrogen $\times$ 6.25 = grams of protein required

In practice, urinary urea is easily measured and forms 80–90% of the total urinary nitrogen.

Protein contains many amino acids, of which at least eight (probably nine) are essential amino acids necessary for protein synthesis and for maintenance of nitrogen balance. The biological value of a protein is defined as the amount of absorbed protein retained by the body, and this primarily depends on the essential amino acids present. Egg and milk have high biological values, whereas plant proteins have low biological values because at least one essential amino acid is missing. Adequate energy is required in addition to protein for the normal diet, otherwise protein will be directed towards oxidative pathways and eventually gluconeogenesis for energy. Alanine is the primary amino acid released from muscle; it is deaminated and converted into pyruvic acid before entering the citric acid cycle.

Fat

The average fat intake per day varies from 90 to 190 g. It has been suggested that the average total fat intake be reduced from 128 g (38% of total energy) to 115 g (34% of total energy). Dietary fat is chiefly in the form of triglycerides. Forty per cent of dietary fat is saturated, but gradually more vegetable oils containing polyunsaturated fats are being introduced into the diet.

Currently the ratio of polyunsaturated to saturated fatty acids in the Western diet is 0.3. Studies, largely epidemiological, suggest that an increase in polyunsaturated fatty acids will decrease the incidence of ischaemic heart disease. However, the advisability of any increase in polyunsaturated fats is still questionable, remembering that it cannot be achieved without a substantial change from meat and dairy products to vegetable fats. A reasonable compromise would be to try to bring the ratio of saturated to polyunsaturated fats nearer to 1.0, which would at least probably do no harm. A reduction in the proportion of saturated fatty acids to 15% of the total energy intake has also been recommended.

Cholesterol is found in all animal products. Eggs are particularly rich in cholesterol, which is virtually absent from plants. The average intake in the UK is 300–500 mg/day. Cholesterol is also synthesized (see p. 239) and only very high or low dietary intakes will significantly affect blood levels.

Essential fatty acids
Only linoleic acid, from which arachidonic acid is derived, is an essential fatty acid. Essential fatty acid deficiency may accompany protein–energy malnutrition but it has only been clearly defined as a clinical entity in patients on long-term parenteral nutrition given glucose and protein and no fat.

Carbohydrate

Carbohydrate intake comprises the polysaccharide starch, some disaccharides (mainly sucrose) and a small amount of lactose. Carbohydrates are cheap compared with other foodstuffs; a great deal is therefore eaten, usually more than required.

Dietary fibre, which is largely non-starch polysaccharide, is removed in the processing of food, leaving highly refined carbohydrate such as sucrose.

The principal classes of dietary fibre are cellulose, hemicelluloses, lignins, pectins and gums—none of which are digested by gut enzymes. However, fibre is partly broken down in the gastrointestinal (GI) tract, mainly by colonic bacteria, producing gas and volatile fatty acids.

All plant food, when unprocessed, contains fibre, so that all unprocessed food eaten will increase the fibre content of the diet. Bran, the fibre from wheat, provides an easy way of adding additional fibre to the diet. It increases faecal bulk and is helpful in the treatment of constipation. Dietary fibre deficiency is now accepted as an entity by many workers in the UK. It is suggested that the total dietary fibre be increased to 25–30 g per day. This could be achieved by increased consumption of bread, potatoes, fruit and vegetables, with a reduction in sugar intake. Each extra gram of fibre daily adds approximately 5 g to the daily stool weight.

Refined carbohydrate, with little or no fibre, is less filling and therefore can be eaten in larger quantities, contributing to obesity.

Recently, pectins and gums have been added to food to slow down monosaccharide absorption, particularly in diabetes.

Protein–energy malnutrition (PEM) as seen in developed countries

Starvation is unusual in developed countries, although some degree of undernourishment is seen in very poor areas. Most nutritional problems occurring in the population at large are due to eating wrong combinations of food, e.g. excess of refined carbohydrate or diets low in fresh vegetables.

Table 3.3 Common conditions associated with protein–energy malnutrition (PEM).

Sepsis
Trauma
Surgery, particularly of gastrointestinal tract, with complications
Gastrointestinal disease, particularly involving small bowel
Psychological—anorexia nervosa
Malignancy
Metabolic disease—renal failure
Any very ill patient

Common causes of protein–energy malnutrition

With the exception of thyrotoxicosis, in which there are increased energy demands, loss of weight leading to malnutrition is almost always due to a poor dietary intake. Table 3.3 gives a list of conditions in which malnutrition is commonly seen. Surgical complications, with sepsis, are the commonest cause in most hospitals. All are associated with a decreased appetite. Malabsorption is sometimes thought to be a cause of weight loss, but failure to absorb nutrient is never so great that it cannot be overcome by increased intake (see p. 201).

Pathophysiology of starvation (Fig. 3.2)

In the first 24 h following low dietary intake, the body relies on the breakdown of hepatic glycogen to glucose for energy. Hepatic glycogen stores are small and therefore gluconeogenesis is soon necessary to maintain glucose levels. Gluconeogenesis takes place mainly from lactate, glycerol and amino acids. All endogenous proteins can be utilized to provide amino acids for gluconeogenesis and loss of muscle bulk eventually occurs.

Lipolysis, the breakdown of the body's fat stores, also occurs. It is inhibited by insulin, but the level of this hormone falls off as starvation continues. The stored triglyceride is hydrolysed by lipase to glycerol, which is used for gluconeogenesis, and non-esterified fatty acids that can be used directly as a fuel or oxidized in the liver to ketone bodies. As starvation continues, adaptive processes take place lest the body's protein be completely utilized.

There is a decrease in metabolic rate and total body energy expenditure. Central nervous metabolism changes from glucose as a substrate to ketone bodies, which now become the main source of energy. Gluconeogenesis in the liver decreases with a consequent reduction of protein breakdown, both being inhibited directly by ketone bodies. Most of the energy at this stage comes from adipose tissue, with some gluconeogenesis from amino acids, particularly glutamine, occurring in the kidney.

Following trauma or surgery adaptation does not take place and there is in addition a rise in glucocorticoid and catecholamine levels. In addition, energy requirements are often increased. These changes all result in continuing gluconeogenesis with massive muscle breakdown.

Regulation of metabolism

The unavailability of the various substrates in starvation produces dramatic changes in hormone levels, these hormones being the main factors in controlling intracellular metabolism.

In the fed state, insulin/glucagon ratios are high. Insulin promotes synthesis of glycogen, protein and fat, and inhibits lipolysis and gluconeogenesis.

In the fasted state, the insulin/glucagon ratios are low. Glucagon acts mainly on the liver and has no action on muscle. It increases glycogenolysis and gluconeogenesis, as well as increasing ketone

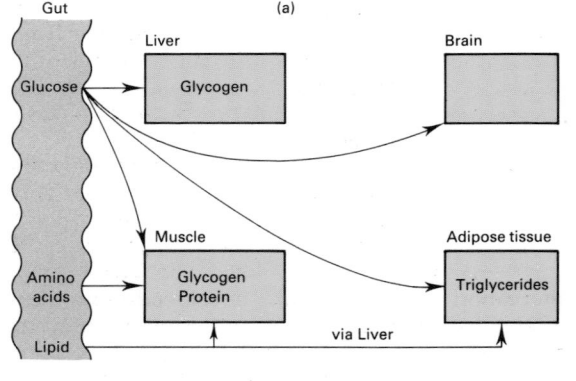
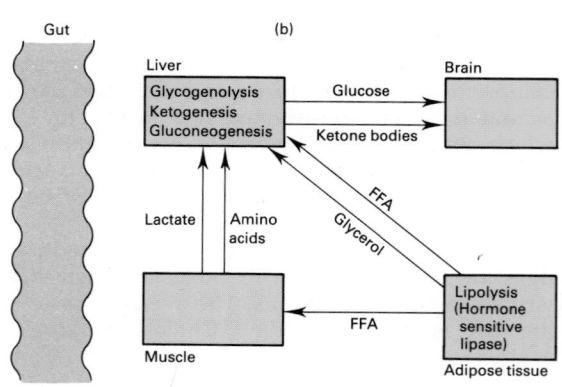

Fig. 3.2 Metabolism in (a) the fed and (b) the fasted state. FFA = free fatty acids.

body production from fatty acids. It also stimulates lipolysis in adipose tissue. Catecholamines have a similar action to glucagon but also affect muscle metabolism. These agents both act via cyclic AMP to stimulate lipolysis, producing free fatty acids that can then act as a major source of energy.

CLINICAL FEATURES

Patients are sometimes seen with loss of weight or malnutrition (failure to thrive in children) as the primary symptom. Mostly, however, malnourishment is only seen as an accompaniment of some other disease process, e.g. malignancy. A careful history may indicate the cause of the weight loss but, if nothing obvious is found, hyperthyroidism must be considered.

Anorexia nervosa commonly occurs in young adolescent females (see p. 995).

Severe malnutrition is mainly seen with advanced organic disease or after surgical procedures followed by complications. PEM leads to a depression of the immunological defence mechanism, leading to decreased resistance to infection (see p. 7).

Table 3.4 Hallmarks of protein–energy malnutrition.

	Males	Females
Weight loss	> 10%	
Triceps skinfold thickness[a]	< 10 mm	< 13 mm
Arm muscle circumference[a]	< 23 cm	< 22 cm
Serum albumin	< 35 g·L^{-1}	
Serum transferrin	< 1.5 g·L^{-1}	
Lymphocyte count	< 1.5 × 10^9/L	
Cell-mediated immunity	Negative *Candida* skin test	

[a] Values obtained in the UK.

Patients who have lost more then 10% of their body weight (unless dieting) suffer from malnutrition. Indicators of malnutrition are given in Table 3.4. The clinician can usually decide whether the patient is malnourished by the patient's general appearance. Retrospective dietary evaluation is not helpful, unfortunately, because of the degree of error in the patients' recollection of their intake.

It is important to establish the cause of the malnutrition, as the treatment often depends on the underlying disease.

TREATMENT

When malnutrition is obvious and the underlying disease cannot be corrected at once, some form of nutritional support is necessary. Nutrition should always be given enterally if the GI tract is

Table 3.5 Clinical features of protein–energy malnutrition in developing countries.

Failure of growth
Apathy, anorexia
Diarrhoea
Hepatomegaly
Muscle wasting
Oedema
Signs of multiple vitamin and mineral deficiency, e.g. corneal keratinization (blindness)
Anaemia
Hair thinning
Angular stomatitis and sore tongue
Skin changes (changes in pigmentation, dryness)

functioning adequately. This can most easily be done by encouraging the patient to eat more often and by giving a high-calorie supplement. If this is not possible, a liquefied diet may be given intragastrically via a fine-bore tube.

If both of these measures fail, parenteral nutrition is given.

Protein–energy malnutrition as seen in developing countries

In many areas of the world, many people border on malnutrition. If events such as drought, war or changes in political climate occur in addition, millions suffer from starvation. Although the basic condition of PEM is the same in all parts of the world from whatever cause, malnutrition due to long periods of near-total starvation produces unique clinical appearances virtually never seen in the Western World (Table 3.5).

The term PEM covers all the clinical conditions seen in adults and children (Table 3.6). It is possible to make a clinical distinction between marasmus and kwashiorkor, but this means very little. The protein content of food has been shown to be the same in both groups and the aetiology of each type is complex. All patients who have a deficiency in protein intake also have deficiencies of total calorie intake and of other, often unspecified, nutrients. It is therefore not possible to be sure which is the most important feature causing any one clinical picture. In addition, infection and diarrhoea with protein loss can affect the clinical picture.

Table 3.6 Wellcome classification of protein–energy malnutrition.

Weight (per cent of standard for age)	Oedema	
	Present	Absent
60–80%	Kwashiorkor	Undernutrition
< 60%	Marasmic kwashiorkor	Marasmus

CLINICAL FEATURES

PEM occurs chiefly in children under 5 years of age but no age is spared; the clinical manifestations in adults are not so severe. Children show failure of growth, often present from the moment of weaning. Oedema is present in kwashiorkor and this hides muscle wasting. The child is usually apathetic, miserable and suffers from anorexia (Fig. 3.3). Diarrhoea is always present and hepatomegaly due to fatty infiltration is often found. Hyper- or hypopigmentation may be present, with skin atrophy and eventually ulceration, particularly of the legs, perineum and buttocks. Hair is very thin and changes colour to red and eventually blond, and nails fail to grow. All tissues and organs malfunction in PEM but most will recover if nutrition is available and the patient is not in the extreme state.

Signs of infection must be looked for carefully, as malnutrition depresses normal responses to infection (see p. 7). Specific nutritional deficiencies of vitamins and trace elements also occur and these produce specific signs (see p. 157).

INVESTIGATION

Investigation is not always practicable. Anaemia due to folate, iron and copper deficiency is often

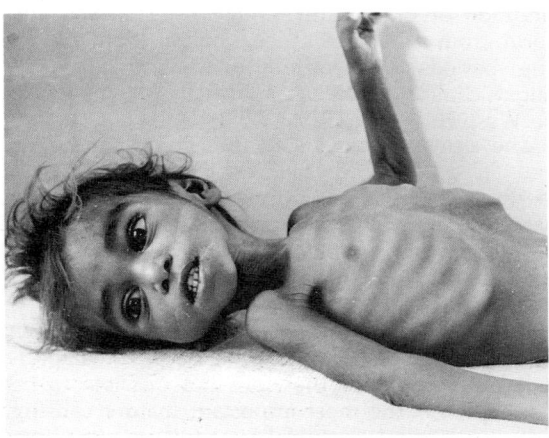

Fig. 3.3 A malnourished child.

present, but the haematocrit may be high owing to dehydration. Electrolyte disturbances are common. Blood should be examined for malarial parasites and the stools for pathogens. Tuberculosis is common and is easily missed if a chest X-ray is not performed.

TREATMENT

Treatment must involve the provision of protein and energy supplements and the control of infection.

The severely ill child will require resuscitation, but intravenous therapy should be avoided if possible because of the danger of fluid overload.

Feeding needs to be carefully planned and during the initial treatment of the acute case only enough energy and protein should be given to maintain a steady state. Large increases in energy lead to heart failure, circulatory collapse and death. A child requires approximately 100 kcal·kg^{-1} (450 kJ·kg^{-1}) daily, which is provided by 0.6 g·kg^{-1} of protein. This is often given as milk with additional water, flour, maize or whatever is available locally. Sugar mixed with dried skimmed milk and small amounts of cottonseed oil (DISCO) is frequently used. Attempts should be made to give the feeds as slowly and as often as possible, although anorexia is often a problem and can be exacerbated by excess feeding. If necessary, fluids and food should be given by nasogastric tube. The child is then gradually weaned to liquids and then solids by mouth.

Hypothermia and hypoglycaemia occur in severely ill children, often with an accompanying infection, and need to be treated urgently. Because of the cold temperatures at night, blankets and sometimes additional heat are necessary. Gradually, as the child improves, more energy can be given and during rehabilitation maximum weight gain is achieved in the shortest time by extra calories ('catch-up weight gain'). Children who have been severely ill need constant attention right through the convalescent period, as often home conditions are poor and feeds are refused.

Supplements of vitamins (A, D, B and C) should always be given, together with folic acid and iron. Many children are deficient in minerals such as zinc, copper and selenium, and supplements should be given if deficiency is suspected.

Diarrhoea can lead to potassium deficiency, and glucose electrolyte mixtures (such as the WHO formulation, p. 33) are sometimes necessary. Diarrhoea is often due to bacterial or protozoal overgrowth and metronidazole is very effective and is often given routinely. Parasites are also common and, as facilities for stool examination are usually not available, mebendazole 100 mg twice daily for 3 days should be given. In high-risk areas, antimalarial therapy is given.

Table 3.7 Fat-soluble and water-soluble vitamins.

Vitamin	Daily requirement	Major clinical features of deficiency
Fat-soluble		
A (retinol)	750 µg	Xerophthalmia, night blindness, keratomalacia, follicular hyperkeratosis
D (cholecalciferol)	2.5–10 µg and sunlight	Rickets, osteomalacia
K	50–150 µg	Coagulation defects
E (α-tocopherol)	8–10 mg	Neurological disorders, e.g. ataxia
Water-soluble		
B_1 (thiamine)	1 mg	Beriberi; Wernicke–Korsakoff syndrome
B_2 (riboflavin)	1–2 mg	Angular stomatitis
Niacin	15–20 equivalents (see text)	Pellagra
B_6 (pyridoxine)	2 mg	Peripheral neuropathy
Pantothenic acid	? 5–10 mg	? No deficiency
Biotin	0.4 mg	Dermatitis
B_{12} (cobalamin)	2–5 µg	Megaloblastic anaemia; neurological disorders
Folic acid	300 µg	Megaloblastic anaemia
C (ascorbic acid)	30 mg	Scurvy

Adults do not usually suffer such severe malnutrition, but the same principles of treatment should be followed.

PROGNOSIS

Children with extreme malnutrition have a mortality of over 50%. By careful management this can be significantly reduced to 1–2%. This will depend on the availability of facilities.

Brain development takes place in the first years of life, a time when severe PEM frequently occurs. There is evidence that intellectual impairment and behavioural abnormalities occur in severely affected children. Physical growth is also impaired. Probably both of these effects can be alleviated if it is possible to maintain a high standard of living with a good diet and freedom from infection over a long period.

PREVENTION

Prevention of PEM depends not only on adequate nutrients being available but also on education of both governments and individuals of the importance of good nutrition. Short-term programmes are useful for acute shortages of food, but long-term programmes involving improved agriculture are equally important.

Bad feeding practices and infections are more important than actual shortage of food in many areas of the world. However, good surveillance is necessary to avoid periods of famine.

Food supplements (and additional vitamins) should be given to 'at-risk' groups by adding high-energy food, e.g. milk powder, meat concentrates, to the diet. Pregnancy and lactation are times of high energy requirement and supplements have

been shown to be beneficial.

Finally, generally good health care with treatment of infections is particularly beneficial in alleviating severe PEM.

Vitamins (Table 3.7)

Deficiencies due to inadequate intake are commonly seen in the developing countries and are always present with protein–energy malnutrition. In the Western World, deficiency of vitamins is rare except in the specific groups shown in Table 3.8. The widespread use of vitamins as 'tonics' is unnecessary and should be discouraged. Toxicity from excess fat-soluble vitamins is occasionally seen.

FAT-SOLUBLE VITAMINS

Vitamin A

Vitamin A (retinol) is found in dairy products, liver and fish, but is also synthesized in the intestinal wall from β-carotene found in green leafy vegetables. This is the main source.

Vitamin A deficiency
Since vitamin A is absorbed in a similar way to all lipids (see p. 198), deficiency can be seen in all chronic conditions where there is fat malabsorption. Nevertheless, the clinical features of vitamin A deficiency are rare in most of these malabsorptive conditions. They are normally only seen

Table 3.8 Some causes of vitamin deficiency in the Western World.

Decreased intake
Alcoholics—chiefly B vitamins, e.g. thiamine
Small bowel disease—chiefly folic acid, occasionally fat-soluble vitamins
Vegans—vitamin D (if no exposure to sunlight), vitamin B_{12}
Elderly with poor diet—chiefly vitamin D (if no exposure to sunlight), folic acid
Anorexia from any other cause—chiefly folate

Decreased absorption
Ileal disease/resection—only vitamin B_{12}
Liver and biliary tract disease—fat-soluble vitamins
Intestinal bacterial overgrowth—vitamin B_{12}
Oral antibiotics—vitamin K

Miscellaneous
Long-term enteral or parenteral nutrition—usually vitamin supplements are given
Renal disease—vitamin D
Drug antagonists, e.g. methotrexate interfering with folate metabolism

associated with severe protein–energy malnutrition and other multiple deficiencies in developing countries. As a result of multiple deficiencies being present, it is not always clear which nutrient deficiency is responsible for any one clinical syndrome.

Clinical features. The clinical features of vitamin A deficiency are impaired dark adaptation followed by night blindness. Later, dryness of the conjunctiva and the cornea (xerophthalmia) occurs as a result of keratinization. Bitot's spots—white plaques of keratinized epithelial cells—are found on the conjunctiva of young children with vitamin A deficiency. These spots can, however, be seen without vitamin A deficiency, possibly due to exposure. Corneal ulceration and dissolution keratomalacia eventually occur; superimposed infection is a frequent accompaniment. Both may lead to blindness. Vitamin A deficiency is a common cause of blindness in developing countries, affecting 250 000 children per year. Follicular hyperkeratosis, in which there is thickening and dryness of the skin, is also seen with vitamin A deficiency. It is also sometimes seen without vitamin A deficiency.

Diagnosis. In parts of the world where the deficiency is common, diagnosis is made on the basis of the clinical features and deficiency should always be suspected if any degree of malnutrition is present. Blood levels of vitamin A will usually be low, but the best guide to the diagnosis is a response to replacement therapy.

Treatment. Retinol palmitate 50 000 i.u. orally should be given on two successive days. In the presence of vomiting and diarrhoea, vitamin A 50 000 i.u. i.m. is given. Associated malnutrition must be treated and superadded bacterial infection should be treated with antibiotics. Referral for specialist ophthalmic treatment is necessary in severe cases.

Prevention. Recommended daily intakes of vitamin A are 750 µg for adults and approximately 500 µg for children, depending on age. Lactating women require 1200 µg. Most Western diets contain enough dairy products and green vegetables but vitamin A is added to foodstuffs in some countries. Vitamin A is not destroyed by cooking. Education of the population is important; in particular, pregnant women and children should be encouraged to eat green vegetables.

Vitamin D

The metabolism and actions of vitamin D are shown in Fig. 3.4. Vitamin D is produced in the skin as cholecalciferol (vitamin D_3) by photoactivation of 7-dehydrocholesterol. This, rather than dietary vitamin D, is the chief source of vitamin D metabolites in humans and poor nutrition is of only small importance in producing vitamin D deficiency. These metabolites are transported in the circulation bound to vitamin D-binding protein.

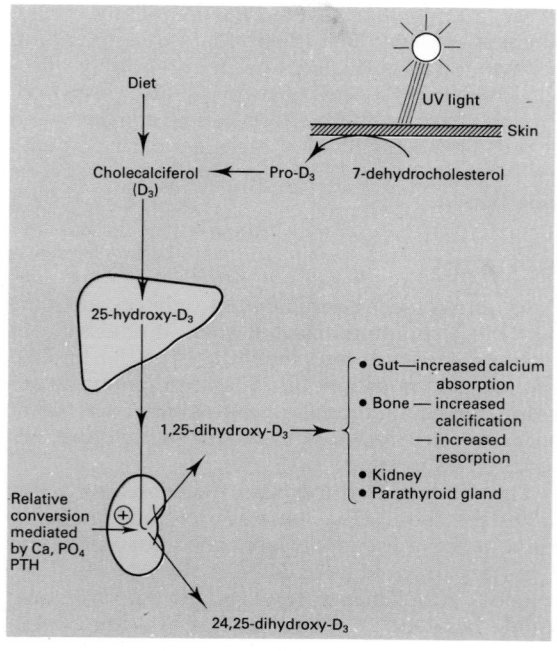

Fig. 3.4 The metabolism and actions of vitamin D. PTH = parathyroid hormone.

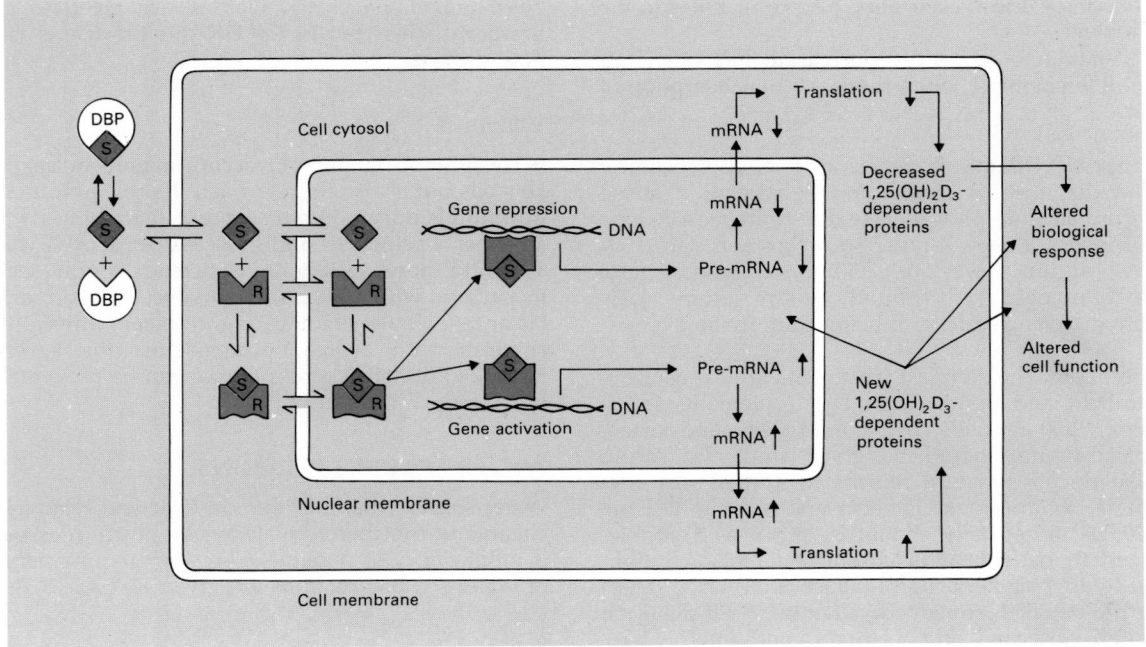

Fig. 3.5 Suggested mode of action of 1,25(OH)₂D₃(S) on target cells (see text). R = receptor protein; DBP = vitamin D serum-binding protein. [Modified with permission from Reichel H, Kaeffler HP, and Norman AW (1989) The role of vitamin D in the endocrine system in health and disease. *N. Eng. J. Med.* **320**, 984.]

In the *liver* cholecalciferol is hydroxylated to 25-hydroxycholecalciferol (25[OH]D₃) and the measurement of this in the blood is a good indicator of vitamin D bioavailability.

The next step in the metabolism occurs in the *kidney* where, in the tubules, the enzyme 1α-hydroxylase is concentrated and the highly biologically active 1,25-dihydroxycholecalciferol (1,25[OH]₂D₃) is produced. The kidney also produces a second metabolite 24,25(OH)₂D₃ as well as 1,25(OH)₂D₃ if vitamin D supplies are adequate. The production of 1,25(OH)₂D₃ is strictly regulated by parathyroid hormone, phosphate and by a feedback inhibition by 1,25(OH₂)D₃ itself. Hypocalcaemia also stimulates 1,25(OH₂)D₃ production probably via parathyroid hormone.

Extra-renal sources of 1,25(OH)₂D₃ production are small under normal conditions but it can be produced in lymphomatous and sarcoid tissue.

The *mode of action* is similar to that of other steroid hormones with interaction with a specific receptor on the target cell (Fig. 3.5). 1,25(OH)₂D₃ acts non-covalently with an intracellular receptor protein. This complex is transported through the cell membrane into the nucleus, where it interacts with DNA to initiate or suppress the synthesis of RNA-encoding proteins. The control of this is regulated by several factors; for example, interleukin, interferons and *c-myc* down-regulate, and

prolactin and fibronectin up-regulate. The biological potencies of the D₃ metabolites influence their ligand affinities for the receptor proteins. Bone, gut, kidney and the parathyroid gland are the prime target organs but many other tissues respond to 1,25(OH)₂D₃, for example, the skin, activated lymphocytes and cancer cells. This suggests a much wider role, e.g. immunoregulation and cellular differentiation, for vitamin D.

The role of vitamin D with parahormone and calcitonin in regulating calcium metabolism is discussed on p. 821.

Vitamin D deficiency
Clinical features. Vitamin D deficiency produces growth failure and rickets in children and osteomalacia in adults (see p. 822). Osteomalacia is common in the elderly population who are immobile and do not go out of their homes. It is also seen frequently in Asians in the UK; Asian women and children are often completely covered by clothes and thus their skin is not exposed to sunlight. Increased melanin in skin decreases vitamin D₃ formation. This is exacerbated by the fact that many Asians are vegans, who take no animal products, and therefore do not benefit from the small amounts of dietary vitamin D found in dairy products. The ingestion of chapatis containing phytates which bind calcium in the gut lumen

reducing calcium absorption also contributes to the problem.

Vitamin D stores are decreased, like other fat-soluble vitamins, when there is a malabsorption of fat.

Diagnosis. Vitamin D deficiency is often subclinical and diagnosis is made on the basis of a raised serum alkaline phosphatase due to increased bone turnover. Bone X-rays show osteomalacia. A low serum level of 25-hydroxycholecalciferol (< 10 nmol·L^{-1}) is found, with serum 1,25-dihydroxycholecalciferol being undetectable.

Treatment. The simplest treatments are exposure to sunlight and oral vitamin D$_2$ supplements (calciferol); 250 µg daily will cure rickets and osteomalacia and should be given until the serum alkaline phosphatase returns to normal. An adequate calcium intake is necessary. Vitamin D 1 mg (40 000 units) daily should be given as a supplement to patients with chronic fat malabsorption. 1α-hydroxycholecalciferol (alfacalcidol) (1 µg daily) is the usual treatment for vitamin D deficiency in renal disease and other conditions. 1,25-dihydroxycholecalciferol (calcitriol) is also available for anephric patients.

All patients receiving pharmacological doses of vitamin D should have their serum calcium measured regularly. Hypervitaminosis D presents with nausea and vomiting and other features of hypercalcaemia.

Prevention. Education to ensure a balanced diet, exposure to sunlight and the taking of vitamin D supplements when necessary will prevent both rickets and osteomalacia.

Vitamin K

Vitamin K is present in many plant foods as phylloquinone (vitamin K$_1$). Intestinal bacteria can synthesize menaquinone (vitamin K$_2$), which may make up an important component of daily requirements. Synthesized vitamin K or that derived from the diet (leafy vegetables) is absorbed in a similar manner to other fat-soluble substances and therefore deficiency occurs with malabsorption of fat. Deficiency is most commonly seen in biliary obstruction, when no bile salts are available to facilitate absorption. Antibacterial drugs also interfere with bacterial synthesis of vitamin K.

Vitamin K is a co-factor necessary for the synthesis of clotting factors (see p. 342) and deficiency will increase the prothrombin time. Vitamin K injection (Phytomenadione 10 mg i.m.) is effective treatment for vitamin K malabsorption. (N.B. An increased prothrombin time due to liver disease does not respond to vitamin K, there being no shortage of vitamin K, just poor liver function.)

Phytomenadione (1 mg) was always given to all newborn babies but in the UK this practice is not now universal.

Vitamin E

α-Tocopherol (vitamin E) occurs mainly in vegetable oils but is also found in fish. Its role in human nutrition is uncertain but severe deficiency leads to anaemia, haemolysis and muscle disorders as well as central nervous lesions. Deficiency is only seen in patients who are virtually unable to absorb any fat or fat-soluble vitamins, e.g. in biliary atresia. In children with abetalipoproteinaemia the severe neurological deficit (gross ataxia) can be prevented by vitamin E injection.

WATER-SOLUBLE VITAMINS

Water-soluble vitamins are non-toxic and relatively cheap and can therefore always be given in excess if a deficiency is possible. The daily requirements of water-soluble vitamins are given in Table 3.7.

Thiamine

Thiamine is a co-factor of many enzyme reactions, particularly in the glycolytic pathway. Body stores are small and signs of deficiency will quickly develop with an inadequate intake. Thiamine is found in many foodstuffs and deficiency is only seen:

- As beriberi, where the only food consumed is polished rice
- In chronic alcoholics who are consuming virtually no food at all
- Rarely in starved patients e.g. with carcinoma of the stomach

Beriberi
This is now confined to the poorest areas of Asia. It can be prevented by eating undermilled or parboiled rice, or by fortification of rice with thiamine. Probably the most important factor in the reduction of beriberi is the general increase in overall food consumption, so that the staple diet is varied and contains legumes and pulses, which contain a large amount of thiamine. There are two main clinical types of beriberi, which, surprisingly, only rarely occur together:

- *Dry beriberi* usually presents insidiously with a symmetrical polyneuropathy. The initial symptoms are heaviness and stiffness of the legs, followed by weakness, numbness, and pins and needles. The ankle jerk reflexes are lost and eventually all the signs of polyneuropathy that may involve the trunk and arms are found (p. 956). Cerebral involvement occurs, producing the picture of the Wernicke–Korsakoff syndrome (p. 956). In endemic areas mild symptoms and signs may be present for years without unduly affecting the patient.

- In *wet beriberi*, oedema occurs. Initially this is of the legs, but it can extend to involve the whole body, with ascites and pleural effusions. The peripheral oedema may mask the accompanying features of dry beriberi.

In thiamine deficiency, glucose is inadequately metabolized and lactate and pyruvate accumulate, producing peripheral vasodilatation and eventually oedema. The heart muscle is also affected and heart failure occurs, causing a further increase in the oedema. Initially there are warm extremities, a full, fast, bounding pulse and a raised venous pressure ('high output state') but eventually heart failure advances and a poor cardiac output ensues. The electrocardiogram may show conduction defects.

Infantile beriberi occurs, usually acutely, in breast-fed babies at approximately 3 months old. The mothers may show no signs of thiamine deficiency but presumably their body stores must be virtually nil. The infant becomes anorexic, develops oedema and has some degree of aphonia. Tachycardia and tachypnoea develop and, unless treatment is instituted, death occurs quickly.

Diagnosis. In endemic areas the diagnosis of beriberi should always be suspected and if in doubt treatment with thiamine should be instituted. A rapid improvement in the heart failure after thiamine (50 mg i.m.) is diagnostic. Other causes of oedema must be considered, e.g. renal or liver disease, and the polyneuropathy is indistinguishable from that due to other causes. The diagnosis is confirmed by measurement of transketolase activity in red cells. This enzyme is dependent on thiamine pyrophosphate (TPP). The assay is performed with and without added TPP; an increase in activity of 30% with TPP indicates deficiency.

Treatment. Thiamine 50 mg i.m. is given for 3 days, followed by 20 mg of thiamine daily by mouth. The response in wet beriberi occurs in hours, giving dramatic improvement, but in dry beriberi improvement is often slow to occur. In most cases all the B vitamins are given because of multiple deficiency. Infantile beriberi is treated by giving thiamine to the mother, which is then passed on to the infant via the breast milk.

Thiamine deficiency in chronic alcoholics
In the Western hemisphere, chronic alcoholics are the only group to suffer from thiamine deficiency. Rarely they develop wet beriberi, which must be distinguished from alcoholic cardiomyopathy. More usually, however, thiamine deficiency presents with polyneuropathy or with the Wernicke–Korsakoff syndrome. This syndrome, which consists of dementia, ataxia, varying ophthalmoplegia and nystagmus (see p. 956), presents acutely and should be suspected in all chronic alcoholics. If treated promptly it is reversible but if left it becomes irreversible; it is a major cause of dementia in the USA.

Treatment is with thiamine 50–100 mg i.m. or i.v., often given in combination with other vitamin B complex vitamins. Thiamine must always be given before any intravenous glucose infusion is given to a chronic alcoholic.

Riboflavin

Riboflavin is widely distributed throughout all plant and animal cells. Good sources are dairy products, offal and leafy vegetables. Riboflavin is not destroyed appreciably by cooking, but is destroyed by sunlight. Riboflavin is a flavoprotein that is a co-factor for many oxidative reactions in the cell.

Riboflavin deficiency is virtually always accompanied by other deficiencies and many features previously attributed to riboflavin deficiency are probably due to multiple deficiencies:

- Angular stomatitis or cheilosis (fissuring at the corners of the mouth)
- A red, inflamed tongue
- Seborrhoeic dermatitis, particularly involving the face (around the nose) and the scrotum or vulva

Riboflavin (5 mg) daily can be tried for the above conditions, usually given as vitamin B complex.

Niacin

This is the generic name for the two chemical forms nicotinic acid and nicotinamide, the latter being found in the two pyridine nucleotides nicotinamide adenine dinucleotide (NAD) and nicotinamide adenine dinucleotide phosphate (NADP). Both act as hydrogen acceptors in many oxidative reactions and in their reduced forms (NADH and NADPH) act as hydrogen donors in reductive reactions. Many oxidative steps in the production of energy require NAD, and NADP is equally important in the hexose monophosphate shunt for the generation of NADPH, which is necessary for fatty-acid synthesis.

Niacin is found in many foodstuffs, including plants, meat (particularly offal) and fish. Niacin is lost by removing bran from cereals but is added to processed cereals and white bread in many countries.

Niacin can be synthesized in humans from tryptophan, 60 mg of tryptophan being converted to 1 mg of niacin (Fig. 3.6). The amount of niacin in food is given as the niacin equivalent which is

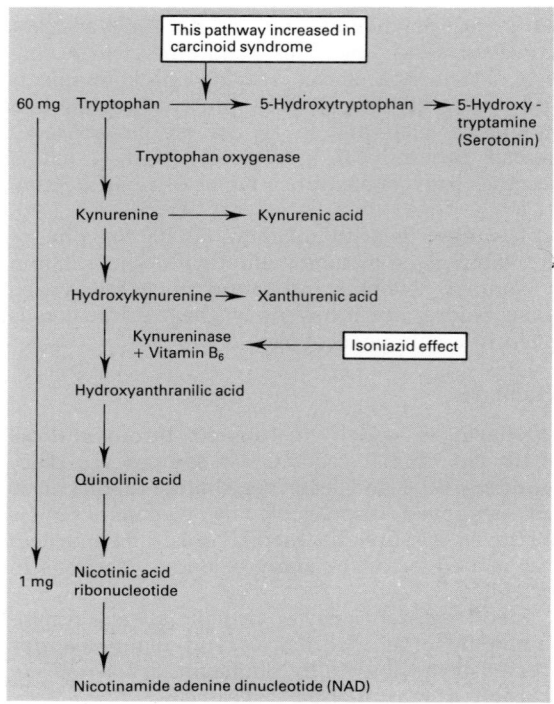

Fig. 3.6 The oxidative pathway of tryptophan metabolism.

equal to the amount of niacin plus one-sixtieth of the tryptophan content.

Pellagra
This is nowadays almost always only found in areas where the main constituent of the diet is maize. It has occurred world-wide, including India, Asia, the southern states of the USA and South America. It is now rarely seen apart from in southern Africa in Bantu homelands and in India. Maize contains niacin in the form of niacytin, which is biologically unavailable, and has a low content of tryptophan. Many of the features of pellagra can be explained purely by niacin deficiency; some, however, are probably due to multiple deficiencies, including proteins and other vitamins.

The clinical features are of dermatitis, diarrhoea and dementia. Although this is an easily remembered triad, not all are always present and the mental changes are not a true dementia.

Dermatitis. Initially there is a redness of the skin in the areas exposed to sunlight. This is followed by cracks in the skin, with occasional ulceration. Chronic thickening, dryness and pigmentation develop. The lesions are always symmetrical and often affect the dorsal surfaces of the hands. The perianal skin and vulva are frequently involved. Casal's necklace or collar is the term given to the

skin lesion around the neck, which is confined to this area by the clothes worn.

Diarrhoea This is often a feature but constipation is occasionally seen. Other GI manifestations include painful red raw tongue, glossitis and angular stomatitis. Recurring mouth infections occur.

Dementia This occurs in chronic disease. In milder cases there are symptoms of depression, apathy and sometimes thought disorders. Tremor and an encephalopathy frequently occur. Hallucinations and acute psychosis are seen with more severe cases.

Pellagra may also occur in (Fig. 3.6):

- Therapy with isoniazid, as this can lead to a deficiency of vitamin B_6, which is needed for the synthesis of nicotinamide from tryptophan; vitamin B_6 is now given concomitantly with isoniazid
- Hartnup disease, a rare inborn error whereby basic amino acids including tryptophan are not absorbed by the gut and there is also loss of this amino acid in the urine
- Generalized malabsorption (rare)
- Chronic alcoholics who do not eat
- Very low-protein diets given for renal disease or taken as a food fad
- Carcinoid syndrome and phaeochromocytoma, in which tryptophan metabolism is diverted away from the formation of nicotinamide to form amines.

Diagnosis. In endemic areas this is based on the clinical features, remembering that other vitamin deficiencies can produce similar changes, e.g. angular stomatitis. Nicotinamide (approximately 300 mg daily by mouth) with a maintenance dose of 50 mg daily is given. Mostly, however, vitamin B complex is given, as other deficiencies are often present.

An increase in the protein content of the diet and treatment of malnutrition and other vitamin deficiencies is essential. Mild cases respond well but dementia is often permanent.

Vitamin B_6

Vitamin B_6 exists as pyridoxine, pyridoxal and pyridoxamine, and is found in plant and animal foodstuffs. Pyridoxal phosphate is involved in the metabolism of amino acids. Dietary deficiency is extremely rare but has been described in coeliac disease and after the administration of drugs antagonistic to B_6, e.g. isoniazid, hydralazine and penicillamine. The peripheral neuropathy occurring after isoniazid usually responds to vitamin B_6. Sideroblastic anaemia occasionally responds to vitamin B_6 (see p. 302).

Biotin

Biotin is involved in a number of carboxylase reactions. It occurs in many foodstuffs and the dietary requirement is small. Deficiency is extremely rare and is confined to a few people who consume raw eggs, which contain an antagonist (avidin) to biotin. It causes a dermatitis that responds to biotin replacements.

Pantothenic acid

Pantothenic acid is necessary for a number of metabolic reactions, including fatty-acid synthesis. It is widely distributed in all foods and deficiency in humans has not been described.

Vitamin C

Ascorbic acid is a simple sugar and a powerful reducing agent, its main role being to control the redox potential within cells. It is involved in the hydroxylation of proline to hydroxyproline, which is necessary for the formation of collagen. The failure of this biochemical pathway in vitamin C deficiency accounts for virtually all of the clinical effects found.

Man, along with a few other animals (e.g. primates and the guinea-pig) is unusual in not being able to synthesize ascorbic acid from glucose.

Vitamin C is present in all fresh fruit and vegetables. Unfortunately, ascorbic acid is easily leached out of vegetables when they are placed in water and it is also oxidized during cooking. Potatoes are a good source as many people eat a lot but, as with other vegetables, vitamin C is lost during storage.

Vitamin C deficiency is mainly seen in infants fed boiled milk and elderly and single people who cannot be bothered to eat vegetables. In the UK it is also seen in Asians eating only rice and chapatis and in food faddists.

Scurvy

In adults the early symptoms may be non-specific, with weakness and muscle pain. Other features are shown in Table 3.9. In infantile scurvy there are irritability, painful legs, anaemia and characteristic

Table 3.9 Clinical features of vitamin C deficiency.

Keratosis of hair follicles with 'corkscrew hair'
Perifollicular haemorrhages
Swollen, spongy gums with bleeding and superadded infection; loosening of teeth
Spontaneous bruising
Spontaneous haemorrhage
Anaemia
Failure of wound healing

subperiosteal haemorrhages, particularly into the ends of long bones.

Diagnosis. The anaemia is usually hypochromic but occasionally a normochromic or megaloblastic anaemia is seen. The type of anaemia depends on whether iron deficiency (due to decreased absorption and loss due to haemorrhage) or folate deficiency (folate is largely found in green vegetables) is present.

Plasma ascorbic acid is very low in obvious deficiency and a vitamin C level of less than $0.1\ \mu g \cdot dl^{-1}$ in the leucocyte-platelet layer (buffy coat) of centrifuged blood indicates deficiency.

Treatment. Ascorbic acid should be given in doses of up to 1 g a day initially and patients should be encouraged to eat fresh fruit and vegetables.

Prevention. Orange juice should be given to bottle-fed infants. The intake of breast-fed infants depends on the mother's diet.

In the elderly, eating adequate fruit and vegetables is the best way to avoid scurvy. Careful surveillance of the elderly, particularly those who live alone, is necessary. Ascorbic acid supplements should only be necessary occasionally.

Ascorbic acid in high dosage has been suggested as a treatment of cancer and the common cold. There is some scientific support for its value; however, clinical trials in the common cold have shown that it is of no help.

Vitamin B$_{12}$ and folate

These are dealt with on p. 303 and in Table 3.7.

Minerals

A number of minerals have been shown to be essential in animals and an increasing number of deficiency syndromes are becoming recognized in humans. Long-term total parenteral nutrition allowed trace-element deficiency to be studied in controlled conditions; now trace elements are always added to long-term parenteral nutrition regimens. It is highly probable (but difficult to study because of multiple deficiencies) that trace-element deficiency is also an important accompaniment of all protein–energy malnutrition states.

Sodium, potassium, magnesium and chloride are discussed in Chapter 10.

COPPER

Deficiency

Menkes' kinky hair syndrome is a rare condition due to malabsorption of copper. Infants with this sex-linked abnormality develop growth failure, mental retardation, bone lesions and brittle hair. Anaemia and neutropenia also occur. This condition, which serves as a model for copper deficiency, supports the idea that some of the clinical features seen in protein–energy malnutrition are due to copper deficiency. Breast and cow's milk are low in copper and supplementation is occasionally necessary when first treating PEM.

Toxicity

Copper toxicity occurs in Wilson's disease—see p. 271.

ZINC

Acrodermatitis enteropathica

This inherited disorder is due to malabsorption of zinc. Infants develop growth retardation, severe diarrhoea, hair loss and associated Candida and bacterial infection. Zinc supplement results in a complete cure.

This condition provides a model for zinc deficiency, which may play a role in protein–energy malnutrition.

Zinc levels have also been shown to be low in a number of conditions associated with malabsorption, skin disease and diarrhoea.

IODINE

The daily intake of iodine varies considerably from approximately 20 µg to 700 µg per day in areas where iodine is added to salt. Endemic goitre occurs in areas where the level is below 150 µg/day (p. 804).

FLUORINE

In areas where the level of fluorine is less than 1 p.p.m. in drinking water, dental caries is more prevalent. Fluoridation of the water seems to reduce this.

Excessive fluorine intake can result in fluorosis, in which there is infiltration of the enamel of the teeth with fluorine, producing pitting and discoloration.

CALCIUM (see p. 821)

This is found in many foods but particularly in milk. Its absorption from the GI tract is vitamin D-

Table 3.10 Other trace elements (see text).

Element	Deficiency
Cadmium	?
Chromium	Glucose intolerance
Cobalt	Anaemia
Manganese	Growth retardation, skeletal abnormalities, glucose intolerance
Molybdenum	? Animals only
Nickel	? Animals only
Selenium	Growth retardation
Vanadium	? Nutritional oedema

dependent. Ninety-nine per cent of body calcium is in the skeleton. Increased calcium is required in pregnancy and lactation, when dietary intake must be increased. Calcium deficiency is usually due to vitamin D deficiency.

PHOSPHATE

Phosphates are present in all natural foods and dietary deficiency has not been described. Patients taking large amounts of aluminium hydroxide can, however, develop phosphate deficiency owing to binding in the gut lumen. It can also be seen in total parenteral nutrition. Symptoms include anorexia, weakness and osteoporosis.

Other trace elements of possible significance are shown in Table 3.10.

Obesity

Some degree of obesity is almost invariable in the Western World and almost all people develop some obesity as they get older. Obesity implies the excess storage of fat and this can most easily be detected by looking at the undressed patient.

Tables of desirable weights for a given height can be found in the Appendices, 10% greater than the ideal weight being described as overweight, 20% or more than the ideal weight as morbid obesity. Another way of classifying grades of obesity is the Body Mass Index (BMI):

$$\text{BMI} = \text{weight (kg)}/(\text{height in metres})^2$$

which is a more accurate measurement of obesity.

Causes of obesity

There are a few unusual causes (Table 3.11) but

Table 3.11 Unusual causes of obesity.

Genetic syndromes associated with hypogonadism, e.g. Prader–Willi syndrome, Laurence–Moon–Biedl syndrome

Hypothyroidism

Cushing's syndrome

Stein–Leventhal syndrome

Drug-induced, e.g. corticosteroids

Hypothalamic damage, e.g. due to trauma, tumour

most patients suffer from simple obesity. Hormonal imbalance is often incriminated in women, e.g. post-menopause or when taking contraceptive pills, but most weight gain in such cases is usually small and due to water retention.

SIMPLE OBESITY

Not all obese people eat more than the average but all obviously eat more than they need.

Suggested mechanisms
Genetic and environmental factors. These are difficult to separate, but obese children mostly have obese parents (usually the mother). The relative importance of genetic make-up compared with the importance of food-eating patterns is complex. It has been suggested that body size is determined in the first few months of life, but not all obese children become obese adults. On the other hand, obese teenagers often remain obese.

Obesity starting in early life is associated with an increased number of fat cells, while in adult obesity ('middle-age spread') there is an increased amount of fat in each fat cell. However, in morbid obesity there is both an increased number and increased amount of fat in cells.

Food intake. Many factors related to the home environment, e.g. finance and the availability of sweets and snacks, will affect food intake. Some patients eat more during periods of heavy exercise or during pregnancy and are unable to get back to their former eating habits. The increase in obesity in social class 5 can usually be related to the type of food consumed, i.e. food containing sugar and fat. The underlying mechanisms for controlling satiety are ill-understood; psychological factors and how food is presented may override complex biochemical interactions.

Despite the above, over the years the obese person does not eat much more than the non-obese when calculated per unit lean-body mass.

Energy expenditure. This is reduced in many obese subjects, partly owing to decreased physical activity. It is unclear whether the latter is a primary event or a result of the obesity. The energy expended on walking at 3 miles per hour is only $3.7\ kcal\cdot min^{-1}$ $(15.5\ kJ\cdot min^{-1})$ and therefore increasing exercise plays only a small part in losing weight. Nevertheless, as increased body fat develops insidiously over many years, any discrepancy in energy balance is important.

Thermogenesis. Brown adipose tissue in animals when stimulated by cold or food dissipates the energy derived from ingested food as heat. This can be a major component of overall energy balance and it has been suggested that this may also apply to man. A defect in thermogenesis would explain why some obese patients require a very low calorie intake to maintain any weight loss achieved and gain weight easily after only small calorie increases. This mechanism may play some role in the development of obesity.

CLINICAL FEATURES

Most patients recognize their own problems, although often they are unaware of the main foods that cause obesity. Many symptoms are related to psychological problems, e.g. in women who cannot find fashionable clothes to wear. Social pressures are also important.

The degree of obesity is assessed by comparison with tables of ideal weight for height (see Appendices) and also by measuring skinfold thickness. This should be measured over the middle of the triceps muscle; normal values are 20 mm in a man and 30 mm in a woman.

Table 3.12 shows the conditions and complications that are associated with obesity. The relation-

Table 3.12 Conditions and complications associated with obesity.

Psychological

Osteoarthritis

Varicose veins

Hiatus hernia

Gallstones

Postoperative problems

Back strain

Accident proneness

Hypertension

Breathlessness

Ischaemic heart disease

Stroke

Diabetes mellitus

Hyperlipidaemia

Menstrual abnormalities

ship between cardiovascular disease (hypertension or ischaemic heart disease), hyperlipidaemia, smoking, physical exercise and obesity is complex. Difficulties arise in interpreting mortality figures because of the number of factors involved. Many studies of obesity do not, for instance, differentiate between smokers and non-smokers or between the types of physical exercise that are taken. Many do not take into account the cuff-size artefact in the measurement of blood pressure; an artefact will occur if a large cuff is not used in patients with a large arm. Nevertheless, obesity almost certainly plays a part in all of these diseases and should be treated. The only exception is that stopping smoking, even if accompanied by weight gain, is more important than any of the other factors.

TREATMENT

This largely depends on a reduction in calorie intake. The commonest diets allow an intake of approximately 1000 kcal (4200 kJ) per day, although this may need to be nearer 1500 kcal (6300 kJ) per day for someone engaged in physical work. A diet that is too low in total calories will usually result in the patient cheating and keeping to the diet only for short periods.

Patients must realize that prolonged dieting is necessary for large amounts of fat to be lost. Furthermore, a permanent change in eating habits is required to maintain the new low weight. It is relatively easy for most patients to lose the first few kilograms, but long-term success in moderate obesity is poor, with an overall success rate of no more than 10–20%.

The aim of any dietary regimen is to lose approximately 1 kg per week, which corresponds to a loss of 7700 kcal (3200 kJ) from adipose tissue. Weight loss will be greater initially owing to accompanying protein and glycogen breakdown and consequent water loss. After 3–4 weeks, weight loss may be very small as only adipose tissue is broken down and there is no accompanying water loss.

Patients must understand the principles of energy intake and expenditure and the best results are obtained in educated, well-motivated patients. Constant supervision, either by a doctor, close relatives or through slimming societies (e.g. WeightWatchers) helps to encourage compliance.

An increase in exercise will increase energy expenditure and should be encouraged, as long as there is no contraindication such as cardiovascular disease. Weight cannot be lost by exercise alone. Nevertheless, a 15-minute brisk daily walk will use the energy contained in a small slice of bread and butter.

The diet should contain adequate amounts of each nutrient; a diet of 1000 kcal (4200 kJ) per day should be made up of approximately 100 g of carbohydrate, 50 g of protein and 40 g of fat. The carbohydrate should be in the form of complex carbohydrates such as vegetables and fruit rather than simple sugars. Alcohol cointains 7 kcal·g^{-1} and should be discouraged. It can be substituted for other foods in the diet but it often reduces the willpower. With a varied diet, vitamins and minerals will be adequate and supplements are not necessary. A balanced diet, attractively presented, is of much greater value and safer than any of the slimming regimens often advertised in women's magazines.

Unfortunately, after a few years most obese persons have regained the weight lost.

Drug therapy

Drugs can be used as an adjunct to the dietary regimen but they do not substitute for strict dieting. Amphetamine is addictive, although some less-stimulating derivatives are now available that produce anorexia. However, their use should be discouraged as they cause dependency and psychotic states. The most commonly used drugs are diethylproprion (75 mg daily) and fenfluramine. The latter differs in that it acts on the serotoninergic system rather than the catecholaminogenic pathway, which is affected by the amphetamine derivatives. It can be given in doses up to 100 mg daily but side-effects are frequent. None of the drugs should be given long-term; they should be withdrawn slowly.

Surgical treatment

Operations involving bypass of parts of the small intestine have fallen out of favour because of their side-effects and cannot now be recommended. Jejunoileal bypass was the commonest operation and involved the anastomosis of approximately 18 cm of jejunum to the terminal 18 cm of the ileum. Complications are chiefly those of intestinal resection (see p. 208). A fatty liver often occurs and in a few patients cirrhosis is seen.

Three procedures are still performed in cases of severe morbid obesity:

- *Wiring the jaws* to prevent eating and allow liquid feeds only. This can be used as a temporary measure but good dental hygiene is essential. Weight gain usually occurs after the wires have been removed.
- *Gastric plication,* in which a small gastric pouch is created by stapling across the wall of the stomach. Good results are claimed without the side-effects of bypass operations.
- *Gastric balloon.* Here a balloon is placed endoscopically inside the stomach and inflated. Its value has been over-exaggerated and complications include intestinal obstruction.

MORBIDITY AND MORTALITY

There is an increase in death in obesity, mainly from diabetes, coronary heart disease and cerebrovascular disease. The greater the obesity the higher the morbidity and mortality figures. For example, men who are 10% overweight have a 13% increased risk of death, whilst the increase in mortality for those 20% overweight is 25%. The rise is less in women. Weight reduction reduces this mortality and therefore should be strongly encouraged.

Nutritional support in the hospital patient

Nutritional support is now recognized as being necessary in many hospitalized patients. The pathophysiology and hallmarks of malnutrition have been described earlier (p. 155); here the forms of nutritional support that are available are discussed.

Principles
Some form of nutritional supplemention is required in those patients who cannot eat, should not eat, will not eat or cannot eat enough. It is necessary to provide nutritional support for:

- All severely malnourished patients on admission to hospital
- Moderately malnourished patients who, because of their physical illness, are not expected to eat for 3–5 days
- Normally nourished patients not expected to eat for 7–10 days

If the gastrointestinal tract is functioning normally, enteral rather than parenteral nutrition should always be used.

Enteral feeding

Feeds can be given by:

- Mouth.
- Fine-bore nasogastric tube (commonest method).
- Percutaneous endoscopic gastrostomy; this is useful for patients who need enteral nutrition for an indefinite period, e.g. motor neurone disease with swallowing problems. A catheter is placed percutaneously into the stomach, which has been dilated with air via a gastroscope.
- Needle catheter jejunostomy. A fine catheter is inserted into the jejunum at laparotomy and brought out through the abdominal wall.

Table 3.13 Standard enteric diet (2000–3000 kcal, approximately 12 000 kJ) per day.

Energy
  Carbohydrate as glucose polymers (70%)
  Fat as triglycerides (30%)
Nitrogen
  Whole protein (9–15 g)
  Ratio of energy to nitrogen (kcal : g) = 150 : 1
Osmolality = 285–300 mosmol·kg^{-1}
Additional electrolytes, vitamins and trace elements

Diet formulation (Table 3.13)
In most patients these standard enteric feeds should be given via a narrow-bore nasogastric tube. Whole-protein and fat can be given except in patients with severely impaired gastrointestinal function who may require predigested diets.
These contain:

Carbohydrate	Glucose polymers
Fat	Medium chain triglycerides
Nitrogen	Purified low-molecular-weight peptides or amino-acid mixtures

The aim of the regimen is to achieve a positive nitrogen balance, which can usually be obtained by giving 3–5 g of nitrogen in excess of output. Nitrogen loss can be calculated using the formula:

N_2 loss (g per 24 h)
= urinary urea (mmol per 24 h) × 0.028 + 2

the 2 representing non-urinary nitrogen excretion.
  Hypercatabolic patients require a high supply of nitrogen (15 g per day) and often will not achieve

Enteral feeding
- Fine bore tube with wire stylet inserted intranasally
- Confirm position of tube in stomach by aspiration of gastric contents and auscultation of the epigastrium
- Check by X-ray if aspiration or auscultation unsuccessful

Problems
No satisfactory way of keeping tubes in place (up to 60% come out).

Main complications
- Regurgitation and aspiration into bronchus
- Gastrointestinal side-effects, the most common being diarrhoea
- Metabolic complications including hyperglycaemia and low levels of potassium, magnesium, calcium and phosphate.

positive nitrogen balance until the primary injury is resolved.

The success of enteral feeding depends on careful supervision of the patient. Any patient requiring long-term therapy will need vitamin and essential trace metal supplements.

Parenteral nutrition

Parenteral nutrition is much more complicated and potentially more dangerous than enteral nutrition. It should therefore not be used unless absolutely necessary. It is seldom necessary for periods of less than 14 days.

Catheter placement (see box)
A silicon catheter is placed into a central vein, usually using the infraclavicular approach to the subclavian vein. The skin-entry site should be dressed carefully and not disturbed unless there is a suggestion of catheter-related sepsis.

Complications of catheter placement include central vein thrombosis, pneumothorax and embolism, but the major problem is catheter-related sepsis. Organisms, mainly staphylococci, enter along the side of the catheter, leading to septicaemia. Sepsis can be prevented by careful and sterile placement of the catheter, by not removing the dressing over the catheter entry site, and by not giving other substances (e.g. blood products, antibiotics) via the central vein catheter.

Catheter placement for parenteral nutrition

This should be performed only by experienced clinicians under aseptic conditions in an operating theatre.

- The patient is placed supine with 5° of head down tilt to avoid air embolism.
- The skin below the midpoint of the left clavicle is infiltrated with 1–2% lignocaine and a 1 cm skin incision made.
- A 20-gauge needle on a syringe is inserted beneath the clavicle and first rib and angled towards the tip of finger held in the suprasternal notch.
- When blood is aspirated freely, the needle is used as a guide to insert the cannula through the skin incision and into the subclavian vein.
- The catheter is advanced so that its tip lies in the distal part of the superior vena cava.
- A skin tunnel is created under local anaesthetic using an introducer inserted through a point about 10 cm below and medial to the incision and passed upwards to the incision.
- The proximal end of the catheter (with hub removed) is passed backwards through the introducer to emerge 10 cm below the clavicle, where it is sutured to the chest wall.
- The original infraclavicular entry incision is now sutured.

Sepsis should be suspected if the patient develops fever and leucocytosis. In two-thirds of cases, organisms can be grown from the catheter tip. Treatment involves removal of the catheter and appropriate systemic antibiotics.

Nutrition
With parenteral nutrition it is possible to provide sufficient nitrogen for protein synthesis and calories to meet energy requirements. Electrolytes, vitamins and trace elements are also necessary. All of these substances are infused simultaneously.

Nitrogen source. Synthetic L-amino acid solutions are used, which contain between 9 and 17 g of nitrogen per litre. Most patients require at least 14 g of nitrogen per day.

Energy source. This is mainly provided by glucose as a 20% solution, with additional calories provided by a fat emulsion. Fat infusions provide a greater number of calories in a smaller volume than can be provided by carbohydrate. They are not hypertonic and they also prevent essential fatty-acid deficiency.

Essential fatty-acid deficiency has been reported in long-term parenteral nutritional regimens without fat emulsions. It causes a scaly skin, hair loss and a delay in healing.

The calorie-to-nitrogen ratio in parenteral nutrition should be approximately 150 : 1.

Electrolytes and trace elements (Table 3.14)
The electrolyte status should be monitored on a daily basis and electrolyte solutions given as appropriate. Water-soluble vitamins can be given daily but fat-soluble vitamins should be given weekly, as overdose can occur. A trace-metal solution is available for patients on long-term parenteral nutrition, but if the patient requires blood transfusions trace-metal supplements are not needed.

Table 3.14 Daily dietary electrolytes and trace elements required for long-term maintenance.

Na^+	70–220 mmol
K^+	60–120 mmol
Mg^{2+}	5–20 mmol
Ca^{2+}	5–10 mmol
Zn^{2+}	50 μmol
Mn^{2+}	7 μmol
Fe^{3+}	70 μmol
Cu^{2+}	8 μmol
Cl^-	70–220 μmol
PO_4^{3-}	20–40 mmol
F^-	50 μmol
I^-	1–8 μmol

Most hospitals now administer parenteral nutrition using 3-litre bags pre-mixed under sterile conditions by the pharmacy. A standard parenteral nutrition regimen is given in the Appendices.

COMPLICATIONS

- Metabolic, e.g. hyperglycaemia—insulin therapy may be necessary
- Electrolyte disturbances
- Hypercalcaemia
- Liver dysfunction

Monitoring of patients on parenteral nutrition
Essential monitoring includes daily plasma electrolytes and weekly assessments of nutritional status (weight and skinfold thickness). Nitrogen balance should also be measured on a weekly basis. Home parenteral nutrition is occasionally required for patients with virtually no small bowel.

Food allergy and food intolerance

Some patients have allergic reactions to particular foods, e.g. urticaria, vomiting or diarrhoea after eating strawberries or shellfish. Vague, non-specific symptoms such as headaches, panic attacks, palpitations and anxiety, although related to food ingestion, may not be due to an allergic reaction and often have a psychological basis. Unfortunately, as symptoms are usually subjective, differentiating between true food allergy and psychiatric ill-health is often difficult.

Definition

Food intolerance may be due to pharmacological, idiosyncratic or allergic mechanisms (Fig. 3.7):

- Pharmacological reactions to a constituent of food, e.g. the histamine in mackerel or canned food, or the tyramine in cheeses
- Reactions to chemical mediators released by food, e.g. histamine may be released by tomatoes or strawberries
- Reactions to toxic chemicals found in food, e.g. the food additive tartrazine
- Irritation of the GI tract by foods containing spices
- Reactions due to an enzyme deficiency, e.g. milk-induced diarrhoea in alactasia, or fava-bean-induced haemolytic anaemia in glucose-6-phosphate dehydrogenase deficiency

Food allergy. This term should be restricted to

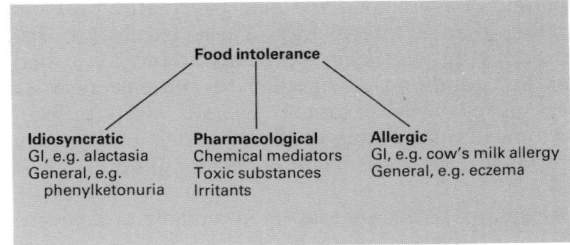

Fig. 3.7 Types of food intolerance.

patients with an immunological hypersensitivity reaction mediated by IgE.

Mechanisms

The exact mechanism of the causation of food allergy is unclear. Antigen food proteins are absorbed across healthy gastrointestinal mucosa and, although small in amount, they are sufficient to immunize and lead to the production of antibodies. This is a normal reaction to the ingestion of foreign material and does not usually lead to symptoms. In some patients, inappropriate allergic reactions to food may lead to local gastrointestinal or distant systematic symptoms.

Excess antigen absorption across an intact gastrointestinal mucosa is prevented by several mechanisms (see p. 200). When an infant first eats a food, a small amount of the antigen appears in the blood and an antibody (usually IgE) is produced. On subsequent ingestion of the antigen, very little enters the blood owing to the protective response (immune exclusion). Ingestion of an antigen also induces partial immunological tolerance to subsequent parenteral contact with the antigen.

The type of antigen absorbed is important. Some foods, e.g. egg, milk, fish and wheat, have a very strong tendency to sensitize, while others are fairly innocuous. Cross-sensitization between related vegetables, e.g. soybean and peas, also occurs. However, the nature of the actual allergen in any particular food is still uncertain.

In certain conditions a genetic predisposition may be important, as there appears to be a familial tendency. In coeliac disease (see p. 204), in which the lesion is produced by gluten ingestion, there is an increase in the incidence of HLA-B8, DR3. Atopic patients with eczema may also have an increase in the incidence of HLA-B8. Environmental factors may also play a part, as concordance of atopic allergic disease in monozygotic twins is not total.

CLINICAL FEATURES

It must be emphasized that of all the many

disorders thought to be due to food allergy, most patients have a food fad or a psychiatric problem rather than a true allergy. These psychiatric disorders may vary from simple avoidance of a food as an attention-seeking ploy to anorexia nervosa associated with extreme weight loss (p. 995). Atopic dermatitis due to allergy to egg and/or dairy products has been documented in children.

Symptoms of allergy may be immediate or delayed:

- *Immediate symptoms* start within a few hours of ingestion of the particular food, with swelling of the lips or tongue, vomiting, rhinorrhoea, urticaria, eczema, asthma or migraine. These reactions are usually thought to be mediated by IgE.
- *Delayed symptoms* are much more difficult to delineate. They may develop hours or even days after the ingestion of food and a causal relationship between the ingestion of the food and the symptoms is often difficult to prove.

Multiple vague symptoms, e.g. tiredness or malaise, are unlikely to be due to food allergy or intolerance and probably have a psychiatric basis.

Migraine, arthritis, behaviour and affective disorders, the irritable bowel syndrome and Crohn's disease have all been suggested to be due to food allergy. However, the results of double-blind studies in adults, in which foods are administered in unmarked capsules, have usually been negative. Nevertheless, cases of immediate food-induced rhinitis and asthma are well-recognized, migraine attacks can be provoked by certain foods in some people, and some cases of urticaria have been shown to be due to certain foods.

INVESTIGATION AND DIAGNOSIS

There are no reliable laboratory tests for food allergy. A careful history may help to delineate the causative agent, particularly if the effects are immediate. Delayed reactions are more difficult to diagnose, as laboratory testing is usually negative. Laboratory tests include:

- Skin-prick testing with allergens—positive results correlate poorly with clinical symptoms.
- Serum IgE—this may be raised in an allergic response (particularly if it is an immediate reaction).
- Radioallergosorbent tests (RASTs) for specific antigen IgE—these may occasionally demonstrate circulating antibody levels to specific foods, but the correlation with symptoms is poor.
- Measurements of circulating immune complexes, leucocyte histamine-release tests, organ culture tests—these have all been performed in various conditions but at the moment are research tools only. Humoral antibodies against various foods are seen in normal individuals but may be helpful in assessing treatment in patients if antibody titres fall.
- 'Fringe' techniques such as hair analysis—although widely advertised, these are valueless and possibly fraudulent.
- Diagnostic exclusion diets—these diets are time-consuming and cumbersome and range from being very simple to extremely tedious. A basic exclusion diet usually excludes colourings, preservatives, milk, eggs, dairy products, fish and nuts. It empirically contains one meat, one vegetable and spring water. Patients are asked to introduce excluded foods one at a time at intervals of 2–7 days; if symptoms do not occur, the food involved is unlikely to be the cause of the symptoms.
- Dietary challenge—this can take various forms. The patients may be 'challenged' with the food under test sublingually, by inhalation, by intragastric or intraduodenal instillation, or by dietary introduction using capsules containing the particular food or a placebo.

MANAGEMENT

- Isolated reactions to particular foods, e.g. strawberries or shellfish, are best managed by simple avoidance. This is usually not a clinical problem, as the patient has already learned to avoid the suspected food.
- Multiple intolerance, if truly suspected, can be managed by a rigorous therapeutic exclusion diet. However, great care must be taken to ensure that the diet is nutritionally adequate.
- Desensitization therapy using injections or oral or nasal administration has been used for immediate reactions, but with little success.
- Treatment of asthma, rhinitis, eczema or migraine is by avoidance of the particular food that the patient has recognized as causing the symptoms.
- In allergic diseases where the antigen is known, e.g. cow's milk protein intolerance in children and coeliac disease, patients should be treated with a milk-free or gluten-free diet, respectively.
- There is no specific drug therapy. Oral *sodium cromoglycate* has been tried and may have some value as an adjunct to a special diet. *Antihistamines*, e.g. terfenadine, brompheniramine, have been tried with some success, and *prostaglandin synthetase inhibitors*, e.g. aspirin, and other non-steroidal anti-inflammatory drugs may be of some use.
- Most patients require only reassurance. Others may need psychiatric help.

Alcohol

Alcohol is a popular 'nutrient' consumed in large quantities all over the world.

Ethanol (ethyl alcohol) is metabolized chiefly in the liver, eventually to carbon dioxide and water, by the following mechanisms:

- Alcohol dehydrogenase, a mitochondrial enzyme, catalyses the oxidation of alcohol to acetaldehyde, which is then further metabolized in the Krebs' cycle.
- Mixed-function oxidases localized in the endoplasmic reticulum can also metabolize alcohol. These enzymes are inducible, which explains why people who often drink alcohol can metabolize alcohol at a faster rate than non-drinkers.

Ethanol itself produces 7 kcal·g^{-1} (297 kJ·g^{-1}), but many alcoholic drinks also contain sugar, which increases their calorific value. For example, one pint of beer provides 250 kcal (2100 kJ). Therefore, the heavy drinker will be unable to lose weight if he or she continues to drink.

Effects of excess alcohol consumption

Excess consumption of alcohol leads to two major problems, both of which can be present in the same patient:

- Alcohol dependence syndrome—see p. 991
- Physical damage to various tissues

Each unit of alcohol, e.g. half a pint of beer, one single spirit, one small glass of wine, contains 8 g of ethanol (Fig. 3.8). All the long-term effects of excess alcohol consumption are due to excess ethanol, irrespective of the type of alcoholic beverage, i.e. beer and spirits are no different in their long-term effects.

Guide to sensible drinking

- Daily maximum:
  3 units for men
  2 units for women
  To help achieve this:
  Use a standard measure
  Do not drink during the day
- Have alcohol-free days each week
- Remember:
  Health can be damaged without being 'drunk'
  Regular heavy intake is more harmful than occasional binges
  Do not drink to 'drown your problems'
- Drinking and driving *limit* is 800 mg·L^{-1} (80 mg%) of blood (in the UK)
  1 unit of alcohol is eliminated per hour, therefore spread drinking time
  Food decreases absorption and therefore results in a lower blood alcohol level
  4–5 units are sufficient to put the blood alcohol level over the legal driving limit in a 70 kg man (less in a lighter person)

Short-term effects, such as hangovers, depend on additional substances, particularly other alcohols such as isoamyl alcohol, which are known as congeners. Brandy and bourbon contain the highest percentage of congeners.

The amount of alcohol that produces damage varies and not everyone who drink heavily will suffer physical damage. For example, only 20% of people who drink heavily develop cirrhosis of the liver.

The effect of alcohol on different organs of the body is not the same; in some patients the liver is affected, in others the brain or muscle. The differences may be genetically determined.

In general the effects of a given intake of alcohol seem to be worse in women. The following figures are for men and should be reduced by 50% for women.

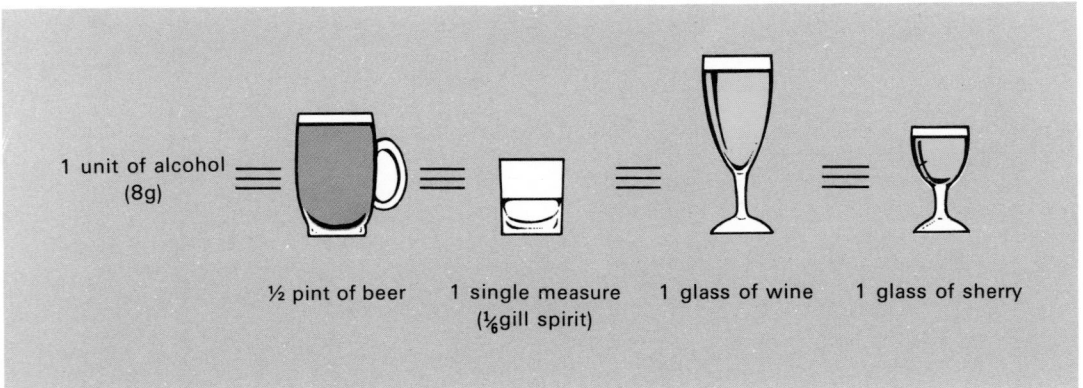

1 unit of alcohol (8g)

½ pint of beer   1 single measure (⅙ gill spirit)   1 glass of wine   1 glass of sherry

Fig. 3.8 Measures of alcohol.

Table 3.15 Physical effects of excess alcohol consumption.

Central nervous system (see Table 18.55)
Epilepsy
Wernicke–Korsakoff syndrome
Polyneuropathy

Muscles
Acute or chronic myopathy

Cardiovascular system
Cardiomyopathy
Beriberi heart disease
Cardiac arrhythmias

Metabolism
Hyperuricaemia (gout)
Hyperlipidaemia
Hypoglycaemia
Obesity

Endocrine system
Pseudo-Cushing's syndrome

Respiratory system
Chest infections

Gastrointestinal system
Acute gastritis
Carcinoma of oesophagus and rectum
Pancreatic disease
Liver disease

Haemopoiesis
Macrocytosis (due to direct toxic effect on bone
   marrow, or folate deficiency)
Thrombocytopenia
Leucopenia

Bone
Osteoporosis
Osteomalacia

For liver disease
- 160 g ethanol per day (20 single drinks) carries a high risk
- 80 g ethanol per day (10 single drinks) carries a medium risk
- 40 g ethanol per day (5 single drinks) carries little risk

Heavy *persistent* drinkers for many years are at greater risk than heavy *sporadic* drinkers.

Susceptibility to damage of different organs is variable and the above figures are only a guide.

Alcohol consumption in pregnancy
Women are advised not to drink alcohol at all during pregnancy as even small amounts of alcohol consumed can lead to 'small babies'.

The fetal alcohol syndrome is characterized by mental retardation, dysmorphic features and growth impairment; it occurs in fetuses of alcohol-dependent women.

A summary of the physical effects of alcohol is given in Table 3.15. Details of these diseases are discussed in the relevant chapters. The effects of alcohol withdrawal are discussed on p. 992.

Further reading

Garrow JS (1988) *Obesity and Related Disorders*. Edinburgh: Churchill Livingstone.
Passmore R & Eastwood MA (1986) *Human Nutrition and Dietetics*, 8th edn. Edinburgh: Churchill Livingstone.
Silk DBA (1983) *Nutritional Support in Hospital Practice*. Oxford: Blackwell Scientific.
Truswell AS (1986) *ABC of Nutrition*. London: British Medical Association.

4

Gastroenterology

Introduction

Gastrointestinal disease is a major cause of ill-health world-wide. In developing countries infection and malnutrition are common. For example, over a billion people are infested with roundworms and hookworms, and amoebiasis affects over 10% of the world's population. Poor hygiene and malnutrition allows the spread of infective organisms and many infections could be prevented by improved sanitation and education.

The developed countries are also affected, as refined diets and food additives may well be causative in such diseases as diverticular disease and cancer. Despite the advances in both diagnosis (e.g. endoscopy and imaging techniques) and treatment (e.g. H_2-receptor antagonists), gastro-intestinal diseases still represent over 15% of the general practitioner's work-load. Much of this load is due to non-organic disorders, which are also becoming a world-wide problem.

Common symptoms (Table 4.1)

Dysphagia

Dysphagia is difficulty in swallowing (see p. 181).

Heartburn

Heartburn is a retrosternal or epigastric burning sensation that spreads upwards to the throat.

Dyspepsia and indigestion

These are terms often used by lay people to describe any symptom, e.g. nausea, heartburn, acidity, pain or distension, that occurs as a result of eating or drinking. They may also be used to describe an inability to digest food. Careful questioning is required to elicit the exact nature of the patient's complaint. 'Indigestion' is common; 80% of the general population will have had indigestion at some time.

Flatulence

Flatulence is the term used to describe excessive wind. It indicates belching, abdominal distension (see below) or the passage of flatus per rectum. Excessive belching is not usually associated with organic disease and is a common functional disorder. It is due to air swallowing (aerophagy), which many people do subconsciously. Some of the swallowed air is passed into the intestines, where most is absorbed. Intestinal bacterial breakdown of food, particularly high-fibre legumes, also produces a small amount of gas. Flatus consists of nitrogen, carbon dioxide, hydrogen and methane. On average, flatus is passed 10 to 20 times per day.

Hiccups

Hiccups are due to involuntary diaphragmatic contractions with closure of the glottis and are extremely common. Rarely, they become continuous, when treatment with chlorpromazine 50 mg three times a day or diazepam 5 mg three times daily may be effective.

Table 4.1 Common gastrointestinal symptoms.

Dysphagia
Heartburn
Dyspepsia/indigestion
Flatulence ('wind')
Vomiting
Diarrhoea/steatorrhoea
Constipation
Abdominal discomfort/pain
Abdominal distension
Anorexia and weight loss
Rectal bleeding

Vomiting

The vomiting centres are located in the lateral reticular formation of the medulla and are stimulated by the chemoreceptor trigger zones (CTZ) in the floor of the fourth ventricle, and also by vagal afferents from the gut. The CTZ are directly stimulated by drugs, motion sickness and metabolic causes. The causes of vomiting are shown in Table 4.2. There are three stages:

- Nausea—a feeling of wanting to vomit often associated with autonomic effects including hypersalivation, pallor and sweating
- Retching—a strong involuntary effort to vomit
- Vomiting—the expulsion of gastric contents through the mouth

Nausea occurs first and is usually associated with decreased gastric motility. This is followed by *retching*, where the glottis remains closed and there is contraction of the diaphragm and the abdominal muscles. Finally, there is a relaxation of the cardia and sustained contraction of the abdominal muscles, which leads to *vomiting*. Vomiting may occur without nausea, particularly in pyloric stenosis.

Most gastrointestinal conditions can cause vomiting, but chronic vomiting with no other abdominal symptoms is not usually due to gastrointestinal disease and is usually due to psychological causes. Early morning vomiting is seen in pregnancy, alcoholism and some metabolic disorders, e.g. uraemia.

Table 4.2 Causes of vomiting.

Any gastrointestinal disease
Acute infections, e.g.
  influenza
  pertussis
Central nervous disease, e.g.
  raised intracranial pressure
  meningitis
  vestibular disturbances
  migraine
Metabolic causes, e.g.
  uraemia
  diabetic ketoacidosis
  hypercalcaemia
Drugs, e.g.
  digitalis toxicity
  opiates
  cytotoxics
Reflex, e.g.
  severe pain—myocardial infarction
Psychogenic
Pregnancy
Alcoholic excess

Diarrhoea

Diarrhoea is extremely common; a single episode is usually due to dietary indiscretion. It is important to establish what the patient means by this symptom. True diarrhoea implies the passing of increased amounts (> 300 g per 24 h) of loose stool and is different from the frequent passage of small amounts of stool, which is commonly seen in functional bowel disease. The consistency of the stools is important; watery stools of large volume are always due to an organic cause. Bloody diarrhoea usually implies colonic disease.

Diarrhoea can be either acute or chronic. If it is acute, infective causes must be looked for.

Steatorrhoea

Steatorrhoea is the passage of pale, bulky stools that contain fat, sometimes float in the lavatory pan and are difficult to flush away. These stools float because of the increased air content. Normally people with steatorrhoea complain of diarrhoea, but occasionally they may pass only one motion per day.

Constipation

This is difficult to define in terms of frequency of bowel action because there is considerable individual and geographical variation. Patients usually consider themselves constipated if their bowels are not opened on most days. The difficult passage of hard stools is also regarded as constipation, irrespective of stool frequency.

Abdominal pain

Pain is stimulated mainly by the stretching of smooth muscle or organ capsules. Severe acute abdominal pain can be due to a large number of gastrointestinal conditions, and normally presents as an emergency. An 'acute abdomen' can occasionally be due to referred pain from the chest, as in pneumonia, or to metabolic causes, such as diabetic ketoacidosis.

In patients with abdominal pain the following should be ascertained:

- The site, intensity, character and periodicity of the pain
- The aggravating and relieving factors
- Associated symptoms, including non-gastrointestinal symptoms

Abdominal pain can very rarely arise from the abdominal wall itself, possibly due to nerve entrapment.

Upper abdominal pain
Epigastric pain. This can be due to many upper and

lower gastrointestinal disorders. It is often a dull ache, but can be severe and sharp. Its relationship to food intake should be ascertained. It is a common feature of peptic ulcer disease.

Gallbladder and biliary pain. This is usually due to gallstones. Gallstones in the gallbladder are asymptomatic unless the cystic duct is obstructed. This obstruction leads to gall-bladder distension and episodes of pain that can go on to acute cholecystitis (see p. 283). Pain can also occur with obstruction of the common bile duct. Clinically the pain is similar in both situations. It occurs in the epigastrium and right hypochondrium, starts suddenly, lasts half an hour to several hours and is not colicky. Biliary 'colic' is therefore a misnomer. The pain may radiate to the back or to the right shoulder. The patient vomits with the severe episodes of pain but when the pain subsides the patient is well until the next episode.

Right hypochondrial pain. Chronic, often persistent, pain in the right hypochondrium is a frequent symptom in healthy females suffering from functional bowel disease. This chronic pain is not due to gallbladder disease. Hepatic congestion, e.g. in hepatitis, and sometimes peptic ulcer can present with pain in the right hypochondrium.

Lower abdominal pain
Pain in the lower abdomen is usually colonic in origin. It is most commonly associated with functional bowel disease (see p. 225). Persistent pain in the right iliac fossa over a long period is not due to appendicitis.

Proctalgia
Proctalgia is a severe pain deep in the rectum that comes on suddenly but lasts only for a short time. It is not due to organic disease.

Abdominal distension

This is a common complaint and often erroneously attributed to wind. There are usually no physical signs and the symptom is due to functional bowel disease. 'Real' distension, see below.

Weight loss

This is due to anorexia (loss of appetite) and is a frequent accompaniment of all gastrointestinal disease. Anorexia is also common in systemic disease and may be seen in psychiatric disorders, particularly anorexia nervosa (see p. 995). Anorexia often accompanies carcinoma but it is a late symptom and not of diagnostic help. Weight loss with a normal or increased dietary intake occurs with hyperthyroidism. Malabsorption is never so severe as to cause weight loss without anorexia.

Weight loss should be assessed objectively as patients often 'think' they have lost weight.

Rectal bleeding (p. 196)

Bright red blood on the toilet paper on wiping the anus is a common symptom of piles (p. 221). There are many other causes, see p. 196.

Clinical examination

A general examination is performed, with particular emphasis on the examination of all lymph nodes and noting the presence of anaemia or jaundice. Detailed examination of the gastrointestinal tract starts with the mouth and tongue, and is followed by:

Examination of the abdomen (Acute abdomen, see p. 226; Liver disease, see p. 246).

Inspection
The organs found in a normal abdomen are shown in Figure 4.1. Figure 4.2 shows a normal CT scan at T12.

Evidence of any abdominal distension, which may be due to flatus, fat, fetus, fluid or faeces, must be looked for. Lordosis may give the appearance of a distended abdomen; it is a common feature of the 'abdominal distension' seen in functional bowel disease.

Palpation
The abdominal organs may be felt in some normal subjects (see Fig. 4.1) but this is not common and such organs are usually only just palpable.

Any palpable mass is carefully felt to decide which organs are involved and also to evaluate its size, shape and consistency and whether it moves with respiration.

The hernial orifices should always be examined.

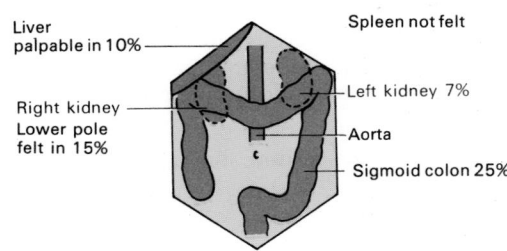

Liver palpable in 10%

Spleen not felt

Right kidney Lower pole felt in 15%

Left kidney 7%

Aorta

Sigmoid colon 25%

Fig. 4.1 Diagram showing the organs sometimes palpable in thin subjects (percentage given).

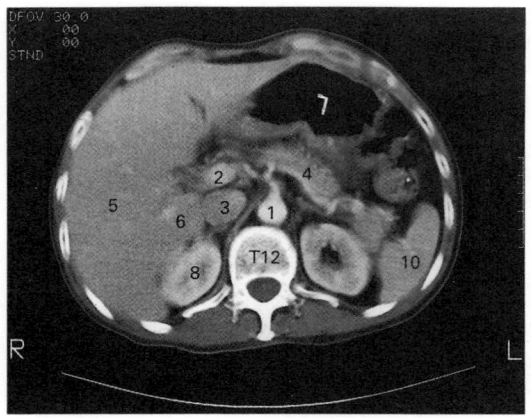

Fig. 4.2 CT scan of normal abdomen at the level of T12. 1 = aorta; 2 = portal vein; 3 = inferior vena cava; 4 = tail of pancreas; 5 = liver; 6 = caudate lobe of liver; 7 = stomach containing air; 8 = right kidney; 9 = left kidney; 10 = spleen.

A strangulated hernia can cause intestinal obstruction.

A succussion splash suggests pyloric stenosis if the patient has not drunk for 2–3 hours; the splash of fluid in the stomach can be heard with a stethoscope laid on the abdomen when the patient is moved.

Percussion
This is performed in the usual way to detect the area of dullness caused by the liver and spleen, and possibly bladder enlargement. The presence of fluid in the abdomen, i.e. ascites, is detected by shifting dullness. The percussion note changes from resonance to dullness when the patient is moved from one side to the other. It is a good physical sign if performed carefully but 1–2 litres of fluid must be present to elicit it. A fluid 'thrill' can be elicited but is not always helpful. A large ovarian cyst can sometimes produce an enlarged abdomen but the dullness is more centrally placed than in ascites.

Auscultation
Apart from in the evaluation of the acute abdomen, auscultation is not of great value in gastrointestinal disease. Abdominal bruits are often present in normal subjects but these are not clinically significant. Intestinal sounds do not help in diagnosis.

Examination of the rectum and sigmoid

Digital examination of the rectum should be performed in most patients with gastrointestinal symptoms and in all patients with a change in bowel habit. The anus should be inspected for anal tags, external haemorrhoids, fissures or fistulas. In males, the prostate projects into the rectum anteriorly and its size and consistency should be noted. In women the cervix or uterus may be felt anteriorly.

Sigmoidoscopy should be part of the routine examination in all cases of diarrhoea and in patients with lower abdominal symptoms such as a change in bowel habit or bleeding. *Proctoscopy* is performed in all patients with a history of bright red blood per rectum; the narrow sigmoidoscope does not distend the lumen and haemorrhoids can be missed.

Sigmoidoscopy

- The technique is easy to learn, provides valuable information and is safe in competent hands.
- The patient is placed in the left lateral position with the knees drawn up and buttocks over the edge of the couch.
- No bowel preparation is usually required.
- Rectal examination is performed initially.
- The sigmoidoscope is pointed towards the symphysis pubis and passed into the anus. The obturator is removed and the instrument passed under direct vision to the rectosigmoid junction and beyond if possible (using air insufflation).
- The mucosa of the anus and rectum is inspected. The normal mucosa is shiny, superficial vessels can be seen, and no contact bleeding should occur.
- Biopsies can be taken from any lesion seen or from apparently normal-looking mucosa which may show histological evidence of inflammation.
- The technique is relatively painless. In the irritable bowel syndrome, the patient's pain is often reproduced by air insufflation.

Proctoscopy

- The proctoscope is passed into the anus directed towards the symphysis pubis; the obturator is removed.
- The patient strains down as the proctoscope is withdrawn. Haemorrhoids are seen as purplish veins in the left lateral, right posterior or right anterior positions.
- Fissures may also be seen.

Flexible-fibre sigmoidoscopy
The rigid sigmoidoscope allows inspection of only the lower 20–25 cm of the bowel but a 70 cm flexible fibre-optic sigmoidoscope allows much more bowel to be visualized. It also can be readily used in the outpatient department after minimal bowel preparation (a disposable enema). Seventy per cent of colonic neoplasms occur within the range of flexible sigmoidoscopy.

Inspection of stools
This is not often performed nowadays. Nevertheless, it can be important to confirm the patient's

symptoms, e.g. of passing blood or steatorrhoea. The shape and size may be helpful, e.g. rabbity stools in the irritable bowel syndrome. Stool charts for recording frequency and volume of defaecation are useful in inpatients to follow the progress of their diarrhoea.

Investigation

Radiology and endoscopy are the principal investigations. These are usually preceded by routine haematology and biochemistry.

Plain X-rays

Plain X-rays of the abdomen are chiefly used in the investigation of the acute abdomen (see p. 226). Areas of calcification can be seen in chronic pancreatitis (see p. 290). Routine abdominal X-rays are of little use in the management of most gastrointestinal disease.

Barium contrast studies

Barium swallow
The oesophagus is visualized as barium is swallowed in the upright and prone positions. Motility abnormalities as well as anatomical lesions can then be observed. Reflux of barium from the stomach into the oesophagus is demonstrated with the patient tipped head down, but minimal reflux under these conditions may well have no clinical significance. Swallowing bread with barium (to add bulk) is sometimes useful in the investigation of undiagnosed dysphagia.

Barium meal
This is performed to examine the stomach and duodenum. A small amount of barium is given together with effervescent granules or tablets to produce carbon dioxide, so that a double contrast between air and barium is obtained. This technique has a high accuracy rate when performed carefully. Single-contrast studies are not recommended.

Small-bowel follow-through
This is used to examine the small bowel and, ideally, should be performed separately from barium meal as a different technique is employed. Barium is swallowed and allowed to pass into the small intestine through the jejunum and into the ileum. This technique is the only way of demonstrating the gross anatomy of the small intestine. It is particularly important to study the terminal ileum using fluoroscopy and to obtain films of the area.

Small-bowel enema (enteroclysis)
A tube is passed through the duodenum and a large volume of dilute barium introduced. This technique is useful for visualizing suspicious areas seen on the follow-through, particularly strictures.

Barium enema
Barium and air are insufflated into the rectum via a retained catheter. A double-contrast view is then obtained of the whole colon, often with views of the terminal ileum as well. The patient must be prepared well with laxatives and wash-outs so that the colon is empty. This technique does not examine the lowest part of the rectum, the rectal examination and sigmoidoscopy should precede this examination.

Barium contrast studies

- Upper GI series patients are fasted overnight.
- Barium enema patients are given a low-fibre diet for three days and laxatives 24 h before the procedure. Washouts are performed immediately before the examination to ensure the colon is empty.
- The radiologist should be given correct clinical information so that he can concentrate on the particular areas under suspicion.
- The radiologist screens the patient so that any suspicious area can be re-examined immediately.
- X-rays should be reviewed by the clinician and the radiologist.

Computed tomography (CT) and ultrasound

These techniques are mainly used in the investigation of the liver and biliary tract, pancreas and retroperitoneal areas (see p. 243). Both techniques are useful in detecting thickened bowel, abscesses and fistula in, for example, Crohn's disease and tuberculosis.

Endoscopy

Video endoscopes producing images of high quality are now available. This technical advance allows easy data collection. *Oesophagogastroduodenoscopy (OGD)* is often used as the investigation of choice for upper gastrointestinal disorders by gastroenterologists because of easy access and the possibility of interventional therapy and obtaining mucosal biopsies. Whether endoscopy or radiology are used depends on availability, local expertise and cost implications. Table 4.3 shows the preferred investigation for various indications.

Colonoscopy allows good visualization of the whole colon and terminal ileum. Biopsies can be obtained and polyps removed. In most institutions work-

Table 4.3 Choice of investigation—barium studies or endoscopy?
(a) UPPER GI

	Barium swallow/ meal	Endoscopy	Reasons
Clinical suspicion of:			
Hiatus hernia and reflux	+	±	
Gastric ulcer or carcinoma		+	Biopsy obtainable
Lesions in postoperative stomach		+	Difficult anatomy
Motility disorders	+		Motility difficult to assess at endoscopy
Extrinsic lesions	+		
For the investigation of:			
Vomiting	+		Gastric outflow obstruction
Dyspepsia	Either		Availability
Oesophagitis		+	Minimal abnormalities can be seen
Dysphagia	+		Probably most useful initially
Upper GI bleeding		+	Barium less able to detect superficial erosions Injection of varices

(b) LOWER GI

	Barium enema (double contrast)	Colonoscopy	Reasons
Sick immobile patient > 70 years		+	Mobility
Rectal bleeding: High-risk (for neoplasia)		+	Biopsies can be taken Small lesions detected Polyps can be removed
Low-risk (for neoplasia)	+		Clinical work-load
Non-specific lower abdominal pain	+		Clinical work-load
Alteration of bowel habit	+		Clinical work-load
Inflammatory bowel disease		+	Multiple biopsies
Polyps and follow-up		+	Removal

loads determine that the barium enema is the primary investigation.

The success rate for reaching the terminal ileum is approximately 80% and the mortality is 1 : 100 000. The major complication is perforation. Table 4.3 gives some indication of the usage of barium studies or endoscopy. The two are frequently complementary and the technique chosen often depends on local expertise.

Endoscopic retrograde cholangiopancreatography (ERCP)

This technique has proved very useful in the investigation of pancreatic and biliary tract disease; it is discussed on p. 244.

Radionuclide imaging

Radionuclides are used for imaging of the liver and

Upper GI endoscopy

- The patient is fasted overnight and the procedure is carried out as an outpatient.
- The mouth is sprayed with lignocaine.
- I.V. sedation for the very anxious patient or for additional procedures.
- O_2 via nasal prongs for elderly patients.
- The instrument is passed into the pharynx with the patient swallowing. It is then passed under direct vision through the oesophagus into the stomach and duodenum.
- The forward-viewing instrument is used for visualization of the oesophagus, stomach and duodenal cap.
- The side-viewing instrument is needed to visualize certain areas, e.g. the ampulla of Vater.

Colonoscopy

- Two days before procedure—low-residue diet started
- One day before procedure—clear fluids only
- Afternoon prior to procedure—71 ml extract of senna with one pint of water given
- Three hours later—one sachet of sodium picosulphate with one pint of water given
- Day of procedure—one sachet of sodium picosulphate with one pint of water given

Alternative preparation consists of giving large volumes of balanced electrolyte solution by mouth on the day of the test.

The instrument is passed under direct supervision and manoeuvred around to the caecum and terminal ileum. Sedation, along with pethidine and hyoscine butyl bromide is required.

biliary tract (see p. 244). Other uses include demonstration of oesophageal reflux and gastric emptying (using technetium-99m sulphur colloid), Meckel's diverticulum (using [^{99m}Tc]pertechnetate, which has an affinity for gastric mucosa) and inflammatory lesions in inflammatory bowel disease (using radiolabelled white cells). All of these techniques require constant evaluation if they are to produce reliable and reproducible results.

The mouth

Mastication of the food takes place in the mouth. The food then passes into the pharynx. Problems in the mouth are extremely common and although they may be trivial they can produce severe symptoms. Poor dental hygiene is often a factor.

Stomatitis

Viral
Herpes simplex virus type I causes an acute stomatitis and recurrent herpes labialis (cold sore) (see p. 1024).

Hand, foot and mouth disease due to Coxsackie A virus produces mouth vesicles, usually in children. No treatment is required.

Herpes zoster involving the fifth cranial nerve can produce unilateral vesicular lesions (see p. 892).

Glandular fever due to the Epstein–Barr virus is associated with palatal petechiae with acute tonsillitis and pharyngitis (see p. 58).

Bacterial
Bacterial stomatitis is not common in Western countries, except as an accompaniment to a sore throat due to *Streptococcus*.

Vincent's stomatitis occurs in the malnourished patient with poor dentition. The sloughing ulceration involves primarily the gums but the whole oral cavity may be affected. The specific causative organisms are not known but it is likely that a number of organisms are responsible. Anaerobic commensals found in normal subjects are present in large numbers in this infectious condition. Treatment is with metronidazole (200 mg three times a day for 4 days) with accompanying good mouth and dental hygiene.

Tuberculosis involving the mouth is very rare and presents as a painful shallow ulcer.

Syphilitic infection due to *Treponema pallidum* is also rare. Primary syphilis produces a chancre; secondary syphilis produces a snail-track ulcer.

Fungal
Fungal infection of the mouth is usually due to *Candida albicans* and in adults it is seen only in the severely ill or immunocompromised patient or after broad-spectrum antibiotics. Infection may be an early manifestation in AIDS. White colonies, often coalescing to form a membrane are seen. The lower pharynx and oesophagus can be involved, producing dysphagia. Treatment (see p. 76).

Angular stomatitis and the stomatitis associated with dentures can sometimes be due to *Candida*.

Non-infective
Recurrent aphthous ulceration is very common. Minor ulcers are superficial and are surrounded by erythema. They are very painful and last 4–14 days. They are usually small, multiple and recur frequently. They start in adolescence and often seem to resolve spontaneously as the patient gets older. The aetiology is unknown. They are sometimes associated with GI disease, notably Crohn's disease, ulcerative colitis and coeliac disease. *Granulomatous ulcers* can also occur in Crohn's disease. *Behçet's disease* presents with deep oral and genital ulceration. Hydrocortisone pellets may help all these conditions and symptomatic treatment with local anaesthetics relieves the pain. However, the efficacy of treatment for this condition has not been proved.

Stomatitis can occur with ill-fitting dentures or with a number of *vitamin deficiencies*, including deficiencies of niacin, riboflavin, folate and B_{12}. Angular stomatitis and glossitis frequently occur together.

Stomatitis is frequently seen in *blood dyscrasias*, particularly acute leukaemia. A blue line on the gums is seen with *lead poisoning*.

Diseases of the tongue

A pale smooth tongue can be seen in iron deficiency. A sore tongue may result from glossitis associated with stomatitis, the various causes of which are described above.

The term 'geographical tongue' describes a migrating glossitis exclusively affecting the dorsum of the tongue. This condition has no clinical significance and the patient should be reassured.

Many patients who complain of a sore tongue do not have an obvious abnormality. Very occasionally this can be due to B_{12} or folate deficiency but mostly there is no organic cause and the symptoms are psychological in origin. A bad taste in the mouth and offensive breath (halitosis), particularly if only noticed by the patient, are also usually psychogenic symptoms. Rarely, patients with pyloric stenosis have halitosis.

Leucoplakia
Leucoplakia consists of white patches that cannot be removed. Any part of the mouth can be involved, particularly the tongue. Often no cause can be found but leucoplakia can be due to viral infections or smoking. Five per cent of cases become malignant. Hairy leucoplakia on the side of the tongue is diagnostic of AIDS and has an ominous prognosis.

Squamous carcinoma
This may be related to smoking and excess alcohol consumption. It may present as a swelling or ulcer on any part of the mouth and tongue. Biopsy of any long-standing ulcer should always be performed. Treatment is with surgery and radiotherapy.

Kaposi's sarcoma (see p. 1044).
This is found on the palate of patients with AIDS and 50% of these patients have visceral involvement.

Lichen planus (see p. 1010).
This can occur in all parts of the mouth and tongue and produces white striae with small papules.

Bullous pemphigus (see p. 1018).
This involves the mouth in all cases at some time. Painful blisters or bullae form and then burst, producing shallow ulcers.

The salivary glands

Xerostomia

Xerostomia means dryness of the mouth. Causes include:

- Psychogenic—anxiety
- Pyrexia
- Drugs—anticholinergics, antihistamines, tricyclic antidepressants and diuretics
- Sjögren's syndrome (see p. 397)
- Diabetic ketoacidosis and dehydration

The sensation of excess salivation (ptyalism) is chiefly psychogenic. It occurs before vomiting and with lesions of the mouth.

Bacterial and viral infections

These can affect any of the salivary glands, the commonest condition being acute parotitis due to the mumps virus. Acute parotitis due to an ascending infection with staphylococci or streptococci occurs often in elderly patients with dehydration and poor oral hygiene. Parotitis is also seen in alcoholics.

Sarcoidosis

This can produce parotid gland enlargement. When combined with lacrimal gland enlargement it is known as Mikulicz's syndrome.

Salivary duct obstruction due to calculus

Obstruction due to calculus usually involves the submandibular gland. There is painful swelling of the gland after eating. The stones can sometimes be felt in the floor of the mouth and their removal is usually followed by complete relief of symptoms.

Tumours

Salivary gland tumours are usually of a mixed type. They may involve any of the salivary glands but usually affect the parotid. The gland becomes swollen but not tender and treatment is by removal, although local recurrences occur.

The pharynx and oesophagus

Structure

The oesophagus is a muscular tube, approximately 25 cm long, connecting the pharynx to the stomach. The muscle coat has two layers—an outer longitudinal layer and an inner circular layer of fibres. In the upper portion both muscle layers are striated. They gradually change to smooth muscle in the lower oesophagus, where they are continuous with the muscle layer of the stomach. The oesophagus is lined by stratified squamous epithelium, except near the gastro-oesophageal junction where columnar epithelium is found.

Function

The oesophagus is separated from the pharynx by the *upper oesophageal sphincter*, which is normally closed by the continuous contraction of cricopharyngeus muscle. The *lower oesophageal sphincter* (*LOS*) consists of an area of the distal end of the oesophagus that has a high resting tone and is largely responsible for the prevention of reflux. The reduction in tone and relaxation that occurs with swallowing is under the control of nervous (vagal) and hormonal mechanisms.

During swallowing, the bolus of food is moved from the mouth to the pharynx voluntarily. Immediately, the upper sphincter relaxes and food enters the oesophagus. A primary peristaltic wave starts in the pharynx at the onset of swallowing and sweeps down the whole oesophagus. Secondary peristalsis occurs locally in response to direct stimulation (e.g. distension by the bolus) and helps to clear food residue from the oesophagus. Non-peristaltic, non-propulsive tertiary waves are frequent in the elderly. The LOS relaxes when swallowing is initiated, before the arrival of the peristaltic wave.

Symptoms of oesophageal disorders

Major oesophageal symptoms are:

- Dysphagia
- Heartburn
- Painful swallowing

Dysphagia
This is either due to a local lesion or is part of a generalized disease. Patients will complain of something sticking in their throat or chest during swallowing or immediately afterwards. It is always a serious symptom and the cause must be found. The causes are shown in Table 4.4. Globus hystericus is the name given to apparent dysphagia —the sensation of a 'lump in the throat' in patients who do not have true dysphagia and can therefore swallow. It has no organic cause and the treatment is reassurance.

Heartburn
Heartburn is a common symptom of acid reflux. The pain can spread to the neck, across the chest, and can be difficult to distinguish from the pain of

Table 4.4 Causes of dysphagia.

Disease of mouth and tongue, e.g. tonsillitis

Neuromuscular disorders
  Pharyngeal disorders
    Bulbar palsy
    Myasthenia gravis
  Oesophageal motility disorders
    Achalasia
    Scleroderma
    Diffuse oesophageal spasm
    Presbyoesophagus
    Diabetes
    Chagas' disease

Extrinsic pressure
  Mediastinal glands
  Goitre
  Enlarged left atrium

Intrinsic lesion
  Foreign body
  Stricture
    Benign—peptic, corrosive
    Malignant—carcinoma
  Lower oesophageal rings
    Oesophageal web
    Pharyngeal pouch

ischaemic heart disease. It occurs at night when the patient lies flat or after bending or stooping. Hot drinks and alcohol often precipitate the pain.

Painful swallowing
Painful swallowing without real difficulty is a symptom of candidiasis and herpes simplex infection. Both these conditions are seen in AIDS patients. Ingestion of tablets such as emepronium and potassium (slow release) will produce local ulceration if they lodge in the gullet when swallowed lying down and without water.

Signs of oesophageal disorders

There are very few signs associated with oesophageal disease, the main one being of weight loss as a consequence of dysphagia.

Investigation of oesophageal disorders

Investigation of oesophageal disorders mainly involves barium contrast studies and oesophagoscopy. Other tests include:

- *Manometry* is performed by passing a fluid-filled catheter through the nose into the oesophagus. Changes in pressure are transmitted up the fluid column and recorded. These studies are useful in motility disorders.
- *Bernstein test*—alternate dilute acid and alkali is

infused into the oesophagus via a nasal tube to try to reproduce or relieve oesophageal pain. A positive test suggests oesophagitis but there are many false negatives.

- *pH monitoring*—24-hour monitoring using a pH sensitive probe positioned in the lower oesophagus is being used increasingly for the identification of reflux episodes (pH < 4). Brief episodes can, however, occur in normal subjects.
- *Radioisotope studies* with technetium sulphur colloid incorporated into food can also be used to study reflux. It is not widely used in the UK.

MOTILITY DISORDERS

Achalasia

DEFINITION

Achalasia is a disease of unknown aetiology that is characterized by aperistalsis in the body of the oesophagus and failure of relaxation of the lower oesophageal sphincter on initiation of swallowing.

PATHOLOGY

Degenerative lesions are found in the vagus as well as a decrease in ganglionic cells in the nerve plexus of the oesophageal wall.

CLINICAL FEATURES

The disease can present at any age but is rare in childhood. The incidence is about 1 per 100 000 per year. Patients usually have a long history of intermittent dysphagia for both liquids and solids. Regurgitation of food from the dilated oesophagus may be induced by the patient or may occur spontaneously, particularly at night, and aspiration pneumonia may result. Occasionally food gets stuck but patients often learn to overcome this by drinking large quantities, thereby increasing the head of pressure in the oesophagus and forcing the food through. Severe retrosternal chest pain occurs particularly in younger patients with vigorous non-peristaltic contraction of the oesophagus. The dysphagia in these patients can be mild and the pain misdiagnosed as cardiac in origin. Weight loss is usually not marked.

INVESTIGATION

A *chest X-ray* may show a dilated oesophagus with occasionally a fluid level behind the heart. The fundal gas shadow is not present.

A *barium swallow* will show dilatation of the oesophagus, lack of peristalsis (see Fig. 4.3) and often synchronous contractions. The lower end gradually narrows (beak deformity); this appear-

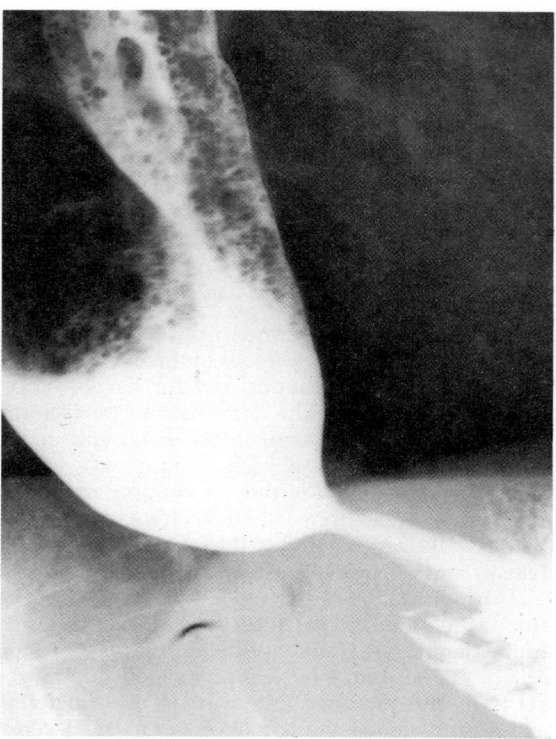

Fig. 4.3 Barium swallow showing achalasia with atonic body of the oesophagus and a narrowed distal end. Note food residue in dilated oesophagus.

ance is due to failure of the sphincter to relax.

Oesophagoscopy is necessary to exclude a carcinoma at the lower end of the oesophagus, which can produce a similar X-ray appearance. When there is marked dilatation, extensive cleansing is necessary to remove food debris in order to obtain a clear view. In achalasia the oesophagoscope easily flops through the apparent narrowing without resistance.

Manometry is used to measure oesophageal motility. It shows aperistalsis of the oesophagus as well as the failure of relaxation of the lower oesophageal sphincter (Fig. 4.4).

Chagas' disease (American trypanosomiasis, see p. 82) damages the neural plexus of the gut and produces a similar clinical picture.

TREATMENT

The lower oesophageal sphincter is dilated forcibly using a pneumatic bag (passed under X-ray control) so as to weaken the sphincter. This is successful in 80% of cases. Forced dilatation is quicker to perform than surgical division of the muscle at the lower end of the oesophagus (cardiomyotomy or Heller's operation), which is now mainly used in patients whose symptoms have not improved after many dilatations. Reflux

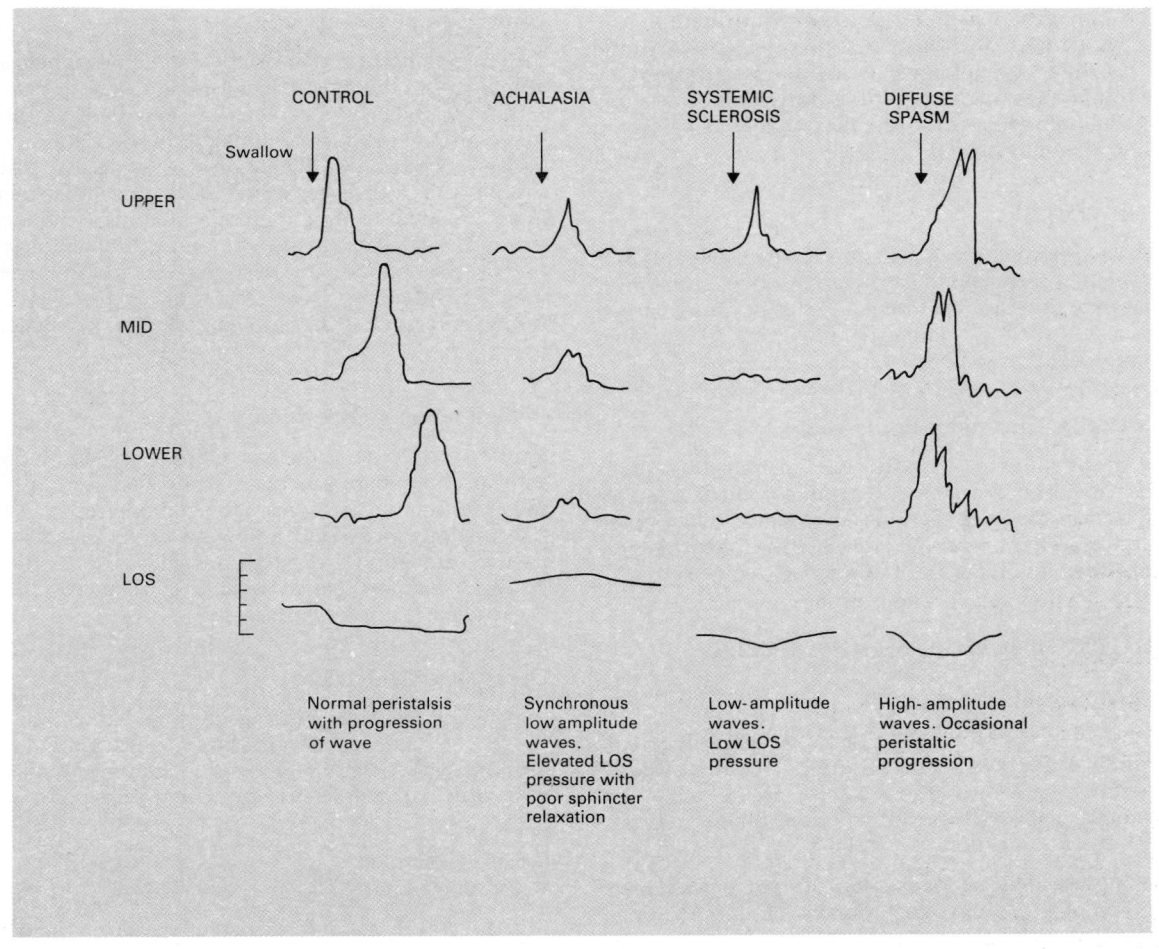

CONTROL   ACHALASIA   SYSTEMIC SCLEROSIS   DIFFUSE SPASM

Swallow

UPPER

MID

LOWER

LOS

Normal peristalsis with progression of wave

Synchronous low amplitude waves. Elevated LOS pressure with poor sphincter relaxation

Low-amplitude waves. Low LOS pressure

High-amplitude waves. Occasional peristaltic progression

Fig. 4.4 Oesophageal manometric patterns. LOS, lower oesophageal sphincter.

oesophagitis complicates both procedures and the aperistalsis of the oesophagus remains.

COMPLICATIONS

There is an increased incidence of 5–10% of carcinoma of the oesophagus in both treated and untreated cases. Recurrent pneumonia may occur due to aspiration of oesophageal contents.

Systemic sclerosis

In 90% or more of patients with this disease there is oesophageal involvement, with diminished peristalsis detected manometrically (Fig. 4.4) or by barium swallow. This is due to replacement of the smooth muscle layers by fibrous tissue. The lower oesophageal sphincter pressure is also decreased, allowing reflux; mucosal damage may occur as a consequence. Strictures may develop. Initially there are no symptoms, but dysphagia and heart-burn occur as the oesophagus becomes severely involved.

Similar motility abnormalities may be found in other connective-tissue disorders, particularly if Raynaud's phenomenon is present. Treatment is as for reflux (see p. 185) and stricture formation (see below).

Diffuse oesophageal spasm

This is a severe form of abnormal oesophageal motility that can sometimes produce retrosternal chest pain and dysphagia. Swallowing is accompanied by bizarre and marked contractions of the oesophagus without progression of the waves (Fig. 4.4). On barium swallow the appearance may be of a 'corkscrew'. However, asymptomatic abnormalities of oesophageal motility are not infrequent, particularly in patients over the age of 60 years (presbyoesophagus). Care must therefore be taken that the symptoms and the X-ray findings of oesophageal spasm are not falsely attributed.

A variant of diffuse oesophageal spasm is the *'nutcracker'* oesophagus, which is characterized by finding very high-amplitude peristalsis (pressures > 200 mm Hg) within the oesophagus. Chest pain and dysphagia occur.

TREATMENT

True oesophageal spasm producing severe symptoms is rare and treatment is often unhelpful. Antispasmodics, nitrates, or calcium-channel blockers such as sublingual nifedipine 10 mg three times daily may be tried.

Miscellaneous motility disorders

Abnormalities of motility that are mostly asymptomatic but occasionally produce dysphagia are found in diabetes mellitus, myotonica dystrophica and myasthenia gravis, as well as any neurological disorder involving the brain stem.

OTHER OESOPHAGEAL DISORDERS

Oesophageal diverticulum

This is a pouch lined with epithelium that can produce dysphagia and regurgitation. It is usually asymptomatic and often detected accidentally on a barium swallow performed for other reasons. Diverticula can occur:

- Immediately above the upper oesophageal sphincter (pharyngeal pouch). If large it may cause dysphagia as well as spillage of contents into the trachea.
- Near the middle of the oesophagus (traction diverticulum produced by extrinsic inflammation).
- Just above the lower oesophageal sphincter (epiphrenic diverticulum)

Only when symptoms are severe should surgery be undertaken.

Rings and webs

A number of rings and webs have been described throughout the oesophagus.

Lower oesophageal or Schatzki ring

This is a narrowing of the lower end of the oesophagus due to a ridge of mucosa or a fibrous membrane. The ring may be asymptomatic, but it can very occasionally produce dysphagia after swallowing a large bolus of bread or meat. The narrowing or ring is seen on a barium swallow, with the oesophagus well distended with barium.

The treatment is reassurance and dietary advice.

Upper oesophageal web

This is a constriction near the upper oesophageal sphincter in the post-cricoid region and appears radiologically as a web. The web may be asymptomatic or may produce dysphagia. In the Plummer–Vinson syndrome (Paterson–Brown–Kelly syndrome) this web is associated with iron-deficiency anaemia, glossitis and angular stomatitis. This rare syndrome affects mainly women and its aetiology is not understood. At oesophagoscopy the web may be difficult to see. Dilatation of the web is rarely necessary. Iron is given for the iron deficiency.

Benign oesophageal stricture

Peptic stricture secondary to reflux is the commonest cause of benign strictures. They also occur after the ingestion of corrosives, after radiotherapy, after sclerosis of varices and following prolonged nasogastric intubation. All strictures give rise to dysphagia. They are usually treated by dilatation, but occasionally surgery is necessary.

Oesophageal infections

Infection is becoming increasingly recognized as a cause of painful swallowing, particularly in immunosuppressed debilitated patients and patients with AIDS. Infection can occur with:

- *Candida*
- Herpes simplex
- Cytomegalovirus

It is difficult to distinguish between these either on barium swallow or oesophagoscopy, as only widespread ulceration is seen. In candidiasis the characteristic white plaques on top of friable mucosa may be found, but oral candidiasis is not always present. The diagnosis of *Candida* can be confirmed by examining a direct smear taken at endoscopy, but often infections are mixed and cultures and biopsies must be performed.

TREATMENT

Most patients on large doses of immunosuppressive agents are treated prophylactically with nystatin or amphotericin. Antifungal or antiviral treatment is given appropriately (Chapter 1).

Mallory–Weiss syndrome

This is described on p. 196.

Oesophageal rupture

This can occur, with violent vomiting producing severe chest pain and collapse. It may follow alcohol ingestion.

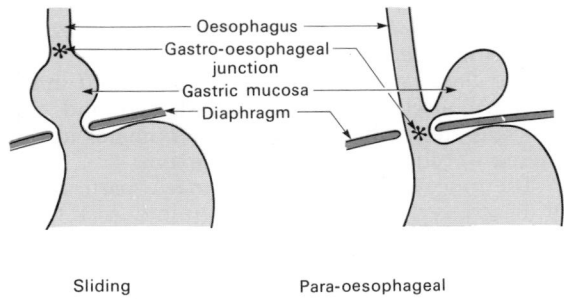

Sliding   Para-oesophageal

Fig. 4.5 Diagrammatic representation of the two types of hiatus hernia.

Carcinoma of the oesophagus

This is discussed on p. 229.

HIATUS HERNIA AND REFLUX OESOPHAGITIS

These will be considered together, as a sliding hiatus hernia on its own does not produce symptoms. The symptoms occur because of the presence of the associated reflux. With a sliding hiatus hernia, the gastro-oesophageal junction 'slides' through the hiatus so that it lies above the diaphragm. With a para-oesophageal or rolling hernia, a small part of the stomach rolls up through the hernia alongside the oesophagus (Fig. 4.5); the sphincter still remains below the diaphragm and remains competent. Occasionally a rolling para-oesophageal hernia will produce pain and need surgical treatment.

Reflux occurs because of failure of the antireflux mechanism, and commonly, but not necessarily, it accompanies a hiatus hernia. The antireflux mechanism includes the local anatomical arrangement of the gastro-oesophageal junction below the diaphragm and, more importantly, the tone of the lower oesophageal sphincter. In the majority of patients with reflux, sphincter pressure will be low. Reflux, however, commonly occurs sporadically in normal subjects several times a day. Presumably the transient nature of this reflux with rapid clearance by secondary peristalsis prevents inflammation in normal subjects. However, if reflux is persistent and prolonged and clearance is poor, inflammation may result. Causes of increased reflux are shown in Table 4.5.

CLINICAL FEATURES

Heartburn is the major feature of reflux oesophagitis. The burning is aggravated by bending, stooping or lying down and may be relieved by antacids. The patient may complain of pain on

Table 4.5 Causes of increased oesophageal reflux.

Pregnancy or obesity
Fat, chocolate or coffee ingestion
Smoking
Anticholinergic drugs
Systemic sclerosis
After treatment for achalasia

drinking hot liquids or alcohol. The correlation between heartburn and oesophagitis is poor. Some patients have little oesophagitis but severe heartburn; others have severe oesophagitis without symptoms and present with an iron-deficiency anaemia due to blood loss. Regurgitation of food into the mouth also occurs, particularly when lying flat. Aspiration into the lungs, producing pneumonia, is unusual without an accompanying stricture, but cough and nocturnal asthma from regurgitation and aspiration can occur.

INVESTIGATION

Barium swallow is still the most widely used investigation. Hiatus hernia occurs in approximately 30% of people of 50 years of age and by itself is of no diagnostic significance. Evidence of free reflux of barium must be demonstrated. Reflux can also be demonstrated with radiolabelled technetium or by using a pH probe when the number of reflux episodes occurring over 24 h is noted. Such reflux episodes can occur with an entirely normal barium swallow. No single test is perfect and often a combination of tests is required.

Oesophagoscopy may show the presence of a red friable mucosa with linear ulceration. A Bernstein test may be helpful in investigating retrosternal chest pain to differentiate oesophageal pain from angina (see p. 181).

TREATMENT

Many patients can be treated successfully with antacids, a reduction in obesity, and raising the head end of the bed at night. Unfortunately, compliance with the latter two treatments is poor. H_2-receptor antagonists are frequently used (see p. 190), to be taken at 6 p.m., doubling the normal dosages if necessary. Proprietary antacids containing alginates (10 ml three times daily) may help. Unfortunately, even with these agents it is difficult to keep a neutral pH in the oesophagus. Metoclopramide, a dopamine antagonist, is helpful as it enhances peristalsis and speeds gastric emptying. Cisapride, a prokinetic agent devoid of dopaminergic activity increases oesophageal peristalsis and is sometimes of value. Omeprazole, which inhibits the $H^+–K^+$ proton pump, produces almost complete reduction of gastric acidity and is extremely effective in patients with severe symptoms.

Surgery is rarely needed and should never be performed for a hiatus hernia alone. The properly selected case with severe reflux and oesophagitis responds well to surgery. Repair of the hernia and some sort of additional antireflux surgery, e.g. Nissen fundoplication, is required.

COMPLICATIONS

The major complication of reflux is peptic stricture, which usually occurs in patients over the age of 60. The symptoms are those of intermittent dysphagia over a long period. Treatment is by dilatation of the stricture and management of the reflux either medically or surgically. There is no increased incidence of carcinoma in hiatus hernia *per se*. However, long-standing acid reflux causes columnization of the oesophageal mucosa (Barrett's oesophagus) which is premalignant. Anaemia and occasionally frank haemorrhage may occur with oesophagitis. Recurrent aspiration pneumonia can occur when stricture formation is present.

The stomach and duodenum

Structure

The *stomach*, which varies considerably in size, is divided into the upper portion—the fundus—the mid-region or body, and the antrum, which extends into the pyloric region.

There are two sphincters—the gastro-oesophageal sphincter and the pyloric sphincter; the latter is largely made up of a thickening of the circular muscle layer. The muscle wall of the stomach has three layers—an outer longitudinal,

an inner circular, and an innermost oblique layer of smooth muscle.

The *duodenum* has outer longitudinal and inner smooth muscle layers. It is C-shaped and the pancreas sits in the concavity. It terminates in the jejunum at the duodenojejunal flexure.

The mucosal lining of the stomach, particularly in the greater curvature, is thrown into thick folds or rugae. The upper two-thirds of the stomach contains parietal cells, which secrete hydrochloric acid, and chief cells, which secrete pepsinogen. The junction between the body and the antrum of the stomach can often be seen macroscopically, but can be confirmed by measuring surface pH. The antrum contains only mucus-secreting and G cells, which secrete gastrin. There are two major forms of gastrin—G17 and G34, depending on the number of amino-acid residues. G17 is the major form found in the antrum.

The duodenal mucosa contains Brunner's glands, which secrete alkaline mucus. This, along with the pancreatic and biliary secretions, helps to neutralize the acid secretion from the stomach when it reaches the duodenum.

Function

Acid secretion
The factors controlling acid secretion are shown in Fig. 4.6. Secretion is under neural and hormonal control. Both stimulate acid secretion through the release of histamine, which acts directly on the parietal cells.

Other major gastric functions

- Reservoir for food
- Absorption (of only minimal importance)
- Emulsification of fat and mixing of gastric contents
- Secretion of intrinsic factor

Gastric emptying depends on many factors. There are osmoreceptors in the duodenal mucosa that

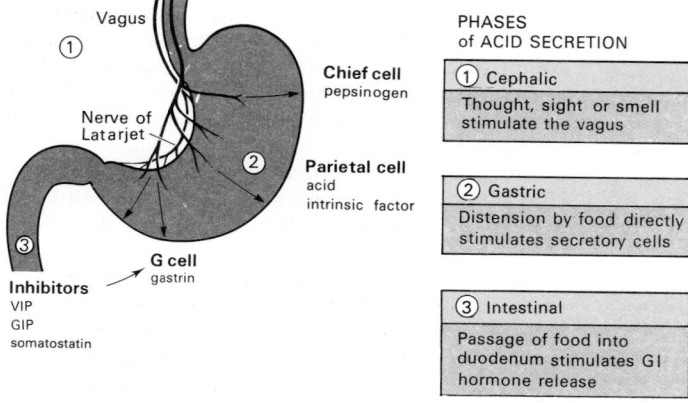

Fig. 4.6 Control of acid secretion.

control gastric emptying by local reflexes and the release of gut hormones. In particular, intraduodenal fat delays gastric emptying by negative feedback through duodenal receptors.

GASTRITIS

This can be divided into acute and chronic. Unfortunately, there is no universally accepted classification of this condition because there is a poor correlation between clinical, pathological and endoscopic findings. Some degree of gastritis can always be found if the stomach is examined by careful histological means but these small areas of gastritis seem to have no signficance.

Acute gastritis, acute ulceration and erosions

In *acute gastritis* there is inflammation of the superficial gastric mucosa.

In *mucosal erosion* there is destruction of small zones of superficial mucosa but healing is complete and there is no subsequent fibrosis. Multiple small erosions, often with an oedematous mucosa, are known as acute erosive gastritis or, if accompanied by extensive intramucosal haemorrhage, as acute haemorrhagic gastritis.

In *acute gastric ulceration* there is destruction of the full thickness of the mucosa; healing occurs with mucosal regeneration and little or no scar formation.

The aetiology of the above is often obscure but gastritis can be produced by drugs such as aspirin and other NSAIDS and alcohol. Aspirin is thought to damage the mucosal barrier by allowing acid to diffuse into the gastric mucosa, where it causes the release of histamine, producing acute inflammation.

Acute ulcers are also seen after severe stress (stress ulcer) and secondary to burns (Curling ulcer), trauma, shock, renal or liver disease. The underlying mechanism for these ulcers is unknown but may be related to an alteration in blood flow.

CLINICAL FEATURES

The correlation between the pathological changes and symptoms is poor, but many patients with acute gastritis will suffer from epigastric pain, indigestion and vomiting, usually for less than 24 h. GI haemorrhage can occur (see p. 191).

DIAGNOSIS

In many patients the diagnosis is obvious (e.g. indigestion after a party) but endoscopy may be performed to confirm the presence of acute ulcers or erosions, particularly in patients admitted with GI haemorrhage.

TREATMENT

No specific therapy is required apart from removal of the offending cause. There is no evidence that acute gastritis will eventually lead to chronic gastritis or peptic ulceration.

Chronic gastritis

Pathogenetically this can be divided into three main categories:

- *Type A (autoimmune) gastritis* is seen in pernicious anaemia (see p. 304) and also in other autoimmune diseases, e.g. thyroid disease, diabetes mellitus. This mainly affects the body of the stomach and is associated with circulating autoantibodies to gastric parietal cells and intrinsic factor. Histologically, there are three stages of mucosal damage:

  Chronic superficial gastritis consists of an infiltration of lymphocytes and plasma cells into the superficial mucosa. The deeper mucosa is unaffected.
  Atrophic gastritis indicates deeper inflammation and loss of parietal and chief cells in the deeper specialized parts of the gland. Intestinal metaplasia is sometimes present.
  Gastric atrophy indicates a thin mucosa with almost complete loss of specialized gastric glands. Intestinal metaplasia is often present and may be premalignant; there is very little mucosal inflammation.

- *Type B (bacterial) gastritis* principally affects the antrum and is associated with the presence of *Helicobacter pylori* (see below) on the surface epithelium. Histologically, all three stages of chronic gastritis described above are seen.

- *Type C (chemical) gastritis* is a recently recognized, histologically distinct lesion, due to repeated injury, e.g. bile reflux or chronic ingestion of NSAIDS (e.g. aspirin). The mucus shows hyperplasia of the necks of the glands, oedema and mild inflammation.

Most chronic gastritis is asymptomatic and requires no treatment. It is found incidentally at endoscopy or barium meal examination of the stomach (absence of mucosal folds). Accompanying pernicious anaemia is investigated and treated (see p. 304). Chronic gastritis associated with *H. pylori* —see p. 188.

MÉNÉTRIER'S DISEASE

Ménétrier's disease is a rare condition in which there is thickening and enlargement of the gastric mucosal folds. Histologically there is hyperplasia of the mucin-producing cells with glandular proliferation and loss of the parietal and chief cells.

The patient may complain of epigastric pain and occasionally peripheral oedema may occur due to hypoalbuminaemia resulting from protein loss through the gastric mucosa. Symptomatic treatment is all that is required for this condition. It is possibly premalignant.

DUODENITIS

Duodenitis is a condition frequently seen at endoscopy. The duodenal mucosa appears inflamed, haemorrhagic and friable. Occasionally small breaks in the mucosa are seen, i.e. erosions. Microscopically there is chronic inflammation.

The condition can occur in asymptomatic individuals and its relationship to symptoms is unknown. Severe inflammation is thought to be one end of the spectrum of chronic duodenal ulcer disease. Treatment is not necessary for the inflammation *per se*.

HELICOBACTER PYLORI (HP) AND THE UPPER GI TRACT

This spiral-shaped urease-producing bacterium (Fig. 4.7), previously known as *Campylobacter pylori*, is found in the upper gastrointestinal tract, but its actual role in the pathogenesis of disease is still being evaluated. Its source is unknown. HP has been found mainly in the antrum of the stomach and in areas of gastric metaplasia in the duodenum. HP is present under the mucous layer attached to cells by pedestals. It is not intracellular and does not colonize the epithelial cells. Intrafamilial clustering suggests person-to-person spread. At present there is no firm correlation between the finding of HP, the presence of symptoms and the pathological lesion. It has been found in:

- *Asymptomatic controls.* 25% of young adults and 60% of patients over 60 years have HP in the stomach with associated gastritis.
- *Chronic gastritis* (bacterial Type B). This has the strongest pathogenetic association with HP (95%). Treatment to eradicate the organism heals the gastritis but the correlation of the gastritis with the symptoms is unclear.
- *Acute gastritis.* Experimentally, 7 days after the ingestion of HP dyspepsia occurred and antral gastritis was found at endoscopy. Treatment with tinidazole cleared symptoms and the lesion.
- *Peptic ulceration.* HP is isolated from the antrum in 70% of patients with gastric ulcer and almost 100% of duodenal ulcer (DU) patients. DU patients have gastric metaplasia in the duodenum and HP is at this site in 50%. The significance of these findings is unclear but may influence the treatment of DU disease.
- *Non-ulcer dyspepsia.* Gastritis associated with HP has been found in this condition but its significance is unclear.
- *Other.* A weak association has been found between HP, gastric carcinoma and hypochlorhydria.

DIAGNOSIS

- Non-invasive
  Serum antibodies—a sensitive specific serological test is now available and will become widely used. Urea breath test with ^{13}C or ^{14}C (see p. 203 but using urea as the substrate). This is a quick and easy way of detecting the presence of HP and is used as a screening test.
- Endoscopic
  HP can be detected histologically. In addition, biopsies are added immediately to a solution of urea and if HP is present the latter is broken down by the urease to produce a colour change in the indicator. Culture takes 3–7 days.

Treatment and eradication of this organism is discussed on p. 190.

CHRONIC PEPTIC ULCER

This is an ulcer of the mucosa in or adjacent to an acid-bearing area. Most ulcers occur in the stomach or proximal duodenum but they can occur in the oesophagus (with oesophageal reflux), in the jejunum in the Zollinger–Ellison syndrome or after a gastroenterostomy, and finally in a Meckel's diverticulum, which contains ectopic gastric mucosa.

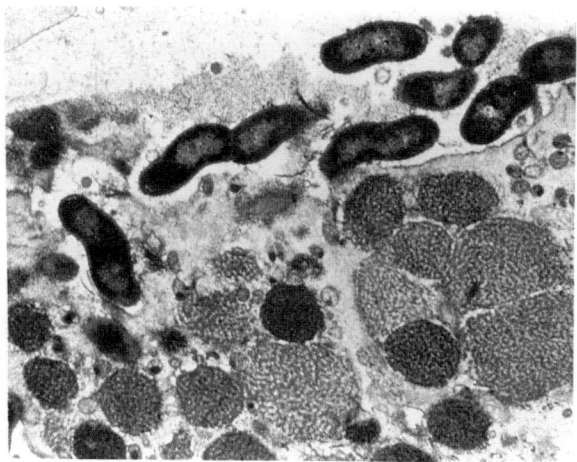

Fig. 4.7 *Helicobacter pylori.* Courtesy of Garnett Keeler Public Relations.

AETIOLOGY

Peptic ulcers occur when the mucosal defences are broken down by various luminal factors. The exact aetiology is unknown but possible aetiological factors are discussed below.

Gastric ulcer

Most patients with gastric ulcers (GU) have normal or low acid outputs. Other factors involved include:

- Alteration in mucus production.
- Duodenogastric reflux with bile damaging the gastric mucosa
- HP is found (see p. 188) but its role is unclear
- Mucosal ischaemia
- Prostaglandins—these play a cytoprotective role in the mucosa.

Thirty per cent of gastric ulcers, mainly prepyloric ulcers, are associated with high acid output and duodenal ulcer disease.

Duodenal ulcer

Most patients with duodenal ulcers (DU) have an increased parietal cell mass and secrete excess acid and pepsinogen, which have always been thought to play a primary aetiological role. Recent evidence has implicated changes in mucosal resistance, as with GU. HP present on foci of gastric metaplasia in the duodenum may make the mucosa more susceptible to damage by acid and pepsin, and thus might play a role in the pathogenesis. Over 90% of patients have HP present in the gastric antrum and its eradication has an implication for healing and recurrence rates.

Epidemiological factors. Duodenal ulceration is common; 15% of the population will suffer from a duodenal ulcer at some time. They are two to three times commoner than gastric ulcers. Duodenal ulcers are commoner in men than women (4 : 1) and both gastric and duodenal ulcers are more common in elderly people. There is considerable geographical variation. Duodenal ulcer is commoner in northern England and Scotland than in other parts of the UK. Southern India has a higher incidence of duodenal ulcer than northern India, and southern Nigeria has more patients with duodenal ulcer than northern Nigeria. Both types of peptic ulcer are common in Australians.

Other aetiological factors of peptic ulcer are shown in Table 4.6. Peptic ulceration is also seen in hyperparathyroidism (since calcium stimulates acid secretion), in the Zollinger–Ellison syndrome and in patients with renal transplants.

PATHOLOGY

Gastric ulcer can occur in any part of the stomach, but is most commonly found on the lesser curve.

Table 4.6 Some other factors involved or thought to be involved in the causation of peptic ulceration.

Factors	Relationship
Diet	Weak
Alcohol	None
Aspirin	Strong association for GU in Australian women
NSAIDS	Damages mucosa but definite ulceration uncertain
Steroid drugs	None
Smoking	Strong for duodenal ulcer
Psychological factors	Weak
Genetic factors	Strong for patients who do not secrete blood group O antigens into gastric secretions
Family history	Strong

Most duodenal ulcers are found in the duodenal cap. Histologically there is a break in the superficial epithelium penetrating down to the muscularis mucosa with a fibrous base and an increase in inflammatory cells. The ulcer heals with fibrosis.

CLINICAL FEATURES

Symptoms

Indigestion is a very common symptom but epigastric pain is the major feature of ulcer disease. The patient who points directly to the epigastrium as the site of the pain is most likely to have an ulcer. The pain of a duodenal ulcer classically occurs at night. In both types of ulcer, pain is helped by antacids. The relationship of the pain to food is variable and on the whole is not helpful in diagnosis. However, patients with a duodenal ulcer may complain of pains when they are hungry.

Nausea may accompany the pain but vomiting is not frequent and when it occurs it may relieve the pain. Other symptoms include flatulence and heartburn, which is due to acid regurgitation. Anorexia and weight loss may occur, particularly with gastric ulcers.

The symptoms of a duodenal ulcer are periodic, with spontaneous relapses and remissions. Sixty per cent of patients will have a recurrence of symptoms within 1 year of the first episode. The natural history appears to be for the disease to remit over many years. Fifty per cent of patients with a gastric ulcer will have a recurrence within 2 years. If the patient complains of persistent and severe pain, complications such as penetration into other organs should be considered. Back pain may suggest a penetrating posterior duodenal ulcer.

Signs
The only signs are those of epigastric tenderness but this is a poor discriminating sign. Tenderness does not necessarily imply disease and is frequently found in non-ulcer dyspepsia.

INVESTIGATION

Many patients, particularly the young presenting with indigestion, can be treated symptomatically for 4–5 weeks without investigation.

- *Blood tests* are unhelpful in uncomplicated cases.
- A *barium meal* (double-contrast technique) or *endoscopy*. A gastric ulcer is shown in Fig. 4.8 and a duodenal ulcer in Fig. 4.9.
- *Gastric function tests.* Secretions from the stomach are collected via a nasogastric tube before (basal secretion) and following stimulation by an injection of pentagastrin. This is a synthetic peptide containing the terminal five peptides of gastrin. The acid status is not useful for the routine case of ulceration because of the overlap with normal values. The main use of this test is in the Zollinger–Ellison syndrome.

TREATMENT

Duodenal ulcer
The symptoms of duodenal ulceration fluctuate and do not correlate with the degree of ulcer healing.

- H_2 *receptor antagonists* are usually the first choice of therapy. They have molecular structures that fit the H_2 receptors on the parietal cells. A single therapeutic dose in the evening produces, at least, an 80% reduction of nocturnal acid production until the following morning. Over 80% of DUs will heal with a 2-month course of this group of drugs (Fig. 4.10), the choice of the drug being often based on the cost. Thereafter patients are advised to either continue on a low-dose maintenance therapy, take tablets when they get symptoms or repeat the course if symptoms recur. The authors usually recommend taking tablets as and when symptoms occur.
- *Tripotassium dicitratobismuthate* (a bismuth chelate) is being increasingly used as, along with antibiotics, it eradicates HP. In one study with eradication of HP only 20% of DUs recurred as opposed to an 80% relapse rate with persistence of infection. Bismuth chelate is given for one month with a simultaneous 2-week course of tetracycline or amoxycillin and metronidazole.

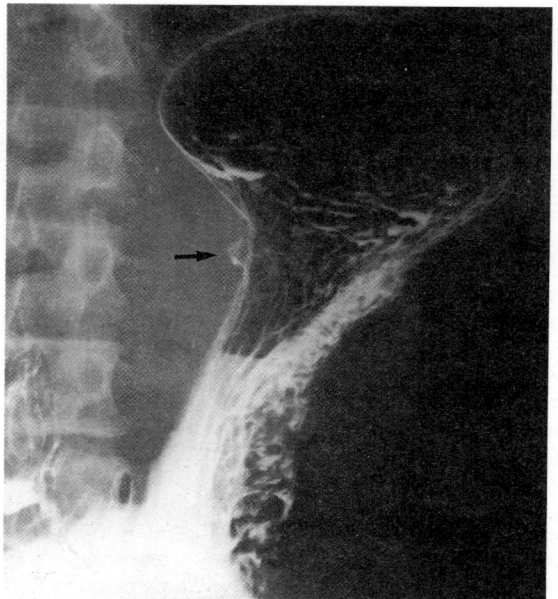

(a)

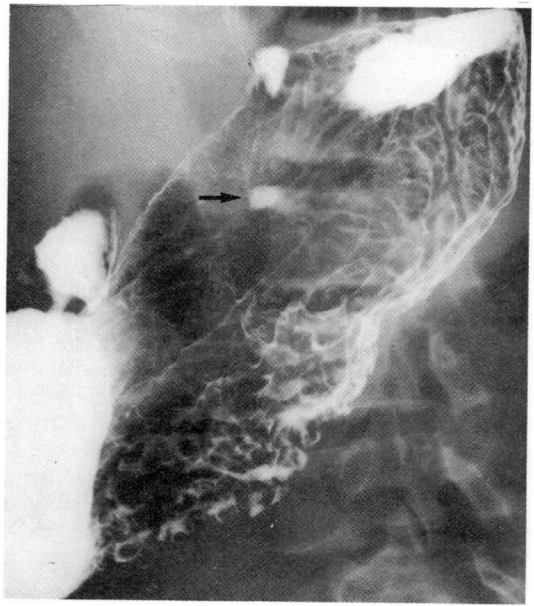

(b)

Fig. 4.8 Double contrast barium meal showing a gastric ulcer (arrow) on the lesser curve. The benign nature of the ulcer is demonstrated by a round niche within the wall of the stomach (a), with mucosal folds radiating to it (b).

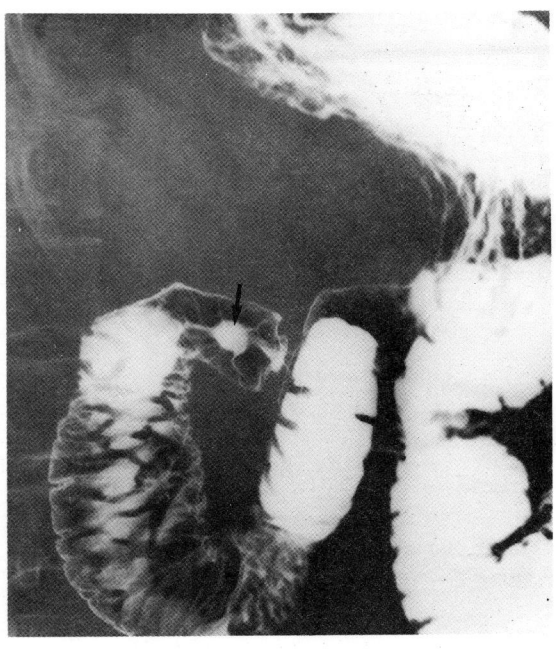

Fig. 4.9 Barium meal showing a large chronic duodenal ulcer (arrow) on the anterior wall of the cap.

Histamine
Cimetidine
800 mg at night

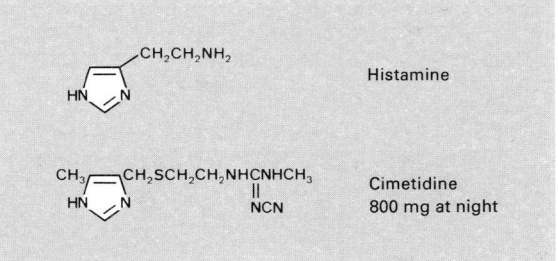

Fig. 4.10 The chemical formula of the first available H_2-receptor antagonist, showing the similarity to histamine.

Other H_2-receptor antagonists

Ranitidine	300 mg at night
Famotidine	40 mg at night
Nizatidine	300 mg at night

- *Omeprazole* produces a 100% inhibition of 24 h intragastric acidity and healing rates of 100% after 4 weeks' treatment (Fig. 4.11). It is used for resistant ulcers.
- *Antacids* are usually prescribed for mild episodes of discomfort and indigestion. The chief antacids are magnesium trisilicate and aluminium hyd-

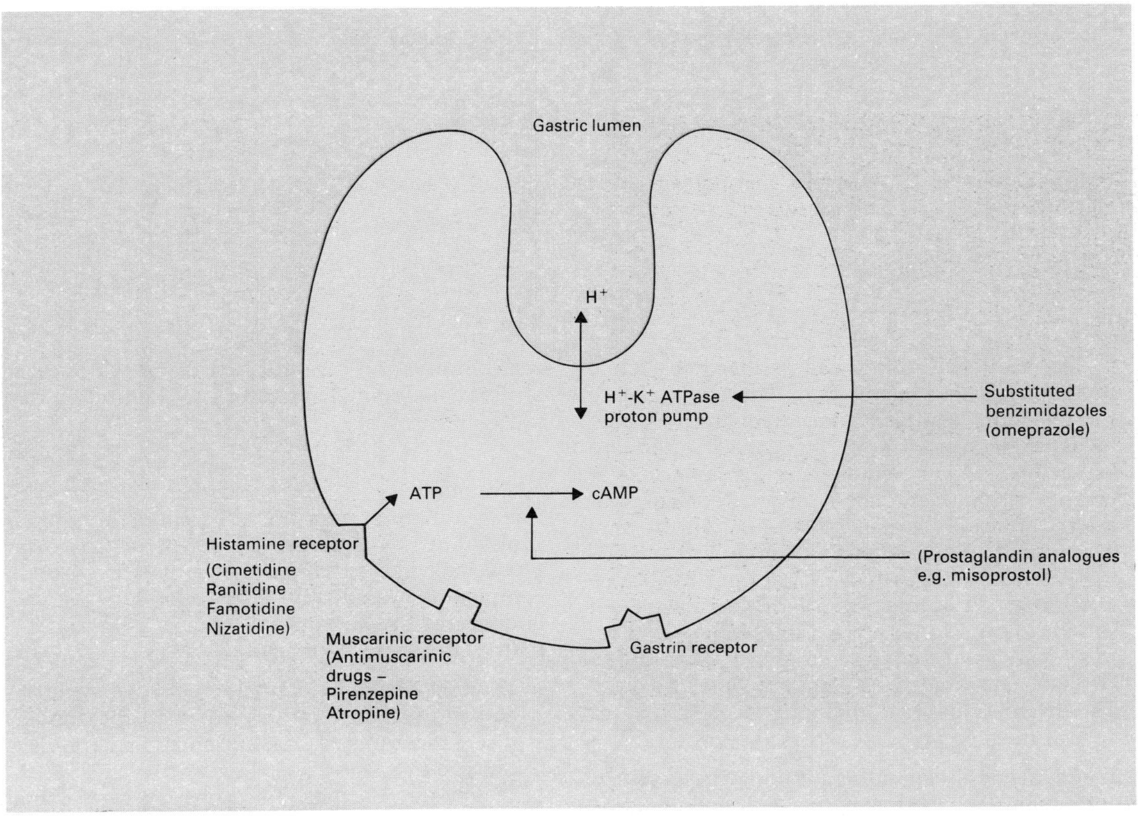

Gastric lumen
H+
H+-K+ ATPase proton pump
Substituted benzimidazoles (omeprazole)
ATP
cAMP
Histamine receptor
(Cimetidine Ranitidine Famotidine Nizatidine)
(Prostaglandin analogues e.g. misoprostol)
Muscarinic receptor (Antimuscarinic drugs – Pirenzepine Atropine)
Gastrin receptor

Fig. 4.11 Diagram of a parietal cell, showing the sites of drug action.

Table 4.7 Drugs other than H$_2$-receptor antagonists and antacids used in the treatment of peptic ulceration.

Drug	Mechanism	Use	Daily dose	Side-effects
Mucosal coating agents				
Bismuth chelate (tripotassium dicitratobismuthate)	Forms protective coating on ulcer	GU and DU; reduces relapses, HP eradicated if antibiotics given as well	15 ml diluted in 15 ml water × 4 or 120 mg tablets × 4 (more palatable)	Unpleasant taste; black tongue, teeth and stools
Sucralfate (aluminium salt of sucrose octasulphate)	Adherence to mucosa	GU and DU	1 g × 4	Constipation
Prostaglandin analogue				
Misoprostol	Cytoprotection plus decreases acid	DU and GU with NSAIDS	200 μg × 4	Diarrhoea
Substituted benzimidazole				
Omeprazole	H$^+$–K$^+$ ATPase pump inhibitor	Resistant PU Z-E syndrome[a]	20 mg	Few. Nausea. Headache
Anti-muscarinic				
Pirenzepine	Reduces acid secretion	Occasionally in DU and GU	50 mg × 2	Occasional dry mouth Blurred vision
Liquorice derivatives (rarely used)				
Carbenoxolone	Affects mucosal resistance	GU	100 mg × 3	Sodium retention with oedema; hypokalaemia; hypertension; do not use in elderly
Deglycyrrhizinized liquorice	? Effect on mucosal resistance	GU and DU	2 tablets × 3	Diarrhoea

[a] Zollinger–Ellison syndrome.

roxide; the former often causes diarrhoea while the latter causes constipation. There is no place for the more complex antacid mixtures, which have no increased buffering capacity and are expensive. Other side-effects of antacids at normal dosages are not a major problem, but many antacids contain sodium, which may exacerbate fluid retention. Aluminium hydroxide has less sodium than magnesium trisilicate.

- *Other drugs.* A number of other drugs have been shown to be effective (see Table 4.7).
- *Miscellaneous.* Stopping smoking should be strongly encouraged as smoking slows healing. The more traditional methods of bed rest or special diets are now never used.

The effectiveness of treatment should be assessed symptomatically. There is no need for follow-up X-rays or endoscopy. If the patient fails to respond, the diagnosis should be reviewed. Duodenal ulcers are common and care must be taken not to falsely attribute abdominal symptoms to the finding of an ulcer.

Gastric ulcer
The treatment of a gastric ulcer differs in approach from that of a duodenal ulcer in that most physicians like to check that a gastric ulcer has completely healed and thus follow-up X-rays or endoscopy are necessary. These differences in management are because:

- There is a better relationship between symptoms and the presence of an ulcer than for duodenal ulcer; nevertheless, asymptomatic gastric ulcers can occur.
- There is a risk that the ulcer may be malignant (see p. 231).

H$_2$-receptor antagonists are the most common

agents used for treatment; follow-up with X-ray or endoscopy at 6 weeks is required. Failure to heal (or to achieve more than a 60% reduction in size) raises the question of malignancy and further endoscopy followed by surgery should be considered.

H$_2$-receptor antagonists are not so successful in the treatment of gastric ulcer as they are for duodenal ulcer but, because of their relative lack of side-effects, are still the drugs of first choice. Omeprazole is being increasingly used and may become the initial therapy. Table 4.7 shows the other drugs that are sometimes used.

Once again, smoking should be strongly discouraged. Dietary changes are unnecessary and there is no reason to avoid spicy foods, coffee or alcohol unless they exacerbate symptoms. Antacids may be necessary to help with symptomatic relief.

Surgical management

Since the introduction of H$_2$-receptor antagonists, surgery for peptic ulceration is rarely performed. Indications for surgery are:

- Failure of medical treatment
- Complications, including recurrent haemorrhage, perforation and outflow obstruction
- Possibility that a GU is malignant

Two types of operation are performed:

- Partial gastrectomy
- Vagotomy

Partial gastrectomy. The principle in both of the two types of gastrectomy performed for peptic ulcer disease is to remove the antral area that secretes gastrin, since this in turn stimulates acid production.

- *Billroth I partial gastrectomy* is now the commonest operation for patients with a gastric ulcer. The lower part of the stomach is removed and the stomach remnant is connected to the duodenum. This operation has a low recurrence rate (< 1%) and low incidence of diarrhoea (< 1%). However, disadvantages include an increased operative mortality, increased complications e.g. metabolic problems, dumping and possible long-term malignancy.
- *Billroth II (Polya gastrectomy)* is now rarely performed, except for duodenal ulceration following a vagotomy. The stomach remnant is connected to the first loop of jejunum (a gastroenterostomy) and the duodenum is closed.

Vagotomy with or without drainage. Vagotomy has the advantage of a decreased operative mortality and further metabolic complications. However, there is a higher recurrence rate of the ulcer (10%) and more than 20% may get diarrhoea. A number of different types of operations have been performed over the years:

- Truncal vagotomy plus gastroenterostomy/pyloroplasty
- Selective vagotomy (preserving the hepatic and coeliac branch of the vagus) plus gastroenterostomy/pyloroplasty
- Highly selective vagotomy or proximal gastric vagotomy, in which only the nerves supplying the parietal cells are transected, and therefore no drainage is required. With this type of operation there is little diarrhoea but the recurrence rate is still 5–10%. This is now the commonest operation for duodenal ulcer.

Complications of surgery. The main complication is recurrent ulcer. This can occur in the stomach, duodenum or jejunum, often at the stoma. The symptoms are similar to those seen in the unoperated stomach, with pain invariably being present, although patients may present with haemorrhage. Because of the deformity of the stomach, investigation by endoscopy is preferred to X-ray examination. Treatment is either medical, using an H$_2$-receptor antagonist (usually long-term) or surgical. Consideration should be given to the possibility of the Zollinger–Ellison syndrome (see p. 235).

The following complications are all becoming less of a clinical problem as fewer and more conservative operations are being performed.

- *Dumping.* This is the term used to describe a number of upper abdominal symptoms, e.g. nausea and distension associated with sweating, faintness and palpitations, that occur in patients following gastrectomy or gastroenterostomy. It is due to 'dumping' of food into the jejunum, which is followed by rapid fluid dilution of the high osmotic load. A number of patients have mild symptoms of dumping but learn to cope with them. It is rare for it to be a clinical problem and, if it is, the symptoms will have a functional element. Treatment should be reassurance and symptomatic treatment. Further operations are rarely needed.
- *Diarrhoea.* This is chiefly seen after vagotomy. Urgency or recurrent severe episodes occur in 1% and can be a major problem. Treatment consists of antidiarrhoeals such as codeine phosphate but is not entirely satisfactory. Cholestyramine—a resin that binds bile salts—helps in some cases. Very occasionally the diarrhoea or steatorrhoea can be due to bacterial overgrowth in the blind loop of a Polya gastrectomy (see p. 207).
- *Vomiting (afferent loop syndrome/bilious vomiting).* The incidence of vomiting has decreased with the more conservative operations. Vomiting occurs because food gets trapped owing to the altered anatomy. Treatment is symptomatic, except on the rare occasions when reconstructive surgery is required.

● *Nutritional complications.* Anaemia is most commonly due to iron deficiency due to poor absorption. Treatment is with oral iron, which may be needed long-term. Megaloblastic anaemia is uncommon but can be due to either folate deficiency (due to poor intake) or B_{12} deficiency (due to long-term atrophic gastritis resulting in intrinsic factor deficiency). Osteomalacia is an uncommon late complication (see p. 822). Patients often fail to gain weight owing to anorexia after gastric surgery and a few suffer from severe protein–energy malnutrition as a result.

COMPLICATIONS OF PEPTIC ULCER

Haemorrhage
This is dealt with below.

Perforation (see also p. 227)
The frequency of perforation of peptic ulcer is decreasing; this is partly attributable to the introduction of H_2-receptor antagonists. Duodenal ulcers perforate more commonly than gastric ulcers, usually into the peritoneal cavity. Perforation into the lesser sac may occur.

Management of perforation. Detailed management is described on p. 228. Surgery is performed to close the perforation and drain the abdomen. Conservative management using nasogastric suction, intravenous fluids and antibiotics is occasionally used in elderly and very sick patients.

Perforation of peptic ulcer

Look for:
● Other acute gastrointestinal conditions, e.g. cholecystitis, pancreatitis (check serum amylase)
● Non GI conditions, e.g. myocardial infarction
● Silent perforations in the elderly or patients on steroids

Remember
● There *is* harm in leaving an undiagnosed perforation
● There is no real harm in operating even if the perforation has occurred at a different site from that expected clinically
● Avoid laparotomy if pancreatitis is diagnosed.

Pyloric stenosis or obstruction
This is more accurately called gastric outflow obstruction, as the obstruction may be prepyloric or in the duodenum. The obstruction occurs either because of an acute ulcer with surrounding oedema or because the healing of an ulcer has been followed by scarring. Occasionally the obstruction is due to a gastric malignancy.

The main symptom of this condition is vomiting, usually without pain as the characteristic ulcer pain has abated owing to healing.

Vomiting is projectile and huge in volume, and the vomitus contains particles of old food. On examination of the abdomen the patient may have a succussion splash.

Severe or persistent vomiting causes loss of acid from the stomach and a metabolic alkalosis occurs (see p. 510).

The diagnosis is made by barium-meal examination but can be suspected when large quantities of fluid are removed by gastric intubation in the fasting state. Fluid and electrolyte replacement is necessary, together with the regular removal of gastric contents via a nasogastric tube. In some patients with oedema rather than scarring, the symptoms will settle with this conservative management. However, most patients require surgery. Postoperative gastric stasis can be a problem, particularly if a vagotomy has been performed, even when accompanied by drainage.

Acute and chronic gastrointestinal bleeding

This section should be read in conjunction with the descriptions of the specific conditions mentioned.

Acute upper gastrointestinal bleeding

Haematemesis is the vomiting of blood. Malaena is the passage of black tarry stools; the black colour is due to altered blood—50 ml or more is required to produce this. Melaena can occur with bleeding from any lesion from areas proximal to and including the caecum. Following a massive bleed from the upper GI tract, unaltered blood (owing to rapid transit) can appear per rectum, but this is rare. The colour of the blood appearing per rectum is dependent not only on the site of bleeding but also on the time of transit in the gut.

AETIOLOGY

Chronic peptic ulceration still accounts for approximately half of all cases of upper GI haemorrhage. This and other causes are shown in Fig. 4.12. The relative incidences of these causes vary depending on the patient population. Aspirin and other non-steroidal anti-inflammatory drugs can undoubtedly produce gastric lesions and probably are the cause of some GI bleeds from acute ulcers. There is doubt, however, whether these agents make

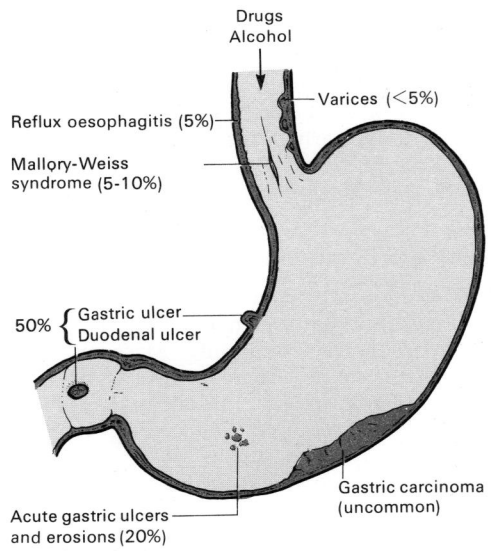

Drugs
Alcohol

Varices (<5%)

Reflux oesophagitis (5%)

Mallory-Weiss
syndrome (5-10%)

50% { Gastric ulcer
Duodenal ulcer

Acute gastric ulcers
and erosions (20%)

Gastric carcinoma
(uncommon)

Other uncommon causes:

Hereditary telangiectasia (Osler-Weber-Rendu syndrome)
Pseudoxanthoma elasticum
Blood dyscrasias

Fig. 4.12 Causes of upper gastrointestinal haemorrhage. The approximate frequency is also given.

chronic ulcers more likely to bleed. Corticosteroids in the usual therapeutic doses probably have no influence on GI haemorrhage.

IMMEDIATE MANAGEMENT

All cases with a recent (i.e. within 48 h) significant GI bleed should be admitted to hospital. In many no further immediate treatment is required as the patient's cardiovascular system can compensate for the blood loss. Approximately 85% of patients stop bleeding spontaneously within 48 h.

Factors affecting management

- Age (see below)
- The amount of blood lost, which may give some guide to the severity
- Continuing visible blood loss
- Signs of chronic liver disease on examination, as the bleeding is often severe and recurrent if it is from varices; liver failure can develop
- Presence of the classical clinical features of shock (i.e. pallor, cold nose, tachycardia and low blood pressure); remember that the peripheral constriction that occurs may keep the blood pressure falsely high

Urgent resuscitation is required in patients with large bleeds and the clinical signs of shock. Details

of the management of shock are given in Chapter 13. The major principle is to restore the blood volume to normal and this can only be satisfactorily achieved by transfusion of whole blood. It may be necessary in a severely shocked patient or in a patient with blood compatibility problems to give a blood substitute initially.

The rate of blood transfusion must be monitored carefully to avoid overtransfusion and consequent heart failure. The pulse rate and venous pressure are the best guides to transfusion rates.

Anaemia does not develop immediately as haemodilution has not taken place and therefore the haemoglobin level is a poor indicator of the need to transfuse. If the level is low (less than 10 g·dl^{-1}) and the patient has either bled recently or is actively bleeding, transfusion may be necessary.

In most patients the bleeding stops, albeit temporarily, so that further assessment can be made.

Important factors in reassessment

- Age—below the age of 60 years mortality from GI bleeding is small. Above the age of 80 the mortality is greater than 20%.
- Recurrent haemorrhage—these patients have an increased mortality.
- Most re-bleeds (approximately 25% of all cases) occur within 48 h.
- Melaena is usually less hazardous than haematemesis.

Taking these factors into account, a decision can be made on future management. In addition, the cause of the haemorrhage should be looked for. The diagnosis may be obvious from the history, e.g. a long history of indigestion or, more significantly, previous haemorrhage from an ulcer. A history of aspirin or non-steroidal anti-inflammatory drug ingestion may suggest acute ulceration.

Signs of chronic liver disease, particularly with splenomegaly, suggest bleeding from oesophageal varices. The source of haemorrhage in most patients with chronic liver disease is their varices, but occasionally they may bleed from an accompanying peptic ulcer. The absence of splenomegaly does not rule out oesophageal varices.

After a careful history and examination, investigations should then be arranged within 12–24 h of admission. Endoscopy will detect the cause of the haemorrhage in 80% or more of cases. If stigmata of a recent bleed are seen, i.e. a visible vessel or adherent clot, the patient is more likely to re-bleed.

TREATMENT

Most conditions require no specific therapy after resuscitation. There is little evidence that H₂-receptor anatagonists affect the mortality rate of GI haemorrhage but these agents are usually given to patients with ulcers because of their longer-term benefits. It may be necessary to operate if the bleeding is persistent or recurrent or if it cannot be controlled. Surgery should be avoided, if at all possible, in patients with acute gastric ulceration. Electrocoagulation and heater probes can be used endoscopically and will usually stop the bleeding.

Specific conditions
Chronic gastric ulcer. These patients may require surgery as they are likely to re-bleed, but omeprazole should be tried first.

Chronic duodenal ulcer. Since the advent of H_2-receptor antagonists and omeprazole, surgery has usually been avoided. When the patient is over his acute episode of haemorrhage, indications for surgery are the same as if the patient had not bled.

Gastric carcinoma. Most patients do not have large bleeds with this condition but surgery may be performed for the lesion *per se*.

Oesophageal varices. These are discussed on p. 263.

Mallory–Weiss tear. This is a linear mucosal tear occurring at the oesophagogastric junction and produced by a sudden increase in intra-abdominal pressure. It often occurs after a bout of coughing or retching and is classically seen in the alcoholic. There may, however, be no antecedent history of retching. The haemorrhage may be large but most patients stop spontaneously. Rarely, surgery with over-sewing of the tear will be required.

PROGNOSIS

The mortality of GI haemorrhage has not changed over the years, despite many changes in management (see above) partly owing to more patients being elderly. Early surgery has not so far reduced the mortality, because of the difficulty in recognizing the patient who will re-bleed.

Acute lower gastrointestinal bleeding

Massive bleeding from the lower GI tract is rare. On the other hand, small bleeds from haemorrhoids occur very commonly. Massive bleeding is usually due to diverticular disease or ischaemic colitis and may require urgent resuscitation. Surgery is rarely required as bleeding usually stops spontaneously. The causes of lower gastrointestinal bleeding are shown in Fig. 4.13.

MANAGEMENT

Resuscitation when required.

Make diagnosis using the following investigations as appropriate:

- Rectal examination, e.g. carcinoma
- Proctoscopy, e.g. haemorrhoids
- Sigmoidoscopy, e.g. inflammatory bowel disease
- Barium enema—any mucosal lesion
- Colonoscopy—diagnosis and removal of polyps
- Angiography—vascular abnormality, e.g. angiodysplasia

Treatment: Individual lesions are treated as appropriate.

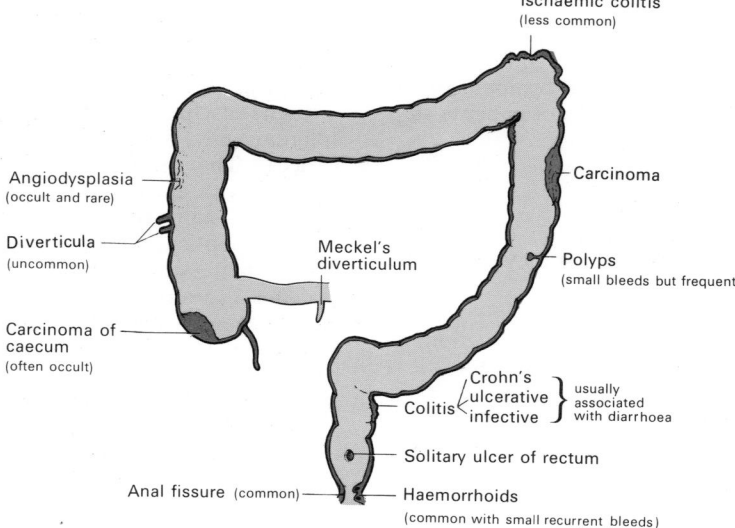

Fig. 4.13 Causes of lower gastrointestinal bleeding. The sites shown are illustrative—many of the lesions can be seen in other parts of the colon.

Chronic gastrointestinal bleeding

Patients with chronic bleeding usually present with iron-deficiency anaemia (see Chapter 6).

Chronic blood loss producing anaemia in all men and all women after the menopause is always due to bleeding from the GI tract, so tests are not required to show this. Occult blood tests are not necessary.

Measurement of faecal occult blood

This is frequently performed *unnecessarily*. It is *only* of value in:

● Premenopausal women: if a history of menorrhagia is uncertain and the cause of iron deficiency is unclear
● As a mass population screening test for large bowel malignancy
   Advantages: cheap and easy to perform
   Disadvantages: high false-positive rate, leading to unnecessary investigations

---

DIAGNOSIS

Chronic blood loss can occur with any lesion of the GI tract that produces acute bleeding (see Figs. 4.12 and 4.13). In addition a Meckel's diverticulum and carcinoma of the caecum may present with an iron-deficiency anaemia. It should be remembered that, world-wide, hookworm is the commonest cause of chronic GI blood loss.

Careful history and examination may indicate the most likely site of the bleeding, but if no clue is available it is usual to investigate the lower bowel first with either a barium enema or colonoscopy (see Table 4.3). The importance of having a clean, well-prepared bowel for both techniques cannot be overemphasized.

If no lesion is found in the lower GI tract, the upper GI tract and small bowel are investigated. If these investigations are also negative, angiography may show up the site of bleeding, particularly when acute bleeding is occurring. Occasionally intravenous technetium-labelled colloid may be used to demonstrate the bleeding site in a Meckel's diverticulum.

The small intestine

Structure

The small intestine extends from the duodenum to the ileum. Its surface area is enormously increased by mucosal folds. In addition, the mucosa has

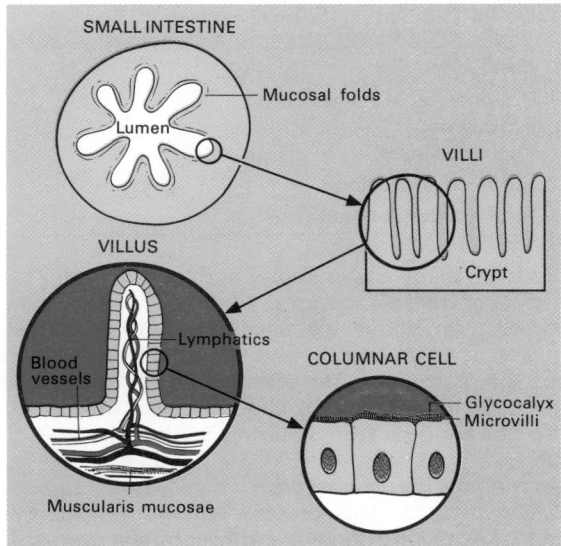

Fig. 4.14 The structure of the small intestine.

numerous finger-like projections called villi, the surface area of which is further increased by microvilli (see Fig. 4.14). Each villus consists of a core containing blood vessels, lacteals (lymphatics) and cells and is covered by epithelial columnar cells that are absorptive. Opening into the lumen between the villi are the crypts of Lieberkühn.

The epithelial cells are formed at the bottom of these crypts and migrate to the tops of the villi, from where they are shed. This process takes 3–4 days. On its luminal side the epithelial cell has a brush border of microvilli that is covered by the glycocalyx. The lamina propria contains plasma cells, lymphocytes, macrophages, eosinophils and mast cells. Scattered throughout the gut are peptide-secreting cells.

Most of the blood supply to the small intestine is via branches of the superior mesenteric artery. The terminal branches are end arteries, i.e. there are no local anastomotic connections.

Histochemically there are three types of nerves in the gut:

● Cholinergic parasympathetic (with muscarinic or nicotinic receptors)
● Adrenergic sympathetic (with both α and β receptors)
● Non-cholinergic, non-adrenergic. The transmitters here are thought to be either cyclic nucleotides and ATP (the purinergic hypothesis) or intestinal hormones, e.g. VIP (peptidergic hypothesis).

Function (Table 4.8)

The small intestine is concerned with the digestion and absorption of nutrients, salt and water. It

Table 4.8 Functions of the small intestine.

Absorption
Defence against antigen entry
Structural
Immunological
Hormone production
Motility—transit of nutrients

produces many enzymes and hormones in order to carry out these processes. Nutrients can be absorbed throughout the small intestine with the exception of vitamin B_{12} and bile salts, which have specific receptors in the terminal ileum. The small intestine also has local defence mechanisms to prevent antigens from entering the body.

General principles of absorption
Simple diffusion. This process requires no energy and takes place if there is a concentration gradient from the intestinal lumen (high concentration) to the bloodstream (low concentration).

Active transport. This requires energy and can work against a concentration gradient. A carrier protein is required and the process is sodium-dependent. For example, glucose enters the enterocyte on the luminal side via a sodium-dependent carrier molecule and leaves on the serosal side via a sodium-independent carrier that is found in the basolateral membrane. A gradient is maintained across the membrane by an energy-dependent sodium pump

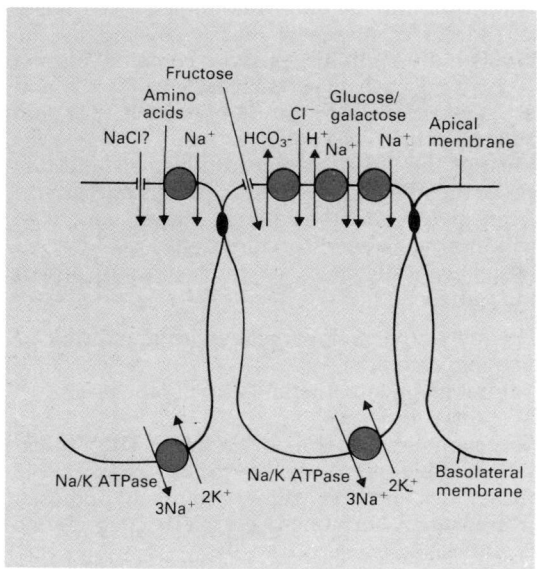

Fig. 4.15 Diagrammatic representation of solute transport across the apical membrane showing glucose/galactose sodium linked transport. The sodium/potassium ATPase pump is located in the basolateral membrane.

(Na^+–K^+ ATPase) that keeps the intracellular sodium concentration low (Fig. 4.15).

Facilitated diffusion. This is an energy-independent carrier-mediated transport system that allows a faster absorption rate than simple diffusion, e.g. fructose absorption.

Absorption in the small intestine
Carbohydrate. Dietary carbohydrate consists mainly of starch with some sucrose and a small amount of lactose. Starch is a polysaccharide made up of numerous glucose units. Its hydrolysis begins in the mouth by salivary amylase. The majority of hydrolysis takes place in the upper intestinal lumen by pancreatic amylase. This hydrolysis is limited by the fact that amylases have no specificity for some glucose/glucose branching links.

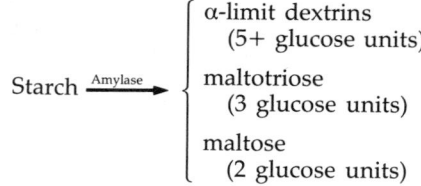

These breakdown products, together with sucrose and lactose, are hydrolysed on the brush border membrane by their appropriate oligo- and disaccharidases to form the monosaccharides glucose, galactose and fructose. These monosaccharides are transported into the cells, largely by sodium-dependent active transport systems.

Protein. Dietary and endogenous proteins (desquamated cells, intestinal secretions) are mainly digested by pancreatic enzymes prior to absorption. These proteolytic enzymes are secreted as proenzymes and transformed to active enzymes in the lumen. The presence of protein in the lumen stimulates the release of enterokinase, which activates trypsinogen to trypsin, and this in turn activates the other proenzymes, chymotrypsin and elastase. These enzymes break down protein into oligopeptides. Some di- and tripeptides are absorbed intact by a carrier-mediated process, while the remainder are broken down into free amino acids by peptidases on the microvillus membranes of the cell, prior to absorption in a similar way to disaccharides. These amino acids are transported into the cell by a number of different carrier systems.

Fat (Fig. 4.16). Dietary fat mainly consists of triglycerides with some cholesterol and fat-soluble vitamins. Emulsification of fat occurs in the stomach and is followed by hydrolysis of triglycerides in the duodenum by pancreatic lipase to yield fatty acids and monoglycerides.

Bile enters the duodenum following gall-bladder

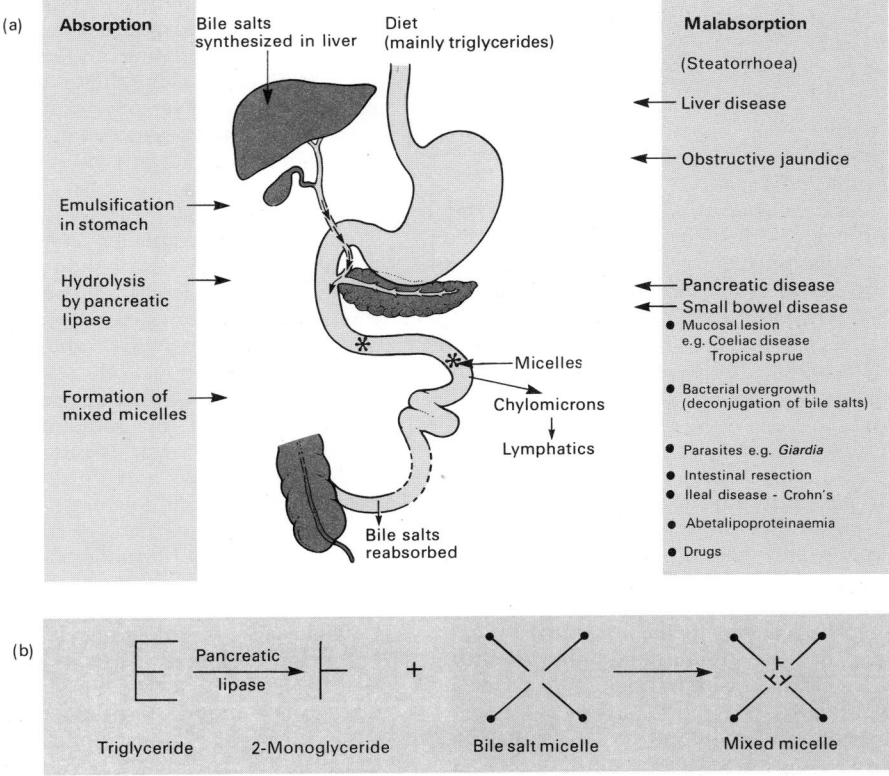

Fig. 4.16 (a) The pathophysiology of fat absorption. (b) Diagram showing the formation of mixed micelles.

contraction. Bile contains phospholipids and bile salts, both of which are partially water-soluble and act as detergents. They aggregate together to form micelles with their hydrophilic ends on the outside. Trapped in the hydrophobic centre of this micelle are the monoglycerides, fatty acids and cholesterol; these are then transported to the intestinal cell membrane. At the cell membrane the lipid contents of the micelle are absorbed, while the bile salts remain in the lumen. Inside the cell the monoglycerides and fatty acids are re-esterified to triglycerides. The triglycerides and other fat-soluble molecules (e.g. cholesterol, phospholipids) are then incorporated into chylomicrons to be transported into the lymph.

Medium-chain triglycerides (which contain fatty acids of chain length 6–12) as well as a small amount of long-chain fatty acid are transported via the portal vein.

Bile salts are not absorbed in the jejunum, so that the intraluminal concentration in the upper gut is high. They pass down the intestine to be absorbed in the terminal ileum and are transported back to the liver. This enterohepatic circulation

prevents excess loss of bile salts (see p. 240).

The pathophysiology of fat absorption is shown in Fig. 4.16. Interference with absorption can occur at all stages, as indicated, giving rise to steatorrhoea.

Water and electrolytes. A large amount of water and electrolytes, partly dietary but mainly from intestinal secretions, are absorbed coupled with monosaccharides and amino acids in the upper jejunum. Some water and electrolytes are absorbed in the ileum and right side of the colon, where active sodium transport occurs but is not coupled to solute absorption. Intestinal secretion also takes place and abnormalities of this mechanism cause secretory diarrhoea (see p. 222).

Water-soluble vitamins, essential metals and trace elements. These all have to be absorbed in the small intestine. It must be remembered that vitamin B_{12} (see p. 303) is the only substance other than bile salts that is specifically absorbed in the terminal ileum alone and malabsorption of both these substances will always occur following ileal resection.

Calcium. See p. 821.

Iron. See p. 299.

Defence against antigens

Structure and immunology. The normal intestinal mucosa forms an intrinsic barrier to the absorption of many antigens such as bacteria, viruses or dietary proteins. It is therefore not surprising that the GI tract acts as an important lymphoid organ. Lymphoid tissue is present either as lymphoid cells scattered throughout the gut mucosa or as lymphoid aggregates, e.g. the tonsils and Peyer's patches (see Fig. 4.17).

A specialized epithelial cell above these Peyer's patches called the M or microfold cell allows antigens to pass through the mucosa. The lymphocytes lying below the epithelium are stimulated by these antigens and pass to the local mesenteric lymph nodes and then, via the thoracic duct, to the circulation. Eventually these sensitized lymphocytes 'home' back again to the intestinal mucosa. Here they become immunoglobulin-producing plasma cells. The major immunoglobulin produced is monomeric IgA.

IgA is secreted into the gut lumen through the epithelial cell layer, where two molecules of IgA are joined together with a J chain. This dimeric IgA then has a 'secretor piece' attached to it. This is a glycoprotein that helps to protect the dimeric IgA from proteolysis by intestinal luminal enzymes.

The function of dimeric IgA is to reduce antigen absorption and to prevent bacteria entering the wall by reducing their adherence to the mucosa. It thus acts as an 'antiseptic paint'. The gut-associated lymphoid tissue (GALT) can also mount a local immune response to an antigen, independent of any circulating antibody. This local antibody production can either protect the host or can produce a hypersensitivity reaction resulting in damage to the mucosa, e.g. cow's milk protein intolerance in children.

Hormone production

The hormone-producing cells of the gut are scattered diffusely throughout its length and also occur in the pancreas. The cells that synthesize these hormones are derived from neural ectoderm and are known as APUD (amine precursor uptake and decarboxylation) cells. Many of these hormones have very similar structures. Although they can be detected by radioimmunoassay in the circulation, their action is often local.

Table 4.9 shows some gut hormones and their possible physiological actions. Many are also found in other tissues, particularly the brain. A number do not act as true hormones but act as neurotransmitters or have local effects on adjacent cells only (paracrine effects).

The exact physiological role of these peptides is still being evaluated. Their importance clinically is that they may be secreted in excess, particularly in endocrine tumours of the pancreas (see p. 235).

Gut motility

This is a complex process and is influenced by both neurological and hormonal factors. Following a meal, food is propelled down the gut by a series of peristaltic contractions. In addition, there are weaker contractions that enable the food to be mixed with the biliary and pancreatic secretions. Peristalsis is initiated by an electrical pacemaker in the lower part of the stomach and duodenum and

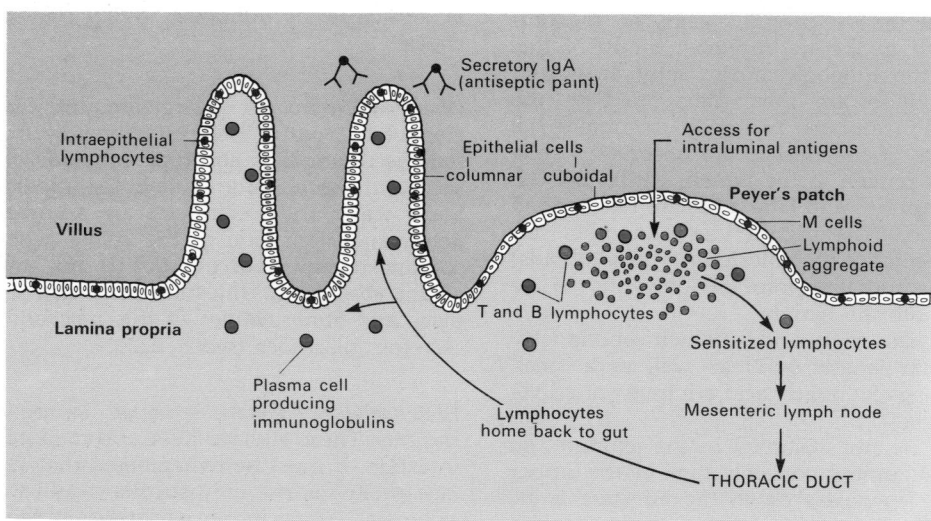

Fig. 4.17 Small intestinal mucosa with a Peyer's patch, showing the gut-associated lymphoid tissue (GALT).

Table 4.9 Gut hormones.

Hormone	Possible physiological action	Main gut localization
Gastrin (G17, 14, 34)	Stimulates acid secretion Stimulates growth of mucosa	Gastric antrum (G17) Small intestine (G34)
Secretin	Stimulates pancreatic secretion (bicarbonate and water)	Duodenum
Cholecystokinin (CCK)	Stimulates gall-bladder contraction and gut motility Role in satiety	Upper small gut
Pancreatic polypeptide (PP)	? Inhibition of pancreatic and biliary secretions	Pancreas
Gastric inhibitory peptide (GIP)	Increases insulin secretion	Upper small gut
Somatostatin	Inhibits release of and antagonizes many hormones	Stomach, pancreas and intestine
Motilin	Increases gut contraction	Upper small gut
Neurotensin	Unclear; possible delaying effect on gastric emptying	Ileum
Enteroglucagon	Unclear	Ileum and colon
Peptide YY	Unclear	Ileum and colon
Substance P	Unclear	Duodenum and colon
Bombesin	Unclear	Stomach and duodenum
Endorphins	Neurotransmitters	Whole gut
Vasoactive intestinal peptide (VIP)	Neurotransmitter; stimulates intestinal secretion	Whole gut
Peptide histidine methionine (PHM)	As for VIP	Whole gut

slow waves progress caudally as far as the ileo-caecal valve.

The pattern of motility is different in the fasting state. It is cyclical and divided into phases. The first phase of motor quiescence lasts about 50 min and is followed by a phase of irregular motor activity lasting about 20 s. This is followed by a period of regular motor activity or a migrating myoelectric complex (MMC) that occurs every 85 min or so. The importance of the MMC is uncertain but it is thought to act as an 'intestinal housekeeper' clearing the lumen of bacteria and other substances; there is a coincidental increase in biliary and pancreatic flow.

Presenting features of small-bowel disease

Regardless of the cause, the common presenting features of small-bowel disease are:

- Diarrhoea/steatorrhoea
- Abdominal pain or discomfort
- Weight loss
- Nutritional deficiencies

Diarrhoea
This is a common feature of small-bowel disease but approximately 10–20% of patients will have no diarrhoea or any other gastrointestinal symptoms.

Abdominal pain and discomfort
Abdominal distension can cause discomfort and flatulence. The pain has no specific character or periodicity and is not usually severe.

Weight loss
Weight loss is due to the anorexia that invariably accompanies small-bowel disease. Although malabsorption occurs, the amount is small relative to intake.

Nutritional deficiencies
Deficiencies of iron, B_{12}, folate or all of these, leading to anaemia, are the only common deficiencies. Occasionally malabsorption of other vitamins or minerals occurs, causing bruising (vitamin K deficiency), tetany (calcium deficiency), osteomalacia (vitamin D deficiency), or stomatitis, sore

tongue and aphthous ulceration (multiple vitamin deficiencies).

Ankle oedema may be seen and is partly nutritional and partly due to intestinal loss of albumin.

Physical signs of small-bowel disease

These are few and non-specific. If present they are associated with anaemia and the nutritional deficiencies described above.

Abdominal examination is often normal, but sometimes distension and, rarely, hepatomegaly or an abdominal mass are found. In the severely ill patient gross malnutrition with muscle wasting is seen. A neuropathy, not always due to B_{12} deficiency, can be present.

Investigation of small-bowel disease (Fig. 4.18)

Blood tests
The following are usually performed in all cases of suspected small-bowel disease:

- *Full blood count and film.* Anaemia can be microcytic (low mean corpuscular volume [MCV]) or macrocytic (high MCV). The blood film may also show other abnormal cells, e.g. Howell–Jolly bodies, which are seen in splenic atrophy associated with coeliac disease. *Serum iron* and *total iron-binding capacity* or *serum ferritin* are then performed if the MCV is low. *Serum B_{12}, serum folate* and *red-cell folate* are performed if the MCV is high. However, with mixed deficiencies, the MCV may be normal.

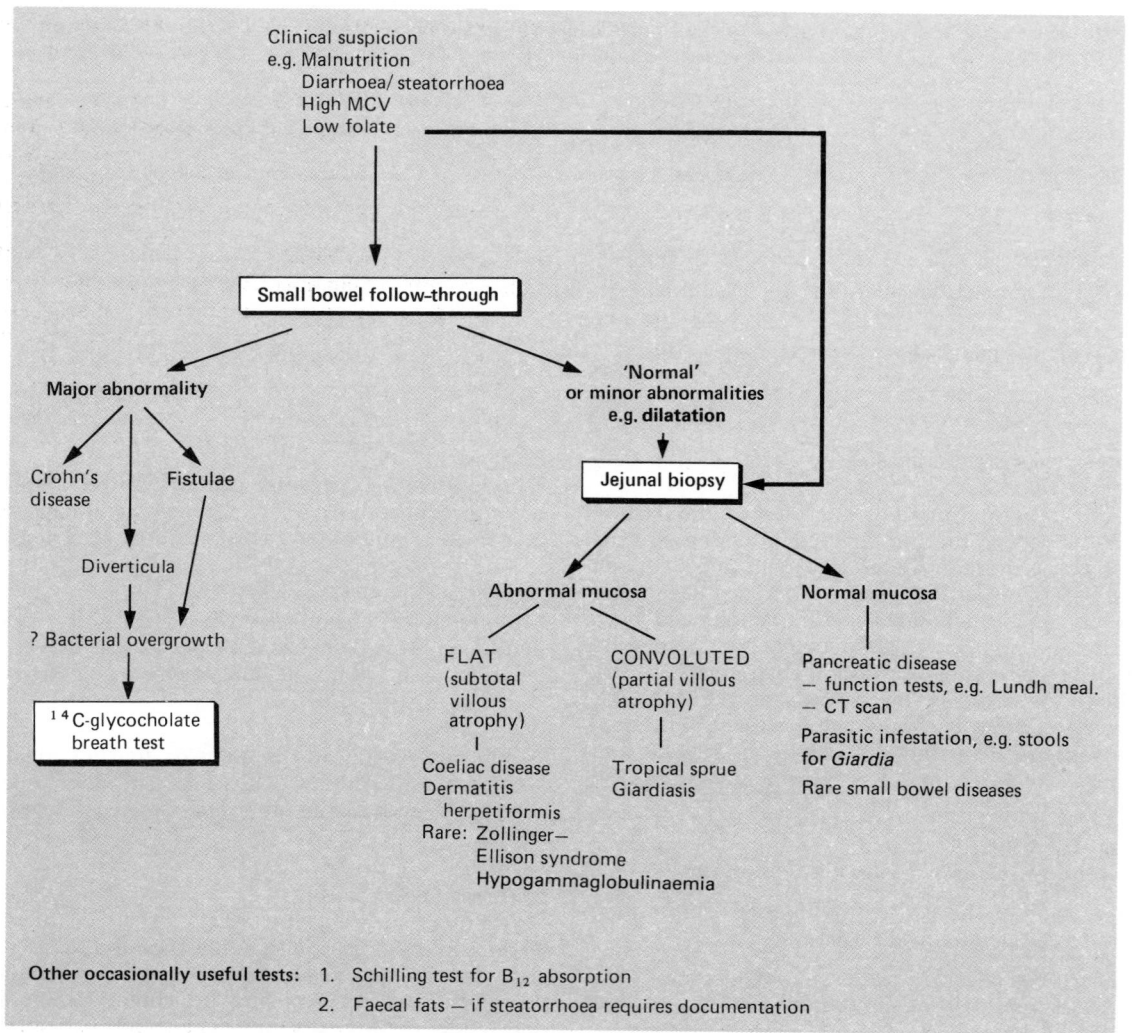

Fig. 4.18 Flow diagram for investigation of patients with suspected small-bowel disease.

- *Serum albumin.* This gives an indication of nutritional status
- *Low serum calcium and raised alkaline phosphatase.* These may indicate the presence of osteomalacia
- *Red-cell folate.* An accurately performed red-cell folate using a microbiological assay is a good indicator of the presence of small-bowel disease. Red-cell folate is frequently low in both coeliac disease and Crohn's disease, which are also the two commonest causes of small-bowel disease

The following non-specific tests of malabsorption are being performed less often and are not always necessary. If the clinical suspicion of malabsorption is high, a definitive test should be performed next.

Non-specific function tests
Fat malabsorption. The fat content of stools is measured using a three-day collection of faeces with the patient on a diet containing 100 g (3.7 mJ) of fat daily. Normal faecal fat excretion is less than 17 mmol (6 g) per day.

To avoid faecal collections, fat absorption can also be measured using breath analysis. Following oral administration of a radiolabelled fat load, the amount of $^{14}CO_2$ in the expired breath gives an indication of the amount of fat malabsorption. Comparison between a labelled triglyceride (^{14}C triolein) and a labelled fatty acid (tritiated oleic acid) is used to diagnose pancreatic disease, when fatty-acid absorption will be normal.

D-Xylose tolerance test. Xylose is a synthetic sugar that is absorbed from the proximal small intestine. The urinary xylose excretion and the blood xylose level following an oral dose reflect its absorption. This test tends to produce many false-positives and should not be used when definitive tests are available.

Lactose tolerance test. This involves the oral ingestion of 50 g of lactose and the measurement of blood glucose. The test is of little use in adults as lactose intolerance is not a clinical problem since these patients avoid milk by choice. There is a high incidence of lactase deficiency in many parts of the world, e.g. the Mediterranean countries, and parts of Africa and Asia. It should be remembered that a glass of milk only contains approximately 11 g of lactose.

A glucose tolerance test should not be performed, as it is influenced by many factors other than absorption.

Definitive tests
Small-bowel follow-through (see p. 177). This detects gross anatomical defects such as diverticula, strictures and Crohn's disease. Dilatation of the folds and a changed fold pattern may suggest malabsorption but, as these are not specific findings, the diagnosis should not be based on these alone. Gross dilatation is seen in pseudo-obstruction.

Jejunal biopsy. This is used to assess the microanatomy of the small bowel. Specimens can be obtained using a Crosby–Kugler capsule. Biopsies can also be obtained via an endoscope passed into the duodenum either with a Crosby–Kugler capsule inserted retrogradely up the endoscope or with a grab biopsy using large biopsy forceps. With either technique, an adequate piece of tissue, well-orientated, is necessary for correct histological evaluation. The histological appearances will be described in the sections on individual diseases.

A smear of the jejunal juice or a mucosal impression can also be made and is helpful in the diagnosis of *Giardia lamblia* (see p. 90).

Other useful tests in specific diseases
^{14}C-glycocholic acid breath test (Fig. 4.19). This is

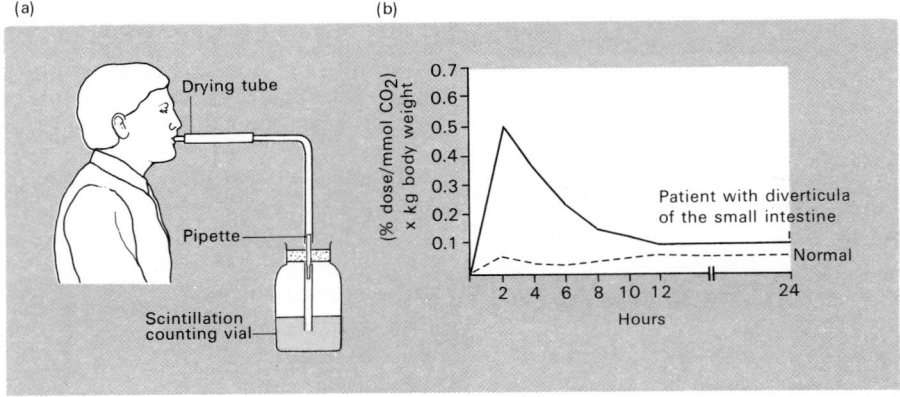

Fig. 4.19 The [^{14}C]glycocholic acid breath test. (a) The apparatus. (b) The amount of $^{14}CO_2$ expired in the breath after an oral dose of [^{14}C]glycocholic acid in a normal subject and in a patient with diverticula of the small intestine.

Jejunal biopsy

- The patient is fasted overnight.
- A Crosby–Kugler capsule is swallowed, guided through the pylorus with screening, and then allowed to pass to just beyond the duodeno-jejunal junction.
- A small piece of mucosa is sucked into the capsule; additional suction triggers the knife to remove a mucosal specimen.
- The capsule is immediately withdrawn.
- The specimen is examined immediately under a dissecting microscope.
- The specimen is then placed in 10% formalin for histological examination.
- Alternatively, biopsies can be obtained via an endoscope.

Complications
- Haemorrhage or perforation (very rare).

---

performed to look for bacterial overgrowth (see below). The patient is given ^{14}C-labelled bile salts by mouth. Bacteria deconjugate the bile salts, releasing [^{14}C]-glycine, which is metabolized and appears in the breath as $^{14}CO_2$. This radioactivity in the breath can easily be measured. An early rise indicates either bacterial overgrowth in the upper small intestine or rapid transit to the colon where, of course, bacteria are normally present.

Direct intubation. Aspiration of intestinal juices is another method by which bacterial contamination can be detected. Bacterial counts are performed on aerobic and anaerobic cultures. Chromatography of bile salts can also be performed on the aspirate to detect evidence of deconjugation by bacteria.

Hydrogen breath test. This can also be used to detect bacterial overgrowth. Oral lactulose is degraded by bacteria, with the production of hydrogen. An early rise in the breath hydrogen will indicate bacterial breakdown of lactulose in the small intestine or rapid transit of the lactulose to the large intestine. As bacteria are present in the oral cavity, the mouth should be rinsed out with an antiseptic mouthwash prior to the test being performed.

Schilling test. This is performed to look for vitamin B_{12} malabsorption. It is described in detail on p. 307. In gastrointestinal disease it is used to detect:

- Pernicious anaemia
- Ileal disease (when oral vitamin B_{12} is given with intrinsic factor)
- Bacterial overgrowth (measurement of vitamin B_{12} plus intrinsic factor absorption is repeated after antibiotics)

Pancreatic tests (see p. 287). These may be required for the differential diagnosis of steatorrhoea.

Other blood tests. Serum immunoglobulins are measured to exclude immune deficiencies. Auto-antibodies to reticulin or gliadin may be measured in suspected coeliac disease but are unhelpful in clinical practice in adult patients. Hormones, e.g. vasoactive intestinal peptide (VIP) are measured in high-volume secretory diarrhoea.

Test for protein-losing enteropathy. Intravenous radio-active chromium chloride ($^{51}CrCl_3$) is used to label circulating albumin. In excess gastrointestinal protein loss, the faeces will contain radioactivity. This test is rarely required unless a low serum albumin is a major clinical feature.

Intestinal permeability tests. These tests can be used for the detection of small-bowel disease but are not in general use. They are based on the fact that the abnormal intestinal mucosa is permeable to large molecules such as lactulose and cellobiose. An oral load of these sugars is given and the sugars are then measured in the urine. Recently, radiolabelled sodium-EDTA has been used in a similar way and is said to be a more accurate investigation.

MALABSORPTION

In many small-bowel diseases, malabsorption of specific substances occurs, but these deficiencies do not dominate the clinical picture. An example is Crohn's disease, in which malabsorption of vitamin B_{12} can be demonstrated, but this is not usually a problem and diarrhoea and general ill-health are the major features. Steatorrhoea—malabsorption of fat—is discussed on p. 199.

The major disorders of the small intestine that cause malabsorption are shown in Table 4.10.

Coeliac disease (gluten-sensitive enteropathy)

Coeliac disease is a condition in which there is an abnormal jejunal mucosa that improves morphologically when the patient is treated with a gluten-

Table 4.10 Disorders of the small intestine causing malabsorption.

Coeliac disease
Dermatitis herpetiformis
Tropical sprue
Bacterial overgrowth
Intestinal resection
Whipple's disease
Radiation enteritis
Parasite infestation, e.g. *Giardia lamblia*

free diet and relapses when gluten is reintroduced. Gluten is contained in the cereals wheat, rye, barley and possibly oats.

Dermatitis herpetiformis is a skin disorder that is associated with a gluten-sensitive enteropathy (see below).

INCIDENCE

Coeliac disease is common in Europe, with an incidence in the UK of approximately 1 in 2000. In Ireland, however, this is 1 in 300. It occurs throughout the world but is rare in the black African.

INHERITANCE

There is an increased incidence of coeliac disease within families but the exact mode of inheritance is unknown; 10–15% of first-degree relatives will have the condition, although it may be asymptomatic. Over 80% of patients have the haplotype HLA-A1, B8, DR3, DR7, DQW2 as compared to 20–30% of the general population. However, the fact that not all patients have this haplotype and that as many as 30% of identical twins are discordant for the condition, suggests an additional factor. This additional factor may be a B-cell antigen or the immunoglobulin heavy-chain allotype.

AETIOLOGY

Gluten is a high-molecular-weight, heterogeneous compound that can be fractionated to produce α, β, γ and ω gliadin peptides. α-Gliadin is injurious to the small-intestinal mucosa although there is some disagreement about the other peptides. The exact mechanism of how the damage is produced is still not understood. There are many immunological abnormalities that revert to normal on treatment. An immunogenetic mechanism may be possible in view of the increased incidence of a particular HLA haplotype. An unconfirmed study has suggested that a viral infection may play a role in view of the amino-acid sequence homology between gliadin and Adenovirus 12.

PATHOLOGY

The mucosa of the proximal small bowel is predominantly affected, the mucosal damage decreasing in severity towards the ileum as the gluten is digested into smaller non-toxic fragments.

Under the dissecting microscope (× 40) there is an absence of villi, making the mucosal surface flat. Histological examination shows that the crypts are elongated, with chronic inflammatory cells in the lamina propria (see Fig. 4.20). The lesion is described as *subtotal villous atrophy*, although true

atrophy of the mucosa is not present because crypt hypertrophy compensates for villous loss and the total mucosal thickness is normal.

The surface cells become cuboidal. There is an increase in the intraepithelial lymphocytes but this change is not specific for coeliac disease. In the lamina propria there is an increase in lymphocytes as well as plasma cells containing IgM.

CLINICAL FEATURES

Coeliac disease can present at any age. In infancy it appears after weaning on to gluten-containing foods. The peak incidence in adults is in the third and fourth decade, with a female preponderance. The symptoms are very variable and often non-specific with tiredness and malaise. Common GI symptoms include diarrhoea or steatorrhoea, abdominal discomfort or pain and weight loss.

Mouth ulcers and angular stomatitis are frequent and can be intermittent. Rare complications include tetany, osteomalacia, neurological symptoms such as paraesthesia, muscle weakness or peripheral neuropathy, or gross malnutrition with peripheral oedema.

There is an increased incidence of atopy and autoimmune disease, including thyroid disease, insulin-dependent diabetes, inflammatory bowel disease, chronic liver disease, and fibrosing allergic alveolitis.

Physical signs are usually few and non-specific and are related to anaemia and malnutrition.

INVESTIGATION

- *Jejunal biopsy*. The mucosal appearance of a jejunal biopsy specimen is diagnostic and this investigation should always be performed in suspected cases. Other causes of a flat mucosa in adults are rare and are shown in Fig. 4.18. If the biopsy is performed endoscopically, a dye can be injected on to the duodenal mucosa to accentuate the smoothness of the mucosa (positive dye test) before the biopsy is taken.
- *Haematology*. A mild or moderate anaemia is present in 50% of cases. Folate deficiency is almost invariably present in coeliac disease, giving rise in most instances to a high MCV. B$_{12}$ deficiency is rare but iron deficiency due to malabsorption of iron and increased loss of desquamated cells is common. A blood film may therefore show micro- and macrocytes as well as hypersegmented polymorphonuclear leucocytes and Howell–Jolly bodies (due to splenic atrophy).
- *Antireticulin antibodies* and *antigliadin antibodies (IgA)* are found in the serum of the majority of cases.
- *Absorption tests* are often abnormal (see p. 203) but are seldom performed.

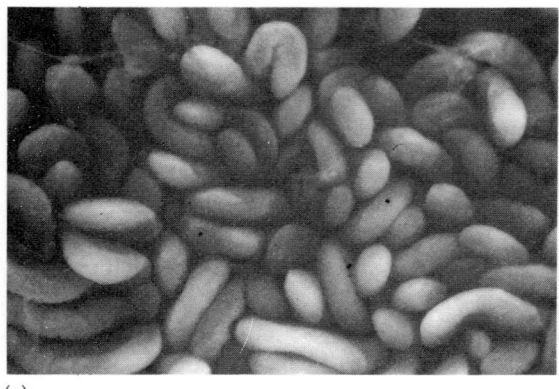

(a)

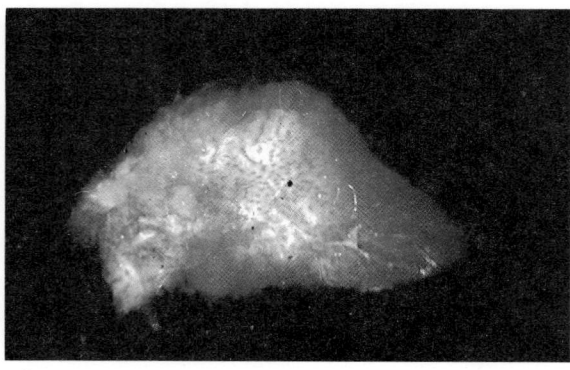

(b)

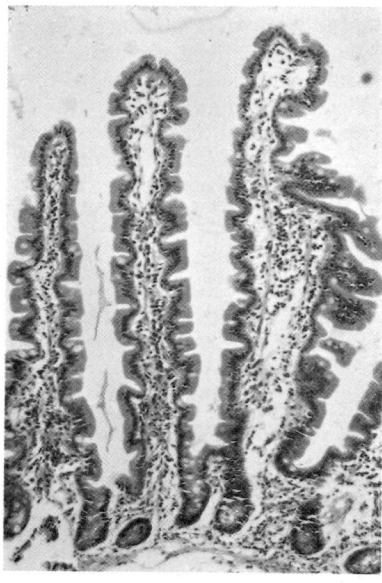

(c)

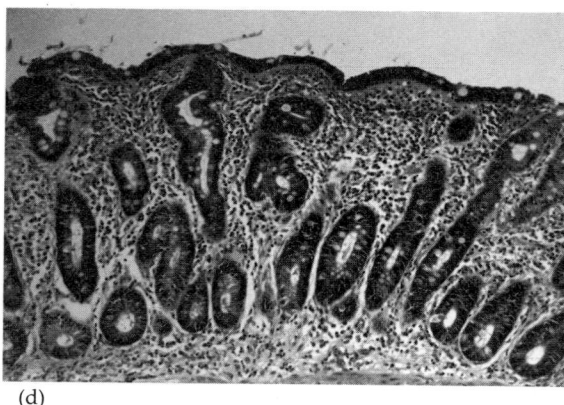

(d)

Fig. 4.20 (*a and b*) The dissecting microscopic appearances of (a) normal mucosa and (b) abnormal mucosa from a patient with coeliac disease. (*c and d*) The histological appearances of (c) normal mucosa and (b) abnormal mucosa from a patient with coeliac disease.

- *A small-bowel follow-through* may show dilatation of the small bowel with a change in fold pattern; folds become thicker and in the severer forms total effacement is seen.
- In the severely ill patient other biochemical abnormalities are seen, e.g. hypoalbuminaemia.

TREATMENT AND MANAGEMENT

A gluten-free diet usually produces a rapid clinical and morphological improvement. Replacement haematinics are given initially to replace body stores. The usual cause for failure to respond to the diet is poor compliance. A gluten challenge, i.e. reintroduction of gluten with evidence of jejunal morphological change, confirms the diagnosis. In the straightforward cases this is not necessary, although transient gluten intolerance has been described in early childhood.

Many patients do not keep to a strict diet but nevertheless maintain good health. The long-term effects of this low gluten intake are uncertain.

COMPLICATIONS

A few patients do not improve on a strict diet (unresponsive 'coeliac disease'). Often no cause for this is found, but intestinal lymphoma or carcinoma are sometimes responsible. The incidence of small-intestinal lymphoma is increased in coeliac disease. Carcinoma of the small bowel and oesophagus as well as extra-gastrointestinal cancers are also seen. Malignancy seems to be unrelated to the duration of the disease but the incidence may be reduced with treatment.

Dermatitis herpetiformis (see p. 1020)

This is an uncommon blistering subepidermal eruption of the skin associated with a gluten-sensitive enteropathy. Rarely there may be gross malabsorption, but usually the jejunal morphological abnormalities are not as severe as in coeliac disease. The inheritance and immunological abnormalities are the same as for coeliac disease. The skin condition responds to dapsone but both the gut and the skin will improve on a gluten-free diet. On this diet the need for dapsone is reduced.

Tropical sprue

This is a condition presenting with malabsorption that occurs in residents or visitors to a tropical area where the disease is endemic.

Malabsorption of a mild degree, sometimes following an enteric infection, is quite common and is usually asymptomatic. The term *tropical sprue* is reserved for severe malabsorption (of two or more substances) that is usually accompanied by diarrhoea and malnutrition. Tropical sprue is endemic in most of Asia, some Caribbean islands, Puerto Rico and parts of South America. Epidemics occur, lasting up to 2 years, and in some areas repeated epidemics occur at varying intervals of up to 10 years.

AETIOLOGY

The aetiology is unknown but is likely to be infective because the disease occurs in epidemics and patients improve on antibiotics.

A number of agents have been suggested but none has been shown to be unequivocally responsible. Different agents could be involved in different parts of the world. An overgrowth of coliforms that produce an enterotoxin has been reported.

CLINICAL FEATURES

These vary in intensity and consist of diarrhoea, anorexia, abdominal distension and weight loss. The onset is sometimes acute and occurs either a few days or many years after being in the tropics. Epidemics can break out in villages, affecting thousands of people at the same time. The onset can also be insidious, with chronic diarrhoea and evidence of nutritional deficiency.

The clinical features of tropical sprue vary in different parts of the world, particularly as different criteria are used for diagnosis.

DIAGNOSIS

- Acute infective causes of diarrhoea must be excluded (see p. 223), particularly *Giardia*, which can produce a syndrome very similar to tropical sprue.
- Malabsorption should be demonstrated, particularly fat and B_{12} malabsorption.
- The jejunal mucosa is abnormal, showing some villus atrophy (partial villus atrophy). In most cases the lesion is less severe than that found in coeliac disease, although it affects the whole small bowel. Mild changes can be seen in asymptomatic individuals in the tropics, so jejunal mucosal changes must be interpreted carefully.

TREATMENT

Many patients improve when they leave the sprue area and take folic acid (5 mg daily). Most patients also require an antibiotic (usually tetracycline 1 g daily) to ensure a complete recovery; it may be necessary to give this for up to 6 months.

The severely ill patient requires resuscitation with fluids and electrolytes for dehydration; any nutritonal deficiencies should be corrected. Vitamin B_{12} (1000 µg) is also given to all acute cases.

PROGNOSIS

The prognosis is excellent. Mortality is usually associated with water and electrolyte depletion, particularly in epidemics.

Bacterial overgrowth

The upper part of the small intestine is almost sterile, containing only a few organisms derived from the mouth. Gastric acid kills most organisms and intestinal motility keeps the jejunum empty. The normal terminal ileum contains faecal-type organisms, mainly *Escherichia coli* and anaerobes.

Bacterial overgrowth is normally only found associated with a structural abnormality of the small intestine, although it can occur alone in the elderly.

Aspiration of the upper jejunum will reveal the presence of *E. coli* and/or *Bacteroides*, both in concentrations greater than 10^6 per ml as part of a mixed flora. These bacteria are capable of deconjugating and dehydroxylating bile salts, so that unconjugated and dehydroxylated bile salts can be detected in aspirates by chromoatography. Steatorrhoea (see p. 199) occurs as a result of conjugated bile salt deficiency.

The bacteria are able to metabolize B_{12} and interfere with its binding to intrinsic factor, thereby leading to B_{12} deficiency; this can be demonstrated using the Schilling test. Conversely some bacteria produce folic acid.

Bacterial overgrowth has only minimal effects on other substances absorbed from the small intestine. The clinical features are chiefly diarrhoea, steatorrhoea and vitamin B_{12} deficiency, although this is not so severe as to produce a neurological deficit.

Although bacterial overgrowth may be responsible for the presenting symptoms, it must be remembered that many of the symptoms may be due to the underlying small-bowel pathology.

TREATMENT

If possible, the underlying lesion should be corrected, e.g. a stricture should be resected. With multiple diverticula, grossly dilated bowel, or in

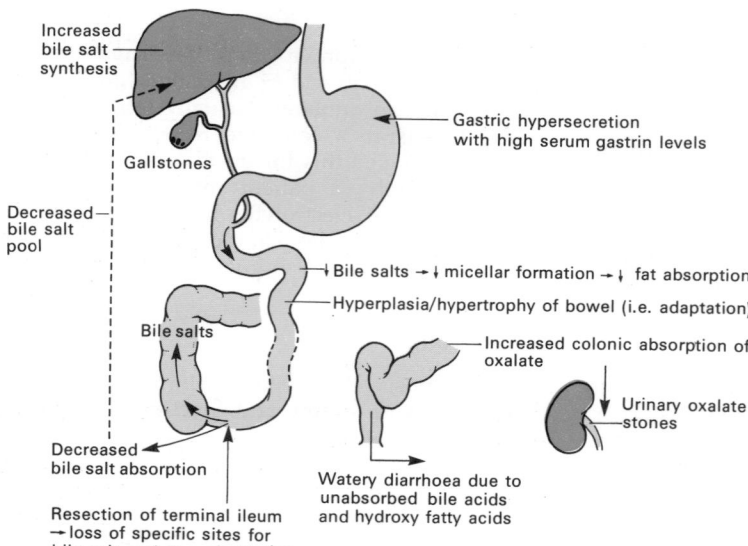

Fig. 4.21 The effects of resection of the distal small bowel.

Crohn's disease, this may not be possible and rotating courses of antibiotics are necessary, such as metronidazole and tetracycline.

Intestinal resection (Fig. 4.21)

Intestinal resection is usually well-tolerated but massive resection is followed by the short-gut syndrome. The effects of resection depend on the extent and the areas involved.

Extent
Because the gut is long, a 30–50% resection can usually be tolerated without undue problems.

Site of resection
The ileum has specific receptors for the absorption of bile salts and vitamin B_{12}, so that relatively small resections will lead to malabsorption of these substances. Removal of the ileocaecal valve increases the incidence of diarrhoea.

In ileal resection:

- Bile salts and fatty acids enter the colon and interfere with water and electrolyte absorption, causing diarrhoea.
- Increased bile salt synthesis can compensate for loss of approximately one-third of the bile salts in the faeces. Greater loss than this results in decreased micellar formation and steatorrhoea, and lithogenic bile and gallstone formation.
- Increased oxalate absorption is caused by the presence of bile salts in the colon. This gives rise to renal oxalate stones.
- There is a low serum B_{12} and macrocytosis.

However, in jejunal resection the ileum can take

over jejunal absorptive function. Jejunal resection may lead to gastric hypersecretion with high gastrin levels; the exact mechanism of this is unclear.

Intestinal adaptation takes place, with an increase in the absorption per unit length of bowel. Patients with massive resection often require parental nutrition initially, but with adaptation most will eventually recover, although continuing to have diarrhoea and having little functional reserve should another GI problem occur. A low-fat diet is often required.

Whipple's disease

This is a rare disease usually affecting males. It presents with steatorrhoea and abdominal pain along with systemic symptoms of fever and weight loss. Peripheral lymphadenopathy, arthritis and involvement of the heart, lung and brain may occur. Histologically, the villi are stunted and contain diagnostic periodic acid–Schiff (PAS)-positive macrophages on electron microscopy; bacilli of an unknown type can be seen 'within' the macrophages.

A dramatic improvement occurs with antibiotic therapy, which should include an antibiotic that crosses the blood–brain barrier, e.g. chloramphenicol.

Radiation enteritis

Radiation of more than 50 Gy will damage the intestine. The ileum and rectum are the areas most often involved, as pelvic irradiation is the common cause. There may be acute signs of diarrhoea and abdominal pain at the time of the irradiation. These usually improve within 6 weeks after completion of therapy. Chronic radiation enteritis is diagnosed if symptoms persist for 3 months or more. The prevalence is more than 15%, although many more patients suffer from an increased bowel frequency.

Rectal damage produces a radiation proctitis with diarrhoea, with or without blood and tenesmus. Treatment is symptomatic; local steroids sometimes help.

Radiation enteritis produces muscle fibre atrophy, ulcerative changes due to ischaemia, and obstruction due to strictures produced by radiation-induced fibrosis. The symptoms are often that of obstruction, which is usually partial but eventually may be complete. Malabsorption due to mucosal damage as well as bacterial overgrowth in dilated segments can occur. Treatment is symptomatic although often unsuccessful in chronic enteritis. Surgery should be avoided if at all possible, being reserved for life-threatening situations such as complete obstruction or occasionally perforation.

Parasite infestation

Giardia lamblia (see p. 90) not only produces diarrhoea but can produce malabsorption with steatorrhoea. Minor changes are seen in the jejunal mucosa and the organism can be found in the jejunal fluid or mucosa.

Cryptosporidiosis (see p. 90) can also produce malabsorption.

Other causes of malabsorption

- *Drugs* that bind bile salts, e.g. cholestyramine, and some antibiotics, e.g. neomycin, produce steatorrhoea.
- Diarrhoea, rarely with steatorrhoea, occurs in *thyrotoxicosis* owing to increased gastric emptying and motility. Steatorrhoea occurs in the *Zollinger–Ellison* syndrome (p. 235).
- *Intestinal lymphangiectasia* produces diarrhoea and rarely steatorrhoea.
- *Lymphoma* that has infiltrated the small bowel mucosa.
- In some patients with *diabetes mellitus*, diarrhoea, malabsorption and steatorrhoea occur, sometimes due to bacterial overgrowth from stasis.
- *Hypogammaglobulinaemia*, which is seen in many conditions including lymphoid nodular hyperplasia, causes steatorrhoea owing either to an abnormal jejunal mucosa or to secondary infestation with *Giardia lamblia*.

MISCELLANEOUS INTESTINAL DISORDERS

Protein-losing enteropathy

Protein-losing enteropathy is seen in many gastrointestinal and systemic conditions. Increased protein loss across an abnormal mucosa causes hypoalbuminaemia. Causes include inflammatory or ulcerative lesions, e.g. Crohn's disease, tumours, Ménétrier's disease, coeliac disease and lymphatic disorders, e.g. lymphangiectasia. Usually it forms a minor part of the generalized disorder but, occasionally hepatic synthesis of albumin cannot compensate for the hypoalbuminaemia, and the peripheral oedema produced may dominate the clinical picture. The investigations are described on p. 204 and treatment is that of the underlying disorder.

Meckel's diverticulum

This is the commonest congenital abnormality of the GI tract, affecting 2–3% of the population. The diverticulum projects from the wall of the ileum approximately 60 cm from the ileocaecal valve. It is usually symptomless but 50% contain gastric mucosa that secretes hydrochloric acid. Peptic ulcers can occur and may bleed (see p. 195) or perforate.

Acute inflammation of the diverticulum also occurs and is indistinguishable clinically from acute appendicitis. Obstruction from an associated band rarely occurs. Treatment is surgical removal.

Tuberculosis

Tuberculosis (TB) can affect the intestine as well as the peritoneum (see p. 229).

Intestinal tuberculosis is due to reactivation of primary disease caused by *M. tuberculosis*. Bovine TB occurs in areas where milk is unpasteurized and is very rare in the UK.

The ileocaecal area is most commonly affected, but the colon, and rarely other parts of the gastrointestinal tract, can also be involved.

CLINICAL FEATURES

These are chiefly diarrhoea and abdominal pain with generalized systemic manifestations, including anorexia and weight loss. Intestinal obstruction may develop.

On examination, a mass may be palpable and 50% have X-ray evidence of pulmonary tuberculosis; this is an important aid to the diagnosis.

DIAGNOSIS

In the Western hemisphere TB must be differentiated from Crohn's disease and should always be considered as a possible diagnosis in Asian immigrants. An ultrasound of the abdomen may show mesenteric thickening and lymph-node enlargement. Histological verification and culture of tissue is highly desirable but it is not always possible to obtain bacteriological confirmation and treatment should be started if there is a high degree of suspicion. Specimens can be obtained by colonoscopy but laparotomy is required in some cases.

TREATMENT

Drug treatment is similar to pulmonary TB, i.e. rifampicin, isoniazid and pyrazinamide (see p. 682) but treatment should last one year.

Amyloid (see p. 869)

In systemic amyloidosis there is usually a diffuse involvement that may affect any part of the GI tract. Occasionally amyloid deposits occur as polypoid lesions. The symptoms depend on the site of involvement; amyloidosis in the small intestine gives rise to diarrhoea.

Connective-tissue disorders

Systemic sclerosis (see p. 394) most commonly affects the oesophagus (see p. 183), although the small bowel and colon are often found to be involved if the appropriate radiological studies are performed. Frequently there are no symptoms of this involvement, but diarrhoea and steatorrhoea can occur. This is usually due to bacterial overgrowth of the small bowel as a result of reduced motility, dilatation and the presence of diverticula.

In *rheumatoid arthritis* (p. 384) and *systemic lupus erythematosus* (p. 391), gastrointestinal symptoms may occur but rarely predominate.

Chronic intestinal ischaemia

This is due to atheromatous occlusion of mesenteric vessels in the elderly, although such occlusion often does not produce clinical effects because of the collateral circulation. The characteristic symptom is abdominal pain occurring after food. This may be followed by acute mesenteric vascular occlusion (see p. 228). Loud bruits may be heard but, as these are heard in normal subjects, they are of doubtful significance. The diagnosis is made using angiography.

The term 'coeliac axis compression syndrome' has been used in young patients with chronic abdominal pain, bruits and minor angiographic changes. Despite its plausible title, it is not an organic syndrome. Its suggested existence results from the false correlation of pain and bruits.

Eosinophilic gastroenteritis

This is a condition of unknown aetiology in which there may be eosinophilic infiltration and oedema of any part of the gastrointestinal mucosa. It usually involves the gastric antrum and proximal small intestine either as a localized lesion (eosino-

philic granuloma) or diffusely with sheets of eosinophils seen in the serosal and submucosal layers. An association with asthma, eczema and urticaria has been described.

The condition may occur at any age but mainly in the third decade. Males are affected twice as often as females. The clinical presentation depends on the site of involvement. Abdominal pain, nausea and vomiting occur. An increased number of eosinophils in the blood is present in only 20% of patients. Radiology or endoscopy will demonstrate the lesion. Steroids are used for the widespread infiltration, particularly if eosinophilia is present.

In some adults the condition appears to be allergic (allergic gastroenteritis) and is associated with peripheral eosinophilia and high levels of blood and tissue IgE.

Intestinal lymphangiectasia

Dilatation of the lymphatics may be primary or secondary to lymphatic obstruction, such as that occurring in malignancy or constrictive pericarditis. In the rare primary form it may be detected incidentally as dilated lacteals on a jejunal biopsy or it can produce steatorrhoea of varying degrees. Hypoproteinaemia with ankle oedema is the main feature. Serum immunoglobulin levels are reduced with low circulating lymphocytes. Treatment is with a low-fat diet.

Abetalipoproteinaemia

In this rare condition there is failure of apo B100 synthesis in the intestinal cell, so that chylomicrons are not formed. This leads to fat accumulation in the intestinal cells, giving a characteristic appearance on jejunal biopsy. Clinical features include acanthocytosis (spiky red cells due to membrane abnormalities), retinitis pigmentosa, and mental and neurological abnormalities. The latter can be prevented by vitamin E injections.

GI problems in patients with HIV infection (see Table 4.18)

Inflammatory bowel disease

Two major forms of *non-specific* inflammatory bowel disease are recognized: Crohn's disease (CD), which can affect any part of the GI tract, and ulcerative colitis (UC), which affects only the large bowel.

There is overlap between these two conditions in their clinical features, and histological and radiological abnormalities; in 10% of cases of colitis a definitive diagnosis of either ulcerative colitis or Crohn's disease is not possible. Currently, it is necessary to distinguish between these two conditions because of certain differences in their managment. However, it is possible that these conditions represent two aspects of the same disease.

EPIDEMIOLOGY AND AETIOLOGY

- The *incidence* of Crohn's disease varies from country to country but is approximately 5–6 per 100 000 with a prevalence of 50–60 per 100 000. The incidence of ulcerative colitis is 5–10 per 100 000 per year with a prevalence of 80–120 per 100 000.
- *Age.* Both conditions can occur at any age. Crohn's disease is uncommon before the age of 10 with a peak incidence between 20 and 40 years. A late peak affecting mainly the colon has been reported in women aged over 60 years. Ulcerative colitis occurs mainly between 20–40.
- *Sex.* Both sexes are affected, but in ulcerative colitis women are more frequently affected than men.
- *Race.* Both conditions have a world-wide distribution but are more common in the Western World. The incidence is lower in the non-white races. Jews are more prone to inflammatory bowel disease than non-Jews; the Ashkenazi Jews have a higher risk than the Sephardic Jews.
- *Familial.* Both conditions are more common amongst relatives of patients than in the general population. There is a tendency for both twins to be affected.
- *Genetic.* There are no HLA markers but HLA-B27 is increased in patients with inflammatory bowel disease and ankylosing spondylitis.
- *Smoking.* Patients with CD are more likely to be tobacco smokers and there is an increased risk of UC amongst non-smokers or exsmokers.
- *Other factors.* The aetiology is unknown but the racial differences and geographical clustering suggest both genetic and environmental causes. A cluster of patients with Crohn's disease has been found in a Cotswold village in England.
- *Infective agent.* In Crohn's disease the most attractive hypothesis is that of a transmissible agent. No bacterium, virus or parasite has been definitely identified.

    Mycobacterium. In cattle and sheep, Johne's disease, which is a chronic inflammatory disorder of the distal ileum, is caused by *M. paratuberculosis.* A mycobacterium has been isolated from Crohn's disease tissue but current evidence is against this being an aetiological agent. Granulomas are character-istic of Crohn's disease but are also seen in tuberculosis and sarcoidosis suggesting a common pathogenetic link, although none has been found.

    Cell wall deficient organism, L-forms, plas-mids may be the transmissible agent but this theory lacks any evidence.
- Viruses have been reported in tissue from UC and CD patients but there is no compelling data.
- *Immunology.* Many immunological abnormalities have been described in IBD. Recent studies show:

    Platelet activating factor (PAF) is increased in active UC tissue. PAF is stimulated by other inflammatory mediators e.g. leukotrienes, interleukins (see p. 137) and is chemotactic for inflammatory cells. A PAF inhibitor may constitute a new treatment in the future.

    Macrophages. Changes in macrophage sub-types in the inflamed tissue have been reported, suggesting defective macrophage function in clearing immune complexes.

    Autoimmunity. The original data suggesting a role has not been confirmed.

These as well as other humoral and cellular mechanisms are being studied but many abnormal-ities may well be secondary to the disease process and play no part in the pathogenesis.

- *Multifocal gastrointestinal infarction* has recently been implicated as a primary event.

PATHOLOGY

Crohn's disease is a chronic inflammatory condi-tion that may affect any part of the GI tract from the mouth to the anus but has a particular tendency to affect the terminal ileum. The disease can involve one small area of the gut such as the terminal ileum, or multiple areas with relatively normal bowel in between ('skip lesions'). It may also be extensive, involving the whole of the colon and/or small bowel.

Ulcerative colitis can affect the rectum alone (proctitis), can extend proximally to involve the sigmoid and descending colon ('left-sided colitis'), or may involve the whole colon ('total colitis'). In some of these patients there is also inflammation of the distal terminal ileum ('backwash ileitis').

Macroscopic changes
In Crohn's disease the involved bowel is usually thickened and narrowed. There are deep ulcers and fissures in the mucosa, producing a cobble-stone appearance. Fistulas and abscesses may be seen. An early sign is aphthoid ulceration that can be seen endoscopically.

In ulcerative colitis the mucosa looks reddened, inflamed and bleeds easily. In severe disease there is extensive ulceration, with the adjacent mucosa appearing as inflammatory polyps. In fulminant disease most of the mucosa is lost, leaving a few islands of oedematous mucosa (mucosal islands) and toxic dilatation occurs. On healing, the mucosa can return to normal, although there is usually some residual glandular distortion.

Microscopic changes

In Crohn's disease the inflammation extends through all layers of the bowel, whereas in ulcerative colitis a superficial inflammation is seen. In Crohn's disease there is an increase in chronic inflammatory cells and lymphoid hyperplasia, and in 50–60% of patients granulomas are present. These granulomas are non-caseating epithelioid cells aggregates with Langhan's giant cells.

In ulcerative colitis the mucosa shows a chronic inflammatory cell infiltrate in the lamina propria. Crypt abscesses and goblet cell depletion are also seen.

The differentiation between these two diseases is made not only on the basis of clinical and radiological data but also on the histological differences seen in the rectal and colonic mucosa obtained by biopsy (Table 4.11).

Table 4.11 Histological differences between Crohn's disease and ulcerative colitis.

	Crohn's disease	Ulcerative colitis
Inflammation	Deep (transmural) Patchy	Superficial Continuous
Granulomas	++	Rare
Goblet cells	Present	Depleted
Crypt abscesses	+	++

CLINICAL FEATURES

Crohn's disease

The major symptoms are of diarrhoea, abdominal pain and weight loss. Constitutional symptoms of malaise, lethargy, anorexia, nausea, vomiting and low-grade fever may be present. Despite the recurrent nature of this condition, many patients remain well and have an almost normal life-style. However, patients with extensive disease may have frequent recurrences necessitating multiple hospital admissions.

The clinical features are very variable and depend partly on the region of the bowel that is affected. The disease may present insidiously or acutely. The abdominal pain may be colicky, suggesting obstruction but it usually has no special characteristics and sometimes in colonic disease only minimal discomfort is present. Diarrhoea is present in 80% of all cases and in colonic disease may contain blood, making it difficult to differen-

tiate from ulcerative colitis. Steatorrhoea can be present in small-bowel disease. Some patients (15%) present with only anorexia, weight loss and general ill-health, with an absence of any other GI symptoms.

Crohn's disease may present as an emergency with acute right iliac fossa pain mimicking appendicitis. If laparotomy is undertaken, an oedematous, reddened terminal ileum is found. There are many other causes of an acute ileitis, e.g. infections such as *Yersinia*. Crohn's disease is the cause of approximately 10% of acute ileitis.

Examination. Physical signs are few, apart from loss of weight and general ill-health. Aphthous ulceration of the mouth is often seen. Abdominal examination is often normal, although tenderness and a right iliac fossa mass are occasionally found. This mass is due either to inflamed loops of bowel that are matted together or to an abscess. A careful examination of the anus should always be made to look for oedematous anal tags, fissures or perianal abscesses. These abnormalities are particularly common (80%) in colonic involvement.

Other extra-gastrointestinal features of inflammatory bowel disease should be looked for, e.g. erythema nodosum, arthritis, iritis (see below).

Sigmoidoscopy should always be performed in a patient with Crohn's disease. With small-bowel involvement the rectum may appear normal but a biopsy must be taken as non-specific histological changes may sometimes be found in the mucosa. Even with extensive colonic Crohn's disease the rectum may be spared and be relatively normal but patchy involvement with an oedematous haemorrhagic mucosa can be present.

Ulcerative colitis

The major symptom in ulcerative colitis is diarrhoea with blood and mucus, sometimes accompanied by lower abdominal discomfort. General features include malaise, lethargy and anorexia. Aphthous ulceration is seen. The disease can be mild, moderate or severe, and runs a course of remissions and exacerbations. Ten per cent of patients have persistent chronic symptoms, although some patients may have only a single attack.

Table 4.12 Definition of a severe attack of ulcerative colitis.

Stool frequency	> 6 stools per day with blood
Fever	> 37.5°C
Tachycardia	> 90 per minute
ESR	> 30 mm per hour
Anaemia	Haemoglobin < 10 g·dl^{-1}
Albumin	< 30 g·L^{-1}

When the disease is confined to the rectum, blood mixed with the stool, urgency and tenesmus are common. There are normally very few constitutional symptoms but patients are nevertheless greatly inconvenienced by the frequency of defaecation.

In an acute attack patients have bloody diarrhoea, passing 10–20 liquid stools per day. Diarrhoea also occurs at night, with urgency and incontinence that is severely disabling for the patient. Occasionally blood and mucus alone are passed.

The definition of a severe attack is given in Table 4.12. The patient may be very ill and needs careful monitoring in hospital with prompt treatment to avoid the development of complications, such as septicaemia, toxic dilatation and perforation.

Examination. In general there are no specific signs in ulcerative colitis. The abdomen may be slightly distended or tender to palpation. The anus is usually normal. Rectal examination will show the presence of blood. Sigmoidoscopy is always abnormal and shows an inflamed, bleeding, friable mucosa. A biopsy should be taken for histological diagnosis.

Extra-gastrointestinal manifestations
These occur with both diseases and some are related to the intestinal disease activity (see Table 4.13). Patients with Crohn's colitis have more extra-gastrointestinal complications than those with small-bowel lesions alone.

INVESTIGATIONS

Blood tests
Anaemia is common and is usually the normocytic, normochromic anaemia of chronic disease. Deficiency of iron and/or folate also occurs. Despite terminal ileal involvement in Crohn's disease, megaloblastic anaemia due to B_{12} deficiency is unusual, although the B_{12} level can be low. There

Table 4.13 Extra-gastrointestinal manifestations of inflammatory bowel disease.

	Per cent of cases	
	Crohn's disease	Ulcerative colitis
Eyes		
Uveitis		
Episcleritis	4	4
Conjunctivitis		
Joints		
Monoarticular arthritis	14	
Ankylosing spondylitis	2–6	11
Sacroiliitis	15–18	
Skin		
Erythema nodosum	5–10	2
Pyoderma gangrenosum	1	3
Vasculitis		
Liver[a,b]		
Fatty change	Common	Common
Pericholangitis	19	25
Sclerosing cholangitis	< 1	12
Chronic active hepatitis	Uncommon	Uncommon
Cirrhosis	7	19
Kidney[a]		
Stones	30	—
Gallbladder[a]		
Stones	30	5 (normal)

[a] These manifestations are not related to disease activity.
[b] Biochemical abnormalities are common, but clinically overt disease is uncommon.

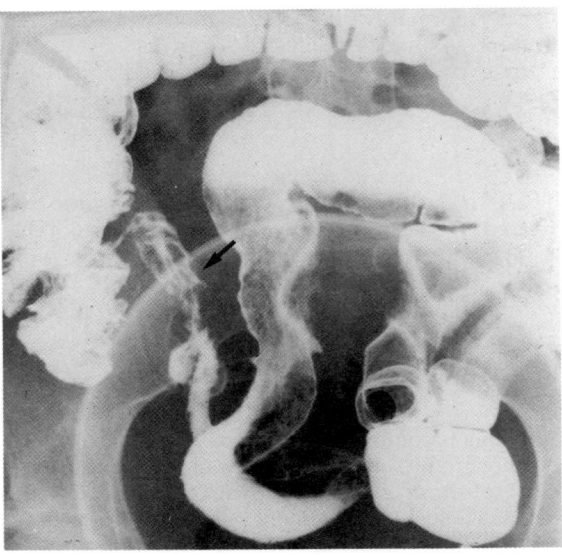

Fig. 4.22 Small-bowel follow-through showing narrowing and ulceration of the terminal ileum (arrow) in Crohn's disease.

is often a raised ESR and CRP and a raised white-cell count. Hypoalbuminaemia is present in severe disease. Liver biochemistry may be abnormal. Blood cultures are required if septicaemia is suspected.

Stool cultures
These should always be performed on presentation if diarrhoea is present.

Radiology
In Crohn's disease a small-bowel follow-through shows an asymmetrical alteration in the mucosal pattern with deep ulceration and areas of narrowing (string sign) largely confined to the ileum (Fig. 4.22). Skip lesions with normal bowel between are also seen. A barium enema is necessary to demonstrate large-bowel involvement. Early changes consist of aphthous ulceration (Fig. 4.23a); this involvement is again usually patchy, with deep ulceration developing later.

In ulcerative colitis a barium enema will show the extent of the disease (Fig. 4.23b) but it is not always possible to distinguish between ulcerative colitis and Crohn's disease. In long-standing disease the colon is shortened and narrowed. A plain abdominal X-ray should be performed if toxic dilatation is suspected.

Ultrasound and CT scanning are helpful in delineating abscesses, masses, thickened bowel wall and mesentery, or other extraluminal problems.

Colonoscopy
This is not always essential but is sometimes necessary to delineate the exact extent of the disease. It is also useful for obtaining biopsies from the whole colon and ileum to differentiate between Crohn's disease and ulcerative colitis. In ulcerative colitis it is used to detect premalignant mucosal dysplasia.

Small-bowel function tests (see p. 203)
When Crohn's disease involves the small bowel, other tests may be necessary, e.g. a breath test for bacterial overgrowth or a test for vitamin B_{12} absorption.

ACTIVITY OF DISEASE

A rough estimate of the activity can be made on the clinical picture and laboratory tests of ESR, serum albumin and acute-phase protein (e.g. CRP or orosomucoids). In some centres scans to localize areas of inflammation are performed using radio-labelled leucocytes injected i.v.; these may help in localizing abscesses.

DIFFERENTIAL DIAGNOSIS

Crohn's disease has to be considered in the differential diagnosis of all chronic diarrhoeas, malabsorption and malnutrition. It is also a differential diagnosis of small stature in children (see p. 795). A small-bowel follow-through usually differentiates it from other forms of small-bowel disease. Ileocaecal tuberculosis is common in Asia and Africa and in Asian immigrants in the UK. Acute ileitis due to *Yersinia* can be distinguished serologically. Lymphomas cause a major diagnostic difficulty.

Colitis, both ulcerative and Crohn's, must be differentiated from amoebic and ischaemic colitidis as well as infective causes of diarrhoea. The latter are becoming commoner in homosexuals (gay bowel disease) and should be suspected if multiple or unusual organisms are found. A rare cause of colitis is Behçet's disease, which also gives oro-genital ulceration.

In a few patients the mucosal appearance on colonoscopy and sigmoidoscopy is macroscopically normal and the inflammation is only detected histologically. This 'microscopic colitis' presents with chronic diarrhoea and is treated as a non-specific colitis. Collagenous colitis also presents as chronic diarrhoea; there is a thick subepithelial deposit of collagen in the macroscopically normal colonic mucosa.

TREATMENT

Medical management
Some patients require only symptomatic treatment.

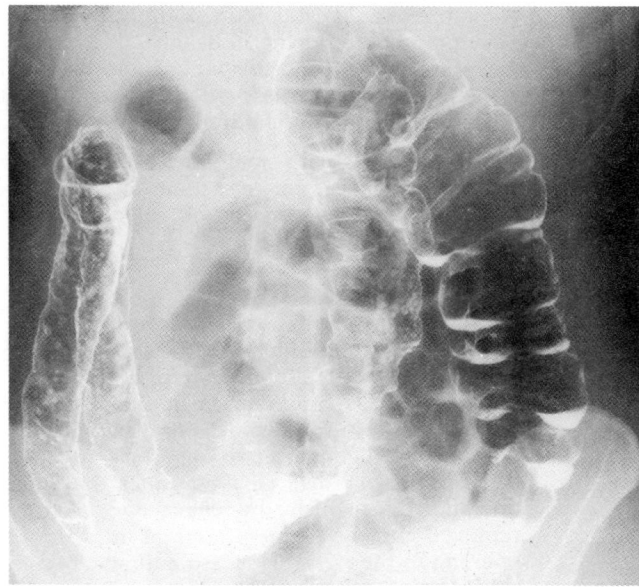

(a)

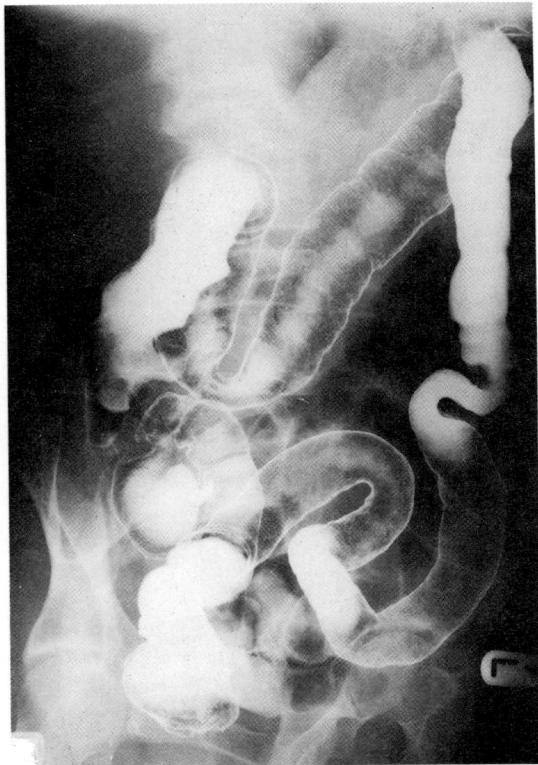

(b)

Fig. 4.23 (a) Double contrast barium enema showing early aphthous ulceration in Crohn's disease. Note the asymmetrical pattern. (b) Double contrast barium enema showing the fine ulceration and tubular colon of ulcerative colitis.

Diarrhoea can be controlled with agents such as loperamide 2–4 mg three times a day, codeine phosphate 30–60 mg three times daily, or diphenoxylate with atropine 1–2 tablets four times daily. Patients with more severe disease require specific medical therapy and acute attacks often require admission to hospital. Medical therapy relies mainly on anti-inflammatory and immunosuppressive drugs. The mechanism of action of these drugs in inflammatory bowel disease is unknown and treatment is largely empirical.

Anaemia will improve as the patient gets better, but appropriate haematinics, e.g. ferrous sulphate 400 mg daily or folic acid 5 mg daily may be required.

Crohn's disease. Acute attacks require oral corticosteroids 30–60 mg daily. On this regimen patients usually improve quickly and the steroid dosage can then be reduced. Mesalazine or sulphasalazine (see below) is used in patients with colonic involvement. Azathioprine ($2 \, \text{mg} \cdot \text{kg}^{-1}$ daily) is an immunosuppressive agent that has been shown to be helpful in maintaining the steroid-induced remission, although it has not gained universal acceptance. Patients with colonic involvement can also be given rectal steroids (see below). Metronidazole (800 mg three times daily) and co-trimoxazole (two tablets twice daily) are useful in severe perianal disease owing to their antibacterial action.

Elemental diets (see p. 167) or parenteral nutrition can induce remissions, usually in small-gut disease and particularly in children. They improve nutrition, allow the bowel to 'rest' and reduce antigen load to the bowel. Their mode of action is unclear and unfortunately most patients relapse on restarting a normal diet.

Some patients in remission may not require therapy but others need small doses of steroids to suppress the disease activity.

Ulcerative colitis. Severe attacks require careful management in hospital as the mortality of this condition is still high.

All patients with ulcerative colitis are treated with sulphasalazine, initially in a dose of 3–4 g daily reducing to a maintenance dose of 2 g daily. In mild cases it may induce a remission. Its main role, however, is to reduce the number of relapses when taken long term. Sulphasalazine consists of a 5-aminosalicylic acid (5-ASA) attached to sulphapyridine as a carrier. This combination is broken down in the colon by bacteria to release the active agent, 5-ASA. Sulphasalazine may induce nausea and has some reversible side-effects, including haemolytic anaemia, skin rashes and infertility in men. These are produced by the sulphapyridine and recently new forms of slow-release 5-ASA without sulphapyridine have been developed and are likely to supersede sulphasalazine. Mesalazine consists of a salicylate radicle attached to an inert compound via an azo bond. A dose of 400–1200 mg three times daily is used. Olsalazine consists of two molecules of 5-ASA linked by an azo bond and can also be used.

Mild attacks and proctitis can be treated with local rectal steroids in the form of enemas (prednisolone-21-phosphate 20 mg) or a 10% hydrocortisone foam. 5-ASA retention enemas are also useful.

Moderate attacks are treated with oral prednisolone 30–40 mg daily. Patients with their first attack or those who do not respond quickly should be admitted to hospital. In severe attacks, high-dose corticosteroids in the form of prednisolone 60 mg, hydrocortisone 100 mg i.v. 6-hourly or corticotrophin (synthetic ACTH) 1–2 mg i.m. are given. In addition, dehydration and electrolyte disturbances should be corrected by intravenous therapy. Accompanying septicaemia, which is usually due to Gram-negative bacteria, should be treated with antibiotics. Surgical treatment may be necessary if there is no improvement.

The main complication of severe ulcerative colitis and Crohn's colitis is toxic megacolon (see below).

Surgical management

Crohn's disease. Approximately 80% of patients will require an operation at some time during the course of their disease. Nevertheless, surgery should be avoided if possible and only minimal resections undertaken, as recurrence (15% per year) is almost inevitable. The indications for surgery are:

- Failure of medical therapy, with acute or chronic symptoms producing ill-health
- Complications, e.g. toxic dilatation, obstruction, perforation, abscesses, enterocutaneous fistula
- Failure to grow in children

In most patients with small-bowel disease, surgical treatment consists of resection and end-to-end anastomosis. The surgery of colonic disease is discussed below.

Ulcerative colitis. This disease is confined to the colon and therefore colectomy is curative.

Indications for surgery are the same as those for Crohn's disease, although complications of the disease are less common. In addition, a prophylactic colectomy is sometimes performed in patients who have a high cancer risk.

Protocolectomy with an ileostomy is the standard operation, in which the colon and rectum are removed and the ileum is brought out through an opening in the right iliac fossa and attached to the skin. The patient wears an ileostomy bag, which is stuck on to the skin over the ileostomy spout. This bag requires to be emptied once or twice daily. This is compatible with a near-normal life-style. Stoma-care therapists are readily available with help and advice.

Problems associated with ileostomies include:

- Mechanical problems
- Dehydration, particularly in hot climates
- Psychosexual problems
- Infertility in men
- Recurrence in Crohn's disease

In ulcerative colitis but *not* in Crohn's disease *colectomy with an ileorectal or ileoanal anastomosis is*

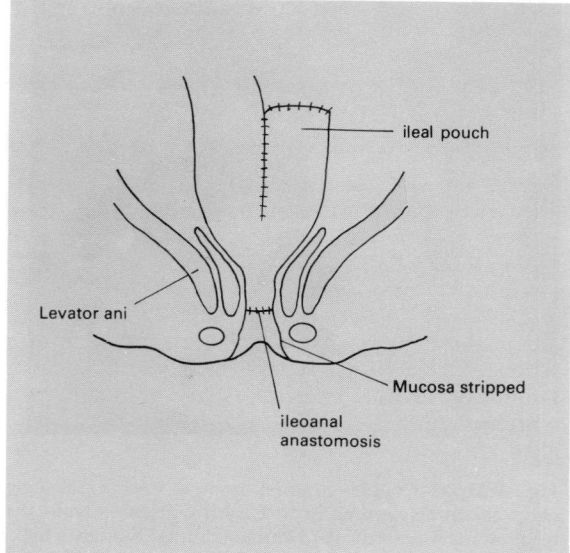

Fig. 4.24 Diagram of an ileoanal pouch for UC.

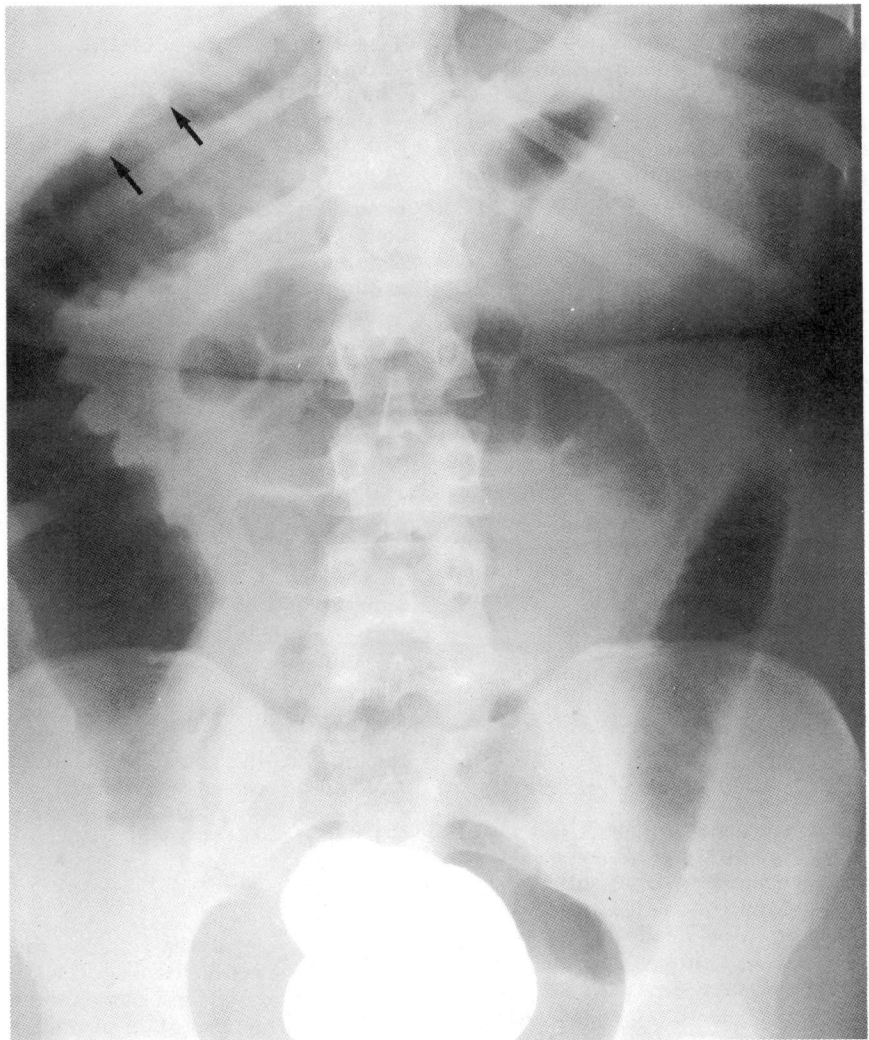

Fig. 4.25 Plain abdominal X-ray showing toxic dilatation in ulcerative colitis. The arrows indicate mucosal islands. Note the barium in the rectum. The enema was stopped because it is contraindicated in toxic dilatation.

used to avoid ileostomy. Ileorectal anastomosis leaves a diseased rectum *in situ* and frequent diarrhoea still occurs. With an ileoanal anastomosis (Fig. 4.24) a pouch of ileum is formed that acts as a reservoir and the patient is continent, with only a few bowel motions per day. The ileoanal operation is being increasingly used but inflammation of the pouch, 'pouchitis', can be a problem. It is not used for Crohn's disease because of the high recurrence rate.

COMPLICATIONS

These are similar in both conditions but vary in frequency. Crohn's disease, with its transmural inflammation, has a higher incidence of fistulas, fissures and abscess formation.

Perforation
This is a rare but serious complication that occurs in association with toxic megacolon. In Crohn's disease local perforations may occur, forming walled-off abscesses, and occasionally small-bowel perforation gives rise to peritonitis.

Haemorrhage
Massive haemorrhage is rare.

Toxic dilatation
Toxic dilatation may occur during an acute severe attack of colitis. The diagnosis should be suspected in a patient with a severe episode (see above) who develops abdominal distension. A plain abdominal X-ray (Fig. 4.25) will show a dilated thin-walled colon with a diameter greater than 5 cm that is gas-

filled and contains mucosal islands. Treatment is as for a severe attack of colitis plus daily abdominal X-rays and measurements of abdominal girth. If the patient does not settle in 48 h with high-dose corticosteroids, emergency surgery should be performed. When mucosal islands are present, the risk of perforation is high, as is the mortality, and many favour immediate surgery without medical therapy.

Carcinoma
The incidence is increased in both conditions (3–5%). In Crohn's disease the incidence of carcinoma is only marginally increased and does not influence management. In ulcerative colitis the risk of carcinoma of the colon in a patient who has had total colitis for more than 10 years is much greater than it is for the general population. It is suggested that regular sigmoidoscopy and colonoscopy with biopsies may detect early premalignant changes. However, the degree of surveillance necessary, or whether surveillance itself is of any benefit, is uncertain.

Amyloid is a rare complication and can affect the bowel or other organs; the kidneys may be affected with a deterioration of renal function.

COURSE AND PROGNOSIS

Crohn's disease
These patients have recurrent relapses and virtually all have a significant relapse over a 20-year period. The mortality rate is variable but generally appears to be at least twice as high as that seen in the normal population. Most deaths are associated with surgery. Despite this, many patients lead a normal life. Crohn's disease in childhood causes growth retardation.

Self-help groups provide patient information and a number of booklets that are invaluable for health staff and patients with inflammatory bowel disease.

Ulcerative colitis
The course and prognosis is variable. In proctitis it is very good; only 10% of these cases go on to develop more extensive disease. On the other hand, severe fulminant disease still carries a 15–25% mortality. The mortality is reduced if the acute attack is treated promptly and surgery is performed if no improvement occurs in the first 2–3 days.

Overall, because many cases are mild, the mortality of this disease is not much greater than the mortality rates for the general population, in contrast to Crohn's disease.

There is no particular risk to mother or child during pregnancy in either form of inflammatory bowel disease.

The colon and rectum

Structure

The large intestine starts at the caecum, on the posterior medial wall of which is the appendix. The colon is made up of ascending, transverse, descending and sigmoid parts, which join the rectum at the rectosigmoid junction.

The muscle wall consists of an inner circular layer and an outer longitudinal layer. The outer layer is incomplete, coming together to form the taenia coli, which produce the haustral pattern seen in the normal colon.

The mucosa of the colon is lined with epithelial cells with crypts but no villi, so that the surface is flat. The mucosa is full of goblet cells. A variety of cells, mainly lymphocytes and macrophages, are found in the lamina propria.

The blood supply to the colon is from the superior and inferior mesenteric vessels. Generally there are good anastomotic channels, but the caecum and splenic flexure are areas where ischaemia can occur.

The rectum is about 12 cm long. Its interior is divided by three crescentic circular muscles producing shelf-like folds. These are the rectal valves and can be seen at sigmoidoscopy.

The anal canal has an internal and an external sphincter.

Physiology

The main role of the colon is the absorption of water and electrolytes (see Table 4.14). Approximately 2 litres of fluid passes the ileocaecal valve each day. The absorption of fluid and electrolytes takes place mainly in the right side of the colon, and only about 150 ml is passed in the faeces.

The role of the rectum and anus in defaecation is complex. The rectum is usually empty and collapsed; the entry of faeces from the colon produces

Table 4.14 Input and output of water and electrolytes in the gastrointestinal tract over 24 h.

	Water (ml)	Sodium (mmol)	Potassium (mmol)
Input			
Diet	1500	150	80
GI secretions	7500	1000	40
Total	9000	1150	120
Output			
Faeces	150	5	12
Ileostomy (adapted)	500–1500	60–120	4

relaxation of the internal sphincter and the pubo-rectalis muscle. This decreases the acute angle between the rectum and the anal canal. When the rectum contains approximately 100 ml of faeces the urge to defecate is experienced. The rectum is emptied by relaxation of the external anal sphincter (under voluntary control) and an increase in intra-abdominal pressure.

Diverticular disease

Diverticula are frequently found in the colon and occur in 50% of patients over the age of 50. They are most frequent in the sigmoid, but can be present over the whole colon.

The term *diverticulosis* indicates the presence of diverticula; *diverticulitis* implies that these diverticula are inflamed. It is perhaps better to use the more general term *diverticular disease*, as it is often difficult to be sure whether the diverticula are inflamed. The precise mechanism of diverticula formation is not known. There is thickening of the muscle layer and, because of high intraluminal pressures, pouches of mucosa extrude through the muscular wall through weakened areas near blood vessels to form diverticula. Diverticular disease seems to be related to the low-fibre diet eaten in the Western hemisphere.

Diverticulitis occurs when faeces obstruct the neck of the diverticulum causing stagnation and allowing bacteria to multiply and produce inflammation. This can then lead to bowel perforation (peridiverticulitis), abscess formation, fistulas into adjacent organs, or even generalized peritonitis.

CLINICAL FEATURES AND MANAGEMENT

Diverticular disease is asymptomatic in 90% and is usually discovered incidentally; no treatment is required.

It may present with pain in the left iliac fossa, sometimes associated with either constipation or the passage of frequent loose stools. On examination there may be tenderness in the left iliac fossa. Rectal examination and sigmoidoscopy are normal. Diagnosis is made on barium enema examination (Fig. 4.26).

Diverticula are often seen and can be an incidental finding, so care must be taken not to miss any other lesion such as a carcinoma. The symptoms are very similar to those of the irritable bowel syndrome and, because both conditions are so common, it is often difficult to distinguish between them. In practice, both conditions are treated symptomatically with a high-fibre diet, antispasmodic drugs (e.g. mebeverine 135 mg three times daily) and agents to regulate the bowel.

Acute diverticulitis almost always affects diverticula in the sigmoid colon. It presents with severe pain in the left iliac fossa, often accompanied by

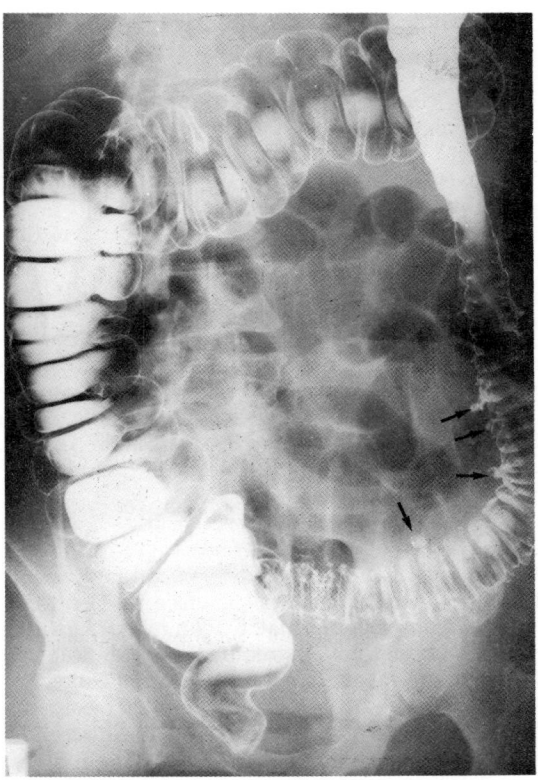

Fig. 4.26 Double contrast barium enema showing diverticular disease (the diverticula are arrowed). Note the mucosal hypertrophy.

fever and constipation. These symptoms and signs are similar to appendicitis but on the left side. On examination there is tenderness, guarding and rigidity on the left side of the abdomen. Tachycardia and pyrexia are present and the white-cell count shows a leucocytosis. An abdominal X-ray is performed to exclude free perforation.

COMPLICATIONS OF ACUTE DIVERTICULITIS

- *Abscess formation*, causing pain, pyrexia, and a palpable tender mass in the left iliac fossa. Ultrasound or CT scanning can show the mass. Surgical drainage with or without a defunctioning colostomy may be required. Antibiotics are always given.
- *Perforation*, leading to generalized peritonitis (see p. 227).
- *Fistula formation* into the bladder, causing dysuria or pneumaturia, or into the vagina, causing discharge; the diverticular disease is often chronic, without evidence of acute inflammation. Surgery is usually required.
- *Intestinal obstruction* (see p. 228). Acute attacks are treated with bowel rest, intravenous fluids

and antibiotics, e.g. ampicillin and metro-nidazole. Most attacks settle on this regimen, but a few require emergency surgery, which usually consists of a defunctioning colostomy to be followed later by resection.

Acute episodes do not necessarily recur and elective surgery is mainly reserved for patients with intestinal obstruction or fistulae.

- *Rectal bleeding.* Diverticular disease can produce rectal bleeding, which is sometimes massive, particularly from right-sided diverticula. In most cases the bleeding stops and the cause of the bleeding can be established by X-ray, colonoscopy and sometimes angiography. In rare cases emergency colectomy is necessary. It is unwise to ascribe an iron-deficiency anaemia to a bleeding diverticulum unless all other causes, e.g. piles or carcinoma, have been excluded.

Simple constipation

This is a major problem that is so common that it need not be considered as a disease. The long-standing constipation that is common in young women does not usually require investigation, but a change in bowel habit in the middle-aged or elderly does need investigation. A rectal examination should always be performed. The differential diagnosis is from other causes of constipation (see Table 4.15). In young women a condition of slow-transit constipation has been identified that is notoriously difficult to treat.

TREATMENT

Laxatives should be avoided if at all possible and the patient should be encouraged to take a high-fibre diet. Glycerol suppositories, which can be used by the patient, are often useful. The types of laxatives available are shown in Table 4.16.

Megacolon

The term megacolon is used to describe a number of congenital and acquired conditions in which the colon is dilated. In many instances it is secondary

Table 4.15 Causes of constipation.

Simple
Obstruction
Painful anal conditions
Drugs, e.g. opiates, aluminium antacids
Hypothyroidism, hypercalcaemia
Depression
Immobility
Hirschsprung's disease (occasionally in the adult)

Table 4.16 Laxatives and enemas.

	Mechanism of action
Bulking agents Dietary fibre Wheat bran Ispaghula husks	Increased faecal mass due to fibre and water

Contact cathartics
Phenolphthalein
Anthraquinones
  senna
  cascara
Dioctyl sodium
  sulphosuccinate
	Stimulate intestinal secretion

Osmotic laxatives Magnesium sulphate Lactulose	Osmotic effect
Suppositories Bisacodyl Glycerol	
Enemas Olive oil Phosphate	

to chronic constipation and in some parts of the world Chagas' disease is a common cause.

All young patients with megacolon should have Hirschsprung's disease excluded. In this disease, which presents in the first years of life, an aganglionic segment of the rectum gives rise to constipation and subacute obstruction. Occasionally Hirschsprung's disease affecting only a short segment of the rectum can be missed in childhood and a rectal biopsy, using special stains for ganglion cells in the submucosal plexus, should be performed in adult patients with megacolon to exclude it; frozen rectal mucosa should be stained for acetyl-cholinesterase. Pressure studies show failure of relaxation of the internal sphincter, which is diagnostic of Hirschsprung's disease. This disease can be successfully treated surgically.

Treatment of megacolon is similar to simple constipation, but saline washouts and manual removal of faeces are sometimes required.

Pneumatosis cystoides intestinalis

This is a rare condition in which multiple gas-filled cysts are found in the submucosa of the intestine, chiefly the colon. The cause is unknown but many cases are associated with chronic bronchitis and some with peptic ulceration. Patients are usually asymptomatic but abdominal pain and diarrhoea do occur and occasionally the cysts rupture to produce a pneumoperitoneum. This condition is diagnosed on X-ray of the abdomen, barium enema or at sigmoidoscopy when cysts are seen.

Treatment is often unnecessary but continuous oxygen therapy will help to disperse the largely nitrogen-containing cysts. Metronidazole may help.

Ischaemic disease of the colon (ischaemic colitis)

This commonly presents in the older age group (over 50 years) with sudden onset of abdominal pain and the passage of bright red blood with or without diarrhoea. There may be signs of shock and there is sometimes evidence of other cardio-vascular disease. This condition has also been described in young women taking the contraceptive pill.

On examination the abdomen is distended and tender. Sigmoidoscopy is normal apart from the presence of blood. Investigations include an abdominal X-ray to exclude perforation. Thumbprinting—a characteristic sign for ischaemic disease—can be seen on a barium enema performed when the patient is well; strictures can also be seen.

The differential diagnosis is of other causes of acute colitis, but these can usually be excluded on the basis of the sigmoidoscopy findings.

TREATMENT

Most patients with this condition settle on symptomatic treatment. A few develop gangrene and perforation and require urgent surgery. Some develop strictures.

Anorectal conditions

These important conditions largely present to surgeons. The major conditions presenting initially to the physicians include the following.

Pruritus ani

Pruritus ani, or an itchy bottom, is common and often no cause is found. Treatment consists of good personal hygiene and keeping the area dry. Secondary causes include any local anal lesions such as haemorrhoids, infestation, e.g. with threadworm (*Enterobius vermicularis*), or fungal infection, e.g. candidiasis. The latter condition often occurs secondary to the use of hydrocortisone creams, which should be avoided.

Haemorrhoids

Haemorrhoids usually produce rectal bleeding and pruritus ani. Patients may notice red blood on the toilet paper on wiping. They are the commonest cause of rectal bleeding (Fig. 4.13) and if minor require no treatment. Diagnosis is made on proctoscopy.

Anal fissures

Anal fissures cause painful defaecation and minor rectal bleeding and can often be seen in the anal margin on inspection. Treatment is by application of a local anaesthetic gel. Dilatation is not required.

Faecal incontinence

This can be a major problem in the elderly, infirm or demented patient. It is often secondary to impaction. Some of the major factors responsible are rectal prolapse, carcinoma of the rectum and diarrhoea from any cause. The patient should be carefully examined and investigation and treatment instituted as appropriate.

Faecal impaction

This occurs in the elderly with constipation. It can lead to overflow incontinence. It usually requires manual removal of faeces, and care to prevent recurrences (see constipation).

Solitary rectal ulcer

These ulcers occur in young adults and produce bowel irregularity and rectal bleeding with the passage of mucus. The cause is unclear but many seem to be due to excess straining at stool with prolapse of the rectal mucosa (descending perineal syndrome).

Rectal examination is usually normal but sigmoidoscopy reveals redness or an ulcer approximately 10 cm from the anal margin on the anterior rectal wall. It often has an appearance not unlike that of a carcinoma.

Histology is diagnostic; there are non-specific inflammatory changes with bands of smooth muscle extending into the lamina propria.

Treatment is unsatisfactory and many cases run an indolent chronic course with continuation of symptoms. Local steroids may help and surgical excision should be avoided. Patients should be advised to stop straining on defecation.

Rectal prolapse

In this common condition affecting children and the elderly the rectal mucosa prolapses through the anus owing to excessive straining. Initially prolapse occurs only during defecation but later ulceration, mucosal discharge and faecal incontinence can occur. Surgical treatment is required in complete prolapse.

Diarrhoea

With true diarrhoea there is an increase in stool weight to greater than 300 g per day. This is usually accompanied by increased stool frequency. Patients often interpret diarrhoea differently (see p. 174).

Mechanisms

Osmotic diarrhoea. The gut mucosa acts as a semi-permeable membrane and fluid enters the bowel if there are large quantities of non-absorbed hypertonic substances in the lumen. This occurs because:

- The patient has ingested a non-absorbable substance, e.g. a purgative such as magnesium sulphate or lactulose.
- The patient has generalized malabsorption.
- The patient has a specific malabsorption, e.g. disaccharidase deficiency or glucose–galactose malabsorption.

The volume of diarrhoea produced by these mechanisms is reduced by the absorption of fluid by the ileum and colon. The diarrhoea stops when the patient stops eating or the malabsorptive substance is discontinued.

Secretory diarrhoea. In this disorder there is both active intestinal secretion of fluid and electrolytes as well as decreased absorption. The mechanism of intestinal secretion is shown in Fig. 4.27a. Common causes of secretory diarrhoea are:

- Enterotoxins, e.g. cholera, *E. coli* (thermolabile or thermostable toxin)
- Hormones, e.g. vasoactive intestinal peptide in the Verner–Morrison syndrome (p. 236)
- Bile salts (in the colon) following ileal resection
- Fatty acids (in the colon) following ileal resection
- Some laxatives, e.g. dioctyl sodium sulphosuccinate

With secretory diarrhoea, the stool volumes may be very high. Food does not affect the diarrhoea and it therefore continues during fasting.

Inflammatory diarrhoea (mucosal destruction). Diarrhoea occurs because of damage to the intestinal mucosal cell so that there is a loss of fluid and blood. In addition, there is defective absorption of

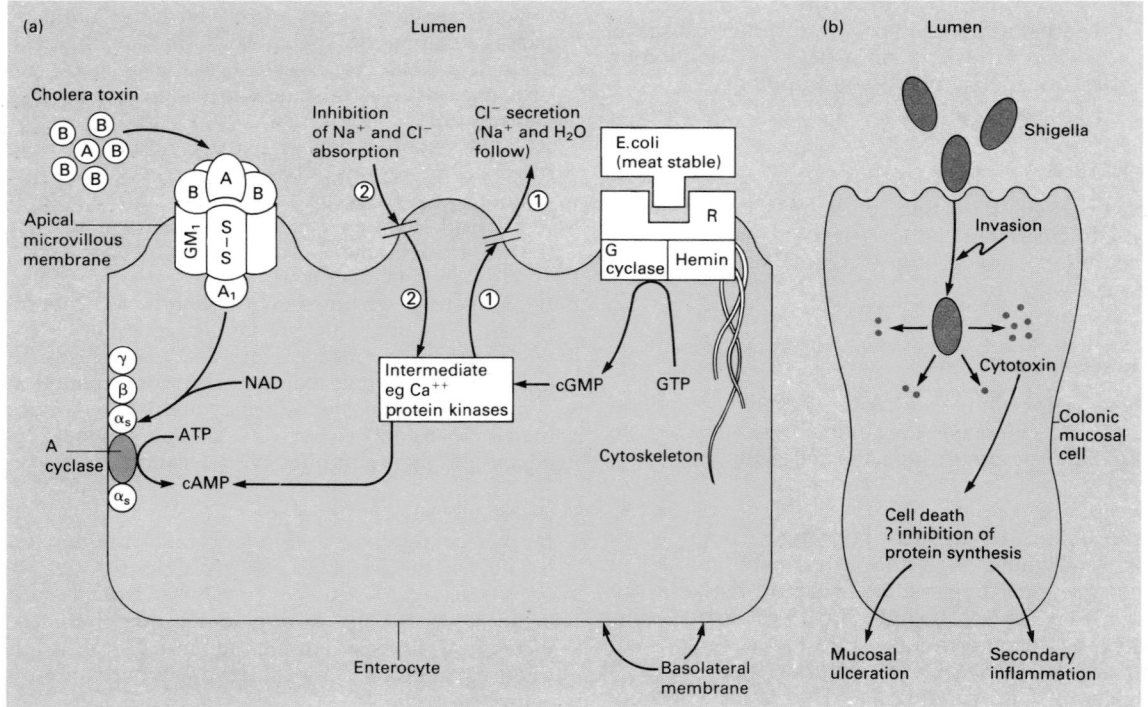

Fig. 4.27 Mechanism of diarrhoea. (a) *Small intestinal cell.* Cholera toxin binds to its receptor (monosialoganglioside GM₁) via its B subunits. The enzymatically active A subunit activates adenylate cyclase (A-cyclase) shown as its three subunits γ, β and α on the basolateral and apical membranes. This, in turn, activates intermediates, e.g. protein kinases and Ca²⁺, which act on the apical microvillous membrane to cause Cl¹ secretion (1) and inhibition of Na⁺ and Cl⁻ absorption (2). Heat labile *E. coli* shares the same receptor as cholera toxin. Heat stable *E. coli* (ST) binds to its receptor protein R and this complex activates guanylate cyclase which produces the same effect. The cytoskeleton and hemin are also actively involved in the binding and activation. The ST receptor is specific for the intestine. In both mechanisms, stimulation occurs without invasion. (b) *Colonic mucosal cell.* This demonstrates one of the mechanisms by which an invasive pathogen, e.g. *Shigella* acts. Following penetration the pathogens generate cytotoxins which lead to mucosal ulceration and cell death.

Table 4.17 Causes of diarrhoea.

Acute
Dietary indiscretion
Infective
    Food poisoning—see p. 34
    Viral gastroenteritis—see p. 62
Traveller's diarrhoea—see p. 34
    e.g. *E. coli*
    Giardia lamblia
    Shigella
    Entamoeba histolytica

Chronic
Inflammatory bowel disease
Parasitic/fungal infections
Gay bowel disease
Malabsorption
Gut resection
Drugs
Colonic neoplasia
Endocrine
    Pancreatic tumours, e.g. gastrinoma
    Thyrotoxicosis
    Diabetic neuropathy
Faecal impaction—in the elderly

fluid and electrolytes. Common causes are infective conditions, e.g. dysentery due to *Shigella*, and inflammatory conditions, e.g. ulcerative colitis (see Fig. 4.27b).

Abnormal motility (usually not true diarrhoea). 'Diarrhoea' in the irritable bowel syndrome is due to abnormal colonic motility. Diabetic, post-vagotomy and hyperthyroid diarrhoea are all due to abnormal motility of the upper gut. In many of these cases the volume and weight of the stool is not all that high, but frequency of defecation occurs; this therefore is not true diarrhoea.

Some causes of diarrhoea are shown in Table 4.17. It should be noted that the irritable bowel syndrome and diverticular disease are not mentioned as they do not cause 'true' diarrhoea, even though the patients may complain of diarrhoea. World-wide, infection and infestation are a major problem and these are discussed under the causative organisms in Chapter 1.

Acute diarrhoea (excluding cholera, which is discussed on p. 32). Diarrhoea of sudden onset is very common, often short-lived and requires no investigation or treatment. This type of diarrhoea is seen after dietary indiscretions, but diarrhoea due to viral agents also lasts 24–48 h (p. 61). The causes of other infective diarrhoeas are shown on p. 34. Traveller's diarrhoea, which affects people travelling outside their own countries, particularly to

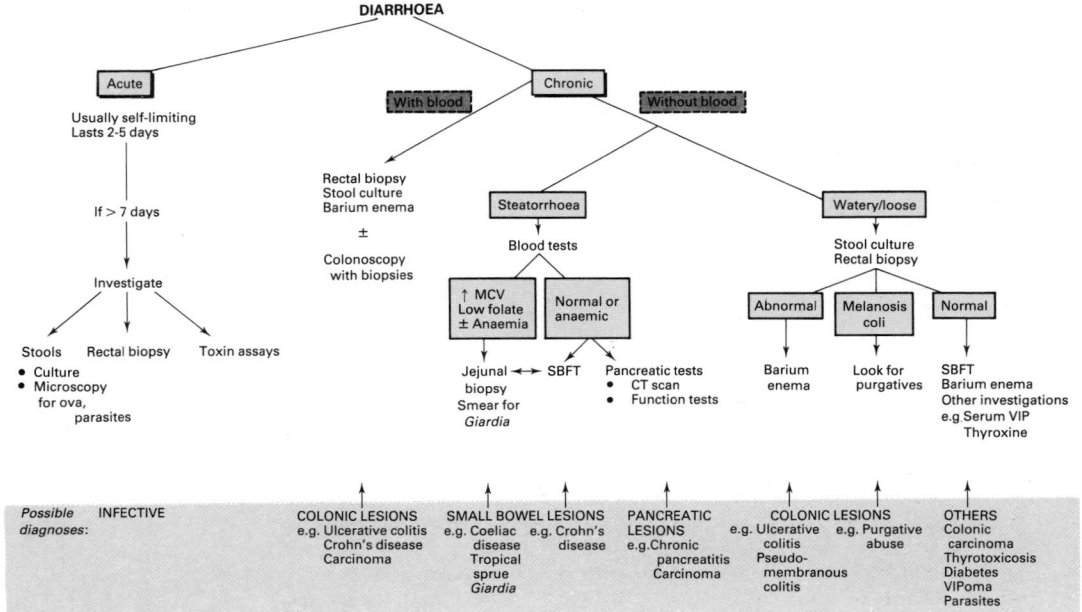

Fig. 4.28 Flow diagram for the investigation of diarrhoea. Rectal biopsies are obtained via a sigmoidoscope, and the macroscopic appearances of the mucosa should be noted. SBFT = small-bowel follow-through; VIP = vasoactive intestinal polypeptide. N.B. Chronic conditions can present as an acute episode.

developing countries, usually lasts 2–5 days; it is discussed on p. 34. Clinical features associated with the acute diarrhoeas include fever, abdominal pain and vomiting. If the diarrhoea is particularly severe, dehydration can be a problem; the very young and very old are at special risk from this. Investigations are necessary if the diarrhoea has lasted more than 1 week. Stools (up to three) should be sent immediately to the laboratory for culture and examination for ova, cysts and parasites. A sigmoidoscopy and rectal biopsy should be performed. If the diagnosis has still not been made, radiological studies should be performed.

Oral fluid replacement is of prime importance in the treatment. Special oral rehydration solutions, e.g. sodium chloride and glucose powder (see Table 1.16), are available for use in severe episodes of diarrhoea in infants. These compounds were initially developed for use in cholera but are valuable in all severe diarrhoeas. Anti-diarrhoeal drugs are thought to impair the clearance of any pathogen from the bowel but may be necessary for short-term relief, e.g. codeine phosphate 30 mg four times daily or loperamide 2 mg three times daily.

Chronic diarrhoea
This always needs investigation (see Fig. 4.28). All patients should have a sigmoidoscopy and rectal biopsy. Whether the large or the small bowel is investigated first will depend on the clinical story of, for example, bloody diarrhoea or steatorrhoea. The investigations and treatment are described under the individual diseases.

Some other causes of diarrhoea
Purgative abuse. This is usually seen in females who surreptitiously take high-dose purgatives and are often extensively investigated for chronic diarrhoea. The diarrhoea is usually of high volume (> 1 litre/day). Sigmoidoscopy may show a pigmented mucosa, a condition known as *melanosis coli*. Histologically the rectal biopsy shows pigment-laden macrophages in patients taking an anthraquinone purgative (e.g. Senokot). Melanosis coli is also seen in people taking regular purgatives in normal doses. Phenolphthalein laxatives can be detected by pouring an alkali, e.g. sodium hydroxide, on the stools, which then turn pink; a magnesium-containing purgative will give a high faecal magnesium content. A barium enema shows

Table 4.18 GI problems in patients with AIDS.

Symptoms	Site	Problems
Dysphagia Retrosternal discomfort Oral ulceration	Mouth/oesophagus	Candidiasis Herpes simplex virus (HSV) Cytomegalovirus (CMV)

Chronic diarrhoea
Steatorrhea
Weight loss
	Small bowel	Parasites
		  Cryptosporidium
		  Isospora belli
		  Microsporidia
		
		Viruses
		  CMV/HSV
		
		Bacteria
		  Salmonella
		  Campylobacter
		  Mycobacterium avium
		    intracellulare
		Non-infective enteropathy—
		  cause unknown

Bloody diarrhoea	Rectum/colon	'Gay bowel disease' (see p. 46) Anorectal warts

Weight loss
Diarrhoea
	Any	Neoplasia
		  Kaposi's sarcoma
		  Lymphoma
		  Hairy leucoplakia
		  Squamous carcinoma

loss of haustral patterns and there may be mild abnormalities of absorption tests and a low serum potassium. Management is difficult as the patient usually denies purgative ingestion. If the diagnosis is suspected, a locker or bed search (while the patient is out of the ward) is occasionally necessary. The patient needs psychiatric help.

Pseudomembranous colitis (antibiotic-associated diarrhoea). This colitis develops following the use of any antibiotic, particularly lincomycin, ampicillin and cephalosporins. Diarrhoea occurs in the first few days after taking the antibiotic or even up to 6 weeks after stopping the antibiotic.

Sigmoidoscopy usually shows multiple yellow plaques and inflammation; histology shows inflammation, sometimes with a pseudomembrane. *Clostridium difficile* (see p. 29) is best detected using a tissue culture assay. Toxin is also detected in the stools but correlation between the two is poor. Treatment, if necessary, is with vancomycin 125–500 mg four times daily for 1–2 weeks or metronidazole 400 mg three times daily.

Diarrhoea in patients with HIV infection

Chronic diarrhoea is a common symptom in HIV infection but its own role in the pathogenesis of diarrhoea is unclear. Cryptosporidium (see p. 90) is the commonest pathogen isolated. Isospora belli and microsporidia have also been found. An enteropathy has been described. The cause of the diarrhoea is often not found and treatment is symptomatic. Table 4.18 shows the conditions affecting the gastrointestinal tract in AIDS.

Functional bowel disease

This is the general term used to embrace two syndromes:

- Non-ulcer dyspepsia
- The irritable bowel syndrome

These conditions are extremely common, making up to 60–80% of patients seen in a gastroenterology clinic. The two conditions overlap, with some symptoms being common to both. In general, however, the term *non-ulcer dyspepsia* is given to patients complaining of indigestion, wind, nausea, heartburn, i.e. dyspepsia, when no ulcer is found. It can be difficult on the history to differentiate it from the symptoms of gastric or duodenal ulceration, but typically patients with ulcers have nocturnal pain and also respond to antacids. Barium studies or endoscopy are often performed to exclude ulceration but are unnecessary in those under 35 years. The relationship between *Helicobacter pylori*, antral gastritis and dyspepsia is controversial and unclear at the present time. Treatment is by reassurance. Antacids and H$_2$-receptor antagonists can be tried but are probably of little benefit apart from the placebo effect. Metoclopramide 10 mg three times daily may be helpful.

The irritable bowel syndrome is the term now used for all other types of functional bowel disease.

The irritable bowel syndrome

CLINICAL FEATURES

The pain is classically situated in the left iliac fossa and is usually relieved by defaecation or the passage of wind. The patient may complain of constipation or diarrhoea with the passage of frequent small-volume stools and a feeling of incomplete emptying of the rectum. Stools may be ribbon-like or rabbity in appearance. True watery diarrhoea suggests organic disease. The pain, however, can be very variable and occur in any part of the abdomen and the bowel habit may be normal.

The length of history is usually long, with frequent recurrent episodes and long symptom-free intervals. The patient may give a history of recurrent episodes of abdominal pain as a child. Mild episodes of pain occur frequently in the normal population and are usually disregarded and therefore undiagnosed. The patient with the irritable bowel syndrome looks well despite frequent episodes of pain, some of which can be very acute and require hospital admission to rule out an acute abdominal condition.

AETIOLOGY

The exact cause of the irritable bowel syndrome is not known but the symptoms do seem to be produced by a combination of disordered gut motility and increased tenderness of the gut.

Psychological factors are important and most patients find the symptoms are exacerbated by stress. Some patients are depressed, and this fact may be missed unless carefully looked for.

EXAMINATION

Examination reveals no abnormality. Rectal examination and sigmoidoscopy should be performed. Although sigmoidoscopy shows a normal mucosa, air insufflation may reproduce the pain. If diarrhoea is a feature, a rectal biopsy should be performed, even if the mucosa looks normal, to help rule out inflammatory bowel disease.

INVESTIGATION

The amount of investigation varies in individual patients. A young girl with pain in the left iliac fossa exacerbated by stress will require no investigation. Conversely, an elderly person who has developed pain or diarrhoea for the first time must be investigated, with a full radiological assessment, before the diagnosis of functional bowel disease is made.

Traps for the unwary

- *Beware of false correlations.* Diverticular disease is common in the elderly and because diverticular disease is seen on the barium enema it must not be assumed to be the cause of the pain. Hiatus hernias are also common findings and are also often asymptomatic.
- *Gynaecological problems* must be excluded; on the other hand, it must not be assumed that all lower abdominal pain in women is due to some gynaecological problem. Many unnecessary operations are carried out as a consequence.
- *Recurrent pain in the right iliac fossa* is not due to chronic appendicitis but to the irritable bowel syndrome.
- *Recurrent pain in the right hypochondrium* is usually not due to gall-bladder disease but to the irritable bowel syndrome.
- *Abdominal bruits* are common and abdominal pain should not be ascribed to ischaemic bowel on this basis alone.

MANAGEMENT

- Explanation of the symptoms and their mechanism often helps and patients must be reassured of the benign nature of the condition. Cancer phobia must be dispelled. Patients have to learn to live with their symptoms, as they tend to be recurrent.
- A high-fibre bran diet may help some patients.
- Antispasmodics, e.g. mebeverine, may be given.
- Underlying stress and depression should be treated.

The acute abdomen

This section deals with acute abdominal conditions that cause the patient to be hospitalized within a few hours of the onset of their pain. It is important to make the diagnosis as quickly as possible to reduce morbidity and mortality. Although a specific diagnosis should be attempted, the immediate problem in management is to decide whether an 'acute abdomen' exists or not.

History

Pain
The onset, site, type and subsequent cause of the pain should be determined as accurately as possible.

Usually the pain is fairly rapid in onset, but if there is a perforation of a hollow viscus, e.g. a perforated duodenal ulcer, the pain is particularly sudden in onset. Acute intestinal ischaemia also presents with acute pain, whereas inflammatory conditions, e.g. appendicitis, produce a more gradual onset of pain. In intestinal obstruction the pain is typically colicky in nature, whereas with peritonitis the pain is continuous and may be made worse by movement.

The site of the pain can help in determining the organ involved: generally upper abdominal pain is produced by lesions of the upper GI tract and lower abdominal pain by lesions of the lower GI tract. It must, however, be remembered that the GI tract is not fixed and, for example, the appendix may not always be in the right iliac fossa.

Vomiting
Vomiting accompanies any acute abdominal pain: it is persistent with a high obstructive lesion of the gut.

Physical examination

The general condition of the patient should be noted. Does he look ill? Is he shocked? Because fluid is lost from the vascular compartment into the peritoneal cavity or into the lumen of the bowel, hypovolaemia frequently occurs, causing a pale, cold skin, especially on the nose, a weak rapid pulse, and hypotension.

Abdomen
Signs of peritonitis. The abdomen should be examined gently. Sites of tenderness and the presence or absence of guarding should be noted. Guarding is involuntary spasm of the abdominal wall and it indicates peritonitis. This can be localized to one area or it may be generalized, involving the whole abdomen.

Rebound tenderness occurs when the palpating hand is removed from the abdomen suddenly. The pain is due to sudden movement of the inflamed peritoneum.

Signs of obstruction. The main findings are distension of the abdomen due to gas in the bowel and increased bowel sounds due to increased bowel movement. High-pitched (tinkling) bowel sounds indicate small-bowel obstruction.

Absent bowel sounds suggest peritoneal involvement (peritonitis) in addition to obstruction and may be seen in intestinal ischaemia or strangulated bowel.

It is essential that the hernial orifices are examined if intestinal obstruction is suspected.

Pelvic and rectal examination. These can be very helpful, particularly in diagnosing gynaecological causes of an acute abdomen, e.g. a ruptured ectopic pregnancy. Rectal examination may detect localized tenderness or blood in the stools, which is suggestive of a vascular lesion.

Other observations

- Tongue—furred in most acute abdominal disease.
- Temperature—fever is more common in acute inflammatory processes.
- Urine—examine for:
    (a) Glucose and ketones (ketoacidosis can present with acute pain).
    (b) White cells (to exclude acute pyelonephritis).
    (c) Porphyrins (porphyria is a rare cause of abdominal pain).
- Think of other conditions, e.g.
    (a) Diabetes mellitus (ketoacidosis).
    (b) Pneumonia (referred pain).
    (c) Myocardial infarction (referred pain).
    (d) Lead poisoning.
    (e) The irritable bowel syndrome (this can produce acute severe pain).

Investigation

- *Blood count*—raised white-cell count likely in inflammatory conditions
- *Serum amylase*—high levels of greater than 5 times normal indicate acute pancreatitis. Raised levels below this can occur in any acute abdomen and should not be considered diagnostic of pancreatitis
- *Serum electrolytes*—not particularly helpful for diagnosis, but useful for general evaluation of the patient
- *X-ray of the abdomen*—an erect and a supine X-ray of the abdomen are useful to detect air under the diaphragm (perforation) or dilated loops of bowel or fluid levels suggestive of obstruction
- *Ultrasound*—to assess any palpable masses, e.g. abscesses

SPECIFIC CONDITIONS

Acute appendicitis

This is the commonest surgical emergency. It affects all age groups from the very young to the very old and appendicitis should always be considered in the differential diagnosis if the appendix has not been removed.

Acute appendicitis mostly occurs when the lumen of the appendix becomes obstructed with a faecolith; however, in some cases there is only generalized acute inflammation. If the appendix is not removed at this stage, gangrene occurs with perforation, leading to a localized abscess or to generalized peritonitis.

CLINICAL FEATURES

All patients have abdominal pain; in many it starts vaguely in the centre of the abdomen, becoming localized to the right iliac fossa in the first few hours. There is nausea, some vomiting and occasional diarrhoea. Because of the variable position of the appendix, symptoms and signs differ.

Examination of the abdomen reveals tenderness in the right iliac fossa, with guarding due to the localized peritonitis. Rectal examination reveals tenderness to the right. There may be a tender mass in the right iliac fossa.

Laboratory tests are unhelpful, except that the white-cell count may be raised. An ultrasound is accurate for the detection of an inflamed appendix and will also indicate an appendix mass or other localized lesion.

In the differential diagnosis all abdominal conditions must be considered, and in children and young adults non-specific mesenteric lymphadenitis may mimic appendicitis. Acute terminal ileitis (see p. 212) also gives similar symptoms and signs. The exact diagnosis may be difficult to make, but if there is a reasonable possibility of it being acute appendicitis, laparotomy should be performed.

Generalized peritonitis still causes a significant mortality and morbidity and early surgery is a better option in suspected acute appendicitis than a 'wait and see' policy. Nevertheless, functional bowel disease can present acutely and must always be considered.

If an appendix mass is present, the patient is treated conservatively. The pain subsides over a few days and the mass usually disappears over a few weeks. Appendectomy is recommended at a later date to prevent further acute episodes.

Acute peritonitis

Localized peritonitis
This is still a serious condition resulting from irritation of the peritoneum due to infection, e.g. perforated appendix, or from chemical irritation due to leakage of intestinal contents, e.g. perforated ulcer. In the latter case, superadded infection gradually occurs; *E. coli* and *Bacteroides* are the commonest organisms.

The peritoneal cavity becomes acutely inflamed with production of an inflammatory exudate that spreads throughout the peritoneum leading to intestinal dilatation and paralytic ileus.

Acute peritonitis should not be allowed to

develop and will not do so if the underlying conditions are treated promptly.

CLINICAL FEATURES AND MANAGEMENT

In perforation the onset is sudden with acute severe abdominal pain, followed by general collapse and shock. The patient may improve temporarily, only to become worse later as generalized toxaemia occurs.

When the peritonitis is secondary to inflammatory disease, the initial features are those of the underlying disease. Peritonitis is always treated surgically, with initial treatment of the patient's general condition, including insertion of a nasogastric tube, intravenous fluids and antibiotics. Surgery has a twofold objective:

- Drainage of the abdominal cavity
- Specific treatment of the underlying condition

COMPLICATIONS

Any delay in treatment of peritonitis produces more profound toxaemia and septicaemia. In addition, local abscess formation occurs and should be suspected if the patient continues to remain unwell with a swinging fever, high white-cell count and continuing pain. Abscesses are commonly pelvic or subphrenic. Both are now localized chiefly by ultrasound examination; treatment is with antibiotics and drainage is often required.

Intestinal obstruction

Most intestinal obstruction is due to a mechanical block. Sometimes the bowel does not function, leading to a paralytic ileus. This occurs temporarily after most abdominal operations and with peritonitis. Some causes of intestinal obstruction are shown in Table 4.19.

Obstruction of the bowel leads to bowel distension above the block, with increased secretion of fluid into the distended bowel. Bacterial contamin-

Table 4.19 Some causes of intestinal obstruction.

Constriction from the outside, e.g.
    bowel entrapped in a hernia
    adhesions
    volvulus, particularly of sigmoid colon

Bowel disease obstructing the lumen, e.g.
    carcinoma
    Crohn's disease
    diverticular disease

Luminal obstruction, e.g.
    foreign body
    gallstones

ation occurs in the distended stagnant bowel. In strangulation the blood supply is impeded, leading to gangrene, perforation and peritonitis unless urgent treatment of the condition is undertaken.

CLINICAL FEATURES

The patient complains of colicky abdominal pain, vomiting and constipation without passage of wind. In upper gut obstruction the vomiting is profuse but in lower gut obstruction it may be absent.

Examination of the abdomen reveals distension, with increased bowel sounds. Examination of the hernial orifices must be performed.

X-ray of the abdomen reveals distended loops of bowel with fluid levels.

MANAGEMENT

Initial management is by nasogastric intubation to decompress the bowel and replacement of fluid loss by intravenous fluids (mainly isotonic saline).

Laparotomy with removal of the obstruction is necessary in most instances and if the bowel is gangrenous owing to strangulation, gut resection will be required.

A few patients, e.g. those with Crohn's disease, may have recurrent episodes of subacute intestinal obstruction that can be managed conservatively.

Rarely the clinical features of obstruction are produced by a condition in which the nerve plexuses of the bowel are damaged—intestinal pseudo-obstruction. This condition is managed conservatively.

Volvulus of the sigmoid colon can be managed by the passage of a rectal tube to unkink the bowel, but recurrent volvulus may require sigmoid resection.

Acute intestinal ischaemia

Mesenteric artery occlusion, either from an embolus or from thrombosis in an arteriosclerotic artery, leads to gut ischaemia and, if not dealt with promptly, necrosis of the intestine.

The patient presents with severe abdominal pain and vomiting. Bloody diarrhoea is a helpful indicator of the diagnosis but does not occur for some time. The abdomen is usually tender and bowel sounds are absent. The diagnosis must be considered in any elderly patient with arteriosclerotic disease or in patients with atrial fibrillation. Early surgery may prevent gut necrosis but sometimes massive resection of the dead gut is required to save the patient's life.

Mesenteric venous thrombosis occurs mainly in patients who have circulatory failure and can lead to gut necrosis. Often the patient is extremely ill from his underlying condition but surgery may be necessary if the patient is fit enough.

The peritoneum

The peritoneal cavity is a closed sac lined by mesothelium. It normally contains a little fluid that allows the intra-abdominal organs to move freely. Some conditions that can affect the peritoneum are shown in Table 4.20.

Table 4.20 Diseases of the peritoneum.

Infective (bacterial) peritonitis
Secondary to gut disease, e.g. appendicitis,
perforation of any organ
Chronic peritoneal dialysis
Spontaneous, usually in ascites with liver disease
Tuberculosis
Neoplasia
Secondary deposits, e.g. from ovary, stomach
Primary mesothelioma
Vasculitis
Connective tissue disease

Peritonitis can be acute or chronic, as seen in tuberculosis. Most cases of infective peritonitis are secondary to gastrointestinal diseases but it occasionally occurs without intra-abdominal sepsis in ascites due to liver disease. Very rarely, fungal and parasitic infections can also cause primary peritonitis, e.g. amoebiasis, candidiasis. Peritonitis is discussed further on p. 227.

The peritoneum can be involved by *secondary malignant deposits* and the commonest cause of ascites in a young to middle-aged woman is an ovarian carcinoma.

A *subphrenic abscess* is usually secondary to infection in the abdomen and is characterized by fever, malaise, pain in the right or left hypochondrium and shoulder-tip pain. A plain abdominal X-ray shows gas under the diaphragm, impaired movement of the diaphragm on screening and a pleural effusion. Ultrasound is usually diagnostic.

Ascites is associated with all diseases of the peritoneum. The fluid that collects is an exudate with a high protein content. It is also seen in liver disease. The mechanism, causes and investigation of ascites are discussed on p. 265.

Tuberculous peritonitis

This is usually due to reactivation of a tuberculous focus in the peritoneum with concurrent pulmonary, intestinal or genital TB. It is often seen in debilitated patients, alcoholics and certain racial groups e.g. Asians. Usually the onset is insidious, with fever, anorexia and weight loss. Abdominal pain is common, accompanied by ascites (75%) or an abdominal mass caused by an inflamed mesentery.

Diagnosis is made by examination of the peritoneal fluid, if present, which shows an increase in lymphocyte count; occasionally tubercle bacilli are seen on staining. Culture of the fluid should be performed. Ultrasound shows mesenteric thickening and enlargement of lymph nodes. At laparoscopy the peritoneum is seen to be studded with tubercles that can be biopsied and sent for culture and histology. Treatment is with conventional chemotherapy (see p. 682) for 18 months to 2 years.

Retroperitoneal fibrosis

This is a rare condition in which there is a marked fibrosis over the posterior abdominal wall and retroperitoneum. The aetiology is usually unknown but it has been associated with the drug methysergide and occasionally with the carcinoid syndrome. The disease usually presents in middle-age with malaise, fever, and loss of weight. There is often anaemia and a raised ESR. The major complication is urinary tract obstruction from ureteric involvement, which may require surgery.

Tumours of the gastrointestinal tract

THE OESOPHAGUS

Benign tumours

Leiomyomas are the commonest benign tumours. They are usually discovered accidentally and they do not often produce symptoms.

Carcinoma

The majority of malignant tumours occur in the middle (50%) and lower third (25%) of the oesophagus. The tumours are usually squamous but adenocarcinoma occurs in the lower third and at the cardia, arising from the fundus of the stomach or from localized areas of columnar epithelium in the lower oesophagus resulting from long-standing reflux (Barrett's oesophagus). The incidence of carcinoma varies throughout the world, being high in China, parts of Africa and in the Caspian regions of Iran (where the incidence is the highest observed for any type of cancer anywhere in the world). In the UK it is 5–10 per 100 000 and represents 2.5% of all malignant disease. The variation in incidence throughout the world is greater than for any other carcinoma and is unusual in that sharp differences occur in regions very close to one another. Dietary and other environmental causes have been looked for, but so far none has been unequivocally proved. Carcinoma of the oesophagus is commoner in men and there is an increased incidence in heavy drinkers of alcohol as well as heavy smokers. Predisposing factors include Plummer–Vinson syndrome, achalasia, Barrett's oesophagus and the familial condition of tylosis (hyperkeratosis of palms and soles).

CLINICAL FEATURES

Carcinoma of the oesophagus occurs mainly in those aged 60–70 years. Dysphagia is the commonest single symptom and is progressive. Initially there is difficulty in swallowing solids, but eventually dysphagia for liquids also occurs. Benign strictures, on the other hand, initially produce intermittent dysphagia. Impaction of food causes pain, but more persistent pain implies infiltration.

The lesion is usually ulcerative, extending around the wall of the oesophagus to produce a stricture. Direct invasion of the surrounding structures rather than widespread metastases occurs, and at presentation 50% have regional lymph node involvement. Weight loss, due to the dysphagia as well as to anorexia, frequently occurs. The oesophageal obstruction eventually causes difficulty in swallowing saliva, and coughing and aspiration into the lungs is common.

Signs are often absent. Weight loss, anorexia and lymphadenopathy are occasionally found.

INVESTIGATION

Barium swallow is the initial investigation (Fig. 4.29). Oesophagoscopy provides histological or cytological proof of the carcinoma; 90% of oesophageal carcinomas can be confirmed with this technique. Computed tomography is useful to outline the size of the tumour and to evaluate mediastinal spread. Endoscopic ultrasound and MRI are also being used to evaluate tumour spread.

TREATMENT

The overall results are poor (2% 5-year survival) and only symptomatic and palliative treatment is a realistic possibility. Dilatation of the stricture and the placing of a tube to keep the oesophagus open is the usual therapy and can be performed via an endoscope.

Tumours can be photocoagulated using a laser beam directed through an endoscope or sloughed using alcohol injections. Both are useful to improve

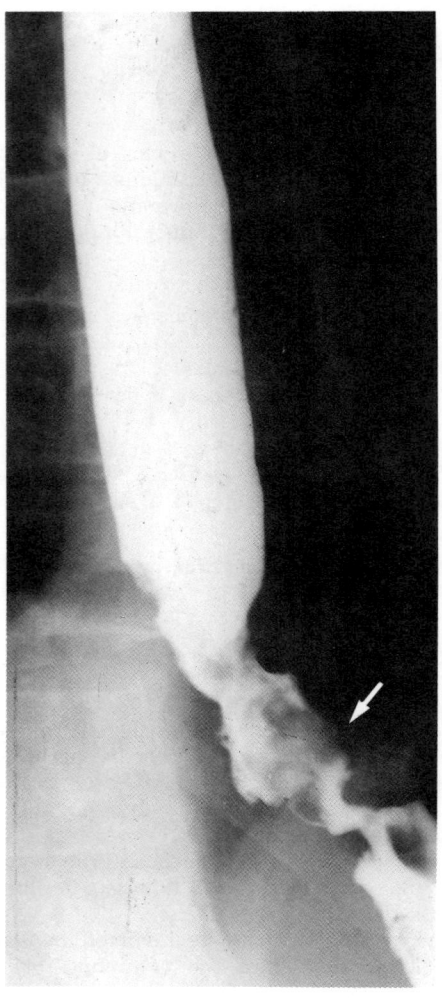

Fig. 4.29 Barium swallow showing carcinoma of the oesophagus. There is an irregular narrowed area (arrow) at the lower end of the oesophagus.

dysphagia. Surgery carries a high morbidity and mortality and little chance of anything but palliation. Radiotherapy and chemotherapy can be used for squamous carcinoma with limited success.

THE STOMACH

Benign tumours

The commonest benign tumour is a leiomyoma. This tumour is usually discovered by chance but it can occasionally ulcerate and produce haematemesis. Treatment is surgical removal.

Gastric polyps are uncommon and are again found usually by chance. They produce no symptoms. The commonest are regenerative or hyperplastic polyps, which are often multiple and require no treatment. Rarely adenomatous polyps are found and endoscopic removal is recommended because of possible malignant potential. Most gastric cancers appear not to arise from pre-existing adenomas (in contrast to colonic carcinomas).

Lymphoma

Lymphoma of the stomach can be primary (10% of all gastric malignancies) or secondary from systemic involvement. Clinical presentation is the same as gastric carcinoma. Treatment is surgical with post-operative radiotherapy and chemotherapy. Prognosis is good with a 50% 5-year survival.

Carcinoma

Carcinoma of the stomach is one of the commonest malignant tumours of the GI tract and is the third most common fatal cancer in the UK. The frequency varies throughout the world, being high in Japan and Chile and relatively low in the USA.

In the UK, 20 per 100 000 males are affected per year. The world-wide incidence of gastric carcinoma appears to be falling, even in Japan, for no obvious reason. The incidence increases with age and more men than women are affected. The reason for the difference in incidence is unclear but it may be due to genetic, dietary or environmental factors:

● Carcinoma is more common in people of blood group A.
● Japanese who emigrate to the USA still have a high incidence, but this decreases in succeeding generations.
● The incidence is higher in lower socioeconomic groups.
● Dietary factors that have been suggested include alcohol, spicy foods and more recently nitrate ingestion. Nitrates can be converted into nitrosamines by bacteria at neutral pH and nitrosamines are known to be carcinogenic in animals. Nitrosamines are present in the stomach of patients with achlorhydria, who have an increased cancer risk.

Possible pre-cancerous conditions
Benign gastric ulcers do not develop into gastric cancer. It can, however, be difficult to differentiate a benign ulcer from a malignant ulcer, as even malignant ulcers can partially heal on medical treatment. For these reasons it was originally thought that gastric ulcers could become malignant.

Pernicious anaemia carries a small increased risk of developing gastric carcinoma. Gastric atrophy/ present in the body and fundus of the stomach of these patients may be a precancerous lesion.

Many gastric cancers develop in areas of *atrophic gastritis* and also areas of *intestinal metaplasia*. Intestinal metaplasia and chronic gastritis are also found in the resected stomach and there is an increased incidence of gastric cancer after *partial gastrectomy* (especially with a gastrojejunostomy). This increased incidence is the same whether the gastric resection was for a gastric or duodenal ulcer.

Screening
Gastric cancer has an appalling prognosis despite treatment, and earlier diagnosis has been advocated in an attempt to improve this. Unfortunately, earlier diagnosis does not necessarily mean longer survival. The patient is merely operated on at an earlier date and, although the survival may appear longer, death will still occur at the same time from the point of genesis of the cancer (called lead time bias) (Fig. 4.30). With length time bias a greater number of slowly growing tumours are detected when screening asymptomatic individuals. In Japan, mass screening with mobile X-ray units has increased the proportion of early gastric cancers diagnosed. Early gastric cancer is defined as a carcinoma that is confined to the mucosa or submucosa. It is associated with 5-year survival rates of approximately 90%. In a large series of patients with gastric cancer from the UK, only 0.7% were identified as having early gastric cancer and therefore screening would not be warranted.

An effective screening procedure should:

● Be cheap
● Be acceptable to all social groups so that they attend for examination

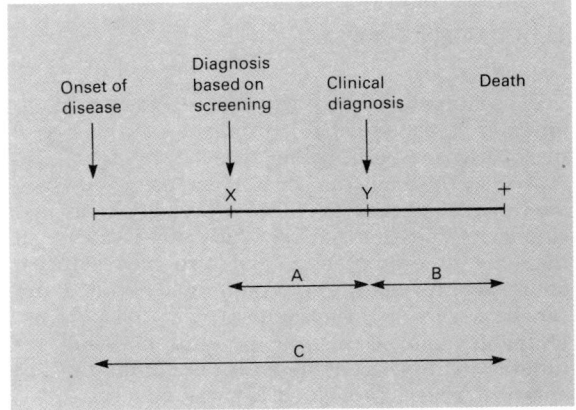

Fig. 4.30 Lead time bias. Earlier diagnosis (X) made by screening tests before clinical diagnosis at Y suggests prolonged survival (A) in comparison to B, but actual survival (C) is unchanged.

- Have a good discriminatory index from benign lesions
- Result in an improvement in prognosis

Unless all these criteria are fulfilled, screening is unwarranted except possibly in individuals with an increased risk for the disease. Nevertheless, even in this high-risk group, screening asymptomatic subjects is not justified as the overall benefit is minimal.

An alternative approach to screening asymptomatic patients is to investigate symptomatic patients as quickly as possible. At the present time the mean interval between the onset of symptoms and attendance at hospital is approximately 6–9 months. However, dyspepsia is very common in the general population without any gastric lesions and it would obviously be impractical for every dyspeptic member of the general population to consult a physician. Even if they did, most primary physicians would think it unjustified to arrange a complicated series of investigations on the first visit.

Thus, the detection of early gastric cancer in symptomatic patients is not a feasible proposition at present.

PATHOLOGY

Most gastric cancers occur in the antrum and are almost invariably adenocarcinomas. The tumours are usually ulcerating lesions with heaped-up, rolled edges. Sometimes they may be fungating polypoid lesions and if present in the fundus may infiltrate into the oesophagus and cause dysphagia. Lastly, the carcinoma may be diffuse with extensive submucosal spread, which may result in the picture of 'linitis plastica'.

CLINICAL FEATURES

Symptoms

The commonest symptom is epigastric pain, which is indistinguishable from the pain of peptic ulcer disease, both being relieved by food and antacids. The pain can vary in intensity, but may be constant and severe. Most patients with carcinoma of the stomach have advanced disease at the time of presentation, and also have nausea, anorexia and weight loss. Vomiting is frequent and can be severe if the tumour is near the pylorus. Dysphagia can occur with tumours involving the fundus. Gross haematemesis is unusual, but anaemia from occult blood loss is frequent.

Patients can present with metastases causing abdominal swelling due to ascites or jaundice due to liver involvement. Metastases also occur in bone, brain and lung, producing appropriate symptoms.

Signs

Nearly 50% of patients have a palpable epigastric mass with abdominal tenderness. Often weight loss is the only feature. A palpable lymph node is sometimes found in the supraclavicular fossa (Virchow's node) and signs of metastases are present in up to one-third of patients. Carcinoma of the stomach is the cancer most frequently associated with dermatomyositis and acanthosis nigricans.

INVESTIGATION

Blood count—this may show anaemia.

Barium meal

A good quality, double contrast barium meal has a diagnostic accuracy of up to 90%. The carcinoma is usually seen as a filling defect or an irregular ulcer with rolled edges. With the infiltrating type, the X-ray may show a rigid stomach.

Gastroscopy

Gastroscopy is sometimes performed as the primary procedure and has the advantage that biopsies can be performed for histological assessment and to exclude lymphoma. Positive biopsies can be obtained in almost all cases of obvious carcinoma, but a negative biopsy does not necessarily rule out the diagnosis. For this reason, 8–10 biopsies should be taken from around the ulcer margin and its base. Superficial brushings for cytology will further improve the diagnostic rate.

Evaluation of metastases is carried out with ultrasound and CT if primary tumour resection is being considered.

TREATMENT

Surgery for stomach cancer gives only a 10% 5-year survival rate; this figure has not changed over the past 25 years. Total gastrectomy is now seldom performed since the operative morbidity is high and the 5-year survival rate no better than subtotal or partial gastrectomy. Sixty-five per cent of cases are found to be inoperable at the time of surgery but a palliative resection is usually performed to prevent obstruction and haemorrhage and to relieve the patient's immediate symptoms.

Treatment with chemotherapy has made little impact and is currently not justifiable apart from in clinical trials. Survival may be prolonged by a few months but the toxicity of the drugs limits their use. Recently, cimetidine has been used in trials.

THE SMALL INTESTINE

The small intestine is relatively resistant to the development of neoplasia and only 3–6% of all GI tumours and fewer than 1% of all malignant lesions occur in the small bowel. The reasons for the rarity of tumours is unknown. Explanations include the fluidity and relative sterility of small-bowel contents and the rapid transit time, reducing the time of exposure to potential carcinogens. It is also possible that the high population of lymphoid tissue and secretion of IgA in the small intestine protects against malignancy.

Benign tumours

Adenomas, leiomyomas or lipomas are rarely found and are usually asymptomatic and picked up incidentally. In familial adenomatous polyposis the upper gut is affected in one-third of patients. Peutz–Jeghers syndrome consists of mucocutaneous pigmentation (circumoral, hands and feet) and gastrointestinal polyps and has a Mendelian dominant inheritance. The brown buccal pigment is characteristic of this condition. The polyps, which are hamartomas, can occur anywhere in the GI tract but are most frequent in the small bowel. They may bleed or cause intussusception. They virtually never become malignant. Treatment is by individual polypectomy. Multiple polypectomies may have to be performed, but bowel resection should be avoided.

Malignant tumours

Adenocarcinoma of the small intestine is rare and found most frequently in the duodenum in the periampullary region and in the jejunum. Lymphomas are most frequently found in the ileum. These are of the non-Hodgkin's type and must be distinguished from peripheral or nodal lymphoma involving the gut secondarily.

Predisposing factors
Coeliac disease. There is an increased incidence of lymphoma and adenocarcinoma of the small bowel in coeliac disease. There are no identifiable risk factors predisposing to malignancy, although the increased cell turnover found may be important. There is some inconclusive evidence that treatment with a gluten-free diet protects against the development of malignancy.

Crohn's disease. There is a small increase in the incidence of adenocarcinoma of the small bowel in Crohn's disease.

Alpha-chain disease. This occurs mainly in areas surrounding the Mediterranean, in South America and in the Far East. It is related to poor hygiene and intestinal infestation. There is a proliferation of plasma cells in the lamina propria of the small bowel. These produce IgA heavy chains that can be detected in the gut mucosa by immunofluorescence as well as in the serum. The disease initially responds to broad-spectrum antibiotics but eventually becomes lymphomatous, when chemotherapy is required.

CLINICAL FEATURES

Patients present with abdominal pain, diarrhoea, anorexia, weight loss and symptoms of anaemia.

There may be a palpable mass and a small-bowel follow-through will detect most lesions. Laparotomy is required on many occasions to help with the diagnosis and to obtain tissue for histology and sometimes for resection. Treatment is often with resection, radiotherapy and chemotherapy.

Carcinoid tumours

These are discussed on p. 236.

THE LARGE INTESTINE

Colon polyps and polyposis syndromes (see Table 4.21)

A polyp is an elevation above the mucosal surface. The majority of colorectal polyps are adenomas with malignant potential. Polyps range in size from a few millimetres to 10 cm in diameter. They may be single or multiple and in the polyposis syndromes hundreds may be found. Not all colorectal polyps are adenomas.

In adults, 2–5 mm polyps in the rectum are often found: 90% of these will be of the innocent metaplastic type. Larger polyps in the rectum and 70–80% of all polyps in the colon are adenomas and 5% (20% of those 2 cm or greater in diameter) will contain invasive carcinoma at discovery. Most polyps are asymptomatic and found by chance when patients are investigated for pain, altered bowel habit, bleeding haemorrhoids or some other cause.

Hamartomatous polyps are commonly large and stalked and are either juvenile or Peutz–Jeghers in type.

Juvenile polyps (occurring in children and teenagers) are confined to the colon and histologically show mucus-retention cysts. They are inherited as an autosomal dominant and are a cause of bleeding, diarrhoea and intussusception, often in the first year of life. There is no evidence that they have a malignant potential.

Peutz–Jeghers polyps are usually multiple and have characteristic fibromuscular fronds radiating between disorganized mucosal crypts. They can occur in the large intestine, producing chronic anaemia. Other non-neoplastic polyps are less

Table 4.21 Classification of colorectal polyps.

	Solitary	Multiple (polyposis syndromes)
Non-neoplastic		
Hamartomas	Peutz–Jeghers	Peutz–Jeghers syndrome
	Juvenile (mucus retention)	Juvenile polyposis
Inflammatory	Lymphoid	Benign lymphoid polyposis
	Inflammatory	Inflammatory polyps, e.g.
		Ulcerative colitis
		Crohn's disease
		Schistosomiasis
Miscellaneous	Metaplastic (hyperplastic)	Metaplastic polyposis
	Connective tissue polyps	Cronkhite–Canada syndrome
	Fibroma	
	Leiomyoma	
	Lipoma	
	Neurofibroma	
Neoplastic		
	Adenomas	Familial adenomatous polyposis
	Tubular	
	Tubulovillous	
	Villous	
	Carcinoid	
		Malignant lymphomatous polyposis

common and are shown in Table 4.21.

In the Cronkhite–Canada syndrome, polyps are associated with ectodermal abnormalities such as alopecia, nail dystrophy and skin hyperpigmentation.

All of these polyps must be distinguished from adenomas, which have malignant potential.

Neoplastic polyps
Adenomas occur in about 10% of the population in the Western World but are rare elsewhere in the world. Genetic and environmental factors have been implicated but no definite aetiological factors have been identified.

Polyps rarely produce symptoms and most are diagnosed on X-ray or on colonoscopy performed for other reasons. Large polyps may bleed intermittently and cause anaemia. Large sessile villous adenomas of the rectum can present with profuse diarrhoea and hypokalaemia.

The frequency with which invasive carcinoma occurs in adenomas increases with the size of the polyp and most, if not all, colonic carcinomas originate as adenomas. Once a polyp has been found on X-ray or endoscopy it is usually removed endoscopically. Further polyps may develop (30–50% probability) and continuous surveillance is necessary.

Familial adenomatous polyposis (FAP) is inherited as an autosomal dominant trait; there is an abnorma-

lity of chromosome 5. Linkage studies in families have shown that the gene involved (apc) is on the long arm of chromosome 5 (between q21–22). Some sporadic colon cancers also have a deletion involving the *apc* gene. This gene therefore acts as a tumour suppressor, but it is unclear whether one or both copies of *apc* require deletion before a carcinoma develops. In FAP, multiple polyps are found in the large intestine and constant surveillance is necessary. For this high-risk group a prophylactic proctocolectomy with ileoanal anastomosis is performed. Screening of relatives is essential from the age of 12 years and if polyps are found proctocolectomy is performed at 20 years of age. One-third of patients have polyps in the upper gut that can also become malignant.

Gardner's syndrome is a variant of this condition in which, in addition to adenomatosis, there are mesodermal tumours (e.g. dermoid tumours, osteomas of the skull) and pigmented ocular fundal lesions.

Colorectal carcinoma

Adenocarcinoma of the large bowel is the second commonest tumour in the UK. The incidence increases with age, the average age at diagnosis being 60–65 years. The disease is rare in Africa and Asia and this difference is thought to be largely environmental rather than racial. There is a correlation between the consumption of meat and animal fat and colonic cancer. Western diets are low in fibre and the resulting intestinal stasis increases the time for which any potential carcinogen is in contact with the bowel wall. The bacterial flora in the colon is also affected by different diets, particularly in amount of fibre present, and it is speculated that certain bacteria convert bile acids to potential carcinogens. Ulcerative colitis (see p. 218) and familial polyposis are predisposing factors.

PATHOLOGY

Two-thirds of carcinomas occur in the rectosigmoid area. The tumour, which is usually a polypoid mass with ulceration, spreads by direct infiltration through the bowel wall. It then invades the lymphatics and blood vessels with early spread to the liver. Widespread metastases, e.g. to the lung, can occur.

CLINICAL FEATURES

Alteration in bowel habit, with or without abdominal pain, is a common symptom of left-sided colonic lesions. Rectum and sigmoid carcinomas usually bleed, blood being mixed in with the stool. Carcinoma of the caecum may become large and still remain asymptomatic. It can present simply as an iron-deficiency anaemia.

Any change in bowel habit or bleeding per rectum must be investigated, particularly in the older age group.

Clinical examination is usually unhelpful, but a mass may be palpable. With liver metastases, hepatomegaly is found. Digital examination of the rectum is essential and sigmoidoscopy should be performed in all cases. Flexible sigmoidoscopy can be performed on an out-patient basis.

INVESTIGATION

A blood count and routine biochemistry are performed. A double contrast barium enema is still the investigation of choice but good preparation to ensure that the colon is free of faeces is essential. Colonoscopy is used for confirmation of doubtful lesions and to obtain specimens for histological examination.

Occult blood tests have been used for mass screening but are of no value in hospital practice (see p. 197). Evaluation of secondary spread is performed prior to surgery with abdominal ultrasound and rectal ultrasound, which is valuable to indicate tumour size and local spread.

TREATMENT

This is surgical, with resection and end-to-end anastomosis if possible. Anastomosis is now pos-

sible with all but the most distal rectal carcinomas, when colostomy is necessary. The 5-year survival rate is 50% overall, but in tumours confined to the bowel wall (i.e. not reaching the serosa—Dukes grade A), the 5-year survival is over 95%.

Chemotherapy is sometimes used when metastases are present, but results are poor.

ENDOCRINE TUMOURS

Most tumours arise in the pancreas from APUD (*a*mine *p*recursor *u*ptake and *d*ecarboxylation) cells and are sometimes called apudomas.

Pancreatic endocrine tumours can occur in association with other endocrine tumours, particularly parathyroid adenoma and pituitary adenoma, as part of multiple endocrine neoplasias (see p. 830).

Endocrine tumours predominantly secrete one hormone that produces its clinical effect, but other hormones are often synthesized and can be detected either in the blood or in the resected tumour.

Gastrinoma (Zollinger–Ellison syndrome)

These tumours mainly arise from G cells in the pancreas and secrete large amounts of gastrin. This stimulates maximal gastric acid secretion, so that the main clinical problem is peptic ulceration. Peptic ulcers occur in the usual areas of the stomach and duodenum and also in the jejunum. The ulcers are often large and deep and sometimes multiple. Haemorrhage and perforation can occur, particularly immediately after surgery has been performed for an apparently straightforward duodenal ulcer.

Diarrhoea due to the low pH in the upper intestine is also a common feature. Jejunal mucosal abnormalities are also seen. A high serum gastrin confirms the diagnosis. Acid studies show high acid output.

Treatment was revolutionized with the introduction of H_2-receptor antagonists. These were given in high doses to reduce acid output. Omeprazole (which inhibits the $H^+–K^+$ proton pump necessary for acid secretion) has replaced them in ZE. Surgery is reserved for removal of the primary tumour only. The tumour may be demonstrated by scans or local venous sampling for gastrin. These tumours are malignant and although they grow slowly the patients now die of malignancy rather than gastrointestinal problems.

Carcinoid tumours

These originate from the argentaffin cells (serotonin producing) of the intestine. They make up 10% of all small-bowel neoplasms, the commonest sites being in the appendix, terminal ileum and the rectum. It is often difficult to be certain histologically whether a particular tumour is benign or malignant. Clinically most carcinoid tumours are asymptomatic until metastases are present. Ten per cent of carcinoid tumours in the appendix present as acute appendicitis, the inflammation being secondary to obstruction.

Carcinoid syndrome

This syndrome occurs in only 5% of patients with carcinoid tumours and only when there are liver metastases. Patients complain of spontaneous or induced bluish-red flushing, predominantly on the face and neck. This can lead to permanent changes with telangietasis. Gastrointestinal symptoms consist of abdominal pain and recurrent watery diarrhoea. Cardiac abnormalities are found in 50% of patients and consist of pulmonary stenosis or tricuspid incompetence.

Examination of the abdomen reveals hepatomegaly, and ultrasound examination confirms the presence of secondary deposits.

Biochemical abnormalities. Some of the features of the carcinoid syndrome are partly due to the tumour's producing serotonin (5-hydroxytryptamine; 5HT). Its breakdown product 5-hydroxyindoleacetic acid is readily measured in the urine.

The diarrhoea and cardiac complications are probably caused by this agent but the cutaneous flushing is thought to be produced by one of the kinins, such as bradykinin, which is known to cause vasodilatation, bronchospasm and increased intestinal motility. Octreotide is an octapeptide somatostatin analogue that has been shown to inhibit the release of many gut hormones. It alleviates the flushing and diarrhoea and can control a carcinoid crisis. It is given subcutaneously in doses up to 200 μg three times daily. The serotonin antagonist cyproheptadine and parachlorophenylalanine, an inhibitor of tryptophan-5-hydroxylase, may also help the diarrhoea.

Surgery is the best treatment for localized carcinoid tumours and can be used for liver involvement to reduce the bulk of tumour and symptoms. Selective embolization of hepatic metastases via the hepatic artery can be used, but may be accompanied by massive liver necrosis and release of 5HT. Chemotherapy is also used with some reduction in tumour bulk initially. Most patients survive for 5–10 years after diagnosis.

Other endocrine tumours

Vipomas. These rare pancreatic tumours produce severe intestinal secretion and watery diarrhoea leading to dehydration. Vasoactive intestinal peptide (VIP) is a neurotransmitter that stimulates adenyl cyclase to produce intestinal secretion.

Plasma concentrations of VIP are very high and are diagnostic. Levels of pancreatic polypeptide (PP) hormone are also raised. The role of peptide histidine methionine (PHM), levels of which are also raised in this condition, is uncertain but this hormone may be involved in secretion.

Corticosteroids help reduce the stool volume but octreotide is the most effective agent. An attempt should be made to localize the tumour and, if possible, it should be resected.

Glucagonomas. These are alpha-cell tumours of the pancreas that produce pancreatic glucagon. The patients have diabetes mellitus and a unique characteristic necrolytic migratory erythematous rash. The diagnosis is made by measuring pancreatic glucagon in the serum.

Enteroglucagonoma. A tumour originating in the right kidney has been described that produces marked hypertrophy of the villi in the jejunum.

Somatostatinomas. These have also been described; they produce diabetes, steatorrhoea and weight loss.

Medullary carcinoma of the thyroid. This tumour secretes calcitonin (see p. 805) and is a rare cause of diarrhoea.

Islet cell tumours. These are described on p. 858.

Further reading

Baillière's Clinical Gastroenterology—quarterly reviews of gastroenterology published by Baillière Tindall, London.

Booth CC & Neale GR (1985) *Disorders of the Small Intestine*. Oxford: Blackwell Scientific.

Bouchier IAD, Allan RN, Hodgson HJF & Keighley MRB (1984) *Textbook of Gastroenterology*. London: Baillière Tindall.

Johnson LR (ed.) (1987) *Physiology of the Gastrointestinal Tract*, 2nd edn, 2 volumes. New York: Raven Press.

Kirshner JB & Shorter RG (eds) (1988) *Inflammatory Bowel Disease*. Philadelphia: Lea & Febiger.

Misiewicz JJ, Pounder RE & Venables CW (1987) *Diseases of the Gut and Pancreas*. Oxford: Blackwell Scientific.

Morson BC & Dawson IMP (1989) *Gastrointestinal Pathology*. 3rd edn. Oxford: Blackwell Scientific.

Sleisenger MH & Fordtran JS (1989) *Gastrointestinal Disease: Pathophysiology, Diagnosis, Management*, 4th edn. Philadelphia: WB Saunders.

Turnberg LA (ed.) (1989) *Clinical Gastroenterology*. Oxford: Blackwell Scientific.

5

Liver, Biliary Tract and Pancreatic Diseases

The liver and biliary tract

Structure

Liver

The liver, the largest organ in the body, is situated in the right hypochondrium. Its upper border lies between the fifth and sixth ribs and its lower border can sometimes be palpated below the right costal margin on inspiration. The liver is divided into two main lobes—right and left. The right is larger and also contains the quadrate and caudate lobes. Riedel's lobe is an extension of the lateral portion of the right lobe and it can occasionally be felt in a normal abdomen.

The blood supply to the liver is via two main vessels:

- The hepatic artery, which is a branch of the coeliac axis and supplies 25% of the total blood flow
- The portal vein, which drains the gastrointestinal tract and the spleen

Both vessels enter the liver at the porta hepatis and the blood is distributed via the portal tracts into the sinusoids throughout the liver. Fifty per cent of the total oxygen supply is via the portal venous system.

Each liver lobe consists of polyhedral lobules containing a central vein and peripheral portal triads (or tracts). Functionally, however, the liver is divided into acini (see Fig. 5.1), each of which lies between a number of central veins with the portal triad (portal vein radicles, hepatic arterioles and bile ductules) in the middle. The hepatocytes near the triad (zone 1) are well supplied with oxygenated blood and are more resistant to damage than the cells nearer the central veins (zone 3). Blood passes from the central vein via the sinusoids to the hepatic vein. These sinusoids are lined by endothelial cells, Kupffer's cells (phagocytic cells) and fat-storage cells (Ito cells) and are separated by plates of liver cells

Introduction

In the Western World alcohol is the major cause of liver disease, while elsewhere the hepatitis B virus is still the most significant factor. Vaccines against hepatitis B viruses have been developed and hold a promise for possible eradication of this disease. Health education and the improvement of social conditions should also help stop the spread of other viral infections.

New imaging techniques such as ultrasound, CT scanning and endoscopic retrograde cannulation of the biliary tree enable the liver and biliary tree to be visualized with precision, resulting in earlier diagnosis and the avoidance of exploratory laparotomy.

Results of liver transplantation continue to improve and transplantation can be of value in the treatment of both acute and chronic liver failure.

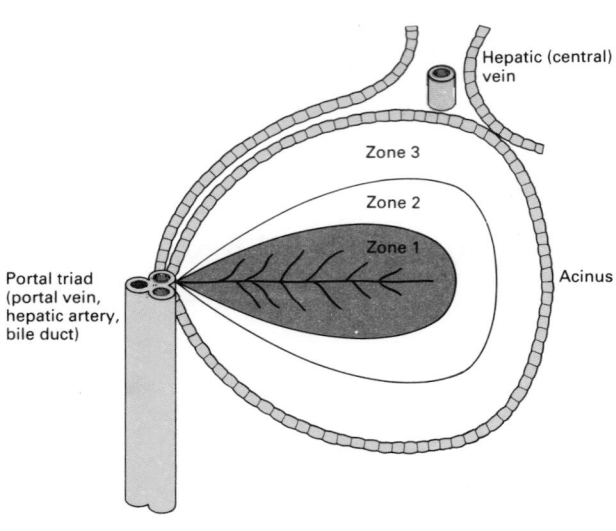

Fig. 5.1 Diagram of an acinus.

(hepatocytes). The space that lies between the sinusoids and hepatocytes (space of Disse) contains fluid that drains to the lymphatics in the portal tracts.

Biliary system

Bile canaliculi form a network between the hepatocytes. These join at the periphery of the hepatic lobules to form thin intralobular bile ductules, which in turn enter the interlobular bile ductules in the portal tracts. These then combine to form the right and left hepatic ducts that leave each liver lobe. The hepatic ducts join at the porta hepatis to form the common hepatic duct. The cystic duct connects the gall-bladder to the lower end of the common hepatic duct. The gall-bladder lies under the right lobe of the liver and stores and concentrates hepatic bile; it has a capacity of approximately 50 ml. The common bile duct is formed by the combination of the cystic and hepatic ducts and is approximately 8 mm wide, narrowing at its distal end to pass into the duodenum. The common bile duct and pancreatic duct open into the second part of the duodenum through a common channel at the ampulla of Vater. The lower end of the common bile duct contains the muscular sphincter of Oddi, which contracts rhythmically and prevents bile entering the duodenum in the fasting state.

Functions of the liver

Protein metabolism

Synthesis

The liver is the principal site of synthesis of all circulating proteins apart from gammaglobulins, which are produced in the reticulo-endothelial system. Plasma contains $60-80$ g·l^{-1} of protein, mainly in the form of albumin, globulin and fibrinogen.

Albumin has a half-life of 16–24 days and 10–12 g are synthesized daily. Its main functions are first to maintain the intravascular oncotic (colloid osmotic) pressure, and second to transport water-insoluble substances, e.g. bilirubin, hormones, fatty acids and drugs. Reduced synthesis of albumin over prolonged periods produces hypoalbuminaemia and is seen in chronic liver disease and malnutrition. Hypoalbuminaemia is also found in hypercatabolic states, e.g. trauma with sepsis, and with excessive loss, e.g. nephrotic syndrome, protein-losing enteropathy.

Transport or carrier proteins such as transferrin and caeruloplasmin, and other proteins, e.g. alpha-1-antitrypsin and alpha-fetoprotein, are also produced in the liver.

The liver also synthesizes all coagulation factors (see Chapter 6) apart from factor VIII, i.e. fibrinogen, prothrombin, factors V, VII, IX, X, XIII, and components of the complement system. Most factor VIII is produced in the reticuloendothelial system.

Degradation (nitrogen excretion)

Amino acids, the products of protein digestion, are degraded by transamination and oxidative deamination to produce ammonia, which is then converted to urea and excreted by the kidneys. This is a major pathway for the elimination of nitrogenous waste. Failure of this process occurs in severe liver disease.

Carbohydrate metabolism

Glucose homeostasis and the maintenance of the blood sugar is an important function of the liver. It stores approximately 80 g of glycogen. In the immediate fasting state, blood glucose is maintained either by glucose released from the breakdown of glycogen (glycogenolysis) or by newly synthesized glucose (gluconeogenesis). Sources for gluconeogenesis are lactate, pyruvate, amino acids from muscles (mainly alanine and glutamine) and glycerol from lipolysis of fat stores. In prolonged starvation, ketone bodies and fatty acids are used as alternative sources of fuel and the body tissues adapt to a lower glucose requirement (see Chapter 3).

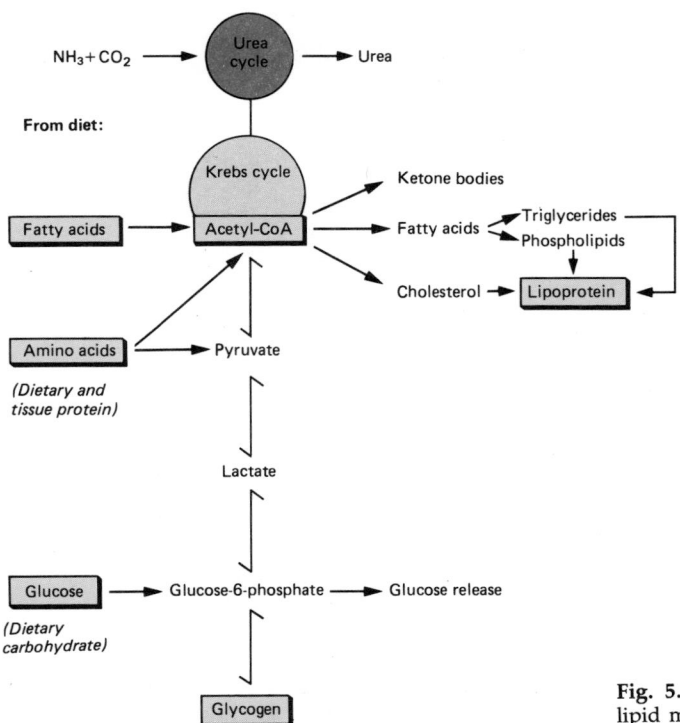

Fig. 5.2 Interrelationships of protein, carbohydrate and lipid metabolism in the liver.

Lipid metabolism

Fats are insoluble in water and are transported in the plasma as protein/lipid complexes (lipoproteins). These are discussed in detail on p. 861.

The liver plays a major role in the metabolism of lipoproteins. It synthesizes very low-density lipoproteins (VLDLs) and high-density lipoproteins (HDLs). HDLs are the substrate for lecithin–cholesterol acyltransferase (LCAT), which catalyses the conversion of free cholesterol to cholesterol ester (see below). Hepatic lipase catabolizes chylomicrons and VLDL remnants and is also involved in the metabolism of HDL phospholipid and triglycerides. The liver and kidney are the major sites of HDL catabolism. Low-density lipoproteins (LDLs) are degraded by the liver after uptake by specific cell-surface receptors.

Triglycerides may be of dietary origin but are also formed in the liver from circulating free fatty acids (FFA) and glycerol and incorporated into VLDLs. Oxidation or *de novo* synthesis of FFA also occurs in the liver, depending on the availability of dietary fat. Cholesterol may also be of dietary origin but most is synthesized from acetyl-CoA mainly in the liver, intestine, adrenal cortex and skin. It occurs either as free cholesterol or esterified with fatty acids, this reaction being catalysed by LCAT. This enzyme is reduced in severe liver disease, increasing the ratio of free cholesterol to

ester, which alters membrane structures. One result of this is the red cell abnormalities, e.g. burr cells, seen in chronic liver disease. Phospholipids, e.g. lecithin, are also synthesized in the liver.

The complex interrelationships between protein, carbohydrate and fat metabolism are shown in Fig. 5.2.

Bile acid metabolism

Bile acids are synthesized in hepatocytes from cholesterol. The rate-limiting step in their production is that catalysed by cholesterol-7α-hydroxylase. They are excreted into the bile and then pass into the duodenum. The two primary bile acids—cholic acid and chenodeoxycholic acid (see Fig. 5.3)—are conjugated with glycine or taurine (in a ratio of 3 : 1 in man) and this process increases their solubility. Intestinal bacteria convert these acids into secondary bile acids—deoxycholic acid and lithocholic acid. Approximately 95% of the bile acids are reabsorbed in the terminal ileum, pass back to the liver in the portal blood, and are re-excreted into the bile (the enterohepatic circulation) (Fig. 5.4). As the bile acid pool is relatively small (3–5 g) and up to 40 g are excreted daily into the bile, the entire bile pool recycles through the enterohepatic circulation six to eight times a day. Approximately 10–20% of the pool is lost daily and synthesis of new bile acids only compensates for this loss.

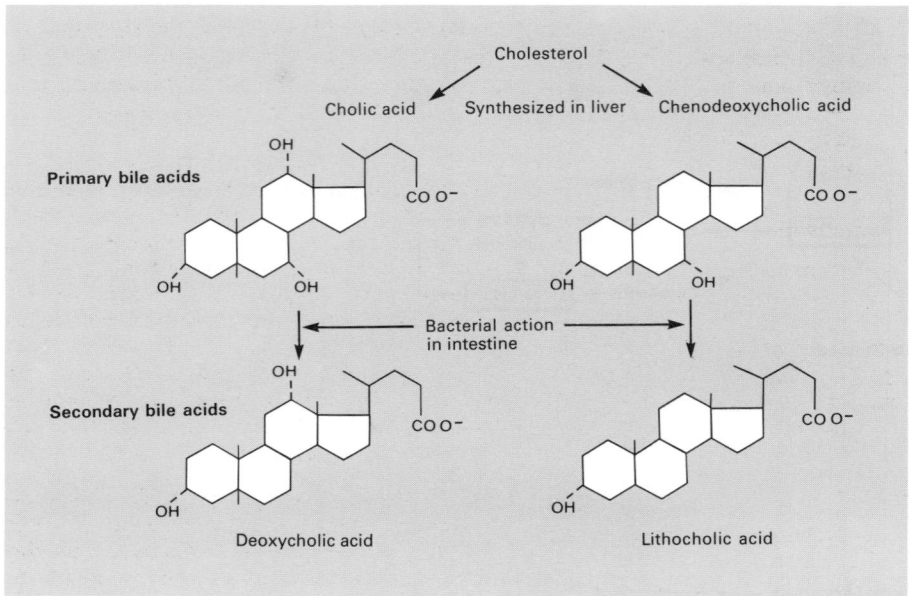

Fig. 5.3 Primary and secondary bile acids. All bile acids are normally conjugated with glycine or taurine.

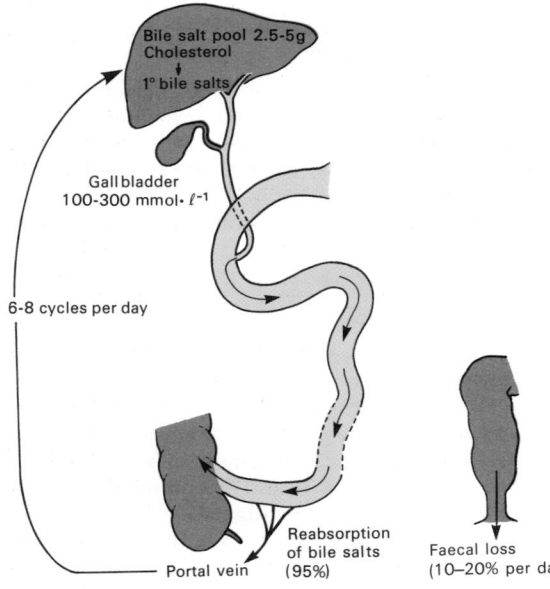

Fig. 5.4 Recirculation of bile acids.

Bile acids act as detergents; their main function is lipid solubilization. Bile acid molecules contain both a hydrophilic and a hydrophobic end. In aqueous solutions they aggregate to form micelles, with their hydrophobic (lipid-soluble) ends in the centre. Micelles are expanded by cholesterol and phospholipids (mainly lecithin), forming mixed micelles.

Bilirubin metabolism

Bilirubin is produced mainly from the breakdown of mature red cells in the Kupffer's cells of the liver and in the reticuloendothelial system. Fifteen per cent of bilirubin comes from the catabolism of other haem-containing proteins, such as myoglobin, cytochromes and catalases.

Normally, 250–300 mg of bilirubin are produced daily. The iron and globin are removed from the haem and are re-utilized. Biliverdin is formed from the haem and this is reduced to form bilirubin. The bilirubin produced is unconjugated and water-insoluble, and is transported to the liver attached to albumin. Bilirubin dissociates from albumin and is taken up by the hepatic cell membrane and transported to the endoplasmic reticulum by cytoplasmic proteins, where it is conjugated with glucuronic acid and excreted into bile. The microsomal enzyme uridine diphosphoglucuronyl transferase catalyses the formation of bilirubin mono- and then di-glucuronide. This conjugated bilirubin is water-soluble and is actively secreted into the bile canaliculi and excreted into the intestine with the bile. It is not absorbed from the small intestine because of its large molecular size. In the terminal ileum, bacterial enzymes hydrolyse the molecule, releasing free bilirubin, which is then reduced to urobilinogen. Some of this is excreted in the stools as stercobilinogen. The remainder is absorbed by the terminal ileum, passes to the liver via the enterohepatic circulation, and is re-excreted into the bile. Urobilinogen bound to albumin enters the circulation and is excreted in the urine via the kidneys. When hepatic excretion of conjugated bilirubin is impaired, a small amount of conjugated bilirubin is found strongly bound to serum albumin. It is not excreted by the kidney and accounts for the continuing hyperbilirubinaemia for a short time after cholestasis has resolved.

Hormone and drug inactivation

The liver catabolizes hormones such as insulin, glucagon, oestrogens, growth hormone, glucocorticoids and parathormone. It is the most important site for the metabolism of drugs (see p. 278) and alcohol (see p. 171). Fat-soluble drugs are converted to water-soluble substances that facilitates their excretion in the bile or urine.

Immunological function

The reticuloendothelial system of the liver contains many immunologically active cells, such as the phagocytic Kupffer's cells, and also a little lymphoid tissue in the portal tracts. The liver acts as a 'sieve' for the bacterial and other antigens carried to it via the portal tract from the gastrointestinal tract. These antigens appear to be phagocytosed and degraded without the production of antibody. This process does not allow the antigens to reach other antibody-producing sites in the body and thereby prevents adverse immunological reactions. The reticuloendothelial system is also thought to play a role in tissue repair, T and B lymphocyte interaction, and cytotoxic activity in disease processes.

Investigation

Investigative tests can be divided into:

- Routine biochemistry
- Additional blood investigations
- Imaging techniques to define gross anatomy
- Liver biopsy for histology

Routine biochemistry

Most liver function tests are markers of liver disease and not actual tests of 'function' *per se*. These tests are usually abnormal in hepatobiliary disease but normal values do not necessarily exclude severe disease. Recognized patterns of test abnormalities may occur in some diseases but considerable overlap occurs.

A routine blood sample sent to the laboratory for liver function tests will be processed by an automated multichannel analyser to produce serum levels of bilirubin, aminotransferases, alkaline phosphatase, gamma glutamyl transpeptidase (γGT) and serum proteins. Subsequent investigations are often based on these tests.

Bilirubin. In the serum, bilirubin is normally almost all unconjugated. Increased serum bilirubin is usually accompanied by other abnormalities in liver biochemistry. Determination of whether the bilirubin is conjugated or unconjugated is only necessary in congenital disorders of bilirubin metabolism (see below) or to exclude haemolysis.

Aminotransferases. These enzymes (often referred to as transaminases) are present in hepatocytes and leak into the blood with liver cell damage. The two enzymes measured are:

- *Aspartate aminotransferase* (AST), which was previously known as serum glutamic oxaloacetic transaminase (SGOT). This is a mitochondrial enzyme and is also present in heart, muscle, kidney and brain. High levels are seen in hepatic necrosis, cardiac infarction, muscle injury and congestive cardiac failure.
- *Alanine aminotransferase* (ALT), which was previously known as serum glutamic pyruvic transaminase (SGPT). This is a cytosol enzyme and is more specific for the liver than AST.

Alkaline phosphatase (AP). This is present in the canalicular and sinusoidal membranes of the liver, but is also present in many other tissues, e.g. bone, intestine and placenta. If necessary, its origin can be determined by electrophoretic separation of isoenzymes or, alternatively, if there is also an abnormality of, for example, the γGT, the alkaline phosphatase can be presumed to come from the liver.

Serum alkaline phosphatase is raised in cholestasis from any cause, whether intra- or extrahepatic disease. Increased alkaline phosphatase is synthesized and leaks into the blood. In cholestatic jaundice, levels may be up to 4–6 times the normal limit. Raised levels may also occur in conditions with infiltration of the liver, e.g. metastases, and in cirrhosis, frequently in the absence of jaundice. The highest serum levels due to liver disease (> 1000 i.u.) are seen with hepatic metastases and primary biliary cirrhosis.

Gamma glutamyl transpeptidase (γGT). This is a microsomal enzyme that is present in many tissues as well as the liver. Its activity can be induced by such drugs as phenytoin and by alcohol. If the alkaline phosphatase is normal, a raised γGT is a good guide to alcohol intake and can be used as a screening test (see p. 991). Mild elevation of the γGT is common even with a small alcohol consumption and does not necessarily indicate liver disease if the other liver biochemical tests are normal. In cholestasis the γGT rises in parallel with the alkaline phosphatase as it has a similar pathway of excretion. This is also true of the *5-nucleotidase*, another microsomal enzyme that can be measured in blood.

Serum proteins. Serum albumin is a sensitive marker of synthetic function and is a valuable guide to the severity of chronic liver disease. A falling serum albumin is a bad prognostic sign.

Hyperglobulinaemia occurs in chronic liver disease. This is thought to be due to reduced phagocytosis by sinusoidal and Kupffer's cells of the antigens absorbed from the gut, which then stimulate antibody production in the spleen and lymph nodes. In chronic liver disease, immunoglobulins are formed by lymphoid and plasma cells that infiltrate the portal tracts. The routine plasma electrophoretic strips contain immunoglobulins in the beta and gamma regions. In cirrhosis there is beta–gamma fusion due to an increase in the faster-moving globulins; the diagnostic value of these strips is, however, limited. In primary biliary cirrhosis the predominant serum immunoglobulin that is raised is IgM, and in autoimmune chronic active hepatitis it is IgG. This latter finding is of help in the diagnosis.

Additional blood investigations

Haematological tests

Anaemia may be present. The red cells are often macrocytic and can have abnormal shapes—target cells and spur cells—owing to membrane abnormalities. Vitamin B_{12} levels are normal or high, and folate levels are often low owing to poor dietary intake.

- Bleeding produces a hypochromic, microcytic picture.
- Alcohol causes macrocytosis, sometimes with leucopenia and thrombocytopenia.
- Hypersplenism results in pancytopenia.
- Cholestasis can often produce abnormal-shaped cells and also deficiency of vitamin K.
- Haemolysis accompanies acute liver failure and jaundice.
- Aplastic anaemia is present in up to 2% of patients with acute viral hepatitis.

Prothrombin time (PT). This is a marker of synthetic function. Because of its short half-life it is a sensitive indicator of both acute and chronic liver disease. It is important to exclude vitamin K deficiency as the cause of a prolonged PT by giving an intravenous bolus (10 mg) of vitamin K. Vitamin K deficiency commonly occurs in biliary obstruction, as the low intestinal concentration of bile salts results in poor absorption of vitamin K.

Viral markers. These are available for most of the common viruses that cause hepatitis (see p. 251).

Alpha-fetoprotein. This is normally produced by the fetal liver. With the more sensitive radioimmunoassay techniques, very low levels can be detected in normal individuals and moderately raised levels in patients with hepatitis or chronic liver disease. Its reappearance in increasing and high concentrations in the adult indicates hepatocellular carcinoma. Increased concentrations in pregnancy in the blood and amniotic fluid suggest neural-tube defects of the fetus. Blood levels are also raised in teratomas.

Immunological tests

There are no specific antibodies to the liver itself that are routinely measured. Autoantibodies found are:

- *Antimitochondrial antibody* (AMA) is found in the serum in over 95% of patients with primary biliary cirrhosis. Many different AMA subtypes have been described, depending on their antigen specificity. AMA is demonstrated by an immunofluorescent technique and is neither organ- nor species-specific. Some subtypes are occasionally found in autoimmune chronic active hepatitis and other autoimmune diseases.
- *Nucleic, actin, liver/kidney microsomal antibodies* can be found in the serum in high titre in patients with autoimmune chronic active hepatitis. These

Table 5.1 Useful blood tests for certain liver diseases.

Test	Disease
Antimitochondrial antibody	Primary biliary cirrhosis
Antinuclear, smooth muscle (actin), liver kidney microsomal antibody	Autoimmune chronic active hepatitis
Raised serum immunoglobulins:	
IgG	Autoimmune chronic active hepatitis
IgM	Primary biliary cirrhosis
Viral markers (IgG and IgM)	Hepatitis A, B, C and others
Alpha-fetoprotein	Primary hepatocellular carcinoma
Serum iron, saturated iron binding capacity, ferritin	Haemochromatosis
Serum and urinary copper, serum caeruloplasmin	Wilson's disease
Alpha-1-antitrypsin	Cirrhosis (± emphysema)

antibodies can be found in the serum in other autoimmune conditions and other liver diseases.

Bromsulphthalein (BSP) test. This is now very rarely performed. The liver normally clears BSP from the blood. The level of BSP in the blood after an intravenous injection of BSP is a guide to hepato-cellular damage. A second recirculation peak occurs in the congenital hyperbilirubinaemia of the Dubin–Johnson syndrome. Anaphylactic reactions may occur.

Useful blood tests for certain liver diseases are shown in Table 5.1

Imaging techniques

The main aim of these investigations is to delineate the anatomy and to look for any abnormality in the liver or biliary tree.

Plain X-rays of the abdomen
These are rarely requested but may show:

- Gallstones (10% contain enough calcium to be seen)

- Air in the biliary tree owing to its recent instrumentation, surgery or to a fistula between the intestine and the gall bladder
- Pancreatic calcification
- Calcification of the gall bladder (porcelain gall bladder)—rare.

Ultrasound examination
This non-invasive, safe and relatively cheap technique is usually the first investigation of choice if hepatobiliary or pancreatic disease is suspected. It involves the analysis of the reflected ultrasound beam detected by a probe moved across the abdomen. The normal liver appears as a relatively homogeneous structure. The gall bladder, common bile duct, pancreas, portal vein and other structures in the abdomen can be visualized.

This technique is most valuable in the jaundiced patient. The size of the common bile duct and intrahepatic ducts can be accurately estimated, thereby distinguishing extra-hepatic biliary obstruction from other intra-hepatic causes of jaundice. Gallstones can be detected in the gall bladder with 98% accuracy (Fig. 5.5) but may be missed in the common bile duct. The size and patency of the

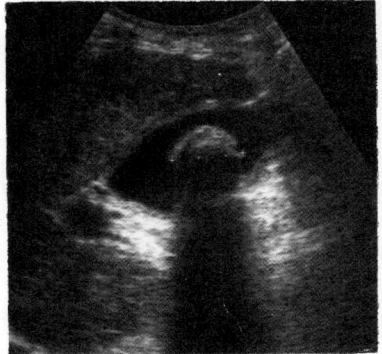

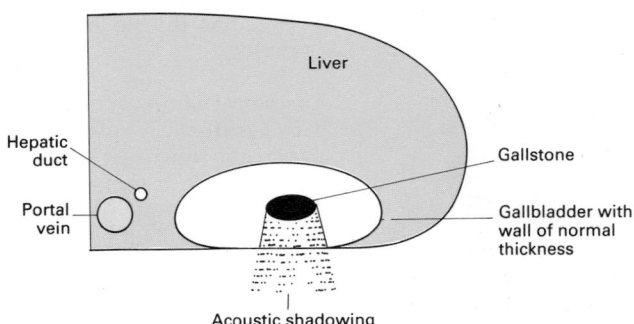

Fig. 5.5 Ultrasound showing a large gallstone (arrow) with acoustic shadowing.

portal and hepatic veins can be assessed. Changes in liver architecture, e.g. cirrhosis, can be detected, as well as space-occupying lesions of more than 1 cm diameter. Other abdominal masses can be delineated and biopsies can be obtained under ultrasonic control.

Computed tomography (CT)
This is useful in all hepatobiliary problems and is complementary to ultrasound. Pancreatic disease, enlargement of regional lymph nodes, and lesions in the porta hepatis can be visualized. Abnormalities of size, shape and density as well as focal lesions of the liver can be detected. CT can detect calcification not seen on plain X-rays. It is not as useful as ultrasound for biliary tract disease but has advantages in obese subjects. As with ultrasound, biopsies can be taken under CT control.

Cholecystogram
This has now been replaced as the first investigation for gall-bladder disease in most centres by ultrasound examination. Tablets of iopanoic acid are taken the night before the X-ray. This is absorbed from the gut, conjugated in the liver, secreted in bile and concentrated in the gall

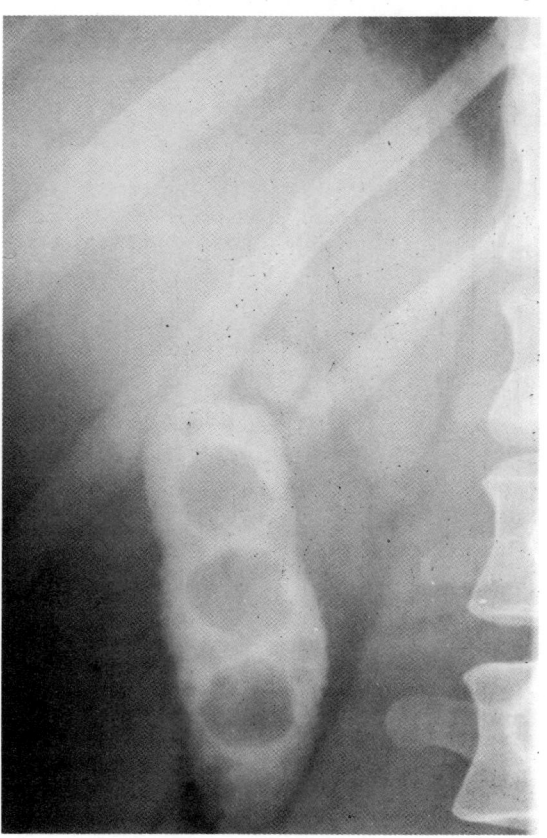

Fig. 5.6 Cholecystogram showing gallstones.

bladder, which opacifies homogeneously. Radiolucent gallstones are shown in Fig. 5.6. A fatty meal is given that makes the gall bladder contract. The bile ducts can be outlined on some occasions.

The gall bladder is frequently not visualized with this technique owing to disease, a blocked cystic duct, or because the contrast medium has not been absorbed. The dye is excreted by the liver via the same mechanism as bilirubin, so that non-visualization will also occur in the jaundiced patient and in the patient with liver disease. A cholecystogram should not be performed in these situations. If non-visualization occurs, an ultrasound examination should be performed.

Intravenous cholangiography
This has been replaced by ultrasound and endoscopic retrograde cholangiopancreatography (ERCP). It was used in patients after cholecystectomy to visualize the biliary duct.

Scintiscanning
Technetium-99m (^{99m}Tc) colloid scan. This colloid, when injected intravenously, is taken up by the reticuloendothelial cells of the liver and spleen. It can show space-occupying lesions and a generalized decrease in uptake is found in parenchymal disease of the liver.

Since the introduction of ultrasound this technique is used less frequently. Currently its main uses are in:

- Advanced cirrhosis in which there is poor uptake in the liver and most of the colloid is taken up in the spleen and bone marrow
- Alcoholic hepatitis in which there is virtually no uptake in the liver owing to Kupffer's cell damage by alcohol

^{99m}Tc-HIDA scan. ^{99m}Tc-HIDA (an imino-diacetic acid derivative) is taken up by the hepatocytes and excreted rapidly into the biliary system. Its main uses are in the diagnosis of:

- Acute cholecystitis
- Hepatitis due to biliary atresia in the neonatal period

Endoscopic retrograde cholangiopancreatography (ERCP)
This technique is used to outline the biliary and pancreatic ducts. It involves the passage of an endoscope into the second part of the duodenum and cannulation of the ampulla. Contrast is injected into both systems and the patient is screened radiologically. Contrast medium with a low iodine content of 1.5 mg·ml^{-1} is used for the common bile duct so that gall-stones are not obscured; a higher iodine content of 2.8 mg·ml^{-1} is used for the pancreatic duct. In addition, other diagnostic and therapeutic procedures can be carried out:

- Removal of common bile duct stones after a diathermy cut to the sphincter has been performed to facilitate their withdrawal
- Draining the biliary system by passing a tube (stent) through an obstruction

Complications include cholangitis, and broad-spectrum prophylactic antibodies should be given to all patients with suspected biliary obstruction. Pancreatitis can occur and ERCP is performed with caution if a pseudocyst of the pancreas is suspected.

Percutaneous transhepatic cholangiography (PTC)

Under a local anaesthetic a fine, flexible needle is passed into the liver. Contrast is injected slowly until a biliary radicle is identified and then further contrast is injected to outline the whole of the biliary tree. The main use of PTC is in jaundiced patients who have been shown to have dilated intrahepatic ducts demonstrated on ultrasound. The choice of ERCP or PTC often depends on local expertise. Sometimes the two techniques are complementary, PTC showing the biliary anatomy leading to an obstruction, while the ERCP shows the more distal anatomy. If an obstruction in the bile ducts is seen, a bypass stent can sometimes be inserted either draining externally or, for long-term use, internally. Contraindications are as for liver biopsy (see below). The main complications are bleeding and cholangitis with septicaemia, and prophylactic antibiotics should be given as for ERCP.

Angiography

This can be performed by selective catheterization of the coeliac axis and hepatic artery, and is useful for detecting the abnormal vasculature of hepatic tumours. The portal vein can be demonstrated with increased definition using subtraction techniques, and splenoportography (by direct splenic puncture) is now rarely performed. In digital vascular imaging (DVI), contrast given intravenously or intra-arterially can be detected in the portal system using computerized subtraction analysis. Attempted visualization of the hepatic veins by venography is particularly important in the diagnosis of the Budd–Chiari syndrome. Hepatic venous cannulation also allows an indirect measurement of portal pressure to be made, although this has seldom been shown to be of any diagnostic or therapeutic value.

Magnetic resonance imaging

This technique is being used for the detection of liver masses.

Liver biopsy

This is the only means by which a diagnosis of intrinsic liver disease can be confirmed. It is a simple, relatively safe procedure that can be performed either on a day-case or overnight-stay basis. The indications and contraindications are shown in Table 5.2. There are many contraindications, and a biopsy should not be undertaken lightly. The mortality rate is less than 0.02%.

Table 5.2 Indications and contraindications for liver biopsy.

Indications
Liver disease
  Unexplained hepatomegaly
  Some cases of jaundice (see p. 251)
  Persistently abnormal liver function tests
  Occasionally in acute hepatitis (see p. 252)
  Cirrhosis
  Drug-related liver disease
  Infiltrations
  Tumours—primary or secondary
  Systemic disease
Screening relatives of patients with certain diseases, e.g. haemochromatosis
Pyrexia of unknown origin

Usual contraindications to needle biopsy
Uncooperative patient
Prolonged prothrombin time (by more than 3 s)
Platelets $< 80 \times 10^9$ litre
Ascites
Extra-hepatic cholestasis

Liver biopsy can also be performed under ultrasound or CT control when specific lesions need to be biopsied.

Liver biopsy is sometimes performed during laparoscopy under local or general anaesthesia through a small incision in the abdominal wall. This procedure has the advantage that the whole peritoneum can be inspected after CO_2 insufflation (pneumoperitoneum). Biopsies can be taken from diseased peritoneal areas as well as from the liver.

Liver biopsies can also be performed via the inferior vena cava using the transjugular route in patients with a prolonged prothrombin time.

COMPLICATIONS

These are usually minor and include abdominal or shoulder pain which settles with analgesics. Minor intraperitoneal bleeding is common but this settles spontaneously. Rare complications include major intraperitoneal bleeding, pleurisy and perihepatitis, biliary peritonitis, haemobilia and transient septicaemia. Haemobilia produces biliary colic, jaundice and melaena within 3 days of the biopsy.

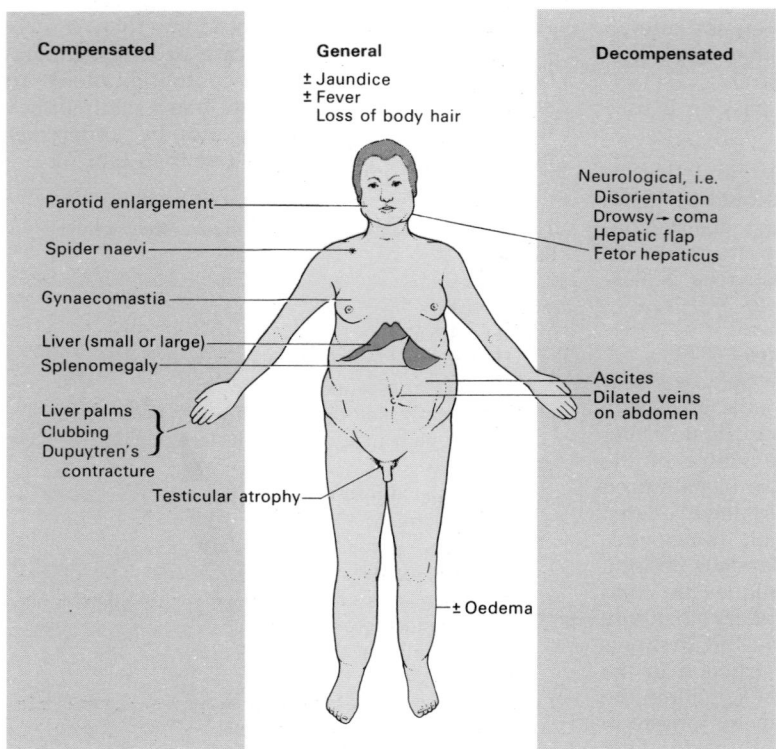

Fig. 5.7 Physical signs in chronic liver disease.

Symptoms of liver disease

Acute liver disease

Acute liver disease may be asymptomatic and anicteric. For example, an abnormality such as raised aminotransferases may be found during a routine biochemical screen.

Symptomatic acute liver disease, which is often viral, produces generalized symptoms of malaise, anorexia and fever. Jaundice may appear as the illness progresses.

Chronic liver disease

Patients may be asymptomatic or complain of non-specific symptoms. Specific symptoms include:

- Abdominal distension due to ascites, ankle swelling and fluid retention
- Haematemesis and melaena from gastro-intestinal haemorrhage
- Pruritus due to cholestasis; this is often an early symptom of primary biliary cirrhosis
- Breast swelling, loss of libido and amenorrhoea due to endocrine dysfunction
- Confusion and drowsiness due to neuro-psychiatric complications

Signs of liver disease

Acute liver disease

There may be few signs apart from jaundice and an enlarged liver. Jaundice is a yellow coloration of the skin and mucous membranes and is best seen in the conjunctivae. In the cholestatic phase of the illness, pale stools and dark urine are seen. Spider naevi and liver palms usually indicate chronic disease but they can occur in severe acute disease.

Chronic liver disease

The possible physical signs are shown in Fig. 5.7. However, it is possible for the physical examination to be normal in patients with advanced chronic liver disease.

Common signs
The skin. The chest and upper body may show spider naevi. These are telangiectases that consist of a central arteriole with radiating small vessels. They are found in the distribution of the superior vena cava, i.e. above the nipple line. They are also found in pregnancy. In haemochromatosis the skin may have a slate-grey appearance.

The hands may show palmar erythema, which is a non-specific change indicative of a hyper-dynamic circulation; it may also be seen in pregnancy, thyrotoxicosis or rheumatoid arthritis. Clubbing occasionally occurs, and a Dupuytren's contracture is often seen in alcoholic cirrhosis.

Xanthomas (cholesterol deposits) may be seen in the palmar creases or above the eyes in primary biliary cirrhosis.

The abdomen. Initial hepatomegaly will be followed by a small liver in well-established cirrhosis.

Splenomegaly is usually taken as an indication of portal hypertension.

The endocrine system. Gynaecomastia (occasionally unilateral) and testicular atrophy may be found in males. The cause of gynaecomastia is complex, but it is probably related to altered oestrogen metabolism or to treatment with spironolactone.

In *decompensated cirrhosis*, additional signs that can be seen are:

- Jaundice
- Ascites with or without peripheral oedema
- Evidence of portosystemic encephalopathy (PSE) (see p. 267) including drowsiness, stupor, fetor hepaticus and a flapping tremor of the out-stretched hands
- Collateral veins and veins around the umbilicus (caput medusae) (rare)

Jaundice

Jaundice (icterus) is detectable when the serum bilirubin is greater than 30–60 mmol·L^{-1} (> 3 mg per 100 ml). The usual division of jaundice into pre-hepatic, hepatocellular and obstructive (cholestatic) is an oversimplification, as mixed pictures are often seen; the latter two in particular often occur together. Jaundice will therefore be considered under the following headings:

- Haemolytic jaundice
- Congenital hyperbilirubinaemias
- Cholestatic jaundice, including parenchymal liver disease and large duct obstruction

Haemolytic jaundice

The increased breakdown of red cells (see p. 309) leads to an increase in production of bilirubin. The resulting jaundice is usually mild (serum bilirubin of 68–102 mmol·L^{-1} [4–6 per 100 ml]) as normal liver function can easily handle the increased bilirubin derived from excess haemolysis. Unconjugated bilirubin is not water-soluble and therefore will not pass into the urine, hence the term 'acholuric jaundice'. Urinary urobilinogen is increased.

The causes of haemolytic jaundice are those of haemolytic anaemia (see p. 311). The clinical features depend on the cause; anaemia, jaundice, splenomegaly, gallstones and leg ulcers may be seen.

Investigations show features of haemolysis (see p. 311). The level of unconjugated bilirubin is raised but the serum alkaline phosphatase, transferases and albumin are normal. Serum haptoglobulins are low.

The differential diagnosis is from other forms of jaundice (see p. 249).

Congenital hyperbilirubinaemias (non-haemolytic)

The commonest is Gilbert's syndrome. The others —Crigler–Najjar, Dubin–Johnson and Rotor syndromes—are rare (see Table 5.3).

Gilbert's syndrome

This is the commonest familial hyperbilirubinaemia and affects 2–5% of the population. It is asymptomatic and is usually detected as an incidental finding of a slightly raised bilirubin (3–5 mg·dl^{-1}; 51–85 mmol·L^{-1}) on a routine check. No signs of liver disease are seen. There is a family history of jaundice in 5–15% of patients. The aetiology of the syndrome is multifactorial and many abnormalities of bilirubin handling have been demonstrated. It is possible that this condition merely represents one end of the normal distribution curve.

The major importance of establishing this diagnosis is to inform the patient that this is not a serious disease and to prevent unnecessary investigation in the future. Investigations show only a raised unconjugated bilirubin, which rises on fasting and during a mild illness. The reticulocyte count is normal. Rarely, a liver biopsy needs to be performed to exclude intrinsic liver disease; this will be normal. No treatment is necessary.

Cholestatic jaundice

This can be divided into:

- *Intrahepatic cholestasis,* due to the swelling of hepatocytes and oedema in parenchymal liver damage (hepatocellular) or to an excretory dysfunction of the bile canaliculi at a cellular level
- *Extrahepatic cholestasis,* due to large duct obstruction of bile flow at any point in the biliary tract distal to the bile canaliculi

The causes are shown in Table 5.4.

Table 5.3 Congenital hyperbilirubinaemias.

	Inheritance	Age at presentation	Prognosis	Defect	Liver histology	Bilirubin in urine	Other findings	Treatment
Unconjugated bilirubin								
Gilbert's syndrome	Autosomal dominant	Mainly young adult, but can be any	Excellent	→ Bilirubin uptake → Glucuronyl transferase → Red cell survival	Normal	No	—	None
Crigler–Najjar syndrome								
Type I	Autosomal recessive	Neonate	Fatal (due to kernicterus)	No glucuronyl transferase	Normal	No	—	None
Type II	Autosomal dominant	Neonate	Survive to adult life	→ Glucuronyl transferase	Normal	No	—	Phenobarbitone if necessary
Conjugated bilirubin								
Dubin–Johnson syndrome	Autosomal recessive	Any	Good	→ Bilirubin excretion	Melanin deposition	Yes	Non-filling gall bladder. BSP test shows secondary rise at 2 h	None
Rotor syndrome	? Autosomal dominant	Variable (usually childhood)	Good	→ Bilirubin uptake → Storage of bilirubin	Normal	Yes	Non-filling gall bladder BSP test abnormal at 45 min; no secondary rise	None

Clinically there is jaundice with pale stools and dark urine. The bilirubin in the serum is conjugated.

Intrahepatic and extrahepatic cholestatic jaundice must be differentiated, as their clinical management is entirely different.

THE DIFFERENTIAL DIAGNOSIS OF JAUNDICE

HISTORY

A careful history may give a clue to the diagnosis. Patients should be asked a series of questions, keeping in mind that certain causes of jaundice are more likely in particular categories of people. A young person is more likely to have hepatitis and therefore questions about drug and alcohol abuse and homosexuality are important. An elderly person with gross weight loss is more likely to have a carcinoma.

All patients may complain of malaise, but abdominal pain only occurs in biliary obstruction with gallstones or sometimes with an enlarged liver, when the pain is due to distension of the capsule.

The following aspects of the history should be covered. Questions should be appropriate to the particular situation.

- *Duration of illness*—a history of jaundice with prolonged weight loss in an older patient suggests malignancy; a short history, particularly with a prodromal illness of malaise, suggests a hepatitis.
- *Recent outbreak* of jaundice in the community—suggests hepatitis A.
- *Recent consumption* of shellfish—suggests hepatitis A.

Table 5.4 Causes of cholestatic jaundice.

Extrahepatic
Common duct stones
Carcinoma
   Head of pancreas
   Ampulla
   Bile duct
Biliary stricture
Pancreatitis ± pseudocyst
Sclerosing cholangitis

Intrahepatic
Viral hepatitis
Drugs
Alcoholic hepatitis
Cirrhosis—any type
Pregnancy
Recurrent idiopathic cholestasis
Some congenital disorders

- *Intravenous drug* abuse, male homosexuality, recent injections or tatoos—all increase chance of hepatitis B.
- *Blood transfusions* or infusion of pooled blood products. In developed countries all are screened for hepatitis B virus (HBV) and more recently for hepatitis C virus (HCV).
- *Alcohol consumption*—a careful history of drinking habits is important, although many patients often lie about the actual amount they drink.
- *Drugs taken*, particularly in the previous 2–3 months—many drugs cause jaundice (see p. 278).
- *Travel abroad* to areas with increased hepatitis risk.
- *Recent anaesthetics*—e.g. halothane may cause jaundice.
- *Family history*—patients with, for example, Gilbert's disease may have family members who get recurrent jaundice.
- *Recent surgery* on the biliary tract or for carcinoma.
- *Occupation*—farm and sewage workers are at risk for leptospirosis as well as swimmers in unchlorinated water.
- *Fevers or rigors*—suggestive of cholangitis or possibly a liver abscess.

CLINICAL EXAMINATION

The signs of acute and chronic liver disease should be looked for (see p. 246). Certain additional signs may be useful:

- *Hepatomegaly*—a smooth tender liver is seen in hepatitis and with extrahepatic obstruction, but a knobbly irregular liver suggests metastases. Causes of hepatomegaly are shown in Table 5.5.
- *Splenomegaly* indicates portal hypertension in patients when signs of chronic liver disease are present. It is also seen occasionally in viral hepatitis.
- *Ascites* is found in cirrhosis but can also be due to carcinoma (particularly ovarian) and many other causes (see Table 5.12).
- *A palpable gall bladder* can suggest a carcinoma of the pancreas obstructing the bile duct.
- *Generalized lymphadenopathy* suggests a lymphoma.

INVESTIGATION

Jaundice is not a diagnosis and the cause should always be sought.

An ultrasound should always be performed to exclude an extra-hepatic obstruction unless the patient is young and the diagnosis of hepatitis is supported by viral markers.

An ultrasound will demonstrate:

- The size of the bile ducts (Fig. 5.8).
- The level of the obstruction

Table 5.5 Causes of hepatomegaly.

'Apparent'
   Low-lying diaphragm
   Reidel's lobe

Cirrhosis—early

Inflammation
   Hepatitis
   Schistosomiasis
   Abscesses—pyogenic or amoebic

Cysts
   Hydatid
   Polycystic

Metabolic
   Fatty liver
   Amyloid
   Glycogen storage disease

Haematological
   Leukaemias
   Lymphoma
   Myeloproliferative disorders

Tumours—primary and secondary carcinoma

Venous congestion
   Heart failure
   Hepatic vein occlusion

Biliary obstruction—particularly extrahepatic

● The cause of the obstruction in virtually all tumours and in 75% of patients with gallstones
● The diagnosis of the lesion by fine-needle aspiration cytology (sensitivity approximately 60%)

Most lesions seen can be biopsied. Using a spring-loaded device, a percutaneous guided needle biopsy can be obtained and an exact diagnosis can be made in approximately 90% of cases.

A flow diagram for the general investigation of the jaundiced patient is shown in Fig. 5.9.

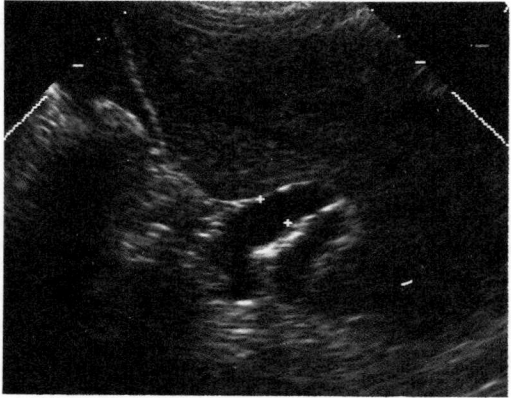

Fig. 5.8 Ultrasound showing a dilated common bile duct, in front of the portal vein, at the porta hepatis.

Liver biochemistry
In hepatitis the serum AST tends to be high early in the disease with only a small rise in the alkaline phosphatase. Conversely, in extra-hepatic obstruction the serum alkaline phosphatase is high with a smaller rise in AST. These findings cannot, however, be relied on alone to make a diagnosis in an individual case. The prothrombin time is often prolonged in longstanding liver disease, and the serum albumin is low.

Haematological tests
These are helpful in haemolytic jaundice. A raised white count may indicate infection, e.g. cholangitis. A leucopenia often occurs in viral hepatitis, while abnormal mononuclear cells suggest infectious mononucleosis or toxoplasmosis; a Monospot test should be performed for the former.

Other blood tests
These include viral studies for hepatitis, e.g. hepatitis A, B and C, cytomegalovirus, auto-immune antibodies, e.g. ANF, AMA (for primary biliary cirrhosis) and α-fetoprotein for a hepatoma.

Acute liver disease

Acute parenchymal liver damage can be caused by many agents (Fig. 5.10). If there is widespread damage of hepatocytes, the normal liver architecture may collapse. The extent of hepatocellular damage may be extremely variable.

PATHOLOGY

Histological changes are essentially similar whatever the cause. Hepatocytes show degenerative changes (swelling, cytoplasmic granularity, vacuolation), undergo necrosis (becoming shrunken, eosinophilic Councilman bodies) and are rapidly removed. The distribution of these changes varies somewhat with the aetiological agent, but necrosis is usually in zone 3. The extent of the damage is very variable between individuals affected by the same agent: at one end of the spectrum, single and small groups of hepatocytes die (spotty or focal necrosis), while at the other end whole lobules are destroyed (massive hepatic necrosis) resulting in fulminant hepatic failure. Between these extremes one sees limited confluent necrosis of hepatocytes with collapse of the reticulin framework resulting in linking (bridging) between central veins, central veins and portal tracts, and portal tracts.

Centrilobular cholestasis is common, but fatty change is usually absent apart from certain types of

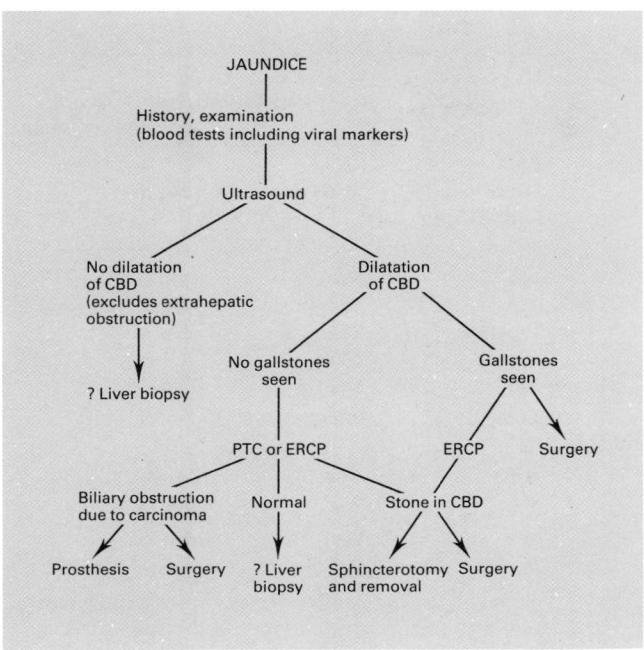

Fig. 5.9 Investigation of cholestatic jaundice. PT = percutaneous trans-hepatic cholangiography; ERCP = endoscopic retrograde cholangiopancreatography; CBD = common bile duct.

hepatitis owing to toxins such as alcohol or that seen in pregnancy. The extent of the inflammatory infiltrate is also variable, but portal tracts and lobules are infiltrated mainly by lymphocytes.

VIRAL HEPATITIS

The differing features of the common forms of viral hepatitis are summarized in Table 5.6.

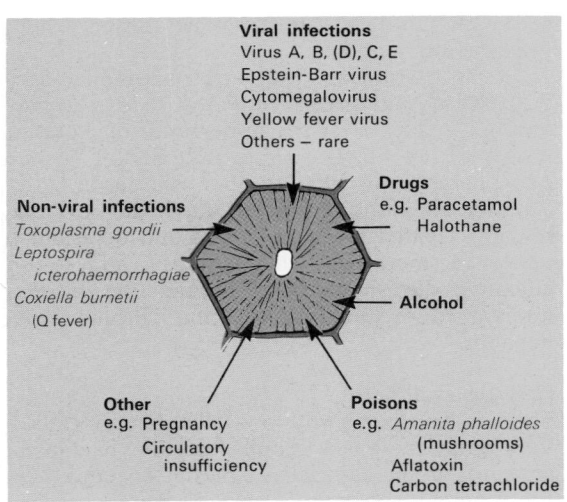

Fig. 5.10 Some causes of acute parenchymal damage.

In hepatitis A the damage is due to the virus itself, but in hepatitis B it is due to an immunological reaction to the virus.

Hepatitis A

EPIDEMIOLOGY

This is the commonest type of viral hepatitis and causes 20–40% of clinically apparent hepatitis. It occurs world-wide, often in epidemics. The disease is commonly seen in the autumn and affects children and young adults. Spread of infection is mainly by the faecal–oral route and arises from the ingestion of contaminated food (e.g. shellfish, clams) or water. Lower socioeconomic classes are affected more frequently, possibly owing to overcrowding and poor sanitation. There is no carrier state.

Hepatitis A virus
Hepatitis A virus (HAV) (Fig. 5.11) is excreted in the faeces of infected persons for about 2 weeks before the onset of the illness and for up to 7 days after. The disease is maximally infectious just before the onset of jaundice. HAV particles can be demonstrated in the faeces by electron microscopy. The disease affects other parts of the body as well as the liver, e.g. the heart, pancreas, gastrointestinal tract and spleen.

Table 5.6 Some features of hepatitis viruses.

	A	B	D	C (post-transfusion)	E (Non-A Non-B epidemic/enteral)
Virus	RNA 27 nm	DNA 42 nm	RNA 36 nm (with HB$_s$Ag coat)	RNA 30–60 nm	? 27 nm
Spread:					
Faecal	Yes	No	No	No	Yes
Blood	Rare	Yes	Yes	Yes	No
Vertical	No	Yes	Probable	Yes	No
Saliva	Yes	Yes	Yes	? Yes	?
Sexual	Occasionally	Yes	Yes	Yes	No
Incubation	Short (2–3 weeks)	Long (1–5 months)	Long	Intermediate	Short
Age	Young	Any	Any	Any	Any
Carrier state	No	Yes	Yes	Yes	No
Chronic liver disease	No	Yes	Yes	Yes	No
Liver cancer	No	Yes	Rare	Yes	No
Mortality (acute)	< 0.5%	< 1%		< 1%	1–2% (pregnant women 10%)
Immunization:					
Passive	Normal immunoglobulin i.m. (0.04–0.06 ml·kg^{-1})	Hyperimmune serum	—	—	—
Active	Available soon	Vaccine	HBV vaccine	—	—

CLINICAL FEATURES

The pre-icteric or prodromal phase lasts up to 2 weeks. The viraemia causes the patient to feel unwell with nausea, vomiting, diarrhoea, anorexia, headaches, malaise and a distaste for cigarettes. Fever is usually mild and there may be upper abdominal discomfort. There are few physical signs at this stage; the liver is tender but not enlarged initially.

After 1 or 2 weeks the patient becomes icteric (although some may never do so) and symptoms often improve. The appetite returns and the patient feels better. As the jaundice deepens the urine becomes dark and the stools pale owing to intrahepatic cholestasis. The liver is moderately enlarged and the spleen is palpable in about 10% of patients. Occasionally, tender lymphadenopathy is seen, with a transient rash in some cases. Thereafter the jaundice lessens and in the majority of cases the illness is over within 3–6 weeks. Relapses occasionally occur, with the return of jaundice. Rarely the disease may be very severe with fulminant hepatitis, liver coma and death. The sequence of events after hepatitis A exposure is shown in Fig. 5.12.

INVESTIGATION

Liver biochemistry
In the prodromal stage the serum bilirubin is usually normal. However, there is bilirubinuria and increased urinary urobilinogen. A raised serum AST, which can sometimes be very high, precedes the jaundice.

In the icteric stage the serum bilirubin reflects the level of jaundice. Serum AST reaches a maximum 1–2 days after the appearance of jaundice, and may rise above 500 i.u.·L^{-1}. Serum alkaline phosphatase is usually less than 300 i.u.·L^{-1}.

After the jaundice has subsided, the AST may remain elevated for some weeks and occasionally up to 6 months; a liver biopsy and serum autoantibodies should be performed after this time interval to exclude autoimmune chronic active hepatitis.

Haematological tests
There is leucopenia with a relative lymphocytosis. Very rarely there is a Coombs' positive haemolytic anaemia or an associated aplastic anaemia. The prothrombin time is prolonged in severe cases. The ESR is raised.

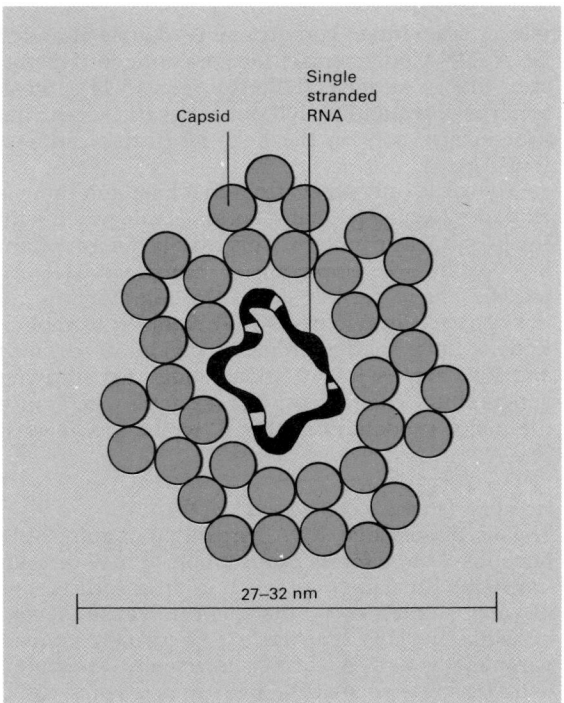

Fig. 5.11 The virion consists of four polypeptides (VP1–VP4) which form a tight protein shell, or capsid, containing the RNA. The major antigenic component is associated with VP1.

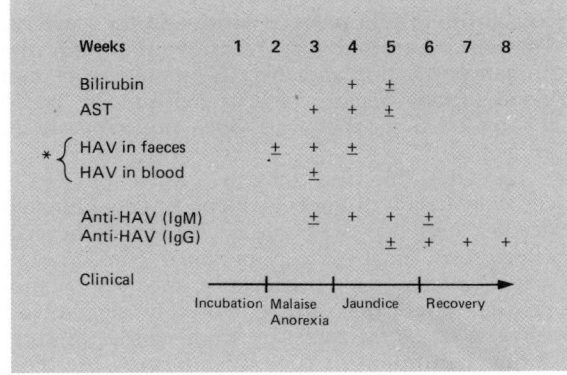

Fig. 5.12 The sequence of events after exposure to the hepatitis A virus (HAV). *Not available routinely.

Viral markers

- *Antibodies to HAV.* IgG antibodies are common in the general population over the age of 50 years but an anti-HAV IgM means an acute infection.

Other tests

- *Ultrasound.* In an older patient, bile duct obstruction should be excluded.
- *Liver biopsy.* This is only indicated when there is doubt about the diagnosis.

DIFFERENTIAL DIAGNOSIS

This is from all other causes of jaundice but, in particular, from other types of viral and drug-induced hepatitis. Ultrasound is performed to exclude biliary obstruction.

COURSE AND PROGNOSIS

The prognosis is excellent, with most patients making a complete recovery. The mortality in young adults is 0.1% but it increases with age. Death is due to fulminant hepatic necrosis. During convalescence 5–15% of patients may have relapse of the hepatitis but this settles spontaneously.

Occasionally a more severe jaundice with cholestasis will run a prolonged course of 7–20 weeks and is called cholestatic viral hepatitis.

There is no reason to stop alcohol consumption other than for the few weeks when the patient is ill. Patients may complain of debility for several months following resolution of the symptoms and biochemical parameters. This is known as the post-hepatitis syndrome; it is a functional illness. Treatment is by reassurance. Hepatitis A never progresses to chronic liver disease.

TREATMENT

There is no specific treatment; rest and dietary measures are unhelpful. Corticosteroids have no benefit. Admission to hospital is not usually necessary. The condition is notifiable in the UK.

PREVENTION AND PROPHYLAXIS

Contacts and persons without antibodies travelling to endemic areas abroad may be protected for approximately 3 months by an injection of normal immunoglobulin (0.04–0.06 ml·kg^{-1} i.m.), which should be repeated on continued exposure. The most effective prophylactic measure is good hygiene and improved sanitation, as the virus is excreted in the faeces. The virus is resistant to chlorination but is killed by boiling water for 10 minutes. A vaccine will soon be commercially available.

Hepatitis B

EPIDEMIOLOGY

The virus (HBV) is present world-wide with an estimated 300 million carriers; the incidence of this carrier state varies from country to country. Britain and the USA have a carrier rate of nearly 1%, but it rises to 10–15% in parts of Africa and the Far East. The virus can only be transmitted within the human population and there is little evidence that blood-sucking vectors such as mosquitoes spread the infection as the virus does not replicate in arthropods.

Spread of this virus is by the intravenous route, e.g. transfusion of infective blood or contaminated needles used by drug addicts, tattooists or acupuncturists, or by close personal contact, e.g. sexual intercourse, particularly in male homosexuals. The virus can be found in semen and saliva. Vertical transmission from mother to child during parturition or soon after birth is the most important means of transmission world-wide.

Hepatitis B virus

Under electron microscopy a number of particles are seen (Fig. 5.13). The whole virus is the Dane particle, which consists of an inner core formed by the liver cell nucleus and an outer surface coat (HBsAg) produced by multiplication in the cyto-plasm. The inner core contains double-stranded DNA, DNA polymerase, the core antigen (HBcAg) and the e antigen (HBeAg) (Fig. 5.14). Small spheres and tubules (100 nm long) of excess viral protein also contain the hepatitis surface antigen (HBsAg).

The virus only replicates in the liver and there is evidence to suggest that it becomes integrated with the host nuclear protein. This may be an important link in the development of hepatoma. HBsAg particles have further antigenic determinants on their surface known as a, d, y, w and r. Combinations of these subdeterminants, e.g. adw, adr, ayw and ayr, are useful in epidemiology for studying geographical differences. For example, in France the major subdeterminant is b, whilst in Greece it is y.

Hepatitis D virus (Delta agent, HDV)

This is a defective RNA virus that requires the hepatitis B virus for its propagation. It may be seen transiently in acute hepatitis B in drug addicts, but its major interest is that it can cause severe hepatitis in HBV carriers. It is usually spread parenterally and if chronic is usually associated with progressive disease with a poor prognosis. Antibodies to the delta virus, both total anti-HDV and anti-HDVIgM (indicating a recent infection) as well as HDVAg can be measured.

CLINICAL FEATURES

The sequence of events following infection are shown in Fig. 5.15. Clinical features are the same as those found in hepatitis A infection. In addition, a serum sickness-like immunological syndrome may be seen with transient rashes, e.g. urticaria or a maculopapular rash and polyarthritis affecting small joints occurs in up to 25% of cases in the prodromal period. Fever is usual. The illness may be more severe than hepatitis A. Extra-hepatic immune complex-mediated conditions such as an arteritis or glomerulonephritis are occasionally seen.

INVESTIGATION

This is generally the same as for hepatitis A.

Specific tests

The markers for HBV are shown in Fig. 5.13. HBsAg is looked for routinely. If it is found, a full viral profile is then performed. In acute infection HBsAg may be cleared rapidly and in such cases IgM anti-core antibodies are helpful.

COURSE

The majority of patients recover completely, fulminant hepatitis occurring in up to 1%. Some

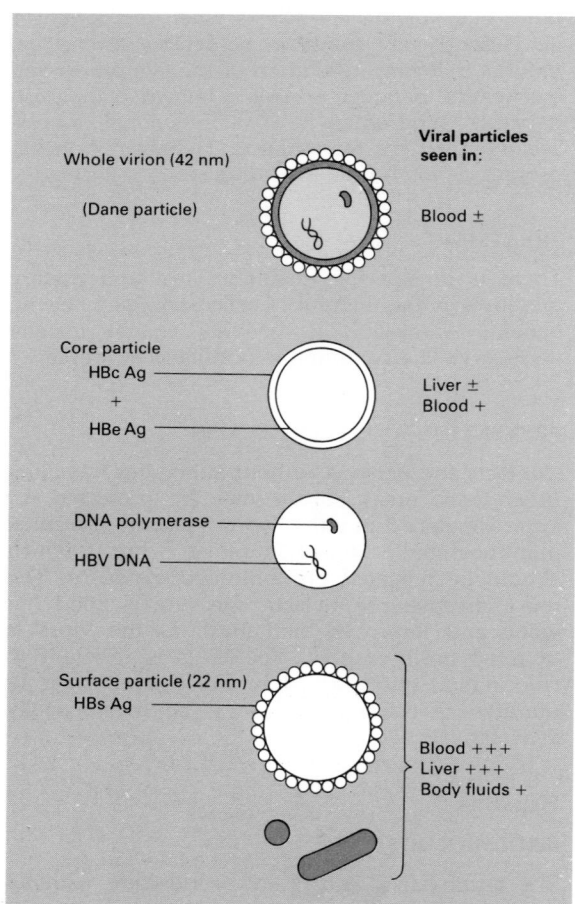

Fig. 5.13 Hepatitis B virus—the antigenic components.

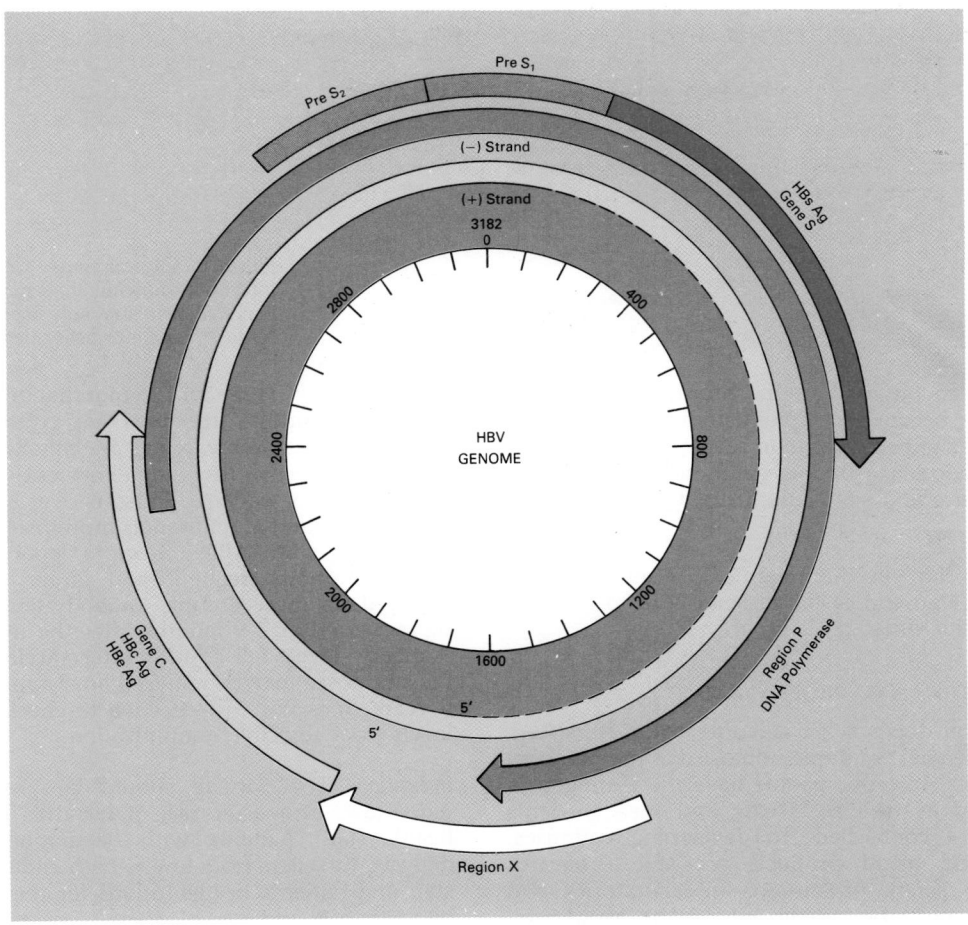

Fig. 5.14 Schematic diagram of the hepatitis B virus.

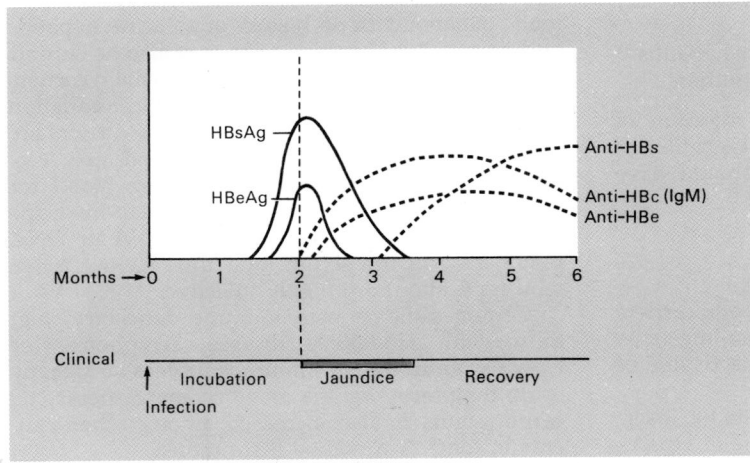

Fig. 5.15 Time course of the events and serological changes seen following infection with hepatitis B virus.

Antigens: HBsAg appears in the blood from about 6 weeks to 3 months after an acute infection. It may then disappear or persist. Its presence indicates a current or chronic infection as well as a carrier state. HBcAg is not usually seen in the blood. HBeAg rises early and usually declines rapidly. It correlates with increased severity and infectivity of the disease and its persistence correlates with the development of chronic liver disease or the carrier state.

Antibodies: Anti-HBs appears late and indicates immunity. Anti-HBc is the first antibody to appear and high titres of IgM anti-HBc suggest an acute and continuing viral replication. It persists for many months. Anti-HBe appears after anti-HBc and its appearance relates to a decreased infectivity, i.e. a low risk.

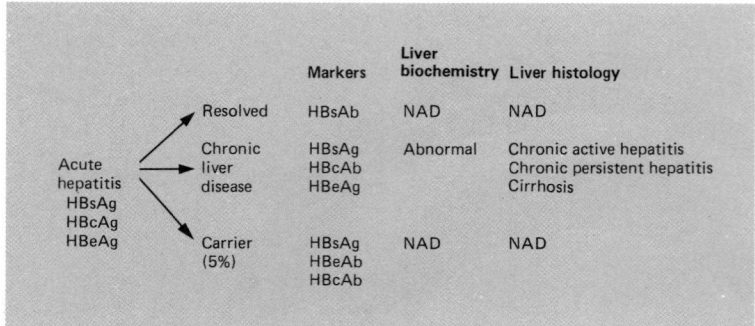

		Markers	Liver biochemistry	Liver histology
	Resolved	HBsAb	NAD	NAD
Acute hepatitis HBsAg HBcAg HBeAg	Chronic liver disease	HBsAg HBcAb HBeAg	Abnormal	Chronic active hepatitis Chronic persistent hepatitis Cirrhosis
	Carrier (5%)	HBsAg HBeAb HBcAb	NAD	NAD

Fig. 5.16 Clinical course of hepatitis B infection, showing the blood markers, liver biochemistry and liver histology. NAD = no abnormality detected.

patients go on to develop chronic hepatitis (see p. 258) or become asymptomtic carriers (Fig. 5.16). The outcome depends upon several factors, including the virulence of the virus and the immunocompetence and age of the patient.

TREATMENT

There is no specific treatment. There is some evidence that corticosteroids may lead to a failure to clear the virus.

PREVENTION AND PROPHYLAXIS

Prevention depends on avoiding risk factors, e.g. shared needles, multiple homosexual partners and prostitutes. Infective people have the e antigen in the blood as well as HBsAg and these patients should be counselled. In developing countries, blood and blood products are still a hazard. Standard safety precautions in laboratories and hospitals must be strictly enforced to avoid accidental needle punctures and contact with infected body fluids.

Passive and active immunization
Prophylactic treatment is given to:

- Persons acutely punctured by an infected needle or exposed to body fluids in a laboratory accident
- Sexual partners of patients with acute hepatitis B
- Babies born to hepatitis B-positive mothers

Treatment consists of an immediate injection of immune serum globulin containing a high titre of anti-HBs. In addition, all the above should have active immunization at the same time.

Active immunization
Two vaccines are available:

- Plasma-derived vaccine prepared from carriers of hepatitis B and consisting of non-infectious subunits of HBsAg that have been inactivated of all known viruses including HIV
- Recombinant yeast vaccine produced by insertion of a plasmid containing the gene of HBsAg into a yeast. This vaccine is cheaper.

Dosage regimen. Three (0, 1, 6 months) or four (0, 1, 6 and 12 months) injections are given into the deltoid muscle. Both vaccines are equally immunogenic and effective in giving short-term protection in over 90% of patients. Persons over 50 years or clinically ill and/or immunocompromised (including those with AIDS) have a poor antibody response; more frequent and larger doses are required. In these groups, antibody levels should be measured at 7–9 months after the initial dose. Antibody levels fall steadily after vaccination and booster doses may be required after approximately 5 years. It is not cost-effective to check antibody levels prior to active immunization.

Indication. The vaccine should be given to all individuals at specific risk of hepatitis B, e.g. all health staff, patients with haemophilia or on dialysis, travellers from low to high endemic areas, staff and patients in institutions for the medically handicapped and sexual contacts of HBsAg carriers. In the future the vaccine may well be given to all people at birth.

Chronic asymptomatic carriers
Following an acute hepatitis B infection, approximately 5–10% of patients will not clear the virus and will become carriers. Alternatively, asymptomatic patients with no history of an acute hepatitis and normal liver function tests may also be chronic carriers. Children are more likely to remain carriers than adults. There is a vast geographical variation in the incidence of carriers. In the UK, carriers are usually discovered incidentally on blood tests, e.g. when they are screened for donating blood for transfusion or when attending genital medicine clinics. Carriers with HBeAg viral DNA or DNA polymerase in the serum (and thus having active viral replication) are highly infective.

Certain patients with immune deficiency, e.g. those with Hodgkin's disease, lymphomas or Down's syndrome, or immunosuppressive therapy or on long-term dialysis may become carriers. The carrier status is also increased among other patients in long-term mental institutions.

The prognosis of the carriers is uncertain but

most remain HBsAg positive. Some may sero-convert, i.e. develop HBe antibodies, and therefore are a lower infective risk to others. Some patients may carry the virus for many years without developing chronic liver disease, whereas others, particularly those with the e antigen may go on to develop chronic hepatitis and cirrhosis and there is an increased risk of hepatocellular carcinoma. Treatment will be discussed on page 259.

Hepatitis C

This is due to an RNA virus (HCV) and is responsible for the majority of post-transfusion hepatitis in all countries where blood is tested for hepatitis B markers. It is also seen in intravenous drug abusers and male homosexuals. An acute hepatitis occurs, generally less severe than in hepatitis A or B. Extra-hepatic manifestations are seen, including arthritis, agranulocytosis and aplastic anaemia, as well as diffuse neurological problems. Rarely, fulminant hepatic failure occurs but progression to chronic liver disease is common. A chronic carrier state occurs. HCV antibodies can be measured in the serum and, in some countries, blood donors are screened for this virus.

Fifty per cent of patients go on to develop chronic liver disease, and cirrhosis develops in 20% of these.

Non-A, non-B hepatitis

Heparidides not due to the above viruses are found world-wide but particularly in India and South America. One variety is an epidemic form of hepatitis, thought to be water-borne (and is now termed HEV). It produces an illness like hepatitis A and it does not go on to chronic liver disease. There is a mortality of 1–2%, which rises to nearly 10% in pregnant women.

Fulminant hepatic failure

This is a rare but often life-threatening syndrome due to acute hepatitis from any cause. Acute viral hepatitis and drugs, e.g. paracetamol overdose (see p. 748) monoamine oxidase inhibitors, isoniazid, halothane anaesthesia, are the commonest aetio-logical factors. Rarely it occurs in pregnancy, Wilson's disease or Reye's syndrome in children, or following poisons, e.g. carbon tetrachloride. The reason why fulminant hepatic failure develops is unknown.

Histologically there is massive necrosis of the whole liver lobule. Severe fatty degeneration is seen in pregnancy, Reye's syndrome or lymphoma or following tetracycline administration.

CLINICAL FEATURES

Examination shows a jaundiced patient with the physical signs of hepatic encephalopathy. The mental state varies from slight drowsiness, confusion and disorientation (grades I and II) to unresponsive coma (grade IV) with convulsions. Ascites and oedema may occur; splenomegaly is uncommon. A small liver is usually found, but hepatomegaly may occur with a fatty liver or lymphoma. Neurological examination shows spasticity and extensor plantar responses. Fever, sweating, hypotension and renal failure also occur.

INVESTIGATION

This is as for acute liver disease. The prothrombin time is the most useful index of severity and when very high indicates a poor prognosis. The AST is high initially but is not a useful indicator of the course of the disease since it falls with progressive liver damage. The serum albumin falls and an EEG is sometimes helpful in grading the encephalopathy.

TREATMENT

There is no specific treatment. Supportive therapy as for hepatic encephalopathy (see p. 268) is necessary. Cerebral oedema is the major cause of death and when signs of raised intracranial pressure are present 20% mannitol (1 g·kg^{-1} body weight) should be infused intravenously; this dose may need to be repeated. Dexamethasone is of no value. Hypoglycaemia, hypokalaemia and hypocalcaemia should be anticipated and corrected with 10% dextrose infusion (checked by 2-hourly Dextrostix testing), potassium and calcium. Haemorrhage may be a problem and patients are given H$_2$-receptor antagonists to prevent gastrointestinal bleeding. Infection should be treated with suitable antibiotics, and renal and respiratory failure treated as appropriate. Charcoal haemoperfusion has been used, but its value has not been proved and it may be hazardous.

Fulminant hepatic failure should be treated in an intensive care unit.

COURSE AND PROGNOSIS

In mild cases (grades I and II), two-thirds of the patients will survive. The outcome of severe cases (grades III and IV) is related to the aetiology. In special units 70% of patients with paracetamol overdosage and grade IV coma survive, as do 30–40% of patients with hepatitis A or B. The survival is almost nil in those with HCV hepatitis and these patients should have liver transplantation.

Acute hepatitis due to other viruses

Infectious mononucleosis (see p. 58)
Infectious mononucleosis is due to the Epstein–

Barr virus. Mild jaundice associated with minor abnormalities of liver biochemistry is extremely common but 'clinical' hepatitis is rare. The patient complains of sore throat, fever and malaise. Lymphadenopathy and splenomegaly may be present. A Paul–Bunnell or Monospot test is usually positive and atypical lymphocytes are present in the peripheral blood. Treatment is symptomatic. Splenic rupture is a rare complication. Toxoplasmosis produces a similar clinical picture to infectious mononucleosis with abnormal liver biochemistry but the Paul–Bunnell test is negative.

Cytomegalovirus (see p. 58)
Cytomegalovirus can cause acute hepatitis, particularly in patients with poor immune responses. The virus may be isolated from the urine. The liver biopsy shows intranuclear inclusions and giant cells.

Yellow fever (p. 63)
This viral infection is carried by the mosquito *Aedes aegypti* and causes acute hepatic necrosis. There is no specific treatment.

Herpes simplex (see p. 56)
Very occasionally the herpes simplex virus causes a generalized acute infection, particularly in the immunosuppressed patient. Liver biopsy shows extensive necrosis. Acyclovir is used for treatment.

Other infectious agents
Abnormal liver biochemistry is frequently found in a number of acute infections. The abnormalities are usually mild and have no clinical significance.

Chronic hepatitis

This is defined as any hepatitis lasting 6 months or longer and the classification is usually based on histological grounds. There are three forms:

- Chronic persistent hepatitis
- Chronic lobular hepatitis
- Chronic active hepatitis

CHRONIC PERSISTENT HEPATITIS

Chronic persistent hepatitis (CPH) is a benign condition with a good prognosis and must be distinguished from the more serious chronic active hepatitis (CAH). Patients are often male and are usually asymptomatic. Physical examination shows minimal hepatomegaly but no signs of chronic liver disease. Laboratory findings show a moderately raised AST but the alkaline phosphatase, albumin and globulin are normal. HBsAg may be positive, but the HBeAg is usually negative. Diagnosis is made on a liver biopsy that shows a marked chronic inflammatory cell infiltrate in enlarged portal tracts. Slender septa may extend into the parenchyma. The basic liver architecture is undisturbed and piecemeal necrosis does not occur (see below). Treatment is unnecessary. Months or years may pass before spontaneous resolution occurs. The majority of patients do not develop CAH or cirrhosis.

CHRONIC LOBULAR HEPATITIS

Chronic lobular hepatitis is an uncommon condition. Patients present with acute hepatitis, and the course is one of remissions and exacerbations. The condition can follow a type B or C hepatitis. Autoantibodies may be present. Histology of the liver resembles acute viral hepatitis and there is intralobular inflammation and necrosis. The condition often responds to corticosteroids but the course is variable and cirrhosis can sometimes develop.

CHRONIC ACTIVE HEPATITIS

Chronic active hepatitis (CAH) was formerly called aggressive hepatitis. The causes are shown in Table 5.7. There are four distinct types although the histological lesion is very similar.

CAH due to hepatitis B virus

This group makes up 20% of all cases of CAH. Three per cent of patients with acute viral hepatitis B progress to CAH. The cause of continued liver damage is unknown but defective immunological responses, mainly 'T' cell responses, are thought to be involved. There is no association with autoimmune disease or any particular genetic markers.

Table 5.7 Causes of chronic active hepatitis.

Viral
Hepatitis B ± delta virus
Hepatitis C
Other
Autoimmune
Drugs, e.g. methyldopa, oxyphenisatin (withdrawn in UK)
Hereditary
Alpha-1-antitrypsin deficiency
Wilson's disease
Others
Inflammatory bowel disease—ulcerative colitis
Alcohol—rarely

It occurs mainly in men and it is often not preceded by an acute attack. The condition may be asymptomatic or may present as a mild, slowly progressive hepatitis. Fifty per cent present with established chronic liver disease.

Investigations show a moderately raised bilirubin and AST and a slightly raised alkaline phosphatase. HBsAg is positive and e antigen is usually present.

Histologically the hallmark of CAH is piecemeal necrosis. This is defined as the destruction of liver cells at an interface between parenchyma and connective tissue, together with a predominantly lymphocytic or plasma cell infiltrate. One sees disruption of the limiting plates of hepatocytes around portal tracts (zone 1), spread of the inflammatory cells and fibrous tissue from portal tracts into the lobules with associated degenerative changes in liver cells. Small groups of hepatocytes become isolated by fibrous septa. A minority of the hepatocytes show a ground-glass appearance to the cytoplasm on haematoxylin and eosin staining owing to the presence of excess HBsAg. This can be confirmed on orcein or immunoperoxidase staining. HBcAg can be demonstrated in hepatocyte nuclei by appropriate immunoperoxidase staining.

TREATMENT

Indications

Ideally, patients with CAH and asymptomatic carriers who have the HBe antigen and HBV-DNA in the serum should be treated. All patients with progressive liver disease should also be treated but decompensated cirrhosis is a contraindication.

The aim of the treatment is to inhibit HBV replication. It is, however, difficult to achieve the eradication of HBsAg once it has been integrated into the host genome and most patients will have a biochemical and histological remission once the HBe antigen, viral DNA and DNA polymerase has disappeared from the sera with seroconversion to anti-HBe.

Antiviral agents

Many antiviral agents have been tried but currently interferon seems to be the most successful. Even so, the response rate is disappointingly low, 10–30%, with untreated patients seroconverting at a rate of 15% per year. In addition, all patients have to be treated over several months with intravenous therapy. During therapy patients often have a clinical relapse of their liver disease, suggesting an immunomodulatory effect of interferon. Drug trials are still being performed.

PROGNOSIS

The progression is slow and remission may occur. Established cirrhosis is associated with a poor prognosis. Primary liver cell carcinoma is a frequent association and is one of the commonest carcinomas in hepatitis B endemic areas such as the Far East.

Autoimmune CAH (HBsAg negative)

This was called 'lupoid' hepatitis because LE cells were found in the blood in 15% of cases. It occurs more frequently in young (10–20 years) and middle-aged women. There is an association with other autoimmune diseases, e.g. pernicious anaemia, thyroiditis and Coombs' positive haemolytic anaemia, and 60% are associated with HLA-B8, DR3.

The cause is unknown, but many immunological abnormalities are seen. Humoral disturbances are associated with a hypergammaglobulinaemia (mainly IgG) and nuclear, smooth muscle (actin), liver/kidney microsomal antibodies are found in the serum. The association with other diseases (see above) suggests immune complex formation and deposition. CAH produced by some drugs (see below) may also be associated with the production of autoantibodies. Suppressor T cell function is impaired and this may play a part in the pathogenesis.

The onset may be insidious but 25% present as acute hepatitis. Alternatively, patients can be asymptomatic for years and the signs of chronic liver disease are discovered on a routine examination. Amenorrhoea is common. Examination shows the signs of chronic liver disease, hepatosplenomegaly, cutaneous striae, acne, hirsuties and bruises. Jaundice may be present. In advanced cases the complications of cirrhosis occur. An ill patient can also have features of an autoimmune disease with a fever, migratory polyarthritis, glomerulonephritis, pleurisy, pulmonary infiltration or fibrosing alveolitis. The 'sicca' syndrome can occur (see p. 387).

INVESTIGATION

The hallmark of this condition is positive antibodies against nuclei, smooth muscle (actin) and occasionally mitochondria. Liver/kidney microsomal antibodies are found in some patients and additional antibodies to a soluble liver antigen and the measles virus have recently been recognized. Serum bilirubin, globulins and aminotransferases are very high. Histology of the liver biopsy shows the changes found in hepatitis B positive CAH with piecemeal necrosis but without the hepatitis B staining.

TREATMENT

Prednisolone 30 mg is given daily for 2 weeks followed by a maintenance dose of 10–15 mg daily.

Azathioprine 2.0 mg·kg^{-1} daily is added to allow the prednisolone dosage to be reduced and in many cases discontinued. With our current knowledge, azathioprine should be continued indefinitely.

COURSE AND PROGNOSIS

Remissions and exacerbations occur, and 50% of patients will die of liver failure within 5 years if no treatment is given. The prognosis can be considerably improved with steroid and azathioprine therapy (90% five-year survival), underlining the importance of establishing this diagnosis by liver biopsy and immune markers. Most patients, nevertheless, develop cirrhosis.

CAH due HCV

CAH can occur following HCV infection. HCV antibodies can be measured. Recombinant interferon α produces chemical and histological improvement but relapse occurs following cessation of therapy.

CAH due to other causes

Viruses other than the above may cause CAH. CAH can also be caused by other agents, e.g. drugs (Table 5.14).

Table 5.8 Causes of cirrhosis.

Common
Alcohol
Chronic active hepatitis due to
  hepatitis B
  hepatitis C
  ? other non-A, non-B viruses

Others
Biliary cirrhosis
  Primary
  Secondary
Autoimmune chronic active hepatitis
Haemochromatosis
Hepatic venous congestion
Budd–Chiari syndrome
Wilson's disease
Drugs, e.g. methotrexate
Alpha-1-antitrypsin deficiency
Cystic fibrosis
Intestinal bypass operations for obesity
Galactosaemia
Glycogen storage disease
Veno-occlusive disease
Idiopathic (cryptogenic)

Cirrhosis

Cirrhosis results from the necrosis of liver cells followed by fibrosis and nodule formation. The liver architecture is distorted and this interferes with the liver blood flow and function. This derangement produces the clinical features of portal hypertension and impaired liver cell function.

AETIOLOGY

The causes of cirrhosis are shown in Table 5.8. Alcohol is now the commonest cause in the Western World but hepatitis B is the commonest cause world-wide. With the increasing identification of new hepatic viruses, idiopathic or cryptogenic cirrhosis is less commonly diagnosed. Young patients with cirrhosis must be carefully investigated as the cause may be treatable, e.g. Wilson's disease.

PATHOLOGY

Histologically two types have been identified:

- *Micronodular cirrhosis*, in which regenerating nodules are usually less than 3 mm in size and are surrounded by fibrous septa and the condition uniformly involves all lobes. This type is often caused by alcohol damage.
- *Macronodular cirrhosis*, in which the nodules are of variable size and normal lobules may be seen within the larger nodules. This type is often seen following hepatitis B infection.

A mixed picture with small and large nodules is sometimes seen and an aetiological cause cannot necessarily be inferred from the pathological picture.

SYMPTOMS AND SIGNS

These are described on p. 246.

INVESTIGATIONS

These are performed to assess the severity and type of liver disease.

Severity

- Liver biochemistry. This can be normal depending on the severity of cirrhosis. In most cases there is at least a slight elevation in the serum alkaline phosphatase and serum aminotransferases. In decompensated cirrhosis all biochemistry is deranged. The serum albumin is the best indicator of liver function.

Table 5.9 Poor prognostic indicators in cirrhosis.

Blood tests
Low albumin (< 25 g·L^{-1})
Low serum sodium (< 120 mmol·L^{-1})
Prolonged prothrombin time

Clinical
Persistent jaundice
Failure of response to therapy
Ascites
Haemorrhage from varices, particularly with poor
   liver function
Neuropsychiatric complications developing with
   progressive liver failure
Small liver
Persistent hypotension
Aetiology, e.g. alcoholic cirrhosis (if the patient
   continues drinking)

- Serum electrolytes. A low sodium indicates severe liver disease because of dilution secondary to free water clearance or to excess diuretic therapy.
- Haematology (see p. 242). The prothrombin time is prolonged commensurate to the severity of the liver disease.
- Serum α-fetoprotein is a useful screening test for a hepatoma.

Type. This can be determined by the following:

- Viral markers
- Serum autoantibodies
- Serum immunoglobulins
- Miscellaneous: serum copper (see p. 271) and serum α$_1$ antitrypsin (see p. 272) should always be measured in young cirrhotics. Serum Fe, TIBC and ferritin should be measured to exclude haemochromatosis.

Liver biopsy is also necessary to confirm the severity and type of liver disease. The core of liver often fragments and sampling errors occur in macronodular cirrhosis. Special stains may be required for iron and copper.

Imaging

- Ultrasound can demonstrate changes in size and shape of the liver. Fatty change and fibrosis produce a diffuse increased echogenicity. The patency of the portal and hepatic veins can be evaluated. Hepatomas can be detected.
- CT is seldom necessary but can detect a fatty liver as well as excess iron deposition.
- Barium swallow and meal are performed to look for oesophageal or gastric varices.
- Endoscopy is performed, particularly if bleeding from varices is suspected.

- Scintiscanning is helpful in advanced cirrhosis when clotting abnormalities preclude a biopsy.

MANAGEMENT

Management is that of the complications seen in decompensated cirrhosis and patients should be followed up in order to detect complications as early as possible.

There is no treatment that will arrest or reverse the cirrhotic changes, although progression may be halted by correcting the underlying cause (see below). Patients with compensated cirrhosis should lead a normal life and no particular diet is helpful. Alcohol should be avoided, although if the cirrhosis is not due to alcohol, small amounts are not harmful.

COURSE AND PROGNOSIS

This is extremely variable, depending on many factors, including the aetiology and the presence of complications. Poor prognostic indicators are given in Table 5.9. Development of any complication usually worsens the prognosis. In general, the 5-year survival rate is approximately 50% but this also varies depending on the aetiology and the stage at which the diagnosis is made. There are a number of prognostic classifications based on modifications of Child's grading (A, B and C). This is based on the presence of jaundice, ascites, encephalopathy and the level of serum albumin. Patients with good liver function—Child's Grade A—do better than patients with poor liver function (albumin < 30 g·L^{-1}, bilirubin > 50 mmol·L^{-1} and ascites)—Child's Grade C.

Liver transplantation

This is now an established treatment for a number of liver diseases and is becoming widely available in the Western hemisphere.

- In *acute* liver disease, patients with fulminant hepatic failure, particularly due to HCV which has a very poor prognosis, should be transplanted.
- In *chronic* liver disease, the indications for transplantation vary and the timing of the transplant is often difficult.
- *Primary biliary cirrhosis*—patients with this disease should be transplanted when their serum bilirubin rises above 100 μmol·L^{-1}.
- *Hepatitis B*—recurrence of the hepatitis occurs in some transplanted cases but this is not an absolute contraindication.
- *Hepatocellular- and cholangiocarcinomas*—recurrence rate is high. Transplantation is not usually indicated.
- *Alcoholic liver disease*—well-motivated patients who have stopped drinking can be offered a transplant.

Table 5.10 Complications and effects of cirrhosis.

Portal hypertension and gastrointestinal haemorrhage
Ascites
Portosystemic encephalopathy
Renal failure
Hepatoma (primary liver cell carcinoma)

The operative mortality is low but postoperative complications include sepsis and acute and chronic rejection. The latter has been reduced using cyclosporin, but opportunistic infections (see p. 6) are still a problem.

Prognosis. The 1-year survival now approaches 75% with a 5-year survival of 50%.

COMPLICATIONS AND EFFECTS OF CIRRHOSIS

These are shown in Table 5.10.

Portal hypertension

The portal vein is formed by the union of the superior mesenteric and splenic veins. The pressure within it is normally 5–8 mm Hg with only a small gradient across the liver to the hepatic vein in which blood is returned to the heart via the inferior vena cava. The development of portal hypertension is mainly due to resistance to flow, although increased flow in conditions such as tropical splenomegaly can also produce portal hypertension.

Portal hypertension can be classified according to the site of obstruction:

- Pre-hepatic due to blockage of the portal vein before the liver
- Intra-hepatic due to distortion of the liver architecture, which can be pre-sinusoidal, e.g. in schistosomiasis, or post-sinusoidal, e.g. in cirrhosis
- Post-hepatic due to venous blockage outside the liver (rare)

As portal pressure rises above 10–12 mm Hg the compliant venous system dilates and collaterals with the systemic venous system occur.

The main sites of the collaterals are at the gastro-oesophageal junction, the rectum, the left renal vein, the diaphragm, the retroperitoneum and the anterior abdominal wall via the umbilical vein.

The collaterals at the gastro-oesophageal junction (varices) are superficial in position and tend to rupture. Portosystemic anastomoses at other sites seldom give rise to symptoms. Rectal varices are

Table 5.11 Causes of portal hypertension.

Pre-hepatic
Portal vein thrombosis
Intra-hepatic
Cirrhosis
Hepatitis (alcoholic)
Idiopathic non-cirrhotic portal hypertension (subtle liver disease)
Schistosomiasis
Partial nodular transformation
Congenital hepatic fibrosis
Myelosclerosis (extramedullary haemopoiesis)
Granulomata
Post-hepatic
Budd–Chiari syndrome
Veno-occlusive disease
Right heart failure—rare
Constrictive pericarditis

frequently found (30%) if carefully looked for and can be differentiated from haemorrhoids, which are lower in the anal canal.

Causes of portal hypertension (see Table 5.11)
The commonest cause is cirrhosis. Other causes are the following:

Pre-hepatic causes. Extrahepatic blockage is due to portal vein thrombosis. The cause is usually unidentifiable but there may be a history of neonatal sepsis of the umbilical vein. Patients usually present with bleeding, often at a young age. They have normal liver function and, because of this, their prognosis following bleeding is excellent. A splenectomy should never be performed, as it may be possible to perform a splenorenal shunt in adult life. Treatment is usually with repeated sclerotherapy.

Intra-hepatic causes. Although cirrhosis is the commonest intrahepatic cause of portal hypertension, other causes include:

- *Non-cirrhotic portal hypertension* or subtle change liver disease. Patients present with portal hypertension and variceal bleeding but without cirrhosis. Histologically, the liver shows broad fibrous bands. The aetiology is unknown, but arsenic, vinyl chloride and other toxic agents have been implicated in some cases. A similar disease is found frequently in India. The liver lesion does not progress and the prognosis is therefore good.
- *Partial nodular transformation.* This is a very rare condition of unknown aetiology. Portal hypertension may arise due to non-cirrhotic nodules in the hilar region. It is not progressive and the

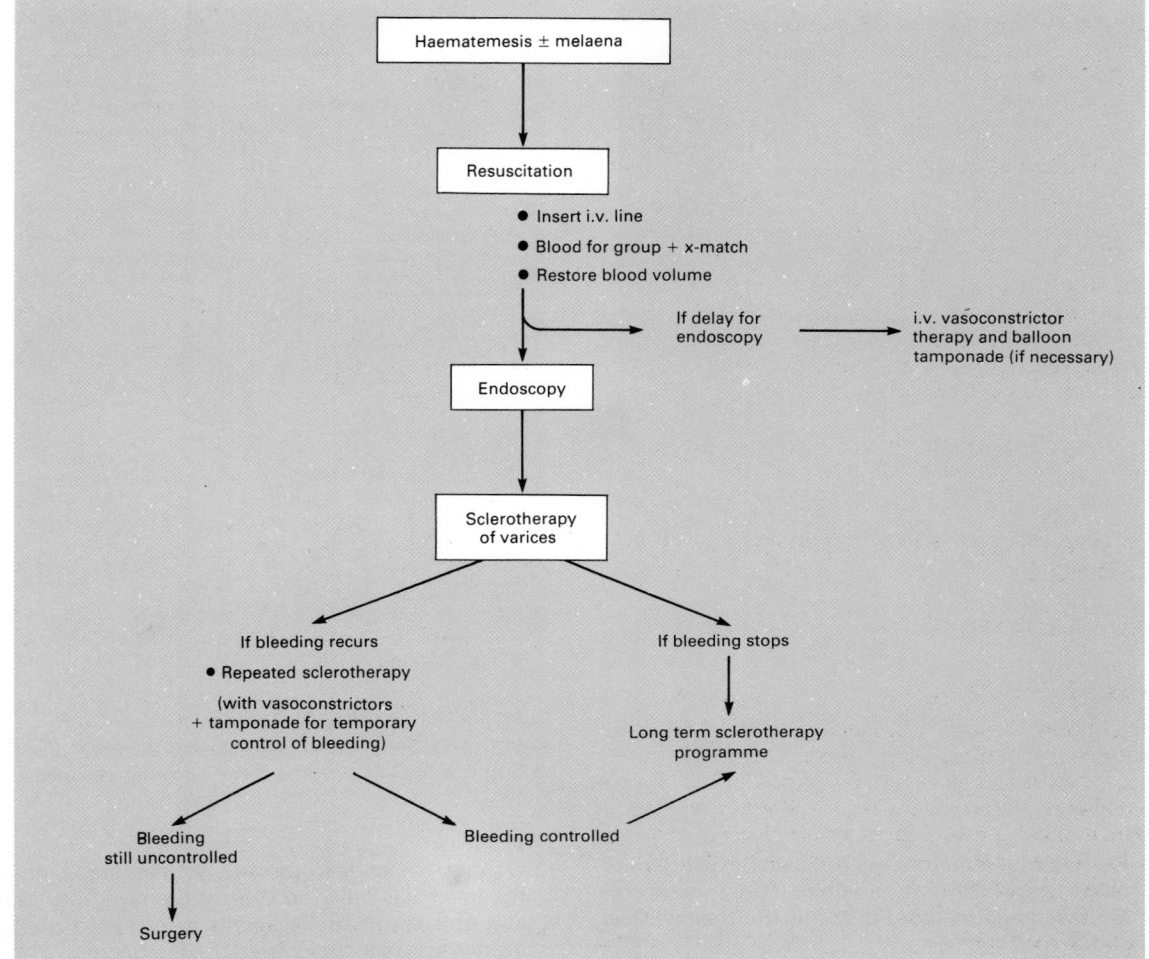

Fig. 5.17 Management of gastrointestinal haemorrhage due to oesophageal varices.

prognosis is better than in patients with cirrhosis.

Post-hepatic causes. Prolonged severe heart failure with tricuspid incompetence and constrictive pericarditis can both lead to portal hypertension. The Budd–Chiari syndrome is described on p. 274.

Clinical features of portal hypertension
Patients with portal hypertension are often asymptomatic and the only clinical evidence of portal hypertension is splenomegaly. Presenting features are:

- Haematemesis or melaena from rupture of gastro-oesophageal varices
- Ascites and/or
- Encephalopathy

Variceal haemorrhage

Approximately 70% of patients with cirrhosis will develop gastro-oesophageal varices but only one-third of these will bleed from them. Bleeding is likely to occur with large varices, high pressure and in the more severe liver disease.

MANAGEMENT

The management can be conveniently divided into the active bleeding episode, the prevention of re-bleeding and prophylactic measures to prevent the first haemorrhage.

Acute variceal bleeding (Fig. 5.17)
INITIAL MANAGEMENT

- Assess the general condition of the patient—pulse and blood pressure.
- Insert an intravenous line and obtain blood for grouping and cross-matching, haemoglobin, urea, prothrombin time, electrolytes and liver biochemistry.

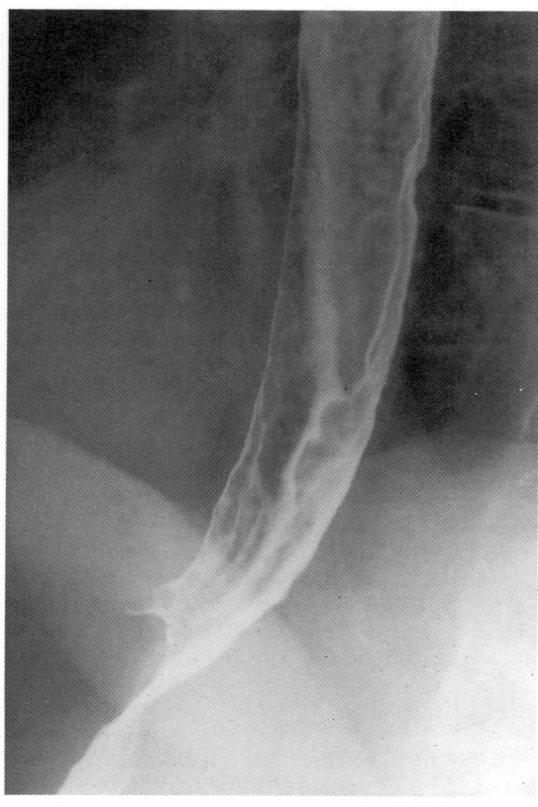

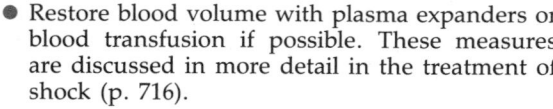

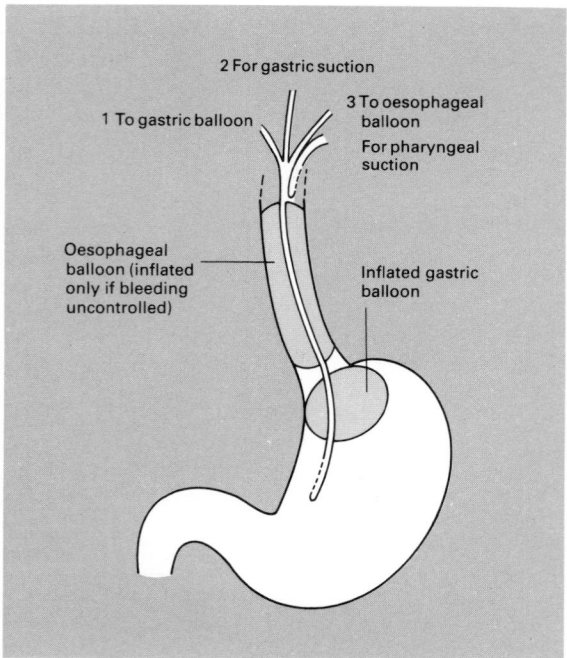

Fig. 5.18 Diagram of a Sengstaken–Blakemore tube *in situ*, and a barium swallow X-ray showing oesophageal varices.

- Restore blood volume with plasma expanders or blood transfusion if possible. These measures are discussed in more detail in the treatment of shock (p. 716).

Prompt correction of hypovolaemia in patients with cirrhosis is particularly important.

- *Endoscopy* should be performed to confirm the diagnosis and to exclude bleeding from other sites (i.e. gastric erosions or ulceration), which are rarely the source of haemorrhage in these patients.
- *Injection sclerotherapy.* The varices should be injected with a sclerosing agent that may arrest bleeding by producing vessel thrombosis. This can be achieved in most cases except when major bleeding occurs. A needle is passed down the biopsy channel of the endoscope and a sclerosant agent is injected into the varices. Complications include oesophageal ulceration and mediastinitis and strictures occur in about 10% with repeated sclerotherapy.

OTHER MEASURES AVAILABLE

- *Vasoconstrictor therapy.* The main use of this is for emergency control of bleeding either whilst waiting for endoscopy and sclerotherapy or if the latter has failed to control the bleeding. The aim of vasoconstrictor agents is to restrict portal inflow by splanchnic arterial constriction.
- *Vasopressin* An infusion of 25 units per hour should be administered by a central venous catheter (if possible) to avoid the risks of local leakage and necrosis. The addition of nitrates either by intravenous, sub-lingual or patch route has been shown to reduce the cardiac complications of vasopressin, which is particularly important in patients with ischaemic heart disease. The patient will complain of abdominal colic, evacuate his bowels and have facial pallor due to the generalized vasoconstriction. Vasoconstrictor therapy is thus only used as a temporizing measure to establish initial haemostasis.
- Octreotide, a *somatostatin* analogue (250 µg bolus followed by an infusion of 250 µg per hour) will also produce splanchnic vasoconstriction without significant systemic vascular effect or complications. The clinical efficacy of somatostatin is in doubt.

The above agents should control the bleeding in approximately 60% of cases.

- *Balloon tamponade* is used mainly to control

bleeding if sclerotherapy or vasoconstrictor therapy has failed or if the latter is contra-indicated. The tube should be left in place for up to 12 h and removed in the endoscopy room prior to sclerotherapy. The usual tube is a Sengstaken–Blakemore (Fig. 5.18). The tube is passed into the stomach and the gastric balloon is inflated with air. It should be positioned in close apposition to the gastro-oesophageal junction to prevent the cephalad variceal blood flow to the bleeding point. The oesophageal balloon should only be inflated if bleeding is not controlled by the gastric balloon alone. This technique is successful in up to 90% of patients but serious complications such as aspiration pneumonia, oesophageal rupture and mucosal ulceration produce a 5% mortality with this technique. The procedure is very unpleasant for the patient.

- *Emergency surgery* is used when sclerotherapy fails to control bleeding, particularly if the bleeding is from gastric fundal varices. Oeso-phageal transection and ligation of the feeding vessels to the bleeding varices is the most common surgical technique.

Portosystemic shunt surgery (see below) involving decompression of the portal vein is performed acutely, but rarely in the UK. Surgical techniques have a high operative mortality in cases of Child's grade C.

ADDITIONAL MANAGEMENT OF ACUTE EPISODE

- *Repeated sclerotherapy* to control recurrent bleeding.
- *Measures to prevent encephalopathy.* Portosystemic encephalopathy (PSE) can be precipitated by a large bleed (since blood contains protein). The management is described below.
- *Nursing.* Patients require high-dependency/intensive-care nursing. They should have nil by mouth until bleeding has stopped.
- Sucralfate 1 g × 4 daily is given to reduce oesophageal ulceration following sclerotherapy

PREVENTION OF RECURRENT VARICEAL BLEEDING

Following an episode of variceal bleeding, the risk of recurrence is 60–80% over a 2-year period with an approximate mortality of 20% per episode; these facts justify the use of measures to prevent such re-bleeding.

- *Long-term injection sclerotherapy.* The use of repeated courses of injection sclerotherapy at weekly intervals leads to the obliteration of the varices by fibrous tissue. This is now the method of choice. Follow-up sclerotherapy should be performed at intervals to keep varices ablated.
- *Surgical procedures.* Portosystemic shunting is associated with an extremely low risk of re-bleeding but the diversion of portal blood away from the liver produces significant encephalopathy. Operative mortality is low in patients with Child's grade A (0–5%) but encephalopathy still occurs. Child's grade C has a very poor prognosis. The 'shunts' performed today are usually an end-to-side portacaval anastomosis or a selective distal splenorenal shunt (Warren shunt), which maintains hepatic blood flow via the superior mesenteric vein. Oesophageal transection does not produce encephalopathy but re-bleeding does eventually occurs.
- *Beta-adrenoreceptor blockade.* Oral propranolol is a dose sufficient to reduce resting pulse rate by 25% has been shown to decrease portal pressure. Portal inflow is reduced by two mechanisms: a decrease in cardiac output (β1) and also by the blockade of β2 vasodilator fibres on the splanchnic arteries, leaving an unopposed vasoconstrictor effect. This has been shown to decrease the frequency of re-bleeding in patients with well-compensated liver disease.

PROPHYLACTIC MEASURES

The prevention of the first variceal haemorrhage (and therefore the approximate 50% associated mortality) has been attempted using medical and surgical therapy. At the present time, no prophylactic measures have been shown to reduce mortality, but beta-adrenoreceptor blockade has been shown to reduce the frequency of the first haemorrhage and should be prescribed.

Ascites

Ascites is the presence of fluid within the peritoneal cavity and is a common complication of cirrhosis of the liver. The development of ascites is secondary to renal sodium and water retention. The importance of portal hypertension is that it exerts a local hydrostatic pressure and leads to transudation of fluid into the peritoneal cavity. A low serum albumin as a consequence of poor synthetic liver function may further contribute by a reduction in plasma oncotic pressure. The factors leading to sodium and water retention are believed to be a consequence of the systemic haemodynamic disturbances associated with cirrhosis—in particular, the low peripheral vascular resistance. These changes are believed to be due to circulating vasodilator factors that closely reflect the severity of the underlying liver disease. These factors include prostaglandins and atrial natriuretic peptide. As perfusion pressure of the kidney falls, the renin–angiotensin–aldosterone system is activated as a primary homeostatic response so as to expand

Table 5.12 Causes of ascites divided according to the type of ascitic fluid.

Straw-coloured
Malignancy—commonest cause
Cirrhosis
Infective
    Tuberculosis
    Following intra-abdominal perforation—any bacteria may be found, e.g. *E. coli*
    'Spontaneous' in cirrhotics
Hepatic vein obstruction (Budd–Chiari syndrome)—protein level high in fluid
Chronic pancreatitis
Constrictive pericarditis
Meigs' syndrome (ovarian tumour)
Hypoproteinaemia, e.g. nephrotic syndrome

Chylous
Obstruction of main lymphatic duct, e.g. by carcinoma—chylomicrons are present

Haemorrhagic
Malignancy
Ruptured ectopic pregnancy
Abdominal trauma
Acute pancreatitis

the circulating volume. Much of the retained fluid is then redistributed into the peritoneal cavity under the influence of the raised portal pressure and as such does not suppress the activated renin–angiotensin system and the stimulus for fluid retention persists.

In patients with ascites, urine sodium excretion rarely exceeds 5 mmol/24 h. Loss of sodium from extra-renal sites accounts for approximately 30 mmol/24 h. Dietary sodium intake may vary between 120–200 mmol/24 h resulting in a positive sodium balance of approximately 90–170 mmol/24 h (equivalent to 600–1300 ml of fluid retained).

CLINICAL FEATURES

The abdominal swelling associated with ascites may accumulate over many weeks or as rapidly as in a few days. The presence of fluid is confirmed by the demonstration of shifting dullness. Mild generalized abdominal pain and discomfort are common but, if more severe, should raise the suspicion of spontaneous bacterial peritonitis (see below). Respiratory distress may accompany tense ascites. Many patients will also have peripheral oedema. A pleural effusion (usually on the right side) may infrequently be found and is believed to arise from the passage of ascites through congenital defects in the diaphragm.

INVESTIGATION

A diagnostic aspiration of 10–20 ml of fluid should be obtained under strict aseptic conditions:

- Cell count: a neutrophil count > 250 cells/mm^3 is indicative of an underlying (usually spontane-

ous) bacterial peritonitis.
- Gram stain and culture for bacteria and acid fast bacilli.
- Albumin and protein: the ascites albumin level enables a division into transudative and exudative ascites. For this division the serum albumin must be used as a reference point. An ascitic albumin 11 g·L^{-1} or more below the serum albumin level suggests a transudate. The level of ascites protein provides an indirect estimate of opsonization capacity and thereby the risk of developing spontaneous bacterial peritonitis. Patients at most risk are those with ascitic protein levels < 10 g·L^{-1}.
- Cytology for malignant cells.
- Amylase: to exclude pancreatic ascites.

The differential diagnosis of ascites is listed in Table 5.12.

MANAGEMENT

The aim is to both reduce sodium intake and increase renal excretion and by doing so produce a net reabsorption of fluid from the ascites back into the circulating volume. The maximum rate at which ascites can be mobilized is 500–700 ml/24 h (see below).

- *Dietary sodium restriction* should always be a part of the management. It is possible to reduce sodium intake to 22 mmol in 24 hours and still maintain an adequate protein and calorie intake. Many patients find this difficult and a 40 mmol diet is frequently an adequate compromise.
- *Bed-rest* alone, probably by improving renal perfusion, may lead to a diuresis in a small proportion of patients.

● *Diuretics*. The diuretics of choice are those acting on the distal nephron, namely spironolactone 200 mg daily, triamterene or amiloride 10 mg daily. These agents have only mild diuretic potency and provide flexibility in dosage without major risks of overdiuresis and renal impairment. The potassium-sparing action of these agents may give rise to hyperkalaemia. Loop diuretics, such as frusemide, have several potential disadvantages. In approximately 50% of patients with cirrhosis they do not cause a diuresis—firstly because the drug may not be secreted into the tubule (the site of action) and, secondly because avid reabsorption of fluid may occur distal to the site of action of frusemide under the influence of aldosterone, thereby negating the diuretic effect (the latter problem may be overcome in selected cases by combining frusemide with a distal nephron diuretic). In those cases in which frusemide does exert a diuretic effect, frequent problems are encountered with respect to hypokalaemia and volume depletion.

The aim of diuretic therapy should be to produce a net loss of fluid approaching 700 ml/24 h (0.700 kg weight loss or 1.5 kg if peripheral oedema is present). At the outset, serum electrolytes and renal function should be estimated two to three times per week. Diuretics should be temporarily discontinued if a rise in creatinine level (to approximately 160 μmol·L^{-1}) occurs, representing overdiuresis and hypovolaemia. Hyponatraemia occurring during therapy almost always represents haemodilution secondary to a failure to clear free water (usually a marker of reduced renal perfusion) and should be treated by water restriction (1000–1500 ml/24 h) and stopping the diuretics if the sodium level falls below approximately 128 mmol·L^{-1}.

A regime including dietary restriction and a titrated dose of a distal nephron diuretic will be successful in 90% of cases.

● *Paracentesis*. The removal of ascites has been reintroduced as means of rapid therapy, thus avoiding prolonged hospital stay. The main danger of this approach is the production of hypovolaemia as the ascites reaccumulates at the expense of the circulating volume. In patients with normal renal function and in the absence of hyponatraemia, this has largely been overcome by the administration of albumen to maintain the plasma volume. In practice, up to 20 L can be removed over 3 h. This should always be followed by 40 g of salt-poor albumin given over ½ h, 3 h after the paracentesis.

● *Peritoneo-venous shunt*. The introduction of a catheter from the peritoneal cavity (subcutaneously) to the internal jugular vein, incorporating a one-way valve, allows passage of the ascites directly into the circulation. This is rarely used except for patients with resistant ascites.

Spontaneous bacterial peritonitis

This condition represents the most serious complication of ascites. The infecting organisms are believed to gain access to the peritoneum by haematogenous spread. The most frequently incriminated bacteria are *E. coli*, *Klebsiella* and non-enteric streptococci. The condition should be suspected in any patient with ascites with evidence of clinical deterioration. Features such as pain and pyrexia are frequently absent and cannot be relied upon. Diagnostic aspiration should always be performed (see above). The raised neutrophil count in the ascites is alone sufficient evidence to instigate treatment. A third-generation cephalosporin, such as cefotaxime or ceftazidine, provides adequate cover in most circumstances and may be modified on the basis of culture results. Early diagnosis and prompt therapy have significantly reduced the hospital mortality of this condition (previously reported as 50%).

Portosystemic encephalopathy (PSE)

The term portosystemic encephalopathy (PSE) refers to a chronic neuropsychiatric syndrome secondary to chronic liver disease. This condition occurs with cirrhosis, but a similar acute encephalopathy can occur in acute fulminant hepatic failure (see p. 257). PSE is seen in patients with portal hypertension due to spontaneous 'shunting' or in patients following a portacaval shunt operation. Encephalopathy is potentially reversible. The mechanism is unknown but several factors are thought to play a part. In cirrhosis, the blood bypasses the liver via the collaterals and the 'toxic' metabolites pass directly to the brain to produce the encephalopathy. Many 'toxic' substances have been suggested as the causative factor, including ammonia, free fatty acids, mercaptans and accumulation of false neurotransmitters (octopamine) or activation of the GABA inhibitory neurotransmitter system. Increased blood levels of aromatic amino acids (tyrosine and phenylalanine) and reduced branch-chain amino acids (valine, leucine and isoleucine) also occur. Nevertheless, ammonia seems to play a major role. Ammonia is produced by the breakdown of protein by intestinal bacteria and a high blood ammonia is seen in most patients. It may alter the blood–brain barrier and allow 'toxins' to interfere with cerebral metabolism. The factors that can precipitate PSE are shown in Table 5.13.

CLINICAL FEATURES

An acute onset often has a precipitating factor (see Table 5.13). The patient becomes increasingly drowsy and comatose.

Chronically, there is a disorder of personality, mood and intellect, with a reversal of normal sleep rhythm. These changes may be fluctuating and a

Table 5.13 Factors precipitating portosystemic encephalopathy.

High dietary protein

Gastrointestinal haemorrhage

Constipation

Infection

Fluid and electrolyte disturbance due to:
    diuretic therapy
    paracentesis

Drugs, e.g. narcotics

Portosystemic shunt operations

history from a relative must be obtained. The patient is irritable, confused, disorientated and has slow slurred speech. General features include nausea, vomiting and weakness. Convulsions and coma occur as the encephalopathy becomes more marked. Hyperventilation and pyrexia are seen.

Signs include fetor hepaticus (a sweet smell to the breath) and a coarse flapping tremor seen when the hands are outstretched and the wrists hyperextended (asterixis). There is a constructional apraxia and the patient cannot write or draw, for example, a five-pointed star. Mental function can be assessed by using the serial-sevens test (see p. 966). A trail-making test (the ability to join numbers and letters with a pen within a certain time—a standard psychological test for brain dysfunction) is prolonged and is a useful bedside test to assess encephalopathy.

Diagnosis is clinical and routine liver biochemistry merely confirms the presence of liver disease, not the presence of encephalopathy.

Additional investigations include:

- *Electroencephalogram (EEG).* This shows a decrease in the frequency of the normal alpha waves (8–13 Hz) to delta waves (1.5–3 Hz). These changes occur before coma supervenes.
- *Visual evoked responses* (p. 879) also detect subclinical encephalopathy.
- *Blood ammonia.* This is occasionally useful in the differential diagnosis of the cause of the coma and to follow the course of the PSE, but is not readily available.

MANAGEMENT

Management consists of restricting protein intake and sterilizing the bowel.

Immediate

- Identify and remove the possible precipitating cause, e.g. drugs with cerebral depressant properties.
- Give purgation and enemas to empty the bowels of nitrogenous substances. Lactulose (10–30 ml three times daily) is an osmotic purgative that

reduces the colonic pH and limits ammonia absorption. Hypernatraemia can result from water loss.

- Institute a protein-free diet, with adequate calories, given if necessary via a fine-bore nasogastric tube.
- Oral neomycin 1 g 6-hourly can be used if lactulose fails. Neomycin can also be used in retention enemas. It is mainly unabsorbed, but in the long-term it can produce deafness.
- Stop or reduce diuretic therapy.
- Correct any electrolyte imbalance.
- Give intravenous fluids as necessary (beware of too much sodium).
- Treat any infection.

Long-term

- Increase protein in the diet to the limit of tolerance (20–50 g) as the encephalopathy improves.
- Avoid constipation.
- Give lactulose 10–30 ml three times daily.
- Avoid precipitating factors, e.g. narcotic drugs, which depress cerebral function, overdiuresis producing electrolyte imbalance.

COURSE AND PROGNOSIS

Acute encephalopathy, often seen after fulminant hepatic failure, has a very poor prognosis as the disease itself has a high mortality. In cirrhosis, chronic PSE is very variable and the prognosis is that of the underlying liver disease.

Renal failure (hepatorenal syndrome)

Renal failure occurs in severe liver disease and is characterized by an extremely low sodium excretion with a residual capacity to concentrate urine (i.e. tubular function is intact). As in ascites there is a low peripheral vascular resistance and a low arterial pressure that lead to increased secretion of the vasoconstrictors noradrenaline, angiotensin and vasopressin.

The initial effect of these vasoconstrictors on the renal vasculature is to cause post-glomerular constriction with little or no impact upon the preglomerular arterioles, thus maintaining perfusion pressure. This 'protection' of the pre-glomerular arterioles, however, is not absolute and constriction may occur, leading to a reduction in renal plasma flow, and the characteristic abnormalities of the hepatorenal syndrome. A number of other mediators have been incriminated in the pathogenesis of the hepatorenal syndrome, in particular the eicosanoids. This has been supported by the precipitation of the syndrome by inhibitors of prostaglandin synthetase such as the non-steroidal anti-inflammatory agents. The kidneys are histologically normal.

This condition usually occurs in the deeply jaundiced patient and must be distinguished from pre-renal failure, which is often precipitated by diuretic therapy.

The patient should be treated for pre-renal failure and diuretic therapy stopped. The prognosis is poor.

Primary hepatocellular carcinoma

This is dealt with on p. 277.

TYPES OF CIRRHOSIS

Alcoholic

This is discussed in the section on alcoholic liver disease (see p. 272).

Primary biliary cirrhosis (PBC)

This is a chronic disorder in which there is a progressive destruction of bile ducts, eventually leading to cirrhosis. It predominantly affects women (female to male ratio = 6 : 1) who are middle-aged. It used to be considered rare but is now being diagnosed more frequently in its milder forms. PBC has been called 'chronic non-suppurative destructive cholangitis'; this term is more descriptive of the early lesion and emphasizes that true cirrhosis only occurs in the later stages of the disease.

AETIOLOGY

The aetiology is unknown, but immunological mechanisms are thought to play a part. Antibodies to mitochondria (AMA) are almost invariable. Three mitochondrial proteins with molecular weights of 74, 52 and 39 kD have been identified. In PBC, specific antibodies to the first two proteins are seen in 80–95% and 30–50% of patients. The 74 kD factor (subtype M2) has been characterized as dihydrolipoamide acetyltransferase of the pyruvate dehydrogenase complex of the mitochondrial membrane. However, the presence of AMA in high titre is unrelated to the clinical or histological picture and may play no part in its pathogenesis. Although damage to bile ducts is a feature, antibodies to bile ductules are not specific to PBC. Cell-mediated immunity is impaired (demonstrated both in vitro and by skin testing) and this suggests that sensitized T lymphocytes might be involved in producing damage. There may be a defect in immunoregulation as a decrease in T suppressor cells may allow cytotoxic T and B cells to produce damage to the bile ducts. There is an increased synthesis of IgM thought to be due to a failure of the switch from IgM to IgG antibody synthesis.

CLINICAL FEATURES

Asymptomatic patients may be discovered on routine examination to have hepatomegaly, a raised serum alkaline phosphatase or autoantibodies.

The earliest symptom is pruritus, often preceding jaundice by a few years. When jaundice appears, hepatomegaly is usually found.

In the later stages there is jaundice with severe pruritus. On examination the patient is jaundiced and pigmented, xanthelasma or other deposits of cholesterol may be seen, usually around the eyes and in the creases of the hands, and there is hepatosplenomegaly.

ASSOCIATIONS

Connective tissue diseases occur with increased frequency. Renal tubular acidosis and membranous glomerulonephritis may occur.

Keratoconjunctivitis sicca (dry eyes and mouth) is seen in 70% of cases.

INVESTIGATION

- Mitochondrial antibodies are present in over 95% of patients. Other non-specific antibodies, e.g. antinuclear factor and smooth muscle, may also be present.
- A high serum alkaline phosphatase is often the only abnormality in the liver biochemistry.
- Serum cholesterol is raised.
- The serum IgM may be very high.
- An ultrasound shows diffuse alteration in liver architecture.
- Liver biopsy shows characteristic histological features of a dense portal tract infiltrate mainly of lymphocytes and plasma cells, sometimes with granulomas, damage to and loss of small bile ducts, predominantly periportal cholestasis, portal tract fibrosis and, eventually, cirrhosis. Most changes are in zone 1.

Hepatic granulomas are also seen in sarcoidosis, tuberculosis, schistosomiasis, drug reactions (e.g. phenylbutazone), brucellosis, parasitic infestation (e.g. strongyloidiasis) and other conditions.

DIFFERENTIAL DIAGNOSIS

The classical picture presents little difficulty with diagnosis, which is confirmed by the characteristic features on liver biopsy and the presence of AMA in the sera.

In the jaundiced patient, extrahepatic biliary obstruction should be excluded by ultrasound and, if there is doubt about the diagnosis, ERCP should be performed to make sure that the bile ducts are normal.

TREATMENT

There is no specific therapy of proven benefit. Azathioprine, corticosteroids and penicillamine have all been tried without beneficial effect, and corticosteroids are contraindicated because of bone thinning. Colchicine (0.6 mg twice daily) has been shown to improve liver function and enhance

Ursodeoxycholate has been tried but with minimal benefit.

Malabsorption of fat-soluble vitamins (A, D and K) occurs and supplementation is required when deficiency is detected and in the jaundiced patient prophylactically. Elemental calcium is required for osteoporosis. Hyperlipidaemia producing symptoms should be treated (p. 863).

Pruritus is difficult to control but cholestyramine, one 4 g sachet three times daily, can be helpful, although it is unpalatable.

Transplantation, see below.

COMPLICATIONS

The complications are those of cirrhosis. In addition, osteoporosis, osteomalacia and a peripheral neuropathy can also occur.

COURSE AND PROGNOSIS

This is very variable. Asymptomatic patients and those presenting with pruritus will survive for more than 20 years. Symptomatic patients with jaundice have a more rapidly progressive course and die of liver failure or bleeding varices in approximately 5 years. Liver transplantation should therefore be offered when the serum bilirubin reaches 100 $\mu mol \cdot L^{-1}$.

Secondary biliary cirrhosis

Cirrhosis can result from prolonged (for months) large duct biliary obstruction. Causes include bile duct strictures, gallstones and sclerosing cholangitis. An ultrasound examination, followed by ERCP or PTC is performed to outline the ducts and any remedial cause is dealt with.

Haemochromatosis

Idiopathic haemochromatosis (IHC) is an inherited disease characterized by excess iron deposition in various organs leading to eventual fibrosis and functional organ failure.

AETIOLOGY

The underlying metabolic defect is unknown, but abnormal enterocyte function resulting in inappropriate levels of iron absorption has been suggested. IHC is inherited as an autosomal recessive with only homozygotes manifesting the clinical features of the disease. It is associated with HLA-A3 and B14. Dietary intakes of iron and chelating agents (ascorbic acid) are probably also important. Iron overload may be present in alcoholics, but alcohol excess *per se* does not cause IHC. There is a history of excess alcohol intake in 25% of patients. The iron accumulation is gradual and occurs throughout life.

PREVALENCE

Prevalence of homozygotes varies between 0.3 and 0.5%, with a heterozygote frequency of 9–14%.

PATHOLOGY

In symptomatic patients the total body iron content is 20–40 g compared to 3–4 g in a normal person.

The iron content is particularly increased in the liver and pancreas (50–100 times normal) but is also increased in all other organs, e.g. the endocrine glands, heart and skin. Gonadal function is impaired despite a low testicular iron content.

Histologically the liver shows extensive pigmentation and fibrosis with iron deposition in dense, fibrous septae forming a network surrounding groups of lobules. Early in the disease, iron is deposited in the periportal hepatocytes (in pericanalicular lysosomes). Later it is distributed widely throughout the lobules, biliary duct epithelium, Kupffer's cells and connective tissue. Cirrhosis with nodularity is a late feature.

CLINICAL FEATURES

The course of the disease depends on a number of features including sex, dietary iron intake, presence of associated hepatotoxins (especially alcohol) and genotype. Overt clinical manifestations occur more frequently in men; the reduced incidence in women is probably explained by physiological blood loss and a smaller dietary intake of iron. Most affected individuals present in the fifth decade. The classic triad of bronze skin pigmentation (due to melanin deposition), hepatomegaly and diabetes mellitus is only present in cases of gross iron overload. Other more common features include gonadal atrophy and loss of libido.

Hypogonadism secondary to pituitary dysfunction is the commonest endocrine feature. Deficiency of other pituitary hormones is also found, but symptomatic endocrine deficiencies are exceedingly rare. Cardiac manifestations, particularly heart failure and arrhythmias, are common, especially in younger patients. Calcium pyrophosphate is deposited asymmetrically in both large and small joints (chondrocalcinosis) leading to an arthropathy. The exact relationship of chondrocalcinosis to iron deposition is uncertain.

COMPLICATIONS

Thirty per cent of patients with cirrhosis will develop primary hepatocellular carcinoma (HCC). HCC has only rarely been described in non-cirrhotic patients in whom the excess iron stores have been removed. This has important implications for early diagnosis.

INVESTIGATION

Homozygotes

● The serum iron is elevated (> 30 $\mu mol \cdot L^{-1}$), with a reduction in the total iron-binding capacity and complete or almost complete transferrin saturation (> 70%).

- The serum ferritin is elevated (usually > 500 $\mu g \cdot L^{-1}$) and there is evidence of excessive parenchymal deposition in the liver.
- Liver biochemistry is often normal, even with established cirrhosis.

Heterozygotes
Heterozygotes may have normal biochemical tests or modest increases in serum iron transferrin saturation (> 50%) or serum ferritin (usually < 400 $\mu g \cdot L^{-1}$).

Liver biopsy
This is important in defining the extent of tissue damage, assessing tissue iron, and measuring the hepatic iron concentration (> 180 $\mu mol \cdot g^{-1}$ dry weight of liver indicates haemochromatosis).

Mild degrees of parenchymal iron deposition in patients with alcoholic cirrhosis can often cause confusion with true homozygous IHC. It is highly likely that many of this former group are heterozygotes for the haemochromatosis gene.

Magnetic resonance imaging is still being investigated for use as a screening test and shows early promise.

Causes of secondary iron overload such as multiple transfusions must be excluded.

TREATMENT AND MANAGEMENT

Venesection
Venesection prolongs life and may reverse tissue damage; the risk of malignancy still remains. All patients should have excess iron removed as rapidly as possible. This is achieved using venesection of 500 ml performed twice weekly for up to 2 years, i.e. 160 units × 250 mg of iron per unit, which equals 40 g removed. During venesection, serum iron and ferritin and the MCV should be monitored. These fall only when available iron is depleted. Three or four venesections per year are required to prevent reaccumulation of iron. Serum ferritin should remain within the normal range. Liver biopsy is repeated to ensure removal of iron and to assess progress of hepatic disease.

Manifestations of the disease usually improve or disappear, except for diabetes, testicular atrophy and chondrocalcinosis. The requirements for insulin often diminish in diabetic patients. Testosterone replacement is often helpful.

Chelation therapy
In rare patients who cannot tolerate venesection (because of severe cardiac disease or anaemia), chelation therapy with desferrioxamine either intermittently or continuously by infusion has been successful in removing iron.

Screening of relatives
In all cases of IHC it is important to screen all first-degree family members to detect early and asymptomatic disease. Serum ferritin is an excellent test with only occasional false-positives in hepatocellular necrosis and rare false-negatives in some family studies.

Wilson's disease (hepatolenticular degeneration)

This is a very rare inborn error of copper metabolism that results in copper deposition in various organs to produce cirrhosis and degeneration of the basal ganglia of the brain. It is potentially treatable and all young patients with cirrhosis must be screened for this condition.

Copper metabolism. Dietary copper is absorbed from the stomach and upper small intestine. It is transported to the liver loosely bound to albumin. Here it is incorporated into caeruloplasmin, a glycoprotein synthesized in the liver, and secreted into the blood. Copper is normally excreted in the bile.

AETIOLOGY

It is inherited as an autosomal recessive gene located on chromosome 13. It occurs world-wide, particularly in countries where consanguinity is common. The basic problem is a failure to excrete copper but, although there is a low serum caeruloplasmin, the precise defect remains unknown.

PATHOLOGY

The histology is not diagnostic and varies from that of chronic active hepatitis to macronodular cirrhosis. Stains for copper show a periportal distribution but this can be unreliable (see below). The basal ganglia are damaged and show cavitation, the kidneys show tubular degeneration, and erosions are seen in bones.

CLINICAL FEATURES

Children usually present with hepatic problems, whereas young adults have more neurological problems, such as tremor, dysarthria, involuntary movements and eventually dementia (see p. 925).

Signs are of chronic liver disease with neurological signs of basal ganglia involvement. A specific sign is the Kayser–Fleischer ring, which is due to copper deposition in Descemet's membrane in the cornea. It appears as a greenish brown pigment at the corneoscleral junction just within the cornea. Identification of this ring frequently requires slit-lamp examination. It may be absent in young children. Very rarely the Kayser–Fleischer ring may be seen in cryptogenic cirrhosis.

INVESTIGATION

The serum copper and caeruloplasmin are usually reduced but can be normal. The 24-hour urinary copper is usually increased. The diagnosis depends on the measurement of the amount of copper in the liver, although high levels of copper are also found in the liver in chronic cholestasis. Measurement of ^{64}Cu incorporation into the liver may be helpful. Haemolysis and anaemia may be present.

TREATMENT

Long-term penicillamine, approximately 1 g daily, is effective in chelating copper and leads to clinical and biochemical improvement. Serious side-effects of the drug occur in 10% and include skin rashes, leucopenia and renal damage. Urine copper levels should be monitored. All siblings and children of patients should be screened. Homozygotes may have the above physical signs, Kayser–Fleischer rings and a low serum caeruloplasmin. Symptomless homozygous relatives should be treated.

PROGNOSIS

Early diagnosis and effective treatment have improved the outlook. Neurological damage is, however, permanent. Death is from liver failure, bleeding varices or intercurrent infection.

Alpha-1-antitrypsin deficiency (see also p. 657)

A deficiency of alpha-1-antitrypsin (α_1AT) is sometimes associated with liver disease and pulmonary emphysema (particularly in smokers). α_1AT is a glycoprotein and part of a family of protease inhibitors (Pi) that control various inflammatory cascades, e.g. complement (C_1 inhibitor), coagulation (antithrombin). It is synthesized in the liver and comprises 90% of the serum α-1-globulin seen on electrophoresis. The genetic variants of α_1AT are characterized by their electrophoretic mobilities as medium (M), slow (S) or very slow (Z). The normal genotype is PiMM, the homozygote for Z is PiZZ and the heterozygotes are PiMZ and PiSZ. S and Z variants are due to a single amino-acid replacement of glutamic acid at positions 264 and 342 of the polypeptide, respectively, and this results in decreased synthesis and secretion of the normal protease inhibitor. S thus forms about 60% of that produced normally by M, whilst the Z variant forms only 15%.

α_1AT is inherited as an autosomal dominant and 1 : 10 of northern Europeans carry a deficiency gene.

INVESTIGATION

- The serum α_1AT is low.
- *Liver biopsy.* Periodic acid–Schiff (PAS)-positive, diastase-resistant globules are seen in the hepatocytes. These can be shown to be α_1AT using immunodiagnostic techniques.
- *Phenotypes.* The PiM is associated with serum levels of α_1AT of 2–4 g·l^{-1}. Homozygotes for the protease inhibitor Z (i.e. PiZZ) have low α_1AT levels and are seriously affected with liver disease. Heterozygotes (e.g. PiSZ, PiMZ) exist and may develop signs of deficiency.

TREATMENT

There is no treatment apart from dealing with the complications of liver disease. Patients should be advised to stop smoking (see p. 657).

Alcoholic liver disease

In this section only a description of the pathology and clinical features of the liver disease will be given. The amounts needed to produce liver damage, alcohol metabolism, and other clinical effects of alcohol are described on page 171.

Ethanol is metabolized in the liver by two pathways (p. 171) resulting in an increase in the NADH/NAD ratio. The altered redox potential results in increased hepatic fatty-acid synthesis with decreased fatty-acid oxidation, both events leading to accumulation of fatty acid that is then esterified to glycerides.

The changes in oxidation–reduction also impair carbohydrate and protein metabolism and are also the cause of the centrilobular necrosis of the hepatic acinus typical of alcohol damage.

Acetaldehyde is formed by the oxidation of ethanol and its effect on hepatic proteins may well be an important factor in producing liver-cell damage. The exact mechanism of alcoholic hepatitis and cirrhosis is unknown, but since only 10–20% of people who drink excessively will suffer from cirrhosis, a genetic predisposition is proposed. Immunological mechanisms have also been proposed.

PATHOLOGY

Alcohol can produce a wide spectrum of liver disease from fatty change to hepatitis and cirrhosis.

Fatty change

The metabolism of alcohol invariably produces fat in the liver, mainly in zone 3. This is minimal with small amounts of alcohol, but with larger amounts the cells become swollen with fat (steatosis) giving, eventually, a Swiss-cheese effect on haematoxylin and eosin stain. Steatosis can also be seen in obesity, diabetes, starvation and occasionally in chronic illness. There is no liver-cell damage and therefore in general this is not precirrhotic. The fat disappears on stopping alcohol.

In some cases collagen is laid down around the central hepatic veins (perivenular fibrosis) and this can sometimes progress to cirrhosis without a preceding hepatitis.

Alcoholic hepatitis
Here there is necrosis of liver cells and infiltration with polymorphonuclear leucocytes mainly in zone 3. A dense perinuclear eosinophilic material called Mallory's hyaline is sometimes seen in hepatocytes. Steatosis is also present and an established cirrhosis is often seen. Mallory's hyaline is suggestive of but not specific for alcoholic damage as it can also be found in other liver diseases, such as Wilson's disease and PBC. Alcoholic hepatitis usually goes on to become cirrhosis if alcohol consumption continues.

Alcoholic cirrhosis
Destruction and fibrosis with regenerating nodules produces cirrhosis. There is bridging fibrosis between portal tracts and terminal hepatic veins. Fat may be present with the additional features of alcoholic hepatitis.

CLINICAL FEATURES

Fatty liver
There are often no symptoms or signs. Vague abdominal symptoms of nausea, vomiting and diarrhoea are due to the more general effects of alcohol on the GI tract. Hepatomegaly, sometimes huge, can occur together with other features of chronic liver disease.

Alcoholic hepatitis
The clinical features vary in degree:

- The patient may be well, with few symptoms, the hepatitis only being apparent on the liver biopsy in addition to fatty change.
- Mild to moderate symptoms of ill-health, occasionally with mild jaundice, may occur. Signs include all the features of chronic liver disease. Liver biochemistry is deranged and the diagnosis is made on a liver biopsy.
- In the severe case, usually superimposed on patients with alcoholic cirrhosis, the patient is ill, with jaundice and ascites. Abdominal pain is frequently present, with a high fever associated with the liver necrosis. On examination there is deep jaundice, hepatomegaly, sometimes splenomegaly, and ascites with ankle oedema. The signs of chronic liver disease are also present.

Alcoholic cirrhosis
This represents the final stage of liver disease from

alcohol abuse. Nevertheless, patients can be very well with few symptoms. On examination, there are usually signs of chronic liver disease. The diagnosis is confirmed by liver biopsy.

Usually the patient presents with one of the complications of cirrhosis. In many cases there are features of alcohol dependency (see p. 991) as well as evidence of involvement of other symptoms, e.g. polyneuropathy.

INVESTIGATION

Fatty liver
An elevated MCV often indicates heavy drinking. Liver biochemistry shows mild abnormalities with elevation of both aminotransferase enzymes. The γ-GT level is a sensitive test for determining whether the patient is taking alcohol. With severe fatty infiltration, marked changes in all liver biochemistry can occur. Ultrasound or CT will demonstrate fatty infiltration.

Liver biopsy is the only way to assess the degree of liver damage.

Alcoholic hepatitis
Investigations show a leucocytosis with markedly deranged liver biochemistry with elevated:

- Serum bilirubin
- Serum aspartate and alanine aminotransferases
- Serum alkaline phosphatase
- Prothrombin time

A low serum albumin may also be found. Rarely, hyperlipidaemia with haemolysis (Zieve's syndrome) may occur.

The prolonged prothrombin time makes liver biopsy impossible in the severe form. In these severe cases the mortality is at least 50%, and with a prothrombin time twice the normal, progressive encephalopathy and renal failure, the mortality approaches 90%.

Alcoholic cirrhosis
Investigations are as for cirrhosis in general.

MANAGEMENT AND PROGNOSIS

Fatty liver
In all but the mildest cases the patient is advised to stop drinking; the fat will disappear and the liver biochemistry usually returns to normal. Small amounts of alcohol can be drunk subsequently as long as the patient is aware of the problems and can control his consumption.

Alcoholic hepatitis
In severe cases the patient is confined to bed. Treatment for encephalopathy and ascites is commenced. Patients should be fed either by a fine bore nasogastric tube or intravenously. Nitrogen solutions enriched with branched-chain amino

acids, e.g. leucine, isoleucine and valine, may be helpful. Vitamins B and C should be given by injection. Corticosteroids are often given, but controlled trials have shown them to be of little benefit.

Patients are advised to stop drinking for life, as this is undoubtedly a precirrhotic condition. The prognosis is variable and, despite abstinence, the liver disease is progressive in many patients. Conversely, a few patients continue to drink heavily without developing cirrhosis.

Alcoholic cirrhosis

The management of cirrhosis is described on p. 261.

Again, all patients are advised to stop drinking for life. Abstinence from alcohol results in an improvement in prognosis, with a 5-year survival of 90%, but with continued drinking this falls to 60%. With advanced disease (i.e. jaundice, ascites and haematemesis) the 5-year survival rate falls to 35%, with most of the deaths occurring in the first year.

Hepatoma is a complication in men in approximately 10–15% of cases.

Budd–Chiari syndrome

In this condition there is obstruction to the venous outflow of the liver owing to occlusion of the hepatic vein. In one third of patients the cause is unknown, but specific causes include hypercoagulability states, such as polycythaemia vera, taking the contraceptive pill, or leukaemia. Other causes include occlusion of the hepatic vein owing to posterior abdominal wall sarcomas, renal or adrenal tumours, hepatomas, hepatic infections (e.g. hydatid cyst), congenital venous webs, radiotherapy, or trauma to the liver.

The acute form presents with abdominal pain, nausea, vomiting, tender hepatomegaly and ascites. The liver biopsy shows centrilobular congestion. In the chronic form there is an enlarged liver, mild jaundice, ascites, a negative hepatojugular reflex, and splenomegaly with portal hypertension.

INVESTIGATION

Investigations show a high protein content in the ascitic fluid and characteristic histology on liver biopsy. Ultrasound or CT will demonstrate hepatic vein occlusion and are now the investigations of choice. With isotopic scanning of the liver there is uptake only in the caudate lobe, which has a different venous drainage. Venography may demonstrate the thrombosed vein.

TREATMENT

Ascites should be treated as well as any underlying cause, e.g. polycythaemia. Congenital webs should be resected surgically. A side-to-side portacaval or splenorenal anastomosis may decompress the congested liver, with considerable improvement in the clinical state of the patient. A peritoneal–jugular LeVeen shunt for resistant ascites is occasionally useful. Liver transplantation is becoming the treatment of choice.

DIFFERENTIAL DIAGNOSIS

A similar clinical picture can be produced by inferior vena caval obstruction, right-sided cardiac failure or constrictive pericarditis, and appropriate investigations should be performed.

PROGNOSIS

The prognosis depends on the aetiology, but some patients can survive for several years.

Veno-occlusive disease

This is due to injury of the hepatic veins and presents clinically like the Budd–Chiari syndrome. It was originally described in Jamaica, where the ingestion of the toxic alkaloids in bush tea (made from plants of the genera *Senecio*, *Heliotropium* and *Crotolaria*) caused toxic damage to the hepatic veins. It can be seen in other parts of the world and nowadays is also associated with the use of antimitotic drugs and hepatic irradiation.

Fibropolycystic diseases

These diseases are usually inherited and lead to the presence of cysts or fibrosis in the liver, kidney and occasionally the pancreas, and other organs.

Polycystic disease of the liver

Adult

This usually presents in middle age with abdominal swelling or right hypochondrial discomfort. It can also be detected by ultrasound scanning or may only be discovered at autopsy. There may or may not be hepatomegaly and bilateral irregular palpable kidneys. It is inherited as an autosomal dominant. The cysts are of variable size and consist of thin-walled cavities containing clear fluid or altered blood. Liver function is normal and complications such as oesophageal varices are very rare. The prognosis is excellent and is often dependent on whether the kidneys are involved.

Child

Childhood polycystic disease is inherited in a different way from the adult type. It is an autosomal recessive condition presenting in the first few months of life. Renal involvement is common, with cystic changes in the renal tubules.

Congenital hepatic fibrosis

In this rare condition the liver architecture is normal but there are broad collagenous fibrous bands extending from the portal tracts. It is often inherited as an autosomal recessive condition but can also occur sporadically. It usually presents in childhood with hepatosplenomegaly, and portal hypertension is common. It may present later in life and can be misdiagnosed as cirrhosis. A wedge biopsy of the liver may be required to confirm the diagnosis. The outlook is good and the condition should be distinguished from cirrhosis. Patients who bleed do well after variceal sclerotherapy or a portacaval anastomosis because of their good liver function.

Congenital intrahepatic biliary dilatation (Caroli's disease)

In this rare, non-familial disease there are saccular dilatations of the intra- or extra-hepatic ducts. It can present at any age (although usually in childhood) with fever, abdominal pain and recurrent attacks of cholangitis with Gram-negative septicaemia. Jaundice and portal hypertension are absent. Diagnosis is by ultrasound, PTC or ERCP.

Solitary non-parasitic cysts

These are rare and probably a variant of polycystic disease.

Liver abscess

Pyogenic abscess

These abscesses are uncommon, but may be single or multiple. The commonest cause used to be a portal pyaemia from intra-abdominal sepsis, e.g. appendicitis or perforations, but now in many cases the aetiology is not known. Biliary sepsis, particularly in the elderly, is a common cause. Other causes include trauma, bacteraemia and direct extension from, for example, a perinephric abscess.

The commonest organism found is *Escherichia coli*. Other organisms include *Streptococcus faecalis*, *Proteus vulgaris* and *Staphylococcus aureus*. *Streptococcus milleri* and anaerobic organisms such as *Bacteroides* are now more frequently seen. Often the infection is mixed. Failure to culture an organism may be due to previous antibiotic therapy or inadequate anaerobic culture.

CLINICAL FEATURES

Some patients are not acutely ill and present with malaise lasting several days or even months. Others can present with fever, rigors, anorexia, vomiting, weight loss and abdominal pain. In these patients a Gram-negative septicaemia with shock can occur. On examination there may be little to find. Alternatively, the patient may be toxic, febrile and jaundiced. In such patients, the liver is tender and enlarged and there may be signs of a pleural effusion or a pleural rub in the right lower chest.

INVESTIGATION

Patients are often investigated as a 'pyrexia of unknown origin' (PUO) and in the mild chronic case most investigations will be normal. Often the only clue to the diagnosis is a raised serum alkaline phosphatase.

The serum bilirubin is raised in 25%. There is a normochromic normocytic anaemia, usually accompanied by a polymorphonuclear leucocytosis. The ESR is often raised. The serum B_{12} is very high, as vitamin B_{12} is stored in and subsequently released from the liver.

Blood cultures are positive in only 30% of cases.

Imaging

Ultrasound has superseded radionuclide scans for detecting filling defects. A chest X-ray will show elevation of the right hemidiaphragm with a pleural effusion in the severe cases.

MANAGEMENT

Aspiration of the abscess should be attempted under ultrasound control. Antibiotics should initially cover Gram-positive, Gram-negative and anaerobic organisms until the causative organism is identified.

Further drainage via a large-bore needle under ultrasound control or surgically should almost always be performed if a localized abscess is found. The underlying cause must also be treated.

PROGNOSIS

The overall mortality depends on the nature of the underlying pathology and is approximately 50% in the ill elderly patient. A unilocular abscess in the right lobe has a better prognosis. Scattered multiple abscesses have a very high mortality, with only one in five patients surviving.

Amoebic abscess (see p. 89)

This condition occurs world-wide and must be considered in patients travelling from endemic areas. *Entamoeba histolytica* (see p. 88) can be carried from the bowel to the liver in the portal venous system. Portal inflammation results, with the development of multiple microabscesses and eventually single or multiple large abscesses.

Clinically the onset is usually gradual but may be sudden. There is fever, anorexia, weight loss and malaise. There is often no history of dysentery. On examination the patient looks ill and has tender hepatomegaly and signs of an effusion or consolidation in the base of the right side of the chest. Jaundice is unusual.

INVESTIGATION

This is as for pyogenic abscess, plus:

- Serological tests for amoeba, e.g. haemagglutination inhibition, amoebic complement-fixation test, ELISA. These are always positive, particularly if there are bowel symptoms, and remain positive after a clinical cure and therefore do not indicate current disease. A repeat negative test, however, is good evidence against an amoebic abscess.
- Diagnostic aspiration of fluid looking like anchovy sauce.

TREATMENT

Metronidazole 800 mg three times daily is given for 10 days. Some physicians recommend repeated aspirations in addition. Surgical drainage is used in patients failing to respond, in multiple and large abscesses, and in those with abscesses in the left lobe of the liver.

COMPLICATIONS

Complications include rupture, secondary infection and septicaemia.

Other infections of the liver

Schistosomiasis (see p. 98)

Schistosoma mansoni and *S. japonicum* affect the liver, but *S. haematobium* rarely does so. During their life-cycle the ova reach the liver via the portal system and obstruct the portal branches, producing granulomas, fibrosis and inflammation but not cirrhosis. Clinically there is hepatosplenomegaly and presinusoidal portal hypertension, which is particularly severe with *S. mansoni*.

Investigations show a raised alkaline phosphatase, and ova can be found in the stools (centrifuged deposits) and in rectal and liver biopsies. Skin tests and other immunological tests often have false results and may also be positive because of past infection.

Treatment is with praziquantel, which still leaves fibrosis and potential portal hypertension.

Hydatid disease (see p. 103)

Cysts caused by *Echinococcus granulosus* are single or multiple. They usually occur in the lower part of the right lower lobe. The cyst has three layers: an outside layer derived from the host, an intermediate laminated layer, and an inner germinal layer that buds off brood capsules to form daughter cysts.

Clinically there may be no symptoms or a dull ache and swelling in the right hypochondrium. Investigations show a peripheral eosinophilia and usually a positive hydatid complement-fixation test or haemagglutination. The Casoni skin test is no longer used because of its lack of specificity. Plain abdominal X-ray may show calcification of the outer coat of the cyst. Ultrasound and CT scan demonstrate a space-occupying lesion and may show diagnostic daughter cysts.

Needle aspiration should *not* normally be performed because of the risk of dissemination or fatal anaphylaxis. Fine-needle aspiration under ultrasound control with chemotherapeutic cover is being used in some centres. Treatment is usually surgical, with removal of the cyst intact if possible after first sterilizing the cyst with formalin or alcohol. Medical treatment, e.g. with albendazole, which penetrates into large cysts, is being evaluated. Chronic calcified cysts can be left.

Complications include rupture, secondary infection and involvement of other organs.

The prognosis without any complications is good, although there is always the risk of rupture. Preventative measures are important, including deworming of pet dogs and prevention of pets from eating infected carcasses where possible.

Acquired immune deficiency syndrome (see p. 68)

The liver is often involved but rarely causes significant morbidity or mortality. The HIV virus itself is probably not the cause of the liver abnormalities. The following are seen:

- Pre-existing/coincidental viral hepatitis (HBV, HCV, HDV)

- Neoplasia—Kaposi's sarcoma and non-Hodgkin's lymphoma
- Opportunistic infection, e.g. *Mycobacterium avium intracellulare, Cryptococcus, Candida albicans*
- Drug hepatotoxicity
- Sclerosing cholangitis (see p. 286)

Clinical hepatomegaly is common in 60% of patients.

Jaundice in pregnancy

Liver function is not impaired in pregnancy. Any liver disease from whatever cause can occur incidentally and coincide with pregnancy. For example, viral hepatitis accounts for 40% of all cases of jaundice during pregnancy. Pregnancy does not necessarily exacerbate established liver disease, but it is uncommon for women with advanced liver disease to conceive. There are, however, three main types specifically associated with pregnancy.

Acute fatty liver of pregnancy

This is a rare, serious condition of unknown aetiology. It presents in the last trimester with symptoms of fulminant hepatitis, i.e. jaundice, vomiting, abdominal pain, possibly haematemesis and coma. Liver histology shows fine droplets of fat (microvesicles) in the liver cells with little necrosis. Immediate delivery of the child may save both baby and mother, but the maternal and fetal mortality is about 75%. The prognosis is good for those who survive. Treatment is as for acute liver failure.

Recurrent intrahepatic cholestasis

Patients present with pruritus and a mild jaundice, usually during the last trimester of pregnancy. There is a cholestatic jaundice with dark urine and pale stools. It does not affect the health of the mother or fetus and disappears within 2 weeks of delivery. Jaundice will recur during subsequent pregnancies and may also occur if the patient takes the contraceptive pill. The aetiology is unknown but it may be a cholestatic response to a steroid produced in pregnancy. A particularly high incidence is seen in South America and Scandinavia.

Toxaemias of pregnancy

Raised serum alkaline phosphatase and aminotransferases are common but jaundice is rare; if it occurs it is mainly haemolytic. Occasionally fulminant hepatic failure can occur.

Liver tumours

The commonest liver tumour is a secondary (metastatic) tumour (Fig. 5.19), particularly from the gastrointestinal tract, breast or bronchus. Clinical features are variable but usually include hepatomegaly. MRI is better than CT at detecting metastases. However, ultrasound is cheaper and more readily available. Primary liver tumours may be benign or malignant. The commonest are malignant.

MALIGNANT TUMOURS

Hepatocellular carcinoma (HCC)

This is one of the commonest cancers world-wide, although it is uncommon in the Western Hemisphere.

AETIOLOGY

Carriers of HBV have an extremely high risk of developing HCC. In areas where HBV is prevalent, 90% of patients with this cancer are hepatitis B-positive. Cirrhosis is present in over 80% of these patients. The development of HCC is related to the integration of viral DNA into the genome of the host hepatocyte. Primary liver cancer is also associated with other forms of cirrhosis, e.g. alcoholic cirrhosis and haemochromatosis. Males are affected more than females; this may account for the high incidence seen in haemochromatosis and low incidence in PBC. Other suggested aetiological factors are aflatoxin (a metabolite of a fungus found in groundnuts) and androgenic steroids, and there is an association with the contraceptive pill.

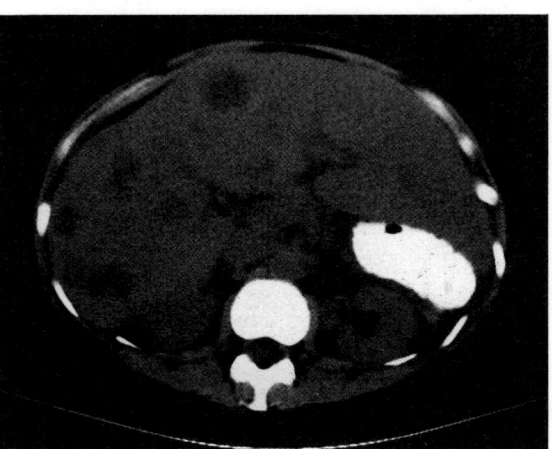

Fig. 5.19 CT scan showing liver metastasis.

PATHOLOGY

The tumour is either single or occurs as multiple nodules throughout the liver. Histologically it consists of cells resembling hepatocytes. It can metastasize via the hepatic or portal veins to the lymph nodes, bones and lungs.

CLINICAL FEATURES

HCC usually presents below the age of 50 years. The clinical features include weight loss, anorexia, fever, an ache in the right hypochondrium and ascites. The rapid development of these features in a cirrhotic patient is suggestive of HCC. On examination, an enlarged, irregular, tender liver may be felt.

INVESTIGATION

Alpha-fetoprotein is raised. Radioisotope or ultrasound scans show large filling defects in 90% of cases. A liver biopsy, particularly under ultrasonic control, is performed for diagnosis.

TREATMENT

Surgical resection is occasionally possible. Chemotherapy and radiotherapy are unhelpful.

PROGNOSIS

Survival is seldom more than 6 months.

Cholangiocarcinoma

Cholangiocarcinomas can be extra-hepatic (see p. 287) or intra-hepatic. Intra-hepatic adenocarcinomas arising from the bile ducts account for approximately 10% of primary tumours. They are not associated with cirrhosis or hepatitis B. In the Far East they may be associated with infestation with *Clonorchis sinensis*. The clinical features are similar to primary hepatocellular carcinoma except that jaundice is frequent with hilar tumours. Treatment is unsuccessful and patients usually die within 6 months.

BENIGN TUMOURS

The commonest benign tumour is a haemangioma. This is usually found incidentally on ultrasound or CT and requires no treatment.

Hepatic adenomas are associated with oral contraceptives. They can present with abdominal pain or intraperitoneal bleeding. Resection is required for symptomatic patients.

Miscellaneous conditions of the liver

Reye's syndrome

This syndrome is of unknown aetiology but recently it has been associated with aspirin consumption in childhood. It consists of an acute encephalopathy with cerebral oedema and diffuse microvesicular fatty infiltration of the liver. It occurs mainly in children and the mortality rate is 50%.

Benign recurrent intra-hepatic cholestasis

This condition often presents in children and consists of bouts of cholestatic jaundice with pruritus. Jaundice may last for weeks or months. There is no treatment; cholestyramine 12 g daily may help relieve the itching.

Indian childhood cirrhosis

This condition of children is seen in the Indian subcontinent. The cause is unknown. Eventually there is development of a micronodular cirrhosis with excess copper in the liver.

Hepatic porphyrias

These are dealt with on p. 871.

Cystic fibrosis (see p. 663)

This disease mainly affects the lung and pancreas, but patients can develop fatty liver, cholestasis and cirrhosis. The aetiology of the liver involvement is unclear.

Drugs and the liver

Drug metabolism

The liver is the major site of drug metabolism. Drugs are converted from fat-soluble to water-soluble substances that can be excreted in the urine or bile. This metabolism of drugs is mediated by a group of mixed-function enzymes, including cytochrome P450, located on the smooth endoplasmic reticulum of the liver cell. It takes place in two stages:

● Phase I metabolism involves oxidation, reduction or demethylation of the drug.
● Phase II involves the conjugation of the deriva-

tives produced in Phase I with glucuronide, sulphate and glutathione. These conjugates are excreted in the urine and bile as they cannot be reabsorbed by renal tubular or bile ductular cells.

Factors affecting drug metabolism
The microsomal enzyme system. The *speed* of metabolism of drugs is dependent on the microsomal enzyme system. Certain drugs, e.g. phenytoin, barbiturates and alcohol, can themselves increase the activity of these enzymes such as cytochrome P450, i.e. cause 'enzyme induction', and are known as 'inducing agents'. Therapy with any of these drugs will produce increased metabolism of the drug and consequently a reduction in its effectiveness. Equally, if two drugs are metabolized by the same microsomal enzymes, metabolism of both drugs will be reduced, prolonging their actions.

Route of administration. Many drugs are partially inactivated on passage through the liver (first-pass effect). If this is pronounced, drugs taken orally are inactive.

Liver blood flow. The rate of removal of the drug from the liver is influenced by the liver blood flow.

Competitive inhibition. Some drugs compete with bilirubin at various stages:

- Uptake by the liver, e.g. rifampicin
- Conjugation, e.g. novobiocin
- Excretion into the bile canaliculus, e.g. oral contraceptives

Drug hepatotoxicity

Many drugs impair liver function and drugs should always be considered as a cause when mildly abnormal liver tests are found. Damage to the liver by drugs is usually classified as being either predictable (or dose-related) or non-predictable (not dose-related) (see p. 732). This classification should not be used rigidly, as there is considerable overlap and many mechanisms may be involved in the production of damage.

Biochemical pathways
When a small amount of hepatotoxic drug whose effect is dose-dependent, e.g. paracetamol, is ingested, a large proportion of it undergoes conjugation with glucuronide and sulphate, whilst the remainder is metabolized by microsomal enzymes to produce toxic derivatives that are immediately detoxified by conjugation with glutathione. If larger doses are ingested, the former pathway becomes saturated and the toxic derivative is produced at a faster rate. Once the hepatic

glutathione is depleted large amounts of the toxic metabolites accumulate and produce damage.

The 'predictability' of drugs to produce damage can, however, be affected by metabolic events preceding their ingestion. For example, chronic alcoholics may become more susceptible to liver damage because of the enzyme-inducing effects of alcohol, or ill or starving patients may become susceptible because of the depletion of hepatic glutathione produced by starvation. Many other factors such as environmental or genetic effects may be involved in determining the 'susceptibility' of certain patients to certain drugs.

Immunological mechanisms
These can be involved in the production of hepatic cell damage by certain drugs. The toxic metabolite produced by the microsomal enzymes may bind to the liver cell protein, thereby altering its antigenicity. The production of antibody against this will lead to immunologically mediated damage. An example of this mechanism is halothane-induced hepatic necrosis, which requires prior sensitization of the patient to halothane, although direct toxicity may also play a part.

Other pointers for the involvement of immunological mechanisms are the development of skin rashes, fever and arthralgia (serum-sickness syndrome) following ingestion of certain drugs. Eosinophilia and circulating immune complexes and antibodies may occasionally be detected.

Hepatic damage

The type of damage produced by various drugs is shown in Table 5.14. The diagnosis of these conditions is usually by exclusion of other causes. Most reactions occur within 3 months of starting the drug. Monitoring liver biochemistry in patients on long-term treatment, e.g. antituberculosis therapy, is advisable. If a drug is suspected to be causing hepatic damage, it should be stopped immediately. Liver biopsy is of limited help in confirming the diagnosis but occasionally hepatic eosinophilia may be seen. Sometimes diagnostic challenge with subtherapeutic doses of the drug is required after the liver biochemistry has returned to normal to prove the diagnosis.

Individual drugs

Paracetamol
In high doses paracetamol produces liver-cell necrosis (see above). The toxic metabolite binds irreversibly to liver cell membranes. Overdosage is discussed on p. 748.

Halothane
This commonly used anaesthetic agent rarely produces a hepatitis in patients having repeated

Table 5.14 Some drugs producing hepatic damage. Percentages indicate the proportion of patients who develop abnormal liver biochemistry.

Type of reaction	Drug
Hepatocellular damage:	
Dose-dependent	Paracetamol Salicylates Tetracycline

Dose-independent	Antidepressants:
	    Monoamine-oxidase inhibitors (1%)
	    Tricyclic antidepressants (< 1%)
	Antituberculous drugs
	    Isoniazid (10–20%)
	    Para-aminosalicylic (PAS) (5%)
	    Pyrazinamide (10%)
	    Rifampicin
	Anticonvulsants and antispasmodics
	    Phenytoin
	    Dantrolene (1–2%)
	    Carbamazepine
	    Phenobarbitone
	    Sodium valproate
	Anti-inflammatory drugs
	    Non-steroidals
	Antibiotics (uncommon)
	    Penicillins
	    Sulphonamides
	Anaesthetics
	    Halothane (20% with repeated exposures)
	Cardiovascular drugs
	    Amiodarone
	    Methyldopa (5%)
	    Perhexiline maleate
	Antifungal drugs
	    Ketoconazole

Cholestasis	
Pure cholestasis	Oral contraceptives Synthetic anabolic steroids
Cholestatic hepatitis	Chlorpromazine (1%) Erythromycin estolate (38%) Antirheumatic drugs, e.g. sodium aurothiomalate Antithyroid drugs, e.g. carbimazole Hypoglycaemic drugs, e.g. chlorpropamide (25%), glibenclamide
Fatty change	Tetracycline
Hepatic fibrosis	Methotrexate Amiodarone
Chronic active hepatitis	Methyldopa Nitrofurantoin Sulphonamides
Granulomatous reaction	Sulphonamides (long-acting) Methotrexate Hydralazine Allopurinol Chlorpropamide
Liver tumours and peliosis hepatis	17α-Alkylated synthetic androgens (hepatocellular carcinomas) Oral contraceptives (benign adenomas)

exposures. The mechanism is thought to be a hypersensitivity reaction. An unexplained fever occurs approximately 10 days after the second or subsequent halothane anaesthetic and is followed by jaundice, typically with a hepatitic picture. Most patients recover spontaneously but there is a high mortality in severe cases. There are no chronic sequelae.

Steroids
Cholestasis is caused by natural and synthetic oestrogens as well as methyltestosterone. These agents interfere with canalicular biliary flow and cause a pure cholestasis. Cholestasis is rare with the contraceptive pill because of the low dosage used. However, the contraceptive pill is associated with an increased incidence of gallstones, hepatic adenomas (rarely hepatocellular carcinomas), the Budd–Chiari syndrome and peliosis hepatis. The latter condition, which also occurs with anabolic steroids, consists of dilatation of the hepatic sinusoids to form blood-filled lakes.

Phenothiazines
Phenothiazines, e.g. chlorpromazine, can produce a cholestatic picture owing to a hypersensitivity reaction. It occurs in 1% of patients, usually within 4 weeks of starting the drug. Typically it is associated with a fever and eosinophilia. Recovery occurs on stopping the drug.

Anti-tuberculous chemotherapy
Isoniazid produces elevated aminotransferases in 10–20% of patients. Hepatic necrosis with jaundice occurs in a smaller percentage. The hepatotoxicity of isoniazid appears to be related to acetylator status, as the damage is due to the metabolites.

Rifampicin produces a hepatitis, usually within 3 weeks of starting the drug, particularly in patients on high doses.

Pyrazinamide produces abnormal liver biochemical tests and, rarely, liver cell necrosis.

Drug prescribing in patients with liver disease

The metabolism of drugs is impaired in severe liver disease (with jaundice and ascites) as the removal of many drugs depends on liver blood flow and the integrity of the hepatocyte. In general, therefore, the effect of drugs is prolonged by liver disease and also by cholestasis. This is further accentuated by portosystemic shunting, which diminishes the first-pass extraction of drugs. With hypoprotein-aemia there is decreased protein-binding of some drugs and bilirubin competes with many drugs for the binding sites on serum albumin. In patients with portosystemic encephalopathy, care must be taken in prescribing drugs with a central depressant action.

Gallstones

Bile secretion

Bile consists of water, electrolytes, bile acids, cholesterol, phospholipids and bilirubin. Two processes are involved in bile secretion across the canalicular membrane of the hepatocyte:

- In the *bile salt-dependent process* there is active secretion of bile salts; water and electrolytes follow down an osmotic and electrical gradient.
- In the *bile salt-independent process*, bile flow is linked to sodium transport, which is dependent on Na^+–K^+ ATPase activity.

One third of the bile flow emanates from the epithelial cells of the bile ductules. Secretion, particularly of bicarbonate, is stimulated mainly by secretin.

The average total bile flow is approximately 1 litre per day. In the fasted state half of the bile flows directly into the duodenum, half being diverted into the gall bladder. The mucosa of the gall bladder absorbs 80–90% of the water and electrolytes, but is impermeable to bile acids and cholesterol. Following a meal, cholecystokinin is secreted by the duodenal mucosa and stimulates contraction of the gall bladder and relaxation of the sphincter of Oddi, so that bile enters the duodenum. An adequate bile flow is dependent on bile salts being returned to the liver by the entero-hepatic circulation.

Prevalence of gallstones

Gallstones are present in 10–20% of the population in the Western Hemisphere, but the exact prevalence is unknown. Gallstones are rare in the Far East and Africa. They occur twice as frequently in young women than in men but this difference decreases with increasing age.

Types of gallstones

Gallstones can be divided into those composed of cholesterol and those composed of bile pigment. Cholesterol stones, which account for 80% of all gallstones in the Western Hemisphere, contain more than 70% cholesterol, often with some bile pigment and calcium (mixed stones). Pure cholesterol stones are often solitary.

Cholesterol gall-stones. Cholesterol is partly derived from dietary sources. In addition, it is synthesized, chiefly in the liver, but also in the small intestine, skin and adrenals. The rate-limiting step in cholesterol synthesis is β-hydroxy-β-methyl-glutaryl-CoA(HMGCoA) reductase, which catalyses the first step, i.e. the conversion of acetate to meva-lonate. The cholesterol formed is secreted into bile. Unesterified cholesterol is insoluble in water and is held in solution in bile by the formation of mixed micelles composed of cholesterol, bile salts and phospholipid.

Cholesterol stones only develop in bile that has an excess of cholesterol relative to bile salts and phospholipids (supersaturated bile). This could occur because of excess of cholesterol or because of a decrease in bile salts. There is a reduced bile salt pool in some patients with cholesterol gallstones and the pool circulates more frequently. This may account for the reduction in the rate-limiting cholesterol-7α-hydroxylase found in some patients (feedback inhibition).

Diminished bile salt synthesis is not the only cause of supersaturated bile; there appears to be an increase in HMGCoA reductase with an increase in cholesterol secretion into bile in some patients.

Factors other than cholesterol saturation are required to form gallstones, as supersaturated bile is found in normal subjects during an overnight fast. The rate of cholesterol crystallization and the state of the gall bladder also play a role. Glyco-proteins in bile promote nucleation of cholesterol crystals, leading to stone formation, but why this occurs only in bile from patients with gallstones is unclear. It may depend on the presence or absence of solubilizing factors. The role of infection is unknown. Definite risk factors for gallstones are shown in Table 5.15.

Bile pigment stones. Black pigment stones contain calcium salts of bilirubin, phosphate and carbonate in addition to bilirubin polymers and mucin glycoproteins. The biliary lipids are normal. They form in the gall bladder but, except in haemolysis, where there is increased bilirubin production, the pathogenesis is unclear.

Brown pigment stones have layers of choles-terol, calcium salts of fatty acids and calcium bilirubinate. They tend to form in the CBD after cholecystectomy and are due to precipitation of bilirubin with calcium. In the Far East these stones are associated with biliary tract infection.

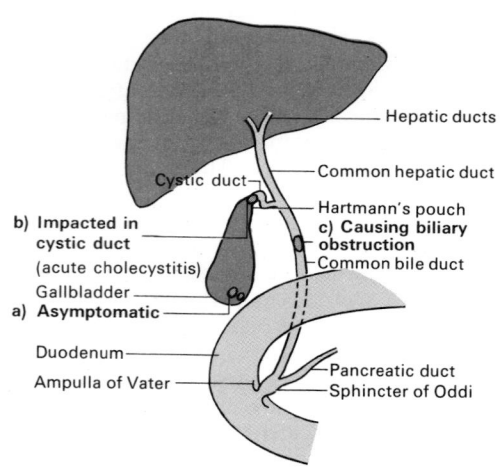

Fig. 5.20 Clinical presentation of gallstones.

Clinical presentation of gallstones (Fig. 5.20)

The majority of gallstones remain in the gall bladder and are asymptomatic.

A gallstone may impact in the neck of the gall bladder or in the cystic duct, giving biliary pain or acute cholecystitis.

Finally, gallstones may pass into the common bile duct, giving rise to biliary obstruction that produces severe biliary pain and sometimes choles-tatic jaundice. Bacterial infection can occur and produce cholangitis.

Rarely a gallstone may perforate through the wall of an inflamed gall bladder into the intestine, producing a fistula.

Gallstones do not give rise to any other symp-tom complex, and the idea that they produce indigestion, chronic right hypochondrial pain or intolerance to fatty food is based on a false correlation. Gallstones and upper abdominal symp-toms are both common, so great care must be taken to establish that the two are truly related. Fair, fat, fertile females of 40 have the same chance of having gallstones as the rest of the general population (10–20%). Thus, if they are investigated regardless of symptoms, gallstones will obviously be seen frequently by chance alone.

Table 5.15 Risk factors for cholesterol gallstones.

Age
Sex (F > M)
Multiparity
Obesity
Diet, e.g. high in animal fat
Drugs, e.g. contraceptive pill
Ileal disease or resection

Asymptomatic (silent) gallstones

Gallstones may be discovered accidentally when a patient is being investigated for some other reason. They require no treatment since the natural history is for them to remain asymptomatic, with only 18% having symptoms over a 15-year period.

Acute cholecystitis

PATHOPHYSIOLOGY

In over 90% of cases the gall bladder contains gallstones. Initially there is obstruction to the neck of the gall bladder or the cystic duct by an impacted stone, leading to distension and inflammation. The inflammation is usually sterile, but within 24 h gut organisms can be cultured from the gall bladder. Occasionally the inflammation may be mild and quickly subsides, leaving a gall bladder distended by mucus (mucocele). In this situation the patient may only have slight abdominal pain with a palpable gall bladder.

More commonly, however, the inflammation is more severe, involving the whole wall and giving rise to localized peritonitis and acute pain. The gall bladder may be distended by pus (an empyema). Very occasionally, acute gangrenous cholecystitis occurs with perforation and a more generalized peritonitis.

CLINICAL FEATURES

The disease is classically seen in females aged 20–40 years but it can occur at any age. The main symptoms are severe pain in the epigastrium and right hypochondrium. The pain is continuous, increasing in intensity over 24 h. It can radiate to the back and shoulder. It may be accompanied by nausea and vomiting. Mild jaundice occurs in 20% of cases owing to accompanying common duct stones.

EXAMINATION

The patient is usually ill with a fever and shallow respirations. Right hypochondrial tenderness is present, being worse on inspiration (Murphy's sign). There is guarding and rebound tenderness. Jaundice is occasionally present but usually this implies a stone in the common duct.

INVESTIGATION

- *Blood count.* A moderate leucocytosis is found.
- *Biochemistry.* The serum bilirubin, alkaline phosphatase and aspartate aminotransferase may be slightly raised.
- *X-ray.* A plain abdominal X-ray shows gallstones in 10% of cases.
- *Ultrasound examination* (Fig. 5.21). The detection of gallstones alone is insufficient for a diagnosis. Additional criteria are:
  - sonographic Murphy's sign (focal tenderness directly over the visualized gall bladder)
  - gall bladder wall thickening—not specific for acute disease
  - distension of gall bladder
  - biliary sludge
- *HIDA scintiscan.* This is extremely valuable and shows blockage of the cystic duct with the bile duct but not the gall bladder visualized. It is gradually being superseded by ultrasound.

DIFFERENTIAL DIAGNOSIS

The differential diagnosis includes other abdominal emergencies, such as a perforated peptic ulcer, retrocaecal appendicitis and acute pancreatitis. Right basal pneumonia and myocardial infarction must also be considered.

MANAGEMENT

The majority of patients improve with conservative management consisting of bed-rest, nil by mouth and intravenous fluids, with the addition of an antibiotic, usually amoxycillin or co-trimoxazole. In all but the mild cases, pain relief with an opiate is required.

In the absence of vomiting, the patient can soon tolerate oral fluids and nasogastric aspiration is not often required. Signs of complications such as generalized peritonitis or gangrene of the gall

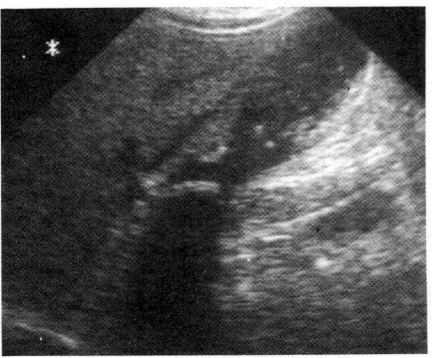
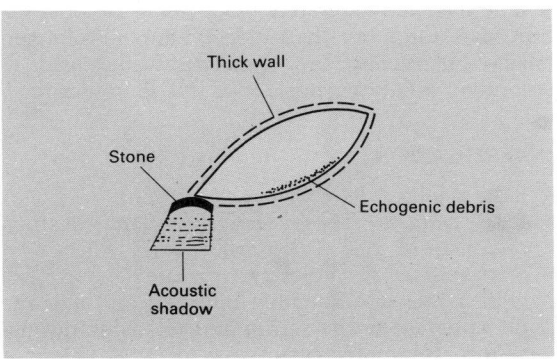

Fig. 5.21 Ultrasound and diagram showing acute cholecystitis with impacted stone. Note distension of gall bladder with thickened wall and sludge.

bladder (which causes increasing pain and fever) are an indication for surgery, particularly in the elderly.

Cholecystectomy within days of the acute attack has been advocated for all patients who are not an anaesthetic risk. A firm diagnosis can usually be made using a HIDA scan or ultrasound. Alternatively, cholecystectomy can be performed 2–3 months later. There is little to choose between the two approaches, although early surgery means only one hospital visit and no possibility of a recurrent attack while awaiting surgery to be performed, and does not increase operative morbidity or mortality.

Chronic cholecystitis

There is no doubt that gall bladders studied histologically can show signs of chronic inflammation and occasionally a small, shrunken gall bladder is found either radiologically or on ultrasound examination. There are, however, no symptoms or signs that can conclusively be shown to be due to chronic cholecystitis and this clinical diagnosis should therefore not be made. Most patients with chronic right hypochondrial pain suffer from functional bowel disease.

Common bile duct stones

These may be asymptomatic or they may present with any one or all of the triad of abdominal pain, jaundice and fever. The pain is usually severe and situated in the epigastrium and right hypochondrium (see p. 175).

The pain may be accompanied by vomiting. It usually lasts for a few hours and then clears up, only to return days, weeks or even months later. Between attacks the patient is well.

The jaundice is variable in degree, depending on the amount of obstruction. The urine is dark and the stools are pale. High fevers and rigors indicate cholangitis.

The liver is moderately enlarged if the obstruction lasts for more than a few hours. Prolonged biliary obstruction or repeated attacks lead to secondary biliary cirrhosis, but this is now rare.

INVESTIGATION

- *Blood count.* A leucocytosis is present.
- *Blood cultures.* These may grow an intestinal organism (*E. coli, S. faecalis*).
- *Biochemistry.* A cholestatic picture (see p. 250) with a raised conjugated bilirubin and alkaline phosphatase in the serum and relatively normal serum aminotransferases.
- *Prothrombin time.* This may become elevated over a few weeks owing to poor vitamin K absorption.

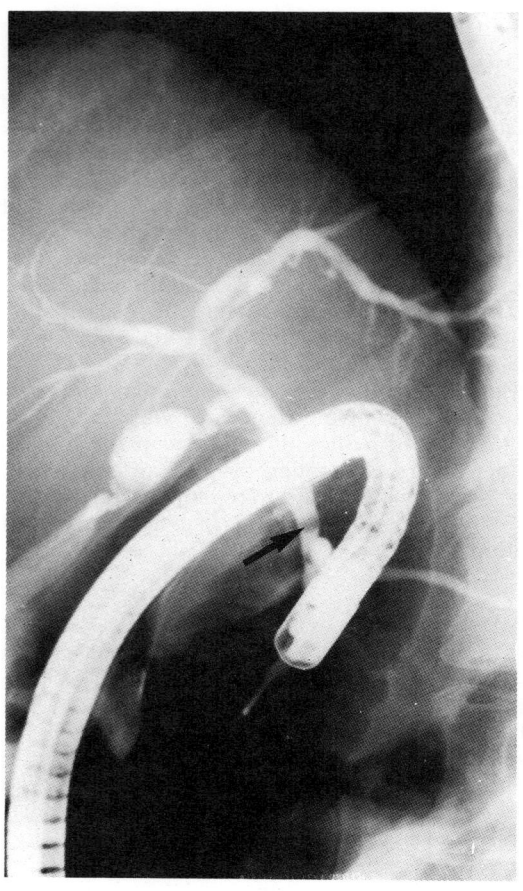

Fig. 5.22 ERCP showing gallstones in CBD.

- *X-ray.* A plain abdominal X-ray may reveal gallstones.
- *Ultrasound examination.* This may reveal a dilated common bile duct and sometimes gallstones (see Fig. 5.8).
- *ERCP.* This may be needed to confirm the diagnosis (Fig. 5.22).

DIFFERENTIAL DIAGNOSIS

The differential diagnosis includes all causes of jaundice.

MANAGEMENT

The acute episode is allowed to settle and the serum bilirubin usually falls to normal levels. During this stage the patient normally only requires pain relief but occasionally antibiotics are necessary.

The serum alkaline phosphatase falls more slowly than the serum bilirubin, and if the patient is seen some time after an acute attack elevation of this enzyme may be the only evidence of biliary tract disease.

Following ultrasonic examination, surgery or endoscopic removal of the stones should then be considered (see below).

Acute cholangitis

Acute cholangitis is due to bacterial infection of the bile ducts and is always secondary to bile duct abnormalities. The common causes are common duct stones, biliary strictures, neoplasms, or following ERCP in the presence of large duct obstruction.

The symptoms are fever, often with a rigor, upper abdominal pain and jaundice. All three symptoms are present in 70% of cases. Older patients can present with collapse and Gram-negative septicaemia.

Specific signs may be minimal but tenderness over the liver occurs.

When all three symptoms are present the diagnosis is not difficult, but the patient can present with only a fever and an accompanying leucocytosis. Blood cultures are often positive (usually for *E. coli*) and a severe Gram-negative septicaemia can occur.

Treatment is with intravenous amoxycillin 1 g 6-hourly with intravenous gentamicin 2–5 mg·kg^{-1} daily in divided doses for severe cases.

Suppurative cholangitis can occur as a complication. The fever continues and shock develops despite adequate antibiotics. Urgent decompression of the duct should be performed, usually endoscopically with placement of a nasobiliary drain. The subsequent treatment of the obstruction is either endoscopic or surgical (see below). Acute renal failure is a recognized complication in the jaundiced patient and all patients should be given intravenous mannitol during the surgical operation.

MANAGEMENT OF GALLSTONES

Stones in the gall bladder

Cholecystectomy is still the treatment of choice for most patients with gall bladder stones and symptoms. It is a safe procedure with a mortality of less than 0.1% in experienced hands. An increased mortality occurs in obese and elderly patients. It is these patients and those who refuse surgery in whom dissolution therapy (see below) can be considered.

Post-cholecystectomy syndrome. Some patients continue to complain of right hypochondrial pain, flatulence, indigestion and intolerance to fatty foods after cholecystectomy, despite a normal radiological appearance of the biliary tree. In the vast majority of these patients the original diagnosis was incorrect and the patient was suffering from functional bowel disease, the gallstones being an incidental finding. The occurrence of severe pain with jaundice suggests a retained stone in the common duct.

Gallstone dissolution or disruption
Cholesterol gallstones can be dissolved by the bile acids chenodeoxycholic acid and ursodeoxycholic acid, which increase cholesterol solubility in bile. They only dissolve radiolucent stones in a functioning gall bladder and not calcified stones. This makes only about 10% of patients suitable for this therapy.

Gallstone dissolution takes anything from 6 months to 2 years and when the treatment is stopped 50% of the gallstones recur. Chenodeoxycholate also produces diarrhoea. For these reasons, as well as the cost, medical therapy is not recommended for the majority of patients with symptoms of gallstone disease and dissolution is rarely advocated.

Shock-wave treatment of gallstones can be carried out using ultrasound-guided lithotripters that do not require a general anaesthetic or water bath. It is still only useful for non-calcified stones in a functioning gall bladder. Patients are placed on dissolution therapy after shock-wave treatment. Its exact role is being evaluated.

Stones in the common bile duct (CBD) with the gall bladder *in situ*

Cholecystectomy with exploration of the CBD is still the optimal treatment in all but the very sick or elderly. In the latter group, endoscopic sphincterotomy with removal of the CBD stone (see below) is a reasonable alternative, but recurrences may well occur. This can be followed by a cholecystectomy when the patient is well.

The duct should be explored at operation in all patients with a history of jaundice or in whom the history suggests biliary colic. The duct is opened and examined with a choledochoscope, if available, and cholangiography is performed. This procedure increases the mortality of the operation over that of simple cholecystectomy. All stones must be removed.

A T-tube is placed in the common bile duct at operation and bile is allowed to drain through it. Prior to removal of the T-tube, further cholangiography is performed to see whether any stones remain.

Retained stones can be treated by:

● Removal via the T-tube: this is possible if the T-tube is large (14 French gauge) using a steerable

catheter under fluoroscopic control
- Chemical dissolution by infusion of mono-octanoin down the T-tube
- Endoscopic removal—see below
- Further surgery if the above fail

Recurrent stones in CBD with the gall bladder previously removed

Endoscopic removal is now the preferred way. Stones can be removed from the common bile duct following a sphincterotomy in three ways:

- They can be allowed to pass naturally through the enlarged opening.
- They can be removed endoscopically using a Dormia basket.
- Instillation of methyl-*t*-butyl ether into the CBD dissolves cholesterol stones in 1–2 days. Its role is still being evaluated.

Shock-wave lithotripsy is now being used for recurrent CBD stones.

COMPLICATIONS OF GALLSTONES

- Cholangitis and cholestatic jaundice (see above)
- Pancreatitis (p. 289)
- Gallstone ileus and biliary enteric fistula. Gallstones can occasionally erode through the wall of the gall bladder into the intestine. They can cause obstruction, mainly in the terminal ileum but occasionally in the duodenum.

Carcinoma of the gall bladder may be causally related.

Miscellaneous conditions of the biliary tract

Primary sclerosing cholangitis

Primary sclerosing cholangitis results from inflammation and fibrosis of the bile ducts leading to multiple areas of narrowing throughout the biliary system. The cause is unknown.

Fifty per cent of patients have inflammatory bowel disease. Patients with AIDS have been found to have sclerosing cholangitis. The cause here is unclear but infection particularly with *Cryptosporidium* is a possible factor.

There may be no symptoms and the diagnosis is suggested by a raised serum alkaline phosphatase. Symptoms that may fluctuate are pruritus, jaundice and occasionally abdominal pain. Portal hypertension can develop. Liver biopsy shows a fibrous obliterating cholangitis with eventual loss of interlobular and adjacent septal bile ducts. An ERCP will show the multiple strictures. Treatment is unsatisfactory. In half of the patients the disease runs a benign course over many years. Steroids and azathioprine are of unproven value but seem to help some patients. Obvious extra-hepatic biliary strictures can sometimes be dilated or stented at endoscopy. Liver transplantation is now being performed for this condition.

Non-calculous cholecystitis

Occasionally cholecystitis occurs in diabetes mellitus, polyarteritis nodosa and systemic infections.

Cholesterolosis of the gall bladder

In this condition, deposits of cholesterol are seen in the mucosal wall, producing a fine yellow pattern on a red background (strawberry gall bladder). Cholesterol stones may or may not be present. The relationship to symptoms is unclear.

Adenomyomatosis of the gall bladder

This may be found as an incidental finding on a cholecystogram and consists of thickening of the mucosal and muscle layers with the presence of Rokitansky–Aschoff sinuses, often associated with small gallstones. It does not usually produce symptoms.

Choledochal cyst

This is a congenital cystic dilatation of the extra-hepatic ducts producing jaundice and abdominal pain. Fifty per cent of the patients do not present until early adult life. Treatment is surgical.

Haemobilia

Haemobilia can occur owing to hepatic trauma, sometimes owing to a tumour, and rarely after liver biopsy. Blood enters the biliary tree and produces either obstructive jaundice or gastro-intestinal bleeding.

Tumours of the biliary tract

Primary carcinoma of the gall bladder

This adenocarcinoma represents < 1% of all cancers. It occurs chiefly in those over 70 years of age and is commoner in females. Gallstones are usually present but a definite relationship is uncertain. The presenting features are of jaundice and occasionally right hypochondrial pain. A mass may be palpable in the right hypochondrium. The diagnosis is often made at operation and cholecystectomy is performed if possible. Few patients survive 1 year.

Cholangiocarcinoma (see p. 278)

This sometimes affects the extrahepatic biliary tree, giving rise to jaundice. Surgery, if possible, is the only effective treatment. Alternatively, a stent or tube can be passed through the obstruction during PTC or ERCP. The prognosis is poor.

Periampullary tumours

These tumours arise from the common bile duct, the ampulla of Vater or the head of the pancreas. All give rise to cholestatic jaundice. Carcinoma of the ampulla can sometimes be resected with a 40% five-year survival rate (compare with pancreatic carcinoma, p. 292).

The pancreas

Structure and function

The pancreas extends retroperitoneally across the posterior abdominal wall from the second part of the duodenum to the spleen. The head is encircled by the duodenum; the body, which forms the main bulk of the organ, ends in a tail that lies in contact with the spleen. The main pancreatic duct usually joins the common bile duct to enter the duodenum as a single duct at the ampulla of Vater. The main pancreatic duct has many tributary ductules and gradually tapers towards the tail of the pancreas. Pancreas divisum is an anatomical variant in which a small proportion of the pancreas drains through an accessory duct into the duodenum.

Exocrine cells form 98% of the human pancreas. The pancreatic acinar cells synthesize the pancreatic enzymes and form a ductal system that eventually joins into the main pancreatic duct.

The main regulators of pancreatic exocrine secretion are the hormones secretin and cholecystokinin (CCK). Secretin is released when acid enters the duodenum; it stimulates pancreatic juice containing water, electrolytes, chiefly bicarbonate. CCK is released when fatty acids and amino acids enter the duodenum but its exact role in stimulating pancreatic enzyme secretion is unclear. Enzymes produced are amylase, lipase, colipase, phospholipase and proteases (trypsinogen and chymotrypsinogen). The proteases are secreted in the inactive form but are then activated in the duodenum by enterokinase.

The endocrine pancreas consists of hormone-producing cells arranged in nests or islets—the islets of Langerhans. They do not connect directly to the duct system. There are four main types of islet cell and these have different secretory granules in their cytoplasm:

- The beta cell, which is the commonest cell, produces insulin.
- Alpha cells produce glucagon.
- D cells produce somatostatin.
- PP cells produce pancreatic polypeptide (PP).

Investigation (see Table 5.16)

Exocrine function

- *Serum amylase measurement* is useful in acute disease but is of no value in chronic disease.
- *Measurement of duodenal enzymes,* either after hormone stimulation or after food, is only sometimes helpful in the diagnosis of chronic pancreatitis because of the large reserve in enzyme capacity. A tube is passed into the duodenum and pancreatic secretions are collected after stimulation. Stimulation with secretin or CCK causes a rise in bicarbonate and enzyme, e.g. trypsin levels, which are low with chronic disease. The differential diagnosis between pancreatic tumour and pancreatitis is difficult. These tests have been largely superseded by imaging techniques. The Lundh test is performed in a similar fashion, the stimulation being produced by a meal. Measurement of trypsin and lipase is undertaken. These are low in chronic pancreatitis. The Lundh meal test is particularly useful in the investigation of steatorrhoea.
- *PABA test.* N-benzoyl-L-tyrosyl p-aminobenzoic acid is a synthetic peptide hydrolysed by pancreatic chymotrypsin to release free PABA, which is absorbed, metabolized and excreted in the urine. Reduction in absorption of free PABA occurs (after an oral load of the peptide) in pancreatic insufficiency and the test is highly specific in expert hands, although not widely utilized.
- *Faecal fat estimation* is performed to demonstrate steatorrhoea. A breath test can also be used; here the amount of $^{14}CO_2$ in expired air is measured following oral ingestion of a labelled fatty acid compared with that after a labelled

Table 5.16 Investigations available for the assessment of pancreatic disease.

Exocrine
Serum amylase
Duodenal enzymes after:
   Hormone stimulation with CCK and secretin
   Food stimulation (Lundh meal)
PABA test
Fat excretion
   Faecal fat (see p. 203)
   Breath tests

Endocrine
Serum levels of:
   Insulin
   Glucagon
   Pancreatic polypeptide
Glucose tolerance test measuring glucose and insulin

Visualization of the pancreas
Abdominal x-ray—to detect calcification
Barium meal—to show an abnormal duodenal loop
Ultrasound ⎱ To demonstrate size and presence of calcification, tumours,
CT scan   ⎰ pseudocyst (NB. Percutaneous biopsies can be taken.)
ERCP—to examine the ductular system
Angiography—to detect tumours

triglyceride (e.g. [^{14}C] oleic acid compared with [^{14}C]triolein). Impaired triglyceride absorption with normal fatty-acid absorption indicates that pancreatic disease is the cause of the steatorrhoea.

Endocrine function

Assessment of endocrine function is only useful if a hormone-secreting tumour is suspected and the serum measurements are often diagnostic. Plasma PP is raised with all endocrine tumours. The glucose tolerance test is seldom performed as it is affected by so many parameters.

Visualization of the pancreas

This now largely depends on ultrasound examination and CT scan to detect pancreatic size and shape, and the presence of cysts or tumours. An ERCP can be used to outline the pancreatic ducts. Selective catheterization of the splenic artery shows irregularity and encasement in carcinoma.

A combination of two or three tests is often necessary and none of the investigations is diagnostic. Fine-needle aspiration of any abnormality discovered can be performed under ultrasound or CT scan control. The presence of malignant cells in the aspirate indicates tumour but, of course, a negative sample does not exclude malignancy.

Pancreatitis

Classification
The Marseilles classification divides pancreatitis into:

- Acute pancreatitis ⎱ Full recovery
- Acute recurrent pancreatitis ⎰ of the gland to normal

- Chronic pancreatitis ⎱ Permanent
- Chronic relapsing pancreatitis ⎰ damage

Aetiology
Acute pancreatitis is associated with gallstone disease, possibly alcohol, and a number of less common causes, as shown in Table 5.17.

Alcohol undoubtedly damages the pancreas and clinically can cause an acute 'episode' of pancreatitis. However, the gland has almost invariably been previously damaged by alcohol, so that it is more correct to use the term 'chronic relapsing pancreatitis' for acute episodes seen in heavy alcohol consumers. In contrast, gallstones cause acute pancreatitis that may be recurrent, but they are rarely associated with chronic pancreatitis with permanent damage to the gland. In some cases of unexplained pancreatitis, pancreas divisum has been found, but the relationship is unclear.

Table 5.17 Causes of pancreatitis.

Acute
Gallstones
? Alcohol (see text)
Viral infections, e.g. coxsackie B, mumps
Ischaemia
Pancreatic tumours
Hyperparathyroidism
Hyperlipidaemia
Drugs, e.g. corticosteroids, azathioprine,
    L-asparaginase
Iatrogenic, e.g. post-surgical, post-ERCP
Idiopathic
Hypothermia

Chronic
Alcohol (> 85%)
Protein–energy malnutrition
Hyperlipidaemia
Idiopathic

Table 5.18 Complications of acute pancreatitis.

Pancreatic
    Phlegmon
    Pseudocyst
    Abscess
    Ascites

Intestinal
    Paralytic ileus
    GI haemorrhage

Hepatobiliary
    Jaundice
    Obstruction of CBD
    Portal vein thrombosis

Systemic
    Metabolic
        Malnutrition
        Hypocalcaemia
        Hypoglycaemia
    Haematological
        Disseminated intravascular coagulation
        Portal vein thrombosis
    Renal
        Acute renal failure
    Cardiovascular
        Circulatory failure (shock)
    Respiratory
        Hypoxic acute respiratory failure

Fat necrosis

Acute pancreatitis

PATHOGENESIS

The exact mechanism by which pancreatic necrosis occurs is unclear. Associated gallstones are mainly found in the gall bladder and only occasionally in the common bile duct. Reflux of bile up the pancreatic duct associated with occlusion of the ampulla may play a role in the pathogenesis. Autodigestion of the pancreas by proteolytic enzymes (particularly trypsin and phospholipase A) released in the pancreas rather than in the intestinal lumen may also be involved in the pathogenesis. Active enzymes could digest cell membranes, leading to proteolysis, oedema, vascular damage and necrosis. The mildest form of pancreatitis is characterized by intestinal oedema with an inflammatory exudate (oedematous pancreatitis), while in the severe form there is pancreatic necrosis and haemorrhage (haemorrhagic pancreatitis).

CLINICAL FEATURES

These vary depending on the severity of the attack. In all patients the principal symptom is abdominal pain that is usually localized to the epigastrium or upper abdomen. It may radiate to the back between the scapulae. The pain will vary from mild discomfort to excruciating pain in severe cases. Rarely, acute pancreatitis can occur in the absence of pain.

Nausea and vomiting accompany the pain in most cases.

Physical examination may reveal tenderness, guarding and rigidity of the abdomen, with varying degrees of shock depending on the severity of the attack. Rarely, body wall ecchymoses occur, e.g. umbilical (Cullen's sign) or in the flanks (Grey–Turner's sign). The remaining clinical features depend on the local and systemic complications that occur (Table 5.18).

Local pancreatic complications can occur with mild attacks of pancreatitis but systemic complications only occur with severe attacks.

INVESTIGATION AND DIAGNOSIS

The clinical manifestations are so varied that pancreatitis must be considered in the differential diagnosis of all causes of upper abdominal pain. Most present as an acute abdomen and differentiation from an acute perforated ulcer is the most difficult, as both may give rise to abdominal rigidity.

The diagnosis of acute pancreatitis depends on the serum amylase. A raised serum amylase level can be seen in other acute abdominal emergencies such as acute cholecystitis and perforated peptic ulcer, but if the serum amylase level is 5 times greater than normal, acute pancreatitis is very likely. However, the serum amylase cannot be entirely relied upon and must be evaluated in conjunction with the history and physical signs; if

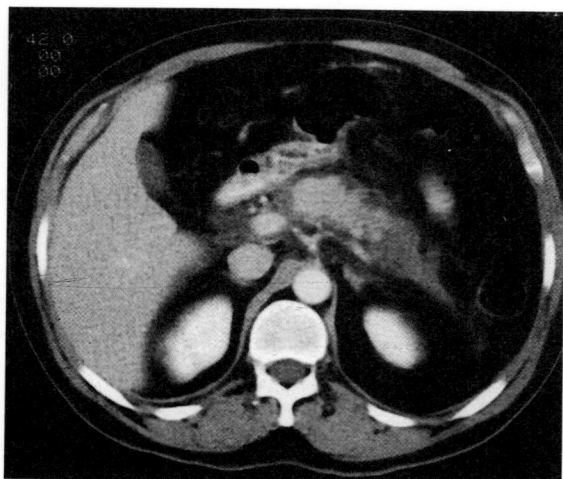

Fig. 5.23 CT showing severe acute pancreatitis with a small effusion around the pancreas.

there is doubt about the diagnosis, exploratory laparotomy must be performed to exclude a potentially fatal but treatable non-pancreatic lesion.

Peritoneal aspiration and lavage, with estimation of amylase in the peritoneal fluid obtained, is particularly useful in difficult cases. Ultrasound or CT scan (Fig. 5.23) may reveal a swollen pancreas, sometimes with peripancreatic fluid collections and gallstones, all of which help with the diagnosis.

The differential diagnosis includes all acute abdominal conditions.

Factors indicating the severity, which is assessed chiefly on blood investigations, are given in Table 5.19.

TREATMENT

Nasogastric suction is necessary to reduce vomiting and abdominal distension even in mild cases. All feeding is stopped and in severe cases nothing is given by mouth for weeks and intravenous nutrition is required (see p. 168). Water and electrolyte replacement and analgesia with an opiate (other than morphine) are necessary. No form of drug therapy has been shown to help and the efficacy of peritoneal lavage, which is sometimes used for severe cases, is in doubt.

Table 5.19 Factors indicating severe pancreatitis and a poor prognosis.

Age	> 55 years
WBC	$> 16 \times 10^9/\text{L}$
Blood urea	$> 16 \text{ mmol·L}^{-1}$
Serum albumin	$< 30 \text{ g·L}^{-1}$
Serum calcium	$< 2 \text{ mmol·L}^{-1}$
$P_a\text{O}_2$	$< 60 \text{ mm Hg (8.0 kPa)}$

Management of shock plus respiratory failure (see p. 716) is required.

LOCAL COMPLICATIONS

Phlegmon. This is a solid inflammatory mass of pancreatic tissue that usually resolves spontaneously.

Pseudocysts (see also p. 291). These are uncommon in the acute attacks and do not usually require treatment *per se*. Large collections persisting for weeks can be aspirated under ultrasonic control or removed surgically.

Pancreatic abscesses. Secondary infection of a peripancreatic collection of fluid may occur, usually after about 2 weeks. The clinical features are persistent fever, leucocytosis and abdominal distension, with a possible palpable mass. Patients are usually very ill with the accompanying respiratory, cardiac and renal problems.

Surgical drainage with vigorous antibiotic therapy and general support of the patient is required, as the disease has a long clinical course of several months.

Pancreatic ascites. This is usually associated with chronic pancreatitis and has a high amylase content.

PROGNOSIS

The mortality rate varies from 1% in mild cases to 50% in severe cases. With multiple complications and the presence of all the bad prognostic signs, the mortality is nearer 100%. The patients who recover may have recurrent attacks, depending on the aetiology and whether accompanying gallstones are dealt with.

Chronic pancreatitis

PATHOGENESIS

The majority of cases occur as a result of high alcohol consumption and it is in these cases that the pathology has been most studied. The earliest change appears to be deposition of protein plugs within pancreatic ducts. These then lead to ductular dilatation followed by acinar atrophy. There is some accompanying infiltration but this is variable. Extensive fibrous tissue is deposited near the pancreatic ducts. Eventually only a few acinar and islet cells remain, with widely dilated pancreatic ducts. Intraluminal calcification of the protein plugs occurs, leading to stone formation.

Chronic pancreatitis is not reversible, but it is possible that the disease will arrest if the patient stops drinking. However, because patients often continue to take small amounts of alcohol, the disease is most often progressive.

CLINICAL FEATURES

The major symptom is abdominal pain situated mainly in the epigastrium and upper abdomen and radiating to the back. The pain can be severe; in some cases it is comparable to that occurring in acute pancreatitis.

Continuing episodes of pain may occur; sometimes these are mild and of brief duration. In other cases there may be chronic pain interspersed with acute episodes (relapsing pancreatitis). The relationship to alcohol is variable; nevertheless, some acute episodes seem to be precipitated by heavy alcohol consumption.

The abdominal pain is accompanied by severe weight loss due to anorexia.

Steatorrhoea occurs when the secretion of pancreatic lipase is reduced by 90%. It occurs in about half the patients. The development of diabetes is more common. The steatorrhoea is often severe and the patient may notice drops of oil in the lavatory pan. Both diabetes and steatorrhoea occur more commonly with calcified pancreatitis.

Less common presentations include biliary obstruction with jaundice and occasionally cholangitis. Obstruction of the splenic vein can lead to portal hypertension.

INVESTIGATION

This includes assessment of some of the endocrine and exocrine functions as outlined earlier, as well as visualization of the pancreas. The serum amylase is of little value in chronic pancreatitis but may be raised during an acute episode of pain.

Patients with pain are investigated using ultrasound or CT scan, which show abnormalities in size and duct dilatation or the presence of calcification (Fig. 5.24) not seen on a plain X-ray. An ERCP is also useful in these patients to confirm the diagnosis. A dilated pancreatic duct, sometimes associated with stones or stenotic areas, can be identified. Early cases are difficult to diagnose and a combination of all tests with a strong clinical suspicion is necessary.

Patients presenting with steatorrhoea require a Lundh test to estimate exocrine function (see p. 287).

DIFFERENTIAL DIAGNOSIS

Carcinoma of the pancreas must be suspected, particularly when the history is short; occasionally laparotomy may be necessary to distinguish between these two conditions.

TREATMENT

In alcoholic pancreatitis the patient should stop drinking alcohol.

The pain needs to be controlled, often with narcotics, with the problem of addiction. Surgery is used for the treatment of intractable pain, pancreatic resection combined with drainage of an obstructed pancreatic duct into the small bowel being required. The use of surgery is controversial; good results are only obtained in a small number of cases, usually those who stop drinking.

Steatorrhoea is treated with a low-fat diet, pancreatic supplements, e.g. pancreatin 2–4 g with each meal, and cimetidine 400 mg twice daily. Diabetes mellitus is treated with diet, oral hypoglycaemic agents and/or insulin as appropriate. The insulin requirement is greater than in idiopathic diabetes, and patients may experience frequent or severe hypoglycaemia. This may be because pancreatic glucagon is lacking.

COMPLICATIONS

The commonest complication is a pancreatic pseudocyst. These are found very frequently if careful ultrasound examinations are performed. Small cysts require no treatment. Large cysts can give rise to increased pain, nausea and vomiting 3–4 weeks after the onset of the most recent attack of pain. A smooth, tender mass may be palpable and the cyst can be easily identified using ultrasound. Surgical treatment has been used for most large pseudocysts but a more conservative approach, with aspiration and close follow-up using ultrasound examination, can now be advocated.

Pancreatic ascites occurs, usually in alcoholic pancreatitis, when there is a communication between the pancreatic duct and the peritoneal

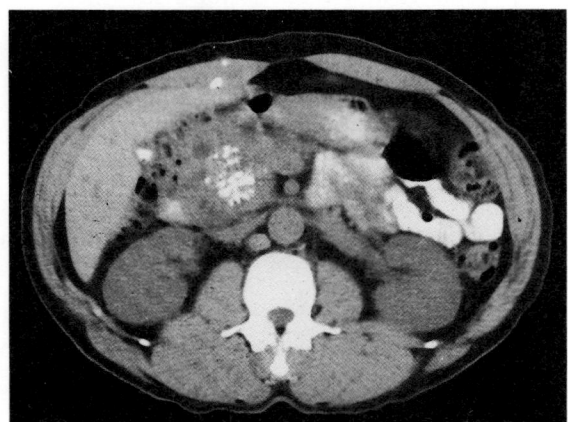

Fig. 5.24 CT showing chronic calcific pancreatitis.

cavity. The amylase content of the ascitic fluid is high.

A good prognosis depends on complete abstention from alcohol.

Carcinoma of the pancreas

The incidence of pancreatic carcinoma is steadily increasing in Western countries. This tumour is now the fourth commonest cause of cancer death in the UK and USA. The incidence increases with age and most patients are over 60 years of age. Males are affected more than females.

There are no known aetiological factors, but the increasing incidence has been attributed to an increase in both smoking and the consumption of alcohol. Excessive coffee ingestion has also been implicated.

Most carcinomas of the pancreas are adeno-carcinomas arising from duct epithelium. In 60% of cases the tumour is in the head of the pancreas. The tumour spreads locally to involve lymph nodes and the liver.

CLINICAL FEATURES

Carcinoma of the head of the pancreas or the ampulla of Vater presents with painless jaundice due to obstruction of the common duct. However, most patients will have pain at some time in the course of their disease. Weight loss also occurs.

Carcinoma of the body or tail of the pancreas presents with abdominal pain, anorexia and weight loss. The pain is often a dull, boring pain that radiates through to the back. It may be relieved by sitting forward. Jaundice is rare. Diabetes may occur and there is an increased incidence of thrombo-phlebitis.

In carcinoma of the head of the pancreas, examination will reveal jaundice with the dilated gall bladder sometimes being palpable (Courvoisier's sign). A dilated gall bladder is not found with gall stone disease because of the accompanying chronic inflammation of the gall bladder.

A palpable mass can be felt in 20% of patients, with hepatomegaly being present in most cases eventually.

INVESTIGATION

Haematological or biochemical tests (including blood glucose) are not helpful.

Diagnosis is usually made using ultrasound

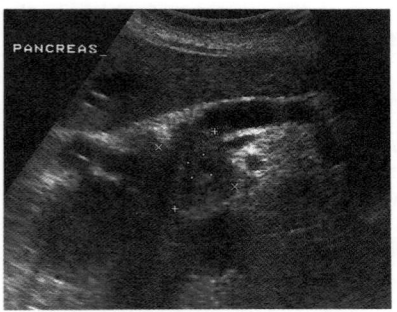

Fig. 5.25 Ultrasound showing carcinoma of head of pancreas with dilated pancreatic duct.

(Fig. 5.25) or CT scan and confirmed by fine-needle or trucut biopsy. However, in almost all cases, by the time the tumour is detected resection is impossible. Duodenoscopy with ERCP may detect tumour of the head of the pancreas or of the ampulla.

DIFFERENTIAL DIAGNOSIS

The differential diagnosis includes all causes of painless jaundice and persistent upper abdominal pain in the elderly.

MANAGEMENT

The 5-year survival rate is miserably low at 1%. Resection of the tumour with total pancreatectomy is not usually possible, and, as this operation carries a very high mortality (20%) and morbidity, it is seldom attempted. Jaundice from carcinoma of the head of the pancreas is usually relieved by a bypass procedure. This is now performed endo-scopically with the placement of a stent through the narrowed area of the CBD to allow drainage. Surgical bypass where the CBD is anastomosed to the jejunum is now reserved for cases where the tumour has obstructed the duodenum. Ampullary tumours have a better prognosis than pancreatic carcinomas and every attempt should be made to diagnose these rare lesions, as a resection in these cases can be performed. Pain and symptoms of anxiety and depression are an important part of management and analgesia with long-acting oral morphines should be used liberally. Addiction is not a problem in these terminally ill patients.

Cystic fibrosis (see p. 663)

This is the commonest cause of pancreatic disease in childhood. It is inherited as an autosomal recessive condition and a specific gene deletion has been identified in 70% of cases (see p. 663). It has been suggested that the resultant protein defect produces an abnormality in the regulation of a β-adrenergic gated chloride channel in the cell membrane. This cystic fibrosis gene product has been named cystic fibrosis transmembrane conductance regulator (CFTR). This basic defect in all exocrine glands produces thick viscoid secretions causing cystic dilatation of the ducts. Increased numbers of patients are now surviving into adult life because of improved therapy.

CLINICAL FEATURES

See p. 663.

DIAGNOSIS

- Sweat testing (p. 664) of symptomatic people and siblings of patients with cystic fibrosis identifies 77% by 2 years of age and 95% by the age of 12.
- In infants, immunoreactive-trypsin assay in dried blood.
- Pancreatic function tests (p. 287).

TREATMENT

Treatment is required for pancreatic insufficiency and respiratory problems (p. 663). Steatorrhoea is treated with a low-fat diet, pancreatic supplements and an H_2-receptor antagonist. Optimal nutrition has been recognized as improving prognosis and a high calorie intake (150% of recommended daily allowance) with vitamin supplements should be given.

Further reading

Schiff L (1987) *Diseases of the Liver*, 6th edn. Philadelphia: Lippincott.

Sherlock S (1989) *Diseases of the Liver and Biliary System*, 8th edn. Oxford: Blackwell Scientific.

Sleisenger MH & Fordtran JS (1988) *Gastrointestinal Disease*, Part VII *The pancreas*. 4th edn. Philadelphia: WB Saunders.

Wright R, Millward-Sadler GH, Alberti KGMM & Karran S (1985) *Liver and Biliary Disease*, 2nd edn. London: Baillière Tindall.

6

Diseases of the Blood

Introduction

Blood disorders are widely prevalent throughout the world. In the United Kingdom anaemia is seen mainly in:

- Children under 5 years of age
- Pregnant women
- Social classes 4 and 5
- The elderly

Anaemia is frequent in tropical and developing countries and the cause is often multiple; iron-deficiency anaemia is widely distributed, particularly in association with malnutrition and hookworm infestation. Hereditary anaemias are also very common. Thalassaemias affect populations originating from an area eastwards from the shores of the Mediterranean Sea through the Middle East to the Indian subcontinent and south-east Asia (see Fig. 6.16). Sickle cell anaemia is found frequently in the black African population throughout the world.

Blood

Blood consists of:

- Red cells
- White cells
- Platelets
- Plasma, in which the above elements are suspended

Plasma is the liquid component of blood, which contains soluble fibrinogen. Serum is what remains after the formation of the fibrin clot.

The formation of the blood
Around the third week of development of the embryo, blood islands are formed in the yolk sac. These produce primitive blood cells, which become the first haemoglobin-synthesizing cells or erythroblasts. In the second month these cells migrate to the liver and spleen, which become the chief sites of erythropoiesis until after birth. Erythropoiesis starts in the bone marrow from about the fifth month in utero; this is known as *medullary erythropoiesis*. Red cells made elsewhere are produced by *extramedullary erythropoiesis*.

At birth erythropoiesis occurs in the marrow of nearly every bone. As the child grows, the marrow cavity starts to be replaced by fat so that in the adult, red cell production is confined to the ends of the long bones, the axial skeleton, the ribs and the skull. Only if the demand for red cells increases and persists do the areas of red marrow extend once again. Pathological processes that obliterate the bone marrow cause extramedullary erythropoiesis to recommence in the liver and spleen.

All peripheral blood cells are derived from a single stem cell (a pluripotential stem cell) (Fig. 6.1). The stem cells have the capability for *self-renewal*, maintaining a constant cellularity in a normal healthy marrow and for *differentiation* into mature cells. The presence of the stem cells can be shown by bone-marrow culture techniques. The earliest detectable colony-forming unit (CFU) is CFU-S (spleen); this gives rise to CFU-GEMM, which produces CFU 'committed' for the production of:

- Granulocytes
- Erythroid cells
- Monocytes
- Megakaryocytes

The stem cell also divides to produce lymphoid cells.

Haemopoietic growth factors
Many haemopoietic growth factors have been identified (Fig. 6.1). All are glycoproteins with a polypeptide chain length of similar length and are

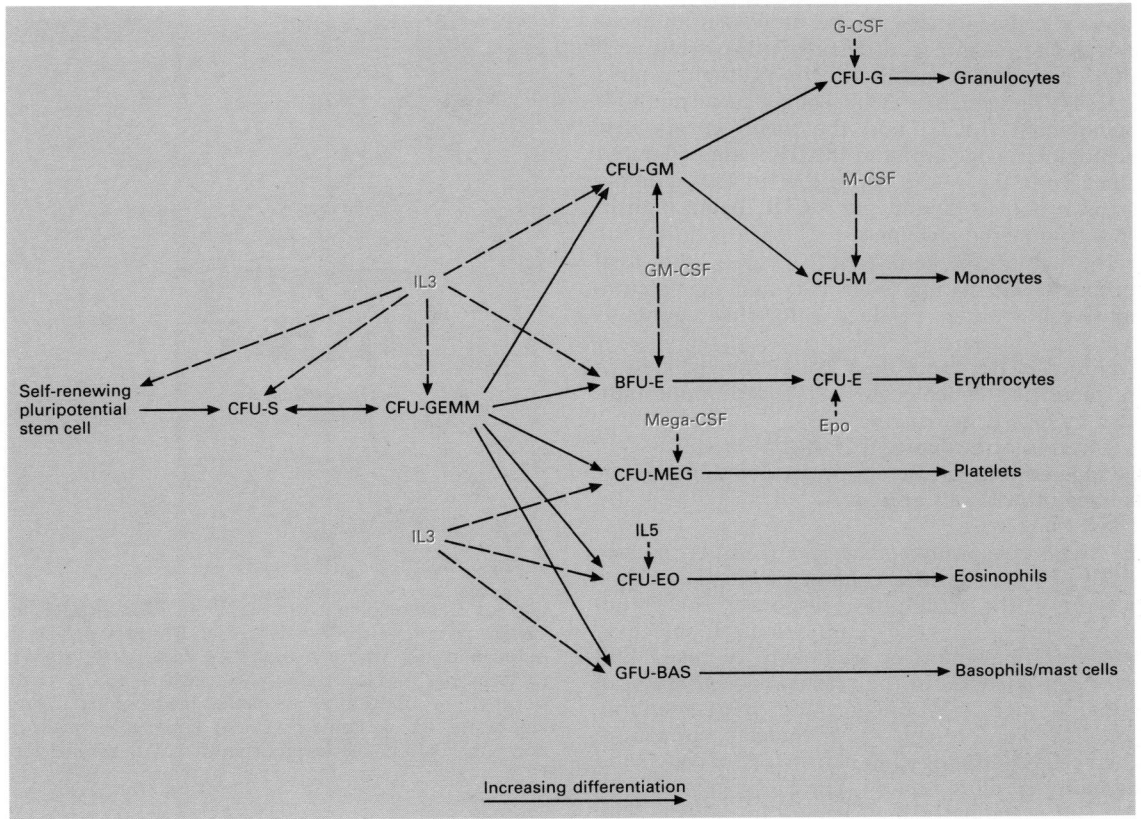

Fig. 6.1 The influence of cytokines on haemopoietic development. The direction of normal haemopoietic growth and differentiation is shown in unbroken arrows; the influence of factors in broken arrows. *Key*: CFU = colony-forming unit (or cell); CFU-S = spleen CFU; CFU-GEMM = mixed CFU having potential to develop into granulocyte, erythroid, monocyte or megakaryocyte lineage; BFU-E = burst forming unit for erythroid lineage; CFU-E = erythroid CFU; CFU-GM = granulocyte/monocyte CFU; CFU-G = granulocyte-CFU; CFU-M = monocyte CFU; CFU-Meg = megakaryocyte CFU; CFU-Eo = eosinophil CFU; CFU-BAS = basophil CFU; Epo = erythropoietin. (From Galvani DW (1988) *Journal of the Royal College of Physicians of London* **22** (4), with permission.)

produced by many cell types. They rapidly increase in response to stresses such as blood loss and anaemia. These factors include erythropoietin, colony-stimulating factors (CSFs—here the prefix indicates the cell type, see Fig. 6.1) and interleukins (IL). The genes for many of these have been localized to the long arm of chromosome 5, viz. multi-CSF (IL-3), GM-CSF, M-CSF, M-CSF receptor and IL-5, suggesting that their transcription is coordinated. Many growth factors can now be assayed and some have been produced by recombinant DNA techniques, for example GM-CSF which has been used after autologous bone marrow transplantation to accelerate neutrophil recovery, see p. 362. The erythropoietin gene, in contrast, is on chromosome 7. Erythropoietin was the original factor characterized and is produced primarily in the kidneys. Its production is mainly regulated by tissue oxygen tension, but increased 'inappropriate' production is also seen in renal tumours and cysts and some rare central nervous tumours producing polycythaemia (see Table 6.16). Human erythropoietin is used to treat secondary anaemias due to an inadequate erythropoietin production, e.g. chronic renal failure.

Peripheral blood—normal values (Table 6.1)
Automated cell counters are used to measure the number and size of red cells, white cells and

Table 6.1 Normal values for peripheral blood.

	Male	Female
Hb (g·dl^{-1})	13–18	11.5–15.5
PCV (haematocrit) (L·L^{-1})	0.42–0.53	0.36–0.45
RCC ($\times 10^{12}$/L)	4.5–6.0	3.9–5.1
MCV (fl)	80–96	
MCH (pg)	27–33	
MCHC (g·dl^{-1})	32–35	
WCC ($\times 10^9$/L)	4.0–11.0	
Platelets ($\times 10^9$/L)	150–400	
ESR (mm·h^{-1})	< 20	
Reticulocytes (%)	0.2–2	

platelets. Other indices can be derived from these values. The mean corpuscular volume of red cells (MCV) is the most useful of the indices and is used to classify anaemias (p. 300). The mean corpuscular haemoglobin (MCH) and the mean corpuscular haemoglobin concentration (MCHC) are of limited value, with the MCH being low in thalassaemia and iron deficiency and the MCHC being high in some haemolytic anaemias.

The white-cell count (WCC) gives the total number of circulating leucocytes and many automated cell counters produce differential counts as well.

Normally not more than 2% of the red cells in the blood are reticulocytes. A raised count indicates increased marrow activity.

A carefully evaluated blood film is still a very valuable adjunct to the above, as definitive abnormalities of cells can be seen.

The Erythrocyte Sedimentation Rate (ESR) is the rate of fall of red cells in a column of blood and is a measure of the acute-phase response. The pathological process may be immunological, infective, ischaemic, malignant or traumatic. A raised ESR reflects an increase in the plasma concentration of proteins, such as fibrinogen and some immunoglobulins. The proteins cause rouleaux formation, when cells clump together like a stack of coins, and therefore fall more rapidly. The ESR increases with age, and is higher in females and in patients with anaemia.

C-reactive protein is one of the proteins produced in the acute phase response (see p. 4). It is being increasingly used instead of the ESR. Its measurement is easy and quick to perform using an immunoassay that can be automated. It is synthesized exclusively in the liver and rises within 6 hours of an acute event. It rises with temperature (possibly triggered by IL-1) and all inflammatory conditions as well as trauma. It follows the clinical state of the patient much more rapidly than the ESR and is unaffected by the haemoglobin, normally it is less than 10 mg·L^{-1}.

The red cell

Erythropoiesis

In the marrow, red cells pass through several stages to maturity. They begin as pronormoblasts, develop into basophilic normoblasts and then, as haemoglobin synthesis starts within them, they start to become polychromatic and finally orthochromatic normoblasts. As the cells develop they become smaller and the nucleus is lost. Reticulocytes contain residual ribosomal RNA and are still

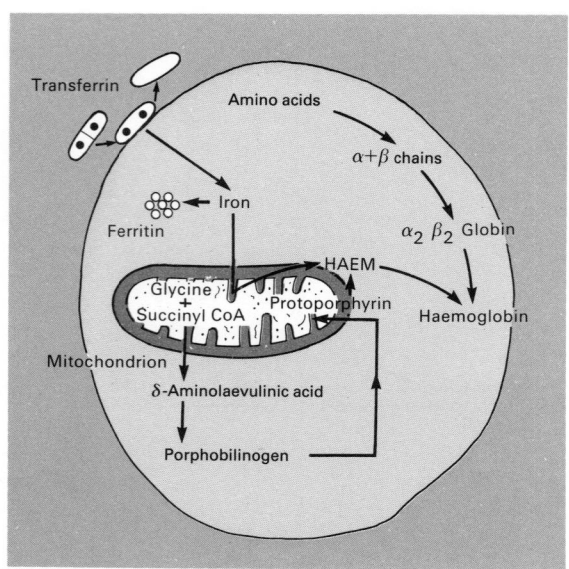

Fig. 6.2 Haemoglobin synthesis. Transferrin attaches to a surface receptor. Iron is released and transported to the mitochondrion, where it combines with protoporphyrin to form haem. Haem combines with α and β chains (formed on ribosomes) to make haemoglobin. (From Hoffbrand AV & Pettit JE (1984) *Essential Haematology*, 2nd edn. Oxford: Blackwell Scientific. With permission.)

able to synthesize haemoglobin. These reticulocytes remain in the marrow for about 24 h and then are released into the circulation, where they lose their RNA and become mature erythrocytes, which are non-nucleated biconcave discs. Throughout the maturation of red cells some 10% of the cells are lost; these lost cells are the result of 'ineffective erythropoiesis'.

Other requirements for normal erythropoiesis

- Iron for haemoglobin synthesis
- Vitamin B$_{12}$ and folate for normal DNA synthesis
- Other vitamins—B$_6$, ascorbic acid and riboflavin
- Trace metals (zinc, copper and cobalt)
- Hormones—androgens and thyroxine

Haemoglobin synthesis

Each red cell contains haemoglobin, which is a special protein able to carry oxygen to the tissues and return carbon dioxide from the tissues to the lungs. The binding of oxygen to haemoglobin is regulated by 2,3-diphosphoglycerate (2,3-DPG), which is an intermediate in red cell glycolysis. The concentration of 2,3-DPG affects the haemoglobin oxygen dissociation curve (see Fig. 13.5); an increased concentration shifts the curve to the right.

Haemoglobin synthesis occurs in the mito-

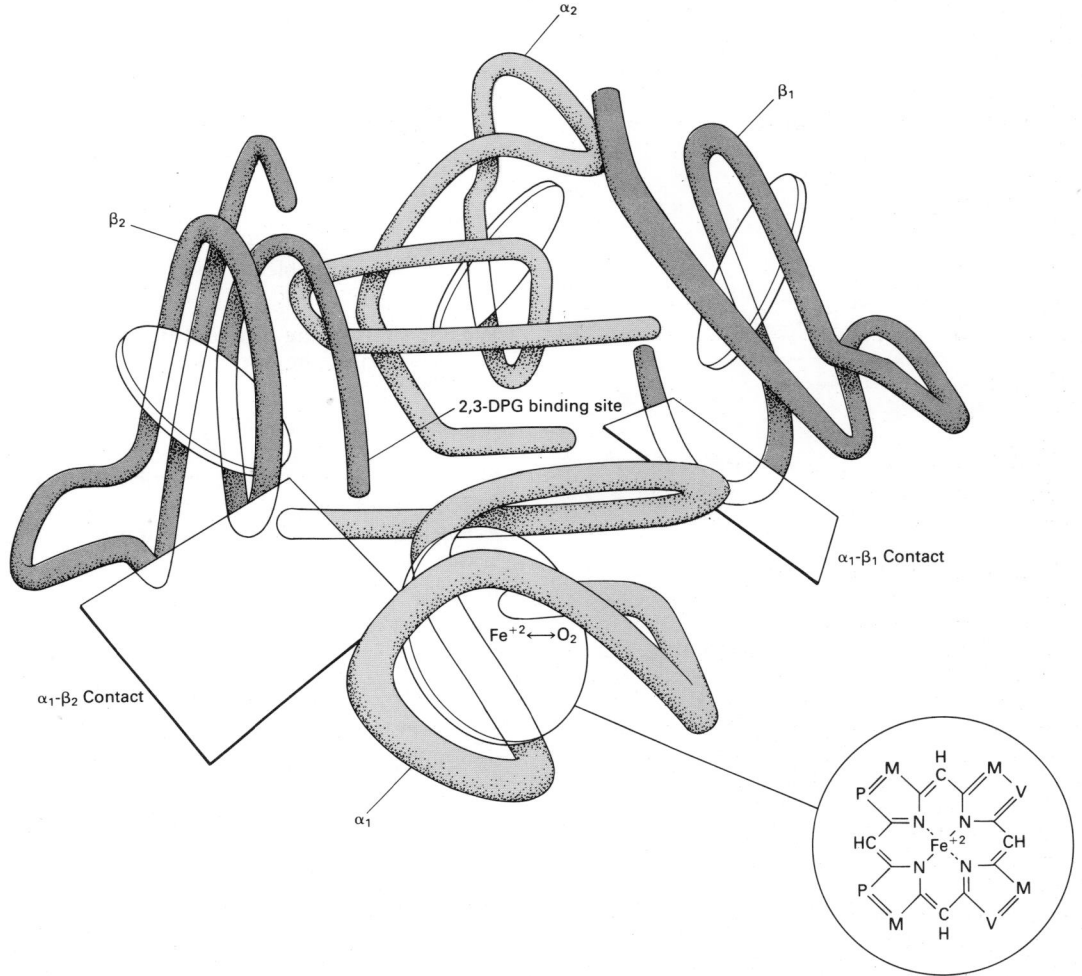

Fig. 6.3 Model of the haemoglobin molecule showing α (red) and β (blue) chains. 2,3-DPG binds in the centre of the molecule and stabilises the deoxygenated form by cross-linking the β chains. M = methyl; V = vinyl; P = propionic acid. (Redrawn from *Scientific American* 5 Hema 1 Hematopoiesis-6, with permission.)

chondria of the developing red cell. The complex biochemical reactions that occur are shown in Fig. 6.2. The major rate-limiting step is the formation of δ-aminolaevulinic acid (ALA) by ALA synthetase, which converts glycine and succinic acid to ALA. This reaction is inhibited by haem and stimulated by erythropoietin. Pyrrole rings are formed and then grouped in fours to produce protoporphyrins. Finally, iron is inserted to form haem. Haem is then inserted into the globin chains to form haemoglobin.

Each normal adult haemoglobin molecule, Hb A, has a molecular weight of 68 000 and consists of two alpha and two beta polypeptide chains. Two other haemoglobins, Hb F and Hb A_2 are found in small amounts in the blood of adults (see Table 6.11). The structure of Hb and its interaction with 2,3-DPG is shown in Fig. 6.3.

A summary of normal red cell production, function and destruction is given in Fig. 6.4.

Anaemia

Anaemia is present when there is a decrease in haemoglobin in the blood below the reference level for the age and sex of the individual (Table 6.1). Alterations in the haemoglobin may occur as a result of changes in the plasma volume, as shown in Fig. 6.5. A reduction in the plasma volume will lead to a spuriously high haemoglobin—this is seen in the clinical condition of stress polycythaemia. A high plasma volume, such as in pregnancy, may produce a spurious anaemia.

After a major bleed, anaemia may not be apparent for several days until the plasma volume returns to normal.

CLINICAL FEATURES

Patients with anaemia may be asymptomatic. A very slowly falling haemoglobin allows for haemo-

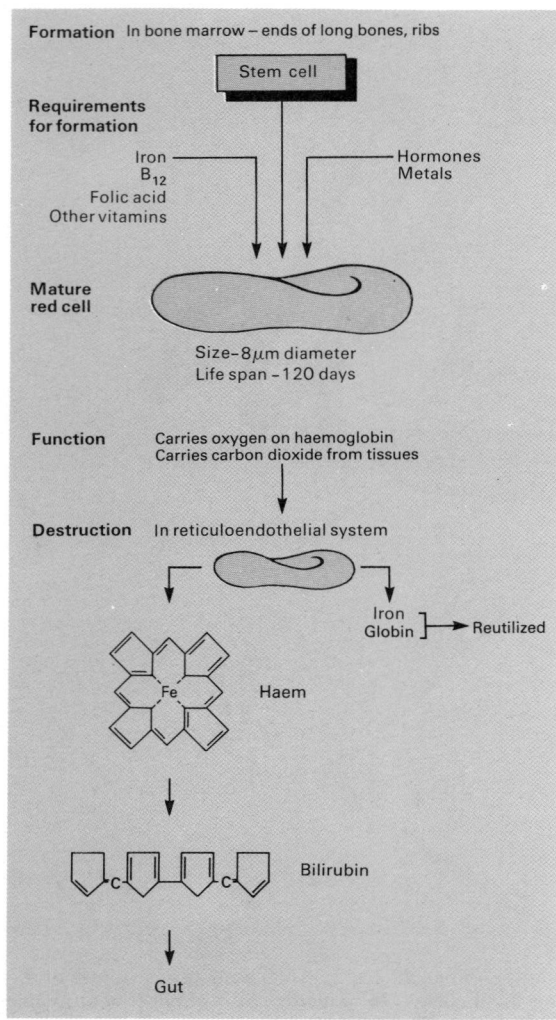

Formation In bone marrow – ends of long bones, ribs

Stem cell

Requirements for formation

Iron
B₁₂
Folic acid
Other vitamins

Hormones
Metals

Mature red cell

Size – 8μm diameter
Life span – 120 days

Function Carries oxygen on haemoglobin
Carries carbon dioxide from tissues

Destruction In reticuloendothelial system

Iron
Globin] → Reutilized

Fe   Haem

Bilirubin

Gut

Fig. 6.4 Red-cell production, function and breakdown.

dynamic compensation and enhancement of the oxygen-carrying capacity of the blood. A rise in 2,3-DPG causes a shift of the oxygen dissociation curve to the right, so that oxygen is more readily given up to the tissues. Where blood loss is more rapid or severe, particularly in elderly people, symptoms may occur.

Symptoms (all non-specific)

- Fatigue   } NB—Very common in the normal
- Headaches } population
- Faintness
- Breathlessness
- Angina of effort
- Intermittent claudication
- Palpitations

Signs
Non-specific signs include:

- Pallor
- Tachycardia
- Systolic flow murmur
- Cardiac failure
- Ankle oedema
- Rarely papilloedema and retinal haemorrhages after an acute bleed (can be accompanied by blindness)

Specific signs of the different types of anaemia will be discussed in the appropriate section. Examples include:

- Koilonychia—spoon-shaped nails seen in iron-deficiency anaemia
- Jaundice—found in haemolytic anaemia
- Bone deformities—found in thalassaemia major
- Leg ulcers—occur in association with sickle cell disease

It must be emphasized that anaemia is not a diagnosis, and a cause must be found.

CLASSIFICATION

The various types of anaemia, classified in terms of the appearance of the red cells, are shown in Fig. 6.6. There are three major types of anaemia:

- Hypochromic microcytic with a low mean corpuscular volume (MCV)
- Normochromic normocytic with a normal MCV
- Macrocytic with a high MCV

Where there are both large and small red cells, a dimorphic anaemia is said to be present. This may,

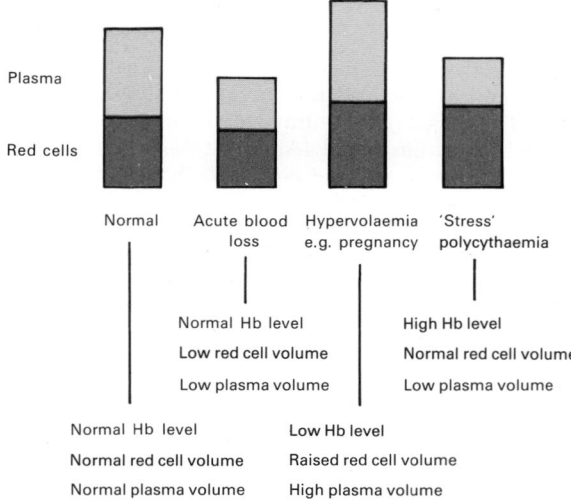

Plasma

Red cells

Normal   Acute blood loss   Hypervolaemia e.g. pregnancy   'Stress' polycythaemia

Normal Hb level
Low red cell volume
Low plasma volume

High Hb level
Normal red cell volume
Low plasma volume

Normal Hb level
Normal red cell volume
Normal plasma volume

Low Hb level
Raised red cell volume
High plasma volume

Fig. 6.5 Alterations of haemoglobin in relation to plasma.

for example, be seen in coeliac disease due to a combination of iron and folate deficiency.

INVESTIGATIONS

Peripheral blood

A low haemoglobin should always be considered in relation to:

- The white cell count
- The platelet count
- The reticulocyte count (as this indicates marrow activity)

Bone marrow

A bone marrow aspiration or trephine is performed to further investigate abnormalities found in the peripheral blood. The following are assessed:

- Cellularity of the marrow fragments
- Type of erythropoiesis, e.g. normoblastic or megaloblastic
- Cellularity of the various cell lines
- Infiltration of the marrow
- Assessment of iron stores
- Special tests may be performed: cytogenetic, immunological, cytochemical markers, biochemical analyses (deoxyuridine suppression test), microbiological culture

Microcytic anaemia

Iron deficiency is the commonest cause of this type of anaemia in the world. Thalassaemia also causes a microcytic hypochromic anaemia and is described on p. 313.

Iron

Dietary intake

The average daily diet in the United Kingdom contains 15–20 mg of iron but normally only 10% of this is absorbed. Absorption is increased, however, in iron deficiency. Iron is contained in many foods, e.g. liver, green vegetables, flour, eggs, meat and milk. Inorganic iron is usually present in the diet in the ferric form, whilst most organic iron is contained in haem.

Absorption

This takes place in the duodenum and jejunum. The absorption of iron is a complex process; some of the factors influencing it are shown in Table 6.2.

The iron content of the body is kept within narrow limits and its loss and intake are finely balanced. The precise mechanisms by which iron is absorbed and transported across the epithelial cell

---

TECHNIQUES FOR OBTAINING BONE MARROW

Aspiration

- Site—usually iliac crest
- Give local anaesthetic injection
- Use special bone marrow needle (e.g. Salah)
- Aspirate marrow
- Make smear on a glass slide
- Stain with:
  (a) Romanowsky technique
  (b) Perls' reaction (Prussian blue) for iron

Trephine

Indications include:

- 'Dry tap' obtained with aspiration
- Better assessment of cellularity, e.g. aplastic anaemia
- Better assessment of presence of infiltration or fibrosis

Technique

- Site—usually posterior iliac crest
- Give local anaesthetic injection
- Use special needle (e.g. Jamshidi—longer and wider than for aspiration)
- Obtain core of bone
- Fix in formalin; decalcify—this takes a few days
- Stain with:
  (a) Haematoxylin and eosin
  (b) Reticulin stain

---

are uncertain but its absorption appears to be closely related to the total iron stores of the body.

Haem iron is absorbed directly into the intestinal cell, where iron is released by haem oxygenase. Non-haem iron is taken up into the intestinal epithelial cell and enters a labile pool

Table 6.2 Factors influencing iron absorption.

- Ferrous iron is absorbed better than ferric.
- Gastric acidity helps to keep iron in the ferrous state and soluble in the upper gut.
- Reducing agents, e.g. ascorbic acid, increase iron absorption.
- Inorganic iron is absorbed better than organic iron.
- Iron absorption is increased with low iron stores and decreased in iron overload.
- Increased erythropoietic activity, e.g. bleeding, haemolysis, high altitude, increases absorption.
- Alcohol increases absorption.
- Formation of insoluble complexes with phytate or phosphate decreases iron absorption.
- There is increased absorption in idiopathic haemochromatosis.

where it is available for transfer to plasma. Excess iron in the intestinal cell is joined to apoferritin to form ferritin. Ferritin is lost into the gut lumen when the intestinal cell is shed. In iron deficiency, the amount of iron in the labile pool is low and more iron enters the cell and is transported to the portal vein. In iron overload, the amount of iron in the labile pool is high and therefore less iron is absorbed and more ferritin is formed and shed into the lumen. Iron enters the plasma in the ferric form and becomes bound to transferrin.

Transport in the blood
Normal serum iron is about 11–30 µmol·L^{-1}; there is a diurnal rhythm with higher levels in the morning. Iron is transported in the plasma bound to transferrin, a beta globulin that is synthesized in the liver. Each molecule binds two atoms of ferric iron and normally transferrin is one third saturated. Most of the iron bound to transferrin comes from macrophages in the reticuloendothelial system and not from iron absorbed by the intestine. Transferrin-bound iron becomes attached by specific receptors to erythroblasts and reticulocytes in the marrow and the iron is removed (Fig. 6.2).

Ferritin is only present in the plasma in small amounts.

Iron stores
Iron is stored in the tissues as ferritin and haemosiderin; stores normally amount to 1000–1500 mg. In an average man, 20 mg of iron, chiefly obtained from red cell breakdown, is incorporated into haemoglobin every day. About two thirds of the total body iron is in the circulation as haemoglobin (2.5–3 g in normal adult man); small amounts are found free in the plasma, with some in myoglobin and enzymes.

Requirements
Each day 0.5–1 mg of iron is lost in the faeces, urine and sweat. Menstruating women lose 40 ml of blood per menstrual period, an average of about 0.7 mg of iron per day of menstruation. Blood loss through menstruation in excess of 100 ml will usually result in iron deficiency as it cannot be compensated for by increased iron absorption from the gut. The demand for iron also increases during growth and pregnancy.

In the normal adult the iron content of the body remains relatively fixed. Increases in the body iron content (haemochromatosis) are classified into primary and secondary forms. Primary (idiopathic) haemochromatosis is discussed on p. 270. Secondary haemochromatosis (transfusion siderosis) is due to iron overload in conditions where repeated transfusion is the only therapy.

Iron deficiency

Iron-deficiency anaemia develops when there is an inadequate amount of iron for haemoglobin synthesis. A normal level of haemoglobin is maintained for as long as possible until all the iron stores are depleted; during this time *latent iron deficiency* is said to be present.

CAUSES OF IRON DEFICIENCY

- Poor intake
- Decreased absorption
- Increased demands
- Blood loss

Most iron deficiency occurs from *blood loss*. Premenopausal women are always in a state of precarious iron balance owing to menstruation. Nutritional iron deficiency is rare in developed countries. In the UK it is sometimes seen in vegetarian Asian women eating chapattis containing phytate. The commonest cause of iron deficiency world-wide is blood loss from the gastrointestinal tract due to hookworm infestation.

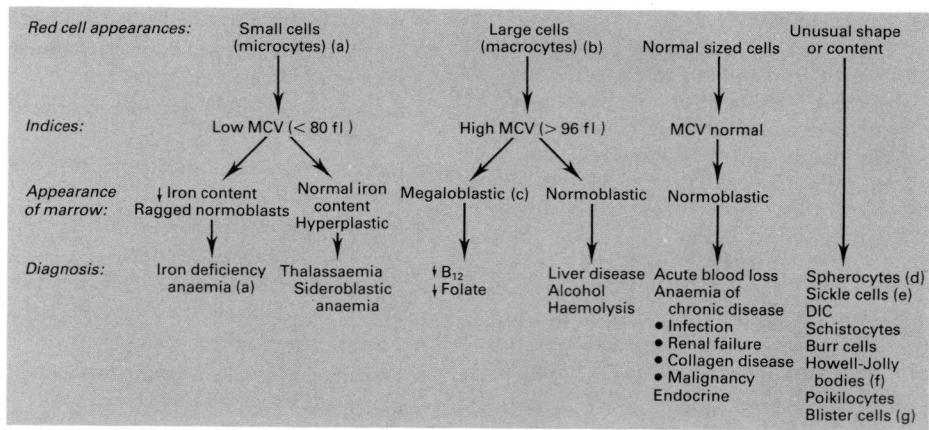

Fig. 6.6 Classification of red-cell appearances: (a)–(g) refer to Fig. 6.7.

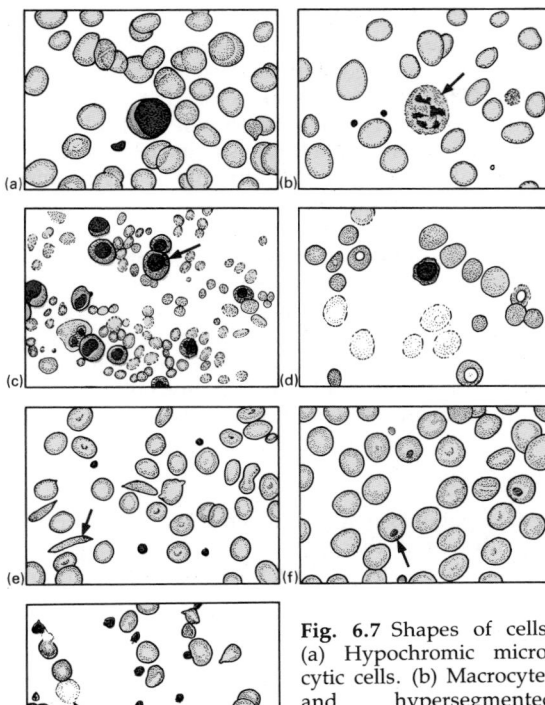

Fig. 6.7 Shapes of cells. (a) Hypochromic microcytic cells. (b) Macrocytes and hypersegmented neutrophils (arrowed). (c) Megaloblasts and giant metamyelocytes (arrowed) in the bone marrow. (d) Spherocytes and reticulocytes (polychromasia). (e) Sickle cells (arrowed) and target cells. (f) Post-splenectomy film with Howell–Jolly bodies (arrowed). (g) 'Blister' cells (arrowed) in G6PD deficiency.

CLINICAL FEATURES

The symptoms of anaemia are described on p. 298. Other clinical features occur as a result of tissue iron deficiency. These are mainly epithelial changes induced by the effect of inadequate iron in the cells:

● Brittle nails
● Spoon-shaped nails (koilonychia)
● Atrophy of the papillae of the tongue
● Angular stomatitis
● Brittle hair
● A syndrome of dysphagia and glossitis (Plummer–Vinson or Paterson–Brown–Kelly syndrome)
● Rarely, in severe iron deficiency, parotid gland enlargement, splenomegaly and failure to grow

The diagnosis of iron-deficiency anaemia relies on a good clinical history with questions about dietary intake, regular self-medication with aspirin (which may give rise to gastrointestinal bleeding) and the presence of blood in the faeces (which may be a sign of haemorrhoids or carcinoma of the lower bowel). No examination of an iron-deficient patient is complete without a rectal examination and proctoscopy. In women, a careful inquiry about the duration of periods, the occurrence of clots and the number of sanitary towels or tampons used should be made.

INVESTIGATION

Blood count and film
A characteristic blood film is shown in Fig. 6.7a. The red cells are microcytic (MCV < 80 fl) and hypochromic (MCH < 27 pg). There is poikilocytosis (variation in shape) and anisocytosis (variation in size). Target cells are seen.

Serum iron and iron-binding capacity
The values for serum iron and iron-binding capacity in iron deficiency are included in Fig. 6.8; the serum iron falls and the total iron-binding capacity rises compared with normal. Iron deficiency is regularly present when the percentage saturation (i.e. serum iron divided by total iron-binding capacity) falls below 19%.

Serum ferritin
The level of serum ferritin reflects the amount of stored iron, probably more accurately than the saturation of the serum iron-binding capacity. The normal value for serum ferritin is 5.8–120 nmol·L^{-1} (15–250 μg·L^{-1}); it is usually lower in females than in males.

Bone marrow
Erythroid hyperplasia with ragged normoblasts are seen in the marrow in iron deficiency. Staining with potassium ferrocyanide does not show the characteristic blue granules of stainable iron in the erythroblasts.

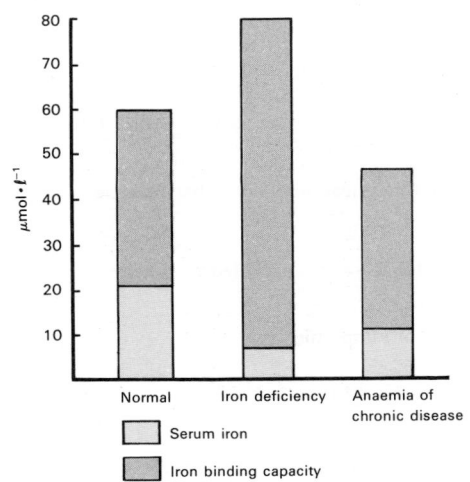

Fig. 6.8 Serum iron and total iron-binding capacity. Chronic diseases causing anaemia include renal failure, carcinoma and connective-tissue disorders.

Examination of the bone marrow is not essential for the diagnosis of iron deficiency except in complicated cases.

Other investigations
These will be indicated by the clinical history and examination; investigations of the gastrointestinal tract are often required (see p. 197).

DIFFERENTIAL DIAGNOSIS

The presence of anaemia with microcytosis and hypochromia does not necessarily indicate iron deficiency. The commonest other causes are thalassaemia, sideroblastic anaemia and anaemia of chronic disorder. In all of these disorders the iron stores are normal or increased.

TREATMENT

The correct management of iron deficiency is to find and treat the underlying cause.

Enough iron must be given not only to restore the haemoglobin level to normal but also to replace the body's iron stores. Oral iron is all that is required in most cases. Preparations such as ferrous sulphate 600 mg daily (120 mg ferrous iron) and ferrous gluconate 600 mg daily (70 mg ferrous iron) are both absorbed well. Various additions such as ascorbic acid and succinic acid bring no clinical benefit. If the patient has side-effects from iron medication, reducing the dose is all that is required. Prescribing expensive iron compounds, particularly the slow-release ones, is a waste of money.

Patients who have general intolerance of oral preparations, even at low doses, and who have chronic diseases, may require parenteral iron. Iron dextran can be given in doses of 50–250 mg daily by deep intramuscular injections. There is no justification for large intravenous infusions of iron, which are dangerous and unnecessary.

The response to iron therapy can be monitored using the reticulocyte count and haemoglobin level.

Table 6.3 Classification of sideroblastic anaemia.

Inherited
X-linked disease—transmitted by females
Acquired
Primary or idiopathic
Secondary:
Drugs, e.g. isoniazid, phenacetin
Alcohol
Lead
Myeloproliferative disorders
Leukaemias
Secondary carcinoma
Other systemic disorders, e.g. connective tissue diseases

Sideroblastic anaemia

Sideroblastic anaemias are inherited or acquired disorders characterized by dyserythropoiesis, iron overload and the presence of ring sideroblasts. They can be classified as shown in Table 6.3. In sideroblastic anaemia there is a disordered accumulation of iron in mitochondria in the erythroblasts. A ring of iron is formed round the nucleus that can be seen with Perls' reaction.

In sideroblastic anaemia, a dimorphic peripheral blood film with both normal and microcytic cells is usually seen. The small cells result from the ineffective synthesis of haemoglobin as a result of failure in the formation of haem. Failure to produce protoporphyrin results in iron not being taken up to form haem, and iron accumulates in the cell.

TREATMENT

Some patients respond when drugs or alcohol are withdrawn if these are the causative agents. In some cases folic acid or pyridoxine may improve iron utilization.

Lead poisoning

The causes, clinical features and treatment are discussed on p. 751. The characteristic haematological features include:

- Sideroblastic anaemia, due to inhibition by lead of several enzymes involved in haem synthesis including δ-aminolaevulinic acid synthetase.
- Haemolysis, which is usually mild, due to damage to the red-cell membrane.
- Punctate basophilia (the blood film shows red cells with small, round blue particles). This appearance is due to aggregates of RNA in red cells due to inhibition by lead of pyrimidine-5-nucleotidase, which normally disperses residual RNA to produce a diffuse blue staining seen in reticulocytes on blood films (polychromasia).

Normocytic anaemia

Normocytic, normochromic anaemia is seen in chronic diseases (see Table 6.4), in some endocrine disorders (e.g. hypopituitarism, hypothyroidism and hypoadrenalism) and in some haematological disorders (e.g. aplastic anaemia and some haemolytic anaemias). In addition, this type of anaemia is seen acutely following blood loss before iron stores are depleted.

The mechanism of the 'anaemia of chronic disease' is unclear but, in chronic renal disease, there is a reduction of erythropoietin and, in other

Table 6.4 Some causes of 'anaemia of chronic disease'

Chronic renal failure

Liver disease

Inflammatory disease
   rheumatoid arthritis
   Crohn's disease

Neoplastic disease

Chronic infections
   infective endocarditis
   tuberculosis

Vasculitis—polymyalgia rheumatica

Connective tissue disease—systemic lupus
erythematosus

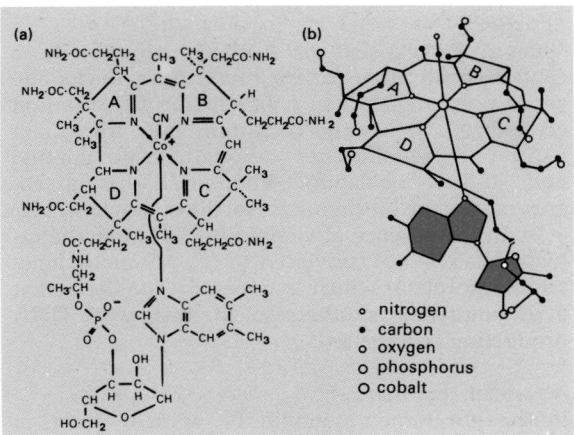

Fig. 6.9 The chemical structure of vitamin B_{12} (cyanocobalamin). (a) The molecular structure. (b) A three-dimensional representation. (From Beck WS (1962) *New England Journal of Medicine* **266**: 708. With permission.)

anaemias of chronic disorder, there is an inadequate erythropoietin response to the anaemia. Other factors include decreased red-cell survival and a decreased release of iron from the bone marrow to developing erythroblasts. The serum iron is low and the total iron-binding capacity (TIBC) is also low, in contrast with a low serum iron and a raised TIBC seen in iron-deficiency anaemia. Serum ferritin is normal or raised, in contrast with the low levels seen in iron deficiency. There is stainable iron present in the bone marrow and, therefore, not surprisingly, patients do not respond to iron therapy. Treatment is that of the underlying disorder.

Macrocytic anaemia

MEGALOBLASTIC ANAEMIA

Megaloblastic anaemia is characterized by the presence in the bone marrow of erythroblasts with delayed nuclear maturation because of defective DNA synthesis (megaloblasts). These megaloblasts are large and have a large immature nucleus; the cytoplasm stains dark blue with a Romanowsky stain. The nuclear chromatin pattern has an open stippled appearance. Associated with this abnormality of the red cell series is a characteristic abnormality of white cells, giant metamyelocytes. Megaloblastic changes occur in:

- Vitamin B_{12} deficiency
- Folic acid deficiency
- Conditions with neither B_{12} nor folate deficiency, e.g. orotic aciduria, where there is a defect in pyrimidine synthesis, therapy with drugs interfering with DNA synthesis and myelodysplasia.

Haematological values
Anaemia may be present. The MCV is characteristically > 96 fl unless there is a co-existing cause of microcytosis. The peripheral blood film shows macrocytes with hypersegmented polymorphs (Fig. 6.7). If severe, there may be leucopenia and thrombocytopenia.

Vitamin B_{12}

Vitamin B_{12} is synthesized by certain microorganisms, and animals and humans are ultimately dependent on this source. It is found in meat, fish, eggs and milk, but not in plants. Vitamin B_{12} is not usually destroyed by cooking. The average daily diet contains 5–30 μg of vitamin B_{12}, of which 1–5 μg are absorbed. The average adult stores some 1000 μg in the liver and, as the daily loss is small, it may take up to 5 years after absorptive failure before B_{12} deficiency develops.

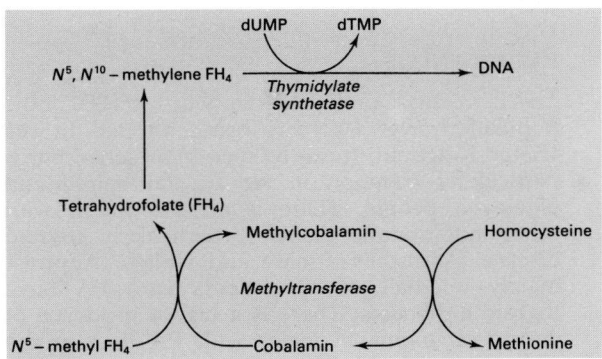

Fig. 6.10 Important biochemical reactions of vitamin B_{12}. dUMP = deoxyuridine monophosphate. dTMP = deoxythymidine monophosphate.

Structure

Vitamin B_{12} consists of a planar group with a central cobalt atom (corrin ring) and a nucleotide set at right angles (Fig. 6.9). Vitamin B_{12} was first crystallized as cyanocobalamin but the main natural cobalamins are deoxyadenosyl, methyl and hydroxycobalamin. Vitamin B_{12} is a co-enzyme for the biochemical reactions shown in Fig. 6.10. In the absence of vitamin B_{12}, N^5-methyltetra-hydrofolate is not converted to N^5, N^{10}-methylene-tetrahydrofolate, which is necessary for the action of thymidylate synthetase. In this way DNA production is impaired.

Absorption and transport

In the gut lumen, vitamin B_{12} initially forms a complex with an 'R' binder. This is broken down by pancreatic juice to liberate B_{12}, which then binds with intrinsic factor. Intrinsic factor is a glyco-protein with a molecular weight of over 44 000 that is secreted from the gastric parietal cell with H^+ ions. It combines with vitamin B_{12} and carries it to specific receptors on the surface of the mucosa of the ileum. B_{12} is then liberated and binds to these receptors, but intrinsic factor remains in the lumen. B_{12} is then transported from the enterocytes by the glycoprotein transcobalamin II (TC II) to the marrow. In serum, B_{12} is mainly bound to TC I (70–90%) and some to TC III (< 10%) but neither protein plays a role in delivering B_{12} to the marrow. TC I and TC III are derived from granulocytes and thus a rise in serum B_{12} is seen in myeloproliferative disorders.

Pernicious anaemia

There are a number of causes of B_{12} deficiency (Table 6.5). The commonest in adults is pernicious anaemia (PA).

Pernicious anaemia is a condition in which there is atrophy of the gastric mucosa with consequent failure of intrinsic factor production and vitamin B_{12} malabsorption.

PATHOGENESIS

This is a disease of the elderly, with 1 in 8000 of the population over 60 years being affected in the United Kingdom. It can be seen in all races, but is particularly common in Nordic, fair-haired and blue-eyed people. There is an association with other autoimmune diseases, particularly thyroid disease, Addison's disease and vitiligo. Approximately one-half of all patients with PA have thyroid antibodies. There is a higher incidence of gastric carcinoma in males with PA than in the general population; females have a normal life expectancy with replacement therapy.

Parietal cell antibodies are present in virtually all patients with PA—and in many older patients with

gastric atrophy (p. 187). Conversely, intrinsic factor antibodies, although found in only 50% of patients with PA, are specific for this diagnosis. Two types of intrinsic factor antibodies are found but their role is uncertain:

- Type 1 or blocking antibody, which inhibits binding of intrinsic factor to B_{12}
- Type 2 or precipitating antibody, which inhibits the binding of the B_{12}-intrinsic factor complex to its receptor site in the ileum

B_{12} deficiency may rarely occur in children due to abnormal or absent intrinsic factor.

PATHOLOGY

Gastric atrophy (see p. 187) is present, with plasma cell and lymphoid infiltration. The histological abnormality can be improved by corticosteroid therapy, which supports an autoimmune basis for the disease.

CLINICAL FEATURES

The clinical features are those of anaemia, weight loss and neurological syndromes. The onset of PA is insidious and patients frequently have a very low haemoglobin before symptoms develop. The neurological changes are of greatest importance; if left untreated, the changes can be irreversible. The neurological abnormalities only occur with very low levels of serum B_{12} (less than 60 ng·L^{-1}) and occasionally occur in patients who are not clinically anaemic.

Table 6.5 Causes of vitamin B_{12} deficiency.

Low dietary intake
Vegans

Impaired absorption
Stomach
    Pernicious anaemia
    Gastrectomy

Small bowel
    Ileal disease or resection
    Bacterial overgrowth
    Tropical sprue
    Coeliac disease

Pancreas
    Chronic pancreatic disease
    Zollinger–Ellison syndrome

Miscellaneous and rare
Fish tapeworm (*Diphyllobothrium latum*)
Congenital deficiency
    Intrinsic factor
    Transcobalamin II
Nitrous oxide (inactivates B_{12})

The classical neurological features are those of polyneuropathy progressively involving the posterior and lateral columns of the spinal cord (subacute combined degeneration). Patients present with symmetrical paraesthesia in the fingers and toes, early loss of vibration sense and proprioception, and progressive weakness and ataxia. Paraplegia may result. Dementia and optic atrophy also occur.

Examination reveals an anaemic patient. Occasionally the skin has a lemon-yellow tint due to the combination of anaemia and hyperbilirubinaemia. There may be signs of bleeding and heart failure, and hepatosplenomegaly is occasionally found. The patient often has a low-grade fever; the reason for this is unknown.

A red sore tongue (glossitis) and angular stomatitis are sometimes present. Purpura may be seen if there is severe thrombocytopenia. Neurological examination may reveal the signs of a polyneuropathy and, less often, the signs of subacute combined degeneration of the cord (see p. 956).

INVESTIGATION

- The peripheral blood film shows the features of a megaloblastic anaemia as described on p. 303.
- The serum vitamin B_{12} is below the normal level of 160 ng·L^{-1}.
- The serum bilirubin is often raised as a result of haemolysis.
- The bone marrow shows the typical features of megaloblastic erythropoiesis (Fig. 6.7c).

Serum vitamin B_{12} can be assayed using microbiological or radioisotope dilution techniques. Concurrent estimation of the serum folate and serum iron will show normal or high levels and the red-cell folate is sometimes reduced. A rapid fall in either the serum iron or folate following the administration of vitamin B_{12} is an early indication of successful B_{12} therapy. Treatment is monitored using the reticulocyte count and haemoglobin levels. The serum potassium and iron can fall with the massive reticulocytosis seen with B_{12} therapy.

In an elderly patient with clinical features of pernicious anaemia, a macrocytic blood film and a low vitamin B_{12} level are sufficient evidence to make the diagnosis and to start treatment. In the younger patient, full investigations are required.

Absorption tests
The absorption of B_{12} can be measured using the Schilling test. This test is satisfactory if a complete 24-hour collection of urine is completed, but this may not be the case, particularly in the elderly. It may also give an inaccurate result when renal function is poor. An alternative to the Schilling test is whole-body counting. A radioactive dose of B_{12} is given orally and the total body activity is

---

Schilling test

Part I

- Give 1 μg ^{58}Co–B_{12} orally to fasting patient.
- Give 1000 μg B_{12} (non-radioactive) by intramuscular injection to saturate B_{12}-binding proteins and to flush out ^{58}Co–B_{12}.
- Collect urine for 24 h.
- Normal subjects excrete more than 10% of the radioactive dose.

If abnormal:

Part II

- Repeat part I after giving oral intrinsic factor capsules.

Result

- If excretion still abnormal, lesion is in the terminal ileum or there is bacterial overgrowth.
- If excretion now normal, diagnosis is pernicious anaemia.

---

measured. The level of radioactivity is counted no less than 7 days later to measure how much vitamin B_{12} has been retained. A normal result is retention of 50% or more of the 1 μg dose of radioactive B_{12}.

Gastrointestinal investigations
In PA there is marked gastric atrophy with achlorhydria and intubation studies can be performed to confirm this. Endoscopy or barium-meal examination of the stomach are performed only if gastric symptoms are present.

DIFFERENTIAL DIAGNOSIS

Vitamin B_{12} deficiency must be differentiated from other causes of megaloblastic anaemia, principally folate deficiency, but usually this is quite clear from the blood level of these two vitamins. PA must also be distinguished from other causes of vitamin B_{12} deficiency, which are briefly indicated below:

- *Vegans.* These are patients who are strict vegetarians and eat no meat or animal products. A careful dietary history should be obtained.
- *Gastrointestinal disease.* Any disease involving the terminal ileum or bacterial overgrowth in the small bowel can produce vitamin B_{12} deficiency (see p. 199).
- Rarely patients can develop IF deficiency after a gastrectomy.

FOLIC ACID

Folic acid was first found in spinach leaves and is widely distributed in plants. It is formed from

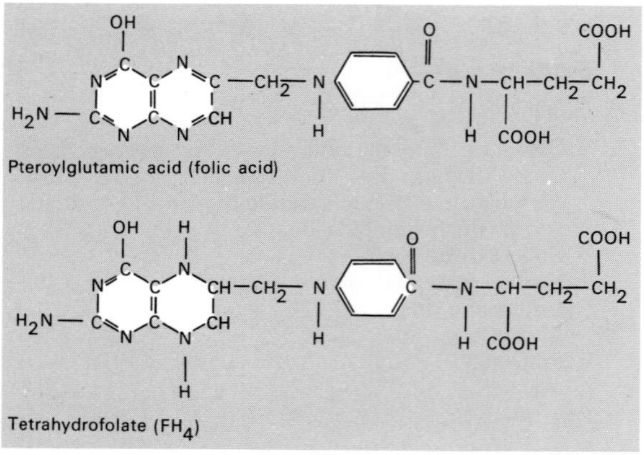

Fig. 6.11 The structure of folic acid and tetrahydrofolate.

three building blocks: a pteridine (similar to xanthopterin), *p*-aminobenzoic acid and glutamic acid (Fig. 6.11). Folates with additional glutamate radicals (polyglutamates) are the form of folate present in most foods. Polyglutamates are broken down to monoglutamates in the upper gastrointestinal tract and during the absorptive process these are then converted to methyltetrahydrofolate.

The biochemistry of tetrahydrofolate is very important because it serves as an intermediate carrier of hydroxymethyl ($-CH_2OH$), formyl ($-CHO$) and methyl ($-CH_3$) groups, which take part in a large number of enzyme reactions. The mechanisms of action of antimetabolite and immunosuppressive drugs depend on the inhibition of these reactions.

Dietary intake

The body obtains its folate from green vegetables such as spinach or broccoli, and offal, such as liver or kidney. Folate is destroyed by cooking. The daily requirement is about 100 µg.

Folate deficiency

The causes of folate deficiency are shown in Table 6.6. The main cause is poor intake. Folate stores are not usually reduced by excessive utilization or malabsorption, but both these mechanisms can precipitate folate deficiency in a patient with an inadequate diet. Unlike vitamin B_{12} reserves, body reserves of folate are low; on a deficient diet, folate deficiency rapidly develops over the course of about 4 months.

Approximately one-fifth of the cases of megaloblastic anaemia occurring in Great Britain are due to folic acid defciency associated with factors such as old age, poverty, alcoholic abuse or regular medication with antiepileptic drugs, such as phenytoin (Table 6.6). The use of parenteral feeding without folic acid supplementation may lead to the development of severe folate deficiency.

Table 6.6 Causes of folate deficiency.

Nutritional (major cause)
Poor intake:
  Old age
  Poor social conditions
  Starvation
  Alcohol excess (also causes impaired utilization)

Poor intake due to anorexia:
  Gastrointestinal disease, e.g.
    partial gastrectomy
    coeliac disease
    Crohn's disease
  Cancer

Excess utilization
Physiological:
  Pregnancy
  Lactation
  Prematurity

Pathological:
  Haematological disease with excess red cell
    production, e.g. haemolysis
  Malignant disease with increased cell turnover
  Inflammatory disease
  Metabolic disease, e.g. homocystinuria
  Haemodialysis or peritoneal dialysis

Malabsorption
Occurs in small bowel disease, but the effect is minor compared with that of anorexia

Antifolate drugs
Anticonvulsants
  Phenytoin
  Primidone
Methotrexate
Pyrimethamine
Trimethoprim

CLINICAL FEATURES

Patients with folate deficiency may be asymptomatic. Symptoms, if present, are those of anaemia. Polyneuropathy is seen rarely.

INVESTIGATION

The blood count shows a raised MCV with or without accompanying anaemia.

The bone marrow shows characteristic megaloblastic erythropoiesis.

Blood measurements

Serum folate can be assayed microbiologically using the *Lactobacillus casei* method. Contamination of specimens with other bacteria or with antibiotics leads to false results. Normal levels of serum folate are 4–18 $\mu g \cdot L^{-1}$. The amount of folate in the red cells is a better measure of tissue folate; the normal range is 160–640 $\mu g \cdot ml^{-1}$.

Deoxyuridine suppression test
Folate and vitamin B_{12} are needed in order to be able to use deoxyuridine to produce DNA. A single carbon unit is added to deoxyuridine monophosphate to form deoxythymidine monophosphate, which is then used to build DNA (see Fig. 6.10). If necessary, preformed thymidine can be used to form DNA via the so-called salvage pathway.

The uptake of tritiated thymidine added to marrow *in vitro* can give an indication of the severity and type of deficiency. In a normoblastic marrow, the thymidine requirement is supplied by the methylation of deoxyuridine and this 'suppresses' the requirement for preformed tritiated thymidine to less than 5%. In a megaloblastic marrow, however, much more tritiated thymidine is used (5–50%). If the addition of B_{12} corrects the abnormality, it suggests that B_{12} is the cause of the deficiency. The addition of folate corrects the abnormality in both vitamin B_{12} and folate deficiency. This is a useful method for rapidly determining the nature and severity of the vitamin deficiency that is causing megaloblastosis.

Further investigations
In many cases of folate deficiency the cause is not obvious from the clinical picture or dietary history. Occult gastrointestinal disease should then be suspected and appropriate investigations, such as jejunal biopsy, should be performed (p. 204).

TREATMENT AND PREVENTION OF MEGALOBLASTIC ANAEMIA

Treatment depends on the type of deficiency. Blood transfusion is not indicated in chronic anaemia; indeed, it is dangerous to transfuse elderly patients, as heart failure may be precipitated.

Vitamin B_{12} deficiency
This is treated with hydroxycobalamin 1000 μg intramuscularly to a total of 5000–6000 μg over the course of 3 weeks; 1000 μg is then necessary every 3 months for the rest of the patient's life. Clinical improvement may occur within 48 h and a reticulocytosis can be seen some 5–7 days after starting therapy. Neurological improvement may take 6–12 months, but long-standing lesions may be irreversible.

In patients who have had a total gastrectomy or an ileal resection, vitamin B_{12} should be monitored, and if low levels occur, prophylactic vitamin B_{12} injections should be given.

Folate deficiency
This is corrected by giving 5 mg of folic acid daily; the same haematological response occurs as seen after treatment of vitamin B_{12} deficiency.

Prophylactic folate is justifiable in pregnancy, and in chronic haematological disorders where there is rapid cell turnover.

MACROCYTOSIS WITHOUT MEGALOBLASTIC CHANGES

A raised MCV with macrocytosis on the peripheral blood film can occur with a normoblastic rather than a megaloblastic bone marrow. Common causes of macrocytosis include:

Physiological
- Pregnancy
- Newborn

Pathological
- Alcohol excess
- Liver disease
- Reticulocytosis
- Hypothyroidism
- Some haematological disorders, e.g. aplastic anaemia, sideroblastic anaemia

Macrocytosis occurs in chronic liver disease and with alcohol due to interference with red-cell membrane formation. Alcohol is a frequent cause of a raised MCV in an otherwise normal individual. An increased number of reticulocytes leads to a raised MCV because they are large cells.

In all these conditions, normal levels of vitamin B_{12} and red-cell folate will be found.

Stomatocytes are red cells in which the central area appears slit-like. Their appearances in large numbers may occur in a hereditary haemolytic anaemia associated with a membrane defect but excess alcohol intake is a common cause.

Anaemia due to marrow failure (aplastic anaemia)

Aplastic anaemia is defined as peripheral blood pancytopenia with aplasia of the bone marrow. It is an uncommon but serious condition that may be inherited but is more commonly acquired.

MECHANISMS

Aplastic anaemia is due to a reduction in the number of stem cells (see Fig. 6.1) together with a

Table 6.7 Causes of aplastic anaemia.

Congenital
Fanconi's anaemia

Acquired
Chemicals, e.g. benzene
Drugs—see Table 6.8
Insecticides
Ionizing radiation
Infections, e.g. viral hepatitis, measles
Miscellaneous infections, e.g. tuberculosis
Thymoma
Pregnancy
Unknown (50% of cases)

fault in differentiation. Suppression of stem cells by subsets of the lymphocyte series, in particular T suppressor cells, has been implicated in some aplastic anaemias.

Failure of a 'committed' cell can lead to decreased cell production or cell renewal, resulting in such isolated deficiencies as the absence of red-cell precursors (pure red-cell aplasia).

CAUSES

A list of causes of aplasia is given in Table 6.7. There is good circumstantial evidence to incriminate a number of drugs in the development of aplastic anaemia; these probably account for the gradual increase in the incidence of this condition in recent times. Table 6.8 shows some of the responsible drugs but the list is ever-increasing.

With aplastic anaemia associated with pregnancy and viral hepatitis, the prognosis is grave, with a mortality rate of 90% in the former and 60% in the latter. In patients with tuberculosis, successful treatment of the infection leads to haematological recovery. In thymoma, removal of the tumour may be effective in restoring the blood count to normal. Congenital aplastic anaemias are rare. Fanconi's anaemia is inherited as an autosomal recessive and is associated with skeletal, renal and central nervous system abnormalities.

CLINICAL FEATURES

The clinical manifestations of marrow failure are anaemia, bleeding and infection. Physical findings include ecchymoses, bleeding gums and epistaxis. Mouth infections are common, particularly fungal infections. Lymphadenopathy, splenomegaly and hepatomegaly are rare in aplastic anaemia.

INVESTIGATION

The laboratory diagnosis is made on the basis of:

- Pancytopenia
- The virtual absence of reticulocytes
- A hypocellular or aplastic bone marrow with increased fat spaces

DIFFERENTIAL DIAGNOSIS

This is from other causes of pancytopenia (Table 6.9).

TREATMENT AND PROGNOSIS

The course of aplastic anaemia can be variable, ranging from a rapid spontaneous remission to a persistent increasingly severe deficiency of all formed elements in the blood, which may lead to

Table 6.8 Some drugs associated with marrow aplasia.

Anticancer drugs (always cause aplasia if dose high enough)
Mercaptopurine
Busulphan
Cyclophosphamide
Doxorubicin
Methotrexate

Anti-inflammatory and anti-rheumatic drugs
Phenylbutazone ⎫ Withdrawn in the UK
Oxyphenbutazone ⎭
Gold compounds
Indomethacin

Anti-epileptic drugs
Phenytoin
Troxidone
Primidone

Antidiabetic drugs
Tolbutamide
Chlorpropamide

Antithyroid drugs
Carbimazole
Methylthiouracil
Propylthiouracil
Potassium perchlorate

Psychotropics
Chlorpromazine
Prochlorperazine
Promazine
Mianserin

Antihistamines
Chlorpheniramine

Antibiotics
Chloramphenicol
Sulphonamides

Table 6.9 Causes of pancytopenia.

Aplastic anaemia (Table 6.7)

Megaloblastic anaemia

Bone marrow infiltration or replacement
  Hodgkin's and non-Hodgkin's lymphoma
  Acute leukaemia
  Myeloma
  Secondary carcinoma
  Myelofibrosis

Hypersplenism

Systemic lupus erythematosus

Disseminated tuberculosis

Paroxysmal nocturnal haemoglobinuria

Overwhelming sepsis

death through haemorrhage or infection. The most reliable determinants for the prognosis are the number of neutrophils, reticulocytes, platelets, and non-myeloid cells present.

Bad prognostic features

- A neutrophil count $< 0.5 \times 10^9/L$
- A platelet count of $< 20 \times 10^9/L$
- A reticulocyte count of $< 10 \times 10^9/L$ (0.1%)
- Non-myeloid cells comprising $> 80\%$ of the cells in the bone marrow

The cause of aplastic anaemia must be eliminated if possible. Supportive care (transfusion of red cells and platelets as well as antibiotics) should be given as necessary.

In mild to moderate cases, androgens or steroids are tried. In severe aplastic anaemia (with three of the four bad prognostic features) there is less than 50% chance of survival beyond 6 months. Bone marrow transplantation (see p. 362) is the treatment of choice for patients under 20 years of age who have an HLA-matched sibling donor; a successful graft occurs in 70% of patients. Older patients are initially treated with antilymphocyte globulin (ALG) with consideration of transplantation for patients failing to respond. ALG produces a haematological recovery in 50–60% of cases, and androgens are used in addition to ALG in some cases, although their effectiveness is uncertain. ALG causes serum sickness in 75% of patients.

Steroids are used to treat children with congenital pure red-cell aplasia (Diamond–Blackfan syndrome) and are occasionally useful in adults. Adult pure red-cell aplasia is associated with a thymoma (30%) and thymectomy may induce a remission. Recently, injections of recombinant colony-stimulating factors (see Fig. 6.1) have been given with promising results.

Haemolytic anaemia

The normal red cell is a remarkably pliable, biconcave disc that is capable of changing shape as it circulates in the bloodstream. The red cell normally survives about 120 days, but in haemolysis the cell survival times are considerably shortened (Fig. 6.12).

Mechanisms of haemolysis

Abnormalities of the red-cell membrane

The red-cell membrane is constantly being renewed and changed in its lipid composition. In addition, red cells can alter their shape by gaining surface or volume, or by losing surface or volume. The conditions and types of cells produced by such changes are shown diagrammatically in Fig. 6.13. For example, in liver disease there is reduction in the volume relative to the surface area, and target cells result. In hereditary spherocytosis the red cell loses membrane, so that the ratio of surface area to volume decreases and the cells become spherocytes. Such cells cannot pass through the reticuloendothelial system of the spleen with ease, and are therefore sequestrated there. If red cells become coated with antibodies they are also sequestrated in the spleen owing to interaction with Fc receptors on macrophages.

Abnormal haemoglobin

Red cells with abnormal haemoglobins, for example in sickle cell disease or thalassaemia, are all much less deformable than normal cells, and are consequently sequestrated in the spleen. In glucose-6-phosphate dehydrogenase deficiency, the red cells are unable to prevent the oxidation of haemoglobin and the red-cell membrane by certain drugs; again the red cell is less deformable.

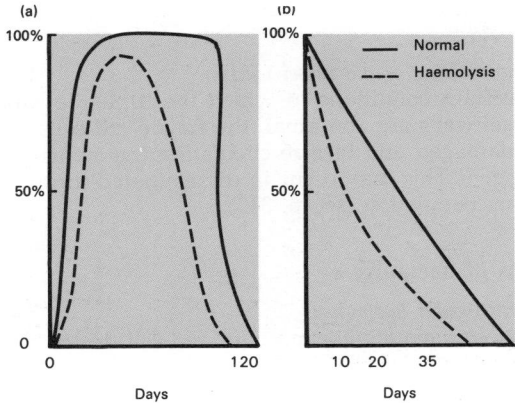

Fig. 6.12 Patterns of survival of normal red cells and cells affected by haemolysis. (a) Cohort of red cells labelled with [^{14}C]glycine. (b) Red cells of mixed ages labelled with ^{51}Cr.

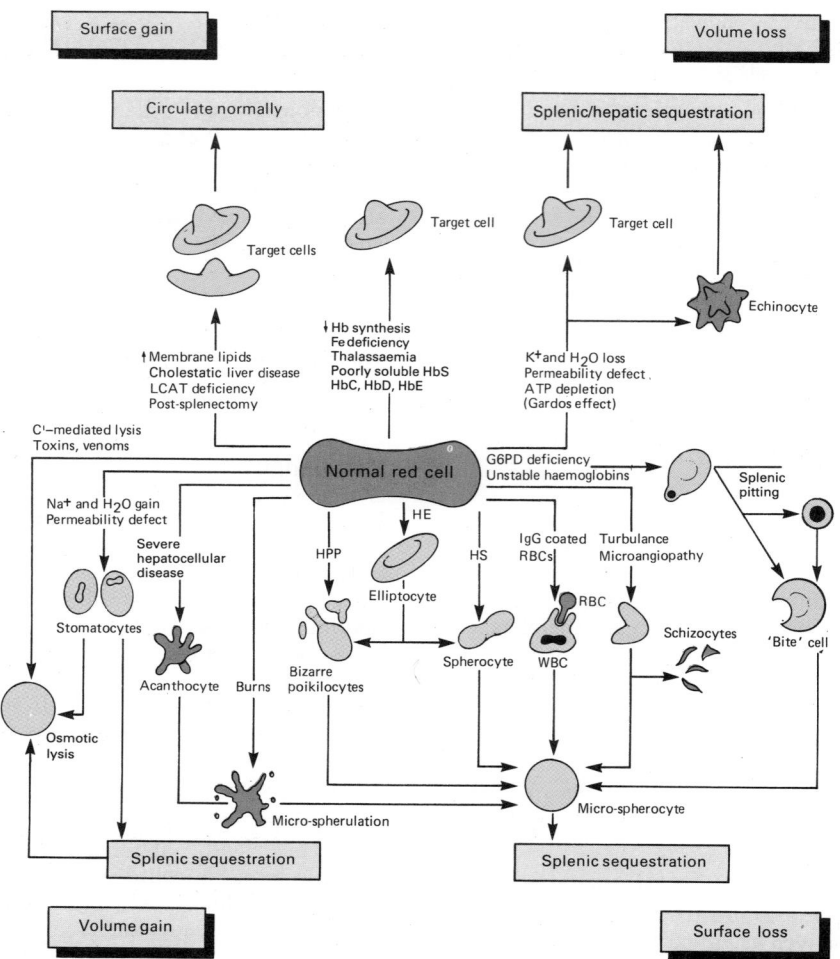

Fig. 6.13 Abnormalities of red cell surface area, volume and shape. HE = hereditary elliptocytosis; HS = hereditary spherocytosis; HPP = hereditary pyropoikilocytosis; LCAT = lecithin cholesterol acyltransferase. (From Beck WS (ed) (1984) *Hematology*, 3rd edn. Massachusetts: MIT Press. With permission.)

Abnormalities of the vessel wall

In certain conditions in which the capillaries and vessel walls are abnormal, the fragile red cells can be damaged and bizarre circulating fragments can be seen. This may occur in disseminated intravascular coagulation (see p. 343).

Sites of haemolysis

Extravascular haemolysis

In most haemolytic conditions red-cell destruction is extravascular. Here, the red cells are removed from the circulation by macrophages in the reticuloendothelial system, particularly the spleen. The haemolysis is variable in severity. When it occurs chronically it may lead to hypertrophy of the spleen, which may become palpable.

Intravascular haemolysis

When red cells are rapidly destroyed within the circulation, haemoglobin is liberated. This is removed by circulating haptoglobin and also haemopexin until these are used up. Any remaining haemoglobin circulates partly as free haemoglobin and as methaemoglobin attached to albumin, forming methaemalbumin. On spectrophotometry of the plasma, methaemalbumin forms a characteristic band; this is the basis of Schumm's test.

Some free haemoglobin is lost in the urine, although small amounts are reabsorbed by the renal tubules. In the renal tubular cell, haemoglobin is broken down and the iron combines with a storage protein to form haemosiderin. This is of low molecular weight and can be excreted in the urine, where it can be detected in the spun sediment using Perls' reaction.

Erythrocytes contain high concentration of lactic dehydrogenase (LDH) and this enzyme is raised in the serum in intravascular haemolysis.

Consequences of haemolysis

The shortening of red-cell survival can lead to anaemia. However, compensatory mechanisms result in an increase in red cell production. If the red cell loss can be contained within the marrow's capacity for increased output (which is usually eight times normal or more), then a haemolytic state can exist without the presence of anaemia. In chronic conditions the area and volume of bone marrow can gradually be increased. In both acute and chronic haemolysis, red cells are released prematurely and therefore contain remnants of RNA (reticulocytes).

Evidence for haemolysis

Increased red cell breakdown leads to:

- Elevated serum bilirubin
- Excess urinary urobilinogen (resulting from bilirubin breakdown in the intestine)
- Abnormalities of the blood film such as spherocytes or red cell precursors
- Reduced plasma haptoglobin

Increased red cell production leads to:

- Reticulocytosis
- Erythroid hyperplasia of the bone marrow

Raised levels of plasma haemoglobin, haemosiderinuria, very low or absent haptoglobin and the presence of methaemalbumin will suggest an *intravascular* site for haemolysis.

Red cell survival studies using ^{51}Cr-labelled red cells are useful in complicated cases and also for quantitation of the severity of haemolysis. The dominant site of red-cell destruction can be shown with external body counting.

Various laboratory studies will be carried out to determine the type of haemolytic anaemia. The causes of haemolytic anaemias are shown in Table 6.10.

Inherited haemolytic anaemias

RED-CELL MEMBRANE DEFECTS (Fig. 6.14)

Hereditary spherocytosis (HS)

Hereditary spherocytosis is a disease in which the cell membrane has a defect in the structural protein

Table 6.10 Causes of haemolytic anaemia.

INHERITED

Red cell membrane defect
Hereditary spherocytosis
Hereditary elliptocytosis

Haemoglobin abnormalities
Thalassaemia
Sickle cell disease

Metabolic defects
Glucose-6-phosphate dehydrogenase deficiency
Pyruvate kinase deficiency

ACQUIRED

Immune
Autoimmune:
    warm
    cold
    drugs
Isoimmune:
    Rh or ABO incompatibility

Non-immune
Membrane defects:
    Paroxysmal nocturnal haemoglobinuria
    Liver disease
    Renal disease
Mechanical:
    Microangiopathic haemolytic anaemia (MAHA)
    Valve prosthesis
    March haemoglobinuria

Miscellaneous
Infections
Drugs and chemicals
Hypersplenism

spectrin, resulting in the cell losing membrane as it passes through the spleen. The surface-to-volume ratio is decreased, and the cells become spherocytic. The red cell membrane is more permeable to sodium ions and the intracellular concentration of potassium ions is low, but these abnormalities are not of primary pathological importance. HS is a relatively common haemolytic anaemia, affecting 1 in 5000 Caucasians. It is inherited in an autosomal dominant manner but in 25% of patients neither parent is affected. This is explained by incomplete penetrance, spontaneous mutation or possibly some form of additional recessive inheritance.

CLINICAL FEATURES

The condition may present with jaundice at birth. However, the onset of jaundice can sometimes be delayed for many years and some patients may go

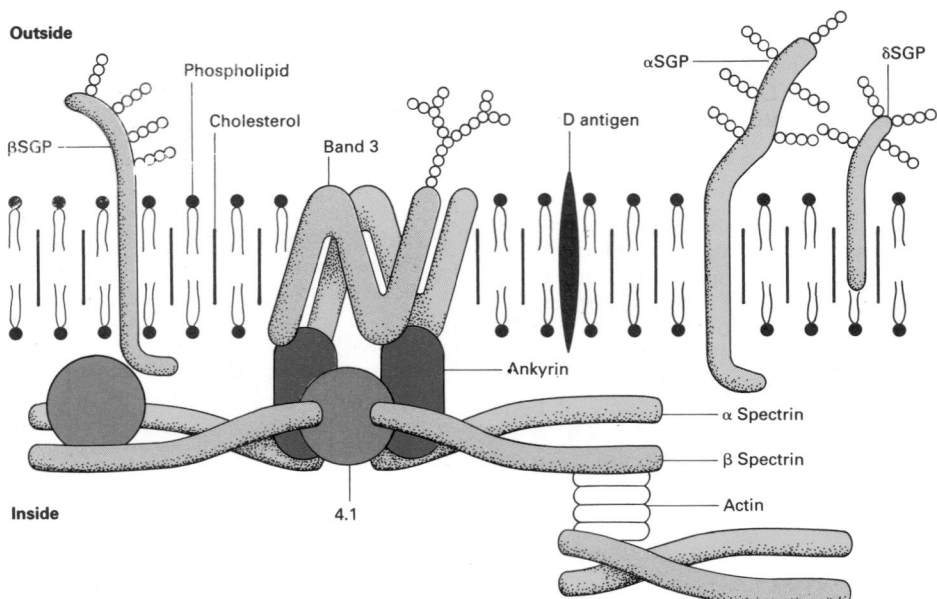

Fig. 6.14 Red cell membrane. Integral membrane proteins, band 3, sialoglycoproteins (α, β, γ SGPs) are within the lipid bi-layer. The structural proteins, septrin and actin, interact with protein 4.1 and this complex is attached to the overlying lipid layer by ankyrin. From *Postgraduate Haematology* (eds Hoffbrand and Lewis), Oxford: Heinemann, with permission.

through life asymptomatic and are only detected during family studies. The patient may eventually develop anaemia, splenomegaly and ulcers on the leg. As in many haemolytic anaemias, the course of the disease may be interrupted by aplastic and megaloblastic crises. Aplastic anaemia usually occurs after infections, particularly with parvovirus, whereas megaloblastic anaemia is the result of folate depletion due to the hyperactivity of the bone marrow. Chronic haemolysis leads to the formation of pigment gallstones (see p. 282).

INVESTIGATION

- Anaemia is usually mild, but occasionally can be severe.
- The blood film shows spherocytes and reticulocytes.
- There is evidence of haemolysis, e.g. the serum bilirubin and urinary urobilinogen will be raised.
- Osmotic fragility: when red cells are placed in solutions of increasing hypotonicity, they take in water, swell, and eventually lyse. Spherocytes tolerate hypotonic solutions less well than normal biconcave red cells. This increased osmotic fragility can also be demonstrated when the cells are incubated in their own plasma for 48 h (autohaemolysis) and this can be corrected by the addition of glucose which indicates that glucose metabolism is normal and that there is a red cell membrane defect. The direct antiglobulin (Coombs') test is negative in spherocytosis, virtually ruling out autoimmune haemolytic anaemia where spherocytes are also seen.

TREATMENT

The spleen, which is the site of cell destruction, is removed in all but the mildest cases. The decision about splenectomy in symptomless patients is difficult, but a raised bilirubin and especially the presence of gallstones should encourage splenectomy. In childhood it is best to avoid splenectomy, as sudden overwhelming fatal infections, usually due to encapsulated organisms such as pneumococci, may occur (see p. 328).

Following splenectomy, the spherocytosis is reduced and the haemoglobin usually returns to normal as the red cells are no longer destroyed. Folate deficiency often occurs in chronic haemolysis with rapid cell turnover. Folate levels should be monitored, or folic acid can be given prophylactically.

Hereditary elliptocytosis

This disorder of the red-cell membrane is inherited in an autosomal dominant manner. The red cells are elliptical. It is similar to HS but milder. Only a minority of patients have anaemia and only occasional patients require splenectomy.

HAEMOGLOBIN ABNORMALITIES

Normal haemoglobin

Normal adult haemoglobin is made up of two polypeptide globin chains, the α and β chains, which have 141 and 146 amino acids, respectively. These are folded so that haem molecules can be held within the fold and are yet able to combine

Table 6.11 Types of haemoglobin.

	Haemoglobin	Structure	Comment
Normal	A	$\alpha_2\beta_2$	Comprises 92% of adult haemoglobin
	A_{1c}	$\alpha_2\beta_2$ (β-NH glucose)	Comprises 5% of adult haemoglobin. This glycosylated haemoglobin is increased in patients with uncontrolled diabetes
	A_2	$\alpha_2\delta_2$	Comprises 2% of adult haemoglobin. Elevated in β-thalassaemia
	F	$\alpha_2\gamma_2$	Normal haemoglobin in fetus from 3rd to 9th month. Increased in β-thalassaemia
Abnormal chain production	H	β_4	Found in α-thalassaemia. Biologically useless
	Barts	γ_4	Comprises 100% of haemoglobin in homozygous α-thalassaemia. Biologically useless
Abnormal chain structure	S	$\alpha_2\beta_2$	Substitution of valine for glutamic acid in position 6 of β chain
	C	$\alpha_2\beta_2$	Substitution of lysine for glutamic acid in position 6 of β chain

reversibly with oxygen. Adult haemoglobin has two α chains and two β chains. In early embryonic life, haemoglobins Gower 1, Gower 2 and Portland are produced. Later, fetal haemoglobin (HbF), which has two α and two γ chains, is produced (Table 6.11). There is increasing synthesis of β chains from 13 weeks' gestation and at term there is 80% fetal haemoglobin and 20% adult haemoglobin. After birth, the genes for γ chain production are further suppressed and there is rapid increase in the synthesis of β chains; there is little HbF produced (normally less than 1%) from 6 months after birth. The δ chain is synthesized just before birth and HbA2 ($\alpha_2\delta_2$) remains at a level of about 2%.

Globin chains are synthesized in the same way as any protein (see Chapter 2). Four globin chain genes are required to control α chain production (see Fig. 6.15). Two are present on each haploid genome (genes derived from one parent). These are situated close together on chromosome 16. The genes controlling the production of ε, γ, δ and β chains are close together on chromosome 11.

Normally there is balanced (1 : 1) production of α and β chains. The defective synthesis of globin genes in thalassaemia leads to 'imbalanced' globin chain production, leading to the precipitation of these chains within the red cell precursors, resulting in ineffective erythropoiesis. Precipitation of abnormal haemoglobin in the mature red cells leads to reduced red-cell survival.

Abnormal haemoglobins
Abnormalities occur in:

- Globin chain production, e.g. thalassaemia
- Structure of the globin chain, e.g. sickle cell disease

These inherited defects can occur together.

THALASSAEMIA

The thalassaemias (Greek *thalassa* = sea) are anaemias originally found in people living on the shores of the Mediterranean but now known to affect people throughout the world (Fig. 6.16).

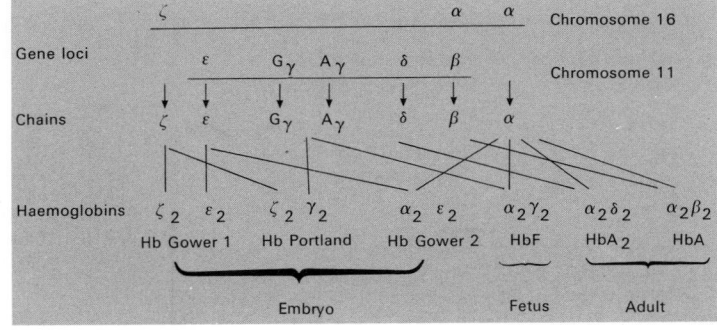

Fig. 6.15 Genetic control of human haemoglobin. (From Weatherall DJ & Bunch C (1985) The blood and blood-forming organs. In Smith LH & Thier SO (eds) *Pathophysiology: The Biological principles of Disease*, pp. 173–320. Philadelphia: WB Saunders. With permission.)

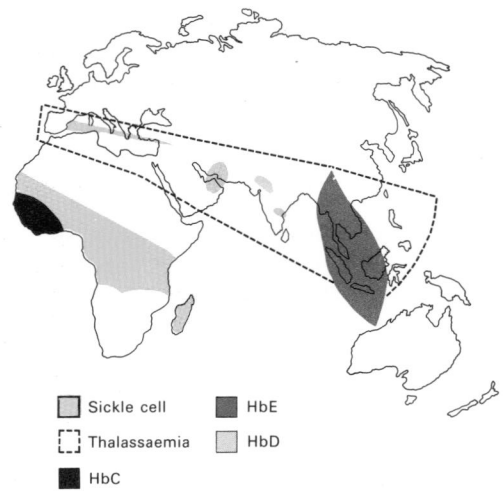

Fig. 6.16 Geographical distribution of the major haemoglobin abnormalities.

β-Thalassaemia

Three per cent of the world's population, or 150 million people, carry the β-thalassaemia gene.

MOLECULAR GENETICS (see Chapter 2)

Over the last few years the molecular defects accounting for 99% of β-thalassaemia genes have been characterized by genetic analysis. Over 50 point mutations and some deletions have been determined. The mutations, mainly single-nucleotide substitutions, produce defects in transcription, RNA splicing and modification, translation via frame shifts and nonsense codons or highly unstable β-globin which cannot be utilized.

In β-thalassaemia either no normal β chains are produced (β^0) or β-chain production is impaired (β^+). Since α-chain production is normal, α chains will combine with any β chains available, leaving the excess α chains to combine with whatever δ or γ chains are produced, resulting in increased quantities of HbA_2 and HbF (Table 6.11). Table 6.12 shows the findings in the homozygote and heterozygote for the common types of β-thalassaemia.

CLINICAL SYNDROMES

The severity of the thalassaemia depends on the amount of HbA_2 and HbF present. Clinically, β-thalassaemia can be divided into the following:

- Thalassaemia major with severe anaemia requiring regular transfusions
- Thalassaemia intermedia, with moderate anaemia, rarely requiring transfusions
- Thalassaemia minor, the symptomless heterozygous carrier state

β-Thalassaemia trait (heterozygous thalassaemia minor)
This common carrier state is asymptomatic. Anaemia is mild or absent. The red cells are hypochromic and microcytic with a low MCV and MCH. It may, therefore, be confused with iron deficiency. However, it can easily be distinguished by the fact that the serum iron, the serum ferritin and the iron stores are normal. Iron must not be given to these patients. Haemoglobin electrophoresis usually shows a raised HbA_2 and often a raised HbF (Fig. 6.17).

β-Thalassaemia intermedia
In thalassaemia intermedia the symptoms vary from virtually none to severe anaemia with spleno-

Table 6.12 Findings in β, δβ and γδβ thalassaemias.

Type of thalassaemia	Findings in homozygote	Findings in heterozygote
β^+	Thalassaemia major Hb A + F + A_2	Thalassaemia minor Hb A_2 raised
β^0	Thalassaemia major Hb F + A_2	Thalassaemia minor Hb A_2 raised
δβ	Thalassaemia intermedia HbF only	Thalassaemia minor HbF 5–15% HbA_2 normal
δβ (Lepore)	Thalassaemia major or intermedia HbF and Lepore	Thalassaemia minor Hb Lepore 5–15% HbA_2 normal
γδβ	Not viable	Neonatal haemolysis Thalassaemia minor in adults with normal Hb F and A_2

From Weatherall DJ (1988) Disorders of the synthesis or function of haemoglobin. In Weatherall DJ, Ledingham JGG & Warrell DA (eds) *Oxford Textbook of Medicine* pp. 19.108–19.130. Oxford: Oxford University Press. With permission.

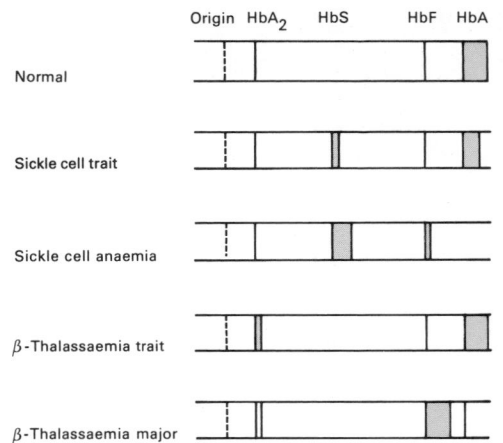

Fig. 6.17 Patterns of haemoglobin electrophoresis.

megaly and bone deformities—i.e. more severe than in β-thalassaemia heterozygotes but milder than in transfusion-dependent thalassaemia major. Thalassaemia intermedia may be due to homozygous mild β^+ and α-thalassaemia or hereditary persistence of HbF with homozygous β-thalassaemia. Recurrent leg ulcers, gallstones and infections are also seen.

β-Thalassaemia major
Children affected by severe β-thalassaemia (thalassaemia major) present during the first year of life with:

- Failure to thrive
- Intermittent infection
- Severe anaemia
- Extramedullary haemopoiesis that soon leads to hepatosplenomegaly and bone expansion, giving rise to the classical thalassaemic facies (Fig. 6.18).

Bone X-rays in these children show the 'hair on end' arrangement of bony trabeculation (Fig. 6.18).
  There is wide variation in the severity of these clinical features.

INVESTIGATION

The following are found:

- The blood count shows a moderate to severe anaemia with reduced MCV and MCH. The reticulocyte count is raised. The white-cell count and the number of platelets are normal unless hypersplenism is present.
- The blood film shows a hypochromic and predominantly microcytic picture. Postsplenectomy features may be present (Fig. 6.7f).
- The iron-binding capacity is saturated, with high serum ferritin levels (after multiple transfusions).

- Haemoglobin electrophoresis shows an increase in HbF, markedly reduced or absent HbA and HbA2 is normal or slightly increased (Fig. 6.17).

MANAGEMENT

The aim of the treatment is to suppress ineffective erythropoiesis, prevent bony deformities and allow normal activity and development. Children should be transfused regularly to keep the haemoglobin above 10 g·dl^{-1}. Febrile transfusion reactions can be prevented by the use of leucocyte-poor blood (p. 331). Blood transfusion may be required every 4–6 weeks. If transfusion requirements increase, splenectomy should be considered. Following splenectomy, prophylaxis against infection is required (see p. 328).
  Iron overload caused by repeated transfusions may lead to damage to the endocrine glands, liver, pancreas and the myocardium by the time patients reach adolescence. The iron-chelating agent of choice remains desferrioximine. This is given as an overnight subcutaneous infusion, the total dose being dependent on the age and size of the child. Iron overload should be periodically assessed by measuring the serum ferritin and assessing organ damage. It is important to monitor the condition of the lens, as reversible cataract may occur with desferrioxamine treatment. There are some promising reports of the use of oral iron-chelating agents. Ascorbic acid is also given, as it helps to increase iron chelation. With current therapy children usually survive to adult life. Bone marrow transplantation has been used but there is often severe graft-versus-host disease (GvHD) and this treatment should be limited to patients who, for some reason, cannot receive adequate symptomatic treatment.
  Gene therapy may become possible with the insertion of intact globin genes into the bone marrow of patients with severe disease.

δβ-Thalassaemias, Hb Lepore and hereditary persistence of fetal haemoglobin (HPFH) (see Table 6.12)
These variants are due to deletions of the δ- and β-globin genes and produce a milder form of thalassaemia than homozygous β^0 thalassaemia because the reduced β-chain production is partially compensated by increased γ-chain synthesis.

α-Thalassaemia

MOLECULAR GENETICS (see Chapter 2)

The abnormalities in α-thalassaemia are complex but, again, there are two main forms. In one there is a deletion of only one α-chain gene and therefore some α chains are produced (α^+). In the other there is deletion of both α-chain genes (α^0) and no α chains are produced (Table 6.13). In heterozygous α^0-thalassaemia, some α chains are pro-

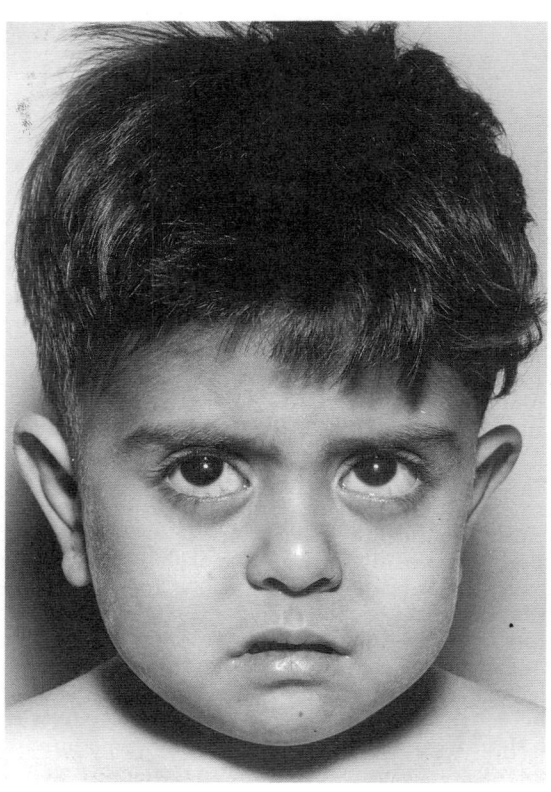

(a)

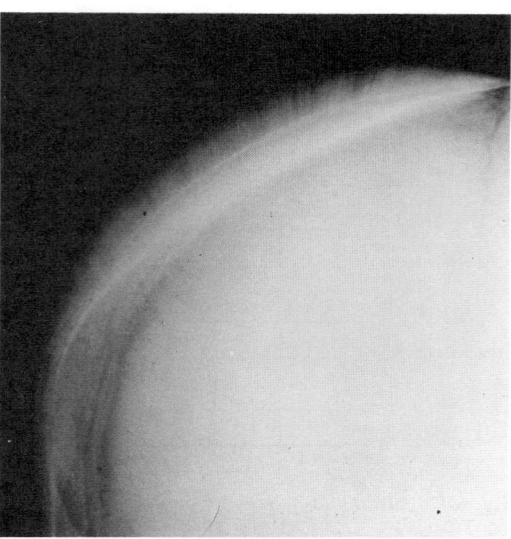

(b)

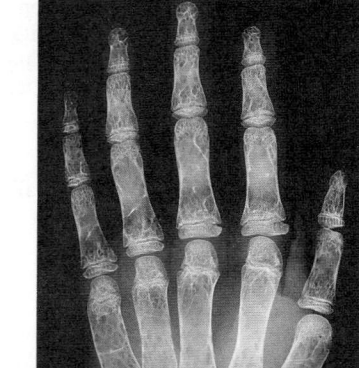

(c)

Fig. 6.18 (a) A child with thalassaemia, showing the typical features. (b) Skull X-ray of a child with β-thalassaemia, showing the 'hair on end' appearance. (c) X-ray of hand, showing expansion of the marrow and a thinned cortex.

duced, but in the homozygous state only haemoglobin Barts (γ_4) is present. Haemoglobin Barts cannot carry oxygen and is therefore incompatible with life (Tables 6.11 and 6.13).

Less commonly, an abnormal α chain with many extra amino acids is produced (haemoglobin Constant Spring) (Table 6.13). In some patients with a marked reduction in α chains (α^+), more β chains are produced. There is therefore some physiologically normal haemoglobin A but also some haemoglobin H(β_4) that is physiologically useless.

CLINICAL SYNDROMES

The above abnormalities give rise to:

Homozygous α^0-thalassaemia. This is incompatible with life—the haemoglobin is Hb Barts (80%) and Hb Portland (20%). Infants are either stillborn at 28–40 weeks or die very shortly after birth. They are pale, oedematous and have enormous livers and spleens—a condition called *hydrops fetalis*.

Haemoglobin H disease. HbH precipitates in red cells and is removed by the spleen. There is moderate

Table 6.13 The α-thalassaemias.

Type of thalassaemia	Findings in homozygote	Findings in heterozygote
α$^+$	Thalassaemia minor 5–10% HB Barts at birth. Normal HbA$_2$	Thalassaemia minor 1–2% Hb Barts
α^0	Hydrops 80% Hb Barts at birth. Fatal	Thalassaemia minor 5–10% Hb Barts at birth. Normal HbA$_2$
Hb Constant Spring	Thalassaemia minor 5–6% Hb Constant Spring. Moderate anaemia	≅ 1% Hb Constant Spring. No clinical abnormality

From Weatherall DJ (1988) Disorders of the synthesis or function of haemoglobin. In Weatherall DJ, Ledingham JGG & Warrell DA (eds) *Oxford Textbook of Medicine*, pp. 19.108–19.130. Oxford: Oxford University Press. With permission.

anaemia (Hb 7–10 g·dl^{-1}) and splenomegaly. The patients are not usually transfusion dependent.

OTHER THALASSAEMIA SYNDROMES

There are many other thalassaemic-like disorders in which the genetics are as yet unclear. These result in globin chain imbalance and varied clinical manifestations. Haemoglobin E thalassaemia (a β-chain variant that is inefficiently synthesized) is widespread throughout south-east Asia and clinically resembles a mild form of β-thalassaemia. Abnormalities of haemoglobin structure, e.g. Hb S, C can also occur with thalassaemia.

PRENATAL DIAGNOSIS OF THALASSAEMIA

Recognition of the heterozygous states and family counselling should provide a basis for reducing the incidence of thalassaemia major. For example, 25% of the offspring of two parents with thalassaemia trait will have severe thalassaemia. Screening programmes, using samples of fetal blood for the investigation of the rate of globin chain synthesis, can pick up homozygous fetuses and abortion can be offered. Alternatively, fetal DNA analysis of chorionic villus samples can be used; this technique can be used in the first trimester and thus second trimester abortions can be avoided.

SICKLE SYNDROMES

The most important structural abnormality of the haemoglobin chain is haemoglobin S. Sickle cell disease is caused by a single-base mutation of adenine to thymine that results in a substitution of valine for glutamine at the sixth codon of the β-globin chain. In the homozygous state (sickle cell anaemia) both genes are abnormal (HbSS), whereas in the heterozygous state (sickle cell trait HbAS) only one chromosome carries the gene. As the

synthesis of HbF is normal, the disease usually does not manifest itself until the HbF decreases to adult levels at about 6 months of age.

The disease occurs mainly in Africans (25% carry the gene) but is also found in India, the Middle East, the Caribbean and Southern United States (Fig. 6.16).

PATHOGENESIS

With deoxygenation, the HbS molecules polymerize, so that the intracellular contents become more viscous. The flexibility of the cells is decreased, so that they become rigid and sickle during their passage through the microcirculation. This process is initially reversible but, with repeated sickling, the cells eventually lose their membrane flexibility and remain in the sickle form. Sickling can produce:

- a shortened red-cell survival
- impaired passage of cells through the microcirculation leading to obstruction of small vessels and tissue infarction

Sickling is *precipitated* by infection, dehydration, cold, acidosis or hypoxia. In many cases the cause is unknown. HbS releases its oxygen to the tissues more easily than normal haemoglobin and patients therefore feel well except during crises or complications.

CLINICAL SYNDROMES

Sickle cell trait These individuals have no symptoms unless they are subjected to anoxia, e.g. poor anaesthesia and post-operative dehydration. Sickle cell trait protects against *Plasmodium falciparum* malaria (see p. 86). Typically there is 60% HbA and 40% HbS. The blood count and film are normal. The diagnosis is made by a positive sickle test or by haemoglobin electrophoresis (see Fig. 6.17).

Sickle cell anaemia

This is a homozygous state and more than 80% of haemoglobin is HbS. Symptoms vary from a mild asymptomatic disorder to a severe haemolytic anaemia and recurrent severe painful crises. The condition usually presents in childhood with anaemia and mild jaundice. The hand-and-foot syndrome is quite common in children and here there are painful swellings of the fingers and toes.

In the older patient, vaso-occlusive problems occur owing to sickling in the small vessels of any organ, mimicking many medical and surgical emergencies.

Typical sickle crises include:

- Bone pain (commonest)
- Chest—pleuritic pain
- Cerebral—hemiparesis, fits
- Kidney—papillary necrosis causing haematuria
- Spleen—painful infarcts
- Penis—priapism
- Liver—pain with abnormal biochemistry

Attacks of pain with low-grade fever last from a few hours to a few days. In a given patient the degree of anaemia is usually stable and during a crisis the haemoglobin does not fall unless there is one or more of the following:

- *Aplasia*: due to decreased erythropoiesis, often associated with infection.
- *Acute sequestration*: the liver and spleen become engorged with sickle cells.
- *Haemolysis*: due to drugs, acute infection or an associated G6PD deficiency.

Long-term problems

- Susceptibility to infections: particularly to Parvovirus and *Streptococcus pneumoniae*, which can give a fatal meningitis. Osteomyelitis can occur in necrotic bone, often due to *Salmonella*
- Chronic leg ulcers: due to ischaemia
- Gallstones: pigment stones from persistent haemolysis
- Aseptic necrosis: particularly of the femoral heads
- Blindness: due to retinal detachment and proliferative retinopathy
- Chronic renal disease

INVESTIGATION

- Blood count: haemoglobin may be 6–8 g·dl^{-1} with a high reticulocyte count (10–20%)
- Blood films can show post-splenectomy features (see p. 301 Fig. 6.7f)
- Sickling can be induced in the presence of sodium metabisulphite
- Haemoglobin electrophoresis (Fig. 6.17) confirms the diagnosis in HbSS, no HbA is found, but HbF is present. The parents of the affected child will show features of sickle cell trait.

MANAGEMENT

The 'steady state' anaemia requires no treatment. No specific medication has been found to prevent sickling. Precipitating factors (see above) should be avoided or treated quickly. Acute attacks require supportive therapy with intravenous fluids, oxygen, antibiotics and adequate analgesia. Transfusions are given only if there is severe anaemia or if patients are having frequent crises in order to suppress the production of HbS. Prophylaxis is given to prevent pneumococcal infection (see p. 328). Folic acid is given to pregnant women and those with severe haemolysis.

Before elective operations and during pregnancy repeated transfusions may be used to reduce the proportion of circulating haemoglobin S to less than 20% to prevent sickling. In these situations, as well as in patients with many recurrent episodes, exchange transfusions are being used. The sudden increase in spleen and liver size due to sequestration can be watched for in babies known to be suffering from sickle cell anaemia. Transfusion and splenectomy may be life-saving.

PROGNOSIS

Some patients with HbSS die in the first few years of life from either infection or episodes of sequestration. There is, however, marked individual variation in the severity of the disease and some patients have a relatively normal life-span with few complications.

Careful genetic counselling is required. When both parents have sickle cell trait, one in four offspring will develop sickle cell anaemia. If analysis of fetal DNA indicates that the fetus has inherited two sickle genes, the parents have the option of abortion or of preparing for the problems of the disease.

Other haemoglobinopathies

There are many haemoglobin variants (e.g. Hb C, D), many of which are not associated with clinical manifestations. Haemoglobin C disease may be associated with haemoglobin S (haemoglobin SC disease) and it is associated with an increased likelihood of thrombosis. This may lead to life-threatening episodes of thrombosis in pregnancy as well as retinopathy. Haemoglobin variants may be associated with thalassaemia, for example, sickle cell thalassaemia, producing variable clinical manifestations.

METABOLIC DISORDERS OF THE RED CELL

It has already been noted how important it is for the red cell to 'keep its figure' if it is to perform satisfactorily. If the sodium or potassium content of

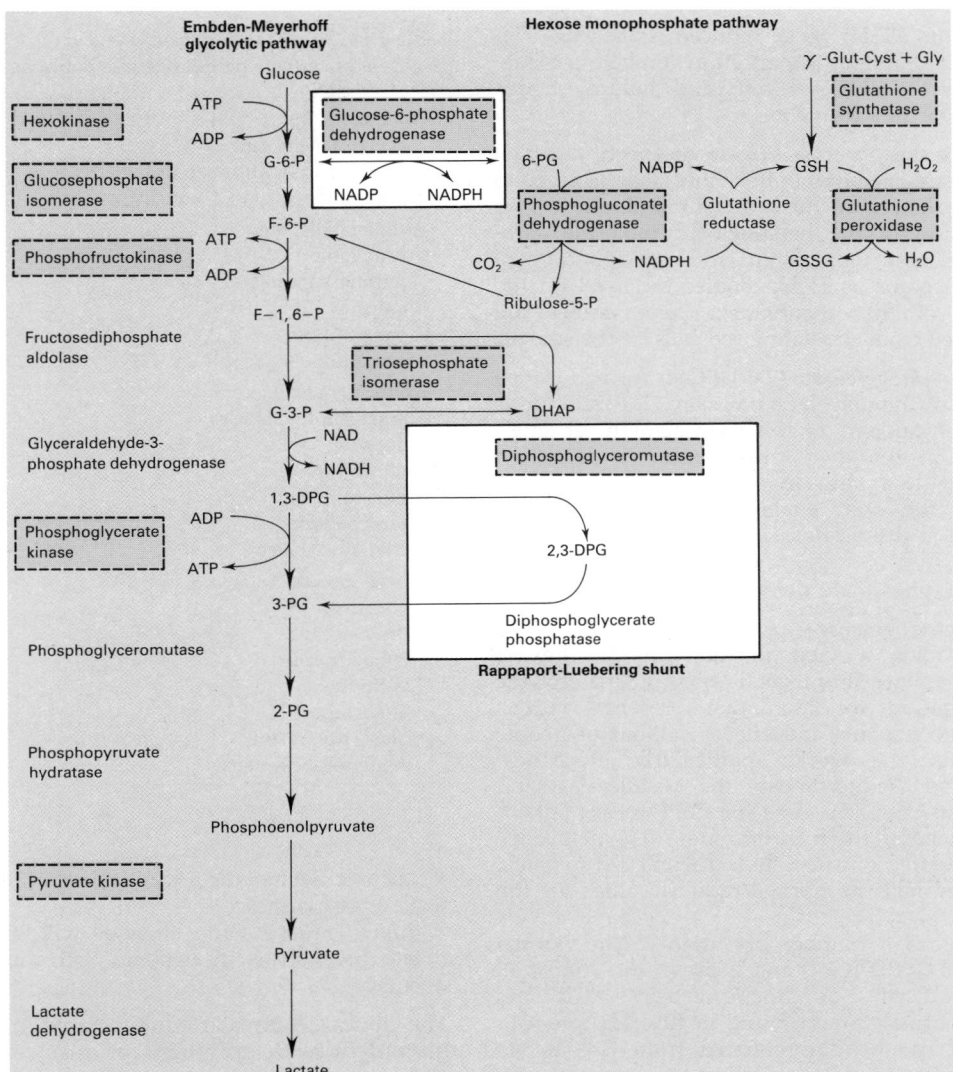

Fig. 6.19 Metabolic pathways (simplified) in the red cell. Enzymes enclosed by dotted lines indicate documented hereditary deficiency diseases. G = glucose; F = fructose; P = phosphate; DPG = diphosphoglycerate; PG = phosphoglycerate; DHAP = dihydroxyacetone phosphate; GSH = reduced glutathione; GSSG = oxidized gluthathione.

the cell varies, then the water content, and consequently the shape, will also alter. Cation 'pumps' in the cell wall maintain the correct balance by the outward transport of sodium at a rate of approximately 3 mmol·L^{-1}·h^{-1}. These cation pumps require ATP. The concentration of calcium is also regulated by a pump that requires ATP. The intracellular calcium is almost undetectable normally, but if the pump fails, calcium accumulates and a spiculated cell is formed that then dies.

Red-cell metabolism
The mature red cell has no nucleus, mitochondria

or ribosomes and is therefore unable to synthesize proteins. Red cells have only limited enzyme systems but they are of major importance in maintaining the viability and function of the cells:

- *Glycolytic (Embden–Meyerhof) pathway* (see Fig. 6.19), in which glucose is metabolized to pyruvate and lactic acid with production of ATP
- *Hexose monophosphate (pentosephosphate) pathway* (see Fig. 6.19), which provides reducing power for the red cell in the form of NADPH

About 90% of glucose is metabolized by the former and 10% by the latter. The importance of the hexose monophosphate shunt is that it maintains glutathione (GSH) in a reduced state (see Fig. 6.19). Glutathione is important in combating oxidative stress to the red cell, and failure of this mechanism may result in:

- Rigidity due to cross-linking of spectrin, which decreases membrane flexibility (see Fig. 6.14) and 'leakiness' of the red cell membrane.
- Oxidation of the haemoglobin molecule, producing methaemoglobin and precipitation of globin chains as Heinz bodies localized on the inside of the membrane. These bodies are removed from circulating red cells by the spleen.

2,3-Diphosphoglycerate (2,3-DPG) is formed from a side-arm of the glycolytic pathway. 2,3-DPG binds to the central part of the haemoglobin tetramer, fixing it in the low-affinity state. A decreased affinity with a shift in the oxygen dissociation curve to the right enables more oxygen to be delivered to the tissues.

Glucose-6-phosphate dehydrogenase deficiency

The enzyme glucose-6-phosphate dehydrogenase (G6PD) holds a vital position in the hexose monophosphate shunt. Deficiency of this enzyme is a common condition that presents with a haemolytic anaemia and affects millions of people throughout the world, particularly in Africa, around the Mediterranean, the Middle East and south-east Asia. The gene for G6PD is sex-linked, being carried on the X chromosome. The deficiency therefore affects males. It is carried by females, who show half the normal red-cell values for the enzyme.

G6PD has a number of variants. The normal enzyme is $G6PD^B(Gd^B)$ and is present in almost all whites and 70% of American blacks. Gd^{A+} is another normal variant found in 20% of American blacks. It can be differentiated from Gd^B by its greater electrophoretic mobility due to the substitution of an asparagine for aspartic acid in the amino-acid sequence. Gd^{A-} is similar to Gd^{A+} but because its catalytic activity is markedly reduced it is associated with haemolysis.

In Gd^{A-}, young cells have normal enzyme activity, whilst older cells are grossly deficient. Haemolysis is self-limiting as the bone marrow compensates by increasing its output. On the other hand, in the variety seen in Mediterranean peoples, G6PD Gd^{Med}, both the young and old red cells have very poor catalytic activity, and following an oxidant shock the haemoglobin level may fall precipitately; death may follow unless the condition is recognized and the patient is transfused urgently.

CLINICAL SYNDROMES

- Acute drug-induced haemolysis (Table 6.14)
- Favism (ingestion of fava beans)

Table 6.14 Drugs causing haemolysis in glucose-6-phosphate dehydrogenase deficiency.

Analgesics, e.g.
  acetylsalicylic acid
  phenacetin (withdrawn in the UK)
  acetanilide

Antimalarials, e.g.
  primaquine
  pyrimethamine
  quinine
  chloroquine
  pamaquin

Antibacterials, e.g.
  most sulphonamides
  dapsone
  nitrofurantoin
  nitrofurazone
  furazolidone
  chloramphenicol

Miscellaneous drugs, e.g.
  vitamin K
  probenecid
  nalidixic acid
  quinidine
  dimercaprol
  phenylhydrazine
  p-aminosalicylic acid

- Chronic haemolytic anaemia
- Neonatal jaundice
- Infections and acute illnesses will also precipitate haemolysis in patients with G6PD deficiency.

The clinical features are due to rapid intravascular haemolysis with symptoms of anaemia, jaundice and haemoglobinuria.

INVESTIGATION

- The blood count is normal between attacks.
- During an attack the blood film may show irregularly contracted cells, bite cells (cells with an indentation of the membrane), blister cells (cells in which the haemoglobin appears to have become partially detached from the cell membrane) (Fig. 6.7g), Heinz bodies (best seen on films stained with methyl violet) and reticulocytosis.
- There is evidence of haemolysis (see p. 311).
- G6PD deficiency can be detected using several screening tests, such as demonstration of the decreased ability of G6PD-deficient cells to reduce dyes, producing a change in colour. The level of the enzyme may also be directly assayed.

TREATMENT

- Any offending drugs should be stopped.
- Underlying infection should be treated.
- Blood transfusion may be life-saving.
- Splenectomy is not usually helpful.

Pyruvate kinase deficiency

This is the most common deficiency after G6PD deficiency, affecting thousands rather than millions of people. The site of the defect is shown in Fig. 6.19. It is inherited in an autosomal recessive manner. Homozygotes have haemolytic anaemia, splenomegaly and a low pyruvate kinase activity; this may be present at birth and continues throughout life.

INVESTIGATION

- The patients have anaemia of variable severity (Hb 5–10 g·dl^{-1}). The oxygen dissociation curve is shifted to the right as a result of the rise in intracellular 2,3-diphosphoglycerate (Fig. 6.19), and this reduces the severity of symptoms due to anaemia.
- The blood film shows distorted ('prickle') cells and a reticulocytosis.
- Autohaemolysis is increased; this is not prevented by the addition of glucose to the red cells, in contrast to hereditary spherocytosis.
- Pyruvate kinase, if assayed, is low (affected homozygotes have levels of 5–20%).

TREATMENT

Where anaemia is causing severe symptoms, a splenectomy may be helpful. Blood transfusions may be necessary during infections and pregnancy.

In addition to G6PD and pyruvate kinase deficiencies, there are a number of rare enzyme deficiencies that need specialist investigation.

Acquired haemolytic anaemia

These anaemias may be divided into those due to immune, non-immune, or other causes (Table 6.10).

- Immune destruction of red cells by autoantibodies, alloantibodies, haemolytic disease of the newborn (HDN) or drug-induced antibodies.
- Non-immune destruction of red cells may be due to acquired membrane defects e.g. paroxysmal nocturnal haemoglobinuria (PNH), liver and renal disease, mechanical factors e.g. prosthetic heart valves, or microangiopathic haemolytic anaemia (MAHA), where fragmentation of red cells occurs in an abnormal microcirculation caused by vasculitis or disseminated intravascular coagulation.
- *Miscellaneous*: Various toxic substances can disrupt the red-cell membrane and cause haemolysis e.g. arsenic, products of *Clostridium welchii*. Anaemia is frequent in malaria and this is due to a combination of a reduction in red cell survival and reduced production of red cells. Hypersplenism (p. 328) results in a reduced red-cell survival, which may also contribute to the anaemia seen in malaria. Extensive burns result in denaturation of erythrocyte membrane proteins and reduced red-cell survival.

IMMUNE HAEMOLYTIC ANAEMIA

Autoimmune haemolytic anaemias are acquired disorders resulting from increased red cell destruction due to red cell autoantibodies. Antibody and/or components of complement bind to the

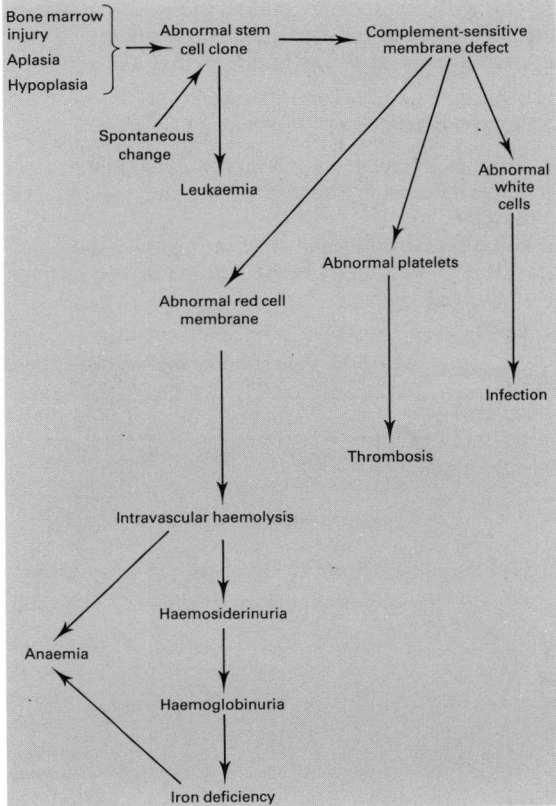

Fig. 6.20 Diagrams of (a) production of Coombs' serum and (b) the principles of the antiglobulin test.

patient's red cells, which are then phagocytosed and removed from the circulation by macrophages of the reticuloendothelial system (see p. 128). These anaemias are characterized by the presence of a positive direct antiglobulin (Coombs') test, which detects the antibody on the surface of the patient's red cells (Fig. 6.20).

Autoimmune haemolytic anaemias are divided into 'warm' or 'cold' types, depending on whether the antibody attaches better to the red cells at body temperature (37°C) or at lower temperatures. The major features and the causes of these two forms of autoimmune haemolytic anaemia are shown in Table 6.15.

'Warm' autoimmune haemolytic anaemias

CLINICAL FEATURES

These anaemias may occur at all ages and in both sexes. They can present as a short episode of anaemia or jaundice or may progress to an intermittent chronic pattern. The spleen may become palpable. Infections or folate deficiency may provoke a profound fall in the haemoglobin level. In more than 30% of cases, the cause remains unknown. These anaemias may be associated with lymphoid malignances or diseases such as rheumatoid arthritis and systemic lupus erythematosus or drugs (Table 6.15).

INVESTIGATION

- There is evidence of haemolytic anaemia.
- Spherocytosis is present as a result of red cell damage.
- The direct antiglobulin test is positive, with IgG and/or complement being found on the surface of the red cells.

- The condition may be associated with auto-immune thrombocytopenia and/or neutropenia (Evans' syndrome).

TREATMENT AND PROGNOSIS

Corticosteroids (e.g. prednisolone in doses of 40–60 mg daily) are effective in inducing a remission in about 80% of patients. Steroids reduce both production of the red-cell antibody and destruction of antibody-coated cells. Splenectomy may be necessary if there is no response to steroids or if the remission is not maintained when the dose of prednisolone is reduced. Other immunosuppressive drugs, such as azathioprine and cyclophosphamide, may be effective.

'Cold' autoimmune haemolytic anaemias

These disorders are due to antibodies, usually of the IgM type, that attach to red cells at low temperatures and produce complement-mediated intravascular haemolysis. Low titres of IgM cold agglutinins reacting at 4°C are normally present in serum and are harmless. After certain infections (such as *Mycoplasma*, cytomegalovirus, EB virus) or protozoa (e.g. malaria, trypanosomiasis) there is increased synthesis of polyclonal cold agglutinins with a higher thermal range and they may produce transient mild to moderate haemolysis.

Chronic cold haemagglutinin disease (CHAD) usually occurs in the elderly with a gradual onset of haemolytic anaemia due to the production of monoclonal IgM cold agglutinins. After exposure to cold the patient develops an acrocyanosis similar to Raynaud's (see p. 624).

Table 6.15 Causes and major features of autoimmune haemolytic anaemias.

	Warm	Cold
Temperature at which antibody attaches best to red cells:	37°C	Lower than 37°C
Type of antibodies:	IgG	IgM
Direct Coombs' test:	Strongly positive	Positive
Causes of primary condition:	Idiopathic	Idiopathic
Causes of secondary condition:	Autoimmune disorders, e.g. systemic lupus erythematosus Lymphomas Chronic lymphatic leukaemias Hodgkin's disease Carcinomas Drugs, e.g. methyldopa	Infections, e.g. infectious mononucleosis, *Mycoplasma pneumoniae* Other viral infections (rare) Lymphomas Paroxysmal cold haemoglobinuria (IgG)

INVESTIGATION

- Red cells agglutinate in the cold or at room temperature. Agglutination is sometimes seen in the sample tube after cooling or in the peripheral blood film made at room temperature.
- Serum antibodies are IgM in type and usually show specificity to the Ii blood group system.
- The direct antiglobulin test shows only complement on red cells.

TREATMENT

The underlying cause should be treated, if possible. Patients should avoid exposure to cold. Treatment with steroids, alkylating agents and splenectomy is usually ineffective. Blood transfusions may be required.

Paroxysmal cold haemoglobinuria (PCH) is a rare condition associated with common childhood infections, such as measles, mumps or chickenpox and syphilis. Intravascular haemolysis is associated with polyclonal complement-fixing antibodies. These react with red cells in the cold in the peripheral circulation and lysis occurs due to complement activation when the cells return to the central circulation. The IgG antibodies react with the P red-cell antigen. The lytic reaction is demonstrated *in vitro* by warming blood to 37°C after antibody fixation at 0°C, the Donath–Landsteiner test.

Drug-induced haemolytic anaemia

Drugs may cause immune haemolytic anaemia by the following mechanisms:

- *Immune complex*. The formation of drug–antibody immune complexes that are attached to red cells, activating complement and resulting in cell destruction. Example: quinine.
- *Membrane adsorption*. An antigenic drug–red-cell complex is formed. Production of IgG antibodies results in cell destruction. Example: penicillin.
- *Autoantibody*. The drug induces the production of a red-cell autoantibody by a direct effect on the immune system. Example: methyldopa.

Haemolytic disease of the newborn (HDN)

This is an *isoimmune* haemolytic anaemia that is due to the passage of IgG antibodies from the maternal circulation via the placenta into the fetus, where they destroy the fetal red cells. HDN is due to fetomaternal incompatibility for ABO, Rh and other blood group antigens. Rh(D) HDN is less common following the introduction of prophylactic IgG anti-D to susceptible mothers (see below). Sensitization usually occurs at delivery, so that first pregnancies are rarely affected.

CLINICAL FEATURES

These vary from a mild haemolytic anaemia of the newborn to intrauterine death from the eighteenth week gestation with the characteristic appearance of hydrops fetalis (hepatosplenomegaly, oedema and cardiac failure). With severe jaundice where the unconjugated (lipid-soluble) bilirubin exceeds 250 mmol·L^{-1}, bile pigment deposition occurs in the basal ganglia, giving rise to *kernicterus*. This results in mental deficiency, deafness, epilepsy and spasticity.

INVESTIGATION

Prenatally
Mothers should have their serum tested for atypical antibodies at the antenatal booking clinic and then monthly during the third trimester. If an antibody is detected, its specificity should be determined and the mother's serum should be tested more frequently; a rising titre is an indication for amniocentesis to assess the level of jaundice in the fetus. A fetus severely affected before 33 weeks may need intrauterine blood transfusions carried out in a special unit.

At birth
A sample of cord blood is obtained. This shows:

- Anaemia with a high reticulocyte count
- A positive direct antiglobulin test
- A raised bilirubin

TREATMENT

Management of the baby
In mild cases phototherapy may be used to convert bilirubin to water-soluble biliverdin. Biliverdin can be excreted by the kidneys and this therefore reduces the chance of kernicterus.

In severe cases, after 33 weeks, induction of labour with postnatal exchange transfusion may be indicated. The blood used should be ABO compatible with the mother and fetus, lack the antigen against which the maternal antibody is directed, be as fresh as possible and seronegative for cytomegalovirus.

Prevention of rhesus immunization in the mother
Anti-D should be given after delivery when all of the following are present:

- The mother is Rh(D) negative.
- The fetus is Rh(D) positive.
- There is no maternal anti-D detectable in the mother's serum, i.e. mother not already immunized.

The dose is 500 i.u. intramuscularly within 48 h of delivery. The Kleihauer test is used to assess the number of fetal cells in the maternal circulation. A blood film prepared from maternal blood is treated with acid, which elutes adult haemoglobin. Fetal haemoglobin is resistant to this treatment and can be seen when the film is stained with eosin. If large numbers of fetal red cells are present in the maternal circulation, a higher dose of anti-D is necessary.

NON-IMMUNE HAEMOLYTIC ANAEMIA

Paroxysmal nocturnal haemoglobinuria (PNH)

This is a rare acquired red-cell defect in which a clone of red cells is particularly sensitive to destruction by activated complement, mainly via the alternative pathway. C3b uptake by the cells is enhanced and there is decreased C3b inactivation. These cells are continually haemolysed intravascularly. There is an association with aplastic anaemia and acute myeloid leukaemia. Platelets and granulocytes are also affected and there may be thrombocytopenia and neutropenia (see Fig. 6.21).

CLINICAL FEATURES

Patients present with haemolysis that may be precipitated by infection, iron therapy or surgery. Because intravascular haemolysis is more common during sleep, the urine voided in the morning may be dark in colour. The condition may be compli-cated by thrombotic episodes, giving acute abdominal pain, myocardial infarction or stroke. The Budd–Chiari syndrome (hepatic vein occlusion) can occur.

INVESTIGATION

- There is evidence of intravascular haemolysis (see p. 311).
- Cells from a patient with PNH lyse more readily in acidified serum than do normal cells (Ham's test). PNH cells also lyse in solutions of sucrose.
- The bone marrow is sometimes hypoplastic despite haemolysis.

TREATMENT

There is no specific treatment for PNH. Very occasionally, if the abnormal cell clone disappears, complete spontaneous recovery may occur.

In severe anaemia, blood transfusion may be necessary. Filtered (leucocyte-depleted) blood is used in order to prevent transfusion reactions resulting in complement activation and acceleration of the haemolysis. The use of bone-marrow transplantation is being explored.

Anticoagulants are used in thrombotic episodes.

Non-leukaemic myeloproliferative disorders

In these disorders there is uncontrolled proliferation of each of the bone-marrow elements, viz. erythroid, myeloid, megakaryocyte lines, owing to malignant transformation of the pluripotential stem cell. This may result in either polycythaemia vera, or essential thrombocythaemia. Also included in this group is myelofibrosis, in which there is variable marrow fibrosis and myeloid metaplasia in the liver and spleen. These disorders are grouped together as there can be transition from one disease to another, for example, polycythaemia vera can lead to myelofibrosis. They may also transform to acute leukaemia.

Polycythaemia

Polycythaemia is defined as an increase in Hb, PCV and red-cell count. PCV is a more reliable indicator of polycythaemia than Hb, which may be disproportionately low in iron deficiency. Polycythaemia can be divided into an absolute erythro-

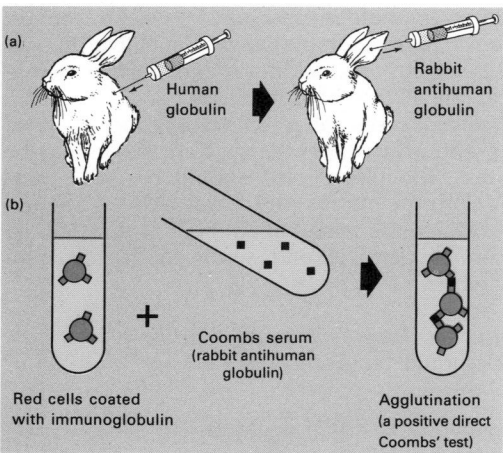

Fig. 6.21 Pathophysiology of paroxysmal nocturnal haemoglobin. (From Beck WS (ed) (1984) *Haematology*, 3rd edn. Massachusetts: MIT Press. With permission.)

Table 6.16 Causes of polycythaemia.

PRIMARY

Polycythaemia vera

SECONDARY

Due to an appropriate increase in erythropoietin
High altitude
Lung disease
Cardiovascular disease (right-to-left shunt)
Heavy smoking
Increased affinity of haemoglobin, e.g. familial
    polycythaemia

Due to an inappropriate increase in erythropoietin
Renal disease, renal cell carcinoma, Wilms' tumour
Hepatocellular carcinoma
Adrenal tumours
Cerebellar haemangioblastoma
Massive uterine fibroma

RELATIVE

Stress or spurious polycythaemia
Dehydration
Burns

cytosis where there is a true increase in red cell volume or relative erythrocytosis where the red cell volume is normal but there is a decrease in the plasma volume (Fig. 6.5).

Absolute erythrocytosis may be due to primary polycythaemia (PV) or secondary polycythaemia.

Secondary polycythaemia may be due to an appropriate increase in red cells in response to anoxia, or may be due to an inappropriate increase associated with tumours, such as a renal carcinoma. The causes of polycythaemia are given in Table 6.16. The serum erythropoietin level is not diagnostic but may be helpful. In PV the levels are low or normal; in secondary polycythaemia the level may be raised, as expected, but may be normal.

PRIMARY POLYCYTHAEMIA

Polycythaemia vera (PV)

PV is a clonal stem-cell disorder in which there is an alteration in the pluripotent progenitor cell leading to excessive proliferation of erythroid, myeloid and megakaryocytic elements. The main clinical problems are due to the increased volume and viscosity of the blood and to the bone-marrow overactivity.

CLINICAL FEATURES

The onset is insidious. It usually presents in patients over 60 with tiredness, depression,

vertigo, tinnitus and visual disturbance. It should be noted that these symptoms are also common in the normal population over the age of 60 and consequently PV is easily missed. These features, together with hypertension, angina, intermittent claudication and a tendency to bleed are suggestive evidence for PV. Severe itching after a hot bath or when the patient is warm is common. Gout due to increased cell turnover may be a feature and peptic ulceration occurs in a minority of patients. Thrombosis and haemorrhage are major complications.

Physical signs
The patient is usually plethoric and has a deep dusky cyanosis of the tongue. Injection of the conjunctivae is commonly seen. The spleen is palpable in 70% and is useful in distinguishing PV from secondary causes. The liver is enlarged in 50% of patients.

INVESTIGATION

- The haemoglobin and PCV are high but the precise upper limit is difficult to define. A haemoglobin > 18 $g \cdot dl^{-1}$ and a PCV > 0.60 $L \cdot L^{-1}$ is good evidence of polycythaemia. Elevated granulocyte count (in 70%). Elevated platelet count (in 50%).
- The bone marrow shows erythroid hyperplasia and increased numbers of megakaryocytes.
- The red-cell volume is measured using ^{51}Cr-labelled red cells is increased (> 36 $ml \cdot kg^{-1}$ in males and 32 $ml \cdot kg^{-1}$ in females). Measurement of plasma volume shows normal or increased values (normal range is 45 ± 5 $ml \cdot kg^{-1}$).
- Serum uric acid levels may be raised.
- The leucocyte alkaline phosphatase (LAP) is high.
- Serum vitamin B_{12} and vitamin B_{12}-binding protein (TCI) levels may be high.

DIFFERENTIAL DIAGNOSIS

An increase in red-cell volume should be established. Raised WCC and platelet count with splenomegaly makes PV very likely. The principal secondary causes can often be excluded by the history and examination but a renal ultrasound, an arterial pO_2 and carboxyhaemoglobin levels are also helpful.

COURSE AND MANAGEMENT

Treatment is designed to maintain a normal blood count and to prevent the complications of the disease, particularly thromboses and haemorrhage. Treatment is now aimed at keeping the PCV below 0.45 $L \cdot L^{-1}$. There are three types of treatment:

- *Venesection.* This will successfully relieve many of the symptoms of PV. Iron deficiency limits erythropoiesis. Venesection may often be used as the sole treatment. Other therapy is often required only to control the thrombocytosis.

- *Chemotherapy.* An alkylating agent (e.g. busulphan) or hydroxyurea are effective. Hydroxyurea is now being used quite frequently because of ease of control and general safety. Alkylating agents carry the risk of leukaemia.
- *Radioactive* ^{32}*phosphorus.* One dose may give control for up to 18 months but the administration of ^{32}P makes the patient liable to radiation-induced acute leukaemia.

There is no generally agreed scheme for the use of these treatment modalities in PV. One current policy is to manage polycythaemia with venesection alone if possible. However, if there is a high platelet count, this can be treated initially with a chemotherapeutic agent (preferably hydroxyurea). ^{32}P may be given in doses of 5–7 mCi (1.8–2.6 × 10^8 Bq) but is usually confined to the over-70 age group.

Allopurinol is given to block uric acid production. The pruritus is lessened by avoiding very hot baths. Sometimes cimetidine is very effective in relieving distressing pruritus. Antihistamines have largely proved unsuccessful.

It should be noted that patients with uncontrolled PV have a high operative risk; 75% of patients have severe haemorrhage following surgery and 30% of these patients die. If the surgery is elective, the polycythaemia should be controlled first. In an emergency, reduction of the haematocrit by venesection and fluid replacement must be carried out.

PROGNOSIS

Polycythaemia frequently develops into myelofibrosis or acute myeloid leukaemia as part of the natural history of the disease.

SECONDARY POLYCYTHAEMIAS

The causes of these are shown in Table 6.16. The treatment is that of the precipitating factor; for example, renal or posterior fossa tumours need to be resected. Heavy smoking can produce as much as 10% carboxyhaemoglobin and this can produce polycythaemia because of a reduction in oxygen-carrying capacity of the blood. Complications are similar to those seen in PV, including thrombosis, haemorrhage and cardiac failure, but myeloproliferative disease does not develop. Venesection may be symptomatically helpful in the hypoxic patient, particularly if the PCV is above 0.55.

'Relative' or 'stress' polycythaemia (Gaisböck's syndrome)

This condition was originally thought to be stress-induced. The red-cell volume is normal but, as the result of a decreased plasma volume, there is a 'relative' polycythaemia. 'Stress' polycythaemia is commoner than PV and occurs in middle-aged men, particularly those who are obese and hypertensive and who smoke. The higher the PCV, the greater the risk of arterial thrombotic episodes; the condition may present as cardiovascular problems such as myocardial or cerebral ischaemia. For this reason, it may be justifiable to venesect the patient until the PCV is normal. Sometimes the PCV then remains stabilized. Smoking must be stopped.

Myelofibrosis (myelosclerosis)

The terms myelosclerosis and myelofibrosis are interchangeable. In this condition there is fibrosis and collagen deposition in the bone marrow and extramedullary haemopoiesis in the liver and spleen. The increased fibrosis is due to fibroblastic proliferation that appears to be secondary to the malignant proliferation of stem cells.

CLINICAL FEATURES

The disease presents insidiously with lethargy, weakness and weight loss. Patients often complain of a 'fullness' in the upper abdomen due to the large spleen. Severe pain related to respiration may indicte perisplenitis secondary to splenic infarction, and pain in the bones and attacks of gout can complicate the illness. Bruising and bleeding occur in the thrombocytopenic patient.

Physical signs

- Anaemia
- Fever
- Massive splenomegaly

Other conditions that must be considered when massive splenomegaly is seen are chronic myeloid leukaemia, chronic malaria, kala-azar or, rarely, Gaucher's disease.

INVESTIGATION

- There is anaemia with leucoerythroblastic features. Poikilocytes and red cells with characteristic tear-drop forms are seen. The white cell count may be over 100 × 10^9/L, and the differential white cell count may be very similar to that seen in chronic granulocytic leukaemia; later leucopenia may develop.
- The platelet count may be very high but, in later stages, thrombocytopenia occurs.
- Bone marrow aspiration is often unsuccessful and this gives a clue to the presence of the

condition. A bone marrow trephine is necessary to show the markedly increased fibrosis and islands of hypercellularity.

- The Philadelphia chromosome is absent; this helps to distinguish myelofibrosis from most cases of chronic myeloid leukaemia.
- The leucocyte alkaline phosphatase is normal or high.
- A high serum urate is present.
- Low serum folate levels may occur owing to the increased activity of marrow tissue.

DIFFERENTIAL DIAGNOSIS

Fibrosis of the marrow, often with a leucoerythroblastic anaemia, can occur secondary to malignant infiltration with metastatic carcinoma, chronic myeloid leukaemia or lymphoma. It can also occur post-irradiation. These secondary causes of myelofibrosis should be excluded.

TREATMENT

This consists of general supportive measures such as blood transfusion, folic acid, analgesics and allopurinol. Cytotoxics and radiotherapy are used to reduce splenic size. Drugs such as busulphan, chlorambucil and hydroxyurea are used to reduce metabolic activity and high leucocyte and platelet levels; hydroxyurea is the commonest drug used. If the spleen becomes very large and painful, and transfusion requirements are high, it may be advisable to perform splenectomy. Splenectomy may also result in relief of severe thrombocytopenia.

PROGNOSIS

Patients may survive for 10 years or more; median survival is 3 years. Death may occur from leukaemic transformation. The most common causes of death are cardiovascular disease, infection and gastrointestinal bleeding.

Essential thrombocythaemia

Essential thrombocythaemia is a rare condition that is closely related to PV. The patient has $> 1000 \times 10^9$/L platelets in the peripheral blood. It presents with bruising, bleeding and cerebrovascular symptoms. Initially splenic hypertrophy may be seen but, as the condition progresses, recurrent thromboses due to the increased number of platelets reduce the size of the spleen and it may atrophy.

Essential thrombocythaemia has to be distinguished from secondary thrombocythaemia that is seen in haemorrhage, connective tissue disorders, malignancy, post-splenectomy and in other myeloproliferative disorders.

Treatment is with hydroxyurea or busulphan.

The spleen

The spleen is the largest lymphoid organ in the body and is situated in the left hypochondrium. There are two anatomical components:

- The red pulp, consisting of sinuses lined by endothelial macrophages and cords (spaces)
- The white pulp, which has a structure similar to lymphoid follicles (p. 125)

Blood enters via the splenic artery and is eventually delivered to the red and white pulp. During the flow the blood is skimmed, with leucocytes and plasma passing to white pulp. Some red cells pass rapidly through into the venous system while others are held up in the red pulp.

Functions

- *Sequestration and phagocytosis.* Normal red cells, which are flexible, pass through the red pulp into the venous system without difficulty. Old or abnormal cells are damaged by the hypoxia, low glucose and low pH found in the sinuses of the red pulp and are therefore removed by phagocytosis along with other circulating foreign matter. Howell–Jolly and Heinz bodies and sideroblastic granules have their particles removed by 'pitting' and are then returned to the circulation.
- *Extramedullary haemopoiesis.* Pluripotential stem cells CFU-S and BFU-E are present and proliferate during severe haematological stress, e.g. haemolytic anaemia, thalassaemia.
- *Immunological function.* IgG-coated red cells are removed through their Fc receptors by macrophages.
- *Blood pooling.* Up to one third of the platelets are sequestrated in the spleen and can be rapidly mobilized. Enlarged spleens pool a significant percentage of the red-cell mass.
- *Miscellaneous.* Other functions include plasma volume control and generation of humoral factors controlling haemopoiesis.

SPLENOMEGALY

A clinically palpable spleen has many causes including:

- *Infection*:
   acute—viral, bacterial
   chronic—tuberculosis and brucellosis
   parasitic—malaria, kala-azar and schistosomiasis
- *Inflammation*: rheumatoid arthritis, sarcoidosis,
   SLE
- *Haematological*: haemolytic anaemia, haemoglo-
   binopathies and the leukaemias
- *Neoplastic*: lymphomas and myeloproliferative
   disorders
- *Portal hypertension*: liver disease
- *Miscellaeneous*: storage diseases, amyloid, primary and secondary neoplasias; Tropical splenomegaly

Massive splenomegaly (see p. 326).

Investigation is that of the primary disorder. The
spleen can be visualized by ultrasound or CT
scanning. Splenic function can be assessed with
isotope scanning.

HYPERSPLENISM

This can result from splenomegaly due to any
cause. It is commonly seen with splenomegaly due
to haematological disorders, portal hypertension,
rheumatoid arthritis (Felty's syndrome) and
lymphoma. Hypersplenism produces:

- Pancytopenia
- Haemolysis due to sequestration and destruction
   of red cells in the spleen
- Increased plasma volume due to pooling of red
   cells in the enlarged spleen

Treatment is often dependent on the underlying
cause but splenectomy is sometimes required for
severe anaemia or thrombocytopenia.

SPLENECTOMY

Splenectomy is performed mainly for:

- Trauma
- Idiopathic thrombocytopenic purpura (p. 339)
- Haemolytic anaemias (p. 309)
- Hodgkin's—staging (p. 367)
- Hypersplenism

Post-splenectomy problems

- Immediate: increased platelet count (usually
   600–1000 × 10^9/L) for 2–3 weeks, thromboembolic phenomena may occur.
- Long-term: increased risk of overwhelming infections, particularly pneumococcal, and parasitic infection, particularly falciparum malaria.

All children should be given long-term prophylactic penicillin (250 mg × 2 daily). All patients
should also receive the polyvalent antipneumo-
coccal vaccine; it should be given 2–3 weeks before
splenectomy, if possible.

Splenic atrophy is seen in sickle cell disease due to
infarction. It is also seen in coeliac disease,
dermatitis herpetiformis and occasionally in ulcerative colitis and essential thrombocythaemia.
Haematological features include thrombocytosis,
Howell–Jolly bodies, Pappenheimer bodies, target
cells and irregular contracted red cells.

Blood groups

The blood groups are determined by antigens on
the surface of red cells; more than 400 blood
groups have been found. The ABO and Rh systems
are the two most important blood groups but
incompatibilities involving many other blood
groups (such as Kell, Duffy, Kidd, Lewis) may
cause haemolytic transfusion reactions and/or
haemolytic disease of the newborn.

ABO system

This is the most important blood group system
because naturally acquired IgM anti-A and anti-B
antibodies are capable of producing rapid and
severe intravascular haemolysis of incompatible
red cells.

The ABO system is under the control of a pair of
allelic genes, *H* and *h*, and also three allelic genes,
A, *B*, and *O*, producing the genotypes and
phenotypes shown in Table 6.17. The A, B and H
antigens are very similar in structure; differences in
the terminal sugars determine their specificity. The
H gene codes for enzyme H, which attaches

Table 6.17 Antigens and antibodies in the ABO system.

Phenotype	Genotype	Antigens	Antibodies	Frequency (UK)
O	OO	None	Anti-A and anti-B	44%
A	AA or AO	A	Anti-B	45%
B	BB or BO	B	Anti-A	8%
AB	AB	A and B	None	3%

fructose to the basic glycoprotein backbone to form H substance, which is the precursor for A and B antigens.

The *A* and *B* genes control specific enzymes responsible for the addition to H substance of *N*-acetylgalactosamine for Group A and D-galactose for Group B. The *O* gene is amorphic and does not transform H substance and therefore O is not antigenic. The A, B and H antigens are present on most body cells. These antigens are also found in soluble form in tissue fluids such as saliva and gastric juice in the 80% of the population who possess secretor genes.

Rh system

This is the second most clinically important blood group system because of the high frequency of development of IgG Rh(D) antibodies in Rh(D) negative individuals after exposure to Rh(D) positive red cells following blood transfusions or during pregnancy. The antibodies formed are of major importance in causing haemolytic disease of the newborn and haemolytic transfusion reactions.

There are thought to be three pairs of allelic genes, *D* and *d*, *C* and *c*, and *E* and *e*; they are inherited as triplets on each chromosome, one from each pair of genes, i.e. *CDE/cde*. The presence of the d antigen has not been demonstrated and the presence or absence of the D antigen determines whether an individual is characterized as Rh(D) positive or negative.

Blood transfusion

The safety of blood transfusion depends on meticulous attention to detail at each stage leading to the transfusion. Prevention of simple errors of identification would avoid most serious haemolytic transfusion reactions, almost all of which involve the ABO system. About 50% of fatalities associated with blood transfusion are due to 'clerical' errors; the remainder are mainly due to post-transfusion hepatitis.

SELECTION AND CROSS-MATCHING OF BLOOD FOR TRANSFUSION

- The ABO and Rh(D) group of the patient is determined.
- The patient's serum is screened for atypical antibodies that may cause a significant reduction in the survival of the transfused red cells.

The patient's serum is tested against red cells from

at least two Group O donors, expressing a wide range of red-cell antigens, using an indirect antiglobulin test. A further test is performed against enzyme-treated red cells, which enhances the reactions of some antibodies, e.g. Rh antibodies and diminishes others, such as Duffy antibodies.

A positive result requires precise identification of the specificity of the antibody using a comprehensive panel of typed red cells.

- Donor blood of the same ABO and Rh(D) group as the patient is selected.
- The patient's serum is 'cross-matched' against the donor red cells suspended in saline in a direct agglutination technique and in an indirect antiglobulin test.

Many hospitals have guidelines for blood ordering for elective surgery, aiming to reduce unnecessary cross-matching and the amount of blood that eventually becomes outdated. Many operations in which blood is only occasionally required for

Table 6.18 Complications of blood transfusion.

Immunological

Alloimmunization

Incompatibility
- *Red cells*
  Immediate haemolytic transfusion reactions
  Delayed haemolytic transfusion reactions
- *Leucocyte and platelets*
  Non-haemolytic (febrile) transfusion reactions
  Post-transfusion purpura
  Poor survival of transfused platelets and
  granulocytes
  Graft-versus-host disease
- *Plasma proteins*
  Urticarial and anaphylactic reactions

Non-immunological

Transmission of infection
  Hepatitis
  HIV
  Other viruses—CMV, EBV, HTLV-1
  Parasites—malaria, trypanosomiasis,
    toxoplasmosis
Syphilis

Transfusion of blood contaminated with bacteria

Circulatory failure due to volume overload

Iron overload due to multiple transfusions

Massive transfusion of stored blood may cause
  bleeding and electrolyte changes

Thrombophlebitis

Air embolism

unexpectedly high blood loss can be classified as 'group and save serum'; this means that, where the antibody screen is negative, blood is not reserved in advance but can be made available quickly if necessary. If a patient has atypical antibodies, compatible blood should be reserved in advance.

THE COMPLICATIONS OF BLOOD TRANSFUSION (Table 6.18)

Immunological

- *Alloimmunization.* All transfusions carry a risk of immunization to the many antigens on red cells, leucocytes, platelets and plasma proteins. Alloimmunization does not usually cause clinical problems with the first transfusion but these may occur with subsequent transfusions. There may also be important delayed consequences of alloimmunization such as haemolytic disease of the newborn and rejection of tissue transplants.
- *Incompatibility.* This may result in poor survival of transfused cells, such as red cells and platelets, and in harmful effects of the antigen–antibody reaction.

Haemolytic transfusion reactions
Immediate. This is the most serious complication of blood transfusion and is usually due to ABO incompatibility. There is complement activation by the antigen–antibody reaction, usually due to IgM antibodies, leading to rigors, lumbar pain, dyspnoea, hypotension, haemoglobinuria and renal failure. Activation of coagulation may also occur; bleeding due to disseminated intravascular coagulation (DIC) is a bad prognostic sign. Emergency treatment may be needed to maintain the blood pressure and renal function.

The diagnosis is confirmed by finding evidence of haemolysis, such as haemoglobinuria, and of incompatibility between donor and recipient. All documentation should be checked to detect clerical errors and blood grouping of both old and new patient samples and the donor units should be performed. At the first suspicion of any transfusion reaction the transfusion should always be stopped and the donor units returned to the blood transfusion laboratory with a new blood sample from the patient to exclude a haemolytic transfusion reaction.

Delayed. This may occur in patients alloimmunized by previous transfusions or pregnancies. The antibody level is too low to be detected by pretransfusion compatibility testing but a secondary immune response occurs after transfusion, resulting in destruction of the transfused cells, usually by IgG antibodies. Haemolysis is usually extravascular and the patient may develop anaemia

and jaundice about a week after the transfusion, although most are clinically silent. The blood film shows spherocytosis and reticulocytosis. The direct antiglobulin test is positive and detection of the antibody is usually straightforward.

Non-haemolytic (febrile) transfusion reactions
Febrile reactions are a common complication of blood transfusion in patients who have previously been transfused or pregnant. Antileucocyte antibodies in the recipient act againt transfused leucocytes, leading to release of pyrogens. Typical signs are flushing and tachycardia, fever ($> 38°C$), chills and rigors. Aspirin may be used to reduce the fever, although it should not be used in patients with thrombocytopenia. Febrile reactions may be prevented by the use of leuocyte-poor red-cell concentrates for subsequent transfusions. Potent leucocyte antibodies in the donor's plasma may cause severe reactions.

Urticaria and anaphylaxis
Urticarial reactions are often attributed to plasma protein incompatibility but, in most cases, they are unexplained. They are common but rarely severe; stopping or slowing the transfusion and administration of chlorpheniramine 10 mg i.v. are usually sufficient treatment. Anaphylactic reactions (see p. 733) occasionally occur; severe reactions may be seen in patients lacking IgA who produce anti-IgA that reacts with IgA in the transfused blood. The transfusion should be stopped and adrenaline 0.5 mg i.m. and chlorpheniramine 10 mg i.v. should be given immediately; endotracheal intubation may be required. Washed red cells should be used for subsequent transfusions in patients who have had severe urticarial or anaphylactic reactions.

Non-immunological

Transmission of infection
The incidence of post-transfusion hepatitis is estimated to be 1–3% in the UK and most cases are due to HCV. This incidence will fall as HCV antibody testing becomes widespread. Each donation is now tested for HB_sAg and HIV antibodies. However, it is mandatory in the USA to test each donation for indirect ('surrogate') markers, such as serum alanine aminotransferase and anti-HBc; high levels of such markers may indicate an increased risk of transmitting HCV hepatitis.

In the UK the incidence of transmission of HIV by blood transfusion is extremely low, probably considerably less than one in one million units. Prevention is based on self-exclusion of donors in 'high-risk' groups and testing each donation for anti-HIV. There is an increased risk of HIV transmission from coagulation factor concentrates prepared from large pools of plasma; these are now heat-treated to inactivate the HIV virus.

Transfusion-transmitted syphilis is now very rare in the UK. Spirochaetes do not survive for more than 72 h in blood stored at 4°C and each donation is tested using the TPHA.

BLOOD, BLOOD COMPONENTS AND BLOOD PRODUCTS

Blood collected from donors is either used 'whole' or processed into blood components and blood products.

- *Whole blood.* The average volume of blood withdrawn is 450 ml, taken into 63 ml of anticoagulant. Blood stored at 4°C has a 'shelf-life' of 5 weeks.
- *Red-cell concentrates.* 200–250 ml of plasma are removed from whole blood to be frozen as FFP or to be further processed.
- *Red cells suspended in optimal additive solutions.* Virtually all the plasma is removed and it is replaced by about 100 ml of an additive solution, such as SAG-M which contains sodium chloride, adenine, glucose and mannitol. The PCV is about 0.65 but the viscosity is low as there is no protein in the additive solution, and this allows fast administration if necessary.
- *Leucocyte-poor red-cell concentrates* are usually prepared by filtration. They are used in patients who have had febrile transfusion reactions and to prevent alloimmunization to leucocyte antigens in patients likely to receive repeated transfusion.
- *Washed red-cell concentrates* are preparations of red cells suspended in saline, produced by cell separators to remove all but traces of plasma proteins. They are used in patients who have had anaphylactic reactions.
- *Platelet concentrates* are prepared either from whole blood by centrifugation or by plateletpheresis of single donors using cell separators. They may be stored for up to 5 days at 22°C. They are used to treat bleeding in patients with severe thrombocytopenia and prophylactically to prevent bleeding in patients with bone-marrow failure.
- *Granulocyte concentrates* are prepared from single donors using cell separators. They are used for patients with severe neutropenia with definite evidence of bacterial infection where antibiotic therapy has failed. They are rarely used now.
- *Fresh frozen plasma (FFP)* is prepared by freezing the plasma from one unit of blood at −30°C within 6 h of donation. The volume is approximately 200 ml. It contains all the coagulation factors present in fresh plasma. It is mostly used for replacement of coagulation factors in acquired coagulation-factor deficiencies.
- *Cryoprecipitate* is obtained by allowing the frozen

plasma from a single donation to thaw at 4–8°C and removing the supernatant. The volume is about 20 ml and it is stored at −30°C. It contains Factor VIII:C, Factor VIII:vWF and fibrinogen.
- *Factor VIII and IX concentrates* are freeze-dried preparations of specific coagulation factors prepared by fractionation of large pools of plasma. They are used for treating patients with haemophilia.
- *Albumin.* There are two preparations:
    Plasma protein fraction (PPF) contains approximately 45 g·L^{-1} albumin and 160 mmol·L^{-1} sodium. It is produced in 50, 100, 250 and 500 ml bottles.
    'Salt-poor' albumin contains approximately 200 g·L^{-1} albumin and 130 mmol·L^{-1} sodium and is produced in 50 and 100 ml bottles.
PPF is indicated for treatment of hypoproteinaemia following burns and as the replacement fluid for plasma exchange. It is also used in the treatment of shock (p. 716). Salt-poor albumin is used for patients with severe hypoproteinaemia due to acute nephrotic syndrome or acute liver disease.
- *Normal immunoglobulin* is prepared from normal plasma. It is used in patients with hypogammaglobulinaemia to prevent infections and in patients with idiopathic thrombocytopenic purpura.
- *Specific immunoglobulins* are obtained from donors with high titres of antibodies. Many preparations are available, such as anti-D, anti-hepatitis B, anti-varicella-zoster.

The white cell (see also Chapter 2)

The five types of leucocytes found in peripheral blood are polymorphonuclear leucocytes (neutrophil granulocytes), eosinophil granulocytes, basophil granulocytes, lymphocytes and monocytes. These cells (apart from lymphocytes) are all derived from the colony-forming unit CFU-GEMM in the bone marrow. The lymphocytes, although derived from the same pluripotential stem cell, have a different lineage (see Fig. 6.1).

NEUTROPHILS

The neutrophil granulocyte is derived by further differentiation of CFU-GEMM to form a myeloblast under the influence of multi-CSF (IL-3) (see Fig. 6.1). This large undifferentiated cell is the earliest morphologically identifiable precursor in the bone marrow. The cytoplasm is scanty and contains a few primary granules, which increase in number as the cell matures. Promyelocytes have more abundant cytoplasm and secondary granules and retain

Table 6.19 Causes of neutrophil leucocytosis.

Bacterial infection
Tissue necrosis, e.g. myocardial infarction
Inflammation
Corticosteroid therapy
Leukaemia
Myeloproliferative disease
Leukaemoid reaction
Leucoerythroblastic anaemia
Acute haemorrhage or haemolysis

nucleoli. Myelocytes are smaller cells, without nucleoli but with even more abundant cytoplasm. Indentation of the nucleus marks the change from myelocyte to metamyelocyte. The mature neutrophil is a smaller cell with a segmented nucleus with primary and secondary granules in the cytoplasm. Neutrophils are stored in the marrow for up to 10 days before release. Peripheral blood neutrophils are equally distributed into a circulating pool and a marginating pool lying along the endothelium of blood vessels. The half-life of neutrophils in the peripheral blood is extremely short, only 6–8 h. In response to stimuli (e.g. infection, corticosteroid therapy) neutrophils are released into the circulating pool from both the marginating pool and the marrow. Immature white cells (occasionally metamyelocytes and myelocytes) are released from the marrow when a rapid response (within hours) occurs in acute infection (described as a 'shift to the left' on a blood film).

Function
The prime function of the neutrophil granulocyte is to ingest and kill bacteria. Neutrophil migration is directed *in vivo* by chemotaxins. Bacteria are first coated with complement. They are ingested into vacuoles where they are subjected to enzymic destruction, which requires the generation of hydrogen peroxide. An accumulation of degenerate neutrophils gives rise to pus.

Neutrophil leucocytosis

A rise in the number of circulating neutrophils to > 10 × 10⁹/L occurs in bacterial infections or as a result of tissue damage. This may also be seen in pregnancy, during exercise and after corticosteroid administration (Table 6.19). In any tissue necrosis there is a release of various soluble factors, causing a leucocytosis. Interleukin-I is also released in tissue necrosis and causes a pyrexia. The pyrexia and leucocytosis accompanying a myocardial infarction are a good example of this and may be wrongly attributed to infection. A *leukaemoid reaction* (an overproduction of white cells, with many immature cells) may occur in severe infec-

tions, tuberculosis, malignant infiltration of the bone marrow and occasionally after haemorrhage or haemolysis. In *leucoerythroblastic anaemia*, erythroblasts and primitive white cells are found in the peripheral blood; causes include marrow infiltration with metastatic carcinoma, myelofibrosis, osteopetrosis, myeloma, lymphoma and occasionally a severe haemolytic or megaloblastic anaemia.

Neutropenia and agranulocytosis

Neutropenia is defined as a circulatory neutrophil count below 1.5 × 10⁹/L. A virtual absence of neutrophils is called agranulocytosis. The causes are given in Table 6.20.

CLINICAL FEATURES

Infections may be frequent, often serious, and are more likely as the neutrophil count falls. A characteristic glazed mucositis occurs in the mouth and ulceration is common.

INVESTIGATION

The blood film shows marked neutropenia. The bone marrow determines whether the neutropenia is due to depressed production or increased destruction of neutrophils. Neutrophil antibody studies may be performed if an immune mechanism is suspected.

TREATMENT

All current drug therapy should be stopped. Antibiotic therapy should be given as necessary.

EOSINOPHILS

Eosinophils are derived by differentiation of CFU-EO under the influence of IL-3 and -5. They are characterized by large cytoplasmic granules that

Table 6.20 Causes of neutropenia.

Racial (neutropenia is common in black races)
Viral infection
Severe bacterial infection, e.g. typhoid
Felty's syndrome
Megaloblastic anaemia
Drugs (for drugs causing marrow aplasia, see Table 6.8)
Autoimmune neutropenia
Pancytopenia from any cause (see Table 6.9)
Cyclic (genetic defect with neutropenia every 2–3 weeks)

Table 6.21 Causes of eosinophilia.

Parasitic infestations, e.g.
  Ascaris
  Strongyloides
Allergic disorders, e.g.
  Hayfever (allergic rhinitis)
  Other hypersensitivity reactions, including drug
    reactions
Skin disorders, e.g.
  Urticaria
  Pemphigus
  Eczema
Pulmonary disorders, e.g.
  Bronchial asthma
  Tropical pulmonary eosinophilia
  Allergic bronchopulmonary aspergillosis
  Polyarteritis nodosa (Churg–Strauss syndrome)
Malignant disorders
  Lymphoma
  Carcinoma
  Melanoma
  Eosinophilic leukaemia
Miscellaneous, e.g.
  Hypereosinophilic syndrome
  Sarcoidosis
  Hypoadrenalism
  Eosinophilic gastroenteritis

stain brightly with eosin. The eosinophil seems to play some part in the hypersensitivity response to infections with helminths and protozoa. Eosinophilia is said to occur when the number of eosinophils is $> 0.4 \times 10^9$/L in the peripheral blood. It is associated with a wide variety of disorders. The causes of eosinophilia are listed in Table 6.21.

BASOPHILS

The physiological role of the basophil is not known. It is, however, associated with acute hypersensitivity reactions and life-threatening urticaria, asthma, and anaphylactic shock. Basophils are usually few in number but are significantly increased in chronic myelocytic leukaemia and myelofibrosis.

MONOCYTES

Monocytes are derived from CFU-GM under the influence of IL-3 and GM-CSF. They are precursors of tissue macrophages and are often involved in immune responses. Monocytes spend only a few hours in the blood but can continue to proliferate in the tissues for many years. Macrophages are widely distributed through the reticuloendothelial system.

LYMPHOCYTES

Lymphocytes form nearly half the circulating white cells. They descend from pluripotential stem cells. Circulating lymphocytes are small cells, a little larger than red cells, with a dark-staining central nucleus. There are two main types: the thymus-dependent or T lymphocytes, which are concerned with cellular immunity and form about 70% of the circulating lymphocytes, and the 'bursa dependent' or B lymphocytes, which are concerned with humoral immunity (see p. 129).

Lymphocytosis (lymphocyte count $> 5 \times 10^9$/L) occurs in response to viral infections, particularly Epstein–Barr virus, which causes the illness known as infectious mononucleosis. It may occur following immunization against various childhood illnesses, and is seen in chronic infections such as tuberculosis and syphilis, and in chronic lymphocytic leukaemia and in some lymphomas.

Bleeding disorders

Blood is normally separated from the activators of haemostasis by the endothelial cell. Injury to the vessel wall exposes collagen and sets in motion a series of events leading to haemostasis.

Haemostasis

Haemostasis is a complex process depending on interactions between the vessel wall, platelets and coagulation factors (Fig. 6.22).

Vessel wall
An immediate reflex vasoconstriction of the injured vessel and adjacent vessels results in a transient reduction of blood flow to the affected area. Damage to the endothelium of the vessel results in activation of platelets and coagulation; release of serotonin and thromboxane A_2 (TXA$_2$) from activated platelets contributes to the vasoconstriction.

Platelets
Platelet adhesion to collagen is dependent on a platelet membrane receptor, glycoprotein Ib, and the presence in the plasma of von Willebrand factor (VIII:vWF). Following adhesion, platelets undergo a shape change from a disc to a sphere, spread along the subendothelium and *release* the contents of their cytoplasmic granules, i.e. the dense bodies (containing ADP and serotonin) and the α-granules (containing platelet-derived growth factor, platelet factor 4, β-thromboglobulin, fibrinogen, VIII:vWF and other factors). The release of ADP leads to exposure of a fibrinogen receptor, the glycoprotein IIb–IIIa complex, on surfaces of

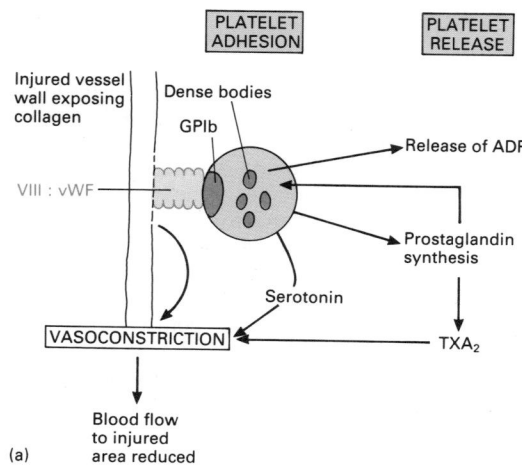

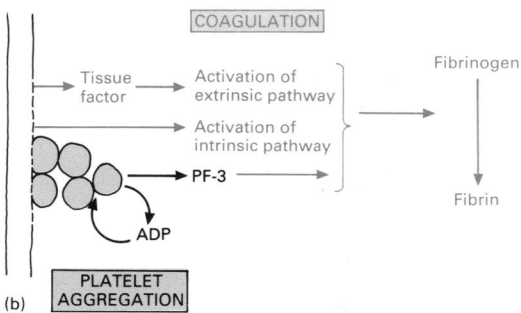

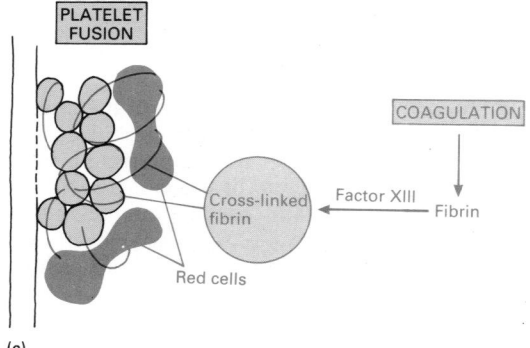

Fig. 6.22 Formation of the haemostatic plug. Sequential interactions of the vessel wall, platelets and coagulation factors. (a) Contact of platelets with collagen, via the platelet receptor GPIb and factor VIII:vWF in plasma, activates platelet prostaglandin synthesis which stimulates release of ADP from the dense bodies. Vasoconstriction of the vessel occurs as a reflex and by release of serotonin and TXA_2 from platelets. (b) Release of ADP from platelets induces platelet aggregation and formation of the platelet plug. The coagulation pathway is stimulated leading to formation of fibrin. (c) Fibrin strands are cross-linked by factor XIII and stabilize the haemostatic plug by binding platelets and red cells.

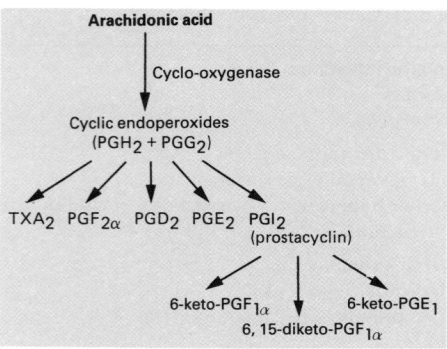

Fig. 6.23 Prostaglandin synthesis (simplified).

adherent platelets; fibrinogen binds platelets into activated aggregates (*platelet aggregation*) and further platelet release occurs. A self-perpetuating cycle of events is set up leading to formation of a platelet plug at the site of the injury. Further platelet membrane receptors are exposed during aggregation, providing a surface for the interaction of coagulation factors; this platelet activity is referred to as platelet factor 3 (PF-3) (Fig. 6.23). The presence of thrombin encourages *fusion of platelets*, and fibrin formation reinforces the stability of the platelet plug.

Central to normal platelet function is platelet prostaglandin synthesis, which is induced by platelet activation and leads to the formation of TXA_2 (Fig. 6.23). TXA_2 is a powerful vasoconstrictor and also lowers cyclic AMP levels and initiates the platelet release reaction. Prostacyclin (PGI_2) is synthesized by vascular endothelial cells and opposes the actions of TXA_2. It produces vasodilatation and increases the level of cyclic AMP, preventing platelet aggregation on the normal vessel wall as well as limiting the extent of the initial platelet plug after injury.

Coagulation and fibrinolysis
Coagulation involves a series of enzymatic reactions leading to the conversion of soluble plasma fibrinogen to fibrin clot (Fig. 6.24). The coagulation factors are either enzyme precursors (factors XII, XI, X, IX and thrombin) or co-factors (V and VIII), except for fibrinogen, which is the subunit of fibrin. The enzymes apart from factor XIII are serine proteases and hydrolyse peptide bonds.

Extrinsic pathway. Tissue factor released from damaged cells together with factor VII and calcium ions activates factor X.

Intrinsic pathway. Factor XII is activated by 'contact' with the injured surface and initiates a series of reactions leading to activation of factor X. Activated factor XII also converts prekallikrein to kallikrein, which leads to further activation of

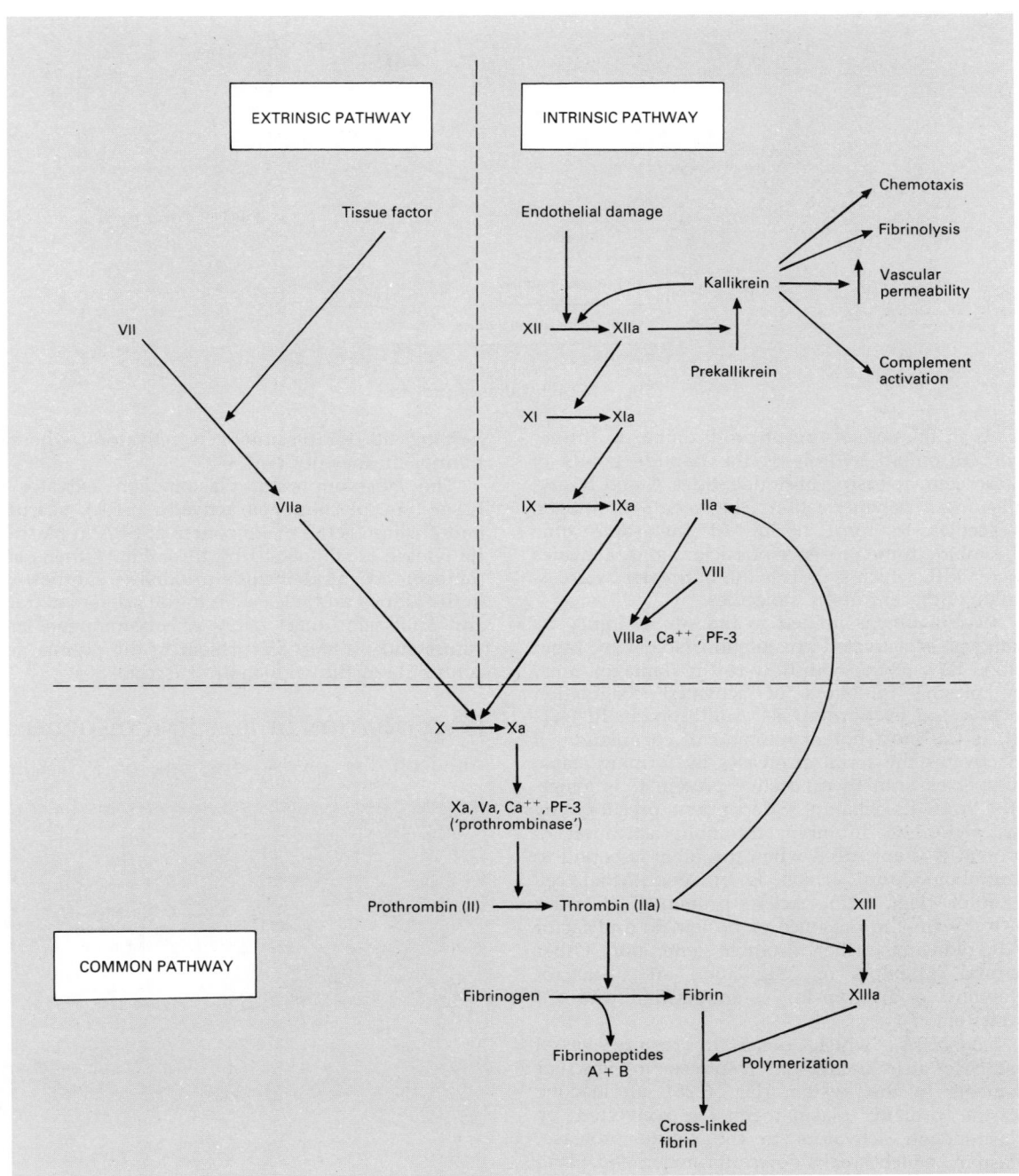

Fig. 6.24 Coagulation sequence.

factor XII and activation of the fibrinolytic pathway. Activated factor IX together with factor VIII, calcium ions and PF-3 activate factor X.

Factor VIII is a complex protein consisting of a small molecule with coagulant activity (VIII:C) and a larger part, von Willebrand factor (VIII:vWF), associated with platelet adhesion. VIII:vWF is a glycoprotein with a molecular weight of about 200 000. It readily forms multimers in the circulation with molecular weights of up to 20 million daltons. The high-molecular-weight multimeric forms of VIII:vWF are the most effective in producing platelet adhesion.

Common pathway. Activated factor X eventually

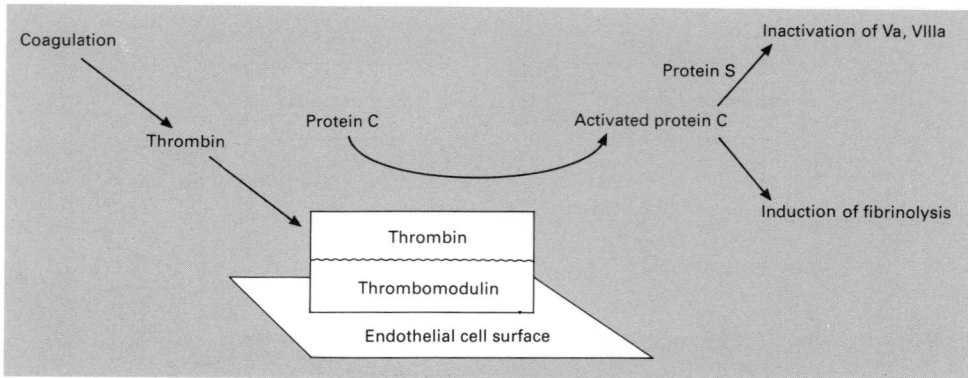

Fig. 6.25 Activation of protein C.

leads to the conversion of prothrombin to thrombin. Thrombin hydrolyses the peptide bonds of fibrinogen, releasing fibrinopeptides A and B, and allowing polymerization between fibrinogen molecules to form fibrin. At the same time thrombin, in the presence of calcium ions, activates factor XIII, which stabilizes the fibrin clot by cross-linking adjacent fibrin molecules.

Coagulation is limited to the site of injury by removal of activated coagulation factors by rapid blood flow at the periphery of the damaged area, by plasma inhibitors of activated coagulation factors and by fibrinolysis. Antithrombin III (AT-III) is the most potent inhibitor of coagulation; it inactivates the serine proteases by forming stable complexes with them. Active protein C is generated from its vitamin K-dependent precursor by the action of thrombin; thrombin activation of protein C is enhanced when thrombin is bound to thrombomodulin, which is an endothelial cell receptor (Fig. 6.25). Active protein C destroys factor V (in the presence of protein S) and factor VIII, reducing further thrombin generation. Other natural inhibitors of coagulation are α_2-macroglobulin, α_1-antitrypsin, α_1-antiplasmin and C1 inhibitor.

Fibrinolysis, which helps to restore vessel patency, also occurs in response to vascular damage. In this system (Fig. 6.26), an inactive plasma protein, plasminogen, is converted by plasminogen activators to the serine protease, plasmin, which breaks down fibrinogen and fibrin into fragments X, Y, D and E, collectively known as fibrin (and fibrinogen) degradation products (FDPs). Degradation of cross-linked fibrin also yields D-dimer and D-dimer-E fragments. Plasmin is also capable of breaking down coagulation factors such as factors V and VIII.

The fibrinolytic system is activated by the presence of fibrin. Plasminogen is specifically adsorbed to fibrin and fibrinogen by lysine-binding sites. However, little plasminogen activation occurs in the absence of fibrin, as fibrin also has a specific binding site for plasminogen activators, whereas fibrinogen does not (Fig. 6.27).

The most important plasminogen activator is tissue-type plasminogen activator (t-PA); vascular endothelium is the major source of t-PA in plasma. Its release is stimulated by thrombin. Other plasminogen activators include urokinase, synthesized in the kidney and released into the urogenital tract, and kallikrein. Inactivators of plasminogen activators and plasmin are present in the plasma and contribute to the regulation of fibrinolysis.

INVESTIGATION OF BLEEDING DISORDERS

Although the precise diagnosis of a bleeding

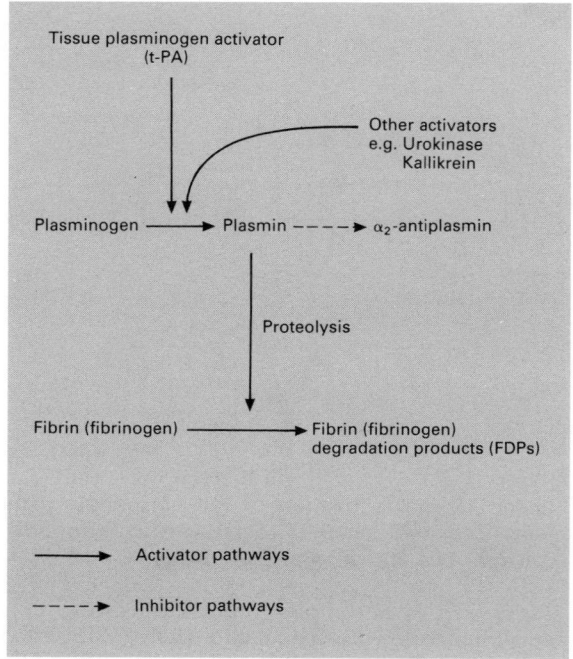

Fig. 6.26 Fibrinolytic system.

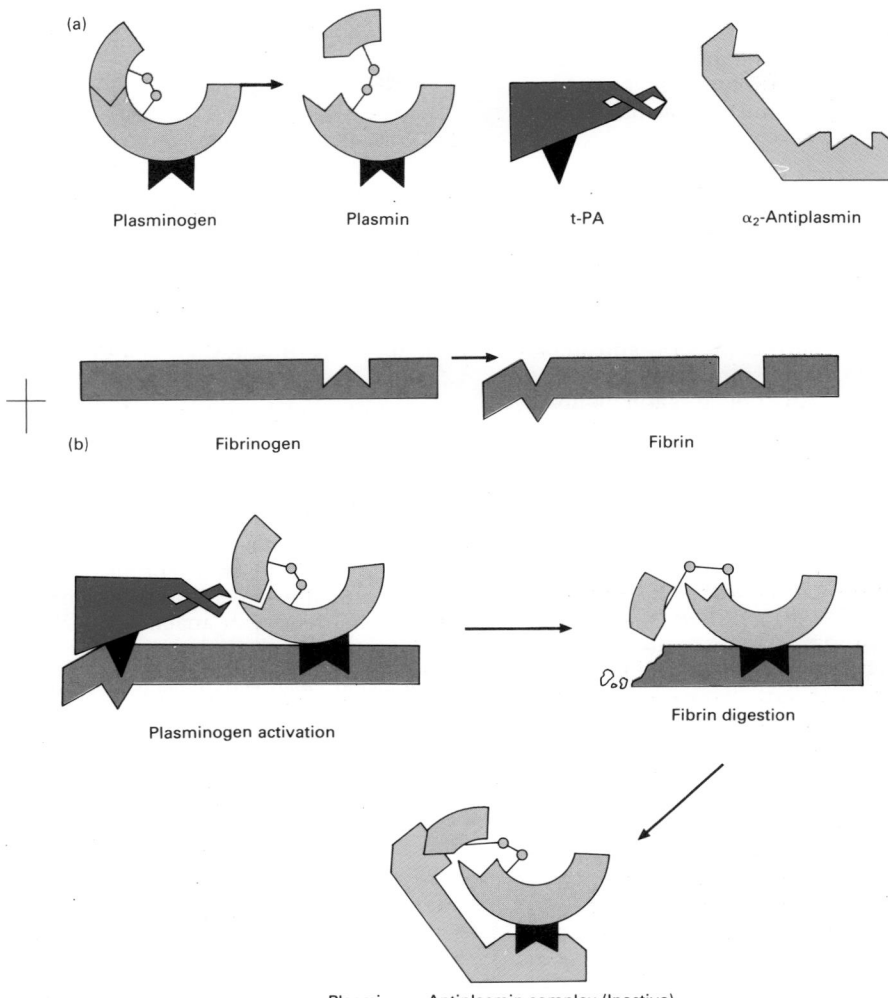

Fig. 6.27 (a) Diagrammatic representation of various factors involved in fibrinolysis. (b) The conversion of plasminogen to plasmin by plasminogen activator (t-PA) occurs most efficiently on the surface of fibrin which has binding sites for both plasminogen and t-PA. Free plasmin in the blood is rapidly inactivated by α_2-antiplasmin but plasmin generated on the fibrin surface is partially protected from inactivation. The lysine-binding sites on plasminogen (represented as ▼▼) are important for the inactivation between plasmin(ogen) and fibrin and between plasmin and α_2-antiplasmin. (Modified from Fibrinolysis by D. Collen in *Hemostasis and Thrombosis* (1985). Ed by Bowie EJW and Sharp AA. Butterworths.)

disorder may depend on laboratory tests, much information may be obtained from the history and physical examination, which should aim to determine the following:

- Is there a generalized haemostatic defect? Supportive evidence for this includes bleeding from multiple sites, spontaneous bleeding and bleeding into the skin.
- Is the defect inherited or acquired? A family history of a bleeding disorder should be sought. A severe inherited defect usually becomes

apparent in infancy, while in mild inherited defects there may be excessive bleeding after previous surgery, childbirth, dental extractions and trauma.
- Is the bleeding suggestive of a vascular/platelet defect or a coagulation defect? Vascular/platelet bleeding is characterized by easy bruising and spontaneous bleeding from small vessels. The bleeding is mainly into the skin (the term purpura includes both petechiae, which are small skin haemorrhages varying from pinpoint size to a few millimetres in diameter and which

do not blanch on pressure, and ecchymoses, which are small bruises) and from mucous membranes, often from the nose and mouth. Coagulation disorders are typically associated with haemarthroses and muscle haematomas.

LABORATORY INVESTIGATION

- The blood count and film show the number and morphology of platelets and any blood disorder such as leukaemia.
- The bleeding time measures platelet plug formation *in vivo*. It is determined by applying a sphygmomanometer cuff to the arm and inflating it to 40 mm Hg. Two 1 mm deep, 1 cm long incisions are made in the forearm with a template. Each wound is blotted every 30 s and the time taken for bleeding to stop is recorded, normally between 3 and 10 min. The Hess or capillary resistance test parallels the bleeding time but is unreliable and is not routinely used.
- Coagulation tests are performed using blood collected into citrate solution, which neutralizes calcium ions and prevents clotting.

The prothrombin time (PT) is measured by adding tissue thromboplastin in the form of animal brain extract and calcium to patient's plasma. The normal PT is 16–18 s and it is prolonged with abnormalities of either the extrinsic or common pathways (Fig. 6.24).

The partial thromboplastin time with kaolin (PTTK) is performed by adding a surface activator, kaolin, phospholipid (as platelet substitute) and calcium to patient's plasma. The normal PTTK is 30–50 s depending on the exact methodology, and it is prolonged with abnormalities of either the intrinsic or common pathways (Fig. 6.24).

The thrombin time (TT) is performed by adding thrombin to patient's plasma. The normal TT is 10–12 s, and it is prolonged with fibrinogen deficiency, dysfibrinogenaemia (normal level of fibrinogen but abnormal function) or inhibitors such as heparin or FDPs.

Prolonged times in the PT, PTTK and TT due to coagulation factor deficiencies may be corrected by addition of normal plasma to the patient's plasma; no correction of an abnormal result after the addition of normal plasma is suggestive of the presence of an inhibitor of coagulation.

Special tests of coagulation will often be required to confirm the precise haemostatic defect, including estimation of fibrinogen and FDPs, assays of coagulation factors, platelet function tests such as platelet aggregation and tests of the fibrinolytic pathway.

Vascular disorders

The vascular disorders, sometimes previously classified as non-thrombocytopenic purpuras, are characterized by easy bruising and bleeding into the skin. Bleeding from mucous membranes sometimes occurs but the bleeding is rarely severe. Laboratory investigations are normal apart from the bleeding time, which may occasionally be prolonged. The vascular disorders are shown in Table 6.22; they include the following.

Hereditary haemorrhagic telangiectasia. This is a rare disorder with autosomal dominant inheritance. Dilatation of capillaries and small arterioles produces characteristic small red spots that blanch on pressure in the skin and mucous membranes, particularly the nose and gastrointestinal tract. Recurrent epistaxis and chronic gastrointestinal bleeding are the major problems and may cause chronic iron-deficiency anaemia.

Easy bruising syndrome. This is a benign disorder occurring in otherwise healthy women. It is characterized by bruises on the arms, legs and trunk with minor trauma, possibly due to skin vessel fragility. It may give rise to the suspicion of a serious bleeding disorder.

Senile purpura and purpura due to steroids. These are both due to atrophy of the vascular supporting tissue.

Purpura due to infections. This is mainly due to damage to the vascular endothelium.

Henoch–Schonlein purpura. This usually occurs in children. It is a Type III hypersensitivity reaction that is often preceded by an acute upper respiratory tract infection. Purpura is mainly seen on the legs and buttocks. Abdominal pain, arthritis, haematuria and nephritis also occur. Recovery is usually spontaneous.

Factitial purpura. Episodes of inexplicable bleeding or bruising may represent abuse, either self-inflicted or caused by others. These various forms of artificial or factitious purpuras are often expressions of severe emotional or psychiatric disturbances.

Table 6.22 Vascular disorders.

Congenital
Hereditary haemorrhagic telangiectasia
  (Osler–Weber–Rendu disease)
Connective tissue disorders (Ehlers–Danlos
  syndrome, osteogenesis imperfecta,
  pseudoxanthoma elasticum, Marfan's syndrome)

Acquired
Severe infections:
  Septicaemia
  Meningococcal infections
  Measles
  Typhoid

Allergic
  Henoch–Schönlein purpura
  Connective tissue disorders (SLE, rheumatoid
    arthritis)

Drugs
  Steroids
  Sulphonamides

Others
  Senile purpura
  Easy bruising syndrome
  Scurvy
  Factitial purpura

Platelet disorders

Bleeding due to thrombocytopenia or abnormal platelet function is characterized by purpura and bleeding from mucous membranes. Bleeding is uncommon with platelet counts above 50×10^9/L, and severe spontaneous bleeding is unusual with platelet counts above 20×10^9/L.

THROMBOCYTOPENIA

This is caused by reduced platelet production in the bone marrow or excessive peripheral destruction of platelets (Table 6.23). A bone marrow aspirate to assess whether the numbers of megakaryocytes are reduced or normal/increased is an essential part of the investigation.

Idiopathic thrombocytopenic purpura (ITP)

Thrombocytopenia is due to immune destruction of platelets. The sensitized platelets are removed by the reticuloendothelial system. There are two distinct clinical syndromes.

Acute ITP is usually seen in children, often following a viral infection. Immune complex deposition on platelets with complement activation is probably responsible for the shortened platelet survival.

Chronic ITP is an autoimmune disorder, characteristically seen in adult women. Platelet autoantibodies are detected in about 60–70% of patients, and are presumed to be present, although not detectable, in the remaining patients.

CLINICAL FEATURES

Major haemorrhage is rare and is only seen in patients with severe thrombocytopenia. Easy bruising, purpura, epistaxis and menorrhagia are common.

Physical examination is normal except for evidence of bleeding. Splenomegaly is rare.

INVESTIGATION

The only blood count abnormality is thrombocytopenia. Normal or increased numbers of megakaryocytes are found in the bone marrow, which is otherwise normal. The detection of platelet anti-

Table 6.23 Causes of thrombocytopenia.

Impaired production
Generalized bone-marrow failure
  Leukaemia
  Aplastic anaemia
  Megaloblastic anaemia
  Myeloma
  Myelofibrosis
  Marrow infiltration by solid tumours

Selective reduction in megakaryocytes
  Drugs, e.g. co-trimoxazole
  Chemicals

Excessive destruction
Immune
  Idiopathic thrombocytopenic purpura
  Secondary immune thrombocytopenia (SLE, CLL,
    viral infections, drugs)
  Alloimmune neonatal thrombocytopenia
  Post-transfusion purpura

Coagulation
  Disseminated intravascular coagulation
  Thrombotic thrombocytopenic purpura
  Haemolytic uraemic syndrome (see p. 442)

Sequestration
Hypersplenism

Dilutional loss
Massive transfusion of stored blood

bodies is not essential for confirmation of the diagnosis, which often depends on exclusion of other causes of excessive destruction of platelets.

TREATMENT

Acute ITP in children usually remits spontaneously. It is still not clear whether treatment in the acute phase with steroids or high-dose intravenous immunoglobulin is effective in minimizing the period of thrombocytopenia or in reducing the incidence of chronic ITP, which develops in 5–10% of children.

Spontaneous remissions are rare in chronic ITP. The main aims of treatment are to reduce the production of platelet autoantibodies and the removal of antibody-coated platelets. Initial treatment is with prednisolone, 40–60 mg daily in adults with cautious reduction of the dose after remission has occurred.

Twenty per cent of patients have a complete response and require no further treatment; 60% have a partial response, and half of these have little bleeding associated with mild or moderate thrombocytopenia (platelet count 30–100 $\times$ 10^9/L) and may require small doses of steroids, prednisolone 5–15 mg daily, or no further treatment. The other half of the partial responders eventually relapse and require splenectomy, as do the 20% of patients who failed to respond to steroids at all.

Splenectomy should be avoided in young children because of the subsequent risk of severe pneumococcal infection (see p. 328). There is a 90% response rate to splenectomy, although about 30% of responders eventually relapse. Some of these refractory patients may respond to immunosuppressive drugs such as azathioprine, cyclophosphamide or vincristine or to danazol, which is a non-virilizing androgen.

Intravenous infusion of high-dose immunoglobin produces a rapid rise in platelet count owing to blocking of Fc receptors in the spleen. The increase in platelet count is usually transient but may be useful in preparing patients with chronic ITP for surgery.

Transfused platelets survive no longer than the patient's own platelets but may sometimes be beneficial in patients with life-threatening bleeding.

Other immune thrombocytopenias

Platelet autoantibodies causing thrombocytopenia may often be associated with other autoimmune disorders such as SLE, thyroid disease, rheumatoid arthritis and haemolytic anaemia (Evans' syndrome). Autoimmune thrombocytopenia also occurs in patients with chronic lymphocytic leukaemia and solid tumours, and in association with viral infections, especially in children; it is a feature of infection with HIV.

Drugs cause immune thrombocytopenia by the same mechanisms as described for drug-induced immune haemolytic anaemia (p. 321). The same drugs may be responsible for immune haemolytic anaemia, thrombocytopenia or neutropenia in different patients; it is not known what determines the target cell in each case.

Alloimmune neonatal thrombocytopenia is due to fetomaternal incompatibility for platelet-specific antigens, usually Pl^{A1}, and is the platelet equivalent of haemolytic disease of the newborn. Thrombocytopenia is self-limiting after delivery, but platelet transfusions may be required to prevent or treat bleeding associated with severe thrombocytopenia; platelet donors may either be Pl^{A1}-negative volunteers or the mother (whose platelets lack the Pl^{A1} antigen). Recently, it has been recognized that severe bleeding such as intracranial haemorrhage may occur *in utero*.

Post-transfusion purpura (PTP) is rare, occurring 2–12 days after a blood transfusion. It is associated with a platelet-specific alloantibody, usually anti-Pl^{A1} in a Pl^{A1}-negative individual who has been previously immunized by pregnancy or blood transfusion. The cause of the platelet destruction is uncertain. PTP is self-limiting but high-dose IgG may limit the period of thrombocytopenia.

Platelet function disorders

These are usually associated with excessive bruising and bleeding and, in some of the acquired forms, with thrombosis. The platelet count is normal or increased and the bleeding time is prolonged. The rare inherited defects of platelet function require more detailed investigations such as platelet aggregation studies and factor VIII:C and VIII:vWF assays, if von Willebrand's disease is suspected.

Acquired forms of platelet dysfunction include:

- Myeloproliferative disorders
- Uraemia and liver disease
- Paraproteinaemias
- Drugs, e.g. aspirin and dipyridamole

Treatment depends on managing the underlying disease and platelet transfusions may be required for bleeding. The use of desmopressin (DDAVP) may be helpful for bleeding associated with uraemia and liver disease.

Coagulation disorders

Coagulation disorders may be inherited or acquired. The inherited disorders are uncommon and

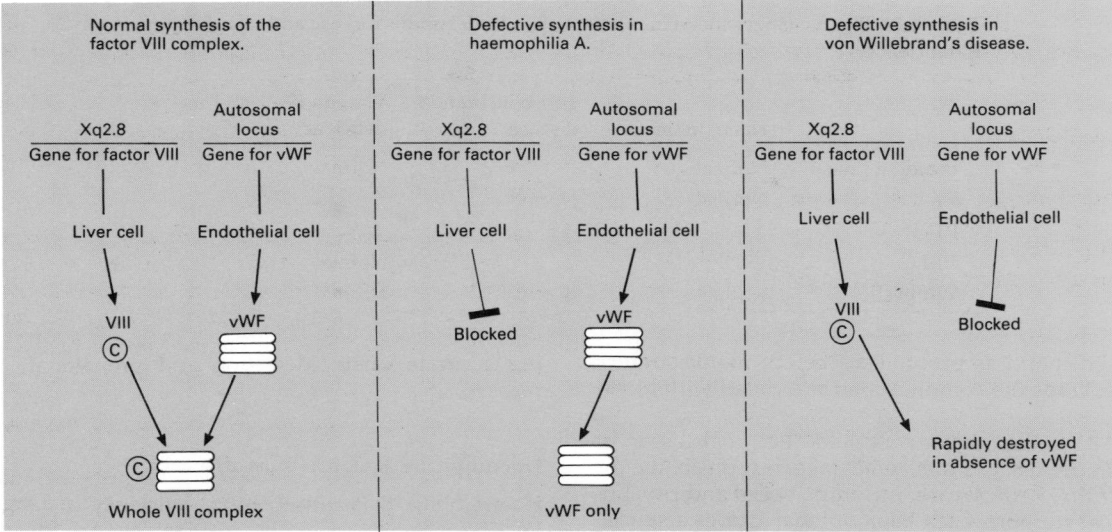

Fig. 6.28 Normal factor VIII synthesis and defective synthesis in Haemophilia A and von Willebrand's disease. (Modified from Tuddenham EGD (1984) The varieties of von Willebrand's disease. *Clinical and Laboratory Haematology* **6**, 307–323, with permission.)

usually involve deficiency of one factor only. The acquired disorders occur more frequently and almost always involve several coagulation factors.

INHERITED COAGULATION DISORDERS

Deficiencies of all factors have been described, but 90% are due to factor VIII deficiency.

Haemophilia A

In haemophilia A, the level of factor VIII:C is reduced but the level of factor VIII:vWF is normal (Fig. 6.28). It is inherited as an X-linked recessive. The incidence of haemophilia A varies from 1 in 5000 to 1 in 10 000 of the male population.

The human factor VIII gene was cloned in 1984. The gene is enormous, constituting about 0.1% of the X chromosome, encompassing 190 kilobases of DNA. Various genetic defects have been found, including deletions, point mutations and insertions. There is a high mutation rate with one third of cases being apparently sporadic.

CLINICAL FEATURES

The clinical features depend on the level of factor VIII:C. Levels of less than 1% are associated with frequent spontaneous bleeding from early life. Haemarthroses are common and may lead to joint deformity and crippling if adequate treatment is not given. Bleeds into muscles are also common.

Levels of less than 5% are associated with severe bleeding following injury and occasional spontaneous episodes, and levels above 5% with milder disease usually with post-traumatic bleeding only.

LABORATORY FEATURES

The main laboratory features of haemophilia A are shown in Table 6.24. The abnormal findings are a prolonged PTTK and a reduced level of factor VIII:C; the PT, bleeding time and factor VIII:vWF level are normal.

TREATMENT

Bleeding is treated by administration of factor VIII concentrate by intravenous injection. For minor bleeding the factor VIII level should be raised to 20–30% of normal, and for severe bleeding episodes it should be raised to at least 50%. For major surgery the level should be raised to 100% preoperatively and maintained above 50% until healing has occurred.

Factor VIII has a half-life of 12 h and therefore must be administered twice daily to maintain the required therapeutic level. Factor VIII concentrate may be stored in domestic refrigerators and so may be given immediately after bleeding has started, reducing the likelihood of chronic damage to joints and the need for inpatient care. Cryoprecipitate is an alternative source of factor VIII but the risk of infection is higher than with factor VIII concentrates; it is not as convenient to use because it is bulky and needs to be stored frozen. Factor VIII:C produced by genetic engineering is undergoing clinical trials.

DDAVP (i.v.) produces a rise in factor VIII. It is useful in mild haemophiliacs for treating bleeding

Table 6.24 Blood changes in haemophilia A, von Willebrand's disease and vitamin K deficiency.

	Haemophilia A	von Willebrand's disease	Vitamin K deficiency
Bleeding time	Normal	↑	Normal
PT	Normal	Normal	↑
PTTK	↑ +	↑ ±	↑
VIII:C	↓ + +	↓	Normal
VIII:vWF	Normal	↓	Normal

episodes and as prophylaxis before minor surgery and avoids the complications associated with blood products.

All haemophiliacs should be registered at Haemophilia Centres, who take responsibility for their full medical care, including social and psychological support. Each haemophiliac carries a special medical card giving details of the defect and treatment.

COMPLICATIONS

About 10% of severe haemophiliacs develop antibodies to factor VIII:C. Inhibitors develop almost exclusively in patients with no detectable VIII:C. Management of such patients may be very difficult, and extremely high doses of factor VIII may be needed to produce a rise in the plasma level of factor VIII:C. Alternative treatment includes purified porcine factor VIII, which may not cross-react with the patient's antibody, and prothrombin complex concentrates containing activated factor X, which may 'bypass' the inhibitor and stop bleeding. Following numerous transfusions there is a high risk of acquiring transfusion-transmitted infections, particularly hepatitis and HIV. The risk has been reduced by excluding high-risk blood donors, testing all donations for hepatitis B surface antigen and anti-HIV, and by heat treatment of plasma.

Carrier detection
Determination of carrier status in females requires detailed information from the family history, results of coagulation factor assays and DNA analysis. Antenatal diagnosis may be carried out by DNA analysis of fetal tissue obtained by chorionic villus biopsy at 9–11 weeks' gestation. Since each family with haemophilia A usually has a different mutation in the factor VIII gene, it is almost impossible to identify directly the molecular defect using restriction endonuclease analysis. However, indirect detection of the abnormal gene can be achieved using DNA polymorphisms as markers within or adjacent to the factor VIII gene, providing accurate carrier detection and prenatal diagnosis.

Haemophilia B (Christmas disease)

Haemophilia B is caused by a deficiency of factor IX. The inheritance and clinical features are identical to haemophilia A, but the incidence is only about 1 : 30 000 males. It is treated with factor IX concentrates.

von Willebrand's disease (vWD)

In vWD, there is defective platelet function as well as factor VIII:C deficiency and both are due to a deficiency or abnormality of factor VIII:vWF (Fig. 6.28). Factor VIII:vWF plays a role in platelet adhesion to damaged subendothelium as well as stabilizing factor VIII:C in plasma. Inheritance is autosomal, usually dominant. The VIII:vWF gene is on chromosome 12.

The clinical features of vWD are usually less severe than those of haemophilia. Bleeding follows minor trauma or surgery and epistaxis and menorrhagia often occur. Haemarthroses are rare.

Characteristic laboratory findings are shown in Table 6.24, and also include defective platelet aggregation with ristocetin.

Treatment depends on the severity of the condition and may be similar to that of mild haemophilia, including the use of DDAVP for minor surgery. Factor VIII concentrates should be used to treat bleeding or to cover surgery in patients with more severe vWD.

ACQUIRED COAGULATION DISORDERS

Vitamin K deficiency

Vitamin K is necessary for the γ-carboxylation of glutamic acid residues on factors II, VII, IX and X; without it, these factors cannot bind calcium and form complexes with PF-3 to exert their coagulant effect.

Deficiency of vitamin K may be due to:

- Inadequate stores, as in haemorrhagic disease of the newborn and protein–energy malnutrition (see p. 155).
- Malabsorption of vitamin K, which particularly occurs in cholestatic jaundice as it is a fat-soluble vitamin.
- Oral anticoagulant drugs, which are vitamin K antagonists.

The PT and PTTK are prolonged (Table 6.24) and there may be bruising, haematuria and gastro-intestinal or cerebral bleeding. Minor bleeding is treated with phytomenadione (vitamin K₁) 10 mg subcutaneously. Some correction of the PT is usual within 6 h but it may not return to normal for 2 days. Severe or prolonged bleeding should be treated by transfusion of fresh frozen plasma for immediate replacement of coagulation factors. Vitamin K deficiency occurs in neonates, and premature infants may have severe deficiency causing bleeding; many centres give prophylactic vitamin K to all neonates, whereas at others it is only given to premature infants.

Liver disease

Liver disease may result in a number of defects in haemostasis:

- Vitamin K deficiency due to intra- or extra-hepatic cholestasis.
- Reduced synthesis of coagulation factors due to severe hepatocellular damage. The use of vita-min K does not improve the results of abnormal coagulation tests, but it is generally given because of the accompanying malabsorption.
- Thrombocytopenia may result from hypersplen-ism due to splenomegaly associated with portal hypertension.
- Functional abnormalities of platelets and fibrino-gen are found in many patients with liver failure.
- Disseminated intravascular coagulation may occur in acute liver failure.

Disseminated intravascular coagulation (DIC)

There is widespread generation of fibrin within blood vessels, due to activation of the extrinsic pathway by release of coagulant material, activa-tion of the intrinsic pathway by diffuse endothelial damage or generalized platelet aggregation. There is consumption of platelets and coagulation factors and secondary activation of fibrinolysis leading to production of FDPs, which may contribute to the coagulation defect by inhibiting fibrin polymeriza-tion (Fig. 6.29).

CAUSES

These are numerous and include septicaemia, disseminated malignant disease, haemolytic trans-fusion reactions, obstetric conditions such as abruptio placentae and amniotic fluid embolism, falciparum malaria and snake bites.

CLINICAL FEATURES

The underlying disorder is usually obvious. The patient is often acutely ill and shocked. The clinical presentation of DIC varies from no bleeding at all to complete haemostatic failure with widespread haemorrhage. Bleeding may occur from the mouth, nose and venepuncture sites and there may be widespread ecchymoses.

Thrombotic events may occur as a result of vessel occlusion by fibrin and platelets; any organ may be involved but the skin and kidneys are most often affected.

INVESTIGATIONS

The diagnosis is often suggested by the underlying condition of the patient. In severe cases with haemorrhage, the PT, PTTK and TT are usually very prolonged and the fibrinogen level markedly

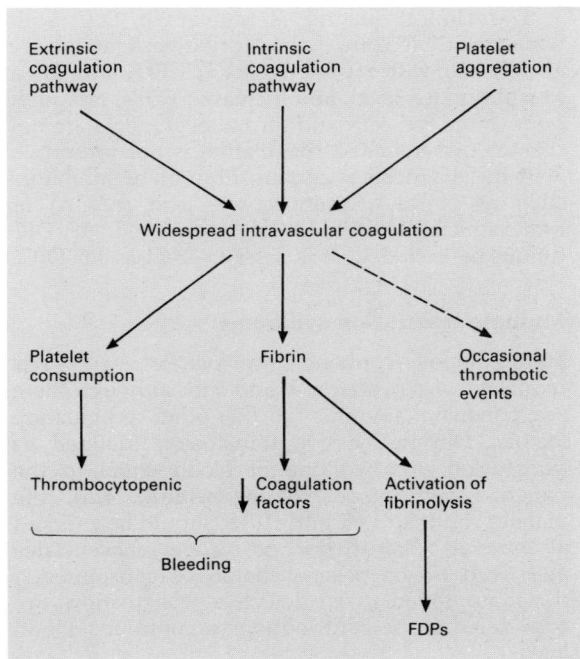

Fig. 6.29 Disseminated intravascular coagulation (DIC). FDP, fibrin degradation products.

reduced. High levels of FDPs are found. There is severe thrombocytopenia and the blood film may show fragmented red blood cells. In mild cases without bleeding, increased synthesis of coagulation factors and platelets may result in normal PT, PTTK, TT and platelet counts, although FDPs will be raised.

TREATMENT

Treatment of the underlying condition is most important and may be all that is necessary in non-bleeding patients. Transfusions of platelet concentrates, fresh frozen plasma and red cell concentrates may be indicated in patients with bleeding. The use of heparin to prevent intravascular coagulation remains controversial but it is now rarely given. Inhibitors of fibrinolysis such as tranexamic acid should not be used in DIC as dangerous fibrin deposition may result.

Excessive fibrinolysis

Activation of fibrinolysis occurs in DIC as a secondary event in response to intravascular deposition of fibrin. Primary hyperfibrinolysis is very rare. It may occur during surgery involving tumours of the prostate, breast, pancreas and uterus owing to release of tissue plasminogen activators.

The clinical picture is similar to DIC with widespread bleeding. Laboratory investigations are also similar with a prolonged PT, PTTK and TT, a low fibrinogen level, and increased FDPs, although fragmented red cells and thrombocytopenia are not seen as disseminated coagulation is not present.

If the diagnosis is certain, fibrinolytic inhibitors such as episolon aminocaproic acid (eACA) or tranexamic acid should be considered. If DIC cannot be excluded, it is safer to treat as for DIC.

Multiple transfusion syndrome

Stored blood contains few platelets and has reduced levels of factors V and VIII, although there are adequate amounts of the other coagulation factors. During massive transfusion (defined as transfusion of a volume of blood equal to the patient's own blood volume within 24 h), the platelet count and PT and PTTK should be checked at intervals. Transfusion of platelet concentrates and fresh frozen plasma should be considered if thrombocytopenia or defective coagulation are considered to be contributing to continued blood loss.

Inhibitors of coagulation

In addition to the factor VIII:C alloantibodies that

arise in a proportion of severe haemophiliacs, factor VIII:C autoantibodies occasionally arise in patients with autoimmune disorders such as systemic lupus erythamatosus and after childbirth. Severe bleeding may occur. The antibodies may disappear spontaneously but treatment such as plasmapheresis and immunosuppressive drugs may be required.

Lupus anticoagulants are IgG autoantibodies directed against phospholipids. They are found in about 10% of patients with SLE and may also occur in otherwise healthy individuals. They lead to prolongation of phospholipid-dependent coagulation tests, particularly the PTTK, but do not inhibit coagulation factor activity and therefore bleeding does not occur unless there is co-existent severe immune thrombocytopenia. The main clinical problems are thrombosis, perhaps due to platelet activation due to inhibition of prostacyclin, and recurrent abortion.

Thrombosis

A thrombus is defined as a solid mass formed in the circulation from the constituents in the blood. Fragments of thrombi (emboli) may break off and block vessels downstream. Thromboembolic disease is much more common than abnormal bleeding; nearly half of adult deaths in England and Wales are due to coronary artery thrombosis, cerebral artery thrombosis or pulmonary embolism.

A thrombus results from a complex series of events involving coagulation factors, platelets, red blood cells and the vessel wall.

Arterial thrombosis

This is usually the result of atheroma, which tends to form in areas of turbulent blood flow such as at the bifurcation of arteries. Platelets adhere to the damaged vascular endothelium and aggregate in response to ADP and TXA_2 to form a 'white thrombus'. The growth of the platelet thrombus is limited at its margins by PGI_2. Eventually blood coagulation may be activated at the site of the thrombus, resulting either in complete occlusion of the vessel or embolization that produces distal obstruction.

The risk factors in arterial thrombosis are related to the development of atherosclerosis (p. 622).

Arterial thrombi may form in the heart, from mural thrombi in the left ventricle after myocardial infarction, from the left atrium in mitral valve disease or from the surfaces of prosthetic valves.

Venous thrombosis

Unlike arterial thrombosis, venous thrombosis often occurs in normal vessels. Important causes are stasis and hypercoagulability. The majority of venous thrombi occur in the deep veins of the leg, originating around the valves as 'red thrombi' consisting mainly of red cells and fibrin. The propagating thrombus is formed of fibrin and platelets and is particularly liable to embolize. Chronic venous obstruction in the deep veins of the leg results in a permanently swollen limb and may lead to ulceration (post-phlebitic syndrome).

Risk factors for venous thrombosis include increasing age, obesity, immobility, past history or family history of venous thrombosis, varicose veins, malignancy, surgery, pregnancy and oestrogen therapy or contraceptive medication. Inherited deficiencies of natural inhibitors of coagulation such as AT-III, protein C and protein S are associated with venous thrombosis (see below). Both arterial and venous thrombosis may also occur with changes in blood cells such as polycythaemia, thrombocythaemia and sickle cell anaemia.

The clinical features and diagnosis of venous thrombosis are discussed on p. 625.

Thrombophilia

Thrombophilia is a term describing inherited or acquired defects of haemostasis leading to a predisposition to venous or arterial thrombosis. It should be considered in patients with recurrent venous thrombosis, venous thrombosis for the first time under 40, a family history of venous thrombosis, an unusual venous thrombosis such as mesenteric vein thrombosis, neonatal thrombosis, recurrent abortion and in patients with arterial thrombosis in the absence of arterial disease.

Laboratory investigation of such patients includes a full blood count including platelet count, coagulation screen including a fibrinogen level and screen for a coagulation factor inhibitor including a lupus anticoagulant, assays for coagulation inhibitors such as AT-III, protein C and protein S, and tests of the fibrinolytic pathway including assays for plasminogen, t-PA and plasminogen-activator inhibitors.

Prevention and treatment of arterial thrombosis

Attempts to reduce arterial thrombosis should be mainly directed at minimizing factors predisposing to atherosclerosis.

Anti-platelet drugs

Platelet activation at the site of vascular damage is crucial to the development of arterial thrombosis,

Table 6.25 Drugs used in the treatment of thrombotic disorders.

Antiplatelet drugs	Aspirin
	Dipyridamole
	Ticlopidine
Thrombolytic therapy	Streptokinase
	Anisoylated plasminogen streptokinase activator complex (APSAC or antistreplase)
	Urokinase
	Single-chain urokinase-type plasminogen activator (scu-PA)
	Tissue-type plasminogen activator (t-PA or alteplase)
Anticoagulant drugs	Heparin
	Warfarin

and this can be altered by the following drugs (Table 6.25):

- *Aspirin* inhibits the enzyme cyclo-oxygenase (Fig. 6.23) and this results in reduced platelet production of thromboxane A_2.
- *Dipyridamole*, which inhibits platelet phosphodiesterase causing an increase in cyclic AMP with potentiation of the action of prostacyclin, has been widely used as an antithrombotic agent but there is little evidence that it is effective.
- *Ticlopidine* inhibits platelet aggregation induced by adenosine diphosphate, collagen and adrenaline. It has no effect on cyclic AMP.

The indications for and results of anti-platelet therapy are discussed in the appropriate sections.

Thrombolytic therapy

Streptokinase is a purified fraction of the filtrate obtained from cultures of haemolytic streptococci. It forms a 1 : 1 complex with plasminogen, resulting in a conformational change in plasminogen. An active site is revealed in plasminogen and this activates other plasminogen molecules to form plasmin. Streptokinase is given i.v. or as an infusion.

A disadvantage of streptokinase is its indiscriminate activation of plasminogen so that both fibrin in clots and free fibrinogen are lysed, leading to low fibrinogen levels and the risk of haemorrhage.

Anisoylated plasminogen streptokinase activator complex (APSAC) is a complex of plasminogen and an anisoylated form of streptokinase. The complex binds to any fibrin within intravascular clots where the anisoyl group is hydrolysed and the streptokinase–plasminogen complex produces fibrinolysis. The advantage of APSAC over streptokinase is its more sustained duration of action and it is given as a single bolus dose.

Urokinase is produced naturally by the kidney. It cleaves plasminogen directly to produce plasmin.

Tissue-type plasminogen activator (t-PA) and *single-chain urokinase-type plasminogen activator (scu-PA)* are produced using recombinant gene technology. They are relatively 'clot-specific', i.e. they have a greater affinity for fibrin-bound plasminogen than circulating plasminogen, although the use of these thrombolytic agents has not yet been proved to produce fewer bleeding episodes than streptokinase.

Indications and results of the use of thrombolytic therapy in myocardial infarction are discussed on p. 579.

The main risk of thrombolytic therapy is bleeding and treatment should not be given to patients who have had recent bleeding, uncontrolled hypertension or a stroke, or surgery or other invasive procedures within the previous 10 days.

PREVENTION AND TREATMENT OF VENOUS THROMBOSIS

Venous thromboembolism is a common problem after surgery, particularly in high-risk patients such as elderly patients and those with malignant disease. The incidence is also high in patients confined to bed following trauma, myocardial infarction or other illnesses.

Prophylactic measures are aimed at methods for preventing stasis, such as elevation of the legs, compression stockings, calf-muscle stimulation and passive calf-muscle exercises during surgery, and early mobilization and methods for preventing hypercoagulability, usually using low-dose heparin. Low-dose heparin is given at a dose of 5000 units subcutaneously every 8 or 12 h until the patient is ambulatory; no laboratory monitoring is required. Some operations such as hip arthroplasty are associated with a very high risk of venous thrombosis and a combined approach such as low-dose heparin and compression stockings or alternative approaches may be considered such as low-dose anticoagulation with warfarin or higher doses of subcutaneous heparin to keep the PTTK at between 1.25 and 1.5 times the control value.

Anticoagulant treatment aims to prevent further thrombosis and pulmonary embolization while resolution of venous thrombi occurs by natural fibrinolytic activity. Six weeks' anticoagulation is sufficient for patients after their first thrombosis as long as there are no persisting risk factors. Long-term treatment should be considered in patients with repeated episodes or continuing risk factors.

Heparin is not a single substance but a mixture of polysaccharides. Commercially available unfractionated heparin consists of components with molecular weights varying from 3000 to 40 000 daltons and an average of about 15 000. It was extracted initially from liver, hence its name, but it is now prepared from hog gastric mucosa or beef lung.

It has an immediate effect on coagulation by potentiation of the formation of irreversible complexes between AT-III and activated serine protease coagulation factors (thrombin, XIIa, XIa, Xa, IXa and VIIa).

For treatment of established thrombosis, an intravenous loading dose of 10 000 units is given followed by a continuous infusion of 20 000 to 30 000 units daily to prolong the PTTK to between 1.5 and 2.5 times the control value. It has been shown recently that a satisfactory alternative is subcutaneous heparin given twice daily, beginning with a dose of 15 000 units, and then adjusting the dose to maintain the PTTK at the same level as for the intravenous route. There is no evidence that it is necessary to use heparin for any longer than it takes for simultaneously administered warfarin to produce an anticoagulant effect, usually about 3–4 days.

The main complication is bleeding. This is managed by stopping heparin. Very occasionally it is necessary to neutralize heparin with protamine. Other complications include osteoporosis with prolonged therapy and thrombocytopenia.

Attempts have been made to find heparin derivatives with a maintained or improved efficacy but with a reduced risk of bleeding. There has been interest in the use of low-molecular-weight heparins because of initial observations that they had little effect on tests of overall coagulation, such as the PTTK, but maintain their potency in more specific assays e.g. anti-factor Xa assays. Clinical trials to date suggest that, although low-molecular-weight heparins are as effective as unfractionated heparin in preventing post-operative thromboses, they are no safer. However, it is likely that new heparins will be developed over the next few years and make its administration easier and less hazardous.

Oral anticoagulants. These act by interfering with

vitamin K metabolism. There are two types of oral anticoagulants, the coumarins and indanediones. The coumarin warfarin is most commonly used because it has a low incidence of side-effects other than bleeding.

The dosage is controlled by PT tests. Thromboplastin reagents for PT testing are derived from a variety of sources and give different PT results for the same plasma. It is now standard practice to compare each thromboplastin with an international reference preparation so that they can be assigned an international sensitivity index (ISI). The international normalized ratio (INR) is the ratio of the patient's PT to a normal control when using the international reference preparation. Most manufacturers supply a chart adapted to the ISI of their thromboplastin to convert the patient's PT to the INR. The use of this system means that PT tests on a given plasma sample using different thromboplastins result in the same INR and that anticoagulant control is comparable in different hospitals across the world.

The following therapeutic ranges for oral anticoagulant control have been proposed by the British Society for Haematology.

INR	Clinical state
2.0–2.5	Prophylaxis of deep venous thrombosis including high-risk surgery. INR 2.0–3.0 for hip surgery and operations for fractured femur.
2.0–3.0	Treatment for deep venous thrombosis, pulmonary embolism and transient ischaemic attacks.
3.0–4.5	Recurrent deep venous thrombosis and pulmonary embolism; arterial disease including myocardial infarction; arterial grafts; cardiac prosthetic valves and grafts.

The initial dose of warfarin is usually 5 or 10 mg for the first 2–3 days, and maintenance doses are usually 1–10 mg daily. The PT is measured daily for the first few days until stability is achieved, and after this the maximum interval between tests is 8 weeks. Outpatient anticoagulation is best supervised in Anticoagulant Clinics.

Contraindications to the use of oral anticoagulants are seldom absolute; they include severe hypertension, non-embolic strokes, peptic ulceration, pregnancy, severe liver and renal disease and a pre-existing haemostatic defect.

Many drugs interact with warfarin (see Chapter 14). More frequent PT testing should accompany changes in medication, which should occur with the full knowledge of the Anticoagulant Clinic. An *increased anticoagulant effect* is usually produced by drugs causing a reduction in the metabolism of warfarin such as tricyclic antidepressants, cimetidine, sulphonamides, phenothiazines and amiodarone and by drugs (such as clofibrate) that increase the sensitivity to the amount of warfarin already present at its site of action. Drugs interfering with vitamin K absorption (such as broadspectrum antibiotics and cholestyramine) may also potentiate the action of warfarin. The displacement of warfarin from its binding site on serum albumin by other drugs is not responsible for clinically important interactions. Drugs that inhibit platelet function (such as aspirin) increase the risk of bleeding. Alcohol excess, cardiac failure, liver or renal disease, thyrotoxicosis and febrile illnesses may result in potentiation of the effect of warfarin. *A decreased anticoagulant effect* is usually produced by drugs that increase the clearance of warfarin by induction of hepatic enzymes that metabolize warfarin, such as rifampicin and barbiturates.

Side-effects of warfarin other than bleeding are rare. A prolonged PT without bleeding may be managed by withholding warfarin for 1–2 days and consideration of the use of a small dose of vitamin K (1 mg intravenously), which will not make the patient resistant to further warfarin therapy for more than a few days. If there is bleeding, rapid reversal of the anticoagulant effect may be achieved by transfusion of fresh frozen plasma. The cause of the loss of anticoagulant control should be determined. Bleeding from single sites, e.g. haematuria and rectal bleeding, during periods of adequate anticoagulant control should be investigated in the usual way to exclude local lesions.

The role of *thrombolytic therapy* in the treatment of venous thrombosis is not established. It is sometimes used in patients with massive pulmonary embolism and in patients with extensive deep venous thrombi.

For these conditions it is necessary to give a bolus dose of streptokinase, 250 000 units over 30 min to inactivate antibodies formed by previous streptococcal infection followed by a continuous infusion, approximately 100 000 units every hour, for 24–72 hours. The dose of streptokinase is adjusted to maintain the TT between 2–4 times the control value.

Thrombolytic therapy should be followed by anticoagulation (see below) with heparin for a few days and then by oral anticoagulants for a few months to prevent rethrombosis.

Further reading

Beck WS (1985) *Hematology*, 4th edn. Cambridge, Massachusetts: MIT Press.

Bloom AL & Thomas DP (1987) *Haemostasis and Thrombosis*, 2nd edn. Edinburgh: Churchill Livingstone.

Bothwell TH, Charlton RW, Cook JD & Finch EA (1980) *Iron Metabolism in Man*. Oxford: Blackwell Scientific.

Chanarin I (1990) *The Megablastic Anaemias*, 3rd edn. Oxford: Blackwell Scientific.

Dacie JV (1985) *The Haemolytic Anaemias*, 3rd edn (volumes 1 & 2). Edinburgh: Churchill Livingstone.

Firkin F, Chesterman C, Pennington D, & Rush B (eds) (1989) *de Gruchy's Clinical Haematology in Medical Practice*, 5th edn. Oxford: Blackwell Scientific.

Mollison PL, Engelfret CP, & Contreras M (1987) *Blood Transfusion in Clinical Medicine*, 8th edn. Oxford: Blackwell Scientific.

Weatherall DJ & Clegg JB (1981) *The Thalassaemia Syndromes*, 3rd edn. Oxford: Blackwell Scientific.

Williams WJ, Beutler E, Erslev AJ, & Lichtman MA (1990) *Hematology*, 4th edn. New York: McGraw-Hill.

7

Medical Oncology

Introduction

Cancer is a widely prevalent disease and is second only to cardiovascular disease as a cause of death in Western countries. Our increasing knowledge of cellular biology has opened up a new era of cancer research. Unfortunately, to date, this has not had a major impact on therapy. The management of cancer frequently involves more than one specialist, including the surgeon, radiotherapist and medical oncologist.

Aetiology and epidemiology

A wide variety of factors have been identified as being associated with cancer, but in the vast majority of commonly occurring neoplasms a single cause has not been defined. Table 7.1 shows a list of possible factors; their role in producing cancers is discussed in the appropriate chapters. It is very likely that more than one factor is involved in tumour induction; for example, it has been shown that asbestos and cigarette smoking are synergistic in the causation lung cancer.

The changing incidence of three major cancers is shown in Fig. 7.1. The increase in lung cancer is directly related to the number of cigarettes smoked. The reason for the decline in stomach cancer is unknown.

Table 7.1 Possible factors in the causation of cancer.

Inheritance
Abnormal gene (e.g. dominant inheritance in retinoblastoma)

Environmental
Smoking
Ionizing radiation
Drugs—alkylating agents
Diet—aflatoxins
Alcohol
Occupation and chemicals (see Table 7.3)
Viruses

Geographical factors
Geographical factors may play a part in determining the incidence of cancer. Scotland, England and Wales have the highest death rate from cancer in the world, largely as a result of the contribution made by carcinoma of the bronchus. Table 7.2 shows the variation in incidence of different tumours related to their geographical site. An example is the very high incidence of liver cancer (hepatoma) seen in parts of Mozambique; this has been traced to the ingestion of a toxic material called aflatoxin, which is formed by a mould on the groundnuts that form part of the diet.

Clustering of certain malignancies may give vital clues as to the aetiology of the condition. For example, the T-cell leukaemia described in the southern part of Japan and in the West Indies has been shown to be associated with the virus HTLV-1.

Occupational factors
The first description of occupation playing a role in the development of cancer was by Percival Pott in 1775, who described scrotal epitheliomas in young chimney sweeps. The tumour was subsequently shown to be associated with carcinogenic hydrocarbons in soot and poor personal hygiene. A list of some of the most important industrially related cancers is given in Table 7.3.

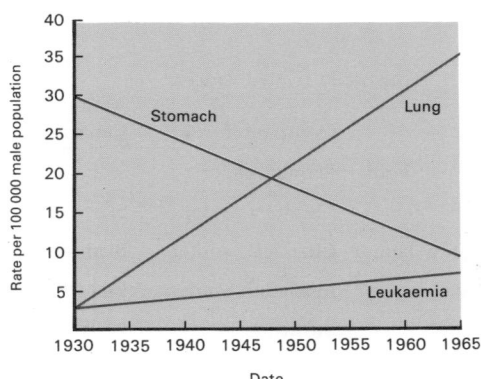

Fig. 7.1 The changing incidences of three major cancers.

Table 7.2 Variations in cancer incidence.

Types of primary cancer	Ratio of incidences	High incidence area	Low incidence area
Liver	1000 : 1	Lourenço Marques Mozambique	Birmingham, UK
Oesophagus	200 : 1	Ghurjen in Kazakhstan	Netherlands
Nasopharynx	100 : 1	Chinese in Singapore	Chile
Bronchus	40 : 1	Liverpool, UK Birmingham, UK	Uganda
Stomach	30 : 1	Japan	Mozambique
Melanoma	10 : 1	New Zealand	Iceland

Pathology of malignancy

The diagnosis of malignancy must be based on a biopsy of the tumour. The differences between the malignant cell and its normal counterpart are given in Table 7.4. Virtually all tumours begin as one abnormal cell. A single cell that transforms into a malignant cell may grow slowly in the epithelium over a number of years, giving rise to a carcinoma *in situ* (as occurs in carcinoma of the cervix). Invasive tumour cells then penetrate the basement membrane; they carry receptors for laminin and fibronectin, which are present on this membrane. The growth may then become more aggressive and invade blood vessels. The next stage involves tumour-induced angiogenesis which allows the tumour to grow rapidly so that eventually it becomes clinically detectable.

Tumours invade their local surroundings; as they do so, they infiltrate blood vessel walls and liberate cells into the circulation that are then deposited in tissues such as the liver and lungs to form micrometastases. The continuing growth of a tumour and the burden of metastatic deposits eventually kill the patient. However, it is important to remember that people with cancer often die of

Table 7.3 Industrially related cancers.

Agent	Occupation	Cancer
Ultraviolet light	Farmer, sailor	Skin
Soot, tar, oil	Chimney sweep	Skin
β-Naphthylamine	Chemical worker	Bladder
Asbestos	Insulation worker	Mesothelioma
Benzene	Varnisher, glueworker	Leukaemia
Vinyl chloride	PVC manufacturer	Liver

Table 7.4 Differences between benign and malignant cells.

Benign	Malignant
Non-invasive	Invasive
Highly differentiated	Poorly differentiated
Mitoses rare	Mitoses common
Slow growth	Rapid growth
No anaplasia	Anaplasia
No metastases	Metastases

infection, for example pneumonia, owing to a combination of factors predisposing to its development. Figure 7.2 shows how a relatively short interval may exist between clinically demonstrable disease and death, and how difficult it is, theoretically, to detect cancer early.

Staging malignant diseases

To the patient, prognosis is of equal importance to diagnosis. One of the major determinants of prognosis in most tumours is the stage that has been reached by the tumour when treatment is being considered. Staging is · essentially a shorthand notation that describes whether the tumour is confined to the tissue of origin, has spread locally, or has metastasized. One of the most widely adopted staging systems is the TNM (tumour, node, metastasis) classification, which can be applied to the majority of so-called 'solid' tumours. Specific staging classifications have been developed for some tumours; for example, Hodgkin's disease is classified according to the Ann Arbor staging scheme, which incorporates not only the stage of the disease, but also the accompanying symptoms (see Table 7.14).

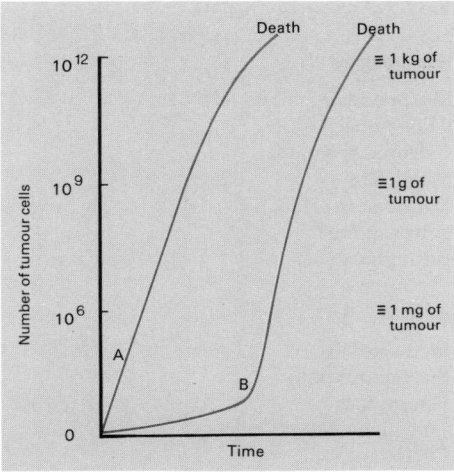

Fig. 7.2 Theoretical growth curves of two tumours. A = rapid growth; B = dormant phase.

Table 7.5 Karnowsky performance status.

100	Normal; no complaints
90	Able to carry on normal activity. Minor symptoms of disease
80	Normal activity with effort. Some symptoms of disease
70	Cares for self. Unable to carry on normal activity or to work
60	Requires occasional assistance but is able to care for most of own needs
50	Requires considerable assistance and frequent medical care
40	Disabled. Requires special care and assistance
30	Severely disabled. Hospitalization indicated, although death not imminent
20	Very sick. Hospitalization necessary, active supportive treatment necessary
10	Moribund. Fatal processes progressing rapidly

The TNM and allied methods of staging have been of great value in an era when surgery has dominated the diagnosis and treatment of patients with cancer. It is likely that, as surgery becomes less important as the initial treatment, such staging classifications will be modified.

Although anatomical staging is important, the effect of the tumour on the person as a whole also needs to be taken into account, as this proves to be a powerful determinant of survival. David Karnofsky introduced the idea of a performance scale, shown in Table 7.5. The so-called Karnofsky performance status is thus an indicator of prognosis, it also allows the patient's general condition as a result of treatment to be monitored and gives a measure of the treatment's toxicity.

Measuring response to treatment

Response to treatment can be subjective or objective. A subjective response is one perceived by the sufferer, in terms of, for example, relief of pain or general malaise. An objective response is one that the observer makes, and is usually associated with some form of measurement, such as the size of a lump, the size of the spleen, or the width of a mediastinal shadow on a chest X-ray. Terms used to evaluate the responses of tumours are given in Table 7.6.

The aim of all treatment for malignant disease is to produce a complete response in a solid tumour, or complete remission in a haematological malignancy, for without these patients will never be cured. A complete response in a solid tumour is defined as the clinical disappearance of all evidence of malignancy, with no evidence of tumour using the appropriate investigations. Complete remission is a term more commonly used in haematological malignancies, e.g. leukaemia, where, in addition to the absence of symptoms and signs of leukaemia, return of the bone marrow to normal is required to confirm complete remission.

Assessing cure rates

Survival of a patient for 5 years used to be equated with cure, particularly when tumours were amenable to surgery, e.g. carcinoma of the colon. Recently, the terms 'median survival' and 'median duration of remission' have come into use; examples of these are shown in Fig. 7.3. The curve in Fig. 7.3b shows a plateau in the remission duration curve, which would imply that a proportion of the patients treated by that particular therapy are being cured. Statistical methods using life-table curves are now of great importance in the assessment of therapeutic programmes.

Table 7.6 Definitions of response.

Complete response	Complete disappearance of all detectable disease
Partial response	More than 50% reduction in the size of the tumour
No response	No change or less than 50% reduction
Progressive disease	Increase in size of tumour at any site

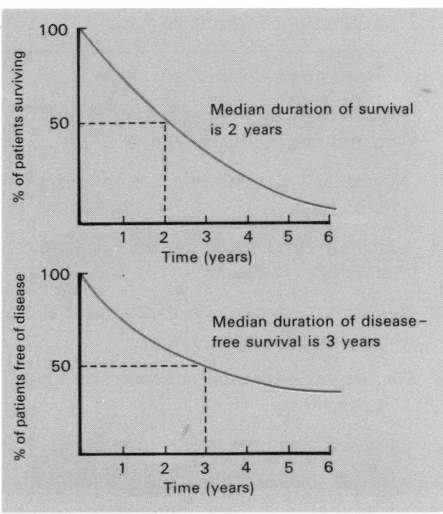

Fig. 7.3 Graphs showing examples of 'median survival' and 'median duration of remission'.

Principles of chemotherapy

The use of drugs to attempt to cure cancer is relatively recent.

Alkylating agents
The discovery that nitrogen mustard, a derivative of the sulphur mustard gases used in World War I, could cause regression in the size of lymphoid tumours opened the era of chemotherapy. Various congeners of nitrogen mustard were produced, all with the ethylenimine group, which is able to alkylate a wide variety of intracellular substances, including DNA. Most of the available alkylating agents are listed in Table 7.7. These drugs are 'radiomimetic', i.e. they damage DNA by breaking up the molecule and by causing cross-linkages, so preventing cell division.

Antimetabolites
Another group of agents are the so-called 'antimetabolic' drugs. Methotrexate, a compound very similar to folic acid, combines with the enzyme dihydrofolate reductase, thus inhibiting the enzyme that is concerned with initiating DNA production. Methotrexate was the first of a large number of synthetic antimetabolic agents, and was originally shown to produce temporary remission in childhood lymphoblastic leukaemia. More recently, the administration of very high doses of

Table 7.7 Antitumour agents.

Alkylating agents

Mustine hydrochloride (HN$_2$)
Chlorambucil
Cyclophosphamide
Melphalan
Dacarbazine (DTIC)
Nitrosoureas
Busulphan

Antimetabolites

Methotrexate
Mercaptopurine
Fluorouracil
Thioguanine
Cytarabine

Antitumour agents derived from plants

Vinblastine ⎫
⎬ Vinca alkaloids
Vincristine ⎭
Etoposide

Antitumour antibiotics

Actinomycin D
Daunorubicin
Doxorubicin
Bleomycin
Mitomycin C

Miscellaneous drugs of importance

Cisplatin/carboplatin
Hexamethylmelamine
Procarbazine
Hydroxyurea
Asparaginase

Hormones and antihormones

Oestrogens
Progestagens
Steroids
Tamoxifen
Aminoglutethimide
Buserelin

methotrexate in order to achieve a high degree of cell kill has been made possible by the discovery that folinic acid can 'rescue' normal cells. A number of antimetabolites are listed in Table 7.7. These agents act by interrupting metabolic pathways or by substitution of various key sites in the DNA molecule.

Drugs derived from plants
The two vinca alkaloids vinblastine and vincristine

are derived from the periwinkle plant (Table 7.7). They are poisons that damage the protein tubules of the spindle of the cell during mitosis. Other powerful anticancer agents derived from plants include the epipodophyllotoxins such as etoposide.

Agents derived from bacteria

In the search for antibacterial agents, some species of *Streptomyces* were found to produce antitumour substances. The most important of these anti-tumour antibiotics are listed in Table 7.7. They are thought to impair cell division by damaging DNA. Actinomycin D, for example, forms complexes in the DNA helix, preventing separation and replication.

Miscellaneous drugs

Some other important drugs are also listed in Table 7.7.

Combinations of anticancer drugs

In many experimental tumours it has been shown that the proportion of cells killed is directly related to the dose of the anticancer drug. Reduction of the number of cancer cells is usually measured in 'logs' (e.g. a decrease from 10^{12} to 10^{11} tumour cells is a decrease of one log) or in millions of cells killed. It is usual for the proportion of cells killed to remain constant with each dose of the anticancer drug. Thus, a number of doses of drug are needed in order to achieve elimination of the cancer.

Anticancer drugs also have a powerful effect on normal tissues. It is therefore beneficial to combine two drugs that are addictive or synergistic in their antitumour effect but that have different toxicities. A good example of this is the combination of vincristine, which is neurotoxic, and prednisolone, which has no neurotoxicity; the resulting summation of their antitumour properties is shown in Fig. 7.4. Multidrug regimens have become widely used in leukaemia, lymphoma and solid tumours such as testicular teratoma and the common childhood malignancies. Since the major dose-limiting factor is damage to the haemopoietic system, recent techniques in which a proportion of the patient's bone marrow is aspirated under general anaesthetic, stored and then administered after the cessation of chemotherapy have enabled larger doses of cytotoxic drugs to be given.

Intermittent drug administration

The administration of chemotherapeutic drugs in 'pulses' allows the restoration of normal tissues between doses, as normal tissues repair more rapidly than tumour tissue. With 'pulses' of drugs, recovery and growth of the tumour will lag behind normal tissue repair, and each course can have

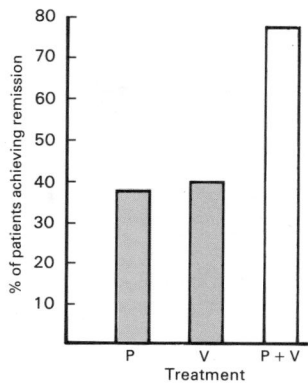

Fig. 7.4 Remission rates in children with acute lympho-blastic leukaemia, showing the summation of antitumour properties when two drugs are combined. P = predniso-lone: V = vincristine.

additive effect despite the relatively narrow therapeutic index for anticancer drugs (Fig. 7.5).

Exploitation of the action of drugs on cell kinetics

On first principles, it would appear to be an advantage for drugs used in combination to affect different parts of the cell cycle. The cell, after dividing, rests for a while (Fig. 7.6); the interval, or gap, between mitosis and the onset of synthesis of the double quantity of DNA required for cell division is called G_1. Combining of drugs that affect G_1, synthesis and mitosis might thus be more effective in killing the tumour. However, early attempts to exploit cell kinetics in this way have not been very successful.

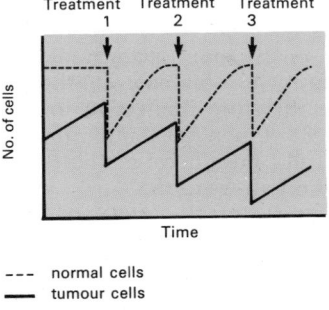

- - - normal cells
——— tumour cells

Fig. 7.5 Effects of multiple courses of cytotoxic chemo-therapy (see text). (From Priestman TJ (1977) *Cancer Chemotherapy—An Introduction*. Barnet: Montedison Pharmaceuticals. With permission.)

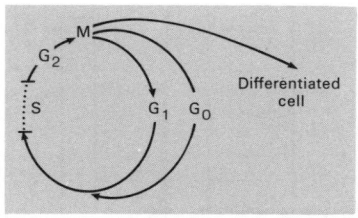

Fig. 7.6 Diagram showing cell kinetics. M = mitosis; G_1 = gap 1; G_2 = gap 2; G_0 = phase out of cycle; S = synthesis.

Adjuvant therapy

When a patient first presents with a tumour, it is very likely that small amounts of tumour tissue have already spread to the lungs, liver, bone marrow and other sites. This micrometastatic disease consists of relatively few cells with a good blood supply, and might be particularly amenable to the action of anticancer drugs. If, therefore, the primary tumour is removed, and chemotherapy is given to destroy the residual micrometastatic disease, the chance of long-term survival and cure might be improved. This was dramatically demonstrated in the childhood renal sarcoma, Wilms' tumour, when the use of actinomycin D given after nephrectomy resulted in a doubling of the number of children who survived. Chemotherapy used in this way is known as adjuvant therapy, and has been employed in a number of other childhood tumours and in breast cancer.

Treatment of malignancy in sanctuary sites

A 'sanctuary site' is the term used to indicate that metastatic disease has involved a site that is not accessible to conventional drug therapy. An example of this is leukaemic infiltration of the meninges in children with acute lymphoblastic leukaemia (Fig. 7.7). Because of the blood–brain barrier, agents such as vincristine and prednisolone do not enter the subarachnoid space in sufficient quantity to eliminate all the leukaemic cells, and are therefore ineffective in preventing the development of meningeal infiltration. In order to treat these cells, intrathecal methotrexate and/or cranial irradiation are required.

Drug toxicity

Chemotherapeutic agents cause a wide variety of toxic side-effects, sometimes of considerable severity. It is very important to be aware of these and to explain them to the patient prior to starting treatment. A useful classification of such reactions

depends on whether they are early, intermediate or late, and whether they are general or specific (Table 7.8). Most chemotherapeutic drugs affect rapidly dividing tissues and consequently are toxic to the bone marrow, the lining of the gut and the hair follicles.

Drug resistance

Drug resistance is said to occur when a tumour is no longer sensitive to a drug and starts to regrow. Drug resistance is one of the major obstacles to curing cancer by chemotherapy. Inherently resistant tumours are colon cancers and melanomas. Small-cell lung cancer shows a high response rate initially, but then acquires resistance.

Drug resistance is genetically determined, cells becoming resistant from generation to generation. The altered gene products responsible for resistance can be identified, and DNA from resistant cells can be experimentally transfected into the DNA of sensitive cells, rendering them resistant. A good example is multidrug resistance (MDR), in which cells acquire resistance for a series of naturally occurring cytotoxic agents, such as the antracyclines, vinca alkaloids and etoposides. The MDR cells have the ability to excrete these agents rapidly through their cell walls owing to an excess

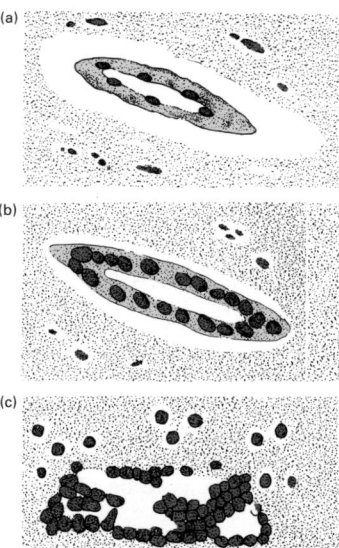

Fig. 7.7 The leukaemic infiltration of the meninges in acute lymphoblastic leukaemia. (a) A post-capillary venule, showing the pial–glial membrane. (b) Blast cells are seen in the vessel wall. (c) The pial–glial membrane is destroyed and blast cells are seen in the grey matter.

Table 7.8 Classification of therapeutic toxicity.

Problems seen with most drugs	Specific problems (causative drugs in parentheses)
Immediate (hours)	
Nausea and vomiting	Haemorrhagic cystitis (cyclophosphamide)
Local tissue necrosis	Hypocalcaemia (mithramycin)
Phlebitis	Facial flushing (mithramycin)
Hyperuricaemia	Radiation reaction (actinomycin D, doxorubicin)
Anaphylaxis	Fever and chills (bleomycin)
Early (days to week)	
Leucopenia	Paralysis (vinca alkaloids)
Thrombocytopenia	Hypercalcaemia (oestrogen, tamoxifen)
Alopecia	Psychosis (steroids)
Stomatitis	Disseminated intravascular coagulation (asparaginase)
Diarrhoea	Pancreatitis (asparaginase)
	Fluid retention (steroids)
	Influenza syndrome (dacarbazine [DTIC])
	Pulmonary fibrosis (methotrexate, bleomycin)
	Cerebellar ataxia (fluorouracil, cytarabine in high doses)
	Ototoxicity (platinum compounds)
	Renal toxicity (platinum compounds)
Delayed (weeks to months)	
Anaemia	Peripheral neuropathy (vinca alkaloids)
Aspermia	Cardiac necrosis (anthracyclines)
Hepatocellular damage	Constipation (vinca alkaloids)
Hyperpigmentation	Cushing's syndrome (steroids)
Pulmonary fibrosis	Inappropriate ADH secretion (cyclophosphamide, vinca alkaloids)
	Masculinization (androgens)
	Feminization (oestrogens)
	Jaundice (6-mercaptopurine)
	Addisonian symptoms (busulphan)
Late	
Sterility	Hepatic fibrosis (methotrexate)
Hypogonadism	Encephalopathy (methotrexate)
Acute leukaemia	Carcinoma of bladder (cyclophosphamide)
Lymphoma	Osteoporosis (steroids)
Other second primary malignant tumours	

of p-glycoprotein. Drugs such as verapamil that check the action of p-glycoprotein have been shown to restore sensitivity of these cells to cytotoxic drugs. A method for detection of p-glycoprotein in the cell wall is now available and this may enable new therapeutic strategies to be developed.

Another mechanism of resistance is that of gene amplification, producing an enzyme that is necessary for malignant cell growth. As mentioned above, methotrexate acts principally by inhibiting the enzyme dihydrofolate reductase (DHFR). If the cell can start to produce DHFR by amplifying many hundreds of times the gene that is responsible for its production, it becomes resistant to methotrexate. A similar mechanism is seen in resistance to cytosine arabinoside, where deaminases are produced in large quantities by the resistant cell.

Currently, the only method of overcoming this resistance is to give massive doses of the drug.

Principles of endocrine therapy

Many organs, particularly those associated with reproduction, are under hormonal control. Consequently, when tumours develop in such organs, manipulation of the hormonal environment may result in regression of the tumours. 'Hormone therapy' may involve removal of the source of a normal hormone, the administration of 'antihormone' or the administration of other hormone substances. In general, hormonal therapy is not curative. It does, however, have the advantage of achieving long-term control with few or no unpleasant side-effects.

Tumours of the breast, prostate, endometrium and thyroid respond to specific hormones. Carcinoma of the prostate responds to orchidectomy, which removes the source of testosterone, but this tumour will also respond to oestrogens, and more recently has been shown to be responsive to buserelin (see below). Endometrial carcinomas can be treated with medroxyprogesterone, and some thyroid cancers respond to thyroid hormone, which causes suppression of thyroid-stimulating hormone. Leukaemia and lymphoma may respond to steroid hormones because of the general, and poorly understood, lympholytic effect of these agents.

The presence of cell-surface receptors for the hormone in question is a prerequisite for the therapy to be effective. The binding of hormone to the receptor and translocation of the hormone–receptor complex into the nucleus, where it reacts with the DNA, is shown diagrammatically in Fig. 7.8. This mechanism can be seen in the 80% of patients with breast cancer who have receptors for oestrogens and progesterone. Hormone manipulation of breast cancer includes the administration of oestrogen, the use of the antioestrogen tamoxifen, the eradication of endogenous oestrogen production by oophorectomy and the use of aminoglutethimide, which produces a 'medical' adrenalectomy. More recently, buserelin, a long-acting analogue of gonadotrophin-releasing hormone, which 'down-regulates' pituitary gonadotrophin production and consequently depresses the level of gonadal hormones, has been shown to have an effect in pre-menopausal women with breast cancer.

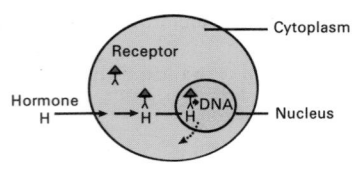

Fig. 7.8 Mechanism of the cell-receptor system. A hormone H combines with a receptor and the complex is transported to the nucleus, where it reacts with DNA.

Principles of biological therapy

An increase in the understanding of normal cell function, together with the development of recombinant DNA technology that has made it possible to synthesize naturally occurring substances such as the interferons, has led to an increased interest in biological therapy. The mechanism of action of interferon is unknown; responses may be due to its direct antiproliferative effect, or to an immunologically mediated mechanism involving the stimulation of immunocompetent cells such as natural killer cells and cytotoxic T cells. With the exception of hairy-cell leukaemia, the role of interferon in malignancy has yet to be established. It is currently being investigated in chronic myeloid leukaemia, myeloma, follicular lymphoma and renal cell carcinoma. Various other naturally occurring substances known as lymphokines, e.g. TNF (tumour necrosis factor) and IL-2 (interleukin-2 or T-cell growth factor) are also being evaluated in clinical studies.

Another experimental 'biological' approach involves the administration of monoclonal antibodies directed against cell-surface antigens found on tumour cells. The antibody can be conjugated to a radioactive compound or to a toxin, thus, theoretically at least, providing a highly tumour-specific compound.

Monoclonal antibodies and complement are being used as a means of removing residual tumour cells from autologous bone marrow in patients with leukaemia and lymphoma undergoing very intensive therapy supported by autologous bone marrow transplantation. Monoclonal antibodies directed against T cell antigens can also be used in conjunction with complement to deplete donor marrow of the cells that cause graft-versus-host-disease (GVHD—see p. 36) in the context of allogeneic bone-marrow transplantation.

The colony-stimulating factors (CSFs) are a quite different group of naturally occurring compounds that are currently the subject of much interest. It is hoped that their use may abrogate or at least reduce the degree of cytopenia associated with chemotherapy.

Haematological malignancy

THE LEUKAEMIAS

These diseases are characterized by the proliferation of a single malignantly transformed progenitor cell in the haemopoietic system. Acute leukaemia is a condition that, untreated, has a rapidly fatal course. Chronic leukaemia has a more prolonged natural history but patients invariably die from it unless another cause of death supervenes. However, with modern effective treatment many patients with acute leukaemia survive for long periods, and a proportion are cured.

CLASSIFICATION

Leukaemia is classified, as shown below, according to the morphological cell type involved and the speed of evolution of the disease.

- Acute lymphoblastic leukaemia (ALL)
- Acute myelogenous leukaemia (AML)
- Chronic lymphatic leukaemia (CLL)
- Chronic myeloid leukaemia (CML)

INCIDENCE

The overall incidence of leukaemia is approximately 5/100 000 per year. Whereas the commonest childhood leukaemia is acute lymphoblastic in type, AML predominates in adults. With increasing age, CLL becomes more prevalent. The relative frequencies of acute and chronic leukaemias at different ages are shown in Table 7.9.

Table 7.9 Percentage of leukaemia at different ages.

Type	Percentage of patients in age group		
	0–14 years	15–49 years	50+ years
All leukaemias	20	20	60
Acute	35	23	42
Chronic	4	15	81

From Gunz FW & Henderson ES (eds) (1983) *Leukemia*, 4th edn. New York: Grune and Stratton. With permission.

AETIOLOGY

The aetiology of the majority of leukaemias in humans remains unknown.

Genetic factors
There is a low frequency of ALL in black children, a high incidence of concordance of leukaemia in identical twins, and an increased risk in patients with chromosomal abnormalities, e.g. Down's Syndrome.

The Philadelphia (Ph) chromosome (Fig. 7.9) is present in granulocytes, erythrocytes and platelet precursors in 95% of patients with CML. It is also occasionally found in ALL, when its presence is associated with a poor prognosis. The long arm (q) of chromosome 22 is shortened by reciprocal translocation with chromosome 9, i.e. t(9;22) (q34;q11). The molecular consequences of the translocation can be summarized as follows. The oncogene *c-abl* (which is analogous to the viral oncogene *v-abl* associated with a murine leukaemia virus) is situated near the break point on chromosome 9. On translocation, *c-abl* fuses at the break point cluster region (*bcr*) of chromosome 22, to form a chimaeric gene, *bcr-abl*. On transcription, a new protein results; the precise function of this protein in man is unknown but the juxtaposition of *c-abl* and *bcr* are thought to be critical for the development of CML. Another consistent translocation between chromosome 15 and 17 is seen in promyelocytic leukaemia.

Many other chromosomal alterations (translocations or deletions), though not as consistent as the Ph chromosome have been found in acute leukaemia, e.g. t(8;21)(q22.1;q22.3) in AML M2, or del(7)(q33;q36) in AML M1, M2, M4, M5, M6 (see over).

Environmental factors
These include:

- *Radiation.* There is an increased incidence of leukaemia (predominantly CML) in survivors of the atomic bomb in Hiroshima and of AML in patients with ankylosing spondylitis who were treated with radiotherapy. A small proportion of patients with Hodgkin's disease treated with radiotherapy (particularly when used in addition to chemotherapy) develop so called 'secondary' AML.
- *Chemicals*, e.g. benzene.
- *Drugs* (phenylbutazone) and chemotherapeutic agents, e.g. alkylating drugs.
- *Viruses*, e.g. human T-cell leukaemia virus type I (HTLV-I) which was first discovered in Japanese patients with T cell leukaemia. HTLV-II has been isolated from some patients with hairy-cell leukaemia.

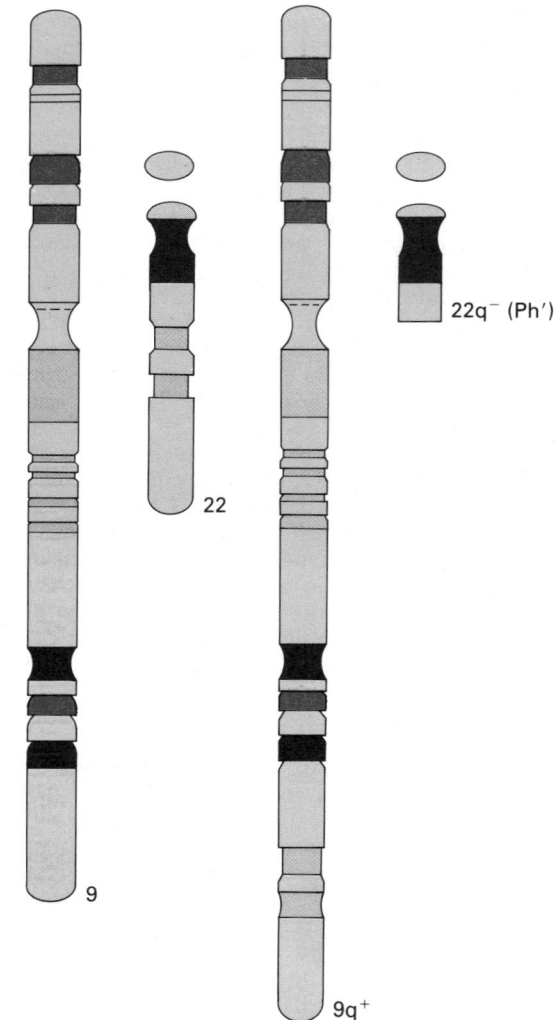

Fig. 7.9 The Philadelphia chromosome (Ph'). The long arm (q) of chromosome 22 has been shortened by the reciprocal translocation with chromosome 9.

PATHOPHYSIOLOGY

In *acute* leukaemia the malignant cells are unable to differentiate normally and proliferate rapidly. This leads to bone-marrow failure resulting in the clinical features of the disease as a consequence of anaemia, neutropenia and thrombocytopenia.

In *chronic* leukaemia there are very few normal cells but the malignant cells are able to differentiate to some degree. Marrow failure is therefore not a feature until late in the course of the disease and the clinical manifestations are predominantly due to the mass of cells produced, e.g. splenomegaly, lymphadenopathy.

Acute leukaemia

Acute lymphoblastic leukaemia (ALL)
The blast cells have been classified morphologically into L1, L2 and L3 subtypes as shown in Fig. 7.10. There are certain differences between the clinical presentation and prognosis of ALL L3 compared with the other two forms, the former having a considerably worse prognosis. In addition to the morphological classification, ALL can be further defined in terms of the different antigenic markers on the surface of the leukaemic blast cell (Table 7.10). These indicate the immunological origin of the cells and have proved to be of considerable prognostic importance in assessing the likelihood of response and the long-term outlook.

Acute myelogenous leukaemia (AML)
In this condition the morphology and cyto-chemistry of the leukaemic blasts have been more helpful than cell-surface phenotype in differentiating the subtype, which to some extent correlates with the clinical form of the disease. The French–American–British (FAB) classification of AML is given in Table 7.11.

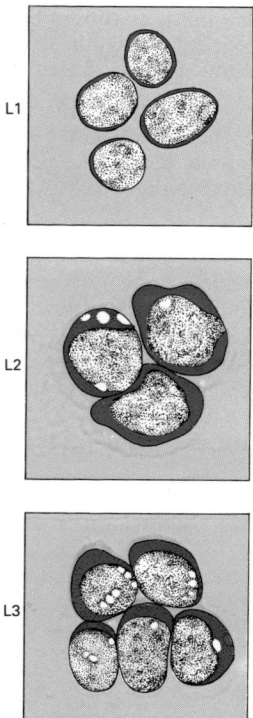

Fig. 7.10 The FAB classificationof lymphoblastic leukaemia. In L1 the cells are small with scanty cytoplasm. In L2 the cells are larger with more abundant cytoplasm. In L3 the cells are large with characteristic vacuolation.

Table 7.10 Immunological classification of acute lymphoblastic leukaemia.

Subtype	Immunophenotype[a]
C-ALL	CD10+, HLA-DR+, CD19+, CD20−, TdT+, CD7−, sIg−
Null-ALL	CD10−, HLA-DR+, CD19−, CD20−, TdT+, CD7−, sIg−
T-ALL	CD10−, HLA-DR−, CD19−, CD20−, TdT+, CD7+, sIg−
B-ALL	CD10−, HLA-DR+, CD19−, CD20+, TdT−, CD7−, sIg+

[a] CD = cluster designation number for cell surface antigens. TdT = terminal deoxynucleotidyl transferase. sIg = surface immunoglobulin.

CLINICAL FEATURES OF ACUTE LEUKAEMIA

Symptoms
The history is usually short and consists of:

- Symptoms of anaemia and malaise
- Repeated acute infections such as mouth ulceration, sore throat, pneumonia, perianal and skin infections
- Bruising and bleeding
- Painful and enlarging lymphadenopathy

- Bone pain—this is particularly common in children with ALL
- Symptoms due to infiltration of tissues with leukaemic blast cells, e.g. gum hypertrophy in AML (M5)
- Headache, nausea, vomiting and blurred vision, as a result of raised intracranial pressure in patients with CNS involvement

Signs
These may be absent or relatively few, but commonly they are:

- Pallor
- Bruising, petechial haemorrhages, bleeding gums and gum hypertrophy
- Lymphadenopathy
- Splenomegaly and/or hepatomegaly
- Haemorrhages in the optic fundi, occasionally with a characteristic central white deposit in the centre of the haemorrhage, a classic feature of leukaemic retinopathy

Rarely, the patient may present with signs of meningeal leukaemia. In boys, hard enlarged testicles indicate that the testes have become infiltrated with leukaemic tissue.

INVESTIGATION

Examination of a peripheral blood film and of the

Table 7.11 FAB Classification of acute myelogenous leukaemia.

FAB class	Common name	Morphology
M1	Acute myelocytic leukaemia without differentiation	Myeloblasts predominant; distinct nucleoli; few granules
M2	Acute myelocytic leukaemia with differentiation	Myeloblasts and promyelocytes predominant; further maturation abnormal
M3	Acute promyelocytic leukaemia	Promyelocytes predominate; hypergranular
M4	Acute myelomonocytic leukaemia	Myelocytic and monocytic maturation evident; may be peripheral
M5	Acute monocytic leukaemia with differentiation	Promonocytes predominant; large cerebriform nuclei
M5A	Acute monoblastic leukaemia with differentiation	Completely undifferentiated blast cells
M6	Erythroleukaemia	Bizarre, multinucleated, megaloblastic erythroblasts predominate; myeloblasts also present
M7	Acute megakaryocytic leukaemia	Pleomorphic, undifferentiated cytoplasmic blebs

bone marrow are essential. Because the disease may spread to the meninges, the CSF should also be examined, either at diagnosis or early in the course of treatment. Tests of renal function, serum uric acid, calcium and electrolytes should be performed, together with blood grouping and coagulation studies. Blood cultures are mandatory if the patient is febrile and a chest X-ray is required to determine the presence of a mediastinal mass.

DIAGNOSTIC FEATURES

- There is a normochromic/normocytic anaemia.
- The white cell count may be normal or raised; very occasionally, only a few blast cells may be seen in the peripheral blood, or none at all.
- The platelet count is usually reduced.
- Bone-marrow examination shows a hypercellular marrow with characteristic blasts in the trails of the fragments on the microscopic slide.
- The CSF should be examined on a cytospin. The prepared sediment will contain blast cells if meningeal leukaemia is present.

TREATMENT

The decision to treat a patient with curative intent will depend on the person's age, their general state of health, their point in the course of the disease (first presentation or relapse), and their wishes. Intensive combination chemotherapy may, for example, be totally inappropriate at the time of relapse in an older person.

The diagnosis, its implications, the treatment option being considered and the likely outcome of such treatment, together with its side-effects, need to be explained to the patient and to the family. People often find it difficult to assimilate all of this information on one occasion; it is therefore essential to give the patient and the family the opportunity to ask questions about the illness and the treatment, particularly as circumstances change.

Specific treatment programmes for the various forms of leukaemia will be considered briefly, but it is well to remember that they are steadily evolving. The supportive care and preparation of the patient before specific therapy is instigated are probably as important to the patient's survival as the precise combination of drugs that is used.

Where there is the potential for rapid destruction of leukaemic cells (e.g. B-ALL, T-ALL) liberation of phosphates and other intracellular components may result in hyperphosphataemia, hypercalcaemia, hyperkalaemia and hyperuricaemia—the so-called tumour lysis syndrome. It is avoided by hyperhydration before administering chemotherapy and careful biochemical monitoring at frequent intervals. Patients may require haemodialysis. However, despite these measures, it may be rapidly fatal.

Therapeutic strategy for all
This includes:

- Correction of dehydration.
- Treatment of hyperuricaemia with intravenous fluids and allopurinol, a xanthine oxidase inhibitor.
- Correction of anaemia and thrombocytopenia by red-cell and platelet transfusions.
- Leukapheresis may be necessary if the blast count is very high ($> 100 \times 10^9/l$) because leukaemic blast cells can infiltrate the brain and the lungs leading to coma and respiratory failure, respectively.
- Control of infection with the appropriate intravenous antibiotics.

Specific therapy. This should only be given in units with experience of managing acute leukaemia and where a particular programme is being followed.

Treatment comprises four phases:

1 *Induction of remission.* A combination of four drugs is usually used: vincristine, prednisolone, an antitumour antibiotic such as doxorubicin or daunorubicin, and asparaginase.
2 *Consolidation.* When remission is achieved there is likely to be morphologically undetectable leukaemia still present, further eradication of these residual lymphoblasts is therefore attempted by consolidation therapy, which may involve giving the same drugs that were given to induce remission or the addition of others.
3 *Cranial prophylaxis.* ALL has a propensity for involving the CNS; this can usually be prevented by giving intrathecal methotrexate and cranial irradiation. Chemotherapy alone using methotrexate, cytarabine and corticosteroids has also been used. In very young children, in whom there is evidence that cranial irradiation may cause brain damage, radiation is only given after completion of treatment.
4 *Continuation or maintenance therapy.* Once the bulk of tumour is reduced to a minimum, and disease is abolished in sanctuary sites, continuation or maintenance therapy is given for a period of about 2 years. This comprises methotrexate and mercaptopurine given orally on an outpatient basis. During this time children are encouraged to lead a normal life, returning to school and all normal activities.

Management of relapse. Relapse of ALL can occur in three sites:

● *Bone-marrow relapse*. This is the major cause of failure of therapy and, if it occurs while the child is on continuation therapy, the outlook is grave. The reinduction of remission and subsequent use of high-dose chemotherapy and total-body irradiation supported by allogeneic or autologous bone-marrow transplantation (BMT) is the only therapy known to produce long-term survival and possible cure. However, at best, such treatment is effective in only 30% of patients.

● *Relapse in the central nervous system*. This is much less frequent. Treatment comprises intrathecal drugs and craniospinal irradiation. If the blasts can be cleared from the cerebrospinal fluid and bone marrow remission maintained, then about one-third of patients may become long-term survivors.

● *Testicular relapse*. This is sometimes seen as an isolated phenomenon, particularly during the first year off therapy, but it is usually a warning of general systemic relapse and has to be treated promptly. The outlook is good if the testes are treated with irradiation and the patient is given reinduction therapy and a further period of maintenance treatment.

Prognostic factors. In childhood ALL the following are poor prognostic factors:

● The height of the initial leucocyte count, i.e. the greater the number of cells present, the worse the prognosis
● The presence of central nervous system involvement at diagnosis
● Massive enlargement of nodes, liver or spleen
● Age below 2 years, or above 10 years
● Thymic enlargement
● The presence of T or B cell markers on the blast cells. (These are probably not independent of the features recorded above.)

All these factors must be taken into account in assessing the outlook in a particular child, but of particular importance is the use of appropriate specific treatment and good supportive care.

Therapeutic strategy for AML
AML has to be distinguished from other haematological conditions in which the bone marrow is infiltrated with myeloid leukaemic blast cells, e.g. 'refractory anaemia with an excess of blasts' (RAEB). The latter condition, which is an example of a myelodysplastic syndrome, is most frequently seen in elderly patients and is generally managed by supportive care with blood transfusions and antibiotics because chemotherapy is rarely effective.

Principles of therapy. The aim is to restore the bone marrow to normal and the patient to a normal state of health. In AML this means temporarily ablating the bone marrow, and thereafter a period of intensive support, with blood products and antibiotics. Remission induction therapy usually includes an antitumour antibiotic, such as doxorubicin or daunorubicin, in conjunction with cytosine arabinoside. As in ALL, some form of consolidation therapy is essential, but long-term maintenance therapy is generally considered to be less effective. The survival curves in a series of patients treated for AML in one unit are shown in Fig. 7.11. The best survival was achieved with the most intensive 'short-term' chemotherapy.

Ablative therapy supported by allogeneic bone-marrow transplantation should be considered in young patients (< 20 years of age) in first remission. Such very intensive treatment certainly results in the lowest rate of recurrence; however, the transplant procedure is itself associated with an appreciable mortality (up to 25%), predominantly due to Graft-versus-host disease, the risk of which increases with increasing age, and infection. Since the majority of patients with AML are older than 20, and do not have an HLA identical donor, ablative therapy with autologous bone-marrow transplantation is currently being evaluated as an alternative means of giving very intensive consolidation therapy.

Therapy for acute promyelocytic leukaemia (APML). Patients with acute promyelocytic leukaemia (M3 in the FAB classification, see Table 7.11) often present with severe bleeding problems due to disseminated intravascular coagulation (DIC) (see p. 343). It may be present at diagnosis but can also be precipitated by therapy, when breakdown of the

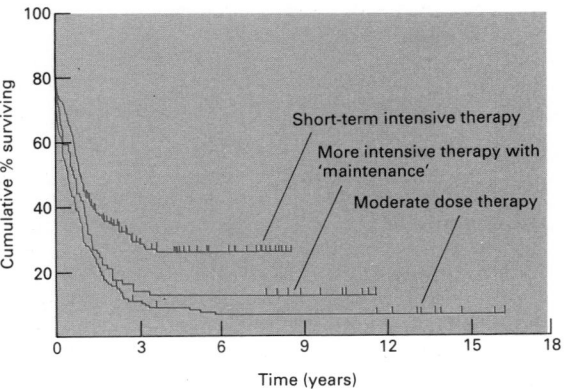

Fig. 7.11 Survival of patients treated at St Bartholomew's Hospital between 1969 and 1985 (censored for patients dying of causes unrelated to leukaemia or its treatment).

Bone Marrow Transplantation (BMT)

Allogeneic BMT

Indications
- Aplastic anaemia
- Acute leukaemia and chronic myeloid leukaemia
- Others—genetic disorders, e.g. thalassaemia

Donor must be closely HLA matched—usually a sibling or an identical twin. Mismatch increases graft rejection and graft-versus-host disease (GVHD). Approximately 1 litre of BM is aspirated under general anaesthetic from the posterior iliac crests.

Recipient is prepared with intensive chemotherapy, usually high doses of cyclophosphamide. Total body irradiation is also given in all cases apart from aplastic anaemia. This treatment kills residual malignant cells, ablates the patient's own bone marrow and prevents rejection of donor bone marrow.

Age. Children and young adults are usually selected.

Prior transfusion should be avoided because of sensitization and increased graft rejection in aplastic anaemia.

Procedure. Intravenous infusion of donor bone-marrow cells (usual dose 2–6×10^8 cell·kg^{-1} body weight; volume up to 1 litre). After the patient has received the ablative therapy these cells repopulate the marrow cavity and peripheral blood counts rise within 2–4 weeks.

Complications
- *Immediate.* Bleeding, infection, drug toxicity
- *GVHD.* This is an immune reaction involving donor T lymphocytes and affecting skin, liver and the gastrointestinal tract. Cyclosporin is used for prevention. GVHD occurs acutely within 2–3 months post-transplantation and may run a chronic course.
- *Infection.* Bacterial, fungal or viral (e.g. cytomegalovirus or herpes). Commonest interstitial pneumonia is due to CMV.

Autologous BMT. Involves re-infusing the patient's own bone marrow to support intensive chemotherapy and radiotherapy. A litre of bone marrow is removed and stored in liquid nitrogen prior to the patient receiving ablative therapy. The marrow mononuclear cell fraction may be treated *in vitro* in an attempt to remove morphologically undetectable tumour cells prior to re-infusion.

---

promyelocytes within the circulation results in an explosive production of fibrin, depletion of fibrinogen, and platelet aggregation.

Initially treatment consists of:

- Platelet transfusion
- Maintenance of the fibrinogen level with fresh frozen plasma
- Heparin

It is important to control the condition before specific cytotoxic therapy is started.

Treatment at relapse. Second remissions are more difficult to achieve and are virtually never durable. The decision to treat a person at the time of relapse will therefore, as at presentation, depend on the patient's overall situation and his or her wishes.

In younger patients, if second remission can be achieved, cure is still a possibility for a proportion, with the use of ablative therapy supported by allogeneic or autologous bone-marrow transplantation (BMT). With regard to allogeneic BMT, such treatment is only appropriate for patients under the age of 40 who have an HLA identical sibling. In the case of autologous BMT, the technique can probably be extended to patients under the age of 50. However, it has to be remembered and explained to patients and their families that the transplant procedure itself carries with it an appreciable morbidity and potential mortality. These risks obviously need to be balanced against the virtual certainty of death from leukaemia without such intensive therapy.

In older patients the options lie between further intensive combination chemotherapy similar to or different from that originally given to induce first remission, in the hope of achieving a second remission, which is, however, unlikely to last more than a few months. Alternatively, it may be more appropriate to try to keep the person well for as long as possible with supportive measures such as blood transfusions for anaemia, antibiotics for infections and the judicious use of palliative oral drugs that help to lower the circulating blast cell count.

SURVIVAL

Children

Remission is achieved in more than 90% of children with ALL, but that is no longer the only criterion by which success is measured. Disease-free survival after 5–6 years is a much better indication of the success of any treatment programme. The overall survival of children with all types of lymphoblastic leukaemia varies between 40% and 60%. Children with blast cells showing the common ALL antigen, so-called CALLA-positive acute leukaemia, may have survival rates in the region of 70%, while children with T cell leukaemia have a worse prognosis.

Adults

The remission rate in adults with ALL is of the order of 70%. Long-term survival is, however, much less satisfactory than in children, with only

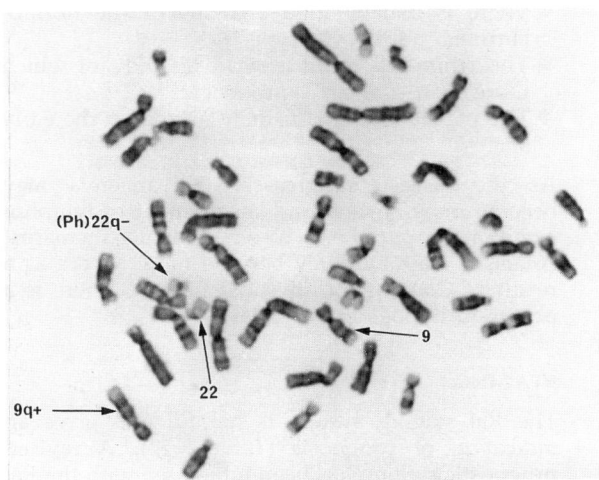

(Ph)22q−

9q+

22

9

Fig. 7.12 Philadelphia chromosome. This is formed by a reciprocal translocation of part of the long arm (q) of chromosome 22 to chromosome 9. It is seen in 90–95% of patients with chronic granulocytic leukaemia. The karyotype is expressed as 46XX, t(9,22)(q34;q11).

15–20% surviving more than 5 years. In AML, complete remission can be achieved in up to 80% of patients and in major centres using intensive chemotherapy overall survival at 4 years is of the order of 30%. Since relapses are rare after that time, these patients are almost certainly cured.

Chronic myeloid leukaemia (CML)

This is a relatively uncommon form of leukaemia characterized by the presence of the Philadelphia chromosome that occurs in middle-aged and elderly people. It is part of a spectrum of myeloproliferative disorders.

CLINICAL FEATURES

- Often of insidious onset (may only be discovered on a routine blood count)
- Anaemia
- Pain or discomfort due to a very large spleen, which may cause gastrointestinal disturbance
- Sweating, fever and loss of weight as the result of a high metabolic rate

Physical signs

- Anaemia
- A large spleen (common)
- Priapism may occur
- Gout (due to a raised serum level of uric acid)

INVESTIGATION

- The blood count initially may show a normal haemoglobin level, but eventually a normocytic, normochromic anaemia develops.
- The white-cell count is greater than 50×10^9/L.
- The blood film shows an abundance of neutrophils, but the whole spectrum of myeloid precursors including a few blast cells may be present.
- The platelet count is normal or sometimes elevated.
- The bone marrow shows a hypercellular marrow with a marked increase in granulocyte precursors.
- A chromosome preparation shows the Philadelphia chromosome (Fig. 7.12).
- The leucocyte alkaline phosphatase (LAP) is very low.
- Levels of serum vitamin B_{12} and B_{12}-binding proteins are elevated.

PROGNOSIS

CML has a relatively slow progression with a median survival of about 35 months. Usually within 5 years of diagnosis, the disease terminates with a blastic phase when acute transformation occurs with either myeloid or lymphoid blast cells predominating. Occasionally, myelofibrosis becomes the dominant picture.

TREATMENT

The treatment of choice is hydroxyurea or busulphan, given to relieve symptoms, control the blood count and reduce the spleen size. Although these drugs are effective, the median survival of patients with CML has not altered in the last 30 years. Allogeneic BMT in patients under the age of 50 years has improved the prognosis with a disease-free survival of 50% at 3 years when performed in the chronic phase. Treatment with interferon has been shown to reduce the percentage of Philadelphia-positive cells in the bone marrow and is currently being evaluated to determine whether this will translate into prolongation of survival.

The management of the blast crisis is very

unsatisfactory. Treatment programmes used in AML may achieve remission but these are always of short duration. Splenectomy does not alter the course of the disease, but can relieve discomfort.

Chronic lymphatic leukaemia (CLL)

This is a disease of late middle-aged and elderly people, and is responsible for the overall rise in leukaemia that is being seen in the increasingly aged population in the Western World. It is a rare disease in the Far East, even in Japan where the proportion of elderly people resembles that seen in the West. None of the environmental factors mentioned earlier plays a role in aetiology, but there is some genetic predisposition. The disorder involves mature lymphocytes that are found in the tissues and peripheral blood. The lymphocytes are almost always of B-cell origin with monoclonal surface immunoglobulins present on the cell surface, albeit in reduced amounts.

CLINICAL FEATURES

The onset is insidious, with:

- Lethargy
- Fever and sweating
- Loss of weight
- Infections

Signs

- Moderate enlargement of lymph nodes in the neck, axilla and groin
- Splenic and hepatic enlargement, but not usually massive

INVESTIGATION

- CLL is often picked up on a 'routine' blood count.

- There is usually mild anaemia of the normochromic, normocytic type.
- The white-cell count is $> 15 \times 10^9$/L, of which more than 40% are lymphocytes.
- The platelet count is usually normal in the early stages.

As the disease progresses, the anaemia may become more severe, and the number of lymphocytes in the peripheral blood gradually increases. Anaemia may suddenly become more severe as a result of Coombs' positive haemolysis. There is a profound hypoglobulinaemia.

STAGING

The Rai staging system is helpful and gives an indication of prognosis (Table 7.12). A revised prognostic staging has been integrated with the Rai classification with Rai I and II incorporated into clinical stages A and B and Rai III and IV into stage C. In A and B there is no anaemia or thrombocytopenia.

TREATMENT

Patients in the early stage of the disease may not need any therapy. When symptoms develop, single-drug therapy with oral chlorambucil is effective. Other useful drugs are cyclophosphamide and prednisolone. Intensive chemotherapy does not benefit patients with CLL.

Radiotherapy should be avoided in the early stages of the disease, unless there is a specific indication, e.g. mediastinal obstruction, as it may result in loss of bone-marrow reserve.

Patients with CLL are very susceptible to infections because of neutropenia and also because the B-cell malignancy suppresses normal immunoglobulin production. Infection is therefore the major cause of death. Potent intravenous prepara-

Table 7.12 The Rai staging system in chronic lymphatic leukaemia.

Stage	Definition	Mean survival (years)
0	Lymphocytes 15×10^9/L Lymphocytes 40% or more No enlarged lymph nodes, splenomegaly or hepatomegaly Normal Hb and platelets	
I	Stage 0 + enlarged lymph nodes	8
II	Stage 0 + enlarged lymph nodes, splenomegaly or hepatomegaly	6
III	As Stage 0, I or II, but Hb < 11 g·dl^{-1}	2
IV	As Stage 0, I, II or III + platelets $< 100 \times 10^9$/L	

tions of gamma globulin are now available and are being assessed as prophylactic therapy.

Hairy-cell leukaemia (HCL)

This is due to clonal proliferation of abnormal B cells. It accounts for 2% of all leukaemias and is commoner in men, with a median age of diagnosis of 50 years. Symptoms are due to neutropenia, thrombocytopenia and anaemia but may be non-specific. There is invariably splenomegaly, often massive. The blood film shows pancytopenia and typical 'hairy' lymphocytes with spiky projections. Until recently, treatment was limited to splenectomy but α-interferon and 2-deoxycoformycin have produced significant responses.

THE LYMPHOMAS

Lymphomas are malignant tumours of the lymphoreticular system that are classified on the basis of histological appearance into Hodgkin's disease and the various subtypes of non-Hodgkin's lymphoma.

Hodgkin's disease (HD)

Hodgkin's disease is characterized by enlargement of the lymph nodes, with hyperplasia, infiltration by histiocytes and lymphocytes and the presence of characteristic cells described by Sternberg and Reed (Fig. 7.13).

EPIDEMIOLOGY

It is a rare disease in children, where it affects boys twice as often as girls, but with increasing age both sexes become equally affected. It has an early peak of incidence in the twenties and a later peak in middle-age.

CLINICAL FEATURES

Hodgkin's disease commonly presents with enlargement of the cervical lymph nodes. However,

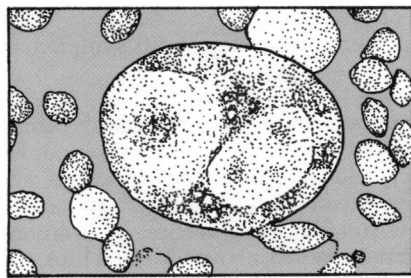

Fig. 7.13 The Sternberg–Reed cell.

Table 7.13 Differential diagnosis of cervical lymph node enlargement.

Infections
Acute
  Pyogenic infections
  Infective mononucleosis
  Toxoplasmosis
  Cytomegalovirus infection
  Infected eczema
  Cat scratch fever
  Acute childhood exanthema

Chronic
  Tuberculosis
  Syphilis
  Sarcoidosis
  HIV infection

Connective tissue disorders
Rheumatoid arthritis

Drug reactions
Phenytoin

Primary lymph node malignancies
Hodgkin's disease
Non-Hodgkin's lymphoma
Chronic lymphocytic leukaemia
Acute lymphoblastic leukaemia

Secondary malignancies
Nasopharyngeal
Thyroid
Laryngeal
Lung
Breast
Stomach

Miscellaneous
Sinus histiocytosis

cervical lymphadenopathy is a relatively common finding in children and adults; the differential diagnosis is shown in Table 7.13. Glands elsewhere may also become enlarged, e.g. in the axillae or inguinal regions, and are classically painless and 'rubbery'. Patients may also present with constitutional symptoms of weakness, fatigue and anorexia. Other clinical features of Hodgkin's disease are:

- Fever*
- Drenching night sweats*
- Loss of weight*
- Pruritus
- Alcohol-induced pain at the site of the enlarged node

*B-symptoms, see Table 7.14.

Table 7.14 Ann Arbor staging classification for Hodgkin's disease. The absence or presence of fever, night sweats, and/or unexplained loss of 10% or more of body weight in the 6 months preceding admission are indicated in all stages by the suffix letters A or B, respectively.

Stage	Definition
I	Involvement of a single lymph node region (I) or a single extralymphatic organ or site (I_E)
II	Involvement of two or more lymph node regions on the same side of the diaphragm (II) or localized involvement of an extralymphatic organ or site and of one or more lymph node regions on the same side of the diaphragm (II_E)
III	Involvement of lymph node regions on both sides of the diaphragm (III), which may also be accompanied by involvement of the spleen (III_S) or by localized involvement of an extralymphatic organ or site (III_E) or both (III_{SE})
IV	Diffuse or disseminated involvement of one or more extralymphatic organs or tissues, with or without associated lymph node involvement

B symptoms are usually seen in more advanced stages of the disease. To so-called classical Pel–Ebstein fever, which consists of a few days of high pyrexia followed by apyrexia for a few days, is very rarely seen. Symptoms due to involvement of other organs, e.g. bone, lung and skin, may also be seen.

Examination reveals lymphadenopathy, sometimes with hepatomegaly and splenomegaly depending on stage.

INVESTIGATION

Haematological findings may be unhelpful in the early stages. Later, a normochromic, normocytic anaemia with a raised ESR is characteristic. With marrow infiltration, a leucoerythroblastic anaemia may occur.

Biochemical findings may show hyperuricaemia and abnormal liver biochemistry due to liver involvement. A chest X-ray and/or chest CT may show mediastinal lymphadenopathy or pulmonary infiltration. Lymphangiography or abdominal CT scanning is used to show infiltration of the iliac, para-aortic and coeliac nodes. When it is intended to proceed to staging laparotomy (see below), lymphangiography should still be carried out.

The diagnosis of Hodgkin's disease rests on the biopsy of a suitable node. If possible, a whole node should be removed, handled as little as possible, and placed immediately into fixative after incising the capsule.

Histological classification

There are four histological subtypes of Hodgkin's disease:

- Lymphocyte-predominant, where there is heavy lymphocytic infiltration of the node
- Nodular sclerosing, where the gland is infiltrated with fibrous tissue
- Mixed cellularity, in which both lymphocytes and histiocytes are present

- Lymphocyte-depleted, in which there may be few or no lymphocytes present

STAGING

The standard Ann Arbor staging classification for Hodgkin's disease is shown in Table 7.14. Recently, it has been modified to take into account the volume or 'bulk' of lymph node masses and the use of modern imaging techniques such as CT scanning. Staging has been of great value in determining the prognosis and appropriate treatment.

TREATMENT

Over the past 50 years, the prognosis for patients with Hodgkin's disease has changed from being almost invariably fatal to being potentially curable for the majority. There are two effective treatments for Hodgkin's disease:

- Radiotherapy
- Combination chemotherapy

The choice of treatment depends on:

- Stage
- Site of disease
- Bulk of disease
- The presence or absence of B symptoms

Radiotherapy

Radiotherapy is curative in Hodgkin's disease if all the involved sites can be encompassed within a radiation field and an adequate dosage given. In preparing a patient for radiotherapy alone, therefore, it is still common practice, in addition to the investigations noted above, to carry out a staging laparotomy with sampling of the paraortic, iliac and coeliac nodes, removal of the spleen and a liver biopsy. Lymphangiography or CT scanning

Table 7.15 Combination chemotherapy for Hodgkin's disease.

Combination therapy regimen	Dosage	Route	Days when administered
MOPP			
Mustine (HN_2)	6 mg·m^{-2}	i.v.	1 and 8
Vincristine (Oncovin)	1.0–1.4 mg·m^{-2}	i.v.	1 and 8
Procarbazine	100 mg·m^{-2} daily	oral	1–14
Prednisolone	40 mg·m^{-2} daily	oral	1–14
14-day cycles separated by 14-day rest periods. Usually 6 cycles. Prednisolone in 1st and 4th cycles only.			
MVPP			
Mustine (HN_2)	6 mg·m^{-2}	i.v.	1 and 8
Vinblastine	6 mg·m^{-2}	i.v.	1 and 8
Procarbazine	100 mg·m^{-2} daily	oral	1–14
Prednisolone	40 mg·m^{-2} daily	oral	1–14
14-day cycles separated by 28-day rest periods. Usually 6 or more cycles. Prednisolone given in all cycles.			
ABVD			
Doxorubicin (Adriamycin)	25 mg·m^{-2}	i.v.	1 and 14
Bleomycin	10 mg·m^{-2}	i.v.	1 and 14
Vinblastine	6 mg·m^{-2}	i.v.	1 and 14
Dacarbazine (DTIC)	150 mg·m^{-2} daily	i.v.	1–5
14-day cycles separated by 14-day rest periods.			
Chl.VPP			
Chlorambucil	6 mg·m^{-2} daily	oral	1–14
Vinblastine	6 mg·m^{-2}	i.v.	1 and 8
Procarbazine	100 mg·m^{-2} daily	oral	1–14
Prednisolone	40 mg daily	oral	1–14[a]
14-day cycles separated by a 14-day rest period.			

[a] Reduced appropriately in children.

alone do not obviate the necessity for a laparotomy to obtain pathological staging of the disease. However, since a large proportion of patients who relapse within the abdomen following radiotherapy given for localized supra-diaphragmatic disease can be 'salvaged' with combination chemotherapy, there is currently debate about the need for staging laparotomy. Treatment of stage IA or IIA disease with radiotherapy has an excellent prognosis, with more than 80% of patients surviving long-term.

Chemotherapy

Patients who have evidence of disseminated disease, i.e. stage IIIB or IV, should be treated with chemotherapy. Complete responses are seen in approximately 70% overall; in patients in whom a complete response is achieved, 80% with stage IIIB disease and 60% with stage IV disease, respectively, are alive after 10 years.

A number of drug regimens for the treatment of Hodgkin's disease are now available and are listed in Table 7.15. It is hoped that some of the more recent regimens, i.e. those that contain less mustine will be more effective and will also be associated with a lower incidence of second malignancy and preservation of fertility.

Failure to achieve a complete response and early relapse are both associated with a very bad prognosis, and there are few long-term survivors in this group.

In children, the danger of splenectomy producing susceptibility to overwhelming and fatal infection and the gross disturbance produced by extended-field high-dose radiotherapy have resulted in the use of combined modality therapy, i.e. chemotherapy and lower-dose radiotherapy, with the avoidance of laparotomy. Centres using such treatment report a greater than 95% overall survival at 5 years.

Non-Hodgkin's lymphoma

These lymphomas are tumours of lymphoreticular tissue derived from malignant clones of B or T cells. Extranodal sites such as Waldeyer's ring (tonsils, adenoids and nasopharyngeal glands), the gut or skin may also be involved.

CLINICAL FEATURES

Lymphadenopathy is again the outstanding feature, but the involved sites may be non-contiguous. Mediastinal lymph-node involvement is less common, except in the T-cell type of lymphoma. Abdominal lymph node involvement is common, and splenomegaly and hepatomegaly may occur.

Wasting, fever and sweating may occur. Pruritus is uncommon, but nodular infiltration of the skin may be seen. Mycosis fungoides (p. 1043) and the Sézary syndrome characteristically involve the skin.

INVESTIGATION

- A normochromic, normocytic anaemia is seen with a raised ESR. Advanced cases show a leucoerythroblastic picture with circulating lymphoma cells.
- Liver biochemistry may be abnormal if there is liver involvement.
- A chest X-ray, CT scan of the abdomen and, if necessary, a CT scan of the chest will show lymph-node involvement.
- A bone-marrow biopsy may show infiltration by lymphoid tissue.

As in Hodgkin's disease, the most important investigation is the biopsy of a lymph node from an accessible site, with careful preservation of its architecture. In addition to formalin fixation, imprints of the gland may be prepared. Cell-surface phenotyping with monoclonal antibodies will determine the immunological origin of the cells.

Histological classification

The Kiel classification is currently the most used in the UK and Western Europe. This was proposed by Karl Lennert in 1978 and updated in 1988 to the form shown in Table 7.16a.

The Kiel classification, in common with others, makes a fundamental subdivision of non-Hodgkin's lymphomas into low- and high-grade. Low-grade tumours tend to be composed of relatively small cells, while high-grade tumours are generally composed of larger, more rapidly dividing 'blast' cells.

The other major subdivision is into tumours of B-cell and T-cell origin. Most non-Hodgkin's lymphomas are B-cell although T-cell tumours are increasingly being recognized. The latter show remarkable morphological diversity and have proved very difficult to classify.

One of the commonest low-grade lymphomas—centroblastic/centrocytic—usually shows a follicular growth pattern, while most other lymphomas show a diffuse pattern of infiltration. Lymphoplasmacytoid lymphomas in particular sometimes produce monoclonal paraproteins.

The Working Formulation for non-Hodgkin's lymphoma (Table 7.16b) for clinical use was devised in 1981, to give some indication of the likely prognosis and to provide a widely accepted basis for comparison of different treatment approaches. There are still problems with classification that remain to be resolved.

TREATMENT OF LOCALIZED DISEASE

Patients who have been found to have stage I disease may be cured by local radiotherapy to the involved area and adjacent nodes.

TREATMENT OF GENERALIZED DISEASE

Low-grade lymphoma
Follicular lymphoma. Repeated remissions can usually be achieved with single-agent chlorambucil but are hardly ever more than temporary; clinical trials have shown no survival advantage for the use of combination chemotherapy or total nodal irradiation. The median survival is 9 years, the response rate at presentation, first and second relapse being approximately 75%. With conventional therapy, patients with follicular lymphoma are thus incurable. New approaches such as the use of chlorambucil in combination with interferon and the use of ablative therapy supported by autologous bone-marrow transplantation are therefore being investigated.

Lymphoplasmacytoid and centrocytic lymphoma. These two subtypes are considered together because of similarities in presentation and response to therapy. The majority of patients present with advanced disease, the bone marrow frequently being involved. In the small proportion of patients who present with localized disease, the site is often extranodal, most frequently the gastrointestinal

Table 7.16a Updated Kiel classification of non-Hodgkin's lymphomas.

B	T
Low-grade	
Lymphocytic (CLL and others)	Lymphocytic (CLL and others)[a]
Lymphoplasmacytoid	Small cerebriform cell (mycosis
Plasmacytic	fungoides, Sézary's syndrome)
Centroblastic/centrocytic (follicular or	Lymphoepithelioid (Lennert's)
diffuse)	Angioimmunoblastic
Centrocytic	T-zone
	Pleomorphic, small cell
High-grade	
Centroblastic	Pleomorphic, medium and large cell
Immunoblastic	Immunoblastic
Large cell anaplastic (Ki-1+)[b]	Large cell anaplastic (Ki-1+)[b]
Burkitt's lymphoma	Lymphoblastic
Lymphoblastic	

[a] CLL = chronic lymphatic leukaemia.
[b] Ki-1 is an activation marker; + indicates expression of this marker.
From Stansfeld AG (1988) *Lancet* **1**, 292–293, 603.

Table 7.16b Working formulation for non-Hodgkin's lymphoma.

Low-grade		High-grade	
A	Small lymphocytic	G	Diffuse large-cell
B	Follicular small-cleaved	H	Immunoblastic
C	Follicular mixed histiocytic	I	Lymphoblastic
D	Follicular large-cell	J	Small non-cleaved
E	Diffuse small-cleaved		
F	Diffuse mixed histiocytic		

tract. The outcome for patients with localized disease is excellent, in contrast to that of patients presenting with disseminated disease, the median survival of the latter group being 3½ years and fewer than 20% patients surviving more than 5 years.

Clinical remission can be achieved in approximately 50% of patients using chlorambucil alone; however, complete remissions are infrequent and the remissions are not durable. The median remission duration is just over a year; relapse and eventual death from lymphoma are virtually inevitable. More intensive therapy results in complete remission being achieved in a greater proportion of patients but has not necessarily improved overall survival.

Lymphomas of T-cell origin. These are pleomorphic in terms of histology and very variable in their clinical course. Remissions can be achieved with chlorambucil but are usually short-lived, and more intensive therapy with adriamycin-containing regimens is currently being evaluated.

High-grade lymphomas of B- and T-cell origin
The majority of patients have B-cell lymphomas. Patients with stage I disease of small volume can be cured with local radiotherapy.

Achievement of complete remission is a prerequisite for cure. With intensive combination chemotherapy (Table 7.17) complete remission can be achieved in 60–70% of patients presenting with advanced disease and about one-third of patients overall are cured. Such chemotherapy is toxic and has a potential treatment-related mortality, particularly in older patients and those with poor performance status. Relapse is virtually synonymous with eventual death from lymphoma. It is, however, becoming apparent that in patients who respond to further chemotherapy at the time of relapse the use of ablative therapy supported by autologous bone-marrow transplantation can result in long-term second remissions and possible cure for approximately one-third. After much intensive treatment, particularly with total-body irradiation and BHT, there is a low but significant risk of secondary cancers.

Table 7.17 Therapy for high-grade non-Hodgkin's lymphoma.

Drug	Dose	Route	Administered
CHOP Chemotherapy			
Cyclophosphamide	600 mg·m^{-2}	i.v.	Day 1
Doxorubicin (hydroxydaunorubicin)	40 mg·m^{-2}	i.v.	Day 1
Vincristine (oncovin)	1.4 mg·m^{-2}	i.v.	Day 1
Prednisolone	40 mg·m^{-2} daily	oral	Day 1 to day 5
Courses are given every 21 days			
MACOP Chemotherapy			
Cyclophosphamide	1 g·m^{-2}	i.v.	Day 1
Doxorubicin (adriamycin)	50 mg·m^{-2}	i.v.	Day 1
Vincristine (oncovin)	1.6 mg·m^{-2}	i.v.	Day 1
Prednisolone	100 mg·m^{-2} daily	oral	Day 1 to day 5
Methotrexate	12.5 mg·m^{-2}	i.t.[a]	Day 7
Methotrexate[b]	300 mg·m^{-2}	i.v.	Day 10

[a] i.t. = intrathecal.
[b] With folinic acid rescue: 15 mg folinic acid 6-hourly after 24 h for eight doses.

Burkitt's lymphoma

Burkitt's lymphoma was first described in African children presenting with massive jaw lesions, extranodal abdominal involvement, and ovarian tumours. It is endemic in areas of central Africa where there is a high incidence of the Epstein–Barr virus (EBV) and in those areas where insect vectors and malaria are rife. EBV antibodies are found in the serum of most cases. There is commonly a chromosome abnormality, most frequently t(8;14)(q4;q32). A child with African Burkitt's lymphoma is shown in Fig. 7.14.

The tumour is very sensitive to radiation and chemotherapy but has a tendency to relapse.

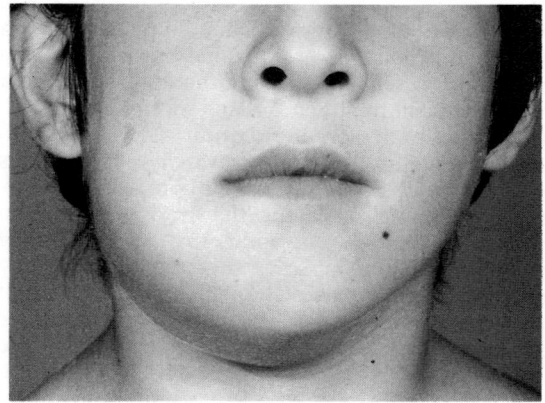

Fig. 7.14 A child with Burkitt's lymphoma.

Paraproteinaemias

Clinical conditions associated with paraproteinaemia are:

- Multiple myeloma
- Waldenstrom's macroglobulinaemia
- Monoclonal gammopathy of undetermined significance (MGUS)
- Plasma-cell leukaemia (very rare)

Paraproteinaemias are usually but not always associated with the presence of circulating paraprotein that is homogeneous and biologically inactive. Paraproteins are demonstrated by a single dark-staining band on serum electrophoresis, which is referred to as an 'M' or monoclonal band. The relative frequencies of these so-called monoclonal gammopathies are given in Table 7.18.

The paraprotein is produced by abnormal cells that arise from a single clone and therefore produce monoclonal immunoglobulin. When there is an accumulation in the serum of either IgG-, IgA- or rarely IgD-producing cells, the disease is known as multiple myeloma and the abnormal cells producing these immunoglobulins are plasma cells. The frequency with which the different immunoglobulins are produced in myeloma is given in Table 7.19. An excess of light chains, which are either kappa or lambda in type may be

Table 7.18 Relative frequencies of monoclonal gammopathies.

	Percentage of total
Plasma cell myeloma:	
Multiple myeloma—symptomatic	60
Multiple myeloma—indolent	3
Localized plasmacytoma	2
Waldenström's macroglobulinaemia	10
Heavy chain disease	< 1
Monoclonal gammopathy of undetermined significance (MGUS)	20
Primary amyloidosis	< 5

excreted in the urine as Bence Jones protein.

In Waldenström's macroglobulinaemia there is an accumulation of IgM, which is produced by plasmacytoid lymphoctyes. Excess monoclonal immunoglobulins may also be seen in lympho-plasmacytoid lymphoma and in MGUS, where there is a monoclonal spike on electrophoresis but no evidence of malignancy.

Multiple myeloma

CLINICAL FEATURES

Multiple myeloma is a disease of the elderly, the median age at presentation being 60 years. Men are affected slightly more often than women, and it occurs three times as often in blacks as in Caucasians.

Symptoms

- Backache occurring in more than 80% of patients. Vertebral collapse may lead to loss of height and paraplegia.
- Symptoms of anaemia.
- Recurrent infections.
- Renal failure, sometimes secondary to hyper-calcaemia, hyperuricaemia and dehydration.

Table 7.19 Relative frequencies of paraproteins in myeloma.

Paraprotein	Percentage of cases of myeloma
IgG	55
IgA	25
Light chain	18
IgD	1
Biclonal	1

- A bleeding diathesis, due either to thrombocytopenia or to the interference of the circulating paraprotein with clotting.
- Associated amyloid disease.
- Symptoms of hyperviscosity, with pre-coma or coma, visual failure or heart failure. Hyperviscosity is particularly common in IgG myeloma, but may also occur in IgA or IgD myeloma.

INVESTIGATION

Three criteria required for the diagnosis of myeloma are:

- The presence of paraprotein in the serum
- The presence of Bence-Jones protein in the urine
- The presence of lytic bone lesions

The presence of any two of these features makes the diagnosis of myeloma very likely. Infiltration of the bone marrow with plasma cells may occur in myeloma, but is not diagnostic. Figure 7.15 shows myeloma cells.

Other investigations
There may be neutropenia and thrombocytopenia. The ESR is elevated, usually above 100 mm·h^{-1}. A normochromic normocytic anaemia is common, with rouleaux formation.

A raised serum calcium is seen in one-third of patients on presentation. The serum alkaline phosphatase is normal in the majority of patients; a raised alkaline phosphatase is a bad prognostic feature, as also is a low serum albumin. About 20% of patients have evidence of renal failure at presentation; this is usually associated with heavy excretion of light chains in the urine, though other factors such as hypercalcaemia, hyperuricaemia, amyloidosis and infiltration of the kidney with myeloma tissue may contribute to the renal failure.

Radiology
Radiology in myeloma may show characteristic features, e.g. the appearance of the skull shown in

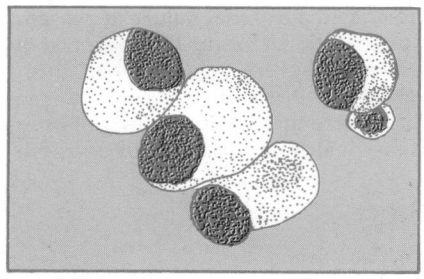

Fig. 7.15 Myeloma cells. Large cells with an eccentric nucleus and a perinuclear halo.

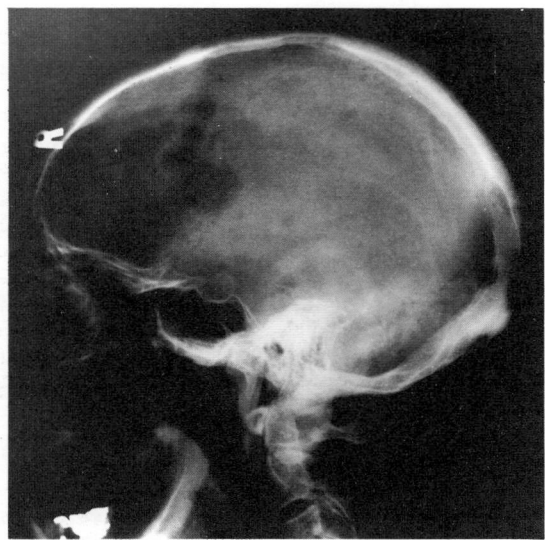

Fig. 7.16 Myeloma affecting the skull. Note the rounded lytic translucencies produced by infiltration of the skull with myeloma cells.

Fig. 7.16. The lytic lesions are caused by an osteoclast-activating factor (OAF) produced by the myeloma cell. OAF also inhibits osteoblastic activity. Lytic lesions in bone may also be caused by the common carcinomas of breast and bronchus, and the rarer carcinomas of thyroid and kidney.

PATHOLOGY

The comple pathology of myeloma is summarized in Fig. 7.17.

PROGNOSIS

The prognosis will depend on the amount of tumour present. Myeloma is difficult to stage, but schemes dependent on radiology and quantification of 'M' protein, the presence of anaemia, renal failure and hypercalcaemia have been devised and give a good indication of the outlook. The presence of severe anaemia or renal failure at presentation is a poor prognostic factor: in the presence of severe renal failure or severe anaemia, half the patients are dead after 9 months. In 'good prognosis' myeloma, where these features are not present, the median survival is of the order of 5 years.

TREATMENT

General management
Pain may be severe and require urgent treatment. If it is due to a local lesion, radiotherapy will give prompt relief.

Lytic lesions in bone may predispose to patho-logical fractures; these may be prevented by the insertion of metal pins.

Patients presenting with severe renal failure often have hypercalcaemia that requires correction with rehydration by intravenous fluids (more than 3 litres daily), and steroids; with such treatment, restoration of renal function is usually prompt and successful. Other agents used to treat hyper-calcaemia, such as calcitonin, mithramycin and diphosphonates, should be considered if the serum calcium fails to be controlled.

Anaemia and thrombocytopenia should be treated by transfusions of blood and platelets, but are more likely in the long term to respond to specific measures.

If the patient presents with paraplegia with bone destruction and the diagnosis is unknown, it is usual for surgery to be carried out in order to make a histological diagnosis. If the diagnosis is already known, the immediate use of dexametha-sone in high dosage (12 mg in 24 h) is the treatment of choice. A myelogram is then per-formed to delineate the extent of the block and is followed by radiotherapy.

Hyperviscosity syndromes are treated using plasmapheresis.

Specific therapy
Specific chemotherapy with melphalan or cyclo-phosphamide has been shown to increase the median duration of survival from 7 to 30 months for large numbers of patients. Melphalan is given in courses at 3-weekly intervals, starting with 10 mg daily together with prednisolone 40 mg daily for 5 days. The courses can be gradually extended until further increase is prevented by the falling white cell count. Intensive multidrug regimens that have included doxorubicin, nitro-soureas and vincristine have been shown to produce slightly better response rates, but current-ly the evidence that they increase survival is

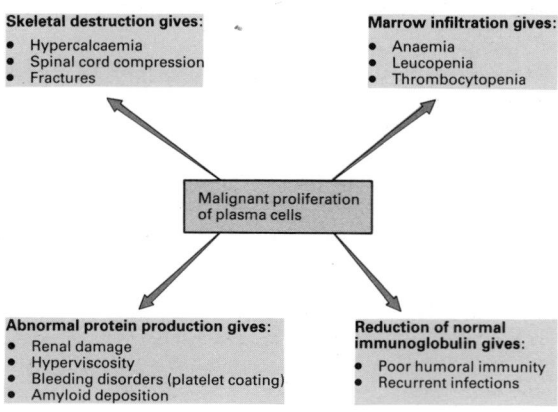

Fig. 7.17 The pathological consequences of plasma cell proliferation in myeloma.

dubious. In special centres with supportive care, the intensive use of high doses of melphalan has produced complete remissions with the reappearance of normal immunoglobulins.

Waldenström's macroglobulinaemia

This is a condition commonly seen in elderly men. It is more benign than myeloma, and is characterized by the production of monoclonal IgM paraprotein.

CLINICAL FEATURES

- Fatigue and weight loss of insidious onset
- Hyperviscosity
- Bleeding tendency
- Anaemia
- Hepatomegaly and splenomegaly

INVESTIGATION

- There is usually a normochromic, normocytic anaemia with rouleaux formation.
- IgM paraprotein is found in the serum.
- The bone marrow shows infiltration with lymphoplasmacytoid cells.
- The ESR is often raised to over 140 mm·h^{-1}.
- Radiology shows an absence of lytic lesions.

TREATMENT

The progress of this disease can be very slow and specific treatment may not be required immediately. Supportive care with blood transfusion and antibiotics for infections will be needed. Specific treatment with alkylating agents such as cyclophosphamide or chlorambucil is usually given. Plasmapheresis is required for the symptoms of hyperviscosity.

Monoclonal gammopathy of undetermined significance (MGUS)

MGUS used to be referred to as 'benign monoclonal gammopathy', but since a proportion of these patients go on to develop lymphoma or myeloma, this term is no longer appropriate. Patients are usually elderly. A paraprotein is present in the blood, but the level is $< 2 \text{ g·L}^{-1}$. Patients are usually well, with no anaemia, renal impairment, skeletal lesions or Bence–Jones protein in their urine. Serial estimations of the paraprotein should show no further increase. Specific therapy is not necessary and, as these patients are often elderly, it is important to recognize this condition and not put them at risk by giving them chemotherapy. The condition has to be distinguished from the rare form of indolent myeloma, which may also not need immediate specific therapy.

Treatment of solid tumours

Some non-haematological tumours can be cured by chemotherapy. They include choriocarcinoma, testicular cancer and a number of childhood tumours such as Wilms' tumour, rhabdomyosarcoma, Ewing's sarcoma and osteosarcoma. Symptoms from such tumours as breast cancer, small-cell lung cancer and ovarian cancer can be relieved, and in small-cell lung cancer (for example) a modest but useful prolongation of life can be achieved.

CARCINOMA OF THE BREAST

Breast cancer is probably a disseminated disease from its clinical onset, and medical treatment is appropriate from an early stage in the majority of patients. Drugs of proven efficacy in the treatment of breast cancer are the alkylating agents, anthracyclines, vinca alkaloids and antimetabolites.

Adjuvant therapy produces a small but significant prolongation of life, when all the results of world-wide trials are examined together. Adjuvant therapy with cytotoxic drugs is indicated in:

- Premenopausal women with positive axillary nodes at operation
- Postmenopausal women who are considered at high-risk for relapse

Cyclophosphamide, methotrexate and 5-fluorouracil (CMF) is one of the most commonly used combinations. In women under 50 or premenopausal, there has been a significant reduction in mortality and this has amounted to 35% in some studies. Endocrine manipulation has also been used in adjuvant therapy. One of the most successful and least-toxic agents currently available is tamoxifen, and this is indicated for adjuvant endocrine therapy in postmenopausal women with positive axillary nodes and positive hormone receptor levels (p. 356).

DISSEMINATED BREAST CANCER

Endocrine manipulation and chemotherapy given for advanced disease probably do not improve survival, but can bring marked relief of symptoms. Endocrine manipulation should be attempted first; when and if this fails, the least-toxic chemotherapy combination should be started. Indications for the use of chemotherapy in disseminated breast cancer are:

- Failure to respond to prior endocrine therapy
- A short disease-free interval from primary treatment

● Rapidly progressing metastatic disease with visceral involvement

Radiotherapy also has a role in the management of advanced disease; for example, useful pain relief can be achieved by irradiating bone deposits.

OVARIAN CANCER

Ovarian cancer is the commonest gynaecological cancer. Patients usually present with an abdominal mass or ascites. Surgery is important not only to diagnose and delineate disease, but also to remove as much tumour as possible. In patients with disease limited to the ovary, surgery may itself be curative.

The drugs that have been of greatest value in treating advanced disease are melphalan, chlorambucil and cisplatin. Meaningful responses are seen and in some patients these have been complete. A few patients in whom complete response has been achieved have remained free of disease long-term. Alternatively radiotherapy can be used.

LUNG CANCER

Small-cell

The problem is that the disease is almost always disseminated at the time of presentation, liver, bone and bone marrow involvement being the most common and brain secondaries being seen not infrequently.

Chemotherapy relieves symptoms and improves survival to some extent. Single agents are often as effective as combination therapies, and are better tolerated. High-dose chemotherapy supported by autologous bone-marrow transplantation has not in general been of benefit. At the present time, the best palliative treatment is the use of short, moderately intensive courses of single agents such as etoposide with intensive chemotherapy reserved for limited disease. Radiotherapy may also be useful in specific situations, such as relieving superior vena caval obstruction or in patients with distressing haemoptysis.

Adenocarcinoma and squamous-cell carcinoma

Unlike small-cell cancer, these subtypes remain localized to the lung and hilar lymph nodes for an appreciable length of time; however, chemotherapy in general is not effective. Useful palliation can be achieved with radiotherapy given to alleviate specific distressing symptoms.

TESTICULAR CANCER (see p. 486)

The disseminated form of the disease, either seminoma or malignant teratoma, used to be almost universally fatal, but the introduction of effective chemotherapy has produced a dramatic change in outcome. Vinblastine, bleomycin, cisplatin are all effective and, when used in combination, result in survival rates of 60–80%.

Terminal care and pain control

In many types of cancer the time comes when specific treatment is no longer effective and therapy intended to cure has to be abandoned. It is important not to look on this phase as the end of treatment; indeed, surgery, chemotherapy or radiotherapy may still be required for palliation, but the focus of treatment becomes symptom control.

Pain relief is a matter of skill. Local lesions in bone may respond dramatically to radiotherapy, while generalized bone pain may be relieved by steroids. Pain related to compression of nerves may be helped by local nerve blocks or cordotomy; newly developed techniques of epidural infusions or injections of steroid are also promising. Analgesia must be given regularly and in sufficient dosage. Addiction is not a problem in the terminally ill and medical and nursing staff should not be inhibited in giving diamorphine or morphine in adequate amounts to control pain. The patient should not have to ask for analgesia, as the principle of administration is that analgesia should be given to prevent the onset of pain. It therefore needs to be given regularly, and the dose and time interval adjusted so that the patient remains pain-free. Drugs ascending in potency can be used; paracetamol and dihydrocodeine may be used initially, when these become ineffective, dipipanone with cyclizine may be substituted, moving on to morphine or heroin for severe pain. Long-acting oral morphines are now available and are useful in patients to whom it is difficult to give parenteral therapy. It should be remembered that pain relief is not only a matter of giving analgesic drugs—sometimes a frank talk with an explanation of the reason for the pain and of the various measures that can be used to suppress it may give considerable benefit.

Anorexia, nausea and vomiting are often troublesome symptoms in the terminally ill. Obstructive vomiting should be relieved by a nasogastric tube. Metoclopramide, cyclizine or chlorpromazine may be helpful in preventing nausea. Small doses of steroid may be of value, and the appetite-inducing effects of drugs like medroxyprogesterone are under study. Constipation is a symptom that causes considerable misery, particularly in the elderly, and this may be made worse by analgesia. Regular mild aperients may help, but enemas may be necessary at the beginning of treatment with analgesics. Cough is relieved by methadone or diamorphine. Dyspnoea is a very difficult symptom to control and is often related to anxiety. Diazepam and reassurance may be helpful.

The aim of terminal care is constantly to assist the patient. The first question should be 'What is the cause of the symptom and is it related to the cancer?' If it is not, then it may well be alleviated. Heart failure, asthma and other common medical conditions can occur in a cancer patient as in any other and these conditions should be treated. If the symptoms are due to the cancer, then it is important to identify the most distressing and to relieve them rapidly. Terminal care is exacting for the doctor and nursing staff but can be rewarding if carried out effectively.

Psychological management of the dying patient

Among patients dying in hospital, up to half manifest significant anxiety and depression. Guilt and anger are also common, with or without depressive symptoms. Guilt is often related to the demands the patient makes on his/her family. Anger at dying may be displaced on to the doctors, nurses and relatives trying to help the patient. Depression can be understood as a form of mourning for the impending loss of friends and family, anxiety as an understandable reaction to the uncertainties posed by dying and death, and the possibilities of pain, incontinence and helplessness.

Dying patients use a number of psychological defence mechanisms against being overwhelmed by depression and anxiety—the three commonest being denial, dependency and displacement. Denial, usually the initial reaction to the news of impending death, may lead to a period of calm. As denial diminishes, the patient slowly comes to terms with the situation. Denial can return from time to time during the course of the illness, such that at times the patient appears to realize the nature of his illness and at other times appears unaware of and uninformed about it. A degree of dependency is inevitable during the final stages of a serious illness but may be exaggerated so that the patient makes extreme demands on others. Displacement occurs when the patient directs angry feelings inappropriately at others.

The management of the dying patient is aimed at ensuring that the patient is relatively free from pain, functions at the most effective level possible, and is able to recognize and resolve remaining conflicts and difficulties and able to yield control to others in whom he/she has confidence. Staff, therefore, need to be aware of the feelings and fears of dying patients and need to take active measures of management. Isolation in a side-ward and management based on denial of death by medical and nursing staff and the family are only likely to increase the fear, anxiety, sadness and sense of isolation of the dying person.

The most important factors in the management include:

- The relief of distressing physical symptoms (see above)
- The forming of a supportive and trusting relationship between the patient and the medical and nursing staff
- The provision of counselling to family members
- The protection of the ties between the patient and his/her family
- The symptomatic relief of extreme psychological symptoms by the judicious use of tranquillizers or sedatives and the use of antidepressants when the usual indications are present
- The prudent provision of information concerning the nature and prognosis of the patient's underlying condition

Further reading

DeVita V, Hellman S & Rosenberg SA (1989) *Principles and Practices of Oncology*. Philadelphia: JB Lippincott.

Garrod IF & Hill RP (1987) *The Basic Science of Oncology*. Oxford: Pergamon Press.

Henderson ES & Lister TA (1989) *Leukaemia*, 5th edn. New York: Grune & Stratton.

Kaplan HS (1980) *Hodgkin's Disease*, Cambridge, Massachusetts: Harvard University Press.

Wiernik PH (ed) (1985) *Contemporary Issues in Clinical Oncology. Leukaemias and Lymphomas*. New York: Churchill Livingstone.

Williams C & S (1986) *Cancer—A Guide for Patients and Their Families*. Wiley.

Yarbro JW (ed) *Seminars in Oncology*. Orlando, Florida: Grune & Stratton.

Saunders C & Baines M (1983) *Living with Dying, The Management of Terminal Disease*. Oxford: Oxford University Press.

8

Rheumatology and Bone Disease

Introduction

Rheumatology is concerned with medical disorders of the locomotor system, which can be divided into three categories: arthritis, back pain and soft-tissue rheumatism. Most of these diseases are seen world-wide, although the prevalence of individual conditions varies. Rheumatological diseases constitute a major part (approximately 20%) of the workload of a primary-care physician. The major complaints are pain and disability, arising not only from the joints, but also from the surrounding soft tissues.

The normal joint

The structure of a typical synovial joint is shown in Fig. 8.1. The joint itself is made up of two articulating bone surfaces, each covered with articular cartilage, and a fibrous capsule lined by synovium. The space within the joint is filled with synovial fluid that acts as a lubricant. Inflammation of the above structures is described as arthritis. The term arthropathy is sometimes used to describe joint disease of any type. The joint is surrounded by so-called 'soft tissues', including tendons, ligaments and bursae. The specialized junction of tendon and bone is called an enthesis; this can also become inflamed.

Table 8.1 Rheumatological terms.

Term	Meaning
Monarticular	One joint involved
Polyarticular	Many joints involved
Oligoarticular or pauciarticular	Two, three or four joints involved
Migratory	Arthritis moving from joint to joint
Arthralgia	Joint pain without swelling
Small joints	Joints of hands and wrists
Large joints	Any other joint
Seropositive arthritis	Rheumatoid factor present in serum
Seronegative arthritis	Rheumatoid factor absent in serum
Seronegative spondyloarthropathies	HLA-B27 associated diseases, e.g. ankylosing spondylitis, Reiter's disease, psoriatic arthritis

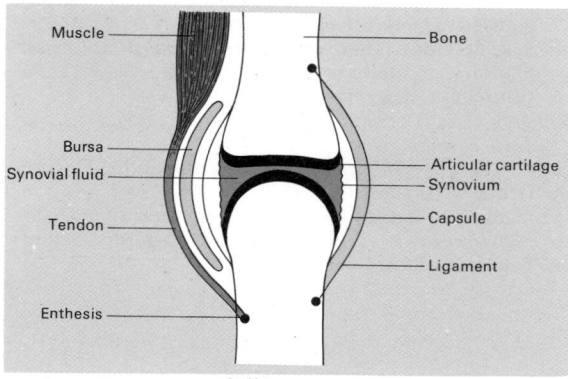

Fig. 8.1 A typical synovial joint.

Rheumatological terminology
The main terms used in rheumatology are outlined in Table 8.1.

CLINICAL FEATURES

History
The main features are listed in Table 8.2 and some of these points are discussed below.

Background information. This may be helpful in assessing the type of arthritis. For example:

- *Age.* Osteoarthritis commonly presents at 50 years of age.
- *Sex.* Rheumatoid arthritis is commoner in women, whilst Reiter's syndrome is commoner in men.
- *Race.* Some arthropathies are particularly associated with diseases occurring in particular races, e.g. in sickle cell disease.
- *Occupation.* This can be an important factor in soft-tissue rheumatism or osteoarthritis.

Joint pain. The type of pain is of little help as all joint pains feel much the same to the patient. The following points are of some value:

- *Duration.* For example, a long history is suggestive of rheumatoid arthritis, whilst a short history may suggest gout.
- *Onset.* Some conditions like gout start suddenly.
- *Precipitating factors.* For example, injury may lead to arthritis, diuretic therapy can precipitate gout, and a sore throat precedes rheumatic fever.
- *Characteristics*
  (a) Site of the pain—this usually indicates the site of the pathology (although hip disease may present with knee pain).
  (b) Radiation—a lesion of the cervical or lumbar spine will give pain in the distribution of the affected roots.

Table 8.2 Main features in the history of a patient with arthritis.

Background information—age, sex
Main complaint
Pain—situation, radiation
Other symptoms, e.g. stiffness
Resultant problems
Pattern of joint involvement
Associated symptoms
Past medical history
Family history
Social history
Previous treatment

(c) Severity—excruciating pain is characteristic of acute gout.
(d) Activity—joint pains are often made worse by activity and relieved by rest.
(e) Diurnal variation—pain due to inflammation is characteristically worst in the mornings and improves during the day.
(f) Episodic nature—the frequency, regularity and duration of attacks should be noted.

Other joint symptoms. Enquire about:

- *Morning stiffness.* This is characteristic of inflammatory arthropathies. The duration of stiffness gives some guide to the activity of the inflammatory process.
- *Joint swelling.* This always indicates local disease.
- *Pattern of joint involvement.* For example, recurrent attacks in the big toe are suggestive of gout.
- *Clicking and creaking of the joint.* These are not important and can be felt in normal joints.
- *Disability.* This is a very individual problem. One patient may continue all activities, whilst another with the same degree of pain may be confined to bed or chair.

Associated non-articular symptoms. These are seen in many types of arthritis; for example, nodules or pleural effusions are seen in rheumatoid arthritis. Alternatively, systemic diseases such as ulcerative colitis may have an associated arthritis.

Past medical history. This may be helpful in the diagnosis, e.g. trauma or psoriasis.

Family history. Some conditions run in families, e.g. diseases associated with HLA-B27. Patients with ankylosing spondylitis may have relatives with ulcerative colitis. Patients with psoriatic arthritis do not necessarily have psoriatic skin lesions but may give a family history of psoriasis.

Social history. The occupation of the patient may have a bearing on his arthritis. In addition, the development of a chronic arthritis has a major influence on the life-style of the patient and his family.

Treatment record. A record of the previous treatments tried and their success is important for the future management.

Examination of joints
There are three stages in the examination of an individual joint: *look at it*, *feel it* and *move it*.

Inspection will reveal swelling, deformities, changes in the overlying skin (e.g. erythema) and abnormalities of the surrounding structures, e.g. wasting of muscle or swelling of bursae.

Palpation will reveal the nature of any observed

swelling as well as the presence or absence of warmth and tenderness, which are cardinal signs of inflammation. There are three types of joint swelling:

- A hard or bony swelling
- An effusion
- Synovial thickening

The presence of an effusion can be demonstrated by fluctuation or by a patellar tap in the knee joint. A firm non-fluctuant swelling is characteristic of synovial thickening.

Movement of a joint may produce pain or crepitus—a sensation of grating that is characteristic of osteoarthritis. The range of movement should be noted. Excessive abnormal movement is called instability. Posture and gait should also be assessed.

Movement of joints is described in terms of flexion, extension, abduction, adduction and rotation. Deformities are described as valgus (like knock knees) or varus (like bow legs).

A system of examination should be followed so that no joint is missed.

INVESTIGATION (see Table 8.3)

Investigations are often unnecessary in patients with rheumatic complaints. In patients with tennis elbow, osteoarthritis and many other conditions, the diagnosis can be made on the basis of history and examination findings. There are no diagnostic tests in osteoarthritis and tests are only requested to exclude some other condition.

Table 8.3 Investigations in rheumatic diseases. (Most diagnoses are made on the history and examination.)

Useful tests
ESR
Rheumatoid factor
Antinuclear antibodies
Serum uric acid
Synovial fluid examination
X-rays

Occasionally useful tests
White blood cell count
CRP
Alkaline phosphatase
ASO titre—in rheumatic fever
Protein electrophoresis, immunoglobulin, urinalysis
  for Bence Jones protein, bone marrow—for
  myeloma
Complement
Arthroscopy ± synovial biopsy
Arthrogram
Bone scan
HLA-B27

Table 8.4 Conditions in which rheumatoid factor is found in the serum.

Diseases involving joints
Sjögren's syndrome (90%)
Rheumatoid arthritis (80%)
Systemic lupus erythematosus (50%)
Systemic sclerosis (30%)
Polymyositis/dermatomyositis (50%)
Mixed connective tissue disease

Chronic infections (low titres), e.g.
Tuberculosis
Leprosy
Infective endocarditis
Kala-azar

'Normal' population
Elderly
Relatives of patients with rheumatoid arthritis

Miscellaneous
Autoimmune chronic active hepatitis
Fibrosing alveolitis
Sarcoidosis
Waldenstrom's macroglobulinaemia

Erythrocyte sedimentation rate (ESR) and C-reactive protein (CRP)
These provide a guide to the activity of inflammation and are characteristically raised in inflammatory conditions such as rheumatoid arthritis but are normal in osteoarthritis.

Tests for rheumatoid factor
Rheumatoid factors are autoantibodies found in the serum, usually of the IgM class, which are directed against human IgG. They are detected by agglutination of either latex particles (the latex test) or sheep red cells (the Rose-Waaler test) (Fig. 8.2). The major value of rheumatoid factor tests is in the

Table 8.5 Conditions in which antinuclear antibodies are found.

Systemic lupus erythematosus (95%)
Systemic sclerosis (80%)
Sjögren's syndrome (60%)
Polymyositis and dermatomyositis (30%)
Rheumatoid arthritis (30%)
Still's disease (30%)

Occasionally seen in:
  Autoimmune chronic active hepatitis
  Primary biliary cirrhosis
  Infections e.g. infective endocarditis
  Normal elderly people

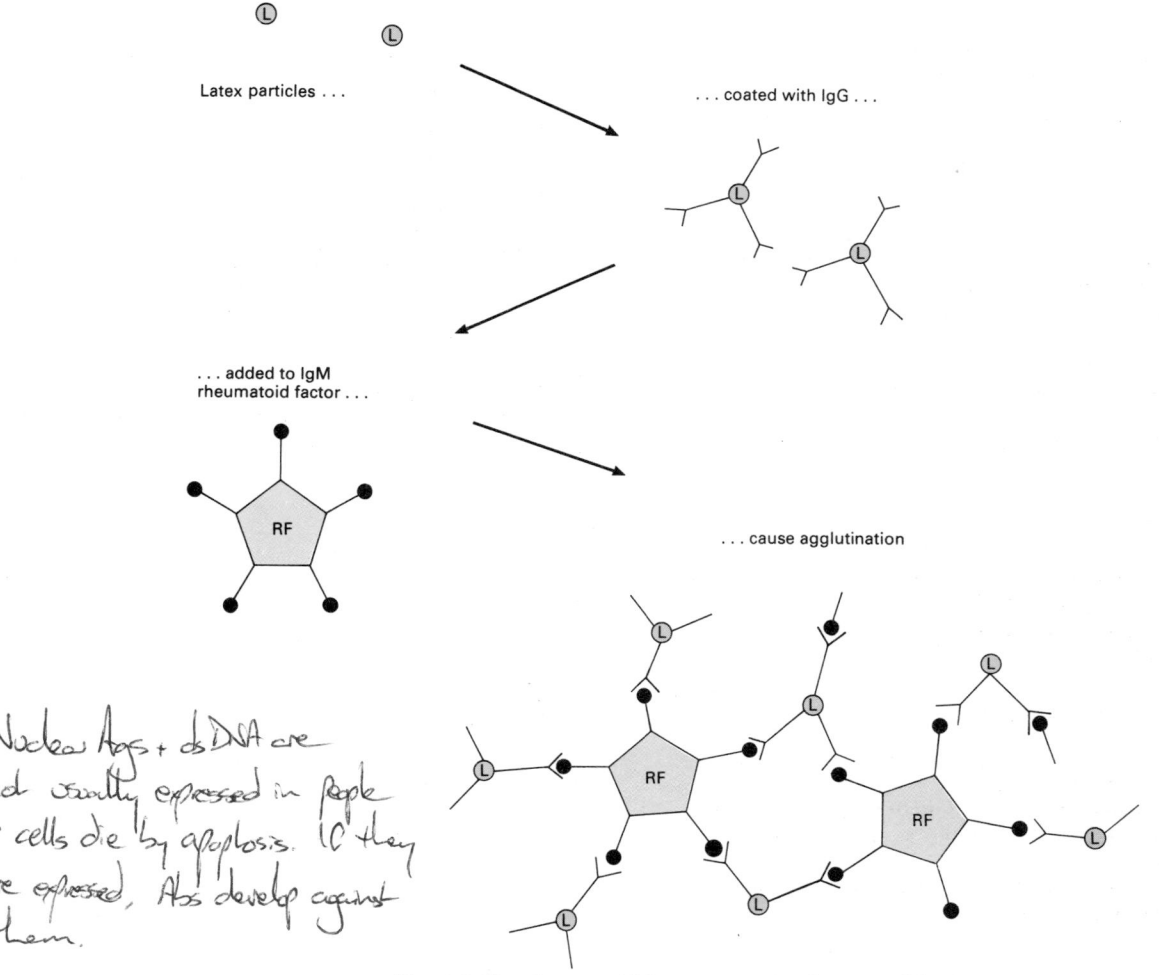

Latex particles . . .

. . . coated with IgG . . .

. . . added to IgM
rheumatoid factor . . .

RF

. . . cause agglutination

Handwritten note: Nuclear Ags + dsDNA are not usually expressed in people ∴ cells die by apoptosis. IC they are expressed, Abs develop against them.

Fig. 8.2 The rheumatoid factor test using latex particles.

diagnosis of rheumatoid arthritis (Table 8.4). The latex test is quicker and easier to perform; it is more sensitive, and therefore more often positive, but is less specific than the sheep red cell test.

Antinuclear antibodies (see Fig. 8.3 and Table 8.5) Antinuclear antibodies in the serum are detected using immunofluorescent staining of the nuclei of a tissue such as rat liver or human cells in tissue culture. A low titre of 1 : 10 is weakly positive and of little significance.

Antibodies to other nuclear antigens. A variety of antinuclear antibodies have been described with particular disease associations that are summarized in Table 8.6. It seems likely that the pattern of disease is determined by the nature of the auto-antibodies produced.

Antibodies against double-stranded DNA (ds DNA). These can be detected using the FARR test, a radioimmunoassay measuring the percentage anti-

Table 8.6 Antinuclear antibodies (ANA) and their clinical associations.

Antibody to	Clinical association
ds DNA	SLE[a]
ENA; ribonucleoprotein (RNP)	Mixed connective tissue disease and SLE
Ro (SSA)[b]	SLE and primary Sjögren's syndrome
La[b]	Primary Sjögren's syndrome
Sm[b]	SLE
Centromere	CREST syndrome
Nucleolus	Systemic sclerosis
ScL-70[b]	Systemic sclerosis
Jo-1[b]	Polymyositis
Cardiolipin	SLE and cardiolipin syndrome

[a] SLE = systemic lupus erythematosus.
[b] Fractions of nuclear material.

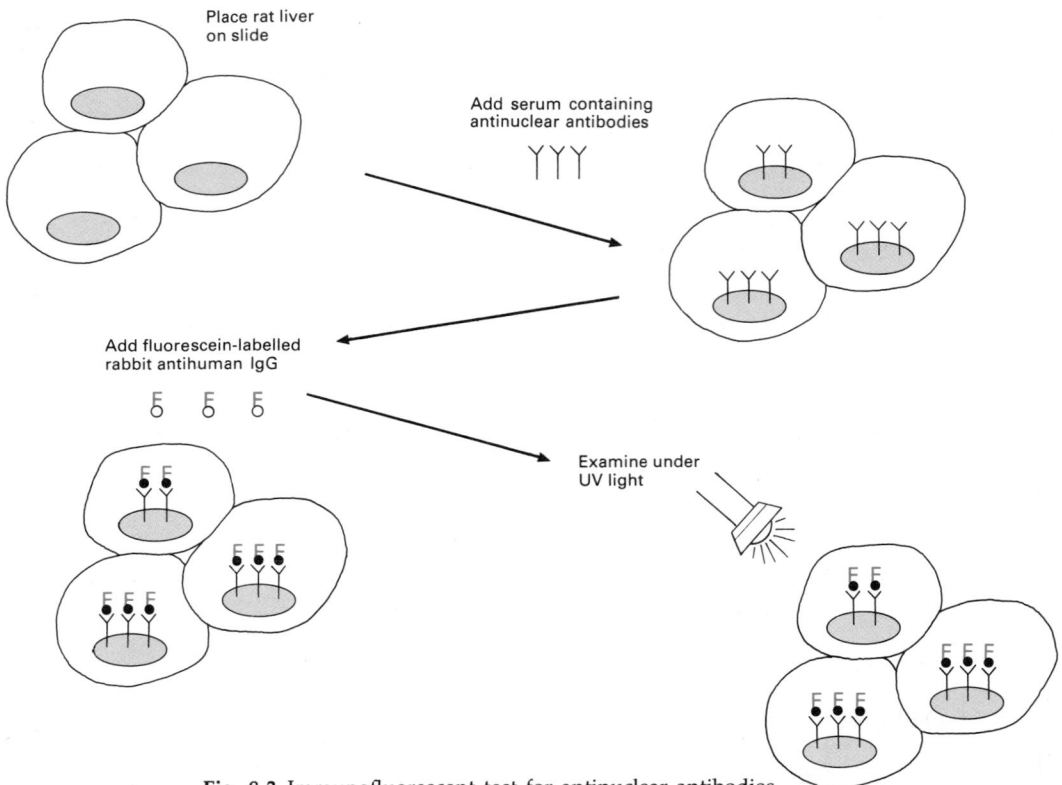

Place rat liver
on slide

Add serum containing
antinuclear antibodies

Add fluorescein-labelled
rabbit antihuman IgG

Examine under
UV light

Fig. 8.3 Immunofluorescent test for antinuclear antibodies.

body binding of added labelled double-stranded DNA. Antibodies are found in about 50% of cases of systemic lupus erythematosus (SLE) but seldom in any other condition. They are therefore a much more specific test than antinuclear antibodies. They are also associated with more severe disease and renal involvement.

Antibodies against extractable nuclear antigen (ENA). IgG class antibodies against soluble nuclear anti-

gens are characteristic of mixed connective-tissue disease, the overlap syndrome described on p. 396, but are also found in patients with SLE.

Serum uric acid
A raised serum uric acid is a good confirmatory test for gout, but is not diagnostic. A low level of uric acid excludes gout. In known cases of gout, the uric acid level is helpful in deciding treatment (see p. 406).

Table 8.7 Typical synovial fluid changes in some rheumatic diseases.

	Normal	Osteoarthritis	Rheumatoid arthritis	Septic arthritis	Gout	Pyrophosphate arthropathy
Appearance:	Clear viscous fluid	Increased volume; viscosity retained	Sometimes turbid, yellow or green in colour; viscosity lost	Turbid; low viscosity	Clear; low viscosity	Clear; low viscosity
White blood cells (× 10⁶/L):	< 200 Mononuclear	3000 Mononuclear	30 000 Neutrophils	100 000 Neutrophils	10 000 Neutrophils	10 000 Neutrophils
Crystals:	None	5% have pyrophosphate	None	None	Needle-shaped, negatively birefringent	Brick-shaped, positively birefringent
Culture:	Sterile	Sterile	Sterile	Positive	Sterile	Sterile

Joint puncture

Indications

- Diagnosis—particularly septic arthritis and crystal deposition disease.
- Drainage—in septic arthritis and to relieve pain from tense effusions.
- Drugs—intra-articular steroids for rheumatoid and other inflammatory arthropathies.

Risks

- Infection—1 in 10 000 punctures with luck and care!
- Destruction—deterioration of cartilage reported in weight-bearing joints of patients given frequent injections who increased their activities.
- Inflammation—some preparations of steroids contain crystals that may cause a transient inflammatory reaction.

Precautions

- Asepsis—no-touch technique
- Advice to patients
  report at once if symptoms worsen
  avoid weight-bearing for 2 days—care for 2 weeks after injection
- Administer only three steroid injections in one joint in one lifetime

Procedure

- Wash hands thoroughly.
- Examine joint and identify correct site for puncture. Clean the skin and do not touch it again.
- Draw up steroid if required.
- Infiltrate with local anaesthetic if necessary, for nervous patients or difficult joints.
- Insert untouched sterile needle into joint.
- Aspirate and inject through same needle.

Synovial fluid handling

- *Inspect* for volume, colour and viscosity.
- Divide into three portions for
  (a) WBC and differential (sequestrene tube)
  (b) Polarized-light microscopy for crystals (slide or plain tube)
  (c) Gram stain and culture (sterile bottle)

Synovial fluid examination

The characteristics of synovial fluid in normal and diseased joints are shown in Table 8.7.

Polarized-light microscopy reveals the presence of negatively birefringent crystals in gout. In pyrophosphate arthropathy, crystals of calcium pyrophosphate, which are weakly positively birefringement, are seen. Crystals of hydroxyapatite are too small to be seen in polarized light microscopy and need to be identified using electron microscopy. Gram stain may identify organisms in septic arthritis but the fluid should also be cultured.

X-rays

X-rays show characteristic abnormalities in many rheumatic conditions; these are described in the appropriate sections. Degenerative changes are present in almost everyone by the age of 65 years and their presence on an X-ray therefore does not necessarily have clinical significance.

X-rays are of little value in acute conditions such as septic arthritis.

Occasionally useful tests (see Table 8.3)

- The white blood cell count is useful in cases of infections and leukaemia presenting with arthritis.
- A raised serum alkaline phosphatase is characteristic of Paget's disease (p. 42) but is also sometimes seen in active rheumatoid arthritis and polymyalgia rheumatica.
- A monoclonal protein band on electrophoresis is found in myeloma (see p. 371).
- A raised antistreptolysin-O (ASO) titre indicates recent streptococcal infection. Very high levels are characteristic of rheumatic fever.
- A high serum iron or ferritin level occurs in haemochromatosis, which may present with arthritis.
- A low serum complement may be found in the active phase of systemic lupus erythematosus (SLE).
- Arthroscopy is useful for the demonstration of mechanical lesions in the knee joint such as a torn meniscus and if necessary a synovial biopsy can be obtained during the procedure. This investigation is particularly useful in persistent monoarticular arthritis, e.g. in tuberculosis.
- An arthrogram can also be used to visualize the meniscus or to demonstrate knee-joint rupture.
- A bone scan is useful in demonstrating malignant deposits. Increased uptake also occurs around osteoarthritic joints and also in inflammatory arthropathies, but these abnormalities can usually be distinguished from malignant disease.
- The histocompatibility antigen HLA-B27 is found in 96% of patients with ankylosing spondylitis and only 5% of normal people in the UK. There are marked differences between the incidence of the antigen in different populations that roughly parallel the frequency of ankylosing spondylitis. In addition, about 60% of patients with Reiter's disease are B27 positive.

Arthritis

The causes of arthritis are given in Table 8.8.

Table 8.8 Main causes of arthritis.

Osteoarthritis

Rheumatoid arthritis

Connective tissue disorders
  Systemic lupus erythematosus
  Polymyositis/dermatomyositis
  Systemic sclerosis

Polymyalgia rheumatica

Crystal deposition diseases
  Gout
  Pyrophosphate arthropathy
  Acute calcific periarthritis

Infective arthritis

Reactive arthritis

Ankylosing spondylitis

Juvenile arthritis, e.g. Still's disease

Arthritis associated with other diseases, e.g.
  psoriasis

Rare rheumatic diseases

Osteoarthritis

Osteoarthritis (OA) is the commonest type of arthritis, occurring in about 10% of the population as a whole and in 50% of those aged over 60. It is a disease of cartilage, which becomes eroded and progressively thinned as the disease proceeds.

The pattern of development of joint disease in osteoarthritis is additive. The disease moves slowly from joint to joint and also progresses very slowly (in most cases) within individual joints. Its greatest impact is on weight-bearing joints such as the hips and knees, and involvement of these joints is the commonest cause of disability in an elderly population.

EPIDEMIOLOGY

OA occurs throughout the world and has occurred throughout the history of mankind. It is twice as common in women as in men. It is particularly common in British populations but this has nothing to do with climate, latitude or longitude and is therefore presumably genetic. OA is uncommon in black populations; when it does occur it usually affects the knees and hand involvement is rare.

PATHOGENESIS

Osteoarthritis is a disease of cartilage. Normal cartilage is composed of a matrix of collagen fibres stuffed with proteoglycan molecules that attract water and thereby maintain a positive pressure within the structure. There are just a few chondrocytes scattered within normal cartilage. It is likely that different stimuli can start off the degenerative process but the two most obvious are:

- Mechanical insults
- Biochemical abnormalities of cartilage

The chondrocyte is believed to initiate the deterioration, releasing enzymes that degrade collagen and proteoglycans. Breaks in the collagen fibres allow the uptake of water; cartilage swells and splits. Crystals are released into the joint and are one of the mechanisms of the synovial inflammation that

Table 8.9 Causes of secondary osteoarthritis.

Congenital abnormalities of joints
Hypermobility
Congenital dysplasias

Structural disorders in children
Slipped femoral epiphysis
Perthes' disease

Trauma and mechanical problems
Intra-articular fractures
Meniscectomy
Obesity
Recurrent dislocation
Occupational hazards (e.g. repetitive actions)

Crystal deposition disease and metabolic abnormalities of cartilage
Pyrophosphate arthropathy
Ochronosis
Haemochromatosis

Avascular necrosis, e.g.
Sickle cell disease
Corticosteroid therapy
Caisson disease

Other conditions in which cartilage is destroyed, e.g.
Septic arthritis
Recurrent haemarthrosis
Inflammatory arthropathy such as rheumatoid arthritis

Neuropathic causes
Diabetes mellitus
Peripheral nerve lesions
Tabes dorsalis
Syringomyelia

---

follows and which may perpetuate the destruction of cartilage. Attempts at repair include remodelling of bone, which produces the characteristic osteophytes.

Identifiable aetiological factors in primary osteoarthritis include:

- *Age*. The disease tends to start at the age of 50.
- *Genetics*. There is a strong familial tendency.
- *Obesity*. Particularly related to osteoarthritis of the knees.
- *Mechanical abnormalities*. The incidence of osteoarthritis is increased by insults such as meniscectomy or fracture through the joint surface.
- *Biochemical abnormalities*. Conditions like haemochromatosis and ochronosis can initiate the process of cartilage degeneration and it seems likely that further research will reveal similar abnormalities in many cases of primary osteoarthritis.

Most OA is primary but in a small proportion of patients there is an obvious cause. The causes of secondary OA are listed in Table 8.9.

PATHOLOGY

There is fibrillation of the superficial layer of cartilage with fissures (splits) developing and extending into the deeper layers. The bases of these fissures contain clusters of chondrocytes, which are increased in number. As the disease advances there is progressive cartilage loss until hard eburnated bone is all that remains. The synovial membrane is heavily infiltrated with mononuclear cells. There is thickening of subchondral bone with cyst formation.

CLINICAL FEATURES

Symptoms

- Pain, typically in the knees, hips or hands, worst in the evenings and aggravated by use and relieved by rest. Sometimes intermittent at first but later chronic with inflammatory exacerbations in particular joints.
- Morning stiffness, usually lasting up to half an hour and stiffness after sitting.
- Disability depends upon the joints affected.

Signs

- Swelling: characteristically hard and bony, sometimes with associated effusion.
- Crepitus on movement.
- Signs of inflammation, warmth in the knees and erythema in the small joints of the hands, particularly in the early stages and during exacerbations.
- Limitation of movement follows with wasting of muscles around the affected joint.
- Joint deformities are particularly important in

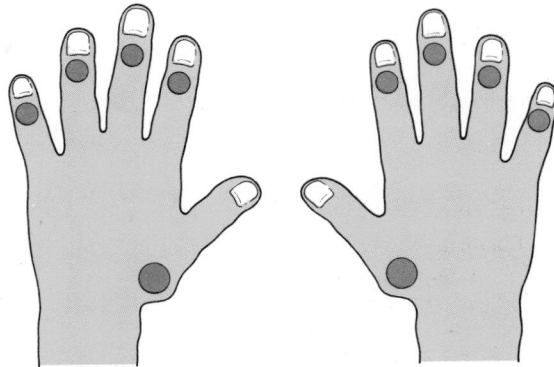

Fig. 8.4 The pattern of hand involvement in osteoarthritis. Bony swelling of the first carpometacarpal joints gives rise to the appearance of 'square hands'.

the knee. Valgus, varus or flexion deformities are seen with instability in the later stages of the disease.

Pattern of disease

Occasionally monarticular; usually one, two, three or four sites including knees (commonest), hands, hips, feet, ankles and lumbar spine; bilateral and symmetrical.

Hands. Bony swellings occur at the distal interphalangeal joints of the fingers (Heberden's nodes) and also at the proximal interphalangeal joints (Bouchard's nodes). At first the joints are often red, warm, swollen and very tender ('hot Heberden's nodes'). Later the inflammation disappears, leaving knobbly but often painless swellings. The pattern of hand involvement is shown in Fig. 8.4; the distal interphalangeal and first carpometacarpal joints are most often affected.

Feet. The metatarsophalangeal joint is often affected, sometimes called 'poor man's gout'. Problems may arise from valgus deformity (hallux valgus) or progressive restriction of movement (hallux rigidus).

Osteoarthritis is characterized by inflammation of joints but, unlike rheumatoid arthritis, there is no systemic involvement. Thus there are no nonarticular features and there is no systemic illness.

DIFFERENTIAL DIAGNOSIS

The pattern of hand involvement should be contrasted with that of rheumatoid arthritis (see later), in which metacarpophalangeal and proximal interphalangeal joint involvement is usual and the distal interphalangeal joints are characteristically spared. The pattern of involvement of other joints in OA is contrasted with that in rheumatoid arthritis in Fig. 8.5. The number of joints affected in OA is much less than in rheumatoid arthritis.

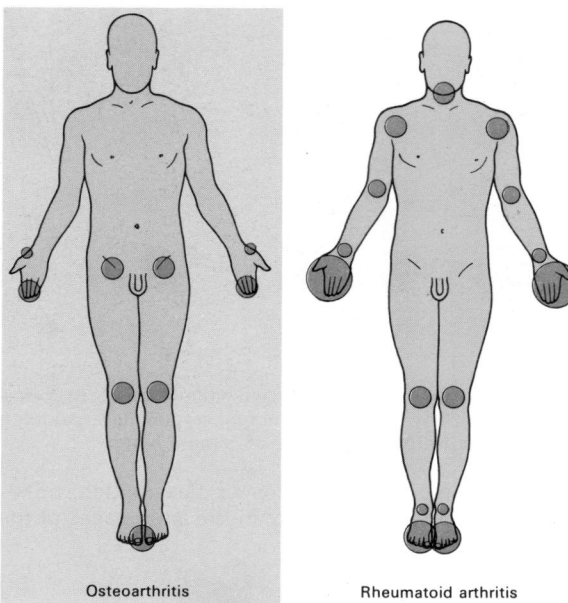

Osteoarthritis   Rheumatoid arthritis

Fig. 8.5 The pattern of joint involvement in osteoarthritis compared with rheumatoid arthritis. Both conditions are usually bilateral and symmetrical in distribution.

Apophyseal joints in the cervical and lumbar spine are not uncommonly involved but it is difficult to distinguish OA at this site from chronic disc disease.

INVESTIGATION

X-ray changes
The X-ray changes in osteoarthritis are shown in Fig. 8.6. Narrowing of the joint space is due to loss of cartilage and is the most important change. It is accompanied by the formation of osteophytes at the margin of the joints, sclerosis of the underlying bone and cyst formation. In addition, in secondary OA there is often calcification, which takes one of two forms:

- Linear calcification, which is characteristic of pyrophosphate deposition
- Spotty calcification, which is characteristic of hydroxyapatite deposition

Blood tests
There are no diagnostic markers for OA. The ESR is normal and there are no biochemical abnormalities. Rheumatoid factor and antinuclear antibodies are negative but, remember that positive tests can occur in the elderly.

Synovial fluid—see Table 8.7.

MANAGEMENT

The nature of the condition, treatment and prognosis should be discussed with the patients.

There are three main types of treatment: drugs, physical measures and surgery. Obese patients should be encouraged to lose weight but, apart from this, it is seldom possible to alter the aetiological factors of the disease.

Drug treatment
There is no specific therapy to control the disease process. Simple analgesics and non-steroidal anti-inflammatory drugs (NSAIDs) are used to control symptoms. The latter are more effective because of the part played by inflammation in OA. Systemic corticosteroid therapy is not used. Drugs such as gold and pencillamine that are used for rheumatoid arthritis are not effective in OA.

Intra-articular corticosteroids can be used for inflammatory exacerbations. Injection should be preceded by aspiration of any fluid in the joint.

Physical therapy
The application of heat to an osteoarthritic joint may provide pain relief. Exercises are useful to maintain muscle power and are especially required for the quadriceps muscle in patients with knee involvement. Hydrotherapy is particularly useful for the hip joint, sometimes enabling a stiff joint to be mobilized and providing symptomatic relief. A walking stick may be useful for a patient with involvement of one hip or knee and should be held in the opposite hand.

Surgery
The greatest advance in the management of osteoarthritis has been joint replacement. Many joints can be successfully replaced. For example, a total hip replacement offers a 99% chance of almost complete pain relief and increased mobility. For disease of the first carpometacarpal joint, the trapezium can be removed or replaced with a plastic prosthesis. The first metatarsophalangeal joint can also be removed (excision arthroplasty) or replaced.

Rheumatoid arthritis

Rheumatoid arthritis (RA) is a common, chronic, systemic disease producing:

- A symmetrical inflammatory polyarthritis
- Extra-articular involvement, e.g. in the lungs and many other organs
- Progressive joint damage causing severe disability in young people, demanding considerable resources in terms of doctors, drugs and surgery.

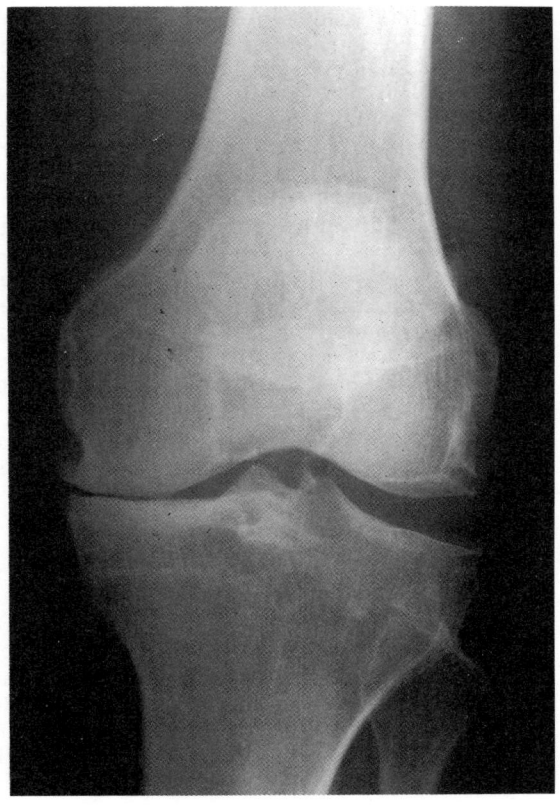

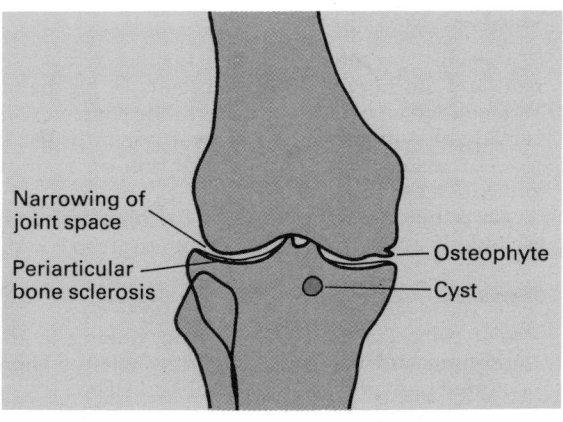

Fig. 8.6 X-ray changes of osteoarthritis of the knee.

EPIDEMIOLOGY

RA affects about 2% of the population world-wide and is just as common in tropical countries as in cold, damp Britain. It is about three times as common in women as in men. It can begin at any age from 10 to 70 years but it most often starts between the ages of 30 and 40. There is an increased incidence in those with a family history of RA (5–10%) and an association with HLA–DR4 (70%).

PATHOGENESIS

The cause of RA is unknown. Toxic substances produced by the inflammatory reaction in the synovium are thought to lead to the destruction of cartilage, the characteristic feature of progressing RA.

Many immunological disturbances are seen and RA is considered to be an autoimmune disease for the following reasons.

- Autoantibodies are seen. Rheumatoid factor is also found in other diseases and therefore may play little part in the pathogenesis of RA.
- Immune complexes are common in the synovial fluid and the circulation.
- Synovial fluid also contains locally synthesized immunoglobulins and lymphokines.

- There is a defect in cell-mediated immunity.
- Association of other organ-specific autoimmune diseases such as primary hypothyroidism and pernicious anaemia.

A likely hypothesis for the chronicity of the inflammatory process is a persistent foreign antigen, perhaps a bacterium or virus, that is taken up by macrophages but not destroyed or removed. This leads to a systemic inflammatory reaction not unlike adjuvant arthritis in rats mediated by the immune system and characterized by an inflammation of many joints, vasculitis and granuloma formation (nodules).

PATHOLOGY

RA is a disease of the synovium. There are two main pathological characteristics—inflammation and proliferation. The synovium shows signs of a chronic inflammatory reaction, with infiltration of lymphocytes, plasma cells and macrophages. It then proliferates and grows out over the surface of the cartilage, producing a tumour-like mass called 'pannus'.

The subcutaneous nodules seen in RA have a central area of necrosis surrounded by a palisade of macrophages and fibrous tissue. Similar lesions occur in the pleura, pericardium and lung. The lymph nodes are often hyperplastic.

CLINICAL FEATURES

RA usually presents with the insidious onset of pain and stiffness in the small joints of the hands and feet, which eventually leads to the characteristic 16bilateral symmetrical peripheral polyarthritis. In 25% of cases it presents as arthritis of a single joint, such as the knee.

An acute onset of the disease is characteristic in the elderly and is sometimes called 'explosive RA'.

Symptoms

- *Joint pain.* The pain is worst on waking in the morning and may improve with activity. There is often pain at night and disturbed sleep.
- *Morning stiffness*, often lasting for several hours.
- *General symptoms.* Fatigue and general malaise are common.
- Disability depends upon the changes in individual joints.
- Non-articular symptoms are discussed below. Patients may present with carpal tunnel syndrome or disease of other systems.

Signs

- Swelling: soft swelling caused by effusion or synovial proliferation
- Warmth
- Tenderness on pressure or movement
- Limitation of movement with muscle wasting around affected joints
- Deformities occurring in the later stages of the disease
- Nodules and other extra-articular features

Pattern of joint involvement

The characteristic pattern of joint involvement is shown in Fig. 8.5. Most patients eventually have many joints involved, including the hands, wrists, elbows, shoulders, cervical spine, knees, ankes and feet. The dorsal and lumbar spines are not involved.

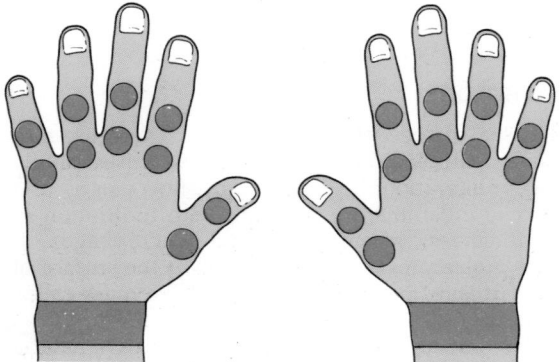

Fig. 8.7 The pattern of hand involvement in rheumatoid arthritis.

The hips. The hip joint is involved in about 50% of patients. This seldom occurs at the onset of the disease but usually develops within the first few years.

The hands and wrists. The pattern of joint involvement is shown in Fig. 8.7. In contrast to OA the distal interphalangeal joints are only involved in 30% of cases. Early in the disease there is spindling of the fingers with swellings of the metacarpophalangeal and wrist joints. Tenosynovitis at the wrists can produce the carpal tunnel syndrome owing to entrapment of the median nerve. Later, with progressive disease activity, there is weakening of joint capsules, muscle wasting and joint instability. These changes may produce the characteristic deformities shown in Fig. 8.8.

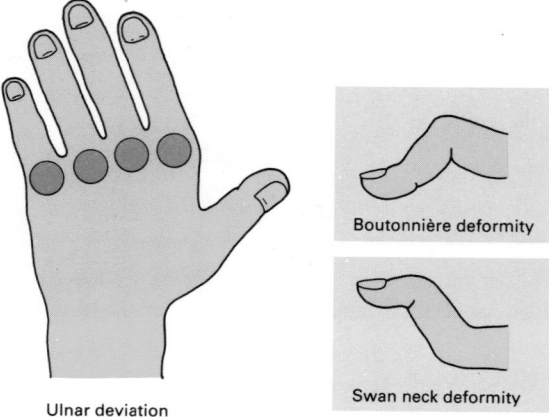

Fig. 8.8 Characteristic hand deformities in rheumatoid arthritis.

The feet and ankles. Deformities occur similar to those seen in the hands and wrists. There is lateral deviation of the toes and subluxation of the metatarsophalangeal joints so that the heads of the metatarsals become palpable in the soles of the feet. Patients often describe a sensation of walking on marbles.

The knees. Synovial effusions and quadriceps wasting are early features. Later flexion, valgus or varus deformities appear with joint instability. The pressure of fluid within the knee leads to the formation of a Baker's cyst in the popliteal fossa. With the increased pressure, the knee joint may rupture, releasing irritant synovial fluid into the muscles of the calf. The sudden onset of pain with swelling of the ankle and a positive Homan's sign may be mistaken for deep vein thrombosis but the correct diagnosis can be confirmed by an arthrogram.

Progression and prognosis of joint involvement

The activity and rate of progression of joint

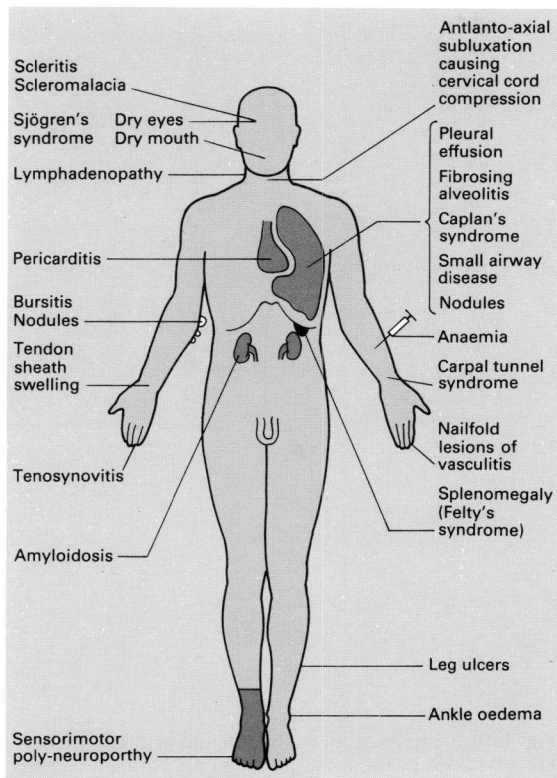

Fig. 8.9 The non-articular manifestations of rheumatoid arthritis.

changes in RA are very variable. New joints are involved in an additive pattern in most cases. The pattern of joint involvement is established within months of its onset. Partial remissions and relapses follow. In some, the disease is mild with little or no progression. In others, the characteristic deformities and complications occur. About 10% of patients become seriously disabled and 40% develop significant disability.

Palindromic rheumatism. Episodes of arthritis may precede the development of chronic RA. Palindromic rheumatism is described on p. 410.

Non-articular features (Fig. 8.9)

Soft tissues surrounding joints

- *Nodules* are found in about 20% of cases. They are most often felt on the surface of the ulnar just below the elbow but they can appear almost anywhere.
- *Bursitis.* The olecranon and other bursae may be swollen and a tendon sheath swelling over the dorsal surface of the wrist is not uncommon.
- *Tenosynovitis.* Tenosynovitis, particularly affecting the flexor tendons in the palm of the hand,

can cause trigger finger and may contribute to flexion deformities.
- *Muscle wasting.* There is wasting of muscles around affected joints, particularly in the hands.

The eyes

- The commonest eye problem in RA is *secondary Sjögren's syndrome*, occurring in about 15% of cases. It comprises dry eyes (keratoconjunctivitis sicca), a dry mouth (xerostomia) and rheumatoid arthritis. This syndrome is also seen in other connective-tissue disorders, e.g. systemic lupus erythematosus. The lacrimal and salivary glands are infiltrated with lymphocytes and plasma cells, suggesting that this syndrome is part of the immunological process of rheumatoid disease. The development of dry eyes is particularly important because tear production protects the cornea. Artificial tears such as hypromellose 0.3% eye drops should be prescribed. Primary Sjögren's is described on p. 397.
- *Scleritis* may occur, causing a painful red eye. Scleromalacia presents as a bluish discoloration of the sclera around the iris; perforation rarely occurs.

The nervous system

- Carpal tunnel syndrome is the commonest neurological abnormality (see p. 953).
- Atlanto-axial subluxation is the most serious neurological abnormality. In this condition rheumatoid involvement of an adjacent bursa leads to weakening of the transverse ligament of the atlas. This in turn allows the odontoid process to separate from the anterior arch of the atlas and to move posteriorly on flexion of the cervical spine with potential infringement on the cervical cord. Atlanto-axial subluxation is a common X-ray finding but cervical cord compression is fortunately rare.
- Polyneuropathy occurs rarely causing glove and stocking sensory loss and sometimes motor weakness. It is usually symmetrical and often involves the legs.

Multiple mononeuropathy (mononeuritis multiplex) can also occur as a result of vasculitis.

The spleen, lymph nodes and blood

- Palpable lymph nodes are common, usually in the distribution of affected joints.
- The spleen may be enlarged. RA and splenomegaly with neutropenia that leads to repeated infections and weight loss is known as *Felty's syndrome.* HLA DRW4 is found in 95% of such patients compared with 70% of patients with RA and 30% of controls. Skin pigmentation also occurs.
- Anaemia is almost universal in RA and is proportional to the activity of the inflammatory

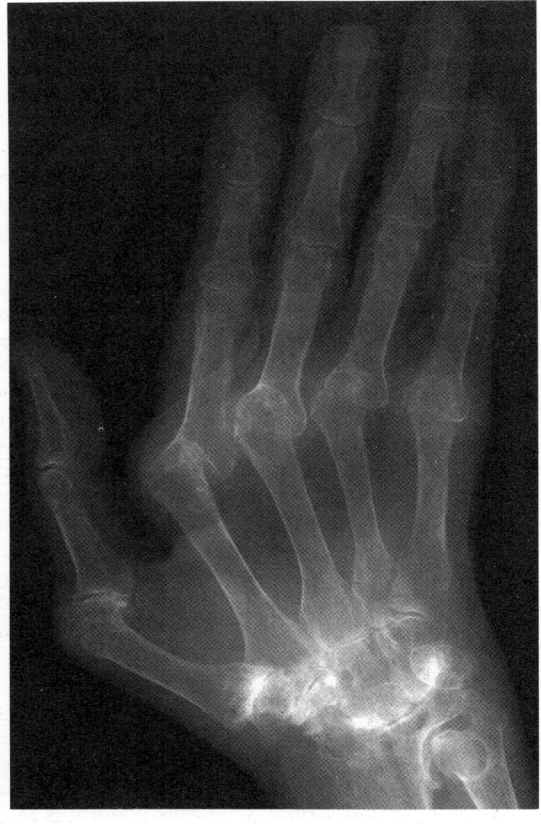

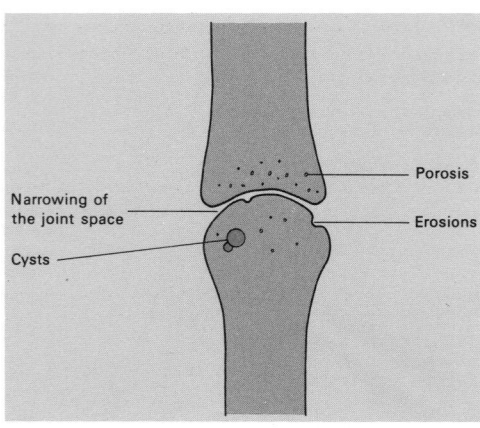

Fig. 8.10 X-ray changes in rheumatoid arthritis. Erosions are best seen in the small joints of the hands and feet.

process. The anaemia may be normochromic normocytic—the anaemia of chronic disease; iron-deficient—due to gastrointestinal blood loss from analgesic ingestion, or rarely, haemolytic (positive Coombs' test) or part of a pancytopenia due to hypersplenism in Felty's syndrome.

● Thrombocytosis correlates with disease activity.

The lungs. The lung is commonly affected; the abnormalities are described in detail on p. 686. They include:

● Pleural effusion—this is the commonest lung problem and occurs in approximately 10% of men but is less common in women. It may occur before the onset of RA.
● Diffuse fibrosing alveolitis—rare.
● Rheumatoid nodules in the lungs—can be up to 3 cm in diameter and mistaken for carcinoma.
● Caplan's syndrome—the occurrence of nodular pulmonary fibrosis in patients with RA exposed to various industrial dusts.
● Small airway disease is commoner in patients with RA who smoke than in healthy smokers.

The heart. A pericardial rub is often heard in patients with RA (up to 30%). Pericarditis is seldom a clinical problem but occasionally a large pericardial effusion causes tamponade. Constrictive pericarditis is rare.

The kidneys. RA is a common cause of amyloidosis affecting the kidneys. It usually presents as proteinuria and may go on to renal failure or to the nephrotic syndrome. Analgesic nephropathy is also seen (see p. 452).

The skin. The skin is not directly involved in RA but leg ulcers may occur, particularly in patients with Felty's syndrome and in those with a vasculitis. Vasculitis most often appears as nail fold lesions in the hands and, very occasionally, it produces gangrene of the fingers or toes. Ankle oedema is often seen in active RA and is due to increased vascular permeability.

INVESTIGATION

X-ray changes
The X-ray changes of RA are shown in Fig. 8.10. The characteristic lesion is an erosion that has the appearance of a mouse-bite on the surface of the affected bone. Erosions are best seen in X-rays of the hands and feet. Other changes include loss of joint space, which indicates thinning of the cartil-

age, porosis of the periarticular bone and cysts. In advanced disease, destruction of bone ends and occasionally ankylosis occur.

Full blood count

A full blood count in RA shows anaemia (see above) and ESR and CRP are raised in proportion to the activity of the inflammatory process.

Other tests

Tests for rheumatoid factor are positive in about 80% of cases and for antinuclear antibodies in about 30%.

Aspirated synovial fluid will show the changes outlined in Table 8.7. Fluid from a suddenly painful rheumatoid joint should always be aspirated and cultured, as septic arthritis can occur in patients with RA.

MANAGEMENT (see Table 8.10)

Stage 1

Many patients have already heard tales of horrific disabilities and should therefore be reassured that only a few patients suffer from severe problems and that the prospects of treatment are good. All the aspects of a patient's life-style should be reviewed, including home, work and leisure activities. In general, a patient's life-style should not be disrupted and he should be encouraged to continue a full, normal and busy life.

Physical activity does not increase the rate of deterioration of joints in RA and since patients are particularly at risk of developing progressive joint stiffness and deformity, they should undertake simple exercises to maintain joint mobility and

Table 8.10 Stages in the management of rheumatoid arthritis.

Stage 1
Making the diagnosis, telling the patient
Joint protection and maintenance
Management planning

Stage 2
Symptomatic treatment with NSAIDs and other
    measures

Stage 3
The control of the disease with long-term
    suppressive drugs

Stage 4
Regular supervision and the management of
    complications

Stage 5
Rehabilitation of the disabled patient

---

muscle power. Restriction of movement is particularly likely to occur in the shoulders, while flexion deformities are more likely to occur in the knees. Both of these problems are easier to prevent than correct.

Plans must be made for the continuing care of a patient with RA. Most will require some supervision for many years, even if the disease is mild.

Stage 2

The second stage of treatment is devoted to the relief of symptoms. NSAIDs are the mainstay of such treatment and are more effective than simple analgesics.

● There is a large variation in an individual's response to NSAIDs. It is often necessary to try a number of different drugs for a particular patient before finding one that provides adequate relief of symptoms. Each compound should be given for about one week to assess its efficacy. Drugs with a low incidence of side-effects, a good safety record and a convenient dosage schedule should be tried first. Aspirin no longer fulfils these requirements and has been replaced as a first line of treatment by newer NSAIDs, e.g. piroxicam 20 mg daily.

The relief of night pain and morning stiffness is particularly important in RA. A single capsule of slow-release indomethacin (75 mg) or a suppository taken on retiring usually produces dramatic relief of symptoms on the following day. This can be given in addition to regular daytime therapy or may be sufficient alone. If patients require additional relief, a simple analgesic can be taken as required. Aspirin or paracetamol are ideal for this purpose but many patients prefer to use a combination such as dextropropoxyphene and paracetamol.

● Corticosteroids are effective but are seldom used because of their side-effects. In explosive RA in the elderly, small doses of prednisolone (less than 10 mg daily) are effective; the dose can be reduced over the years. In the younger patient, however, much larger doses of prednisolone, often for long periods, are necessary to control symptoms and because of side-effects such treatment should not be used.

● Rest in hospital is often useful, either to produce a remission of the disease or to encourage a dispirited disabled patient. Localized rest for individual joints can be provided with splints, which are particularly useful for the wrist.

● Intra-articular corticosteroid injections are of value for particularly troublesome joints to avoid the risk of systemic steroids.

Stage 3

The third stage consists of long-term suppressive drug therapy with drugs such as penicillamine

Table 8.11 Drugs used in long-term suppressive therapy for rheumatoid arthritis.

Drug	Usual dose	Side-effects
Penicillamine	250 mg daily	Rash Loss of taste Thrombocytopenia Proteinuria
Gold (sodium aurothiomalate)	50 mg weekly i.m.	Rash Thrombocytopenia
Oral gold (auranofin)	3 mg twice daily	Diarrhoea Rash
Azathioprine	50 mg twice daily	Neutropenia Nausea and vomiting Infections
Methotrexate	7.5 mg weekly	As for azathioprine
Hydroxychloroquine	400 mg daily	Retinopathy
Sulphasalazine	1 g twice daily	Nausea Mild depression Male infertility

(Table 8.11). The indications for this type of treatment are:

- Progressive disease
- Troublesome extra-articular problems
- Failure of NSAIDs to control symptoms
- Excessive corticosteroid requirements

The characteristics of long-term suppressive therapy are:

- A slow action: these drugs start to work after 4–6 weeks and take 6 months to produce their full effect. For this reason, NSAIDs should be continued for a few months at least.
- Improvement in joint symptoms is accompanied by a fall in ESR and the titre of rheumatoid factor.
- Complete remission or very effective suppression of disease can be achieved, delaying or preventing joint destruction. This type of treatment should therefore be considered early in the course of the disease before joint deformities and irreversible damage have developed.

The mode of action of these drugs is unknown and it is impossible to predict which patient will respond to a particular compound. It is often necessary to try several, as with NSAIDs.

Penicillamine is usually used as the first line of treatment in severe cases; hydroxychloroquine, sulphasalazine or auranofin, which are safer but less effective, are used for milder disease in younger patients. Immunosuppressive drugs such as azathioprine are as effective as penicillamine but, because of their potential side-effects, are usually only used in patients over the age of 45 and in those who have failed to respond to gold or penicillamine. All of these drugs have side-effects and patients require regular supervision, including blood and sometimes urine checks. Patients should be informed of the potential for side-effects and told to report new symptoms immediately. The antimalarial drug hydroxychloroquine may affect the eyes and vision must be checked regularly.

Stage 4
Regular supervision is required to assess the course of the disease and to treat complications.

Articular complications. Joints may become stiff and painful and require intra-articular injections of corticosteroids and exercises to mobilize the joint and improve muscle power. Deformities can also sometimes be corrected by steroid injections and exercises.

Rupture of the knee joint is treated with aspiration, injection of corticosteroid and rest. A Baker's cyst behind the knee does not itself require treatment since it merely reflects inflammatory changes in the knee joint. Steps should be taken to control the activity of the disease in the affected knee.

Painful feet may be treated with insoles; metatarsal bar insoles are particularly useful for subluxed metatarsal heads. More complex foot deformities may require special shoes such as space shoes.

At this stage in the disease replacement surgery plays an increasingly important role in the management of a patient with a wrecked joint. Not only can hips be replaced, but also knees, shoulders, elbows and the small joints of the hands.

Excision arthroplasty is of value in two situations. First, the painful subluxed metatarsal heads in the feet can be excised (Fowler's operation) and

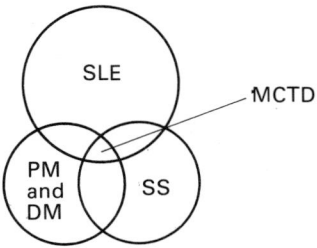

Fig. 8.11 The family of connective-tissue diseases: systemic lupus erythematosus (SLE); polymyositis (PM); dermatomyositis (DM); systemic sclerosis (SS); and mixed connective-tissue disease (MCTD).

the lateral deviation of the toes corrected at the same time. Second, the head of the ulnar can be excised at the wrist, often relieving pain and allowing better movement. Osteotomy is occasionally used at the knee joint to relieve pain and correct deformity.

Non-articular complications. Many different symptoms require treatment. For example, the patient who develops carpal tunnel syndrome will require an injection of corticosteroid or surgical decompression of the median nerve.

Social and domestic complications. RA strains relationships and makes life difficult. Crises arise in these matters and patients often turn to a sympathetic physician for advice and help.

Stage 5
Despite all treatments, the disease may continue to progress and become disabling. Priorities in treatment then change. It is no longer relevant to control the disease and the aims of treatment become relief of symptoms and maintenance of a reasonable life-style. It may be useful to visit a patient's home with a view to making life easier. A wheelchair may be required and many other aids and appliances can be used to reduce disability. Steps should be taken to preserve as much as possible of all aspects of the patient's life. Successful management can make an enormous difference to the quality of life of rheumatoid patients.

Connective tissue diseases

The term connective tissue disease is used for three diseases—systemic lupus erythematosus, systemic sclerosis and polymyositis and dermatomyositis, whose relationship is illustrated in Fig. 8.11. The collective term 'connective tissue disease' means little but, since the aetiology of these conditions is

unknown, it is difficult to suggest a better alternative. The diseases have a number of features in common, including the occurrence of arthritis or arthralgia, multisystem involvement, vasculitis and immunological abnormalities such as circulating autoantibodies and immune complex deposition. Features of all three diseases appear in mixed connective tissue disease.

Systemic lupus erythematosus (SLE)

Systemic lupus erythematosus is the commonest of the connective tissue disorders and is characterized by the presence in the serum of antibodies against nuclear components (ANA). It is a multisystem disease, with arthralgia and rashes as the commonest clinical features, and cerebral and renal disease as the most serious problems.

EPIDEMIOLOGY

The disease probably affects about 0.1% of the population and is thus about 20 times less common than RA. It is much commoner in black women in USA, with a prevalence of up to 1 in 250. It is about nine times as common in women as men, with a peak age of onset between 20 and 40 years.

PATHOGENESIS

The cause of SLE is unknown but is probably multifactorial, including a variable genetic predisposition and environmental factors that trigger the disease. In some cases, genetic predisposition is so strong that minor additional triggers are sufficient. Known predisposing factors include:

● Heredity: the identical twin of a patient with SLE has a 30% chance of developing the disease; first degree relatives have a 5% chance. Certain races are especially prone, including Sioux Indians, Africans and Polynesians.
● Complement deficiencies of all types.
● Sex hormone status: women are much more often affected than men.

Known environmental triggers include:

● Drugs such as hydrallazine
● Ultraviolet light
● Infection: a virus infection is a popular theory for the cause of lupus and it is easy to see how a DNA virus could lead to the production of antibodies to nuclear material.

The immunological mechanisms of the disease include:

● Polyclonal B-cell activation. Increased numbers of B cells lead to hyperglobulinaemia
● The production of ANA and other autoantibodies

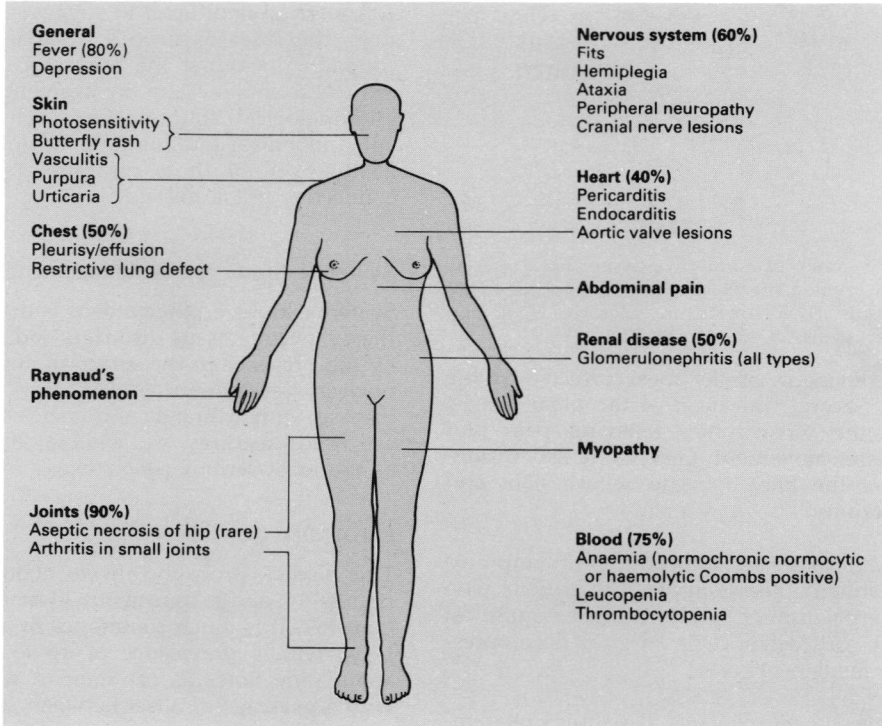

General
Fever (80%)
Depression

Skin
Photosensitivity ⎫
Butterfly rash ⎭
Vasculitis ⎫
Purpura ⎬
Urticaria ⎭

Chest (50%)
Pleurisy/effusion
Restrictive lung defect

**Raynaud's
phenomenon**

Joints (90%)
Aseptic necrosis of hip (rare)
Arthritis in small joints

Nervous system (60%)
Fits
Hemiplegia
Ataxia
Peripheral neuropathy
Cranial nerve lesions

Heart (40%)
Pericarditis
Endocarditis
Aortic valve lesions

Abdominal pain

Renal disease (50%)
Glomerulonephritis (all types)

Myopathy

Blood (75%)
Anaemia (normochronic normocytic
or haemolytic Coombs positive)
Leucopenia
Thrombocytopenia

Fig. 8.12 Clinical features of systemic lupus erythematosus.

- Impaired T cell regulation of the immune response
- Failure to remove immune complexes from the circulation. Circulating immune complexes cause arthralgia; deposition of immune complexes in tissues causes vasculitis and many other features of the disease, including glomerulonephritis.

Many immunological abnormalities are seen, including antibodies to human IgG, nuclear protein, smooth muscle, cytoplasm, organ-specific antibodies, e.g. thyroid, leucocytes, platelets, red cells, clotting factors and cryoglobulins with varying clinical effects. Their role in the pathogenesis, if any, is unknown.

PATHOLOGY

SLE is characterized by a widespread vasculitis affecting capillaries, arterioles and venules. Fibrinoid (an eosinophilic amorphous material) is found along blood vessels and tissue fibres. The synovium of joints may be oedematous and may contain fibrinoid deposits. Haematoxylin bodies (rounded blue homogenous haematoxylin-stained deposits) are seen in inflammatory infiltrates and are thought to result from the interaction of antinuclear antibodies and cell nuclei.

Lesions of other organs are described in the appropriate chapters.

CLINICAL FEATURES (Fig. 8.12)

SLE is extremely variable in its manifestation and most of the clinical features are due to the consequences of vasculitis. Mild cases may present only with arthralgia, whilst in severe cases there may be multisystem involvement.

General features. Fever is common in exacerbations, occurring in up to 80% of cases. Patients complain of malaise and tiredness.

The joints. Joint involvement is the commonest clinical feature (> 90%). Patients often present with symptoms that sound like rheumatoid arthritis. Joints are painful but characteristically appear clinically normal, although sometimes there is slight soft-tissue swelling surrounding the joint. Aseptic necrosis affecting the hip or knee is a rare complication of the disease.

The skin. This is affected in 80% of cases (see p. 1031). Erythema in a butterfly distribution on the cheeks of the face and across the bridge of the nose is characteristic. Vasculitic lesions on the fingertips and around the nail folds, purpura and urticaria occur. In one-third of cases there is photosensitivity and prolonged exposure to sunlight can lead to exacerbations of the disease. Livedo reticularis, palmar and plantar rashes, pigmentation and alopecia may be seen. Raynaud's phenomenon is common and may precede the development of arthralgia and other clinical problems by years.

Discoid lupus. See p. 1032.

The lungs. Up to two-thirds of patients will have lung involvement sometime during the course of the disease (see p. 686). Recurrent pleurisy and pleural effusions (exudates) are the commonest manifestations. Pneumonitis and atelectasis may be seen; eventually a restrictive lung defect develops. Rarely, pulmonary fibrosis occurs.

The heart. This is involved in over 40% of cases. Pericarditis, with small pericardial effusions detected by echocardiography, is common. A mild myocarditis also occurs. Aortic valve lesions and a cardiomyopathy can rarely be present. Endocarditis involving the mitral valve (Libman–Sacks syndrome) is very rare.

The kidneys. These are affected in 30–50% of cases. Proteinuria (> 1 g per 24 h) is common. The renal histological lesions consist of minimal change, proliferative changes (either focal, diffuse or crescentic) or a membranous glomerulonephritis (see p. 438). Most patients with or without renal disease have immune complex deposits in their kidneys.

Hypertension may occur owing to progression to either the nephrotic syndrome or renal failure.

The nervous system. Involvement of the nervous system occurs in 60% of cases. There may be a mild depression but occasionally more severe psychiatric disturbances occur. Epilepsy, cerebellar ataxia, aseptic meningitis, cranial nerve lesions, cerebrovascular accidents or peripheral neuropathy may be seen. These lesions may be due to vasculitis or immune-complex deposition.

The eyes. Retinal lesions include cytoid bodies, which appear as hard exudates, and haemorrhages. Blindness is uncommon. Secondary Sjögren's syndrome may be seen.

The gastrointestinal system. SLE often causes gastrointestinal symptoms, although these are usually not a major presenting feature. Symptoms include nausea, vomiting, anorexia and diarrhoea.

Lupus variants

Discoid lupus is a benign variant of the disease in which skin involvement is often the only feature, although systemic abnormalities may occur with time. The rash is characteristic and appears on the face as well-defined erythematous plaques that progress to scarring and pigmentation (see p. 1032).

Drug-induced SLE. This is usually characterized by arthralgia and mild systemic features, rashes and pericarditis, but seldom renal or cerebral disease. It usually disappears when the drug causing it is stopped. Hydralazine and procainamide are the most likely causes, but other drugs have occasionally been implicated.

Cardiolipin syndrome. This rare condition is characterized by recurrent thromboses and abortions, thrombocytopenia and cerebral disease, particularly strokes. Other features of SLE may occur. The serological characteristic is the presence of antibodies directed against phospholipids such as cardiolipin. False positive serological tests for syphilis and the lupus anticoagulant may also be found.

Mixed connective tissue disease. See p. 396.

INVESTIGATION

- A full blood count usually shows an anaemia (usually normochromic normocytic), neutropenia and thrombocytopenia. An autoimmune haemolytic anaemia may occur. The ESR is raised in proportion to the disease activity. In contrast, the CRP is normal.
- Antinuclear antibodies are positive in almost all cases. Double-stranded DNA binding is specific for SLE, although it is only present in 50% of cases, particularly those with severe systemic involvement, e.g. renal disease.
- Rheumatoid factor is positive in half of the patients.
- Serum complement levels are reduced during active disease. Immunoglobulins are raised (usually IgG and IgM).
- Characteristic histological abnormalities are seen in biopsies from, for example, the kidney.
- Immunofluorescence of skin will show immunoglobulin and complement deposition at the dermoepidermal junction, which is known as the positive band test.

MANAGEMENT

Drug therapy

Systemic corticosteroid therapy is the mainstay of treatment in SLE, although patients with mild disease and arthralgia can be managed with

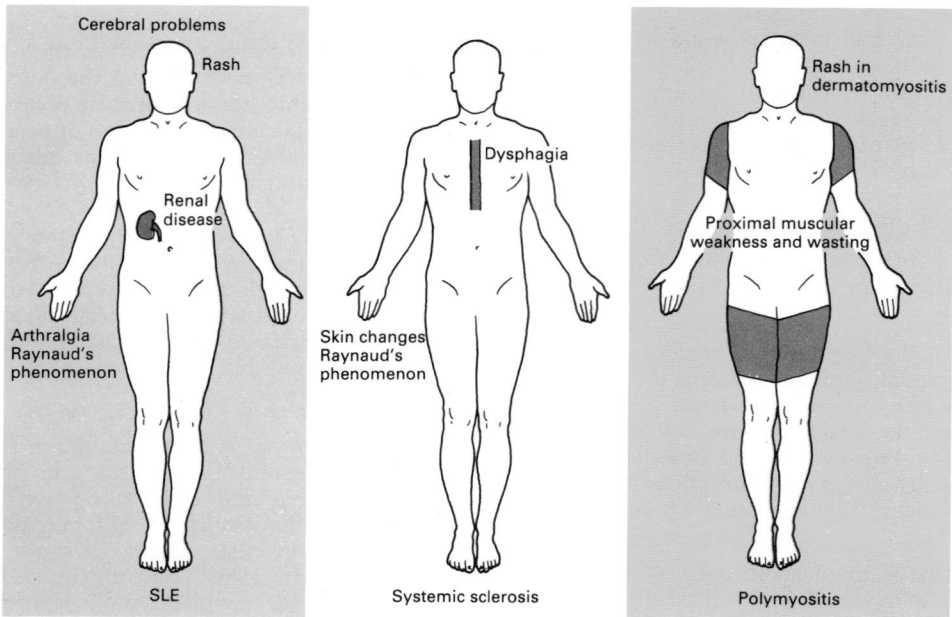

Fig. 8.13 Major clinical features distinguishing various connective-tissue diseases.

NSAIDs. In cases where steroids are required, they should be used in small doses for short periods just sufficient to suppress the disease in order to minimize complications. Active SLE, with fever and pleurisy, should be treated with prednisolone 30 mg daily, the dose being reduced over the course of a few weeks to a maintenance level of around 5–10 mg daily. It may be possible to stop treatment in such a patient within a few months.

Two other types of drug are used in the management of SLE:

- The antimalarial drug hydroxychloroquine (400 mg daily) is useful for suppressing the disease activity in patients with minor manifestations such as arthralgia that cannot be controlled with NSAIDs or troublesome skin lesions. Ocular toxicity may occur.
- Immunosuppressive drugs are used for patients with more serious disease manifestations such as renal disease, usually in combination with steroids. Azathioprine (2 mg·kg^{-1} daily) is most often used; chlorambucil is an alternative and cyclophosphamide is reserved for patients with life-threatening disease. Immunosuppressive drugs also have a useful steroid-sparing effect.

General management
Patients should be told about their disease and its management. Patients with photosensitivity problems should avoid excessive exposure to sunlight.

There is no major contraindication to pregnancy. However, there is an increased rate of fetal loss and complications may arise during the pregnancy; specialist care should therefore be available.

COURSE AND PROGNOSIS

An episodic course is characteristic, with exacerbations and complete remissions that may last for long periods of time. These remissions may occur even in patients with renal disease. A chronic course is occasionally seen. Earlier estimates of the mortality in SLE were exaggerated; 5-year survival rate is about 95%. In most cases the pattern of the disease becomes established in the first few years; if serious problems have not developed in this time, they are unlikely to do so. The arthritis is usually intermittent. Chronic progressive destruction of joints as seen in RA and OA does not occur, but a few patients develop deformities such as ulnar deviation.

Systemic sclerosis

Systemic sclerosis is a multisystem disease that predominantly affects the skin and presents with Raynaud's phenomenon in over three-quarters of cases. It is less common than SLE. The major features distinguishing systemic sclerosis from polymyositis and SLE are shown in Fig. 8.13. It is commoner in women than men (3 : 1) and can appear at any age under 50 years.

AETIOLOGY

The aetiology of systemic sclerosis is unknown. Abnormalities in both humoral and cellular immunity have been documented. A positive speckled or nucleolar antinuclear antibody is found in up to 60% of patients. Familial cases have been documented and HLA-B8,DR3 has been reported to occur with greater frequency in systemic sclerosis. A similar syndrome can be produced by certain chemicals, including polyvinyl chloride, and in poisoning with adulterated oil (toxic epidermal syndrome).

PATHOLOGY

In the early phase the skin is oedematous, with perivascular lymphocyte infiltration and degeneration of collagen fibres. Later there is an increase in collagen. Small blood vessels show intimal proliferation and obliteration. Progressive fibrosis is the major feature of visceral involvement.

CLINICAL FEATURES

The involvement of various organs is shown in Table 8.12.

The skin. The cutaneous changes that occur are described on p. 1033. Sclerosis of the skin can lead to beaking of the nose and difficulty in opening the mouth. Other changes seen in the skin include telangiectasis, pigmentation or depigmentation, ulceration and calcinosis. Raynaud's phenomenon often occurs; it is described on p. 624.

The gastrointestinal system (p. 183). Oesophageal involvement is almost invariable, although only half of these patients will have symptoms of heartburn or dysphagia. A barium swallow may show delayed peristalsis, dilatation or stricture formation, but oesophageal manometry is the most sensitive test. This shows lack of distal oesophageal peristalsis and a reduced oesophageal sphincter pressure.

Table 8.12 Involvement of various organs in systemic sclerosis.

Organ	Involved in
Skin	90%
Vascular system— Raynaud's phenomenon	80%
Oesophagus	80%
Lungs	45%
Heart	40%
Kidneys	35%
Joints	25%
Muscle	20%

The small bowel can be involved, producing malabsorption from bacterial overgrowth due to dilatation and atony. Dilatation and atony may also affect the colon.

The joints and muscles. The fibrotic process can affect tendons, causing flexion deformities of the fingers. The small joints of the hands are affected in 25% of patients, particularly in the early stages of the disease. Soft-tissue swelling of the fingers produces 'sausage fingers'. Progressive changes in joints are not seen.

Myopathy and myositis occur and EMG abnormalities are common.

The lungs (see also p. 686). Lower-lobe fibrosis leads to cyst formation and honeycombing in advanced cases. Gas transfer and restrictive ventilatory defects are seen. Aspiration pneumonia and pulmonary hypertension may occur.

The heart. Diffuse myocardial fibrosis with arrhythmias (in 25%) and conduction defects may occur. Effusions accompany pericardial disease.

The kidneys. This is the most serious manifestation of the disease and is caused by an obliterative endarteritis of renal vessels. It can cause renal failure and malignant hypertension.

The eyes. Sjögren's syndrome with keratoconjunctivitis sicca may be seen.

VARIANTS OF SYSTEMIC SCLEROSIS

- Morphoea—see p. 1032.
- CR(E)ST syndrome consists of calcinosis (C), Raynaud's phenomenon (R), oesophageal involvement (E), sclerodactyly (S) and telangiectasia (T). Antinuclear antibodies to the centromere are found in the blood.
- Mixed connective tissue disease—see p. 396.

INVESTIGATION

Antinuclear antibodies are often positive. Antinucleolar and anticentromere antibodies are specifically elevated. A positive rheumatoid factor is found in 30% of cases.

- A normochromic normocytic anaemia can be seen. An acquired haemolytic anaemia with 'cold' agglutinins may occur. The ESR may be raised.
- X-rays of the hands may show deposits of calcium around the fingers. In severe cases there is erosion and resorption of the tufts of the distal phalanges.
- A barium swallow to detect oesophageal involvement is often a useful confirmatory test.

TREATMENT

No treatment has been shown to influence the progress of this condition. Management is therefore symptomatic.

PROGNOSIS

In some patients the disease is mild, whilst in others it is severe and complicated by systemic features such as renal disease. The mean 5-year survival rate is 50%.

Polymyositis and dermatomyositis

Polymyositis is a disorder of muscle in which the pathological features are necrosis of muscle fibres together with evidence of regeneration and inflammation, particularly around blood vessels. It presents with proximal muscular weakness and wasting. When this is accompanied by a rash, it is called dermatomyositis. Its incidence is comparable with that of systemic sclerosis, i.e. it is less common than SLE. It occurs at any age, even in children, but with a peak incidence in adults aged between 30 and 60 years. It is twice as common in women as in men.

AETIOLOGY

The aetiology is unknown, but immunological and viral factors have been suggested. Dermatomyositis is associated with an increased incidence of carcinoma of the bronchus in men or of the ovary in women, mainly in patients presenting after 50 years.

CLINICAL FEATURES

The major feature of polymyositis is muscle weakness and wasting affecting the proximal muscles of the shoulder and pelvic girdles. It may be very acute in onset, particularly in children, and is sometimes accompanied by myoglobinuria. In the chronic form there is gradually progressive muscular weakness. Muscle pain and tenderness are found in about one-half of the cases, but weakness is the chief complaint. The rash of dermatomyositis is characteristic (see p. 1033). As in other connective tissue diseases, systemic features are often found:

- Arthralgia or arthritis occur in about half of all patients and may be the presenting feature, occurring before the onset of the muscular symptoms. The small joints of the hands are particularly affected but the arthritis may extend in a distribution resembling that of rheumatoid arthritis. Joints are often swollen but the arthritis is intermittent and not progressive.
- Dysphagia is found in 50% of cases and is due to oesophageal muscle involvement.
- Raynaud's phenomenon is common.
- Sjögren's syndrome and respiratory problems may occur.

INVESTIGATION

The diagnosis of polymyositis is made on the basis of three tests, two of which at least should be positive:

- *Muscle enzymes.* Serum creatine phosphokinase and aldolase are raised and can be used to follow the progress of the disease during treatment.
- *Electromyography (EMG).* Short polyphasic motor potentials, sometimes spontaneous fibrillation and high-frequency repetitive discharges (see p. 960) are almost pathognomonic of polymyositis.
- *Muscle biopsy.* This shows necrosis of muscle fibres with swelling and disruption of muscle cells. Vacuolation, fragmentation and fibrosis of the fibres are seen, with thickening of the blood vessels. There are also inflammatory changes.

Other tests

- The ESR is usually raised. A normochromic normocytic anaemia and a polymorphonuclear leucocytosis are seen in acute cases.
- Serum antinuclear antibodies and tests for rheumatoid factor may be positive.

MANAGEMENT

Systemic corticosteroids, starting with 60 mg of prednisolone daily and reducing to a maintenance dose of about 15 mg daily are used. In most cases this produces a gradual remission of the disease. Physiotherapy may be required to restore muscle power. Treatment is required for a variable period, usually months but sometimes years. Some patients fail to respond to steroids, and immunosuppressive drugs such as methotrexate or occasionally azathioprine may be required.

PROGNOSIS

Fifty per cent of affected children die within 2 years. In adults the prognosis is better, except in association with malignancy.

Mixed connective tissue disease

The existence of this rare disorder emphasizes the overlap between the connective tissue diseases, although it may not itself be a distinct entity. It is a useful term for cases with features of more than one of the connective tissue diseases together with high titres of antibody to extractable nuclear antigens such as RNA. Like the other conditions, it affects women more often than men and presents in young adults.

Clinical features include arthralgia, Raynaud's phenomenon, proximal muscle weakness and wasting, and a puffy swelling of the skin of the hands that somewhat resembles the changes occurring in scleroderma. Other features of systemic lupus erythematosus, polymyositis or scleroderma may appear, but serious problems such as renal disease are unusual.

The condition tends to be benign and often responds well to small doses of prednisolone.

Primary Sjögren's syndrome

The syndrome of dry eyes (keratoconjunctivitis sicca), in the absence of rheumatoid arthritis, is known as primary Sjögren's syndrome. Dryness of the mouth, skin or vagina may also be a problem.

Systemic associations include:

- Arthralgia and occasionally non-progressive polyarthritis like that seen in SLE
- Raynaud's phenomenon
- Dysphagia and abnormal oesophageal motility as seen in systemic sclerosis
- Other organ-specific autoimmune diseases, including thyroid disease, myasthenia gravis, primary biliary cirrhosis and chronic active hepatitis
- Renal tubular defects causing nephrogenic diabetes insipidus and renal tubular acidosis
- Pulmonary hypertension, diffusion defects and fibrosis
- Peripheral neuropathy, fits and depression
- Vasculitis

DIAGNOSIS

- The Schirmer tear test, in which a standard strip of filter paper is placed on the inside of the lower eye lid; wetting of less than 10 mm in 5 min indicates defective tear production
- Rose Bengal staining showing punctate or filamentary keratitis

Laboratory abnormalities include raised immunoglobulin levels, circulating immune complexes and many autoantibodies. Rheumatoid factor is usually positive, antinuclear antibodies are found in 70% and antimitochondrial antibodies in 10% of cases. Anti-Ro (SSA) antibodies are found in 70% of cases compared with 10% of cases of rheumatoid arthritis and secondary Sjögren's syndrome. This antibody is of particular interest because it can cross the placenta and cause congenital heart block.

Vasculitis

The 'vasculitides' encompass a wide range of diseases with considerable overlap between them. Many classifications have been suggested; one of these is based on the size of the vessels. Large-vessel disease includes giant-cell arteritis (see below) and Takayasu's disease (p. 624). Polyarteritis nodosa is a systemic arteritis involving medium-sized vessels. Small vessel vasculitis occurs in the connective tissue diseases such as SLE and rheumatoid arthritis as well as in infections such as infective endocarditis. This vasculitis may be responsible for some of the clinical features of these conditions. Skin lesions are usually associated with small-vessel vasculitis.

Polyarteritis nodosa (PAN)

Polyarteritis nodosa is a rare condition and, unlike other connective tissue diseases, it usually presents in middle-aged men. Pathologically there is a fibrinoid necrosis of blood-vessel walls and microaneurysm formation. These changes give rise to the clinical manifestations of multisystem disease with progressive organ failure, infarction and haemorrhage.

CLINICAL FEATURES

Initial features are non-specific, being fever, malaise, weight loss, myalgia and arthralgia. Later the most characteristic features are renal impairment, hypertension, peripheral neuropathy, lung disease and cardiac problems, including arrhythmia, heart failure and myocardial infarction. The peripheral neuropathy in vasculitic disorders characteristically takes the form of a mononeuritis multiplex (p. 952). A migratory arthralgia or arthritis and fever are seen, and abdominal pain, with evidence of vasculitis in the liver and gastrointestinal tract, is common. Death is usually from renal disease.

INVESTIGATION

The ESR is raised but the diagnosis depends upon either histological examination of biopsy material from an affected organ or angiographic demonstration of microaneurysms in hepatic, intestinal or renal vessels.

TREATMENT

Treatment is with corticosteroids, usually in combination with immunosuppressive drugs such as azathioprine.

Essential mixed cryoglobulinaemia

In this disorder a cutaneous vasculitis is associated with cryoglobulinaemia. It is exacerbated by exercise and the cold, and there is an association with hepatitis B infection. Multisystem involvement occurs as in other connective tissue disorders.

Vasculitis associated with granulomas

Two forms of vasculitis associated with granulomas also occur. *Wegener's granulomatosis* classically consists of the triad of upper respiratory tract granuloma, fleeting pulmonary shadows, and glomerulonephritis; it is discussed on p. 442. The *Churg–Strauss syndrome*, in which there is eosinophilic infiltration, mainly of the lungs, is described on p. 389.

Polymyalgia rheumatica and giant-cell arteritis

Polymyalgia rheumatica and giant-cell arteritis (also known as temporal or cranial arteritis) can be regarded as two conditions at the ends of a spectrum, with giant-cell arteritis as the basic pathological lesion (see Fig. 8.14). The cause is unknown. Occasionally the syndrome of polymyalgia is due to some underlying condition, e.g. a severe infection or a malignancy.

CLINICAL FEATURES

Polymyalgia rheumatica is characterized by pains and morning stiffness in the proximal muscles of the shoulder and pelvic girdle, and a high ESR.

The onset is sudden. It is rare before the age of 50 years and usually occurs in those aged 60–70 years. Women are three times more commonly affected than men. Severe pains and stiffness occur in the girdle muscles and also in the muscles of the cervical and lumbar spines. The hands and feet are never affected. Early morning stiffness often causes difficulty in getting out of bed. Systemic symptoms include malaise, anorexia, weight loss and a low-grade fever. Painful restriction of movement of the shoulders and hips is characteristic. The distribution of joint involvement is bilateral and symmetrical. Occasionally knees and wrists are involved. There may be no physical signs if the patient is examined in the afternoon when the stiffness has worn off.

Headache, particularly if localized and accompanied by temporal tenderness and loss of pulsation, suggests a temporal arteritis (see p. 942), which can occur with polymyalgia.

INVESTIGATION

- The ESR is usually raised to a very high level (around 100 mm·h^{-1}) but returns to normal with treatment.
- There is a mild normochromic normocytic anaemia.
- Tests for rheumatoid factor are negative, though false-positive results are found particularly in older people.
- Serum alkaline phosphatase levels are sometimes raised but return to normal with treatment.

There is no specific test. It is not usual to carry out a temporal artery biopsy in polymyalgia, although a giant-cell arteritis can be demonstrated in 20% of cases. Temporal artery biopsy is often performed in temporal arteritis, but is not necessary in classic cases.

MANAGEMENT

Corticosteroids are the treatment of choice in polymyalgia rheumatica, starting with 15 mg of prednisolone daily. NSAIDs are less effective and, as they do not control the arteritis, should not be used. Treatment should be started immediately the diagnosis is made and before waiting for the results of tests, in order to prevent irreversible blindness, although this is rare in the absence of temporal arteritis. With steroid therapy, patients feel better within days, though mobilization of stiff shoulders may take a month or two. The dose of prednisolone is slowly reduced over the course of the next 2 years in increments not exceeding 1 mg and at intervals not exceeding one month. Relapses are common. In most patients it is possible to stop treatment after 2–4 years.

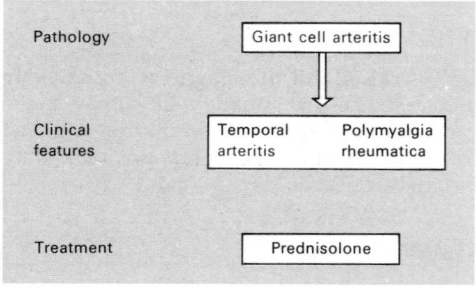

Fig. 8.14 The spectrum of diseases associated with giant-cell arteritis.

Differential diagnosis of arthritis in the elderly

Common conditions are summarized in Fig. 8.15. Osteoarthritis is common from the age of 50

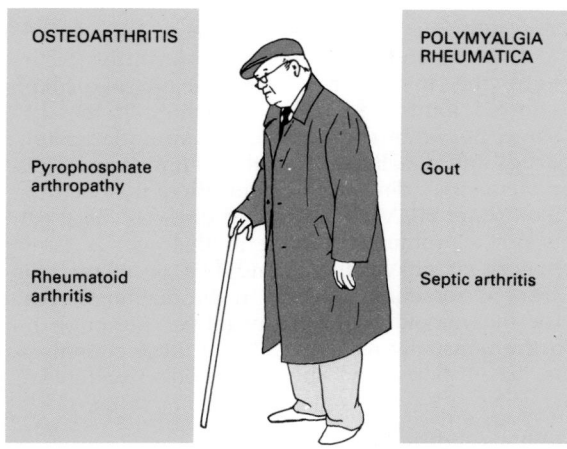

OSTEOARTHRITIS

Pyrophosphate
arthropathy

Rheumatoid
arthritis

POLYMYALGIA
RHEUMATICA

Gout

Septic arthritis

Fig. 8.15 The differential diagnosis of arthritis in the elderly.

onwards but is easily distinguished from poly-myalgia rheumatica by its less-dramatic onset, peripheral distribution and normal ESR; if there is any doubt, a one-week trial of prednisolone should be given.

Rheumatoid arthritis can begin in elderly patients. It is often sudden in onset, with very dramatic joint inflammation ('explosive' rheumatoid arthritis). Unlike the disease in young patients, it often responds very well to small doses of steroids (prednisolone 10–15 mg daily) and has a good prognosis.

Pyrophosphate deposition is common in elderly patients, typically presenting as a painful swollen knee.

Gout and septic arthritis are other causes of acute problems in the elderly.

Arthritis in children (see Fig. 8.16)

Joint pain is a common problem in childhood but arthritis is fortunately rare. Benign limb pain in childhood is sometimes called 'growing pain' and, though meaningless, this is probably a convenient term that parents readily accept.

Juvenile chronic arthritis is a general term used to cover a group of diseases in which an exact diagnosis is not always possible. There are three main types: Still's disease, juvenile rheumatoid arthritis and juvenile ankylosing spondylitis.

Still's disease

This is the commonest type of juvenile chronic arthritis, accounting for about 70% of cases. It is entirely distinct from rheumatoid arthritis, being distinguished by a number of clinical features and negative tests for rheumatoid factor. There are two peaks in the age of onset: the first and largest is between the ages of 2 and 5 years, and the second between the ages of 10 and 15. Still's disease occasionally begins after the age of 16, and rarely in the 20s. The disease is often episodic, with bouts of fever and arthritis. It can be divided into three subtypes:

- *The systemic type* is usually seen in children under the age of 5. They present with a high fever, a characteristic rash and various other features, including lymphadenopathy, spleno-megaly and pericarditis. The rash is character-ized by patches of erythema on the trunk or limbs, often appearing in the evening and brought out by warmth. Arthritis or arthralgia are minor features of the illness and may be

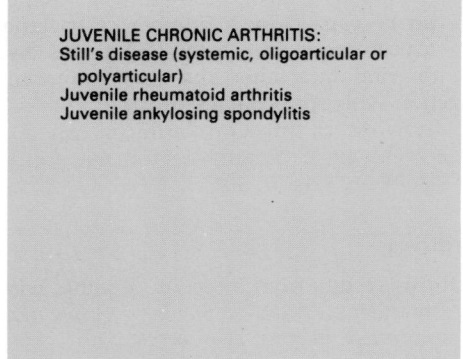

JUVENILE CHRONIC ARTHRITIS:
Still's disease (systemic, oligoarticular or
    polyarticular)
Juvenile rheumatoid arthritis
Juvenile ankylosing spondylitis

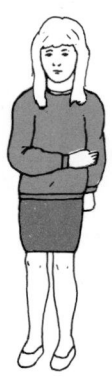

OTHER TYPES:
Infections, e.g. tuberculosis, rubella
Rheumatic fever
Henoch-Schönlein purpura
Traumatic arthritis
Hypermobility syndrome
Leukaemia
Sickle cell disease
Psoriatic arthritis
SLE and connective tissue disorders
Transient synovitis of the hip

Fig. 8.16 The differential diagnosis of arthritis in children.

absent. Arthritis may, however, develop later in the course of the disease.

- *The pauciarticular or oligoarticular type* of Still's disease affects up to four of the large joints such as the hips, knees or ankles. These patients are particularly liable to chronic iritis, which may lead to blindness without any preceding symptoms. Antinuclear antibodies are often positive and provide a useful warning that iritis may develop. Slit-lamp examination should be performed at regular intervals in these patients.
- *Polyarticular Still's disease* presents with a bilateral symmetrical polyarthritis not unlike that of rheumatoid arthritis, but with less-prominent and less-frequent involvement of the small joints of the hands and feet.

The characteristic systemic features described above may be associated with arthritis, whether polyarticular orpauciarticular.

DIAGNOSIS

The non-articular features of Still's disease are often helpful in making a diagnosis. A high swinging fever is also characteristic. This can be misleading to the unwary, as it suggests the possibility of infection.

The joints themselves are swollen, but pain and tenderness are much less prominent than in adult rheumatoid arthritis. The ESR is usually raised and there is frequently an anaemia.

TREATMENT

Treatment is with NSAIDs as in rheumatoid arthritis. Gold and penicillamine are effective but probably in a smaller proportion of cases than in rheumatoid arthritis. Corticosteroids should be avoided because of their effect on growth. It is important to protect the joints and prevent deformity during relapses, particularly as spontaneous remissions occur in 85% of patients before the age of 20 years. Long periods of rest and splinting of joints may be necessary. The patient's education and normal life-style should be continued if possible.

Juvenile rheumatoid arthritis

Rheumatoid arthritis may begin before the 16th birthday. The clinical features are identical to those of adults and tests for rheumatoid factor are usually positive. However, the prognosis is much worse than in adults. Juvenile rheumatoid arthritis accounts for about 15% of cases of juvenile chronic arthritis.

Juvenile ankylosing spondylitis

This accounts for the remaining 15% of cases of juvenile chronic arthritis. It is the most benign of the subtypes and usually presents between the ages of 10 and 15. A peripheral arthritis occurs, with the lower limb joints being particularly affected. Joints are swollen and painful in the acute stage, but often respond well to anti-inflammatory drugs and usually settle within a few years. These patients may develop iritis and there may be other features of HLA-B27 associated diseases. Back pain is not a prominent feature at this age. A family history of ankylosing spondylitis or related diseases is sometimes helpful in the diagnosis. Tests for rheumatoid factor are negative. Although the arthritis usually resolves, 50% of these patients go on to develop ankylosing spondylitis in adult life.

Other conditions

Other types of arthritis that are seen in childhood are summarized in Fig. 8.16.

Some soft-tissue syndromes particularly affect children; one of these is Osgood–Schlatter's disease, which is characterized by localized pain over the tibial tubercle and is often seen in athletic teenagers.

A mysterious condition called transient synovitis of the hip, which causes hip pain, may give rise to concern because of the possibility of tuberculosis or other serious conditions. It presents as painful limitation of movement of one hip, and usually resolves within a few weeks or months.

Infective arthritis

Infection of joints is fortunately uncommon but is important because of the damage it produces. The possibility of infection as a cause of arthritis must always be kept in mind. If its presence is suspected, synovial fluid must be obtained for culture. Infection with pyogenic organisms (septic arthritis) can be caused by a number of bacteria, including mycobacteria (see below). Arthritis also occurs with viral infections and less commonly from infection with spirochaetes or fungi.

Apart from direct infection, arthritis can also occur as a result of an immunological reaction to infection elsewhere (see p. 404).

Septic arthritis

Septic arthritis results from infection of joints with pyogenic organisms, of which *Staphylococcus aureus* is the commonest. It can also occur with other types of staphylococci, pneumococci, gonococci or Gram-negative bacilli.

Organisms reach the joint in septic arthritis via

the bloodstream, sometimes from an identifiable site of infection such as otitis media or a boil. Less commonly, infection spreads from osteomyelitis adjacent to the joint or the organism is introduced directly as a result of trauma, surgery or intra-articular injection.

Septic arthritis particularly occurs at the extremes of life and in immunologically compromised individuals, e.g. patients receiving immunosuppressive drugs or with rheumatoid arthritis.

CLINICAL FEATURES

The clinical features of septic arthritis are similar for all the different causative organisms. The presentation is usually dramatic. The patient typically presents with a single painful joint, often the knee. The joint is red, warm and swollen, with a demonstrable effusion. Fever is usual and there may be evidence of infection elsewhere.

In rheumatoid arthritis, the presentation may be misleading; patients are often afebrile and do not necessarily have a systemic reaction or a leucocytosis. Any suddenly painful joint in a patient with rheumatoid arthritis should be aspirated to exclude infection.

Systemic and local reactions can also be absent in patients receiving corticosteroids.

INVESTIGATION

- Aspiration of the joint is the only important diagnostic manoeuvre (Table 8.7). The synovial fluid is often purulent and typically contains about $100\,000 \times 10^6/l$ white blood cells, predominantly neutrophils. A Gram stain may show the presence of organisms. Culture of the fluid, including special techniques for detecting anaerobes and gonococci, usually gives a definite answer.
- There may be a leucocytosis.
- Blood culture may be positive.
- X-rays are of no value in the diagnosis of septic arthritis; they become abnormal only when joint destruction is advanced.

TREATMENT

This should be started immediately the diagnosis is made, as cartilage destruction can occur within a few days of the onset of the joint infection and the situation can be life-threatening. The joint should be immobilized.

Antibiotic therapy
The choice of antibiotic will depend upon the organism concerned. If the identification of this is delayed, 'blind' therapy should be started immediately with a slow i.v. infusion of flucloxacillin 500 mg 6-hourly together with clindamycin 300 mg

i.v. 6-hourly or fusidic acid 500 mg 8-hourly by mouth. Antibiotics given by the intramuscular or intravenous route will pass into joints, especially when they are inflamed; antibiotics should not be injected intra-articularly. Antibiotic levels in the synovial fluid should be checked during the acute illness. Antibiotics should be continued for 6 weeks.

Drainage
Drainage of infected joints is best achieved by needle aspiration, which should be performed daily until no further fluid is obtainable. For inaccessible joints such as the hip, surgical drainage may be required. If infection is allowed to continue, debris that cannot be removed with a needle collects within the joint and this delays recovery. In these circumstances, the effusion will fail to resolve and surgical debridement will be required.

PROGNOSIS

The resolution of septic arthritis with complete recovery usually occurs within a few days or weeks.

SPECIFIC TYPES OF BACTERIAL ARTHRITIS

Tuberculous arthritis

One per cent of patients with tuberculosis have skeletal involvement. Tuberculous arthritis affecting children usually occurs in the primary stage of the disease. In adults, it is invariably secondary to pulmonary or renal disease and is due to haematogenous spread to the subchondral bone or the spinal intervertebral discs. Predisposing factors for tuberculous arthritis are those for developing TB anywhere in the body, e.g. alcoholism, diabetes mellitus or any other chronic debilitating disease.

PATHOLOGY

The synovial membrane and periarticular tissues become inflamed and oedematous; histologically caseating granulomas are seen. Later there is destruction of cartilage and this may lead to fibrous ankylosis. When the spine is involved, the infection may track along the fascial planes to produce a psoas abscess.

CLINICAL FEATURES

There is usually a monarticular arthritis affecting the hip or knee (30%) or the sacroiliac or other joints (20%); in 50% of patients there is spinal involvement. There is an insidious onset of pain and dysfunction of the joint, with swelling and synovial proliferation very like that seen in rheumatoid arthritis, and restriction of movement associated with general symptoms of malaise, anorexia and night sweats.

DIAGNOSIS

The mycobacterium may be cultured from the synovial fluid; however, negative results do not exclude the diagnosis and if suspicion remains, synovial biopsy is required. X-rays are at first normal but later there is narrowing of the joint space and bony erosions.

TREATMENT

Drug treatment is as for tuberculosis elsewhere (see p. 682). The joint should be immobilized in the acute phase. If infection is allowed to continue, the effusion cannot be aspirated via a needle because of debris and surgical debridement is necessary.

Meningococcal arthritis

Meningococcal arthritis usually occurs as part of a generalized meningococcal septicaemia. It is a migratory polyarthritis and organisms cannot usually be recovered from the synovial fluid. Joint destruction does not occur. This type of arthritis is due to circulating immune complexes containing meningococcal antigens. Occasionally the effusion is purulent and contains meningococcal organisms. Treatment is with penicillin.

Gonococcal arthritis

Gonococcal arthritis is similar to meningococcal arthritis. It particularly affects young adult females and also homosexual men. It presents with a mildly inflammatory polyarthritis. It is usually asymmetrical and occasionally migratory. A useful clue to the diagnosis is the presence of small pustular skin lesions, often near the affected joints. The organism can be recovered from the bloodstream and in 25% of cases from the joints. In the remainder the arthritis is a reaction to the infection, and is probably immunologically mediated.

If neglected, gonococcal septicaemia may go on to produce a typical septic arthritis. Treatment is with penicillin 1 g orally, daily for 2 weeks.

Salmonella arthritis

Salmonella infection differs from septic arthritis in being polyarticular. It is also less dramatic than septic arthritis and is therefore easily missed. It occurs with types of *Salmonella* that invade the bloodstream rather than staying within the gastrointestinal tract. Gastrointestinal features may therefore be minor or absent, deflecting attention away from the correct diagnosis.

Treatment with systemic antibiotics, e.g. amoxycillin 500 mg 6-hourly, is curative.

Lyme disease (see p. 52)

Arthritis is seen in patients with Lyme disease in the USA. It occurs mainly in children and is easily mistaken for Still's disease. It is characteristically episodic with attacks of arthritis affecting about three large joints and lasting one week.

Infective endocarditis

Infective endocarditis (p. 596) may present with arthritis, which occurs particularly in the early stages of the disease. Like other clinical features, the arthritis may be due to circulating immune complexes; direct infection of the joints is much less common. Asymmetrical arthritis of a few large joints is characteristic, but other patterns may occur. Localized back pain associated with fever is another manifestation.

VIRAL ARTHRITIS

A number of different viral infections cause arthritis. The commonest and most important is *rubella*, where the virus can occasionally be isolated from the joint. Arthritis is particularly a complication of the disease in young adult females, occurring in 15% of cases. Arthritis may follow either rubella or the rubella vaccine. It begins a few days after development of the rash, or 2 weeks after vaccination. It may be associated with other complications such as lymphadenopathy. It presents as a bilateral, symmetrical polyarthritis, closely resembling rheumatoid arthritis, for which it is often mistaken. However, it resolves within a few weeks in most cases. Occasionally there is persistent or recurrent arthralgia that may continue for years. Treatment is symptomatic.

Arthritis may also complicate *mumps*. A few large joints are typically affected and, as in rubella, the condition is self-limiting.

Arthralgia and sometimes arthritis may be features of the prodromal stage of *hepatitis B infection*, but resolve when the jaundice appears. As in meningococcal arthritis, this prodromal syndrome is associated with circulating immune complexes.

Transient polyarthritis is also seen in *infectious mononucleosis, chickenpox* and other viral infections.

FUNGAL INFECTIONS

Fungal infections of joints occur rarely. Actinomycosis can affect the mandible or vertebrae. Bone abscesses may be seen. Destructive joint lesions

Table 8.13 Classification of arthropathies following infections.

HLA-B27 association:	HLA-B27 associated	Not associated with HLA-B27
Type of infection:	Enteric or venereal	Streptococcal
Resulting arthropathies:	Reactive arthritis Reiter's syndrome	Rheumatic fever Henoch–Schönlein purpura

can also occur with blastomycosis. A benign polyarthritis accompanied by erythema nodosum occasionally occurs in coccidioidomycosis and histoplasmosis. Culture of purulent synovial fluid and skin tests for fungi may help the diagnosis.

Arthritis following infection

Much more common than direct infection of joints is a condition in which arthritis is associated with an immunological reaction to infection. There are two different types, which are summarized in Table 8.13. Rheumatic fever and Henoch–Schönlein purpura follow streptococcal infections and predisposition to these disorders is not related to the presence of the antigen HLA-B27. By contrast, HLA-B27-positive individuals are particularly likely to develop reactive arthritis following enteric or venereal infection.

Reiter's syndrome

This syndrome consists of the triad of a seronegative reactive arthritis, non-specific urethritis and conjunctivitis. Two types are recognized:

- Following a gastrointestinal infection with *Shigella, Salmonella, Yersinia* or *Campylobacter*
- Following non-specific urethritis

The male-to-female ratio is 20 : 1 and most cases occur in young adults. HLA-B27 is present in up to 80% of cases.

CLINICAL FEATURES (Fig. 8.17)

- The *arthritis* begins within 2 weeks of the enteric or venereal infection, which may have been mild and asymptomatic. The joints of the lower limbs are particularly affected in an asymmetrical pattern; the knees, ankles and feet are the commonest sites. The wrists and other joints of the upper limbs are occasionally involved, and there may be localized pain and tenderness in the spine due to sacroiliitis. The arthritis is often very acute at presentation but resolves over the course of a few months. It is occasionally associated with non-articular inflammatory lesions, including plantar fasciitis and Achilles tendinitis.
- The *urethritis* is associated with a sterile urethral discharge and mild dysuria. Prostatism can occur. Circinate balanitis, a superficial penile lesion characterized by a circle of erythema with a pale centre, is rare.
- The *conjunctivitis* is usually mild and bilateral, resolving spontaneously. It occurs in only one-third of patients. Acute anterior uveitis develops later in the disease, in approximately 10% of patients.
- *Keratoderma blennorrhagica* is seen in 10% of patients with post-venereal Reiter's syndrome. It is characterized by intense scaling of the skin of the soles of the feet, resembling pustular psoriasis. Nail dystrophy with subungual keratosis may lead to shedding of the nails.

Patients with Reiter's syndrome may have a low-grade fever. Very rarely cardiac (e.g. pericarditis,

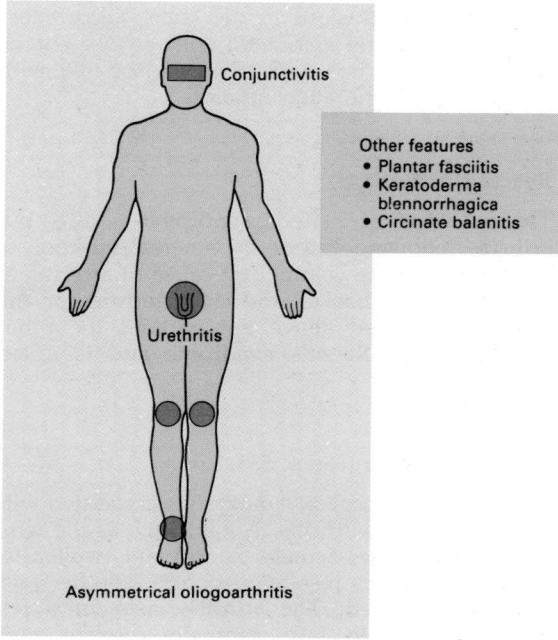

Fig. 8.17 The clinical features of Reiter's syndrome.

aortitis), respiratory (mainly pleurisy) or neurological (peripheral neuropathy) complications occur.

DIAGNOSIS

The diagnosis in these conditions is entirely clinical; there are no diagnostic blood tests. The ESR is raised in the acute stage. Tests for rheumatoid factor and other autoantibodies are negative. X-rays are of no value in the acute stage of the disease, though signs of sacroiliitis may appear with the development of ankylosing spondylitis. Aspirated synovial fluid is inflammatory in nature, with a high polymorphonuclear leucocyte count; it is sterile.

TREATMENT

Treatment is with NSAIDs such as indomethacin. It is often useful to aspirate acutely inflamed joints and to inject them with a corticosteroid preparation.

PROGNOSIS

Although the acute arthritis resolves within a few months, there is a very high incidence of long-term problems. About 50% of patients with Reiter's syndrome will go on to develop recurrences of arthritis, iritis or ankylosing spondylitis. Recurrent synovitis is the commonest problem and typically presents with effusions in the knee. Recurrences are not necessarily associated with further enteric or venereal infection and are not associated with progressive deterioration of joints.

Reactive arthritis

The full triad of Reiter's syndrome is rare, but arthritis following enteric or venereal infection is common. It is the commonest cause of arthritis in young men. It has all the characteristics of the arthritis described above but without the other associations of Reiter's syndrome and is called reactive arthritis.

Rheumatic fever (see p. 583)

This post-streptococcal condition is associated with a migratory polyarthritis. A joint such as the wrist or elbow becomes acutely painful and swollen for about 2 days. As resolution occurs, another joint becomes involved. The arthritis lasts for a few weeks or months but eventually resolves completely without any long-term problems. Its importance is the association of carditis in 40% of cases.

Henoch–Schönlein purpura (see p. 338)

This childhood condition also follows a streptococcal infection. It presents as a generalized purpuric rash associated with abdominal pain or a symmetrical polyarthritis, and lasts for a few weeks. Its importance is the association of glomerulonephritis in 40% of cases.

Crystal deposition diseases

Three types of crystal are deposited in joints; each is associated with a characteristic clinical syndrome (Fig. 8.18):

- *Monosodium urate deposition* is associated with acute gout, typically affecting the big toe.
- *Calcium pyrophosphate deposition* causes many different syndromes including pseudogout, which most often affects the knee.
- *Hydroxyapatite deposition* causes acute calcific periarthritis and most often affects the shoulder.

In addition, calcium pyrophosphate and hydroxyapatite crystals are found in the joints of patients with osteoarthritis and may contribute to the inflammation.

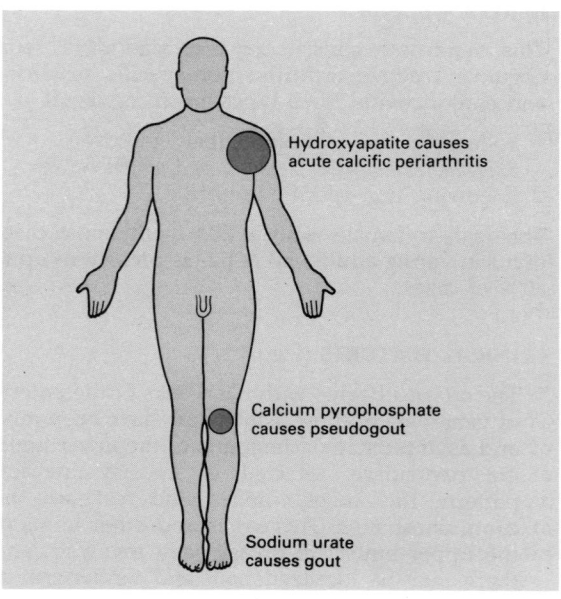

Hydroxyapatite causes acute calcific periarthritis

Calcium pyrophosphate causes pseudogout

Sodium urate causes gout

Fig. 8.18 The typical patterns of joint involvement seen in crystal deposition disease.

Gout

Gout is an abnormality of uric acid metabolism that results in the deposition of sodium urate crystals in:

- *Joints*—causing acute gouty arthritis
- *Soft tissue*—causing tophi and tenosynovitis
- *Urinary tract*—causing urate stones

EPIDEMIOLOGY

The prevalence varies from approximately 0.2% in Europe and USA to 10% in the adult male Maori of New Zealand. Filipinos have high prevalences in the USA but not in the Philippines, suggesting an environmental factor. Gout is commoner in the upper social classes and one-third of patients give a family history. At least 50% are regular alcohol drinkers.

PATHOGENESIS

The biochemical abnormality is hyperuricaemia resulting from overproduction or underexcretion of uric acid. A high dietary intake of purines can be an additional factor, but does not in itself produce hyperuricaemia.

Uric acid production
Uric acid is the last step in the breakdown pathway of nucleoprotein and purines. The last two steps—the conversion of hypoxanthine to xanthine and of xanthine to uric acid—are catalysed by the enzyme xanthine oxidase.

Uric acid excretion
Uric acid is completely filtered by the glomerulus; 100% is then reabsorbed in the proximal tubule and 75% is secreted by the distal tubule. Some post-secretory reabsorption also takes place.

Causes of hyperuricaemia
In most patients with idiopathic (primary) gout the major cause of the hyperuricaemia is impaired renal excretion; but increased synthesis also occurs. Conditions in which hyperuricaemia occur are shown in Table 8.14.

CLINICAL FEATURES

Gout is predominantly a disease of men. Hippocrates was the first to note that it does not occur in men before puberty or in women until after the menopause. It is a disease that mostly begins in middle life. Asymptomatic hyperuricaemia is 10 times more common than gout.

There are two stages in the natural history of the disease. First, recurrent acute attacks of arthritis occur. Secondly, the attacks fail to resolve completely and there are persistent symptoms

Table 8.14 Causes of hyperuricaemia.

Impaired excretion of uric acid
Idiopathic (primary) gout
Chronic renal disease (clinical gout unusual)
Drug therapy, e.g. thiazide diuretics, low-dose aspirin
Hypertension
Lead toxicity
Primary hyperparathyroidism
Hypothyroidism
Increased lactic acid production from alcohol, exercise, starvation
Glucose-6-phosphatase deficiency (interferes with renal excretion)

Increased production of uric acid
Idiopathic (primary) gout
Increased purine synthesis de novo due to:
  Hypoxanthine-guanine-phosphoribosyl transferase (HGPRT) reduction (an X-linked inborn error causing the Lesch–Nyhan syndrome)
  Phosphoribosyl-pyrophosphate synthetase overactivity
  Glucose-6-phosphatase deficiency with glycogen storage disease type I (patients who survive develop hyperuricaemia due to increased production as well as decreased excretion)
Increased turnover of purines due to:
  Myeloproliferative disorders, e.g. polycythaemia vera
  Lymphoproliferative disorders, e.g. leukaemia
  Others, e.g. carcinoma, severe psoriasis

associated with the permanent deposition of urate in and around joints; this stage is known as chronic tophaceous gout.

The typical acute attack begins suddenly in the early hours of the morning with excruciating pain in the big toe. Attacks may be precipitated by events such as:

- A surgical operation (hence postoperative arthritis is usually gout)
- Dietary or alcoholic excess
- Starvation
- Drugs, e.g. thiazide diuretics

In 25% of attacks, a joint other than the big toe is the site of the disease. Joints of the lower limb are most often affected, including the toes, ankles and knees. Occasionally attacks occur in the upper limb, particularly in the distal interphalangeal joints of the fingers. One joint only is affected in 90% of attacks.

SIGNS

The typical gouty joint is red, warm, swollen and exquisitely tender. The presence of tophi in the ear lobes or around joints may provide a clue to the correct diagnosis, but they usually occur in the later stages of the disease, by which time the nature of the problem is obvious.

ASSOCIATED FEATURES

Patients with gout have a higher than expected incidence of vascular disease, hypertension and renal disease. Renal disease may be due to uric acid stones or very rarely to deposition of uric acid in the kidney itself, a condition known as chronic hyperuricaemic nephropathy (see p. 453). However, most often the renal disease is due to hypertension and vascular disease, which are genetic associations of gout rather than complications of hyperuricaemia.

INVESTIGATION

- The affected joint is aspirated and the synovial fluid is examined under polarized-light microscopy. In acute gout, the presence of long, needle-shaped, negatively birefringent crystals is diagnostic. The test takes just a few minutes and is the best way to make the diagnosis.
- The serum uric acid has a number of limitations as a diagnostic test. It takes time, and a high incidence of false-positive and false-negative results makes interpretation difficult. Acute gout never occurs with a serum uric acid in the lower half of the normal range. However, in the first few attacks, which are the most difficult to diagnose, the serum uric acid is often below the upper limit of normal. The level also falls after an acute attack. Thus, a normal serum uric acid does not exclude the diagnosis of gout. Similarly, a high level alone is not diagnostic. However, the serum uric acid is useful in monitoring treatment.

MANAGEMENT

Acute attacks
Acute gout is treated with anti-inflammatory drugs:

- Indomethacin 50 mg three to four times daily should produce substantial relief within 24–48 h, when the dose should be reduced to 25 mg three to four times daily. The attack should resolve completely within a few weeks. Azapropazone 600 mg twice daily, is an alternative.
- Colchicine works slowly and produces diarrhoea; it is now rarely used.
- Intramuscular ACTH (corticotrophin) is very effective in difficult cases.
- Effusions in large joints should be aspirated and a corticosteroid injected to reduce inflammation.

Long-term therapy
Long-term therapy should be considered when the acute attack has settled. Simple measures to reduce uric acid levels include:

- Weight reduction
- Reduction in alcohol intake
- Avoidance of foods containing high levels of purine, e.g. game
- Good fluid intake
- Withdrawal of drugs such as salicylates and thiazides

Drugs. Allopurinol (a xanthine oxidase inhibitor) is the drug of choice. Indications include:

- Frequent acute attacks
- Tophi or chronic gouty arthritis
- Renal stones
- Very high serum uric acid levels (> 9 mg/ 100 ml^{-1} or 0.55 mmol·L^{-1})
- Prophylaxis when treating malignant disease

Allopurinol should not be started for 4 weeks after the last acute attack. It may precipitate acute gout and should be given with a prophylactic to prevent attacks. Colchicine in a dose of 0.5 mg twice daily is ideal for this purpose and should be continued for 6 months.

The dosage of allopurinol is 300 mg daily, which should be sufficient to bring the serum urate down to normal levels. In renal disease 100 mg daily is given. Side-effects are uncommon and include skin rashes. The tophi disappear with the reduction in serum urate.

Probenecid, a uricosuric drug, is occasionally used as an alternative to allopurinol.

Pyrophosphate arthropathy

This condition is associated with the deposition of calcium pyrophosphate dihydrate in joints. The acute attacks of crystal synovitis that occur in about 25% of patients with the disease are known as pseudogout.

The aetiology of pyrophosphate arthropathy is unknown but there is an association with primary hyperparathyroidism, haemochromatosis, hypothyroidism, hypophosphatasia and true gout.

Pyrophosphate arthropathy is a disease of older people, with the typical age of onset being 60 years. It is equally common in men and women.

CLINICAL FEATURES

The commonest manifestation of pyrophosphate arthropathy is osteoarthritis; this occurs in about 50% of cases. It is not dissimilar to primary osteoarthritis but tends to be polyarticular, sometimes with involvement of unusual joints such as the wrist. The course of osteoarthritis associated with pyrophosphate deposition may be punctuated by attacks of pseudogout.

Acute attacks most commonly affect the knee but they can affect other joints, usually large ones and mainly one at a time. The attacks begin suddenly with pain and swelling. The affected joint is warm and swollen with a large effusion. The attack resolves within weeks or months but recurs at irregular intervals. Patients may have other changes associated with osteoarthritis, such as Heberden's nodes.

Occasionally, pyrophosphate deposition is entirely asymptomatic. Rarely, it causes a polyarthritis resembling rheumatoid arthritis, a severe destructive arthritis of weight-bearing joints, an acute spinal syndrome or polymyalgia rheumatica.

INVESTIGATION

- The serum calcium is normal.
- The ESR may be raised during an attack.
- Aspiration of synovial fluid and identification of crystals by polarized-light microscopy is diagnostic. Calcium pyrophosphate crystals are smaller than urate crystals. They are brick-shaped and postively birefringent, and are therefore easily distinguished from urate crystals.
- X-rays of the knee and occasionally the wrist may show linear calcification lying between and parallel to the articular surfaces (chondrocalcinosis articularis). X-rays may also show changes of osteoarthritis, with joint space narrowing and osteophyte formation.

MANAGEMENT

Pyrophosphate arthropathy is not as easy to treat and control as gout. Rest and aspiration of as much fluid as possible from an affected joint and an injection of corticosteroid are helpful. NSAIDs are less dramatic in their effects than in gout but are, nevertheless, useful.

Acute calcific periarthritis

This syndrome is associated with deposition of hydroxyapatite in the soft tissues around joints. It is the least common of the crystal deposition diseases, but is by no means rare. It typically occurs in adults aged above 40 years and is equally common in men and women.

The shoulder joint is the commonest site, but it can affect the small joints of the hands and feet, the wrists, the knees and other joints. When the big toe is affected, the condition is often confused with gout. There is a sudden onset of pain, which is often very severe. The affected joint is red, warm and swollen, and there is sometimes a small effusion. The attack resolves within days or weeks,

but attacks recur at irregular intervals.

X-rays are diagnostic: there is a rounded well-defined radiopaque deposit in the soft tissue adjacent to the joint.

Treatment is with NSAIDs such as indomethacin. Potent analgesics such as opiates are sometimes required in the acute stage. It is often useful to inject the affected joint or soft tissues with a combination of local anaesthetic and corticosteroid. It is seldom, if ever necessary to remove the calcific deposit.

Arthritis associated with other diseases

Gastrointestinal and liver disease

Enteropathic synovitis occurs in 11% of patients with ulcerative colitis and 14% of patients with Crohn's disease. This type of arthritis is always related to the activity of the underlying disease, although in a small proportion of cases it is the first manifestation of underlying bowel problems. The aetiology is unknown but deposition of immune complexes in the joint may play a part. Enteropathic synovitis usually affects the knees and ankles as a monoarthritis or asymmetrical oligoarthritis. It presents with painful swollen joints and large effusions. Attacks last for a few months only and resolve without joint damage. Enteropathic synovitis should be distinguished from ankylosing spondylitis. The latter occurs in about 5% of patients with inflammatory bowel disease but is an associated lesion rather than a complication of the bowel disease and therefore is not related to disease activity. Other non-articular features of inflammatory bowel disease, e.g. iritis, may be present.

X-rays of affected joints are normal and investigations are otherwise unhelpful. The first priority for treatment is to control the underlying inflammatory bowel disease. Aspiration and injection of affected joints and oral anti-inflammatory drugs may help the symptoms while the underlying disease is being brought under control.

Autoimmune chronic active hepatitis (see p. 259) may be accompanied by an arthralgia that is like that seen in systemic lupus erythematosus. Joint pain occurs in a bilateral, symmetrical distribution, with the small joints of the hands being prominently affected. Joints usually look normal but sometimes there is a slight soft-tissue swelling. These patients often have positive tests for antinuclear antibodies and sometimes other features of connective tissue disorders such as Sjögren's syndrome.

Whipple's disease (see p. 208) is accompanied by a fever and an arthralgia.

Malignant disease

Hypertrophic pulmonary osteoarthropathy

Hypertrophic osteoarthropathy is most often associated with carcinoma of the bronchus. It is a non-metastatic complication and may be the presenting feature of the disease. It occurs only rarely with other conditions that cause clubbing. It is seen most often in middle-aged men, who present with pain and swelling of the wrists and ankles. Other joints are occasionally involved.

The diagnosis is made on the presence of clubbing of the fingers, which is usually gross, and periosteal new bone formation along the shafts of the distal ends of the radius, ulna, tibia and fibula seen on X-ray. A chest X-ray usually shows the malignancy.

Treatment should be directed at the underlying carcinoma; if this can be removed, the arthropathy disappears. NSAIDs may help to relieve the symptoms.

Other disorders

Secondary gout occurs in conditions such as chronic myeloid leukaemia. Pain in the shoulder or back may be referred from malignant disease of the chest or abdomen. Secondaries around the joints may present with pain, but primary joint tumours are very rare. A synovioma presents as a painless soft-tissue swelling adjacent to joints. It is highly malignant but extremely rare.

Skin disease

Psoriatic arthritis

This is a seronegative arthritis occurring in 10% of patients with psoriasis. The aetiology is unknown, but there is an increased incidence of HLA-B27 and of a history of psoriasis in the family.

The skin lesion, which is described on p. 1007, may be minimal. The nail changes of psoriasis are usually present (85%). Differing patterns of arthritis are seen:

- The commonest pattern of psoriatic arthropathy is a polyarthritis affecting the small joints of the hands, including the distal interphalangeal joints, in an asymmetrical pattern. This is a mild but chronic condition, and in most cases is benign. It can usually be controlled with analgesics but NSAIDs are sometimes necessary.
- Less often the pattern of the arthritis is similar to that in rheumatoid arthritis, i.e. a bilateral, symmetrical polyarthritis.
- Rarely the disease is rapidly progressive, producing destruction of the ends of the small bones of the hands and feet (arthritis mutilans), a condition that can also occur in rheumatoid arthritis. Because of the shortening of the bones of the fingers there is an excess of soft tissue and the fingers can be pulled in and out like an opera glass, after which the condition is sometimes named.
- Finally, patients with psoriasis have an increased incidence of ankylosing spondylitis.

Blood tests are unhelpful in the diagnosis. The ESR is often normal and tests for rheumatoid factor are negative. X-rays may show characteristic changes in the terminal interphalangeal joints, with erosions and periarticular osteoporosis.

Treatment is with analgesic and anti-inflammatory drugs. In progressive cases, immunosuppressive drugs such as azathioprine are particularly effective. Gold is sometimes effective in psoriatic arthropathy, but penicillamine is not.

Erythema nodosum

Erythema nodosum (p. 1016) can be due to several conditions, e.g. sarcoid and is accompanied by arthritis in over 50% of cases. The knees and ankles are particularly affected and are swollen, red and tender. The arthritis subsides, along with the skin lesions, within a few months. Treatment is with NSAIDs or occasionally steroids.

Neurological disease

Neuropathic joints (Charcot's joints) are joints damaged by trauma as a result of the loss of the protective pain sensation. They were first described by Charcot in relation to tabes dorsalis. They are also seen in syringomyelia, diabetes mellitus and leprosy. The site of the neuropathic joint depends upon the localization of the pain loss:

- In tabes dorsalis, the knees and ankles are most often affected.
- In diabetes mellitus, the joints of the tarsus are involved.
- In syringomyelia, the shoulder is involved.

Neuropathic joints are not painful, although there may be painful episodes associated with crystal deposition. Presentation is usually with swelling and instability and eventually grotesque deformities appear.

The characteristic finding is a swollen joint with abnormal but painless movement. This is associated with neurological findings that depend upon the underlying disease, e.g. dissociated sensory loss in syringomyelia or peripheral neuropathy in diabetes. X-ray changes are characteristic, with gross joint disorganization and bony distortion.

Treatment is symptomatic; surgery may be required in advanced cases.

Blood disease

Arthritis due to haemarthrosis is a common presenting feature of *haemophilia*. Attacks begin in early childhood in most cases and are recurrent. The knee is the commonest affected joint but the elbows and ankles are sometimes involved. The arthritis can lead to bone destruction and disorganization of joints. Apart from replacement of factor VIII, affected joints require initial immobilization followed by physiotherapy to restore movement and measures to prevent and correct deformities.

Sickle cell crises are often accompanied by joint pain that particularly affects the hands and feet in a bilateral, symmetrical distribution. Affected joints usually look normal but are occasionally swollen. This condition may also be complicated by avascular necrosis (see below) and by *Salmonella osteomyelitis*.

Arthritis can also occur in *acute leukaemia*; it may be the presenting feature in childhood. The knee is particularly affected and is very painful, warm and swollen. Treatment is directed at the underlying leukaemia. Arthritis may also occur in chronic leukaemia, with leukaemic deposits in and around the joints.

Endocrine disorders

Hypothyroid patients may complain of pain and stiffness of proximal muscles, resembling polymyalgia rheumatica. They may also have carpal tunnel syndrome. Less often, there is an arthritis accompanied by joint effusions, particularly in the knees, wrist and small joints of the hands and feet. These problems respond rapidly to thyroxine.

In acromegaly an arthritis occurs in about 50% of patients. It resembles osteoarthritis and particularly affects the small joints of the hands and knees. It may be associated with the carpal tunnel syndrome.

In Cushing's disease back pain is common.

Diabetes mellitus-related joint disorders are described later (see p. 856).

Less-common arthropathies

Amyloidosis (see p. 869)

Primary amyloidosis causes a polyarthritis that resembles rheumatoid arthritis in distribution and it is also often associated with carpal tunnel syndrome and subcutaneous nodules.

Ankylosing vertebral hyperostosis (Forrestier's disease)

This is a condition of elderly people in which exuberant osteophytes are found in the spine, particularly the dorsal region. It is often asympto-matic, but it may be confused with ankylosing spondylitis. Sometimes there is stiffness and occasionally some discomfort. It may be associated with peripheral soft-tissue problems associated with calcification, ossification and spur formation, when it is called diffuse idiopathic skeletal hyperostosis (DISH).

Avascular necrosis

In this condition, bone infarction disrupts the surface of the joint and often leads to changes resembling osteoarthritis. The hip is particularly affected, for example, following fractures of the neck of the femur, perhaps because of its precarious blood supply. It also occurs in various systemic conditions, including sickle cell disease, prolonged steroid therapy, systemic lupus erythematosus, alcohol abuse and Gaucher's disease. It occurs in deep-sea divers (caisson disease). It may occur for no obvious reason, particularly in middle-aged men.

Avascular necrosis presents with a single painful joint. X-rays are usually diagnostic in the latter phases, showing rarefaction and dense bone in the subcortical areas with distortion of the epiphysis.

Behçet's syndrome

This is a rare condition characterized by oral and genital ulceration, iritis, and a polyarthritis of variable distribution that may be either chronic or episodic. There are many less-common features of the disease, including erythema nodosum, pustular skin lesions, and neurological and gastrointestinal manifestations. Treatment is with oral steroids but response is variable.

Drugs

Drugs may cause arthritis. Systemic lupus erythematosus may be induced by procainamide, hydralazine and other drugs. Certain drugs may also precipitate or aggravate gout.

Familial Mediterranean fever

This condition occurs in certain ethnic groups, particularly Jews and Arabs. The aetiology is unknown. It is characterized by recurrent attacks of fever, arthritis and abdominal or chest pain due to pleurisy. The arthritis is usually monoarticular and attacks last up to 1 week. The condition may be mistaken for palindromic rheumatism, but such attacks are not usually accompanied by fever. In familial Mediterranean fever, attacks can usually be prevented by regular treatment with colchicine 1.0–1.5 mg daily. In general the disorder is benign but in some cases amyloidosis develops.

Hypermobility syndrome

Hypermobility syndrome occurs in children or young adults with lax joints. The musculoskeletal manifestations of this syndrome include recurrent attacks of joint pain and effusion, dislocation, ligamentous injuries, low back pain and premature osteoarthritis. Hypermobility is also associated with some rare congenital disorders such as the Ehlers–Danlos syndrome. Joints become stiffer with increasing age. Treatment should be directed at improving muscle power.

Osteochondritis dessecans

This is a rare condition of adolescent sportsmen in which there is separation of an avascular osteochondral fragment in the knee joint. It results in disruption of the joint surface and the formation of loose bodies within the joint. Osteoarthritis may develop.

Osteochondromatosis

In this condition, foci of cartilage form within the synovial membrane. These foci become calcified and then ossified (osteochondromas). They may give rise to loose bodies within the joint. The condition occurs in a single joint of a young adult and X-rays are usually diagnostic. Treatment involves removal of loose bodies and synovectomy.

Palindromic rheumatism

This condition is a variant of rheumatoid arthritis, characterized by recurrent attacks of arthritis. They occur at irregular intervals, sometimes with long periods of freedom between them, begin suddenly, reach a peak after a few hours and fade over the course of the next 2 days. A single joint is affected in each attack and during the attack it is red, warm, swollen and very painful. Between attacks the joints are normal. Tests for rheumatoid factor are positive in 50% and one-third of cases go on to develop chronic rheumatoid arthritis.

Pigmented villonodular synovitis

This is characterized by exuberant synovial proliferation that occurs either in joints or in tendon sheaths. The main manifestation in joints is recurrent haemarthrosis. Treatment is synovectomy. In tendons, the condition gives rise to a nodular mass that requires excision.

Relapsing polychondritis

Relapsing polychondritis is a rare condition of cartilage. It gives rise to a polyarthritis accompanied by chest disease due to tracheal or bronchial involvement. The diagnosis is often made on the basis of recurrent attacks of pain and swelling of the nose or external ear.

Temporomandibular pain dysfunction syndrome

This is a functional disorder of the temporomandibular joint associated with abnormalities of bite. It particularly occurs in anxious people who grind their teeth at night. It gives rise to pain and clicking in one or both temporomandibular joints. Treatment is dental correction of the bite.

Sarcoidosis

- The commonest type of arthritis is that associated with erythema nodosum, which occurs in 20% of cases of sarcoidosis at or soon after the onset of the disease. The most useful diagnostic test is a chest X-ray, which shows hilar lymphadenopathy in 80% of cases.
- Other patterns of arthritis including a transient rheumatoid-like polyarthritis and an acute monarthritis that can be mistaken for gout occur later in the course of the disease. If NSAIDs fail to control the symptoms, corticosteroids are usually very effective.

Hyperlipidaemia type II (see p. 864)

This is associated with xanthomas in the tendons and a migratory polyarthritis.

Back pain

Back pain is extremely common. It can be mild and transient, or chronic and disabling. In many cases, the exact cause is not established. In Britain 375 000 people lose some time from work each year because of back pain, an annual loss of 11.5 million working days, and back pain accounts for 6% of general-practice consultations. Back pain is not usually serious and mostly resolves; in one survey 44% of cases resolved within a week and 12% within 2 months.

Most back pain can be readily diagnosed from a simple clinical history and physical examination. A diagnostic approach to back pain is shown in Table 8.15.

In many patients (30%) no cause will be found. It is foolish to label such patients as having 'spondylosis' or arthritis of the spine, terms that merely cause anxiety. It is better to use a term such as non-specific low back pain and explain to the patient what this means.

The back is a common site of psychogenic pain. If possible a positive diagnosis of psychogenic back

Table 8.15 A diagnostic approach to back pain.

	Possible causes
1 Is it serious?	Infection
	Septic discitis
	Tuberculosis
	Malignancy
	Metastases
	Myeloma
	Spinal tumour
	Referred pain
2 Is it inflammatory?	Ankylosing spondylitis
3 Is it disc disease? or osteroarthritis?	Acute disc prolapse
	Chronic disc disease/ osteoarthritis (spondylosis)
4 Is it bone disease?	Osteoporosis
	Osteomalacia
	Paget's disease
	Hyperparathyroidism
	Renal osteodystrophy
5 Is it a mechanical problem—perhaps amenable to surgery?	Spondylolisthesis
	Spinal stenosis
	Posture
	Pregnancy
	Obesity
	Congenital abnormalities
6 Is it a soft tissue problem?	Fibrositis, sprains and strains
7 Is it psychogenic?	

If not, it is non-specific back pain.

pain, rather than a diagnosis by exclusion, should be made. Supportive treatment can then be given.

HISTORY

The following factors should be considered:

Site

- *Lumbar pain.* This is usually due to degenerative disease, disc prolapse and OA, which are almost never seen in the thoracic spine.
- *Thoracic pain.* This is a characteristic site of osteoporotic crush fractures.

Radiation

Sciatic radiation of pain suggests root compression; however, sacroiliac pain can also radiate down the back of the thigh to the knee.

Table 8.16 Points of distinction between inflammatory and mechanical back pain.

	Inflammatory	Mechanical
Onset	Gradual	Sudden
Worst pain	In the morning	In the evening
Morning stiffness	Present	Absent
Effect of exercise	Relieves pain	Aggravates pain

Onset

- Sudden, e.g. disc prolapse or mechanical injury
- Gradual, e.g. ankylosing spondylitis

Aggravating factors
Pain in the back and leg on walking and relieved by stopping, suggestive of intermittent claudication, can be due to spinal stenosis.

Time pattern

- Disc disease is recurrent.
- Ankylosing spondylosis is chronic.

Inflammatory vs. mechanical
The differences in the history given in inflammatory and in mechanical back pain are shown in Table 8.16.

EXAMINATION

Examination of the patient is summarized in Table 8.17.

INVESTIGATION (see Table 8.18)

In back pain, investigations are less important than the history and examination. They can also be misleading; for example, degenerative changes on X-ray are virtually always present in older people and may not be the cause of the pain.

Table 8.17 Examination of patients with back pain.

The back
Appearance—deformity
Movement
Palpation for tenderness

The nerve roots
Straight leg raising; femoral stretch test
Sensation; weakness
Reflexes; plantar responses

Complete physical examination ESSENTIAL
Look for abdominal masses, lymph nodes, iritis

Table 8.18 Investigations to consider in a patient with back pain.

Plain X rays
Blood count and ESR
Serum calcium, phosphate, alkaline phosphatase
Serum acid phosphatase
Protein electrophoresis; immunoglobulins
HLA-B27
Bone scan
Radiculogram
EMG
CT scan/magnetic resonance imaging

X-rays are particularly useful for excluding serious bone disease. Normal X-rays usually exclude metastases but not invariably. They are of little value in acute disc disease, although a narrowed disc space is suggestive of disc involvement.

A radiculogram can be performed to demonstrate the spinal cord and nerve roots. It will detect large disc prolapses and spinal stenosis. However, it does not show the lateral recess that is the region of the intervertebral foramen in which osteophytes may compress the nerve root, giving rise to sciatica.

A CT scan or magnetic resonance imaging are being used more often for the detection of disc lesions.

Bone scans are useful to detect metastases; 'hot spots' will also appear at sites of degenerative disease.

Blood tests

- ESR or CRP is a particularly useful investigation. A normal ESR or CRP makes a serious disease unlikely. A very high ESR suggests myeloma.
- Calcium, phosphate and alkaline phosphatase levels are measured to look for bone disease.
- Acid phosphatase is measured to look for secondary prostatic disease.
- Protein electrophoresis, immunoglobins and bone marrow aspiration are performed to look for myeloma.

Table 8.19 Features that suggest that back pain is serious.

Recent onset
Weight loss
Symptoms elsewhere, e.g. cough
Localized pain in the dorsal spine
Fever
Raised ESR

Back pain due to serious disease

Back pain is seldom serious but, nevertheless, is important because conditions such as infection are readily treatable. Some features that suggest serious back pain are shown in Table 8.19.

Spinal infections

Spinal infections include osteomyelitis, discitis and epidural abscess. Infections tend to affect the disc, while malignant processes affect the vertebra itself.

Discitis can be due to pyogenic organisms such as *Staphylococcus aureus*, *Mycobacterium tuberculosis* or rare organisms such as *Brucella*.

INVESTIGATION

- X-rays and bone scan to confirm the diagnosis
- Blood count—leucocytosis, high ESR
- Blood culture
- Needle aspiration of disc for culture

TREATMENT

Immobilization in the acute stage and prolonged appropriate antibiotic therapy are required.

Malignant disease

Bone metastases are classically from primaries in the bronchus, breast, kidney, thyroid or prostate. These are discussed on p. 423. Multiple myeloma produces osteolytic lesions of the spine (see p. 371). Primary tumours of the spinal cord are rarely causes of back pain (see p. 945).

Referred pain

Sources of referred pain are shown in Table 8.20.

Inflammatory back pain

Ankylosing spondylitis

Ankylosing spondylitis is the most important cause of inflammatory back pain. It affects young adults, with men more severely afflicted than women. It presents with back pain and morning stiffness, and is typically associated with sacroiliitis on X-ray. Other important associations include peripheral arthritis and non-articular features such as iritis.

It is a genetically-determined disease, susceptibility to which is related to the presence of HLA-B27. This antigen is found in about 5% of European people and 95% of patients with anky-

Table 8.20 Sources of referred pain in the back.

Kidney	Stomach and duodenum
Stones	Peptic ulcer
Tumours	Carcinoma
Infection	
Hydronephrosis	**Pancreas**
	Pancreatitis
Uterus	Carcinoma
Dysmenorrhoea	
Pelvic infection	**Aorta**
Tumours	Aneurysm
Ovary	**Bowel**
Tumours	Diverticulitis
Cysts	Abscess
	Tumour
Oesophagus	
Oesophagitis	**Gallbladder**
Carcinoma	Cholecystitis
Hiatus hernia	

losing spondylitis. Studies of large populations of B27-positive subjects such as blood donors suggest that about 20% of B27-positive individuals have ankylosing spondylitis or a related disease. The prevalence of ankylosing spondylitis in the population can thus be calculated as 1%. Since B27 is found equally in men and women, the incidence of the disease should also be equal. Population surveys using radiological sacroiliitis as the main criterion for diagnosis have shown both a much lower incidence than 1% and a male preponderance. It is now clear that there are many mild cases, especially in women, that present as pain and stiffness but with no other features. The disease is probably almost as common in men as in women and the presence of X-ray changes are not essential to the diagnosis.

The frequency of ankylosing spondylitis in different populations is roughly paralleled by the incidence of HLA-B27. Africans and Japanese have a low incidence of both B27 and ankylosing spondylitis. Some Indian tribes in America have a correspondingly higher incidence of both. HLA-B27 is the genetic marker of a family of diseases that includes Reiter's disease, iritis, inflammatory bowel disease, one type of juvenile chronic arthritis, and psoriasis. These associations are often helpful in the diagnosis of ankylosing spondylitis, since patients may give a family history of B27-related disorders.

CLINICAL FEATURES

The typical case presents with an insidious onset of low back pain in the late teens or early twenties. The pain is typically inflammatory in type (see Table 8.16). The first symptoms may arise from sacroiliitis, with pain in the buttocks radiating down the back of both legs. Peripheral polyarthritis

may also occur; the joints of the lower limbs are particularly affected. Plantar fasciitis may cause heel pain. Iritis occurs at some time in 30% of cases.

Inspection of the spine in a patient with ankylosing spondylitis reveals two characteristic abnormalities:

● Loss of lumbar lordosis and increased kyphosis
● Variable limitation of spinal flexion and a reduction in chest expansion

In addition, tenderness is commonly found around the pelvis and chest wall.

INVESTIGATION

● The ESR and CRP are often raised.
● X-rays of the lumbar spine and pelvis are almost always abnormal. In the early stages, the sacro-iliac joints are eroded, with irregular margins, and there is sclerosis of adjacent bone. As the disease advances, the sacroiliac joints may fuse. In the spinal column, the characteristic abnormality is a syndesmophyte that grows between the margins of the vertebrae. There is calcification and ossification of the interspinous ligaments so that with the syndesmophytes the PA X-ray shows three continuous lines, the so-called tramline appearance. Vertebrae appear square as a result of the erosion of their corners. These changes are particularly seen at the dorsilumbar junction, but may occur throughout the spine (Fig. 8.19).

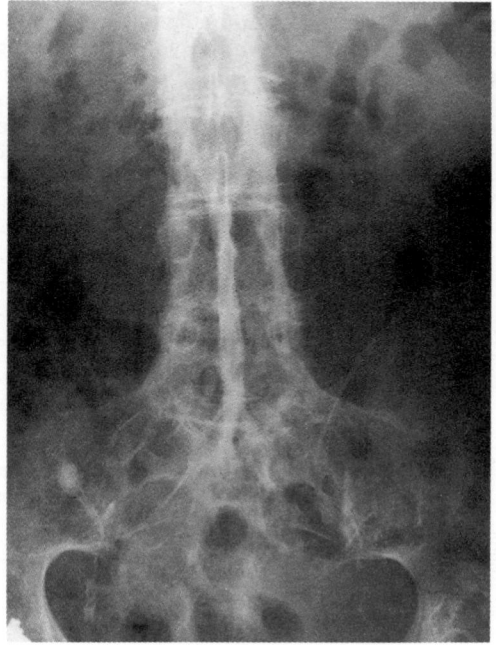

Fig. 8.19 X-ray of ankylosing spondylitis with and without sacroiliitis.

- HLA-B27 is useful supporting evidence in the difficult case but one must remember that many normal people carry the gene.

COURSE AND PROGNOSIS

In all but the mild case there is progressive limitation of spinal movement over the course of a few years. In severe cases the spine becomes completely fused. There is a tendency for patients to develop a kyphosis, but this can usually be prevented. Despite the limitation of spinal movement, most patients are able to lead a normal active life and remain at work. In women, the disease is usually mild, with little restriction and no deformity.

MANAGEMENT

- NSAIDs are very effective; slow-release indomethacin is often the best choice (75 mg at night). It is particularly useful in relieving night pain and morning stiffness. Useful alternatives include piroxicam or flurbiprofen.
- An exercise programme is essential to maintain movement, relieve symptoms and prevent deformity, particularly kyphosis. Exercises should be carried out at least twice daily. In addition, patients should be encouraged to take part in whatever sports they like.
- Sulphasalazine is useful as a long-term suppressive drug in the difficult case but there is no evidence that penicillamine, gold or immunosuppressive drugs are effective in the management of ankylosing spondylitis. Radiotherapy has been used but should seldom be necessary and carries a small risk of leukaemia. Surgery plays little part, but hip replacement is occasionally required.

Disc disease

The term 'disc disease' is used to describe an acute syndrome in which disc prolapse causes conditions that are known to the layman as either lumbago or sciatica, depending upon the presence or absence of radiation of the pain to the areas supplied by the sciatic nerve. It is also used to describe a chronic syndrome in which back pain is associated with 'degenerative changes' on X-ray. This chronic syndrome is sometimes called spondylosis. Chronic disc disease is often associated with osteoarthritis of the apophyseal joints of the spine and it is difficult or impossible to separate the role of these two pathologies in the pathogenesis of symptoms. There is a very poor correlation between the presence of radiological changes and symptoms. Severe X-ray changes can be seen in patients without any appropriate symptoms and chronic back pain may also occur in patients with little radiological change.

Acute disc disease

Acute disc disease causes acute back pain (lumbago) with or without sciatic radiation (sciatica). The severity of this syndrome is enormously variable, from a brief and trivial episode to a long and difficult illness that occasionally requires surgical intervention. It is predominantly a disease of younger people with a peak incidence between the ages of 20 and 40, since the disc degenerates with age and is no longer capable of prolapse in the elderly. In older patients, sciatica is more likely to be due to compression of the nerve root by osteophytes in the lateral recess of the spinal canal.

Table 8.21 Symptoms and signs of common root compression syndromes produced by lumbar disc prolapse.

Root lesion	Pain	Sensory loss	Motor weakness	Reflex lost	Other signs
S1	From buttock down back of thigh and leg to ankle and foot	Sole of foot and posterior calf	Plantar flexion of ankle and toes	Ankle jerk	Diminished straight-leg raising
L5	From buttock to lateral aspect of leg and dorsum of foot	Dorsum of foot and anterolateral aspect of lower leg	Dorsiflexion of foot and toes	None	Diminished straight-leg raising
L4	Lateral aspect of thigh to medial side of calf	Medial aspect of calf and shin	Dorsiflexion and inversion of ankle; extension of knee	Knee jerk	Femoral stretch test (hyperextension of hip with patient lying prone)

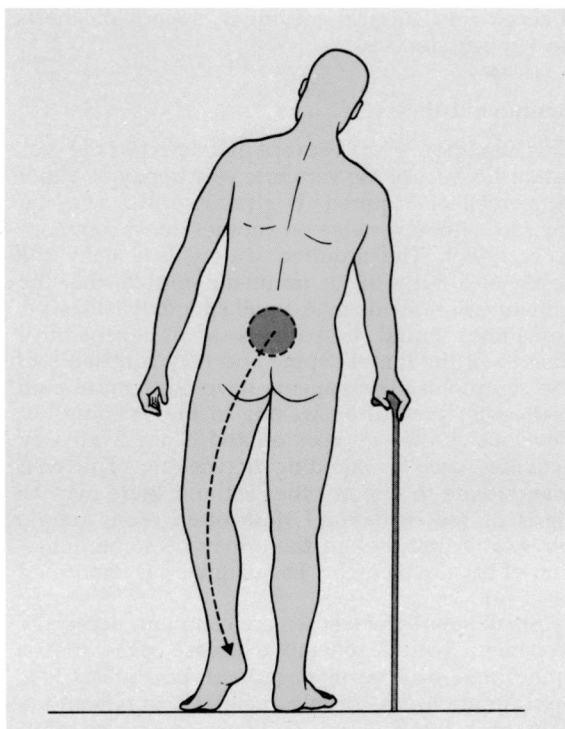

Fig. 8.20 Acute lumbar prolapse and sciatica, showing the area of the pain and the compensatory scoliosis.

CLINICAL FEATURES

The back pain is sudden, often severe and often continuous at first. Its onset may be associated with a feeling that something has 'gone' in the back. This may occur after some strenuous activity, typically with the back in forward flexion. The pain is often clearly related to position and at first the back may be fixed in forward flexion. The pain is aggravated by movement and by certain activities. The radiation of the pain and various examination findings are dependent upon the disc affected; these features are summarized in Table 8.21. The three lowest discs account for most cases of disc disease; in order of frequency, they are the L5/S1, L4/L5 and L3/L4 discs.

In a mild case there may be no signs at all, but characteristic findings include loss of lumbar lordosis, sometimes a compensatory scoliosis (Fig. 8.20) and limitation of movement in all directions. Severe neurological problems such as foot-drop or bladder or bowel dysfunction are fortunately rare.

INVESTIGATION

Investigations are of very limited value in acute disc disease. X-rays do not visualize the disc itself, although there may be narrowing at the level of the lesion. Radiculography and CT scan are usually reserved for patients in whom surgery is being considered.

MANAGEMENT

Treatment probably has little effect on the duration of the disease and is therefore aimed at the relief of symptoms and the maintenance of a reasonable way of life for the duration of the illness.

In the *acute* stage:

- *Rest* for a few days on a firm bed. Longer periods of rest are unnecessary except in the most severe cases.
- *Corsets* may be used in the acute stage.
- *Drugs*: analgesics to relieve pain; anti-inflammatory drugs if required, for example for pain at night or morning stiffness; diazepam for short periods as a muscle relaxant.
- *Epidural corticosteroid injection* reduces pain and speeds recovery but is unpleasant and requires hospitalization. It is worth considering for acute sciatica that is not responding to simpler measures.
- *Surgery* is required in the acute stage only for severe or increasing neurological impairment, e.g. foot-drop or bladder symptoms.

In the *recovery* stage, which usually begins within a few days of the acute episode:

- *Physiotherapy* to relieve pain, correct posture and restore movement. A particularly useful technique is Maitland mobilization, which begins with careful assessment by the therapist to determine levels involved and restriction of movement. Applied movements with local pressure are then used to mobilize individual segments of the lumbar spine. An exercise programme is often useful at this stage. The MacKenzie approach to back care is a self-help system of exercises that emphasize extension, and includes advice about everyday activities that is useful both in treatment and in the prevention of recurrence.
- *Surgery* will be required for a small proportion of patients (less than 1%) who fail to recover after an adequate period of conservative therapy.

COURSE AND PROGNOSIS

Most cases of acute lumbar disc prolapse recover completely, though the process may take as long as a year. A small proportion of patients fail to recover and may require surgery. Further investigations, including a radiculogram and perhaps EMG, are required to pinpoint the lesion as closely as possible, thus improving the prospects of surgery. The simplest operation is removal of the prolapsed disc.

Chronic disc disease and osteoarthritis

This very common syndrome is characterized by

the presence of chronic low back pain associated with 'degenerative' changes in the lower lumbar discs and apophyseal joints. Pain in these cases is of the mechanical type and is typically aggravated by exercise, although there may be an inflammatory component, reflected in a brief period of morning stiffness. Sciatic radiation of the pain may occur and there may be a past history of acute disc prolapse. In many cases, the pain is long-standing and the prospects for cure are very limited. Nevertheless, there are measures that will alleviate a difficult situation:

- *Drugs*. Analgesic or anti-inflammatory drugs to relieve pain. Diflunisal 500 mg twice daily has good analgesic properties but there are many alternatives.
- *Physiotherapy*. The same techniques are used as in acute disc prolapse, described above, and with the same aims. Maitland mobilization is useful when there is restriction of movement. An exercise programme, such as the MacKenzie approach is usually required and it may be necessary to try different types of programme to achieve the desired result.
- *Back care*. Advice about way of life, lifting, firm beds and other aspects of daily living is essential to identify and remove aetiological factors as well as preventing recurrence. Many physiotherapy departments have 'back' schools for this purpose.
- *Corsets* should be avoided. They may be useful for patients with mechanical abnormalities, such as instability, or a spondylolisthesis, but are grossly overprescribed. Fortunately, many patients have the good sense not to wear them!
- *Surgery* should be considered especially for a patient with severe pain of mechanical origin, arising from a single identifiable level, that has failed to respond to conservative measures. Fusion at this level would be appropriate together with decompression of affected nerve roots. The results of surgery for chronic disc disease are not particularly good—about 50% of patients recovering completely—and a failed operation is a demoralizing event in the course of a chronic illness.
- *Weight reduction* may help obese patients.
- *Pain relief* can be achieved in many other ways including acupuncture, transcutaneous nerve stimulation, massage, hypnosis and faith healing.

Mechanical problems

There are two mechanical problems in the spine that are of particular importance because they are amenable to surgical treatment: spondylolisthesis and spinal stenosis.

Spondylolisthesis

This condition arises because of a defect in the pars interarticularis of the vertebra, which may be either congenital or acquired. It gives rise to a slipping forward of one vertebra on another, most commonly at L4/L5. The acquired variety is usually the result of a fairly major traumatic episode that the patient will remember. A small spondylolisthesis is sometimes found in patients with degenerative disease of the lumbar spine and may contribute to the symptoms. The patients have mechanical pain that is not present on waking in the morning but develops as the day goes on and is aggravated by activities such as standing or walking. The pain may radiate to one or other leg and there may be signs of root irritation. More often there are no physical signs, though there may be some limitation of back movement. The diagnosis is confirmed by X-ray.

Small spondylolistheses are common, especially in patients with degenerative disease of the lumbar spine, and may be managed conservatively. It is appropriate to use simple analgesics to relieve the pain and there is no particular need for anti-inflammatory agents. A corset may provide support; this is one of the few indications for its use. A large spondylolisthesis causing severe pain, especially in a younger patient without associated degenerative changes, requires spinal fusion. This is usually a very successful procedure.

Spinal stenosis

This is sometimes called spinal claudication because of the resemblance of the symptoms to those of intermittent claudication due to vascular occlusion. The anatomical change in spinal stenosis is narrowing of the central canal, compressing the cauda equina. This can result from a variety of causes:

- Disc prolapse
- Degenerative osteophyte formation
- Tumour—rare
- Congenital narrowing of the spinal canal

The patient typically presents with pain in one or sometimes both legs. The absence of back pain makes the diagnosis difficult. The pain comes after a period of walking that tends to diminish with the passage of time. The symptoms are relieved by rest and occasionally by leaning forward. Signs of root compression such as limitation of straight-leg raising or absent reflexes may be precipitated by exertion.

If spinal stenosis is suspected, a CT scan and in addition a radiculogram will be required to confirm the diagnosis. Treatment is by surgical decompression.

Other mechanical problems

Bad posture is sometimes the cause of back pain. An exercise programme designed to improve posture will also therefore improve the pain. Such postural problems may be precipitated by congenital abnormalities of the spine such as a minor kyphoscoliosis. Obesity and presumably lack of activity sometimes appear to be relevant and weight-loss combined with an exercise programme may help.

Soft-tissue problems

Back pain can arise from soft tissues, including the muscles, tendons and ligaments.

Sprains and strains

The relationship of symptoms to some unusual physical activity will usually make the diagnosis obvious. Spontaneous resolution is usual and may be aided by the use of a NSAID and soothing pressures such as heat, ice packs or massage. Injection of tender areas with steroid–local anaesthetic combinations may also be of value.

Sacroiliac strain
This usually results from some physical activity and is particularly common in people whose occupation requires lifting, such as nurses. The pain radiates from the sacroiliac joint to the buttock and sometimes down the back of the thigh. It is a sudden acute problem that usually resolves within a few weeks with rest, avoidance of lifting and NSAIDs. Unfortunately, it has a great tendency to recur.

Coccyodynia

This is a soft-tissue problem in which pain arises from the region of the coccyx, often in anxious women. Reassurance and protection with a soft ring cushion are usually sufficient treatment since the condition is self-limiting.

Fibrositis/fibromyalgia

This is described on p. 420.

Psychogenic back pain

Diagnostic points include:
- Young adult females predominantly affected
- Continuous unvarying pain, often described in vivid terms; no relief from rest, which usually helps even the most severe organic conditions
- Long history of treatment failures, including with analgesics
- Associated symptoms, e.g. headaches; history of fruitless investigation of symptoms from other systems
- Sometimes depression but more often difficult life situations
- No signs—normal tests

MANAGEMENT
- Reassure and explain.
- Explore causes.
- Treat depression if appropriate.
- Avoid inappropriate diagnoses, e.g. 'arthritis of the spine' and repeated referrals.
- Avoid confrontation.
- Avoid prescribing drugs or predicting cures. The drugs won't work and the cures won't happen.

Non-specific low back pain

This is an appropriate term for those cases that defy diagnosis with current knowledge and techniques. Patients will vary from those with acute pain that will quickly resolve to those with long-standing symptoms and little prospect of recovery. Without the possibility of definitive treatment, one must rely on simple symptomatic measures such as analgesic drugs.

Neck pain

Pain in the neck may be caused by rheumatoid arthritis, ankylosing spondylitis, soft-tissue rheumatism or fibrositis. In addition, disc disease, both acute and chronic, the latter in association with osteoarthritis, may occur in the neck as well as in the lumbar spine. The three lowest cervical discs are most often affected and there is pain and stiffness of the neck with or without root pain radiating to the arm (see p. 957). Chronic cervical disc disease is known as cervical spondylosis.

Painful stiff necks are common clinical problems, often attributed, without much evidence, to disc disease. The essence of treatment is to mobilize the neck with physiotherapy techniques such as traction or Maitland mobilization. Pain may be relieved with simple analgesics. While cervical collars may be required in the acute stage of cervical disc prolapse and occasionally in patients with cervical spondylosis, they can also perpetuate the problem of a painful stiff neck when the right treatment is mobilization.

Soft-tissue rheumatism

Soft-tissue rheumatism is a convenient term for a number of conditions with similar features (Table 8.22). They cause musculoskeletal or joint pain that arises, not from the joint itself, but from surrounding structures such as the tendon sheaths and bursae. These conditions are benign and in most cases self-limiting. They are often regarded as trivial except by those who have them. Many are best treated by local corticosteroid injection rather than by anti-inflammatory drugs. It is also important to remove aetiological factors whenever possible; mechanical factors such as over-use and repetitive strain are probably particularly important.

Common soft-tissue rheumatic syndromes are shown in Fig. 8.21.

Bursitis

There are numerous bursae around the body and any of these can become inflamed; olecranon bursitis (student's elbow) and prepatellar bursitis (housemaid's knee) are two examples. Bursitis may appear for no obvious reason or it can be secondary to trauma, repetitive injury or an arthritis such as rheumatoid arthritis or gout. Occasionally, bursitis is due to infection, when aspiration may be necessary. In many cases no treatment is required other than protection of the inflamed site. Injection

Table 8.22 Mechanisms of soft-tissue rheumatism.

Bursitis

Tenosynovitis or peritendinitis

Enthesitis

Nerve compression

Periarthritis or capsulitis

Muscle tension and dysfunction

of corticosteroid may be useful and, very occasionally, large and troublesome bursae may require excision. Ischial bursitis causes pain over the ischial tuberosity and makes sitting difficult. A ring cushion is usually helpful.

Tenosynovitis

Tenosynovitis can occur in any tendon sheath. The flexor tendons of the fingers are often affected and cause the condition known as trigger finger. Patients characteristically wake with one finger fixed in flexion. Some force is needed to extend the finger and this produces pain. There is a palpable nodule in the flexor tendon. Injection of this nodule with a corticosteroid preparation usually provides relief.

De Quervain's tenosynovitis gives rise to pain in the anatomical snuff box and may be mistaken for osteoarthritis of the first carpometacarpal joint. The point of maximum tenderness should be injected with a combination of corticosteroid and local anaesthetic.

Enthesitis

The enthesis is the specialized area at the junction of tendons or ligaments and bone.

Inflammation of the junction of the common extensor origin of the muscles of the forearm and the lateral humeral epicondyle results in 'tennis elbow'. This condition is seldom due to tennis, more often it is caused by housework or some repetitive manual occupation. Often there is no obvious cause. There is pain in the elbow, but it is not clearly localized. However, on examination, the joint is normal and there is an area of exquisite tenderness over the lateral epicondyle. It is usually treated by injecting this tender area with a combination of corticosteroid and local anaesthetic. Since the condition resolves within a year or two whatever is done, in mild cases it may be best ignored.

Golfer's elbow is a similar problem at the junction of the origin of the flexor muscles of the forearm and the medial humeral epicondyle. Another common site is the greater trochanter of the femur (trochanteric syndrome).

In plantar fasciitis, the inflammation arises on the undersurface of the heel at the origin of the plantar fascia. This common condition is best treated with an injection of corticosteroid and a protective heel pad; it normally resolves within a year or two.

Nerve compression syndromes

Carpal tunnel syndrome is described on p. 953. A similar condition in the foot, tarsal tunnel syndrome, gives rise to burning pain with pins and

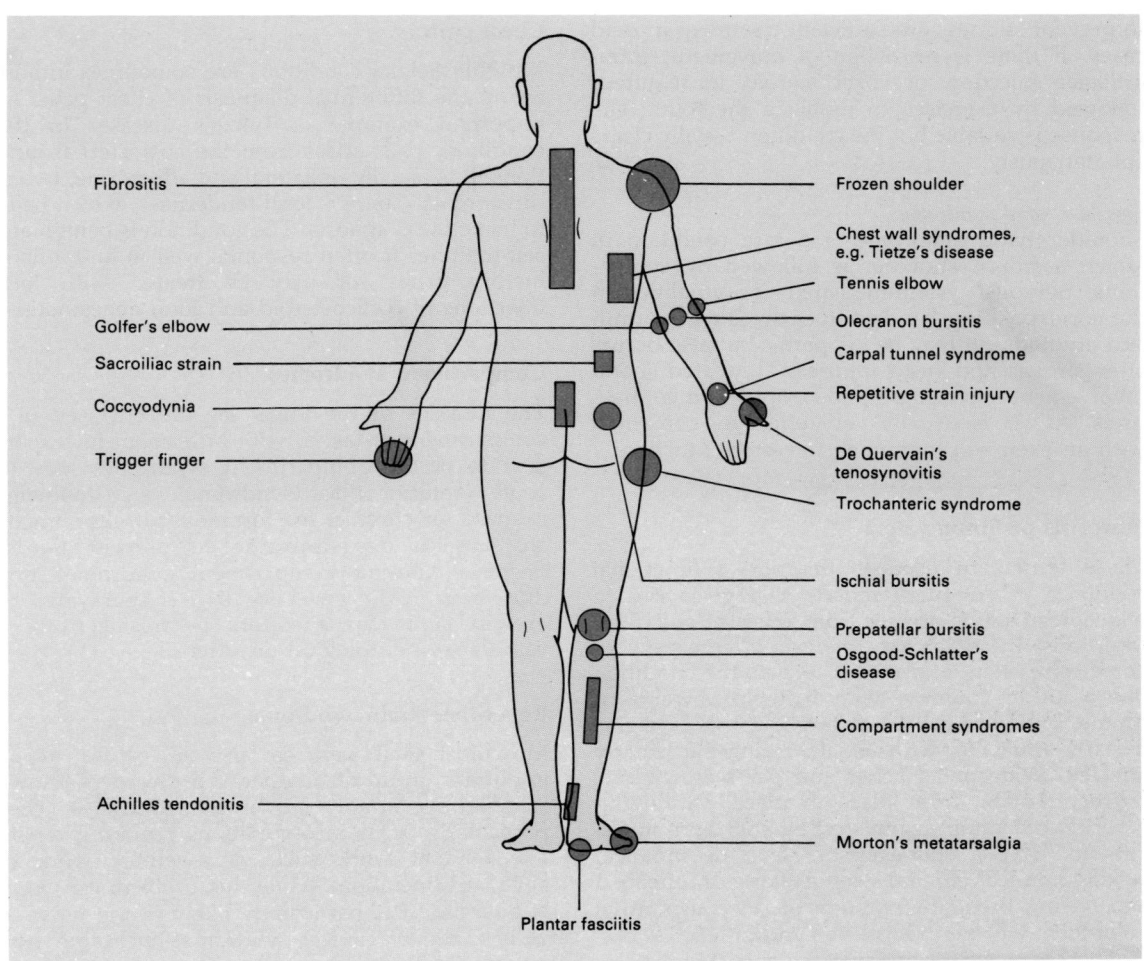

Fibrositis

Golfer's elbow

Sacroiliac strain

Coccyodynia

Trigger finger

Achilles tendonitis

Plantar fasciitis

Frozen shoulder

Chest wall syndromes,
e.g. Tietze's disease

Tennis elbow

Olecranon bursitis

Carpal tunnel syndrome

Repetitive strain injury

De Quervain's
tenosynovitis

Trochanteric syndrome

Ischial bursitis

Prepatellar bursitis

Osgood-Schlatter's
disease

Compartment syndromes

Morton's metatarsalgia

Fig. 8.21 Common soft-tissue rheumatic syndromes.

needles in the sole of the foot and toes. As in carpal tunnel syndrome, the pain is often worse at night and may wake the patient from sleep. In cases of diagnostic difficulty, nerve conduction studies will show a block at the appropriate level.

In Morton's metatarsalgia, pain arises from a digital nerve in the foot, usually between the third and fourth metatarsal heads. It is due either to a neuroma or to compression by a bursa. There is pain in the forefoot that radiates into the toes. It is usually aggravated by wearing shoes and relieved by removing them. Manual compression of the forefoot reproduces the symptoms. The condition sometimes responds to local injection and to the use of a metatarsal pad. If not, surgical exploration and excision of the bursa or digital nerve is required.

Frozen shoulder

This is a convenient term for a group of soft-tissue syndromes that produce the same clinical picture—

a painful stiff shoulder. Some people reserve the term for the later stage of the disease when the glenohumeral joint is completely immobile. Many other terms, such as periarthritis or capsulitis, are used to describe this condition, but without much pathological justification. In some cases, local tenderness points to a lesion such as supraspinatus tendinitis, bicipital tendinitis or subacromial bursitis. In most cases, however, it is not possible to identify a specific cause and differentiation makes little difference to the outcome or treatment.

Frozen shoulder is a common condition occurring in adults at any age. It is usually but not always unilateral. There is pain in the shoulder that may radiate to the arm and is usually most troublesome at night. In most cases the condition appears without obvious cause but it may occasionally be related to overuse or injury. A similar clinical picture is produced by acute calcific periarthritis (see p. 407). Examination shows restriction of glenohumeral movement. Analgesics and exercises to prevent stiffness are sufficient treatment in mild cases. If there is restriction of movement, intra-articular injection of corticosteroid is required, followed by exercises to mobilize the joint. The response is variable but the condition usually clears spontaneously.

Shoulder hand syndrome

Shoulder hand syndrome is a rare condition in which a frozen shoulder is followed by sympathetic nervous system-mediated abnormalities in the corresponding hand, diffuse swelling, warmth and erythema. It may be idiopathic but also occurs after strokes and head injuries. Untreated, hand involvement may progress to atrophy and contractures. ACTH is usually very effective, combined with an exercise programme to restore function.

Fibrositis or fibromyalgia

These terms are used to describe a functional condition of voluntary muscle that gives rise to widespread pains arising from muscles and their insertions. In some cases there is a large psychogenic component and in this respect the condition has a lot in common with irritable bowel syndrome, with which it is often associated. It begins in early adult life, with females being particularly affected. Widespread aches and pains are characteristic, moving from place to place, varying in severity and often aggravated by cold and stress. Patients have a characteristic sleep disturbance, lacking non-REM (delta) sleep, waking unrefreshed and feeling tired. Interruption of sleep in normal volunteers will reproduce the syndrome.

The characteristic physical sign in fibrositis is multiple areas of localized soft-tissue tenderness known as trigger points. They are particularly found around the dorsal spine in the interscapular region, around the base of the neck, over both sacroiliac joints, over the lateral epicondyles of the elbows (resembling tennis elbows), and over the medial sides of the knees. In some patients, crops of nodules appear on the muscles, but these have no consistent pathological basis and are believed to be part of the functional abnormality. Blood tests and X-rays are normal.

The condition is chronic or recurrent but entirely benign. Treatment measures include:

- An exercise programme. The rationale for this is the observation that it is difficult to induce fibrositis experimentally in trained athletes.
- Measures to improve sleep. Amitriptylline at night is particularly useful.
- Heat, massage and local ointments to relieve pain. Analgesic and anti-inflammatory drugs are seldom helpful.
- Local injection of trigger points.
- Reassurance and explanation.

Chest pain

Musculoskeletal conditions are sometimes important in the differential diagnosis of chest pain. An important example is Tietze's disease. In this condition, pain arises from the costosternal junctions. It is usually unilateral and affects one, two or three joints. There is local tenderness, which helps to make the diagnosis. The condition is benign and self-limiting. It often responds well to anti-inflammatory drugs, or may be treated with local injections of corticosteroid and local anaesthetic.

Compartment syndromes

The muscles of the lower leg are enclosed in a compartment of fascia, with little room for expansion to occur. Compartment syndromes may be acute (anterior tibial syndrome), e.g. following exercise, or chronic, the former requiring immediate surgical decompression to prevent muscle necrosis. Chronic compartment syndromes produce pain in the lower leg that is aggravated by exercise and may therefore be mistaken for a vascular or neurological disorder.

Repetitive strain syndrome

Musculoskeletal pain is also a feature of an important group of occupational disorders known as repetitive strain or overuse syndromes. They particularly occur in occupations requiring repetitive manual work such as assembly work or keyboard operation. While this problem can occur at any site, it is particularly likely in the wrist. A wide range of clinical syndromes including conditions similar to frozen shoulder or tennis elbow can occur. It is important to recognize the nature of the problem as early as possible so that measures

Table 8.23 Diseases of bone.

Osteomalacia and rickets (see p. 822)
Osteoporosis (see p. 823)
Paget's disease
Hyperparathyroidism (see p. 825)
Other hypercalcaemias
Disorders of collagen, e.g. Marfan's syndrome (see p. 1049)
Renal bone disease (see p. 476)
Infections
Neoplastic disease
Disorders of mucopolysaccharides, e.g. Hurler's syndrome (see p. 868)
Skeletal dysplasias (achondroplasia)
Other hereditary diseases
    Osteogenesis imperfecta
    Osteopetrosis
    Hypophosphatasia

can be taken to prevent it by varying the nature of the patient's work, providing adequate breaks and correcting faulty equipment.

Bone disease

The structure, physiology and function of bone are described on p. 820. Table 8.23 shows the diseases of bone. Osteomalacia and osteoporosis are two important diseases and are described in Chapter 16.

Paget's disease

PATHOPHYSIOLOGY

There is greatly increased bone turnover with excessive osteoclastic resorption followed by increased osteoblastic activity producing new bone. Fibrosis occurs in narrow spaces. The cause of these changes is unknown but a viral aetiology is possible.

INCIDENCE

The disease is common, affecting 0.5% of the population at the age of 40 and 10% at the age of 90. It is twice as common in men as in women. It is common in Europe with an increased incidence in Lancashire (UK).

CLINICAL FEATURES

- 95% asymptomatic, discovered by X-ray or raised serum alkaline phosphatase.
- Joint pain when bone adjacent to joints is involved; usually hips or knees. Stiffness after sitting as in osteoarthritis.
- Bone pain, usually dorsal or lumbar spine.
- Deformities and complications. Enlarged skull and bowed tibia are characteristic (Fig. 8.22).

COMPLICATIONS

- Fracture
- High-output cardiac failure
- Nerve compression, particularly causing deafness, occasionally spinal nerve root or cord compression
- Osteogenic sarcoma

INVESTIGATION

X-rays

- Changes best seen in skull or pelvis, sometimes

spine; can be anywhere
- Expansion of bone
- Abnormal trabeculae (coarse and dense)
- Areas of porosis (osteoporosis circumscripta) and sclerosis
- Joint space narrowing and periarticular calcification

Bone scan

- Isotope bone scanning identifies affected bones, showing localized 'hot' areas but does not differentiate Paget's disease from other disorders (e.g. metastatic disease).

Biochemical abnormalities

- Serum alkaline phosphatase of bone origin is increased (often to very high levels > 1000 i.u.$\cdot$L^{-1}) owing to the excessive bone turnover. This increase may be minimal if bone involvement is very localized.
- Urinary hydroxyproline excretion, another marker of bone turnover, is also increased.
- Calcium and phosphate levels are normal, except occasionally during immobilization; the parathormone level and vitamin D metabolism are also normal (Table 8.24).

TREATMENT

The incidental finding of asymptomatic Paget's disease does not require treatment. When pain is present, several lines of therapy are possible:

- Simple analgesics or anti-inflammatory drugs may be sufficient in mild cases.
- The diphosphonate disodium etidronate (5–10 mg$\cdot$kg^{-1} daily) is thought to be adsorbed on to hydroxyapatite crystals, preventing osteoclastic activity. It has the advantage of oral administration but because of poor absorption must be given several hours away from food and is often taken during the night for this reason. A course of 6–12 months' treatment is usually sufficient and the serum alkaline phosphatase is a good guide to progress; prolonged treatment may lead to bone pain and fractures.
- Calcitonin (100 units s.c., two or three times weekly) inhibits bone resorption and turnover. It is extremely expensive, and clinical resistance because of antibody formation to the salmon and porcine preparations may limit its use. Side-effects following injection are flushing and mild nausea, sometimes accompanied by diarrhoea and vomiting, and can be disabling.
- Mithramycin 15 µg$\cdot$kg^{-1} i.v. daily for up to 10 days is worth considering in the severe case. Careful monitoring of serum calcium and liver biochemistry is required.

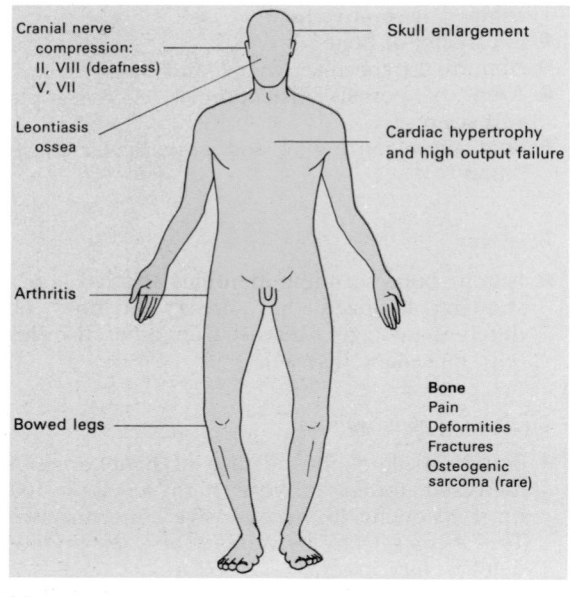

(a)

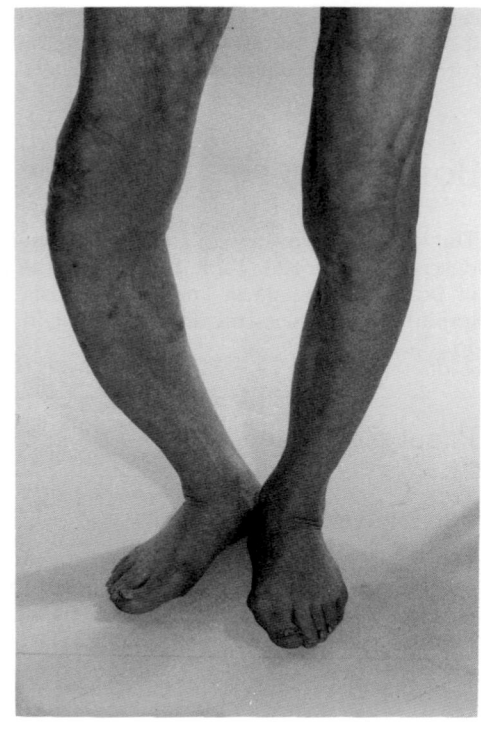

(b)

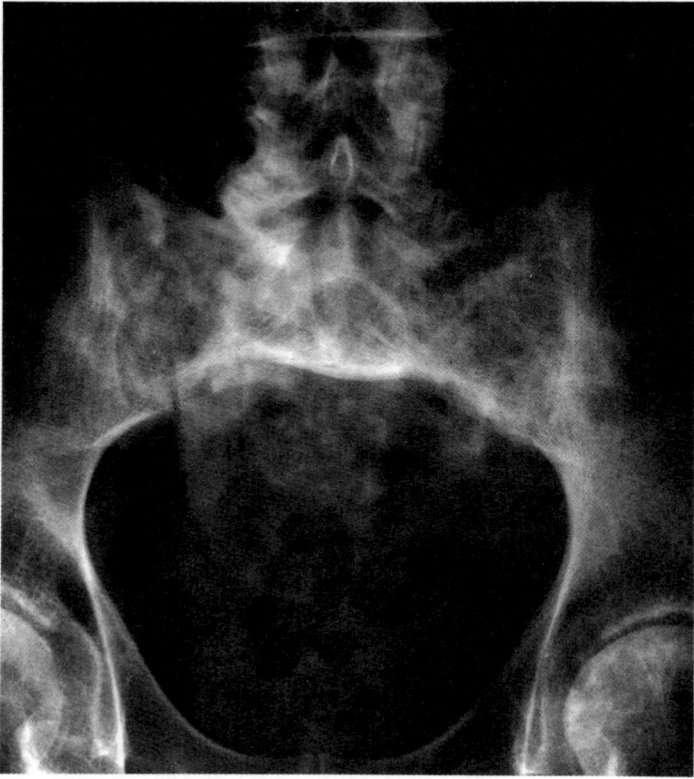

(c)

Fig. 8.22 Paget's disease. (a) Clinical features. (b) Paget's disease of the tibia, showing bowing due to increased bone growth. (c) X-ray appearance of Paget's disease of the pelvis.

Table 8.24 Serum biochemical findings in some bone diseases.

	Calcium	Phosphate	Alkaline phosphatase
Osteoporosis	N	N	N
Osteomalacia (and rickets)	N or ↓	N or ↓	↑
Paget's disease	N	N	↑ ↑
Hyperparathyroidism (and bone disease)	↑	↓	↑
Multiple myeloma	N or ↑	↓ , N or ↑	N

N = normal; ↓ = low; ↑ = high.

Infections of bone

Osteomyelitis

Staphylococcus is the organism responsible for 90% of cases of acute osteomyelitis (see p. 22). Other organisms include *Haemophilus influenzae* and *Salmonella*; infection with the latter may occur as a complication of sickle cell anaemia.

Osteomyelitis can be due either to metastatic haematogenous spread (e.g. from a boil) or to local infection. Malnutrition, debilitating disease and decreased immunity may play a part in the pathogenesis.

Chronic osteomyelitis may follow an acute infection. Another variety of chronic osteomyelitis is due to infection being localized to form a chronic abscess within the bone (Brodie's abscess). Patients may be asymptomatic for months or years or may have intermittent local pain.

Treatment of osteomyelitis is with immobilization and antibiotics.

Tuberculous osteomyelitis. This is usually due to haematogenous spread from a primary focus in the lungs or gastrointestinal tract. The disease starts in intra-articular bone. The spine is commonly involved (Pott's disease), with damage to the bodies of two neighbouring vertebrae leading to vertebral collapse and later abscess formation ('cold abscess'). Pus can track along tissue planes and discharge at a point far from the affected vertebrae. Symptoms consist of local pain and later swelling if pus has collected. Systemic symptoms of malaise, fever and night sweats occur. Treatment is as for pulmonary tuberculosis (see p. 682), together with immobilization.

Neoplastic disease

Malignant tumours of bone are shown in Table 8.25. The most common tumours are *metastases* from the bronchus, breast and prostate. Metastases from kidney and thyroid are less common. Symptoms are usually related to the anatomical position of the tumour, with local bone pain over the area. Systemic symptoms including malaise and pyrexia, and aches and pains occur and are sometimes related to the hypercalcaemia (see p. 825). The diagnosis of metastases can often be made from the history and examination, particularly if the primary has already been diagnosed. Symptoms from bony metastases may, however, be the first presenting feature.

INVESTIGATION

- Skeletal isotope scans can pick up bony metastases as 'hot' areas before radiological changes occur.
- X-rays may show metastases as osteolytic areas with bony destruction. Osteosclerotic metastases are characteristic of prostatic metastases.
- Serum alkaline phosphatase (from the bone) is usually raised.
- Hypercalcaemia is seen in 10–20% of patients with malignancies. It is chiefly associated with metastases, but can also result from ectopic parathormone secretion.
- Serum acid phosphatase is raised in prostatic metastases.

Table 8.25 Malignant neoplasms of bone.

Metastases (osteolytic):
  Bronchus
  Breast
  Prostate (often osteosclerotic as well)
  Thyroid
  Kidney

Multiple myeloma

Primary bone tumours (rare; seen in the young), e.g.
  Osteosarcomas
  Fibrosarcomas
  Chondromas
  Ewing's tumour

TREATMENT

Treatment is usually symptomatic with analgesics and anti-inflammatory drugs like indomethacin. Local radiotherapy over bone metastases may be the best way of relieving pain. Depending on the tumour, cytotoxic chemotherapy is occasionally helpful. Some tumours are hormone-dependent and a remission can be obtained by hormonal therapy. Occasionally pathological fractures require internal fixation.

Primary bone tumours are rare and usually seen in children and young adults.

Skeletal dysplasia

This is a heterogeneous group of disorders that affect the normal development of bone and cartilage and sometimes lead to shortness of stature.

Achondroplasia

Achondroplasia (dwarfism) is diagnosed in the first years of life. The disease is inherited in an autosomal dominant manner. The trunk is of normal length but the limbs are very short and broad. The vault of the skull is enlarged, the face is small and the nose bridge is flat. Intelligence is normal.

Other hereditary diseases

Osteogenesis imperfecta (fragilitas ossium, brittle bone syndrome)

This rare group of inherited disorders is due to an abnormality of connective tissue. The major feature is very fragile and brittle bones; other collagen-containing tissues are also involved, such as tendons, the skin and the eyes. Osteogenesis imperfecta tarda is a mild, dominantly inherited condition with milder bony deformities, blue sclerae, defective dentine, early-onset deafness, hypermobility of joints, and heart valve disorders. More severe forms present with multiple fractures and gross deformities. Prognosis is variable, depending on the severity of the disease.

Osteopetrosis (marble bone disease)

This condition may be inherited in either an autosomal dominant or an autosomal recessive manner; the recessive type is severe and the dominant type is mild. In the severe form, bone density is increased throughout the skeleton but bones tend to fracture easily. Involvement of the bone marrow leads to a leucoerythroblastic anaemia. There is mental retardation and early death.

In the mild form there may only be X-ray changes, but fractures and infection can occur. The acid phosphatase level is raised.

Hypophosphatasia

This rare autosomal recessive condition is due to a deficiency of alkaline phosphatase and pyrophosphatase. It is not known where the primary defect lies, but it may be in the osteoblasts. It varies in severity from unmineralized bones *in utero* resulting in death, to rickets in infancy or recurrent fractures in adults.

Further reading

Currey HLF (1985) *Mason and Currey's Clinical Rheumatology*, 4th edn. London: Pitman Medical.

Huskisson EC & Hart FD (1987) *Joint Disease: All the Arthropathies*, 4th edn. Bristol: John Wright.

Kelly WN, Harris ED Jr, Ruddy S & Sledge CD (1989) *Textbook of Rheumatology* 3rd edn. Philadelphia: WB Saunders.

McCarty DJ (1989) *Arthritis and allied conditions*, 11th edn. Lea & Febiger, Philadelphia.

Scott JT (ed) (1986) *Copeman's Textbook of the Rheumatic Diseases*, 6th edn. Edinburgh: Churchill Livingstone.

Renal function and structure

The kidneys' principle role is the elimination of waste material and the regulation of the volume and composition of body fluid (Table 9.1). The kidneys have a unique system involving the free ultrafiltration of water and non-protein-bound low-molecular-weight compounds from the plasma and the selective reabsorption and/or excretion of these as the ultrafiltrate passes along the tubule.

The functioning unit is the *nephron*, of which there are approximately one million in each kidney. A conventional diagrammatic representation is shown in Fig. 9.1a and a physiological version in Fig. 9.1b.

An essential feature of renal function is that a large volume of blood—25% of cardiac output or approximately 1300 ml of blood per minute—passes through the two million glomeruli.

A hydrostatic pressure gradient of approximately 10 mm Hg (a capillary pressure of 45 mm Hg minus 10 mm Hg of pressure within Bowman's

Table 9.1 Functions of the kidney.

Excretory—excretion of waste products, drugs

Regulatory—control of body fluid volume and composition

Endocrine—production of erythropoietin, renin, prostaglandins

Metabolic—metabolism of vitamin D, small-molecular weight proteins

space and 25 mm Hg of plasma oncotic pressure) provides the driving force for ultrafiltration of virtually protein-free and fat-free fluid across the glomerular capillary wall into Bowman's space and so into the renal tubule (Fig. 9.2).

The ultrafiltration rate (glomerular filtration rate; GFR) varies with age and sex but is approximately 120–130 ml per minute per 1.73 m^2 surface area in adults. This means that each day ultrafiltration of between 170 and 180 litres of water and unbound small-molecular-weight constituents of blood occurs. The 'need' for this high filtration rate relates to the elimination of compounds present in relatively low concentration in plasma (e.g. urea). If these large volumes of ultrafiltrate were excreted unchanged as urine, it would be necessary to ingest huge amounts of water and electrolytes to stay in balance. This is avoided by the selective reabsorption of water, essential electrolytes and other blood constituents, such as glucose and amino acids, from the filtrate in transit along the nephron. Thus, 60–80% of filtered water and sodium are reabsorbed in the proximal tubule along with virtually all the potassium, bicarbonate, glucose and amino acids (Fig. 9.1b). Further water and sodium chloride are reabsorbed more distally, and fine tuning of salt and water balance is achieved in the distal and collecting tubules under the influence of aldosterone and anti-diuretic hormone (ADH). The final urine volume is thus 1–2 litres/day. Calcium, phosphate, and magnesium are also selectively reabsorbed in proportion to need to maintain a normal electrolyte composition of body fluids.

The urinary excretion of some compounds is more complicated. For example, potassium is freely filtered at the glomerulus, almost completely absorbed in the proximal tubule, and excreted in the distal tubule and collecting ducts. An important clinical consequence of this is that the ability to eliminate unwanted potassium is less dependent on glomerular filtration rate (GFR) than is the elimination of urea or creatinine. Other compounds filtered and reabsorbed or excreted to a variable extent include urate and many organic acids, including many drugs or their metabolic breakdown products. The more tubular secretion of a compound occurs, the less dependent is elimination on the GFR; penicillin and cephradine are examples of compounds secreted by the tubules.

Tubular function is also critical to the control of

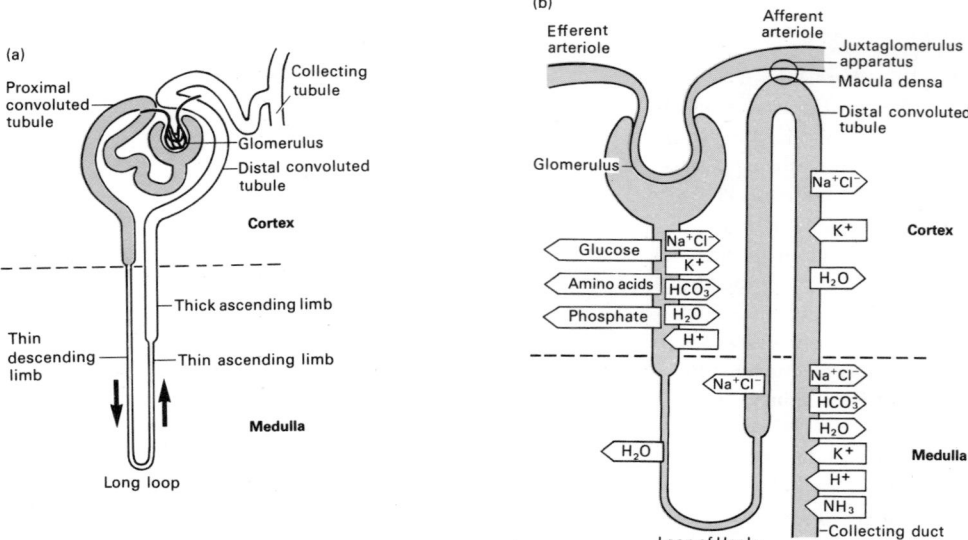

Fig. 9.1 (a) The principal parts of the nephron. (b) Sites of removal or addition of electrolytes from or into tubular fluid.

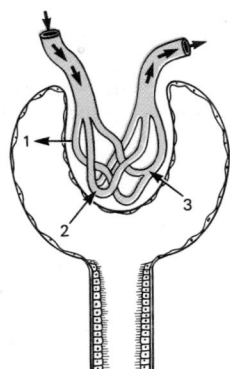

Fig. 9.2 Pressures controlling glomerular filtration. 1 = capillary hydrostatic pressure (45 mm Hg). 2 = hydrostatic pressure in Bowman's space (10 mm Hg). 3 = plasma protein oncotic pressure (25 mm Hg). Arrows indicate direction of pressure gradient.

acid–base balance. Thus, filtered bicarbonate is largely reabsorbed and hydrogen ion is excreted either buffered by ammonia or phosphate (p. 503).

Glomerular filtration rate (GFR)

In health the GFR remains remarkably constant owing to intrarenal regulatory mechanisms. In disease, with a reduction in intrarenal blood flow, damage to or loss of glomeruli, or obstruction to the free flow of ultrafiltrate along the tubule, the GFR will fall and the ability to eliminate waste material and to regulate the volume and composition of body fluid will decline. This will be manifest as a rise in the blood level of urea or the plasma

level of creatinine and in a reduction in *measured* GFR.

Uraemia

The concentration of urea or creatinine in blood or plasma, respectively, represents the dynamic equilibrium between production and elimination. In healthy subjects there is an enormous reserve of renal excretory function and blood urea and serum creatinine do not rise above the normal range until there is a reduction of 50–60% in the GFR. Thereafter, the level of urea depends both on the GFR and the production rate (Table 9.2). The latter is heavily influenced by protein intake and tissue catabolism. The level of creatinine is much less dependent on diet but is more related to age, sex and muscle mass. Once it is elevated, serum creatinine is a better guide to GFR than urea and, in general, measurement of serum creatinine is a good way to monitor further deterioration in the GFR.

It must be re-emphasized that a normal blood urea or serum creatinine is *not* synonymous with a normal GFR.

Measurement of GFR

Measurement of the GFR is necessary to define the exact level of renal function. It is essential when the blood urea or serum creatinine are within the normal range.

Inulin clearance—the gold standard of physiologists—is not practical or necessary in clinical practice. The most widely used measurement is creatinine clearance, which closely approximates to inulin clearance (Fig. 9.3).

The use of creatinine clearance is dependent on the fact that daily production of creatinine (principally from muscle cells), is remarkably constant

Table 9.2 Factors influencing blood urea levels.

Production	Elimination
Increased by	**Increased by**
High-protein diet	Elevated GFR
Increased catabolism	e.g. pregnancy
Surgery	
Infection	**Decreased by**
Trauma	Glomerular disease
Steroid therapy	Reduced renal blood flow
Tetracyclines	Hypotension
	Dehydration
Decreased by	Urinary obstruction
Low-protein diet	Tubulo-interstitial nephritis
Reduced catabolism	
e.g. old age	

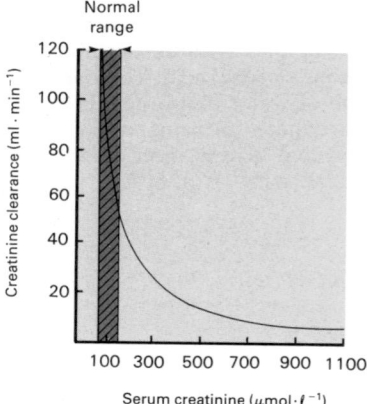

Fig. 9.3 Creatinine clearance versus serum creatinine. Note that the serum creatinine does not rise above the normal range until there is a reduction of 50–60% in the glomerular filtration rate (creatinine clearance).

and little affected by protein intake. Serum creatinine and urinary output thus vary very little throughout the day. This permits the use of 24-hour urine collections, which reduce collection errors, and the measurement of a single serum creatinine value during the 24 hours.

Creatinine excretion is, however, by both glomerular filtration and tubular secretion, although at normal serum levels the latter is relatively small. As most laboratory methods for measurement of serum creatinine give slight overestimates, the calculation of clearance fortuitously gives a value close to that of inulin.

With progressive renal failure, creatinine clearance may overestimate GFR but, in absolute terms, this is seldom important. Certain drugs—for example cimetidine, trimethoprim, spironolactone and amiloride—reduce tubular secretion of creatinine, leading to a rise in serum creatinine and a fall in measured clearance.

Given these observations, creatinine clearance, nevertheless, is a reasonably accurate measure of GFR in those situations in which it is most required—normal or near normal renal function.

Where urine collections are difficult (e.g. with ileal conduits) or deemed inaccurate, the GFR may be measured by the single injection of compounds such as [51Cr]EDTA (ethylene diamine tetra-acetic acid) or [99mTc]DTPA (diethylene triamine penta-

acetic acid), their excretion being primarily by glomerular filtration. Following intravenous injection of the compound, three blood samples are obtained at 2, 3 and 4 h (or rather longer intervals if the patient is oedematous or if renal failure is suspected). The GFR may then be calculated from the slope of the exponential fall in blood level of the compound.

TUBULAR FUNCTION

The major function of the tubule is the selective reabsorption or excretion of water and various cations and anions to keep the volume and electrolyte composition of body fluid normal (see Chapter 10).

The active reabsorption from the glomerular filtrate of compounds such as glucose and amino acids also takes place. Within the normal range of blood concentrations these substances are completely reabsorbed by the proximal tubule. However, if blood levels are elevated above the normal range, the amount filtered (filtered load = GFR × plasma concentration) may exceed the maximal absorptive capacity of the tubule and the compound 'spills over' into the urine. Examples of this occur with hyperglycaemia in diabetes mellitus or elevated plasma phenylalanine in phenylketonuria.

Conversely, inherited or acquired defects in tubular function may lead to incomplete absorption of a *normal* filtered load, with loss of the compound in the urine (a lowered 'renal threshold'). This is seen in renal glycosuria, in which there is a genetically determined defect in tubular reabsorption of glucose. It is diagnosed by demonstrating glycosuria in the presence of normal blood sugar levels. Inherited or acquired defects in the tubular reabsorption of amino acids, phosphate, sodium,

---

Measurement of creatinine clearance

- Urine is collected over 24 h for measurement of urinary creatinine; a 24-hour collection diminishes collection errors.
- A plasma level of creatinine is measured sometime during the 24-hour period.
- Given the rate of urine flow (V), the urine (U) and plasma (P) concentrations of creatinine, clearance is obtained from the formula:

$$\frac{U \times V}{P} \times 100$$

potassium and calcium also occur, either singly or in combination. Examples include cystinuria and the Fanconi syndrome (see p. 866). Tubular defects in the reabsorption of water (nephrogenic diabetes insipidus) or bicarbonate (proximal renal tubular acidosis) and defective acidification of the urine (distal RTA) are dealt with on p. 507.

ENDOCRINE FUNCTION

Renin–angiotensin system

The juxtaglomerular apparatus is made up of specialized arteriolar smooth muscle cells that are sited on the afferent glomerular arteriole as it enters the glomerulus (Fig. 9.1b). These cells secrete renin, which converts angiotensinogen in blood to angiotensin I. Renin release is controlled by:

- Pressure changes in the afferent arteriole
- Sympathetic tone
- Chloride and osmotic concentration in the distal tubule via the macula densa (Fig. 9.1b)
- Local prostaglandin release

Angiotensin II is generated from angiotensin I by angiotensin-converting enzyme (ACE). Angiotensin II is both a vasoconstrictor and the most important stimulus for the release of aldosterone by the adrenal cortex. It also modifies intra-renal blood flow.

Erythropoetin (see p. 295)

Erythropoietin is a glycoprotein produced principally by the kidney and is one of the major stimuli for erythropoiesis. Loss of renal substance, with decreased erythropoietin production, results in a normochromic, normocytic anaemia. Conversely, erythropoietin secretion may be increased, with resultant polycythaemia in patients with polycystic renal disease, benign renal cysts or renal cell carcinoma.

Recombinant human erythropoieten has now been biosynthesized and is available for clinical use, particularly in patients with renal failure (see p. 478).

Prostaglandins

Prostaglandin E_2 is the primary prostaglandin produced by the kidney and is known to be a powerful vasodilator agent. Its precise role in regulating intrarenal blood flow and its interaction with renin release remains unclear. It may also have some direct or indirect role in the renal handling of sodium and water.

Kallikrein–kinin system

The role of this system is not fully understood but it probably also plays a part in the control of the distribution of renal blood flow and in salt and water excretion.

Natriuretic hormones (see p. 828)

There is now considerable evidence that atrial tissue contains a group of peptides, one of which is a regulator of sodium balance—atrial natriuretic peptide (ANP). Intravenous infusion of ANP is followed by a marked natriuresis with a rise in GFR and a fall in blood pressure. This peptide appears to have four antirenin/angiotensin system actions: reduced renin secretion, reduced aldosterone secretion and opposition to the action of angiotensin II and to the sodium-retaining action of aldosterone on the renal tubule. Its role in the long-term regulation of sodium balance and blood pressure in man remains to be clarified.

METABOLIC FUNCTION

Vitamin D metabolism (see p. 159)

Naturally occurring vitamin D_3 requires hydroxylation in the liver and again by the kidney to produce the metabolically active 1,25- or 24,25-dihydroxycholecalciferol. Loss of this metabolic activity in diseased kidneys results in renal osteodystrophy.

Protein and polypeptide metabolism

It is now clear that the kidney is a major site for the catabolism of many small-molecular-weight proteins and polypeptides, including many hormones such as insulin, parathyroid hormone and calcitonin. In renal failure the metabolic clearance of these substances is reduced and their half-life is prolonged.

Tests for renal disease or malfunction

Renal disease is suspected if there are:

- Symptoms referable to the urinary tract
- Hypertension
- An elevated blood urea
- Abnormalities on urinalysis

THE URINE

Appearance

This is of little value in the differential diagnosis of renal disease except in the diagnosis of haematuria. Overt 'bloody' urine is usually unmistakable but should be checked using dip sticks (Stix testing).

Very concentrated urine or urine containing pigments ingested in food or medicines may also appear as dark or smoky urine. Urine that becomes dark on standing suggests the relatively rare condition of porphyria.

Smell

This is rarely important except in patients with infection, when a typical fishy odour may be noted.

Volume

In health, the volume of urine passed is primarily determined by diet and fluid intake. In temperate climates it lies within the range of 800–2500 ml per 24 h. The minimum amount passed to stay in fluid balance is determined by the amount of solute—mainly urea and electrolytes—being excreted and the maximum concentrating power of the kidneys. Thus, on a normal diet, some 800 mosmol of solute are passed daily. Since the maximum urine concentration is approximately $1200 \text{ mosmol} \cdot \text{L}^{-1}$, the minimum volume of urine obligated by excretion of 800 mosmol of solute would thus be approximately 650 ml (Table 9.3). Fluid intake is generally greater than this, so that larger volumes of more dilute urine are passed. A diet rich in carbohydrate and fat and low in protein and salt results in a lower solute excretion and as little as 300 ml of urine per day may be required. Conversely, a high-salt, high-protein intake obligates a larger urine flow and, via the thirst mechanism, a higher fluid intake. The appropriateness of a given daily urine output must therefore be related to factors such as diet, body size and fluid intake.

In disease, impairment of concentrating ability requires increased volumes of urine to be passed, given the same daily solute output (Table 9.3). An increased solute output, e.g. in glycosuria or increased protein catabolism following surgery or associated with sepsis, also demands increased urine volumes.

The maximum urine output depends on the ability to produce a dilute urine. Intakes of 10 or even 20 litres daily can be tolerated by normal man but, given a daily solute output of 800 mosmol, require the ability to dilute to 80 and 40 $\text{mosmol} \cdot \text{l}^{-1}$, respectively. Where diluting ability is impaired, the ability to excrete large volumes of ingested water is also impaired.

Oliguria

Oliguria, usually defined as the excretion of less than 300 ml of urine per day, may be 'physiological', e.g. in patients with hypotension and hypovolaemia, where urine is maximally concentrated in an attempt to conserve water. More often, it is due to intrinsic renal disease or obstructive nephropathy (see p. 462).

Anuria (no urine) suggests urinary tract obstruction until it is proved otherwise; bladder outflow obstruction must always be considered first.

Polyuria

Polyuria is a persistent, large increase in urine output, usually associated with nocturia. It must be distinguished from frequency of micturition with the passage of small volumes of urine. Documentation of fluid intake and output may be necessary. Polyuria is the result of an excessive (hysterical) intake of water, an increased excretion of solute (as in hyperglycaemia and glycosuria), or a defective renal concentrating ability.

Specific gravity and osmolality

The time-honoured measurement of specific gravity is of little value in clinical practice. Measurement of urine concentration is best done by osmometry and is only required under limited circumstances, such as the differential diagnosis of oliguric renal failure or the investigation of polyuria or inappropriate ADH secretion.

pH

Measurement of urinary pH is unnecessary except in the investigation and treatment of renal tubular acidosis (see p. 507).

Table 9.3 Relationship between diet, kidney function and urine volume.

Diet	Approximate solute output (mosmol/24 h)	Minimum urine volume required to excrete solute load (ml/24 hr)	
		With normal urine concentration (maximum $1200 \text{ mosmol} \cdot \text{kg}^{-1}$)	In disease (impaired urine concentration—maximum $300 \text{ mosmol} \cdot \text{kg}^{-1}$)
Normal	800	667	2667
High-protein/salt	1200	1000	4000
Low-protein/salt	360	300	1200

Chemical (Stix) testing

Routine Stix testing of urine for blood, protein and sugar is obligatory in all patients suspected of having renal disease.

Blood

Haematuria may be overt, with bloody urine, or microscopic and found only on chemical testing. A positive Stix test must always be followed by urine microscopy to confirm the presence of red cells and so exclude the relatively rare condition of haemoglobinuria (or the even rarer myoglobinuria). Bleeding may come from any site within the urinary tract (Fig. 9.4):

- Overt bleeding from the urethra is suggested when blood is seen at the start of voiding and then the urine becomes clear.
- Blood diffusely present throughout the urine comes from the bladder or above.
- Blood only at the end of micturition suggests bleeding from the prostate or bladder base.

Careful urine microscopy is mandatory as the presence of red-cell casts is diagnostic of bleeding from the kidney, most often due to glomerulonephritis. In the absence of red-cell casts, further investigations, such as urine cytology, intravenous urography and cystoscopy, are required to define the site of bleeding. Rarely, renal biopsy may be required (see p. 434).

Protein

Proteinuria is one of the most common signs of renal disease. Detection is now primarily by Stix testing. Most reagent strips can detect a concentration of 20 mg·dl^{-1} or more in urine. They react primarily with albumin and are relatively insensi-

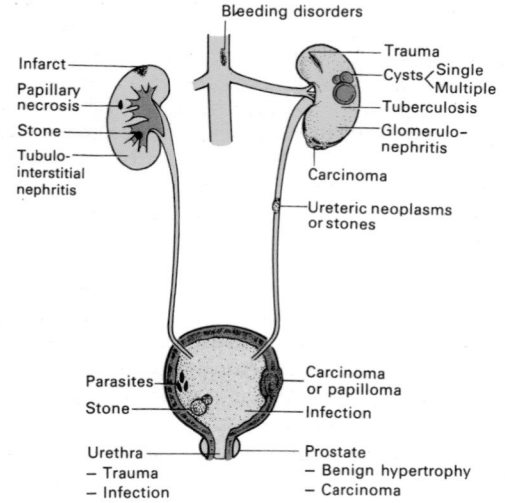

tive to globulin and Bence–Jones proteins.

If proteinuria is confirmed on repeated Stix testing, it should be quantitated by measurement of daily protein excretion in 24-hour urine collections.

Normal values for urinary protein excretion are dependent on the laboratory methods used and in particular whether or not the method measures Tamm–Horsfal glycoprotein, which is a normal constituent of urine. Results must therefore take account of the laboratory's normal reference range. Given this caveat, healthy adults excrete approximately 60–100 mg of protein per day but up to 150–200 mg per day is within the acceptable range. Slightly higher values—up to 300 mg daily—may be excreted by adolescents. Proteinuria, while occasionally benign, always requires further investigation.

Glucose

Renal glycosuria is uncommon, so that a positive test for glucose always requires exclusion of diabetes mellitus.

Bacteriuria

Dip sticks are available for testing for bacteriuria based on detection of nitrite produced from the reduction of urinary nitrate by bacteria. Unfortunately, there is an unacceptable false-negative detection rate and urine culture is still required.

Microalbuminuria

Normal urine contains albumin in a concentration of less than 20 mg·L^{-1}. Dip sticks, however, only detect albumin in a concentration around 150 mg·L^{-1}. An increase in albumin between these two levels—so-called microalbuminuria—is now known to be an early indicator of diabetic glomerular disease. It is now widely used as a predictor of the development of nephropathy in diabetics and may be extended to other conditions.

Measurement is done by radioimmunoassay. Timed or 24-hour urinary excretion may be measured. Microalbuminuria is then defined as an excretion rate between 30–150 micrograms per minute. Equally reliable results may be more conveniently obtained using random samples in which albumin concentration is related to urinary creatinine concentration (normal range < 0.2–2.8 mg of albumin per mmol·L^{-1} creatinine).

Enzymuria and excretion of small-molecular-weight proteins

Tubular damage can be detected by the presence in the urine of various enzymes normally present in tubular cells. The most popular is measurement of the excretion of N-acetyl-β-glucosaminidase (NAG) for which a dip stick is available. Increased urinary excretion of NAG undoubtedly indicates tubular damage, but the test suffers from too great sensitivity and lack of specificity. Thus, enzymuria may be induced even by non-specific pyrexial illnesses.

Fig. 9.4 Sites and causes of bleeding from the urinary tract.

The urinary excretion of small-molecular-weight proteins normally filtered but largely reabsorbed and metabolized by the tubule has also been studied. These include B2 microglobulin and retinol-binding protein (RBP). Increased excretion of either indicates proximal tubular damage.

Microscopy

Urine microscopy should be carried out in all patients suspected of having renal disease. Care must be taken to obtain a 'clean' sample of midstream urine. The presence of numerous skin squames suggests a contaminated, poorly collected sample that cannot be properly interpreted.

If a clean sample of urine cannot be obtained, suprapubic aspiration is required in suspected urinary-tract infections.

White cells
The presence of 10 or more white blood cells (WBC) per mm^3 in fresh unspun midstream urine samples is abnormal and indicates an inflammatory reaction within the urinary tract. Most commonly it is due to urinary tract infection (UTI) but it may also be found in sterile urine in patients during antibiotic treatment of urinary infection or within 14 days of treatment. Sterile pyuria also occurs in patients with stones, tubulo-interstitial nephritis, papillary necrosis, tuberculosis, and interstitial cystitis (Hunner's ulcer).

Red cells
The presence of one or more red cells in unspun

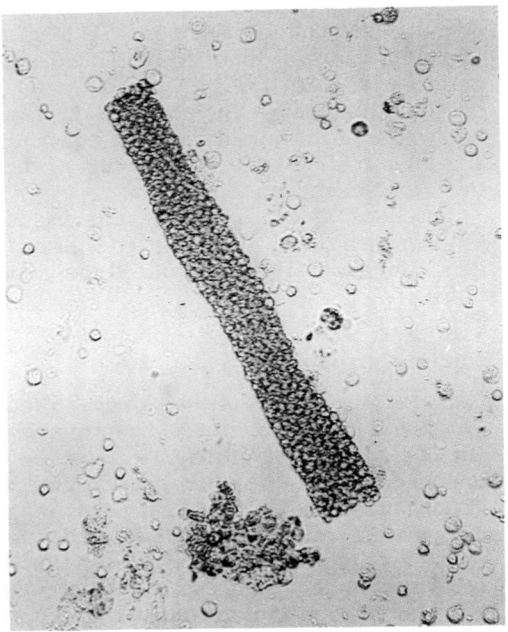

Fig. 9.5 Red cell cast. Note aggregation of red cells as a 'cast' of the tubule.

urine samples results in a positive Stix test for blood and is abnormal. It is claimed that red cells of glomerular origin can be identified by their dysmorphic appearance, especially on phase-contrast microscopy, but this is not yet generally available or accepted.

Casts (Fig. 9.5)
These cylindrical bodies, which are moulded ('cast') in the shape of the distal tubular lumen, may be hyaline, granular or cellular. Hyaline casts and fine granular casts represent precipitated protein and may be seen in normal urine, particularly after exercise. More coarsely granular casts occur with pathological proteinuria in glomerular and tubular disease. Red-cell casts—even one—always indicate renal disease. If red cells degenerate, a rusty-coloured 'haemoglobin' granular cast is seen. White-cell casts may be seen in acute pyelonephritis. They may be confused with the tubular cell casts that occur in patients with acute tubular necrosis.

Bacteria
The demonstration of bacteria on Gram staining of the centrifuged deposit of a clean-catch midstream urine sample is highly suggestive of urinary infection and can be of value in the *immediate* differential diagnosis of UTI. If accompanied by pyuria it may be accepted as evidence of UTI in the ill and febrile patient and treatment should be initiated.

Urine for quantitative culture (see p. 449) must always be obtained prior to starting antibiotic

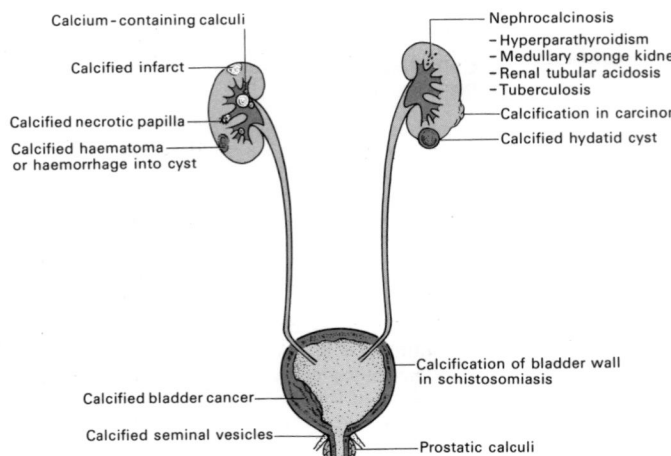

Fig. 9.6 Calcification in the renal tract. Calculi can occur at any site.

treatment in order to confirm the diagnosis and to allow definition of bacterial antibiotic sensitivities.

Stix testing for blood or protein is of no value in the diagnosis of UTI, as both are absent from the urine of many patients with bacteriuria.

QUANTITATIVE TESTS OF RENAL FUNCTION

The use of blood urea, serum creatinine and GFR as measures of renal function is discussed on p. 426. Quantitation of proteinuria, including the investigation of selective proteinuria, is discussed on p. 445. Other quantitative tests of disturbed renal function such as measurements of urine output of calcium, sodium or potassium or urine acidification are described under the relevant disorders.

IMAGING TECHNIQES

Plain X-ray

A plain radiograph of the abdomen is always taken prior to urography. Its main value is to identify renal calcification or radiodense calculi in the kidney pelvis, line of the ureters or bladder (Fig. 9.6). Care must be taken in viewing the X-ray in order not to miss calculi obscured by bowel shadows or bone. Renal size and outline are best assessed during excretion urography or by ultrasound.

Excretion urography

This is also known as intravenous urography (IVU) or intravenous pyelography (IVP). If carefully executed and properly interpreted, the urogram is one of the most valuable diagnostic tools for the investigation of renal disease. Carefully timed serial X-rays are taken of the kidneys and the full length of abdomen following a slow intravenous

injection of an organic iodine-containing contrast medium. Films taken at the end of the injection show opacification of the parenchyma, allowing definition of size and renal outline. The kidneys are normally smooth in outline. In adults they measure 11–14 cm in length, differing by less than 2 cm. An irregular outline, whether due to local bumps or to cortical scarring, is abnormal. Reduction in size indicates chronic parenchymal disease.

The application of a compression band to the abdomen, designed to partially obstruct ureteral emptying, helps distension of the upper tracts. Special attention is paid to the size, shape and disposition of the calyces and pelvis for evidence of anatomical abnormality such as calyceal clubbing, abnormal dilatation, cavitation or filling defects. The significance of these are described under the particular diseases.

After 10–20 min, the compression bands are removed and full-length films are obtained before and after voiding to study emptying of the upper tract, ureters and bladder.

Reactions to the contrast media include anaphylactic reactions and rarely convulsions. Nonionic contrast media have reduced these complications.

Ultrasonography

Ultrasonography (US) of the kidneys, bladder and prostate is well-established. Unfortunately, it is often used indiscriminately. It must be clearly understood that it cannot provide the detailed visualization of the calyces and pelvis required to demonstrate pelvicalyceal abnormalities such as reflux nephropathy or papillary necrosis. It does not visualize the greater part of the ureter and gives no functional information on the upper tract. It requires considerable operator skill in performance. For the general investigation of suspected renal disease, intravenous urography remains the imaging technique of first choice.

The particular value of ultrasound is in defining:

- Renal masses or cystic disease
- The presence or absence of obstruction in patients with renal failure when intravenous urography is unlikely to provide calyceal detail and the administration of contrast medium may be less safe
- Renal size in a patient with renal failure

and for the study of:

- Bladder emptying combined with urodynamic studies
- The prostate by means of a rectal transducer

Computed tomography (CT)

Computed tomography has a valuable role in the diagnosis of renal tumours when this is not possible by ultrasound or excretion urography, and in the diagnosis of retroperitoneal masses. It is also valuable in defining the presence and spread of bladder or prostatic tumours.

Antegrade urography (Fig. 9.7)

Antegrade urography involves percutaneous puncture of a renal calyx, with the insertion of a fine catheter and the injection of contrast medium in an antegrade fashion. It is now the procedure of choice in patients with upper urinary tract obstruction demonstrated by ultrasound. Not only does it allow definition of the site of obstruction but also the catheter may be left *in situ* to allow urine drainage in oliguric patients.

Retrograde urography

Following cystoscopy, preferably under screening control, a catheter is either impacted in the ureteral orifice or passed a short distance up the ureter, and contrast medium is injected; this is followed by X-ray filming.

This investigation is now less often used as it is invasive, commonly requires a general anaesthetic and may result in the introduction of infection. It is mainly used to investigate lesions of the ureter and to define the lower level of ureteral obstruction shown on excretion urography or ultrasound plus antegrade studies.

Micturating cystourography (MCU)

This involves catheterization and the instillation of contrast medium into the bladder. The patient is then screened and filmed during voiding to demonstrate or exclude vesicoureteric reflux and to study bladder emptying. It is primarily used in children with recurrent infection (see p. 450) and in adults with disturbed bladder function, when it may be combined with urodynamic studies of bladder pressure and urethral flow.

The presence or absence of vesicoureteric reflux may also be investigated by scintigraphy.

Aortography or renal arteriography

These may be required to investigate extra- or intrarenal arterial disease and to investigate the presence and extent of renal tumours.

Increasing use is made of digital subtraction angiography (DSA) as this allows the use of smaller doses of contrast medium which can be injected via a central venous catheter (venous DSA) or via a fine transfemoral arterial catheter (arterial DSA).

Renal scintigraphy

Renal scintigraphy using a gamma camera is divided into:

- Dynamic studies in which the function of the kidney is examined serially over a period of time, most often using a radiopharmaceutical excreted by glomerular filtration
- Static studies involving imaging of tracer that is taken up and *retained* by the renal tubule

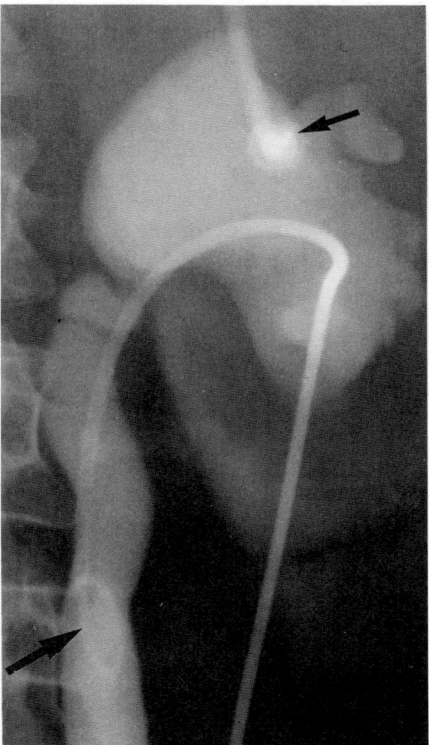

Fig. 9.7 Antegrade pyelography via percutaneous catheter (small arrows) of obstructed system. Percutaneous drainage catheter (large arrow) has been inserted.

Dynamic scintigraphy

The radiopharmaceutical most often used is [^{99m}Tc] DTPA (diethylene triamine penta-acetic acid). It is excreted by glomerular filtration. ^{123}I-labelled ortho-iodohippuric acid (hippuran) is both filtered and secreted by the tubules and is also used but is more expensive and not generally available. Following venous injection of a bolus of tracer, emissions from the kidney can be recorded and stored on computer for analysis of time–activity curves. Analogue images can also be generated at intervals as the study proceeds. This information allows examination of blood perfusion of the kidney, uptake of tracer as a result of glomerular filtration, transit of tracer through the kidney and the outflow of tracer-containing urine from the collecting system.

Dynamic studies are used for:

● *Renal blood flow.* To investigate patients in whom renal artery stenosis is suspected as a cause for hypertension and in patients with severe oliguria (post-traumatic, post-aortic surgery, or after a kidney transplant) to establish whether and to what extent there is renal perfusion.

In patients with unilateral renal artery stenosis there is, typically, a slowed and reduced uptake of tracer with delay in reaching a peak. Studies carried out before and after administration of an angiotensin-converting enzyme may demonstrate a fall in uptake that is highly suggestive of functional arterial stenosis.

In patients with total renal artery occlusion, no kidney uptake of tracers is observed.

● *Investigation of obstruction.* Renography can demonstrate the severity of obstruction. The results obtained from overall uptake and outflow curves must be treated with caution because of the large 'dead space' commonly contributed by dilated calyces and pelves. Dynamic scintigraphy combined with the injection of frusemide can commonly distinguish functional obstruction from a dilated non-obstructed system.

● *Bladder emptying.* At the end of dynamic studies, bladder emptying may be investigated and any post-micturition residual quantitated. Vesicoureteric reflux may be observed, although the sensitivity for detection of this is low. Increased sensitivity can be obtained by direct isotope cystograpy when a dilute isotope solution is instilled into the bladder by catheter.

● *Glomerular filtration rate* (see p. 426).

Static renal scintigraphy

This is usually performed using ^{99m}Tc[DMSA] (dimercaptosuccinic acid), which is taken up by tubular cells. Uptake is proportional to renal function. Static studies are used for:

● *Relative renal function.* Function is normally evenly divided between the kidneys with a range of 45–55%. Static studies are particularly useful in unilateral renal disease, where the relative uptake of the two kidneys can be calculated.

● *Kidney visualization.* Normal kidneys show a uniform uptake with a smooth renal outline. Scars can be identified as photon-deficient 'bites'. Static scintigraphy is of considerable value in identifying ectopic kidneys or 'pseudo-tumours' of the kidneys—i.e. normally functioning renal tissue abnormally placed within the kidney.

● *Localization of infection.* The use of citrate labelled with gallium-67 or isotopically labelled leucocytes that are taken up by inflammatory tissue may be of value in defining localized infection, such as renal abscesses or infection within a renal cyst.

TRANSCUTANEOUS RENAL BIOPSY

Indications and contraindications for renal biopsy are shown in Table 9.4.

The biopsies are carried out under ultrasound control. The biopsy may be carried out manually or using a 'Biopty gun' that automatically controls the actual biopsy procedure. Tissue must be examined by conventional histochemical staining, by electron microscopy and by immunofluorescence.

The complications of transcutaneous renal biopsy are shown in Table 9.5.

Table 9.4 Renal biopsy.

Indications

Nephrotic syndrome (with some exceptions)

Unexplained renal failure with normal-sized kidneys

Failure to recover from assumed reversible acute renal failure

Diagnosis of systemic disease with renal involvement such as sarcoidosis, amyloidosis (occasional indication only)

Asymptomatic proteinuria or haematuria (very occasional indication—justified only if knowledge of prognosis is essential)

Contraindications

Uncooperative patient

Single kidney (with the exception of transplant kidney, when biopsy is acceptable)

Small kidneys (technically difficult, histology hard to interpret, prognosis cannot be altered)

Haemorrhagic disorders (unless correctable temporarily or permanently, e.g. by Factor VIII administration in haemophilia)

Gross obesity or oedema (technical difficulties)

Uncontrolled hypertension

Table 9.5 Complications of transcutaneous renal biopsy.

Macroscopic haematuria—about 20%

Pain in the flank, sometimes referred to shoulder tip

Peri-renal haematoma

Arteriovenous aneurysm formation—about 20%, almost always of no clinical significance

Profuse haematuria demanding blood transfusion—1–3%

Profuse haematuria demanding occlusion of bleeding vessel at angiography or nephrectomy—approximately 1 in 400

Introduction of infection

The mortality rate is about 0.1%

Glomerulonephritis

Glomerulonephritis is a general term for a group of disorders in which:

- There is immunologically mediated injury to glomeruli.
- The kidneys are involved symmetrically.
- Secondary mechanisms of glomerular injury come into play following an initial immune insult (see below).
- The renal lesion may be part of a generalized disease, e.g. systemic lupus erythematosus

---

Transcutaneous renal biopsy

Before biopsy
- A coagulation screen is performed.
- The serum is grouped and saved for cross-matching.
- The patient is given a full explanation of what is involved.

During biopsy
- The patient lies prone with a hard pillow under his abdomen.
- The kidney is localized by ultrasound.
- Local anaesthetic is injected along the biopsy track.
- The patient holds his breath when the biopsy is performed.

After biopsy
- A pressure dressing is applied to the biopsy site and the patient rests in bed for 24 h.
- The fluid intake is maximized to prevent clot colic.
- The pulse and blood pressure are checked regularly.
- The patient is advised to avoid heavy lifting or gardening for 2 weeks.

PATHOGENESIS

Two chief pathogenetic mechanisms are recognized:

- Deposition or *in situ* formation of immune complexes (most human glomerulonephritides)
- Deposition of antiglomerular basement membrane antibody (less than 5% of glomerulonephritides)

Both of these pathogenetic mechanisms activate secondary mechanisms that produce glomerular damage.

Immune complex nephritis. Circulating antigen–antibody complexes (see p. 143) are deposited in the kidney or complexes are formed locally when circulating free antigen has become trapped in the glomerulus. The nature of the antigen involved in the complex formation is important in many instances.

The antigen may be:

- *Exogenous* (e.g. bacterial). For example, a nephritogenic Lancefield group A beta-haemolytic Streptococcus can cause glomerulonephritis in previously healthy individuals.
- *Endogenous.* For example, patients with systemic lupus erythematosus may form antibodies to host DNA, leading to a glomerulonephritis.

Harmful immune complexes can also occur when there is impaired host ability to produce appropriate antibody. Certain strains of black mice regularly develop glomerulonephritis as a result of an impaired ability to produce antibody of appropriate quality or quantity, and it is possible that there may be human counterparts of this phenomenon. There is an association between HLA markers and certain nephritides.

Impaired ability on the part of the host to clear immune complexes from the circulation and deficiencies in the complement system are each associated with an increased incidence of glomerulonephritis.

Antiglomerular basement membrane (anti-GBM) antibody. Anti-GBM antibody reacts with an antigen in the glomerular basement membrane, producing a rare form of glomerular damage. It is of the IgG type. The antibody can also react with alveolar capillary basement membrane (owing to shared antigens) and can cause both lung haemorrhage and glomerulonephritis (Goodpasture's syndrome).

Secondary mechanisms of glomerular injury
Several events can be triggered by the above immunological insults:

- Complement activation

- Fibrin deposition
- Platelet aggregation
- Inflammation with neutrophil-dependent mechanisms
- Activation of kinin systems

Immune complex or anti-GBM antibody deposition trigger these mechanisms to varying degrees, resulting in an increase in capillary permeability and glomerular damage.

In experimentally induced glomerulonephritis in animals, prior anticoagulation, prevention of complement activation, and depletion of polymorphonuclear leucocytes have all been shown to reduce the severity of the induced glomerular injury. However, in humans presenting with most forms of glomerulonephritis these measures do not help.

T-cell dysfunction may play a part in the production of lesions when immune complexes are not seen. There is as yet no direct evidence for this mechanism in man.

CAUSES

In the majority of patients with immune complex-mediated glomerulonephritis, the cause is unknown, i.e. the nature of the antigen involved is not determined. Antigen derived from viruses, bacteria, parasites, drugs and from the host may be involved (Table 9.6). The reasons for the development of anti-GBM antibody are not known; viral damage to alveolar capillary basement membrane,

Table 9.6 Some causes of immune complex mediated glomerulonephritis.

Viruses:
  Mumps
  Measles
  Hepatitis B
  Epstein–Barr virus
  Coxsackie virus

Bacteria:
  Lancefield group A beta-haemolytic streptococci
  Streptococcus viridans (infective endocarditis)
  Staphylococci
  Treponema pallidum

Parasites:
  Plasmodium malariae
  Schistosoma

Host antigens:
  DNA (systemic lupus erythematosus)
  Cryoglobulin
  Malignant tumours

Drugs:
  Penicillamine

rendering it antigenic, has been suggested as a possible cause.

PATHOLOGY

Macroscopic appearances
In acute glomerulonephritis, the kidneys are normal in size or enlarged and oedematous, and the surface of the kidney may show punctate haemorrhages.

In long-standing progressive chronic glomerulonephritis the kidneys may be normal in size or small with finely granular cortical scarring.

Microscopic appearances
Different immunological insults may induce similar or identical histological changes. For example, the immune complex-mediated glomerulonephritis in mumps is not distinguishable from that following beta-haemolytic streptococcal infection. Conversely, different histological responses may occur in the same disease process in different individuals, e.g. in systemic lupus erythematosus (see below).

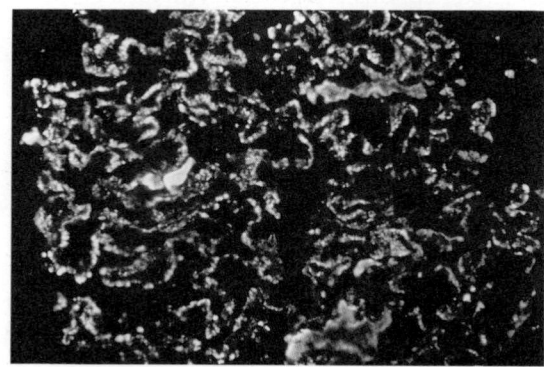

Fig. 9.8 Immunofluorescence showing immune complex deposition in a diffuse granular pattern.

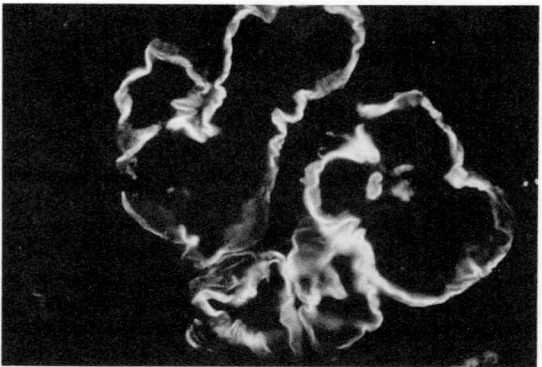

Fig. 9.9 Immunofluorescence showing antiglomerular basement membrane antibody deposition in a linear pattern typical of Goodpasture's syndrome.

The histological response to immune complex deposition probably depends on the size of the complexes, their rate of deposition and the efficiency of host clearance mechanisms.

Renal tissue, obtained at transcutaneous renal biopsy, is examined by:

- *Light microscopy* to assess the extent and histological type of disease. Immunoperoxidase methods may also be applied.
- *Electron microscopy* to define the type of disease and to correlate with immunofluorescence, e.g. to see the exact sites of deposits.
- *Immunofluorescence* to assess the type of immunological injury.

All three methods of examination are necessary for proper histopathological assessment.

Immune complex deposition results in a diffuse granular pattern of staining, with IgG, IgM, IgA components of the complement system and, in addition, fibrin and fibrinogen all present (Fig. 9.8).

The presence of anti-GBM antibody produces a smooth linear pattern of staining for IgG (Fig. 9.9).

Histopathological types
There is not a complete correlation between the histopathological types and the clinical features of the disease; Table 9.7 shows the commonest associations.

Proliferative glomerulonephritis. Proliferative changes occur in many immune complex-mediated nephritides and also in anti-GBM nephritis. It has the following subtypes:

- *Diffuse proliferative glomerulonephritis.* All the glomeruli are similarly affected; Fig. 9.10 shows the typical histological appearances. There is proliferation of endothelial and mesangial cells and several polymorphonuclear leucocytes are present. The glomerulus is swollen, packed with cells and bulges into the opening of the proximal tubule. A normal glomerulus is shown in Fig. 9.11 for comparison. Electron microscopy of the lesions shows subepithelial humps present on

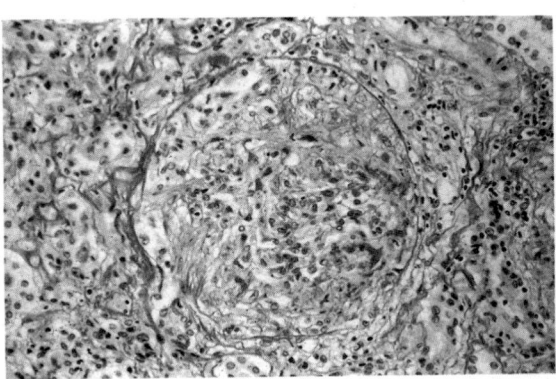

Fig. 9.10 A glomerulus showing proliferative glomerulonephritis.

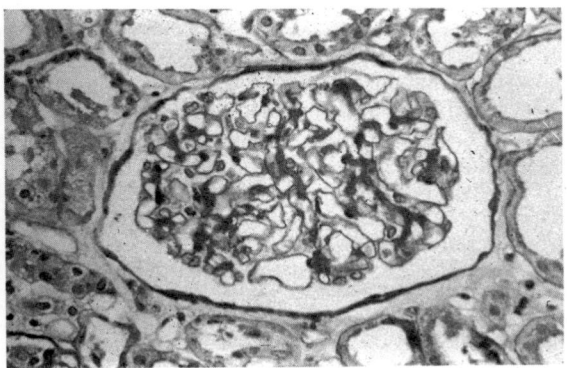

Fig. 9.11 A normal glomerulus.

Table 9.7 Correlation between the histological type of glomerulonephritis and the clinical picture.

Histological type	Most common clinical presentation
Proliferative glomerulonephritis:	
Diffuse	Acute nephritis
Focal segmental	Haematuria, proteinuria
With crescent formation (rapidly progressive glomerulonephritis)	Progressive renal failure
Mesangiocapillary (membranoproliferative)	Haematuria, proteinuria, nephritis or nephrotic syndrome
Membranous glomerulonephritis	Nephrotic syndrome in adults
Minimal-change nephropathy	Nephrotic syndrome especially in children
Idiopathic focal glomerulonephritis with mesangial deposits of IgA	Asymptomatic haematuria
Focal glomerulosclerosis	Proteinuria or nephrotic syndrome

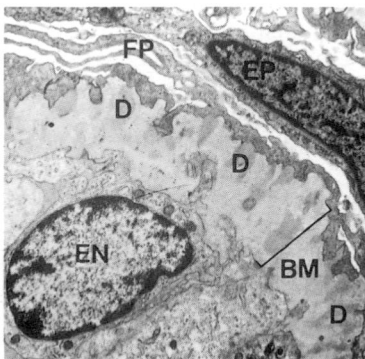

Fig. 9.12 An electron micrograph showing immune complex-mediated glomerulonephritis. EN = endothelial cell; FP = foot process; BM = basement membrane; EP = epithelial podocyte; D = electron-dense deposits (antigen–antibody complexes).

the glomerular basement membrane (Fig. 9.12) and immunofluorescence shows granular deposits of immunoglobulin and C3.

This type of glomerulonephritis, presenting as an acute nephritis, is commonly seen after a streptococcal infection (see below).

- *Focal segmental glomerulonephritis.* Only some of the glomeruli here show proliferative changes whilst others are normal, hence the term focal. The affected glomeruli show segmental involvement of the tufts, i.e. changes are present in one or more parts of the glomerulus.

This condition may occur as a primary renal disease, but it is also seen in systemic lupus erythematosus, subacute infective endocarditis, with infected atrioventricular shunts (shunt nephritis), and in disorders with IgA deposits, e.g. Henoch–Schönlein purpura and IgA disease. A severe focal necrotizing form is seen in polyarteritis nodosa and Wegener's granulomatosis. Special subtypes (IgA disease and focal glomerulosclerosis) are discussed below.

- *Proliferative glomerulonephritis with crescent formation (rapidly progressive glomerulonephritis; RPGN)* (Fig. 9.13). The term 'crescent' is applied to an aggregate of macrophages and epithelial cells in Bowman's space. Crescents are associated with severe damage to the glomerular tuft and are seen in occasional glomeruli in several types of glomerulonephritis. However, if most glomeruli show crescents the glomerulonephritis is usually placed in this subtype, as clinical progression to renal failure is rapid.

This condition is seen in both immune complex and anti-GBM antibody-mediated nephritis. It particularly occurs in polyarteritis, Wegener's granulomatosis and Goodpasture's syndrome.

- *Mesangiocapillary (membranoproliferative) glomerulonephritis (MCGN).* In *type 1* there is mesangial cell proliferation, with mainly subendothelial immune-complex deposition and apparent splitting of the capillary basement membrane, giving a 'tram-line' effect. It may be idiopathic or may occur with shunt nephritis. It can be associated with persistently reduced levels of C3 and normal levels of C4.

In *type 2* there is mesangial cell proliferation with electron-dense, linear intramembranous deposits that usually stain for C3 only. This type may be idiopathic or may occur after measles. Partial lipodystrophy (loss of subcutaneous fat in various parts of the body) may be seen.

MCGN affects young adults. Patients present with haematuria, proteinuria, the nephrotic syndrome or renal failure. Most patients eventually go on to develop renal failure over several years.

Membranous glomerulonephritis (Fig. 9.14). Thickening of the capillary basement membrane due to immune complex deposition is the main feature of this disease. In the majority of patients the antigenic component of the complex is unknown. Associations include systemic lupus erythematosus

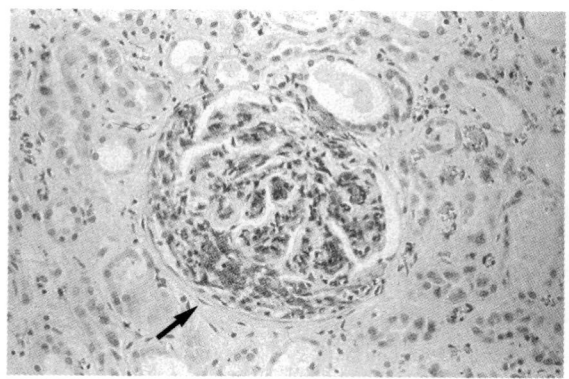

Fig. 9.13 Crescentic glomerulonephritis. Note 'epithelial' crescent at the periphery of the glomerulus (arrow).

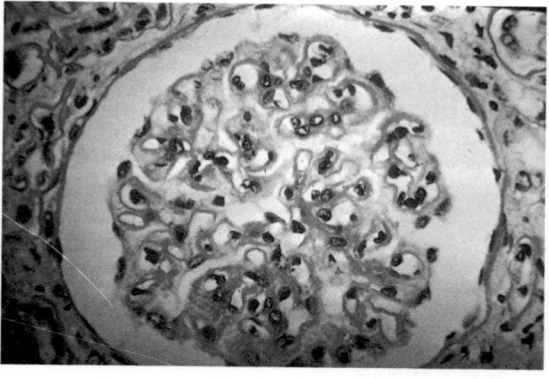

Fig. 9.14 Membranous glomerulonephritis showing thickened basement membrane.

(where the antigen is host DNA), malignancy of the bowel and bronchus (tumour-derived antigen) and penicillamine therapy. *Plasmodium malariae* is a common cause in the tropics. Recently a strong association with HLA-DR3 has been found.

This condition occurs mainly in adults, predominantly in males. Patients present with proteinuria or frank nephrotic syndrome. Thirty per cent of patients undergo spontaneous remission, but the remainder eventually go on to develop chronic renal failure.

Minimal change glomerular lesion (minimal change nephropathy). This is not a true glomerulonephritis and is included here for convenience. In this condition the glomeruli appear normal on light microscopy. The only abnormality seen on electron microscopy is fusion of the foot processes of epithelial cells (podocytes). This is a non-specific finding and is seen in many conditions associated with proteinuria.

Neither immune complexes nor anti-GBM antibody can be demonstrated by immunofluorescence. However, the immunological pathogenesis of this condition is suggested by:

- Its response to steroids and immunosuppressive drugs
- Its occurrence in Hodgkin's disease, with remission following successful treatment
- Patients with the condition and family members having a higher incidence of asthma and eczema. Remission following desensitization or antigen avoidance has been described.

A suggested explanation for the proteinuria is the production by lymphocytes of a factor that increases glomerular permeability to protein.

Minimal change nephropathy occurs chiefly in children ages 2–4 years but it can occur in adults. Patients present with the nephrotic syndrome (see below). It does not lead to chronic renal failure.

Idiopathic focal glomerulonephritis with mesangial deposits of IgA (IgA disease, Berger's disease). This disease consists of focal proliferative glomerulonephritis and mesangial deposits of IgA. In some cases IgG, C3 and properdin may also be seen in the glomerular mesangium.

Glomerulonephritis in Henoch–Schönlein purpura has a similar pathological picture.

This type of glomerulonephritis tends to occur in children and young adults. They present with recurrent haematuria, which is sometimes related to infection. The prognosis is usually good, but up to 10% of patients eventually develop renal failure.

Focal segmental glomerulosclerosis (FSGS). This is a disease of unknown pathogenesis. It may recur in kidneys transplanted into affected individuals, sometimes within hours of transplantation. A circulating factor may be involved. It presents as proteinuria or nephrotic syndrome and is usually resistant to steroid therapy. All age groups are affected.

On light microscopy, segmental glomerulosclerosis is seen, which later progresses to global sclerosis. The deep glomeruli at the corticomedullary junction are affected first. These may be missed on transcutaneous biopsy, leading to a mistaken diagnosis of minimal change glomerular lesion. Immunofluorescence may show deposits of C3 and IgM in affected portions of the glomerulus, but non-specific fixation to damaged tissue, rather than immune-complex deposition, may well be the explanation for this.

About 50% of patients progress to end stage renal failure within 10 years of diagnosis.

CLINICAL FEATURES

Glomerulonephritis presents in one of four ways:

- Asymptomatic proteinuria and/or microscopic haematuria
- Acute nephritic syndrome (see below)
- Nephrotic syndrome (see p. 443)
- Chronic renal failure (see p. 468)

Asymptomatic proteinuria and/or microscopic haematuria is discovered incidentally, e.g. at a routine medical examination. Some causes of haematuria are shown in Fig. 9.4. Overt haematuria may occur after exercise.

INVESTIGATION

Since false positives are often obtained using Stix methods, the presence of significant proteinuria must be demonstrated by measuring the 24-hour urinary output of protein on two consecutive occasions (see p. 430).

Urinary protein loss increases when in the erect position and 'postural' proteinuria can occur. Stix testing gives a negative result on urines passed early in the morning after rising, but positive results are seen during the day when the patient is mainly erect. Insurance companies do not tend to discriminate against those with postural proteinuria, as the prognosis is usually good. Nevertheless, the majority of individuals with this condition have glomerulonephritis of some sort on renal biopsy.

Urine microscopy is performed to look for haematuria. A positive Stix test for blood may result from haematuria or haemoglobinuria. These can be differentiated on microscopy since red cells are only seen in patients with haematuria. Red cell morphology may provide a guide to diagnosis (see p. 430).

Further investigations will include:

- Urine microscopy for red cell casts

- Assessment of renal function by estimation of blood urea, serum creatinine and endogenous creatinine clearance
- Renal imaging, usually by excretion urography

Acute nephritic syndrome

This comprises:

- Haematuria (macroscopic or microscopic). Red cell casts are typically seen on urine microscopy.
- Proteinuria
- Hypertension
- Oedema (periorbital, leg or sacral) } owing to salt and retention.
- Oliguria.
- Uraemia.

CLINICAL FEATURES

In classical post-streptococcal glomerulonephritis the patient, usually a child, will have suffered a streptococcal infection 1–3 weeks before the onset of the acute nephritic syndrome. Streptococcal tonsillitis or pharyngitis, otitis media or cellulitis may be responsible.

The infecting organism is a Lancefield group A beta-haemolytic streptococcus of a nephritogenic type. The latent interval between the infection and development of symptoms and signs of renal involvement reflects the time taken for immune-complex formation and deposition and glomerular injury to occur.

INVESTIGATION

A list of investigations is given in Table 9.8.

If the clinical diagnosis of a nephritic illness is clear-cut, e.g. in post-streptococcal glomerulonephritis, renal imaging and renal biopsy are usually unnecessary. A biopsy is required if the diagnosis is uncertain, if the clinical features are unusual, or if renal failure is rapidly progressive, suggesting the presence of crescentic glomerulonephritis (RPGN).

MANAGEMENT

In the majority of patients with glomerulonephritis, neither corticosteroid nor immunosuppressive therapy is of benefit. The same applies to treatment with agents that alter coagulation and platelet function. Important exceptions to this general rule include glomerulonephritis complicating systemic lupus erythematosus, polyarteritis nodosa, Wegener's granulomatosis, Goodpasture's syndrome and, in all probability, some forms of rapidly progressive crescentic glomerulonephritis (see later).

As spontaneous remissions usually occur in acute glomerulonephritis, the aim of managment is to prevent patients dying from pulmonary oedema, uraemia or hypertensive encephalopathy while awaiting improvement in renal function.

Hospital admission is advisable for all adults and for children with oliguria and marked hypertension; levels of blood pressure that are of no risk

Table 9.8 Investigation of acute nephritic syndrome.

Investigations	Positive findings
Urine microscopy	Red cells, red-cell casts
Blood urea	May be elevated
Serum creatinine	May be elevated
Culture (throat swab, discharge from ear, swab from inflammed skin)	Nephritogenic organism—not always
Antistreptolysin-O titre	Elevated in post-streptococcal nephritis
C3 level	May be reduced
Antinuclear antibody	Present in significant titre in systemic lupus erythematosus
Creatinine clearance	Reduced
Urinary protein output	Increased
Chest X-ray	Cardiomegaly Pulmonary oedema } Not always
Renal imaging	Usually normal
Renal biopsy	Glomerulonephritis

to adults may be associated with hypertensive fits in the young.

Otherwise, hospital admission is not mandatory, providing the general practitioner is able to visit daily to examine the patient and check his blood pressure. Blood for measurement of urea or serum creatinine concentrations should be taken every few days.

Management in hospital
Most patients with renal disease who are admitted to hospital require:

- Daily recording of fluid intake and output
- Daily weighing (as a check on change in body fluid status)
- Regular measurement of blood pressure

Strict bedrest is unnecessary unless the patient feels ill, is severely hypertensive or has pulmonary oedema.

Dietary protein restriction is required only if severe uraemia occurs, but salt restriction is always necessary. In oliguric patients, fluid restriction is necessary to maintain body weight at a level at which severe hypertension, pulmonary congestion and gross oedema are prevented.

Mild to moderate hypertension and oedema may respond to salt restriction and diuretic therapy, e.g. frusemide given orally or parenterally. Other hypotensive agents may be required. Beta-adrenergic receptor blocking therapy should be used with caution for hypertension as it may precipitate pulmonary oedema in those on the brink of heart failure due to the salt and water overload.

The prognosis in immune complex-mediated glomerulonephritis is improved if the antigen responsible can be eradicated. In patients with post-streptococcal glomerulonephritis, a course of penicillin should be given.

Management of life-threatening complications
Hypertensive encephalopathy. In this condition the priorities are to maintain the airway and to reduce the blood pressure using a parenteral agent such as hydralazine 5–20 mg by slow intravenous infusion over 20 min. Fits should be controlled with parenteral diazepam (10 mg i.v.), but this may induce respiratory depression and facilities for resuscitation must be available.

Pulmonary oedema. This should be treated in the usual way (see p. 568). Because of the renal failure, high doses of potent diuretics such as frusemide given parenterally may be required. If this fails to produce a diuresis, salt and water may be removed osmotically by peritoneal dialysis, by ultrafiltration of blood alone, or by ultrafiltration combined with haemodialysis (see p. 473).

Severe uraemia. Peritoneal or haemodialysis will be required pending recovery of the renal function.

Outbreak of post-streptococcal glomerulonephritis in a closed community. Prophylactic penicillin (phenoxymethylpenicillin 500 mg daily) should be given to all individuals at risk, providing that they are not allergic to penicillin. If one member of a family living in overcrowded conditions develops the disorder, other members should be treated prophylactically. Evidence in support of long-term penicillin prophylaxis after the development of glomerulonephritis is lacking.

PROGNOSIS

Post-streptococcal glomerulonephritis
The prognosis in children is excellent. A small number of adults develop hypertension and/or renal impairment later in life. Therefore in older patients, an annual blood pressure check, and less frequently an estimation of serum creatinine, is a reasonable precaution, even after apparent complete recovery.

Acute glomerulonephritis of unknown cause
Here the prognosis is less good and the need for follow-up is correspondingly greater.

Rapidly progressive crescentic glomerulonephritis
Severe renal failure with oliguria and hypertension occurs within a few weeks or months of the onset of the illness. Coriticosteroid treatment (to reduce glomerular inflammatory reaction), treatment with agents that prevent platelet aggregation, immunosuppression (e.g. with azathioprine or cyclophosphamide) and anticoagulants are used in combination. Such 'quadruple therapy' carries substantial risk but does appear to be of benefit in some patients. Repeated plasma exchange to remove circulating immune complexes or antibody may also be helpful. The prognosis is poor.

Goodpasture's syndrome (see p. 689)

This rare condition is mediated by anti-GBM antibody. It presents with recurrent haemoptysis and a severe progressive glomerulonephritis. There is a strong association with HLA-DR2. Lung haemorrhage responds to repeated plasma exchange (which removes the anti-GBM antibodies) combined with immunosuppressive therapy. The effect of this treatment upon the glomerulonephritis is less clear-cut; when oliguria occurs or serum creatinine rises above 0.6–0.7 mmol·L^{-1} renal failure is almost always irreversible.

The kidney in systemic disease

GLOMERULONEPHRITIS AS A PART OF SYSTEMIC VASCULITIS

Systemic lupus erythematosus (SLE) (see p. 391)

Renal disease in systemic lupus erythematosus is 10 times as common in women as in men. All varieties of histological abnormality are seen, ranging from a minimal-change lesion to crescentic glomerulonephritis. The prognosis is better in patients with the minimal-change and membranous lesions than in those with proliferative glomerulonephritis.

Whilst corticosteroid therapy improves the extrarenal manifestations of SLE, evidence is lacking that this treatment alters the renal prognosis. Both azathioprine and cyclophosphamide may improve renal function, but long-term studies suggest that cyclophosphamide is better.

The indications for treatment vary. Those whose urine sediment contains many red cells and red-cell casts and those in whome renal function is impaired or is observed to deteriorate are strong candidates for treatment. A histological diagnosis should be obtained before commencing such potentially hazardous treatment.

Polyarteritis nodosa (see p. 397)

In this multisystem disorder, aneurysmal dilatation of medium sized arteries may be seen on renal arteriography. A focal proliferative glomerulonephritis with or without crescents can be present. The condition is commoner in men and in the elderly.

Corticosteroid therapy and immunosuppression with azathioprine or cyclophosphamide are of benefit.

Wegener's granulomatosis (see p. 398)

In this condition, microscopic polyarteritis occurs together with necrotizing granulomatous lesions affecting the nasopharynx, lungs and kidneys. The necrotizing glomerular lesions do not appear to be due to immune complex deposition.

Corticosteroid treatment and cyclophosphamide are of benefit.

Systemic sclerosis (see p. 394)

Interlobular renal arteries are affected with intimal thickening and fibrinoid changes occur in afferent glomerular arterioles. Glomerular changes are non-specific. The pathogenesis is unknown and neither steroid nor immunosuppressive therapy is of value.

RENAL INVOLVEMENT IN OTHER DISEASES

Diabetes mellitus

Renal disease is a major complication of diabetes; it is discussed on p. 852.

Amyloidosis

The kidney is often affected in amyloidosis (see p. 869). Presentation is with asymptomatic proteinuria, nephrotic syndrome or renal failure.

PATHOLOGY

On light microscopy eosinophilic deposits are seen in the mesangium, capillary loops and arteriolar walls. Staining with Congo red renders these deposits pink and they show green birefringence under polarized light. Immunofluorescence is unhelpful but on electron microscopy the characteristic fibrils of amyloid can be seen. Primary and secondary renal amyloid are indistinguishable.

DIAGNOSIS

The diagnosis can often be made clinically when features of amyloidosis are present elsewhere. On excretion urography or ultrasound the kidneys are usually large. Renal biopsy is necessary in doubtful cases.

TREATMENT

Treatment of the underlying cause should be undertaken. Steroids and immunosuppression are of no proven value. The prognosis for renal function is poor in primary amyloid as well as in amyloid secondary to myelomatosis. The success of dialysis and kidney transplantation is dependent upon the extent of amyloid deposition in extrarenal sites, especially the heart.

Haemolytic uraemic syndrome (HUS)

HUS is a disorder of infancy and childhood that is characterized by intravascular haemolysis with red-cell fragmentation (microangiopathic haemolysis), thrombocytopenia and acute renal failure. The syndrome often follows a febrile illness, particularly gastroenteritis or upper respiratory tract infection. A few particular strains of pathogenic *Escherichia coli* have been isolated in many cases. Clustering of cases and the occurrence of 'epidemics' of HUS provide further support for an infective aetiology. It has been suggested that infection triggers endothelial damage and that derangements of the coagulation system then occur in susceptible individuals. Recurrent episodes of HUS have been described in the same individual. Fibrin deposition is seen in the vascular endothelium, particularly in the renal arterioles and glomerular capillaries. Most children recover spontaneously.

Treatment with heparin, inhibitors of platelet aggregation, synthetic prostacyclins, infusion of fresh frozen plasma and plasma exchange have been employed, but controlled trials of treatment are lacking.

Thrombotic thrombocytopenic purpura (TTP)

TTP is characterized by the presence of widespread hyaline thrombi in small vessels. Young adults are most commonly affected. Microangiopathic haemolysis, renal failure and evidence of neurological disturbance are characteristically found. The pathogenesis is unknown. Some patients with TTP have underlying systemic lupus erythematosus or polyarteritis nodosa and there is clearly considerable overlap between HUS, TTP and the connective-tissue disorders.

Multiple myeloma

Acute renal failure is relatively common in myeloma, occurring in 2–8% of affected individuals. Histological appearances may be simply those of acute tubular necrosis; tubular blockage by Tamm–Horsfall glycoprotein, light chains and immunoglobulin may also be apparent. Dehydration and the administration of intravenous or intraarterial contrast medium to the volume-depleted patient with myeloma predispose to the development of actue renal failure.

In myeloma, free kappa and lambda light chains are excreted. Blockage of tubules by casts composed in part at least of light chains and perhaps their toxic effects upon tubular cells account for the proteinuria and chronic renal impairment associated with 'myeloma kidney'. Renal amyloid deposition often complicates myelomatosis, accounting both for proteinuria—sometimes of nephrotic proportions—and chronic renal failure.

Hypercalcaemia, renal sepsis and—rarely—urinary tract obstruction due to bulky myeloma deposits are further causes of renal impairment in myelomatosis.

Nephrotic syndrome

The nephrotic syndrome consists of heavy urinary protein loss, hypoalbuminaemia and oedema. Hypercholesterolaemia is almost always present.

PATHOPHYSIOLOGY

Urinary protein loss of the order of 3–5 g per day or more in an adult is required to cause hypoalbuminaemia. In children, proportionately less proteinuria results in hypoalbuminaemia.

The normal dietary protein intake in the UK is of the order 70 g daily and the normal liver can synthesize albumin at a rate of 10–12 g daily. How then does a urinary protein loss of the order of 3–5 g daily result in hypoalbuminaemia? The explanation appears to be that in normal individuals there is some catabolism within the kidney of albumin filtered at the glomeruli. In nephrotic patients with heavy proteinuria, catabolism is substantially increased, limiting the amount of protein appearing in the urine and concealing the extent of protein loss through the glomerulus.

The mechanism of the proteinuria is complex. It occurs partly because structural damage to the glomerular basement membrane leads to an increase in the size and numbers of pores, allowing passage of more and larger molecules. Electrical charge is also involved in glomerular permeability. Fixed negatively charged components are present in the glomerular capillary wall, which repel negatively charged protein molecules. Reduction of this fixed charge occurs in glomerular disease and appears to be an important factor in the genesis of heavy proteinuria.

Pathogenesis of oedema in hypoalbuminaemia
The pathogenesis of the oedema is incompletely understood. A reduction in the concentration of osmotically active albumin molecules in the blood results in a reduction in the oncotic force that retains fluid within blood vessels, and salt and water escapes into the extravascular compartment, i.e. oedema occurs. Such loss of salt and water results in a fall in blood volume and a reduction in pressure within afferent glomerular arterioles. This activates the renin–angiotensin–aldosterone system (see p. 828). The consequent hyperaldosteronism promotes sodium and water reabsorption in the distal nephron, increasing the tendency to oedema. However, measurements of these various parameters do not always support this concept. The plasma renin activity in nephrotic patients is often normal and measured blood volume may be normal or high in nephrotic patients, even those without renal failure.

Table 9.9 Causes of the nephrotic syndrome.

All glomerulonephritides and minimal-change glomerular lesions

Systemic vasculitides, mainly systemic lupus erythematosus

Diabetic glomerulosclerosis

Amyloidosis

Drugs

Allergies

CAUSES (Table 9.9)

All types of glomerulonephritis can produce the nephrotic syndrome.

Although proliferative glomerulonephritis is commoner than membranous disease, the latter is the commonest cause of nephrotic syndrome in adults in the UK.

Minimal change glomerular disease accounts for more than 50% of cases of the nephrotic syndrome in childhood compared with approximately 20% of adult cases. In tropical areas minimal change is present in fewer than 10% of nephrotic children owing to the high incidence of nephrotic syndrome due to infections such as malaria. Minimal-change disease does not progress to chronic renal failure (see p. 439).

Diabetic glomerular disease can also cause the nephrotic syndrome. The histological lesion seen on light microscopy in diabetes may comprise amorphous nodular deposits, which are not immune complexes, in the glomeruli or a diffuse glomerulosclerosis. There is associated glomerular basement membrane thickening.

Diabetes is also a cause of renal papillary necrosis, but patients with this lesion alone do not have sufficiently heavy proteinuria to become nephrotic.

Drugs

Many drugs can cause sufficiently heavy proteinuria to result in the nephrotic syndrome. Penicillamine, which in all probability combines with a plasma protein to form an antigen hapten, induces an immune complex-mediated membranous glomerulonephritis. Troxidone, used in the treatment of absence seizures, may also cause heavy proteinuria. Various metals, whether used therapeutically (e.g. gold) or in industry (e.g. mercury and cadmium), can induce proteinuria severe enough to cause the nephrotic syndrome.

Allergic reactions

Reactions to many allergens such as poison ivy, pollens, bee stings and cow's milk may be associated with the nephrotic syndrome, but evidence of a causal relationship is lacking in most cases.

Most lists of causes of the nephrotic syndrome include renal vein thrombosis, but this is probably a complication rather than a cause of the syndrome. It is particularly likely to complicate membranous glomerulonephritis. In nephrotic patients the blood is more coagulable than normal and the circulation may be sluggish owing to hypovolaemia, both of which are likely to induce thrombosis. Estimates of the incidence of this complication range from 5% to approximately 50%.

Renal disorders not associated with the nephrotic syndrome

Proteinuria severe enough to cause the nephrotic syndrome is not a feature of reflux nephropathy (chronic atrophic pyelonephritis), chronic tubulointerstitial nephritis, renal tuberculosis, polycystic disease or many other renal disorders.

HISTORY

The history may provide clues to the aetiology, e.g. exposure to a drug or allergen. Patients with minimal-change lesion may give a history of atopy. There may be a family history of renal disease.

Patients with heavy proteinuria may have noted that their urine has been frothy; the onset of the renal lesion can be timed from this observation.

EXAMINATION

Examination will reveal oedema; ascites may also be present, particularly in children. Genital oedema is sometimes seen. The oedema may involve the face (periorbital oedema) and arms. Neither elevation of the jugular venous pressure nor pulmonary oedema are features of the nephrotic syndrome, though either or both may be present if renal and/or cardiac failure are present in the nephrotic patient.

Features of the underlying disorder may be evident, such as the butterfly facial rash of systemic lupus erythematosus or the neuropathy and retinopathy associated with diabetes mellitus.

Exclude:

- Primary cardiac failure: here, the venous pressure is high, oedema is not usually present in the face, and the proteinuria is less severe.
- Liver disease, and other causes of hypoalbuminaemia (Table 9.10), with oedema and ascites.

INVESTIGATION

The presence of the nephrotic syndrome is established by measuring:

- The 24-hour urinary protein—usually more than

Table 9.10 Causes of hypoalbuminaemia.

Inadequate protein intake—protein–energy malnutrition

Failure of protein production—liver disease

Excessive protein loss—nephrotic syndrome, protein-losing enteropathy, extensive burns

3–5 g/day in adults
- The serum albumin concentration—usually less than 30 g·L^{-1}

Increased hepatic albumin synthesis is accompanied by increased cholesterol synthesis and there is an approximate reciprocal relationship between the serum albumin and the serum cholesterol concentration. LDL cholesterol concentrations are elevated but HDL cholesterol is usually normal. Hypertriglyceridaemia is present in about 50% of patients.

Renal function is assessed by measuring:

- The blood urea and serum creatinine
- The creatinine clearance, to determine the GFR

Further investigations are required to elucidate the cause:

- Microscopy of the urine may show red cells and red-cell casts; the latter are virtually diagnositic of glomerulonephritis. Minimal change lesions do not usually result in red cells or red-cell casts in the urine.
- Serum C3 complement concentrations may be decreased in immune complex-mediated glomerulonephritis.
- A throat swab and serum ASO titre may show evidence of streptococcal infection.
- The presence of antinuclear factor and other antibodies may suggest systemic lupus erythematosus.
- In the nephrotic syndrome there is always a reduced serum albumin, commonly with an increase in the alpha- and beta-globulin fractions (Fig. 9.15) on serum electrophoresis. In myeloma, abnormal protein bands may be found, including Bence–Jones protein in the urine. Ten per cent of patients with myeloma have amyloid and can develop the nephrotic syndrome.
- A raised blood glucose indicates diabetes mellitus.
- Selective protein clearance may be measured. Blood and urine samples are taken at the same time; a timed urine collection is not required. The clearance of large-molecular-weight protein such as IgG is compared with that of a smaller molecule such as albumin or transferrin. A low ratio (selective protein leak) is found in minimal-change glomerulopathy, early diabetes and renal amyloidosis. Severe glomerulonephritides, e.g. diffuse proliferative glomerulonephritis with

crescent formation, are more typically associated with an unselective protein leak. Overlap between the groups exists. Measurement of selective protein clearance is unnecessary if renal biopsy is to be carried out. Its main use is in children in whom a minimal change lesion is suspected. An unselective protein leak in such a child would bring this diagnosis into question and might prompt renal biopsy (see below).

Renal biopsy (see p. 434)
Transcutaneous biopsy is performed to make a histological diagnosis when management will be affected, particularly when the major question is whether a steroid-sensitive minimal change lesion is present or not. It is *not* indicated:

- In young children (particularly males) who have a highly selective protein leak, no hypertension and no red cells or red-cell casts in the urine. The diagnosis is almost certain to be a minimal-change lesion, so that a trial of steroids should be instituted first.
- In long-standing, insulin-dependent diabetes with associated retinopathy or neuropathy, since the diagnosis is not in doubt.
- In patients on drugs such as penicillamine, which should be stopped first.

MANAGEMENT

General measures
Initial treatment should be with dietary sodium restriction and a thiazide diuretic, e.g. bendrofluazide 5 mg daily. Unresponsive patients require

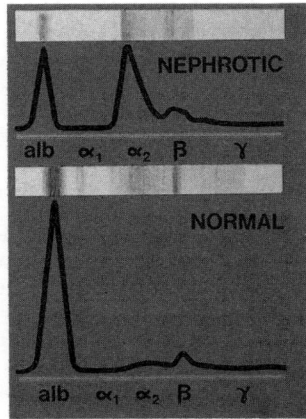

Fig. 9.15 Serum electrophoresis in a normal person and a patient with nephrotic syndrome. Note the reduced albumin and increased alpha- and beta-globulin in the nephrotic patient.

frusemide 40–120 mg daily with the addition of amiloride (5 mg daily), but the serum potassium concentration should be monitored carefully.

Patients are often hypovolaemic, and moderate oedema may have to be accepted in order to avoid postural hypotension.

A high-protein diet (approximately 80–90 g protein per day) is usually given, but the superiority of a high, as opposed to a normal, protein intake is unproven.

Infusion of albumin produces only a transient effect and is normally employed only in diuretic-resistant patients. Such infusion is combined with diuretic therapy. Diuresis, when once initiated, often continues with diuretic treatment alone.

Specific measures
The aim is to reverse the abnormal urinary protein leak.

Minimal-change glomerular lesion. High-dose corticosteroid therapy with prednisolone 60 mg per day (dose corrected to a normal body surface area of 1.73 m^2) for 8 weeks corrects the urinary protein leak in more than 95% of children. Response rates in adults are significantly lower and response may occur only after many months of steroid therapy. Spontaneous remission also occurs and steroid therapy should, in general, be withheld if urinary protein loss is insufficient to cause hypoalbuminaemia or oedema.

In both children and adults, if remission lasts for 4 years after steroid therapy, further relapse is very rare. In children, approximately one-third do not subsequently relapse, but in the remainder further courses of corticosteroids are indicated. A third of these patients relapse regularly on steroid withdrawal and in these patients remission is induced with steroid therapy once more and a course of cyclophosphamide 3 mg·kg^{-1} daily is given for 6–8 weeks. This increases the likelihood of long-term remission. Steroid-unresponsive patients may also respond to cyclophosphamide. No more than two courses of cyclophosphamide should be prescribed in children because of the risk of side-effects, which include azoospermia.

Membranous glomerulonephritis. Spontaneous remission does occur in this condition, particularly in women. Nevertheless, more than 50% of nephrotic patients with idiopathic membranous glomerulonephritis develop end-stage renal failure within 10 years of diagnosis. Some nephrologists believe that corticosteroid therapy combined with azathioprine chlorambucil or cyclophosphamide may protect against deterioration in renal function to some extent in idiopathic membranous glomerulonephritis, though this remains controversial. Such treatment may best be reserved for patients in whom glomerular filtration rate is known to have declined rapidly.

Other causes. Remission occurs if the underlying disease can be treated. In patients with systemic lupus erythematosus, treatment with steroids and cyclophosphamide or azathioprine usually induces long-term remission. Amyloidosis does not usually respond to therapy.

When the glomerular lesion causing the nephrotic syndrome progresses and the GFR declines, the degree of proteinuria often diminishes so that the hypoalbuminaemia and oedema improve.

Prevention and management of complications
Venous thrombosis. Hypovolaemia and a hypercoagulable state predispose to venous thrombosis. Prolonged bed rest should therefore be avoided.

Once renal vein thrombosis has occurred, prolonged anticoagulation is required. Thromboembolism is particularly common in nephrotic syndrome due to membranous glomerulonephritis and prophylactic anticoagulation may be warranted.

Sepsis. Sepsis is an important cause of death in nephrotic patients. The increased susceptibility to infection is partly due to loss of immunoglobulin in the urine. Pneumococcal infections are particularly common.

Early detection and aggressive treatment of infections, rather than long-term antibiotic prophylaxis, is the best approach.

Oliguric renal failure. A low blood volume and hypotension may lead to underperfused kidneys. Acute tubular necrosis may therefore readily develop when renal ischaemia occurs from other complications such as blood loss or septicaemia. In some patients, uraemia appears to result from derangements in renal perfusion in the absence of hypotension.

Albumin infusion combined with mannitol or another diuretic may initiate a diuresis in oliguric renal failure.

Lipid abnormalities. Proof that these are responsible for any increase in risk of myocardial infarction or peripheral vascular disease is lacking and there is no consensus on whether lipid-lowering agents should be prescribed.

Urinary tract infection

Urinary tract infection (UTI) is common in women, uncommon in men and of special importance in children. If recurrent, it may be a cause of considerable morbidity; if complicated, it can cause severe renal disease including 'end-stage renal failure'. It is also a common source of life-threatening Gram-negative septicaemia.

PATHOGENESIS

Infection is most often due to bacteria from the patient's own bowel flora (Table 9.11) but in 20–30% of young women it is due to *Staphylococcus saprophyticus* or *S. epidermidis*. Transfer to the urinary tract may be via the bloodstream, the lymphatics or by direct extension (e.g. from a vesicocolic fistula), but is most often via the ascending transurethral route (Fig. 9.16). For the latter route, three important steps are involved:

1 The periurethral area is heavily colonized with bacteria. This may be facilitated by the adhesion of bacteria to uroepithelial surfaces by pili or fimbriae present on their surface. Previous UTIs may also predispose to further colonization, initiating a vicious circle. Other factors involved are unclear, although gross lack of personal hygiene, the wearing of nappies or sanitary towels, local infection (e.g. vaginitis) and the use of bubble baths or chemicals in bath water have all been incriminated.

Table 9.11 Organisms causing urinary tract infection in domiciliary practice.

Organism	Approximate frequency
Escherichia coli and other 'coliforms'	68% +
Proteus mirabilis	12%
Klebsiella aerogenes[a]	4%
Streptococcus faecalis[a]	6%
Staphylococcus saprophyticus or epidermidis[b]	10%

[a] More common in hospital practice.
[b] More common in young women (20–30%).

2 Bacteria are transferred along the urethra to the bladder. This step is facilitated by catheterization or sexual intercourse. Spontaneous transfer along the short female urethra is easy, while the longer male urethra protects against transfer of bacteria to the bladder; in addition, prostatic fluid has defensive bactericidal properties.

3 The most important step is the *establishment* and *multiplication* of bacteria within the bladder. Bladder urine is normally sterile, owing to bladder defence mechanisms that are the main protection against UTI. These include hydrokinetic and bladder mucosal factors. A low flow rate and infrequent and poor bladder emptying predispose to infection.

Mucosal defence mechanisms are poorly understood. The establishment of infection may be facilitated by fimbriated bacteria adhering to the bladder uroepithelium or previous damage to this epithelium. Neither humoral nor cell-mediated immune mechanisms have been shown to play any part in maintaining the sterility of bladder urine.

The first critical phase in the development of UTI is thus the entry and establishment of bacteria within the bladder. Extension of infection up the ureters to the kidneys is relatively easy and is facilitated by vesicoureteric reflux and dilated hypotonic ureters. In terms of infection, and with the possible exception of renal carbuncles (see below), the urinary tract can be thought of as a continuous functional unit from the bladder to the kidney. Once infection is established it can pass up or down the system quite readily.

NATURAL HISTORY

UTI is commonly an isolated, never (or rarely) repeated event (Fig. 9.17). At least 50% of women will experience an episode of 'cystitis' at some time in their lives. Although often unpleasant, such single episodes of UTI rarely result in significant kidney damage. Recurrent or persistent infections are much more important.

Complicated versus uncomplicated infection (Fig. 9.18) It is important to distinguish between UTI occurring in patients with:

● Functionally normal urinary tracts (with normal

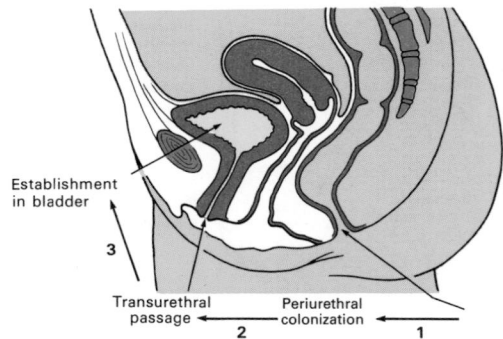

Fig. 9.16 Ascending infection of the urinary tract.

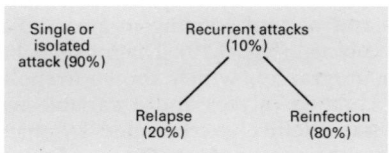

Fig. 9.17 The natural history of urinary tract infection.

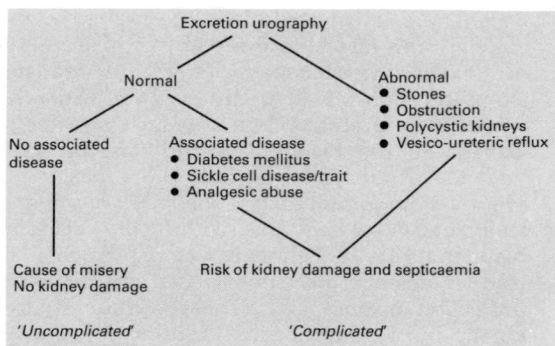

Fig. 9.18 Complicated versus uncomplicated urinary tract infection.

excretion urography). Here, persistent or recurrent infection rarely results in serious kidney damage (*uncomplicated UTI*).

● Abnormal urinary tracts (e.g. with stones) or associated diseases (e.g. diabetes mellitus) which themselves cause kidney damage may be made worse with infection (*complicated UTI*). UTI, particularly with *Proteus*, may predispose to stone formation. The combination of infection and obstruction results in severe, sometimes rapid, kidney damage (obstructive pyonephrosis) and is an important cause of Gramnegative septicaemia.

Chronic pyelonephritis
Chronic pyelonephritis (also called atrophic pyelonephritis or reflux nephropathy) is now known to result from a combination of:

● Vesicoureteric reflux, and
● Infection acquired in infancy or early childhood

Normally the vesicoureteric junction acts as a oneway valve (Fig. 9.19), urine entering the bladder from above; the ureter is shut off during bladder contraction, thus preventing reflux of urine. In some infants and children—possibly even *in utero*—this valve mechanism is incompetent, bladder voiding being associated with variable reflux of a jet of urine up the ureter. A secondary consequence is incomplete bladder emptying, as refluxed urine returns to the bladder after voiding. This latter event predisposes to infection, and the reflux of infected urine leads to kidney damage. Typically there is papillary damage, interstitial nephritis and cortical scarring in areas adjacent to 'clubbed calyces' (Fig. 9.19). Diagnosis is based on excretion urography, which shows irregular renal outlines, clubbed calyces and a variable reduction in renal size. Reflux is confirmed by micturating cystourography (see p. 433). The condition may be unilateral or bilateral and affect all or part of the kidney.

Reflux usually ceases around puberty with growth of the bladder base. Damage already done persists and progressive renal fibrosis and further loss of function occurs in severe cases even though there is no further infection. This condition does not develop in the absence of reflux and does not begin in adult life. Chronic pyelonephritis acquired in infancy predisposes to hypertension in later life and, if severe, is a relatively common cause of endstage renal failure in childhood or adult life. Early detection and treatment of infection, with or without ureteral reimplantation to create a competent valve, can prevent further scarring and allow normal growth of the kidneys.

Reinfection versus relapsing infection
When UTI is recurrent it is important to distinguish between relapse and reinfection.

Relapse is diagnosed by recurrence of bacteriuria with the *same* organism within 7 days of treatment and implies failure to eradicate infection (Fig. 9.20). It usually occurs in conditions in which it is difficult to eradicate the bacteria, e.g. stones, scarred kidneys, polycystic disease or bacterial prostatitis.

By contrast, in reinfection bacteriuria is absent after treatment for at least 14 days, usually longer, followed by recurrence of infection with the same or different organisms. This is not due to failure to eradicate infection, but is the result of reinvasion of a susceptible tract with new organisms. Approximately 80% of recurrent infections are due to reinfection.

SYMPTOMS AND SIGNS

The most typical symptoms of UTI are:

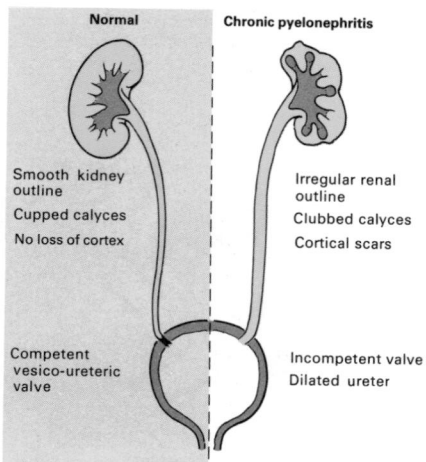

Fig. 9.19 Chronic pyelonephritis with vesicouretic reflux compared with the normal state.

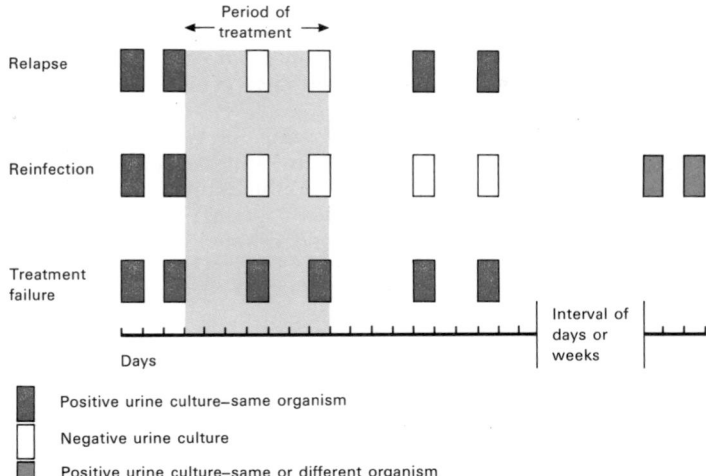

Period of treatment

Relapse

Reinfection

Treatment failure

Days

Interval of days or weeks

■ Positive urine culture–same organism

□ Negative urine culture

▨ Positive urine culture–same or different organism

Fig. 9.20 A comparison of reinfection, relapse and treatment failure in urinary tract infection.

- Frequency of micturition by day and night
- Painful voiding (dysuria)
- Suprapubic pain and tenderness
- Haematuria
- Smelly urine

These symptoms relate to bladder and urethral inflammation, commonly called 'cystitis', and suggest lower urinary tract infection. Loin pain and tenderness, with fever and systemic upset, suggest extension of the infection to the pelvis and kidney, known as pyelitis or pyelonephritis. However, localization of the site of infection on the basis of symptoms alone is unreliable.

UTI may also be present with minimal or no symptoms or may be associated with atypical symptoms such as abdominal pain, fever or haematuria in the absence of frequency or dysuria.

In small children, who cannot complain of dysuria, symptoms are often 'atypical'. The possibility of UTI must always be considered in the fretful, febrile sick child who fails to thrive.

Abacteriuric frequency or dysuria ('the urethral syndrome')
Symptoms of frequency and/or dysuria are *not* synonymous with UTI and 50% of symptomatic young women may have no demonstrable bacteriuria. Alternative causes include post-coital bladder trauma, vaginitis, atrophic vaginitis or urethritis in the elderly, and interstitial cystitis (Hunner's ulcer).

Interstitial cystitis is an uncommon but distressing complaint, most often affecting women over the age of 40 years. It presents with frequency, dysuria and often severe suprapubic pain. Urine cultures are sterile. Cystoscopy shows typical inflammatory changes with ulceration of the bladder base. The cause is unclear but it is commonly thought to be an autoimmune disorder.

Various treatments are advocated with variable success. These include oral prednisolone therapy, bladder instillation of sodium cromoglycate and bladder stretching under anaesthesia.

Careful history-taking will identify a group with predominant frequency and passing small volumes of urine who have 'irritable bladders', possibly consequent on previous UTI or conditioned by psychosexual factors. Such patients must be distinguished from those with frequency due to polyuria. Repeated courses of antibiotics in patients with abacteriuric frequency or dysuria are quite inappropriate and detract from identifying the true nature of the problem.

DIAGNOSIS

The diagnosis must be based on *quantitative* culture of a clean-catch midstream specimen of urine. Details on the collection of urine samples are given on p. 431. Once collected, samples must be sent to the laboratory immediately or refrigerated pending despatch in order to prevent further multiplication of bacteria. More than 100 000 of the same organism per millilitre of urine indicates bladder infection ('significant bacteriuria'). Lower counts may be accepted as evidence or infection in patients passing large volumes of urine. If in doubt, urine must be obtained by suprapubic bladder aspiration, when any growth of a uropathogenic organism is evidence of infection. Pyuria is not a constant feature of UTI and its absence does not exclude the diagnosis (see p. 431). Dipstick tests for nitrite have a high false-negative detection rate (p. 430).

SPECIAL INVESTIGATIONS

Excretion urography
Excretion urography is not indicated in women

with one or two isolated episodes of UTI if post-treatment urinalysis, including microscopy and urine culture, are normal. If there are further attacks or if post-treatment urinalysis is abnormal, excretion urography should be performed to identify or exclude anatomical or functional abnormalities predisposing to or complicating infection, e.g. impaired bladder emptying.

Excretion urography should be carried out in all males and children following a first proven episode of bacteriuria to identify complicating factors.

Micturating cystourography

Micturating cystourography is indicated in children with abnormal excretion urograms and may be required to evaluate abnormal bladder emptying at any age. Otherwise it is of no value in the management of UTI.

Cystoscopy

Cystoscopy in patients with known UTI has a very limited role. It is indicated only to investigate abnormal bladder or ureteral emptying, or haematuria in bacteriuric women over the age of 40 years, bladder cancer becomes more common with age. It is more commonly performed in abacteriuric frequency or dysuria to exclude bladder lesions such as carcinoma or interstitial cystitis (Hunner's ulcer).

TREATMENT

Single isolated attack

Pre-treatment urine cultures are desirable.

- If *symptoms are mild*, symptomatic treatment with potassium citrate mixture (10 ml three times daily) can be given pending the result of urine culture.
- If *symptoms are severe*, treatment with 3–5 days of amoxycillin (250 mg three times daily), nitrofurantoin (50 mg three times daily) or trimethoprim (200 mg twice daily) should be started immediately without waiting for the result of urine culture. A high (2 litres daily) fluid intake should be encouraged during treatment and for some weeks following.

  Urinalysis, microscopy and culture should be repeated 5 days after treatment. 'Single-shot' treatment with 3 g of amoxycillin, 1.92 g of co-trimoxazole or 2 g of sulphafurazole can be used for patients with bladder symptoms of less than 36 h duration who have no previous history of UTI.
- If *the patient is acutely ill* with high fever, loin pain and tenderness (acute pyelonephritis), intravenous ampicillin or amoxycillin (1 g 6-hourly) or intravenous gentamicin (2–5 mg·kg^{-1} daily in divided doses) should be given switching to a further 7 days' treatment with oral

therapy as symptoms improve. Intravenous fluids may be required to achieve a good urine output.

In patients presenting for the first time with high fever, loin pain and tenderness, urgent renal ultrasound examination is required to exclude an obstructed pyonephrosis. If this is present it should be drained by percutaneous nephrostomy.

Recurrent infection

Pre- and post-treatment urine cultures are mandatory to confirm the diagnosis and identify whether recurrent infection is due to relapse or reinfection.

In *relapse*, a search should be made for a cause, e.g. stones or scarred kidneys, and this should be eradicated if possible, for example by the removal of stones. Intense or prolonged treatment—intravenous or intramuscular aminoglycoside for 7 days or oral antibiotics for 4–6 weeks—is required. If this fails, long-term antibiotics are required.

Reinfection implies that the patient has poor defence systems; such patients must undertake prophylactic measures:

- A 2-litre daily fluid intake
- Voiding at 2–3 h intervals with double micturition if reflux is present
- Voiding before bedtime and after intercourse
- Avoidance of bubble baths and other chemicals in bath water
- Avoidance of constipation, which may impair bladder emptying

Evidence of impaired bladder emptying on excretion urography requires urological assessment. If UTI continues to recur, treatment for 6–12 months with low-dose prophylaxis (trimethoprim 100 mg, co-trimoxazole 480 mg, or nitrofurantoin 50 mg) is required; it should be taken last thing at night when urine flow is low.

Bacteriuria in pregnancy

The urine of pregnant women must always be cultured as 2–6% have asymptomatic bacteriuria. Failure to treat this may result in severe symptomatic pyelonephritis later in pregnancy, with the possibility of premature labour. Asymptomatic bacteriuria, particularly in the presence of previous renal disease, may predispose to pre-eclamptic toxaemia, anaemia of pregnancy, and small or premature babies. Therefore bacteriuria must always be treated and be shown to be eradicated. Reinfection may require prophylactic therapy. Tetracycline drugs must be avoided in pregnancy, as should trimethoprim in the first trimester and sulphonamides in the third.

Bacterial prostatitis

Bacterial prostatitis may cause relapsing infection and is difficult to treat. It presents as perineal pain, recurrent epididymo-orchitis and prostatic tenderness, with pus in expressed prostatic secretion. Treatment is with drugs that penetrate the prostate —trimethoprim, tetracylines or erythromycins—for 4–6 weeks. Long-term low-dose treatment may be required.

Renal carbuncle

Renal carbuncle is an abscess in the renal cortex caused by a blood-borne staphylococcus, usually from a boil or carbuncle of the skin. It presents with high swinging fevers, loin pain and tenderness, and fullness in the loin. The urine shows no abnormality as the abscess does not communicate with the renal pelvis, more often extending into the perirenal tissue. Staphylococcal septicaemia is common. Diagnosis is by ultrasound. Treatment involves antibacterial therapy with flucloxacillin and surgical drainage.

Tuberculosis of the urinary tract

Tuberculosis of the urinary tract should still be kept in mind in patients presenting with frequency, dysuria or haematuria, particularly in the Asian immigrant population of the UK. Cortical lesions result from haematogenous spread in the primary phase of infection. Most heal, but in some infection persists and spreads to the papillae, with the formation of cavitating lesions and the discharge of mycobacteria into the urine. Infection of the ureters and bladder commonly follows, with the potential for the development of ureteral stricture and a contracted bladder. Rarely, cold abscessses may form in the loin. In males the disease may present with testicular or epididymal discomfort and thickening.

Diagnosis depends on constant awareness, especially in patients with sterile pyuria. Excretion urography may show cavitating lesions in the renal papillary areas, commonly with calcification. There may also be evidence of ureteral obstruction with hydronephrosis. Diagnosis of active infection depends on culture of mycobacteria from early-morning urine samples.

The treatment is as for pulmonary tuberculosis (see p. 682); follow-up with excretion urography must be carried out as ureteral strictures may first develop in the healing phase.

Xanthogranulomatous pyelonephritis

This is an uncommon chronic interstitial infection of the kidney, most often due to *Proteus* spp., in which there is fever, weight loss, loin pain and a palpable enlarged kidney. It is usually unilateral and associated with staghorn calculi. CT scanning shows up intrarenal abscesses as lucent areas within the kidney. Nephrectomy is the treatment of choice; antibacterial treatment rarely, if ever, eradicates the infection.

Tubulo-interstitial nephritis

Interstitial inflammation with tubular damage is a regular feature of bacterial pyelonephritis but, contrary to former belief, it rarely, if ever, leads to chronic renal damage in the absence of reflux, obstruction or other complicating factors. However, there is growing concern that tubulo-interstitial disease due to other causes is more common than was previously diagnosed. The major stimulus for this interest came from recognition that it could be due to analgesic abuse. Subsequently, tubulo-interstitial disease due to a variety of drugs has been recognized and this condition should be considered in all patients presenting with otherwise unexplained renal failure. Presentation may be with acute, often oliguric renal failure or more commonly as chronic slowly progressive renal disease.

ACUTE TUBULO-INTERSTITIAL NEPHRITIS

Acute tubulo-interstitial nephritis is most often due to a hypersensitivity reaction to drugs (Table 9.12), most commonly drugs of the penicillin family and non-steroidal anti-inflammatory drugs (NSAIDs). Patients present with fever, arthralgia, skin rashes and acute oliguric or non-oliguric renal failure. Many have eosinophilia and eosinophiluria. Renal biopsy shows an intense interstitial cellular infiltrate, often including eosinophils, with variable tubular necrosis.

Treatment involves withdrawal of offending drugs. High-dose steroid therapy (prednisolone 60 mg daily) is commonly given but its efficacy has not been proved. Patients may require dialysis for management of the acute renal failure. Most

Table 9.12 Common causes of acute tubulo-interstitial nephritis.

Penicillins
Sulphonamides
Non-steroidal anti-inflammatory drugs
Phenindione
Allopurinol

Table 9.13 Causes of chronic tubulo-interstitial nephritis.

Common
Chronic pyelonephritis
Non-steroidal anti-inflammatory drugs
Diabetes
Sickle cell disease or trait
Cadmium or lead intoxication

Uncommon
Alport's syndrome
Balkan nephropathy
Irradiation
Sjögren's syndrome
Hyperuricaemic nephropathy

patients have good recovery of kidney function, but some may be left with significant interstitial fibrosis.

CHRONIC TUBULO-INTERSTITIAL NEPHRITIS

The major causes of chronic tubulo-interstitial nephritis are set out in Table 9.13. The patient usually either presents with polyuria and nocturia, or is found to have proteinuria or uraemia. Proteinuria is usually slight (less than 1 g per day). Papillary necrosis with ischaemic damage to the papillae occurs in a number of interstitial nephritides, e.g. in analgesic abuse, diabetes mellitus, sickle cell disease or trait. The papillae can separate and be passed in the urine. Chronic tubulo-interstitial nephritis may be associated with micro-

scopic or overt haematuria or sterile pyuria, and occasionally a sloughed papilla may cause ureteral colic or produce acute ureteral obstruction. The radiological appearances must be distinguished from those of chronic pyelonephritis (Fig. 9.21).

Tubular damage to the medullary area of the kidney leads to defects in urine concentration and sodium conservation with polyuria and salt wasting. Fibrosis progressing into the cortex leads to loss of excretory function and uraemia.

Analgesic nephropathy

The chronic consumption of *large* amounts of analgesics (especially those containing phenacetin) leads to chronic tubulo-interstitial nephritis and papillary necrosis. This also seems to be true of NSAIDs. In Australia, 20% of patients with end-stage renal failure have analgesic nephropathy.

CLINICAL FEATURES

Analgesic nephropathy is twice as common in women as in men and presents typically in middle-age. Patients are often depressed or neurotic. Presentation may be with anaemia, chronic renal failure, symptoms of urinary infection (which may be difficult to eradicate), haematuria, or urinary tract obstruction (due to sloughing of a renal papilla). Salt- and water-wasting renal disease may occur.

Chronic analgesic abuse also predisposes to the development of uroepithelial tumours.

MANAGEMENT

The consumption of analgesics should be discouraged. If necessary, dihydrocodeine, or paracetamol are reasonable alternative choices. This may result in the arrest of the disease and even in improvement in function.

Urinary tract infection, hypertension (if present) and saline depletion will require appropriate management.

The development of flank pain or an unexpectedly rapid deterioration in renal function should prompt ultrasonography or urography to screen for urinary tract obstruction due to a sloughed papilla.

Balkan nephropathy

This is a chronic tubulo-interstitial nephritis endemic in the central Danube basin in Yugoslavia, Bulgaria and Rumania. Primarily restricted to rural areas, its cause is unknown. The disease is insidious in onset, with mild proteinuria progressing to renal failure in 3 months to 10 years. Patients exhibit a high incidence of uroepithelial tumours. There is no treatment.

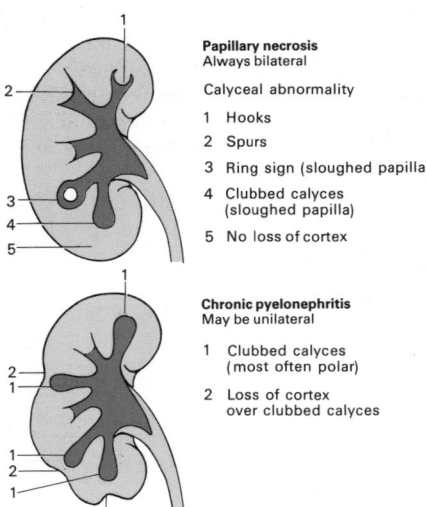

Papillary necrosis
Always bilateral

Calyceal abnormality

1 Hooks
2 Spurs
3 Ring sign (sloughed papilla)
4 Clubbed calyces (sloughed papilla)
5 No loss of cortex

Chronic pyelonephritis
May be unilateral

1 Clubbed calyces (most often polar)
2 Loss of cortex over clubbed calyces

Fig. 9.21 A comparison of radiological appearances of chronic pyelonephritis and papillary necrosis.

Other forms of chronic tubulo-interstitial nephritis are rare (see Table 9.13). Diagnosis of all forms depends on a careful history being taken, with special attention to drug taking and industrial exposure to nephrotoxins. In patients with un-explained renal impairment with normal-sized kidneys, renal biopsy must always be undertaken to exclude a treatable interstitial nephritis.

Hyperuricaemic nephropathy (gouty nephropathy)

Three patterns of renal disease have been des-cribed in patients with hyperuricaemia or hyper-uricosuria:

- Gouty or chronic hyperuricaemic nephropathy
- Acute hyperuricaemic nephropathy
- Uric acid stone formation (see p. 405)

Chronic hyperuricaemic nephropathy

Considerable controversy surrounds the possible role of chronic hyperuricaemia as a cause of tubulo-interstitial disease and progressive renal damage. While uric acid 'tophi' may be found in the kidneys of patients with gout, there is no convincing evidence that chronic hyperuricaemia *per se* causes progressive renal failure, nor that allopurinol treatment improves renal function. There is one important exception: a rare form of familial hyperuricaemia and gout occurring in adolescence is associated with renal impairment and allopurinol therapy both improves and pro-tects kidney function.

Acute hyperuricaemic nephropathy

This is a well-recognized cause of acute renal failure in patients with marked hyperuricaemia due to lympho- or myeloproliferative disorders. This may occur prior to treatment but most often occurs on commencement of treatment, when there is rapid lysis of malignant cells, release of large amounts of nucleoprotein and increased uric acid production. Renal failure is due to intra- and extrarenal obstruction caused by deposition of uric acid crystals in the collecting ducts, pelvis and ureters. The condition is manifest in oliguria or anuria with increasing uraemia. There may be flank pain or colic. Plasma urate levels are above 0.75 mmol·L^{-1} and may be as high as 4.5 mmol·L^{-1}. Diagnosis is based on the hyper-uricaemia and the clinical setting. Ultrasound demonstrates extrarenal obstruction due to stones

but a negative scan does not exclude this where there is coexistent intrarenal obstruction.

PREVENTION

It is now regular practice to prescribe allopurinol 100–200 mg three times daily for 5 days prior to and continuing throughout treatment with radio-therapy or cytotoxic drugs. A high rate of urine flow must be maintained by oral or parenteral fluid and the urine kept alkaline by the administration of sodium bicarbonate 600 mg four times daily and acetazolomide 250 mg three times daily.

TREATMENT

Allopurinol treatment should be commenced im-mediately and a forced alkaline diuresis attempted with intravenous 1.26% sodium bicarbonate plus acetazolomide (500 mg dose, then 250 mg three times daily). In severely oliguric or anuric patients, dialysis is required to lower the plasma urate, which allows urate to diffuse out of the obstructed collecting ducts into the peritubular capillaries. Percutaneous nephrostomy (see p. 464) may be required to relieve extrarenal obstruction due to stones in the pelvis or ureters. Such stones may subsequently be passed spontaneously or may require surgical removal (see p. 460).

Hypertension and the kidney

Hypertension can be the cause or the result of renal disease. It is often difficult to differentiate between the two on clinical grounds. Routine tests as described on p. 617 should be performed on all patients, but an IVU is usually unnecessary. A guide to which patients should be fully investi-gated is given on p. 827.

ESSENTIAL HYPERTENSION

PATHOPHYSIOLOGY

In *benign essential hypertension*, arteriosclerosis of major renal arteries and changes in the intrarenal vasculature (nephrosclerosis) occur as follows.

- In small vessels and arterioles, intimal thicken-ing with reduplication of the internal elastic lamina occurs and the vessel wall becomes hyalinized.
- In large vessels, concentric reduplication of the internal elastic lamina and endothelial prolifera-tion produce an 'onion skin' appearance.

- Reduction in size of both kidneys may occur; this may be asymmetrical if one major renal artery is more affected by atheromatous change than the other.
- The proportion of sclerotic glomeruli is increased compared with age-matched controls.

Deterioration in excretory function accompanies these changes, but severe renal failure requiring protein restriction is unusual in Whites. In Afro-Caribbeans, by contrast, such hypertension much more often results in the development of renal failure.

In *accelerated, or malignant phase hypertension*:

- Arteriolar fibrinoid necrosis occurs, probably as a result of plasma entering the media of the vessel through splits in the intima.
- Fibrinoid necrosis in afferent glomerular arterioles is a prominent feature.
- Fibrin deposition within small vessels is often associated with thrombocytopenia and red-cell fragmentation seen in the peripheral blood film (microangiopathic haemolytic anaemia).

Microscopic haematuria, proteinuria, usually of modest degree (1–3 g daily), and progressive uraemia occur. If untreated, fewer than 10% of patients survive 2 years.

MANAGEMENT

Management of benign essential and malignant hypertension is described on p. 617.

If treatment is begun before renal impairment has occurred, the prognosis for renal function is good. Stabilization or improvement in renal function with healing of intrarenal arteriolar lesions and resolution of microangiopathic haemolysis occur with effective treatment of malignant phase hypertension. Life-long follow-up of the patient is mandatory.

RENAL HYPERTENSION

Bilateral renal disease

Hypertension commonly complicates bilateral renal disease such as chronic glomerulonephritis, bilateral reflux nephropathy (chronic atrophic pyelonephritis of childhood), polycystic disease and analgesic nephropathy.

Two main mechanisms are responsible:

- Activation of the renin–angiotensin–aldosterone system
- Retention of salt and water with impairment in excretory function leading to an increase in blood volume and hence blood pressure

The second of these assumes greater importance as renal function deteriorates.

Hypertension occurs earlier, is more common and tends to be more severe in patients with renal cortical disorders such as glomerulonephritis than in those with disorders affecting primarily the renal interstitium, such as reflux or analgesic nephropathy.

Management is described on p. 617. Good control of the blood pressure is necessary to prevent further deterioration of renal function secondary to vascular changes produced by the hypertension itself.

Unilateral renal disease

A small proportion of cases of hypertension are due to unilateral renal disease. The main causes are:

- Unilateral renal artery stenosis due to fibromuscular hyperplasia or atheroma
- Unilateral reflux nephropathy (atrophic pyelonephritis)

Mechanism of hypertension
Unilateral renal ischaemia results in a reduction in the pressure in afferent glomerular arterioles. This leads to an increase in the production and release of renin from the juxtaglomerular apparatus (see p. 827).

Physiological changes in renal artery stenosis
In unilateral renal artery stenosis, renal perfusion pressure is reduced and nephron transit time is prolonged on the side of the stenosis; salt and water reabsorption is therefore increased. As a result, urine from the ischaemic kidney is more concentrated but has a lower sodium concentration than urine from the contralateral kidney. Inulin, creatinine and *para*-amino hippuric acid (PAH) clearances are decreased on the ischaemic side.

Screening for unilateral renovascular disease
- Rapid sequence excretion urography is still widely employed.
- Intravenously injected contrast medium is filtered at the glomerulus more slowly and concentrated within the nephron to a greater extent on the side of the stenosis. Rapid sequence films taken after injection of contrast may show a small kidney and a delayed and denser pyelogram on the side of the stenosis.
- Radionuclide studies (see p. 433) using labelled DTPA can demonstrate decreased renal perfusion on the affected side.
- Divided renal function studies that involve ureteric catherization are seldom used.
- Renal arteriography remains the gold standard for the diagnosis of renal artery stenosis.

TREATMENT

Surgical options in renal artery stenosis include transluminal angioplasty to dilate the stenotic region, reconstructive vascular surgery and nephrectomy. With good selection of patients, more than 50% are cured or improved by intervention. In recent years, increasing interest has focused upon the diagnosis and correction of unilateral and bilateral renal arterial disease with a view to improving renal perfusion and excretory function rather than to correcting hypertension alone. No test can predict the results of vascular surgery and many patients will do well on hypotensive therapy with or without surgery.

Unilateral atrophic pyelonephritis. In this condition prediction of the outcome after nephrectomy is currently not possible. The case for nephrectomy is strengthened if isotope renography demonstrates the abnormal kidney to be making an insignificant contribution to overall excretion function, particularly if the patient is young and medical treatment has proved unsatisfactory. About one-third of patients with unilateral atrophic pyleonephritis benefit from nephrectomy.

Calculi and nephrocalcinosis

RENAL AND VESICAL CALCULI

Approximately 2% of the population in the UK have a urinary tract stone at any given time. A much higher prevalence of stone disease has been recorded elsewhere, notably in the Middle East. In the Western World, most stones occur in the upper urinary tract.

The incidence of bladder stones has declined in the UK since the eighteenth and nineteenth centuries, whereas in some developing countries they are still common.

Most stones are composed of calcium oxalate and phosphate; these are commoner in men (Table 9.14). Mixed infective stones, which account for about 20% of all calculi, are twice as common in women as in men. The overall male/female ratio of stone disease is 2 : 1.

Stone disease is frequently a recurrent problem. More than 50% of patients with a calculus will have formed a further stone or stones within 10 years. The risk of recurrence increases if a metabolic or other abnormality predisposing to stone formation is present and is not modified by treatment.

Table 9.14 Type and frequency of renal stones.

Type of renal stone	Approximate frequency (%)
Calcium oxalate	65
Calcium phosphate	15
Magnesium ammonium phosphate	10–15
Uric acid	3–5
Cystine	1–2

AETIOLOGY

It is in a sense surprising that stones are not universal, since some constituents of urine are at times present in concentrations that exceed their maximum solubility in water. The presence of inhibitors of crystal formation in normal urine appears to be of importance in preventing stones.

Most stone-formers have no detectable metabolic defect, although microscopy of warm, freshly passed urine reveals both more and larger calcium oxalate crystals than are found in normal subjects. Factors predisposing to stone formation in these so-called 'idiopathic stone formers' are:

- A chemical composition of urine that favours stone crystallization
- The production of a concentrated urine as a consequence of dehydration associated with life in a hot climate or work in a hot environment
- Impairment of inhibitors that prevent crystallization in normal urine

Recognized causes of stone formation are listed in Table 9.15.

Hypercalcaemia
If the GFR is normal, hypercalcaemia inevitably leads to hypercalciuria. The common causes of hypercalcaemia leading to stone formation are:

- Primary hyperparathyroidism
- Vitamin D ingestion
- Sarcoidosis

Table 9.15 Causes of urinary tract stone formation.

Dehydration
Hypercalcaemia
Hypercalciuria
Hyperoxaluria
Hyperuricaemia and hyperuricosuria
Infection
Cystinuria
Renal tubular acidosis
Primary renal disease (polycystic kidneys, medullary sponge kidneys)

Of these, primary hyperparathyroidism (see p. 825) is the commonest cause of stones.

Hypercalciuria

This is by far the commonest metabolic abnormality detected in calcium stone-formers.

Approximately 8% of men excrete in excess of 7.5 mmol calcium per 24 h. Calcium stone formation is commoner in this group, but as most patients do not form stones the definition of 'pathological' hypercalciuria is arbitrary. A reasonable definition of pathological hypercalciuria is excretion of more than 7.5 mmol calcium per 24 h in males and more than 6.25 mmol calcium per 24 h in female stone formers.

Causes of hypercalciuria are:

- Hypercalcaemia
- An excessive dietary intake of calcium
- Excessive resorption of calcium from the skeleton, such as occurs with prolonged immobilization or weightlessness
- Idiopathic hypercalciuria

The majority of patients with idiopathic hypercalciuria can be shown to have increased absorption of calcium from the gut. Dietary calcium restriction in this group markedly reduces urinary calcium excretion. However, a proportion of these patients appear to have a renal tubular calcium leak with secondary compensatory hyperabsorption of calcium from the gut. Calcium restriction has less effect on urinary calcium excretion in this group.

Hyperoxaluria

Two inborn errors of glyoxalate metabolism that cause increased endogenous oxalate biosynthesis are known. Both are inherited in an autosomal recessive manner. In type I (primary hyperoxaluria) there is increased glycolate excretion as well as hyperoxaluria. In type II L-glycerate excretion is increased. In both types, calcium oxalate stone formation occurs.

The prognosis is poor owing to widespread calcium oxalate crystal deposition in the kidneys. Renal failure typically develops in the late teens or early twenties.

Much commoner causes of mild hyperoxaluria are:

- Excess ingestion of high oxalate-containing food, such as spinach, rhubarb and tea
- Dietary calcium restriction, with compensatory increased absorption of oxalate
- Gastrointestinal disease, such as Crohn's disease, usually with an intestinal resection and/or an ileostomy with associated increased absorption of oxalate from the gut. Dehydration secondary to fluid loss from the gut also plays a part in stone formation.

Hyperuricaemia and hyperuricosuria

Uric acid stones account for 3–5% of all stones in the UK, but in Israel the proportion is as high as 40%.

Uric acid is the end-point of purine metabolism. Hyperuricaemia (see p. 405) can occur as a primary defect in idiopathic gout, and as a secondary consequence of increased cell turnover, e.g. in myeloproliferative disorders. Increased uric acid excretion occurs in these conditions, and stones will develop in some patients. Some uric acid stone formers have hyperuricosuria without hyperuricaemia.

Dehydration alone may also cause uric acid stones to form. Patients with ileostomies are at particular risk both from dehydration and from the fact that loss of bicarbonate from gastrointestinal secretions results in the production of an acid urine (uric acid is more soluble in an alkaline than an acid medium).

Some patients with calcium stones also have hyperuricaemia and/or hyperuricaciduria; it is believed the calcium salts precipitate upon an initial nidus of uric acid in such patients.

Urinary tract infection

Mixed infective stones are composed of magnesium ammonium phosphate together with variable amounts of calcium. Such stones are often large, forming a cast of the collecting system (staghorn calculus). They are believed to form as a result of infection of the urinary tract with organisms such as *Proteus mirabilis* that hydrolyse urea, with formation of the strong base ammonium hydroxide.

$$\begin{aligned} NH_2 \\ {\large\diagdown}\; C{=}O + HOH &\rightleftharpoons 2NH_3 + CO_2 \\ NH_2 \diagup \end{aligned}$$

$$NH_2 + HOH \rightleftharpoons NH_4OH \rightleftharpoons NH_4^+ + OH^-$$

The availability of ammonium ions and the alkalinity of the urine favour stone formation. An increased amount of mucoprotein resulting from infection also creates an organic matrix on which stone formation can occur.

Cystinuria (see p. 866)

Cystinuria results in the formation of cystine stones. About 1–2% of all stones are composed of cystine.

Primary renal diseases

There is a moderate increase in prevalence of stone disease in patients with polycystic renal disease (see p. 482).

Medullary sponge kidney is another primary renal disorder associated with stones. In this congenital (though not inherited) condition there is dilatation of the collecting ducts with associated

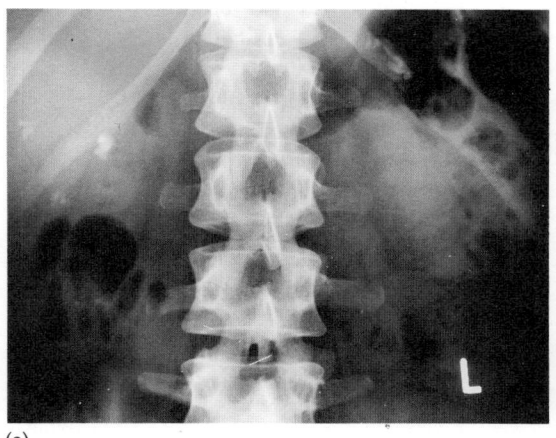
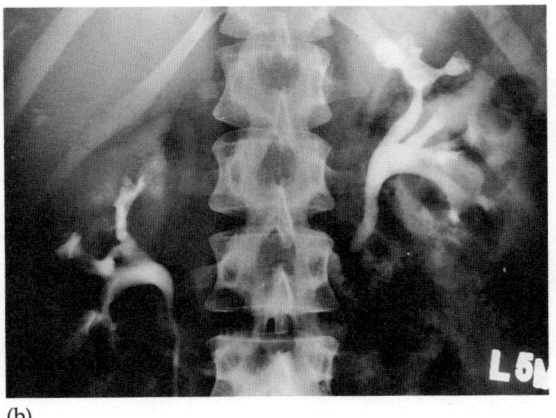

(a)   (b)

Fig. 9.22 Medullary sponge kidney. (a) Plain film showing 'spotty' calcification in the renal areas. (b) After injection of contrast, the calcification is shown to be small calculi in the papillary zones.

stasis and calcification (Fig. 9.22). Approximately 20% of these patients have hypercalciuria and a similar proportion have a renal tubular acidification defect.

The renal tubular acidoses, both inherited and acquired, are associated with nephrocalcinosis and stone formation owing, in part at least, to the production of a persistently alkaline urine and reduced urinary citrate excretion (see p. 508).

Aetiology of bladder stones
Bladder stones are endemic in some developing countries. The cause of this is unknown but dietary factors are probably important.

Stones forming in the bladder do so as a result of:

- Bladder outflow obstruction, e.g. urethral stricture, neuropathic bladder, prostatic obstruction
- The presence of a foreign body, e.g. catheters, non-absorbable sutures

Significant bacteriuria is usually found in patients with bladder stones.

Some stones found in the bladder have been passed down from the upper urinary tract.

PATHOLOGY

Stones may be single or multiple and vary enormously in size from sand-like minute particles to staghorn calculi or large stone concretions in the bladder. They may be located within the renal parenchyma or within the collecting system. Pressure necrosis from a large calculus may cause direct damage to the renal parenchyma and stones regularly cause obstruction, leading to hydronephrosis. They may ulcerate through the wall of the collecting system, including the ureter. A combination of obstruction and infection accelerates damage to the kidney.

CLINICAL FEATURES (Table 9.16)

Most people with urinary tract calculi are asymptomatic. Pain is the commonest symptom and may be sharp or dull, constant, intermittent or colicky.

When urinary tract obstruction is present, measures that increase urine volume, such as copious fluid intake or diuretics, including alcohol, make the pain worse. Physical exertion may cause mobile calculi to move, precipitating pain and, occasionally, haematuria. Calyceal colic, i.e. pain resulting from movement of stones within the calyces, is a real entity, but whether small calyceal calculi are the cause of backache or not is often difficult to decide.

Ureteric colic occurs when a stone enters the ureter and either obstructs it or causes spasm during its passage down the ureter (Fig. 9.23). This is one of the most severe pains known. Radiation from the flank to the iliac fossa and testis or labium in the distribution of the first lumbar nerve root is common. Pallor, sweating and vomiting often occur and the patient is restless, tending to assume a variety of positions in an unsuccessful attempt to obtain relief from the pain. Haematuria often occurs. Untreated, the pain of ureteric colic typically subsides after a few hours.

When urinary tract obstruction and infection are present, the features of acute pyelonephritis or of a

Table 9.16 Clinical features of urinary tract stones.

Asymptomatic
Pain—renal colic
Haematuria
Urinary tract infection
Urinary tract obstruction
Strangury

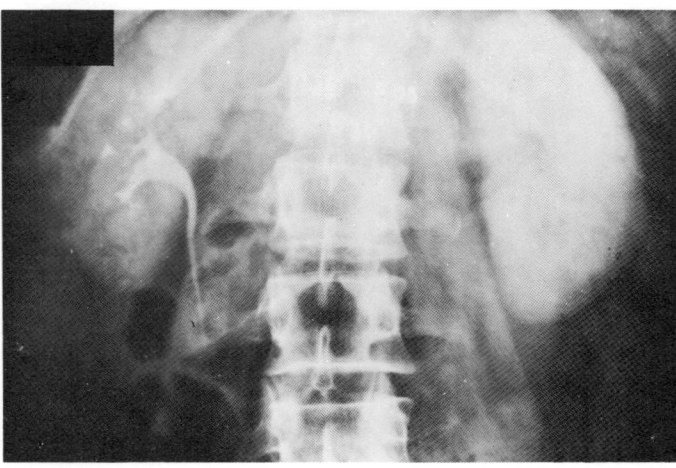

Fig. 9.23 X-ray showing acute left ureteric obstruction. Note the increased density of the nephrogram and the absence of a pyelogram on the left side 15 min after contrast injection. (From Weatherall DJ, Ledingham JGG & Warrell DA (eds) (1987) *Oxford Textbook of Medicine*, 2nd edn. Oxford: Oxford University Press. With permission.)

gram-negative septicaemia may dominate the clinical picture.

Vesical calculi associated with bladder bacteriuria may present with frequency, dysuria and haematuria; severe introital or perineal pain may occur if trigonitis is present. A calculus at the bladder neck or an obstruction in the urethra may cause bladder outflow obstruction, resulting in anuria and painful bladder distension.

Physical examination should include a search for corneal or conjunctival calcification, gouty tophi and arthritis and features of sarcoidosis.

DIAGNOSIS AND INVESTIGATION

A history of possible aetiological factors should be obtained, including:

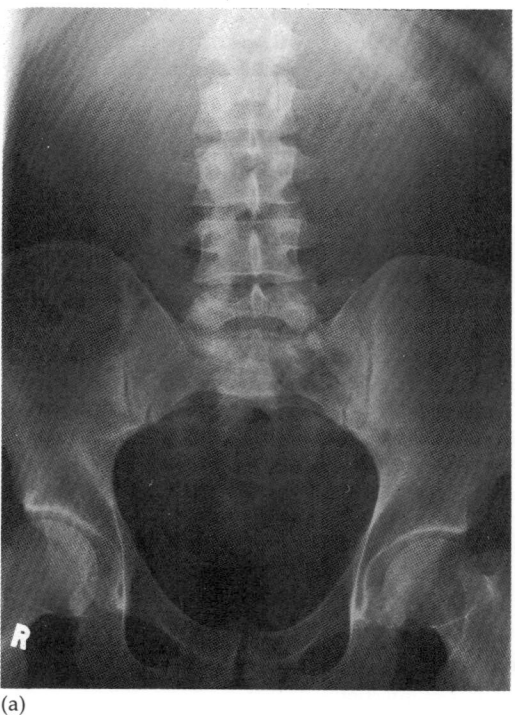

(a)

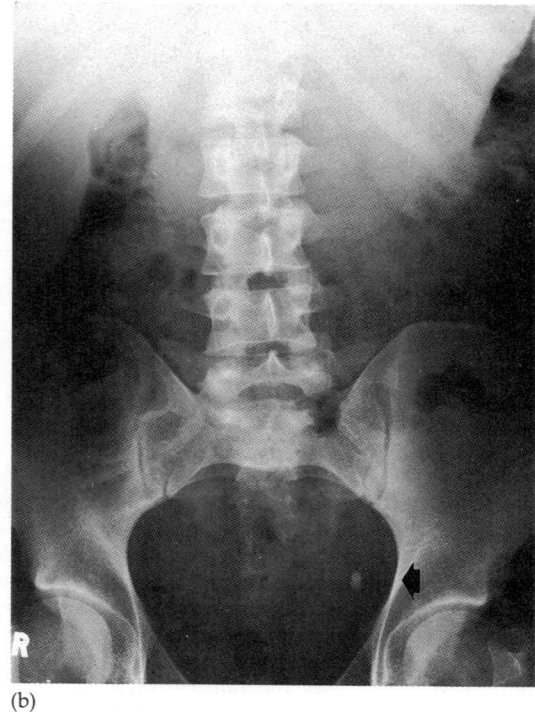

(b)

Fig. 9.24 X-rays showing calculus. (a) The calculus is overlying bone on the left (easily missed). (b) The same patient 1 week later. The calculus has descended and is easily seen in the pelvis of the left side (arrowed).

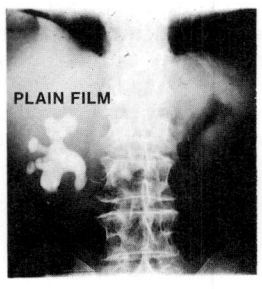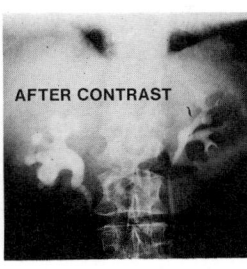

Fig. 9.25 Staghorn calculus. X-ray appearances before and after contrast on the right side are identical owing to a staghorn calculus in a non-functioning right kidney. A plain film may be confused with those taken after contrast injection.

- Occupation and residence in hot countries likely to be associated with dehydration
- A history of vitamin D consumption
- Gouty arthritis

Calcified papillae may mimic ordinary calculi, so that causes of papillary necrosis such as analgesic abuse should be considered.

Investigations should include a mid-stream specimen of urine for culture and measurement of the blood urea and electrolytes and serum creatinine and calcium levels.

Plain abdominal X-ray, renal tomography and excretion urography are the mainstay of diagnosis.

Pure uric acid stones are radiolucent. Mixed infective stones in which organic matrix predomin-ates are barely radiopaque. Calcium-containing and cystine stones are radiopaque. Calculi overlying bone are easily missed (Fig. 9.24). Staghorn calculi may be missed on excretion urography (Fig. 9.25). Uric acid stones may present as a filling defect after injection of contrast medium (Fig. 9.26). Such stones are readily seen on CT scanning (Fig. 9.27).

Excretion urography is carried out during the episode of pain; a normal urogram excludes the diagnosis of pain due to calculous disease. The urographic appearances in a patient with acute left ureteric obstruction are shown in Fig. 9.23. The urine of the patient should be passed through a sieve to trap any calculi passed for chemical analysis.

MANAGEMENT

Adequate analgesia should be given, e.g. morphine 15–30 mg i.m. repeated as necessary. Alternatively an NSAID can be tried. A high fluid intake is recommended but its efficacy is in doubt.

Stones less than 0.5 cm in diameter usually pass spontaneously and can be left. Stones greater than 1 cm in diameter usually require surgery.

Persistent pain, frequent bouts of severe pain, or anuria, are indications for operation. Intervention is also required if a stone is not moving though causing only partial obstruction in the absence of infection. With the advent of percutaneous surgery and extracorporeal shock-wave lithotripsy (see below) there has developed a trend towards earlier intervention in such cases. Complete obstruction or the coexistence of urinary tract infection with partial obstruction should prompt even earlier intervention owing to the increased risk of permanent kidney damage in these circumstances.

Stones may be removed by a cutting operation:

- Nephrolithotomy for renal calculi
- Pyelolithotomy for stones in the renal pelvis
- Ureterolithotomy for ureteric stones

Cutting operations can now be avoided by using

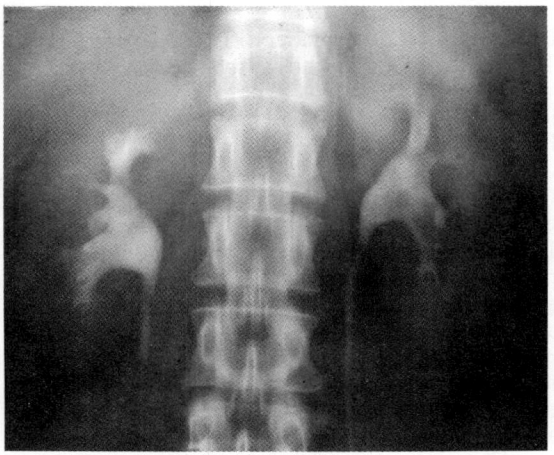

Fig. 9.26 An excretion urogram showing a lucent filling defect (uric acid stone) in the left renal pelvis. The differential diagnosis includes a sloughed papilla and a transitional cell tumour.

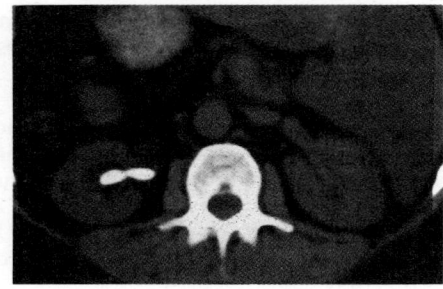

Fig. 9.27 CT scan showing a uric acid stone, which appears as a bright lesion in the left kidney.

either percutaneous nephrolithotomy or extracorporeal shock-wave lithotripsy. In the former, stones in the calyces and renal pelvis are removed by creating a percutaneous track down to the collecting system followed by endoscopic removal along this track. In the latter, shock waves generated under water are focused upon the renal calculi, causing them to fragement. Most of the fragments then pass spontaneously via the urethra. Fragments that do not pass can be removed percutaneously.

Ureteric stones may be removed endoscopically or may be pushed up into the upper urinary tract, to allow percutaneous nephrolithotomy or extracorporeal shock-wave lithotripsy.

Large renal stones need to be reduced in bulk by percutaneous means before lithotripsy can be expected to be successful. Some staghorn calculi are best dealt with by open operation.

Bladder stones can be removed endoscopically. They may be dealt with by direct electrohydraulic disintegration at cystoscopy or may be gripped in a lithotrite and crushed, the stone fragments then being washed out. Open cystotomy is required for very large bladder stones.

INVESTIGATING THE CAUSE OF STONE FORMATION

In an elderly patient who has had a single episode with one stone, further investigation is not required. Younger patients and those with recurrent stone formation require detailed investigation.

- An excretion urogram is necessary to define the presence of a primary renal disease predisposing to stone formation.
- Significant bacteriuria may indicate mixed infective stone formation but relapsing bacteriuria may be a consquence of stone formation rather than the original cause.
- Chemical analysis of any stone passed may be of great value and may be all that is required to make a diagnosis of cystinuria or uric acid stone formation.
- Serum calcium concentration should be estimated and corrected for serum albumin concentration (see p. 822). Hypercalcaemia, if present, should be investigated further (see p. 825).
- Serum urate concentration is often, but not invariably, elevated in uric acid stone formers.
- A screening test for cystinuria should be carried out by adding sodium nitroprusside to a random unacidifed urine sample; a purple colour indicates that cystinuria may be present. Urine chromatography is required to define the diagnosis precisely.

Urinary calcium, oxalate and uric acid output should be measured in two consecutive carefully collected 24-hour urine samples. After withdrawing aliquots for estimation of uric acid, it is necessary to add acid to the urine in order to prevent crystallization of calcium salts upon the walls of the collection vessel, which would give falsely low results for urinary calcium and oxalate.

- Plasma bicarbonate is low in renal tubular acidosis. The finding of a urine pH that does not fall below 5.5 in the face of metabolic acidosis is diagnostic of this condition (see p. 507).

PROPHYLAXIS

The age of the patient and the severity of the problem affect both the need for and the type of prophylaxis.

Idiopathic stone formers

Where no metabolic abnormality is present, the mainstay of prevention is maintenance of a high intake of fluid throughout the day and night. The aim should be to ensure a daily urine volume of 2–2.5 litres, which requires a fluid intake in excess of this, substantially so in the case of those who live in hot countries or work in a hot environment. A large glass of water should be drunk before retiring for the night and on waking during the night if this occurs. Special dietary measures are not warranted, although avoidance of excessive consumption of calcium-rich dairy products seems sensible.

Idiopathic hypercalciuria

Dietary calcium restriction is the first measure to be taken; particular emphasis is placed on the restriction of milk, cheese, and white bread if this is fortified (as it is in the UK) with calcium and vitamin D. Vitamin D supplements should be avoided. Dietary calcium restriction results in hyperabsorption of oxalate and foods containing large amounts of oxalate should also be limited. The advice of a dietitian is invaluable.

A high fluid intake should be advised as for idiopathic stone formers. Patients who live in a hard-water area may benefit from drinking softened water.

If hypercalciuria persists and stone formation continues, a thiazide, e.g. bendrofluazide 5 or 10 mg each morning, or sodium cellulose phosphate is used. The former reduces urinary calcium excretion by a direct effect upon the renal tubule and the latter binds calcium in the gut, thereby reducing calcium absorption. Bendrofluazide occasionally causes side-effects but is convenient to take and is inexpensive. Cellulose phosphate is not absorbed. Side-effects are mild diarrhoea and the consequences of absorption of sodium in patients with, for example, heart failure. For most patients, thiazide prophylaxis taken once daily proves more practicable than ingestion of sodium cellulose phosphate two or three times daily.

Mixed infective stones
Recurrent stones should be prevented by maintenance of a high fluid intake and meticulous control of bacteriuria. This will require long-term follow-up and may demand the use of long-term low-dose prophylactic antibacterial agents.

Uric acid stones
Dietary measures are probably of little value and are difficult to implement. Effective prevention can be achieved by the long-term use of the xanthine oxidase inhibitor allopurinol to maintain the serum urate and urinary uric acid excretion in the normal range. A high fluid intake should also be maintained. Uric acid is more soluble at alkaline pH and long-term sodium bicarbonate supplementation to maintain an alkaline urine is an alternative approach in those few patients unable to take allopurinol. However, alkalinization of the urine facilities precipitation of calcium oxalate and phosphate.

Cystine stones
These can be prevented and indeed will dissolve slowly if there is obsessional attention to maintenance of a high fluid intake—5 litres of water must be drunk each 24 h, and the patient must wake twice during the night to ingest 500 ml or more of water. Many patients cannot tolerate this regimen. An alternative, though potentially more troublesome, option is the long-term use of the chelating agent penicillamine; this causes cystine to be converted to the more soluble penicillamine–

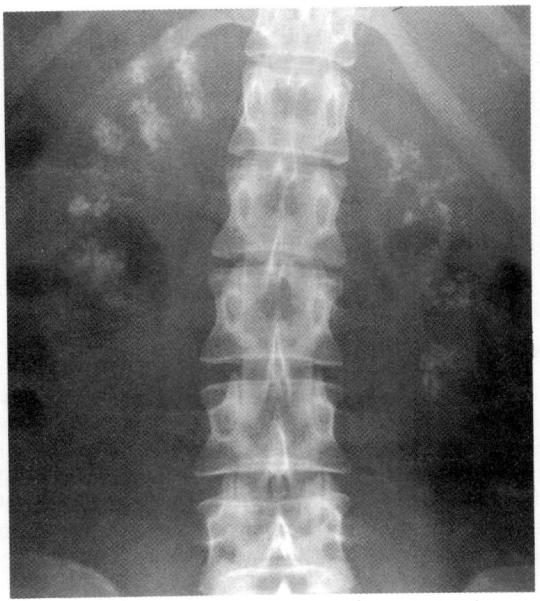

Fig. 9.28 An X-ray of nephrocalcinosis.

Table 9.17 Common causes of nephrocalcinosis.

Mainly cortical (rare)
Renal cortical necrosis (tram-line calcification)

Mainly medullary
Hypercalcaemia (primary hyperparathyroidism, hypervitaminosis D, sarcoidosis)
Renal tubular acidosis (inherited and acquired)
Primary hyperoxaluria
Medullary sponge kidney

cysteine complex. Side-effects include drug rashes, blood dyscrasias and immune complex-mediated glomerulonephritis and are by no means uncommon. In addition, the drug is expensive. It is, however, especially effective in promoting dissolution of cystine stones already present.

Mild hyperoxaluria with calcium oxalate stones
A high fluid intake and dietary oxalate restriction are required.

NEPHROCALCINOSIS

The term nephrocalcinosis means diffuse renal parenchymal calcification detectable radiologically (Fig. 9.28). The condition is typically painless. Hypertension and renal impairment commonly occur.

The main causes of nephrocalcinosis are listed in Table 9.17.

Dystrophic calcification occurs following renal cortical necrosis. In hypercalcaemia and hyperoxaluria, deposition of calcium oxalate results from the high concentration of calcium and oxalate within the kidney.

In renal tubular acidosis (see p. 507) failure of urinary acidification and a reduction in urinary citrate excretion both favour calcium phosphate and oxalate precipitation, since precipitation occurs more readily in an alkaline medium and the calcium-chelating action of urinary citrate is reduced.

Treatment and prevention of nephrocalcinosis consists of treatment of the cause.

Urinary tract obstruction

The urinary tract may be obstructed at any point between the kidney and the urethral meatus. This results in dilatation of the tract above the obstruction. Dilatation of the renal pelvis is known as hydronephrosis.

Table 9.18 Causes of urinary tract obstruction.

Within the lumen
Calculus
Blood clot
Sloughed papilla (diabetes; analgesic abuse; sickle
   cell disease or trait)
Tumour of renal pelvis or ureter
Bladder tumour

Within the wall
Pelvi-ureteric neuromuscular dysfunction
   (congenital, 10% bilateral)
Ureteric stricture (tuberculosis, especially after
   treatment; calculus; after surgery)
Ureterovesical stricture (congenital; ureterocele;
   calculus; schistosomiasis)
Congenital megaureter
Congenital bladder neck obstruction
Neuropathic bladder
Urethral stricture (calculus; gonococcal; after
   instrumentation)
Congenital urethral valve
Pin-hole meatus

Pressure from outside
Pelvi-ureteric compression (bands; aberrant vessels)
Tumours (e.g. retroperitoneal tumour or glands,
   carcinoma of colon, diverticulitis, aortic aneurysm)
Retroperitoneal fibrosis
Accidental ligation of ureter
Retrocaval ureter (right-sided obstruction)
Prostatic obstruction
Tumours in pelvis (e.g. carcinoma of cervix)
Phimosis

AETIOLOGY

Obstructing lesions may lie within the lumen, in the wall of the urinary tract, or outside the wall, causing obstruction by external pressure. The major causes of obstruction are shown in Table 9.18. Overall the frequency is the same in men and women. However, in the elderly, urinary tract obstruction is more common in men owing to the frequency of bladder outflow obstruction.

PATHOPHYSIOLOGY

Obstruction with continuing urine formation results in:

- Progressive rise in intraluminal pressure
- Dilatation proximal to the site of obstruction
- Compression and thinning of the renal parenchyma, eventually reducing it to a thin rim and resulting in a decrease in the size of the kidney

CLINICAL FEATURES

Symptoms
Upper tract obstruction. Loin pain occurs and can be dull or sharp, constant or intermittent. It may be provoked by measures that increase urine volume and hence distension of the collecting system, such as a high fluid intake or diuretics, including alcohol.

Complete anuria is strongly suggestive of complete bilateral obstruction or complete obstruction of a single kidney.

Conversely, polyuria may occur in partial obstruction owing to impairment of renal tubular concentrating capacity. Intermittent anuria and polyuria indicates intermittent complete obstruction.

Infection complicating the obstruction may give rise to malaise, fever and septicaemia.

Bladder outflow obstruction. Symptoms may be minimal. Hesitancy, narrowing and diminished force of the urinary stream, terminal dribbling and a sense of incomplete bladder emptying are typical features. The frequent passage of small volumes of urine occurs if a large volume of residual urine remains in the bladder after urination. Incontinence of such small volumes of urine is known as 'overflow incontinence' or 'retention with overflow'.

Infection commonly occurs, causing increased frequency, urgency, urge incontinence, dysuria and the passage of cloudy smelly urine. It may precipitate acute retention.

Signs
Loin tenderness may be present. An enlarged hydronephrotic kidney may be palpable.

In acute or chronic retention the enlarged bladder may be felt or percussed.

Examination of the genitalia, rectum and vagina are essential, since prostatic obstruction and pelvic malignancy are common causes of urinary tract obstruction. However, the apparent size of the prostate on digital examination is a poor guide to the presence of prostatic obstruction.

INVESTIGATION

Routine blood and biochemical investigations may be abnormal, e.g. there may be a raised blood urea or serum creatinine, hyperkalaemia, anaemia of chronic disease or blood in the urine, but the diagnosis of obstruction cannot be made on these tests alone and further investigations must be performed.

Ultrasonography (see p. 432)
This is a reliable means of ruling out upper urinary tract dilatation. Ultrasound cannot distinguish a

baggy, low-pressure unobstructed system from a tense, high-pressure obstructed one, so that false-positive scans are seen. However, a normal scan does rule out urinary tract obstruction.

Radionuclide studies (see p. 434)

In obstructive nephropathy, the relative uptake may be normal or reduced on the side of obstruction, peak activity may be delayed and parenchymal (as distinct from pelvic) transit time prolonged. If doubt exists as to whether obstruction at the pelviureteric junction is present, frusemide may be administered; satisfactory 'washout' of radionuclide rules out obstruction and vice versa. In general, absence of uptake of radiopharmaceutical indicates renal damage sufficiently severe to render correction of obstruction unprofitable.

Excretion urography

This is the most widely used investigation. Urography can usually exclude obstruction even in the presence of severe renal failure, provided that a high dose of contrast medium, renal tomography and, if necessary, delayed films are employed.

A plain film is necessary to detect calcification. However, calculi overlying bone are easily missed.

In recent unilateral obstruction, the affected kidney is enlarged and smooth in outline. The nephrogram is delayed due to a reduction in the GFR. The calyces and pelvis fill with contrast medium later than on the normal side.

In time the nephrogram on the affected side becomes denser than normal, owing to the prolonged nephron transit time, which allows greater than normal concentration of contrast medium within the tubules. Later, the site of obstruction may be seen, with dilatation of the system proximal to the level of the block (Fig. 9.29).

A full-length film should be taken after an attempt at bladder emptying by the patient. Complete emptying indicates either that no obstruction to bladder outflow exists or that intravesicular pressure can be raised sufficiently to overcome it. Apparent bladder outflow impairment may be the result of nervousness or embarrassment on the part of the patient or failure to carry out the X-ray before the bladder has refilled with contrast medium from above, or may be due to an atonic but non-obstructed bladder. Vesicoureteric reflux can result in contrast medium returning to the bladder from above, giving the appearance of a partially full bladder.

Antegrade pyelography and ureterography (see p. 433)

This defines the site and cause of obstruction. It

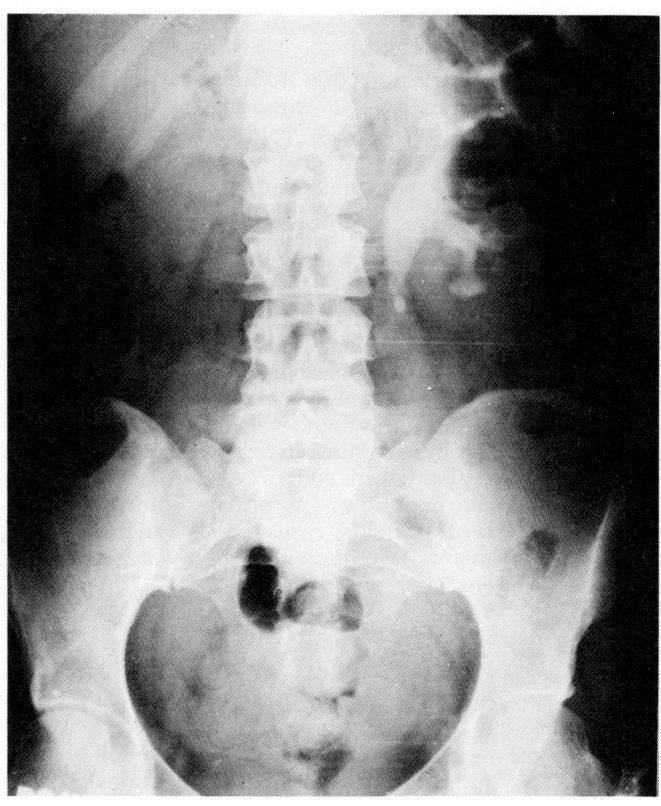

Fig. 9.29 An X-ray taken 24 h after injection of contrast, showing a delayed nephrogram and pyelogram on the left side and dilatation of the system to the level of the block. By this time contrast medium has disappeared from the normal right side. (From Weatherall DJ, Ledingham JGG & Warrell DA (eds) (1987) *Oxford Textbook of Medicine*, 2nd edn. Oxford: Oxford University Press. With permission.)

can be combined with drainage of the collecting system by percutaneous needle nephrostomy.

Retrograde ureterography (see p. 433)

This is indicated if antegrade examination cannot be carried out or if there is the possibility of dealing with ureteric obstruction from below at the time of examination. The technique carries the risk of introducing infection into an obstructed urinary tract.

In obstruction due to neuromuscular dysfunction at the pelviureteric junction or retroperitoneal fibrosis, the collecting system may fill normally from below.

Cystoscopy, urethroscopy and urethrography

Obstructing lesions within the bladder and urethra can be seen directly by endoscopic examination.

Urethrography involves introducing contrast medium into the bladder by catheterization or suprapubic bladder puncture, and taking X-ray films during voiding to show obstructing lesions in the urethra. It is of particular value in the diagnosis of urethral valves and strictures.

Pressure-flow studies

Pressure changes within the bladder during filling and emptying can be recorded. Demonstration that a high voiding pressure is required to maintain urine flow is indicative of bladder outflow obstruction. This may be combined with video cystography and urethrography to define the site of obstruction.

Normally, while the bladder is being filled there is only a small pressure rise before the voluntary initiation of urination. Uninhibited contractions of the detrusor muscle during filling may be seen in upper motor neurone bladder neuropathy, such as occurs in multiple sclerosis. Less commonly, a neuropathic bladder may be 'hypotonic', readily accepting large volumes of fluid before the initiation of weak contractions at a low intravesical pressure. A common cause of such lower motor neurone bladder neuropathy is diabetes mellitus.

Pressure-flow and video studies may enable a logical decision to be taken as to whether surgery to relieve bladder outflow impairment should be carried out.

TREATMENT

Aims

Treatment involves:

- Relieving the obstruction
- Treating the underlying cause
- Preventing and treating infection

The ultimate aim of treatment is to relieve symptoms and to preserve renal function.

Temporary external drainage of urine by neph-

rostomy may be valuable, as this allows time for further investigation when the site and nature of the obstructing lesion is uncertain and doubt exists as to the viability of the obstructed kidney, or when immediate definitive surgery would be hazardous.

Recent, complete upper urinary tract obstruction demands urgent relief to preserve kidney function, particularly if infection is present.

In contrast, with partial urinary tract obstruction, particularly if spontaneous relief is expected, e.g. by passage of a calculus, there is no immediate urgency.

Surgical management

This depends on the cause of the obstruction (see below). Dialysis may be required in the ill patient prior to surgery.

Nephrectomy or nephroureterectomy is justified when obstruction is due to malignant disease or when it is judged that no worthwhile amount of renal excretory function will be conserved by, or will return after, relief of obstruction.

Permanent urinary diversion is required when the obstruction cannot be relieved; in such cases malignant disease is usually present. Ureteric anastomosis to an ileal conduit opening on to the abdominal wall is often a satisfactory method of diversion. In some patients, obstruction is best relieved by the insertion of indwelling catheters or stents into the ureter. An obstruction high in the urinary tract may require a permanent nephrostomy.

In obstruction due to untreatable malignant disease it is wise to consider carefully whether urinary diversion is justified, since this may exchange a pain-free death from renal failure for a painful one with malignant invasion of bones or nerves.

Diuresis usually follows relief of obstruction at any site in the urinary tract. Massive diuresis may occur due to previous sodium and water overload and the osmotic effect of retained solutes combined with a defective renal tubular reabsorptive capacity (as in the diuretic phase of recovering acute tubular necrosis). This diuresis is associated with increased blood volume and high levels of ANP. The diuresis is usually self-limiting, but a minority of patients will develop severe sodium, water and potassium depletion requiring appropriate intravenous replacement. In milder cases oral salt and potassium supplements together with a high water intake are sufficient.

Specific causes of obstructions

Calculi

These are discussed on p. 455.

Pelvi-ureteric junction obstruction (Fig. 9.30)

This appears to result from a functional disturbance in peristalsis of the collecting system in the absence of mechanical obstruction. Typically, a circular inelastic ring of collagen tissue is present at the pelviureteric junction. Surgical attempts at correction of the obstruction by open or percutaneous pyeloplasty should be limited to patients with recurrent loin pain and those in whom serial excretion urography, background-subtraction isotope renography or measurements of GFR indicate progressive kidney damage. Nephrectomy to remove the risk of developing pyonephrosis and septicaemia is indicated if long-standing obstruction has destroyed kidney function.

Obstructive megaureter

This childhood condition may only become evident in adult life. It results from the presence of a region of defective peristalsis at the lower end of the ureter adjacent to the ureterovesical junction. The condition is commoner in males. It presents with urinary tract infection, flank pain or haematuria.

The diagnosis is made on excretion urography or, if necessary, ascending ureterography. Excision of the abnormal portion of ureter with reimplantation into the bladder is always indicated in children, and is indicated in adults when the condition is associated with evidence of progressive deterioration in renal function, bacteriuria that cannot be controlled by medical means or recurrent stone formation.

Retroperitoneal fibrosis

In this condition the ureters become embedded in dense retroperitoneal fibrous tissue with resultant unilateral or bilateral obstruction. The condition may extend from the level of the second lumbar vertebra to the pelvic brim. The incidence of the condition in men is three times that in women. The majority of cases are of unknown aetiology; it has been suggested that the fundamental problem is immunologically mediated peri-aortitis. Recognized associations are with retroperitoneal lymph-

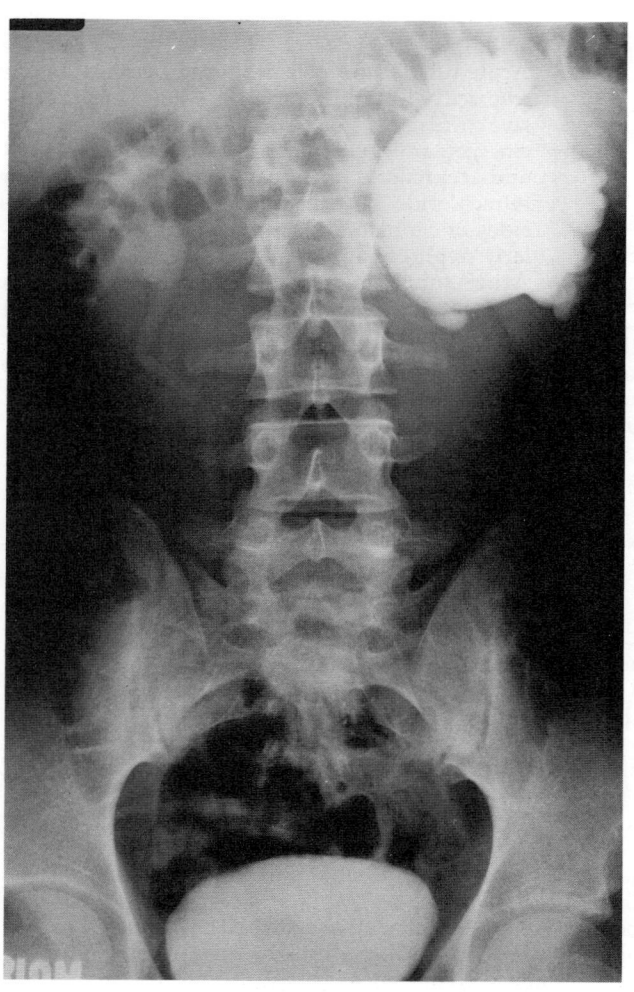

Fig. 9.30 An X-ray showing left pelvi-ureteric junction obstruction.

oma, carcinoma of the bladder or colon, abdominal aortic aneurysm and prolonged exposure to the drug methysergide.

Malaise, back pain, normochromic anaemia, uraemia and a raised ESR are typical features. Excretion urography shows bilateral but usually asymmetrical obstruction to the ureter commencing at the level of the pelvic brim. A peri-aortic mass may be seen on a CT scan.

Obstruction is relieved surgically by ureterolysis. Biopsy should be performed at operation to determine whether there is an underlying lymphoma or carcinoma. Corticosteroids are of benefit, and in bilateral obstruction in frail patients it may be best to free only one ureter and to rely upon steroid therapy to induce regression of fibrous tissue on the contralateral side, since bilateral ureterolysis is a major operation. In some patients, surgery alone or steroid therapy alone may suffice, but in the majority both surgery and subsequent corticosteroid therapy appear to be necessary.

Response to treatment and disease activity are assessed by serial measurements of ESR and GFR supplemented by isotopic and imaging techniques including CT scanning. The latter method enables the size of the retroperitoneal mass to be assessed. Relapse after withdrawal of steroid therapy may occur and treatment may need to be continued for years. Long-term follow-up is mandatory.

Benign prostatic hypertrophy
Benign prostatic hypertrophy is a common cause of urinary tract obstruction. It is described on p. 486.

Prognosis of urinary tract obstruction

The prognosis depends upon the cause and the stage at which obstruction is relieved. In obstruction, four factors influence the rate at which kidney damage occurs, its extent and the degree and rapidity of recovery of renal function after relief of obstruction. These are:

- Whether obstruction is partial or complete
- The duration of obstruction
- Whether or not infection occurs
- The site of obstruction

Complete obstruction for several weeks will lead to irreversible or only partially reversible kidney damage. If the duration of complete obstruction is several months, total irreversible destruction of the affected kidney will result.

Partial obstruction carries a better prognosis, depending upon its severity.

Bacterial infection coincident with obstruction rapidly increases kidney damage.

Obstruction at or below the bladder neck may induce hypertrophy and trabeculation of the bladder without a rise in pressure within the upper urinary tract, in which case the kidneys are protected from the effects of back-pressure.

Drugs and the kidney

Drug-induced impairment of renal function

Prerenal
Impaired perfusion of the kidneys can result from drugs that cause:

- Hypovolaemia due to:
    potent loop diuretics such as frusemide, especially in elderly patients
    renal salt and water loss, e.g. from hypercalcaemia induced by vitamin D therapy (since hypercalcaemia affects adversely renal tubular salt and water conservation)
- Decrease in cardiac output, which impairs renal perfusion, e.g. due to beta-blockers
- Decreased renal blood flow, e.g. angiotensin-converting enzyme inhibitors

Renal
Several mechanisms of drug-induced renal damage exist and may co-exist. These include:

- Acute tubular necrosis produced by direct nephrotoxicity. Examples include prolonged or excessive treatment with aminoglycosides (kanamycin, gentamicin, streptomycin), amphotericin B and cephaloridine, heavy metals or carbon tetrachloride. The combination of aminoglycosides or cephaloridine with frusemide is particularly nephrotoxic (see p. 739).
- Acute tubulo-interstitial nephritis (see p. 451) with interstitial oedema and inflammatory cell infiltration. This cell-mediated hypersensitivity nephritis occurs with many drugs, including penicillins, particularly methicillin, sulphonamides and some NSAIDS.
- Chronic tubulo-interstitial nephritis due to drugs (see p. 452).
- Immune complex-mediated glomerulonephritis. Examples include penicillamine.

Postrenal
Retroperitoneal fibrosis with urinary tract obstruction may result from the use of methysergide.

Use of drugs in patients with impaired renal function

Many aspects of drug handling are altered in patients with renal impairment.

Absorption. This may be unpredictable in uraemia as nausea and vomiting are frequently present.

Metabolism. Oxidative metabolism of drugs by the liver may be altered in uraemia. This is rarely of clinical significance.

The rate of drug metabolism by the kidney may be reduced as a result of:

- *Reduced drug catabolism.* Insulin, for example, is in part catabolized by the normal kidney. In renal disease, insulin catabolism is reduced. The insulin requirements of diabetics decline as renal function deteriorates for this reason.
- Reduced conversion of a precursor to a more active metabolite, e.g. the conversion of 25-hydroxycholecalciferol to the more active 1,25-dihydroxycholecalciferol. The 1-hydroxylase enzyme responsible for this conversion is located in the kidney. In renal disease, production of the enzyme declines and deficiency of 1,25 dihydroxycholecalciferol results.

Protein binding. Reduced protein binding of a drug potentiates its activity and increases the potential for toxic side-effects. Measurement of the total plasma concentration of such a drug can give misleading results. For example, the serum concentration of phenytoin required to produce an antiepileptic effect is much higher in normal individuals than in those with renal failure, since in the latter proportionately more drug is present in the free form.

Some patients with renal disease are hypoproteinaemic and reduced drug-binding to protein results. This is not the sole mechanism of reduced drug-binding in such patients. For example, hydrogen ions, which are retained in renal failure, bind to receptors for acidic drugs such as sulphonamides, penicillin and salicylates, thus enhancing their potential for causing toxicity.

Volume of distribution. Salt and water overload or depletion may occur in patients with renal disease. This affects the concentration of drug obtained from a given dose.

End organ sensitivity. The renal response to drug treatment may be reduced in renal disease. For example, mild thiazide diuretics have little diuretic effect in patients with severe renal impairment.

Renal elimination. By far the most important problem in the use of drugs in renal failure concerns the reduced elimination of many drugs normally excreted by the kidneys.

Water-soluble drugs such as gentamicin that are poorly absorbed from the gut, typically given by injection and are not metabolized by the liver give rise to far more problems than lipid-soluble drugs such as propranolol, which are well-absorbed and principally metabolized by the liver. Metabolites of lipid-soluble drugs, however, may themselves be water-soluble and potentially toxic.

Safe prescribing in renal disease

Safe prescribing in renal failure demands knowledge of the clinical pharmacology of the drug and its metabolites in normal individuals and in uraemia. The clinician should ask the following questions when prescribing:

1 Is treatment mandatory?
  Unless it is, it should be withheld.
2 Can the drug reach its site of action?
  For example, there is little point in prescribing the urinary antiseptic nitrofurantoin in renal failure since bacteriostatic concentrations will not be attained in the urine.
3 Is the drug's metabolism altered in uraemia?
4 Will accumulation of the drug or metabolites occur?
  Even if accumulation is a potential problem owing to the drug or its metabolites being excreted by the kidneys, it is not necessarily an indication to change the drug given. The size of the loading dose will depend upon the size of the patient and is unrelated to renal function. Avoidance of toxic levels of drug in blood and tissues subsequently requires the administration of normal doses of the drug at longer time intervals than usual or smaller doses at the usual time intervals.
5 Is the drug toxic?
6 Are the effective concentrations of the drug in biological tissues similar to the toxic concentrations?
7 Should blood levels of the drug be measured?
8 Will the drug worsen the uraemic state by means other than nephrotoxicity, e.g. steroids, tetracycline?
9 Is the drug a sodium or potassium salt?
  These are potentially hazardous in uraemia.

Not surprisingly, adverse drug reactions are more than twice as common in renal failure as in normal individuals. Careful attention to the above and careful titration of the dose of drugs employed should reduce this problem.

The dose may be titrated by:

- Observation of its clinical effect, e.g. hypotensive agents
- Early detection of toxic effects
- Measurement of drug levels in the blood, e.g. gentamicin levels

---

Drugs causing uraemia by effects upon protein anabolism and catabolism

Tetracyclines with the exception of doxycycline, have an antianabolic effect and as a result the concentration of nitrogenous waste products is increased. They may also cause impairment of GFR by a direct effect. Corticosteroids have a catabolic effect and so also increase the production of nitrogenous wastes. A patient with moderate impairment of renal function may therefore become severely uraemic if given tetracyclines or corticosteroid therapy.

Drugs and toxic agents causing specific renal tubular syndromes include mercury, lead, cadmium and vitamin D.

Problem patients

Particular problems are presented by patients in whom renal function is altering rapidly, such as those with recovering acute tubular necrosis and those on regular dialysis treatment. In addition, drugs may be removed by dialysis, which will affect the dosage required.

Renal failure

Renal impairment describes a reduction in renal excretory or regulatory function without elevation of the blood urea or serum creatinine. *Renal failure* or *uraemia* describe more severe functional impairment when blood urea and serum creatinine are elevated. The development of 'renal hypertension' can occur early in renal disease, but disturbances of endocrine or metabolic function are usually only seen in renal failure.

Acute renal failure (ARF) is the loss of renal function developing over days or a few weeks. *Chronic renal failure (CRF)* is the loss of function developing over a period of months or years.

Acute deterioration in function may occur on a background of known or unknown chronic renal failure and is known as 'acute-on-chronic' renal failure.

Causes of renal failure

Renal failure, whether acute or chronic, may be due to prerenal, renal or postrenal causes or some combination of these:

- *Prerenal* causes are a reduction in renal blood flow, for a variety of reasons, increased production of waste products, or both (Table 9.19).
- *Renal* causes are intrinsic diseases of the kidneys themselves. These can be subdivided into glomerular, tubulo-interstitial or vascular disease (Table 9.20).

  Also included under this heading are functional disturbances of intrarenal blood flow. Thus, certain drugs such as angiotensin-converting enzyme (ACE) inhibitors or non-steroidal anti-inflammatory drugs (NSAIDs) may affect intrarenal blood flow and reduce GFR. This is usually only functionally significant in the presence of established intrinsic renal disease or renal artery stenosis.
- *Postrenal* causes are diseases leading to obstruction to urine outflow (obstructive nephropathy; Fig. 9.31).

Table 9.19 Pre-renal causes of renal failure.

Circulatory failure
Volume depletion with inadequate replacement
  Vomiting and diarrhoea
  Fistula drainage
  Polyuria (diuretics, diabetic ketoacidosis, post-
    obstruction)
Shock
  Haemorrhage
  Septicaemia
  Extensive burns
Cardiac failure
Severe liver failure (hepato-renal syndrome)
Renal artery obstruction

Increased production of waste products (urea)

Infection/tissue damage	Uraemia unusual
Upper gastrointestinal bleeding	unless there is
Steroid therapy	also failure of
Tetracyclines	excretion

Table 9.20 Renal causes of renal failure.

Glomerular
Glomerulonephritis
  Primary
  Part of a systemic vasculitis (systemic lupus
    erythematosus, polyarteritis nodosa, Wegener's
    granulomatosis)
Diabetic nephropathy
Amyloidosis

Tubulo-interstitial
Acute tubular necrosis
  Shock
  Ischaemia/hypoxia
  Drugs
  Chemical poisons
Acute cortical necrosis
Acute and chronic tubulo-interstitial nephritis
Congenital/inherited
  Medullary cystic disease
  Polycystic disease

Vascular
Hypertensive nephrosclerosis
Polyarteritis
Atheroma kidney

Functional
ACE Inhibitors
NSAIDs

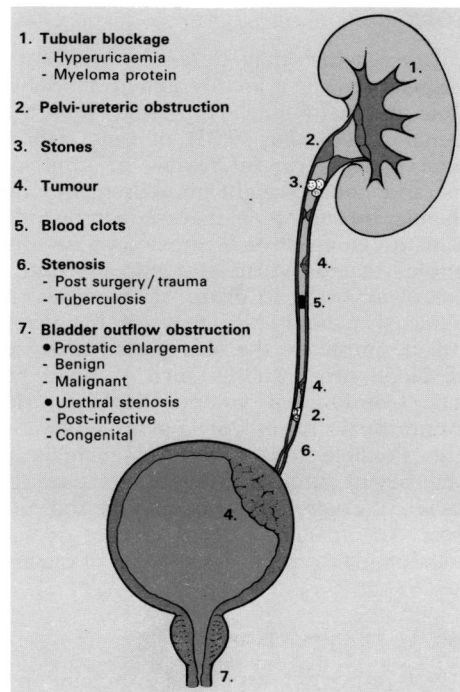

1. **Tubular blockage**
   - Hyperuricaemia
   - Myeloma protein

2. **Pelvi-ureteric obstruction**

3. **Stones**

4. **Tumour**

5. **Blood clots**

6. **Stenosis**
   - Post surgery / trauma
   - Tuberculosis

7. **Bladder outflow obstruction**
   ● Prostatic enlargement
   - Benign
   - Malignant
   ● Urethral stenosis
   - Post-infective
   - Congenital

Fig. 9.31 Postrenal causes of renal failure (obstructive nephropathy).

Acute or acute-on-chronic renal failure

Glomerulonephritis, acute tubulo-interstitial nephritis and obstructive nephropathy are the commonest causes of acute renal failure (ARF) in domiciliary practice, while acute volume depletion and acute tubular necrosis are more often seen in hospital practice.

The major functional and clinical sequelae of ARF are set out in Table 9.21.

In *domiciliary practice* ARF most often presents:

● As acute oliguria with or without haematuria
● With fluid retention (peripheral oedema or increasing breathlessness)
● With uraemia, giving rise to anorexia, nausea and vomiting

Occasionally the picture is dominated by symptoms of hypertension such as headaches and impaired vision. The clinical features may also be related to any systemic disease causing the renal failure. Examples include:

● The generalized rash and polyarthropathy occurring with drug hypersensitivity
● The muscle pain due to rhabdomyolysis occurring with heroin abuse
● The dyspnoea and haemoptysis occurring in Goodpasture's syndrome

In *hospital practice* ARF usually presents with increasing uraemia or with oliguria. It most often develops in a setting of severe illness in association with shock, recent major surgery or trauma, or sepsis.

Prerenal causes are common from fluid loss due to:

● Diuretics
● Gut losses
● Polyuria following the relief of urinary obstruction

The various diseases causing *intrinsic* renal failure are discussed under their relevant sections. Special mention must at this point be made of acute tubular necrosis and acute cortical necrosis.

Table 9.21 Major functional and clinical sequelae of acute renal failure.

Functional changes	Clinical sequelae
Loss of excretory function	
Retention of waste products (e.g. urea, creatinine, phosphate)	Uraemic symptoms (anorexia, nausea, vomiting) Bleeding tendency Impaired resistance to infection Reduced wound healing
Retention of drugs	Drug toxicity
Loss of regulatory function	
Retention of sodium chloride and water	Oedema (peripheral, pulmonary, cerebral) Hypertension
Retention of potassium	Cardiac arrhythmias
Retention of fixed acid	Acidotic breathing Arrhythmia in patients with ischaemic heart disease

Acute tubular necrosis (ATN)

ATN is a condition in which there is acute tubular cell damage. It accounts for some 75% of cases of ARF seen in hospital practice. Known as the 'crush syndrome' in World War II, it was originally ascribed to a mixture of hypoxic damage to the metabolically active tubular cells during periods of shock and reduced renal blood flow plus tubular cell injury due to myoglobin released from crushed muscle. It is now known to occur in a variety of situations where there is reduced renal perfusion with or without major trauma or sepsis, as well as following the administration of certain drugs or exposure to chemical toxins.

ATN is characterized by acute, usually oliguric, potentially reversible renal failure. The oliguria is due to a variable combination of tubular cell necrosis, tubular obstruction caused by cell debris and, possibly most importantly, reduced cortical perfusion due to arteriolar vasoconstriction. Urine output decreases over 1–5 days to severe oliguria (< 300 ml urine per day). Urine osmolality is low (< 350 mosmol·kg^{-1}). There is commonly mild proteinuria on Stix testing and microscopy shows granular or tubular cell casts. The urine/plasma creatinine concentration ratio is usually less than 20 and the urinary sodium concentration more than 50 mmol·L^{-1}. Serial measurement shows a rise in blood urea and serum creatinine and, in oliguric patients with tissue injury, there may be a rapid rise in serum potassium.

Symptoms and signs of uraemia and fluid overload are often dominated by those of the causal condition, e.g. major trauma or septicaemia. Occasionally urine output is maintained (non-oliguric ATN), the dominant features being progressive moderate uraemia. Hyperkalaemia and fluid overload are less likely to occur in this situation.

Acute cortical necrosis

Acute cortical necrosis may be considered a more extreme form of ATN due to more severe and prolonged ischaemia. It mainly occurs in association with abruptio placentae, but it also occurs occasionally (1–2%) as a result of other circumstances that may cause ATN. It is characterized by extensive necrosis of the cortical tissue and acute oliguric renal failure. There is little potential for recovery; limited recovery of function, depending on subcapsular or juxtamedullary nephrons, may be achieved, but many cases require permanent renal replacement therapy. The diagnosis of acute cortical necrosis is usually suspected if there is a history of abruptio placentae or if there is failure to recover renal function after 30 days of suspected ATN. It can be confirmed by renal biopsy. Occasionally X-ray evidence of linear cortical calcification may develop after 4–8 weeks.

HISTORY

The history, which may be taken from the patient or his relatives, is primarily aimed at identifying possible prerenal (Table 9.19), renal (Table 9.20) or postrenal causes (Fig. 9.31) of renal failure. In hospital patients careful review of input–output charts and serial weight measurements can be invaluable. Intrinsic renal disease may be indicated by a history suggestive of previous renal disease, symptoms suggestive of systemic vasculitis or a history of exposure to drugs or chemicals. In the hospitalized patient ARF may be insidious and identified simply by the observation of a steadily rising blood urea. Causes such as heart failure, diuretic overdose or volume depletion due to gastrointestinal losses or polyuria should be sought. Possible causes of ATN such as severe trauma, recent surgery, or septicaemia are usually self-evident. Postrenal causes may be indicated by a history of prostatism, stone disease or haematuria, abdominal or pelvic surgery, or of cancer (Fig. 9.31).

PHYSICAL EXAMINATION

The first important aspect of examination is to define the presence or absence of circulatory failure due to volume depletion. This includes:

- Measurement of blood pressure (lying and standing if possible)
- Assessment of central venous pressure (CVP)
- Assessment of the presence or absence of oedema
- Assessment of the state of the peripheral circulation

In overt hypovolaemic shock there will be pallor, hypotension, cold peripheral parts and tachycardia. More often, circulatory failure is less obvious. Lack of a visible venous pulsation in the neck when supine indicates a low CVP and circulatory volume depletion. When in doubt, measurement of the CVP by insertion of a central venous line is immensely valuable (see p. 713). If associated with postural hypotension (a fall in standing systolic pressure of more than 20 mm Hg from the recumbent value, or to less than 100 mm Hg) and no oedema, a low CVP is good evidence of volume depletion. Conversely, the presence of oedema, an evaluated jugular venous pressure (JVP) and evidence of pulmonary congestion indicates heart failure or primary fluid overload.

Equally important is the exclusion of bladder outflow obstruction by careful examination for a large bladder or, if doubt exists, by aseptic bladder catheterization. A self-retaining catheter with continuous closed-seal drainage is instituted if bladder outflow obstruction is confirmed. If obstruction is not confirmed, the catheter should be removed after 50 ml of 1% noxythiolin has been instilled to prevent catheter-induced infection.

Rectal examination must always be performed to assess the prostate in males for size and possible malignancy, to identify the presence of pelvic cancer in either sex, and to look for melaena.

Acute tenderness in the renal angles or over the lower poles of the kidney anteriorly suggests acute tubulo-interstitial nephritis, whether due to infection or other causes (Table 9.20). This sign may also be found with acute glomerulonephritis.

A more general examination may be helpful in making the diagnosis; for example:

- The presence of jaundice or the stigmata of liver failure suggests hepatorenal failure.
- The presence of skin lesions may suggest a systemic hypersensitivity reaction, vasculitis, septicaemia or allergy, which may have resulted in tubulo-interstitial nephritis.
- The retinal lesions of diabetes or malignant hypertension may be found.

INVESTIGATION

Chemical and microscopic examination of the urine is essential.

Proteinuria. In pure prerenal or postrenal failure proteinuria is usually absent or slight (+) at most. Conversely, heavy proteinuria (++ or more) suggests intrinsic renal disease, most often glomerular in nature.

Haematuria. Haematuria is uncommon in prerenal failure. It may occur with postrenal disease (tumours, stones), and is usual in intrinsic renal disease.

Urine microscopy. The presence of red-cell casts on microscopy is highly suggestive of glomerulonephritis, but they may also be seen in acute tubulo-interstitial disease.

The presence of bacteria and pyuria suggest infection.

Urine culture. Culture of clean-catch midstream urine or catheter specimens must always be carried out.

Chemical testing of urine. With prerenal 'circulatory' failure the *healthy* kidney responds with avid retention of salt and water. The urine is thus concentrated (osmolality > 500 mosmol·kg^{-1}), low in sodium (< 20 mmol·L^{-1}), with a urine/plasma concentration ratio of more than 8 : 1 for urea or more than 40 : 1 for creatinine. Similar urinary findings may be observed in acute glomerulonephritis. In patients with acute tubulo-interstitial disease, urine-concentrating ability is lost, as is the ability to conserve sodium, the urine being isosmolar with plasma and the urinary sodium usually

being greater than 50 mosmol·kg^{-1}. A similar pattern is usually seen in chronic glomerular disease and obstructive nephropathy. Thus, urine osmolality, sodium concentration and urine/plasma concentration ratio of creatinine or urea may be of value in distinguishing prerenal from other forms of renal failure.

Diagnosis of prerenal 'circulatory' ARF
If, on the basis of the history and clinical examination, prerenal (volume depletion) circulatory failure is diagnosed or strongly suspected, the effect of volume repletion on renal function must be tested. Volume repletion should be with an appropriate fluid: blood should be used in the case of post-haemorrhagic shock (or human albumin in an emergency) and normal saline if fluid depletion is due to vomiting, diarrhoea or polyuria. Fluid replacement is most safely given with simultaneous measurement of the CVP. With pure prerenal failure, urine output should increase with volume replacement.

Forced diuresis in 'incipient ATN'
It has been postulated that early renal damage due to ATN may be reversible ('incipient ATN') if the kidneys are subjected to a powerful diuretic stimulus. When the CVP or JVP returns to normal with fluid replacement but urine output does not increase, or in patients who are not volume depleted but have been exposed to conditions predisposing to ATN, it is usual to give a powerful diuretic combination of 20% mannitol 100 ml i.v. over 5–10 min followed by frusemide 120 mg i.v. over 5–10 min. A satisfactory response is a urine output of more than 40 ml·h^{-1}. If the response is equivocal (10–40 ml·h^{-1}), the diuretic stimulus may be repeated *once* after 2 h. If there is no increase in urine output, this procedure should not be repeated a third time. The administration of more than 40 g of mannitol per day to the oliguric patient is potentially harmful. The urine flow rate in response to forced diuresis may be monitored in the unconscious patient by bladder catheterization, but the catheter must be removed as soon as possible in diuresing patients and immediately if no diuresis occurs.

If these measures do not induce a diuresis, the diagnosis of prerenal circulatory failure or incipient ATN has been excluded. The differential diagnosis then lies between intrinsic renal disease and obstructive nephropathy.

Dopamine infusion in ATN
Infusion of dopamine hydrochloride in low dosage (1–2 µg·kg^{-1}·min^{-1}) causes renal vasodilatation and a sodium diuresis. It also increases cardiac output by its positive inotropic action. In large doses, dopamine causes vasoconstriction. Because of these actions in *normal subjects*, infusion of 'renal

doses' of dopamine is widely practised in intensive care units in circumstances in which acute renal failure is likely to develop (acute heart failure, post-cardiac surgery, or septicaemia) or in patients with incipient or established ATN. It may be combined with large doses of frusemide. Despite its popularity there is no good evidence that this prevents or alters the degree or duration of ATN. It may increase urine flow rates, so making control of fluid balance more easy but this is not usually associated with an increase in excretory function.

Distinction between renal and postrenal failure

Clues may be provided by the history and clinical examination, including urinalysis. Haematuria with red-cell casts, recent trauma or sepsis with hypotension, and exposure to nephrotoxic drugs or chemicals all suggest intrinsic disease, while a previous history of stone disease or a 'frozen' or solid pelvis on rectal examination (indicating a pelvic carcinoma) suggest obstructive nephropathy. In the absence of obvious acute glomerulonephritis or acute tubulo-interstitial nephritis it is usually necessary to exclude obstruction by renal imaging. Anuria should always be considered to be due to obstruction until proved otherwise.

Renal imaging. This should be carried out as soon as possible both to define or exclude obstruction and to define renal size. Plain abdominal X-rays and renal tomography are performed to exclude radio-dense stones. Ultrasound will define or exclude obstruction and allow measurement of renal size in the majority of patients. Renal scintigraphy can give useful information regarding renal perfusion.

If obstruction is diagnosed, definition of the site of obstruction often requires antegrade or retrograde ureterography (see p. 433).

Diagnosis of renal causes of ARF

If obstruction is excluded, renal failure is due to intrinsic renal disease. Further investigation of the *nature* of the disease depends on the history, urinalysis and renal size. If the kidneys are small on renal imaging, the intrinsic renal disease is long-standing and irreversible. Definition of the precise pathology will not usually influence management. If the kidneys are normal or large and the history and urinalysis, including urine culture, suggest acute glomerulonephritis, acute tubular necrosis or bacterial pyelonephritis, further investigation is rarely necessary for management purposes. If the diagnosis is unclear, renal biopsy should be performed.

MANAGEMENT

Prerenal causes

Diagnosis of prerenal circulatory failure as the cause of ARF requires volume repletion to be carried out (see above), and this is also the first step in management. After this, continuing careful assessment of fluid and electrolyte requirement is necessary, especially in polyuric patients and in those with continuing gastrointestinal losses:

- The patient must be weighed daily to ensure stable fluid balance.
- The JVP must be checked regularly and the presence or absence of peripheral oedema recorded.
- Lying and standing blood pressure must be recorded at least twice daily.
- Careful fluid input–output records are essential.
- Plasma electrolytes must be measured daily to ensure adequate replacement of sodium and potassium. Measurement of the daily excretion of these cations is rarely necessary.

Fluid is always best given by mouth as water. Supplements of sodium or potassium may be required depending on dietary intake and daily measurement of plasma electrolytes.

Oral supplements are best given as Slow Sodium and effervescent potassium (bicarbonate-containing) or Slow-K (chloride-containing). Average daily excretion of these electrolytes is set out in Table 10.3 (see p. 493). If oral replacement is impossible, intravenous infusion is required. The volume of fluid needed is gauged from the urinary output, the daily clinical assessment of fluid balance and daily weighing. The nature of fluid required can be roughly predicted from Table 10.3. Plasma electrolyte levels should be checked daily.

Treatment of symptomatic prerenal uraemia caused by the administration of tetracycline or steroids includes withdrawal of these drugs.

Renal and postrenal causes

The management of renal failure due to intrinsic disease or obstructive nephropathy that cannot be relieved immediately involves the restoration of normal fluid and electrolyte balance and the control of uraemia and acidosis.

Maintaining fluid balance. The principles involved in controlling fluid balance (and uraemia and acidosis) may be summed up succinctly as 'what goes in must come out'. Normally, the kidneys keep the volume of body water constant by increasing or decreasing the urine volume in response to an increased or decreased fluid intake. In acute oliguric or polyuric renal failure this function is lost. It is then necessary to match fluid intake to urine output. Patients with ARF may, at the time of presentation, be hypovolaemic, normovolaemic or fluid overloaded. Treatment of volume depletion is discussed on p. 496.

In patients with ARF who are in normal fluid balance (i.e. who have a normal JVP and no evidence of systemic oedema or pulmonary congestion), fluid balance is maintained by a daily fluid intake of 300–500 ml plus an amount equal to the total fluid output on the previous day, i.e. urine volume plus any losses in vomit, stools, and fistula drainage. Careful records of all fluid intake and output are therefore essential. This is supported by daily weighing, the objective being to keep the patient's weight constant or with daily losses of no more than 0.5 kg in hypercatabolic patients who are losing flesh weight. Twice daily assessment of the JVP, lying and standing blood pressure, the presence or absence of systemic oedema and pulmonary congestion is mandatory. An increase in weight, a rise in JVP or the development of oedema indicates too large a fluid ration, while an excessive fall in weight or the development of postural hypotension indicates the reverse.

In patients presenting with fluid overload (i.e. who have an elevated JVP with systemic or pulmonary oedema), an attempt must be made to get rid of fluid. The effects of large doses of diuretics, e.g. frusemide 180 mg i.v. or 500–1000 mg orally, may be tested. If no diuresis occurs and the patient has clinical or radiological evidence of pulmonary congestion, fluid must be removed during dialysis or by ultrafiltration. Once the fluid balance has been corrected, it must be maintained as described for patients in normal fluid balance.

Electrolyte balance. In general, patients with oliguric renal failure cannot excrete sodium or potassium. Their intake of both must therefore be reduced to a minimum compatible with an adequate diet. Satisfactory control is assessed by daily measurement of the plasma electrolytes.

In polyuric patients, e.g. those in the recovery phase of ATN or following the relief of urinary obstruction, increased amounts of sodium and potassium may be lost in the urine, as shown by falling plasma levels. Such patients need supplements of both (see above).

Hyperkalaemia leading to cardiac arrhythmias and cardiac arrest is a major hazard in oliguric renal failure, especially where there has been extensive trauma or hypoxia, both of which may lead to flooding of the extracellular fluid with potassium from the cells. Acute-onset hyperkalaemia is more dangerous than that developing over weeks or months. The immediate danger of dysrhythmia is best assessed from the ECG when typical changes (Fig. 10.6) indicate the need for immediate and effective control of hyperkalaemia by dialysis (see p. 500). Temporary measures to control hyperkalaemia include the use of ion-exchange resins or the intravenous infusion of glucose and insulin (see p. 500).

Control of uraemia. The retention of waste products is less immediately life-threatening than fluid overload or hyperkalaemia. In otherwise healthy patients (e.g. those with acute glomerulonephritis) the increase in blood urea and serum creatinine are usually gradual and can be controlled by dietary restriction of protein to approximately 40 g per day, 75% of which must be first-class protein. Some 8400–10 000 kJ must be provided in the diet made up from fats and carbohydrate, commonly supplemented by starch hydrolysates such as Caloreen or Hycal. More strict protein restriction to 30 g per day is now rarely used. Diets for such patients should also be low in sodium (< 30 mmol per day) and potassium (< 20 mmol per day).

In patients with oliguric renal failure following sepsis, trauma or major surgery, tissue catabolism is greatly increased and the accumulation of waste products is faster. Again, dietary restriction of protein, sodium, and potassium, but with adequate calories, must be introduced. Such patients commonly require dialysis to control their uraemia. There is no absolute level of blood urea or serum creatinine above which dialysis should be commenced; rather it is the *rate* of rise in urea, plus fluid overload or hyperkalaemia, that indicates the need for dialysis. Overt symptoms of uraemia (anorexia, nausea, vomiting) plus severe acidosis certainly require dialysis. In the absence of these, it is generally felt that dialysis should be used if the blood urea exceeds 40 mmol·L^{-1} or serum creatinine exceeds 800 μmol·L^{-1}. Early dialysis with a protein intake of about 70 g is favoured in surgical or post-trauma cases in the belief that it may reduce the risk of infection and promote wound healing.

Control of acidosis. Acidosis rarely requires treatment *per se* as its severity commonly parallels that of the uraemia, for which dialysis may be indicated. Without removal of fixed acid by dialysis, acidosis is difficult to correct in oliguric patients because of the hazard of fluid overload that is inherent in intravenous infusions of sodium bicarbonate or other buffers. If control of acidosis is essential, as for example in patients with cardiac ischaemia, it is best achieved by dialysis.

General management

Many patients with oliguric renal failure are severely ill and have infections. They require dedicated nursing care and constant supervision. Infection must be controlled, but the choice of antibiotics (and indeed of all drugs) must take account of altered drug excretion due to renal failure.

Blood purification and ultrafiltration

A variety of techniques is now available for the removal of waste products of metabolism, the 'normalization' of plasma electrolytes and the removal of plasma water (ultrafiltration).

Peritoneal dialysis. This is widely available and easily instituted using a hard PVC catheter introduced into the peritoneal space using a trocar through a small scalpel skin stab. In patients who have had abdominal surgery, peritoneal dialysis may not be possible and in hypercatabolic patients it may be insufficient to control the uraemia. The principles of peritoneal dialysis are discussed on p. 480.

Temporary (acute) peritoneal dialysis

Indications

- Severe uraemia
  (a) Used in acute renal failure continuously or intermittently until renal function recovers
  (b) used in chronic renal failure for support until long-term dialysis is instituted

Insertion of catheter

Using a sterile technique:

- Local anaesthetic is injected in the midline below the umbilicus.
- A small cut is made in the skin with a scalpel.
- A rigid plastic catheter is inserted through the abdominal wall into the peritoneal cavity using a trocar.
- The catheter is firmly bound to the abdomen.

The catheter can remain in situ for several days or a few weeks.

Peritoneal dialysis

- In acute renal failure, approximately 2 L of sterile dialysate solution are instilled into and drained out of the abdomen approximately hourly.
- A typical composition of the dialysate is sodium 135 mmol·L^{-1}, chloride 105 mmol·L^{-1}, potassium 0 mmol·L^{-1}, glucose 80 mmol·L^{-1} (1.5%), calcium 1.75 mmol·L^{-1}, magnesium 0.50 mmol·L^{-1}, and lactate 35 mmol·L^{-1}.
- Net fluid removal is achieved by osmosis. 1.5% glucose is approximately isotonic with plasma. Higher concentrations of glucose are used if fluid needs to be removed.

Complications

- Leakage
- Pain—usually short lasting and not severe
- Peritonitis
  (a) Uncommon with careful technique
  (b) Treated with appropriate antibiotics added to the dialysate solution or with withdrawal of the catheter

---

Haemodialysis. This is the most popular alternative to peritoneal dialysis. It is significantly more efficient than peritoneal dialysis for blood purification. It is now most commonly performed using temporary cannulation of the subclavian or femoral veins. It requires quite sophisticated equipment and special expertise in its use. It can therefore only be performed in specialist centres. The principles of haemodiaylsis are discussed on p. 479.

Haemofiltration. This is a third alternative which is becoming increasingly popular for ARF in ITU. In this procedure, which is less likely than haemodialysis to cause acute hypotension in patients with septicaemia or with poor myocardial function, large volumes of plasma water are removed using a porous filter and are replaced by a sterile electrolyte solution. Although, like haemodialysis, it can be carried out intermittently using a machine, it is most popularly performed as continuous 'arteriovenous' haemofiltration (CAVH). The patient's systemic arterial pressure drives blood through the extracorporeal circuit. Between 10 and 20 litres of plasma water are removed daily and replaced by electrolyte solution (Fig. 9.32).

Removal of waste products is relatively inefficient. 'Clearance' is the same as the rate of haemofiltration. Thus, removal of 10–20 litres of plasma water daily is equivalent to a glomerular filtration rate of between 7 and 14 ml·min^{-1}. While adequate to control uraemia in some patients, it is rarely sufficient in hypercatabolic subjects. Its main advantage is in controlling fluid and electrolyte balance and for creating space for intravenous feeding in the severely oliguric patient. Continuous venovenous haemofiltration (CVVH) can be carried out using double lumen central venous lines but requires a blood pump for circulation of the blood and more sophisticated monitoring equipment. A further variation is to combine continuous haemofiltration with continuous dialysis (CAVHD). In this, blood passing through the haemofilter is not only ultrafiltered but also dialysed. Waste material is thus removed both by diffusion and by haemofiltration. Again this requires more sophisticated equipment than does CAVH.

Drawbacks of CAVH and CAVHD include the need to insert cannulas into a major artery (usually the radial artery) and a draining vein to form an arteriovenous shunt and the need for very frequent assessment of fluid balance.

Recovery phase of ARF

Paradoxically, the recovery phase of ARF is often the most dangerous. As glomerular filtration rate increases, large volumes of urine may be passed before the damaged tubules fully recover their ability to retain salt and water. This carries the risk of fluid depletion and hypokalaemia. This so-called 'polyuric phase' of ARF can last for several days and demands careful monitoring of plasma sodium and potassium levels to detect a negative balance of either.

PROGNOSIS

In acute tubular necrosis, the commonest renal

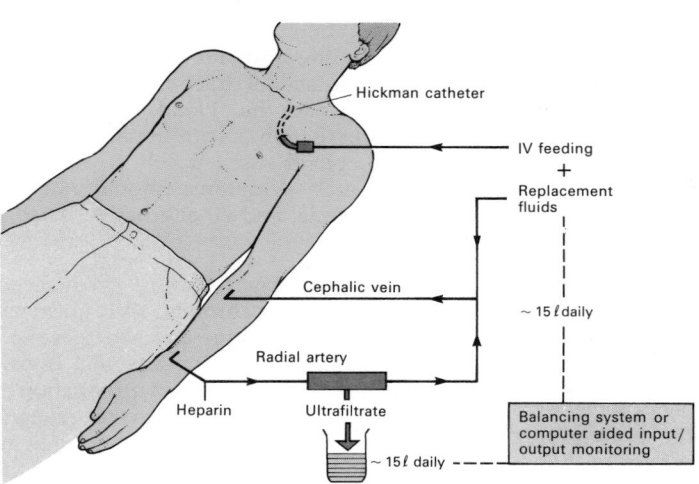

Fig. 9.32 Continuous arterio-venous haemofiltration (CAVH).

lesion, the renal prognosis is excellent; 95% of patients recover satisfactory renal function within 6 weeks. Unfortunately acute tubular necrosis often develops in patients who have a poor chance of survival for non-renal reasons. The outlook is particularly poor in patients with severe trauma, multisystem failure and overwhelming sepsis. In those who survive, renal function usually returns to normal within a few months. In patients with cortical necrosis, only partial recovery of function, if any, can be expected.

The prognosis in patients with acute glomerulonephritis, acute tubulo-interstitial nephritis or obstructive nephropathy is discussed earlier in this chapter.

Chronic renal failure

Although chronic renal failure (CRF) is not common, its impact in fiscal, political and ethical terms has been enormous since the introduction of long-term haemodialysis in the 1960s and increasingly successful transplantation in the 1970s. Long-term dialysis and transplantation together are often referred to as 'renal replacement'.

PREVALENCE AND CAUSES

An indication of the prevalence and causes of CRF is shown in Fig. 9.33. These data are for patients who reach end-stage renal failure (ESRF) and who are accepted for dialysis and renal transplantation.

The distribution of primary renal disease varies little between countries, except for analgesic nephropathy, which is particularly common in Australian women. Glomerulonephritis is the most common cause of ESRF, followed by chronic

atrophic pyelonephritis.

A pessimistic outlook with respect to long-term renal replacement in patients with diabetic nephropathy in the past has given way to a more optimistic and positive approach in these patients. Diabetics now comprise the fastest-growing group of patients accepted for dialysis and transplantation in Europe. Polycystic disease of the kidney is the most common cause of inherited renal disease leading to ESRF. In ESRF a histological diagnosis is often not available as biopsy of small kidneys is not warranted. It is likely therefore that many patients in the 'uncertain' group have chronic glomerulonephritis.

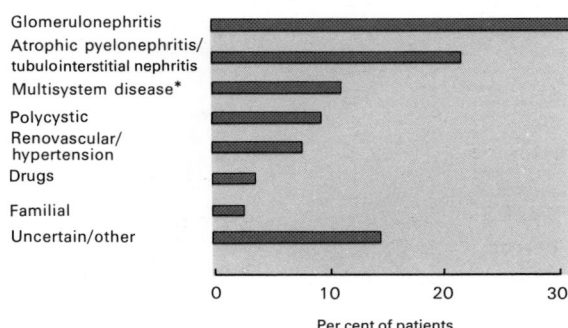

* Diabetes mellitus accounts for most patients in this group.

Fig. 9.33 Distribution of type of primary renal disease in patients accepted for dialysis and transplantation in the years 1980–1982. (Data from the Registry of the European Dialysis and Transplant Association—European Renal Association.)

CLINICAL FEATURES

Asymptomatic CRF may be discovered on routine health screening programmes, as a chance finding in hospitalized patients, or during follow-up of patients known to have had renal disease.

In patients with chronic renal disease, symptomatic uraemia is not uncommonly precipitated by prerenal factors such as increased tissue catabolism associated with infection, tetracycline therapy, volume depletion due to vomiting or diarrhoea, or the development of malignant phase hypertension. A prerenal factor must always be sought and treated if present.

Symptomatic uraemia most often presents with gastrointestinal symptoms (anorexia, nausea, vomiting) but it may manifest as symptoms of anaemia, bone disease, hypertension or hypertensive heart failure. In CRF hypertension has usually been long-standing and frequently severe. Advanced coronary artery and peripheral vascular disease may be present even in young patients.

Symptoms and signs

In severe renal failure, practically every system of the body is affected and leads to symptoms (Fig. 9.34). Minor symptoms such as lethargy, fatigue and nocturia have often gone unnoticed for many months and are only recognized when patients are specifically questioned about them. Menstrual disturbances, particularly amenorrhoea, and erectile impotence are troublesome symptoms. The accumulation of 'toxic metabolites' in uraemia sometimes causes a peripheral neuropathy that is characteristically reversible with dialysis treatment. Yellow-brown pigmentation of the skin, which is often dry and itchy, commonly occurs.

Anorexia, nausea and vomiting. These are the most typical symptoms of uraemia and are usually attributed to the formation of ammonia in the upper gastrointestinal tract from urea. They are uncommon until the blood urea exceeds 30 mmol·L^{-1}. In patients with renal disease but in whom the blood urea level is less than 20 mmol·L^{-1}, such symptoms should not be attributed to 'uraemia' and an alternative cause should be sought.

Anaemia. This is a typical feature of advanced renal disease. It is normochromic and normocytic in type. Symptoms of fatigue and shortness of breath on exertion may occur. The anaemia is primarily due to reduced erythropoietin production by the kidney but, when there is severe uraemia (i.e. blood urea > 30 mmol·L^{-1}), a shortened red-cell life and toxic marrow depression also contribute.

The blood urea must always be measured in patients with unexplained normochromic, normocytic anaemia. It is not uncommon for a uraemic patient to have received courses of iron for anaemia many months before presenting with renal failure. Not surprisingly, the anaemia does not respond.

Renal osteodystrophy

The term renal osteodystrophy embraces the various forms of bone disease that develop in CRF, i.e. osteomalacia and osteoporosis, secondary and tertiary hyperparathyroidism and osteosclerosis (Fig. 9.35). Covert renal osteodystrophy is present in most patients with severe renal failure. Phosphate retention results in hyperphosphataemia, which lowers the concentration of ionized serum calcium.

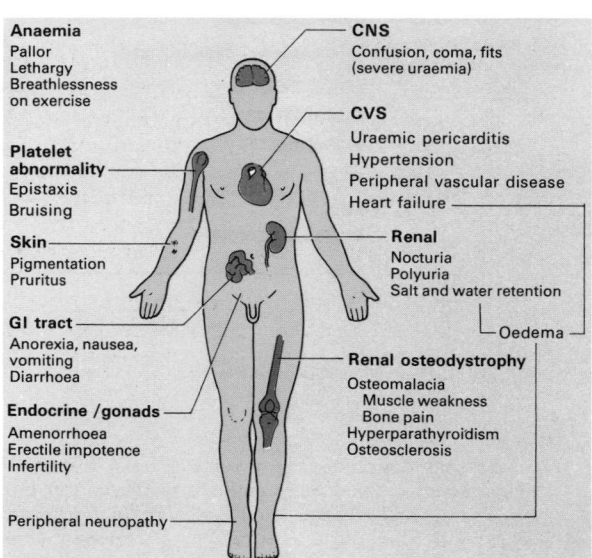

Anaemia
Pallor
Lethargy
Breathlessness
on exercise

Platelet abnormality
Epistaxis
Bruising

Skin
Pigmentation
Pruritus

GI tract
Anorexia, nausea,
vomiting
Diarrhoea

Endocrine /gonads
Amenorrhoea
Erectile impotence
Infertility

Peripheral neuropathy

CNS
Confusion, coma, fits
(severe uraemia)

CVS
Uraemic pericarditis
Hypertension
Peripheral vascular disease
Heart failure

Renal
Nocturia
Polyuria
Salt and water retention

Oedema

Renal osteodystrophy
Osteomalacia
  Muscle weakness
  Bone pain
Hyperparathyroidism
Osteosclerosis

Fig. 9.34 Symptoms and signs of chronic renal failure. Oedema may be due to a combination of primary renal salt and water retention and heart failure.

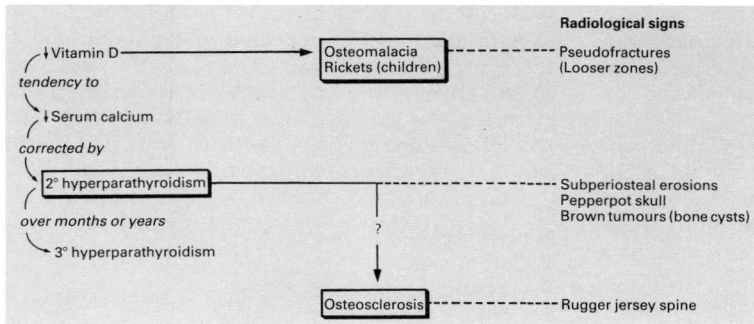

Fig. **9.35** Pathogenesis and radiological features of renal osteodystrophy.

Other effects include decreased renal production of $1,25(OH)D_3$, which leads to decreased calcium absorption and a fall in serum calcium. This in turn stimulates the release of parathyroid hormone, which may already be increased due to the loss of the normal inhibitory effect of $1,25(OH)D_3$.

Osteomalacia and osteoporosis are described on p. 822.

Hyperparathyroidism. Poor absorption of dietary calcium and phosphate retention lowers the serum calcium. Parathyroid hormone is released in response to hypocalcaemia and promotes resorption of calcium from bone and increased proximal tubular reabsorption of calcium in the kidney in an attempt to correct the low serum calcium. Over months or years, this 'secondary' hyperparathyroidism can lead to severe decalcification of the skeleton associated with the classical radiological appearances listed in Fig. 9.35.

A common, but not inevitable, sequel to long-standing secondary hyperparathyroidism is hyperplasia of the glands, leading to autonomous or 'tertiary' hyperparathyroidism. In this condition parathyroid hormone is released inappropriately, resulting in hypercalcaemia and severe bone disease. Hyperparathyroidism causes bone and joint pains and a high serum alkaline phosphatase. Histologically there is increased osteoclastic activity, cyst formation and bone marrow fibrosis (osteitis fibrosa cystica or von Recklinghausen's disease of bone).

Osteosclerosis. This literally means 'hardening of bone' and may be a direct result of excess parathyroid hormone. Alternate bands of sclerotic and porotic bone in the vertebrae produce the characteristic 'rugger-jersey spine' X-ray appearance.

INVESTIGATION

As with ARF it is critical to define renal size and to exclude treatable obstruction. When renal failure is

modest (blood urea $< 20\ mmol\cdot L^{-1}$), high-dose excretion urography can commonly show details of the calyces and allow identification of conditions such as papillary necrosis. With more severe renal impairment, calyceal detail may not be shown. In such cases plain renal tomography plus ultrasonography can identify renal size and define or exclude obstruction, eliminating the need for excretion urography. If the kidneys are not obstructed or shrunken, transcutaneous biopsy is required to exclude treatable tubulo-interstitial disease. An exception to this is where there is a long history of diabetes and evidence of diabetic retinopathy, when the diagnosis of diabetic glomerulosclerosis can be presumed. Conversely, renal failure should not be ascribed to diabetic glomerulosclerosis if there is no retinopathy. If the kidneys are found to be small, smooth and non-obstructed, it is difficult to distinguish between chronic glomerulonephritis, chronic tubulo-interstitial nephritis or nephrosclerosis.

MANAGEMENT

Dietary protein restriction
Protein restriction not only reduces the rate of production of nitrogenous waste products, but there is increasing evidence that it also slows down the rate of decline of function in certain chronic renal diseases. Restricting the amount of protein in the daily diet to between 40 and 50 g strikes a balance between achieving these objectives and avoiding protein malnutrition. Protein restriction should be introduced when the creatinine clearance falls below 30 ml·min^{-1}. Potassium intake may also have to be reduced. Patients with symptomatic uraemia who cannot be controlled on a 40-g protein diet should be considered for renal replacement (see p. 481).

Blood pressure control
Hypertension should always be treated in patients with chronic renal disease, since it will accelerate loss of kidney function if uncontrolled. Initial control of hypertension may be accompanied by some reduction in GFR, but this is preferable to

hypertensive kidney damage. Renal hypertension usually responds to conventional treatment with a diuretic, a beta-blocker and, if necessary, a vasodilator drug (see p. 618). Salt intake should be reduced to 50 mmol per day.

Control of renal hypertension by angiotensin-converting enzyme (ACE) inhibitors would seem logical and it is undoubtedly effective. Care must be taken in introducing treatment with these drugs as they may result in an acute fall in glomerular filtration rate, especially in patients with atheromatous renal artery disease or severe renal vascular disease. There must be close monitoring of blood urea, serum creatinine and serum potassium in the first few days of introducing ACE inhibition.

Some patients with diseases primarily affecting the medulla (e.g. chronic pyelonephritis, papillary necrosis or postobstructive atrophy) may be unable to conserve salt and water and volume depletion, hypotension and prerenal failure may result. This should always be suspected in patients with a normal or low blood pressure who have a normal or low JVP and no oedema. Postural hypotension supports a diagnosis of volume depletion. The diagnosis is confirmed if, after the cautious prescription of salt supplements (Slow Sodium 10–20 mmol three times daily) and a high fluid intake the blood pressure rises, the postural hypotension disappears, the renal function improves and the body weight increases without the development of oedema. Enough salt is given to just avoid causing abnormal elevation of the JVP or the development of oedema. Elimination of prerenal failure in these circumstances may result in a marked improvement in renal function.

Treatment of anaemia

This has changed since the availability of erythropoietin.

Control of severe uraemia (blood urea > 30 mmol·L^{-1}) may reduce haemolysis and marrow depression. Most patients adjust to haemoglobin levels of between 6 and 9 g·dl^{-1}. A policy of minimal blood transfusion was adopted both to minimize the risk of transmission of viral infection and to avoid sensitization to white-cell antigens that may compromise successful transplantation in the future. Such sensitization may be reduced by white-cell filters. However, there is evidence that blood transfusion actually enhances the chances of a successful kidney transplant through mechanisms that are not understood. A compromise is therefore required. Potential transplant recipients are given only the minimum number of transfusions needed but are electively transfused with 3 units of blood if no transfusion has ever been required.

Iron therapy is usually required in patients on:

- A protein-restricted diet that is low in iron

- Haemodialysis, as blood is lost in haemodialysis equipment and by repeated venepuncture

Human recombinant erythropoietin (r-HuEPO;EPO) increases the haemoglobin in patients with CRF and those on regular haemodialysis or CAPD although experience with this therapy is limited.

Complications include:

- Hypertension
- Convulsions
- Hyperkalaemia
- Cerebral ischaemic attacks
- Clotting of A-V fistulae

The mechanism of these complications is unclear but may be due to the removal of hypoxic dilatation, which is believed to be present in anaemic subjects. Dosage regimen is either three times weekly i.v. at the end of the haemodialysis session or subcutaneously in patients with CRF or on CAPD to maintain a haemoglobin between 10 and 11 g·dl^{-1}. It is very expensive.

Treatment of renal osteodystrophy

Treatment is directed at reducing serum phosphate levels by the use of phosphate binders in the gut and by increasing calcium absorption. Historically, binding of phosphate in the gut involved the use of aluminium hydroxide preparations. Recognition that aluminium can be absorbed from the gut and anxiety that oral aluminium therapy might contribute to aluminium bone disease or brain damage has led to more cautious use of aluminium hydroxide. Calcium carbonate (1–2 g elemental calcium a day in divided doses with meals) has been substituted as a gut phosphate binder.

Calcium absorption from the gut is increased by the use of vitamin D preparations—dihydrotachysterol (DHT) 0.2–0.6 mg daily; alfacalcidol (1α-hydroxycholecalciferol) 0.5–2.0 µg daily; calcitriol (1,25-dihydroxycholecalciferol) 1–2µg daily. These preparations are listed in order of increasing potency, which requires increasingly careful monitoring of serum calcium to avoid hypercalcaemia. Serum calcium levels must be measured at least monthly. Combined treatment with both calcium carbonate and vitamin D products increases the risk of hypercalcaemia.

Increasing use is made of 'prophylactic' vitamin D therapy with the object of preventing the development of hyperparathyroidism. Treatment is best monitored by regular measurement of parathyroid hormone levels, which should be kept within the normal range. Prophylactic regimens again require careful monitoring of serum calcium levels.

Tertiary hyperparathyroidism in which parathormone levels cannot be suppressed by raising the serum calcium requires total parathyroidectomy. For some years, subcutaneous implantation of parathyroid tissue was carried out following total parathyroidectomy. Because of recurrence of hypercalcaemia and difficulty in identifying the site of production and hence treatment, this has now been abandoned. Patients undergoing total parathyroidectomy will require life-long treatment with a vitamin D preparation.

Socioeconomic aspects

Because dialysis and/or transplantation are required to replace renal function, forward planning on an individual basis is essential. This includes assessment of the patient's home, which may have to be converted to take dialysis equipment. Job prospects and economic resources need to be considered, given that a certain amount of time will be taken up with self-treatment in the future and mobility will be limited. The prospects for live donor kidney transplantation need to be carefully assessed.

For all these reasons it is customary to transfer patients with progressive kidney failure to their 'local' specialist centre after the initial diagnosis has been made and management implemented. Most centres now employ specially trained personnel to deal with these problems.

Patient education

Involvement in various aspects of treatment at an early stage often helps prepare the way for the complicated specialist training that may lie ahead. Dietary and drug treatment should be explained and the patient should be encouraged to question changes in treatment. Cannulation of forearm veins may prejudice the successful creation of vascular access for dialysis in the future (see below). The responsibility for making sure that this does not happen can largely be passed to the patient.

Replacement of renal function by dialysis

Apart from protein restriction and the control of hypertension there is little that can be done to influence the natural history of chronic renal disease. Tragically, patients all too frequently present with symptoms and signs of ESRF. Since the late 1960s, increasing numbers of patients with ESRF have had 'replacement' of renal function by dialysis and transplantation.

At the end of 1987 there were in Europe 90 924 patients receiving haemodialysis; 10 700 receiving long-term peritoneal dialysis and 38 108 patients with a functioning kidney transplant. This represents 221 per million of population.

Haemodialysis. The principles of haemodialysis are illustrated in Fig. 9.36. Blood is perfused in a thin film across a membrane (usually prepared from cellulose) that has a surface area of approximately 1 m^2 and is permeable to water, electrolytes and small molecules such as urea and creatinine. Dialysate solution flows on the opposite side of the membrane. Diffusion of solutes takes place in both directions. The concentration of potassium in the dialysate is chosen to allow diffusion from the blood at a rate just below that which creates hypokalaemia, and the concentration of ionized calcium is chosen such that there is slow diffusion *into* the blood. This helps to alleviate the problems of calcium balance in ESRF.

Because of difficulty in producing bicarbonate-containing dialysate fluid, for many years acetate was substituted. During dialysis this diffuses into the bloodstream and is usually metabolized to bicarbonate in the body. The rate of metabolism may, however, vary and a significant rise in acetate may occur in serum.

Cardiovascular instability and especially hypotension during haemodialysis have been attributed to the use of acetate. Equipment has now been developed that allows the use of bicarbonate dialysis and this, in general, is now preferred for elderly and cardiovascularly unstable patients.

Ingested water and water produced by metabolism accumulates between dialysis sessions and has

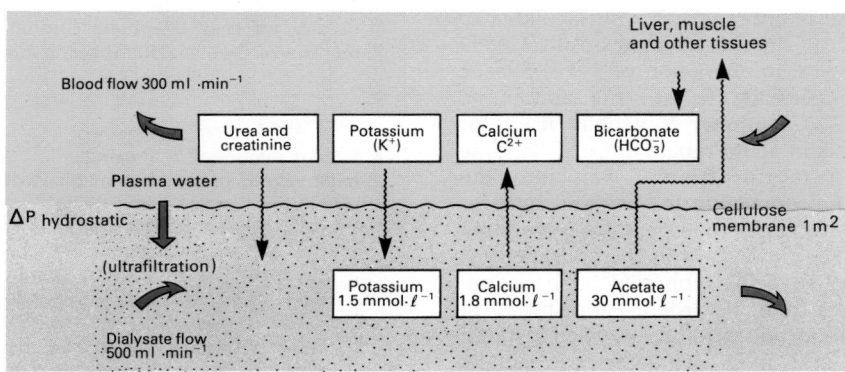

Fig. 9.36 The principles of haemodialysis.

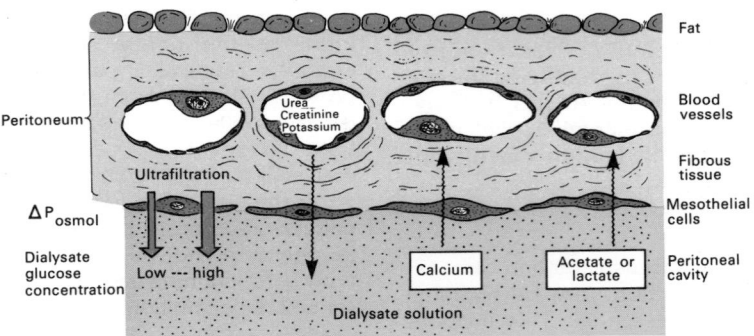

Fig. 9.37 The principles of peritoneal dialysis.

to be removed. Removal of plasma water on dialysis is achieved by creating a hydrostatic pressure gradient across the membrane (ultrafiltration).

Haemodialysis requires easy access to the circulation. This is most commonly achieved by creating a fistula between the radial artery and the cephalic vein at the wrist. For dialysis, needles are inserted into the high-flow 'arterialized' forearm veins that result.

It has been found that patients remain well and can survive many years with between 12 and 21 h of dialysis each week. Usually this is split into three or sometimes two sessions. Hypertension is usually controlled by the gradual removal of salt and water during the first few months of dialysis, hypotensive drugs being gradually withdrawn. Dietary protein intake is increased to about 60 g per day.

Peritoneal dialysis. Continuous 'ambulatory' peritoneal dialysis (CAPD) is the preferred method of dialysis in some centres. Low capital costs and the necessity for only a short training period for the patient are particularly attractive in units with an active transplantation programme, when the need for dependence on dialysis for more than a few years is unlikely for the majority.

The peritoneal membrane has a surface area of approximately 2 m^2 in the average adult. CAPD requires the surgical implantation of a soft Silastic rubber catheter (Tenckhoff) into the abdominal cavity (a hard PVC catheter is usually used for peritoneal dialysis in acute renal failure). Dialysate (usually 2 litres) is run from a bag into the abdomen, the line connecting the bag and catheter is clamped, and the bag is rolled up and placed in a belt or pocket. The fluid stays in the abdomen for several hours before being siphoned off back into the bag, which is then discarded. A fresh bag of dialysate is connected and the cycle restarts. Between three and five exchanges are usually required every day.

The principles employed in peritoneal dialysis

for the diffusion of solutes and electrolytes are the same as for haemodialysis except that potassium-free dialysate is used (Fig. 9.37). Ultrafiltration is effected by osmosis: the dialysate is made hypertonic with respect to plasma by the addition of

---

Home haemodialysis

The majority (56%) of haemodialysis patients in the UK have self-supervised home haemodialysis. The majority (90%) of patients in the rest of Europe have hospital-based dialysis.

Advantages of home haemodialysis

- Confidence in own treatment
- Reduced travelling
- Less time off work
- Dialysis times are at the patient's own choosing—more socially acceptable
- Hepatitis B infection is very rare
- Approximately one-third of the cost of hospital dialysis in the long term.

Requirements

- Suitable home available
- Home conversion—a separate room is needed with special plumbing and drains
- Several months training period in hospital
- Facility for easy telephone communication with dialysis nurses, technicians and doctor if necessary

Disadvantages

- Patient may need rehousing
- Expensive if patient is transplanted within a few months of starting home dialysis

'Minimal care' dialysis units are gaining popularity. Patients supervise their own treatment in small 'satellite' units with minimal supervision. The bed station and equipment are shared by several patients, and it is less expensive than hospital dialysis. In some cases, these units have social advantages over home dialysis.

Continuous ambulatory peritoneal dialysis (CAPD)

Currently more than half the patients accepted for renal replacement therapy in the UK start on CAPD.

Advantages over haemodialysis

- Easy to teach
- Short training period
- Special room/equipment unnecessary—merely a sink and storage space
- Rehousing rarely required
- Low capital cost, and therefore less expensive than haemodialysis if transplanted 'early'
- Continuous corrections of biochemistry are very well tolerated
- Easily carried out away from the home so that holidays are simple to arrange

Disadvantages

- Peritonitis—about half of the patients have to discontinue CAPD within 2 years on account of peritonitis
- Excessive weight gain in some patients
- Hernias and pancreatitis occasionally occur

glucose. The higher the osmolality of the dialysate, the higher the ultrafiltration rate.

Outlook and complications of dialysis. Overall, the 5-year survival rate of patients on haemodialysis is approximately 70%, most of the deaths being due to cardiovascular disease. In many cases this results from hypertension present before the start of dialysis. In the individual patient, haemodialysis is compatible with survival for more than 20 years and a high proportion of patients are successfully rehabilitated. Many return to their previous occupations despite the time needed to perform dialysis (which can often be performed at night).

Patients on long-term dialysis are commonly infertile. Pregnancies are few and successful pregnancy almost unknown in female dialysis patients. Only a small number of babies have been fathered by patients on dialysis. Erectile impotence is a very distressing complication that is estimated to affect approximately 30% of male patients. In general, these problems are reversed by successful transplantation.

Despite a clearer understanding of the role of the kidney in calcium metabolism, bone disease remains an important cause of morbidity in dialysis patients. The likelihood of parathyroidectomy for tertiary hyperparathyroidism increases with time on dialysis: the prevalence of parathyroidectomy in patients who have been on dialysis for less than 5 years is 2%, and 16% in those who have had dialysis for over 10 years. For this reason a more aggressive approach to 'prophylaxis'/treatment for bone disease has been adopted (see above).

While vascular access is the 'Achilles heel' of successful haemodialysis, peritonitis is the major drawback of CAPD and half the patients who start CAPD change to some other treatment within 2 years as a result. On the other hand, very successful rehabilitation is possible using CAPD and this treatment has offered new hope to diabetic patients and elderly patients, in whom problems with vascular access and blood pressure stability on haemodialysis tend to be considerable.

Renal transplantation

Successful renal transplantation offers the potential for complete rehabilitation in ESRF. It allows freedom from dietary and fluid restriction, anaemia and infertility are corrected, and the likelihood of requiring parathyroidectomy is reduced.

Coincident with the use of lower doses of immunosuppressive drugs, patient survival has increased over the years such that the 1-year survival rate is over 95% for live donor recipients and over 85% for cadaver donor recipients. With the use of newer immunosuppressive drugs, the graft survival rate has improved, being approximately 80% at 2 years. For this reason, some patients who are satisfactorily established on dialysis treatment are increasingly electing to undergo transplantation.

Tissue matching of the donor kidney and recipient has become less important with the introduction of cyclosporin A in place of azathioprine. Less-strict matching criteria have therefore been adopted. With the use of cyclosporin A the previously observed protective effect of prior transfusion is less evident (see above).

A transplant operation is relatively straightforward. The donor kidney is placed in an extraperitoneal pouch in the iliac fossa (Fig. 9.38) and the renal artery and vein are anastomosed to the

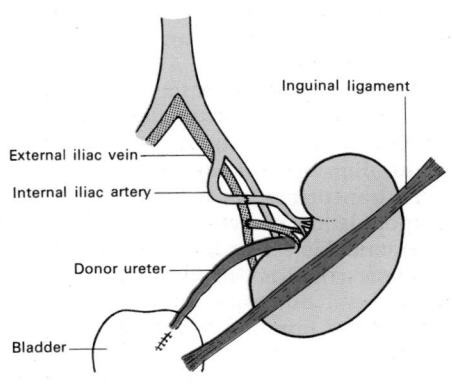

Fig. 9.38 The anatomy of a transplant operation.

recipient's iliac vessels. The donor ureter is implanted into the bladder through a submucosal tunnel designed to prevent reflux. The recipient's own kidneys are left undisturbed unless there is another indication for nephrectomy.

Immunosuppressive drugs are given from the moment of transplantation.

In the past, prednisolone and azathioprine was the immunosuppressive drug combination almost universally used. Cyclosporin A, in spite of its nephrotoxicity and expense, is now employed in the place of azathioprine because of its remarkable immunosuppressant properties. The place of 'triple therapy' (cyclosporin A, azathioprine and prednisolone) remains unclear.

Rejection of the transplant, if it is to take place, usually occurs within the first few months. This is also the period when the patient is at greatest risk from infection. Viral infections (e.g. with cytomegalovirus) that generally produce trivial illnesses in normal people can produce life-threatening infections in immunosuppressed patients. There are also longer-term complications of immunosuppressive therapy: avascular necrosis of the femoral head due to corticosteroid drugs is not uncommon, and there is an increased incidence of squamous-cell carcinoma of the skin and of non-Hodgkin's lymphoma in transplant recipients, although the actual numbers who develop these complications are very small.

Despite the success of cadaveric renal transplantation, the number of patients on dialysis awaiting transplantation continues to increase. At the end of 1987 there were 27 620 patients in Europe on transplant waiting lists. The cause of this was a shortage of cadaver organs. Several studies indicate that throughout the United Kingdom there are many potential donors whose kidneys are not offered for transplantation. The reasons for this are complex but include reluctance on the part of both the public and the medical profession to consider organ donation, insufficiently streamlined organizations for recovery of donor kidneys and continuing unjustified anxiety about the diagnosis of death. Attempts to alter legislation to facilitate the supply of cadaver kidneys have been resisted. Given more complete usage of potential donors, recent experience suggests that no European country can achieve a cadaver graft transplantation rate above 40 grafts per million population per year.

An understandable result has been the increasing use in some countries of live donors. In the past, this has been primarily parents, siblings or offspring. Improved immunosuppressive regimens have led to the use of unrelated volunteers, such as spouses.

Cystic, congenital and familial disease

Cystic renal disease

Solitary or multiple renal cysts are common, especially with advancing age: 50% of those aged 50 years or more have one or more such cysts. They have no special significance except in the differential diagnosis of renal tumours (see p. 486). Such cysts are often asymptomatic and are found on excretion urography or ultrasound examination performed for some other reason. Occasionally they may cause pain and/or haematuria due to their large size or bleeding may occur into the cyst.

Adult polycystic renal disease

Adult polycystic renal disease (APCD) is an important cystic disease of the kidney that is relatively common. Inherited in an autosomal dominant manner as a single gene defect linked to the α-haemoglobin gene locus on the short arm of chromosome 16, it is manifested in infancy as tiny cystic lesions distributed throughout both kidneys and should be distinguished from juvenile nephronophthisis (see below). The precise mechanism for cyst formation is disputed. With advancing age the cysts enlarge at a variable rate, often at the same rate within family groups but at different rates between different families. There is progressive asymmetric renal enlargement, with compression of intervening renal tissue and progressive loss of excretory function.

Clinical presentation may be at any age from the second decade. Presenting symptoms include:

- Acute loin pain and/or haematuria due to haemorrhage into a cyst
- Vague loin or abdominal discomfort due to the increasing size of the kidneys
- The development of hypertension or symptoms of uraemia

Increasingly APCD is diagnosed by ultrasound screening of the children of parents known to have the condition.

The natural history of the disease is one of progressive renal impairment, sometimes punctuated by acute episodes of loin pain and haematuria and commonly associated with the development of hypertension. It is popularly believed that there is an increased incidence of urinary tract infection in patients with APCD. There is little evidence to support this, but if such patients do develop infection it may be more difficult to eradicate. As mentioned earlier, the rate of progression to renal failure is variable but tends to follow the same pattern in families. Some may reach end-stage renal failure at 40 years but others

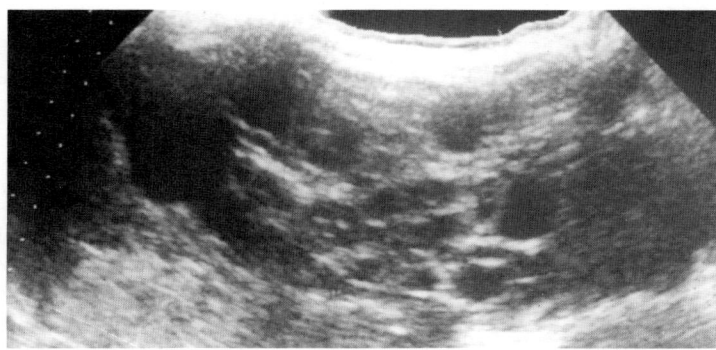

Fig. 9.39 Ultrasound scan of a polycystic kidney showing an enlarged kidney with many cysts of varying size.

survive to 70 years or more.

Approximately 30% of patients with APCD have hepatic cysts; these rarely cause liver dysfunction. Cysts may more rarely develop in the pancreas, spleen, ovary and other organs. Berry aneurysms of the cerebral vessels (10–30%) are not infrequent and may result in subarachnoid or cerebral haemorrhage. Renal neoplasms may develop in polycystic kidneys and are difficult to diagnose.

Polycythaemia and mitral valve prolapse are not uncommon associations.

DIAGNOSIS

Physical examination commonly reveals large, irregular kidneys and possibly hepatomegaly. Definitive diagnosis was previously based on excretion urography, but is now more easily established by ultrasound examination (Fig. 9.39). However, such renal imaging techniques may be equivocal, especially in subjects under the age of 20 years.

TREATMENT

The disease is always progressive. The most important aspect of management is regular blood-pressure recording in affected patients, with control of hypertension as it develops. Uncontrolled hypertension accelerates the loss of kidney function. Some patients may develop salt and water wasting as the disease advances (see p. 496), when salt replacement with Slow Sodium can improve excretory function. Many patients will require renal replacement by dialysis and/or transplantation.

SCREENING

There is debate as to whether the children and siblings of patients with established APCD should be routinely offered screening. We believe that this should be offered to identify patients with this disorder, who must then have regular blood-pressure checks and should be offered genetic counselling in respect of family planning. Screening should not be carried out before the age of 20 years, as excluding the condition may be difficult and hypertension is unusual before this age, as is the start of new families.

Medullary cystic disease ('juvenile nephronophthisis')

Developing early in childhood, juvenile nephronophthisis is commonly inherited in an autosomal recessive manner. A similar condition developing later in childhood (medullary cystic disease) is inherited as an autosomal dominant trait, but sporadic cases occur in both conditions. Despite its name, the dominant histological finding is interstitial inflammation and tubular atrophy, with later development of medullary cysts. Progressive glomerular failure is a secondary consequence.

The dominant features are polyuria, polydipsia and growth retardation. Diagnosis is based on the family history and renal biopsy, the cysts rarely being visualized by imaging techniques.

Medullary sponge kidney

Medullary sponge kidney is an uncommon but not rare condition that usually presents with renal colic or haematuria. Although it is most often sporadic, a few affected families have been reported. The condition is characterized by dilatation of the collecting ducts in the papillae, sometimes with cystic change. In severe cases the medullary area has a sponge-like appearance. The condition may affect one or both kidneys or only part of one kidney. Cyst formation is commonly associated with the development of small calculi within the cyst. In about 20% of patients there is associated hypercalciuria or renal tubular acidosis (see p. 507). Hemihypertrophy of the skeleton has been described in this condition.

The diagnosis is made by excretion urography, which shows small calculi in the papillary zones with an increase in radiodensity *around* these following injection of contrast medium as the dilated or cystic collecting ducts are filled with contrast (Fig. 9.22).

The natural history is one of intermittent colic with passage of small stones or haematuria. Renal function is usually well maintained and renal failure is unusual, except where obstructive nephropathy develops owing to the growth of stones in the pelvis or ureters.

CONGENITAL ABNORMALITIES

Agenesis

Bilateral agenesis is incompatible with extrauterine life. Unilateral agenesis ('a solitary kidney') occurs in 1 in 1000 of the population. It is usually associated with compensatory hypertrophy of the single kidney and normal renal function. Save for the potential hazard of trauma to this solitary kidney, it has no clinical significance.

Hypoplasia

Renal hypoplasia (failed development) of one kidney is uncommon, and hypoplasia of both kidneys is rare. It may be difficult to distinguish unilateral renal hypoplasia from a small kidney due to renal artery stenosis, obstruction or reflux nephropathy in early life. Clinical interest in the condition most often arises in patients with hypertension, where the small kidney may be considered the cause. If the small kidney is shown by radioisotope studies to contribute no useful renal function and if the hypertension has developed in a young subject or is difficult to control by medical treatment, nephrectomy should be undertaken.

Ectopic kidneys

Defects in embryological renal development may lead to ectopic or maldeveloped renal systems. At the risk of oversimplification, the kidneys may be thought of as developing in the embryo as one structure in the 'pelvic' area, migrating upwards and separating with growth. Failure in normal development may result in failure of the kidneys to migrate normally and indeed they may fail to separate. This results in a 'pelvic kidney' when one or both remain in the pelvis, a 'crossed ectopic kidney' when both have moved to the same side of the spine, a horseshoe or discoid kidney when there is partial (usually fusion of the lower poles) or total failure of separation.

In clinical practice the main problem associated with ectopic kidneys usually relates to impaired urinary drainage with secondary obstruction or stone formation. This may be compounded if infection supervenes, the poor drainage making eradication of infection difficult and predisposing to stone formation. Pelvic kidneys may interfere with parturition.

OTHER FAMILIAL RENAL DISEASE

Familial renal disease is in general rare, but there are a number of familial conditions that, among other things, can affect the kidneys.

Alport's syndrome

Alport's syndrome is a rare condition characterized by hereditary nephritis with haematuria, progressive renal failure and high-frequency nerve deafness. It is principally expressed in males and both X-linked and dominant modes of inheritance have been postulated. Some 15% of cases may have ocular abnormalities such as cataract, conical cornea and dislocated small lens. The disease is progressive and accounts for some 5% of cases of end-stage renal failure in childhood or adolescence.

Congenital nephrotic syndrome

This syndrome is rare.

Renal tubular transport defects

Renal tubular transport defects include cystinuria, Hartnup's disease, adult Fanconi syndrome, galactosaemia and fructosaemia. They are discussed in more detail on p. 507.

Renal glycosuria

Renal glycosuria, in which there is glucose in the urine in subjects demonstrated to have normal blood glucose levels, who are not starved and who have no other urinary abnormality, is uncommon. Such patients have either a defect in the tubular threshold for reabsorption of glucose in the proximal tubule (a 'splayed' reabsorption curve) or a defect in the maximal tubular reabsorption of glucose. Both autosomal dominant and recessive inheritance have been postulated. It has no clinical significance except in the differential diagnosis of patients with diabetes mellitus or other tubular disorders such as the Fanconi syndrome.

Tumours of the kidney and genitourinary tract

MALIGNANT RENAL TUMOURS

These comprise 1–2% of all malignant tumours, and the male/female ratio is 2 : 1.

Renal cell carcinoma

Renal cell carcinomas (previously called hyper-nephromas or Grawitz tumours) arise from proximal tubular epithelium. They are the commonest renal tumour in adults. They rarely present before the age of 40, the average age of presentation being 55 years.

PATHOLOGY

The tumours may be solitary, multiple or occasionally bilateral. The tumour lies within the kidney but it may eventually penetrate the capsule. Macroscopically, its cut surface appears as a yellow mass, sometimes containing areas of haemorrhage and cystic degeneration. Local invasion of renal veins and spread to the opposite kidney may occur, as may metastasis to lymph nodes, liver, bone and lung (often as an apparently solitary metastasis). Renal cell carcinomas are highly vascular tumours. Microscopically the tumour is composed of large cells containing clear cytoplasm.

CLINICAL FEATURES

Patients present with haematuria, loin pain and a mass in the flank. Malaise, anorexia and weight loss may occur, and occasionally patients present with polycythaemia (see p. 325). Pyrexia is present in about one-fifth of patients and approximately one-quarter present with metastases. Rarely, a left-sided varicocele may be associated with left-sided tumours that have invaded the renal vein and caused obstruction to drainage of the left testicular vein.

DIAGNOSIS

Excretion urography will reveal a space-occupying lesion in the kidney; 10% of these show calcification.

Ultrasonography is used to demonstrate the solid lesion and to examine the patency of the renal vein and inferior vena cava. CT scanning can also be used to identify the renal lesion and involvement of the renal vein or inferior vena cava. Renal arteriography will reveal the tumour's circulation (Fig. 9.40). Urine cytology for malignant cells is of no value. The ESR is usually raised.

TREATMENT

Treatment is by nephrectomy unless bilateral tumours are present or the contralateral kidney functions poorly, in which case conservative surgery such as partial nephrectomy may be indicated. If metastases are present, nephrectomy may still be warranted since regression of metastases has been reported after removal of the main

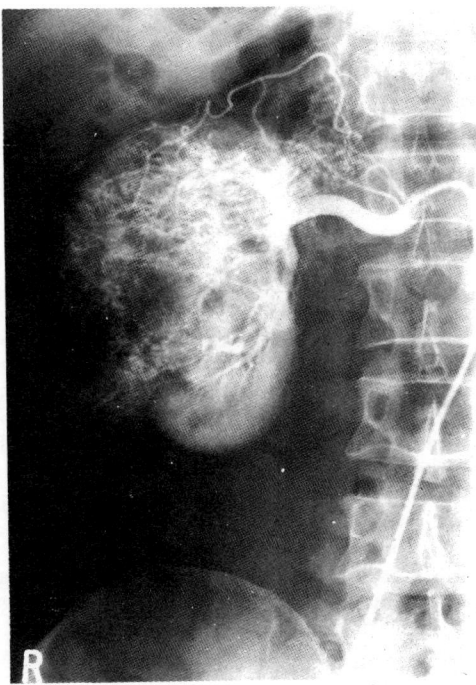

Fig. 9.40 Renal arteriogram in a patient with renal carcinoma. Note the abnormal tumour circulation.

tumour mass. Severe flank pain may also demand nephrectomy despite the presence of metastases. Radiotherapy and chemotherapy have no proven value. Medroxyprogesterone acetate is of some value in controlling metastatic disease. α-Interferon is being used in clinical trials.

PROGNOSIS

The prognosis depends upon the degree of differentiation of the tumour and whether or not metastases are present. In the absence of metastases, the 5-year survival rate exceeds 50%.

Nephroblastoma (Wilms' tumour)

This tumour is seen mainly within the first 3 years of life and may be bilateral. It presents as an abdominal mass, rarely with haematuria. Diagnosis is established by excretion urography followed by arteriography. A combination of nephrectomy, radiotherapy and chemotherapy has much improved survival rates, and the majority of children, even those with metastatic disease, are cured.

BENIGN RENAL TUMOURS

Renal adenoma

Benign adenomas are usually an incidental finding, presenting as a space-occupying lesion on excretion urography. They seldom cause symptoms. On urography they may be difficult to distinguish from a renal cell carcinoma.

Simple cysts

Simple cysts are common. They are discussed in more detail on p. 482.

Differentiation of benign renal cyst from malignant tumour
If a space-occupying lesion is a chance finding on excretion urography in a patient with no relevant symptoms and no haematuria, ultrasonography should be carried out. If the lesion is transonic with no features suggesting a tumour, no further investigation is required. If haematuria has been present, a needle should be inserted into the transonic lesion and cyst fluid aspirated and examined for malignant cells. Contrast medium may be injected to delineate the walls of the cyst. Lesions shown to be solid or non-homogeneous on ultrasonography require further investigation by CT or arteriography.

UROTHELIAL TUMOURS

The calyces, renal pelvis, ureter, bladder and urethra are lined by transitional cell epithelium. Transitional cell tumours account for about 3% of deaths from all forms of malignancy. Such tumours are uncommon below the age of 40 years, and the male/female ratio is 4 : 1. Bladder tumours are about 50 times as common as those of the ureter or renal pelvis.

PREDISPOSING FACTORS

These include:

- Cigarette smoking.
- Exposure to industrial carcinogens such as β-naphthylamine and benzidene. Workers in the chemical, cable and rubber industries are at particular risk.
- Exposure to drugs, e.g. phenacetin, cyclophosphamide.
- Chronic inflammation, e.g. schistosomiasis (usually associated with squamous carcinoma).

PRESENTATION

Painless haematuria is the commonest presenting symptom of bladder malignancy, although pain may occur owing to clot retention. Symptoms suggestive of urinary tract infection may develop in the absence of significant bacteriuria. In patients with bladder cancer, pain may also result from local nerve involvement.

Presenting symptoms may result from local metastases.

Transitional cell carcinomas in the kidney and ureter may present with haematuria. They may also give rise to flank pain, particularly if urinary tract obstruction is present.

INVESTIGATION

Investigation includes:

- Cytological examination of urine for malignant cells
- Excretion urography
- Cystoscopy if no evidence of upper urinary tract pathology has been found

Cytoscopy may be omitted in men under 20 and women under 30 years if significant bacteriuria accompanies the haematuria and both cease following control of the infection, and if urine cytology and excretion urography are normal. With these exceptions, it is essential that haematuria is always investigated.

In cases where the tumour is not clearly outlined on excretion urography, abdominal CT scanning and/or retrograde ureterography may be helpful.

TREATMENT

Pelvic and ureteric tumours
These are treated by nephroureterectomy. Radiotherapy and chemotherapy appear to be of little or no value.

Subsequently cystoscopy should be regularly carried out, since about half the patients will develop bladder tumours.

Bladder tumours
Treatment depends upon the stage of the tumour (in particular whether it has penetrated the bladder muscle) and its degree of differentiation. Treatment options include local cystodiathermy and/or resection with follow-up check cystoscopies, cystectomy, radiotherapy, or local and systemic chemotherapy.

PROGNOSIS

The prognosis ranges from a 5-year survival rate of 80% for lesions not involving bladder muscle to 5% for those presenting with metastases.

BENIGN ENLARGEMENT OF THE PROSTATE GLAND

Benign prostatic enlargement occurs most often in men over the age of 60 years. Such enlargement is much less common in African and Asian individuals. It is unknown in eunuchs. The aetiology of the condition is unknown.

Microscopically, hyperplasia affects the glandular and connective tissue elements of the prostate. Enlargement of the gland stretches and distorts the urethra, obstructing bladder outflow. The bladder musculature hypertrophies so that a higher than usual pressure is generated within the bladder in order to overcome the obstruction and to enable voiding of urine to occur. Bands of muscle fibre are seen at cystoscopy (trabeculation). Eventually the bladder becomes dilated and the muscle hypotonic. The sphincter mechanism at the vesicoureteric junction may be impaired and reflux of urine from the bladder into the ureters and upper urinary tract may occur.

CLINICAL FEATURES

Frequency of urination, usually first noted as nocturia, is a common early symptom. Difficulty or delay in initiating urination, with variability and reduced forcefulness of the urinary stream and post-void dribbling are often present. Suprapubic pain occurs if bladder bacteriuria is present, or if a bladder calculus has formed as a result of stagnation of urine within the bladder, or in acute retention of urine. Flank pain may accompany dilatation of the upper tracts. Acute retention of urine (see p. 487) or retention with overflow incontinence may occur. Occasionally, severe haematuria results from rupture of prostatic veins or as a consequence of bacteriuria or stone disease. Some patients present with severe renal failure.

Abdominal examination for bladder enlargement together with examination of the rectum are essential. A benign prostate feels smooth. An accurate impression of prostatic size cannot be obtained on rectal examination.

INVESTIGATION

This should include urine culture, assessment of renal function by measuring the blood urea and serum creatinine concentrations, a plain abdominal X-ray, and renal ultrasonography to define whether upper-tract dilatation is present. Excretion urography is not usually necessary. If possible, an act of urination should be watched and the flow rate of urine measured. The completeness of bladder emptying after an act of voiding can be assessed by ultrasonography or by inspection of the after-voiding radiograph carried out during excretion urography. Cystourethroscopy is essential.

MANAGEMENT AND PROGNOSIS

Patients with prostatic symptoms who do not have upper tract dilatation require surgery only if symptoms are troublesome or if acute retention has occurred. Eradication of bacteriuria may relieve symptoms originally attributed to outflow obstruction.

Deterioration in renal function or the development of upper-tract dilatation requires surgery. Transurethral resection is usually successful unless the gland is very large. It carries a lower morbidity and mortality with a shorter stay in hospital than open prostatectomy. Very large glands require open transvesical prostatectomy.

In acute retention or retention with overflow, the first priorities are to relieve pain and to establish urethral catheter drainage. The bladder should be decompressed slowly to prevent bleeding from the mucosa. If urethral catheterization is impossible, suprapubic catheter drainage should be carried out. The choice of further management is then between immediate prostatectomy, a period of catheter drainage followed by prostatectomy, or the acceptance of a permanent indwelling suprapubic or urethral catheter.

PROSTATIC CARCINOMA

Prostatic carcinoma accounts for 7% of all cancers in men and is the fourth commonest cause of death from malignant disease in men in England and Wales. Malignant change within the prostate becomes increasingly common with advancing age. By the age of 80 years, 80% of men have malignant foci within the gland, but most of these appear to lie dormant. Histologically, the tumour is an adenocarcinoma. Hormonal factors are thought to play a role in the aetiology.

CLINICAL FEATURES

Presentation is usually with symptoms of lower urinary tract obstruction or of metastatic spread, particularly to bone. The diagnosis may be made by the incidental finding of a hard irregular gland on rectal examination or as an unexpected histological result after prostatectomy for what was believed to be benign prostatic hypertrophy.

INVESTIGATION

A histological diagnosis is essential before treatment is considered. This may be obtained:

- By cytological staining of biopsy material from the prostate
- By histological examination of biopsy material or material obtained at transurethral or open prostatectomy

If metastases are present, serum acid phosphatase may be elevated; it is a myth that elevated levels occur as a result of rectal examination.

Ultrasonography is of value in defining the size

of the gland and staging any tumour present. The upper renal tracts can be examined by ultrasonography for evidence of dilatation. Bone metastases may appear as osteosclerotic lesions on X-ray or may be detected by isotopic bone scans.

TREATMENT

Treatment is by prostatectomy for disease confined to the gland, combined with bilateral orchidectomy or stilboestrol or antiandrogen therapy if metastases are present. External pelvic irradiation is used in some locally infiltrating prostatic malignancies.

PROGNOSIS

The duration of survival depends on the age of the patient and the degree of differentiation and extent of the tumour.

TESTICULAR TUMOURS

Testicular tumours, though uncommon, are the commonest malignant disease in men between the ages of 29 and 34 years. All such tumours should nowadays be regarded as curable. Patient survival depends upon early diagnosis, accurate staging of the tumour and appropriate treatment and follow-up. The expertise of a specialist centre is invaluable.

More than 96% of testicular tumours arise from germ cells. Two main types of tumour exist:

- Seminomas (about one-third)
- Teratomas (about two-thirds)

AETIOLOGY

The aetiology is unknown. The risk of malignant change is much greater in undescended testes and there is a history of orchidopexy in about 10% of patients.

CLINICAL FEATURES

Common presenting symptoms are:

- Testicular swelling, which may be painless or painful
- Symptoms from metastases

DIFFERENTIAL DIAGNOSIS

The differential diagnosis includes:

- Epididymo-orchitis
- Torsion
- Chronic infection, e.g. tuberculosis, syphilitic gumma

INVESTIGATION

Diagnosis may only be possible after surgical exploration of the testis through the groin. Scrotal exploration and scrotal testicular biopsy should be avoided owing to the high incidence of tumour implantation.

Staging of the tumour will require:

- Chest X-ray to look for metastases
- Estimation of α-fetoprotein and β-human chorionic gonadotrophin concentrations (tumour markers)
- Abdominal CT scanning

TREATMENT

Seminomas are radiosensitive, so tumours confined to the testis or with metastases below the diaphragm only are treated by radiotherapy. More widespread tumours require chemotherapy.

Teratomas are treated by orchidectomy if the growth is confined to the testis. Chemotherapy is required for more widespread disease (see p. 374).

Renal disease in the elderly

Renal failure in the elderly more often results from renal vascular disease or urinary tract obstruction than in younger age groups. In males, obstruction is most often due to benign or malignant prostatic enlargement, while in females it results from pelvic cancer.

Progressive sclerosis of glomeruli occurs with ageing and this, together with the development of atheromatous renal vascular disease, accounts for the progressive reduction in glomerular filtration rate seen with advancing years. A glomerular filtration rate of 50–60 ml·min^{-1} (about half the normal value for a young adult) may be regarded as 'normal' in a patient in his or her eighties. The reduction in muscle mass often seen with ageing may mask this deterioration in renal function in that the serum creatinine concentration may be less than 0.12 mmol·L^{-1} in an elderly patient whose glomerular filtration rate is 50 ml·min^{-1} or lower. The use of serum creatinine as a measure of renal function in the elderly must take this into account. This is especially important in the elderly when prescribing drugs whose excretion is in whole or in part by the kidney.

Urinary tract infections are more common in the elderly, in whom impaired bladder emptying due to prostatic disease in males and neuropathic bladder—especially common in females—is frequently found. Symptoms may be atypical, the major complaints being incontinence, nocturia, smelly urine or vague change in well-being with little in the way of dysuria. Demonstration of significant bacteriuria in the presence of such symptoms requires treatment.

Urinary incontinence is one of the major disabilities of the elderly. Correctable factors, such as chronic constipation, bacteriuria and treatable bladder outflow impairment need to be excluded. An expert and committed incontinence advisory and treatment service combining nursing and medical skills is invaluable in elderly patients with this distressing problem.

Further reading

Cattell WR, Webb JAW & Hilson AJW (1989) *Clinical Renal Imaging*. Chichester: John Wiley & Sons.

Massey SG & Glassock RJ (eds) (1983) *Textbook of Nephrology*. Baltimore: Williams & Wilkins.

Schrier RW & Gottschalk CW (eds) (1988) *Diseases of the Kidney*, 4th edn. Boston: Little, Brown and Co.

Wood REM (1983) *Renal Transplantation: A Clinical Handbook*. London: Bailliere Tindall.

10

Water, Electrolyte and Acid–Base Homeostasis

Water and electrolyte homeostasis

In health the volume and composition of body fluids are held remarkably constant from day to day. The end-organ primarily responsible for this is the kidney. In disease this constancy of the 'milieu interieur' can be seriously deranged as a result of:

● Extrarenal factors (e.g. vomiting or diarrhoea)
● Endocrine disturbances
● Intrinsic renal disease

The diagnosis and treatment of fluid and electrolyte imbalance are commonly considered complicated and difficult. This is not the case provided certain basic physiological principles are understood and simple rules for clinical assessment are applied. The aim here is to set these out simply so that control of fluid and electrolyte balance is no longer surrounded by an ill-founded 'mystique'.

Physiological principles

It is helpful in clinical practice to distinguish between the *volume* of any body fluid and its *composition*. These may be disturbed singly or together.

Body fluid volume and distribution

Water is the chief constituent of the body, accounting for 45–80% of the body weight. This percent-

Table 10.1 Body water as a percentage of body weight.

Build	Infants	Men	Women
Thin	80%	65%	55%
Average	70%	60%	50%
Fat	65%	55%	45%

age varies with age, sex and body build (Table 10.1), being greater in men, in thin subjects and in infants. An average 75-kg male has about 45 litres of water. Two thirds of this is intracellular fluid (ICF). The remaining 15 litres is extra-cellular fluid (ECF) and is divided between the interstitial fluid (IF) (10 litres) and the vascular compartment (VC) (5 litres) (see Fig. 10.1). A fourth, 'transcellular' compartment includes cerebrospinal, synovial, pleural and pericardial fluids, plus water in the gut. Normally this is small, but in disease, e.g. in paralytic ileus or massive pleural effusion, it can become important.

Distribution of water between the extracellular and intracellular compartments depends on an osmotic equilibrium between them.

The *osmolality* of a solution is determined by the total concentration of dissolved or colloid particles within the solution. Thus, 1 mol of sodium chloride dissolved in 1 kg of water has an osmolality of 2 osmol·kg^{-1}, as sodium chloride freely dissociates into the two particles, sodium ion and chloride ion.

One millimole of sodium chloride in 1 kg of water gives an osmolality of 2 mosmol·kg. One mole of urea (which does not dissociate) in 1 kg of water has an osmolality of 1 osmol·kg^{-1}.

In a complex solution of several electrolytes, osmolality can be calculated by adding together the molar concentration of all the constituents, taking account of the degree of dissociation. As sodium and chloride are the dominant ECF ions, plasma osmolality is, for practical purposes:

$$\text{sodium concentration (mmol·L}^{-1}) \times 2 + 10$$

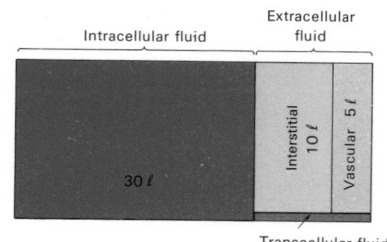

Fig. 10.1 Distribution of body water in a 75-kg man.

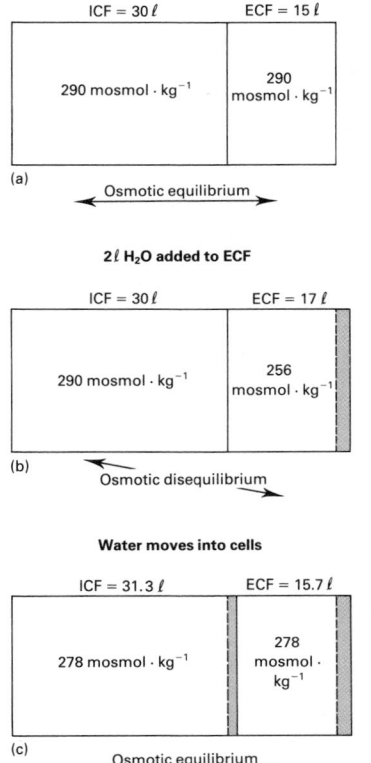

Fig. 10.2 Osmotic equilibrium, showing the changes occurring (a–c) when 2 litres of water are added to the ECF.

The 10 takes into account the osmolality of the glucose and urea in the plasma.

The concentration of particles, i.e. the osmolality, within the ICF and the ECF is always in equilibrium. Addition of water to the ECF reduces its osmolality, causes disequilibrium in osmolality between the two compartments, and leads to water moving into cells until the osmolality equilibrium is re-established (see Fig. 10.2). Loss of water from the ECF would do the reverse.

Partitioning of water between the vascular and interstitial compartments depends on osmotic equilibrium but is also affected by the osmotic pressure exerted by non-diffusible plasma proteins (mainly albumin). This 'oncotic pressure', equal to about 25 mm Hg, is critical to the circulation of fluid between the capillaries and interstitial fluid. Fluid leaves the arteriolar end of capillary beds under the influence of capillary hydrostatic pressure and is 'recaptured' at the low-pressure, venous, end by the oncotic pressure of plasma proteins. In hypoalbuminaemic states this balance is lost and oedema fluid accumulates in the tissues. Conversely, removal of water from plasma, e.g. by ultrafiltration in patients with kidney failure (see p. 474) causes a rise in plasma oncotic pressure that 'sucks' fluid into the vascular compartment.

The balance of fluid between the two compartments is also dependent on the Gibbs–Donnan equilibrium (this explains the unequal distribution of diffusible ions on the two sides of a semipermeable membrane if one side contains a poorly diffusible ion). The result of both these effects is that the osmolality of plasma is marginally greater than that of interstitial fluid and the electrolyte composition of the two compartments is also slightly different (Table 10.2).

The composition of body fluids

The composition of intracellular, interstitial and plasma fluid is set out in Table 10.2. Allowing for the plasma oncotic pressure and the Gibbs–Donnan distribution, plasma and interstitial fluid have, for practical purposes, the same electrolyte content. Intracellular fluid, which constitutes two-thirds of body fluid, is quite different. In particular, sodium and chloride ions are primarily extracellu-

Table 10.2 Electrolyte composition of intracellular and extracellular fluids.

	Plasma (mmol·L^{-1})	Interstitial fluid (mmol·L^{-1})	Intracellular fluid (mmol·L^{-1})
Na$^+$	142	144	10
K$^+$	4	4	160
Ca^{2+}	2.5	1.25	1.5
Mg^{2+}	1.0	0.5	13
Cl$^-$	102	114	2
HCO$_3^-$	26	30	8
PO$_4^{2-}$	1.0	1.0	57
SO$_4^{2-}$	0.5	0.5	10
Organic acid	6	5	
Protein	16	0	55

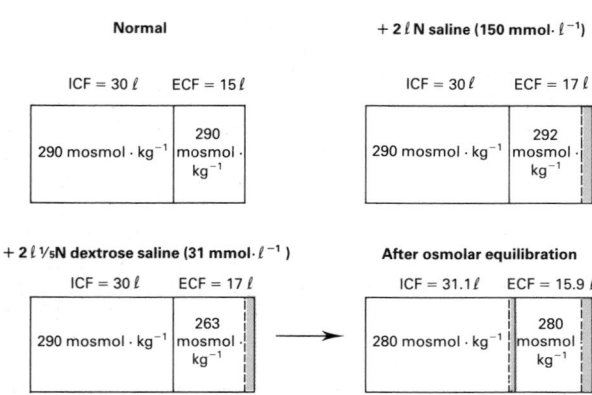

Fig. 10.3 The effect on osmotic equilibrium of adding saline or dextrose saline.

lar, while potassium is the dominant intracellular cation, balanced by phosphate, sulphate and bicarbonate anions and protein. This 'in–out' difference in the distribution of sodium and potassium is a consequence of the metabolic cell pumps and is dependent on normal oxygenation and metabolism. The separation of sodium and potassium outside and inside cells has important consequences in relation to fluid distribution. Since sodium and chloride are extracellular, loss or addition of salt-containing solutions primarily affects the volume of the ECF and only affects the ICF if there is also a change in the osmolality of the ECF.

The intravenous infusion of 'normal' (isotonic) saline (150 mmol sodium and chloride per litre) primarily affects the volume of the ECF, since there is little change in osmolality (see Fig. 10.3). The slight rise in osmolality shown in Fig. 10.3 is due to the fact that the concentration of sodium in normal saline (150 mmol·L^{-1}) slightly exceeds the physiological mean (145 mmol·L^{-1}) in ECF. Any subsequent osmolar equilibration would result in a shift of a mere 40 ml of water into the vascular compartment. Addition of $\frac{1}{5}$-normal saline (30 mmol of sodium and chloride per litre) reduces the osmolality of ECF (Fig. 10.3). Water accompanied by glucose but not sodium enters cells until a new osmolar equilibrium is achieved. The 2 litre infusion thus distributes between both the extracellular fluid and the intracellular fluid compartment. The increase in extracellular fluid volume is significantly less than is seen with infusion of normal saline (see Fig. 10.3).

Factors controlling volume and composition

Body water homeostasis is effected by thirst and the urine-concentrating and diluting functions of the kidney. These in turn are controlled by intracellular osmoreceptors, principally in the hypothalamus, to some extent by volume receptors

in capacitance vessels close to the heart, and possibly via the renin–angiotensin system. Of these, the major and best-understood control is via osmoreceptors.

An increase in intracellular osmolality—for example after water deprivation—stimulates both thirst and release of ADH (arginine vasopressin: AVP) from the posterior pituitary. Thirst stimulates increased water intake while ADH increases the reabsorption of water from the tubular fluid by its action on the distal tubules of the kidney. This causes a reduction in the urine output. The increased intake of water and reduced urinary excretion result in a net gain of water that returns body fluid osmolality to normal. A decrease in intracellular osmolality in the osmoreceptors has the reverse effect. By this means the amount of water in body fluid is adjusted to ensure normal osmolality in the face of varying increase or loss of water or solute.

Non-osmotic release of ADH mediated via baroreceptors (see below) is now well recognized as a further control mechanism for maintaining an effective circulating blood volume both by the antidiuretic and vasopressor effect of arginine vasopressin.

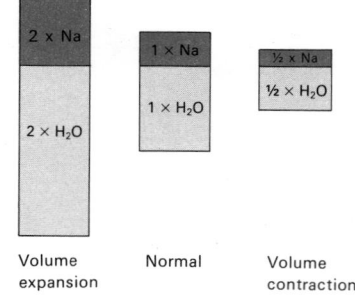

Fig. 10.4 The relationship of sodium to water in normonatraemia.

Control of effective circulating blood volume

For the health of all tissues it is essential that there is a constant circulation of blood, both to supply oxygen and nutrients and to remove waste products. To achieve this there must be an adequate pump (the heart) and an appropriate circulating blood volume. The importance of maintaining the circulating blood volume is reflected in the variety of 'feedback' systems that exist to guard it. Apart from the control of the circulating red cell mass and vasomotor tone, these operate primarily through the control of body sodium and the secondary control of accompanying water.

Control of body sodium and extracellular body fluid

Sodium and its accompanying anions, principally chloride and bicarbonate, are the main extracellular electrolytes. They are the main determinants of plasma osmolality and, through osmoreceptors, they control water homeostasis. It is the *amount* of sodium in the ECF, with adjustment of water balance to a normal body fluid osmolality, that determines the *volume* of the ECF; control of the volume of ECF is thus achieved by controlling the amount of sodium in the ECF.

To understand disturbance of fluid balance, it is essential to distinguish clearly between the *concentration* of sodium in the ECF (in practice, the plasma sodium) and the *amount* of sodium present (see Fig. 10.4). Concentration only tells the relative amounts of sodium to water; it tells nothing about the absolute amount or volume of either. In practice, this requires a separate clinical assessment of the volume of the ECF.

Control of the volume of ECF via control of sodium balance is dependent on a variety of volume receptors or sensors. Volume receptors are believed to be present in the large-capacitance vessels close to the heart and possibly in heart muscle.

Volume receptors in the cardiac atria control the release of a powerful natriuretic hormone—atrial natriuretic peptide—from granules localized in the atrial wall. Atrial natriuretic peptide (ANP) infusion in man also causes hypotension, the precise mechanism for which is unclear.

Receptors in the walls of the afferent glomerular arterioles respond, via the juxtaglomerular apparatus, to changes in renal perfusion, and control the activity of the renin–angiotensin–aldosterone system. Neurogenic reflexes within the kidney may also be involved, and the circulation of a further natriuretic hormone, the source of which is unclear, is postulated. The final common path for such regulatory systems is to increase or decrease the renal excretion of sodium in the event of an increase or decrease in effective circulating blood volume. An increase in the reabsorption of salt, with concomitant retention of water (due to a change in osmolality), expands the vascular and interstitial compartments, while increased sodium excretion has the opposite effects.

Clinical assessment of water and electrolyte balance

The average normal daily intakes of sodium, potassium and water are 100–250 mmol, 40–120 mmol, and 500–2500 ml, respectively. The possible losses from the gut are given in Table 10.3. Daily urinary losses vary greatly; they may be as much as 5 litres or more of water, with loss of 150–200 mmol of sodium and 50–100 mmol of potassium.

HISTORY

The first essential step is a careful history to define circumstances that might lead to fluid and electrolyte imbalance, such as vomiting, diarrhoea or polyuria (see Table 10.4).

PHYSICAL EXAMINATION

Except in severe dehydration, the time-honoured assessment of skin turgor, intraocular pressure and

Table 10.3 Average concentrations and potential daily losses of water and electrolytes from the gut.

	Na$^+$ (mmol·L^{-1})	K$^+$ (mmol·L^{-1})	Cl$^-$ (mmol·L^{-1})	Volume (ml per 24 h)
Stomach	50	10	110	2500
Small intestine:				
Recent ileostomy	120	5	110	1500
Adapted ileostomy	50	4	25	500
Bile	140	5	105	500
Pancreatic juice	140	5	60	2000
Diarrhoea	130	10–15	95	1000–2000+

the state of the tongue is imprecise and of limited value. Of much greater importance is careful assessment of the circulatory status and the presence or absence of oedema. Circulatory failure may be obvious, with recumbent hypotension, tachycardia and cold peripheral parts. When less obvious, particular attention must be paid to the jugular venous pressure (JVP) and to the presence or absence of postural hypotension. Usually a normal or elevated JVP can be defined, but if in doubt, and especially in oliguric patients, a central venous line must be inserted to record central venous pressure (CVP).

An elevated JVP or CVP always indicates fluid overload, except in acute heart failure. A low JVP or CVP in a setting of fluid loss or incomplete replacement must be taken as evidence of volume depletion and is an indication for the administration of fluids. A normal or low blood pressure in a previously hypertensive patient in the absence of drug treatment or evidence of acute myocardial damage is also highly suggestive of fluid depletion.

Postural hypotension (a fall of systolic blood pressure after 5 min of standing of more than 20 mm Hg from the recumbent value or to less than 100 mm Hg) may result from:

- Hypotensive drugs
- Autonomic neuropathy
- Volume depletion

A low JVP plus postural hypotension in an appropriate clinical setting provides very strong evidence for volume depletion.

Sacral or symmetrical peripheral oedema and, less reliably, basal lung crackles are evidence of fluid overload, whether due to oliguric renal failure, heart failure or hypoalbuminaemic states. Only very rarely, and usually in a setting of excessive diuretic therapy for heart failure or gross hypoalbuminaemic states, is it possible to have oedema associated with a *reduced* blood volume due to salt and water depletion.

Evidence of weight loss due to negative fluid balance is rarely available at the time of first presentation, except in severe cases when it has been noted by the patient or his relatives. In hospital, review of weight charts is valuable. An acute increase or decrease in weight always reflects a change in water balance, and in problem cases daily weighing is mandatory. In hospitalized patients, careful review of 'input/output' charts can also give valuable information, but these are often inaccurate.

It should be noted that the physical signs described relate primarily to changes in the ECF volume, especially the intravascular volume. In turn these relate principally to changes in body fluid balance due to salt and water—the most common clinical problem. Pure water loss or excess has much less effect on the circulation, as the

Table 10.4 Causes of fluid and electolyte disturbances.

Losses

Gut
Vomiting
Diarrhoea
Fistula or 'ostomies'
Paralytic ileus

Kidney
Diuretic therapy
Polyuria
   Post-obstructive
   Post-acute tubular necrosis
   Severe renal failure
   Hypokalaemia
   Lithium therapy
   Hypercalcaemia
Diabetes mellitus
Diabetes insipidus
Hypoadrenalism

Reduced intake

Loss of thirst mechanism
Unconscious/confused states
Hypothalamic lesion (rare)

Lack of access to water
Unconscious/confused states
Bedridden
Infants

Inappropriate/inadequate intake
Hospitalized patients, especially on i.v. regimens

Fluid retention

Heart failure
Hypoproteinaemia, e.g. cirrhosis, nephrotic
   syndrome
Oliguric renal failure
Cirrhosis
Excessive fluid replacement
Inappropriate ADH secretion
Idiopathic oedema

altered water volume is 'shared' by all of the 45 litres of body water; quite severe losses or excesses can be tolerated haemodynamically and can be difficult to detect on clinical examination (see Fig. 10.2). Net water loss or gain is more readily identified by the development of hyper- or hyponatraemia. Pure water loss is uncommon; pure water excess is usually iatrogenic.

INVESTIGATION

Haematological investigation
In an appropriate setting an abnormally high haemoglobin or haematocrit suggests fluid deple-

tion. The clinical situation is, however, often complex. Interpretation of haemoglobin level or haematocrit is particularly difficult in patients who are anaemic or who have lost blood as a result of the underlying disease.

Biochemical investigation
Having assessed the volume of body fluid, the nature of the fluid loss or excess can be defined by measurement of plasma electrolytes, particularly the plasma sodium. It must be re-emphasized that sodium concentration does *not* of itself give information as to whether there is sodium depletion or overload. Rather, consideration of plasma sodium concentration taken in conjunction with an assessment of body fluid volume allows definition of the nature of the problem and the measures required to treat it.

Measurement of random urinary sodium concentration or 24-hour urinary sodium excretion is of very little value in the *managment* of salt and water balance. Thus, the urinary sodium concentration and daily output depends both on kidney function and on sodium intake, whether oral or i.v. To challenge the kidney's ability to conserve or excrete sodium (or water), the patient must be deprived or loaded with sodium (or water). Neither is usually appropriate in the *management* of derangements in salt and water balance. Challenges *are* required to prove unequivocally salt-wasting or salt-retaining states but are, for the most part, academic. A low urinary sodium concentration may be diagnostic of acute prerenal failure (see p. 472). Water deprivation is a necessary part of the diagnosis of diabetes insipidus (see p. 819).

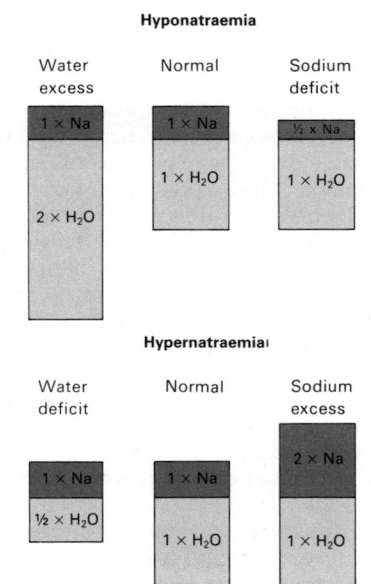

Fig. 10.5 The relationship of sodium to water in hyponatraemia and hypernatraemia.

NORMONATRAEMIC VOLUME OVERLOAD OR DEFICIT

This is the most common disturbance (see Fig. 10.4). The fluid overload or deficit is normally modest. The former may be due to heart failure, oliguric renal failure or hypoalbuminaemic states and the latter to vomiting, diarrhoea or polyuria from whatever cause. It is identified by clinical evidence of fluid overload or deficit plus a serum sodium value within the normal range of 135–150 $mmol \cdot L^{-1}$.

TREATMENT

Treatment may be divided into primary and secondary.

Primary treatment
This is directed at eliminating the cause of the problem, e.g.

- Improvement in cardiac function } overload
- Correction of hypoalbuminaemia
- Arrest of vomiting and diarrhoea } deficit
- Removal of drugs causing polyuria

Secondary treatment
This is concerned with correcting the salt and water abnormality pending the response to primary treatment or alleviating the situation when primary treatment is not possible.

Salt and water overload. This requires:

- Restriction in sodium intake—a 'no added salt

The causes and nature of disturbances in water and electrolyte balance

The major causes for a disturbance in fluid and electrolyte balance are set out in Table 10.4. At the time of presentation the situation is commonly confused by partial correction of the problem by the patient, e.g. thirst and increased water intake in diarrhoea, or by partial or overenthusiastic treatment by attending clinicians.

Following a careful history, the volume of body fluid (especially the ECF) and its composition with respect to sodium and potassium concentrations should be assessed. The ECF volume may be normal, expanded or contracted (see Figs. 10.4 and 10.5). At the same time the serum sodium may be normal, increased or decreased (see Fig. 10.5).

regimen', allowing salt only in cooking with no addition of salt at table and avoidance of salty foods (50 mmol of sodium daily).

- Diuretic (or more correctly natriuretic) treatment with thiazide diuretics (e.g. bendrofluazide 5 mg twice daily). More powerful loop diuretics (frusemide or ethacrynic acid) should only be used when a thiazide diuretic fails *or* where there is severe renal failure or life-threatening pulmonary congestion.
- Modest restriction in water intake (1000 ml per day). This is usually sufficient since, if the sodium overload is corrected, the accompanying water overload will correct itself.

Normonatraemic volume depletion. This requires replacement of salt and water. This is best done orally if possible.

If kidney function is normal, an increased water intake (2–3 litres per day) accompanied by 60–80 mmol of sodium chloride (6–8 tablets Slow Sodium daily in divided doses) will suffice, as sodium retention by the kidneys will be maximal. In the presence of salt-wasting kidney disease, larger amounts of sodium chloride may be required. These are best supplied by the *cautious* infusion of normal saline.

Glucose–electrolyte solutions have been increasingly used to restore fluid balance in patients with diarrhoeal illnesses. This is based on the fact that the presence of glucose stimulates intestinal absorption of salt and water. In patients eating normally, glucose–electrolyte solutions have no special advantage over water and Slow Sodium. They are of value in anorexic patients or in postoperative patients prior to returning to a normal food intake.

HYPONATRAEMIA

Hyponatraemia may be due to an excess of body water with a normal amount of body sodium, a normal amount of water with reduced sodium, or some combination of the two (Fig. 10.5). Rarely it may be pseudohyponatraemia, where in hyperlipidaemia there is a spuriously low measured sodium concentration, the sodium being confined to the aqueous phase but having its concentration expressed in terms of the total volume of plasma.

Salt-deficient hyponatraemia

The commonest sites of large sodium losses (see Table 10.4) are:

- *The gut.* Vomiting, diarrhoea or sequestration of fluid in paralytic ileus can lead to considerable losses of sodium and potassium as well as causing acid–base disturbance.

- *The kidney.* Renal salt loss is usually less obvious than loss from the gut, and occurs as a result of defective tubular reabsorption, whether as a result of:
  (a) Osmotic diuresis (e.g. hyperglycaemia or severe uraemia)
  (b) Excessive use of diuretics
  (c) Adrenocortical insufficiency (see p. 812)
  (d) Tubulo-interstitial renal disease

With the exception of the recovery phase of acute tubular necrosis (see p. 474), salt-wasting renal disease is most often associated with disease of the medullary area, as in:

- Atrophic pyelonephritis
- Obstructive nephropathy
- Tubulo-interstitial disease due to:
  (a) Sickle cell disease or trait
  (b) Analgesic nephropathy
  (c) Diabetes mellitus
- Medullary cystic disease

Hyponatraemia due to salt loss in excess of water initially suppresses ADH secretion via the osmoreceptors, but as fluid volume is lost, volume receptors override the osmoreceptors and stimulate both thirst and the release of ADH. With extrarenal losses and normal kidneys, the urinary excretion of sodium falls in response to the volume depletion, as does water excretion, leading to concentrated urine containing less than 10 mmol·L^{-1} of sodium. However, in salt-wasting kidney disease, renal compensation cannot occur and the only physiological protection is increased water intake in response to thirst.

CLINICAL FEATURES

With sodium depletion the clinical picture is usually dominated by features of volume depletion.

The diagnosis is usually obvious where there is a history of gut losses, diabetes mellitus or diuretic abuse. Losses due to renal or adrenocortical disease may be less easily identified and are suggested by a urinary sodium concentration of more than 20 mmol·L^{-1} in the presence of clinically evident volume depletion.

TREATMENT

This is directed at the primary cause whenever possible. Increased salt intake as Slow Sodium 60–80 mmol daily is all that is required in the relatively healthy patient who can take this by mouth. In the face of vomiting or severe volume depletion, intravenous infusion of normal saline is given. Potassium supplements and correction of acid–base abnormalities may also be required.

Table 10.5 Intravenous fluids in general use for fluid and electrolyte disturbances.

	Na^+ $(mmol \cdot L^{-1})$	K^+ $(mmol \cdot L^{-1})$	HCO_3^- or equivalent $(mmol \cdot L^{-1})$	Cl^- $(mmol \cdot L^{-1})$	Ca^{2+} $(mmol \cdot L^{-1})$	Indication (see footnotes)
Normal plasma values	142	4.5	26	103	2.5	
Sodium chloride 0.9% ('normal saline')	150	—	—	150	—	1
Sodium chloride 0.18% + glucose 4% ('1/5 normal saline')	30	—	—	30	—	2
Glucose 5%	—	—	—	—	—	3
Sodium bicarbonate 1.26%	150	—	150	—	—	4
Sodium bicarbonate 8.4%	1000	—	1000	—	—	5
Compound sodium lactate (Hartmann's)	131	5	29	111	2	6

1. Volume expansion in hypovolaemic patients. Rarely to maintain fluid balance when there are large losses of sodium.
2. Maintenance of fluid balance in normo-volaemic, normo-natraemic patients.
3. To replace *water*. May be alternated with normal saline as an alternative to (2).
4. For volume expansion in hypovolaemic, *acidotic* patients alternating with (1). Occasionally for maintenance of fluid balance combined with (2) in salt-wasting, acidotic patients. To induce forced alkaline diuresis, e.g. in severe salicylate poisoning.
5. Small amounts (100–200 ml) used to correct acidosis following cardiac arrest.
6. Reserve for healthy (e.g. postoperative) patients. *Never* in patients with renal disease because of potassium content. Best avoided.

Guidelines for intravenous fluid administration in fluid and electrolyte disturbances

Only use if not possible to give fluids by mouth or nasogastric tube.

If hypovolaemic, correct with:

- Normal saline
  or
- Normal saline alternating with 1.26% sodium bicarbonate if acidotic

For maintenance fluid balance:

- 'Guesstimate' daily water and salt losses (see Table 10.3)
- Identify appropriate fluid (see Table 10.5)
- Confirm replacement is appropriate by assessing daily body *fluid volume* clinically and fluid composition from plasma electrolytes

If hypervolaemic:

- Give no fluid
- Give minimum fluid required for parenteral drugs in a fluid compatible with drug (usually 5% glucose)

It cannot be overemphasized that, apart from in severe fluid overload or in life-threatening pulmonary congestion or severe volume depletion due to gross salt and water loss (as in infants), aggressive correction of abnormalities of salt and water balance are rarely justified, and are often dangerous. Gradual correction over 48 h is gener-

ally satisfactory. Aggressive volume repletion demands obsessional monitoring of the CVP, which is best done by a CVP line, and regular checks for evidence of pulmonary congestion or peripheral oedema.

Table 10.5 gives a list of fluids and electrolytes available for intravenous use.

Hyponatraemia due to water excess ('dilutional hyponatraemia')

This results from an intake of water in excess of the kidneys' ability to excrete it. It is uncommon with normal kidney function, requiring an intake of approximately $1 \text{ L} \cdot \text{h}^{-1}$. Overgenerous infusion of 5% glucose into postoperative patients is one of the commonest causes, in which situation it is exacerbated by increased ADH secretion in response to stress. Some degree of hyponatraemia is usual in acute oliguric renal failure, while in patients with chronic renal failure it is most often due to ill-advised advice to 'push' fluids.

The commonest presentation of hyponatraemia due to water excess is in patients with severe cardiac failure, hepatic cirrhosis or the nephrotic syndrome. In all these conditions there is usually an element of reduced glomerular filtration rate with avid reabsorption of sodium and chloride in the proximal tubule. This leads to reduced delivery of chloride to the 'diluting' ascending limb of Henle's loop and a reduced ability to generate 'free water', with a consequent inability to excrete dilute urine. This is commonly compounded by the administration of diuretics that block chloride reabsorption and interfere with the dilution of filtrate either in Henle's loop (loop diuretics) or distally (thiazides).

Adrenal insufficiency (see p. 812) also interferes with the renal excretion of water.

CLINICAL FEATURES

Symptoms are common with dilutional hyponatraemia when this develops acutely. They are principally neurological and are due to the movement of water into brain cells in response to the fall in extracellular osmolality. Symptoms rarely occur until the serum sodium is less than 120 mmol·L^{-1} and are more usually associated with values around 110 mmol·L^{-1} or lower. Symptoms include confusion and restlessness leading to drowsiness, myoclonic jerks, generalized convulsions and eventually coma.

TREATMENT

Most cases are simply managed by restriction of water intake with review of diuretic therapy. Hypertonic salt solutions should never be used in oedematous patients. The use of hypertonic saline should be restricted to patients with acute water intoxication and *must* be given slowly (not more than 70 mmol·h^{-1}), the aim being to increase the serum sodium to more than 125 mmol·L^{-1}. Rapid infusion of hypertonic saline carries a risk of acute heart failure due to sodium overload or brain damage due to acute fluid shifts.

In already fluid-overloaded patients 100 ml of 20% mannitol may be infused in an attempt to increase renal water excretion.

Syndrome of inappropriate ADH secretion

This is described in Chapter 16. It is manifest as hyponatraemia with normal or slight expansion of ECF volume.

HYPERNATRAEMIA

This is most often the result of a loss of water in excess of sodium. A true excess of body sodium with normal water (see Fig. 10.5) is rare and is usually iatrogenic. Loss of water from the ECF is buffered by the movement of water from the ICF to maintain osmotic equilibrium. Water losses must therefore be massive to induce a significant rise in serum sodium. Water depletion results either from inadequate intake or losses from the gut, kidneys or via the skin and lungs.

Insufficient intake is most often found in the elderly or neonates or in unconscious patients

when access to water is denied or confusion or coma eliminates the normal response to thirst. Rarely it is due to hypothalamic disease with loss of normal thirst. The situation is exacerbated by increased losses of fluid.

Gastrointestinal fluids are for the most part hypotonic (see Table 10.3). Thus, unreplaced losses due to vomiting or diarrhoea result in hypernatraemia. Similarly, litres of hypotonic fluid can be lost from the skin or lungs, especially in febrile diseases and in hot, dry climates. Infants, because of their large surface area relative to volume, are at special risk. Hypernatraemia due to large water losses is also common in patients with extensive burns.

Renal losses of water in sufficient excess of sodium to induce hypernatraemia occur only in patients with diabetes insipidus or in those undergoing spontaneous osmotic diuresis as in severe hyperglycaemia or (less often) uraemia. The latter mechanism was responsible for the hypernatraemia formerly seen in neurosurgical wards when unconscious patients were tube-fed solutions high in protein and low in water.

Hypernatraemia due to salt excess is virtually always iatrogenic, as the result of a too liberal infusion of hypertonic saline or bicarbonate solution, or the accidental addition of salt rather than sugar to an infant's feed.

CLINICAL FEATURES

Water-depletion hypernatraemia is associated with signs of volume depletion and circulatory failure. If acute, hypernatraemia may lead to venous thrombosis in infants and cerebral symptoms such as lethargy, drowsiness, muscle twitching and coma secondary to brain-cell dehydration.

TREATMENT

The hyperosmolality must be corrected slowly. Water should be given by mouth whenever possible, but intravenous infusion is usually necessary. If the plasma sodium is more than 170 mmol·L^{-1}, normal saline (150 mmol sodium per litre) is given to allow gradual correction. If the plasma sodium is 150 mmol·L^{-1} or less, $\frac{1}{5}$-normal dextrose saline (30 mmol sodium per litre) should be used. The aim is to correct the hypernatraemia over 48 h. Too fast correction can result in cerebral oedema or brain haemorrhage.

IDIOPATHIC OEDEMA OF WOMEN

This condition, also called cyclic or periodic oedema, is a not uncommon condition affecting females after the menarche in whom there is intermittent or constant fluid retention. Typically there are diurnal weight gains exceeding 1.5 kg with day-to-day changes of up to 5 kg. Patients complain of swelling of the face, hands, breasts and thighs and of a feeling of being generally 'bloated'. Pitting oedema is unusual, but tightness and difficulty in removing rings is typical. Weight gain may be unpredictable or related to prolonged standing, emotional stress or a high-carbohydrate diet.

There is no satisfactory explanation for this condition. Rarely hyperprolactinaemia has been observed, but there is no evidence of any primary abnormality of the renin–angiotensin–aldosterone system or abnormality in oestrogen or progesterone metabolism. There is some evidence for 'leaky capillaries' with loss of plasma protein into the interstitial space during standing, but the cause of this is unknown. Many patients have already commenced diuretic therapy when first seen and it has been postulated that diuretic abuse may be a cause. Rebound fluid retention certainly occurs in those patients if diuretics are stopped, but it is doubtful whether it is a primary cause.

Treatment is by explanation and reassurance that there is no heart or kidney disease. Patients should be advised to avoid prolonged standing if at all possible. Obesity exacerbates the condition and should be treated. Supporting elastic stockings may occasionally be helpful. If related to a high-carbohydrate diet, this should be avoided. Diuretics are best avoided as they tend to exacerbate the problem. Other drugs are of doubtful value.

DISORDERS OF POTASSIUM METABOLISM

Physiological considerations
Ninety eight per cent of body potassium is intracellular at a concentration of approximately 160 mmol·L^{-1}, contrasting with an extracellular concentration of 3.5–5.0 mmol·L^{-1} (see Table 10.2). This 'in-out' ratio is critical for the normal activity of all cells. Dietary intake of potassium is normally 80–150 mmol daily and balanced excretion is principally via the kidneys with a small amount (5–15 mmol) excreted in the faeces.

Control of the distribution of potassium between the ECF and the ICF is dependent on metabolic cell pumps and is influenced by:

- *pH*. Potassium moves into cells in alkalosis and out of cells in acidosis.
- *Aldosterone*. An increase or decrease in plasma potassium increases or decreases aldosterone production. It is suspected, but not proved, that aldosterone increases the uptake of potassium into cells.
- *Insulin*. An increase in plasma potassium increases insulin release. Exogenous insulin increases potassium uptake into liver and muscle cells, but the physiological role of endogenous

insulin in potassium metabolism is less clear.
- *Beta-adrenergic nervous actvity*. Hyperkalaemia is seen in treatment with beta-blocking drugs and in autonomic neuropathy, suggesting a role for the beta-adrenergic nervous system in controlling 'in-out' potassium balance.

In the kidney, filtered potassium is normally totally absorbed in the proximal tubule, controlled secretion occurring in the distal tubule and collecting ducts. Several factors control potassium secretion. A high intake leads to adaptive increased potassium secretion. Any condition that increases delivery of sodium to the distal nephron, such as salt loading, loop diuretics or osmotic diuretics, increases potassium secretion. Mineralocorticoids enhance sodium reabsorption and potassium secretion. Systemic alkalosis increases potassium secretion, while acidosis decreases it, probably as a result of a shift of potassium into or out of tubular cells, as occurs with cells generally. Finally, potassium secretion increases with urine flow rate.

Hypokalaemia

Hypokalaemia may result from a shift of potassium into cells (internal imbalance) or from the loss of potassium via the kidneys or the gut (Table 10.6). Vomit contains relatively little potassium (5–10 mmol·L^{-1}), but persistent vomiting leads to a hypochloraemic alkalosis due to loss of chloride and gastric acid, which causes severe renal wasting of potassium and movement of potassium into

Table 10.6 Causes of hypokalaemia.

Intracellular shifts
Alkalosis
High-dose insulin
Periodic paralysis (see p. 963)

Extra renal loss
Diuresis
  Drugs
  Osmotic (e.g. hyperglycaemia, uraemia)
Renal tubular acidosis
Hyperaldosteronism—primary or secondary
Cushing's and adrenogenital syndromes
Bartter's syndrome
Drugs (e.g. liquorice, carbenoxolone sodium, gentamicin toxicity)
Leukaemia

Gastrointestinal loss
Vomiting and diarrhoea
Ileostomy or ureterosigmoidostomy
Purgative abuse
Anorexia nervosa with bulimia
Villous adenoma of rectum

cells. Liquid stool contains 10–50 mmol·L^{-1} of potassium, so profuse diarrhoea can induce marked hypokalaemia. Chronic laxative-induced purgation can also cause hypokalaemia. Much less common is loss of potassium from a villous adenoma of the colon or rectum or loss in patients with ureterosigmoidostomies.

Renal potassium wasting is most often due to diuretic drugs, being more common with large doses and in the presence of secondary hyperaldosteronism, as occurs in severe heart failure, hepatic cirrhosis or the nephrotic syndrome. Severe hypokalaemia, especially in women, may be seen as a result of self-treatment with diuretics for cosmetic reasons and in anorexia nervosa. The other important causes of renal potassium wasting are primary hyperaldosteronism (see p. 828), Cushing's syndrome (see p. 814) or adrenogenital syndromes. Liquorice in large amounts and carbenoxolone sodium (prescribed for peptic ulcer treatment) have an aldosterone-like effect that can lead to hypokalaemia. Rare causes include Bartter's syndrome, renin-secreting tumours and Liddel's syndrome.

CLINICAL FEATURES

Marked hypokalaemia (less than 2.5 mmol·L^{-1}) is associated with impaired muscle function and increased myocardial excitability, and may be immediately life-threatening because of severe cardiac dysrhythmia—a risk increased by digitalization. In skeletal muscle there is weakness, sometimes progressing to paralysis, with absent reflexes. Hypokalaemia may result in ileus of the gut. In the kidney, hypokalaemia impairs concentrating ability (nephrogenic diabetes insipidus), and may reduce the GFR and increase sodium retention. The dominant clinical feature of this renal impairment is polyuria, especially nocturia.

TREATMENT

Treatment must be directed at correcting the hypokalaemia and eliminating the cause of potassium loss. In most cases, withdrawal of oral diuretics or purgation, accompanied by the oral administration of potassium supplements in the form of slow-release potassium or effervescent potassium, is all that is required. Only in severe cases (potassium < 2.5 mmol·L^{-1}) is intravenous potassium replacement required, e.g. where there are cardiac arrhythmias, muscle weakness or severe diabetic ketoacidosis. When used, intravenous therapy must take account of renal function, and replacement at rates greater than 20 mmol·h^{-1} should only be used with hourly monitoring of serum potassium and ECG changes.

The treatment of adrenal disorders is described on p. 813.

Table 10.7 Causes of hyperkalaemia.

Excessive intake

Impaired renal excretion
Oliguric renal failure
Potassium-sparing diuretics, e.g. amiloride
Adrenal insufficiency
Renal tubulo-interstitial disease
ACE inhibitors, e.g. enalapril

Loss of potassium from cells
Acidosis
Crush injury, rhabdomyolysis, burns
Tumour therapy
Suxamethonium

Hyperkalaemia

Hyperkalaemia is much less common than hypokalaemia but is more dangerous, the commonest clinical manifestation being cardiac arrest. It occasionally presents with muscle weakness. Diagnosis depends on clinical awareness of its possible development in certain situations (Table 10.7).

Hyperkalaemia rarely occurs in healthy patients except with gross abuse of potassium-retaining diuretics or overdose with potassium supplements. It may occur in hospital practice if intravenous infusion of potassium exceeds 20 mmol·h^{-1}. It most often develops on a background of renal or adrenal disease. Haemolysed blood samples produce an 'apparent' hyperkalaemia; laboratory reports on blood samples should always indicate whether the specimen received was haemolysed.

In acute or chronic renal failure, hyperkalaemia rarely occurs spontaneously except where there is oliguria. It is more likely to occur if patients with renal disease take food rich in potassium or potassium supplements, or are treated with potassium-sparing diuretics (amiloride, triamterene or spironolactone) or angiotensin converting enzyme (ACE) inhibitors. Hyperkalaemia also occurs if there is a shift of potassium out of cells due to acidosis, crush or ischaemic injuries, burns, rhabdomyolysis from muscle injury, or massive death of tumour cells in response to treatment. Loss of potassium from cells may follow use of certain muscle relaxants, e.g. suxamethonium. Rarely, hyperkalaemia occurs spontaneously in patients with severe renal tubular disorders where there is a defect in potassium secretion (see p. 508).

Addison's disease and isolated hypoaldosteronism are commonly associated with modest (5.0–6.5 mmol·L^{-1}) hyperkalaemia (see p. 814); other clinical features usually suggest the diagnosis.

TREATMENT

A serum potassium of more than 7.0 mmol·L^{-1} is a medical emergency, and is associated with ECG

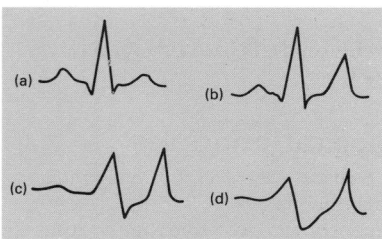

Fig. 10.6 Progressive ECG changes with increasing hyperkalaemia. (a) Normal. (b) Tented T wave. (c) Reduced P wave with increased QRS complex. (d) 'Sine wave' pattern (pre-cardiac arrest).

changes (see Fig. 10.6). Intravenous glucose (50 g) plus 15 units of soluble insulin will lower potassium rapidly, the effect lasting for 1–2 h. 8.4% sodium bicarbonate 50–100 ml i.v. will also reduce the potassium level and help correct acidosis, but must be used sparingly in fluid-overloaded patients. If severe ECG changes are present, intravenous 10% calcium gluconate (10–30 ml over 5–10 min) is required; the effect is short-lived, but the dose can be repeated. These are all emergency measures that 'push' potassium back into cells. Removal of potassium from the body requires either cation exchange resins (e.g. 15–20 g of calcium resonium three times daily by mouth or retention enema) or dialysis. Hyperkalaemia is also helped by mild diarrhoea induced by oral lactulose 10–20 ml three times daily, which also avoids constipation when resins are used.

DISORDERS OF MAGNESIUM METABOLISM

Plasma magnesium levels are normally maintained within the range 0.7–1.1 mmol·L^{-1}. Like potassium, magnesium is principally an intracellular cation (Table 10.2). Regulation of magnesium balance is mainly via the kidney. Primary disturbance of magnesium balance is uncommon, hypo- or hyper-magnesaemia usually developing on a background of more obvious fluid and electrolyte disturbances. Disturbance in magnesium balance should always be suspected in association with other fluid and electrolyte disturbances when the patient develops unexpected neurological signs or symptoms.

Hypomagnesaemia

This most often develops as a result of deficient intake, defective gut absorption, or excessive gut or urinary loss (see Table 10.8). It can also occur with acute pancreatitis, possibly due to the formation of magnesium soaps in the areas of fat necrosis. Calcium deficiency usually develops with hypomagnesaemia.

Table 10.8 Causes of hypomagnesaemia.

Decreased intake
Starvation
Prolonged parenteral feeding

Decreased gut absorption
Small gut disease
Extensive small gut resection

Gut losses
Prolonged nasogastric suction
Excessive purgation
Gastrointestinal/biliary fistula
Severe diarrhoea

Excessive urine losses
Diuretic states due to:
   Loop diuretics
   Post obstruction
   Recovery phase of acute tubular necrosis
   Hyperglycaemia
   Diabetic ketoacidosis
Renal tubular acidosis
Chronic alcohol consumption
Gentamicin toxicity
Primary aldosteronism
Hypothyroidism

Acute pancreatitis

CLINICAL FEATURES

Symptoms and signs include irritability, tremor, ataxia, carpopedal spasm, hyperreflexia, confusional and hallucinatory states and epileptiform convulsions. The serum magnesium is usually less than 0.7 mmol·L^{-1}. An ECG may show a prolonged QT interval, broad flattened T waves and occasional shortening of the ST segment.

TREATMENT

This involves the withdrawal of precipitating agents such as diuretics or purgatives and the parental infusion of 50 mmol of magnesium chloride in 1 litre of 5% dextrose or other isotonic fluid over 12–24 h. This should be repeated daily until the plasma magnesium level is normal.

Hypermagnesaemia

This primarily occurs in patients with acute or chronic renal failure given magnesium-containing laxatives or antacids. It can also be induced by magnesium-containing enemas. Mild hypermagnesaemia may occur in patients with adrenal insufficiency.

Table 10.9 Relationship between [H⁺] and pH.

[H⁺] (nmol·L⁻¹)	pH
100 000	4
10 000	5
1 000	6
100	7
10	8
1	9
Ranges in blood	
126	6.90
100	7.00
79	7.10
63	7.20
50	7.30
40	7.40
32	7.50
25	7.60
20	7.70
16	7.80

CLINICAL FEATURES

Symptoms and signs relate to neurological and cardiovascular depression, and include weakness with hyporeflexia proceeding to narcosis, respiratory paralysis and cardiac conduction defects. Symptoms usually develop when the plasma magnesium level exceeds 2 mmol·L⁻¹.

TREATMENT

Treatment requires withdrawal of magnesium therapy and the intravenous injection of 10 ml of calcium gluconate 10% (which contains 2.25 mmol calcium), to be repeated as necessary to lower the plasma magnesium level. Dialysis may be required in patients with severe renal failure. Respiratory failure requires artificial ventilation until the plasma magnesium level returns to normal levels.

Acid–base homeostasis

Physiological principles

The concentration of hydrogen ions ([H⁺]) is enormously important to most cell metabolism. For this reason intracellular and extracellular [H⁺] is normally controlled very tightly. The negative logarithm of [H⁺] (known as the pH) is commonly measured, but its use may conceal large changes in [H⁺] (Table 10.9); it is therefore better to use [H⁺]. Normal resting arterial blood [H⁺] is approximately 40 nmol·L⁻¹ (pH 7.4). The major source of H⁺ is tissue respiration ($H_2O + CO_2 = H^+·HCO_3^-$). Ten times less H⁺ comes from organic acid production (lactic, hydroxybutyric, acetoacetic and free fatty acids) and ten times less again from the dietary 'fixed acids'—sulphuric and phosphoric acid. H⁺ derived from cell respiration is eliminated via the lungs, organic acids are normally metabolized in liver and other tissues, and fixed acids are excreted via the kidney (Table 10.10).

Between production and excretion there is an extremely efficient buffering system such that the concentration of H⁺ inside and outside cells is very constant. Buffers include haemoglobin, proteins, bicarbonate and phosphate. Most important is the

$$pH = pK + \log \frac{[HCO_3^-]}{[H^+ \cdot HCO_3^-]}$$

Fig. 10.7 The Henderson–Hasselbach equation.

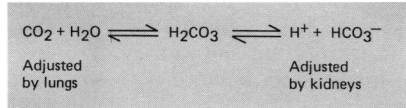

Fig. 10.8 The bicarbonate/carbonic acid buffering system.

Table 10.10 Source and elimination of hydrogen ions.

Nature	Daily production (moles)	Source	Elimination
CO_2 ($H_2O + CO_2 \rightarrow$ $H^+ + HCO_3^-$)	15	Tissue respiration	Lungs
Organic acids	1.5	Liver, muscle, brain	Liver and most tissues
Fixed acids	0.1	Diet	Kidneys

bicarbonate–carbonic acid buffer system expressed in the classic Henderson–Hasselbalch equation (see Fig. 10.7): as $H^+ \cdot HCO_3^-$ (which is dependent on the P_{CO_2}) increases or decreases, bicarbonate also increases or decreases (by renal conservation or secretion) to maintain constant pH.

Capacity in the buffering system is maintained by the ease with which carbonic acid can be disposed of via the lungs and by the excretion of fixed acid by the kidneys (see Fig. 10.8).

RENAL REGULATION OF ACID-BASE BALANCE

The kidney plays a major role in the control of acid–base balance and a clear understanding of the mechanism involved facilitates understanding of the pathophysiology and treatment of metabolic acidosis.

Control of acid–base balance depends on both:

- Reabsorption of filtered bicarbonate *from* tubular fluid
- Excretion of hydrogen ion (H^+) and ammonia (NH_3) *into* tubular fluid

All are interlinked (Fig. 10.9).

Bicarbonate absorption

Some 90% of filtered bicarbonate is 'recaptured' in the proximal tubules and further bicarbonate is reabsorbed distally. Virtually all bicarbonate may be reabsorbed—as for example in acidotic states— or significant amounts may be excreted as, for example, in the recovery phase of respiratory acidosis (see p. 723).

The reabsorption is indirect in that (H^+) excreted into the lumen combines with luminal HCO_3^- to form H_2CO_3. Breakdown of H_2CO_3 to $H_2O + CO_2$ is catalysed by carbonic anhydrase in the tubular cell brush border. The CO_2 enters the cell to combine again with H_2O under the influence of intracellular carbonic anhydrase (on this occasion hydration of CO_2 contrasting with the dehydration within the lumen). H_2CO_3 dissociates to H^+ plus HCO_3^-. H^+ is excreted into the lumen coupled to the reabsorption of sodium, while bicarbonate is returned to the blood by $Na^+ \cdot HCO_3^-$ co-transport. Failure to reabsorb bicarbonate is equivalent to failure to excrete H^+.

Failure in tubular bicarbonate reabsorption is the underlying defect in type 2 renal tubular acidosis (RTA) (see p. 508), while failure of distal tubular reabsorption is found in type 1 (distal) RTA (see p. 507).

Ammonia excretion

The kidney actively produces ammonium ion from the metabolism of glutamine. This occurs primarily in the proximal tubular cell. It should be noted that NH_4^+ (ammonium ion) rather than NH_3 (ammonia) is produced, contrary to previous concepts. However, NH_4^+ dissociates to NH_3, which diffuses out of the tubular cell into the luminal fluid. Ammonia produced in the proximal tubular cells and excreted into the lumen is reabsorbed in the loop of Henle and the main site of final excretion

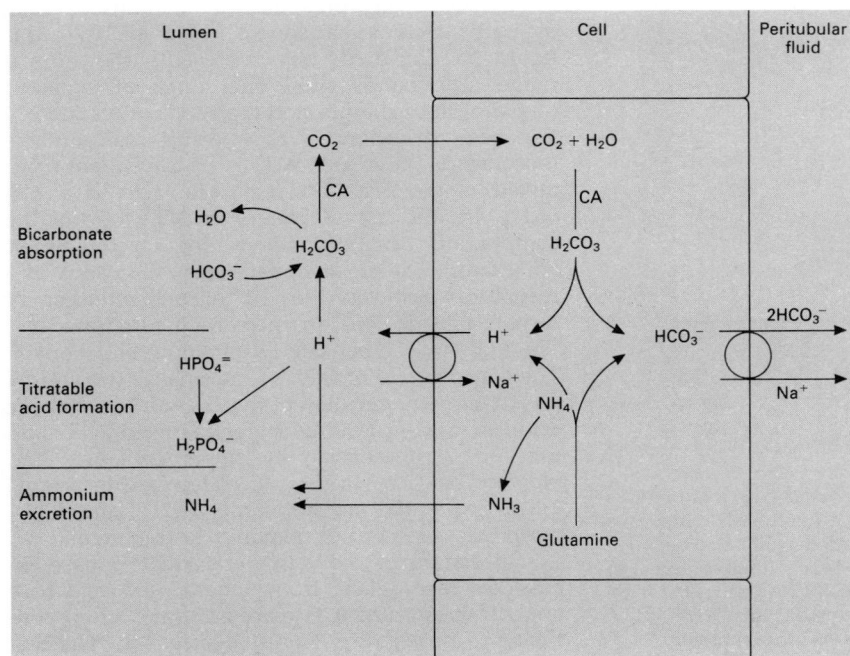

Fig. 10.9 Renal tubular excretion of H^+. CA = Carbonic anhydrase.

is in the distal nephron. NH_3 diffusing into the distal tubule acts as a buffer for acceptance of H^+, thus increasing net excretion of H^+.

Metabolism of glutamine yields α-ketoglutarate, which is in turn metabolized to bicarbonate either in the tubular cell or elsewhere in the body.

Ammoniagenesis is immensely important for the excretion of H^+. It is increased by acidosis and decreased by alkalosis. The ability to excrete NH_3 decreases in progressive renal disease when there is loss of nephrons.

Titratable acid

The third mechanism for the excretion of H^+ is its binding in the lumen by filtered buffer—principally phosphate ($Na_2HPO_4 \rightarrow NaH_2PO_4$). Quantitatively this mechanism for the excretion of H^+ is normally much smaller than either bicarbonate reabsorption or ammonia excretion.

Diagnosis of acid–base disturbances

Except in acute respiratory distress, symptoms are non-specific and are described below. The most definitive means of diagnosing acid–base disorder is by measuring the $[H^+]$ and P_aCO_2 in arterial or arterialized venous blood plus the plasma electrolytes.

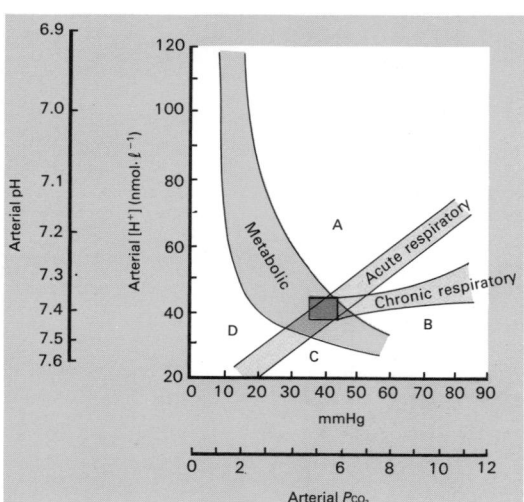

Fig. 10.10 Diagram for analysis of acid–base disturbances from measured $[H^+]$ and P_aCO_2. The cross-hatched area shows the normal range. (From Cohen RD & Woods HF (1987) Disturbances of acid–base homeostasis. In Weatherall DJ, Ledingham JGG & Warrell DA (eds) *Oxford Textbook of Medicine*, 2nd edn., pp. 9.164–9.175. Oxford: Oxford University Press. With permission.)

Table 10.11 Causes of metabolic acidosis with a normal anion gap.

Gastrointestinal bicarbonate loss
Diarrhoea
Pancreatic fistula
Uretero sigmoidostomy

Renal tubular acidosis (RTA)
● Type I distal
  Primary
  Acquired
    Primary biliary cirrhosis
    Chronic active hepatitis
    Obstructive nephropathy
    Vitamin D intoxication
    Hypergammaglobulinaemia
● Type II 'proximal' bicarbonate wastage
  Primary
    Isolated
    Part of Fanconi syndrome
  Acquired
    Hyperparathyroidism
    Heavy metal poisoning (e.g. mercury)
    Paraproteinaemia (e.g. myeloma)
    Acetazolamide therapy

Ingestion/infusion
NH_4Cl or arginine·HCl
Feeding excess cationic amino acids

Dilutional acidosis
Rapid i.v. hydration

Acid–base disorders may be diagnosed using diagrams such as that shown in Fig. 10.10. In this figure the hatched area represents the normal range. The bands show the range of expected response in uncomplicated metabolic or respiratory acid–base disorders. Where results fall outside these bands (in area A, B, C or D) the patient has a mixed respiratory and metabolic acid–base disorder. In the case of areas B and D, one of the components can be compensating for the other. For example, in chronic respiratory disease with a respiratory acidosis (area B) there is retention of carbon dioxide and an increase in arterial PCO_2. The kidneys compensate by retaining bicarbonate. The consequence of this is to normalize the arterial $[H^+]$, but with elevation of the PCO_2. In a metabolic acidosis (area D), the body retains fixed acids and the lungs compensate by hyperventilating and blowing off CO_2, leading to a decrease in arterial PCO_2. Sequential measurement of $[H^+]$ and P_aCO_2 permits assessment of response to treatment.

Calculation of 'standard bicarbonate', 'base excess' or 'base deficit' from widely used acid–base analytical equipment is inaccurate and often confusing or misleading. This stems from the fact that the bicarbonate titration curve of blood measured *in vitro* differs from that *in vivo* and takes no account of interstitial and intracellular fluid buffering. It does not therefore represent the true *in vivo* situation. Further, an 'excess' of bicarbonate may be a desirable compensatory mechanism as, for example, in chronic respiratory acidosis and is then *not* a primary defect. Casual interpretation of these values can be misleading, and their use is best abandoned in favour of the approach outlined above.

Anion gap

The main electrolytes measured in plasma are sodium, potassium, chloride and bicarbonate. The sum of the cations sodium and potassium normally exceeds that of chloride and bicarbonate by 10–18 $mmol \cdot L^{-1}$. This is known as the anion gap. This gap is made up by negative charged proteins, phosphate and organic acids (see Fig. 10.11).

$$Anion\ gap = [Na^+ + K^+] - [HCO_3^- + Cl^-]$$
$$(Normal = 10–18\ mmol \cdot L^{-1})$$

Calculation of this gap is simple and of great value in identifying and managing metabolic acidosis in which the anion gap may be normal or increased.

Normal anion gap acidosis (hyperchloraemic acidosis)
This occurs when bicarbonate is lost via the gut or the kidneys. Rarely it is due to the ingestion of H^+ as ammonium chloride (Table 10.11). Chloride is retained as bicarbonate is lost (see Fig. 10.11).

Increased anion gap acidosis
This results from the retention of 'fixed' or organic acids and is most often seen in uraemia, ketoacidosis, lactic acidosis and salicylate poisoning (Table 10.12). Bicarbonate is utilized to maintain a normal $[H^+]$ and therefore decreases. Chloride may be normal or low (see Fig. 10.11).

Given a careful history and awareness of the causes of acid–base imbalance, diagnosis can be based on these measurements.

Symptoms and systemic effects of acidosis

Severe, chronic metabolic acidosis is commonly associated with no or only non-specific symptoms. When acute and severe, it may be associated with deep sighing respiration (Kussmaul breathing: 'air hunger'). Vasodilatation of the cerebral arterioles may cause headache. Peripheral vasodilatation with warm peripheral parts may be seen but it is usually slight. Severe acidosis may be associated with increasing drowsiness and even coma. Various systems of the body may be affected as follows.

Lungs. Apart from hyperventilation, acute meta-bolic acidosis contributes, in part, to the development of 'shock lung' ARDS (see p. 729).

Heart. Acidosis adversely affects cardiac contractility (negative inotropism) and if severe and prolonged, may lead to circulatory collapse. The cardiac effect of acidosis is offset, to some extent, by increased catecholamine release. In patients with cardiac arrest, defibrillation is facilitated by alkalosis. Thus infusion of bicarbonate is sometimes given prior to attempting defibrillation.

Blood oxygen dissociation curve. Acute acidosis also affects the blood oxygen dissociation curve, moving it to the right (Fig. 13.5). This improves the unloading of oxygen to the tissues but reduces oxygen uptake in the lungs in the presence of pulmonary disease or low inspired oxygen concentrations. After some hours this is offset by a fall in 2,3-diphosphoglycerate (2,3DPG) due to inhibition of its synthesis and increased breakdown due to acidosis. This is only slowly corrected with alkaline treatment, which, if overenthusiastic, may cause an acute shift of the blood oxygen dissociation curve to the left and reduce oxygen delivery to the tissues.

Potassium. Acute acidosis causes a shift of potassium from cells into the ECF (see p. 499). In polyuric states such as diabetic ketosis or renal tubular acidosis this can result in considerable

Table 10.12 Causes of metabolic acidosis with a high anion gap.

Uraemic acidosis
Drug poisoning
Salicylates
Methanol
Ethylene glycol
Paraldehyde
Ketoacidosis
Diabetes
Starvation
Alcohol poisoning
Lactic acidosis
Type A:
Strenuous exercise
Shock
Severe hypoxia
Type B:
Biguanide drugs—metformin
Acute liver failure
Poisoning—ethanol, paracetamol
Leukaemia, lymphoma
Intravenous nutrition with fructose and sorbitol

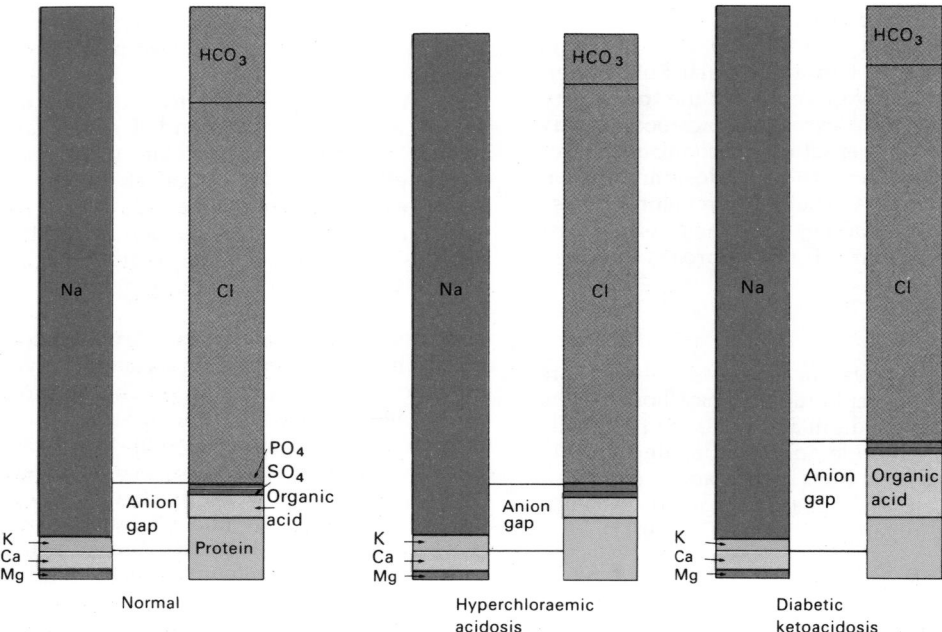

Fig. 10.11 The anion gap in metabolic acidosis.

potassium wastage in the urine and depletion of whole-body potassium. Alkali therapy causes a movement of potassium back into the cells and can result in acute hypokalaemia. Such patients must, therefore, be given potassium replacement *prior* to alkali therapy.

Bone. In patients with chronic metabolic acidosis, bone acts as a buffer. This can result in leaching out of calcium and negative calcium balance. It may contribute to the osteomalacia of chronic renal failure and renal tubular acidosis.

Carbohydrate metabolism. Glycolysis is inhibited by acidosis and stimulated by alkalosis. Hepatic gluconeogenesis from lactate is inhibited by acidosis, which may excerbate lactic acidosis due to shock.

Causes of acid-base disturbances

Since respiratory acidosis and alkalosis are dealt with in Chapter 12, only metabolic acidosis and alkalosis will be discussed in this section.

METABOLIC ACIDOSIS

It is convenient to subdivide metabolic acidosis into:

- Increased acid production or defective excretion (high anion gap) (Fig. 10.11). The causes of retention of 'fixed' or organic acids are shown in Table 10.12.
- Loss of bicarbonate; hyperchloraemic acidosis (normal anion gap) (Fig. 10.11). This occurs when bicarbonate is lost via the gut or the kidneys. Rarely it is due to the ingestion of hydrogen ion as ammonium chloride or the administration of intravenous feeds containing an excess of cationic amino acids (Table 10.11).

Uraemic acidosis

Acute or chronic renal failure is typically associated with a high anion gap metabolic acidosis due to failure by the kidneys to excrete fixed acid. The major functional defect of the kidneys is reduced glomerular filtration. This results in reduced excretion of titratable buffer (see p. 503) and thus reduction in titratable acid (see p. 504). However, depending on the nature and extent of the renal disease, there are commonly additional defects in bicarbonate absorption in the proximal tubule and hydrogen ion secretion and ammoniagenesis in the distal tubule. Retention of acid may therefore be due to a mixture of glomerular failure and renal tubular acidosis (see p. 507).

Most often, however, urine acidification is normal allowing titration of filtered phosphate. In glomerular failure, serum phosphate is usually elevated increasing the filtered load per residual nephron and facilitating net hydrogen ion excretion. Ammonium production and excretion may be increased or decreased depending on the degree and nature of the renal damage.

In general, compensatory mechanisms including buffering of hydrogen ion by bone allow a mild or moderate acidosis to persist as a steady state for long periods in patients with chronic renal failure.

Symptoms are unusual unless the plasma bicarbonate is very low (less than 10 mmol·L^{-1}).

Treatment of uraemic acidosis requires a reduction in the acid load from dietary protein. This is rarely necessary for the acidosis *per se*, protein usually being restricted to control symptoms of uraemia and to reduce the rate of decline in renal function (see p. 477).

Treatment with sodium bicarbonate is potentially dangerous, the sodium load exacerbating hypertension and predisposing to salt and water retention with pulmonary congestion. However, sodium bicarbonate supplements can be very effective in patients with sodium-losing chronic renal disease (see p. 478). Severe acidosis requires removal of fixed acid by dialysis.

Renal tubular acidosis (RTA)

Varying degrees of tubular dysfunction with respect to bicarbonate reabsorption, hydrogen ion excretion and ammoniagenesis may be present in patients with different forms of renal disease. This is especially true of patients with medullary disease such as reflux nephropathy, papillary necrosis or obstructive nephropathy in whom varying degrees of RTA are seen.

A primary abnormality of the renal tubules leading to metabolic acidosis is relatively uncommon.

Three types of RTA are recognized:

- Type 1 (distal tubular, 'gradient' or classical) RTA in which the acidification defect is in the distal tubule.
- Type 2 (proximal tubular 'bicarbonate wasting') RTA in which there is a failure in hydrogen ion excretion into the proximal tubules with consequent wasting of filtered bicarbonate in the urine.
- Type 4 RTA due to aldosterone deficiency or tubular resistance. This is characterized by a hyperkalaemic metabolic acidosis with normal urine acidification.

Type 3 RTA has been dropped from the classification. It referred to a condition usually seen in infants and children in which both proximal bicarbonate wasting and a distal acidification defect were present. It is now believed to be a variant on distal Type 1 RTA.

Type 1 RTA
This may be due to inherited defects—autosomal recessive, autosomal dominant or sex-linked recessive—or secondary to a variety of diseases (see Table 10.11).

CLINICAL PRESENTATION

The condition may present at any age. In children it most often presents with failure to thrive or symptoms due to hypokalaemia. With increasing age, presentation is more often with symptomatic or asymptomatic stone disease, although hypokalaemic symptoms may also be the presenting feature. Occasionally, patients may present with acute acidosis and hyperventilation commonly associated with muscle weakness due to the hypokalaemia.

The diagnosis should be suspected in patients shown to have a hyperchloraemic acidosis with normal or low serum potassium. Diagnosis is confirmed by demonstration of a failure to acidify the urine (see below).

Nephrocalcinosis and renal stone disease may also be associated with an 'incomplete' form of type 1 RTA in which serum bicarbonate and acid–base balance may be normal. However, patients are unable to reduce the urine pH below 5.5 when challenged with an acid load (see below).

Nature of tubular defect. Distal tubular secretion of hydrogen ion depends on a sodium dependent luminal membrane ('secretory') pump and on a voltage-dependent transport system—reabsorption of sodium creating a transepithelial voltage potential leading to hydrogen-ion excretion. It also depends on the ability of the distal nephron to maintain a steep, intraluminal-tubular hydrogen gradient (approximately 800 : 1). Distal RTA may result from a secretory defect, a voltage-dependent defect or a back-leakage due to failure to maintain the normal steep hydrogen-ion gradient.

DIAGNOSIS

This requires demonstration of a failure to acidify urine.

- A urine pH of less than 5.5 in acidotic subjects excludes the diagnosis. A first morning urine sample of pH 5.5 or more confirms the diagnosis. An acid load test is not required in these patients.
- An acid load test is required if the patient does not have a systemic acidosis and RTA is suspected.
- (a) The *short* ammonium chloride test involves giving 100 mg·kg^{-1} of ammonium chloride (preferably in gelatine capsules) over 30–40 min. Serum bicarbonate (and if possible blood pH) should be measured before and 2 h after ingestion of the ammonium chloride

to ensure induction of acidosis. Urine samples are collected at hourly intervals for 4–6 h and either pH-tested immediately or collected under oil. Failure of the urine pH to fall below 5.5 indicates distal RTA.

(b) Some prefer *prolonged* acid loading—100 mg·kg^{-1} daily for 3–5 days—and this is of value when any doubt exists as to the results obtained with the short test. In patients incapable of taking ammonium chloride, calcium chloride (2 mmol·kg^{-1}) may be substituted.

Nephrocalcinosis and nephrolithiasis. Nephrocalcinosis and nephrolithiasis is virtually confined to patients with Type 1 RTA. The reasons for this remain controversial.

Hypercalciuria. Is a common feature of Type 1 RTA but less common and less severe in Type 2. It has been attributed to loss of calcium from bone due to the systemic acidosis, but this alone cannot account for the increased excretion in patients with Type 1 versus Type 2 who have comparable degrees of acidosis. In the case of Type 2 RTA, increased delivery of bicarbonate to the distal tubule may enchance calcium reabsorption and reduce urinary losses.

Urinary citrate excretion. Is determined by the amount of filtered citrate reabsorption in the proximal tubule. Reabsorption is enhanced by acidosis so that citrate excretion is usually low in patients with Type 1 RTA. In patients with Type 2 RTA, proximal reabsorption is reduced as part of the tubular defect and urinary citrate excretion is commonly normal.

Citrate is the major chelating agent for calcium, thus increasing its solubility in the urine. This effect is reduced in Type 1 but increased in Type 2 RTA. This may explain, in part, the different prevalance of nephrocalcinosis and renal stones.

The greater the duration of Type 1 RTA and the more normal glomerular filtration rate the more likely are stones to develop. In *acquired* Type 1 RTA, GFR and so the filtered load of calcium are commonly reduced and the duration of the condition is short. This may explain the infrequent occurrence of stones in this Type 1 RTA.

TREATMENT

This involves administration of sufficient alkali to balance normal hydrogen-ion production from an acid ash diet. This usually amounts to 1–1.5 mmol·kg^{-1} per day (60–80 mmol) of bicarbonate. This is equivalent to 6–12 g per day for a 70 kg man. Alkali treatment increases urinary citrate excretion and potassium excretion. A citrate solution (Shohl's solution) that provides 1 mmol·ml^{-1}

of bicarbonate by hepatic metabolism is often better tolerated, causing less abdominal distention and belching. Potassium citrate administration (1–2 mmol·kg^{-1} per day) has also been reported to reduce calcium excretion, increase citrate excretion and reduce the stone recurrence rate. It has the added advantage of providing supplementary potassium, which is often required.

Type 2 (proximal or bicarbonate wasting) RTA
This is less common than Type 1. It may present as an isolated defect inherited as an autosomal dominant. More often, there is a generalized defect of proximal tubular function with defective absorption of glucose, aminoacids and phosphate—'the Fanconi syndrome' (see p. 866). It may be acquired (see Table 10.11) or be iatrogenic as a result of treatment with acetazolamide.

Clinical presentation is usually with symptomatic acidosis, polyuria and polydypsia, hypokalaemic myopathy, rickets in children or osteomalacia in adults. The last are most often found with the Fanconi syndrome due to associated defects in vitamin D metabolism.

Nature of tubular defect. The basic defect is failure in hydrogen-ion secretion by the proximal tubule with consequent failure of reabsorption of the normally large amount of bicarbonate. This floods the distal tubule, exceeding its relatively limited capacity to reabsorb bicarbonate. Serum bicarbonate falls, leading to a hyperchloraemic normal anion gap acidosis. As serum bicarbonate falls, the filtered load diminishes so that when serum bicarbonate levels fall to approximately 15 mmol·L^{-1} complete reabsorption of the filtered bicarbonate can be achieved. Urine pH may then fall to normal levels of 4.5–5.3.

The large distal load of sodium bicarbonate also leads to sodium wastage, which may, in turn, lead to hypotension. This stimulates the release of aldosterone, which increases sodium/potassium exchange at the distal tubular level, with potassium wasting leading to hypokalaemia. Polyuria results both from the sodium bicarbonate wasting and the hypokalaemia.

TREATMENT

Combination of sodium bicarbonate and potassium citrate are most valuable. Administration of thiazide diuretics, which may enhance proximal tubular reabsorption of bicarbonate, has been suggested. Unfortunately, this commonly increases potassium wastage, which demands increased supplements of potassium.

Type 4 (hyperkalaemic) RTA
This is also rare. Again there is a hyperchloraemic normal anion gap acidosis. As in Type 2, urine

acidification may return to normal if serum bicarbonate falls to low levels. The distinguishing feature is hyperkalaemia. Type 4 RTA is due either to hypoaldosteronism (see p. 829) or to end-organ resistance to the action of aldosterone as in patients with severe medullary disease due to papillary necrosis. The hypoaldesterone may be due to primary adrenal disease or result from reduced renin production in various forms of chronic renal disease.

The acidosis is due to diminished hydrogen-ion exchange for sodium in the distal tubule and the hyperkalaemia to reduced potassium excretion. If the acidosis or hyperkalaemia is severe, treatment is with fludrocortisone (0.05–0.15 mg per day).

Diabetic ketoacidosis

This is dealt with on p. 846. This is a high anion gap acidosis due to the accumulation of organic acids, acetoacetic acid and hydroxybutyric acid due to reduced peripheral utilization and increased production.

Lactic acidosis

Lactic acid (as lactate) is normally present in the venous blood in low concentrations (0.6–1.2 mmol·L^{-1}), increasing up to 10-fold after severe exercise. Lactic acidosis should be suspected in patients with high anion gap metabolic acidosis when there is no uraemia or diabetic ketoacidosis. It most often occurs in association with circulatory failure or shock, with or without severe hypoxia, when peripheral metabolism of lactate is reduced and production is increased (type A). The potential for lactic acidosis increases where there is liver disease (reduced metabolism of lactate) or impaired renal excretion of acid.

The other major cause (type B) is as a result of various drugs or poisons (Table 10.12). With these there is variable increase in the production of lactate and reduced liver metabolism. It may occur *de novo* in severe liver failure. Cases may present acutely with nausea, vomiting, epigastric pain, hyperventilation and impaired consciousness. The diagnosis is based on recognizing a high anion gap acidosis in the absence of uraemia or diabetic ketoacidosis, and can be confirmed by demonstration of a high level of lactate in plasma.

Treatment of lactic acidosis involves correction of the cause. In the case of circulatory failure and hypoxia, correction of these must be pursued, but care should be taken with vasoconstrictor drugs, which may increase lactate production. Causal drugs or poisons must be stopped and measures to accelerate their excretion employed. Because of the negative inotropic effect on cardiac output, intravenous infusion of sodium bicarbonate is necessary; large amounts (500–1000 mmol) may be required. Dialysis may be used if sodium overload is a problem. Trihydroxymethylaminomethane (THAM) buffer 0.3 M solution (pH 10.2) is also an occasionally valuable adjunct to treatment.

Treatment hazards

There are real hazards associated with the over enthusiastic treatment of acidosis. Thus, while correction of acidosis may improve cardiac function and peripheral circulation, alleviate hyperventilation and correct hyperkalaemia, there are real hazards associated with a shift to the left of the blood oxygen dissociation curve. This results in an acute reduction in oxygen delivery. Rapid alkalinization may also reduce cerebral blood flow. The use of sodium bicarbonate as the alkalinizing agent may not only cause sodium overloading, but, because of an acute rise in $P\text{CO}_2$, may acutely *increase* intracellular acidosis—possibly the most important factor in the deleterious effects of acidosis.

In general, if the cause of the acidosis can be removed, acid–base disorders will self-correct. If the clinical situation demands alkalinization, slow infusion of isotonic sodium bicarbonate (150 mmol·L^{-1}) should be used rather than bolus injections of hypertonic solution. A very careful watch must be kept on fluid balance and serial measurements must be made of pH and $P\text{CO}_2$. Calculations of the amount of alkali required on the basis of 'base deficit' are inaccurate.

Table 10.13 Causes and mechanisms of metabolic alkalosis.

Vomiting
Loss of gastric H$^+$ and Cl$^-$
Secondary renal potassium wasting with acid urine

Diuretics
Renal chloride wasting commonly associated with
  hypokalaemia

Hyperaldosteronism
Increased reabsorption of bicarbonate
Hypochloraemic alkalosis

Excess liquorice ingestion

Carbenoxolone sodium

Milk alkali syndrome
Excess intake of calcium and calcium antacids (rare)

Excess i.v. NaHCO$_3$
Treatment of acidosis
Treatment of salicylate/barbiturate poisoning

METABOLIC ALKALOSIS

This is much less common than acidosis and is often associated with potassium or chloride depletion. The main causes are persistent vomiting, diuretic therapy or hyperaldosteronism; other causes are much less common (Table 10.13).

Vomiting
The amount of H^+ and chloride lost in vomitus may be considerable, especially in pyloric stenosis. Hypochloraemic alkalosis develops, leading to hypokalaemia, and considerable loss of potassium in the urine. Symptoms are those of volume depletion and hypokalaemia.

The urine contains very little chloride (< 10 $mmol \cdot L^{-1}$) and is acid despite a systemic alkalosis. Treatment includes intravenous normal saline with potassium supplements to correct first the chloride deficit and then the potassium deficit. The bicarbonate excess will correct itself.

Diuretic therapy
Diuretic therapy, especially with loop diuretics, may induce a hypochloraemic alkalosis, often associated with hypokalaemia, by blocking the renal reabsorption of chloride. Treatment includes review of the diuretic therapy, oral supplments of potassium chloride (Slow-K 2 tablets [16 mmol potassium] three times daily) or the use of potassium-sparing diuretics (amiloride, triamterene or spironolactone).

Hyperaldosteronism or an excessive intake of liquorice or carbenoxolone sodium, which have an aldosterone-like effect, is usually associated with a moderate hypochloraemic alkalosis with potassium depletion. The alkalosis is possibly due to increased renal bicarbonate reabsorption. Treatment is that of the primary cause.

Further reading

Cohen RD & Woods HF (1987) Disturbances of acid-base homeostasis. In Weatherall DJ, Ledingham JGG & Warrell DA (eds) *Oxford Textbook of Medicine*, Vol. 1, pp. 9.164–9.175. Oxford: Oxford University Press.

Schrier RW & Gottschalk CW (eds) (1988) *Diseases of the Kidney*, 4th edn, Vol. 1, pp. 119–309. Boston: Little, Brown and Company.

11

Cardiovascular Disease

Introduction

In the western hemisphere approximately 50% of deaths are related to cardiovascular disease. This is due mainly to ischaemic heart disease that could, perhaps, be significantly reduced if smoking were prohibited, lifestyle moderated (e.g. weight reduction) and the intake of cholesterol and saturated fats reduced. Whilst the incidence of rheumatic heart disease is decreasing in the West, it is still an important problem world-wide, predominantly in countries with poor sanitation, overcrowding and malnutrition. Up to one-third of all cardiac cases admitted to hospital in, for example, India, Jamaica, Egypt or the Philippines are due to rheumatic heart disease. Hypertension is another major cause of mortality, being responsible for 10% of deaths world-wide. The incidence of hypertension usually increases with age and is higher in Western countries. There is also a wide geographical variation in other cardiac diseases: endomyocardial fibrosis is seen in the tropics; cardiac problems associated with protein–energy malnutrition are seen in countries where famine and malnutrition occur; cardiomyopathy is seen with beriberi and myocarditis is seen with other diseases associated with the tropics, e.g. Chagas' disease, typhoid fever and diphtheria.

Congenital heart disease is important in the young and is responsible for approximately 1% of deaths in patients below 15 years of age.

Lastly, pulmonary heart disease is common in countries with a high incidence of smoking.

Essential anatomy, physiology and embryology of the heart

The cellular basis of myocardial contraction

Myocardial fibres consist of bundles of parallel myofibrils. Each myofibril is made up of a series of sarcomeres (Fig. 11.1). A sarcomere is bound by two transverse Z lines to each of which is attached a perpendicular filament of the protein actin. The actin filaments from each of the two Z bands overlap with thicker parallel protein filaments known as myosin. The molecular weight of myosin is approximately 500 000 and that of actin is about 47 000. Actin and myosin molecules are attached to each other by cross-bridges that contain ATPase.

During cardiac contraction the length of the actin and myosin molecules does not change. Rather, the actin molecules slide between the myosin molecules when a high-energy bond of ATP is split by ATPase. This interaction requires magnesium ions. Calcium ions are also required to inactivate another protein called troponin, which ordinarily inhibits the actin–myosin interaction. Calcium is made available during the plateau phase (phase 2) of each action potential (see Fig. 11.33) by calcium ions entering the cell and being mobilized from the sarcoplasm. The force of cardiac muscle contraction ('inotropic state') is thus regulated by the influx of Ca^{2+} into the cell through slow calcium channels (Fig. 11.2).

Starling's law of the heart

The contractile function of an isolated strip of cardiac tissue can be described by the relationship between the velocity of muscle contraction, the load that may be moved by the contracting muscle, and the extent to which the muscle is stretched

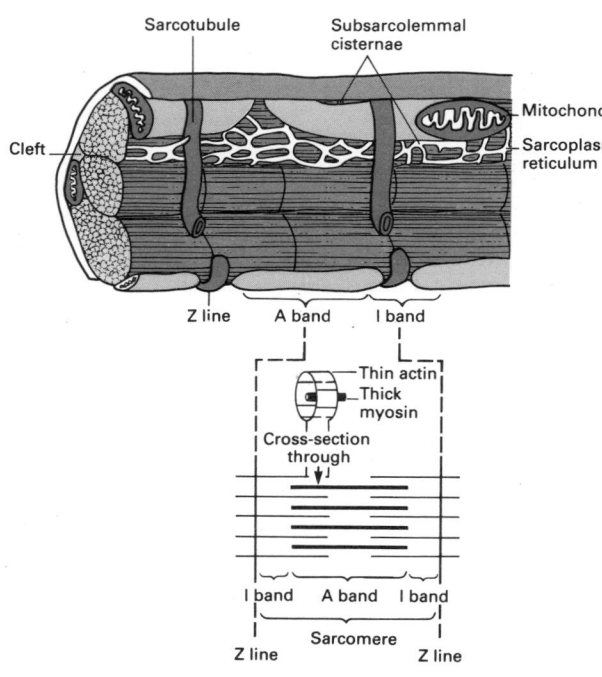

Fig. 11.1 A schematic diagram showing the structure of a myofibril. The myofibrils are made up of a series of sarcomeres joined at the Z line.

before contracting. As with all other types of muscle, the velocity of contraction of myocardial tissue is reduced by increasing the load against which the tissue must contract. However, in the non-failing heart, prestretching of cardiac muscle improves the relationship between the force and velocity of contraction (Fig. 11.3, p. 514).

This phenomenon was described in the intact heart as an increase of stroke volume (ventricular performance) with an enlargement of the diastolic volume (pre-load), and is known as 'Starling's law of the heart' or the 'Frank–Starling relationship'. It has been transcribed into more clinically relevant indices. Thus, stroke work (aortic pressure × stroke volume) is increased as ventricular end-diastolic volume is raised. Alternatively, within certain limits, cardiac output rises as pulmonary capillary wedge pressure increases. This clinical relationship is described by the ventricular function curve (Fig. 11.3, which also shows the effect of sympathetic stimulation).

The conduction system of the heart

Each natural heart beat begins in the heart's pacemaker—the sinoatrial (SA) node. This is a crescent-shaped structure that is located around the medial and anterior aspect of the junction between the superior vena cava and the right atrium (Fig. 11.4, p. 514). Progressive loss of the diastolic resting membrane potential is followed, when the threshold potential has been reached, by a more rapid depolarization of the sinus node

tissue. This depolarization triggers depolarization of the atrial myocardium. The atrial tissue is activated like a 'forest fire', but the activation peters out when the insulating layer between the atrium and the ventricle—the annulus fibrosus—is reached.

The depolarization continues to conduct slowly through the atrioventricular (AV) node. This is a small, bean-shaped structure that lies beneath the right atrial endocardium within the lower inter-atrial septum. The AV node continues as the His bundle, which penetrates the annulus fibrosus and conducts the cardiac impulse rapidly towards the ventricle. The His bundle reaches the crest of the interventricular septum and divides into the right bundle branch and the main left bundle branch.

The right bundle branch continues down the right side of the interventricular apex, from where it radiates and divides to form the Purkinje network, which spreads throughout the subendo-cardial surface of the right ventricle.

The main left bundle branch is a short structure which fans out into many strands on the left side of the interventricular septum. These strands can be grouped into an anterior superior division (the anterior hemibundle) and a posterior inferior division (the posterior hemibundle). The anterior hemibundle supplies the subendocardial Purkinje network of the anterior and superior surfaces of the left ventricle, and the inferior hemibundle supplies the inferior and posterior surfaces. Impulse conduction through the AV node is slow and depends on action potentials largely produced by slow transmembrane calcium flux. In the atria,

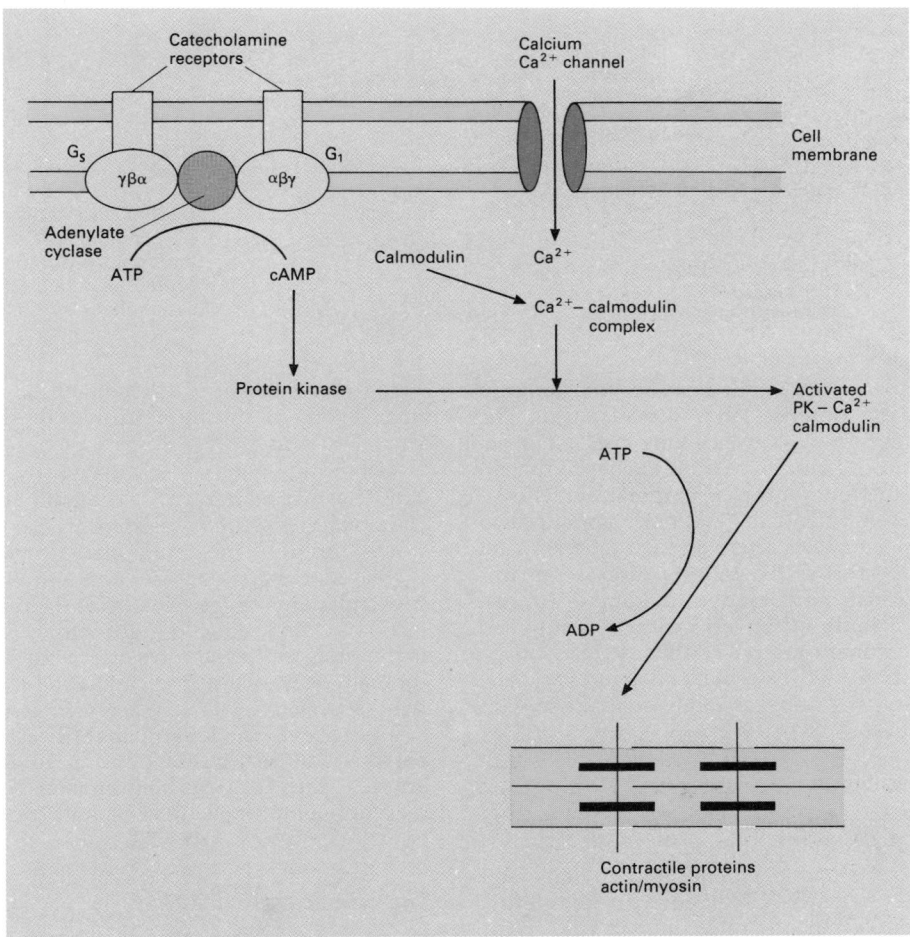

Fig. 11.2 The cell membrane contains calcium channels and catecholamine receptors. The latter after stimulation increases cAMP, which via protein kinase and calmodulin activate the contractile proteins of cardiac muscle. G_S, G_I: stimulatory and inhibitory guanine nucleotide binding proteins. PK: protein kinase.

ventricles and His–Purkinje system conduction is rapid and is due to action potentials generated by rapid transmembrane sodium diffusion.

Nerve supply of the cardiovascular system

Adrenergic nerves supply artrial and ventricular muscle fibres as well as the conduction system. β_1 receptors predominate in the heart with both adrenaline and noradrenaline having positive inotropic and chronotropic effects. β_2 receptors predominate in the vascular smooth muscle.

Cholinergic nerves from the vagus supply mainly the SA and AV nodes via M2 muscarinic receptors. Under basal conditions vagal inhibitory effects predominate over the sympathetic resulting in a slow heart rate. However intrinsic mechanisms also exist as the heart can beat without autonomic control.

The coronary circulation

The coronary arterial system (Fig. 11.5) consists of the right and left coronary arteries. The right coronary artery arises from the right coronary sinus and courses through the right side of the atrioventricular groove, giving off vessels that supply the right atrium and the right ventricle. The vessel usually continues as the posterior descending coronary artery, which runs in the posterior interventricular groove and supplies the posterior part of the interventricular septum and the posterior left ventricular wall.

The left coronary artery arises from the left coronary sinus. The first part is known as the left main coronary artery, and is usually not more than 2.5 cm long. It then divides into the left anterior descending and the left circumflex arteries. The left anterior descending artery runs in the anterior

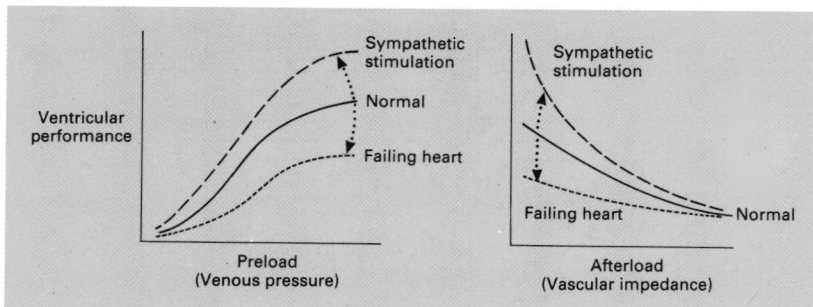

Fig. 11.3 The Frank–Starling mechanism, showing the effect of alterations in pre-load (left) and after-load (right) in the normal and failing heart during sympathetic stimulation.

interventricular groove and supplies the anterior septum and the anterior left ventricular wall. The left circumflex artery travels along the left atrioventricular groove and gives off branches to the left atrium and the left ventricle (marginal branches).

The sinus node and the AV node are supplied by the right coronary artery in 60% and 90% of people, respectively. Therefore, disease in this artery may cause sinus bradycardia and AV nodal block. The majority of the left ventricle is supplied by the left coronary artery, so that stenosis in the left main artery is extremely dangerous; total obstruction of this vessel is rarely compatible with life.

The fetal circulation

In utero, the pulmonary circulation is largely unnecessary because fetal blood is oxygenated by placental blood flow, a parallel and integral element in the systemic circulation. In the fetus, systemic venous blood returning to the right atrium is partly deflected through the foramen ovale to the left atrium. Blood that passes through the right ventricle is diverted away from the pulmonary arteries to the aorta through the ductus arteriosus. Thus, the systemic venous return, which is a mixture of oxygenated and deoxygenated blood, is mostly returned to the systemic arterial system.

At birth, inspiration dilates the pulmonary arterioles, resulting in a dramatic reduction of pulmonary vascular resistance. Blood therefore flows through the pulmonary circulation. The increased oxygen tension and reduced levels of prostaglandins trigger closure of the ductus arteriosus, and the reduced right atrial pressure and increasing left atrial pressure tend to close the foramen ovale. Thus, the circulation is divided into two separate circuits connected in series.

In the fetus the left and right heart both propel blood from the systemic veins to the systemic arteries; thus, severe abnormalities of the heart may not compromise fetal blood flow.

The cardiac cycle (Fig. 11.6)

The first event in the cardiac cycle is atrial depolarization (a P wave on the surface ECG) followed by right atrial and then left atrial contraction. Ventricular activation (the QRS complex on the ECG) follows after a short interval (the PR interval). Left ventricular contraction starts and shortly thereafter right ventricular contraction begins. The increased ventricular pressures exceed the atrial pressures, and close first the mitral and then the tricuspid valves. Until the aortic and pulmonary valves open, the ventricles contract with no change of volume (isovolumetric contraction). When ventricular pressures rise above the aortic and pulmonary artery pressures, the pulmonary valve and then the aortic valve open and ventricular ejection occurs. As the ventricles begin to relax, their pressures fall below the aortic and pulmonary arterial pressures, and aortic valve closure is followed by pulmonary valve closure. Isovolumetric relaxation then occurs after the ventricular pressures have fallen below the right atrial and left atrial pressures and the tricuspid and mitral valves open.

The cardiac cycle determines the sequence of heart sounds (see p. 523).

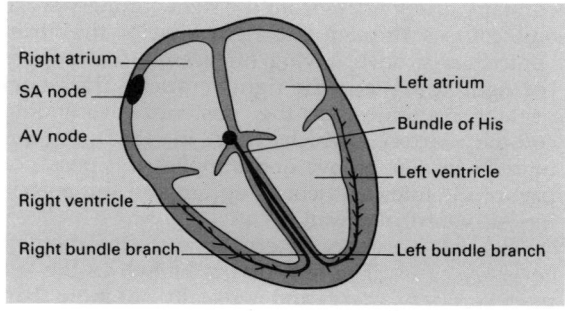

Fig. 11.4 The normal cardiac conduction system. SA = sino-atrial; AV = atrioventricular.

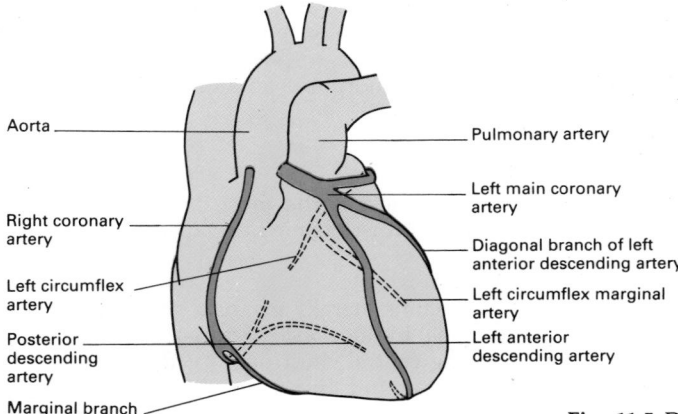

Aorta

Right coronary artery

Left circumflex artery

Posterior descending artery

Marginal branch of right coronary artery

Pulmonary artery

Left main coronary artery

Diagonal branch of left anterior descending artery

Left circumflex marginal artery

Left anterior descending artery

Fig. 11.5 Diagram of the normal coronary arterial anatomy.

Symptoms of heart disease

Dyspnoea, chest pain, palpitations, syncope, fatigue and ankle swelling are the usual symptoms produced by cardiac disease. However, patients are often completely asymptomatic until a relatively late stage in their illness.

Dyspnoea

Dyspnoea is an awareness of breathlessness. It can be due to cardiac or respiratory causes. It is also a symptom during exercise in healthy people.

Breathlessness may occur only on exercise or may be present at rest. The New York Heart Association has graded this symptom (see Table 11.1) but this classification, although often used, has now been officially discontinued and is replaced by a very similar grading known as 'cardiac status' (Table 11.2).

It is also clinically valuable to grade dyspnoea by the amount of physical exertion possible before breathlessness occurs, e.g. climbing 14 stairs or walking 200 yards on the flat.

Left ventricular failure causes dyspnoea because of a rise in left atrial pressure and pulmonary capillary pressure leading to interstitial and alveolar oedema. This makes the lung stiff (less compliant) and this increases the amount of respiratory effort necessary to breathe. Usually a fast breathing rate (tachypnoea) is also present due to stimulation of the pulmonary stretch receptors.

Table 11.1 The New York Heart Association functional and therapeutic classification applied to dyspnoea.

Grade 1	No breathlessness
Grade 2	Breathlessness on severe exertion
Grade 3	Breathlessness on mild exertion
Grade 4	Breathlessness at rest

Table 11.2 The New York Heart Association grading of 'cardiac status'.

Grade 1	Uncompromised
Grade 2	Slightly compromised
Grade 3	Moderately compromised
Grade 4	Severely compromised

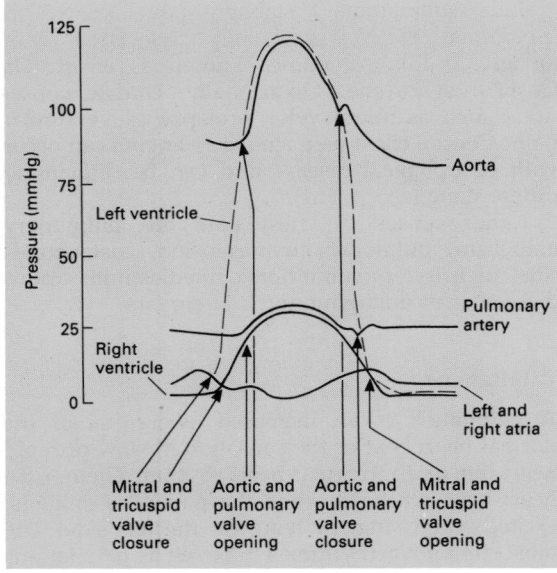

Fig. 11.6 The cardiac cycle.

Orthopnoea

This is a form of breathlessness that occurs when the patient lies flat. Orthopnoea occurs because lying flat results in the redistribution of blood, leading to an increased central and pulmonary blood volume. Recumbancy also causes the abdominal contents to press up against the diaphragm. Both factors increase the difficulty of breathing. Patients usually cope with orthopnoea by propping themselves up with pillows. It is convenient to grade orthopnoea by the number of pillows used, e.g. 'three pillow orthopnoea'. However, patients may also sleep with pillows for comfort.

Paroxysmal nocturnal dyspnoea (PND)

This occurs when there is an accumulation of fluid in the lungs (pulmonary oedema) at night. The mechanism is similar to orthopnoea, but because sensory awareness is depressed during sleep, severe interstitial and alveolar oedema can accumulate. The patient is woken from sleep fighting for breath, a dramatic and frightening experience. The breathlessness may be relieved by sitting on the side of the bed or getting up. Sometimes the patient will get up and open a window to gasp for fresh air. Wheezing, due to bronchial endothelial oedema, is common (cardiac asthma), and a cough, often productive of frothy or blood-tinged sputum, usually occurs. The patient is vasoconstricted and therefore cold and cyanosed. Initially these episodes terminate spontaneously. Episodes of 'PND', often with coughing, can occur in asthma, but conventionally the term is reserved for cardiac problems.

Cheyne–Stokes respiration (see also p. 906)

In very severe heart failure, alternate hyperventilation and apnoea known as Cheyne–Stokes respiration may occur. This may also develop in the elderly without obvious heart failure. It is related to depression of the respiratory centre, which is partly due to prolonged circulation time and cerebrovascular disease. This type of respiration is also seen after morphine administration.

Chest pain

Pain in the chest is the most common symptom associated with ischaemic heart disease.

Angina pectoris

Angina pectoris literally means a strangling sensation (angina) in the chest (pectoris). It is a gripping or crushing central chest pain (or discomfort) that may be felt around the whole chest or deep within the chest. The pain may radiate into the neck or jaw and rarely, into the teeth, back or abdomen. It is associated with heaviness, paraesthesia or pain in one (usually the left) or both arms. It is typically provoked by exercise and is promptly relieved by rest. A pain of similar distribution and type also occurs at rest in myocardial infarction (see p. 575). The mechanism of the pain is myocardial hypoxia secondary to inadequate coronary blood flow. Sharp pains over the heart are not usually angina. Angina should be classified according to the Canadian Cardiovascular Society grading of angina of effort (Table 11.3), although most physicians find that a verbal description is adequate.

Other causes of chest pain

The pain of pericarditis is felt in the centre of the chest and, like that of pleurisy, is aggravated by movement, posture, respiration and coughing. It is sharp and severe.

Left, submammary stabbing pain, known as 'precordial catch', is usually associated with anxiety and is sometimes known as effort (Da Costa's) syndrome. Occasionally, cardiac conditions such as mitral valve prolapse cause similar pain. Central chest pain similar to angina can occur with oesophageal disease and can be difficult to differentiate (see p. 181).

Other causes of chest pain are pulmonary embolism, pulmonary hypertension, costochondritis, pleurisy, pneumothorax, mediastinitis and a dissecting or enlarging aortic aneurysm.

Palpitations

A palpitation is an increased awareness of the normal heart beat or the sensation of slow or rapid heart rate or an irregular heart rhythm. The normal heart beat is sensed when the patient is anxious, excited, exercising, or lying on the left side. The most common arrhythmias to be felt as palpitations are premature ectopic beats and paroxysmal tachycardias.

Table 11.3 The Canadian Cardiovascular Society grading of angina of effort.

Grade I	Ordinary physical activity does not cause angina (strenuous physical activity provokes angina)
Grade II	Slight limitations of ordinary physical activity (climbing more than one flight of stairs or walking uphill provokes angina)
Grade III	Marked limitation of ordinary physical activity (walking on the level or climbing one flight of stairs provokes angina)
Grade IV	Inability to carry on any physical activity (angina may be present at rest)

Table 11.4 Cardiac causes of syncope.

Arrhythmias
Ventricular tachycardia
Rapid supraventricular tachycardia
Sinus arrest
AV block
Artificial pacemaker failure

Obstruction
Aortic/pulmonary stenosis
Hypertrophic obstructive cardiomyopathy
Fallot's tetralogy
Pulmonary hypertension/embolism
Atrial myxoma
Atrial thrombus
Defective prosthetic valve

Premature beats
These are usually felt as 'missed beats' because the premature beat is followed by a pause before the next normal beat, which is rather forceful because of the longer diastolic filling period. Premature beats often occur in clusters and may cause the patient much anxiety.

Paroxysmal tachycardias
These start abruptly and may terminate equally suddenly. Often, however, the tachycardia slows before terminating and therefore seems to fade away. Paroxysmal atrial fibrillation is noticeably irregular, whereas other forms of paroxysmal supraventricular or ventricular tachycardia are regular. Paroxysms of rapid tachycardia, especially when prolonged, may be associated with syncope, presyncope, dyspnoea or chest pain. Palpitations can be graded in a similar way to the grading of dyspnoea or angina. Supraventricular tachycardias, such as atrial fibrillation or junctional tachycardias, may produce polyuria.

Bradycardias
An unduly slow heart rate may be appreciated as slow, regular, 'heavy' or forceful beats. Most often bradycardias are not felt as palpitations.

Syncope

Syncope can be due to many causes (see p. 920). The commonest syncopal attacks are vasovagal in nature (simple faints) and are not due to serious disease. Vasovagal attacks are due to venous pooling (postural hypotension) or may be provoked by fright or shock. They are associated with a prodome, that consists of dizziness, nausea, sweating, ringing in the ears, a sinking feeling and yawning. There is peripheral vasodilatation and a bradycardia. Recovery occurs within a few seconds.

Cardiovascular syncope is usually sudden and brief. The classical variety is known as a Stokes–Adams attack and is due to a disturbance of cardiac rhythm, e.g. a profound bradycardia related to complete heart block. Without warning the patient falls to the ground, pale and deeply unconscious. The pulse is usually very slow or absent. After a few seconds the patient flushes brightly and recovers consciousness as the pulse quickens. If the period of unconsciousness is prolonged the patient may suffer a generalized convulsion but this is not usual. Often there are no sequelae but patients may injure themselves during falls.

Other causes of syncope due to heart disease can be grouped as cardiac arrhythmias or valvular or vascular obstruction (see Table 11.4).

Fatigue

This symptom, which consists of tiredness and lethargy, is associated with heart failure, persistent cardiac arrhythmias and cyanotic heart disease. It is due to poor cerebral and peripheral perfusion and poor oxygenation. When severe cardiac disorders are not present, an active infection such as infective endocarditis may be responsible. However, disorders of most systems may produce this non-specific symptom. Drugs prescribed for angina or hypertension, particularly beta-blockers, may cause fatigue.

Oedema

Heart failure results in salt and water retention. Retained fluid accumulates in the feet and ankles of ambulant patients and over the sacrum of bed-bound patients. The oedema associated with heart failure becomes progressively worse during the day and is often absent on initial rising as the fluid is reabsorbed on lying down. When severe, the calf and thigh may become oedematous and ascites or a pleural effusion may develop.

Examination of the cardiovascular system

GENERAL EXAMINATION

General features of the patient's well-being should be noted as well as the presence of anaemia, obesity, jaundice and cachexia.

Clubbing (see also p. 639)

The most common cardiac causes of severe clubbing are subacute infective endocarditis and congenital cyanotic heart disease, particularly Fallot's tetralogy. Clubbing takes many months to develop and is therefore not seen in acute endocarditis or in neonates or infants with cyanotic heart disease. Clubbing seen in cor pulmonale is due to the underlying pulmonary disease (e.g. bronchiectasis or fibrosing alveolitis).

Splinter haemorrhages

These small, subungal linear haemorrhages are most frequently due to trauma but are also caused by infective endocarditis.

Cyanosis

This is a dusky blue discoloration of the skin (particularly at the extremities) or of the mucous membranes. It is due to the presence of unoxygenated haemoglobin (traditionally at least 5 g·dl^{-1} of blood) and occasionally, of other reduction products of haemoglobin such as sulphaemoglobin or methaemoglobin. Cyanosis is more readily provoked in the presence of polycythaemia and is uncommon when anaemia is present.

Central cyanosis
This is present when the tongue is cyanosed. It is caused by cardiac failure or respiratory disorders. The central cyanosis of pulmonary or cardiac failure is improved by breathing oxygen if the degree of shunting is small.

Peripheral cyanosis
This is due to vasoconstriction and stasis of blood in the extremities, and increased oxygen extraction by peripheral tissues. Peripheral cyanosis occurs in congestive heart failure, shock, exposure to cold temperatures and with abnormalities of the peripheral circulation.

THE ARTERIAL PULSE

A pulse is felt by compressing an artery against a bone. The first pulse to be examined is the right radial pulse. The timing of the left radial and femoral pulses are then compared with that of the right radial pulse. Delayed pulsation occurs because of a proximal stenosis, particularly of the aorta (coarctation). The radial pulse is examined to reveal the pulse rate and the heart rhythm. A large-volume pulse will also be obvious, especially if the arm is raised and the pulse felt by gripping the wrist so that the palm of the examiner's hand is located over the radial pulse.

Rate

The pulse rate should be between 60 and 80 beats per minute (bpm) when an adult patient is lying quietly in bed. Young children may have higher pulse rates and athletes and elderly adults may have slower rates. The exact rate is unimportant but changes (seen on a pulse chart) are helpful. When the pulse is irregular, not all beats may be transmitted to the wrist and it is therefore best to count the pulse whilst at the same time listening to the heart beat with a stethoscope. This apex-radial (pulse) deficit is common in atrial fibrillation.

Rhythm

In normal subjects the pulse is regular except for a slight quickening in early inspiration and a slowing in expiration (sinus arrhythmia). Irregularities of the pulse rhythm are usually due to premature beats, intermittent heart block or atrial fibrillation.

Premature beats occur as occasional or repeated irregularities superimposed on a regular pulse rhythm. Similarly, intermittent heart block is revealed by occasional beats dropped from an

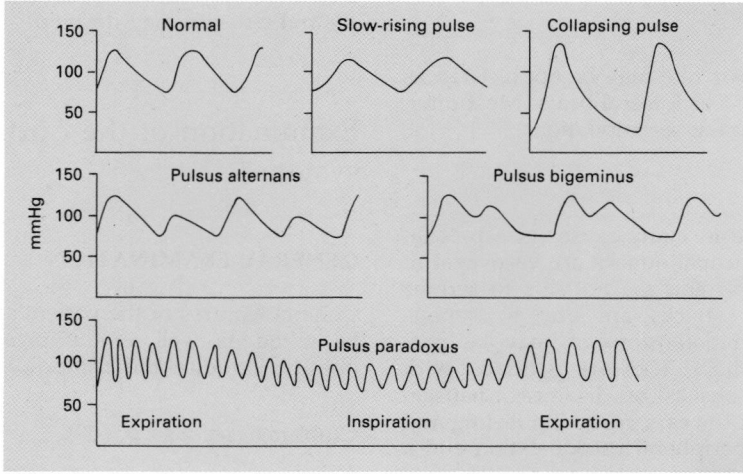

Fig. 11.7 Various arterial wave forms.

otherwise regular rhythm. A totally irregular pattern (irregularly irregular) of heart beats occurs in atrial fibrillation. This irregular pattern persists when the pulse quickens in response to exercise in contrast to pulse irregularity due to ectopic beats, which disappears on exercise. However, this is not a reliable way to distinguish ectopic beats from other causes of pulse irregularity.

Carotid pulse

The amplitude and shape of the carotid pulse is examined. Usually carotid pulsation is not visible, but a very large-volume pulse may be apparent as pulsation of the neck (Corrigan's sign). A large volume pulse occurs in high output states and in aortic regurgitation. The carotid pulse is also visible when the carotid artery is aneurysmal or kinked. The right carotid is palpated lightly in order to detect a thrill.

A large volume pulse with a brisk rise and fall is known as a collapsing or waterhammer pulse (Fig. 11.7). It is found in the elderly when the aorta is rigid, or when the cardiac output is high, e.g. in thyrotoxicosis, anaemia or fever. Aortic valvular regurgitation or a persistent ductus arteriosus also cause a collapsing pulse. A large-volume pulse that is not collapsing in nature is associated with the large stroke volume that is necessary if bradycardia is present.

A small-volume pulse is seen in cardiac failure, shock and obstructive vascular or valvular disease. It is also present when tachycardia occurs. The pulse of aortic stenosis is not only small in volume but is slow in rising to a peak (plateau pulse) and is often associated with a notch on the upstroke (anacrotic pulse) or a systolic shudder or thrill.

Other changes in arterial pulse

Paradoxical pulse (pulsus paradoxus) (Fig. 11.7)
Paradoxical pulse is a misnomer as it is actually an exaggeration of the normal pattern. In normal subjects, the systolic pressure and the pulse pressure (the difference between the systolic and diastolic blood pressures) fall during inspiration. The normal fall of systolic pressure is less than 10 mm Hg and this can be easily measured using a sphygmomanometer. The reason for this fall in pressure is that the right heart responds directly to changes in intrathoracic pressure while the filling of the left depends on the pulmonary intravascular volume. Thus as the return of blood to the left ventricle falls there is a drop in systolic pressure. At high respiratory rates this is exaggerated with the volumes of the right and left ventricles being unequal. In severe air flow limitation (especially severe asthma) there is an increased and sudden negative intrathoracic pressure on inspiration and this will enhance the normal fall in blood pressure.

In patients with cardiac tamponade the fluid in the pericardium increases the intrapericardial pressure thereby reducing the heart's filling capacity. The inspiratory increase in the right ventricle occurs very much at the expense of the left ventricle as both ventricles are confined within a relatively 'fixed' pericardium. Through a similar mechanism, paradox can occur in constrictive pericarditis but is less common.

Alternating pulse (pulsus alternans)
This is characterized by alternate beats that are weak and strong but with a regular rhythm. It is a feature of severe myocardial failure and is due to the prolonged recovery time of damaged myocardium; it indicates a very poor prognosis. It is easily noticed when taking the blood pressure because the systolic blood pressure may vary from beat to beat by as much as 50 mm Hg. Pulsus alternans may also occur when there is rapid, abnormal tachycardia. In this case it acts as a compensatory mechanism and does not indicate a poor prognosis. Pulsus alternans should be distinguished from a bigeminal pulse (see below).

Bigeminal pulse (pulsus bigeminus)
This is due to premature ectopic beats following every sinus beat. The rhythm is not regular (Fig. 11.7) because every weak pulse is premature.

Taking the blood pressure

- The blood pressure is taken in the (right) arm with the patient relaxed and comfortable.
- The sphygmomanometer cuff is wrapped around the upper arm with the inflation bag placed over the brachial artery.
- The cuff is inflated until the pressure exceeds the arterial pressure and the radial pulse is no longer palpable.
- The diaphragm of the stethoscope is positioned over the brachial artery just below the cuff.
- The cuff pressure is slowly reduced until sounds (Korotkoff sounds) can be heard (phase 1). This is the systolic pressure.
- The pressure is allowed to fall further until the Korotkoff sounds become suddenly muffled (phase 4).
- The pressure is allowed to fall still further until they disappear (phase 5).

The diastolic pressure is usually taken as phase 5 because this phase is more reproducible and nearer to the intravascular diastolic pressure. The Korotkoff sounds may disappear (phase 2) and reappear (phase 3) between the systolic and diastolic pressures. It is important not to mistake phase 2 for the diastolic pressure or phase 3 for the systolic pressure.

Pulsus bisferiens

This is a pulse that is found in hypertrophic obstructive cardiomyopathy and in aortic regurgitation combined with aortic stenosis. The first systolic wave is the 'percussion' wave produced by the transmission of the left ventricular pressure in early systole. The second peak is the 'tidal' wave caused by recoil of the vascular bed. This normally happens in diastole (the dicrotic wave), but when the left ventricle empties slowly or is obstructed from emptying completely, the tidal wave occurs in late systole. The result is a palpable double pulse.

BLOOD PRESSURE

The peak systemic arterial blood pressure is produced by transmission of left ventricular systolic pressure. The diastolic blood pressure is maintained by vascular tone and an intact aortic valve.

The normal blood pressure

There is no single blood pressure or limited range of blood pressures that is normal in all subjects and circumstances. However:

● In a resting adult the systolic blood pressure does not usually exceed 150 mm Hg and the diastolic pressure does not exceed 90 mm Hg.
● In children or young adults the pressures are correspondingly less.
● In the elderly the rigidity of the arterial vessels produces an increase, predominantly in the systolic blood pressure.
● There is a diurnal variation of blood pressure, the pressure during the day being greater than at night.
● Anxiety and exertion increase the blood pressure.

Note that a cuff that is too small leads to overestimation of the pressure. For example, if a standard arm cuff size (12 cm) is used in an obese patient, the pressure measured will be too high. Similarly, if an arm cuff is used on the thigh (with the diaphragm of the stethoscope applied over the popliteal artery), the femoral pressure will be overestimated. The usual thigh cuff is 15 cm wide. Smaller cuff sizes are available for children and thin adults.

Variations in blood pressure

The systolic blood pressure varies by up to 10 mm Hg between the right and left brachial arteries. Standing usually causes a slight reduction of the systolic pressure (< 20 mm Hg) and an increase in the diastolic blood pressure (< 10 mm Hg). In postural (orthostatic) hypotension, a large postural fall of both the systolic and diastolic pressures is associated with dizziness. When an irregular heart rhythm such as atrial fibrillation is present, the blood pressure is somewhat variable. Because the blood pressure is normally liable to variation it must be estimated on several occasions before it can be declared elevated.

JUGULAR VENOUS PULSE

There are no valves between the internal jugular vein and the right atrium and observation of the column of blood in the internal jugular system is therefore a good measure of right atrial pressure. The external jugular cannot be relied upon because of its valves and because it may be obstructed by the fascial and muscular layers through which it passes; it can only be used if typical venous pulsation is seen, indicating no obstruction to flow

---

Measurement of the jugular pressure

● The patient is positioned at about 45° to the horizontal (between 30° and 60°, wherever the top of the venous pulsation can be seen).
● The head is supported by a pillow and the neck is slightly flexed to allow the skin and muscle overlying the vein to relax.
● The jugular venous pressure is measured as the vertical distance between the manubriosternal angle and the top of the venous column.
● The normal jugular venous pressure is usually less than 3 cm H_2O, which is equivalent to a right atrial pressure of 8 cm H_2O when measured with reference to a point midway between the anterior and posterior surfaces of the chest. The venous pulsations are not usually palpable (except for the forceful venous distension associated with tricuspid regurgitation).
● Pulsations should be looked for before touching the neck.
● Gentle pressure at the root of the neck may abolish visible venous pulsation and may make a vein visible by causing distension above the occlusion.
● Hepatojugular reflex. Abdominal compression causes a temporary increase in central and hence jugular venous pressure. It is a simple way of confirming the venous nature of a pulsation in the neck.

An abnormally low jugular venous pressure cannot be measured clinically. Causes include haemorrhage and other forms of hypovolaemia.

Elevation of the jugular venous pressure occurs in heart failure (see p. 563). It is also produced by:

● Constrictive pericarditis
● Cardiac tamponade
● Renal disease with salt and water retention
● Overtransfusion or excessive infusion of fluids

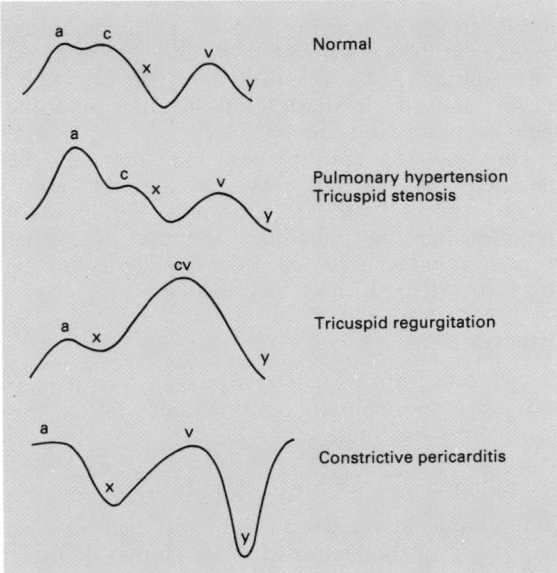

Fig. 11.8 Various jugular venous wave forms.

● Superior vena caval obstruction (but in this case pulsation is absent)

In constrictive pericarditis or cardiac tamponade, ventricular filling is reduced during inspiration because the ventricles are squeezed by the pericardial fluid or non-compliant pericardium, which tightens as the diaphragm descends. Thus, the level of venous pressure increases during inspiration (Kussmaul's sign).

Other causes of an increased jugular pressure also distort the shape of the pressure wave and are considered below.

The jugular venous pressure wave

This consists of three peaks and two troughs (Fig. 11.8). The peaks are described as *a*, *c* and *v* waves and the troughs are known as *x* and *y* descents:

● The *a wave* is produced by atrial systole.
● The *x descent* occurs when the atrial contraction finishes.
● As the pressure falls there is a small transient increase that produces a positive deflection called the *c wave*. This is caused by transmission of the rapidly increasing right ventricular pressure before the tricuspid valve closes.
● The *v wave* develops as the venous return fills the right atrium during continued ventricular systole.
● The *y descent* follows the *v* wave when the tricuspid valve opens.

The *a* wave can be distinguished from the *v* wave by observing the venous pulse while palpating the carotid artery. The *a* wave occurs immediately before carotid pulsation and the *v* wave occurs simultaneously with carotid pulsation.

The main abnormalities of the shape of the jugular venous pressure wave are elevations of the *a* and *v* waves and steepness of the *y* descent (Fig. 11.8).

Large a waves
These are caused by increased resistance to ventricular filling, as seen with right ventricular hypertrophy due to pulmonary hypertension or pulmonary stenosis. They may also be caused by tricuspid stenosis, but this is unusual because patients with tricuspid stenosis are usually in atrial fibrillation and therefore do not have *a* waves.

A very large *a* wave occurs when the atrium contracts against a closed tricuspid valve. This is known as a 'cannon wave'. Cannon waves occur irregularly in complete heart block and in ventricular tachycardia. In both these situations there is atrioventricular dissociation, and by random chance there is occasional simultaneous atrial and ventricular contraction. In junctional rhythms the atria and ventricles usually contract simultaneously and regular cannon waves are produced.

Large v waves
Tricuspid regurgitation results in giant *v* waves (systolic waves) because the right ventricular pressure is transmitted directly to the right atrium and the great veins.

Steep y descent
Diastolic collapse of elevated venous pressure can occur in right ventricular failure but is more dramatic in constrictive pericarditis and tricuspid regurgitation. At the end of the ventricular systole the elevated atrial pressure suddenly falls when the tricuspid valve opens. However, the ventricles are stiff and cannot be distended. The venous pressure therefore rapidly rises again. This rapid fall and rise of the jugular venous pulse is known as Friedreich's sign.

EXAMINATION OF THE PRECORDIUM

Inspection

Deformities should be looked for as they can mimic cardiac abnormalities. For example, pectus excavatum (funnel chest) or kyphoscoliosis may cause an ejection systolic murmur. The position of the apex beat and other cardiac pulsations should be noted; a left ventricular aneurysm may produce an eccentric and abnormal pulsation.

Palpation

The apex beat is defined as the most inferior and most lateral point of cardiac pulsation. It is usually felt just inside the mid-clavicular line at the level of the fourth or fifth left intercostal space. Cardiac enlargement, particularly left ventricular dilatation, displaces the apex beat to the left. The apex beat may also be displaced by a pneumothorax, pulmonary collapse or skeletal abnormalities such as scoliosis. The character of the apex beat is also important. It is normally just palpable and is confined to a point that can be covered by one finger. There are several abnormal forms of pulsation:

- *Tapping apex beat*—a sudden but brief cardiac impulse felt in mitral stenosis
- *Thrusting apex beat*—vigorous but non-sustained pulsation typical of 'volume overload' due to mitral or aortic regurgitation
- *Heaving apex beat*—vigorous and sustained pulsation due to 'pressure overload' as in aortic stenosis and systemic hypertension
- *Impalpable apex beat*—occurs in emphysema, pleural effusion, obesity and pericardial effusion
- *Double apex beat*—two apical pulsations with each heart beat may be felt in hypertrophic cardiomyopathy. This may be due to a palpable atrial impulse. A double apex can also be due to accentuated outward moment in late systole in ventricular aneurysm.

A parasternal heave is elicited by pressing the outstretched hand flat against the sternum or against the costal cartilages just to the left of the sternum. It occurs because of right ventricular hypertrophy. An enlarged left atrium may also cause a parasternal heave. Left atrial pulsation can be distinguished from pulsation due to right ventricular hypertrophy because it occurs before the apex beat or carotid pulsation.

Vigorous pulmonary artery pulsation may be appreciated by palpation in the second left interspace. This is usually due to pulmonary hypertension.

Thrills are palpable murmurs that are most easily appreciated with the flat or ulnar border of the hand rather than with the fingers. A thrill implies a definite abnormality. Systolic thrills in the aortic area are usually due to aortic stenosis, whereas at the apex a systolic thrill is due to mitral regurgitation. A diastolic thrill is usually caused by mitral stenosis; a diastolic thrill due to aortic regurgitation is uncommon.

Heart sounds that are very loud may also be palpated. In systemic hypertension the aortic second sound may be felt, and in pulmonary hypertension the pulmonary component of the second sound may be felt. Occasionally a third or fourth heart sound may be palpated.

Percussion

Percussion is not usually undertaken, but it may allow the approximate position and size of the heart to be determined.

Auscultation

The sounds best heard with the bell or the diaphragm of the stethoscope are shown in Table 11.5. Other heart sounds and murmurs are heard equally well with the bell or diaphragm; most listeners prefer the diaphragm.

Although it is important to auscultate over most of the precordium, there are four areas where the heart sounds and valvular murmurs are best heard:

- The *aortic area* is in the second intercostal space immediately to the right of the sternum. The aorta arches upwards and forwards from the aortic valve and the murmur of aortic stenosis is transmitted best to this area.

Table 11.5 Use of the stethoscope.

Bell (for low-frequency sounds)	Diaphragm (for high-frequency sounds)
Mid-diastolic rumbles of mitral stenosis and tricuspid stenosis	Early diastolic murmurs of aortic and pulmonary regurgitation
Third and fourth heart sounds	Second heart sound Systolic clicks and opening snaps

Table 11.6 Summary of the auscultation procedure.

The mitral, tricuspid, pulmonary and aortic areas should be auscultated in turn.

1 *Supine*
   First heart sound—mitral area
   Second heart sound—pulmonary and aortic areas, during respiration
   Third and fourth heart sounds—mitral and tricuspid areas
   Clicks, snaps, plops, knocks—mitral and tricuspid areas
   Systolic murmurs—all four auscultation areas, also the neck, axilla and back

2 *Sitting forward*
   Aortic diastolic murmur—tricuspid and mitral areas

3 *Lying on left side*
   Mitral diastolic murmur—mitral area (exactly over the apex beat)

4 *During inspiration and expiration*—see Table 11.8

5 *Exercise, squatting, Valsalva manoeuvres*
   Can be used to accentuate murmurs

- The *pulmonary area* is in the second interspace just to the left of the sternum. This is the closest point to the pulmonary valve, where the murmur of pulmonary stenosis and the pulmonary component of the second heart sound are loudest.
- The *tricuspid area* is in the fourth interspace to the left of the sternum (left sternal edge). Not only is this close to the tricuspid valve but is also over the right ventricle. Therefore, as well as the murmurs and sounds from the tricuspid valve, the murmurs of pulmonary and aortic regurgitation and third and fourth right ventricular sounds are heard well here.
- The *mitral area or apex* is the point at which the apex beat is felt. The first heart sound and mitral murmurs are loudest here, and aortic regurgitation and third and fourth left ventricular sounds are often heard best at this point.

The sequence of cardiac auscultation is summarized in Table 11.6.

Heart sounds
The first heart sound. This is caused by the closure of the mitral and tricuspid valves and is best heard at the cardiac apex. The sound is usually single but may be slightly split. If split, this 'double' sound at the beginning of systole must be distinguished from the combination of the first heart sound with a fourth heart sound or with an ejection click.

The first heart sound is loud when the patient is thin and when the circulation is hyperdynamic, e.g. due to anaemia or thyrotoxicosis. The sound is also loud if the valve is still open when ventricular systole begins, e.g. in mitral stenosis.

A soft first heart sound occurs in patients with obesity, emphysema or pericardial effusion. It is also present when the valve leaflets are immobile, e.g. in severe calcific mitral stenosis, or when the leaflets are partly closed when systole begins, which occurs when the PR interval is long. A soft first heart sound also occurs when the valve does not close properly, as in mitral regurgitation. Heart failure and cardiogenic shock are also associated with a soft first heart sound.

The intensity of the first heart sound is variable when the relationship between atrial and ventricular systole is not constant, e.g. during ventricular tachycardia or complete heart block: when the PR interval is short the sound is loud, and when the PR interval is long the sound is soft.

The second heart sound. This is caused by the closure of the aortic and pulmonary valves and is best heard with the diaphragm of the stethoscope placed over the aortic or pulmonary area. Unless excessively loud, the pulmonary component of the second sound is only heard in the pulmonary area. Left heart emptying is usually finished just before

right heart emptying; therefore the pulmonary component of the second sound closely follows the aortic component. Inspiration results in increased venous return to the right heart, which further delays right heart emptying. The pulmonary sound is therefore delayed further on inspiration and the second heart sound becomes audibly split (Fig. 11.9) Splitting of the second heart sound on inspiration is known as normal or physiological splitting and is most commonly heard in children or young adults.

Reversed splitting of the second heart sound (when the aortic component follows the pulmonary component) occurs on expiration. It is due to a fixed delay in left heart emptying caused by aortic stenosis, left bundle branch block or left ventricular failure. Thus, when right heart emptying is delayed during inspiration, the two sounds move together, and when the right heart empties more quickly during expiration, the sounds move apart.

The fixed delay in the emptying of the right ventricle produced, for example, by right bundle branch block or pulmonary stenosis will result in wide splitting of the second heart sound. With an atrial septal defect there is usually some degree of right bundle branch block, and because of shunting of blood from the left to the right atrium the right-sided cardiac output is high and ventricular emptying is further delayed. The second heart sound is therefore widely split. Because communication at atrial level prevents differential changes of the venous return during inspiration and expiration, the wide splitting of the second heart sound is not varied by respiration. This is called fixed splitting.

The aortic second sound is louder in systemic hypertension and when a hyperdynamic circulation is present. It is soft in aortic stenosis because

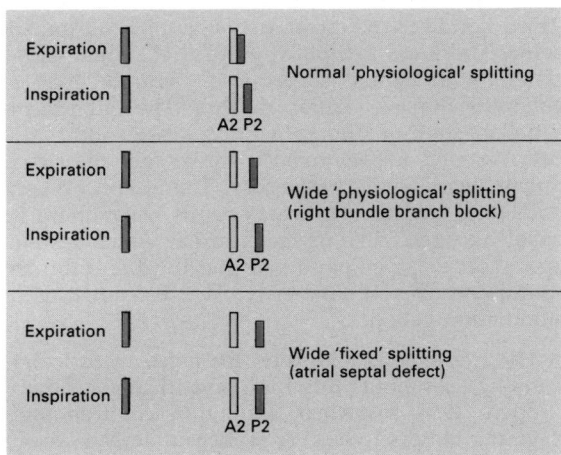

Fig. 11.9 Variations of the second heart sound. A_2 = aortic component; P_2 = pulmonary component.

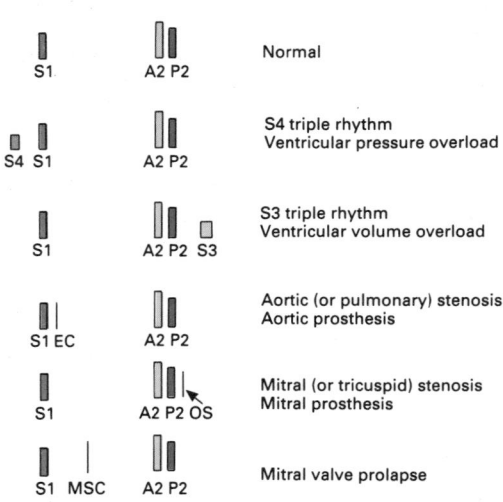

Fig. 11.10 Normal and additional heart sounds and the conditions in which they are found. S_1 = first heart sound; A_2 = aortic component of the second sound; P_2 = pulmonary component of the second sound; S_3 = third heart sound; S_4 = fourth heart sound; EC = ejection click; OS = opening snap; MSC = mid-systolic click.

the valve is relatively immobile, and it is soft in cardiac failure because of low blood flow. Similarly, the pulmonary component of the second heart sound is loud in pulmonary hypertension and soft in pulmonary stenosis.

Additional heart sounds (Fig. 11.10). Third and fourth heart sounds are low-frequency sounds best heard at, and between, the lower left sternal edge and the cardiac apex. They are diastolic in timing, representing ventricular filling, and are heard as soft 'thudding' noises immediately before the first sound (fourth sound) or after the second sound (third sound). The presence of a third or fourth sound produces a triple rhythm that, when associated with sinus tachycardia, sounds like a galloping horse—a gallop rhythm. The cadence of a gallop rhythm due to a third heart sound has been likened to 'Kentucky', whilst that due to a fourth heart sound resembles 'Tennessee'. When both third and fourth heart sounds occur there is usually a marked sinus tachycardia, which results in a short diastolic period so that third and fourth sounds occur simultaneously. This is known as a summation gallop.

- The *third sound* is due to rapid ventricular filling as soon as the miral and tricuspid valves open. It is a normal finding in children and young adults when it is heard at the apex, especially in the left lateral position. In those over 40 years it represents heart failure or volume overload, e.g. due to mitral regurgita-

tion. It is therefore sometimes referred to as a sound of 'distress'. A right ventricular third sound is heard best at the left sternal edge, and a left ventricular third sound is heard at the apex.

- The *fourth sound* is caused by the surge of ventricular filling that accompanies atrial systole. It therefore occurs in late diastole. It may be a normal finding in an elderly subject, but in younger patients it usually indicates increased ventricular stiffness associated with hypertension, aortic stenosis or acute myocardial infarction. It is called the sound of cardiac 'stress', and can sometimes be felt.

- Abnormal heart valves may cause an audible signal when opening. An *ejection click* is a high-frequency sound, best heard with the diaphragm of the stethoscope at the left sternal edge, and occurs immediately following the first heart sound. It is produced by the sudden opening of a deformed but mobile aortic or pulmonary valve. It is most commonly heard in association with a bicuspid aortic valve when it is easily heard throughout the respiratory cycle. A stenotic pulmonary valve also produces an ejection click, but this is best heard on expiration. A dilated aorta or pulmonary artery may also give rise to an ejection click.

- A *stenotic mitral or tricuspid valve* may produce a high-frequency opening snap that occurs just after the second heart sound. It is best heard with the diaphragm of the stethoscope at the left sternal edge or between the left sternal edge and the apex. It can be distinguished from a split second sound or a third sound by the site at which it is best heard, its higher frequency and its lack of respiratory variation.

- A *mid-systolic click (or clicks)* is due to sudden prolapse of the mtiral valve into the left atrium during ventricular systole. It occurs when the mitral valve is congenitally deformed or has undergone myxomatous degeneration, as in the mitral valve prolapse syndrome. These auscultatory features are inconsistent and wax and wane with time.

- *Tumour plops* are low-frequency sounds produced by the sudden checking of the travel of an atrial tumour when it reaches the valve. Such sounds occur after an opening snap, but before a third sound would be expected. The pericardial knock is another sound that occurs in this position in the cardiac cycle. Like a third heart sound, it is low frequency. It is heard in constrictive pericarditis and is due to rather early, sudden and marked halting of ventricular filling due to constriction.

Prosthetic sounds
Mechanical replacement heart valves produce loud clicks due to the opening and closing of the valve.

These prosthetic sounds may be muffled or absent if valve movement is impeded by thrombus or vegetations.

Heart murmurs

Turbulent blood flow causes heart murmurs. Turbulence may be produced when there is high blood flow through a normal valve, or when there is normal blood flow through an abnormal valve or into a dilated chamber. Turbulence is also caused by the regurgitation of blood through a leaking valve. Murmurs produced by high-velocity blood flow (e.g. the systolic murmur of mitral regurgitation) are high frequency and are often described as 'blowing' in quality. The intensity of murmurs is determined not only by the blood velocity but also by the volume of blood producing the murmur and the distance of the source of the murmur from the stethoscope. Right-sided murmurs tend to become louder on inspiration because inspiration increases the venous return to the right heart.

Heart murmurs may occur with a normal or near-normal heart (innocent murmurs). They are usually soft and short, and occur early in systole. Murmurs also occur in the following situations:

- Anaemia, thyrotoxicosis, pregnancy and other causes of a high cardiac output produce flow murmurs, which are usually brief systolic ejection murmurs heard best at the left sternal edge or in the pulmonary area. These murmurs are believed to emanate from the pulmonary or aortic valve. Similar murmurs are heard in association with skeletal abnormalities such as kyphoscoliosis or funnel chest.
- A very small ventricular septal defect may produce a short early systolic murmur, heard well at the left sternal edge. The murmur is short because contraction of the ventricle closes the small defect early in systole.

Table 11.7 The grading of murmur intensity.

Grade	Systolic murmurs	Diastolic murmurs
1	Very soft (heard only in good circumstances)	Very soft (heard only in good circumstances)
2	Soft	Soft
3	Moderate	Moderate
4	Loud	Loud or associated with palpable thrill
5	Very loud	—
6	Very loud (no stethoscope needed) or associated with palpable thrill	—

Table 11.8 Some common structural causes of murmurs.

Murmur	Position where murmur is best heard
SYSTOLIC	
Ejection (mid-) systolic	
Aortic stenosis	Aortic area and clavicles
Pulmonary stenosis ⎫ Atrial septal defect ⎭	Left sternal edge on inspiration
Left (e.g. hypertrophic cardiomyopathy— HOCM) and right (e.g. Fallot's tetralogy) outflow tract obstruction may also cause mid-systolic murmurs	
Pan-systolic	
Mitral regurgitation (blowing)	Apex to axilla
Tricuspid regurgitation (low-pitched)	Left sternal edge
Ventricular septal defect (loud and rough)	Left sternal edge
Late systolic	
Dynamic outflow tract obstruction (HOCM)	Accentuated on standing
Mitral valve prolapse	Apex
Coarctation of the aorta	Left sternal edge
DIASTOLIC	
Mid-diastolic	
Mitral stenosis (low-frequency rumbling)	Apex, patient on left side, accentuated on exertion
Tricuspid stenosis	Left sternal edge, accentuated on inspiration
Austin Flint murmur	Apex
Early diastolic	
Aortic regurgitation (blowing, high-pitched)	Left sternal edge and apex, patient sitting forward and in expiration
Pulmonary regurgitation (blowing, variable pitch)	Right of sternum, louder on inspiration
Graham Steell in pulmonary hypertension (due to mitral stenosis)	Left sternal edge

● A buzzing, twanging or vibratory murmur, called Still's murmur, may be heard at the lower left sternal edge or cardiac apex. It is thought to arise from the region below the aortic valve.

Murmurs are classified as systolic, diastolic or continuous. Another functional classification divides systolic murmurs into ejection or regurgitant. Murmurs should be assessed carefully; a summary of the auscultation procedure is shown in Table 11.6. The intensity of cardiac murmurs can be graded as indicated in Table 11.7.

Systolic murmurs (see Table 11.8). Systolic murmurs occur synchronously with carotid pulsation. There are three main varieties of pathological systolic murmur:

● *Ejection mid-systolic murmurs* are heard separately from the first and second heart sounds. Their intensity rises then falls, being greatest in mid-systole.
● *Pan-systolic murmurs* extend from the first to the second heart sound and tend to be of constant intensity throughout the whole of systole.
● *Late systolic murmurs* are separated from the first sound but extend up to the second sound.

Diastolic murmurs (see Table 11.8). Diastolic murmurs are always associated with cardiac disease. They are of two types:

● *Mid-diastolic murmurs* usually arise from the mitral and tricuspid valves. In aortic regurgitation the flow of blood back into the left ventricle may partially close and obstruct the mitral valve, producing a mitral mid-diastolic murmur

(Austin Flint murmur).
● *Early diastolic murmurs* usually result from aortic regurgitation and rarely from pulmonary regurgitation. These murmurs begin with the second heart sound and are blowing (high-pitched) in quality. Pulmonary hypertension secondary to mitral stenosis may lead to pulmonary valve regurgitation (Graham Steell murmur).

Continuous murmurs. A continuous murmur may occur because of a combination of systolic and diastolic murmurs, due to connections between the aorta and pulmonary artery (e.g. patent ductus arteriosus) or due to arteriovenous anastamoses and collateral circulations such as those associated with coarctation of the aorta. High venous flow, especially in young children, can produce a continuous venous hum in the neck. This is reduced by occluding the vein or by lying the child flat. Similarly, high mammary blood flow in pregnant or lactating women can produce a continuous murmur known as a mammary souffle.

Extra cardiac sounds
Bruits, usually due to arterial stenoses, are murmurs arising from a peripheral artery, including the distal aorta.

A pericardial friction rub is a scratching or crunching noise produced by the movement of inflamed pericardium. Since it is relatively high frequency, it is best heard with the diaphragm. It is most obvious in systole but may also be heard in early diastole or synchronously with atrial contraction. It should be listened for during both held inspiration and expiration.

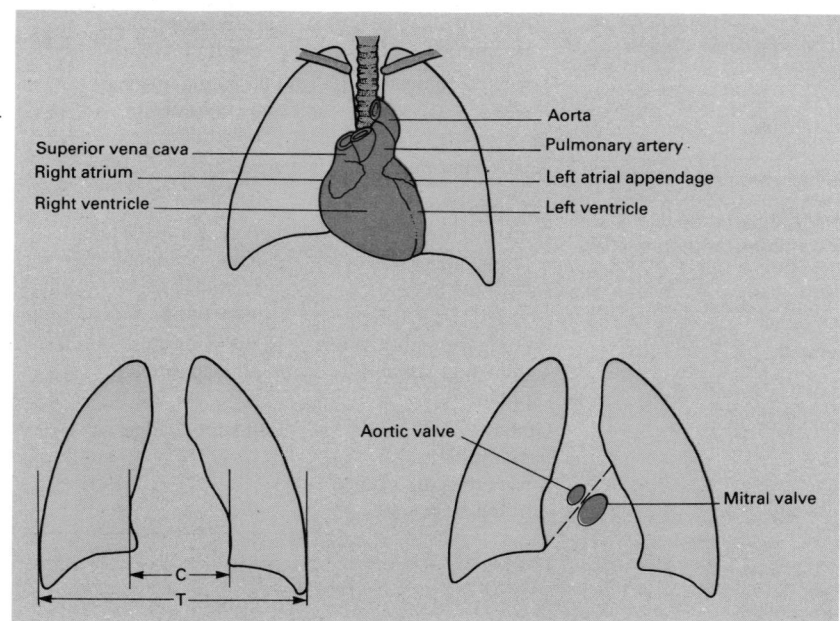

Fig. 11.11 Diagrams to show the heart silhouette on the chest X-ray, measurements of the cardiothoracic ratio (CTR) and the location of the cardiac valves. CTR = (C/T) × 100%; normal CTR < 50%.

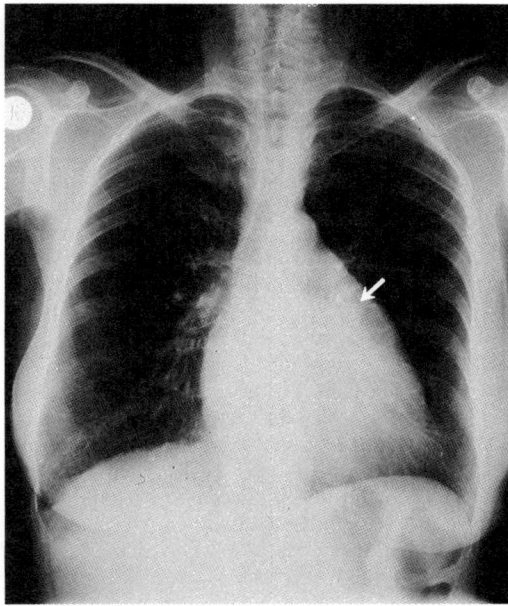

Fig. 11.12 X-ray of mitral stenosis showing left atrial dilatation (arrow).

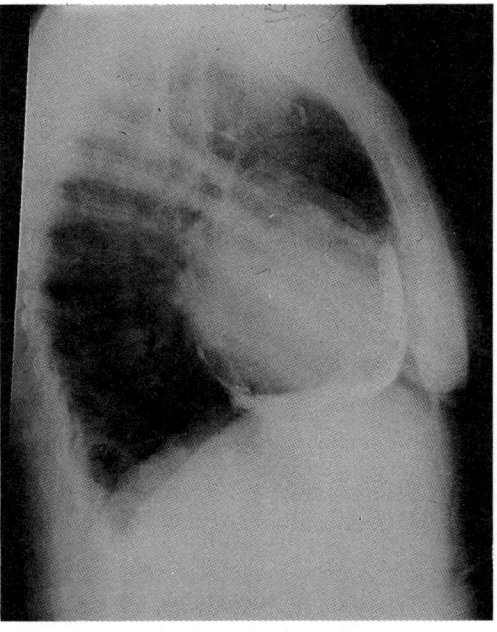

Fig. 11.13 X-ray showing heavy calcification of the pericardium.

Cardiac investigations

Chest X-ray

This is an essential investigation. It is taken in the postero-anterior (PA) direction with the heart close to the X-ray film to minimize magnification with respect to the thorax. A left lateral and a penetrated PA film are also taken in patients with abnormal plain PA films. The cardiac structures and great vessels that can be seen on these X-rays are indicated in Fig. 11.11.

Heart size
Heart size can be assessed from the PA chest film; the maximum transverse diameter of the heart is compared with the maximum transverse diameter of the chest (see Fig. 11.11).

The cardiothoracic ratio (CTR) is usually less than 50%, except in neonates, infants, athletes and patients with skeletal abnormalities such as scoliosis and funnel chest. A transverse cardiac diameter of more than 15.5 cm is abnormal. Pericardial effusion or cardiac dilatation causes an increase in the ratio.

A pericardial effusion produces a globular, sharp-edged shadow. This enlargement may occur quite suddenly and, unlike heart failure, there is no associated change in the pulmonary vasculature. The echocardiogram is more specific than the chest X-ray for the diagnosis of pericardial effusion, particularly because at least 250 ml of fluid must accumulate before X-ray changes are apparent.

Certain patterns of specific chamber enlargement may be seen on the chest X-ray:

- *Left atrial dilatation* results in prominence of the left atrial appendage on the left heart border, a double atrial shadow to the right of the sternum, and splaying of the carina because a large left atrium elevates the left main bronchus (Fig. 11.12). On a lateral chest X-ray an enlarged left atrium bulges backwards, indenting the barium-filled oesophagus.
- *Left ventricular enlargement* results in an increase in the CTR and a smooth elongation and increased convexity of the left heart border. A left ventricular aneurysm may produce a distinct bulge or distortion of the left heart border.
- *Right atrial enlargement* results in the right border of the heart projecting into the right lower lung field.
- *Right ventricular enlargement* results in an increase of the CTR and an upward displacement of the apex of the heart because the enlarging right ventricle pushes the left ventricle leftwards, upwards and eventually backwards. Differentiation of left from right ventricular enlargement may be difficult from the shape of the left heart border alone, but the lateral view shows enlargement anteriorly for the right ventricle and posteriorly for the left ventricle.

- *Ascending aortic dilatation* is seen as a prominence of the aortic shadow to the right of the mediastinum.
- *Enlargement of the pulmonary artery* in pulmonary hypertension and left-to-right shunts produces a prominent bulge on the left hand border of the mediastinum below the aortic knuckle.

Calcification

Calcification in the cardiovascular system occurs because of tissue degeneration. Calcification is visible on a lateral or a penetrated PA film, but is best studied by fluoroscopy. Various types of calcification can occur:

- *Pericardial calcification* (Fig. 11.13) may be seen as plaque-like opacities over the surface of the heart, but particularly concentrated in the AV groove. Such calcification often results from tuberculous pericarditis and may be associated with pericardial constriction.
- *Valvular calcification* may result from long-standing rheumatic or congenital heart disease. The aortic and mitral valves are most commonly affected. On the lateral film, a calcified aortic valve is seen on or above a line joining the carina to the sternophrenic angle. Mitral valvular calcification is seen below and behind this line.
- *Myocardial calcification* may occur in association with a left ventricular aneurysm.
- *Calcification of the aorta* is a common, normal finding in patients over the age of 40 years and appears as a curvilinear opacity around the circumference of the aortic knuckle. Calcification in the ascending aorta usually denotes syphilitic aortitis, whereas in the descending aorta it is due to atheroma or, in the younger patient, to non-specific aortitis.
- *Coronary arterial calcification*, especially of the proximal left coronary artery, is associated with coronary atheroma but does not necessarily correspond to the site of maximal stenosis.

Lung fields

Pulmonary plethora results from left-to-right shunts, e.g. atrial or ventricular septal defects. It is seen as a general increase in the vascularity of the lung fields and as an increase in the right lower lobe artery, which normally should not exceed 16 mm in diameter.

Pulmonary oligaemia is a paucity of vascular markings and a reduction in the width of the arteries. It occurs in situations where there is reduced pulmonary blood flow, such as pulmonary embolism, severe pulmonary stenosis and Fallot's tetralogy.

Pulmonary arterial hypertension may result from pulmonary embolism, chronic lung disease or chronic heart disease such as ventricular septal defect or mitral valve stenosis. In addition to X-ray features of these conditions, the pulmonary arteries are prominent close to the hili but are very reduced in size (pruned) in the peripheral lung fields. This pattern is usually symmetrical.

Pulmonary venous hypertension occurs in left ventricular failure or mitral valve disease. Normal pulmonary venous pressure is 5–14 mm Hg at rest. Mild pulmonary venous hypertension (15–20 mm Hg) produces isolated dilatation of the upper lobe pulmonary veins. Interstitial oedema occurs when the pressure is between 21 and 30 mm Hg. This manifests as fluid collections in the interlobar fissures, interlobular septa (Kerley B lines) and pleural spaces. Alveolar oedema occurs when the pressure exceeds 30 mm Hg, appearing as areas of central consolidation, indistinctness of the hilar regions, haziness and mottling of the lung fields

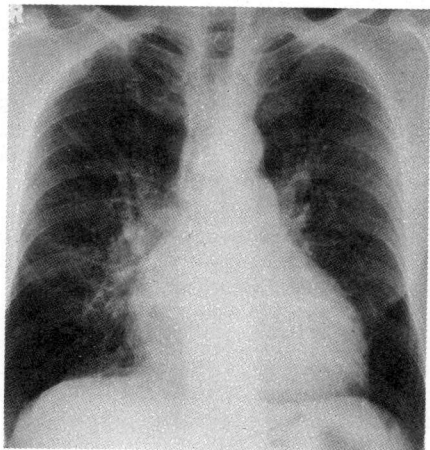 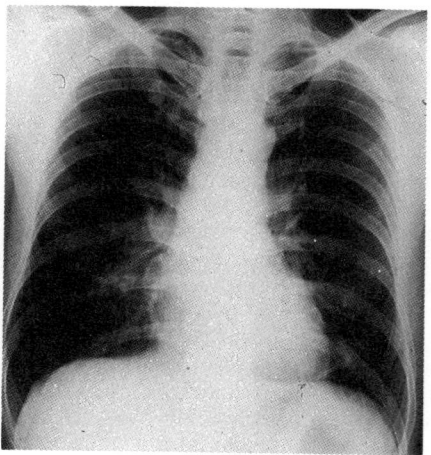

Fig. 11.14 X-rays showing pulmonary oedema before treatment (left) and after treatment (right).

(Fig. 11.14) and pleural effusions. Patients with long-standing elevation of the pulmonary venous pressure have reactive thickening of the pulmonary arteriolar intima, which protects the alveoli from pulmonary oedema. Thus, in these patients the pulmonary venous pressure may increase to well above 30 mm Hg before frank pulmonary oedema develops.

Fluoroscopy

Fluoroscopy has been largely superseded by echo-cardiography. It is essential for the insertion of cardiac catheters and pacemaker electrodes.

Electrocardiography

The electrocardiogram (ECG) is a recording of the electrical activity of the heart. It is the vector sum of the depolarization and repolarization potentials of all myocardial cells (see Fig. 11.33). At the body surface these generate potential differences of about 1 mV and the fluctuations of these potentials create the familiar P–QRS–T pattern. At rest the intracellular voltage of the myocardium is polarized at −90 mV compared with that of the extracellular space. This diastolic voltage difference occurs because of the high intracellular potassium concentration, which is maintained by the sodium-potassium pump despite the free membrane permeability to potassium. Depolarization of cardiac cells occurs when there is a sudden increase in the permeability of the membrane to sodium. Sodium rushes into the cell and the negative resting voltage is lost (Stage 0; see Fig. 11.33). The depolarization of a myocardial cell causes the depolarization of adjacent cells and, in the healthy heart, the entire myocardium is depolarized in a coordinated fashion. During repolarization, cellular electrolyte balance is slowly restored (Stages 1, 2 and 3). Slow diastolic depolarization (stage 4) follows until the threshold potential is reached. Another action potential then follows (see Fig. 11.33).

The ECG is recorded from two or more simultaneous points of skin contact (electrodes). When cardiac activation proceeds towards the positive contact, an upward deflection is produced on the ECG. Correct representation of a three-dimensional spatial vector requires recordings from three mutually perpendicular (orthogonal) axes. The shape of the human torso does not make this easy, so the practical ECG records 12 projections of the vector, called 'Leads' (Fig. 11.15). Six of these are obtained by recording voltages from the limbs (I, II, III, AVR, AVL and AVF). The other six leads record potentials between points on the chest surface and an average of the three limbs: RA, LA and LL. These are designated V_1–V_6 and aim to select activity from the right ventricle (V_1–V_2), interventricular septum (V_3–V_4) and left ventricle (V_5–V_6). Note that leads AVR and V_1 are oriented towards the cavity of the heart, leads II, III and AVF face the inferior surface and leads I, AVL and V6 face the lateral wall of the left ventricle.

The ECG potentials are picked up by electrodes attached to the patient. Limb electrodes are usually plates of nickel-silver attached by rubber straps. Contact is aided by a proprietary cream or jelly (*not* alcohol wipes or K-Y jelly!), or the electrode has a cloth cover soaked in saline. The chest electrodes are attached by suction. Disposable, self-adhesive electrodes are more convenient and hygienic, but do not always achieve such good electrical contact.

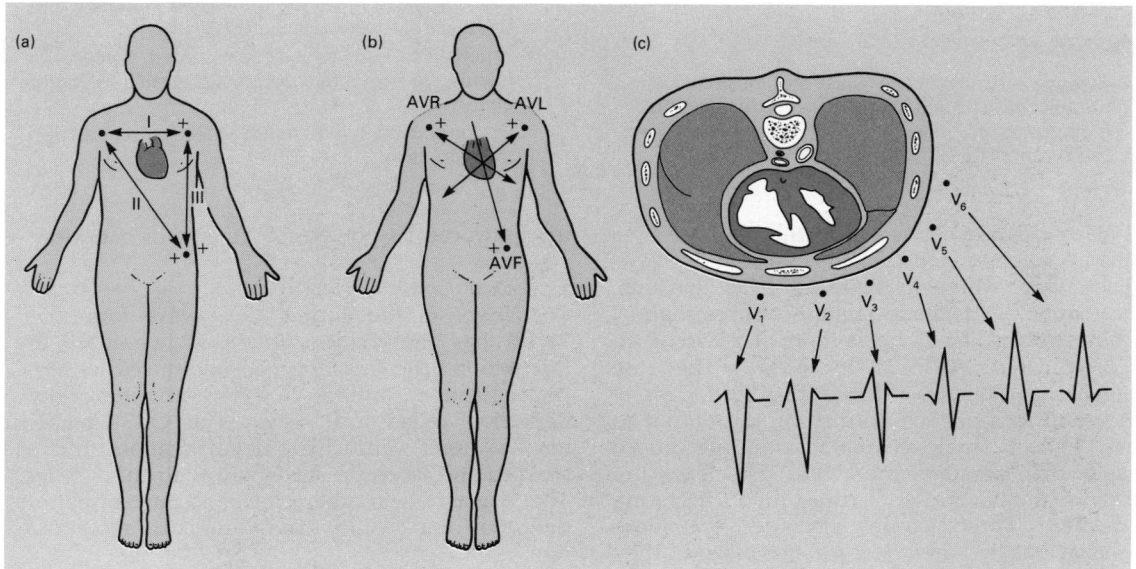

Fig. 11.15 The connections or directions that comprise the 12-lead electrocardiogram. (a) The bipolar leads. (b) The unipolar leads. (c) The chest leads.

HOW TO DO AN ECG

The Machine

- Buttons or a rotary switch for selecting which lead(s) to record.
- Control for paper speed: 25 mm/s (England and N. America) or 50 mm/s (parts of Europe).
- Amplification control. The universal convention is to represent 1 mV as 10 mm on the paper, but sometimes 5 mm/mV (half-standard) is required if large ECG voltages are encountered.
- A means of recording a 1 mV square-wave calibration pulse (sometimes done automatically when the paper drive is started).
- A filter switch. Sometimes interference (see below) is so great as to render the ECG unreadable. Electronic filters can be used to reduce interference, but they do this by limiting the machine's frequency response and this affects the ECG, sometimes masking important diagnostic features. Interference can almost always be controlled by careful technique and use of the electronic filter should be regarded as a last resort, *not* normal practice.
- 'Reset' button to centre the baseline should a large transient wave send the trace off scale.
- Standard ECG paper is illustrated in Fig. 11.16. There are bold lines drawn every 0.2 s and fine lines occur at 40 ms intervals. The usual voltage calibration is 1 mV/cm. The normal 12-lead ECG is shown in Fig. 11.17.
- The ECG voltage is very small and it has to be detected in the presence of other, often larger, signals, e.g. somatic (muscle) tremor, AC interference (due to proximity to main wiring—shows regular 50 Hz waves on baseline) or baseline wander due to respiration or poor electrode contact.

The patient

- Remove clothing above waist and position comfortably on a couch. Explain procedure carefully (patients often think they are about to receive some form of electrical therapy!)

- Turn on machine and apply electrodes to limbs over fleshy areas to ensure good contact. Connect wires.

Lead I	Right arm (−ve) to Left arm (+ve)
Lead II	Right arm (−ve) to Left leg (+ve)
Lead III	Left arm (−ve) to Left leg (+ve)
Lead AVR	Right arm (+ve) to (Left arm & Left leg) (−ve)
Lead AVL	Left leg (+ve) to (Right arm & Left leg) (−ve)
Lead AVF	Left leg (+ve) to (Right arm & Left arm (−ve)

- Identify the sites for the chest electrodes. These are shown in Fig. 11.15 and must be located precisely.

V1	4th intercostal space, just to right of sternal edge
V2	4th intercostal space, just to left of sternal edge
V3	Halfway on a line joining V2 and V4
V4	5th intercostal space, on mid-clavicular line
V5	On same horizontal level as V4, at anterior axillary line
V6	On same horizontal level as V4 and V5, at mid-axillary line

- If a three-channel machine is used, all six chest electrodes are connected. For a single-channel machine, the electrode is positioned at V_1.
- The *recording* commences. In some machines, it is possible to view the pen deflectors without activating the paper drive, in others, the whole recording procedure is automatic. If there is excessive interference, or large voltages are encountered, necessitating use of lower amplification, the recordings may have to be aborted or repeated. Most three-channel machines calibrate with a 1 mV pulse and identify the leads automatically. With single-channel recorders, you will probably have to do the calibration manually and write on the paper to identify leads.
- When all 12 leads have been recorded, inspect the tracings to see if they are of acceptable technical quality.
- Disconnect the wires, remove electrodes and wipe the skin clean.

The electrodes are connected to the machine by a multiwire colour-coded cable.

There are two main types of ECG machine: three-channel and single channel. Three-channel machines record the 12 leads three at a time: I, II, III: AVR, AVL, AVF: V_1–V_3: V_4–V_6. They are usually semiautomatic and record a set length of each group in sequence, formatting the output to fit an A4 sheet. Single-channel machines record on a paper strip about 50 mm wide. The leads are selected manually and each is recorded for as long as desired. Three-channel machines are more expensive but are preferred for hospitals as they are quicker to use and the recordings do not have to be cut up and mounted afterwards. ECG machines can be powered by mains or batteries.

ECG wave form

The shape of the normal ECG wave form (Fig. 11.16) has important similarities, whatever the orientation. The first deflection is caused by atrial depolarization, and it is a low-amplitude slow deflection called a P wave. The QRS complex results from ventricular depolarization and is sharper and larger in amplitude than the P wave. The T wave is another slow and low-amplitude deflection that results from ventricular repolarization.

The atrial repolarization wave is not seen in a conventional ECG because it is low in voltage and

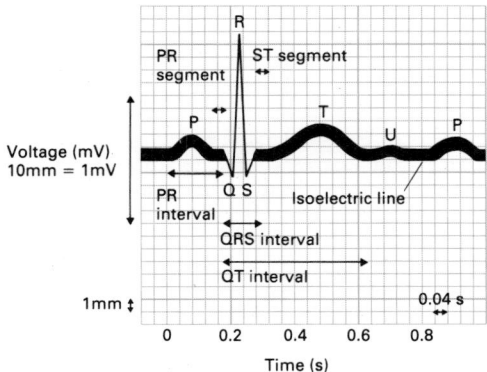

Fig. 11.16 The waves and elaboration of the normal electrocardiogram. (From Goldman MJ (1976) *Principles of Clinical Electrocardiography*, 9th edn. Loas Altos: Lange).

is hidden by the QRS complex.

The *PR interval* is the length of time from the start of the P wave to the start of the QRS complex. It is the time taken for activation to pass from the sinus node, through the atrium, AV node and the His–Purkinje system to the ventricle.

The *QT interval* extends from the start of the QRS complex to the end of the T wave. This interval represents the time taken to depolarize and repolarize the ventricular myocardium.

The *ST segment* is the period between the end of the QRS complex and the start of the T wave. In the normal heart, all cells are depolarized by this phase of the ECG.

The normal values for the electrocardiographic intervals are indicated in Table 11.9. Leads that face the lateral wall of the left ventricle have predominantly positive deflections, and leads looking into the ventricular cavity are usually negative. Detailed patterns depend on the size, shape and rhythm of the heart and the characteristics of the torso.

Cardiac vectors (Fig. 11.18)
At any point in time during depolarization and repolarization, electrical potentials are being propagated in different directions. Most of these cancel each other out and only the net force is recorded. This net force in the frontal plane is known as the cardiac vector.

The mean QRS vector can be calculated from the six standard leads (Fig. 11.18); it normally lies between $-30°$ and $+90°$. Left axis deviation lies between $-30°$ and $-90°$ and right axis deviation between $+90°$ and $+150°$. Calculation of this vector is occasionally useful in the diagnosis of cardiac disorders.

Exercise electrocardiography
This is a technique used to assess the cardiac response to exercise. The ECG is recorded whilst

Table 11.9 Normal ECG intervals.

P wave duration	$\leqslant 0.12$ s
PR interval	$0.12–0.22$ s
QRS complex duration	$\leqslant 0.10$ s
Corrected QT (QT_c)	$\leqslant 0.44$ s

$$QT_c = \frac{QT}{\sqrt{RR\ interval}}$$

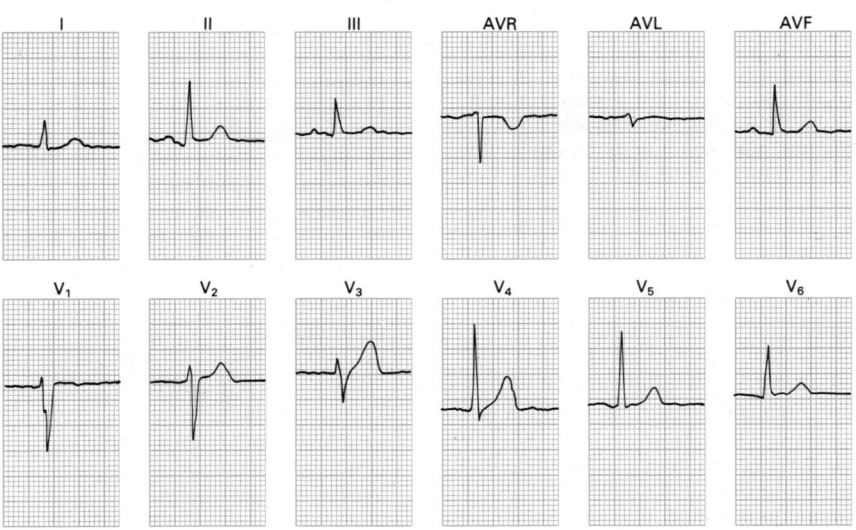

Fig. 11.17 A normal 12-lead electrocardiogram.

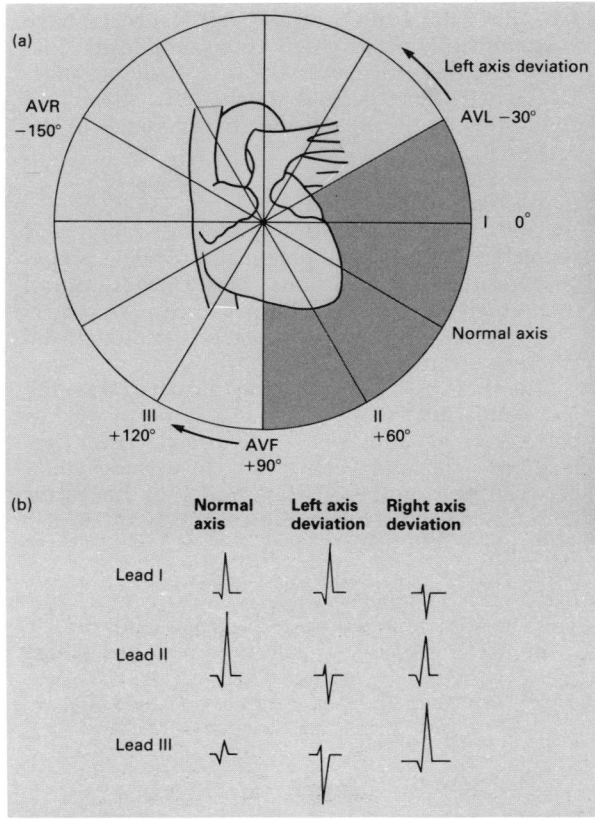

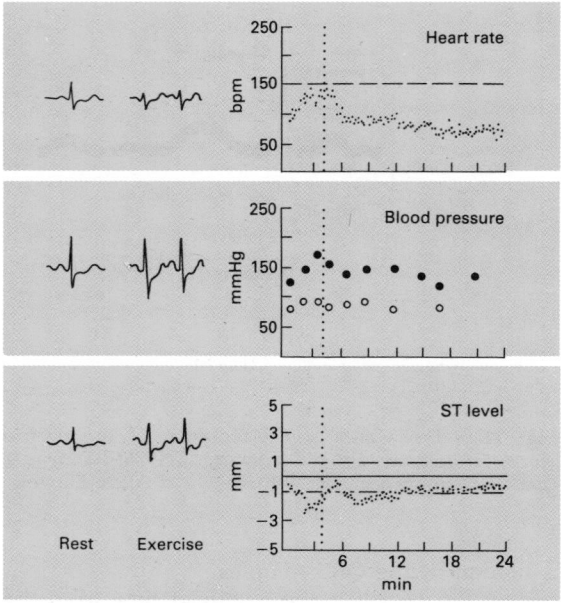

Fig. 11.19 Electrocardiographic, heart rate and blood pressure changes on exercise, showing characteristic down-sloping ST segment depression in response to 4 min of exercise in a patient with myocardial ischaemia. The end of the exercise period is indicated by the dotted line.

exercise test the exercise tolerance, blood pressure and rhythm responses to exercise are also assessed. Exercise causes an increase in heart rate and blood pressure. A sustained fall in blood pressure indicates severe coronary artery disease.

Table 11.10 Indications and contraindications for exercise electrocardiography.

Indications

Diagnosis of chest pain
Provocation of ischaemia
Evaluation of treatment of angina
Provocation of arrhythmia
Evaluation of treatment of arrhythmia
Risk assessment after myocardial infarction
Functional assessment in a patient with heart disease

Contraindications

Recent myocardial infarction (within 1 week); a limited test recommended within 1 month
Unstable angina
Uncompensated heart failure
Severe aortic stenosis
Malignant hypertension

N.B.: Provided that adequate precautions are observed (doctor and resuscitation facilities available, continuous monitoring), the mortality from exercise testing is less than 0.01%. Myocardial infarction occurs in less than 0.05%.

Fig. 11.18 (a) The hexaxial reference system illustrating the six leads in the frontal plane, e.g. lead I is 0°, lead II is +60°, lead III is +120°. (b) Calculating the direction of the cardiac vector. In the first column the QRS complex with zero magnitude (i.e. when the positive and negative deflections are equal) is seen in lead III. The mean QRS vector is therefore perpendicular to lead III and is either −150° or +30°. Lead I is positive, so the axis must be + 30°, which is normal. In left axis deviation (second column) the main deflection is positive (R wave) in lead I and negative (S wave) in lead III. In right axis deviation (third column) the main deflection is negative (S wave) in lead I and positive (R wave) in lead III.

climbing stairs, riding a bicycle ergometer, or walking or running on a treadmill. Recording the ECG after the exercise is not an adequate form of stress test. Normally there is little change in the T wave or ST segment.

Myocardial ischaemia provoked by exertion results in ST segment depression (> 1 mm) in leads facing the affected area. Although most abnormalities are detected in leads V₅ (anterior and lateral ischaemia) or AVF (inferior ischaemia), it is best to record a full 12-lead ECG. The form of ST segment depression provoked by ischaemia is characteristic: it is either planar or shows down-sloping depression (see Fig. 11.19). Up-sloping depression is a non-specific finding. During an

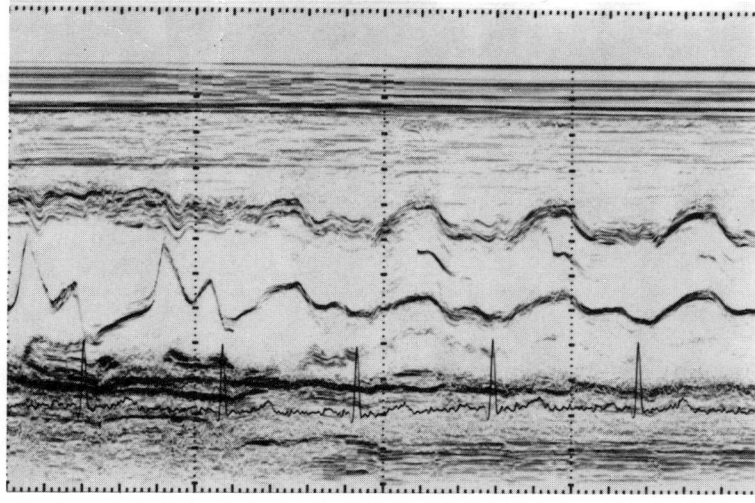

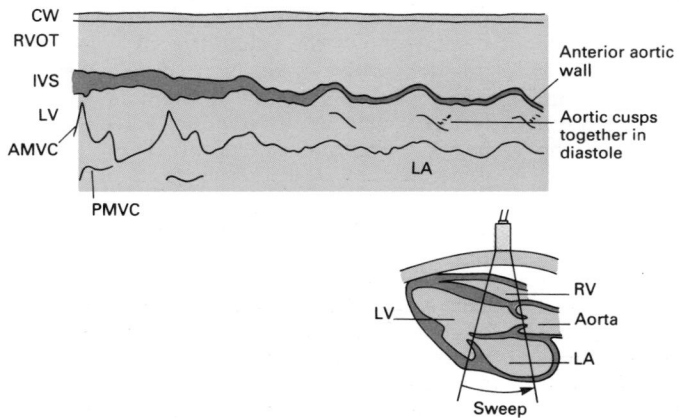

Fig. 11.20 An M-mode echocardiogram. This is a 'sweep' from the left ventricle to the aorta as shown on the inset. CW = chest wall; RVOT = right ventricular outflow tract; IVS = interventricular septum; LV = left ventricle; LA = left atrium; AMVC = anterior mitral valve cusp; PMVC = posterior mitral valve cusp; RV = right ventricle. Note the pattern of movement of the AMVC. At the onset of diastole there is a rapid anterior movement followed by a slower backward movement. It moves sharply anteriorly at the end of diastole owing to atrial contraction. The PMVC moves in the opposite direction to the AMVC.

The usual indications and contraindications for the test are shown in Table 11.10.

Twenty-four hour ambulatory taped electrocardiography This is a technique for recording transient changes such as brief paroxysm of tachycardia, an occasional pause in the rhythm, or intermittent ST segment shifts. A conventional 12-lead ECG is recorded in less than a minute and usually samples approximately 30–50 complexes. In a 24-hour period over 100 000 complexes are recorded. Such a large amount of data must be analysed by automatic or semi-automatic methods. This technique is called 'Holter' electrocardiography after its inventor.

Event recording is another technique that may be used to record rare arrhythmias. The patient is provided with a pocket-sized device that can record and store a short segment of the ECG. The device may be kept for several days or weeks until the arrhythmia is recorded. Most units of this kind will also allow transtelephonic ECG transmission

so that the physician can determine the need for treatment or the continued need for monitoring.

Phonocardiography

The application of a sensitive microphone to the chest wall allows heart sounds and murmurs to be recorded. Usually cardiac, carotid or jugular pulsations are recorded at the same time. The technique is difficult and, except for research purposes, has been largely superseded by echocardiography and other non-invasive techniques.

Echocardiography

Echocardiography uses echoes of ultrasound waves to map the heart and study its function. To provide detailed images, ultrasound wavelengths of 1 mm or less are used, which correspond to frequencies of 2 MHz (1 MHz = 1 000 000 cycles per second) or more. At such high frequencies, the ultrasound waves behave more like light and can be focused into a 'beam' and aimed at a particular region of the heart. The waves are generated in very short bursts or pulses a few microseconds long by a crystal transducer, which also detects returning echoes and converts them into electrical signals.

When the crystal transducer is placed on the body surface, the ultrasound pulses emitted encounter interfaces between various body tissues as they pass through the body. In crossing each interface, some of the wave energy is reflected, and if the beam path is approximately at right angles to the plane of the interface, the reflected waves return to the transducer as an echo. Since the velocity of sound in body tissues is almost constant ($1550 \ \text{m·s}^{-1}$), the time delay for the echo to return measures the distance of the reflecting interface. Thus, if a single ultrasound pulse is transmitted, a series of echoes return, the first from the closest interface, and so on, until the distance becomes too great for further echoes to be detected.

To document in detail the motion patterns of individual structures, a technique called M-mode is used. The echo signals from a particular beam direction are recorded as a column of dots on a roll of photosensitive paper which is pulled past the cathode-ray tube display at constant speed. Stationary structures thus generate straight lines, the distances of which from the top of the paper indicate their depths, and movements, such as those of heart valves, are indicated by zig-zag lines (Fig. 11.20).

Calibration markers indicate depth at 1 cm intervals and lines along the edges of the paper show time intervals of 0.04 s. It is customary to add an ECG trace as an aid to identifying the phases of the heart cycle.

Alternatively a series of views from different positions can be obtained in the form of a two dimensional image (cross-sectional 2D echocardiography). This method is useful for delineating anatomical structures.

Doppler echocardiography

Echocardiography imaging utilizes echoes from tissue interfaces. Using high amplification, it is also possible to detect weak echoes scattered by small targets, including those from red blood cells. If the blood is moving relative to the direction of the ultrasound beam, the frequency of the returning echoes will be changed according to the Doppler phenomenon. The Doppler shift frequency is directly proportional to the blood velocity.

Blood velocity data can be acquired and displayed in several ways. Continuous wave (CW) Doppler collects all the velocity data from the path of the beam and analyses it to generate a spectral display. The outline of the envelope of the spectral display shows the value of peak velocity throughout the cardiac cycle. Normal velocities are of the order of $1 \ \text{m·s}^{-1}$, but if there is an obstructive lesion, such as a stenotic valve, velocities of $5 \ \text{m·s}^{-1}$ or more can occur. These velocities are generated by the pressure gradient that exists across the lesion. According to the Bernoulli equation:

$$\text{Pressure gradient} = 4 \times (\text{velocity})^2.$$

This equation has been validated in a wide variety of clinical situations, including valve stenoses, and ventricular septal defects, and makes it unnecessary to resort to invasive methods to measure intracardiac pressure gradients in many cases.

CW Doppler does not provide any depth information. Pulsed-wave (PW) Doppler extracts

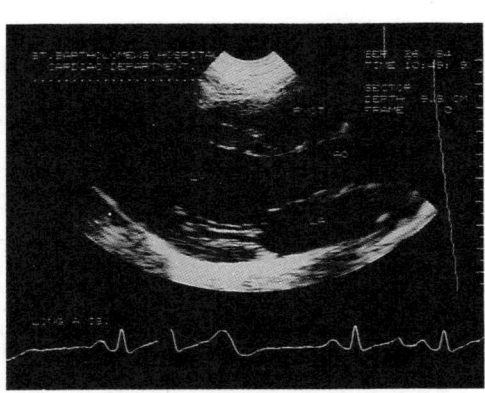
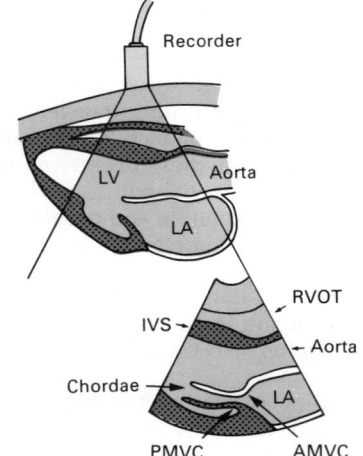

Fig. 11.21 Normal two-dimensional echocardiogram in the parasternal 'long axis'. The diagram shows the anatomy of the area scanned and a diagrammatic representation of the echocardiogram. LV = left ventricle; LA = left atrium; RVOT = right ventricular outflow tract; IVS = interventricular septum; PMVC = posterior mitral valve cusp; AMVC = anterior mitral valve cusp.

velocity data from the pulse echoes used to form a two-dimensional image and gives useful qualitative information. It can be thought of as a small intracardiac 'stethoscope' the location of which can be determined precisely. Doppler colour flow imaging uses one colour for blood flowing towards the transducer and another colour for blood flowing away. This technique allows the direction, velocity and timing of the flow to be measured with a simultaneous view of cardiac structure and function.

The echocardiographic examination

Echocardiography is a 'non-invasive' procedure that causes the patient no discomfort and is harmless. Studies are performed by a physician or technician and a comprehensive examination takes 15–30 min.

The major problem of echocardiography is that access to the heart is restricted by the lungs and rib cage, both of which form impenetrable barriers to ultrasound in the adult subject. Small 'windows' can usually be found in the third and fourth left intercostal spaces (termed left parasternal); just below the xiphoid process of the sternum (subcostal); and, with the subject turned to the left and exhaling, from the point where the apical beat is palpated (apical). By positioning the transducer successively over these sites and angling and rotating it to align the scan plane, a series of standard sectional views is obtained. In children, and some adults, the aortic arch can be visualized from a suprasternal position.

The standard nomenclature for two-dimensional echocardiographic images is shown in Fig. 11.21. The left parasternal position gives access to the long-axis and short-axis planes. The apical approach gives a second view of the long-axis plane, but with the apex in the foreground, and also shows the four-chamber plane. Note that the convention of showing the transducer position at the top of the image results in these views being 'upside-down'.

M-mode recordings are obtained from the parasternal position to document motion patterns of the aorta, aortic valve and left atrium, the mitral valve, and the left and right ventricles (Fig. 11.20).

The 1 cm calibration markers on M-mode recordings permit measurement of cardiac dimensions at any point in the cardiac cycle with an accuracy typically of ± 2–3 mm.

Comparison of end-diastolic and end-systolic values allows some parameters of cardiac function to be derived: for example, the percentage reduction in the left ventricular cavity size ('shortening fraction (SF)') is given by:

$$SF = \frac{LVDD - LVSD}{LVDD} \times 100\%$$

(normal range 30–45%)

LVDD = left ventricular diastolic diameter, LVSD = left ventricular systolic diameter.

Although introduced into clinical practice much more recently than the ECG and chest X-ray, the rapid development of ultrasound techniques and the non-invasive nature of the examination have resulted in echocardiography and Doppler becoming vital aids to the diagnosis of the majority of cardiac disorders.

The echocardiographic findings in particular conditions will be referred to elsewhere, but a brief overview is given below.

- *Valve stenosis.* Congenitally abnormal aortic or pulmonary valves show a characteristic 'dome' shape in systole because the cusps cannot separate fully and a bicuspid configuration may be demonstrated. The presence of calcium in a valve gives rise to intense echoes that generate multiple, parallel lines on M-mode recordings. CW Doppler directed from the apex measures velocity of the jet crossing the diseased valve, from which the pressure gradient can be calculated (Fig. 11.22).

  In mitral stenosis, the M-mode shows restriction and reversal of direction of the posterior leaflet motion (Fig. 11.23). A short-axis view shows the shape of the mitral orifice in diastole and its area can be measured directly from the image. Peak, mean and end-diastolic pressure gradients can be obtained from CW Doppler. Additional imaging views indicate the size of the left atrium, and may show the presence of left atrial thrombus.

- *Valve regurgitation.* Doppler is extremely sensitive for detecting valve regurgitation and, indeed, demonstrates mild physiological regurgitation through the tricuspid and pulmonary valves in the majority of normal subjects. It is hard to quantify the amount of regurgitation with echo Doppler techniques but echocardiography is an excellent way to determine the underlying cause of valve regurgitation, e.g. rheumatic disease or mitral valve prolapse.

- *Aortic aneurysms and dissections.* Dilatation of the aortic root can be measured accurately and the presence of a reflecting structure within the lumen of the aorta is strongly suggestive of an intimal flap associated with dissection.

- *Prosthetic heart valves.* Each type of heart valve prosthesis has characteristic echocardiographic features. Irregularity or restriction of movement can be shown on M-mode recordings. The presence of stenosis or regurgitation may be documented by Doppler.

- *Infective endocarditis.* Vegetations > 2 mm can be detected (Fig. 11.72).

- *Cardiomyopathies.* Dilated cardiomyopathy is characterized by an enlarged, globular-shaped, thin-walled left ventricle with poor function and

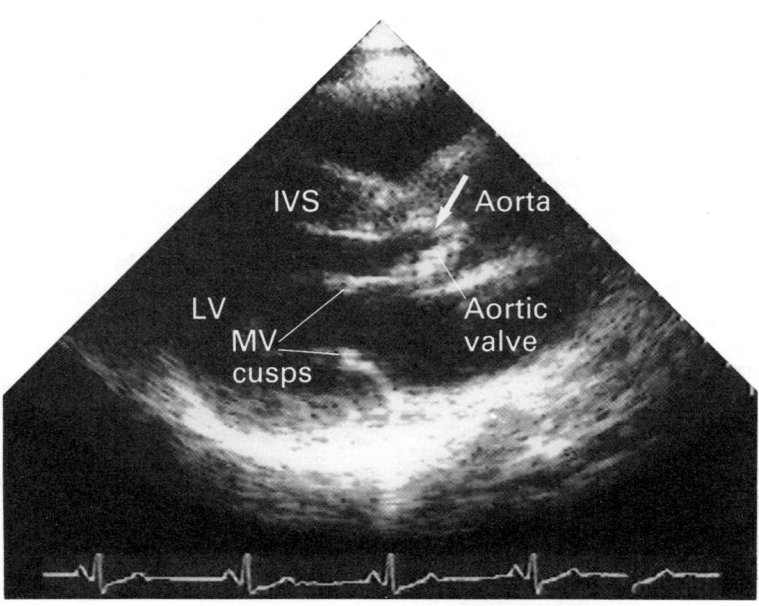

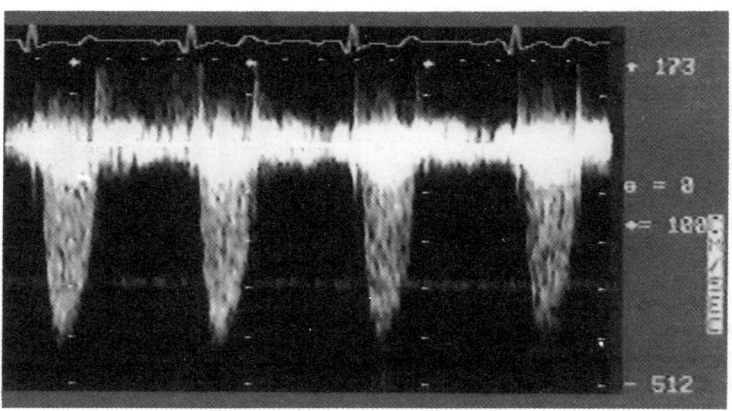

Fig. 11.22 (a) 2-D parasternal long axis echocardiogram from a patient with aortic stenosis. There is gross thickening of aortic valve leaflets and evidence of left ventricular hypertrophy. (b) CW doppler ultrasound showing aortic stenosis. The flow towards the aorta is below the baseline. Abnormally high velocities occur through the narrowed valve corresponding to the instantaneous pressure drop across the stenosis. Systole occurs after each QRS complex of the ECG.

low stroke output shown by reduced movements of the valves (Fig. 11.83).

In hypertrophic cardiomyopathy (see Fig. 11.84), the left ventricle is small, with a grossly thickened, immobile interventricular septum (asymmetric septal hypertrophy—ASH). There is a characeristic, though poorly understood, displacement of the mitral valve apparatus towards the septum in systole (systolic anterior motion—SAM).

- *Pericardial effusion.* Fluid in the pericardial cavity shows as an echo-free region between the myocardium and the intense echo of the parietal pericardium (Fig. 11.24).
- *Masses within the heart.* Echocardiography is a sensitive method for detecting masses within the heart (see Fig. 11.82).
- *Ischaemic disease.* Coronary arteries cannot be

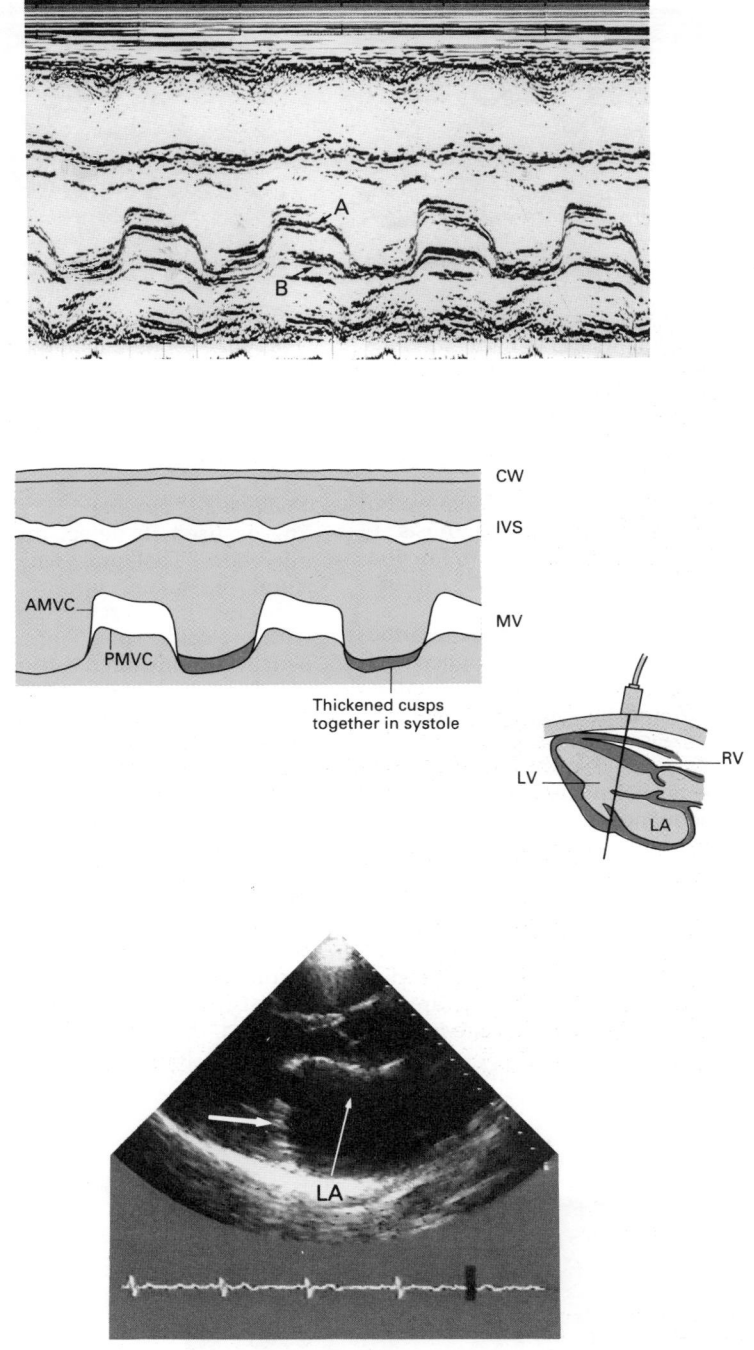

Fig. 11.23 M-Mode (upper panel) and 2-D (lower panel) parasternal long-axis echocardiogram recorded from a patient with rheumatic mitral stenosis. The M-mode trace shows thickened mitral valve leaflets. Note that both the anterior (A) and posterior (B) leaflets move towards the transducer (that is towards the chest wall) during diastole. The 2-D echo shows doming and thickening of the mitral valve leaflets (arrow) and an enlarged left atrium (LA).

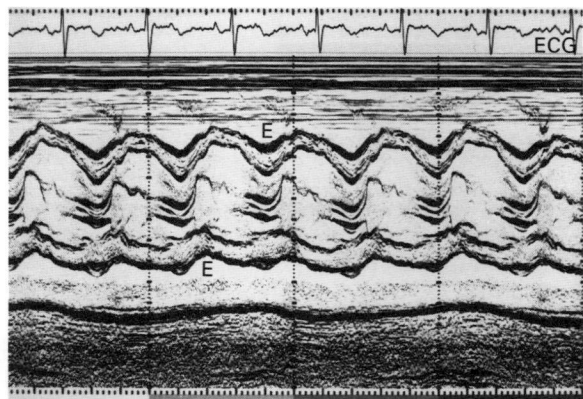
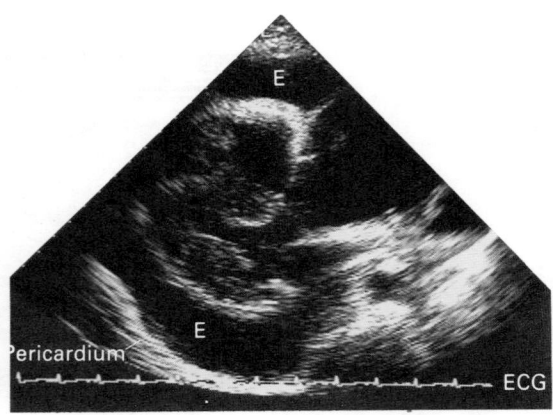

Fig. 11.24 Echocardiograms (M-Mode—left panel, 2-D parasternal long axis—right panel) in a patient with a large pericardial effusion. Note the echo-free spaces occupied by the effusion (E) behind and in front of the heart. Note that the 2-D image demonstrates the extent of the effusion particularly clearly.

imaged adequately using echo techniques but images may be useful for the diagnosis of complications related to myocardial infarction, such as mitral papillary muscle rupture, tamponade or ventricular septal rupture.

In the post-infarction period, echocardiography and Doppler are used to diagnose left ventricular aneurysm, left ventricular thrombus, mitral regurgitation and pericardial effusion.

- *Congenital heart disease.* Echocardiography has largely replaced cardiac catheterization and angiography. The aim of the examination is first to establish the sequence of blood flow through the heart, and to define anatomical abnormalities.

Nuclear imaging

Nuclear imaging techniques are primarily used in ischaemic heart disease. Myocardial structure and function can be assessed by radionuclide-imaging techniques.

Thallium-201 imaging

This is used to detect myocardial ischaemia and infarction. Thallium, which behaves like potassium, is taken up by healthy myocardium. Ischaemia or infarction produces a nuclear image with a 'cold' spot (Fig. 11.25). The isotope is usually administered during exercise and an image is taken soon after the exercise. Three or four hours later the heart is scanned again to obtain a redistribution image. The disappearance of the cold spot on the redistribution image implies ischaemia provoked by exertion and reversed by rest, whereas a persistent cold spot indicates infarction.

Pyrophosphate scan

Pyrophosphate labelled with technetium-99m concentrates in bone and acutely infarcted myocardium. The isotope should be injected intravenously between 1 and 5 days (best on the second or third day) following a myocardial infarction. Imaging a few hours later detects a 'hot spot' (Fig.

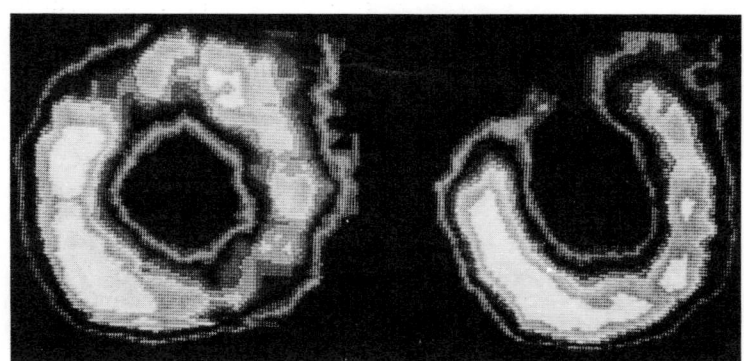

Fig. 11.25 Thallium myocardial perfusion scans using a grey scale (increased activity being whiter). The exercise scan (right) shows a defect at the top (between 10 and 12 o'clock) that fills in after 4 h rest (left). This suggests reversible myocardial ischaemia.

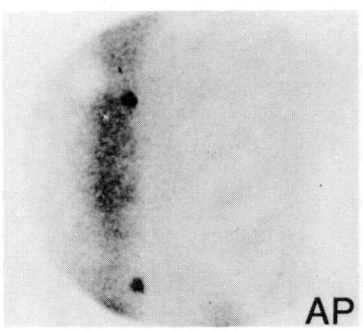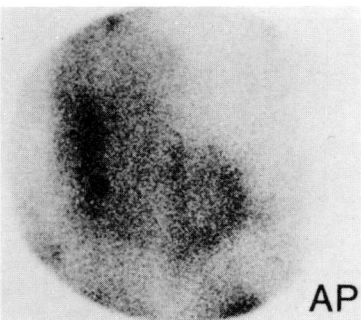

Fig. 11.26 Infarct-avid scans using technetium-labelled pyrophosphate. A negative scan (left) shows bone uptake in the ribs and sternum; the darker circles are position markers. A positive scan (right) shows myocardial uptake with a density greater than the ribs but slightly less than the sternum. AP = anterior-posterior.

11.26) in the region of the infarction. Scans are difficult to interpret because calcified costal cartilage and breast tissue may both concentrate the isotope. On the other hand, infarction may not result in the expected hot spot because the isotope is prevented from reaching the infarct owing to complete occlusion of coronary vessels to the infarcted myocardium. False-positive scans may occur in unstable angina.

Radionuclide ventriculography

Two methods are used to obtain blood pool images:

- A *MUGA* (multigated acquisition) or equilibrium image is obtained by intravenous injection of technetium-99m which attaches to the patient's own red cells *in vivo* and which is therefore retained in the vascular space. Over 200 heart beats are imaged. Comparison of the study with the ECG allows systolic and diastolic points of the cycle to be identified.
- A *first-pass study* images the heart as a bolus of isotope makes a single pass through the circulation.

These techniques are complementary, but both outline the cardiac chambers, particularly the left ventricle, by imaging the isotope within the central circulation during systole and diastole. The percentage of the left ventricular volume ejected with each systole (the ejection fraction) can be accurately measured, and any section of the left ventricular wall that contracts abnormally (a wall motion defect) can be visualized (Fig. 11.27). Radionuclide studies may be performed at rest and during exercise to assess changes in cardiac function. A deterioration on exercise suggests coronary disease or myocardial abnormality.

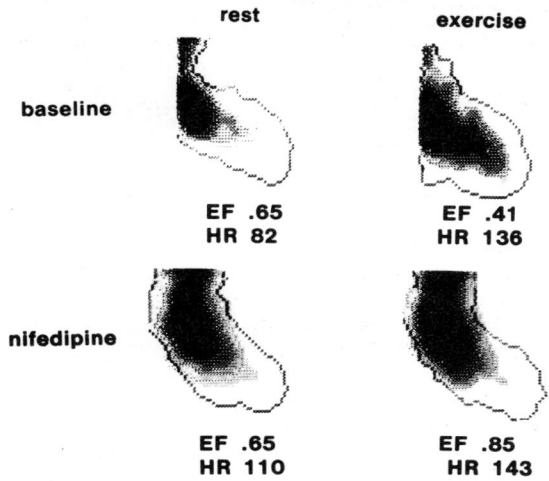

Fig. 11.27 First-pass radionuclide angiograms. The images show the diastolic perimeter surrounding the systolic image. The ejection fraction (EF)—the proportion of diastolic blood ejected during systole—and the heart rate (HR) are shown. These two rest and exercise studies show a control test (top), repeated after nifedipine (bottom). Note the improved exercise EF after nifedipine, suggesting amelioration of ischaemia.

Cardiac catheterization

Cardiac catheterization is the introduction of a thin radiopaque tube (catheter) into the circulation.

The right heart is catheterized by introducing the catheter into a peripheral vein and advancing it through the right atrium and ventricle into the pulmonary artery. The left heart is reached by way of a peripheral artery. The catheter is manipulated through the aortic valve into the left ventricle.

The pressures in the right heart chambers, left ventricle, aorta and pulmonary artery can be measured directly. An indirect measure of left atrial pressure can be obtained by 'wedging' a catheter into the distal pulmonary artery (see also p. 715). In this position the pressure from the right ventricle is obstructed by the catheter and only the pulmonary venous and left atrial pressures are

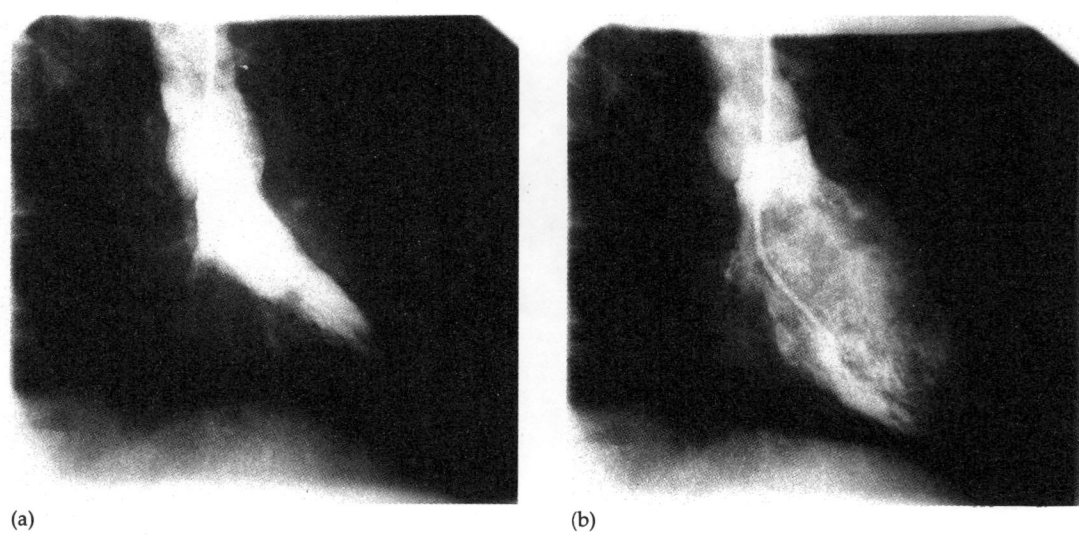

(a)   (b)

Fig. 11.28 Left ventricular angiogram. (a) End-systolic and (b) end-diastolic cine angiogram frames.

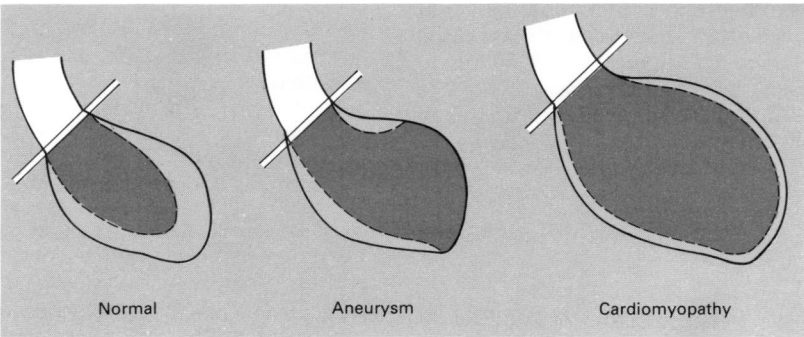

Normal   Aneurysm   Cardiomyopathy

Fig. 11.29 Diagrams showing left ventricular angiograms. A normal picture is compared with those showing an aneurysm and cardiomyopathy. The solid line represents the end-diastolic perimeter and the dotted line the end-systolic perimeter of the left ventricle. The double line marks the plane of the aortic valve.

recorded. Pressure measurements are used to quantify stenoses or measure contractile function.

During cardiac catheterization, blood samples may be withdrawn to measure the concentration of ischaemic metabolites, e.g. lactate, and the oxygen content. These estimations are used to gauge ischaemia, quantify intracardiac shunts, and measure cardiac output.

Contrast cine-angiograms are also taken during catheterization. Radiopaque contrast material is injected into the cardiac chambers (Fig. 11.28), arterial trunks or coronary arteries. Fig. 11.29 shows a normal angiogram compared with angiograms showing an aneurysm and cardiomyopathy.

Digital subtraction angiography
This technique permits the injection of small volumes of radiocontrast agents during cardiac catheterization with the production of computer-

analysed high-quality angiograms.

Unfortunately, peripheral injection of contrast does not give adequate visualization of the coronary arteries, but aortic lesions can be visualized.

CT scanning is particularly useful for showing the size and shape of the cardiac chambers as well as the thoracic aorta and mediastinum.

Magnetic resonance imaging

This non-invasive imaging technique does not involve harmful radiation. A powerful magnetic field is used to line up the protons in the hydrogen atoms of the body, each of which can be thought of as a tiny magnet. A radio-frequency emission distorts this line-up, but when the radio waves are turned off, the atoms return to their previous position and give off energy. This energy can be reconstituted as an image. Magnetic resonance

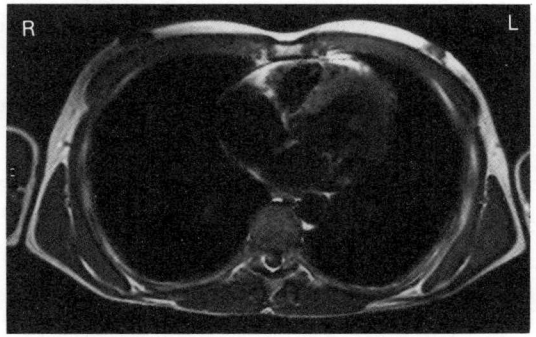 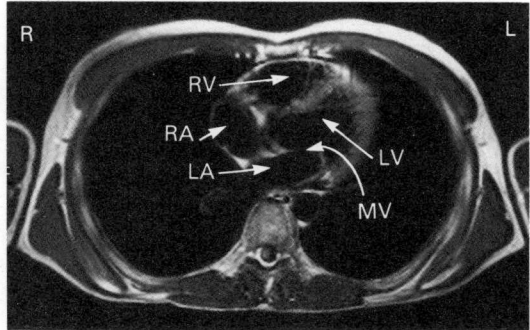

Fig. 11.30 Magnetic resonance image (MRI) showing a pair of axial images taken through the midthorax at the level of the mitral valve. Image (a) is a view of end-systole, image (b) is taken at end-diastole. Note the clear differentiation between the atria and ventricles. This is a normal study.

imaging of the heart is complicated because the heart is a moving structure, but the technique is already finding clinical application for imaging vascular structures.

Synchronization with the ECG allows cardiac images in systole and diastole to be obtained (Fig. 11.30).

Therapeutic procedures

Cardiac resuscitation

No matter where cardiac arrest occurs it is essential that someone close to the victim institutes basic life support. The longer the period of respiratory and circulatory arrest, the less the possibility of restoring healthy life. After 3 min there will be permanent cerebral dysfunction. Because sudden unexpected cardiac arrest is relatively common in the hospital, medical students and all doctors must know what to do. A cardiac arrest usually causes a great deal of excitement and some panic. Therefore, it is very important that the basic procedure is well known. A standard procedure must be used in order that a variety of personnel may work easily together. The scheme that follows is recommended by the UK Resuscitation Council. It should be practised on a resuscitation dummy at least every 6 months.

Basic life support
The first step is to establish whether the victim is unconscious (shake and shout at the patient) and whether there is a pulse. It is best to feel the carotid pulse by pressing backwards just to the side of the thyroid cartilage. If there is no pulse, immediately call for help. Quickly place the victim in an accessible position with firm underlying support (e.g. on his back on the floor), and begin basic life support. This can be remembered as A (airway) and B (breathing) and C (circulation).

Airway. Any loose obstruction (e.g. blood and mucus) in the mouth and pharynx should be quickly removed. Unless already detached, leave false teeth in place because they give form and support to the oral cavity. Open the airway by flexing the neck and extending the head ('sniffing the morning air' position).

Breathing. Look for the rise and fall of the chest and abdomen. If there is no respiration, begin expired air respiration. With the head of the victim tilted backwards and the chin pulled forward the rescuer takes a deep breath and seals his lips around the mouth or nose of the victim. Four quick puffs are given. Expired air respiration is the only method of artificial respiration that successfully ventilates the patient. The mechanical methods of Holger and Neilson, Shaeffer and Sylvester are completely useless because they result in the movement of less air than is required to fill the dead space.

If the airway is obstructed, the head, neck and jaw are readjusted and another check is made for debris in the mouth. If obstruction persists, any foreign body stuck in the larynx or upper airway should be removed by a firm thrust to the epigastrium (the *Heimlich manoeuvre*, see p. 654).

Circulation. Circulation is achieved by external chest compression. The heel of one hand is placed over the lower half of the victim's sternum and the heel of the second hand is placed over the first with the fingers interlocked. The arms are kept straight and the sternum is rhythmically depressed by 1½–2 inches. Chest compression does not massage the heart. The thorax acts as a pump and the heart provides a system of one-way valves to ensure forward circulation.

Respiration and compression is now continued as follows:

- *Single rescuer*—compression at a rate of 80 beats per minute with two respirations after 15 compressions.
- *Two rescuers*—continuous compressions at a rate of 60 beats per minute and one respiration given after every 5 compressions.

If possible, it is better to give compressions without interruption. This maintains adequate cerebral and coronary perfusion pressures. Ventilation can easily be achieved despite continued chest compression.

Advanced cardiac life support
By the time effective life support has been established, more help should have arrived and advanced cardiac life support can begin. This consists of ECG monitoring, endotracheal intubation and setting up an intravenous infusion in a large peripheral vein or a central vein. Immediate therapy includes defibrillation, oxygen and cardioactive drugs. It is not possible to recommend an exact sequence of managment because it will depend on the arrival of skilled personnel and equipment and the nature of the cardiac arrest. However, as soon as possible the ECG should be connected. At first this is easily achieved by monitoring the ECG through the paddles of a defibrillator. Later, electrodes, leads and specific ECG scopes can be set up. If the ECG shows ventricular fibrillation, no time should be lost before defibrillating the patient. If initial defibrillation attempts are unsuccessful, time can then be spent intubating the patient and setting up an intravenous infusion whilst the circulation is supported by external chest compression. If there is any difficulty in intubating the patient, ventilation should be continued by means of an airway, a ventilating bag and oxygen.

There are three main mechanisms of sudden unexpected cardiac arrest:

- Ventricular fibrillation
- Asystole
- Electromechanical dissociation

Three-quarters of arrests are due to ventricular fibrillation. Only a very small proportion are due to electromechanical dissociation, and the remainder are due to asystole. In patients dying of other causes, such as terminal pneumonia, the heart rhythm is described as being agonal. This is characterized by an inexorable slowing and widening of the QRS complexes associated with falling blood pressure and cardiac output. This type of arrhythmia is very difficult to reverse and usually no attempt should be made because it is the result rather than the cause of death.

Arrests are treated in the following ways:

- *Ventricular fibrillation* is readily treated with defibrillation, anti-arrhythmic drugs and cardiac stimulants.
- *Asystole* is more difficult to treat but the heart may respond to atropine or adrenaline. If there is any sign of electrocardiographic activity, emergency pacing should be used.
- *Electromechanical dissociation* is often due to a severe mechanical problem such as pericardial tamponade or massive pulmonary embolism. These conditions should be treated urgently. Toxic levels of cardiodepressant drugs, such as beta blockers, may also cause electromechanical dissociation. If there is an antidote, such as adrenaline, it should be administered.

Fig. 11.31 shows the treatments recommended by the UK Resuscitation Council.

Sudden death

Each year in the UK there are approximately 100 000 unexpected deaths occurring within 24 h of the development of cardiac symptoms. About half of these deaths are almost instantaneous. There are several causes:

- Cardiac arrhythmias (e.g. ventricular fibrillation)
- Sudden pump failure (e.g. acute myocardial infarction)
- Acute circulatory obstruction (e.g. pulmonary embolism)
- Cardiovascular rupture (e.g. dissecting aneurysm of the aorta, myocardial rupture)
- Vasomotor collapse (e.g. pulmonary hypertension)

Most deaths are due to ventricular fibrillation, and a small proportion are due to severe bradyarrhythmias. Although coronary disease is frequent in these victims, acute coronary occlusion and myocardial infarction is relatively uncommon (~ 40%).

Defibrillation
This technique is used for the conversion of ventricular fibrillation to sinus rhythm. Electrical energy is discharged through two paddles placed on the chest wall. Initially 200 J is used for defibrillation.

The paddles are placed in one of two positions:

- One paddle is placed to the right of the upper sternum and the other over the cardiac apex.
- One paddle is placed under the tip of the left scapula and the other is placed over the anterior wall of the left chest.

Electrode jelly or elecrolyte gel pads should be used to ensure good contact between the electrode paddles and the skin. Jelly smeared carelessly across the chest may cause short circuits and arcing of the charge. All personnel should stand clear of the patient.

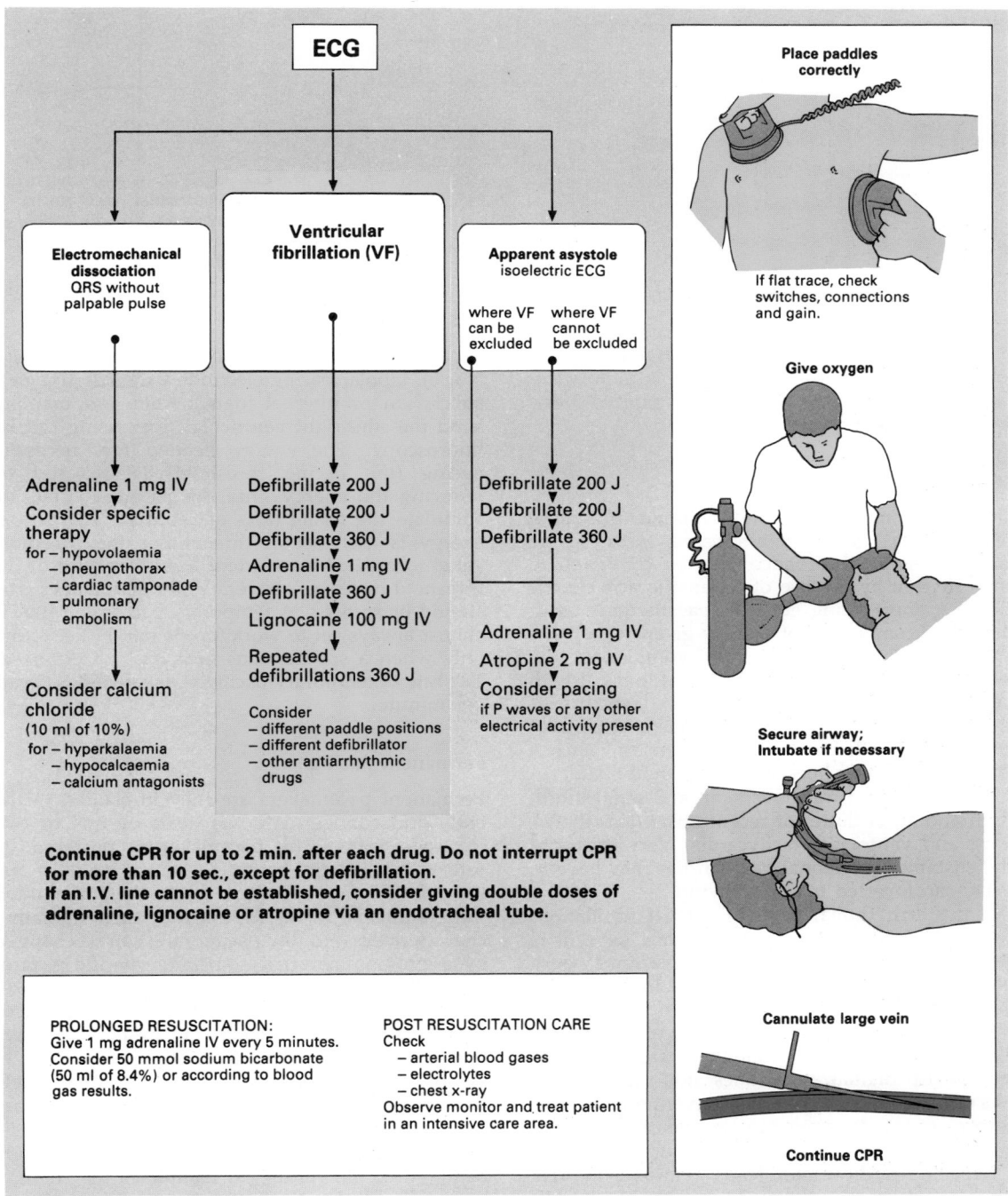

ECG

Electromechanical dissociation
QRS without palpable pulse

Ventricular fibrillation (VF)

Apparent asystole
isoelectric ECG

where VF can be excluded | where VF cannot be excluded

Adrenaline 1 mg IV

Consider specific therapy
for – hypovolaemia
    – pneumothorax
    – cardiac tamponade
    – pulmonary embolism

Consider calcium chloride
(10 ml of 10%)
for – hyperkalaemia
    – hypocalcaemia
    – calcium antagonists

Defibrillate 200 J
Defibrillate 200 J
Defibrillate 360 J
Adrenaline 1 mg IV
Defibrillate 360 J
Lignocaine 100 mg IV

Repeated defibrillations 360 J

Consider
– different paddle positions
– different defibrillator
– other antiarrhythmic drugs

Defibrillate 200 J
Defibrillate 200 J
Defibrillate 360 J

Adrenaline 1 mg IV
Atropine 2 mg IV
Consider pacing
if P waves or any other electrical activity present

Continue CPR for up to 2 min. after each drug. Do not interrupt CPR for more than 10 sec., except for defibrillation.
If an I.V. line cannot be established, consider giving double doses of adrenaline, lignocaine or atropine via an endotracheal tube.

PROLONGED RESUSCITATION:
Give 1 mg adrenaline IV every 5 minutes.
Consider 50 mmol sodium bicarbonate
(50 ml of 8.4%) or according to blood gas results.

POST RESUSCITATION CARE
Check
    – arterial blood gases
    – electrolytes
    – chest x-ray
Observe monitor and treat patient in an intensive care area.

Place paddles correctly

If flat trace, check switches, connections and gain.

Give oxygen

Secure airway; Intubate if necessary

Cannulate large vein

Continue CPR

Fig. 11.31 Schema for management of the three common forms of cardiac arrest: ventricular fibrillation, ventricular asystole, and electromechanical dissociation. (Based on recommendations of the UK Resuscitation Council, 1989.)

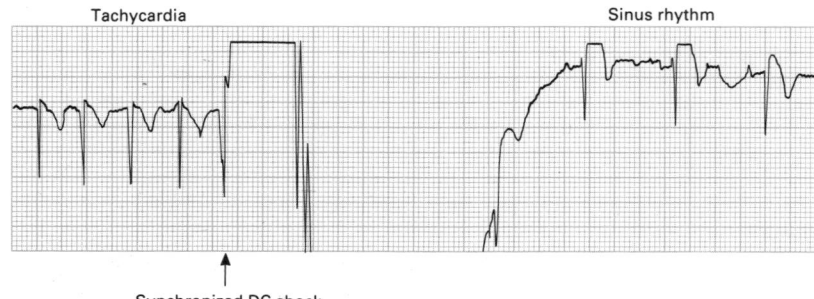

Tachycardia　　　　　　　　　　Sinus rhythm

↑
Synchronized DC shock

Fig. 11.32 DC-cardioversion of a supraventricular tachycardia to sinus rhythm. The direct current shock is delivered synchronously with the QRS complex.

When the defibrillator is discharged, a high-voltage field envelops the heart. This depolarizes the whole heart and allows an organized heart rhythm to emerge.

DC-cardioversion

Tachyarrhythmias that do not respond to medical treatment or that are associated with severe haemodynamic disturbance may be converted to sinus rhythm by the use of a transthoracic electric shock. A short-acting general anaesthetic is used. Muscle relaxants are not usually given. When the arrhythmia has definite QRS complexes, the delivery of the shock should be timed to occur with the downstroke of the QRS complex (synchronization) (Fig. 11.32). This is the major difference between defibrillation and cardioversion, since a non-synchronized shock is used to defibrillate.

Indications for cardioversion are atrial fibrillation and atrial flutter of recent onset (less than 1 year), and ventricular tachycardia. Very occasionally, sustained junctional tachycardias may have to be DC-cardioverted to sinus rhythm.

If the arrhythmia, especially atrial fibrillation, has been present for more than a few days, it is wise to anticoagulate the patient for several weeks before elective cardioversion. This reduces the risk of embolization.

Digoxin toxicity may lead to ventricular arrhythmias or asystole following cardioversion. Therapeutic digitalization does not increase the risks of cardioversion, but it is conventional to omit digoxin several days prior to elective cardioversion in order to be sure that toxicity is not present.

Repeated cardioversion leads to an enzyme rise because of damage to the muscles of the chest wall. Specific cardiac enzymes may increase slightly because of myocardial damage produced by the shock.

Temporary pacing

Symptomatic bradycardias unresponsive to atropine are treated with a cardiac pacemaker. A temporary pacemaker (external unit) may be connected to the myocardium by a thin (French gauge 5 or 6), bipolar pacing electrode wire inserted via a subclavian or internal jugular vein and manipulated into the right ventricular apex using cardiac fluoroscopy. The energy needed for successful pacing (the pacing threshold) is assessed by reducing the energy until the pacemaker fails to stimulate the tissue (loss of capture). The output energy is then set at three times the threshold value to prevent inadvertent loss of capture. If the threshold increases above 5 V, the pacemaker wire should be re-sited. A temporary pacemaker unit is almost always set to work 'on demand', i.e. to fire only when a spontaneous beat has not occurred. The rate of temporary pacing is usually 60–80 beats per minute.

Permanent pacing

Permanent pacemakers are fully implanted in the body and connected to the heart by one or two electrode leads. The pacemaker is powered by solid-state lithium batteries, which usually last from 5–10 years. Modern pacemakers are often 'programmable'. This means that their operating characteristics (e.g. the pacing rate) can be changed by a programmer that transmits specific electromagnetic signals through the skin. The pacemaker leads are passed transvenously to the right heart chambers. Most pacemakers are designed to pace and sense the ventricles. Occasionally, e.g. in symptomatic sinus bradycardia, an atrial pacemaker may be implanted. Pacemakers that are connected to both the right atrium and ventricle ('dual chamber' pacemaker) are now increasingly being used in order to simulate the natural pacemaker and activation sequence of the heart. Another form of 'physiological' pacemaker is the 'rate-responsive' system, which, by measuring activity, respiration, biochemical or electrical indicators, changes its rate of pacing so that it is appropriate to the level of exertion.

Permanent pacemakers are inserted under local anaesthetic using fluoroscopy to guide the insertion of the electrode leads. Antibiotics may be prescribed prophylactically.

Complications are few but include:

- *Infection*. When a pacemaker system is infected, antibiotic treatment is not sufficient and the pacemaker must usually be removed before antibiotics will subdue the infection. Another pacemaker is fitted later.
- *Erosion*. The pacemaker may erode through the skin. This is usually due to a low-grade infection. Mechanical factors may also be responsible.
- *Lead displacement*. In most cases the pacing lead is securely wedged into the trabeculae of the right ventricle. It rarely displaces but when it does it may lead to sudden loss of pacing and a recurrence of pre-pacing symptoms.
- *Pacemaker malfunction*. This is now a very uncommon complication but requires the replacement of the pacemaker.

Pericardiocentesis

A pericardial effusion is an accumulation of fluid between the parietal and visceral layers of pericardium. Fluid is removed to relieve symptoms due to haemodynamic embarrassment or for diagnostic purposes. Pericardial aspiration or pericardiocentesis is performed by inserting a needle into the pericardial space, usually via a subxiphisternal route. If a large volume of fluid is to be removed, a wide-bore needle and cannula are inserted. The needle may be removed and the cannula left *in situ* to drain the fluid. Fluid that is removed is sent for chemical analysis, microscopy, including cytology, and culture. If a reaccumulation of pericardial fluid is anticipated, the cannula may be left in place for several days or an operation can be performed to cut a window in the parietal pericardium (fenestration) or to remove a large section of the pericardium.

Right heart bedside catheterization

Bedside catheterization of the pulmonary artery with a Swan–Ganz catheter is performed in patients with:

- Cardiac failure
- Cardiogenic shock
- Doubtful fluid status

The catheter is used to measure cardiac output, pulmonary artery pressure, right atrial pressure and the pulmonary artery wedge pressure (an indirect measurement of left atrial pressure). The measurement of these pressures and the cardiac output allows appropriate therapy to be prescribed and the effects of that therapy to be monitored. The catheter also provides a route for the delivery of drugs to the central circulation (see Fig. 13.14).

Intra-aortic balloon pumping

This is a technique used to assist temporarily the failing left ventricle. A catheter with a long sausage-shaped balloon at its tip is introduced percutaneously into the femoral artery and manipulated under X-ray control so that the balloon lies in the descending aorta just below the aortic arch. The balloon is rhythmically deflated and inflated with carbon dioxide gas. Using the ECG or intra-aortic pressure changes, the inflation is timed to occur during ventricular diastole to increase diastolic aortic pressure and consequently to improve coronary and cerebral blood flow. During systole the balloon is deflated, resulting in a reduction in the resistance to left ventricular emptying.

Balloon pumping is used:

- To improve cardiac output when there is a transient or reversible depression of left ventricular function, e.g. in a patient with severe mitral valve regurgitation who is awaiting surgical replacement of the mitral valve or in a patient with a ventricular septal defect due to septal infarction
- To treat unstable angina pectoris by improving coronary flow and decreasing myocardial oxygen consumption by reducing the 'afterload'. This technique may be successful, even when medical therapy has failed. It is followed by early arteriography and appropriate definitive therapy such as surgery or coronary angioplasty.

Balloon pumping should not be used when there is no remediable cause of cardiac dysfunction. It is also unsuitable in patients with aortic valve regurgitation or dissection of the aorta.

Complications of balloon pumping occur in about 20% of cases and include aortic dissection, leg ischaemia, emboli from the balloon, and balloon rupture. Embolic complications are reduced by anticoagulation with heparin.

Cardiac arrhythmias

An abnormality of the cardiac rhythm is called a cardiac arrhythmia. Such a disturbance of rhythm may cause sudden death, syncope, dizziness, palpitations or no symptoms at all. There are two main types of arrhythmia:

- *Bradycardia*, where the heart rate is slow (< 60 beats per minute). The slower the heart rate the more likely the arrhythmia will be symptomatic.
- *Tachycardia*, where the heart rate is fast (> 100 beats per minute). Tachycardias are more symp-

tomatic when the arrhythmia is fast and sustained. Tachycardias are subdivided into *supraventricular tachycardias*, which arise from the atrium or the atrioventricular junction, and *ventricular tachycardias*, which arise from the ventricles.

Ventricular tachyarrhythmias tend to be more symptomatic than supraventricular tachycardias. Some arrhythmias occur in patients with apparently normal hearts, and in others arrhythmias reflect underlying cardiac abnormalities. When myocardial function is poor, arrhythmias tend to be more symptomatic and are potentially life threatening.

Mechanisms of arrhythmia production

There are four main mechanisms of tachycardia production:

- Two are abnormalities of automaticity, which might theoretically arise from a single disordered cell.
- Two are abnormalities of conduction, which require abnormal interaction between cells.

Figure 11.33 shows the mechanisms of arrhythmias.

Accelerated automaticity

The normal mechanism of cardiac rhythmicity is slow depolarization of the transmembrane voltage during diastole until the threshold potential is reached and the pacemaker fires. This mechanism may be accelerated by increasing the rate of diastolic depolarization or changing the threshold potential. Such changes are thought to produce sinus tachycardia, escape rhythms and accelerated AV nodal rhythms.

Triggered automaticity

Myocardial damage can result in oscillations of the end of the action potential. These oscillations may reach threshold potential and produce an arrhythmia. The abnormal oscillations can be exaggerated by pacing and by catecholamines and these stimuli can be used to trigger this abnormal form of automaticity. Some of the arrhythmias produced by digoxin toxicity are due to triggered automaticity.

Reflection

If adjacent cells repolarize at different rates, the cells that repolarize more quickly may be restimulated by those cells that have not yet repolarized. The ventricular tachyarrhythmias associated with the long-QT syndrome may result from this mechanism.

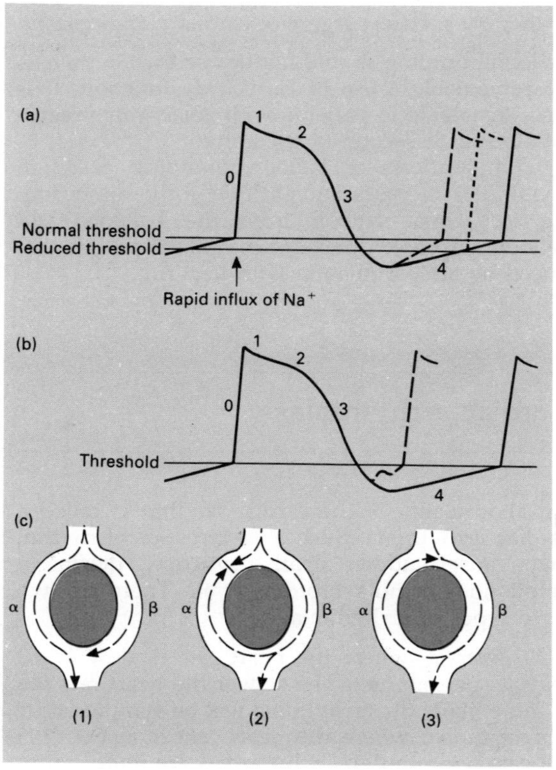

Fig. 11.33 Mechanisms of arrhythmogenesis. (a) and (b) show action potentials (i.e. the potential difference between intra- and extracellular fluid) of ventricular myocardium after stimulation. (a) shows increased automaticity due to a reduced threshold potential or an increased slope of phase 4 depolarization (see p. 529). (b) shows abnormal automaticity due to 'after' depolarizations reaching threshold potential. (c) shows the mechanism of circus movement or re-entry. In panel (1) the impulse passes down both limbs of the potential tachycardia circuit. In panel (2) the impulse is blocked in the alpha pathway but proceeds slowly down the beta pathway and returns along the alpha pathway. In panel (3) the impulse travels so slowly along the beta pathway that when it returns along the alpha pathway to its starting point it is able to travel again down the beta pathway, producing a circus movement tachycardia.

Re-entry (or circus movement)

A wave of depolarization may be forced to travel in one direction around a ring of cardiac tissue. If the time to conduct around the ring is longer than the recovery of any tissue within the ring, circus movement will result, producing a tachycardia. The majority of regular paroxysmal tachycardias are thought to be produced by this mechanism.

SINUS RHYTHMS

The normal cardiac pacemaker is the sinus node and, like most cardiac tissue, it depolarizes spontaneously (see Fig. 11.34). Its rate of discharge is controlled by the autonomic nervous system. Normally the parasympathetic system predominates, resulting in slowing of the spontaneous discharge rate from approximately 100 to 70 beats per minute. A reduction of parasympathetic tone or an increase in sympathetic stimulation leads to tachycardia; conversely, increased parasympathetic tone and decreased sympathetic stimulation produces bradycardia. The sinus rate in women is slightly faster than in men. Normal sinus rhythm is characterized by P waves that are upright in leads I and II of the ECG (Fig. 11.17), but are inverted in the cavity leads AVR + VI (Fig. 11.34).

Sinus arrhythmia

Fluctuations of autonomic tone result in phasic changes of the sinus discharge rate. Thus, during inspiration, parasympathetic tone falls and the heart rate quickens, and on expiration the heart rate falls. This variation is normal, particularly in children and young adults.

Sinus bradycardia

A sinus rate of less than 60 beats per minute during the day or less than 50 beats per minute at night is known as sinus bradycardia. It is usually asymptomatic unless the rate is very slow. It is normal in athletes and in elderly patients. Causes include:

- Hypothermia, hypothyroidism, cholestatic jaundice and raised intracranial pressure
- Drug therapy with beta blockers, digitalis and other anti-arrhythmic drugs
- Acute ischaemia and infarction of the sinus node
- Chronic degenerative changes such as fibrosis of the atrium and sinus node

TREATMENT

Treatment of acute symptomatic sinus bradycardia is atropine 600 µg i.v. If the symptomatic arrhythmia persists, a cardiac pacemaker is required.

Sinus tachycardia

Sinus rate acceleration to more than 100 beats per minute is known as sinus tachycardia. Causes include:

- Fever
- Exercise
- Emotion
- Pregnancy
- Anaemia
- Cardiac failure with compensatory sinus tachycardia
- Thyrotoxicosis
- Catecholamine excess
- Primary sinus tachycardia (rare)

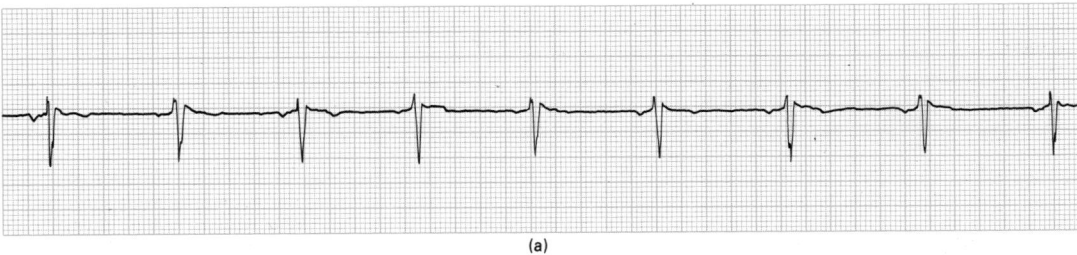

(a)

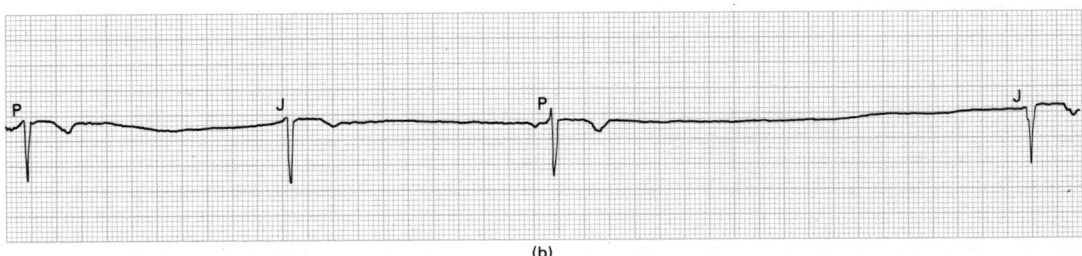

(b)

Fig. 11.34 (a) An ECG showing normal sinus rhythm. (b) An ECG from a patient with sick sinus syndrome. This shows sinus arrest (only occasional sinus P waves) and junctional escape beats (J). P waves are inverted in these cavity leads.

TREATMENT

This involves correction of the condition causing the tachycardia. If necessary, beta-blockers may be used to slow the sinus rate, but not in heart failure.

PATHOLOGICAL BRADYCARDIAS

There are two main forms of severe bradycardia: sinus node disease and atrioventricular block.

Sinus node disease (sick sinus syndrome)

Sinus node disease is caused by ischaemia, infarction or degenerative disease of the sinus node. It is characterized by long intervals between consecutive P waves (> 2 s) on the ECG (see Fig. 11.34). These sinus pauses may be an exact multiple of the basic sinus interval (sinoatrial exit block) or not (sinus arrest). Both conditions have a similar prognosis.

Sinus pauses and sinus bradycardia may allow cardiac tachyarrhythmias to emerge. A combination of fast and slow supraventricular rhythms is known as the tachycardia–bradycardia (tachy–brady) syndrome.

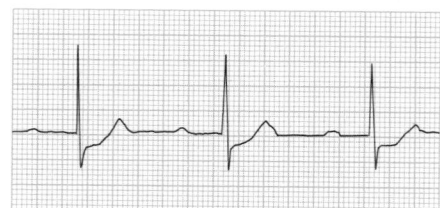

Fig. 11.35 An ECG showing first-degree atrioventricular block with a prolonged PR interval. In this trace ST depression is also present.

TREATMENT

Treatment of chronic symptomatic sick sinus syndrome requires permanent pacing, with additional anti-arrhythmic drugs to manage any tachycardia element. Thromboembolism is common in sick sinus syndrome and patients should be anticoagulated unless there is a contraindication.

Atrioventricular (AV) block

There are three forms: first-degree block, second-degree (partial) block and third-degree (complete) block.

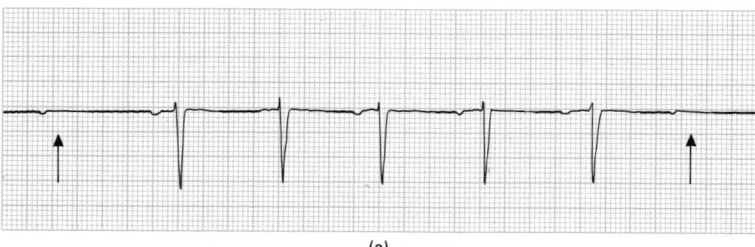

(a)

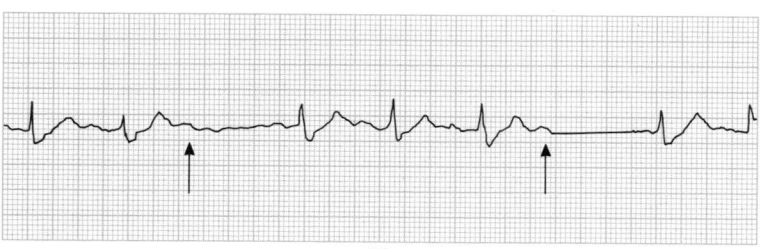

(b)

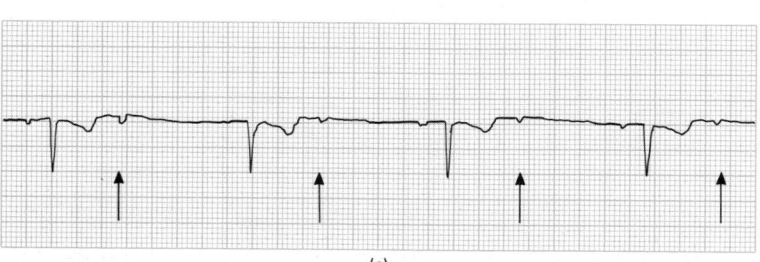

(c)

Fig. 11.36 Three varieties of second-degree atrioventricular (AV) block. (a) Wenckebach (Mobitz type I) AV block. The PR interval gradually prolongs until the P wave does not conduct to the ventricles (arrows). (b) Mobitz type II AV block. The P waves that do not conduct to the ventricles (arrows) are not preceded by gradual PR interval prolongation. (c) Two P waves to each QRS complex. The PR interval prior to the dropped P wave is always the same. It is not possible to define this type of AV block as type I or type II Mobitz block and it is, therefore, a third variety of second-degree AV block.

First-degree AV block

This is simple prolongation of the PR interval to more than 0.22 s. Every atrial depolarization is followed by conduction to the ventricles but with delay (Fig. 11.35).

Second-degree (partial) AV block

This occurs when some P waves conduct and others do not. There are several forms of second degree AV block (Fig. 11.36).

- *Mobitz I block* (Wenckebach phenomenon) is progressive PR interval prolongation until a P wave fails to conduct. The PR interval before the blocked P wave is much longer than the PR interval after the blocked P wave.
- *Mobitz II block* occurs when a dropped QRS complex is not preceded by progressive PR interval prolongation.
- *2 : 1 or 3 : 1 block* occurs when every second or third P wave conducts to the ventricles. This

form of second-degree block is neither Mobitz I nor II. 4 : 1 block, 5 : 1 block, can also occur.

Traditionally, Wenckebach block is said to be more benign than other forms of second-degree block, but recent evidence suggests that all forms of second-degree AV block have a similar prognosis. Patients with this conduction problem are usually asymptomatic. A close watch should be kept on them, although no treatment is necessary unless more serious or symptomatic heart block develops.

Third-degree (complete) AV block

This occurs when no P waves conduct to the ventricles (Fig. 11.37). In this situation life is maintained by a spontaneous escape rhythm that has either broad (> 0.1 s) or narrow (< 0.1 s) QRS complexes.

Narrow complex (Fig. 11.37a). This is due to disease in the AV node or the proximal His bundle. The

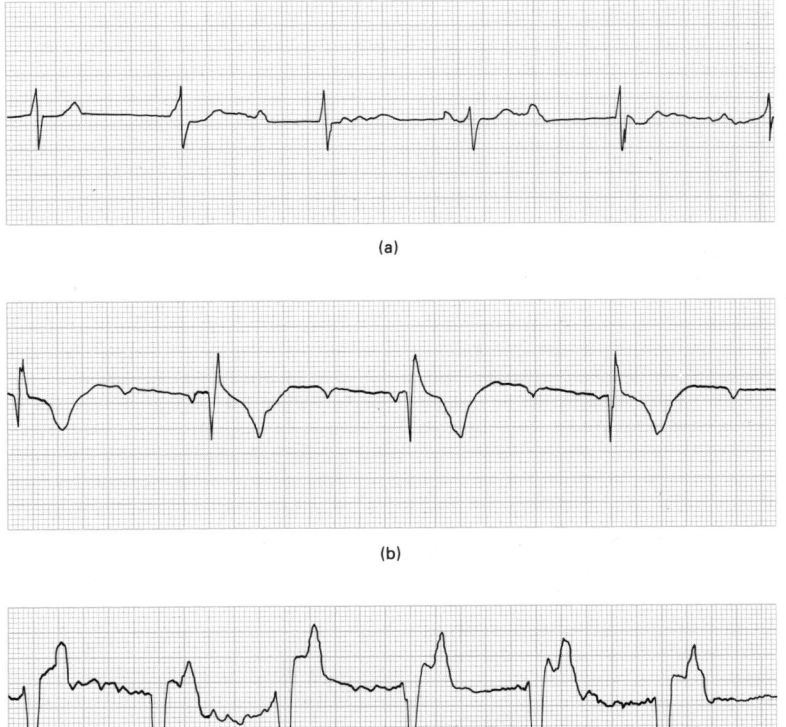

(a)

(b)

(c)

Fig. 11.37 Three examples of complete heart block. (a) Congenital complete heart block. The QRS complex is narrow (0.08 s) and the QRS rate is relatively rapid (52 beats per minute). (b) Acquired complete heart block. The QRS complex is broad (0.13 s) and the QRS rate is relatively slow (38 beats per minute). (c) Drug-induced complete heart block in a patient with atrial fibrillation rather than sinus rhythm (note the undulating baseline but the regular and slow ventricular rate).

escape rhythm occurs with an adequate rate (50–60 beats per minute) and is relatively reliable. It occurs in association with:

- Congenital heart disease (such as transposition of the great arteries)
- An isolated congenital problem (congenital heart block)
- Inferior wall myocardial infarction
- Diphtheria
- Rheumatic fever
- Toxic concentrations of drugs such as digitalis, verapamil or beta-blockers

Treatment is often unnecessary except for the eradication of toxic causes. Recent-onset narrow complex AV block due to acute myocardial infarction may respond to intravenous atropine but a temporary pacemaker may be necessary. Chronic narrow complex AV block requires permanent pacing if it is symptomatic or associated with heart disease.

Occasionally, permanent pacing is advocated for asymptomatic, isolated, congenital AV block.

Broad complex (Fig. 11.37b). This occurs because of disease in the Purkinje system. The escape pacemaker arises from the distal Purkinje network or the ventricular myocardium. The resulting rhythm is slow (15–40 beats per minute) and relatively unreliable. Dizziness and blackouts (Stokes–Adams attacks) often occur. In the elderly, it is usually caused by degenerative fibrosis and calcification of the distal conduction system (Lenegre's disease) or the more proximal conduction system (Lev's disease). In younger patients, broad complex AV block may be caused by ischaemic heart disease.

A permanent pacemaker should always be inserted, as the mortality from the condition, even when asymptomatic, is considerably reduced by pacing.

Intraventricular conduction disturbances

The intraventricular conduction system consists of the His bundle, the right and left bundle branches and the antero-superior and postero-inferior divisions of the left bundle branch. Various conduction disturbances can occur:

- *His bundle delay* may produce a long PR interval but it is often too small a delay to be noticed on the surface ECG.
- *Blocked His bundle conduction* produces AV block.
- *Bundle branch conduction delay* produces trivial widening of the QRS complex (up to 0.11 s). This is known as incomplete bundle branch block.
- *Complete block of a bundle branch* is associated with a wider QRS complex (0.12 s or more). The shape of the QRS depends on whether the right

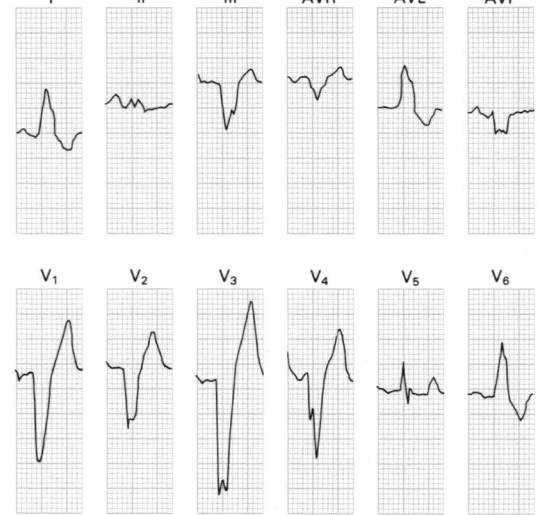

Fig. 11.38 (a) A 12-lead ECG showing left bundle branch block. The QRS duration is greater than 0.12 s. Note the broad notched R waves with ST depression in leads I, AVL and V_6, and the broad QS waves in V_1–V_3.

or the left bundle is blocked. *Right bundle branch block* (an example is shown in Fig. 11.61) produces late activation of the right ventricle. This is seen as deep S waves in leads I and V_6 and as a tall late R wave in lead V_1 (see Fig. 11.78) (late activation moving towards right- and away from left-sided leads). *Left bundle branch block* (Fig. 11.38) produces the opposite, i.e. a deep S wave in lead V_1 and a tall late R wave in leads I and V_6. Because left bundle branch conduction is normally responsible for the initial ventricular activation, left bundle branch block also produces abnormal Q waves.

Delay or block in the divisions of the left bundle branch produces a swing in the direction of depolarization (electrical axis) of the heart. When the antero-superior division is blocked, the left ventricle is activated from inferior to superior. This produces a superior (leftwards) movement of the axis. Delay or block in the postero-inferior division swings the QRS axis inferiorly.

- *Bisfascicular block* (see Fig. 11.61) is a combination of a block of any two of the following: the right bundle branch, the left antero-superior division and the left postero-inferior division. Block of the remaining fascicle will result in complete AV block.

CLINICAL FEATURES

Intraventricular conduction disturbances other than complete block of the His bundle are usually asymptomatic. Sometimes left bundle branch block actually seems to provoke chest pain.

Right bundle branch block causes wide but

Table 11.11 Causes of right bundle branch block. It is also a normal finding in 1% of young adults and 5% of elderly adults.

Congenital heart disease
Atrial septal defect
Fallot's tetralogy
Pulmonary stenosis
Ventricular septal defect

Pulmonary disease
Cor pulmonale
Recurrent pulmonary embolism
Acute pulmonary embolism (transient)

Myocardial disease
Acute myocardial infarction
Cardiomyopathy
Conduction system fibrosis

Drugs and electrolytes
Hyperkalaemia
Class Ia drugs (see p. 560)

Right ventriculotomy

Table 11.12 Causes of left bundle branch block.

Left ventricular outflow obstruction
Aortic stenosis
Hypertension

Coronary artery disease
Acute myocardial infarction
Severe coronary disease (two- to three-vessel disease)

Cardiomyopathy

Conduction system fibrosis

physiological splitting of the second heart sound. Left bundle branch block may cause reverse splitting of the second sound. Patients with intraventricular conduction disturbances may complain of syncope. This is due to intermittent complete heart block or to ventricular tachyarrhythmias. ECG monitoring and electrophysiological study is needed to determine the cause of syncope in these patients.

CAUSES

Right bundle branch block (Table 11.11) occurs as an isolated congenital anomaly or is associated with right ventricular volume overload. Left bundle branch block (Table 11.12) is almost always caused by disease of the left ventricle. All forms of intraventricular conduction disturbance may be caused by ischaemic heart disease and cardiomyopathy.

Table 11.13 Causes of atrial arrhythmias.

Ischaemic heart disease
Rheumatic heart disease
Thyrotoxicosis
Cardiomyopathy
Lone atrial fibrillation (i.e. no cause discovered)
Wolff–Parkinson–White syndrome
Pneumonia
Atrial septal defect
Carcinoma of the bronchus
Pericarditis
Pulmonary embolus
Acute and chronic alcohol abuse

Conduction system fibrosis and calcification (Lenegre's disease and Lev's disease, see above) are progressive conditions that may present with bundle branch block or bifascicular block and eventually lead to complete heart block, when a pacemaker will be required.

PATHOLOGICAL TACHYCARDIAS

Atrial tachyarrhythmias

Ectopic beats, tachycardia, flutter and fibrillation may all arise from the atrial myocardium. They share common aetiologies, which are listed in Table 11.13.

Atrial ectopic beats
These often cause no symptoms although they may be sensed as an irregularity or heaviness of the heart beat. On the ECG they appear as early and abnormal P waves, and are usually, but not always, followed by normal QRS complexes (see Fig 11.40a).

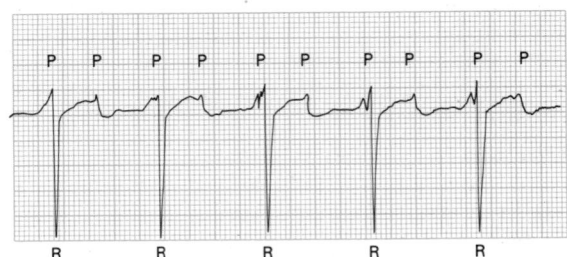

Fig. 11.39 Atrial tachycardia with second-degree atrioventricular block. Note the fast atrial (P wave) rate of 150 per minute and the slower ventricular (R wave) rate of 75 per minute. This arrhythmia is most commonly due to digoxin toxicity.

Treatment is not normally required unless the ectopic beats provoke more significant arrhythmias, when beta-blockade is usually effective.

Atrial tachycardia

This is an uncommon arrhythmia. (Previously, arrhythmias arising from the AV junction were wrongly called 'atrial tachycardias'.) There are three varieties of true atrial tachycardia:

- Paroxysmal tachycardia
- Chronic tachycardia
- Atrial tachycardia with block

All are usually associated with heart disease, but chronic atrial tachycardia may occur in young children with no obvious heart disease. Atrial tachycardia with block is often a result of digitalis poisoning.

Figure 11.39 demonstrates an atrial tachycardia at an atrial rate of 150 beats per minute. The P waves are abnormally shaped and occur in front of the QRS complexes. Carotid sinus massage may increase AV block during tachycardia but does not usually terminate the arrhythmia. Treatment with class Ia, Ic or III drugs (see p. 560) is usually successful, e.g. disopyramide $2 \text{ mg} \cdot \text{kg}^{-1}$ over 10 min.

Atrial flutter

This is a rhythm disturbance that is almost always associated with organic heart disease. The atrial rate varies between 280 and 350 beats per minute but is usually around 300 beats per minute.

Symptoms are largely related to the degree of AV block. Most often, every second flutter beat conducts, giving a ventricular rate of 150 beats per

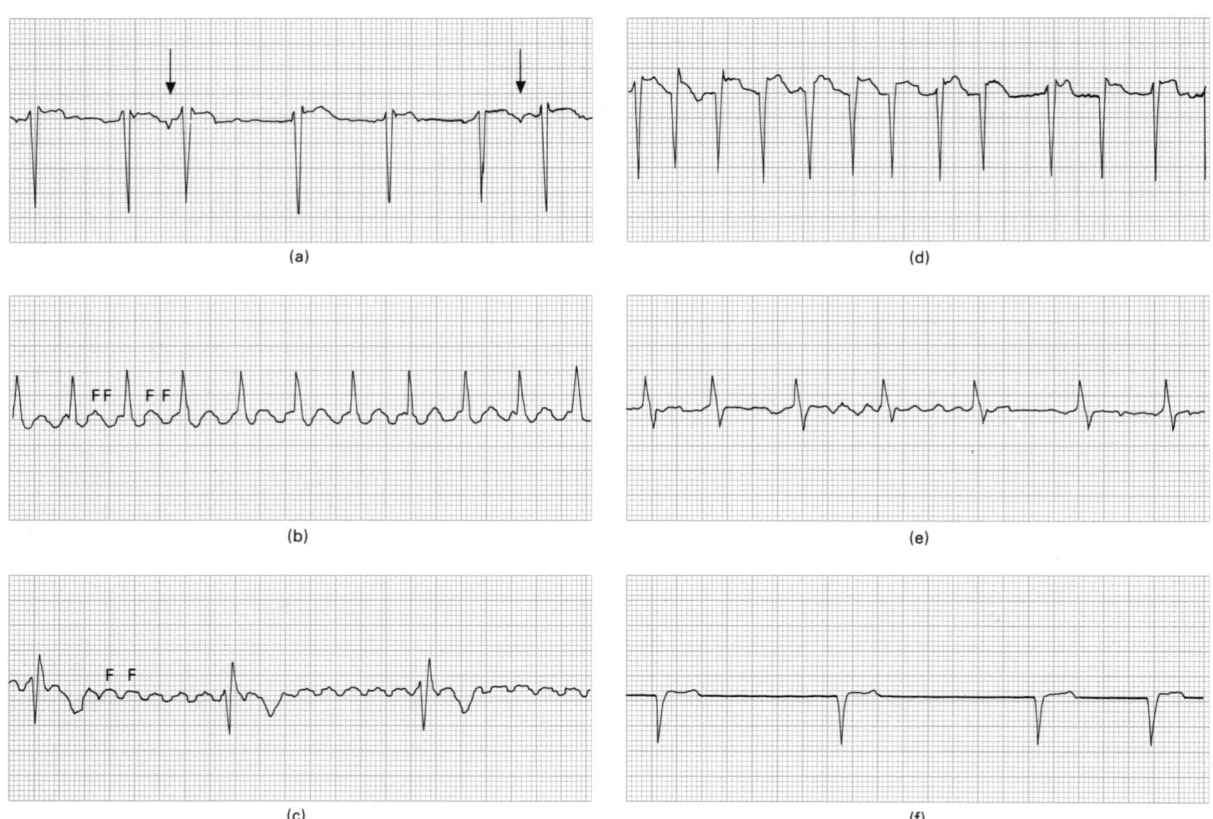

Fig. 11.40 ECGs of a variety of atrial arrhythmias. (a) Atrial premature beats (arrows). The premature P wave is different to the sinus P wave and conducts to the ventricle with a slightly prolonged PR interval. (b) Atrial flutter. The flutter waves are marked with an F. In this case the flutter frequency is 270 per minute. Every second flutter wave is transmitted to the ventricles, and the ventricular rate is therefore 135 per minute. (c) Atrial flutter at a frequency of 305 per minute. The ventricular rate is approximately 38 per minute. Therefore, only one in eight flutter waves is transmitted to the ventricles. (d) Irregular ventricular response. This is typical of rapidly conducted atrial fibrillation. (e) Moderate conduction of atrial fibrillation. The underlying baseline undulations can now be appreciated. (f) So-called 'slow' atrial fibrillation. The ventricular response rate is slow and the underlying atrial fibrillation is seen as minor fluctuations of the baseline.

minute. Occasionally, every beat conducts, producing a heart rate of 300 beats per minute. More often, especially when patients are receiving treatment, AV conduction block reduces the heart rate to approximately 75 beats per minute.

The ECG shows regular sawtooth-like atrial flutter waves (F waves) between QRST complexes (Fig. 11.40b and c). If they are not clearly visible, AV conduction may be transiently impaired by carotid sinus massage or by the administration of AV nodal blocking drugs such as verapamil.

Treatment of an acute paroxysm is electrical cardioversion. Prophylaxis is achieved with class Ia, Ic or III drugs (see p. 560). If the arrhythmia is chronic, AV nodal blocking drugs (classes II or IV, or digitalis) are used.

Atrial fibrillation

This is a common arrhythmia, occurring in between 5 and 10% of patients over 65 years of age. It also occurs, particularly in a paroxysmal form, in younger patients. It is caused by a raised atrial pressure, increased atrial muscle mass, atrial fibrosis, or inflammation and infiltration of the atrium.

Atrial fibrillation is continuous, rapid (400 or more beats per minute) activation of the atria. The atria respond electrically at this rate but there is practically no mechanical action and only a proportion of the impulses are conducted.

The aetiology (see Table 11.13) includes most cardiac disorders, but in some patients no cause can be found—'lone atrial fibrillation'. Thyrotoxicosis may provoke atrial fibrillation, sometimes as virtually the only feature of the disease (apathetic hyperthyroidism). Thyroid function tests are mandatory in any patient with unaccounted atrial fibrillation. When caused by rheumatic mitral stenosis, the onset of atrial fibrillation results in considerable worsening of cardiac failure.

Clinically the patient has a totally irregular pulse, as opposed to a basically regular pulse with an occasional irregularity (e.g. extra-systoles) or recurring irregular patterns (e.g. Wenckebach block). The irregular nature of the pulse in atrial fibrillation is maintained during exercise.

The ECG shows fine oscillations of the baseline (so-called fibrillation or f waves) and no clear P waves. The QRS rhythm is rapid and irregular. Untreated, the ventricular rate is usually 120–180 beats per minute, but it slows with treatment (Fig. 11.40d, e and f).

When atrial fibrillation is due to an acute precipitating event such as alcohol toxicity, chest infection or thyrotoxicosis, the provoking cause should be treated before attempting to convert the arrhythmia. Conversion to sinus rhythm can then be achieved by electrical DC-cardioversion (see p. 544) in about 80% of patients.

Intravenous infusion of some anti-arrhythmic drugs, e.g. classes Ia, Ic and III drugs, is often

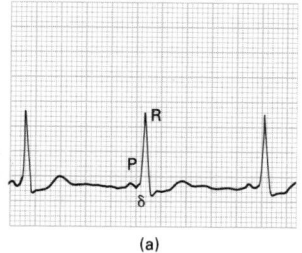

(a)

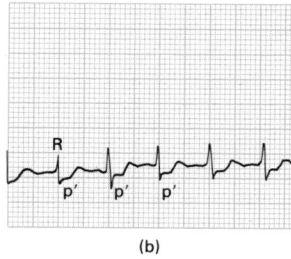

(b)

Fig. 11.41 An ECG showing Wolff–Parkinson–White syndrome. (a) A trace taken during sinus rhythm demonstrating a short PR interval (0.09 s) and broad QRS complex (0.12 s). (b) A trace demonstrating the paroxysmal junctional tachycardia associated with this syndrome. Notice the tachycardia p' waves, which closely follow each QRS complex. δ = delta wave.

used to restore sinus rhythm. This is known as medical cardioversion. Electrical cardioversion is often also necessary. Recurrent paroxysms may be prevented by oral medication with class Ia, Ic or III drugs.

If the arrhythmia is chronic and cannot be converted to sinus rhythm, AV nodal blocking drugs should be used to control the ventricular response rate. The most usual drug for this purpose is digoxin.

Anticoagulation is advised for patients with atrial fibrillation if the cause is mitral valve disease. It is often given for recurrent paroxysms of atrial fibrillation if the cause is alcoholic heart disease (unless the patient is still drinking), thyrotoxicosis or sick sinus syndrome, because of the risk of atrial thrombosis and embolism.

Junctional tachycardia

Almost all junctional tachycardia is paroxysmal in nature. There is usually no associated structural heart disease but there may be demonstrable electrophysiological or electrocardiographic abnormalities such as the Wolff–Parkinson–White syndrome (Fig. 11.41) (see p. 555) or the Lown–Ganong–Levine syndrome (in which there is an anomalous connection between the atrium and the bundle of His).

There are two main varieties of junctional tachycardia:

- Intra-AV nodal tachycardia
- Atrioventricular tachycardia

Both tachycardias are re-entry in type. In the intra-AV nodal re-entry tachycardia the entire tachycardia circuit is confined to the AV node and its surrounding myocardium. In atrioventricular re-entry tachycardia there is a large circuit comprising the AV node, the His bundle, the ventricle, an abnormal connection and the atrium. The abnormal connection linking the ventricle to the atrium completes the circuit necessary to sustain the tachycardia.

Typically, the tachycardia strikes suddenly without obvious provocation, but exertion, coffee, tea and alcohol may aggravate or induce the arrhythmia. The rhythm is rapid (140–280 beats per minute) and regular. An attack may stop spontaneously or may continue indefinitely until medical intervention. The predominant symptom is palpitations, but chest pain, dyspnoea and polyuria may develop. The polyuria occurs because tachycardia leads to an elevated atrial pressure and the release of atrial natriuretic peptide and other hormones.

The rhythm is recognized by normal QRS complexes at a rate of 140–280 beats per minute. Sometimes the QRS complexes will show typical bundle branch block (aberration). The P waves may occur simultaneously with the QRS complex (AV nodal tachycardia) or just after the QRS in the ST segment or the T wave (atrioventricular tachycardia).

TREATMENT

An acute paroxysm of tachycardia is easy to treat.

Carotid sinus massage

Carotid sinus massage is performed for three reasons:

- To break supraventricular tachycardia by blocking AV nodal conduction
- To reveal on the ECG the P wave pattern of an atrial arrhythmia by reducing the frequency of AV nodal conduction during the tachycardia so that the QRS complexes do not mask the atrial activity
- To test for carotid sinus hypersensitivity, which is a severe fall in blood pressure or heart rate in response to carotid sinus stimulation

Carotid sinus massage is performed by locating the carotid pulse, ensuring that no bruit is present, and rubbing the carotid with a circular motion for 5–10 s.

Each carotid should be tried in turn. In general, right carotid pressure tends to slow the sinus rate and left carotid pressure tends to impair AV nodal conduction.

Vagotonic manoeuvres

Most supraventricular arrhythmias require conduction through the AV node for their continuation or their expression at ventricular level. An intense efferent vagal discharge increases AV nodal conduction time and the AV nodal recovery time. Thus, atrial arrhythmias may be revealed by

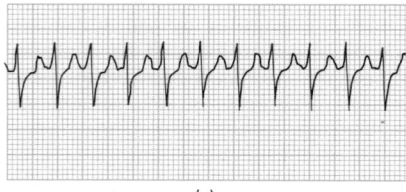

(a)

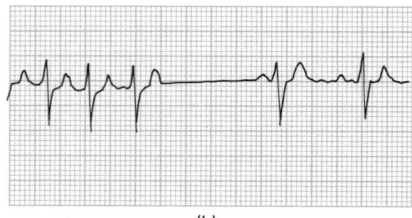

(b)

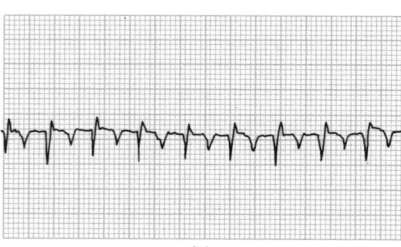

(c)

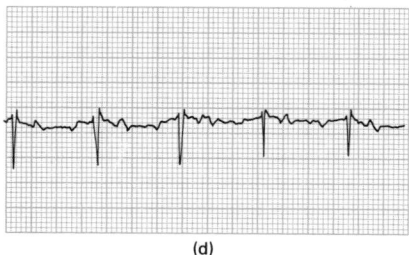

(d)

Fig. 11.42 Two examples of the slowing of tachycardia following the administration of anti-arrhythmic drugs. (a) A supraventricular tachycardia (rate = 205 beats per minute) before treatment with verapamil. (b) The result 60 s later. The tachycardia slows to 130 beats per minute before terminating abruptly and revealing sinus rhythm. (c) Atrial tachycardia at a rate of 170 beats per minute. It is difficult to discern the atrial tachycardia waves. Verapamil is administered and the result is shown in (d). Now the atrial tachycardia is easily seen. The proportion of atrial tachycardia beats transmitted to the ventricles has been reduced following the administration of verapamil.

vagotonic stimulation, which blocks the transmission of these arrhythmias to the ventricles, and junctional tachycardias that involve continuous circulation (circus movement or re-entry) involving the AV node may be terminated by these manoeuvres.

Carotid sinus massage, ocular pressure, immersion of the face in water (diving reflex) and the Valsalva manoeuvre may be used to stimulate the vagal efferent discharge. Of these techniques the Valsalva manoeuvre is the best and often easier for the patient to preform successfully. It should be performed when the patient is resting in the supine position (thus avoiding elevated background sympathetic tone). Several seconds after the release of strain, the resulting intense vagal effect may terminate a junctional re-entry tachycardia or may produce sufficient AV block to reveal an underlying atrial tachyarrhythmia.

Drug treatment

If physical manoeuvres have not been successful, intravenous adenosine (up to 0.25 mg·kg^{-1}) may be tried. This is a very short-acting (half-life = 13 s) naturally occurring purine nucleoside that causes complete heart block for a fraction of a second following intravenous administration. It is highly effective at terminating junctional tachycardias or revealing atrial tachycardias. It rarely affects ventricular tachycardia. The side-effects of adenosine are very brief but include bronchospasm, chest pain and heaviness of the limbs. An alternative treatment is verapamil 10 mg given i.v. over 5–10 min (Fig. 11.42). It is important not to give verapamil if beta-blockers have been previously administered or if the tachycardia presents with broad (> 0.14 s) QRS complexes.

Other treatments

Rarely, medical therapy fails to terminate a tachycardia and rapid atrial pacing (directly or via the oesophagus) or DC-cardioversion may be considered.

Prophylaxis

To prevent recurrences, drugs may be used to impair AV nodal conduction (classes II and IV and digoxin), impair abnormal connection conduction (classes Ia and III) or suppress the ectopic beats that initiate the arrhythmia (classes I, II and III) (see p. 560).

Wolff–Parkinson–White (WPW) syndrome

This is a congenital condition caused by an abnormal myocardial connection between atrium and ventricle (bundle of Kent). During sinus rhythm the electrical impulse can conduct quickly over this abnormal connection to depolarize the ventricles abnormally. This results in the typical ECG pattern of WPW syndrome—a short PR interval and a wide QRS complex that begins as a slurred part known as the delta wave (see Fig. 11.41). About half of those with WPW pattern on the ECG have tachycardias (see Fig. 11.41b). The tachycardias are of two sorts:

- *Atrioventricular re-entry.* This is a circus movement tachycardia in which a depolarization wave travels from the atrium to the ventricle, usually through the AV node, and from the ventricle to the atrium through the abnormal pathway. Intravenous verapamil will terminate most of these tachycardias.
- *Atrial fibrillation.* During atrial fibrillation the ventricles may be depolarized by impulses travelling over both the abnormal and the normal pathways. The conduction ability of the abnormal pathway is depressed by drugs that affect the atrium (e.g. disopyramide and amiodarone) but not by verapamil and digoxin, which, paradoxically , may improve conduction over the abnormal pathway. Therefore, neither verapamil nor digoxin should be used to treat atrial fibrillation associated with the WPW syndrome.

Patients with frequent tachyarrhythmias should have appropriate prophylactic therapy as above, but some require surgery. The operation is designed to locate and destroy the accessory pathway.

Table 11.14 Causes of prolonged repolarization syndrome (long QT interval and torsades de pointes tachycardia).

Congenital syndromes
Jervell–Lange–Nielsen (autosomal recessive)
Romano–Ward (autosomal dominant)

Electrolyte abnormalities
Hypokalaemia
Hypomagnesaemia
Hypocalcaemia

Drugs
Quinidine (and other class 1a anti-arrhythmic drugs)
Amiodarone (and other class III anti-arrhythmic drugs)
Amitriptyline (and other tricyclic antidepressants)
Chlorpromazine (and other phenothiazine drugs)

Poisons
Organophosphate insecticides

Miscellaneous
Bradycardia
Mitral valve prolapse
Acute myocardial infarction
Prolonged fasting and liquid protein diets (long term)
Central nervous system diseases

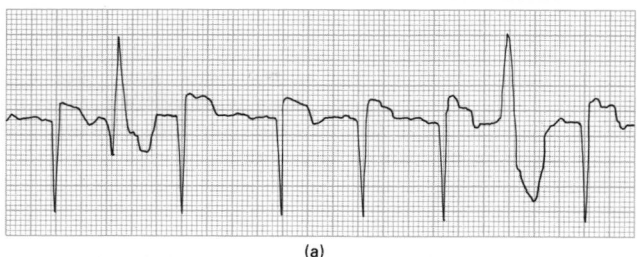

(a)

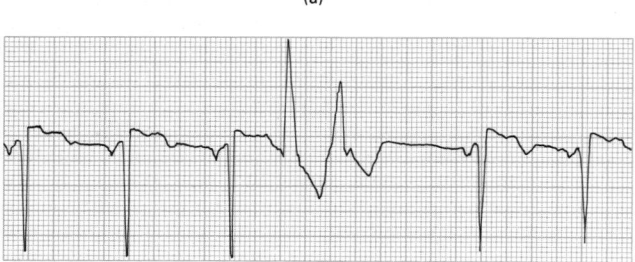

(b)

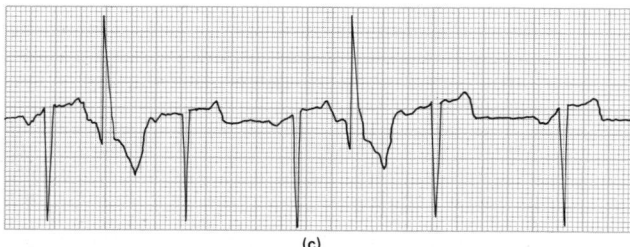

(c)

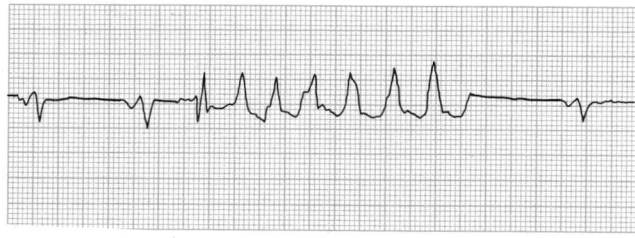

(d)

Fig. 11.43 Varieties of ventricular ectopic activity. (a) Two ventricular ectopic beats of different morphology (multi-morphological). (b) Two ventricular premature beats (VPBs) occurring one after the other (a pair or couplet of VPBs). (c) Frequently repetitive ventricular ectopic activity of a single morphology. (d) A brief run of ventricular tachycardia (non-sustained ventricular tachycardia) that follows previous ectopic activity.

Table 11.15 Grading system for ventricular premature beats (VPBs) following acute myocardial infarction, as proposed by Lown.

Grade	Description
0	No VPBs
1	Occasional VPBs (< 30/h, not > 1/min)
2	Frequent VPBs (≥ 30/h)
3	Multiform VPBs
4A	Couplets (two consecutive VPBs)
4B	Repetitive VPBs (3 or more)
5	Early VPBs (R-on-T)

Ventricular tachyarrhythmias

There are four main types of ventricular tachyarrhythmia:

- Ventricular premature beats
- Ventricular tachycardia
- Ventricular fibrillation
- Torsades de pointes (twisting of points)

Except for torsades de pointes, most ventricular arrhythmias are caused by coronary heart disease, hypertension or cardiomyopathy. Torsades de pointes arises when ventricular repolarization is greatly prolonged (long QT interval). The causes of QT prolongation and torsades de pointes are listed in Table 11.14. Congenital QT prolongation may be associated with syncope, and torsades de pointes which may cause sudden death. Congenital QT prolongation may (Jervell–Lange–Nielsen syndrome) or may not (Romano–Ward syndrome) be associated with congenital deafness.

Ventricular premature beats

These may be uncomfortable, especially when frequent. The patient may complain of extra beats, missed beats or heavy beats because it may be the premature beat, the post-ectopic pause or the next sinus beat that is noticed by the patient. The pulse is irregular owing to the premature beats. Some early beats may not be felt at the wrist. When a premature beat occurs regularly after every normal beat, 'pulsus bigeminus' may occur.

On the ECG (Fig. 11.43) the premature beat has a broad (> 0.12 s) and bizarre QRS complex because it arises from an abnormal (ectopic) site in the ventricular myocardium. Following the premature beat there is usually a complete compensatory pause because the timing of sinus rhythm is not influenced by the premature beat.

Ventricular premature beats have been graded in order of severity. The 'Lown Classification' (Table 11.15) is designed for premature beats occurring in the setting of acute myocardial infarction, but has been wrongly applied to other situations. This is particularly true of R-on-T ventricular premature beats (occurring simultaneously with the upstroke or peak of the T wave of the previous beat). Following myocardial infarction, such premature beats may induce ventricular fibrillation. This is extremely uncommon in other circumstances.

Treatment of ventricular ectopics may be advised because of symptoms or because they may provoke or threaten to provoke more serious arrhythmias. If structural heart disease is present and premature beats are frequent or run together (three or more beats at a time), treatment is offered. Drugs from classes I, II or III (see p. 560) are used. In the absence of heart disease, ventricular premature beats may safely be ignored.

Ventricular tachycardia

This is defined as three or more ventricular beats occurring at a rate of 120 beats per minute or more. Often the patient will be hypotensive and ill but some ventricular tachycardias are well tolerated.

Examination reveals a pulse rate of 120–220 beats per minute. Usually there are clinical signs of atrioventricular dissociation, i.e. intermittent cannon *a* waves and variable intensity of the first heart sound.

Table 11.16 ECG distinction between supraventricular tachycardia (SVT) with bundle branch block and ventricular tachycardia (VT).

VT is more likely than SVT with bundle branch block when there is:

1 A very broad QRS (> 0.14 s)
2 AV dissociation
3 A bifid, upright QRS with a taller first peak in V_1
4 A deep S wave in V_6
5 A concordant (same polarity) QRS direction in all chest leads (V_1–V_6)

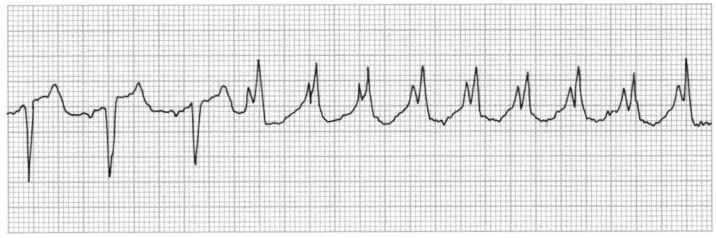

Fig. 11.44 ECG rhythm strip. Ventricular tachycardia at a rate of 140 beats per minute following three sinus beats at a rate of 92 beats per minute.

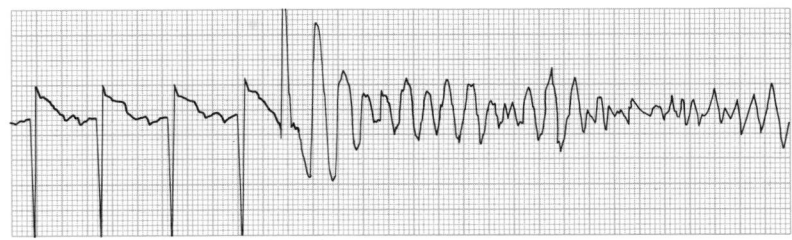

Fig. 11.45 A rhythm strip demonstrating four beats of sinus rhythm followed by a ventricular ectopic beat that initiates ventricular fibrillation. The ST segment during sinus rhythm is elevated owing to acute myocardial infarction.

The ECG shows a rapid ventricular rhythm with broad (often 0.14 s or more), abnormal QRS complexes. Dissociated P wave activity may be seen (Fig. 11.44). Supraventricular tachycardia with bundle branch block (aberration) may resemble ventricular tachycardia on the ECG; the diagnostic features are indicated in Table 11.16. In all cases of doubt, a ventricular tachycardia should be diagnosed.

Treatment may be urgent depending on the haemodynamic situation. If the cardiac output and the blood pressure are very depressed, emergency DC-cardioversion must be considered. On the other hand, if the blood pressure and cardiac output are well maintained, intravenous therapy with class I drugs is usually advised. First-line drug treatment consists of lignocaine (50–100 mg i.v. over 5 min) followed by a lignocaine infusion (2–4 mg·min^{-1} i.v.). DC-cardioversion may be necessary if medical therapy is unsuccessful. The administration of multiple anti-arrhythmic drugs should be avoided.

Prophylaxis against relapse is extremely important. If possible, the likely success of therapy should be judged by Holter monitoring, exercise testing or other provocative techniques. Initial therapy is usually with a beta-blocker if exercise induces the arrhythmia, or a class I drug if exercise is not responsible. If these drugs fail, a class III drug such as amiodarone or sotalol is tried. When severe left ventricular dysfunction is present, most anti-arrhythmic drugs cannot be used because they cause further depression of myocardial function (negative inotropic effect). In such cases amiodarone or mexiletine may be the agent of choice.

Ventricular fibrillation

This is very rapid and irregular ventricular activation with no mechanical effect. The patient is pulseless and becomes rapidly unconscious, and respiration ceases. The ECG shows shapeless, rapid oscillations and there is no hint of organized complexes (Fig. 11.45). It is usually provoked by a ventricular ectopic beat (especially in acute myocardial infarction), ventricular tachyardia or torsades de pointes. Ventricular fibrillation rarely reverses spontaneously. The only effective treatment is electrical defibrillation or, on rare occasions, intravenous bretylium 5–10 mg·kg^{-1} over 5 min. Basic and advanced cardiac life support is needed (see p. 541).

If the attack of ventricular fibrillation occurs during the first day or two of an acute myocardial infarction, it is probable that prophylactic therapy will be unnecessary. If the ventricular fibrillation was not related to an acute infarction, prophylaxis with anti-arrhythmic drugs, especially amiodarone or beta-blockers, and possibly an implantable defibrillator (see p. 560) may be necessary.

Torsades de pointes (see Table 11.14)

This arrhythmia is usually short in duration and spontaneously reverts to sinus rhythm. It does, however, give rise to presyncope or syncope and occasionally converts to ventricular fibrillation, and sudden death may occur. It is characterized on the ECG by rapid, irregular, sharp complexes that continuously change from an upright to an inverted position (Fig. 11.46). Between spells of tachycardia the ECG shows a prolonged QT interval: the corrected QT (see Table 11.9) is equal

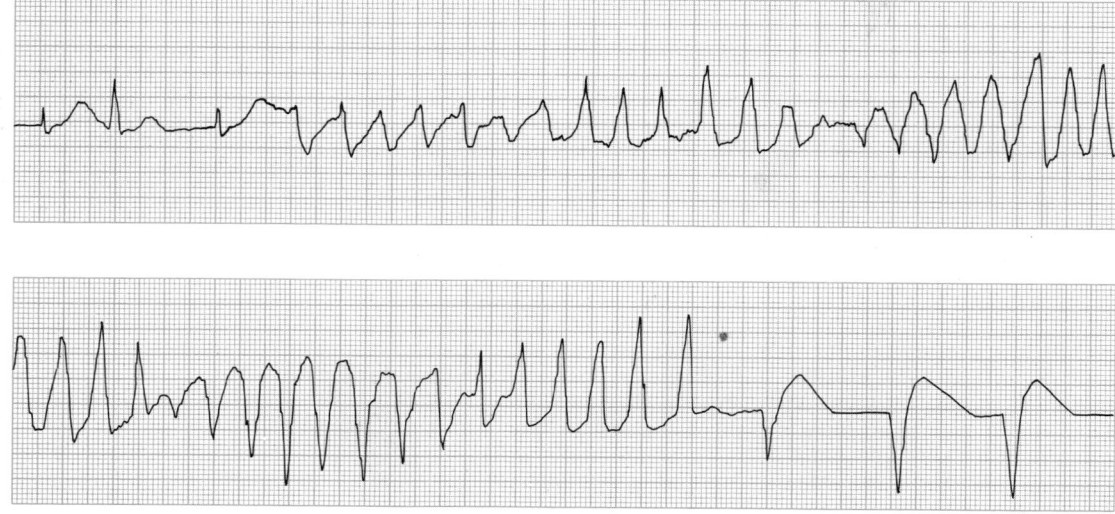

Fig. 11.46 An ECG demonstrating a supraventricular rhythm with a long QT interval giving way to atypical ventricular tachycardia (torsades de pointes). The tachycardia is short-lived and is followed by a brief period of idioventricular rhythm.

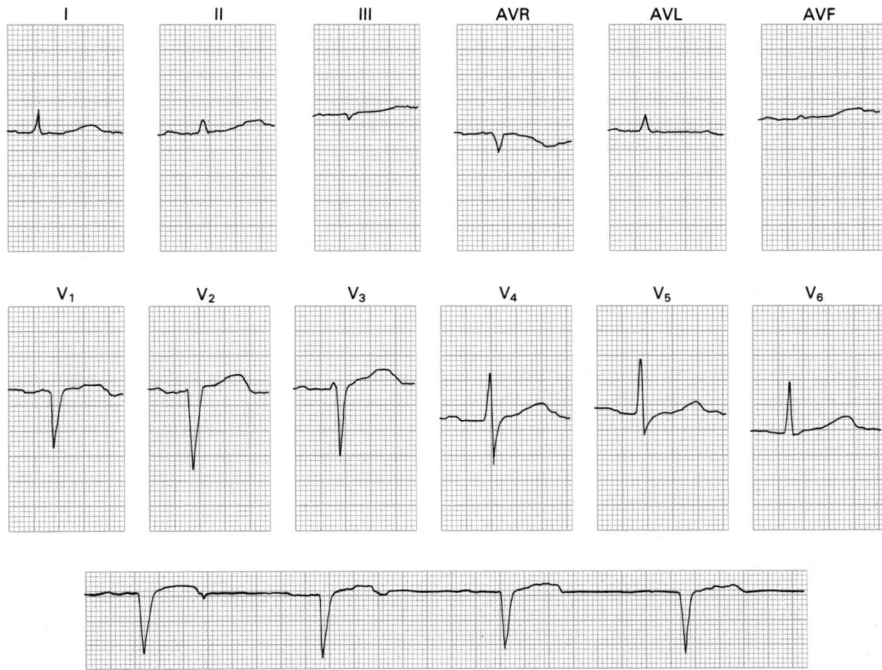

Fig. 11.47 A 12-lead ECG from an 11-year-old child with a history of syncope, demonstrating sinus bradycardia with a long QT interval (560 ms). The ECG is typical of the hereditary long QT syndrome.

to or greater than 440 ms.

Figure 11.47 shows a further example of a prolonged QT interval. The arrhythmia is treated as follows:

● Any electrolyte disturbance is corrected.
● Causative drugs are stopped.
● The heart rate is maintained with atrial or ventricular pacing.
● Intravenous isoprenaline may be effective when QT prolongation is acquired.
● Beta-blockade or left stellectomy is advised if the QT prolongation is congenital. (Isoprenaline is contraindicated for congenital long QT syndrome.)

MANAGEMENT OF ARRHYTHMIAS

Many cardiac arrhythmias are symptomatic, and some are life-threatening. Treatment is directed towards relieving symptoms and removing the threat to life. Usually arrhythmias can only be suppressed, but occasionally, for example with surgical treatment, a complete cure can be effected.

Arrhythmias such as ventricular tachycardia must be terminated, but others, such as atrial fibrillation, may not easily convert to sinus rhythm. In this case, control of the ventricular rate response is the best treatment available.

Arrhythmias can be managed by a wide variety of means (Table 11.17), ranging from simple

techniques that increase vagal tone to expensive and sophisticated treatments such as surgery or implantable electronic devices. Because of the large numbers of patients who suffer from arrhythmias, anti-arrhythmic drugs remain the most important form of treatment.

Anti-arrhythmic drugs

Drugs that modify the rhythm and conduction of the heart may be used to prevent cardiac arrhythmias. It is important to realize that all such drugs may aggravate or produce arrhythmias. They may also depress ventricular contractility and must therefore be used with caution. There are more than 30 anti-arrhythmic drugs. They are classified

Table 11.17 Management of arrhythmias.

Aims
Cure
Prevention (suppression)
Termination
Reduction of ventricular rate

Techniques available
Vagotonic methods
DC cardioversion
Anti-arrhythmic drugs
Pacemakers and other electronic devices
Surgery and other ablation methods

Table 11.18 Vaughan Williams' classification of anti-arrhythmic drugs.

Class I	
Ia	Quinidine, procainamide, disopyramide
Ib	Lignocaine, mexiletine, tocainide
Ic	Flecainide, Propafenone
Class II	Beta-adrenergic blocking drugs
Class III	Amiodarone, sotalol, bretylium
Class IV	Verapamil, diltiazem

according to their effect on the action potential (Vaughan Williams' classification; see Table 11.18 and Fig. 11.48).

Class I drugs
These are membrane-depressant drugs that reduce the rate of entry of sodium into the cell. They may slow conduction, delay recovery or reduce the spontaneous discharge rate of myocardial cells.

Class Ia drugs (e.g. disopyramide) lengthen the action potential, Class Ib drugs (e.g. lignocaine) shorten the action potential, and Class Ic (flecainide, propafenone) do not affect the duration of the action potential.

In one post-infarction study in the USA (cardiac arrhythmia suppression trial—CAST), mortality in the patient group receiving flecainide was twice that of the control group. In view of this, flecainide should be reserved for life-threatening ventricular arrhythmias or supraventricular arrhythmias causing disabling symptoms.

Class II drugs
These anti-sympathetic drugs prevent the effects of catecholamines on the action potential. Most are beta-adrenergic antagonists. Cardioselective beta-blockers (beta-1) include metoprolol, atenolol and acebutalol.

Class III drugs
These prolong the action potential and do not affect sodium transport through the membrane. There are two major drugs in this class: amiodarone and sotalol. Sotalol is also a beta-blocker.

Class IV drugs (Table 11.24)
These are calcium antagonists that reduce the plateau phase of the action potential. They are particularly effective at slowing conduction in nodal tissue. Verapamil is the most important drug in this group. Nifedipine is also a calcium antagonist but has less effect on nodal tissue. Diltiazem has important anti-arrhythmic effects.

Another clinically important classification is based on the part of the heart that is affected by the anti-arrhythmic drug (Fig. 11.49).

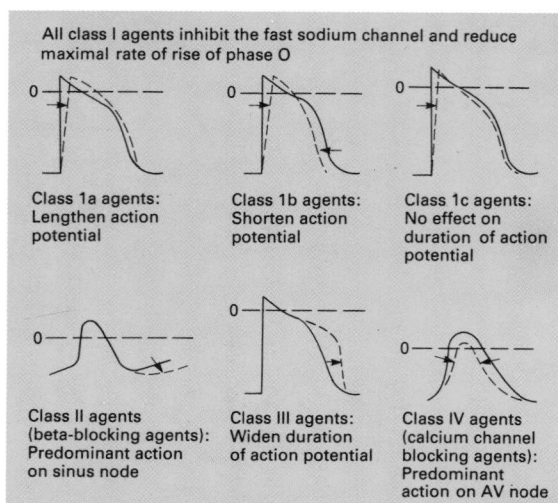

All class I agents inhibit the fast sodium channel and reduce maximal rate of rise of phase O

Class 1a agents: Lengthen action potential

Class 1b agents: Shorten action potential

Class 1c agents: No effect on duration of action potential

Class II agents (beta-blocking agents): Predominant action on sinus node

Class III agents: Widen duration of action potential

Class IV agents (calcium channel blocking agents): Predominant action on AV node

Fig. 11.48 Vaughan Williams' classification of anti-arrhythmic drugs based on their effect on cardiac action potentials. O = 0 mV. The dotted curves indicate the effects of the drugs.

Important features of the major anti-arrhythmic drugs are given in Table 11.19.

Other management techniques

Although anti-arrhythmic drugs are the mainstay of tachycardia treatment, other techniques are sometimes necessary. Surgical division of the anomalous connections responsible for the WPW syndrome is now possible with virtually no surgical mortality and very little morbidity. Ventricular tachycardia can be eradicated by surgical removal of the focus of the arrhythmia, but this operation carries considerable risk and is reserved for very serious problems. It is now possible to destroy the AV node or His bundle by electrical energy delivered through a catheter electrode and discharged close to the AV conduction system. This procedure effectively prevents the conduction of atrial arrhythmias or interrupts the circuit responsible for the arrhythmias. In any case a ventricular pacemaker is then needed to prevent ventricular bradycardia. Pacemakers of another sort can also be used to interrupt repetitive paroxysms of tachycardia.

Implantable automatic cardioverter–defibrillator

Serious ventricular arrhythmias (ventricular fibrillation or rapid ventricular tachycardia with hypotension) carry a mortality within 1 year of up to 40%. Anti-arrhythmic drug therapy, particularly with amiodarone, may reduce the mortality. An important alternative therapy is the implantable cardioverter–defibrillator (ICD), which can recognize ventricular tachycardia or fibrillation and

Table 11.19 Details of anti-arrhythmic drugs. (For class II drugs (beta blockers) see Table 11.37.)

	Quinidine	Disopyramide	Lignocaine	Mexiletine	Flecainide	Propafenone	Amiodarone	Sotalol	Verapamil	Dilitiazem	Digoxin
Class:	Ia	Ia	Ib	Ib	Ic	Ic	III	III	IV	IV	N/A
Daily dose:	250–500 mg ×3 orally	100–250 mg ×3 orally	1–4 mg·min⁻¹ (50–150 mg i.v. loading dose)	400–800 mg orally loading 150–300 mg maintenance	100 mg ×2 orally	150 mg ×3 300 mg ×2 or 300 mg ×3	200 mg ×1–2 orally	80–160 mg ×2–3 orally	0.1 mg·kg⁻¹ i.v. 40–160 mg ×3–4 orally	60–120 mg ×3–4 orally	0.25 mg ×1 orally
Protein binding:	75%	40–90%	50–80%	70%	50%	85%	98%	< 10%	90%	80%	25%
Half-life:	6 h	5 h	1½ h	15 h	18 h	6 h	50 days +	24 h	6 h	2–8 h	36 h
Plasma therapeutic range:	2–5 µg·ml⁻¹	3–6 µg·ml⁻¹	2–6 µg·ml⁻¹	0.5–2.0 µg·ml⁻¹	0.2–0.8 µg·ml⁻¹	0.2–1.5 µg·ml⁻¹	0.2–5.0 µg·ml⁻¹	0.3–1.5 µg·ml⁻¹	0.1–0.3 µg·ml⁻¹	0.02–0.16 µg·ml⁻¹	0.3–2.6 nmol·L⁻¹
Indications:	AF PSVT VT VPBs WPW	AF PSVT VT VPBs WPW	VT/VF associated with myocardial infarction	VT, especially after myocardial infarction	VT PSVT WPW	VT/VF PSVT	VT/VF WPW PSVT AF	VT WPW PSVT	PSVT	PSVT	AF/AFL PSVT
Side-effects:	Nausea Diarrhoea Rash Fever Cinchonism Syncope Blood dyscrasia	Hypotension Anti-cholinergic effects Dry mouth Urinary hesitancy Blurred vision Heart failure AV block	Confusion Convulsions	Confusion Tremor Bradycardia Hypotension	Dizziness Visual disturbance Arrhythmo-genesis	Light-headedness Unusual taste Headache Constipation Arrhythmo-genesis	Corneal deposits Photo-sensitivity Skin pigmentation Thyroid disturbance Pulmonary alveolitis Nightmares Liver disease	Ventricular arrhythmias Bradycardia Heart failure Broncho-spasm	Nausea Vomiting Constipation Flushing Headache Bradycardia Fluid retention	Nausea Vomiting Constipation Flushing Headache Bradycardia Fluid retention	Nausea Anorexia Vomiting Visual disturbance Bradycardia

AF = atrial fibrillation.
PSVT = paroxysmal supraventricular tachycardia.
VT = ventricular tachycardia.
VF = ventricular fibrillation.
WPW = Wolff–Parkinson–White syndrome.
AFL = atrial flutter
VPBs = ventricular premature beats.
N/A = not applicable.

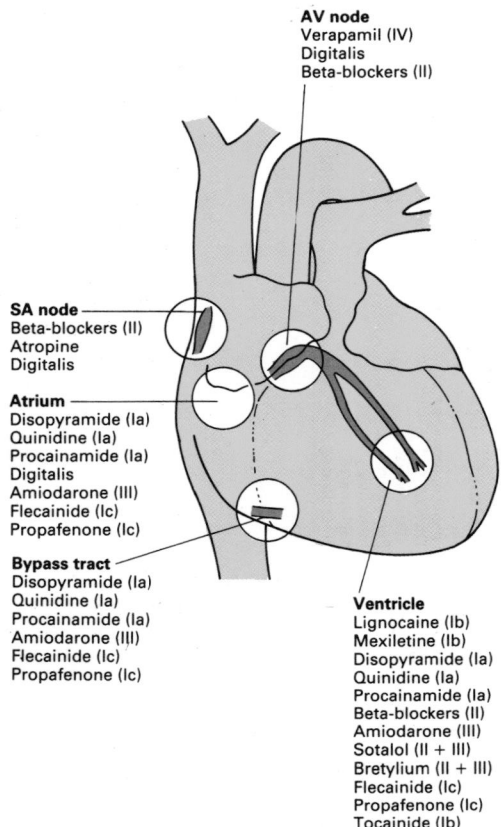

AV node
Verapamil (IV)
Digitalis
Beta-blockers (II)

SA node
Beta-blockers (II)
Atropine
Digitalis

Atrium
Disopyramide (Ia)
Quinidine (Ia)
Procainamide (Ia)
Digitalis
Amiodarone (III)
Flecainide (Ic)
Propafenone (Ic)

Bypass tract
Disopyramide (Ia)
Quinidine (Ia)
Procainamide (Ia)
Amiodarone (III)
Flecainide (Ic)
Propafenone (Ic)

Ventricle
Lignocaine (Ib)
Mexiletine (Ib)
Disopyramide (Ia)
Quinidine (Ia)
Procainamide (Ia)
Beta-blockers (II)
Amiodarone (III)
Sotalol (II + III)
Bretylium (II + III)
Flecainide (Ic)
Propafenone (Ic)
Tocainide (Ib)

Fig. 11.49 Drugs that affect different parts of the heart. The Vaughan Williams class is given in parentheses.

automatically deliver a defibrillating shock to the heart. It is relatively small and is powered by lithium batteries sufficient to provide energy for about 100 shocks each of 25–30 J. The device is usually implanted behind the rectus abdominis muscle and is connected to the heart by several wires and electrodes. When an arrhythmia develops that requires treatment, the device takes about 15 s to recognize the arrhythmia and charge its capacitors. It then delivers the defibrillating discharge. The shock may be painful, particularly if the patient is still fully conscious.

The use of this device has cut the sudden death rate in patients with serious ventricular arrhythmias to between 1 and 2% in the first year. However, because of its expense it is not widely available.

Cardiac failure

Cardiac failure occurs when, despite normal venous pressures, the heart is unable to maintain sufficient cardiac output to meet the demands of the body. The incidence of heart failure is estimated at 10 per 1000 over 65 years of age. Irrespective of the aetiology of heart failure, the prognosis is poor. Approximately 50% of patients with severe heart failure die within 2 years of diagnosis from either progression of heart failure or sudden death. The causes of heart failure include:

● Myocardial dysfunction, e.g. ischaemic heart disease, cardiomyopathy, hypertension
● Volume overload, e.g. valvular regurgitation (aortic and mitral)
● Obstruction to outflow, e.g. aortic stenosis
● Obligatory high-output, e.g. anaemia, thyrotoxicosis, Paget's disease, beri-beri, systemic to pulmonary shunts
● Compromised ventricular filling, e.g. constrictive pericarditis, pericardial tamponade, restrictive cardiomyopathy
● Altered rhythm, e.g. atrial fibrillation

Haemodynamic effects of myocardial failure

When the myocardium begins to fail, its velocity of contraction and the active tension that it is capable of developing are reduced. Factors involved are the venous return, the outflow resistance, the contractility of the myocardium, and salt and water retention.

Venous return (pre-load). In the intact heart, myocardial failure leads to a reduction of the volume of blood ejected with each heart beat and an increase in the volume of blood remaining after systole. This increased diastolic volume stretches the myocardial fibres and, as Starling's law of the heart would suggest, myocardial contraction is restored. However, the failing myocardium results in depression of the ventricular function curve (cardiac output plotted against the ventricular diastolic volume) (see Fig. 11.3).

Slight myocardial depression is not associated with a reduction in cardiac output because it is maintained by an increase in venous pressure (and hence diastolic volume). However, the proportion of blood ejected with each heart beat (ejection fraction) is reduced early in heart failure. Sinus tachycardia also ensures that any reduction of stroke volume is compensated for by the increase in heart rate; cardiac output (stroke volume × heart rate) is therefore maintained.

When there is more severe myocardial dysfunction, cardiac output can only be maintained by a large increase in venous pressure and/or marked sinus tachycardia. This eventually results in further depression of the ventricular function curve and reduced contractility, the resultant increased venous pressure contributes to the development of dyspnoea, owing to the accumulation of interstitial and alveolar fluid, and to the occurrence of hepatic enlargement, ascites and dependent oedema, owing to increased systemic venous pressure. Despite symptoms due to increased venous pressure, the cardiac output at rest may not be much depressed, but myocardial and haemodynamic reserve is so compromised that a normal increase in cardiac output cannot be produced by exercise.

In very severe heart failure the cardiac output at rest is depressed, despite high venous pressures. The inadequate cardiac output is redistributed to maintain perfusion of vital organs, such as the heart, brain and kidneys, at the expense of the skin and muscle.

Outflow resistance (after-load) see Figs 13.2 and 13.4). This is the load or resistance against which the ventricle contracts. It is formed by:

- The pulmonary and systemic resistance
- The physical characteristics of the vessel walls
- The volume of blood that is ejected

An increase in after-load decreases the cardiac output. This decrease in function with further increase of end-diastolic volume and dilatation of the ventricle itself further exacerbates the problem of after-load. This is expressed by Laplace's law: the tension of the myocardium (T) is proportional to the intraventricular pressure (P) multiplied by the radius of the ventricular chamber (R), i.e. $T \propto PR$.

Myocardial contractility (inotropic state). The state of the myocardium also influences performance. Increased contractility (positive inotropism) can result from increased sympathetic drive, and this is a normal part of the Frank–Starling relationship (see Fig. 11.3). Conversely, myocardial depressants (e.g. hypoxia) decrease myocardial contractility (negative inotropism).

Salt and water retention. The increase in venous pressure that occurs when the ventricles fail leads to retention of salt and water and their accumulation in the interstitium, producing many of the physical signs of heart failure. Reduced cardiac output also leads to diminished renal perfusion,

activating the renin–angiotensin system and enhancing fluid retention. This increased salt and water retention further increases venous pressure, which in the early stages of heart failure improves cardiac output by the Starling mechanism. In severe heart failure the ventricular function curve plateaus such that further increases in venous pressure do not provoke an increase in cardiac output. This retention of sodium is in part compensated by the action of circulating atrial naturetic peptides. These are short-chain peptides secreted by the atria in response to distension. These atrial peptides are potent vasodilators with natriuretic properties and levels rise considerably in heart failure. The effect of their action may represent a beneficial, albeit inadequate, compensatory response tending to reduce cardiac load (pre- and after-load) by vasodilatation and by enhancing sodium and water excretion.

Clinical syndromes of heart failure

It is clinically useful to divide heart failure into the syndromes of right, left and biventricular (congestive) but it is rare for any part of the heart to fail in isolation.

Right heart failure
This syndrome occurs in association with:

- Chronic lung disease (cor pulmonale)
- Pulmonary embolism or pulmonary hypertension
- Tricuspid valve disease
- Pulmonary valve disease
- Left to right shunts, e.g. atrial or ventricular septal defects
- Isolated RV cardiomyopathy

The most frequent cause of right heart failure is secondary to left heart failure; other causes being RV infarction, mitral valve disease with pulmonary hypertension.

Symptoms include fatigue, breathlessness, anorexia and nausea and relate to distension and fluid accumulation in areas drained by the systemic veins. The physical signs are usually more prominent than the symptoms, with:

- Jugular venous distension (± v waves of tricuspid regurgitation)
- Tender smooth hepatic enlargement
- Dependent pitting oedema
- Development of free abdominal fluid
- Pleural transudates (commonly right-sided)

Dilatation of the right ventricle produces cardiomegaly and may give rise to functional tricuspid regurgitation. Tachycardia and a right ventricular third heart sound are usual.

Left heart failure
Causes include:

- Ischaemic heart disease (commonest)
- Systemic hypertension (chronic or 'malignant')
- Mitral and aortic valve disease
- Cardiomyopathies

Mitral stenosis causes left atrial hypertension and signs of left heart failure but does not itself cause failure of the left ventricle.

Symptoms are predominantly fatigue, exertional dyspnoea, orthopnoea and paroxysmal nocturnal dyspnoea. Physical signs are few and not prominent until a late stage or if the ventricular failure is acute. Cardiomegaly is demonstrable with a displaced and often sustained apical impulse. Auscultation reveals a left ventricular third or fourth heart sound that, with tachycardia, is described as a gallop rhythm. Dilatation of the mitral annulus results in functional mitral regurgitation. Crackles are heard at the lung bases. In severe left heart failure the patient has pulmonary oedema. In this circumstance a chest X-ray (CXR) is the most useful investigation. Rarely the cause of left ventricular failure is apparent, e.g. ventricular aneurysm at the site of previous infarction.

Biventricular failure (congestive)
This term is used variously but is best restricted to cases where right heart failure is a result of pre-existing left heart failure. The physical signs are thus a combination of the above syndromes.

Acute heart failure
Acute failure of the heart most commonly occurs in the setting of acute myocardial infarction when there is extensive loss of ventricular muscle. The condition may also occur with rupture of the intraventricular septum producing a VSD, or due to acute valvular regurgitation. Common examples are papillary or chordal rupture producing mitral regurgitation or sudden aortic valve regurgitation in infective endocarditis, other causes include obstruction of the circulation due to acute pulmonary embolus and cardiac tamponade. In each case severe cardiac failure can occur with a relatively normal heart size.

High-output heart failure
The heart may not be able to meet the demands placed on it in conditions such as anaemia, thyrotoxicosis, beri-beri, and Gram-negative septicaemia. This form of heart failure presents in much the same manner as low-output states but is associated with tachycardia and a gallop rhythm. Patients are often warm with distended superficial veins. Unlike low-output failure the oxygen content of systemic venous blood is high owing to the delivery of large amounts of arterial blood to non-metabolizing tissues.

Factors aggravating or precipitating heart failure

Any factor that increases myocardial work may aggravate existing heart failure or initiate failure. These factors must be carefully considered in patients who present with heart failure. The most common are arrhythmias, anaemia, thyrotoxicosis, pregnancy, infective endocarditis, pulmonary infection or adjustment of heart failure therapy.

INVESTIGATION

The diagnosis of heart failure is inadequate and a cause should be determined. In many cases the cause will be evident from the clinical history and examination. Investigations are determined by the suspected cause of heart failure and include:

General/diagnostic

- CXR/ECG
- Echocardiography
- Full blood count
- Liver biochemistry
- Urea and electrolytes
- Cardiac enzymes
- Thyroid function
- Cardiac catheterization

Functional/prognostic

- Exercise testing
- Resting and stress radionuclide angiography (MUGA)—ejection fraction, regional wall motion abnormality
- 24–48-hour ambulatory ECG monitoring

Treatment of heart failure

The management of heart failure requires that any factor aggravating the failure should be identified and treated. Similarly the cause of heart failure must be elucidated and where possible corrected. Nursing care of the mouth and pressure areas is necessary and patients should be nursed in a comfortable upright position.

GENERAL TREATMENTS

- *Reduction of physical activity.* Bed rest reduces the demands of the heart and is useful for a few days. Migration of fluid from the interstitium promotes a diuresis, reducing heart failure. Prolonged bed rest may, however, lead to development of deep vein thrombosis; this can be avoided by daily leg exercises, low-dose subcutaneous heparin and elastic support stockings.
- *Dietary modifications.* Large meals should be avoided and if necessary weight reduction instituted. Salt restriction is important and foods rich

in salt or added salt in cooking and at the table should be avoided. A low-sodium diet is unpalatable and of questionable value. Alcohol has a negatively inotropic effect and patients should abstain.

DRUG MANAGEMENT

The pharmacological management of heart failure relies on the following categories of drugs: diuretics; vasodilators; positive inotropic agents, including digitalis glycosides, and antiarrhythmic agents.

Diuretics

Thise form the main basis of treatment of heart failure. They act by promoting the renal excretion of salt and water by blocking tubular reabsorption of sodium and chloride. The resulting loss of fluid reduces ventricular filling pressures (pre-load) and shifts the Starling curve upwards (Fig. 11.3) with an increase in cardiac output. The intravenous administration of loop diuretics such as frusemide relieves pulmonary oedema rapidly by means of arteriolar vasodilatation after-load, an action that is independent of its diuretic effect.

Diuretics act in different ways:
- Loop diuretics such as frusemide and bumetanide act by reducing sodium and chloride reabsorption in the ascending limb of the loop of Henle. They cause a brisk and generally short-lived diuresis as the concentrating power of the kidney is reduced. These agents also produce marked potassium loss and promote hyperuricaemia.
- Thiazide diuretics such as bendrofluazide have a mild diuretic effect and act on the distal convoluted loop, reducing sodium reabsorption. Potassium excretion is enhanced. Metolazone is a powerful thiazide producing profound diuresis acting synergistically with loop diuretics. This combination is useful in treating severe and resistant heart failure.

- Potassium sparing diuretics

Spironolactone is a specific competitive antagonist to aldosterone, producing a weak diuresis but with a potassium-sparing action.

Amiloride and triamterene act at the distal tubule preventing potassium secretion in exchange for sodium. These drugs are weak diuretics but are useful in combination with more powerful loop diuretics. They should be avoided in the presence of renal failure.

Mild heart failure is generally managed with an oral thiazide. Combination with potassium sparing diuretic avoids development of hypokalaemia.

More severe heart failure requires loop diuretics often with the addition of a thiazide (e.g. metolazone) to maintain a diuresis. Too vigorous a diuresis can result in hypovolaemia, hyponatraemia or dilutional hyponatraemia (when sodium is lost in excess of water).

In the presence of acute heart failure or acute or chronic deterioration, diuretics must be administered intravenously because they may not be adequately absorbed.

Vasodilator therapy (Table 11.20)

Diuretics and sodium restriction serve to activate the renin–angiotensin system, promoting formation of angiotensin (a potent vasoconstrictor) and an increase in after-load. A variety of other neural and hormonal reactions also serve to increase pre-load and after-load. These compensatory mechanisms are initially beneficial in maintaining blood pressure and redistributing blood flow, but in the later stages of heart failure they are deleterious and reduce cardiac output. The high venous pressures found in heart failure are also related to the activation of the sympathetic nervous system and the presence of circulating vasoconstrictors, thus shifting the Starling curve to the right.

If diuretics are not sufficient to control heart

Table 11.20 Effects of vasodilator drugs used in heart failure.

	Reduction in	
	Pre-load	After-load
Nitroprusside	+	+++
Glyceryl trinitrate	+++	+
Isosorbide: di/mono nitrate	+++	+
Prazosin	+	++
ACE inhibitors	++	++
Hydralazine	○	+++
Nifedipine	+	++

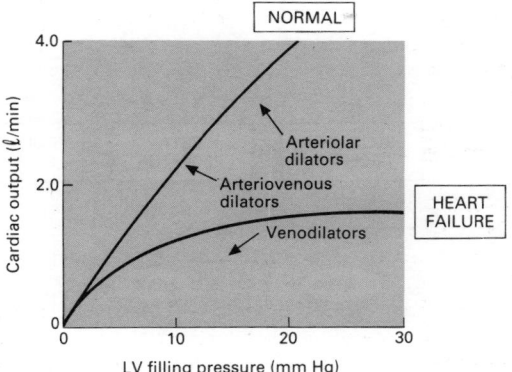

Fig. 11.50 Effect of vasodilators on cardiac output and left ventricular filling pressure. Agents with arteriolar and arteriovenous dilating properties reduce the after-load and increase cardiac output. Venodilators reduce the left ventricular filling pressure (and pulmonary oedema) but do not increase cardiac output.

Table 11.21 Angiotensin converting enzyme inhibitors.

Drug	First dose	Maintenance dose
Captopril	6.25 mg	25–50 mg twice daily
Enalapril	5 mg	10–20 mg daily
Lisinopril	2.5 mg	10–20 mg daily
Perindopril	2 mg	4–8 mg daily

Note:
(a) All ACE inhibitors should be given with caution to patients who have received diuretics when the first dose may cause marked hypotension. It is therefore recommended that the first dose is given at bedtime after witholding diuretics for a few days. In heart failure therapy should be initiated in hospital.
(b) Renal impairment may occur or be aggravated by treatment with ACE inhibitors, particularly when co-administered with non steroidal anti-inflammatory drugs.
(c) Other side effects of ACE inhibitors include: dry cough, loss of taste, rash, abdominal pain and angioedema.

failure, the addition of vasodilators may be beneficial. These agents are now being commenced earlier in the management of heart failure often in place of augmenting the diuretic dose. Many physicians now use an angiotensin converting enzyme inhibitor because long-term therapy with other vasodilators has been disappointing. In addition the CONSENSUS study showed a marked improvement in survival with enalapril.

● *Arteriolar vasodilators* (Fig. 11.50). Drugs such as α-adrenergic blockers (e.g. prazosin), and direct smooth-muscle relaxants (e.g. hydralazine) are potent arteriolar vasodilators. The reduction in after-load that they produce causes an increase in cardiac output. Any tendency to hypotension is usually offset by the increased output.

● *Venodilators* (Fig. 11.50). Short- and long-acting nitrates (e.g. glyceryl trinitrate and isosorbide mononitrate) act by reducing pre-load and lowering venous pressure with resulting reduction in pulmonary and dependant oedema. Reduction of filling pressure does not significantly enhance cardiac output because the heart is operating on the flat portion of the ventricular filling curve. With chronic use, tolerance develops with loss of efficacy and consequent worsening of heart failure.

● *Angiotensin converting enzyme (ACE) inhibitors* (Table 11.21 and Fig. 16.32). ACE inhibitors lower systemic vascular resistance, venous pressure and reduce levels of circulating catecholamines, thus improving myocardial performance. The beneficial haemodynamic effect of these drugs appears to be independent of their inhibition of ACE as they are equally effective when plasma renin activity is normal.

These drugs should be carefully introduced to patients with heart failure because of the risk of first-dose hypotension. This is a particular risk in patients who are receiving large doses of diuretics and in the presence of hyponatraemia (< 130 mmol.L^{-1}). In such cases a test dose of ACE inhibitor should be commenced in hospital and the preceding diuretic dose omitted. Some of these agents are pro-drugs (e.g. enalapril) and require conversion to the active metabolite (enalaprilat) by liver enzymes; these drugs have a delayed onset of action and first-dose hypotension may not occur for several hours. Pro-drugs are best avoided if heart failure results in significantly altered hepatic function. Serious hypotension may result in acute renal failure. Concomitant potassium-sparing diuretics should

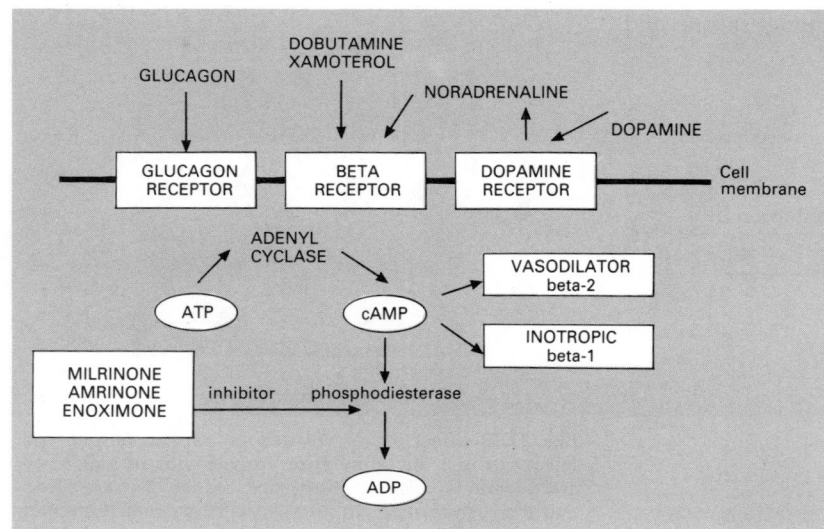

Fig. 11.51 Diagrammatic represenation of the action of inotropic drugs. Dopamine stimulates the myocardium by activating the β₁ adrenergic receptors; it also acts indirectly by releasing noradrenaline from sympathetic nerve terminals. Dopamine is unselective and also activates widespread dopaminergic receptors causing vasodilatation.

Dobutamine and Xamoterol act through the β₁ receptor to produce cAMP.

Phosphodiesterase inhibitors e.g. amrinone prevent the breakdown of cAMP which accumulates and increases contractility and causes vasodilataion by acting on peripheral vascular β₂ receptors.

be discontinued, as ACE inhibitors tend to promote potassium retention.

Inotropic agents (Fig. 11.51)
Recently, several orally active positive inotropic drugs have become available, supplementing those currently available for intravenous use. They can be classified as follows:

- Digitalis glycosides
- Beta-adrenergic agonists
- Phosphodiesterase inhibitors

Efficacy of these agents is variable and must be judged both in terms of objective and symptomatic improvement on an individual patient basis.

- *Digitalis glycosides*. Digitalis glycosides are no longer as extensively used in the management of heart failure, although they remain effective positive inotropic agents in the short term. Digoxin is the most common glycoside in use with a half-life of approximately 36 h. It is highly protein-bound, making it liable to drug interaction. Ninety per cent is excreted unchanged in the urine, causing accumulation in renal failure. Digoxin acts as a positive inotrope by competitive inhibition of sodium–potassium ATPase, producing high intracellular levels of sodium. The intracellular sodium is exchanged for extracellular calcium. High intracellular levels of calcium ions allow increased binding of contractile proteins actin and myosin, enhancing the force of cardiac contractility (Fig. 11.2). Whether this positive inotropic benefit is sustained over time is controversial. Digoxin usage is of particular benefit in congestive heart failure associated with atrial fibrillation when the rapid ventricular response is effectively controlled. Digoxin is usually administered orally (1 mg loading and 0.25 mg daily). In elderly patients and in patients with impaired renal function digoxin may accumulate, resulting in serious toxicity. Careful titration of the dose is important with monitoring of trough serum levels (0.9–2.4 ng·ml^{-1}) and avoidance of hypokalaemia. Patients with hypothyroidism are particularly sensitive to digitalis glycosides. In patients with fluctuating renal function the administration of the liver-metabolized digitoxin may be preferable.

    With improvement in formulation, digoxin toxicity has become less problematic but is prone to occur in the elderly and in patients with renal impairment. The most common features of *digoxin toxicity* are:

    - Anorexia, nausea, altered vision
    - Arrhythmia, e.g. ventricular premature beats especially bigeminy. Ventricular tachycardia and AV block
    - Digoxin levels > 2.5 ng·ml^{-1}

Digoxin toxicity is treated by discontinuing the drug, restoration of serum potassium levels and management of arrhythmias. Digoxin antibodies (Fab fragments) are a specific antidote that may be useful.

- *β-Adrenergic agonists*. Dopamine and dobutamine are adrenergic agonists but are only effective intravenously. Dobutamine is a selective agonist of the beta-1 receptor, increasing intracellular cyclic AMP, which in turn increases calcium availability for the contractile process. Dopamine is a less potent inotrope than dobutamine but because of its unselective action on the adrenergic system it improves renal perfusion. Xamoterol is a beta-blocking drug with high intrinsic sympathomimetic activity (ISA) and is effective in improving cardiac performance. Xamoterol competes competitively with endogenous catecholamines at the beta-1 receptor. At states of low sympathetic tone (rest) this produces a positive inotropic effect together with lowering of filling pressures. At states of high sympathetic tone (e.g. exercise), xamoterol produces a beta-blocking effect, blunting the chronotropic response. In mild to moderate heart failure xamoterol (200 mg twice daily) is as effective as intravenous dobutamine in improving cardiac performance. It is superior to digoxin with respect to improved exercise capacity and symptoms. Chronic high levels of circulating catecholamines in severe heart failure may lead to down-regulation of the beta receptors; the administration of xamoterol to these patients may precipitate acute heart failure.
- *Phosphodiesterase inhibitors*. Amrinone, milrinone and enoximone are in a new class of so called 'inodilator' drugs that act by inhibiting phosphodiesterase, thus preventing breakdown of cyclic AMP. Accumulation of cAMP produces an increase in contractility and also peripheral vasodilatation. The Starling curve is shifted upwards. Although these agents are effective in improving myocardial performance acutely, there is evidence that they have a deleterious effect on myocardial cells when administered in the long term.

Anti-arrhythmic agents
Arrhythmias are frequent in heart failure and are implicated in sudden death. Although treatment of complex ventricular arrhythmias might be expected to improve survival there is conflicting evidence that this is so. Sustained ventricular tachycardia is probably best managed with amiodarone with the addition of a class I agent or a beta blocker with high intrinsic sympathomimetic activity (ISA) such as xamoterol. The use of class I agents may result in deterioration of heart failure owing to their negative inotropic effect. It should be noted that ACE inhibitors probably exert an indirect anti-

arrhythmic effect by reducing high circulating levels of noradrenaline and improving cardiac function. In the future the use of the implantable cardioverter–defibrillator device (ICD) is likely to improve the survival prospects of patients with serious ventricular arrhythmias. Ventricular arrhythmias are frequent occurring in more than 70% of patients with heart failure. The commonest are ventricular ectopics and non-sustained ventricular tachycardia.

CARDIAC TRANSPLANTATION

Since the advent of cyclosporin A in the late 1970s and improved immunosuppression regimens, cardiac transplantation has become the treatment of choice for younger patients with severe intractable heart failure, whose life expectancy is less than 6 months. With careful recipient selection the expected 1-year survival for patients following transplantation is over 80%, and is 70% at 5 years; irrespective of survival, quality of life is dramatically improved for the majority of patients.

PULMONARY OEDEMA

This is a very frightening, life-threatening emergency characterized by extreme breathlessness. The dyspnoea may first occur at night in the form of paroxysmal dyspnoea, when the reabsorption of dependent oedema when lying flat and the relative insensitivity of the respiratory centre at night allow pulmonary congestion to develop. In more severe cases the patient is severely breathless at all times of the day.

PATHOPHYSIOLOGY

Left ventricular failure and mitral valve disease cause pulmonary oedema because of increased pulmonary capillary pressure. A pressure above 20 mm Hg causes increased filtration of fluid out of the capillaries into the interstitial space (interstitial oedema). Further accumulation of fluid disrupts intercellular membranes, leading to the collection of fluid in the alveolar spaces (alveolar oedema). Alveolar oedema occurs when the capillary pressure exceeds the total oncotic pressures (approximately 30 mm Hg).

CLINICAL FEATURES

Patients with alveolar oedema are acutely breathless, wheezing, anxious and perspiring profusely. In addition, they usually have a cough productive of frothy, blood-tinged (pink) sputum, which can be copious. The patient is tachypnoeic with peripheral circulatory shutdown. There is a tachycardia, a raised venous pressure and a gallop rhythm. Crackles and wheeze are heard throughout the chest. The arterial PO_2 falls and initially the P_aCO_2 also falls owing to overbreathing. Later, however, the P_aCO_2 increases because of impaired gas exchange. The chest X-ray shows diffuse haziness due to alveolar fluid and the Kerley B lines of interstitial oedema (see Fig. 11.14). The abnormality can be unilateral, giving the appearance of a tumour that disappears on treatment (a pseudotumour).

TREATMENT

- The patient should be placed in the sitting position.
- High-concentration oxygen (60% via a variable-performance mask) is given unless it is suspected that there is a coexisting chronic hypercapnia due to long-standing respiratory failure. In severe cases it may be necessary to ventilate the patient using positive-pressure techniques (see p. 724).
- Intravenous diuretic treatment with frusemide, bumetanide or ethacrynic acid is given. These diuretics produce *immediate* vasodilatation in addition to the more delayed diuretic response.
- Morphine (10–20 mg i.v. depending on the size of the patient) together with an antiemetic such as metoclopramide (10 mg i.v.) or cyclizine (50 mg i.v.) is given. Morphine sedates the patient and causes systemic vasodilatation; it must be avoided if the systemic arterial pressure is less than 90 mm Hg. Respiratory depression occurs with large doses of morphine.
- Venous vasodilators, such as glyceryl trinitrate, may produce prompt relief by reducing the pre-load. Cardiac output may be increased by using arterial vasodilatation, such as occurs with hydralazine (Table 11.20).
- Aminophylline (250–500 mg or 5 mg·kg^{-1} i.v.) is infused over 10 min. Aminophylline is a phosphodiesterase inhibitor that causes bronchodilatation, vasodilatation and increased cardiac contractility. It must be given slowly because of the risk of precipitating ventricular arrhythmias. It is now only used when bronchospasm is present.
- Venesection and mechanical methods of reducing venous return (e.g. sphygmomanometer cuffs inflated to 10 mm Hg below diastolic blood pressure and placed around the thighs) are rarely used and are usually inefficient.

In a severe case, after the acute emergency is controlled, a pulmonary artery balloon catheter may be inserted to monitor progress and treatment. Any factor that precipitated the heart failure, such as cardiac arrhythmias or chest infection, should be corrected. The underlying cardiac problem should be diagnosed and treated.

CARDIOGENIC SHOCK

Shock is a severe failure of tissue perfusion, usually characterized by hypotension, a low cardiac output and signs of poor tissue perfusion such as oliguria, cold extremities and poor cerebral function. Cardiogenic shock (pump failure) is an extreme type of cardiac failure with a high mortality of approximately 90%. Its most common cause is myocardial infarction.

Cardiogenic shock must be differentiated from other forms of shock. Cardiogenic shock is diagnosed when the shock syndrome occurs despite an adequate or elevated pulmonary capillary wedge pressure and in the absence of mechanical circulatory obstruction. An essential element in this diagnosis is the measurement of the pulmonary capillary wedge pressure (see p. 715). In situations where the vascular capacity has expanded or the circulatory fluid volume has decreased, the wedge pressure will be low. In cardiogenic shock the wedge pressure is normal or elevated.

The mortality rate in cardiogenic shock is so high because of the vicious downward spiral that occurs: hypotension due to pump failure results in a reduction of coronary flow, which results in further impairment of pump function, and so on.

TREATMENT (see also p. 716)

- Patients require intensive care (see Chapter 13).
- General measures such as complete rest, continuous 100% oxygen administration and pain relief are essential.
- The infusion of fluid is necessary if the pulmonary capillary wedge pressure is below 18 mm Hg, which is probably the optimal 'filling pressure' with which to prime a failing heart.
- Short-acting venous dilators such as glyceryl trinitrate or sodium nitroprusside should be administered intravenously if the wedge pressure is 25 mm Hg or more.
- Cardiac inotropes such as dobutamine and dopamine may be used to increase aortic diastolic pressure (coronary perfusion pressure). Dopamine also selectively increases renal perfusion.
- Mechanical assist devices such as an intra-aortic balloon pump may be used (see p. 545). Although leading to a temporary improvement, long-term prognosis is not improved unless there is a surgically correctable cause, such as a ruptured interventricular septum or acute mitral regurgitation.

Ischaemic heart disease

An imbalance between the supply of oxygen (and other essential myocardial nutrients) and the myocardial demand for these substances results in myocardial ischaemia. The causes are as follows:

1 The coronary blood flow to a region of the myocardium may be reduced by an obstruction due to:

- Atheroma
- Thombosis
- Spasm
- Embolus
- Coronary ostial stenosis (e.g. syphilis)
- Coronary arteritis (e.g. polyarteritis)

2 There can be a decrease in the flow of oxygenated blood to the myocardium due to:

- Anaemia
- Carboxyhaemoglobinaemia
- Hypotension causing decreased coronary perfusion pressure

3 An increased demand for oxygen may occur owing to an increase in cardiac output (e.g. during exercise or in thyrotoxicosis) or myocardial hypertrophy (e.g. from aortic stenosis or hypertension).

In types 2 and 3, ischaemia may occur despite normal coronary arteries. In a small number of cases, ischaemia develops despite normal coronary arteries and a normal demand for oxygen. This condition is known as syndrome X and is possibly caused by an abnormality of small coronary vessels, resulting in a reduction of coronary flow reserve.

The most common cause of ischaemic heart disease is coronary atheroma, which causes a fixed obstruction to coronary blood flow. Variations in the tone of smooth muscle in the wall of a coronary artery may add an important element of dynamic or variable obstruction. Sometimes an extreme increase in coronary tone may produce coronary spasm and severely reduced coronary blood flow in the absence of any underlying coronary atheroma.

Atheroma

The word 'atheroma' comes from the Greek word *athere* meaning 'porridge'. It is a condition that affects medium-sized arteries and is characterized by the development of atherosclerotic plaques. Such a plaque consists of a necrotic core, rich in cholesterol and other lipids, surrounded by smooth muscle cells and fibrous tissue. There are two main theories of plaque development:

- Insudation may be due to the accumulation of plasma constituents such as cholesterol in the intima of the arterial wall because of low-grade inflammation. This theory was suggested by Virchow.
- Platelet thrombi may develop on areas of damaged intima. Rokitansky suggested that the organization of these thrombi could lead to atheroma.

AETIOLOGY OF CORONARY ATHEROMA

The immediate cause of this condition is not known. However, a number of 'risk' factors are known to predispose to coronary atherosclerosis. Some of these, such as age, sex and family history, cannot be modified, whereas other major risk factors, such as serum cholesterol, smoking habits and hypertension, can be changed. There are a number of other factors, such as lack of exercise, personality type and stress, that may be implicated in the causation of atherosclerosis (see Table 11.22).

Age
Atherosclerosis develops progressively as age advances. It is rarely present in early childhood, except in familial hyperlipidaemia, but it is often detectable in post-mortem specimens of young men between 20 and 30 years. It is almost universal in the elderly in the Western World.

Sex
Men are more affected than pre-menopausal women. However, after the menopause the incidence of atheroma in women becomes similar to that in men. The cause of this difference in incidence is not clearly understood.

Table 11.22 Risk factors for coronary disease.

Fixed
Age
Male sex
Positive family history
Potentially changeable with treatment
Strong association
Hyperlipidaemia
Cigarette smoking
Hypertension
Diabetes mellitus
Weak association
Personality
Obesity
Gout
Soft water
Lack of exercise
Contraceptive pill
Heavy alcohol consumption

Family history
Coronary artery disease is often found in several members of the same family. Because the disease is so prevalent and because other risk factors are familial, it is uncertain whether family history is an independent risk factor.

Hyperlipidaemia (see p. 862)
Atherosclerotic plaques contain cholesterol. A high serum cholesterol, especially when associated with low values of high-density lipoproteins, is strongly associated with coronary atheroma. High triglyceride levels are less definitely linked with coronary atheroma.

Familial hypercholesterolaemia, familial combined hyperlipidaemia and remnant hyperlipidaemia are associated with an increased risk of coronary atherosclerosis.

Measurement of total cholesterol, HDL cholesterol with calculation of LDL cholesterol and HDL ratio as well as triglycerides should be performed on all patients. Lowering the serum cholesterol has been shown to decrease the incidence of coronary artery disease and slow the progression of coronary atheroma. Management is described on p. 863.

Smoking
In men, the risk of developing coronary artery disease is directly related to the number of cigarettes smoked. This relationship is less certain, but still important, in women and in cigar and pipe smokers. The risk from smoking declines to almost normal after 10 years of abstention.

Hypertension
Both systolic and diastolic hypertension are associated with an increased risk of coronary artery disease. The risk is the same for men and women. Reduction of blood pressure with hypotensive therapy reduces the risks of a cerebrovascular accident but does not affect the risk of cardiac events such as myocardial infarction.

Other factors
Lack of exercise increases the risk of coronary artery disease, and regular exercise probably protects against its development. Diabetes mellitus, or even just an abnormal glucose tolerance test, is associated with vascular disease. Obesity is certainly associated with coronary artery disease, but it is not certain whether obesity itself is independently linked with the condition.

A certain kind of personality type known as 'type A', which is characterized by unsuccessful aggression, ambition, compulsion and competitiveness, is said to be associated twice as frequently with coronary artery disease than is 'type B' (the converse of type A). Gout, oral contraceptives, alcohol and soft water have also been suggested as risk factors for coronary atheroma.

It is clear that many factors influence the development of coronary atheroma. It is not certain that modification of any of these can substantially reverse the established atherosclerotic process.

Angina (see p. 516)

Angina ranges from a mild ache to a most severe pain that provokes sweating and fear. It is generally described as 'heavy', 'crushing' or 'gripping', and the patient may indicate the type of pain by clenching his fist or gripping his hands together. Occasionally these symptoms may occur in the arms without any chest pain.

There are several types of angina; these are described below.

Classical or exertional angina

Physical exertion, especially after a meal, in cold weather or walking against the wind, provokes this pain. It is also aggravated by anger or excitement. The pain usually fades quickly (in less than 3 min) when the patient ceases to exert himself. Sometimes the pain will disappear even though exertion continues ('walking through the pain'); the exertion threshold for the development of pain is very variable. Usually, pain is more easily provoked in the early morning than later in the day. This type of angina can be graded as in Table 11.3.

Decubitus angina

This is angina that occurs when the patient lies down. It usually occurs in association with heart failure because of the increased central blood volume and consequent myocardial tensions that develop in the recumbent position. Patients with this symptom usually have severe coronary artery disease.

Nocturnal angina

This is angina that wakes the patient from sleep. It may be provoked by vivid dreams. Patients with this symptom usually have critical coronary artery disease, or the angina may be associated with coronary spasm.

Variant (Prinzmetal's) angina

A classical attack of variant angina, as described by Prinzmetal, has no obvious provocation. It occurs at rest, especially at night or in the early morning, and is rarely induced by exertion. It occurs more frequently in women and the pain is usually more severe and more prolonged than in classical angina. It produces a characteristic electrocardiographic feature of ST segment elevation developing during the pain. Arrhythmias—both heart block and ventricular tachycardia—are common in the ischaemic episode.

Prinzmetal's angina is caused by spasm of a coronary artery often in association with an eccentric coronary artery atheromatous lesion. More often, variant angina is not classical Prinzmetal's angina but is due to variation in coronary arterial tone rather than frank coronary arterial spasm. Such patients have a varying exercise threshold for the provocation of angina.

Unstable angina

Unstable angina includes angina of very recent onset, worsening angina or angina at rest. A number of terms, such as crescendo angina, pre-infarction angina and intermediate chest pain syndrome, have been used to describe angina that is provoked more easily and persists for a longer duration than ordinary angina or that fails to respond readily to therapy. Whilst the pain is present, myocardial infarction must be considered, but with angina the ECG changes (T wave inversion or ST segment depression) are only transient and cardiac enzyme levels are not elevated. Unless vigorously treated, a large proportion of patients with unstable angina will proceed to develop a myocardial infarction within weeks.

EXAMINATION

There are usually no abnormal findings in angina, although a fourth heart sound may be heard. Any factor responsible for angina (e.g. thyrotoxicosis) or risk factors may lead to physical signs such as nicotine staining, hypertension or xanthelasma.

DIAGNOSIS

The primary diagnosis rests on the description of the chest pain as investigations may be normal.

INVESTIGATION

Resting ECG

This is usually normal between attacks, although an old myocardial infarction, left ventricular hypertrophy or other unrelated heart disease may be present. During an attack, transient ST segment depression, symmetrical T wave inversion or tall, pointed, upright T waves may appear.

A normal ECG between attacks or even during an attack cannot definitely exclude angina pectoris. Typical ECG changes during an attack are strong pointers to the diagnosis of angina.

Exercise ECG (see p. 531)

When angina is provoked by exertion, an exercise stress ECG should be performed. ST segment depression greater than or equal to 1 mm suggests myocardial ischaemia, especially if typical chest pain occurs at the same time. The severity of the electrocardiographic changes indicates the extent of the coronary artery disease. Approximately 75% of patients with severe coronary artery disease will give a positive test. Stress testing is less reliable in women and is confused by electrolyte abnormalities, therapy with digoxin, and intraventricular conduction disturbances. A normal stress test does not definitely exclude coronary disease.

Cardiac scintigraphy
Uptake of thallium-201 (see p. 538). This is useful:

● When the exercise test is equivocal
● In deciding whether stenotic vessels on angiography are giving rise to ischaemic areas on exercise

A normal perfusion scan after exercise makes significant coronary artery disease unlikely.

Radionuclide ventriculography (see p. 539). This can be used to outline the left ventricle. When part of the left ventricular wall is ischaemic it does not contract normally, producing an abnormal image. This test can be performed at rest and during exertion. The ejection fraction is a good index of ventricular function and is useful in the assessment of patients for coronary artery bypass surgery.

Echocardiography (see p. 533)
This can be used to assess ventricular wall involvement and ventricular function. An abnormal resting echocardiogram reflects previous ventricular damage. Exercise echocardiography, although technically difficult, may be useful in patients with an equivocal exercise electrocardiogram.

Coronary angiography
This is occasionally useful in patients with chest pain when the cause is unclear. More often, the test is performed to delineate the exact coronary anatomy (Fig. 11.52) prior to coronary grafting or coronary angioplasty. Coronary angiography should only be performed when the benefit in terms of diagnosis and potential treatment outweighs the small risk associated with the procedure (a mortality of less than 1 in 1000 cases) (see Table 11.23).

Table 11.23 Indications for coronary angiography.

● Angina refractory to medical therapy
● Severely abnormal exercise ECG
● Unstable angina
● Angina occurring after myocardial infarction
● Subendocardial myocardial infarction (non-Q-wave infarction), especially if exercise test is abnormal
● Angina or myocardial infarction in a young (< 50 years) patient, especially if exercise test is abnormal

A coronary angiogram may not reveal coronary spasm unless an intracoronary injection of dihydroergotamine has been given. This test is not often performed because the induction of coronary spasm may prove difficult to reverse and its clinical relevance is uncertain.

TREATMENT

Management of an acute attack
An acute attack is treated by stopping exercise (exertional angina) or by getting up (decubitus angina) and dissolving a fresh glyceryl trinitrate tablet (0.5 mg) under the tongue. After 2–3 min the angina usually recedes. When the pain is relieved the glyceryl trinitrate tablet is spat out or swallowed to inactivate it. This minimizes the main side-effect, which is a severe pounding headache. Some prefer to use an aerosol formulation of glyceryl trinitrate that, unlike the tablets, is stable for a long period. If glyceryl trinitrate cannot be tolerated, a capsule of nifedipine may be chewed or sucked. However, this has similar side-effects to glyceryl trinitrate.

General management
Patients should be reassured that their condition is not uniformly or rapidly fatal. Many have a good prognosis—30% survive for more than 10 years and spontaneous remission does occur. Any underlying problems such as obesity, thyrotoxicosis, anaemia or aortic stenosis should be treated. Risk factors should be evaluated and steps made to correct them. Smoking must be stopped. Patients must be encouraged not to do things that they know provoke their angina, but this must not lead to a severe restriction of lifestyle. Regular exercise sufficient to improve the fitness of the patient will tend to increase the threshold to angina. Exercise is not recommended unless the cardiovascular response to exertion (treadmill ECG test) has been documented. Emotional crises and overexcitement must be minimized.

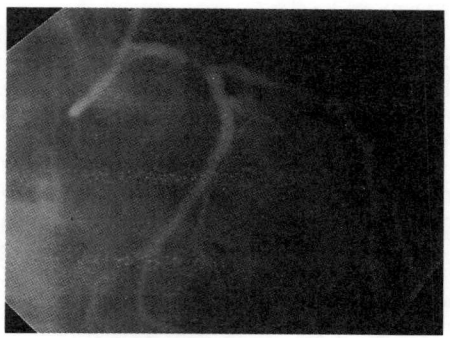

Fig. 11.52 Coronary angiogram demonstrating a tight stenosis in the left main coronary artery.

Medical treatment

Patients should be told to suck a tablet of glyceryl trinitrate before exertion rather than waiting for the pain to commence. They must be specifically encouraged to do this, because many prefer to believe that it is better to suffer the pain than to take more tablets. When angina occurs frequently, or with only modest exertion, regular prophylactic therapy should be advised. This consists of nitrates, beta-adrenergic blocking drugs or calcium antagonists.

Nitrates such as glyceryl trinitrate are available in a variety of slow-release formulations, particularly infiltrated skin plasters and buccal pellets. Alternatively, tablets of long-acting nitrate preparations such as isosorbide dinitrate or isosorbide mononitrate may be used. Nitrates are successful in the treatment of angina pectoris because they reduce venous and hence intracardiac diastolic pressures, they reduce the impedance to the emptying of the left ventricle, and they relax the tone of the coronary arteries.

Beta-adrenergic blocking drugs reduce heart rate (negative chronotropic effect) and the force of ventricular contraction (negative inotropic effect), both of which reduce myocardial oxygen demand, especially on exercise. Sufficient beta-blocker to reduce the resting heart rate to about 60 beats per minute is usually necessary to achieve relief from angina. Very high doses of beta-blockers are no longer used because of side-effects and the possibility of infarction or arrhythmia on withdrawal, and because many alternative therapies are available. Propranolol 40–80 mg three times daily is the most conventional therapy.

Relatively cardioselective beta-blockers (beta-1-antagonists) such as atenolol (50–100 mg daily) or metoprolol (50 mg three times daily) are often preferred because they have fewer side-effects.

Calcium antagonists (Table 11.24) such as nifedipine, nicardipine, amlodipine, verapamil and diltiazem block calcium flux into the cell and the utilization of calcium within the cell. They relax coronary arteries and other vascular systems and also reduce the force of left ventricular contraction, reducing the oxygen demand and improving angina. Nifedipine 20–30 mg daily is the calcium antagonist most commonly used in angina.

Coronary angioplasty

This is a technique of dilating coronary atheromatous obstructions by inflating a balloon against the obstruction (Fig. 11.53). The balloon, which is mounted on the tip of a very thin catheter, is inserted through the obstruction using X-ray fluoroscopy, and it is then inflated with dilute contrast material. Multiple inflations of the balloon using a pressure of several atmospheres will squash and crack the atheroma and relieve the obstruction. This technique is widely applied for the treatment of angina due to isolated, proximal, non-calcified, atheromatous plaques, usually in patients with a relatively short history of coronary ischaemia. Multiple lesions may be treated and repeat procedures can be undertaken. Two complications are acute coronary occlusion (2–4%) and chronic re-stenosis, which occurs in 30% in the first 6 months after angioplasty.

Surgical management

When angina worsens or persists despite general

Table 11.24 Calcium antagonists.

Class	1 (non-dihydropyridine)	2 (dihydropyridine)*
Example	Verapamil Diltiazem	Nifedipine Nicardipine Isradipine
Effects		
Sinus node suppression	+++	+
AV node suppression	+++	+
Myocardial depression	++	++
Arteriolar vasodilatation	+	+++
Side-effects		
Flushing, ankle oedema, palpitations	+	++
Bradycardia, impaired AV conduction	++	+
Aggravation of heart failure	++	+
Combination with beta-blockers	No	Yes

* Nimodipine and amlodipine (single daily dose) have recently been introduced.

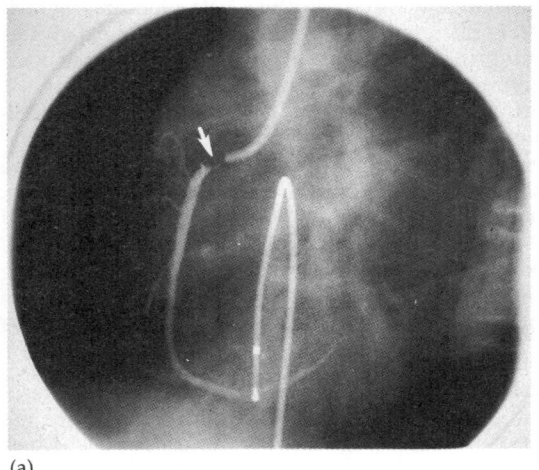

(a)

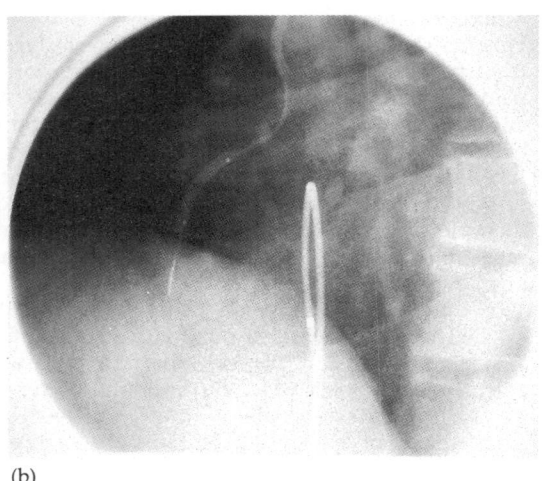

(b)

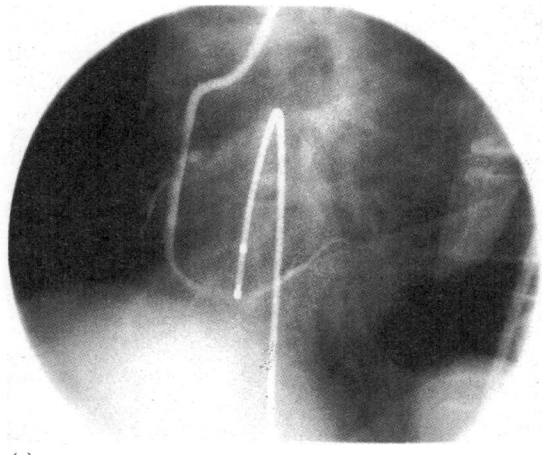

(c)

Fig. 11.53 (a) Stenosis in right coronary artery (arrow). (b) Dilatation of the stenosis using an angioplasty balloon. (c) Post dilatation—the obstruction is no longer seen.

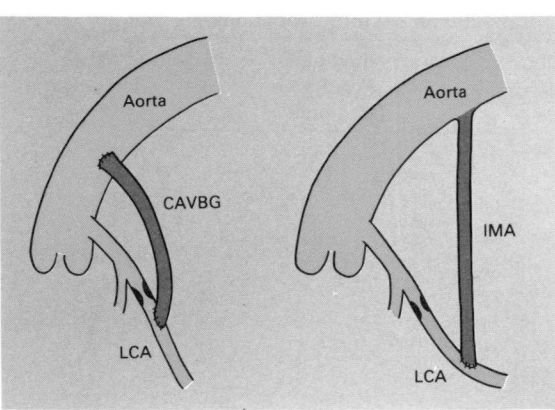

Fig. 11.54 The relief of coronary obstruction by surgical techniques: coronary artery vein bypass grafting (CAVBG) or internal mammary arterial implantation (IMA). In both of these examples, the graft bypasses a coronary obstruction in the left coronary artery (LCA).

measures and optimal medical treatment, the option of surgery should be considered. The patient should be assessed using exercise testing and angiography. Symptomatic patients with left main stem obstructions, two- or three-vessel involvement and good ventricular function are often treated surgically.

There are three operations currently used for the relief of myocardial ischaemia:

- Coronary artery vein bypass grafting (CAVBG) (Fig. 11.54) involves taking a vein, usually from the leg (saphenous) and bypassing the coronary obstruction by suturing the vein (reversed because of the venous valves) between the aorta and the coronary artery distal to the obstruction.
- An internal mammary artery may be mobilized and implanted into the left anterior descending coronary artery distal to an obstruction (Fig. 11.54).
- Endarterectomy (removal of an atheromatous obstruction) can sometimes be successful when

combined with bypass or internal mammary artery grafting.

Surgery provides dramatic relief from angina in about 90% of those operated on. When surgery is performed for left main stem obstruction or for three-vessel disease involvement, an improved life-span and quality of life can be expected. Surgical mortality is well below 1% in patients with normal left ventricular function. Progressive slow occlusion of grafts with atheroma occurs in a significant number of cases (5–10% a year).

Treatment of variant angina

The treatment of variant angina is slightly different. Nitrates and calcium antagonists are useful, but beta-blockers may increase coronary tone and exacerbate the angina, so should not be used. It may be necessary to treat the arrhythmias provoked by the spasm. Surgical relief is rarely necessary or possible.

Treatment of unstable angina

Unstable angina should be managed vigorously. If rest pain persists despite the use of agents such as sublingual glyceryl trinitrate, the patient should be treated with bed rest, mild sedation, intravenous heparin and/or oral aspirin as well as standard medical antianginal therapy. Oxygen may also be beneficial. Calcium antagonists are particularly valuable for the treatment of this condition but usually beta-blockers, nitrates and calcium antagonists are all used in combination. Aspirin decreases both death and myocardial infarction. If medical therapy fails, urgent coronary arteriography is desirable with a view to coronary artery surgery or angioplasty. Fibrinolytic therapy may be of benefit if myocardial infarction is suspected. Alternatively, intra-aortic balloon pumping (p. 545) may help to stabilize the patient.

Irrespective of the immediate success of treatment, early coronary angiography and, depending on the results, urgent referral for surgery are usually advised.

Myocardial infarction

Myocardial infarction is now the most common cause of death in the UK and other developed countries, but was hardly known before 1910. It almost always occurs in patients with coronary atheroma because of sudden coronary thrombosis. This usually develops at the site of a fissure or rupture of the intimal surface of an atheromatous plaque. Haemorrhage may occur into a plaque and local coronary spasm may develop. Sometimes thrombosis results from stasis at a critical stenosis or in association with coronary spasm. About 6 h after the onset of infarction the myocardium is pale and swollen, and at 24 h the necrotic tissue

appears deep red owing to haemorrhage. In the next weeks an inflammatory reaction develops, lymphocytes infiltrate and the infarcted tissue turns grey. Necrotic tissue is replaced by mononuclear cells, and gradually a thin fibrous scar develops.

CLINICAL PRESENTATION

Myocardial infarction presents with chest pain, similar in character to exertional angina pectoris, but usually occurring at rest and lasting for some hours. The pain may be so severe that the patient may fear imminent death ('angor animi'), but it may be less severe and mistaken for indigestion. It is usually sudden in onset, but it may develop gradually. The pain of myocardial infarction is often associated with restlessness and the patients usually cannot remain still. Sweating, nausea and vomiting are often associated with myocardial infarction.

About 20% of patients with myocardial infarction have no pain. Diabetics, hypertensives and elderly patients often have 'silent' myocardial infarctions. In these cases the myocardial infarction may go unnoticed or may produce hypotension, breathlessness or arrhythmias.

Physical signs

Usually there are no abnormal physical signs unless complications develop. Hypotension, which may first occur several hours after the onset of infarction and may increase over the following 3–4 days, abnormal precordial pulsation due to the systolic bulging of the infarcted myocardium, an additional heart sound (particularly a fourth heart sound), and sinus tachycardia may be noted in some patients. A raised venous pressure and basal crackles are common. As the infarction progresses, a modest fever (up to 38°C) due to muscle necrosis and lasting for up to 7 days occurs. A pericardial friction rub may develop.

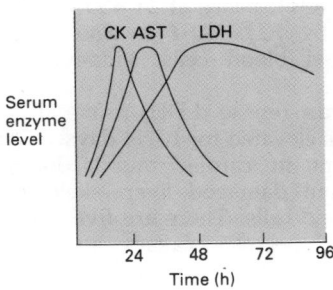

Fig. 11.55 The enzyme profile in acute myocardial infarction. CK = creatine kinase; AST = aspartate aminotransferase; LDH = lactic dehydrogenase.

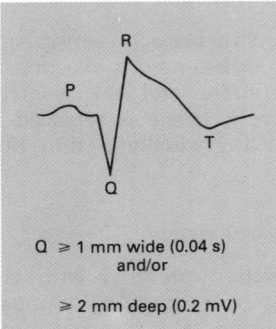

Fig. 11.56 The electrocardiographic features of myocardial infarction, showing a Q wave, ST elevation and T wave inversion.

INVESTIGATION

Non-specific tests
Non-specific abnormalities such as an increased ESR (up to 70 mm in the first hour) and a polymorphonuclear leucocytosis (up to $20 \times 10^9/L$) may occur in the first few days following myocardial infarction.

Cardiac enzymes (Fig. 11.55)
Necrotic cardiac tissue releases cellular enzymes; three of these are commonly assayed.

- Creatine kinase (CK) is released by infarcted myocardium and peaks within 24 h. It is usually back to normal before 48 h. It is also produced by damaged skeletal muscle and brain. The myocardial-bound (MB) isoenzyme fraction of CK is specific for heart muscle damage. A several-fold increase in total CK, but not in MB-CK, can be produced by an intramuscular injection. Cardioversion can increase both the total CK and the MB isoenzyme fraction of CK. The size of the infarction determines the total enzyme release. Large infarcts tend to produce high serum levels of enzymes.
- Aspartate aminotransferase (AST), which was formerly called serum glutamic oxaloacetic transaminase (SGOT), peaks at 24–48 h and may fall to normal by 72 h. AST is also released by damaged red blood cells, kidney, liver and lungs.
- Lactic dehydrogenase (LDH) peaks at 3–4 days and remains elevated for 10–14 days. LDH is not only present in cardiac muscle but is also released from damaged liver, skeletal muscle and red blood cells. There are five isoenzymes, and cardiac necrosis causes a predominant increase of LDH 1, which can also be measured as hydroxybutyrate dehydrogenase (HBD).

Enzymes are usually estimated for the first 3 days following a suspected myocardial infarction. The first assay is often normal and subsequent

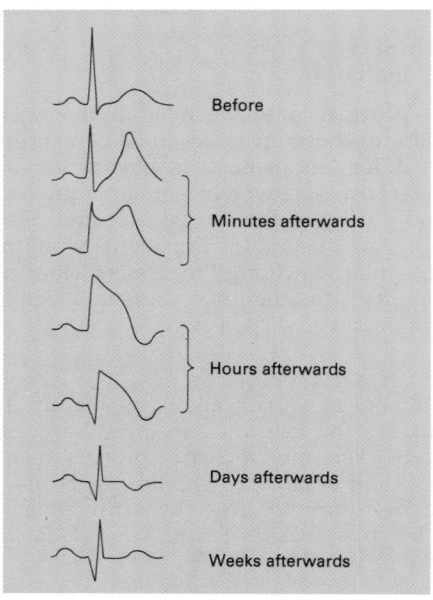

Fig. 11.57 Electrocardiographic evolution of myocardial infarction. After the first few mintues the T waves become tall, pointed and upright and there is ST segment elevation. After the first few hours the T waves invert, the R wave voltage is decreased and Q waves develop. After a few days the ST segment returns to normal. After weeks or months the T wave may return to upright but the Q wave remains.

assays will show a threefold or more increase in the majority of cases. With reperfusion after thrombolytic therapy the enzyme rise may be curtailed.

The ECG
The ECG is particularly valuable for the diagnosis of myocardial infarction. In the majority of cases the development of a full thickness myocardial infarction is associated with evolving electrocardiographic features.

A Q wave (Fig. 11.56) is a broad (> 1 mm) and deep (> 2 mm or more than 25% of the amplitude of the following R wave) negative deflection that starts the QRS complex. It may occur normally in leads AVR and V_1 (and sometimes in lead III), but in other leads it is abnormal. Abnormal Q waves are produced by several abnormalities such as left bundle branch block, ventricular tachycardia and the Wolff–Parkinson–White syndrome. The gradual development of Q waves over minutes or hours suggests the occurrence of a full-thickness (as opposed to a subendocardial) myocardial infarction. They develop because the electrical silence of infarcted cardiac tissue results in a so-called 'window' through which the normal endocardial-to-epicardial activation of the opposite non-infarcted ventricular wall is 'seen' resulting in an unopposed depolarization front moving away from an electrode situated over the epicardial surface of the infarct (Fig. 11.56). Q waves are usually

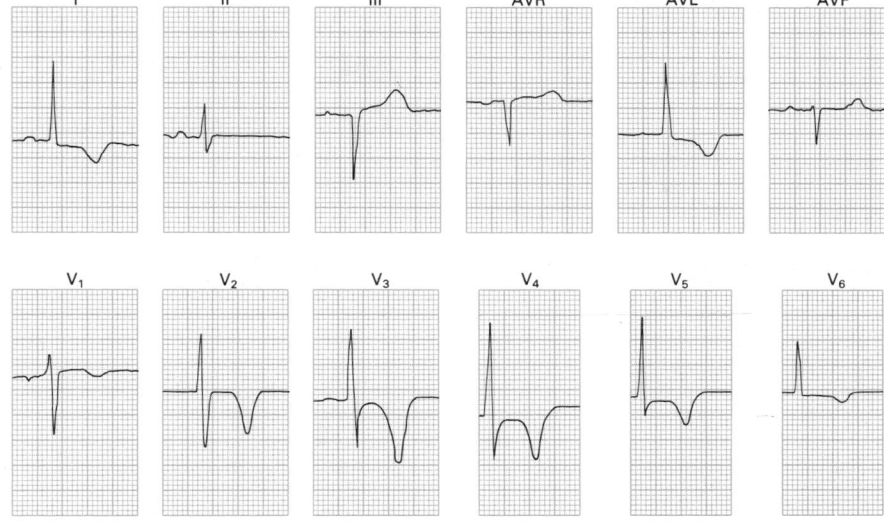

Fig. 11.58 A 12-lead ECG showing a widespread (antero-lateral) subendocardial myocardial infarction. Note the deeply inverted, symmetrical T waves in addition to ST depression.

permanent electrocardiographic features following full-thickness myocardial infarction.

T wave and ST segment changes result from ischaemia and injury. They are therefore often transient, occurring only during the acute attack. The progressive changes or evolution of the ECG during the course of a full-thickness myocardial infarction are illustrated in Fig. 11.57.

With subendocardial infarction (Fig. 11.58) only the endocardial surface is infarcted and Q waves do not develop. ST segment and T wave changes are therefore the only ECG features of a subendocardial infarction. Because the injury is endocardial rather than predominantly epicardial, ST segment depression rather than elevation is usual.

Typically ECG changes (Table 11.25) are usually confined to the ECG leads that 'face' the infarction. Therefore, an inferior wall myocardial infarction is diagnosed when the ECG findings are seen in leads II, III and AVF (Fig. 11.59). Lateral infarction produces changes in leads I, II and AVL. In anterior infarction, leads V_2–V_5 may be affected (Table 11.25). Changes seen in an anterolateral infarction are shown in Fig. 11.60. Because there are no posterior leads, a true posterior wall infarct is usually diagnosed by the appearance of mirror image or reciprocal changes in leads V_1 and V_2, i.e. the development of a tall initial R wave, ST segment depression and tall, upright T waves. These reciprocal changes can also be seen in association with other infarctions. For example, in an inferior wall myocardial infarction, anterior ST segment depression may be seen.

A normal ECG, especially early in the presentation, does not exclude myocardial infarction.

Pyrophosphate scanning (see p. 539)
This test is particularly useful when the ECG is unhelpful because of pre-existing abnormalities such as left bundle branch block. Imaging is performed about 2 h after the injection of the isotope to detect the infarcted area.

MANAGEMENT

During an acute myocardial infarction, lethal arrhythmias may occur. Patients should therefore be admitted to the coronary care unit as soon as possible. Here, the ECG should be monitored continuously for the first 48 h to allow the detection of arrhythmias such as 'R on T' ventricu-

Table 11.25 Typical ECG changes in myocardial infarction.

Infarct site	Leads showing main changes
Anterior	
Small	V_3–V_4
Extensive	V_2–V_5
Anteroseptal	V_1–V_3
Anterolateral	V_4–V_6, I, AVL
Lateral	I, II, AVL
Inferior	II, III, AVF
Posterior	V_1, V_2 (reciprocal)
Subendocardial	Any lead

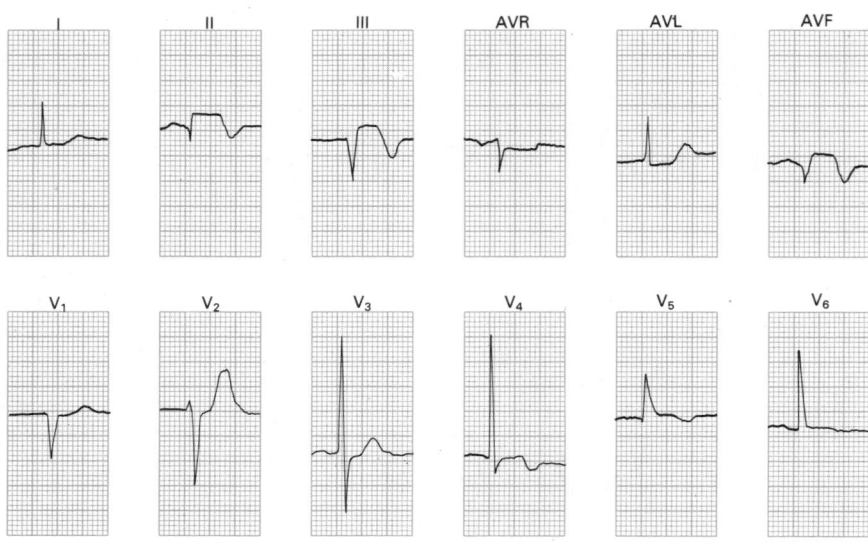

Fig. 11.59 A 12-lead ECG showing an acute inferior wall myocardial infarction. Notice the raised ST segment and Q waves in the inferior leads (II, III and AVF). The additional T wave inversion in V_4 and V_5 probably represents anterior wall ischaemia.

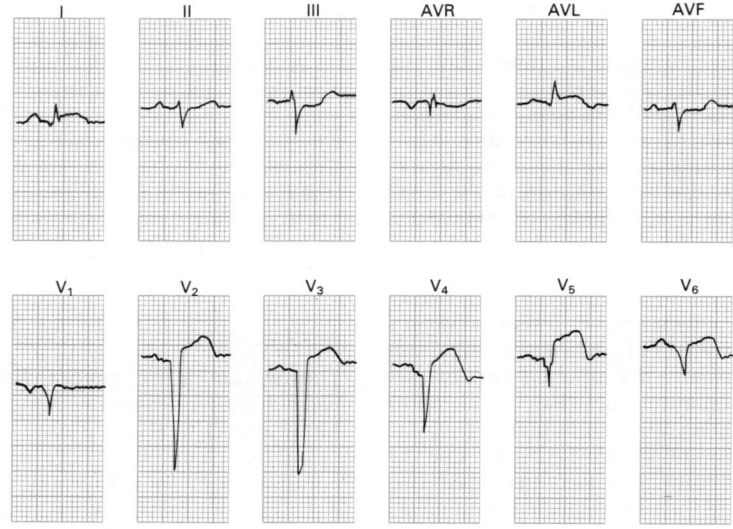

Fig. 11.60 A 12-lead ECG showing an acute anterolateral myocardial infarction. Notice the ST segment elevation in leads I, AVL and V_2 to V_6. The T wave is inverted in leads I, AVL and V_3 to V_6. Pathological Q waves are seen in leads V_2 to V_6.

lar ectopic beats, which may precipitate ventricular fibrillation. Even if these potentially provocative arrhythmias are not seen, it is important that ventricular fibrillation is recognized promptly and that resuscitation is started immediately. Therefore, patients should not be kept in casualty departments waiting for ECGs and chest X-rays but should be admitted immediately to the coronary care unit. If this is not possible then the Accident & Emergency Department must have the staff and

facilities to provide the treatment required in the first few hours.

● An intravenous cannula is always inserted so that emergency intravenous medication can be administered.
● The pain of myocardial infarction should be treated promptly with powerful analgesics such as morphine (10–20 mg i.v. or s.c.) or diamorphine (5–10 mg i.v. or s.c.) combined with

antiemetics such as cyclizine (50 mg i.v.) or metoclopramide (10 mg i.v.).

- Oxygen is usually given routinely because during an acute myocardial infarction the arterial PO_2 is reduced. Oxygen at 60% is usually administered by face mask or nasal cannulae for several hours following myocardial infarction.
- Fibrinolytic therapy should be considered as soon as the diagnosis is suspected. These agents can achieve early reperfusion in 50–70% of patients (compared with a spontaneous reperfusion rate of less than 30%) and have been shown to reduce the extent of ventricular damage, and the early and 1-year mortality rates associated with myocardial infarction. A reduction in expected mortality of up to 25% is possible if these agents are given within the first 3–6 h following infarction, but some benefit is achieved up to 24 h. Although many physicians administer these drugs on the history alone, provided there are no contraindications it is recommended on present evidence that typical electrocardiographic evidence of early infarction should also be available prior to their administration. Oral aspirin therapy (150 mg daily) should accompany the fibrinolytic therapy and be continued for at least 4 weeks after infarction, as shown by ISIS-2 (International Study of Infarct Survival).

Three fibrinolytic agents are currently licensed for use in acute myocardial infarction. Streptokinase is most commonly used. The recommended doses of these drugs are shown in Table 11.26. Recombinant tissue plasminogen activator (rt-PA) achieves slightly higher reperfusion rates than the other two agents, but there is at present no definite evidence that this is associated with a greater reduction in early and late mortality and morbidity rates compared to the others. It is also expensive. Although the single-injection administration of anistreplase confers some advantage over the other two agents (both of which are given as an intravenous infusion of at least 1 h), this is also considerably more expensive than streptokinase. Both streptokinase and anistreplase increase the patient's anti-streptokinase antibody level, which falls to baseline levels afer 3–6 months. These antibodies reduce the effectiveness of a repeat dose and theoretically increase the risk of an anaphylactic reaction. Repeat usage of these drugs within 3 months is therefore not recommended. If repeat administration is deemed necessary, it should be preceded by intravenous methylprednisolone. The use of rt-PA, or even urokinase, (neither of which provokes antibody formation) is preferable in these circumstances. Because of the small risk of bleeding following fibrinolytic therapy, all patients should have their blood group assessed in case of the need for transfusion.

Because of the risk of reperfusion arrhythmias, patients should be monitored during and after fibrinolytic therapy. The ventricular arrhythmias that develop are usually short-lived and do not require treatment, but, rarely, ventricular fibrillation can occur.

- Persistent pain can be treated with nitrates. If there is no hypotension, sublingual glyceryl trinitrate should be given. Alternatively, especially if the haemodynamic situation is not stable, continuous intravenous infusion of either isosorbide dinitrate or glyceryl trinitrate should be considered.
- Sedation is important. Anxious patients should be reassured and mild sedation, in addition to analgesia, may be necessary. A quiet atmosphere should reduce anxiety.
- Bed-rest is advised for the first 24–48 h, after which the patient is progressively mobilized. Smoking is not allowed.
- Anticoagulation is useful for patients who are immobilized for long periods. Usually, heparin (5000 units 8-hourly s.c.) is sufficient. Patients with severe cardiac failure or cardiogenic shock are particularly vulnerable to thromboembolism. In these cases intravenous heparinization by continuous infusion (10 000 units in 6 h) is appropriate. Early mobilization policies have reduced the need for anticoagulation except in high-risk cases.

Home versus hospital care of myocardial infarction victims

Coronary care units were developed to facilitate the detection and treatment of arrhythmias occurring in the immediate post-infarction period. However, it has been suggested that the coronary care ward is a frightening environment that may itself increase the incidence of these arrhythmias. There have been several studies comparing home care and coronary ward care of patients with myocardial infarction. The conclusions have been controversial but home care can be considered if:

- The patient has suffered a myocardial infarction 24 h or more previously

Table 11.26 Fibrinolytic therapy for acute myocardial infarction.

Agent	Intravenous dose regimen
Streptokinase	1.5 million i.u. over 1 h
Anistreplase (APSAC)	30 u. over 4–5 min
Alteplase (rt-PA, recombinant tissue type plasminogen activator)	10 mg bolus, followed by 50 mg in the first hour, and 40 mg over the subsequent 2 h

- There are no complications such as shock or arrhythmia
- The patient is aged 70 years of older
- The patient has concurrent terminal disease

However, most patients suffering from myocardial infarction should be cared for in the coronary care ward of a hospital, where sudden and perhaps fatal complications can be promptly recognized and effectively treated.

Mobile coronary care units

Because a large proportion of deaths from myocardial infarction are due to arrhythmias that occur in the first few minutes of the infarction, it is logical to train ambulance-men in methods of advanced cardiac life support and to provide them with the equipment to perform these techniques (intravenous infusion, endotracheal intubation and ventilation and ECG monitoring and defibrillation). Ambulances manned and equipped in this way are called mobile coronary care units (CCUs), coronary rescue vehicles or cardiac resuscitation vehicles. This kind of ambulance is sent to those patients who have severe chest pain or who have collapsed unconscious. Together with the training in basic life support of a significant proportion (at least one-third) of the general public, mobile CCUs have reduced the incidence of sudden unexpected cardiac death, whether due to myocardial infarction or to arrhythmias unrelated to acute myocardial infarction. The provision of such vehicles is still patchy, but this service is becoming increasingly available throughout the UK.

COMPLICATIONS

In the acute phase, i.e. the first 2–3 days following a myocardial infarction, cardiac arrhythmias, cardiac failure and pericarditis are the most common complications. Later, recurrent infarction, angina, thromboembolism, mitral valve regurgitation, and ventricular septal or free wall rupture may occur. Late complications include the post-myocardial infarction syndrome (Dressler's syndrome), shoulder–hand syndrome, ventricular aneurysm and recurrent cardiac arrhythmias.

Cardiac arrhythmias

These are described in detail on pp. 545–562.

Ventricular extrasystoles. These commonly occur after myocardial infarction. Their occurrence may precede the development of ventricular fibrillation. If they are frequent (more than 5 per minute), multiform (different shapes) or R-on-T (falling on the upstroke or peak of the preceding T wave), they may be treated with lignocaine 50–100 mg i.v. over 5 min followed by 1–4 mg·min^{-1} by continuous infusion, which is slowly reduced and discontinued over 24 h. Such treatment has not been

shown to reduce the likelihood of subsequent ventricular tachycardia or fibrillation.

Ventricular tachycardia. This may degenerate into ventricular fibrillation or may itself produce serious haemodynamic consequences. It is treated with intravenous lignocaine. If haemodynamic deterioration occurs, the tachycardia is immediately treated with synchronized cardioversion (initially 200 J).

Ventricular fibrillation. This may occur in the first few hours or days following a myocardial infarction in the absence of severe cardiac failure or cardiogenic shock. This is known as primary ventricular fibrillation. It is treated with prompt defibrillation (200–400 J). Intravenous lignocaine is usually prescribed in an attempt to prevent recurrences of ventricular fibrillation. The prognosis is usually very good because the electrical derangement is only transient.

When ventricular fibrillation occurs in the setting of heart failure, shock or aneurysm, it is called secondary ventricular fibrillation. It is treated in a similar way to primary ventricular fibrillation, but the prognosis is very poor unless the underlying haemodynamic or mechanical cause can be corrected.

Atrial fibrillation. This occurs in about 10% of patients with myocardial infarction. It is due to atrial irritation caused by heart failure, pericarditis and atrial ischaemia or infarction. It may be managed with intravenous digoxin or intravenous amiodarone and by treatment of the underlying pathology. It is not usually a long standing problem.

Table 11.27 Progression from different types of fascicular block to complete heart block in patients with acute myocardial infarction.

Type of fascicular block	Percentage progressing to complete heart block
LAH	4
LPH	8
Long PR interval	10
LBBB	10
RBBB	20
RBBB + LAH	30
RBBB + LPH	40
RBBB + (LPH *or* LAH) + Long PR interval	40

LAH = left anterior hemiblock.
LPH = left posterior hemiblock.
LBBB = left bundle branch block.
RBBB = right bundle branch block.

Table 11.28 Killip (clinical) classification of heart failure in patients with acute myocardial infarction.

Class	Description	Incidence (%)	Mortality (%)
I	No heart failure	40	5
II	Mild left ventricular failure	40	20
III	Pulmonary oedema	10	40
IV	Cardiogenic shock	10	90

Sinus bradycardia. This is especially associated with acute inferior wall myocardial infarction. Symptoms emerge only when the bradycardia is severe. When symptomatic, treatment consists of elevating the foot of the bed and giving intravenous atropine 600 µg if necessary. When sinus bradycardia occurs, an escape rhythm such as idioventricular rhythm (wide QRS complexes with a regular rhythm at 50–100 beats per minute) or idiojunctional rhythm (narrow QRS complexes) may occur. Usually no specific treatment is required.

It has been suggested that sinus bradycardia following myocardial infarction may predispose to the emergence of ventricular fibrillation. Severe sinus bradycardia associated with symptoms or the emergence of unstable rhythms may need treatment with temporary pacing.

Sinus tachycardia. This is produced by heart failure, fever and anxiety. Usually no specific treatment is needed.

Conduction disturbances. These are common following myocardial infarction. AV nodal delay (first-degree AV block) or higher degrees of block may occur during acute myocardial infarction, especially of the inferior wall. First-degree block does not need treatment, but progressive or complete block may need treatment with atropine or an artificial temporary pacemaker. Such blocks may last for only a few minutes but frequently persist for days or several weeks; they are rarely permanent.

Acute anterior wall myocardial infarction may produce damage to the distal conduction system (the His bundle or the bundle branches). The development of complete heart block usually implies a large myocardial infarction and a poor prognosis. The ventricular escape rhythm is slow and unreliable and a temporary pacemaker is necessary. This form of block is often permanent.

The development of complete AV block (Table 11.27) can be expected in 20–30% of cases where progressive bundle branch block (right bundle branch block and then right bundle branch block with a QRS axis shift) has already occurred (see Fig. 11.61).

Cardiac failure and cardiogenic shock

Heart failure after acute myocardial infarction is graded according to a clinical classification (Table 11.28).

Mild left heart failure (a few basal crackles that persist after coughing, an extra heart sound and upper lobe blood division on the chest X-ray) occur in about 40% of patients with acute myocardial infarction. Treatment for a few days with a mild diuretic such as a thiazide is usually all that is needed.

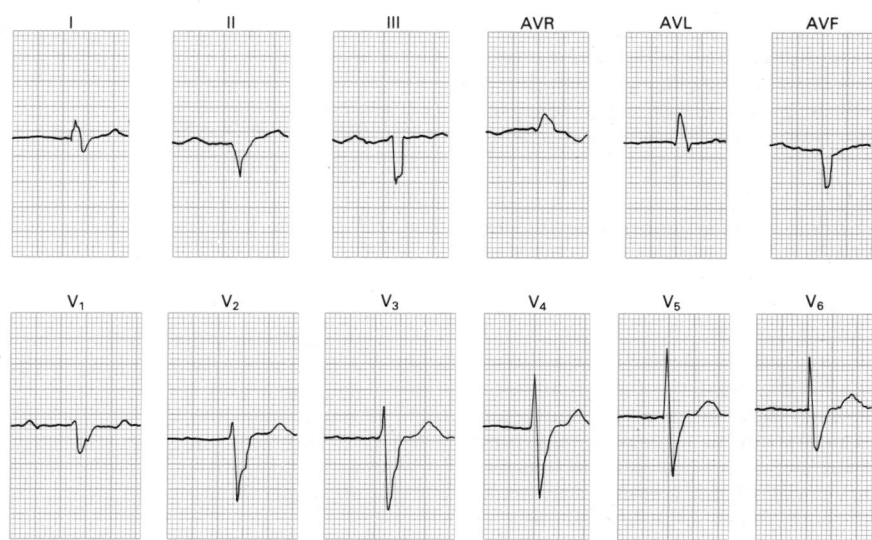

Fig. 11.61 A 12-lead ECG demonstrating a prolonged PR interval (0.32 s), a broad QRS complex with a deep S wave in leads I and V₆ (right bundle branch block) and left axis deviation (−75°). This electrocardiographic picture is consistent with bifascicular block.

A large myocardial infarction may lead to severe heart failure and pulmonary oedema. In such cases more prolonged and powerful diuretics and vasodilator treatment with ACE inhibitors may be necessary.

In very severe cases a pulmonary artery balloon catheter is used to measure the pulmonary artery and 'left atrial' pressures and the cardiac output. Treatment is with loop diuretics, vasodilators (see p. 565) and, occasionally, digoxin.

Severe heart failure may also follow ventricular septal rupture or mitral valve papillary muscle rupture. Both of these conditions present with worsening heart failure, a systolic thrill and a loud pansystolic murmur, widely heard over the precordium. Often, echocardiography and right heart catheterization with a balloon catheter is needed to differentiate between these two conditions. Both are associated with a poor prognosis, but vigorous treatment including early surgical correction may be successful.

Ventricular asynergy and papillary muscle dysfunction (not rupture) may produce mild mitral regurgitation in association with heart failure. This causes a transient, soft, pansystolic murmur in up to half of those with acute myocardial infarction. In these cases no specific treatment is necessary for the mitral regurgitation.

Cardiac rupture results in almost immediate cardiac tamponade and is usually fatal within a few minutes. Electromechanical dissociation, i.e. no pulse or cardiac output but a persistently normal rhythm on the ECG, is the classical presentation. Treatment is rarely successful.

Cardiogenic shock is an extreme form of cardiac failure or circulatory collapse. Its features and management are described on p. 569. The mortality from this condition is about 90%. The majority of those rescued have a complication that can be treated surgically (e.g. left ventricular aneurysm, torrential mitral regurgitation or ventricular septal perforation).

Thomboembolism

Bedrest and cardiac failure contribute to the common occurrence of thrombosis and embolism associated with myocardial infarction. Only 10% of patients have clinical features of thromboembolism, but in almost 50% of patients who die there is evidence of emboli. Deep venous thrombosis (see p. 625) is the most common manifestation, and pulmonary embolism may result from this. A left ventricular mural thrombus may form on the endocardial surface of the infarcted region. Such a thrombus is dislodged, forming a systemic embolus, in 15% of cases. Prophylactic anticoagulation with subcutaneous heparin probably reduces the risk of this complication.

Other complications

The shoulder–hand syndrome. This consists of pain and immobility of the left arm in the weeks and months following an acute myocardial infarction. Early mobilization reduces the incidence of this symptom and physiotherapy improves those symptoms that do occur.

Pericarditis. This is characterized by sharp chest pain and a pericardial rub. It frequently occurs in the first few days after an acute myocardial infarction, especially following anterior wall infarction. Anticoagulation should be avoided in these patients and anti-inflammatory medication is usually a successful treatment.

The post-myocardial infarction syndrome (Dressler's syndrome). This occurs weeks to months after an acute myocardial infarction, and consists of a combination of pericarditis, fever and a pericardial effusion. It is caused by an autoimmune response to damaged cardiac tissue and is more common after second or subsequent myocardial infarction. Anti-inflammatory medication, including systemic corticosteroids, may be necessary. Anticoagulation should be avoided.

Left ventricular aneurysm. This is a late complication. Patients present with heart failure, arrhythmias or emboli. It is characterized by ventricular asynergy, often palpable as a double impulse, a fourth heart sound, persistent ST segment elevation on the ECG and sometimes a visible bulge on the chest X-ray. Diagnosis is confirmed by 2D echocardiography. Treatment includes suitable anti-arrhythmic drugs, anticoagulants and medication for heart failure. Surgical removal of the aneurysm (aneurysmectomy) may be necessary if arrhythmias or embolic or haemodynamic complications occur.

REHABILITATION AND RISK STRATIFICATION

If possible, full mobilization should be achieved within 1 week to 10 days to reduce the degree of physical and mental debility inflicted by this illness. Strong reassurance and constant encouragement are very important. Prior to discharge it is ideal to assess:

- The heart size (chest X-ray)
- The cardiovascular response to stress (limited or submaximal exercise test)
- Signal-averaged ECG
- An arrhythmia profile (24-h taped ECG)
- Ventricular function (echocardiogram or nuclear angiogram)

Any abnormalities that are detected should stimulate further investigations such as coronary angiography and left ventriculography. Baroreceptor sensitivity assessment and attempts to provoke ventricular tachycardia by right ventricular pacing must be considered for identification of patients at high risk of sudden death. Revascularization is probably beneficial for some patients with certain arteriographic patterns of coronary disease (see Table 11.23). The most appropriate therapy for other high-risk patients is under investigation.

After a patient has presented with myocardial infarction every opportunity should be taken to modify risk factors for coronary disease. The patient should be instructed to stop smoking. High blood pressure and lipid abnormalities should be corrected.

The families of young patients who present with myocardial infarction should be screened for lipid abnormalities and other risk factors.

Structured psychological and physical rehabilitation schemes are valuable but are only available in a few centres. The patient may return to work after 3 months. Car driving is not permitted for 6 weeks following myocardial infarction. Heavy goods (and public service) vehicle driving licences are withdrawn pending evaluation of the patient's status.

Follow-up treatment
The patient should be discharged taking regular beta-blockade (e.g. propranolol 80 mg twice daily or metroprolol 50 mg twice daily), which has been shown to reduce the incidence of sudden death in the 6 months following acute myocardial infarction. Timolol 10–20 mg daily and probably other beta blockers are similarly effective. Routine treatment with other anti-arrhythmic drugs has not proved beneficial in reducing the incidence of sudden death following myocardial infarction. Long-term aspirin (150 mg daily) further reduces cardiac events following myocardial infarction, but there is little similar evidence for other antithrombotic and anticoagulant medications. Patients should stop smoking.

PROGNOSIS

Statistics concerning sudden death from acute myocardial infarction and from other cardiac causes are so often combined that it is difficult to accurately assess the mortality specifically from myocardial infarction. Assuming that all sudden unexpected cardiac death is due to myocardial infarction, then about 50% of those who die do so within the first 2–3 h, and 75% of the deaths occur within 24 h. Of those who leave hospital alive, about 15–25% die in the first year, and therefore the annual mortality is 5–10%. Fifty per cent of myocardial infarction victims survive for 10 years. Factors suggesting an unfavourable prognosis include a large myocardial infarction, heart failure, a large heart on chest X-ray, ventricular arrhythmias, multiple infarction, recurrent angina, and an abnormal exercise test.

Rheumatic fever

Rheumatic fever is an inflammatory disease that occurs in children and young adults (the first attack usually occurs between 5 and 15 years of age) as a result of infection with group A streptococci. It affects the heart, skin, joints and central nervous system. It is common in the Middle East, Far East, eastern Europe and South America, but it is now rare in the UK, western Europe and North America. This decline in the incidence of rheumatic fever (from 10% of children in the 1920s to 0.01% today) parallels the reduction in all streptococcal infections and is largely due to improved sanitation and also to the use of antibiotics.

Pharyngeal infection with group A *Streptococcus* may be followed by the clinical syndrome of rheumatic fever. This is thought to develop because of an autoimmune reaction triggered by the infecting *Streptococcus*. The condition is not due to direct infection of the heart or to the production of a toxin.

PATHOLOGY

All three layers of the heart may be affected. The characteristic lesion of rheumatic carditis is the Aschoff nodule, which is a granulomatous lesion with a central necrotic area occurring in the myocardium, particularly in the subendocardium of the left ventricle. Small, warty vegetations may develop on the endocardium, particularly on the heart valves. This leads to some degree of valvular regurgitation. A serofibrinous effusion characterizes the acute pericarditis that occurs.

The synovial membranes are acutely inflamed during rheumatic fever, and subcutaneous nodules (which are also granulomatous lesions) are seen in the acute stage of the disease.

CLINICAL FEATURES

The disease presents suddenly, with fever, joint pains, malaise and loss of appetite. The clinical features depend on the organs that are involved. Diagnosis relies on the presence of two or more major clinical manifestations or one major manifestation plus two or more minor features. These are known as the Duckett–Jones criteria (see Table 11.29).

Carditis manifests as:

● New or changed heart murmurs
● The development of cardiac enlargement or cardiac failure
● The appearance of a pericardial effusion and ECG changes of pericarditis (raised ST seg-

Table 11.29 Revised Duckett–Jones criteria for the diagnosis of rheumatic fever. The diagnosis is made on the basis of two or more major criteria, or one major plus two or more minor criteria.

Major criteria
Carditis
Polyarthritis
Chorea
Erythema marginatum
Subcutaneous nodules
Minor criteria
Fever
Arthralgia
Previous rheumatic fever
Raised ESR/C-reactive protein
Leucocytosis
Prolonged PR interval on ECG

Plus evidence of antecedent streptococcal infection, e.g. positive throat cultures for group A streptococci, elevated ASO titre (> 250 units) or other streptococcal antibodies, or a history of recent scarlet fever

ments) or myocarditis (inverted or flattened T waves), first-degree or greater AV block or other cardiac arrhythmias
- A transient diastolic mitral (Carey–Coombs) murmur due to mitral valvulitis

Non-cardiac features include the following.

- A fever with an apparently excessive tachycardia is usually present.
- The arthritis associated with rheumatic fever is classically a fleeting polyarthritis affecting large joints such as the knees, elbows, ankles and wrists. The joints are swollen, red and tender. As the inflammation in one joint recedes, another becomes affected. Once the acute inflammation disappears, the rheumatic process leaves the joints normal.
- Sydenham's chorea (or St Vitus' dance) (see p. 925) is involvement of the central nervous system that develops late after a streptococcal infection. Sufferers are noticeably 'fidgety' and display spasmodic, unintentional movements. Speech is often affected.
- Skin manifestations include erythema marginatum, a transient pink rash with slightly raised edges, which occurs in 20% of cases. The erythematous areas found mostly on the trunk and limbs coalesce into cresent- or ring-shaped patches. Subcutaneous nodules, which are painless, pea-sized, hard nodules beneath the skin, may also occur, particularly over tendons, joints and bony prominences.

INVESTIGATION

- Throat swabs are cultured for the group A *Streptococcus*.

- Serological changes may indicate a recent streptococcal infection. The antistreptolysin O titre, and sometimes others such as the antistreptokinase titre, are performed.
- Non-specific indicators of inflammation such as the ESR and the C-reactive protein levels are usually elevated.

TREATMENT

Patients with fever, active arthritis or active carditis should be completely rested in bed. When the clinical syndrome has subsided (e.g. no pyrexia, normal pulse rate, normal ESR, normal white count) the patient may be mobilized.

Residual streptococcal infections should be eradicated with a single intramuscular injection of 916 mg of benzathine penicillin or oral phenoxymethyl penicillin 500 mg four times daily for 1 week. This therapy should be administered even if nasal or pharyngeal swabs do not culture the streptococci.

High-dose salicylate (preferably acetyl salicylate, i.e. aspirin) therapy is given to the limit of tolerance determined by the development of tinnitus. If carditis is present, systemic corticosteroids may be given. Prednisolone 60–120 mg in four divided doses each day is administered until the clinical syndrome is improved and the ESR has fallen to normal. Steroids are then tapered off over 2–4 weeks. However, the efficacy of steroids is in doubt.

Recurrences are most common when persistent cardiac damage is present, and are prevented by the continued administration of oral phenoxymethyl penicillin 250 mg daily or by monthly injections of 916 mg of benzathine penicillin until the age of 20 or for 5 years after the latest attack (see p. 12). A sulphonamide (e.g. sulphadimidine) may be used if the patient is allergic to penicillin. Any streptococcal infection that does develop should be very promptly treated.

Chronic rheumatic heart disease

More than 50% of those who suffer acute rheumatic fever *with carditis* will later (after 10–20 years)

Table 11.30 Rheumatic valvular lesions.

Valves involved	Percentage of cases
Mitral valve alone	50
Mitral and aortic valves	40
Mitral, aortic and tricuspid	5
Aortic valve alone	2
All other combinations	3

develop chronic rheumatic valvular disease, predominantly affecting the mitral and aortic valves (see Table 11.30).

Valvular heart disease

MITRAL STENOSIS

Almost all mitral stenosis is due to rheumatic heart disease:

- At least 50% of sufferers have a history of rheumatic fever or chorea.
- The single most common valve lesion due to rheumatic fever is pure mitral stenosis (50%).
- The mitral valve is affected in over 90% of those with rheumatic valvular heart disease.
- Rheumatic mitral stenosis is much more common in women.
- The pathological process results after some years in valve thickening, cusp fusion, calcium deposition, a narrowed (stenotic) valve orifice and progressive immobility of the valve cusps.

Other causes

- Lutembacher's syndrome is the combination of acquired mitral stenosis and an atrial septal defect.
- A rare form of congenital mitral stenosis can occur.
- In the elderly a syndrome similar to mitral stenosis can develop because of calcification and fibrosis of the valve, valve ring and subvalvular apparatus (chordae tendineae).

PATHOPHYSIOLOGY

When the normal valve orifice area of 5 cm^2 is reduced to approximately 1 cm^2, severe mitral stenosis is present. In order that sufficient cardiac output will be maintained, the left atrial pressure increases and left atrial hypertrophy and dilatation

Table 11.31 Complications of mitral stenosis.

Atrial fibrillation
Systemic embolization
Pulmonary hypertension
Pulmonary infarction
Chest infections
Infective endocarditis (rare)
Tricuspid regurgitation
Right ventricular failure

occurs. Consequently, pulmonary venous, pulmonary arterial and right heart pressures also increase. The increase in pulmonary capillary pressure is followed by the development of pulmonary oedema. This is partially prevented by alveolar and capillary thickening and pulmonary arterial vasoconstriction (reactive pulmonary hypertension). Pulmonary hypertension leads to right ventricular hypertrophy, dilatation and failure. Right ventricular dilatation results in tricuspid regurgitation. The complications of mitral stenosis (see Table 11.31) are frequent.

SYMPTOMS

Usually there are no symptoms until the valve orifice is moderately stenosed, i.e. has an area of 2 cm^2. In Europe this does not usually occur until several decades after the first attack of rheumatic fever, but in the Middle or Far East, children of 10–20 years of age may have severe calcific mitral stenosis.

Because of pulmonary venous hypertension and recurrent bronchitis, progressively severe dyspnoea develops. A cough productive of blood-tinged, frothy sputum is quite common, and occasionally frank haemoptysis may occur. The development of pulmonary hypertension eventually leads to right heart failure and its symptoms of weakness, fatigue and abdominal or lower limb swelling.

The large left atrium favours atrial fibrillation, giving rise to symptoms such as palpitations. Atrial fibrillation may result in systemic and pulmonary emboli, which give rise to cerebral, mesenteric, renal and pulmonary infarcts.

SIGNS

Face
Severe mitral stenosis with pulmonary hypertension is associated with the so-called mitral facies or malar flush. This is a bilateral, cyanotic or dusky pink discolouration over the upper cheeks that is due to arteriovenous anastomoses and vascular stasis.

Pulse
At first the pulse is regular (sinus rhythm) but later the irregular pulse of atrial fibrillation usually develops. The onset of atrial fibrillation often causes a dramatic clinical deterioration.

Jugular veins
If right heart failure develops there is obvious distension of the jugular veins. If pulmonary hypertension or tricuspid stenosis is present, the *a* wave will be prominent provided that atrial fibrillation has not supervened.

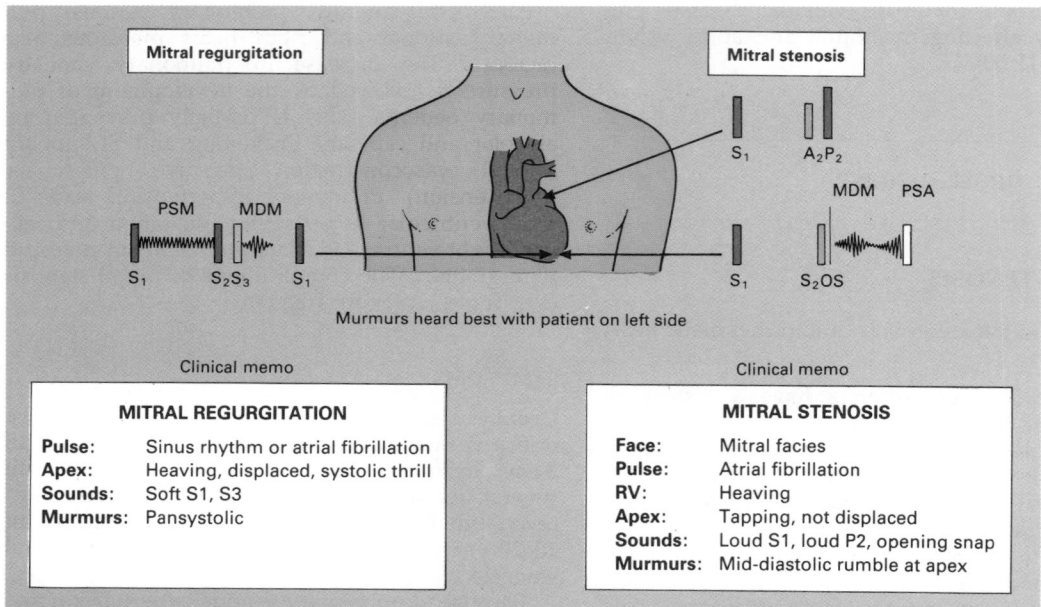

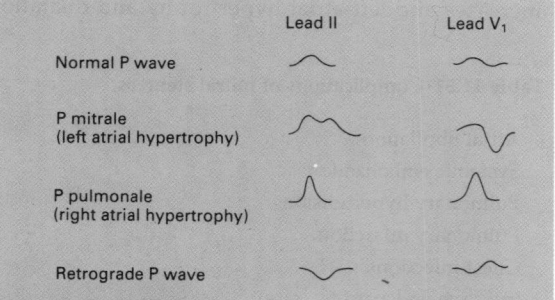

Fig. 11.62 Auscultatory features associated with mitral regurgitation and mitral stenosis. S_1 = first heart sound; S_2 = second heart sound; S_3 = third heart sound; OS = opening snap; A_2 = aortic component of the second heart sound; P_2 = pulmonary component of the second heart sound; PSM = pansystolic murmur; MDM = mid-diastolic murmur; PSA = presystolic accentuation.

Apex beat
The apex beat is 'tapping' in quality. This is the result of a palpable first heart sound combined with left ventricular backward displacement produced by an enlarging right ventricle. A diastolic thrill may be felt at the apex. If pulmonary hypertension is present, the closure of the pulmonary valve may be felt in the second left intercostal space to the side of the sternum. A parasternal heave due to right ventricular hypertrophy may also be felt.

Auscultation
Auscultation (see Fig. 11.62) reveals a loud first heart sound because the cusps are kept open until the beginning of ventricular systole. In early diastole a sound is produced when the mitral valve opens (opening snap). This is followed by a diastolic rumbling murmur, usually localized to the apex and best heard with the patient inclined towards the left. The murmur is due to turbulent blood flow through the narrowed valve. If the patient is in sinus rhythm the murmur becomes louder when atrial systole occurs. This is called pre-systolic accentuation.

The severity of mitral stenosis is judged by the closeness of the opening snap and the following diastolic murmur to the second heart sound. In severe mitral stenosis the very high left atrial pressure opens the mitral valve earlier in diastole.

As the valve cusps become immobile, the loud first heart sound softens and the opening snap disappears. When pulmonary hypertension occurs, the pulmonary component of the second sound is increased in intensity and the mitral diastolic murmur may become quieter because of the reduction of cardiac output.

INVESTIGATION

Chest X-ray
The chest X-ray usually shows a generally small heart with an enlarged left atrium (see Fig. 11.12). Pulmonary venous hypertension (see p. 528) is usually also present. Late in the course of the

Fig. 11.63 A bifid P wave as seen on the ECG in mitral stenosis (P mitrale). Also shown for comparison are other P wave abnormalities.

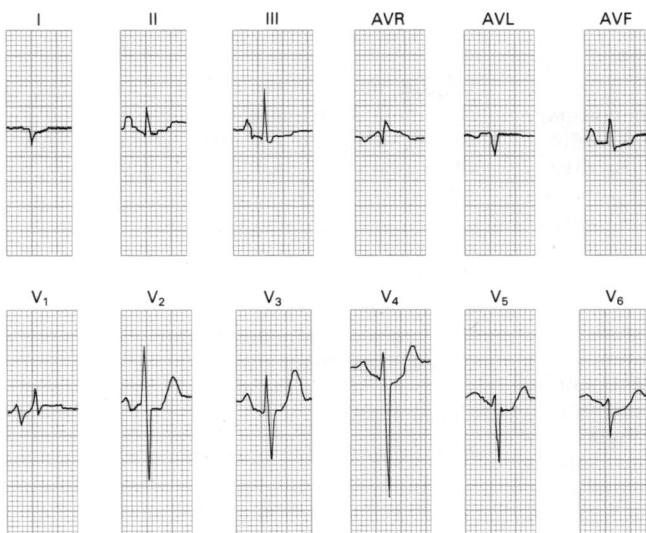

Fig. 11.64 A 12-lead ECG of a patient with severe mitral stenosis. Note the right axis deviation (frontal plane axis = +120°), the left atrial conduction abnormality (large terminal negative component of the P wave in V_1) and the right ventricular hypertrophy (R wave in V_1 and right axis deviation).

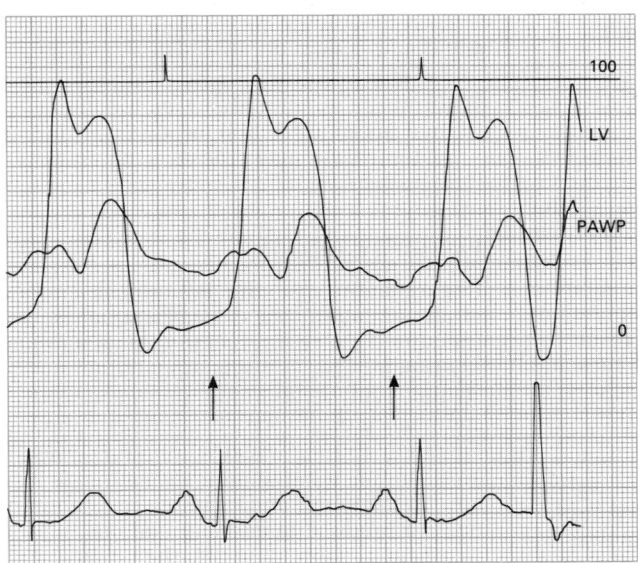

Fig. 11.65 Simultaneous recordings of the ECG, the left ventricular (LV) and the pulmonary arterial wedge pressure (PAWP). The PAWP is almost equivalent to the left atrial pressure. Thus at end-diastole (the onset of the QRS complex) the PAWP is significantly higher than the left ventricular pressure (arrows). The pressure gradient is due to mitral valve stenosis.

disease a calcified mitral valve may be seen on a penetrated or lateral view. The signs of pulmonary oedema or pulmonary hypertension may also be apparent when the disease is severe.

ECG

In sinus rhythm the ECG shows a bifid P wave due to delayed left atrial activation (Fig. 11.63). This double-humped P wave is best seen in leads II, V_3 and V_4. A biphasic P wave with a large late negative component is seen in lead V_1 (Fig. 11.64). However, atrial fibrillation is frequently present. As the disease progresses, the ECG features of right vent-

ricular hypertrophy (right axis deviation and perhaps tall R waves in lead V_1) may develop (Fig. 11.64).

Echocardiogram (see Fig. 11.23)

The movement of the valve cusps and the rate of diastolic filling of the left ventricle may be measured—severe mitral stenosis produces immobility of the valve cusps and slow filling of the ventricles. The echocardiogram appearances are usually sufficiently accurate to allow surgical management to be considered. CW Doppler is used to estimate peak mitral trans-valvular gradient and the valve area.

Cardiac catheterization

This is only required if an adequate echocardiogram is impossible to obtain or if coexisting cardiac problems (e.g. mitral regurgitation or coronary artery disease) are suspected. The typical findings in mitral stenosis are a diastolic pressure that is higher in the left atrium than in the left ventricle (Fig. 11.65). This gradient of pressure is usually proportional to the degree of the stenosis.

TREATMENT

Mild mitral stenosis may need no treatment other than prompt therapy of attacks of bronchitis. Although infective endocarditis in pure mitral stenosis is uncommon, antibiotic prophylaxis is advised (see p. 12). Early symptoms of mitral stenosis such as mild dyspnoea can usually be treated with low doses of diuretics. The onset of atrial fibrillation requires treatment with digoxin and anticoagulation to prevent atrial thrombus and systemic embolization. If pulmonary hypertension develops or the symptoms of pulmonary congestion persist despite therapy, surgical relief of the mitral stenosis is advised. There are three types of operation: closed valvotomy, open valvotomy and mitral valve replacement.

Closed valvotomy

This operation is advised for patients with mobile, non-calcified and non-regurgitant mitral valves. The fused cusps are forced apart by a dilator introduced through the apex of the left ventricle and guided into position by the surgeon's finger inserted via the left atrial appendage. Cardiopulmonary bypass is not needed for this operation. Closed valvotomy may produce a good result for 10 or more years. The valve cusps often re-fuse and eventually another operation may be necessary.

Open valvotomy

This operation is often preferred to closed valvotomy. The cusps are carefully dissected apart under direct vision. Cardiopulmonary bypass is required. Open dissection reduces the likelihood of causing traumatic mitral regurgitation.

Mitral valve replacement

Replacement of the mitral valve is necessary:

● If mitral regurgitation is also present
● If there is a badly diseased or badly calcified stenotic valve that cannot be reopened without producing significant regurgitation

Artificial valves may work successfully for more than 20 years. Anticoagulants are generally necessary to prevent the formation of thrombus, which might obstruct the valve or embolize.

MITRAL REGURGITATION

Of the many causes of mitral valve regurgitation, rheumatic heart disease (50%) and the prolapsing mitral valve are the most common. Any disease that causes dilatation of the left ventricle may cause mild mitral regurgitation, e.g.:

● Aortic valve disease
● Acute rheumatic fever
● Myocarditis
● Cardiomyopathy
● Hypertensive heart disease
● Ischaemic heart disease

Other causes

● In hypertrophic cardiomyopathy, left ventricular contraction is disorganized and mitral regurgitation often results.
● It may follow myocardial infarction or infective endocarditis.
● It may occur in connective tissue disorders such as systemic lupus erythematosus.
● Collagen abnormalities such as Marfan's syndrome and Ehlers–Danlos syndrome may be associated with mitral regurgitation.
● Degeneration of the valve cusps or mitral annular calcification may result in regurgitation.
● Rupture of the chordae tendineae (due to myocardial infarction or trauma) and infective endocarditis may cause very sudden mitral regurgitation.

PATHOPHYSIOLOGY

Regurgitation into the left atrium produces left atrial dilatation but little increase in left atrial pressure if the regurgitation is long-standing as the regurgitant flow is accommodated by the large left atrium. With acute mitral regurgitation the normal compliance of the left atrium does not allow much dilatation and the left atrial pressure rises. Thus, in acute mitral regurgitation the left atrial v wave is greatly increased and pulmonary venous pressure rises to produce pulmonary oedema.

Since a proportion of the stroke volume is regurgitated, the stroke volume increases to maintain the forward cardiac output and the left ventricle therefore enlarges.

SYMPTOMS

Mitral regurgitation can be present for many years and the cardiac dimensions may be greatly increased before any symptoms occur. The increased stroke volume may be sensed as a 'palpitation'. Dyspnoea and orthopnoea may develop owing to pulmonary venous hypertension occurring as a direct result of the mitral regurgitation and secondarily to left ventricular failure. Fatigue and lethargy develop because of the reduced cardiac output. In the late stages of the disease the symptoms of right heart failure also occur and eventually lead to congestive cardiac failure. Cardiac cachexia may develop. Thromboembolism is less common than in mitral stenosis, but subacute infective endocarditis is much more common.

SIGNS (see Clinical Memo)

The physical signs (Fig. 11.62) of uncomplicated mitral regurgitation are:

- A laterally displaced, thrusting, diffuse apex beat and a systolic thrill
- A soft first heart sound because of the incomplete apposition of the valve cusps and their partial closure by the time ventricular systole begins
- A pansystolic murmur due to regurgitation occurring throughout the whole of systole, which is loudest at the apex but radiates widely over the precordium and into the axilla
- A prominent third heart sound occurs because of the sudden rush of blood back into the dilated left ventricle in early diastole. Sometimes a short mid-diastolic flow murmur may follow the third heart sound.

The signs related to atrial fibrillation, pulmonary hypertension, and left and right heart failure may develop later in the disease. The onset of atrial fibrillation has a much less dramatic effect on symptoms than in mitral stenosis.

INVESTIGATION

Chest X-ray
The chest X-ray may show left atrial and left ventricular enlargement. There is an increase in the cardiothoracic ratio, and valve calcification may be seen.

ECG
The ECG shows the features of left atrial delay (bifid P waves) and left ventricular hypertrophy (see Fig. 11.66) as manifest by tall R waves in the left lateral leads, e.g. leads I, AVL and V_6, and deep S waves in the right-sided precordial leads, e.g. leads V_1 and V_2. (SV_1 plus RV_5 or RV_6 > 35 mm indicates left ventricular hypertrophy). Left ventricular hypertrophy occurs in about 50% of patients with mitral regurgitation. Atrial fibrillation may be present.

Echocardiogram
The echocardiogram shows a dilated left atrium and left ventricle. There may be specific features of chordal or papillary muscle rupture. CW Doppler can determine the velocity of the regurgitant jet.

Cardiac catheterization
This demonstrates a prominent left atrial systolic pressure wave, and when contrast is injected into the left ventricle it may be seen regurgitating into an enlarged left atrium during systole.

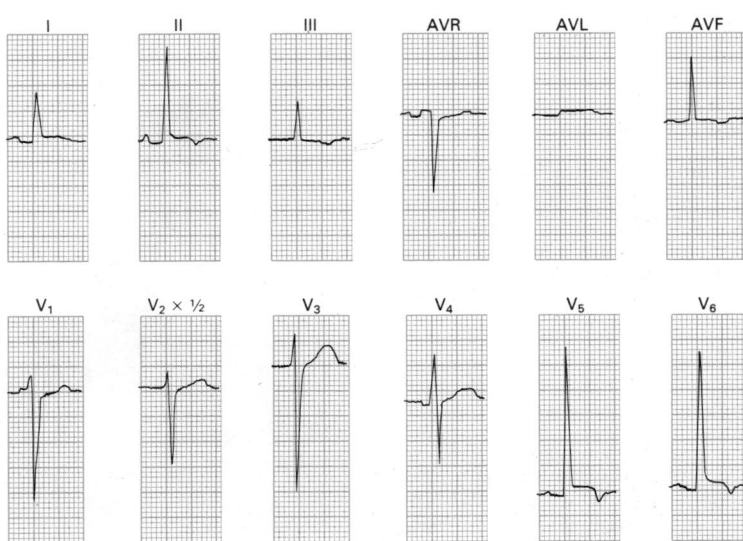

Fig. 11.66 A 12-lead ECG showing features of left ventricular hypertrophy. Note the size of the S wave seen in V_1 (26 mm).

TREATMENT

The development of symptoms usually dictates the need for treatment. Mild mitral regurgitation can usually be managed medically with diuretics for pulmonary congestion, and with digoxin, and possibly anticoagulation, for atrial fibrillation. Antibiotic prophylaxis against infective endocarditis is mandatory (see p. 12).

More severe symptoms that are unresponsive to medical therapy require mitral valve replacement or, occasionally, operative repair of the mitral valve. Rarely, progressive left ventricular enlargement in a relatively asymptomatic patient may indicate that surgery is necessary. Sudden torrential mitral regurgitation, as seen with chordal or papillary rupture or infective endocarditis, may necessitate emergency mitral valve replacement.

Prolapsing (billowing) mitral valve

This is also known as Barlow's syndrome or floppy mitral valve. It is due to excessively large mitral valve leaflets, an enlarged mitral annulus, abnormally long chordae or disordered papillary muscle contraction. Histology may demonstrate myxomatous degeneration of the mitral valve leaflets. It is more commonly seen in young women than in men or older women and it has a familial incidence. Its cause is usually unknown but it may be due to Marfan syndrome, thyrotoxicosis, or rheumatic or ischaemic heart disease. It also occurs in association with atrial septal defect and as part of hypertrophic cardiomyopathy. Mild mitral valve prolapse is so common that it should be regarded as a normal variant.

PATHOPHYSIOLOGY

During ventricular systole, a mitral valve leaflet (most commonly the posterior leaflet) prolapses into the left atrium. This may result in abnormal ventricular contraction, papillary muscle strain and some mitral regurgitation. Usually the syndrome is not haemodynamically serious. Thromboembolism may occur.

SYMPTOMS

Atypical chest pain is the most common symptom. Usually the pain is left submammary and stabbing in quality. Sometimes it is substernal, aching and severe. Rarely it is similar to typical angina pectoris. Palpitations may be experienced because of the abnormal ventricular contraction or because of the atrial and ventricular arrhythmias that are commonly associated with mitral valve prolapse.

SIGNS

The most common sign is a mid-systolic click, which is produced by the sudden prolapse of the valve and the tensing of the chordae tendineae that occurs during systole. This may be followed by a late systolic murmur due to some regurgitation. Sometimes, pan-systolic mitral regurgitation occurs. The signs typically fade quickly but return later.

INVESTIGATION

Chest X-ray
The chest X-ray is usually normal unless significant mitral regurgitation is present.

ECG
The ECG is often abnormal with inverted or biphasic T waves in the inferior leads (leads II, III and AVF) and in the left lateral precordial leads (leads V_5 and V_6). The ST segment may also be slightly depressed in these leads.

Echocardiogram
The diagnosis is confirmed on M-mode echocardiography, which typically shows posterior movement of one or both mitral valve cusps into the left atrium during systole.

Cardiac catheterization
Contrast angiograms performed during cardiac catheterization reveal the systolic prolapse of the mitral valve into the left atrium, and mitral regurgitation, if present, is seen. This investigation is not normally required.

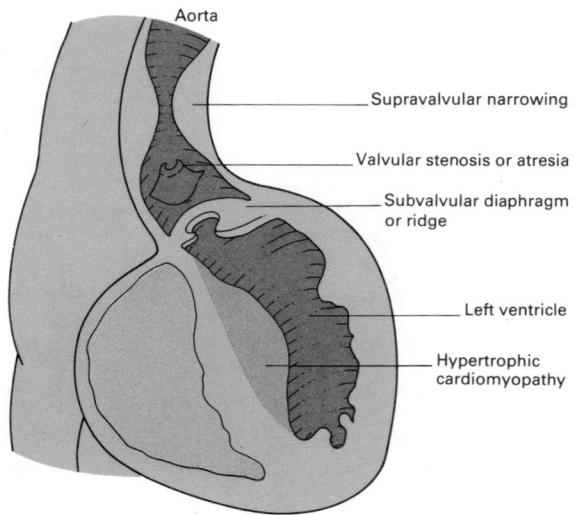

Fig. 11.67 Several forms of left ventricular outflow tract obstruction.

TREATMENT

Usually, beta-blockade is effective for the treatment of the atypical chest pain and palpitations. Sometimes more specific anti-arrhythmic drug treatment is necessary. When a prolapsing mitral valve is associated with significant mitral regurgitation and atrial fibrillation, anticoagulation is advised to prevent thromboembolism. Very occasionally, mitral valve replacement may be necessary for severe regurgitation. Prophylaxis against endocarditis (see p. 12) is advised if there is significant mitral valve regurgitation.

AORTIC STENOSIS

There are three causes of aortic valve stenosis:

- Congenital aortic valve stenosis develops progressively because of turbulent blood flow through a congenitally abnormal (usually bicuspid) aortic valve. Most congenitally abnormal aortic valves occur in men.
- Rheumatic fever results in progressive fusion, thickening and calcification of a previously normal three-cusped aortic valve. In rheumatic heart disease the aortic valve is affected in about 45% of cases and there is usually associated mitral valve disease.
- The wear and tear of age may lead to arterio- sclerotic degeneration and calcification of the aortic valve. It is not usually severely stenotic and symptoms are not usually present.

Valvular aortic stenosis should be distinguished from other causes of obstruction to left ventricular emptying (Fig. 11.67), which include:

- Supravalvular obstruction—a congenital fibrous diaphragm above the aortic valve
- Hypertrophic cardiomyopathy—septal muscle hypertrophy obstructs left ventricular outflow
- Subvalvular aortic stenosis—a congenital condition in which a fibrous ridge or diaphragm is situated immediately below the aortic valve

PATHOPHYSIOLOGY

Obstructed left ventricular emptying leads to increased left ventricular pressure and compensatory left ventricular hypertrophy. In turn, this results in relative ischaemia of the left ventricular myocardium, and consequent angina, arrhythmias and left ventricular failure. The obstruction to left ventricular emptying is relatively more severe on exercise. Normally, exercise causes a many-fold increase in cardiac output, but when there is severe narrowing of the aortic valve orifice the cardiac output can hardly increase. Thus, the blood pressure falls, coronary ischaemia worsens, the myocardium fails and cardiac arrhythmias develop particularly on exercise.

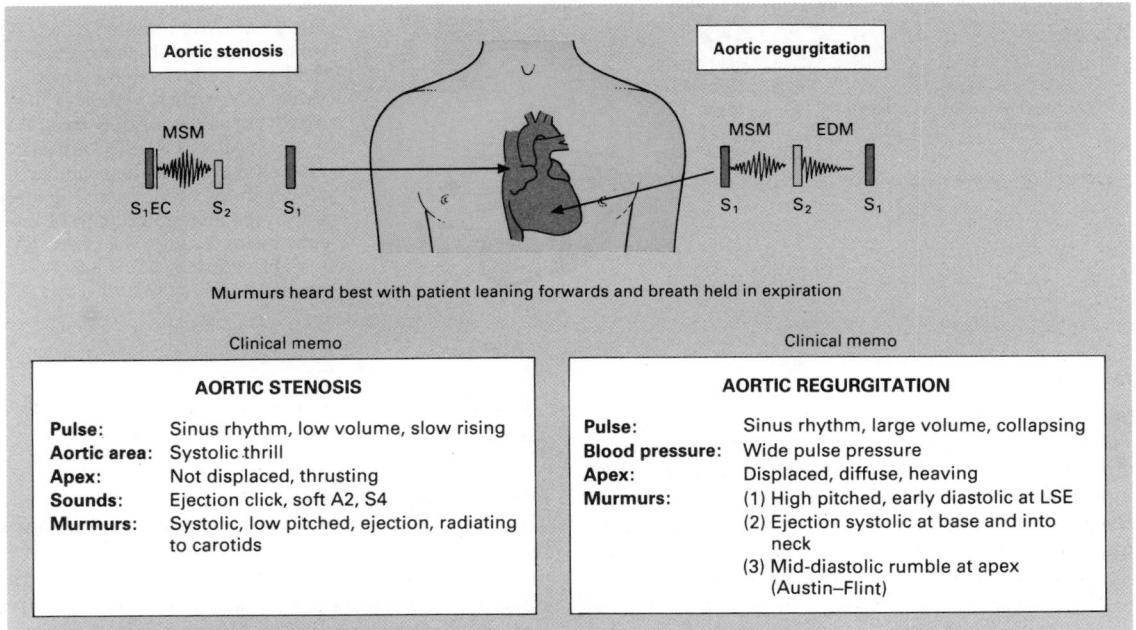

Fig. 11.68 Auscultatory features of aortic stenosis and aortic regurgitation. S_1 = first heart sound; EC = ejection click; MSM = mid-systolic murmur; EDM = early diastolic murmur.

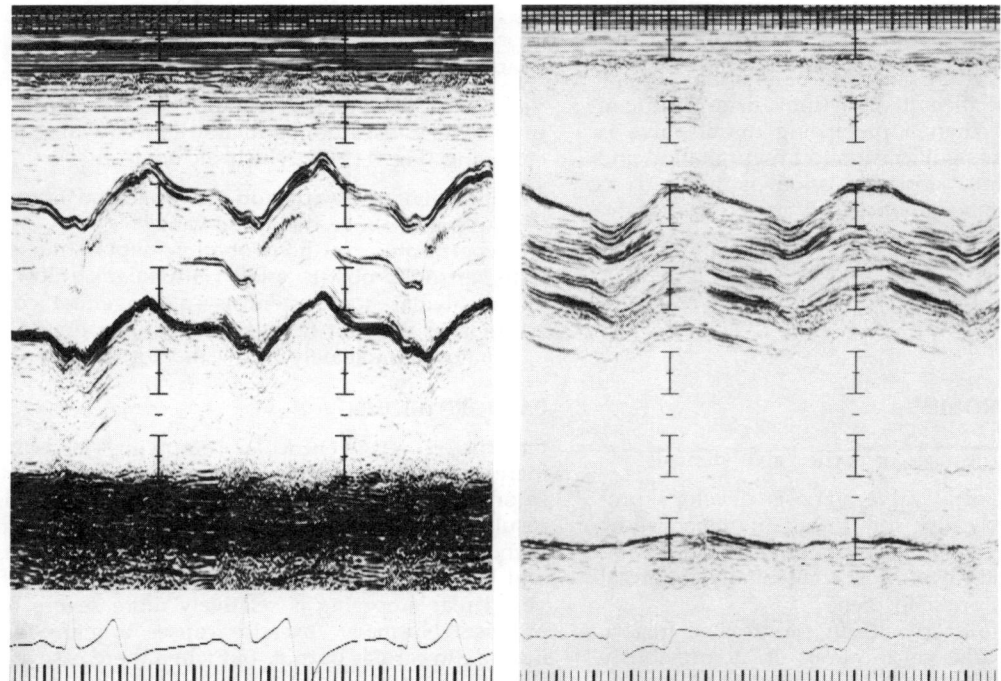

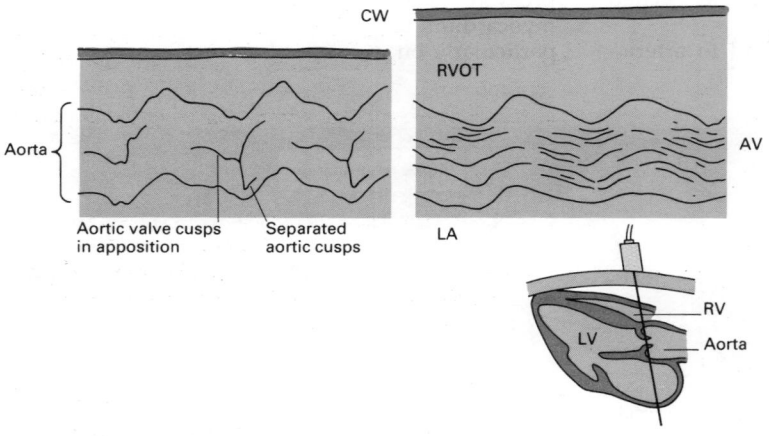

Fig. 11.69 An M-mode echocardiogram showing a normal (left) and stenotic (right) aortic valve. CW = chest wall; RVOT = right ventricular outflow tract; AV = aortic valve; LA = left atrium. There are multiple dense linear echoes in the aortic root. The inset shows the anatomical path of the echo beam through the chest. RV = right ventricle; LV = left ventricle.

SYMPTOMS

There are usually no symptoms until aortic stenosis is moderately severe (when the aortic orifice is reduced to one-third of its normal size). At this stage, exercise-induced syncope, angina and dyspnoea may develop. When symptoms occur, the prognosis is poor—on average, death occurs within 2–3 years if there has been no surgical intervention.

SIGNS (see Clinical Memo)

Aortic stenosis is characterized by abnormalities of the pulse, precordial pulsation and auscultation.

Pulse
The carotid pulse is of small volume and is slow rising or plateau in nature (see p. 518).

Precordial palpation
The apex beat is not usually displaced because hypertrophy (as opposed to dilatation) does not produce noticeable cardiomegaly. However, the pulsation is sustained and obvious—a *heaving apex beat*. A double impulse is sometimes felt because the fourth heart sound or atrial contraction ('kick') may be palpable. A systolic thrill may be felt in the aortic area.

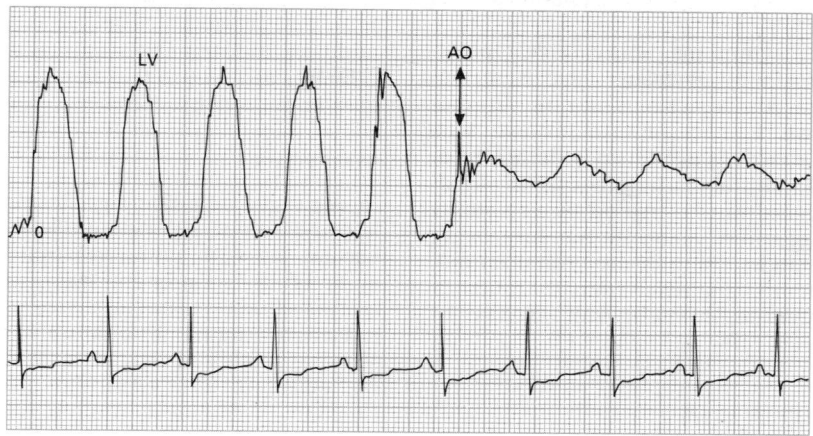

Fig. 11.70 ECG and pressure trace as a cardiac catheter is withdrawn from the left ventricle (LV) to the aorta (AO). Note that the peak systolic pressure changes from 250 to 130 mm Hg (arrow). The 120 mm Hg peak-to-peak systolic gradient indicates severe aortic valvular stenosis.

Auscultation (see Fig. 11.68)
The most obvious auscultatory finding in aortic stenosis is a mid-systolic ejection murmur that is usually 'diamond' shaped (crescendo–decrescendo). The murmur is usually longer when the disease is more severe, as a longer left ventricular ejection time is needed. The intensity of the murmur is not a good guide to the severity of the condition because it is lessened by a reduced cardiac output. The murmur is usually rough in quality and best heard in the aortic area. It radiates widely and is usually easily heard over the clavicles and the carotid arteries.

Other findings

- A systolic ejection click (see p. 524), unless the valve has become immobile and calcified
- Soft or inaudible aortic second heart sound when the aortic valve becomes immobile
- Reversed splitting of the second heart sound (splitting on expiration) (see p. 523)
- A prominent fourth heart sound (see p. 524), unless coexisting mitral stenosis prevents this

Degenerative disease of the aortic valve (aortic sclerosis) results in a loud mid-systolic murmur but, because there is little stenosis, there are no signs of left ventricular hypertrophy or of a slow rising pulse. This murmur can be ignored.

INVESTIGATION

Chest X-ray
The chest X-ray usually reveals a relatively small heart with a prominent, dilated, ascending aorta. This occurs because turbulent blood flow above the stenosed aortic valve produces so-called 'post-stenotic dilatation'. The aortic valve may be calcified. When heart failure occurs, the cardiothoracic ratio increases.

ECG
The ECG shows left ventricular hypertrophy and left atrial delay. A left ventricular 'strain' pattern due to 'pressure overload' (depressed ST segments and T wave inversion in leads orientated towards the left ventricle, i.e. leads I, AVL, V_5 and V_6) is common when the disease is severe. Usually, sinus rhythm is present, but ventricular arrhythmias may be recorded.

Echocardiogram
The echocardiogram readily demonstrates the thickened, calcified and immobile aortic valve cusps (see Fig. 11.69). Left ventricular hypertrophy may also be seen. The gradient across the valve can be estimated by CW Doppler.

Cardiac catheterization
Cardiac catheterization is used to document the systolic pressure difference (gradient) between the aorta and the left ventricle (Fig. 11.70). A gradient of 50 mm Hg or more is usually sufficient to advise surgery. A trivial degree of aortic regurgitation that is undetectable clinically is often demonstrated by contrast aortography. Coronary angiography is important before recommending surgery.

TREATMENT

Patients with aortic stenosis should not overly exert themselves, and in particular they should not compete in strenuous physical games. Angina is best treated with beta-blockade because vasodilators such as glyceryl trinitrate or isosorbide dinitrate may aggravate exertional syncope. Antibiotic prophylaxis against infective endocarditis is essential (see p. 12).

Irrespective of symptoms, aortic valve replacement with a prosthetic or tissue valve is recommended when aortic stenosis is severe. Cardiopulmonary bypass is necessary to achieve this. Provided that the valve is not severely deformed or heavily calcified, critical aortic stenosis in childhood or adolescence can be treated by valvotomy (performed under direct vision by the surgeon or by balloon dilatation using X-ray visualization). This produces temporary relief from the obstruction. Aortic valve replacement will usually be needed a few years later.

AORTIC REGURGITATION

The most common causes of aortic regurgitation are rheumatic fever and infective endocarditis complicating a previously damaged valve. This can be a congenitally abnormal valve (e.g. a bicuspid valve) or one damaged by rheumatic fever. There are numerous other causes and associations (see Table 11.32). The majority of patients with aortic regurgitation are men (75%), but rheumatic aortic regurgitation occurs more commonly in women.

PATHOPHYSIOLOGY

Aortic regurgitation is reflux of blood from the aorta through the aortic valve into the left ventricle during diastole. If net cardiac output is to be maintained, the total volume of blood pumped into the aorta must increase, and consequently the left ventricular size must enlarge. Because of the aortic

Table 11.32 Causes and associations of aortic regurgitation.

Acute aortic regurgitation
Acute rheumatic fever
Infective endocarditis
Dissection of the aorta
Ruptured sinus of Valsalva aneurysm
Failure of prosthetic heart valve
Chronic aortic regurgitation
Rheumatic heart disease
Syphilis
Arthritides
Reiter's syndrome
Ankylosing spondylitis
Rheumatoid arthritis
Hypertension (severe)
Bicuspid aortic valve
Aortic endocarditis
Marfan syndrome
Osteogenesis imperfecta

run-off during diastole, diastolic blood pressure falls and coronary perfusion is decreased. In addition, the larger left ventricular size is mechanically less efficient so that the demand for oxygen is greater and cardiac ischaemia develops.

SYMPTOMS

In aortic regurgitation significant symptoms occur late and do not develop until left ventricular failure occurs. As with mitral regurgitation, a common symptom is 'pounding of the heart' because of the increased left ventricular size and its vigorous pulsation. Angina pectoris is a frequent complaint. Varying grades of dyspnoea occur depending on the extent of left ventricular dilatation and dysfunction. Arrhythmias are relatively uncommon.

SIGNS (see Clinical Memo)

The signs of aortic regurgitation are many and are due to the hyperdynamic circulation, reflux of blood into the left ventricle and the increased left ventricular size.

The pulse is bounding or collapsing (see p. 519). The following signs, which are rare, also indicate a hyperdynamic circulation:

- Quincke's sign—capillary pulsation in the nail beds
- De Musset's sign—head nodding with each heart beat
- Durozier's sign—systolic bruit over the femoral arteries when the stethoscope is lighted applied
- Pistol shot femorals—a sharp bang heard on auscultation over the femoral arteries in time with each heart beat

The apex beat is displaced laterally and downwards and is thrusting in quality.

On auscultation there is a high-pitched diastolic murmur running from the aortic component of the second heart sound (Fig. 11.68). It is loudest in early diastole and is heard best at the lower left sternal edge or the cardiac apex.

INVESTIGATION

Chest X-ray
The chest X-ray features are those of left ventricular enlargement and possibly of dilatation of the ascending aorta. The ascending aortic wall may be calcified in syphilis and the aortic valve may be calcified if valvular disease is responsible for the regurgitation.

ECG
The ECG appearances are those of left ventricular hypertrophy due to 'volume overload', i.e. tall R waves and deeply inverted T waves in the left-sided chest leads, and deep S waves in the right-sided leads. Normally, sinus rhythm is present.

Echocardiogram

The echocardiogram demonstrates vigorous cardiac contraction and a dilated left ventricle. The aortic root may also be enlarged. Diastolic fluttering of the mitral leaflets or septum occurs in severe aortic regurgitation (producing the Austin Flint murmur, see p. 525). The regurgitant jet can be detected by CW Doppler.

Cardiac catheterization

During cardiac catheterization, injection of contrast medium into the aorta (aortography) will outline aortic valvular abnormalities and allow assessment of the degree of regurgitation.

TREATMENT

The underlying cause of aortic regurgitation (e.g. syphilitic aortitis or infective endocarditis) may require specific treatment. The treatment of aortic regurgitation usually requires aortic valve replacement but the timing of surgery is important.

Because symptoms do not develop until the myocardium fails and because the myocardium does not recover fully after surgery, it is important to operate before significant symptoms occur. The timing of the operation is best determined according to haemodynamic, echocardiographic or nuclear angiographic criteria.

Both mechanical prostheses and tissue valves are used. Tissue valves are preferred in the elderly and when anticoagulants must be avoided, but are contraindicated in children and young adults because of the rapid calcification and degeneration of the valves.

Antibiotic prophylaxis against infective endocarditis (see p. 12) is necessary even if a prosthetic valve replacement has been performed.

TRICUSPID STENOSIS

This uncommon valve lesion, which is seen much more often in women than in men, is usually due to rheumatic heart disease and is frequently associated with mitral and/or aortic valve disease. Tricuspid stenosis is also seen in the carcinoid syndrome.

PATHOPHYSIOLOGY

Tricuspid valve stenosis results in a reduced cardiac output, which is restored towards normal when the right atrial pressure increases. The resulting systemic venous congestion produces hepatomegaly, ascites and dependent oedema.

SYMPTOMS

Usually, patients with tricuspid stenosis complain of symptoms due to the associated left-sided rheumatic valve lesions. The abdominal pain (due to hepatomegaly) and swelling (due to ascites) and peripheral oedema that occur are relatively severe when compared with the degree of dyspnoea.

SIGNS

If the patient remains in sinus rhythm, which is unusual, there is a prominent jugular venous *a* wave. This presystolic pulsation may also be felt over the liver. There is usually a rumbling mid-diastolic murmur, which is heard best at the lower left sternal edge and is louder on inspiration. It may be missed because of the murmur of coexisting mitral stenosis. A tricuspid opening snap may occasionally be heard.

Hepatomegaly, abdominal ascites and dependent oedema may be present.

INVESTIGATION

Chest X-ray

On the chest X-ray there may be a prominent right atrial bulge.

ECG

The enlarged right atrium may be manifest on the ECG by peaked, tall P waves ($\geq$ 3 mm) in lead 2.

Echocardiogram

The echocardiogram may show a thickened and immobile tricuspid valve, but this is not so clearly seen as an abnormal mitral valve.

Cardiac catheterization

This demonstrates a diastolic pressure gradient between the right atrium and the right ventricle. Contrast injection will demonstrate a large right atrium.

TREATMENT

Medical management consists of diuretic therapy and salt restriction. Tricuspid valvotomy is occasionally possible, but tricuspid valve replacement is often necessary. Other valves usually also need replacement because tricuspid valve stenosis is rarely an isolated lesion.

TRICUSPID REGURGITATION

Functional tricuspid regurgitation may occur whenever the right ventricle dilates, e.g. in cor pulmonale, myocardial infarction or pulmonary hypertension.

Organic tricuspid regurgitation may occur with rheumatic heart disease, infective endocarditis, carcinoid syndrome, Ebstein's anomaly (a congenitally malpositioned tricuspid valve) and other congenital abnormalities of the atrioventricular valves.

SYMPTOMS AND SIGNS

The valvular regurgitation gives rise to high right atrial and systemic venous pressure. Patients may complain of the symptoms of right heart failure.

Physical signs include a large jugular venous *cv* wave and a palpable liver that pulsates in systole. Usually a right ventricular impulse may be felt at the left sternal edge, and there is a blowing pansystolic murmur, best heard on inspiration at the lower left sternal edge. Atrial fibrillation is common.

TREATMENT

Functional tricuspid regurgitation usually disappears with medical management. Severe organic tricuspid regurgitation may require operative repair of the tricuspid valve (annuloplasty or plication). Very occasionally, tricuspid valve replacement may be necessary. In drug addicts with infective endocarditis of the tricuspid valve, surgical removal of the valve is recommended to eradicate the infection. This is usually well tolerated in the short term. The insertion of a prosthetic valve for this condition is considered later (p. 599).

PULMONARY STENOSIS

This is usually a congenital lesion, but it may rarely result from rheumatic fever or from the carcinoid syndrome. Congential pulmonary stenosis may be associated with an intact ventricular septum or with a ventricular septal defect (Fallot's tetralogy).

Pulmonary stenosis may be valvular, subvalvular or supravalvular. Multiple congenital pulmonary arterial stenoses are usually due to infection with rubella during pregnancy.

SYMPTOMS AND SIGNS

The obstruction to right ventricular emptying results in right ventricular hypertrophy which in turn leads to right atrial hypertrophy. Severe pulmonary obstruction may be incompatible with life, but lesser degrees of obstruction give rise to fatigue, syncope and the symptoms of right heart failure. Mild pulmonary stenosis may be asymptomatic.

The physical signs are characterized by a harsh mid-systolic ejection murmur, best heard on inspiration, to the left of the sternum in the second intercostal space. This murmur is often associated with a thrill. The pulmonary closure sound is usually delayed and soft. There may be a pulmon-

ary ejection sound if the obstruction is valvular. A right ventricular fourth sound and a prominent jugular venous *a* wave are present when the stenosis is moderately severe. A right ventricular heave may be felt.

INVESTIGATION

Chest X-ray
The chest X-ray usually shows a prominent pulmonary artery due to post-stenotic dilatation.

ECG
The ECG demonstrates both right atrial and right ventricular hypertrophy, although it may sometimes be normal even in severe pulmonary stenosis.

Cardiac catheterization
The passage of a catheter through the right heart allows the level and degree of the stenosis to be established by measuring the systolic pressure gradient.

TREATMENT

Treatment of severe pulmonary stenosis requires pulmonary valvotomy (balloon valvotomy or direct surgery).

PULMONARY REGURGITATION

This is the most common acquired lesion of the pulmonary valve. It results from dilatation of the pulmonary valve ring, which occurs with pulmonary hypertension. It is characterized by a decrescendo diastolic murmur beginning with the pulmonary component of the second sound (Graham Steell murmur) that is difficult to distinguish from the murmur of aortic regurgitation. Pulmonary regurgitation usually causes no symptoms and treatment is rarely necessary.

Infective endocarditis

Infective endocarditis is an infection of the endocardium or vascular endothelium. The disease may occasionally occur as a fulminating or acute infection, but more commonly runs an insidious course and is known as subacute (bacterial) endocarditis (SBE). The incidence is 6–7 per 100 000 per year in the UK, but is much more common in developing countries. Endocarditis occurs most commonly on rheumatic or congenitally abnormal valves as well as in mitral valve prolapse and calcified aortic valve disease. It also occurs in association with congenital lesions such as ventricular septal defect or persistent ductus arteriosus. A very similar disease may occur from infection of arteriovenous fistulas. Prosthetic valves or prosthetic vascular material may be similarly infected and this is one of the reasons for the increasing incidence of endocarditis in developed countries. The organisms are often non-virulent.

Virulent organisms may infect normal valves, especially when the victim is generally debilitated or immunologically incompetent.

The term 'infective endocarditis' is preferred because not all the infecting organisms are bacteria.

AETIOLOGY

Many organisms cause infective endocarditis. At the present time the most common organisms are:

- *Streptococcus viridans* (e.g. *S. mitis* and *S. sanguis*) (50% of cases). These organisms are part of the bacterial flora of the pharynx and upper respiratory tract, and the infection may follow dental extraction or cleaning, tonsillectomy or bronchoscopy.
- *Streptococcus faecalis* (found in perineal and faecal bacterial flora). Infections with this organism are more usual in older men with prostatic disease, in women with genitourinary infections, or following pelvic surgery.
- *Staphylococcus aureus*. This organism may cause subacute endocarditis and is responsible for 50%

of the acute forms. Patients with central venous catheters used for parenteral feeding, temporary pacemaker electrode catheters or pulmonary artery (Swan–Ganz) catheters are prone to this infection. Cellulitis or skin abscesses are often the origin of the infection, particularly in drug addicts who 'mainline'.

Infective endocarditis can also be caused by:

- *Staphylococcus epidermidis*, *Histoplasma*, *Brucella*, *Candida* and *Aspergillus*. Infections with these organisms are particularly common in intravenous drug addicts, alcoholics and patients with prosthetic heart valves.
- *Coxiella burnetii* (the causative organism of Q fever, see p. 55). This may cause a subacute infection.

Although Gram-negative bacteraemia/septicaemia frequently occur, endocarditis with these organisms is unusual.

PATHOLOGY

Infection occurs along the edges of the heart valves. It is more common on the left side, with mitral and aortic regurgitation being the commonest valve lesions complicated by endocarditis. In drug addicts the valves in the right heart are usually affected.

The endocardium on the low-pressure side of a shunt such as ventricular septal defect is infected and it is the pulmonary artery that is infected when a persistent ductus arteriosus is present; in both instances the lesions are 'jet lesions' produced on the wall opposite the shunt (Figure 11.71).

Hypertrophic cardiomyopathy, syphilitic aortic regurgitation, prolapsing mitral valve and arteriosclerotic valve lesions may also be rarely complicated by endocarditis.

The lesion of infective endocarditis is a mass of fibrin, platelets and infecting organisms known as a vegetation. The chance of an organism sticking to a vegetation is increased because of the clumping together of bacteria caused by agglutinating antibodies. These can develop because of repeated infection with the bacterium over a period of years. In acute endocarditis, vegetations may be very large and may embolize. Virulent microorganisms may rapidly destroy the valve cusp, producing ulceration and regurgitation.

The extracardiac manifestations result either from embolization or from the deposition of immune complexes. The latter is thought to be responsible for arthralgia, Roth spots and Janeway lesions, focal glomerulonephritis and acute vasculitis (see below).

Splenic and renal infarcts are produced by emboli. Myocardial infarction can result from coronary emboli, and pulmonary infarction may occur if right-sided lesions embolize.

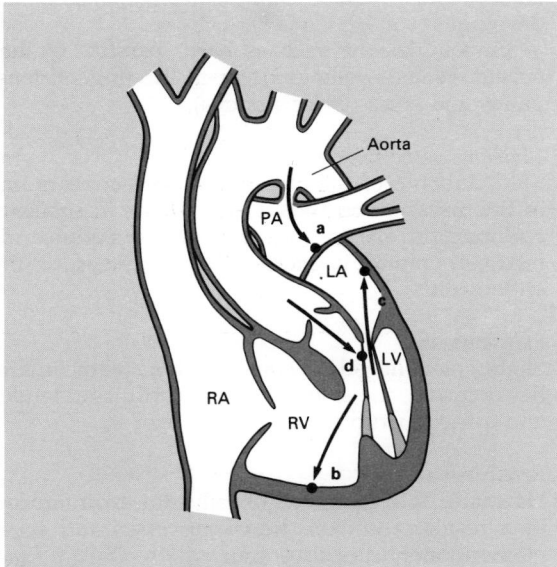

Fig. 11.71 Diagram of jet lesions produced in infective endocarditis. **a** = a lesion in the pulmonary artery (PA) because of a ductus arteriosus. **b** = a lesion in the right ventricle (RV) due to a ventricular septal defect. **c** = a lesion in the left atrium (LA) due to mitral regurgitation. **d** = a lesion in the left ventricle (LV) and on the mitral valve chordae tendineae due to aortic regurgitation. RA = right atrium.

Table 11.33 Clinical features of infective endocarditis.

	Approximate %
General systems	
Malaise	95
Clubbing	10
Cardiac	
Murmurs	90
Cardiac failure	50
Arthralgia	25
Pyrexia	90
Skin lesions	
Osler's nodes	15
Splinter haemorrhages	10
Janeway lesions	5
Petechiae	50
Eyes	
Roth spots	5
Conjunctival splinter haemorrhages	Rare
Splenomegaly	40
Neurological	
Cerebral emboli	20
Mycotic aneurysm	10
Renal	
Haematuria	70

PRESENTATIONS

Subacute endocarditis
The patient presents with fever, night sweats, weight loss, weakness and symptoms due to cardiac failure or embolism. Another important presentation is the combination of renal failure and a heart murmur. It is not usually possible to date the onset of the illness.

Acute endocarditis
In IV drug abusers or following an acute suppurative illness such as pneumonia or meningitis, the development of acute endocarditis is suggested by the persistence of fever and the development of heart murmurs, vasculitis (with petechial haemorrhage) and emboli, including metastatic abscesses. The onset of severe heart failure may indicate chordal rupture or acute valvular destruction.

Prosthetic endocarditis
There are two varieties: the first develops soon after surgery and is due to infection of the prosthesis at surgery, and the second occurs late and follows a bacteraemia. In both cases it is the valve ring that is infected. This produces myocardial abscesses and damage, for example to the

conduction system. Vegetations in the valve may prevent it from opening and closing properly. Emboli are common.

CLINICAL FEATURES (see Table 11.33)

The patients are often elderly. They appear pale (often anaemic) and ill, are intermittently pyrexial and may complain of myalgia and arthralgia. Some of the following signs and symptoms may be present but endocarditis must always be suspected in a patient with a heart murmur and a fever.

Cardiac findings
The signs of any underlying heart disease should be obvious, but occasionally only trivial lesions such as mild aortic regurgitation or a bicuspid aortic valve are present. The development of a new murmur or a change in the character of an existing murmur may warn of the presence of endocarditis.

Vascular lesions
Small petechial or mucosal haemorrhages occur because of vasculitis. They are usually small and red, usually with a pale centre. They frequently appear on the mucosa of the pharynx and conjunctivae. Sometimes they are seen on the retinae (Roth spots). Small, flat, erythematous, non-tender macules are seen mainly on the thenar and hypothenar eminences (Janeway lesions); these blanch with pressure. Splinter haemorrhages may develop.
Embolic lesions such as hard, painful, tender, subcutaneous swellings occur in the fingers, toes, palms and soles (Osler's nodes).

Clubbing of the fingers
Mild clubbing of the fingers and toes appears late in the disease, and thus it only occurs in subacute endocarditis. It is rare nowadays because of relatively rapid diagnosis and treatment of the endocarditis.

Splenomegaly
Slight splenomegaly is common. If a splenic infarct has occurred, the spleen may be painful and tender and a friction rub may be heard over it.

Renal lesions
Haematuria is common, usually due to infarction as a result of emboli. Renal abscesses and acute glomerulonephritis also occur.

Arthritis
Arthritis of the major joints is frequently seen.

Other embolic phenomena
Cerebral emboli can occur, usually to the middle cerebral artery or its branches. Mycotic infected aneurysms are seen and may present after the

endocarditis has healed. Peripheral arterial, pulmonary and coronary infarcts may also occur.

INVESTIGATION

- A normochromic normocytic anaemia is usual and C-reactive protein and the ESR are increased. A polymorphonuclear leucocytosis is common and thrombocytopenia can occasionally occur.
- Liver biochemistry is often mildly disturbed with, in particular, an increased serum alkaline phosphatase.
- Serum immunoglobulins are increased, but total complement and C3 complement are decreased owing to immune complex formation. Circulating immune complexes are present in more than 70% of cases but are not routinely measured.
- Proteinuria may occur and microscopic haematuria is nearly always present.
- Blood cultures are positive in about three quarters of cases. At least six sets of samples are usually taken and cultured in aerobic and anaerobic conditions. Special culture techniques may be necessary for unusual microorganisms such as *Brucella* and *Histoplasma*. Serological tests are needed to incriminate *Coxiella* and *Chlamydia*, and may be helpful for *Candida* and *Brucella*.
- Echocardiography is used to visualize vegetations (Fig. 11.72), but small vegetations typical of the subacute disease can be missed. Echocardiography is useful to document valvular dysfunction and to identify patients in need of urgent surgery. Vegetations may persist despite treatment.
- Chest X-ray may show evidence of heart failure or emboli in right-sided endocarditis.

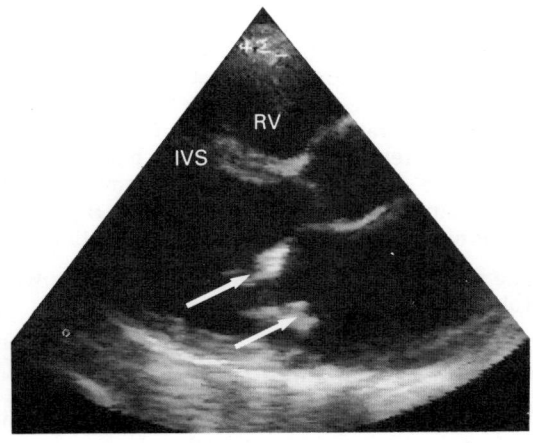

Fig. 11.72 Two-dimensional echocardiogram (long axis parasternal view) which demonstrates vegetations on the leaflets of the mitral valve in a patient with infective endocarditis: CW = chest wall; RV = right ventricle; IVS = interventricular septum; MV = mitral valve.

- ECGs may show evidence of myocardial infarction (emboli) or conduction defects.

TREATMENT

Drug therapy

Any underlying infection should be treated (e.g. a dental abscess should be drained). The endocarditis is treated with bactericidal antibiotics chosen on the basis of the results of the blood culture and antibiotic sensitivity assessment. The treatment should continue for 4–6 weeks. Serum levels are measured and 'back titration' is performed to ensure that sufficient bactericidal antibiotic activity is present to inhibit growth of the organism.

Streptococcus viridans is usually treated with i.v. benzylpenicillin 2.4 g 6-hourly daily and low-dose gentamicin 1 mg·kg^{-1} 8-hourly for the first 2 weeks because of the additive effects of gentamicin and penicillin against *S. viridans*. Oral amoxycillin 6 g daily can replace i.v. therapy after 2 weeks.

Streptococcus faecalis is managed with penicillin and gentamicin (3 mg·kg^{-1} in divided 8-hourly doses). The dosage of penicillin should be higher (up to 24 g daily) than for *S. viridans* because *S. faecalis* is relatively insensitive to penicillin and ampicillin 8 g daily is often substituted. The exact dose of gentamicin depends on renal function and efficacy, and blood levels should be measured at least twice each week.

It is more difficult to choose antibiotics when the infecting organism has not been isolated. However, in the acute form of the disease this is likely to be *Staphylococcus*, and treatment should include flucloxacillin and fusidic acid. In the subacute form, unless it is highly likely that the infecting organism is *Streptococcus viridans*, it is usual to begin treatment with a broad-spectrum combination of antibiotics such as gentamicin and ampicillin. The treatment is adjusted if it is not successful.

The recurrence of fever may suggest that the antibiotic therapy is inadequate, but may also signal a drug reaction. The antibiotics may be omitted for 24–72 h to test this.

Surgery

There are several situations in which surgery is necessary:

- Extensive damage to a valve
- Early infection of prosthetic material
- Worsening renal failure
- Persistent infection but failure to culture an organism
- Embolization
- Large vegetations
- Progressive cardiac failure

The timing of surgery is important. On the one

hand the infection should, if possible, be eradicated before surgery is undertaken, but on the other hand the heart should not be left in a badly compromised haemodynamic state. In general, early surgery is preferable.

PROGNOSIS

The prognosis is worse when the organism cannot be isolated, when cardiac failure is present, when infection occurs on a prosthetic valve, and when the microorganisms found are resistant to therapy. In general, 70% of those affected are treated effectively, but greater awareness of the subacute form of the disease will improve the success rate.

PROPHYLAXIS (see p. 12)

Those at risk of developing endocarditis should receive antibiotic therapy before undergoing a procedure likely to result in a bacteraemia. The form of the prophylaxis depends on the procedure and on the likelihood of endocarditis. High-risk patients are those with a prosthetic heart valve or a previous history of endocarditis.

Congenital heart disease

A congenital cardiac malformation occurs in about 1% of live births. There is an overall male predominance, although some individual lesions (e.g. atrial septal defect and persistent ductus arteriosus) occur more commonly in females. The aetiology of congenital cardiac disease is often unknown but involves:

- Maternal rubella infection (persistent ductus arteriosus, and pulmonary valvular and arterial stenosis)
- Maternal alcohol abuse (septal defects)
- Maternal drug treatment and radiation
- Genetic abnormalities, e.g. the familial form of atrial septal defect and congenital heart block
- Chromosomal abnormalities, e.g. septal defects and mitral and tricuspid valve defects associated with Down's syndrome (trisomy 21) or coarctation of the aorta in Turner's syndrome (45, XO).

Some symptoms and signs are common in congenital heart disease:

- *Central cyanosis* occurs because of right-to-left shunting of blood or because of complete mixing of systemic and pulmonary blood flow.
- *Pulmonary hypertension* results from large left-to-right shunts. The persistently raised pulmonary

Table 11.34 Common congenital lesions.

	Percentage of congenital lesions
Ventricular septal defect	39
Atrial septal defect	10
Persistent ductus arteriosus	10
Pulmonary stenosis	7
Coarctation of the aorta	7
Aortic stenosis	6
Fallot's tetralogy	6
Others	15

flow leads to the development of increased pulmonary artery vascular resistance and consequent pulmonary hypertension. This is known as the Eisenmenger reaction (or the Eisenmenger syndrome when due specifically to a ventricular septal defect). The development of pulmonary hypertension significantly worsens the prognosis.
- *Clubbing of the fingers* may occur in congenital cardiac conditions associated with prolonged cyanosis.
- *Paradoxical embolism* of thrombus from the systemic veins to the systemic arterial system may occur when a communication exists between the right and left heart.
- *Reduced growth* is common in children with cyanotic heart disease.
- *Syncope* is common when severe right or left ventricular outflow tract obstruction is present. Exertional syncope, associated with deepening central cyanosis, may occur in Fallot's tetralogy. Exercise results in increased resistance to pulmonary blood flow but reduced systemic vascular resistance. Thus, the right-to-left shunt increases and cerebral oxygenation falls.
- *Squatting* is the posture adopted by children with Fallot's tetralogy. It results in obstruction of venous return of desaturated blood and an increase in the peripheral systemic vascular resistance. This leads to a reduced right-to-left shunt and improved cerebral oxygenation.

The most common congenital lesions are shown in Table 11.34.

Ventricular septal defect (VSD)

VSD is the most common congenital cardiac malformation (1 in 500 live births). It may occur as an isolated abnormality or in association with other anomalies. Left ventricular pressure is higher than right ventricular pressure; blood therefore moves from left to right and pulmonary blood flow increases. When pulmonary blood flow is very large, obliterative pulmonary vascular changes may cause the pulmonary arterial pressure to equal the systemic pressure (Eisenmenger's syndrome). Consequently, the shunt is reduced or reversed (becoming right-to-left) and central cyanosis may develop.

CLINICAL FEATURES

A small VSD (maladie de Roger) presents with a loud and sometimes long systolic murmur in an asymptomatic patient. Such VSDs usually close spontaneously. Moderate VSDs produce some fatigue and dyspnoea. Physical signs include cardiac enlargement and a prominent apex beat. There is often a palpable systolic thrill at the lower left sternal edge. A loud 'tearing' pan-systolic murmur is heard at the same position.

Large VSDs are associated with increasing pulmonary hypertension (right ventricular parasternal heave and a loud, pulmonary component of the second heart sound). The murmur may be soft because the increased right ventricular pressure may be nearly equal to the left ventricular pressure, so that flow across the VSD is small.

INVESTIGATION

A small VSD produces no abnormal X-ray or ECG findings. On the chest X-ray, larger defects show a prominent pulmonary artery owing to increased pulmonary blood flow. In Eisenmenger's syndrome the radiological signs of pulmonary hypertension (i.e. 'pruned' pulmonary arteries) can be seen. Cardiomegaly occurs when a moderate or a large VSD is present. The ECG shows features of both left and right ventricular hypertrophy. The size and location of the VSD, and its haemodynamic consequences, can be assessed by two-dimensional echocardiography and CW Doppler.

TREATMENT

Moderate and large VSDs should be surgically repaired before the development of severe pulmonary hypertension. Infective endocarditis prophylaxis (see p. 12) should be advised.

Atrial septal defect (ASD)

This congenital condition is often first diagnosed in adults. It is more common in women than in men. There are two types of ASD—ostium secundum and ostium primum. The common form of ASD is ostium secundum. Communication at the level of the atria allows left-to-right shunting of blood. Because the pulmonary vascular resistance is low and the right ventricle is easily distended (i.e. it is compliant), there is a considerable increase in right heart output. Above the age of 30 years there may

---

ATRIAL SEPTAL DEFECT	
Clinical Memo	
Sternal impulse:	RV heave
Sounds:	Loud P$_2$
	Fixed split S$_2$ (A$_2$–P$_2$) .
Murmurs:	Mid-systolic ejection in pulmonary area

be an increase in pulmonary vascular resistance, which gives rise to pulmonary hypertension. Atrial arrhythmias, particularly atrial fibrillation, are common at this stage.

CLINICAL FEATURES (see Clinical Memo)

Most children with ASDs are asymptomatic, although they are prone to pulmonary infection. Some complain of dyspnoea and weakness. Palpitations due to atrial arrhythmias are not uncommon. Right heart failure may develop in later life.

The physical signs of ASD reflect the volume overloading of the right ventricle. Therefore, the splitting of the second sound is wide and fixed (see p. 523). The increased flow through the right heart produces a loud ejection systolic pulmonary flow murmur, and sometimes a diastolic tricuspid flow murmur may be heard. A right ventricular impulse can usually be felt.

INVESTIGATION

- The chest X-ray shows a prominent pulmonary artery and pulmonary plethora (Fig. 11.73). Figure 11.74 shows a more severe case with pulmonary hypertension. There may be noticeable right ventricular enlargement.
- The ECG usually shows some degree of right bundle branch block (because of dilatation of the right ventricle) and right axis deviation.
- The echocardiogram demonstrates right ventricular hypertrophy and pulmonary arterial dilatation. The interventricular septum moves abnormally. Sometimes the ASD is part of a major developmental abnormality and may also involve the ventricular septum and the mitral and tricuspid valves. In this case there is left axis deviation on the ECG. Two-dimensional cardiography will define the site and size of the defect.
- Flow disturbance can be assessed by Doppler.
- Cardiac catheterization is not always necessary with the advent of echocardiography.

TREATMENT

A significant ASD (i.e. a pulmonary flow that is more than 50% increased when compared with

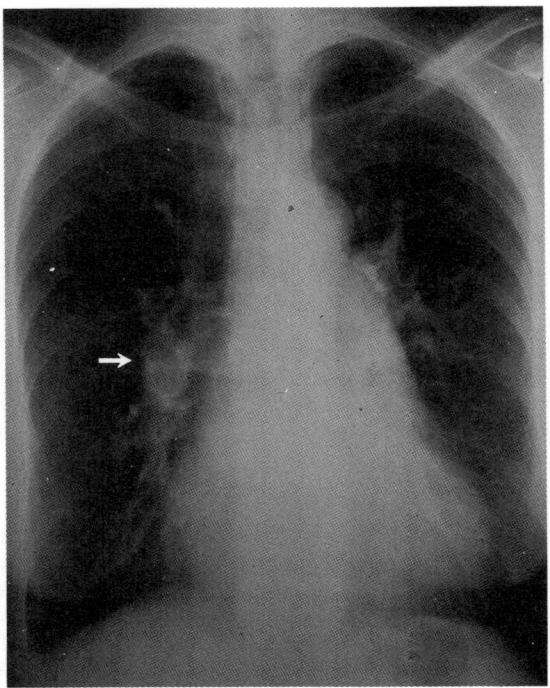

Fig. 11.73 Chest X-ray of a patient with an atrial septal defect. Notice the prominent pulmonary artery (arrow) and the plethoric lung fields.

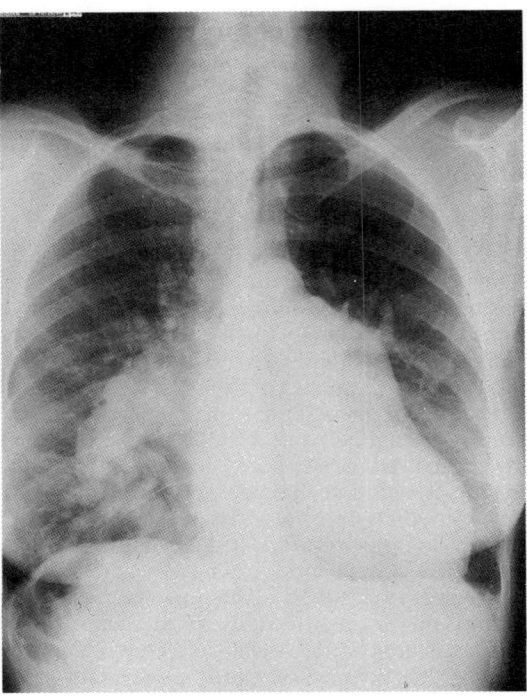

Fig. 11.74 Chest X-ray from a patient with pulmonary hypertension secondary to an atrial septal defect. It shows enlargement of the heart and a prominent pulmonary artery with greatly enlarged proximal branches.

systemic flow) should be repaired before the age of 10 years or as soon as possible if first diagnosed in adulthood. There is a good result from surgery unless pulmonary hypertension has developed.

Persistent ductus arteriosus (PDA)

The ductus arteriosus connects the pulmonary artery at its bifurcation to the descending aorta immediately distal to the subclavian artery. In fetal life the ductus diverts blood away from the unexpanded, and hence high-resistance, pulmonary circulation into the systemic circulation, where the blood is reoxygenated as it passes through the placenta. At birth, the high oxygen in the lungs and the reduced pulmonary vascular resistance triggers closure of the duct. If the duct is malformed, i.e. it does not contain sufficient elastic tissue, it will not close. This is more common in females and is sometimes associated with maternal rubella. Premature babies are often born with persistent ducts that are anatomically normal but are immature in that they lack the mechanism to close.

Because aortic pressure exceeds pulmonary artery pressure throughout the cardiac cycle, a persistent duct produces continuous aorta-to-pulmonary artery shunting. This leads to an increased pulmonary venous return to the left

heart and an increased left ventricular volume load.

CLINICAL FEATURES

If the shunt is large, the left heart volume overload results in severe left heart failure. However, there are often no symptoms until later in life when heart failure or infective endocarditis develop.

The characteristic physical sign is a continuous 'machinery' murmur (due to turbulent aortic-to-pulmonary artery shunting in both systole and diastole), best heard below the left clavicle in the first interspace or over the first rib. A thrill may often be felt. The peripheral pulse is large in volume ('bounding') because of the increased left heart blood flow and the decompression of the aorta into the pulmonary artery.

INVESTIGATION

The aorta and pulmonary arterial system are prominent radiologically. There is both a left atrial abnormality and left ventricular hypertrophy on the ECG. The echocardiogram shows a dilated left atrium and left ventricle.

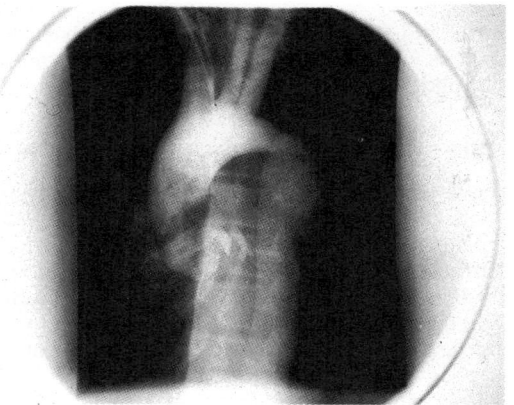
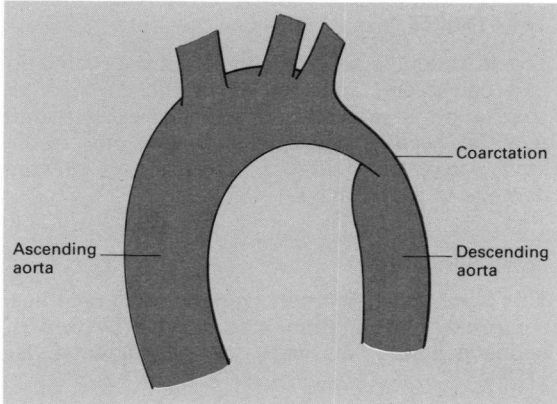

Fig. 11.75 An arch aortogram demonstrating a coarctation of the aorta.

TREATMENT

Premature infants with a persistent duct may be treated medically with indomethacin, which inhibits prostaglandin production and stimulates duct closure. In other cases the duct can be ligated surgically with very little risk. Surgery should be performed as soon as possible and not later than 5 years.

Coarctation of the aorta

Coarctation of the aorta occurs twice as commonly in men as in women. However, it is also associated with Turner's syndrome. The coarctation is a narrowing of the aorta at, or just distal to, the insertion of the ductus arteriosus (Fig. 11.75). In 80% of cases coarctation of the aorta is associated with a bicuspid (and potentially stenotic) aortic valve.

Severe narrowing of the aorta encourages the formation of a collateral arterial circulation involving the periscapular and intercostal arteries. Decreased renal perfusion can led to the development of systemic hypertension that persists even after surgical correction.

CLINICAL FEATURES

Coarctation of the aorta is often asymptomatic for many years. Headaches and nose bleeds (due to hypertension) and claudication and cold legs (due to poor blood flow in the lower limbs) may be present.

Physical examination reveals hypertension in the upper limbs, and weak, delayed (radiofemoral delay) pulses in the legs.

A mid-to-late systolic murmur due to turbulent flow through the coarctation may be heard over the upper precordium or the back. Vascular bruits from the collateral circulation may also be heard.

INVESTIGATION

The chest X-ray may reveal a dilated aorta indented at the site of the coarctation. This is manifested by an aorta (seen in the upper right mediastinum) shaped like a figure '3'. In adults, tortuous and dilated collateral intercostal arteries may erode the undersurfaces of the ribs ('rib notching') (Fig. 11.76). The ECG demonstrates left ventricular hypertrophy. Echocardiography sometimes shows the coarctation and other associated anomalies. Aortography will show the defect and digital vascular imaging allows the coarctation to be visualized after the intravenous injection of contrast. MRI will also demonstrate the coarctation.

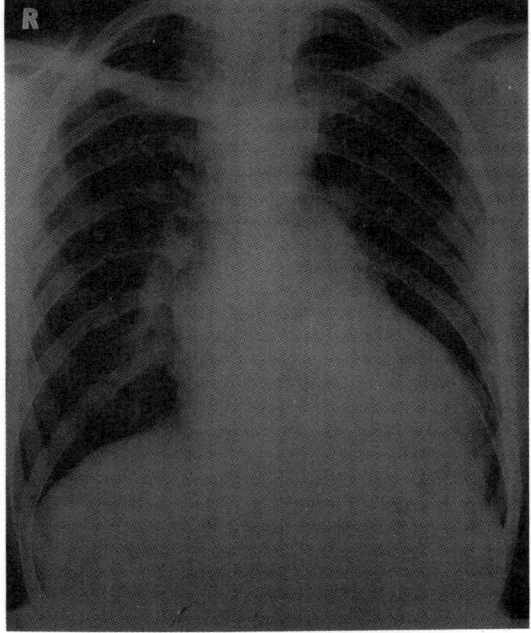

Fig. 11.76 An X-ray from a patient with coarctation of the aorta. Notice the notching of the underside of the upper ribs.

TREATMENT

The treatment is surgical excision of the coarctation and end-to-end anastomosis of the aorta. If the coarctation is extensive, prosthetic vascular grafts may be needed. Hypertension may not resolve after successful surgery because of previous damage to the kidneys.

Fallot's tetralogy

This is the most common cyanotic congenital heart abnormality in children who survive beyond the neonatal period. It consists of the following (Fig. 11.77).

- A ventricular septal defect (VSD)
- Right ventricular outflow obstruction. The level of the obstruction may be subvalvular, valvular or supravalvular. The commonest obstruction is subvalvular, either alone (50%) or in combination with valvular stenosis (25%).
- Positioning of the aorta above the VSD ('overriding arota').
- Right ventricular hypertrophy

This combination of lesions leads to a high right ventricular pressure and right-to-left shunting of blood through the VSD. Thus the patient is centrally cyanosed.

CLINICAL FEATURES

Children with this condition may present with dyspnoea or fatigue or with hypoxic episodes (Fallot's spells), i.e. deep cyanosis and possible syncope, on exertion. Squatting is common.

Physical signs include a parasternal heave and a systolic ejection murmur, often associated with a thrill in the second left interspace close to the sternum. The second heart sound is usually single because the pulmonary component is too soft to be heard. Central cyanosis is commonly present from

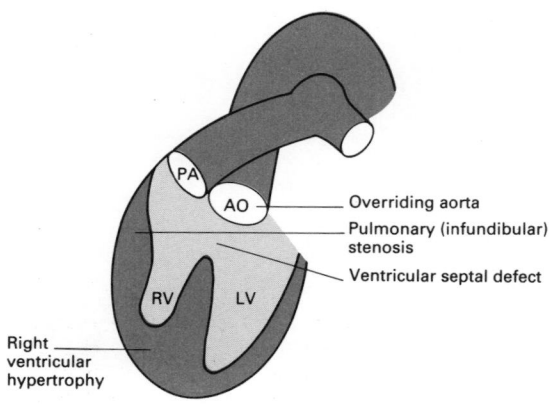

Fig. 11.77 The four features of Fallot's tetralogy.

birth, and finger clubbing and polycythaemia are obvious after about 1 year. Growth may be retarded.

INVESTIGATION

The chest X-ray shows a large right ventricle and a small pulmonary artery. The ECG reveals right ventricular hypertrophy and the echocardiogram demonstrates discontinuity between the aorta and the anterior wall of the ventricular septum. Cardiac catheterization is performed to evaluate the size and degree of the right ventricular outflow obstruction.

TREATMENT

Complete surgical correction of this combination of lesions is possible even in infancy. Often a palliative procedure—an anastomosis between a subclavian artery and a pulmonary artery (Blalock shunt)—is performed on very young infants.

This operation results in an increased blood supply to the lungs. Fallot's spells may need treatment with beta-blockade or, when severe, with diamorphine to relax the right ventricular outflow obstruction.

Pulmonary heart disease

Pulmonary hypertension

An elevated pulmonary arterial pressure, known as pulmonary hypertension, has numerous causes:

- Chronic lung disease, which is diagnosed clinically and by abnormalities of lung function.
- Increased pulmonary blood flow because of left-to-right shunting through a ventricular septal defect, atrial septal defect or persistent ductus arteriosus.
- Left ventricular failure, mitral valve disease, left atrial tumour or thrombus, or pulmonary veno-occlusive disease, which cause an elevation in the pulmonary arterial pressure secondary to an elevation of the pulmonary venous and pulmonary capillary pressure; the pulmonary wedge pressure is elevated in these cases.
- Pulmonary thromboembolic disease.
- Primary pulmonary hypertension, a rare condition seen predominantly in young women. Its aetiology is unknown but recurrent small pulmonary emboli, pulmonary vasoconstriction due to neural, humoral factors or drugs (e.g. oral contraceptives, crotalaria teas and the appetite suppressant fenfluramine), connective-tissue

disease and familial causes have all been suggested.

Pulmonary hypertension leads to enlarged proximal pulmonary arteries, right ventricular hypertrophy and right atrial dilatation. The pulmonary arterial changes depend on the aetiology of the pulmonary hypertension.

Multiple peripheral pulmonary arterial stenoses can produce a syndrome that is similar to pulmonary hypertension, but the pressure in the distal pulmonary bed is normal or low.

CLINICAL FEATURES

Chest pain, exertional dyspnoea, syncope and fatigue are common symptoms, and sudden death may occur. Other symptoms are due to the cause of the pulmonary hypertension.

On physical examination there is a prominent *a* wave in the jugular venous pulse, a right ventricular (parasternal) heave and a loud pulmonary component to the second heart sound. Other findings include a right ventricular fourth heart sound, a systolic pulmonary ejection click, a midsystolic ejection murmur and an early diastolic murmur due to pulmonary regurgitation (Graham Steell murmur). If tricuspid regurgitation develops, there is a pansystolic murmur and a large jugular *v* wave.

INVESTIGATION

The chest X-ray may show right ventricular enlargement and right atrial dilatation. The pulmonary artery is usually prominent and the enlarged proximal pulmonary arteries taper rapidly. Peripheral lung fields are oligaemic.

The ECG demonstrates right ventricular hypertrophy (right axis deviation, possibly a predominant R wave in lead V_1, and inverted T waves in right precordial leads) and a right atrial abnormality (tall peaked P waves in lead II) (Fig. 11.78).

Other investigations are performed to evaluate the cause of pulmonary hypertension. It is particularly important to look for treatable conditions such as left-to-right shunts, mitral stenosis or left atrial tumours with echocardiography. Radioisotope lung scans and sometimes open lung biopsy are performed, e.g. in young patients with severe pulmonary hypertension of unknown cause. Pulmonary angiography is dangerous and is rarely necessary.

TREATMENT

Treatment is determined by the condition underlying pulmonary hypertension. Primary pulmonary hypertension is treated with anticoagulation (because of the possibility of recurrent thromboembolism). Diuretic treatment may be used for right ventricular failure, but care should be taken to avoid reduction of the left ventricular filling pressure. Hypoxia is avoided by the use of oxygen therapy when necessary. Vasodilators including calcium antagonists such as verapamil have been tried, but with little long-term success. Usually there is a progressive downhill course. Heart and lung transplantation is now possible for young patients with this condition.

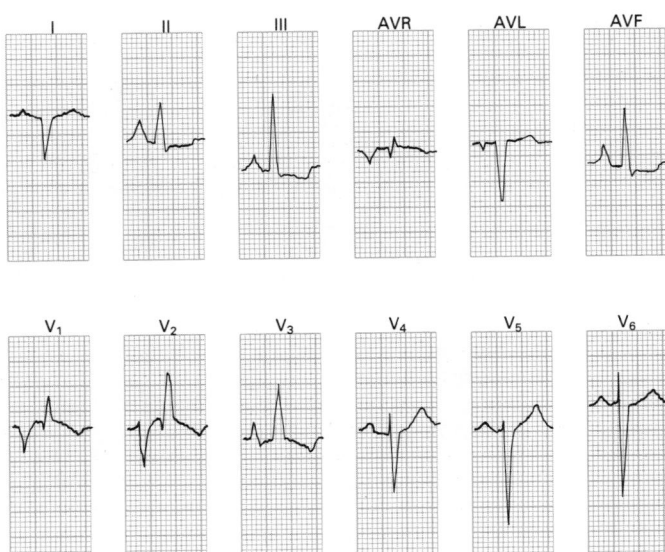

Fig. 11.78 A 12-lead ECG demonstrating pulmonary hypertension. There is right axis deviation (+120°), right ventricular hypertrophy (dominant secondary R wave [R'] in V_1) and a combination of left and right atrial conduction abnormalities.

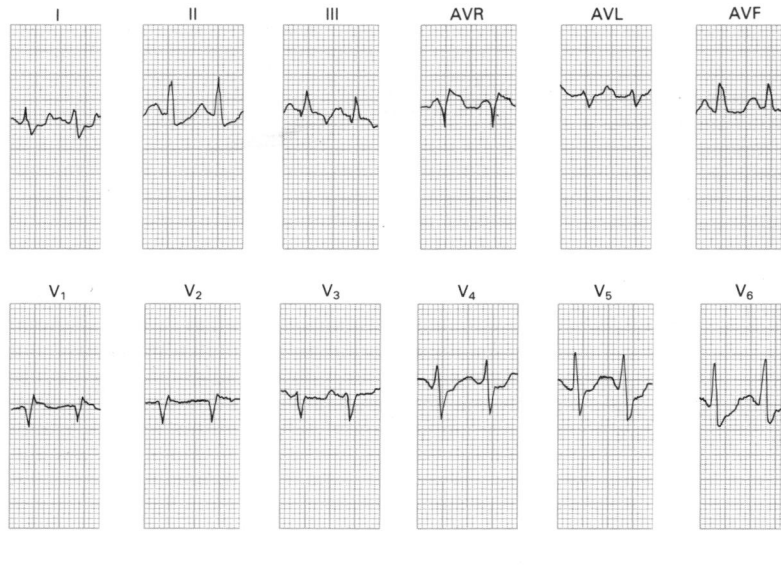

Fig. 11.79 A 12-lead ECG demonstrating some features of acute pulmonary embolism. There is an S wave in lead I, a Q wave in lead III and an inverted T wave in lead III (the S1, Q3, T3 pattern). There is sinus tachycardia (160 beats per minute) and an incomplete right bundle branch block pattern (an R wave in AVR and V_1 and an S wave in V_6).

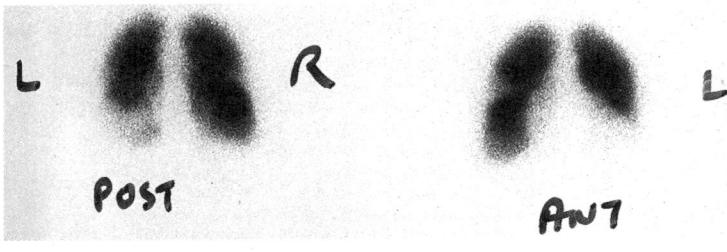

Fig. 11.80 Perfusion lung scan using technetium-labelled macroaggregates. Multiple perfusion defects are seen, the most prominent in the right mid-zone (left). This is suggestive of multiple pulmonary emboli.

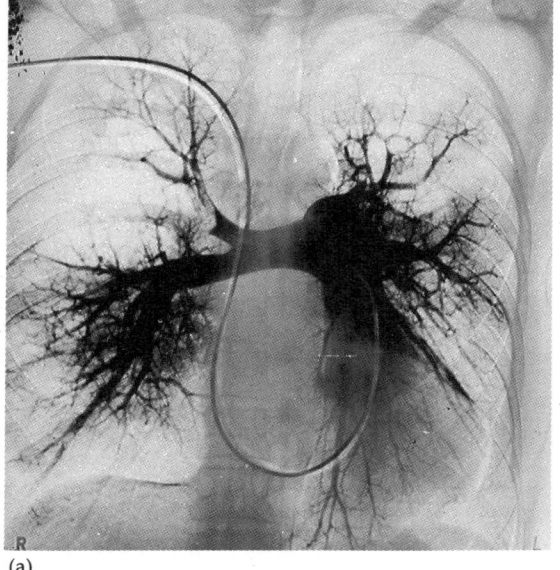

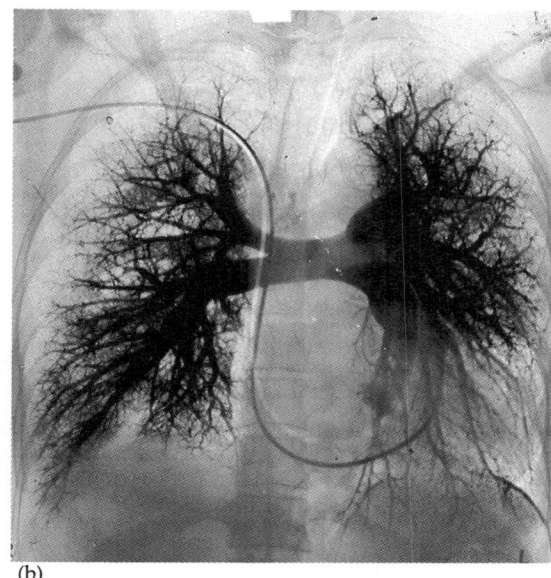

(a)   (b)

Fig. 11.81 Pulmonary arteriogram (subtraction film). (a) Many parts of the lungs are underperfused. An embolus is particularly well seen as filling defects in the vessel to the right upper lobe. (b) Repeat angiogram after treatment with streptokinase.

Pulmonary embolism (acute cor pulmonale)

Thrombus, usually formed in the systemic veins or rarely in the right heart, may dislodge and embolize into the pulmonary arterial system. Post-mortem studies indicate that this is a very common condition (microemboli are found in up to 60% of autopsies) but it is not usually diagnosed this frequently in life. Ten per cent of clinical pulmonary emboli are fatal.

Conditions leading to the formation of clot in the systemic veins (and hence predisposing to pulmonary emboli) include prolonged bed-rest, pelvic and lower limb fractures, pelvic or abdominal surgery, cardiac failure, pregnancy and childbirth, oral contraceptive drugs, malignant disease, chronic pulmonary disease and hypercoagulable states.

Atrial fibrillation may allow thrombus formation in the right atrium, and septal or right ventricular infarction may favour thrombosis in the right ventricle. A small proportion (less than 10%) of pulmonary emboli are due to these cardiac causes.

After pulmonary embolism, lung tissue is ventilated but not perfused, resulting in impaired gas exchange. After some hours surfactant is no longer produced by the non-perfused lung, alveolar collapse occurs and hypoxaemia is the result. The haemodynamic consequence of pulmonary embolism is an elevation of pulmonary arterial pressure and a reduction in cardiac output. The zone of lung that is no longer perfused by the pulmonary artery may infarct but often does not do so because oxygen continues to be supplied by the bronchial circulation and the airways.

CLINICAL FEATURES

A small embolus may present with effort dyspnoea, tiredness, syncope and, occasionally, cardiac arrhythmias.

A medium-sized embolus leading to pulmonary infarction can present with sudden onset of pleuritic pain, cough with haemoptysis, and dyspnoea.

A massive pulmonary embolus presents as a medical emergency: the patient has severe central chest pain and suddenly becomes shocked, pale and sweaty, with marked tachypnoea and tachycardia. Syncope may result if the cardiac output is transiently but dramatically reduced. Death may follow rapidly.

Physical signs vary according to the size of the embolus and the occurrence of pulmonary infarction:

- A small embolus may reveal no abnormal signs apart from a few basal crackles.
- Large emboli lead to a right ventricular heave, a gallop rhythm, tachycardia and a prominent *a* wave in the jugular venous pulse. The second heart sound may be loud because of pulmonary hypertension or soft if the cardiac output is very reduced. Continuous (systolic and diastolic) murmurs may be generated by turbulent blood flow around the embolic obstructions.
- With pulmonary infarction, a pleural rub and pyrexia may also be present.
- In about 50% of cases there is evidence of deep venous thrombosis, especially in the lower limbs or pelvic veins.

INVESTIGATION

The *chest X-ray* is often normal but the abrupt cut-off of a pulmonary artery or a translucency of an underperfused distal zone is occasionally seen. Later, atelectasis leads to opacities. An infarction may be visualized as a wedge-shaped opacity adjacent to the pleural edge, a pleural effusion and a raised hemidiaphragm. Past infarcts may be seen as opaque linear scars.

The *ECG* is usually normal except for sinus tachycardia. In relatively severe cases, however, right atrial dilatation produces tall, peaked P waves in lead II, and right ventricular hypertrophy and dilatation give rise to right axis deviation, some degree of right bundle branch block and T wave inversion in the right precordial leads (Fig. 11.79). The classical pattern of an S wave in lead I and a Q wave and inverted T waves in lead III (S1, Q3, T3), which reflects right ventricular 'strain', is not usually present.

If pulmonary infarction has occurred there will be a polymorphonuclear leucocytosis, an elevated ESR and increased lactate dehydrogenase levels.

Pulmonary embolism usually results in arterial hypoxaemia and hypocapnia.

A *pulmonary technetium-90m* scintigram may demonstrate underperfused areas (Fig. 11.80). The specificity of this technique is greatly improved when combined with a ventilation scintigram performed after inhalation of radioactive xenon gas (p. 643). The finding of a non-perfused but ventilated zone is more suggestive of pulmonary embolism.

Pulmonary *angiography* is sometimes undertaken if surgery is considered in acute massive embolism. The test is performed by injecting contrast material through a catheter inserted into the main pulmonary artery. Filling defects or obstructed vessels can be delineated (Fig. 11.81). Angiography is hazardous but the risk may be reduced if contrast is injected into each pulmonary artery separately. If the patient is in extremis and the diagnosis is obvious, surgery should proceed without prior angiography.

TREATMENT

Prevention of further emboli
The basis of therapy is intravenous heparin,

starting with a bolus of 5000 units and followed by the continuous infusion of 10 000 units every 6 h. Oral anticoagulants are usually begun after 48 h and the heparin is tapered off as the oral anticoagulant becomes effective. Oral anticoagulants are continued for 6 weeks to 6 months, depending on the likelihood of recurrence of venous thrombosis or embolism.

Dissolution of the thrombus

Fibrinolytic therapy such as streptokinase (250 000 units by i.v. infusion over 30 min, followed by streptokinase 100 000 i.v. hourly) is often used following a major embolism. It may also be given into the pulmonary artery.

Surgical embolectomy

This is rarely necessary, but when the haemodynamic circumstances are very severe there may be no alternative. Inferior vena caval interruption or plication, or the insertion of a filter into the inferior vena cava, may occasionally be necessary if anticoagulant or fibrinolytic therapy is contraindicated or fails to prevent recurrences of pulmonary embolism.

Chronic cor pulmonale

Cor pulmonale is the commonest variety of pulmonary hypertensive heart disease.

CAUSES

These are listed in Table 11.35.

PATHOPHYSIOLOGY

Pulmonary vascular resistance is increased because of effective loss of pulmonary tissue and because of

Table 11.35 Causes of cor pulmonale.

Intrinsic lung disease, e.g.
Chronic bronchitis and emphysema
Asthma
Pulmonary fibrosis
Recurrent pulmonary emboli
Skeletal abnormalities, e.g.
Kyphoscoliosis
Hypoventilation, e.g.
Morbid obesity (Pickwickian syndrome)
Neuromuscular disease, e.g.
Poliomyelitis
Myasthenia gravis
Obstruction, e.g.
Sleep-apnoea syndrome

pulmonary vasoconstriction caused by hypoxia and acidosis. The increased pulmonary vascular resistance leads to pulmonary hypertension, which initially occurs only during an acute respiratory infection. Eventually, the pulmonary hypertension becomes persistent and progressively more severe. The pulmonary vascular bed is gradually obliterated by muscular hypertrophy of the arterioles and thrombus formation. Right ventricular function is progressively compromised because of the increased pressure load. Hypoxia further impairs right ventricular function, and, as it develops, left ventricular function is also depressed.

CLINICAL FEATURES

The clinical features are those of pulmonary hypertension and right ventricular failure occurring in patients with chronic chest disease. The dominant clinical picture depends on the type of lung disease.

TREATMENT

Vigorous therapy of the pulmonary condition may lead to marked improvement of blood gases and consequent improvement of the heart failure. Acute chest infections must be treated promptly. Oxygen therapy over a long period may reduce established pulmonary hypertension, with improvement in overall prognosis (see p. 660). Any heart failure should be treated (see p. 564).

Atrial myxoma

This is the commonest primary cardiac tumour. A myxoma usually develops in the left atrium and is a polypoid, gelatinous structure attached by a pedicle to the atrial septum. The tumour may obstruct the mitral valve or may be a site of thrombi that then embolize. It is also associated with constitutional symptoms: the patient may present with dyspnoea, syncope or a mild fever. The most important physical signs are a loud first heart sound, a tumour 'plop' (a loud third heart sound produced as the pedunculated tumour comes to an abrupt halt), a mid-diastolic murmur, and signs due to embolization. A raised ESR is usually present.

The diagnosis is easily made by echocardiography because the tumour is demonstrated as a dense space-occupying lesion (Fig. 11.82). Surgical removal usually results in a complete cure.

Myxomas may also occur in the right atrium or in the ventricles. Other primary cardiac tumours include rhabdomyomas and sarcomas.

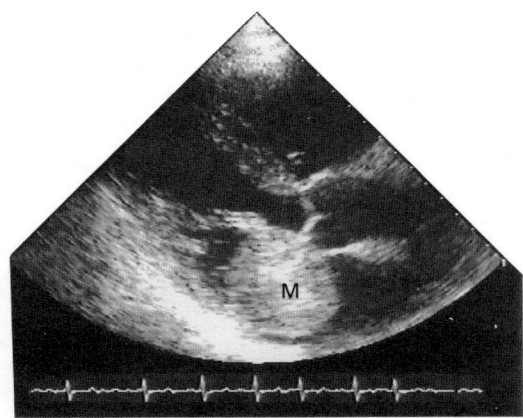

Fig. 11.82 Two dimensional echocardiogram (long axis parasternal view) showing an echo dense mass (M) in the left atrium. This mass proved to be due to an atrial myxoma which was removed surgically.

Myocardial disease

Myocardial disease that is not due to a specific heart muscle disorder or a known infiltrative, metabolic/toxic or neuromuscular disorder may be caused by:

- An acute or chronic inflammatory pathology (myocarditis)
- Idiopathic myocardial disease (cardiomyopathy)

MYOCARDITIS

Myocarditis, whether idiopathic or infective, is the most common form of inflammatory endomyocardial disease. A definitive aetiology with isolation of viruses or bacteria is uncommon. Causative factors include:

- Viruses, particularly coxsackie, influenza, rubella, polio, adeno- and echoviruses
- *Rickettsia, Chlamydia, Coxiella* (the causative agent of Q fever)
- *Toxoplasma gondii*—a common cause of myocarditis in the newborn or in immunologically compromised adults
- Protozoa, e.g. *Trypanosoma cruzi*, which causes Chagas' disease and is endemic in central and South America
- Radiation, chemicals and drugs, e.g. lead poisoning, emetine and chloroquine
- Bacterial infection, e.g. diphtheria, which is due to an exotoxin produced by *Corynebacterium*

CLINICAL FEATURES

Patients present with an acute illness, often characterized by fever and cardiac failure. There may be a history of previous respiratory or febrile illness. Physical examination reveals soft heart sounds, a prominent third sound and tachycardia (gallop rhythm). Often a pericardial friction rub may be heard.

INVESTIGATION

The chest X-ray may show some cardiac enlargement, depending on the stage and virulence of the disease

- The ECG demonstrates ST and T wave abnormalities and arrhythmias. Diphtheritic myocarditis may induce heart block, and Chagas' disease produces both heart block and ventricular tachyarrhythmias.
- Cardiac enzymes are elevated.
- Cardiac biopsy shows acute inflammation.
- Viral antibody titres may be increased.

TREATMENT

General management includes bed rest and the eradication of any acute infection. Therapy is directed towards the management of cardiac failure and the treatment of cardiac arrhythmias. Depending on the aetiology, the prognosis is usually good, although a chronic cardiomyopathy may occasionally ensue.

CARDIOMYOPATHY

These idiopathic conditions are classified according to their clinical presentation as:

- Dilated cardiomyopathy—ventricular dilatation
- Hypertrophic cardiomyopathy — myocardial hypertrophy
- Restrictive cardiomyopathy—impaired ventricular filling

Dilated cardiomyopathy (DCM)

DCM is characterized by dilatation and impaired systolic function of the left ventricle and/or right ventricle. The aetiology of DCM is unknown but there is an association with viral (coxsackie) infection and an immune-mediated pathogenesis is likely. Many cases of specific heart muscle disease present with clinical features of DCM and they include:

- Cardiovascular disease (ischaemic, rheumatic, congenital, systemic hypertension)
- Generalized disease, e.g. haemochromatosis, sarcoidosis
- Connective tissue disorders, e.g. systemic lupus

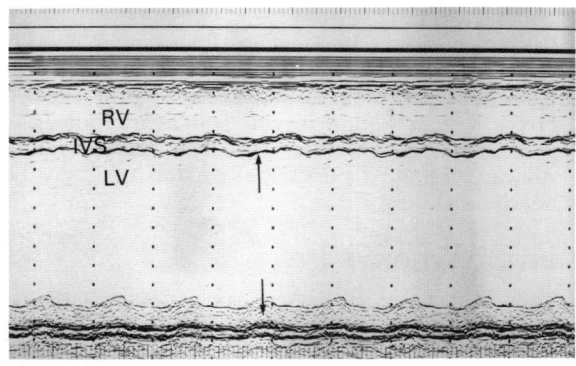
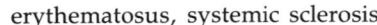
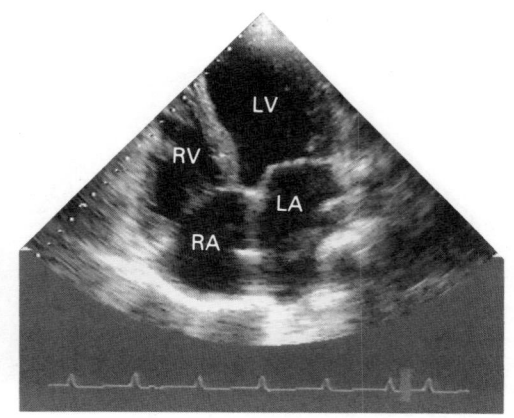

Fig. 11.83 These echocardiograms (left—M-Mode, right—apical 4 chamber 2D) show dilated cardiomyopathy. Note the poor left ventricular wall motion. The 2–D echo image shows dilatation of all four cardiac chambers, particularly the left ventricle (LV).

erythematosus, systemic sclerosis
- Neuromuscular disease, e.g. muscular dystrophy, Friedreich's ataxia
- Glycogen storage disease, e.g. Pompé's disease
- Primary heart muscle disease, e.g. amyloidosis
- Alcohol excess
- Cytotoxic drug therapy, e.g. doxorubicin, cyclophosphamide

CLINICAL FEATURES

Symptoms depend on the relative degree of right and left heart failure and the incidence of cardiac arrhythmias and emboli.

Physical signs reflect heart failure, i.e. cardiomegaly, tachycardia, jugular venous pressure elevation, third or fourth heart sounds and basal crackles. Ventricular dilatation leads to functional mitral or tricuspid valvular regurgitation.

INVESTIGATION

- Generalized cardiac enlargement is demonstrable on the chest X-ray.
- Diffuse non-specific ST segment and T wave changes are seen on the ECG. Conduction disturbances, sinus tachycardia, and arrhythmias (such as atrial fibrillation, ventricular premature contractions or ventricular tachycardia) may also be seen.
- The echocardiogram reveals dilatation of the LV and/or RV with poor global contraction (Fig. 11.83).
- Cardiac biopsy shows variable fibrosis and non-specific leucocyte infiltration. Infiltrative disorders (e.g. amyloid) may be detected in specific cases.

TREATMENT

Management involves the conventional treatment of heart failure and arrhythmias. A history of embolization is an indication for anticoagulant treatment. Prolonged bed-rest, corticosteroid therapy, the avoidance of alcohol, and nutritional supplements may be indicated in special cases. Severe congestive cardiomyopathy in relatively young adults may be treated with cardiac transplantation.

Hypertrophic cardiomyopathy (HCM)

Also known as hypertrophic obstructive cardiomyopathy (HOCM), this is characterized by marked hypertrophy of the left and/or right ventricle, particularly the interventricular septum in the absence of a cardiac or systemic cause. The hypertrophied muscle results in distorted left ventricular contraction and abnormal mitral valve movement during systole. Some degree of mitral regurgitation may develop. Apposition of the anterior cusp of the mitral valve to the hypertrophied septum may cause some obstruction to left ventricular emptying. About half the cases of hypertrophic cardiomyopathy are familial (inherited in an autosomal dominant manner), but the sporadic cases are of unknown aetiology. The failure of hypertrophy to manifest before completion of the adolescent growth phase may make diagnosis difficult in children.

CLINICAL FEATURES

Patients with this condition may present with syncope or pre-syncope (typically exertional),

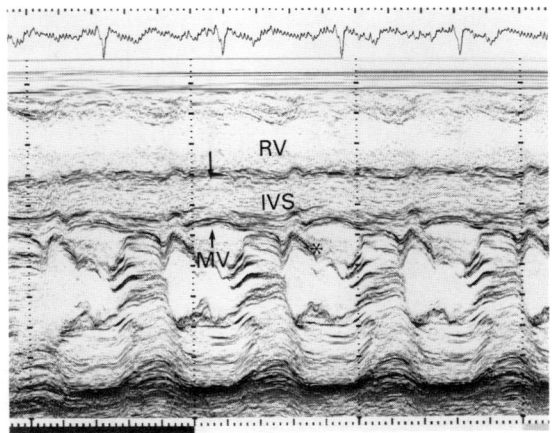 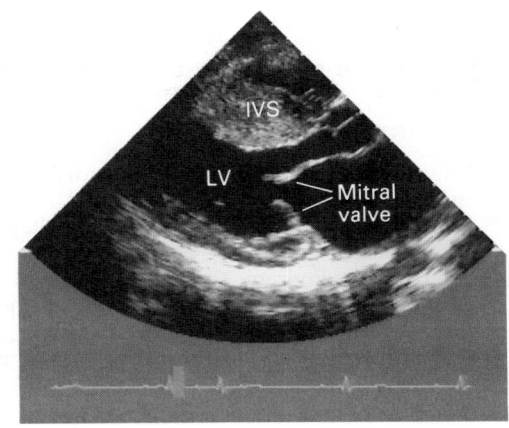

Fig. 11.84 M-Mode (left panel) and 2-D (right panel) parasternal left axis echocardiogram from a patient with hypertrophic cardiomyopathy. The M-Mode demonstrates a thickened intraventricular septum and abnormal mitral valve motion—anterior movement during systole (x) which results in the mitral valve leaflet touching the interventricular septum. The thickened septum (IVS) is very clearly seen on the 2D image.

angina, cardiac arrhythmias or sudden death. As with other cardiomyopathies, dyspnoea due to left ventricular failure is a common but late presentation. In this case left ventricular failure is not due to the failing contractile function of the myocardium; instead, it is due to the inability of the heart muscle to relax. Thus, left ventricular filling and therefore left ventricular emptying is impaired.

The classical physical findings are:

- A double apical pulsation (forceful atrial contraction produces a palpable fourth heart sound)
- A jerky carotid pulse because of rapid ejection and sudden obstruction to left ventricular outflow during asystole
- An ejection systolic murmur because of left ventricular outflow obstruction late in systole that can be increased by physical manoeuvres, e.g., Valsalva, squatting
- A pansystolic murmur due to mitral regurgitation
- A fourth heart sound

INVESTIGATION

- The chest X-ray is usually unremarkable.
- The ECG demonstrates left ventricular hypertrophy (see Fig. 11.66) and ST and T wave changes.
- The echocardiogram is diagnostic because it shows septal hypertrophy (greater than the hypertrophy of the posterior wall), abnormal mitral valve movement and a very vigorously contracting ventricle (Fig. 11.84).

TREATMENT

Firstly, sudden death must be avoided by anti-arrhythmic treatment. Long-term amiodarone treatment is effective. Syncope or chest pain may be treated with beta-blockade. Vasodilators should be avoided because they may aggravate left ventricular outflow obstruction owing to peripheral venous blood pooling. Occasionally, resection of septal myocardium may be indicated.

Restrictive cardiomyopathy

Some cardiomyopathies do not present with muscular hypertrophy or ventricular dilatation. Instead, ventricular filling is restricted (as with constrictive pericarditis).

Conditions associated with this form of cardiomyopathy are amyloidosis, sarcoidosis, Loeffler's endocarditis and endomyocardial fibrosis; in the latter two conditions there is myocardial and endocardial fibrosis associated with eosinophilia. Thrombus formation is common in restrictive cardiomyopathy.

CLINICAL FEATURES

Dyspnoea, fatigue and embolic symptoms may be the presenting features. Restriction to ventricular filling also results in persistently elevated venous pressures and consequent hepatic enlargement, ascites and dependent oedema.

Physical signs are similar to those of constrictive pericarditis, i.e., a high jugular venous pressure with diastolic collapse (Friedreich's sign) and elevation of the jugular venous pressure with inspiration (Kussmaul's sign). Cardiac enlargement with a third or fourth heart sound is common.

INVESTIGATION

- The chest X-ray confirms the cardiac enlargement.
- The ECG usually generally has low-voltage and ST segment and T wave abnormalities.
- The echocardiogram shows symmetrical myocardial thickening and a normal systolic ejection fraction, but impaired ventricular filling.
- Transvenous endocardial biopsy may be useful for more detailed diagnosis.

TREATMENT

There is no specific treatment. Cardiac failure and embolic problems should be treated. Cardiac transplantation should be considered in some severe cases.

Pericardial disease

The normal pericardium lubricates the surface of the heart, prevents sudden deformation or dislocation of the heart, and acts as a barrier to the spread of infection. There are three common presentations of pericardial disease:

- Acute pericarditis
- Pericardial effusion
- Constrictive pericarditis

ACUTE PERICARDITIS

Inflammation of the pericardium gives rise to chest pain that is substernal and sharp. It may be referred to the neck or shoulders. It is relieved by sitting forward and made worse by lying down and, like pleurisy, is aggravated by movement and respiration.

Acute pericarditis has numerous aetiologies, but coxsackie viral infections and myocardial infarction are the commonest causes in the UK. Viral pericarditis can occur in epidemics. Other aetiologies include uraemia, connective tissue disease, trauma, post-pericardiotomy, rheumatic fever, tuberculosis and malignancy.

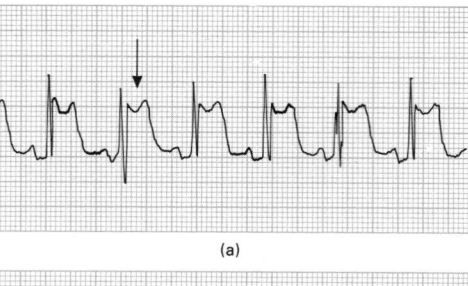

(a)

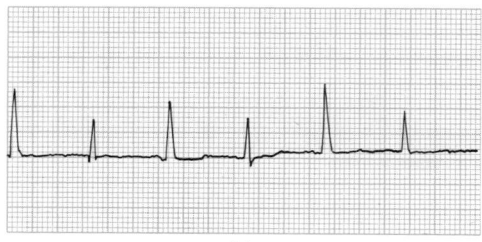

(b)

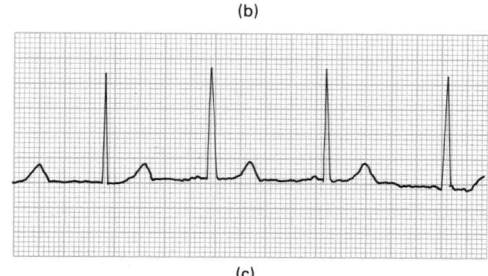

(c)

Fig. 11.85 ECGs associated with pericarditis. (a) Acute pericarditis. Note the raised ST segment, concave upwards (arrow). (b) Chronic phase of pericarditis associated with a pericardial effusion. Note the T wave flattening and inversion and the alternation of the QRS amplitude (QRS alternans). (c) The same patient after evacuation of the pericardial fluid. Note that the QRS voltage has increased and the T waves have returned to normal.

CLINICAL FEATURES

The cardinal clinical sign is a pericardial friction rub. There is usually a fever when pericarditis is due to viral or bacterial infection, rheumatic fever or myocardial infarction.

INVESTIGATION

During the first week of the illness the ECG shows ST segment elevation, concave upwards, in all leads facing the epicardial surface, i.e. the anterior, lateral and inferior leads (Fig. 11.85). ST segment depression is only seen in the cavity leads (AVR and V_1). Later, the ST segment falls and T wave inversion develops. As the illness improves the T waves become normal.

Cardiac enzymes may be elevated if there is associated myocarditis.

TREATMENT

Treatment consists of anti-inflammatory medication such as oral aspirin, naproxen or indomethacin. Occasionally, if pericarditis is severe or recurrent, systemic corticosteroids may be needed.

Varieties of pericarditis

Viral pericarditis
This tends to affect young adults and is sudden in onset. Usually, the illness lasts for only a few weeks and the prognosis is good. However, recurrences do occur.

Bacterial pericarditis
Septicaemia or pneumonia may rarely be complicated by purulent pericarditis. *Staphylococcus* and *Haemophilus influenzae* account for two-thirds of such cases.
   Antibiotics and surgical drainage may be required. This form of pericarditis, especially when due to *Staphylococcus*, is usually fatal.

Tuberculous pericarditis
This is typified by a chronic low-grade fever, especially in the evening, associated with signs and symptoms of acute pericarditis, malaise and weight loss. Pericardial aspiration may be required to make the diagnosis. The pericardial effusion is usually serous but may be blood-stained. Specific antituberculous chemotherapy is needed.

Uraemic pericarditis
This is uncommon and is often asymptomatic. It usually develops in the terminal stages of uraemia.

Pericarditis following myocardial infarction
A pericardial friction rub and the recurrence of chest pain and fever occurs in about 20% of patients during the first few days after myocardial infarction, especially anterior wall infarction.

Dressler's syndrome
This is pericarditis occurring 1 month to 1 year after an acute myocardial infarction (see p. 582).

Malignant pericarditis
Carcinoma of the bronchus, carcinoma of the breast and Hodgkin's disease are the most common tumours to infiltrate the pericardium. Leukaemia and malignant melanoma are also associated with pericarditis. Pericardiocentesis may be useful in diagnosing the malignancy.

PERICARDIAL EFFUSION

Although acute pericarditis is initially dry and fibrinous, almost all aetiologies of this inflammatory reaction also induce the formation of a pericardial effusion. The effusion collects in the closed pericardium. When the pericardium can distend no more, it may produce mechanical embarrassment to the circulation by preventing ventricular filling; this is called cardiac tamponade.

CLINICAL FEATURES

The clinical features include a raised jugular venous pressure, with sharp diastolic collapse (Friedreich's sign), a paradoxical pulse (the blood pressure falls during inspiration), increased neck vein distension during inspiration (Kussmaul's sign) and reduced cardiac output. Because of the effusion, the apex beat may not be palpable and heart sounds are soft. Although a friction rub is often heard, it may be quieter than before the fluid accumulated as the effusion separates the visceral from the parietal pericardium.

INVESTIGATION

The ECG shows reduced voltages, and the chest X-ray may demonstrate an increasingly large globular heart with sharp outlines. The pulmonary veins are typically not distended.
   Echocardiography is the most useful technique for demonstrating a pericardial effusion (see Fig. 11.24).

TREATMENT

When the effusion collects rapidly and the circulation is embarrassed, the effusion must be tapped. Pericardiocentesis is also indicated when a malignant, tuberculous or a purulent effusion is suspected. Reaccumulation may require pericardial fenestration, i.e. the surgical creation of a window in the pericardium.

CONSTRICTIVE PERICARDITIS

Following tuberculous pericarditis, haemopericardium, or acute pericarditis due to viral infection, bacterial infection or rheumatic heart disease, the pericardium may become thick, fibrous and calcified. The heart is then encased in a solid shell and cannot fill properly.

CLINICAL FEATURES

There are signs of systemic venous congestion, i.e. ascites, dependent oedema, hepatomegaly and jugular venous distension, without much breathlessness or pulmonary venous distension. There are also signs of impaired ventricular filling, i.e. Kussmaul's sign, Friedreich's sign and pulsus paradoxus.
   Atrial fibrillation is common (30%) and a loud heart sound, called a pericardial knock, due to

rapid ventricular filling may be heard. This is an early third heart sound.

Other causes of ascites must be excluded (see p. 266).

INVESTIGATION

The chest X-ray shows a relatively small heart with obvious calcification seen on the lateral film and using fluoroscopy.

The ECG shows low QRS voltages and T wave inversion, and the echocardiogram will demonstrate the thickened pericardium and the relative immobility of the heart.

TREATMENT

Treatment involves the surgical removal of a substantial proportion of the pericardium. About half the patients do well, but in the others persistent constriction, atrial fibrillation and myocardial disease prevent full recovery.

The cardiovascular system in systemic disease

The heart can be involved in many diseases (see Table 11.36).

Systemic hypertension

Blood pressure within a population has an individual skewed distribution, i.e. there is a single peak frequency of blood pressure and there are more individuals with high pressures than low pressures. Different populations have different levels of blood pressure, with those of African origin tending to have higher pressure than Caucasians, i.e. the whole distribution is shifted to the left. The distribution curves for systolic and diastolic blood pressure are similar. Risk of mortality and morbidity rises continuously with increasing blood pressure throughout the range. The rise of risk is not linear, however, being steeper at higher pressures.

The level of blood pressure can be said to be abnormal when it is associated with a clear increase in morbidity and mortality. This level varies with age, sex, race and country. For life insurance reasons and for simple clinical purposes, a diastolic

Table 11.36 Cardiac involvement in some systemic disorders.

Disease	Cardiac involvement
Endocrine disorders	
Diabetes mellitus	Coronary artery disease
Thyrotoxicosis	Atrial fibrillation Cardiomyopathy
Hypothyroidism	Bradycardia Heart failure Coronary disease Pericardial effusion
Acromegaly	Cardiomegaly Hypertension Cardiac arrhythmias
Cushing's syndrome	Hypertension
Conn's syndrome	Hypertension
Phaeochromocytoma	Hypertension
Connective-tissue disorders	
Systemic lupus erythematosus	Non-infective endocarditis (Libman Sachs) Myocarditis Pericarditis
Systemic sclerosis	Myocarditis Pericarditis Arrhythmias
Polyarteritis nodosa	Hypertension Pericarditis Arrhythmias
Rheumatoid disease	Aortic and mitral regurgitation Pericarditis
Miscellaneous	
Renal failure	Hypertension Heart failure Pericarditis Infective endocarditis
Morbid obesity	Hypertension Cardiomegaly Associated with atherosclerotic coronary artery disease
Gout	Hypertension
Carcinoid syndrome	Pulmonary stenosis Tricuspid stenosis
Alcohol	Cardiomyopathy Atrial arrhythmias
Syphilis	Aortic regurgitation Coronary arterial stenosis (ostial) Ascending aortic aneurysm

blood pressure in a young adult above 100 mm Hg and/or 160 mm Hg systolic is taken as definitely hypertensive and a diastolic pressure above 95 mm Hg is regarded as probably hypertensive. The World Health Organisation have used a definition of 160/95 mm Hg, and in Framingham (a small town in Massachusetts, USA) where a very detailed population study is being carried out, 160/95 mm Hg was deemed abnormal and 140/90 to 160/95 mm Hg was regarded as borderline. The significance of a single elevated reading is unclear and for a firm diagnosis the blood pressure should be elevated on more than one examination.

It is recommended that blood pressure should be taken on three separate occasions and the mean of these readings used for definition of normality and abnormality. Despite this, several studies suggest that a single elevated blood pressure reading is predictive of future events. Systolic blood pressure relates to prognosis more strongly than diastolic or mean arterial pressure.

CAUSES

In the large majority of cases no cause can be identified, and this form of hypertension is known as primary or essential. A cause of hypertension can be discovered in less than 10% cases; such cases are known as secondary hypertension.

Essential hypertension

No single factor has been found to explain essential hypertension; many factors are probably responsible. The blood pressure is determined by the product of the cardiac output and the peripheral vascular resistance.

In the early stages of essential hypertension the increase of blood pressure is due to a small increase in cardiac output. This could be due to sympathetic overactivity. Later in the disease, the cardiac output is normal but the peripheral resistance is increased. It is possible that the initial increase in cardiac output induces vascular changes that then sustain and increase the blood pressure.

The baroreceptor reflexes operate at a higher pressure in hypertension. An increased blood pressure should stimulate a bradycardia via the carotid sinus baroreceptor mechanism. This does not happen in essential hypertension. This abnormal reflex may be due to the hypertension rather than being its cause.

The causes of essential hypertension include:

1 *Genetic factors*. Racial and familial tendencies to high blood pressure are found.
2 *Environmental factors*. Numerous factors have been related to the development of hypertension but only the following appear to be important.

- *Obesity*. Blood pressure rises with increasing obesity. This relationship persists when errors of blood pressure measurement in obese subjects are taken into account.
- *Alcohol intake*. Ingestion of alcohol acutely raises blood pressure and alcohol intake tends to be higher in individuals with higher pressures. Reduction or withdrawal of regular alcohol intake reduces blood pressure 5–10 mm Hg.
- *Salt intake*. There is much controversy about the role of salt in hypertension. There is some evidence of a relationship between the salt intake of an individual and the level of the blood pressure *within* populations. Similar, but weaker relationships are found between populations. There is less convincing evidence that a moderate reduction of salt intake will reduce blood pressure. Salt intake may increase intravascular volume in the initial stages of the genesis of hypertension, but once peripheral vascular resistance becomes raised, alterations of salt intake may play little part in the regulation of blood pressure.
- *Humoral factors* have been implicated in the genesis of hypertension including catecholamines, the renin–angiotensin system, and atrial natriuretic peptide. Convincing evidence is lacking that any of these are involved.

Secondary hypertension

This should always be considered in patients with hypertension. In particular, a careful search should be made in hypertensive patients presenting under the age of 35 years. The causes of secondary hypertension can be divided into the following.

Renal causes (see p. 454). Renal diseases are the most common causes of secondary hypertension, accounting for over 80% of cases. Chronic glomerulonephritis, chronic atrophic pyelonephritis and congenital polycystic kidneys are the conditions usually involved. It may be difficult to determine whether renal disease has caused hypertension or whether the hypertension has produced the renal disease.

The mechanism by which renal disease causes hypertension is probably related to salt and water retention. Occasionally, renal artery stenosis due to fibromuscular hyperplasia or atheroma may cause hypertension (renovascular hypertension) owing to excess renin production (see p. 454).

Endocrine causes (see Table 16.49). These include:

- Conn's syndrome
- Phaeochromocytoma
- Cushing's syndrome
- Acromegaly
- Hyperparathyroidism

Cardiovascular causes. Renovascular hypertension is discussed above.

Coarctation of the aorta (see p. 603) should be considered in young patients with hypertension and a late systolic murmur.

Pregnancy. Hypertension in the early stages of pregnancy is usually essential hypertension or due to renal disease.

Pre-eclampsia or toxaemia of pregnancy is diagnosed when hypertension develops in the last 3 months of pregnancy and is associated with oedema and proteinuria. The cause of pre-eclampsia is unknown.

Pre-eclampsia may worsen, with the development of severe hypertension, nausea, vomiting, pulmonary oedema and fits. This condition, known as eclampsia, needs urgent treatment (see p. 620).

Drugs. Oestrogen-containing contraceptives, other steroids, carbenoxolone, liquorice and vasopressin may all cause hypertension. Paroxysms of severe hypertension may occur in patients taking mono-amine oxidase inhibitors who eat cheese or other tyramine-containing foods and those who drink wines.

PATHOPHYSIOLOGY

An increase in vascular tone initially accounts for the increased peripheral vascular resistance. As the disease progresses, the walls of small arteries thicken and atheroma develops in larger arteries. Malignant hypertension is characterized by fibrinoid necrosis of the vascular wall.

The increased peripheral vascular resistance leads to a greater impedance to left ventricular emptying. Consequently, left ventricular hypertrophy develops.

A reduction in renal perfusion pressure can occur, leading to decreased glomerular filtration and reduced sodium and water excretion. The renal changes are described in more detail on p. 453. The decreased renal perfusion leads to the production of renin, which converts angiotensinogen to angiotensin I. This is changed to angiotensin II, which stimulates the secretion of aldosterone and further contributes to salt and water retention (see Fig. 16.32).

Secondary aldosteronism, which occurs with severe or accelerated hypertension and with the use of diuretics, is characterized by high serum levels of aldosterone and renin. In primary aldosteronism (Conn's syndrome), only the aldosterone is raised. About 10% of patients with essential hypertension have a high plasma renin level, and 25% have a low renin level.

In some cases the pressure rises rapidly and these patients are said to have 'malignant' hypertension. Without treatment death occurs within 1–2 years.

The accelerated rise in blood pressure produces cerebral oedema, left ventricular failure and severe renal impairment, with proteinuria and microscopic haematuria. Retinal haemorrhages, exudates and papilloedema are also seen and are diagnostic of malignant hypertension.

COMPLICATIONS

Hypertension is a risk factor for developing atheroma and patients may therefore develop thrombotic cerebral vascular disease, coronary artery disease and peripheral vascular disease. The increased pressure in the circulation can result in heart failure, cerebral haemorrhage, renal disease and dissecting aortic aneurysms.

ASSESSMENT OF PATIENTS

The possible causes and consequences of hypertension are assessed. In uncomplicated or essential hypertension, apart from the high blood pressure there are usually no signs, symptoms or abnormal investigations.

History
The patient with mild hypertension is usually asymptomatic. Nose bleeds and headaches have been traditionally regarded as possible symptoms, but are probably no commoner than in the general population. There may be a past history of renal disease or a family history of hypertension.

Secondary causes of hypertension are suggested by a specific history, such as attacks of sweating and tachycardia in phaeochromocytoma.

Angina may occur either because of associated coronary artery disease or because of the high oxygen demand from hypertrophied muscle. If cardiac failure develops, breathlessness occurs.

Accelerated or malignant hypertension presents with visual impairment, nausea and vomiting, fits, transient paralysis, severe headaches, impairment of consciousness, or symptoms of acute cardiac failure.

Examination
In the majority of patients the only sign is the high blood pressure, but in others, features of the cause of hypertension may be noted. For example, there may be abdominal bruit due to renovascular obstruction, or delayed femoral pulses due to coarctation of the aorta.

Hypertensive heart disease presents with a loud aortic second sound, a prominent left ventricular apical heave and a fourth heart sound. Sinus tachycardia and a third heart sound develop if cardiac failure occurs.

Examination of the retina may reveal various abnormalities which are known as Keith–Wagener retinal changes. They are graded as follows:

- *Grade 1*—increased tortuosity of retinal arteries and increased reflectiveness (silver wiring)
- *Grade 2*—grade 1 plus the appearance of arteriovenous (AV) nipping produced when thickened retinal arteries pass over the retinal veins
- *Grade 3*—grade 2 plus flame-shaped haemorrhages and soft 'cotton wool' exudates
- *Grade 4*—grade 3 plus papilloedema (bulging and blurring of the edges of the optic disc)

The presence of haemorrhages, exudates or papilloedema are diagnostic of malignant hypertension which requires urgent treatment.

INVESTIGATION (see also p. 827)

Routine investigation of a hypertensive patient should always include:

- A chest X-ray
- An ECG
- Urinalysis
- Fasting blood lipids
- Urea and electrolytes

If the blood urea is abnormal, the creatinine level, creatinine clearance, intravenous excretion urography, renal ultrasound and other tests of renal function are necessary. If the tests of renal function or an abnormal bruit suggest a renovascular cause, full renal investigation is essential.

If coarctation of the aorta is suspected, digital vascular imaging with intravenous contrast injection or MRI will usually demonstrate the lesion.

If the patient is not taking diuretics, a low serum potassium should suggest an endocrine problem, and aldosterone, cortisol and renin measurements should be performed. A history suggestive of phaeochromocytoma can be investigated with measurement of serum catecholamines or urinary catecholamine metabolites such as vanillylmandelic acid (VMA).

The chest X-ray may show a large heart and pulmonary congestion if heart failure has developed, or rib notching in coarctation of the aorta.

The ECG may show left ventricular hypertrophy or signs of myocardial infarction or ischaemia. Very rarely, ECG features of hyperkalaemia (see Fig. 10.6) (e.g. with renal failure) or hypokalaemia may be detected.

TREATMENT

In the young, the secondary causes of hypertension should be excluded before treatment is commenced. When the blood pressure is only mildly or moderately elevated, it may be difficult to persuade an asymptomatic patient that treatment is necessary. However, there are definite advantages from treating diastolic blood pressures in excess of 100 mm Hg. If the diastolic blood pressure is between 90 and 100 mm Hg it should be carefully reassessed on several occasions with the patient in a comfortable, relaxed position. If it is truly elevated (above 90 mm Hg) it should be actively treated, especially in young men, and particularly so if there is any evidence of hypertensive retinal, cardiac or renal changes. In elderly patients it is probably unnecessary, and possibly unwise, to attempt to treat mild ·hypertension, but more severe hypertension (diastolic pressures greater than 105 mm Hg) should be reduced cautiously. The Framingham studies have shown that the systolic blood pressure is as important as the diastolic blood pressure and is the best guide to the risk of peripheral arterial disease. Thus, a man with a systolic pressure of 170 mm Hg has twice the risk of dying compared with a man with a systolic pressure of 120 mm Hg. Borderline or labile hypertension, where the blood pressure readings are occasionally above normal, was also shown to have an increased mortality of 1.5–2 times in this study.

General measures

A review of the patient's lifestyle and diet may suggest modifications that could lead to some reduction of blood pressure, such as:

- *Weight reduction.* Obese patients should lose weight. This leads to a true fall in blood pressure as well as to a reduction of artefactually increased cuff measurements.
- *Reduction of heavy alcohol consumption.* This also leads to a small reduction in blood pressure of around 5–10 mm Hg.
- *Salt restriction.* This is generally of little effect except in some individuals. Usually, the patient is advised not to add salt at the table.
- *Regular exercise, meditation and biofeedback.* These are all techniques that have been claimed to lead to blood pressure reduction. An attempt should be made to reduce stress and anxiety.

Patients should also be told to stop smoking to reduce their overall coronary risk. It is doubtful whether cessation of smoking reduces the blood pressure except in malignant hypertension. Hyperlipidaemia should also be corrected (see p. 863) to reduce the risk of atheroma.

Drug treatment

A large number of drugs are used to treat hypertension. This reflects the difficulty in finding a single drug that effectively lowers blood pressure without producing side-effects that may be more troublesome or more dangerous than the hypertension itself. Compliance is a problem as the side-effects of drug therapy are frequent and the immediate benefits of treatment are not obvious to the patient.

Available drugs

Diuretics. Loop diuretics (e.g. frusemide 40 mg daily or bumetanide 1–2 mg daily) and thiazide diuretics (e.g. bendrofluazide 5 mg daily or cyclopenthiazide 0.5 mg daily) are equally effective at lowering the blood pressure. Thiazides are usually preferred because the duration of action is longer, the diuresis is not so severe, and they cost less. Loop diuretics are restricted to those with cardiac or renal impairment for whom an additional diuretic effect is required.

Although diuretics may lower blood pressure transiently by sodium and water excretion, they also act by directly dilating arterioles. Oral potassium supplements are often not required. Occasionally, hypokalaemia occurs and this is most effectively treated with a potassium-sparing diuretic.

Potassium-sparing diuretics (e.g. triamterene 150–250 mg daily, spironolactone 50–200 mg and amiloride 5–10 mg daily) are not effective hypotensive agents, with the exception of spironolactone in primary or secondary aldosteronism. These diuretics are combined with others to treat hypokalaemia, which very occasionally occurs in hypertensive patients on diuretics.

Thiazide diuretics may cause hyperuricaemia and may precipitate gout. They may worsen glucose intolerance. Thiazide diuretics increase the serum renin level. Unlike other hypotensives, their effect is not postural.

Beta-adrenergic antagonists (see Table 11.37). The mechanism by which beta-blockers reduce hypertension is unclear. Although they reduce the force of cardiac contraction and renin production, they probably act predominantly via the central nervous system. Beta-blockers also reduce anxiety. Propranolol 80 mg twice daily, atenolol 50–100 mg daily and oxprenolol 80 mg twice daily have been most widely used for the treatment of blood pressure, but there is a wide range of beta-blockers with different properties:

- Cardioselectivity implies a greater effect on beta-1-receptors (cardiac receptors) than on beta-2-receptors. Such a selective effect is preferred when bronchospasm, intermittent claudication or diabetes is present. Metoprolol, atenolol and acebutolol are cardioselective beta-blockers.
- Intrinsic sympathomimetic activity (ISA) is necessary if bradycardia complicates therapy with beta-blockade. Pindolol has the largest degree of ISA.
- Poor lipid solubility (e.g. sotalol) is an advantage if central nervous system side-effects are prominent.

The complications of beta-blockade include aggravation of ventricular failure, bradycardia, cold extremities, aching muscles, fatigue, weakness, bad dreams and hallucinations. Non-selective beta-blockade may lead to elevation of serum potassium and may mask or prolong the effects of hypoglycaemia. Beta-blockers can, however, usefully be used in patients with both hypertension and angina.

Vasodilators. Dilatation of the peripheral arterioles leads to a fall in blood pressure. There are many mechanisms by which vasodilatation can be achieved.

- Calcium antagonists (Table 11.24) such as nifedipine (20 mg twice daily), diltiazem (60 mg three times daily), verapamil (120–240 mg daily in divided doses) and amlodipine (5–10 mg once daily) reduce blood pressure predominantly by arteriolar dilatation but also by reducing the force of cardiac contraction. They have proved to be effective antihypertensive agents with only a few side-effects; those that do occur include bradycardia and conduction defects (verapamil and diltiazem), headaches, constipation, flushing and fluid retention. The routine use of calcium antagonists in the treatment of hypertension has been increasing as they prove to be safe and effective drugs.

Table 11.37 Main properties of beta-blockers.

	Cardiac selectivity	Intrinsic sympathomimetic activity	Lipid solubility	Plasma half-life
Acebutalol	+	+	0	5 h
Atenolol	+	0	0	6 h
Metoprolol	+	0	+	4 h
Nadolol	0	0	0	20 h
Oxprenolol	0	++	+	1.5 h
Pindolol	0	+++	+	4 h
Propranolol	0	0	++	5 h
Sotalol	0	0	0	10 h
Timolol	0	0	+	5 h

- Alpha-1 adrenergic antagonists such as prazosin (500 μg to a maximum of 20 mg daily) and indoramin (25 mg twice daily) are post-synaptic alpha-blockers that produce vasodilatation and are very effective hypotensive drugs. Their main complication is marked hypotension following the first dose, especially when the patient is salt-depleted because of previous diuretic therapy. Pre-synaptic (alpha-2 adrenergic) antagonists such as phentolamine are now used only in combination with beta-blockers in the treatment of phaeochromocytoma. Labetolol (300–600 mg daily in divided doses) is a combined beta- and alpha-blocker but is has little advantage over beta-blockers.

- Angiotensin-converting enzyme (ACE) inhibitors (Table 11.21) such as captopril (50–150 mg daily in divided doses), lisinopril (10–20 mg daily) and enalapril (10–20 mg daily) block the conversion of angiotensin I to angiotensin II, which is a more powerful vasoconstrictor. ACE inhibitors also block the degradation of bradykinin, which is a vasodilator. Their side-effects include first-dose hypotension and cough. A metallic taste, proteinuria, skin rashes and leucopenia occur generally when they are given in very high doses. The use of ACE inhibitors is increasing as they prove to be safe and effective drugs in the treatment of high blood pressure. ACE inhibitors should not be used in the presence of renal artery stenosis since in this situation the renin–angiotensin system is critical to the maintenance of renal blood flow. Blockade of the production of angiotensin II may result in loss of renal blood flow and infarction of the kidney.

- Non-diuretic thiazides, including indapamide (2.5 mg daily in the morning) and diazoxide (250–600 mg i.v. in divided doses), produce vasodilatation but are seldom used. They produce fluid retention and may provoke glucose intolerance.

- Hydralazine (up to 150 mg daily in divided doses) and minoxidil (10 mg or more daily; maximum 50 mg) directly dilate the peripheral arterioles, leading to a fall in blood pressure. Hydralazine, when given in doses greater than 200 mg daily, may provoke a lupus erythematosus-like syndrome, and minoxidil produces fluid retention and an increase in facial and body hair (hypertrichosis) that renders it unsuitable for women. Both drugs are complicated by sinus tachycardia, which may cause uncomfortable palpitations. They are therefore often combined with beta-blockade for the resistant case.

- Sodium nitroprusside is effective as an arterial and venous dilator when given intravenously. However, it is inconvenient to use because it must be protected from light to prevent degradation. It is occasionally used for the treatment of hypertensive emergencies such as dissecting aneurysm.

- Centrally acting drugs such as methyldopa (a false adrenergic transmitter) (750 mg daily in divided doses) and clonidine (an alpha-2 agonist) (0.1–0.3 mg daily in divided doses) reduce the degree of vasomotor tone. Both drugs are complicated by tiredness, fluid retention and mild postural hypotension. Methyldopa may also cause a dry mouth, impotence, pyrexia and a positive Coombs' test. Very rarely, a haemolytic anaemia may be produced. It can also rarely cause chronic active hepatitis. Clonidine may cause depression and it is important that it is not stopped suddenly because severe rebound hypertension may occur.

- Debrisoquine, bethanidine and guanethidine block post-synaptic adrenergic neurones and are powerful hypotensive drugs. Side-effects include marked postural hypotension, bradycardia, diarrhoea, nasal congestion, salivary gland pain and inability to ejaculate. Centrally acting drugs and ganglion blockers are rarely used nowadays.

Stepped care for the control of hypertension

The majority of patients with mild or moderate hypertension can be treated as outpatients. The usual practice is to attempt to reduce the blood pressure to about 150/95 mm Hg. If general adjustment to lifestyle and diet have not led to an adequate fall in the blood pressure, it is conventional to prescribe either a beta-blocker or a diuretic. Diuretics (e.g. bendrofluazide 5–10 mg daily) are preferred if heart failure or peripheral vascular disease is present, but beta-blockers (e.g. propranolol 80 mg twice daily or atenolol 100 mg daily) are more suitable if the patient complains of angina. Calcium antagonists such as nifedipine 10 mg twice daily have also been used as a first-line therapy.

If single drug treatment is unsuccessful, it is appropriate to prescribe both a beta-blocker or a calcium antagonist in combination with a diuretic. The combination of beta-blockers and diuretics is particularly attractive because some of their side-effects are partially antagonistic. For example, beta-blockers lead to potassium retention, aggravation of heart failure and decreased renin secretion, whilst thiazide diuretics induce the opposite changes. If these combined therapies are insufficient, more powerful vasodilators such as hydralazine, prazosin or nifedipine are added to the regimen. ACE inhibitors may be used if these prove inadequate. The hypotensive effect of ACE inhibitors is increased by their use with a diuretic.

It is essential that the patient understands that high blood pressure does not go away after a single course of treatment. It is necessary to continue treatment for many years or for life. In addition, the patient's blood pressure must be checked at regular intervals. Since treatment is life-long the physician must attempt to simplify treatment regimens to improve compliance. Evidence suggests that poor treatment is better than no treatment at all.

Hypertension that is unresponsive to treatment is usually due to the patient not taking the drugs prescribed or to the presence of an underlying primary cause such as coarctation or renal artery stenosis. Such underlying causes must be discovered and corrected before therapy will succeed.

The management of severe or malignant hypertension
Patients with severe hypertension should be admitted to hospital for urgent treatment under close supervision, and frequent blood pressure measurements should be taken. It is unwise to reduce the blood pressure too rapidly because of possible cerebral infarction. Hypertensive emergencies should be treated by bringing the blood pressure back to about 110 mm Hg diastolic over a few hours. This can normally be achieved with oral hydralazine 25 mg or a beta-blocker, e.g. atenolol 25–50 mg. Parenteral treatment is seldom necessary. Oral nifedipine (chewed) or captopril may also be effective. In resistant cases, intravenous nitroprusside, labetalol or diazoxide can be used.

The management of hypertension during pregnancy
Mild hypertension in pregnancy is usual, but more severe hypertension (> 140/90 mm Hg), associated with proteinuria and peripheral oedema, may be a prelude to eclampsia. Pre-eclampsia is treated with bed rest and hypotensive drugs known to be safe in pregnancy. Methyldopa, propranolol, atenolol, nifedipine and hydralazine are usually used. Full-blown eclampsia is treated as a hypertensive emergency with intravenous hydralazine. If the high pressure cannot be reduced, the pregnancy may need to be terminated, and this universally reduces the high blood pressure unless the patient had prior high blood pressure.

PROGNOSIS

Patients with untreated malignant or accelerated hypertension have a very poor prognosis—more than 90% will die within the first year. Effective reduction in the blood pressure leads to a dramatic improvement of prognosis. In general, the risk from hypertension depends on:

- The level of blood pressure
- The presence of retinal changes
- The presence of cardiac or renal complications
- The sex of the patient (men are more at risk than women)

Table 11.38 Congenital and inherited disorders causing cardiovascular abnormalities.

Mode of inheritance	Disorder	Recurrence in first-degree relative
Multifactorial	Ventricular septal defect	4%
	Patent ductus arteriosus	4%
	Fallot's tetralogy	4%
	Aortic stenosis	4%
	Atrial septal defect	2%
	Aortic coarctation	2%
	Early coronary disease	
	Male relative	9%
	Female relative	3%
Chromosomal	Congenital heart disease (see p. 600)	
Trisomy 21		
Trisomy 18		
Turner's syndrome		
Single gene		
Autosomal dominant	Familial hypercholesterolaemia	
	Familial Marfan syndrome	
	Familial hypertrophic obstructive cardiomyopathy	50%
	Familial Wolff–Parkinson–White syndrome	
Autosomal recessive	Jervell–Lange–Neilsen syndrome (long QT)	25%

- The coexistence of coronary disease and risk factors for coronary disease such as high plasma lipids, diabetes and smoking
- The age of the patient (young patients fare worse than the old)

The cause of death in hypertensive patients is usually myocardial infarction, cardiac failure, renal failure or cerebrovascular accident. Effective treatment of moderate hypertension clearly improves the prognosis for each of these causes of death. The treatment of even mild hypertension reduces the likelihood of stroke or cardiac failure.

Genetic aspects of heart disease

As part of total patient care it is essential to take a brief but thorough family medical history of first-degree relatives (parents, siblings and children) and initiate screening, counselling and treatment in appropriate cases. Some chromosomal abnormalities such as Turner's syndrome lead to cardiac malformations, and other cardiac conditions have a genetic basis (Table 11.38). Many cardiovascular disorders, such as coronary disease and hypertension, have a multifactorial aetiology including genetic elements.

Genetic aspects should be considered in the assessment and management of heart disease. For example, parents with a child suffering from Fallot's tetralogy stand a 4% chance of conceiving another child with the disease. Fetal ultrasound screening is therefore important for this couple. A strong family history of coronary disease in a young man who presents with myocardial infarction or angina pectoris strongly suggests that familial hypercholesterolaemia may be present. In this kind of patient lipid analysis should be undertaken and, if the diagnosis is confirmed, treatment with lipid-lowering drugs should be initiated. Young children in the family should also be screened.

Heart disease in the elderly

As the average age of the population increases, cardiac disease predominates. The elderly population are vulnerable to most forms of heart disease, especially coronary artery disease, hypertension, arrhythmias and degenerative pathologies.

Diagnosis of mild forms of heart disease may be difficult in the elderly. The wear and tear of age results in some features that would be regarded as abnormal in the young. For example, a fourth heart sound and a systolic aortic ejection murmur are common findings on examining normal elderly adults. The electrocardiogram often shows slight PR interval prolongation (to 0.22 s), left axis deviation and T wave flattening. On the chest X-ray there may be some aortic, valvular or coronary arterial calcification, but the cardiac silhouette is usually normal. The echocardiogram may show mild myocardial hypertrophy and buckling of the ventricular septum.

It is particularly difficult to diagnose and define hypertension in the elderly. Cuff blood pressure usually overestimates intravascular pressure if the old arterial wall is stiff (pseudo-hypertension). Normally blood pressure steadily increases with age, at least up to the age of 70 years, and blood pressure is particularly labile in the elderly. In old people there is only a weak association between 'hypertension' and diseases such as stroke, myocardial infarction and heart failure. The value of treating marginally high blood pressure is not established.

Cardiac disease may present in unexpected ways in an old person. It is not unusual for significant bradycardia to present as a fractured hip because the fall that caused the fracture resulted from transient asystole. Left heart failure may present as an acute confusional state due to poor cerebral perfusion, rather than with the classical symptom of breathlessness. Myocardial infarction may not cause any chest pain ('silent' myocardial infarction) but may present as weakness or abdominal pain.

The principles of treatment of heart disease in old people are usually no different from those governing treatment in the young. However, it is important to remember that drug pharmacokinetics are changed in the elderly: absorption is reduced, renal and hepatic clearance are delayed, body fat increases and lean body mass decreases. Old people may forget to take their medications or be confused about the correct dose.

Some therapies seem inappropriate or futile in the elderly. For example, it is probably unnecessary to inflict a spartan life style or rigorous uncomfortable drug therapy on an old person in an attempt to modify the risk of developing coronary disease. However, there are treatments that have emerged in recent years that are extremely useful for old people. Coronary angioplasty, and perhaps mitral/aortic valvuloplasty, can be undertaken in patients too frail to consider for surgery. Cardiac surgery does carry a much greater (approximately 2–5 times) risk in the elderly but, as with younger patients, the absolute risk is dependent upon the state of the myocardium, the extent of cardiac disease and the condition of other organ systems.

Age is no bar to effective treatment of heart disease.

There are a few cardiac conditions that are largely confined to the elderly.

- *Aortic sclerosis* results from fibrosis and calcification on the aortic side of an otherwise normal tricuspid aortic valve. This may result in an obstruction to left ventricular outflow but it is often trivial. Aortic valve replacement may be necessary if the obstruction is severe.
- *Mitral annulus calcification* occurs predominantly in old women. It is diagnosed from the chest X-ray and it is not usually responsible for any symptoms.
- A non-infective form of *endocarditis* may occur in the elderly. It is a hypercoagulable state that presents with cachexia, thrombosis and embolization. Anticoagulation may be needed.
- Disruption of His–Purkinje conduction by fibrosis and calcification is most common in the old when it is known as *Lev's disease*. It presents with Adams–Stokes attacks and must be treated by pacemaker insertion.
- Atrial fibrillation is much more common in the old but it is often well tolerated and may not need any active treatment.

The heart in pregnancy

In pregnancy the cardiac output and blood volume increase from the second month up to the thirtieth week to 30–50% above the normal levels. This, along with the increased metabolic work, produces the physical signs of warm extremities, a tachycardia with a large-volume pulse and a slight rise in venous pressure. The apex beat is displaced, owing partly to cardiomegaly and partly to a raised diaphragm. The increased blood flow produces a pulmonary systolic murmur and a third heart sound. The diastolic blood pressure is lower owing to vasodilatation.

The added burden of pregnancy on the cardiovascular system can make underlying, otherwise latent, disease clinically apparent. Ten per cent of maternal deaths in England and Wales are due to heart disease. This is usually rheumatic or congenital in origin, but any heart disease can be seen in pregnancy. Moderate to severe mitral stenosis can cause breathlessness early in pregnancy and may lead to pulmonary oedema later in pregnancy. Pregnancy should be avoided in severe mitral stenosis or delayed until after valvotomy. Termination may be necessary in a severe case occurring before the sixteenth week. Most cases of congenital heart disease have been corrected by the time

women reach the reproductive age. However, patients with small and uncomplicated septal defects usually tolerate pregnancy well. Patients with prosthetic valves are usually on anticoagulant therapy. This may require a change to heparin because warfarin can cause fetal abnormalities. Patients with pulmonary hypertension of any aetiology have an extremely high mortality (up to 50%) either during or immediately after delivery, and termination should be considered.

Post partum or late in pregnancy, a cardiomyopathy of uncertain aetiology is sometimes seen. There is also a rise in thromboembolic complications of cardiac disease owing to the hypercoagulability that exists *post partum*. Sepsis is a risk during delivery, and patients with heart disease may be at risk of developing infective endocarditis.

Peripheral vascular disease

ARTERIAL DISEASE

This can be due to a number of pathological processes.

Arteriosclerosis
This is the term applied to generalized, age-related arterial changes, which are exaggerated in hypertension. In arteries down to 1 mm in diameter these changes initially take the form of compensatory muscular hypertrophy of the media, which is followed by fibrosis and dilatation of the lumen. In hypertensive vessels of this size, atheroma is often superadded.

Smaller arteries show different changes that are usually most marked in the viscera, especially in the kidneys. Here, though there is medial hypertrophy, the predominant change is intimal thickening by concentric layers of connective tissue, with luminal narrowing.

Arterioles undergo hyaline thickening of their walls and luminal narrowing. The narrowing of small vessels in the kidney owing to hypertension causes renal ischaemia, which further promotes hypertension.

In malignant hypertension, arterioles also show fibrinoid necrosis of their walls.

Mönckeberg's sclerosis
This is a degenerative disease of unknown cause, characterized by dystrophic calcification of the media. It is especially common in the major lower limb arteries of the elderly, and there is an increased incidence of this degeneration in diabetics.

Cystic medial necrosis or degeneration

This describes mucoid degeneration of the collagen and elastic tissue of the media, often with cystic changes. It occurs mainly in elderly hypertensives. Dissecting aneurysms of the thoracic aorta are often due to this process. Cystic medial degeneration also occurs in inherited defects of collagen tissue formation (e.g. Marfan syndrome, Ehlers–Danlos syndrome), again resulting in dissecting aneurysms.

Atheroma

The pathogenesis of this condition is described on p. 569. The different vessels which may be involved are shown in Table 11.37. Atheroma seldom involves arteries of less than 2 mm in diameter. Most arterial disease is due to atheromatous degeneration.

Chronic ischaemia of the legs

This is due to atheromatous disease involving the aorta, iliac and/or any other peripheral vessels. It consequently occurs over the age of 50 years, chiefly in men who are smokers.

SYMPTOMS

- Ischaemic, cramp-like pain, usually in the calves during exercise and relieved by rest (intermittent claudication)
- Rest pain
- Non-healing leg ulcers or gangrene

Both limbs are often affected, but usually one is more severely affected than the other.

SIGNS

- A cold limb with dry skin and lack of hair
- Absent pulses to diseased areas
- Ulceration or gangrene

INVESTIGATION

- X-rays may show calcification of the arteries of the leg.
- Doppler ultrasound is of some help in defining the severity of the lesion.
- Aortography by direct injection of contrast

Table 11.39 Common sites of clinically significant atherosclerosis in order of frequency.

Abdominal aorta and iliac arteries
Proximal coronary arteries
Femoral and popliteal arteries, and thoracic aorta
Internal carotid arteries
Vertebrobasilar system

medium into the aorta is used. Angiography is also performed via a percutaneous catheter inserted into the brachial artery and, recently, digital vascular imaging with an intravenous injection has been used. These investigations show narrowing and stenosis of the arteries.

MANAGEMENT

General

- Risk factors should be reduced (e.g. smoking should be stopped, diabetes and hypertension should be treated, and weight should be reduced).
- The limbs should be kept warm but local heat should not be applied.
- Care should be taken to avoid infection, trauma, etc., of the feet. Elderly patients often need regular visits to a chiropodist.
- Regular exercise should be taken to encourage the development of anastomotic vessels.
- Low-dose aspirin should be given.
- Vasodilators should not be used.
- Anticoagulants are of no benefit.

Surgery

- Surgery should not be considered for 3 months after symptoms have developed, to allow time for collaterals to develop. In 75% of patients the disease remains static.
- Aorto-iliac bypass grafts give good results, but reconstructive surgery for blockages below the inguinal ligament is less successful.
- Balloon dilatation via a catheter inserted into the artery is useful for local iliac or femoral stenoses.
- Amputation is necessary for severely ischaemic limbs, usually those with gangrene. Rehabilitation may take months in the elderly and is often unsuccessful.

Many of the patients have generalized atheromatous conditions, so that the overall prognosis often dictates the outcome of localized disease.

Acute ischaemia of the legs

Like chronic ischaemia of the legs, this is mainly due to atheromatous disease with thrombosis, but it can also occur owing to embolism from the heart (e.g. in atrial fibrillation) or from an atheromatous central vessel.

The clinical picture is of an acutely painful, pale, paralysed, pulseless limb.

Treatment is surgical, with removal of the clot. If gangrene develops, amputation is necessary.

Aortic aneurysms

Abdominal aneurysms

The commonest aortic aneurysms are abdominal.

These are usually due to atheroma.

Asymptomatic aneurysms may be found as a pulsatile mass on examination or as calcification on an X-ray. A CT scan or ultrasound of the abdomen will demonstrate the size of the aneurysm, the thickness of the aortic wall and whether any leak has occurred. An expanding aneurysm may cause epigastric or back pain. Rupture presents with epigastric pain radiating through to the back. A pulsatile mass is felt and the patient is shocked.

Treatment of symptomatic aneurysms is surgical. A ruptured aneurysm requires emergency surgery, but even then the mortality is high. Large, asymptomatic aneurysms should also be treated surgically (except in the very old) because those larger than 6 cm in diameter have a high risk of rupture.

Thoracic aneurysms

Most thoracic aneurysms in the past were due to syphilis, but now many are due to atheromatous disease. The aneurysms may affect all parts of the thoracic aorta—the ascending aorta, the arch and the descending aorta.

Most are asymptomatic, but when large they can give rise to chest pain or to evidence of pressure on other organs, such as the superior vena cava or the oesophagus. They can rupture.

Dissecting aortic aneurysms

In the majority of cases, the dissection starts in the ascending aorta. Pain, which is severe and central, often radiating to the back, is the major symptom. The pain radiates down the arms and into the neck and can be difficult to distinguish from myocardial infarction.

On examination, the patient is usually shocked and there may be neurological signs owing to the involvement of the spinal vessels. The peripheral pulses may be absent, but this is not invariable.

The diagnosis is suggested by the presence of back pain with no ECG or enzyme changes of myocardial infarction. The chest X-ray may show a wide mediastinum and CT scanning and ultrasonography are helpful. Aortography may be necessary to confirm the diagnosis.

Half of the patients are hypertensive and this should be controlled immediately. Emergency surgery is necessary for many dissections.

There is an increased risk of dissection in pregnancy.

Thromboangiitis obliterans (Buerger's disease)

This disease, involving the small vessels of the lower limbs, occurs in young men who smoke. It is thought by some workers to be indistinguishable from atheromatous disease. However, pathologically there is inflammation of the vessels that may indicate a separate disease activity. Clinically it presents with peripheral ischaemia and patients must stop smoking.

Takayasu's syndrome

This is rare, except in Japan. It is known as 'pulseless disease' or the aortic arch syndrome. It is of unknown aetiology and occurs in young females. There is a vasculitis involving the aortic arch as well as other major arteries. There is also a systemic illness, with pain and tenderness over the affected arteries. Absent peripheral pulses and hypertension are usually found. Corticosteroids help the constitutional symptoms. Heart failure and cerebrovascular accidents eventually occur, but most patients survive for at least 5 years.

Kawasaki disease (mucocutaneous lymph node syndrome)

This is an uncommon acute febrile illness of early childhood. There is a generalized vasculitis with involvement of the coronary arteries.

Cardiovascular syphilis

This gives rise to

- Uncomplicated aortitis
- Aortic aneurysms, usually in the ascending part
- Aortic valvulitis with regurgitation
- Stenosis of the coronary ostia

The diagnosis is confirmed by serology. Treatment is with penicillin. Aneurysms and valvular disease are treated as necessary by the usual methods.

Connective-tissue disorders

These cause vasculitis and can give rise to peripheral vascular disease. They are discussed on p. 391.

Raynaud's disease and phenomenon

Raynaud's phenomenon consists of spasm of the arteries supplying the fingers or toes and is usually precipitated by cold and relieved by heat. When Raynaud's phenomenon occurs without any underlying disorder, it is then known as Raynaud's disease. This is a common disease affecting 5% of the population and occurring predominantly in young women. The disorder is usually bilateral and fingers are affected more commonly than toes. There is an initial pallor of the skin resulting from vasoconstriction and this is followed by cyanosis due to sluggish blood flow. Redness finally occurs owing to hyperaemia. The duration of the attacks can be variable and can sometimes last for hours. Numbness and burning of the fingers usually occurs and pain can be severe, particularly in the re-warming phase.

Between the attacks the pulses and the digits appear normal, but trophic changes with small areas of gangrene can occur in severe and persistent cases.

DIAGNOSIS

Primary Raynaud's disease must be differentiated from secondary causes of Raynaud's phenomenon, which are chiefly disorders of connective tissue, particularly systemic sclerosis. It can also occur in cryoglobulinaemia and as a side-effect of drug treatment, especially with beta-blocking agents.

TREATMENT

No treatment is usually required for the attacks but any underlying disease must be looked for. The hands and feet should be kept warm, and smoking should be avoided. Beta-blockers should be stopped. Nifedipine 10 mg three times daily may be helpful.

VENOUS DISEASE

Varicose veins

Varicose veins are a common problem, sometimes giving rise to pain. They are treated by injection or surgery.

Venous thrombosis

Thrombosis can occur in any vein, but the veins of the leg and the pelvis are the commonest sites.

Superficial thrombophlebitis
This commonly involves the saphenous veins and is often associated with varicosities. Occasionally the axillary vein is involved, usually as a result of trauma. There is local superficial inflammation of the vein wall, with secondary thrombosis.

The clinical picture is of a painful, tender, cord-like structure with associated redness and swelling.

The condition usually responds to symptomatic treatment with rest, elevation of the limb and analgesics (e.g. non-steroidal anti-inflammatory drugs). Anticoagulants are not necessary, as embolism does not occur from superficial thrombophlebitis.

Deep-vein thrombosis
A thrombus forms in the vein, and any inflammation of the vein wall is secondary to this.

Thrombosis commonly occurs after periods of immobilization, but it can occur in normal individuals for no obvious reasons. The precipitating factors are discussed on p. 345.

Deep-vein thrombosis occurs in 50% of patients after prostatectomy or following a cerebral vascular accident. In addition, one-third of patients with a myocardial infarct have a deep-vein thrombosis.

Thrombosis can occur in any vein of the leg, but is particularly found in veins of the calf. It is often undetected; autopsy figures give an incidence of over 60% in hospitalized patients.

Clinical features. The major presenting features are:

- Asymptomatic, presenting with clinical features of pulmonary embolism (see p. 607).
- Pain in the calf, often presenting with swelling, redness and engorged superficial veins. The affected calf is often warmer and there may be ankle oedema. Homans' sign (pain in the calf on dorsiflexion of the foot) is often present, but is not diagnostic and occurs with all lesions of the calf.

Thrombosis in the iliofemoral region can present with severe pain, but there are often few physical signs apart from occasional swelling of the thigh and/or ankle oedema.

Complete occlusion, particularly of a large vein, can lead to a cyanotic discoloration of the limb and severe oedema, which can very rarely lead to venous gangrene.

Pulmonary embolism can occur with any deep vein thrombosis but is more frequent from an iliofemoral thrombosis and is rare with thrombosis confined to veins below the knee. Spread of thrombosis can occur proximally without clinical evidence, so the extent of the thrombosis must be carefully assessed.

Investigation. Clinical diagnosis is unreliable and confirmation of an iliofemoral thrombosis can usually be made with an ultrasound. Below knee thromboses can only reliably be detected by venography but whether this is necessary is questionable (see treatment). A venogram is performed by injecting a vein in the foot with contrast which will detect virtually all thrombi that are present.

Treatment. The main aim of therapy is to prevent pulmonary embolism and all patients with thrombi above the knee must be anticoagulated. Anticoagulation of below knee thrombi is controversial. Bed rest is advised until the patient is fully anticoagulated. The patient should then be mobilized, with an elastic stocking giving graduated pressure over the leg.

Heparin is given normally for 48 h but how long warfarin should be given is debatable—3 months is the usual recommended period. Anticoagulants do not affect the thrombus that is already present.

Thrombolytic therapy (see p. 345) is occasionally used for patients with a large iliofemoral thrombosis.

Prognosis. Destruction of the deep-vein valves produces a clinically painful, swollen limb that is made worse by standing and is accompanied by oedema and sometimes venous eczema. It occurs in approximately half of the patients with a clinically symptomatic deep-vein thrombosis, and it means that elastic support stockings are then required for life.

Prevention. Subcutaneous low-dose heparin (see p. 346) should be given to patients with cardiac failure, a myocardial infarct or surgery to the leg or pelvis.

Early ambulation is indicated as most thromboses occur within the first 72 h following surgery. Leg exercises should be encouraged and patients should not sit in a chair with their legs immobilized on a stool. An elastic support stocking should be given to patients at high risk, e.g. those with a history of thrombosis or with obesity.

Further reading

Braunwald E (1987) *Heart Disease*, 3rd edn. Philadelphia: WB Saunders.

Chesler E (1981) *Schrire's Clinical Cardiology*, 4th edn. Bristol: John Wright.

Hampton JR (1986) *The ECG Made Easy*, 3rd edn. Edinburgh: Churchill Livingstone.

Hurst JW (1990) *The Heart, Arteries and Veins*, 7th edn. New York: McGraw–Hill.

Julian DG, Camm AJ, Fox KS, Hall RJC & Poole-Wilson PA (1989) *Diseases of the Heart*. London: Ballière Tindall.

Sokolow M & McIlroy MB (1986) *Clinical Cardiology*, 4th edn. New York: Lange.

A glossary of terms and abbreviations used in this chapter is given in the Appendices on p. 1065.

Diseases of the respiratory system are a major cause of morbidity and mortality throughout the world. In the UK, respiratory diseases account for approximately one-fifth of all deaths, exceeded only by heart disease. Respiratory disorders are the single biggest cause of days lost from work and generate the largest number of visits to general practitioners. Some diseases, such as asthma, are probably increasing; chronic bronchitis and emphysema continue to remain a major problem in the UK. Tuberculosis continues to be seen frequently even in the UK, mainly in the Asian population. There is still no cure for the common cold, and, in spite of intense efforts to discourage cigarette smoking, carcinoma of the bronchus remains the commonest cancer.

Structure of the respiratory system

The nose

The anterior one-third of the nasal cavity is divided into right and left halves by the nasal septum (Fig. 12.1). The nasal vestibule leads to the internal ostium (a) which is the narrowest part of the nasal cavity. This causes a resistance to airflow, which is 50% greater when breathing through the nose than through the mouth. The respiratory region (b) is divided by three folds arising from the lateral wall, termed the superior turbinate (ST), middle turbinate (MT) and inferior turbinate (IT). Behind these turbinates are situated the openings of the nasolacrymal duct and the frontal, ethmoidal and maxillary sinuses. The olfactory region for smell is found above the superior turbinate. The nasal cavities communicate with the nasopharynx via the posterior nasal apertures (the choanae (c)), and the eustachian tube opens into this area just above the soft palate.

The pharynx and larynx

The pharynx is divided by the soft palate into an upper nasopharyngeal and lower oropharyngeal region. There are numerous collections of lymphoid tissue arranged in a circular fashion around the nasopharynx; these include the adenoids. The tonsils lie between the anterior and posterior fauces, separating the mouth from the oropharynx.

The larynx consists of a number of articulated cartilages, vocal cords, muscles and ligaments, all of which serve to keep the airway open during breathing and occlude it during swallowing.

The main motor nerve to the larynx is the recurrent laryngeal nerve. The left recurrent laryngeal nerve leaves the vagus at the level of the aortic arch, hooking round it to run upwards through the mediastinum between the trachea and the oesophagus; it can be affected by disease in these areas. The principal tensor of the vocal cords is the external branch of the superior laryngeal nerve, which can be injured during thyroidectomy.

The trachea, bronchi and bronchioles

The trachea is 10–12 cm in length. It lies slightly to the right of the midline and divides at the carina into right and left main bronchi. The carina lies under the junction of the manubrium sternum and the second right costal cartilage.

The right main bronchus is more vertical than the left and, hence, inhaled material is more likely to pass into it.

The right main bronchus divides into the upper lobe bronchus and the intermediate bronchus, which further subdivides into the middle and lower lobe bronchi. On the left the main bronchus divides into upper and lower lobe bronchi only. Each lobar bronchus further divides into segmental and subsegmental bronchi.

There are about 25 divisions in all between the trachea and the alveoli. Of the first seven divisions the bronchi have:

- Walls consisting of cartilage and smooth muscle
- Epithelial lining with cilia and goblet cells
- Submucosal mucus-secreting glands

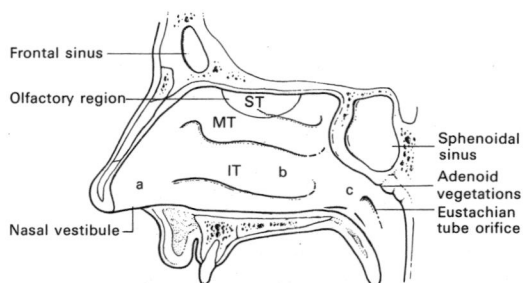

Fig. 12.1 The anatomy of the nose in longitudinal section. ST = superior turbinate; MT = middle turbinate; IT = inferior turbinate. a = internal ostium; b = respiratory region; c = choanae.

- Endocrine cells—Kulchitsky or APUD containing 5-hydroxytryptamine

In the next 16–18 divisions the bronchioles have:

- No cartilage and a muscular layer that progressively becomes thinner
- A single layer of ciliated cells but very few goblet cells
- Granulated Clara cells that produce a surfactant-like substance

The ciliated epithelium is an important defence mechanism. Each cell contains approximately 200 cilia beating at 1000 times per minute in organized waves of contraction. Each cilium consists of nine peripheral parts and two inner longitudinal fibrils in a cytoplasmic matrix (Fig. 12.2). Nexin links join

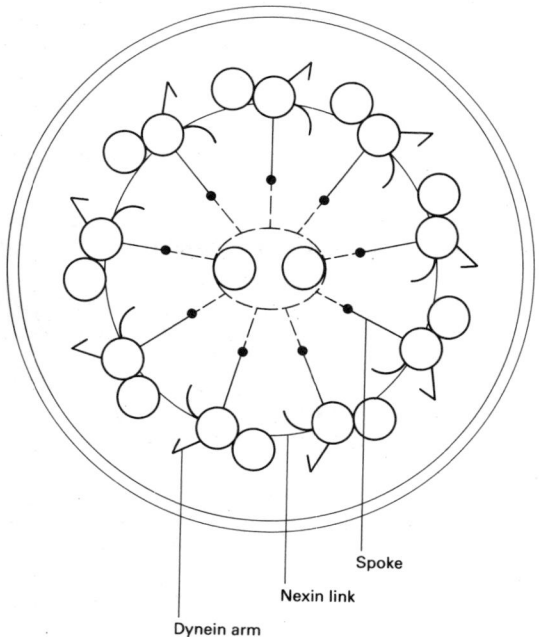

Fig. 12.2 Cross-section of a cilium. Nine outer microtubular doublets and two central single microtubules are linked by spokes, nexin links and dynein arms.

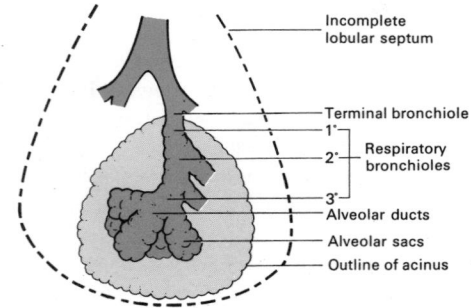

Fig. 12.3 Branches of a terminal bronchiole ending in the alveolar sacs.

the peripheral pairs. Dynein arms consisting of ATP-ase protein project towards the adjacent pairs. Bending of the cilia results from a sliding movement between adjacent fibrils powered by an ATP-dependent shearing force developed by the dynein arms. Absence of dynein arms leads to immotile cilia. Mucus, which contains macrophages, cell debris, inhaled particles and bacteria, is moved by the cilia towards the larynx at about 1.5 cm per minute—the 'mucociliary escalator' (see below).

The bronchioles finally divide within the acinus into smaller respiratory bronchioles that have alveoli arising from the surface (Fig. 12.3). Each respiratory bronchiole supplies approximately 200 alveoli via alveolar ducts. The term 'small airways' refers to bronchioles of less than 2 mm; there are 30 000 of these in the average lung.

The alveoli

There are approximately 300 million alveoli in each lung. Their total surface area is 40–80 m². The epithelial lining consists largely of type I pneumocytes (Fig. 12.4). These cells have an extremely attenuated cytoplasm, and thus provide only a thin barrier to gas exchange.

Type II pneumocytes are slightly more numerous than type I cells but cover less of the epithelial

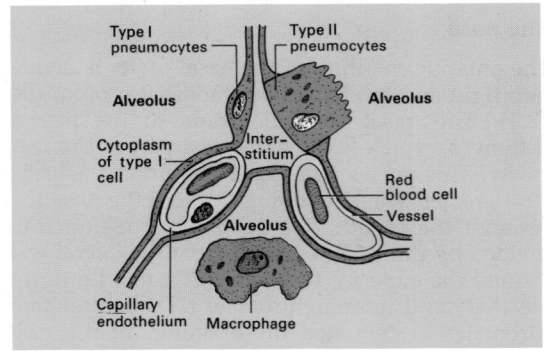

Fig. 12.4 The structure of alveoli, showing the pneumocytes and capillaries.

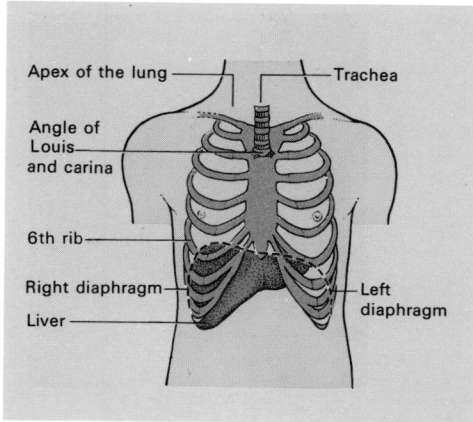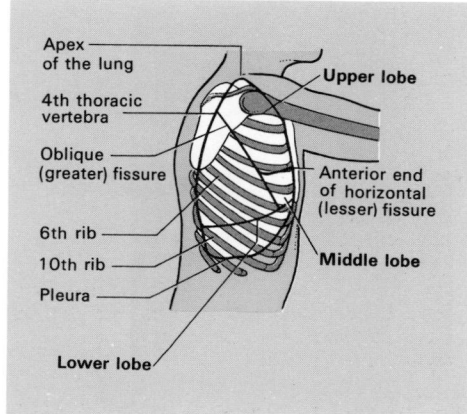

Fig. 12.5 Surface anatomy of the chest.

lining. They are found generally in the borders of the alveolus and contain distinctive lamellar vacuoles, thought to be a source of surfactant. Type II cells are fixed to type I cells by tight junctions that limit the fluid movements in and out of the alveoli. Macrophages are also present in the alveoli and are involved in the defence mechanisms of the lung.

The pores of Kohn are holes in the alveolar wall allowing communication between alveoli of adjoining lobules.

The lungs

The lungs are separated into lobes by invaginations of the pleura, which are often incomplete. The right lung has three lobes, whereas the left lung has two. The position of the oblique fissures and the right horizontal fissure are shown in Fig. 12.5. The upper lobe lies mainly in front of the lower lobe and therefore signs on the right side in the front of the chest found on physical examination are due to lesions mainly of the upper lobe or part of the middle lobe.

Each lobe is further subdivided into bronchopulmonary segments by fibrous septa that extend inwards from the pleural surface. Each segment receives its own segmental bronchus.

The bronchopulmonary segment is further divided into individual lobules approximately 1 cm in diameter and generally pyramidal in shape, the apex lying towards the bronchioles supplying them. Within each lobule a terminal bronchus supplies an acinus and within this structure further divisions of the bronchioles eventually give rise to the alveoli.

A chest X-ray (Fig. 12.6) illustrates the above features.

The pleura

The pleura is a layer of connective tissue covered by a simple squamous epithelium. The visceral pleura covers the surface of the lung, lines the interlobar fissures, and is continuous at the hilum with the parietal pleura, which lines the inside of the hemithorax. At the hilum the visceral pleura continues alongside the branching bronchial tree for some distance before reflecting back to join the parietal pleura. The pleurae are in apposition apart from a small quantity of lubricating fluid, so the pleural cavity is only a potential space.

The diaphragm

The diaphragm is lined by parietal pleura and peritoneum. Its muscle fibres arise from the lower ribs and insert into the central tendon. Motor sensory nerve fibres go separately to each half of the diaphragm via the phrenic nerves. Fifty per cent of the muscle fibres are of the slow-twitch type with a low glycolytic capacity that are relatively resistant to fatigue.

Pulmonary vasculature and lymphatics

The pulmonary artery divides to accompany the bronchi. The arterioles accompanying the respiratory bronchioles are thin-walled and contain little smooth muscle. The pulmonary venules drain laterally to the periphery of the lobules, pass centrally in the interlobular and intersegmental septa, and eventually join to form the four main pulmonary veins.

In addition, a further bronchial circulation arises from the descending aorta. These bronchial arteries supply tissues down to the level of the respiratory bronchiole. The bronchial veins drain into the pulmonary vein, forming part of the physiological shunt observed in normal individuals.

Lymphatic channels lie in the potential interstitial space between the alveolar cells and the capillary endothelium of the pulmonary arterioles.

(a)

(b)

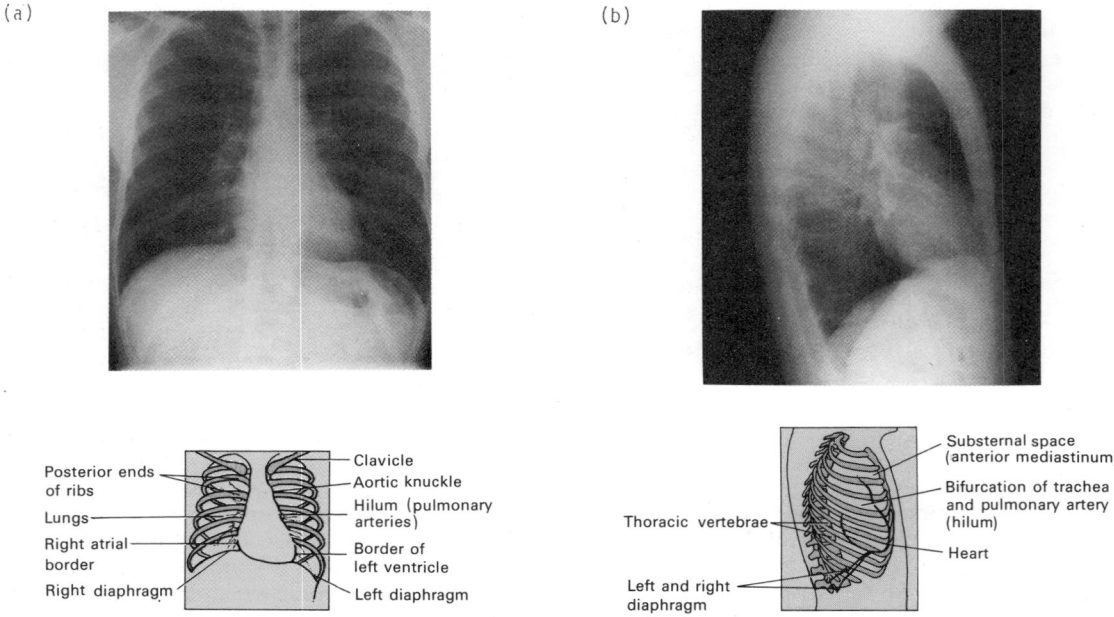

Fig. 12.6 Chest X-rays. (a) PA; (b) lateral.

Physiology of the respiratory system

The nose

The major functions of nasal breathing are:

- To heat and moisten the air
- To remove particulate matter

About 10 000 litres of particle-laden air are inhaled daily. Deposited particles are removed from the nasal mucosa within 15 min, compared with 60–120 days from the alveolus. The relatively low flow rates and turbulence of inspired air are ideal for particle deposition, and few particles greater than 10 μm pass through the nose. For this reason nasal secretion contains many protective proteins in the form of antibodies, lysozymes and interferon. In addition, the cilia of the nasal epithelium move the mucous gel layer rapidly back to the oropharynx where it is swallowed. Bacteria have little chance of settling in the nose. Mucociliary protection against viral infections is more difficult because viruses appear to possess a special affinity for receptors on cilia. Many noxious gases, for example SO_2, are almost completely removed by nasal breathing.

Breathing

Lung ventilation can be considered in two parts:

- The mechanical process of inspiration and expiration

- The control of respiration to a level appropriate for the metabolic needs

Mechanical process
Inspiration is an active process and results from the descent of the diaphragm and movement of the ribs upwards and outwards under the influence of the intercostal muscles. In resting healthy individuals, contraction of the diaphragm is responsible for most of inspiration. Respiratory muscles though similar to other skeletal muscles are less prone to fatigue, though weakness may play a part in respiratory failure resulting from neurological, muscle and possibly severe chronic airflow limitation diseases.

Expiration follows passively as a result of gradual lessening of contraction of the intercostal muscles, allowing the lungs to collapse under the influence of their own elastic forces.

Inspiration against increased resistance may require the use of the accessory muscles of ventilation, such as the sternomastoid and scalene muscles. Forced expiration is also accomplished with the aid of accessory muscles, chiefly those of the abdominal wall, which help to push up the diaphragm.

The lungs have an inherent elastic property that causes them to tend to collapse away from the thoracic wall, generating a negative pressure within the pleural space. The strength of this retractive force relates to the volume of the lung; for example, at higher lung volumes the lung is stretched more, and a greater negative intrapleural pressure is generated.

Lung compliance is a measure of the relationship between this retractive force and lung volume. It is defined as the change in lung volume brought about by unit change in transpulmonary (intrapleural) pressure and is measured in litres per kilopascal ($L \cdot kPa^{-1}$). At the end of a quiet expiration, the retractive force exerted by the lungs is balanced by the tendency of the thoracic wall to spring outwards. At this point respiratory muscles are resting and the volume of the lung is known as the *functional residual capacity* (FRC).

Diseases that can affect the movement of the thoracic cage and diaphragm can have a profound effect on ventilation. These include diseases of the thoracic spine such as ankylosing spondylitis and kyphoscoliosis, neuropathies (e.g. the Guillain–Barré syndrome), injury to the phrenic nerves, and myasthenia gravis.

The control of respiration

Coordinated respiratory movements result from rhythmical discharges arising in an anatomically ill-defined group of interconnected neurones in the reticular substance of the brain stem known as the respiratory centre. Motor discharges from the respiratory centre travel via the phrenic and intercostal nerves to the respiratory musculature.

The pressures of oxygen and carbon dioxide in arterial blood are closely controlled. In a typical normal adult at rest:

- The pulmonary blood flow of $5 \ L \cdot min^{-1}$ carries $11 \ mmol \cdot min^{-1}$ ($250 \ ml \cdot min^{-1}$) of oxygen from the lungs to the tissues.
- Ventilation at about $6 \ L \cdot min^{-1}$ carries $9 \ mmol \cdot min^{-1}$ ($200 \ ml \cdot min^{-1}$) of carbon dioxide out of the body.
- The normal pressure of oxygen in arterial blood (P_aO_2) is between 11 and 13 kPa (83 and 98 mm Hg).
- The normal pressure of carbon dioxide in arterial blood (P_aCO_2) is 4.8–6.0 kPa (36–45 mm Hg).

Neurogenic and chemical factors are involved in the control of ventilation.

Neurogenic factors. Neural stimuli include:

- Consciously induced changes in rate and depth of breathing
- Impulses from limb receptors, as in exercise, which cause respiratory stimulation
- Impulses arising from pulmonary receptors sensitive to stretch and bronchial irritation
- Juxtapulmonary capillary receptors (J receptors) stimulated by pulmonary congestion
- Impulses arising from receptors in muscles and joints of the chest wall

Abnormal stimuli include:

- Lesions in the pons and midbrain, which give rise to central neurogenic hyper- or hypoventilation
- Medullary compression, which leads to respiratory depression

Chemical stimuli. Peripheral and central (in the respiratory centre) chemoreceptors cause an increase in ventilation when they are stimulated by:

- *Carbon dioxide.* The strongest respiratory stimulant to breathing is a rise in P_aCO_2. Sensitivity to this may be lost in chronic bronchitis, so that in these patients hypoxaemia is the chief stimulus to respiratory drive; treatment with oxygen may therefore reduce respiratory drive and produce a further rise in P_aCO_2.
- *Hydrogen ion concentration of arterial blood.* An increase in [H+] due to metabolic acidosis will increase ventilation with a fall in P_aCO_2. In respiratory disease, [H+] and P_aCO_2 rise together.
- *Oxygen.* Peripheral chemoreceptors in the carotid and aortic bodies respond to reduced P_aO_2. The stimulus is not strong unless the P_aO_2 is below 8 kPa. These chemoreceptors also respond to increases in [H+].

The respiratory centre is depressed by severe hypoxaemia and sedatives (e.g. opiates) and stimulated by large doses of aspirin or by pyrexia.

In certain common conditions such as mild asthma, pulmonary embolism and pneumonia there is an increase in ventilation, leading to a reduction in the P_aCO_2. These conditions probably cause this effect through stimulation of irritant receptors in the bronchioles and J receptors stimulated deep in the parenchyma of the lung.

Anxiety or hysteria cause hyperventilation, and increased ventilation is also a prominent feature of metabolic acidosis.

The airways of the lungs

From the trachea to the periphery, the airways become smaller in size (although greater in number). The actual cross-sectional area available for air flow does not decrease as the total number of airways increases. The flow of air is maximum in the trachea and slows progressively towards the periphery (as the velocity of air flow depends on the ratio of flow to cross-sectional area). In the terminal airways, gas flow occurs solely by diffusion. The resistance to air flow is very low— 0.1–0.2 $kPa \cdot L^{-1}$ in a normal tracheobronchial tree.

Airways expand as lung volume is increased and at full inspiration (total lung capacity TLC) they are 30–40% larger in calibre than at full expiration (residual volume RV). In chronic bronchitis and emphysema, which principally affect the smaller airways, the airway narrowing is partially overcome by breathing at a larger lung volume.

Control of airway tone

This is under the autonomic nervous system. Bronchomotor tone is maintained by vagal efferent nerves and, even in a normal subject, is reduced by atropine or β-adrenoreceptor agonists. The many adrenoreceptors on the surface of bronchial muscles respond to circulating catecholamines, although sympathetic nerves do not directly innervate them. Airway tone shows a *circadian rhythm*, which is greatest at 04.00 h and lowest in the mid-afternoon. Tone can be increased briefly by inhaled stimuli acting on cough receptors, which then trigger reflex bronchoconstriction via the vagus. These stimuli include cigarette smoke, inert dust, cold air; airway responsiveness to these increases following respiratory tract infections even in healthy subjects. In asthma, the increased airway responsiveness is an exaggeration of this normal response and, as the circadian rhythm remains the same, asthmatic symptoms are worst in the early morning.

Air flow

Movement of air through the airways results from a difference between the pressure in the alveoli and the atmospheric pressure; a positive alveolar pressure occurs in expiration and a negative pressure occurs in inspiration. During quiet breathing the subatmospheric pleural pressure throughout the breathing cycle slightly distends the airways. With vigorous expiratory efforts (e.g. cough), although the central airways are compressed by positive pleural pressures exceeding 10 kPa, the airways do not close completely because the driving pressure for expiratory flow (alveolar pressure) is also increased. *Alveolar pressure P_{ALV} is equal to the elastic recoil pressure of the lung plus the pleural pressure P_{PL}.* When there is no air flow (i.e. a pause in breathing) the tendency of the lungs to collapse (the positive recoil pressure) is exactly balanced by an equivalent negative pleural pressure.

As air flows from the alveoli towards the mouth there is a gradual loss of pressure owing to flow resistance (Fig. 12.7). In forced expiration, as mentioned above, the driving pressure raises both the alveolar pressure and the intrapleural pressure. Between the alveolus and the mouth, a point will occur (c in Fig. 12.7) where the airway pressure will equal the intrapleural pressure, and airway compression will occur. However, this compression of the airway is temporary, as the transient occlusion of the airway results in an increase in pressure behind it (i.e. upstream) and this raises the intra-airway pressure so that the airways open and flow is restored. The airways thus tend to vibrate at this point of 'dynamic compression'.

The elastic recoil pressure of the lungs decreases with decreasing lung volume and the 'collapse point' moves upstream (i.e. towards the smaller

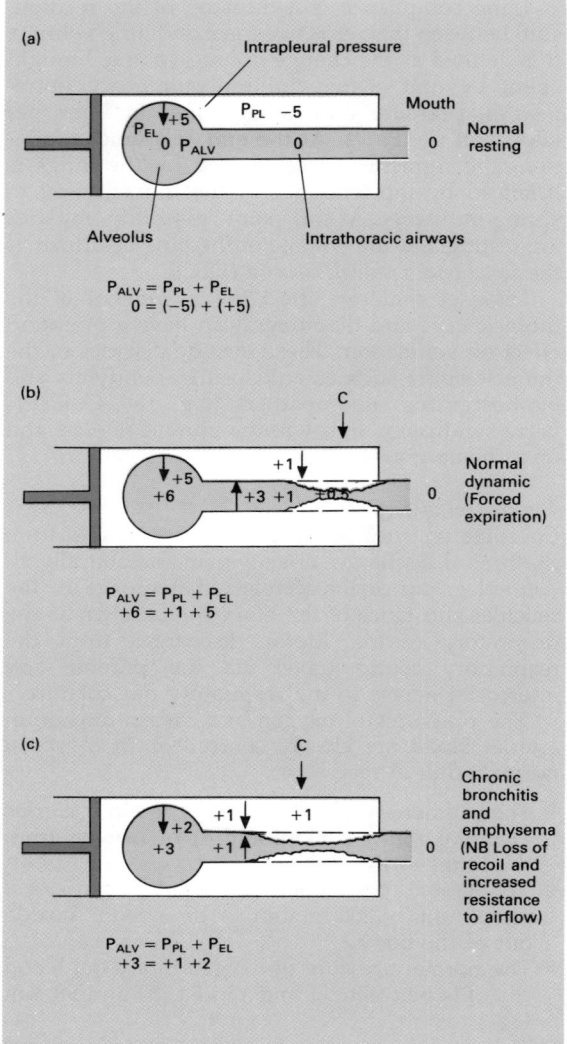

Fig. 12.7 Diagrams showing the ventilatory forces during (a) resting at functional residual capacity, (b) forced expiration in normal subjects, (c) forced expiration in a patient with chronic bronchitis and emphysema. The respiratory system is represented as a piston with a single alveolus and the collapsible part of the airways within the piston (see text). C = compression point.

airways—see Fig. 12.7c). Where there is pathological loss of recoil pressure (as in chronic bronchitis and emphysema), the 'collapse point' starts even further upstream and these patients are often seen to 'purse their lips' in order to increase airway pressure so that their peripheral airways do not collapse. The expiratory airflow limitation is the disordered physiology that underlies chronic airflow limitation. The measurement of the forced expiratory volume in 1 s (FEV) is a useful clinical index of this phenomenon.

On inspiration the intrapleural pressure is

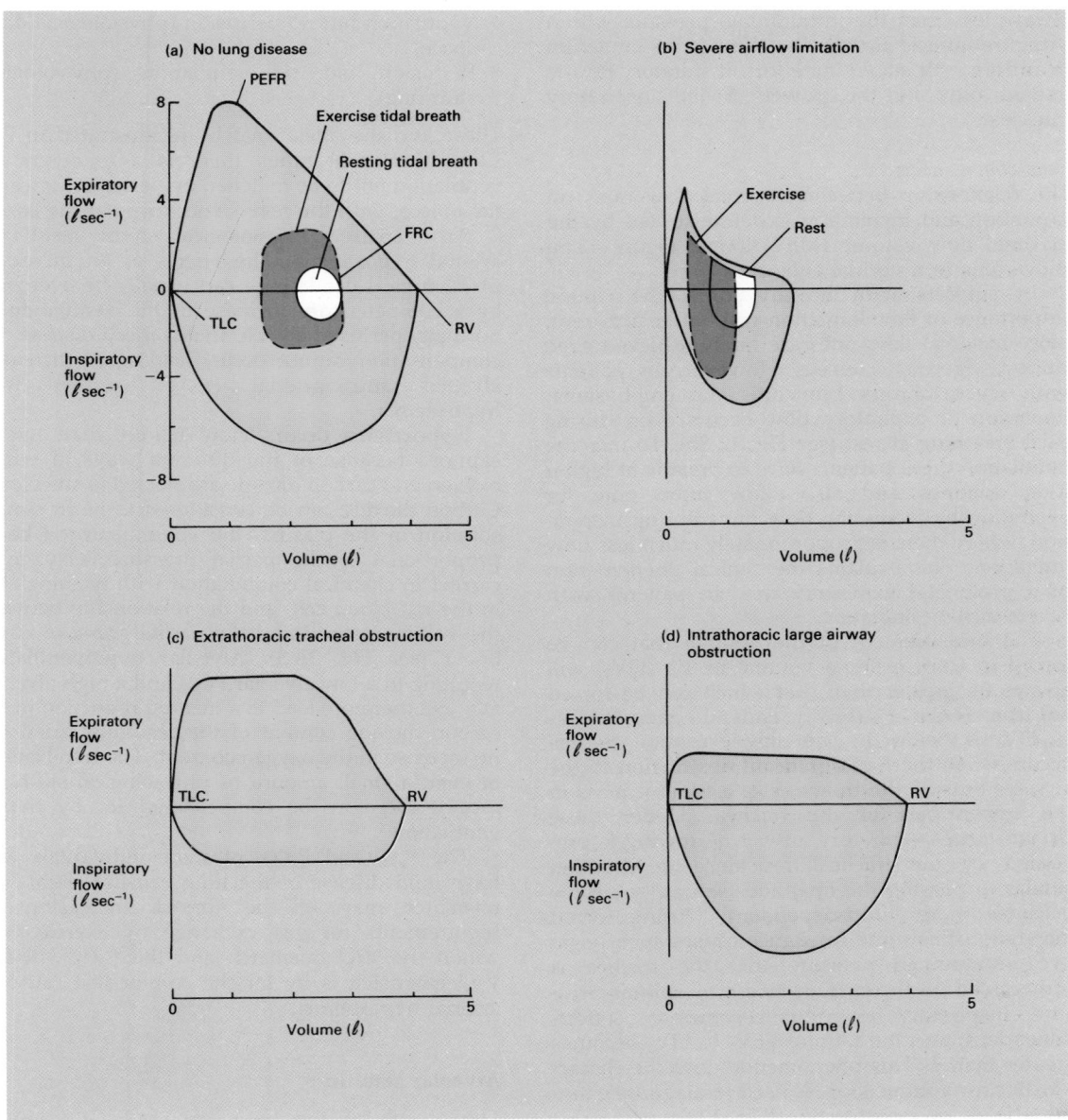

Fig. 12.8 (**a** and **b**) Maximal flow volume loops, showing the relationship between maximal flow rates on expiration and inspiration in (**a**) a normal subject and (**b**) a patient with severe airflow limitation. Flow volume loops during tidal breathing at rest (starting from the functional residual capacity [FRC]) and during exercise are also shown. The highest flow rates are achieved when forced expiration begins at total lung capacity (TLC) and represent the peak expiratory flow rate (PEFR). As air is blown out of the lung, so the flow rate decreases until no more air can be forced out, a point known as the residual volume (RV). Because inspiratory airflow is only dependent on effort, the shape of the maximal inspiratory flow volume loop is quite different, and inspiratory flow remains at a high rate throughout the manoeuvre.

(**c** and **d**) Flow volume loops of patients with large airway (tracheal) obstruction, showing plateauing of maximal expiratory flow high in the lung volume. (**c**) Extrathoracic tracheal obstruction with a proportionally greater reduction of maximal inspiratory (as opposed to expiratory) flow rate. (**d**) Intrathoracic large airway obstruction; the expiratory plateau is more pronounced and inspiratory flow rate is less reduced than in (**c**).

always less than the intraluminal pressure within the intrathoracic airways, so there is no limitation to airflow with increasing effort. Inspiratory flow is limited only by the power of the inspiratory muscles.

Flow volume loops

The relationship between maximal flow rates on expiration and inspiration is demonstrated by the maximal flow volume (MFV) loops. Figure 12.8a shows this in a normal subject.

In subjects with healthy lungs the clinical importance of flow limitation will not be apparent, since maximal flow rates are rarely achieved even during vigorous exercise. However, in patients with severe chronic bronchitis and emphysema, limitation of expiratory flow occurs even during tidal breathing at rest (see Fig. 12.8b). To increase ventilation these patients have to breathe at higher lung volumes and also allow more time for expiration by increasing flow rates during inspiration, where there is proportionately much less flow limitation. This explains the clinical phenomenon of a prolonged expiratory time in patients with severe airflow limitation.

The measurement of the volume that can be forced in from residual volume in 1 s (FIV_1) will always be greater than that which can be forced out from TLC in 1 s (FEV_1). Thus, the ratio of FEV_1 to FIV_1 is below 1. The only exception to this occurs when there is significant obstruction to the airways outside the thorax, e.g. a tumour mass in the upper part of the trachea. Under these circumstances expiratory airway narrowing is prevented by the tracheal resistance (a situation similar to pursing the lips) and expiratory airflow becomes more effort-dependent. During forced inspiration this same resistance causes such negative intraluminal pressure that the trachea is compressed by the surrounding atmospheric pressure. Inspiratory flow thus becomes less effort-dependent, and the ratio of FEV_1 to FIV_1 becomes greater than 1. This phenomenon, and the characteristic flow volume loop, is used to diagnose extrathoracic airways obstruction (Fig. 12.8c).

When obstruction occurs in large airways within the thorax (lower end of trachea and main bronchi), expiratory flow is impaired more than inspiratory flow but a characteristic plateau to expiratory flow is seen (Fig. 12.8d).

Ventilation and perfusion relationships

For efficient gas exchange it is important that there is a match between ventilation of the alveoli ($\dot{V}_A$) and their perfusion ($\dot{Q}$). There is a wide variation in the $\dot{V}_A/\dot{Q}$ ratio throughout both normal and diseased lung. In the normal lung the extreme relationships between alveolar ventilation and perfusion are:

- Ventilation but no perfusion (physiological dead space)
- Perfusion but no ventilation (physiological shunting)

These and the 'ideal' match are illustrated in Fig. 12.9. In normal lungs there is a tendency for ventilation not to be matched by perfusion towards the apices, with the reverse occurring at the bases.

An increased physiological shunt results in arterial hypoxaemia. The effects of an increased physiological dead space can usually be overcome by a compensatory increase in the ventilation of normally perfused alveoli. In advanced disease this compensation cannot occur, leading to increased alveolar and arterial $P\text{CO}_2$, together with hypoxaemia.

Hypoxaemia occurs more readily than hypercapnoea because of the different ways in which oxygen and carbon dioxide are carried in the blood. Carbon dioxide can be considered to be in simple solution in the plasma, the volume carried being proportional to the partial pressure. Oxygen is carried in chemical combination with haemoglobin in the red blood cell, and the relationship between the volume carried and the partial pressure is not linear (see Fig. 13.5). Alveolar hyperventilation resulting in a low alveolar $P\text{CO}_2$ and a high alveolar $P\text{O}_2$ will therefore lead to a marked reduction in the carbon dioxide content of the resulting blood but no increase in the oxygen content. The hypoxaemia of even a small amount of physiological shunting cannot therefore be compensated for by hyperventilation.

The $P_a\text{O}_2$ and $P_a\text{CO}_2$ of some individuals who have mild disease of the lung causing slight $\dot{V}/\dot{Q}$ mismatch may still be normal. Increasing the requirements for gas exchange by exercise will widen the $\dot{V}/\dot{Q}$ mismatch and the $P_a\text{O}_2$ will fall. $\dot{V}/\dot{Q}$ mismatch is by far the commonest cause of arterial hypoxaemia.

Alveolar stability

The alveoli of the lung are essentially hollow spheres. Surface tension acting at the curved internal surface tends to cause the sphere to decrease in size. The surface tension within the alveoli would make the lungs extremely difficult to distend were it not for the presence of surfactant. The type II cells within the alveolus secrete an insoluble lipoprotein largely consisting of dipalmitoyl lecithin, which forms a thin monomolecular layer at the air–fluid interface. Surfactant reduces surface tension so that alveoli remain stable.

Fluid surfaces covered with surfactant exhibit a phenomenon known as hysteresis, i.e. the surface-tension-lowering effect of the surfactant can be improved by a transient increase in the size of the surface area of the alveoli. During quiet breathing,

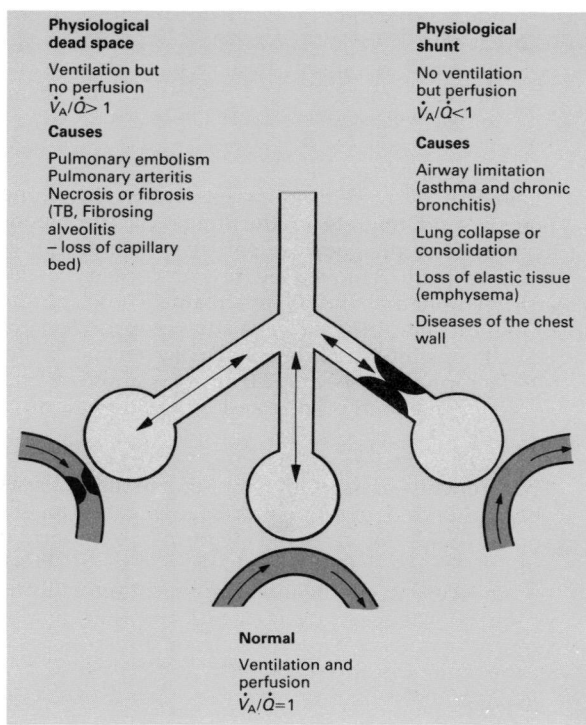

Physiological dead space

Ventilation but no perfusion
$\dot{V}_A/\dot{Q} > 1$

Causes

Pulmonary embolism
Pulmonary arteritis
Necrosis or fibrosis
(TB, Fibrosing alveolitis
– loss of capillary bed)

Physiological shunt

No ventilation but perfusion
$\dot{V}_A/\dot{Q} < 1$

Causes

Airway limitation (asthma and chronic bronchitis)

Lung collapse or consolidation

Loss of elastic tissue (emphysema)

Diseases of the chest wall

Normal

Ventilation and perfusion
$\dot{V}_A/\dot{Q} = 1$

Fig. 12.9 Relationships between ventilation and perfusion: a schematic diagram showing the alveolar–capillary interface. The centre shows normal ventilation and perfusion. On the left there is a block in perfusion (physiological dead space), while on the right there is reduced ventilation (physiological shunting).

small areas of the lung undergo collapse, but it is possible to re-expand these rapidly by a deep breath, hence the importance of sighs or deep breaths as a feature of normal breathing. Failure of such a mechanism, which can occur, for example, in patients with fractured ribs, gives rise to patchy basal lung collapse. Surfactant levels may be reduced in a number of diseases that cause damage to the lung (e.g. pneumonia), and may play a central role in the respiratory distress syndrome of the newborn. Severe reduction in perfusion of the lung causes impairment of surfactant activity and may well account for the characteristic areas of collapse associated with pulmonary embolism.

Defence mechanisms of the respiratory tract

Pulmonary disease often results from a failure of the many defence mechanisms that usually protect the lung in a healthy individual (Fig. 12.10). These can be divided into physical and physiological mechanisms and humoral and cellular mechanisms.

Physical and physiological mechanisms

The following mechanisms are important:

- *Humidification*—prevents dehydration of the epithelium
- *Particle removal*—over 90% of particles greater than 10 µm in diameter are removed in the nostril or nasopharynx. Of the remainder, 5–10 µm particles become impacted in the carina and 1–2 µm particles are deposited in the distal lungs. Most pollen grains (> 20 µm) are deposited in the nose and conjunctiva
- *Particle expulsion*—by coughing, sneezing or gagging
- *Respiratory tract secretions*

The mucus of the respiratory tract is a gelatinous substance consisting chiefly of acid and neutral polysaccharides. The mucus consists of a 5 µm thick gel that is relatively impermeable to water. This floats on a liquid or sol layer that is present around the cilia of the epithelial cells. The gel layer is secreted from goblet cells and mucous glands as distinct globules that coalesce increasingly in the central airways to form a more or less continuous mucus blanket. Under normal conditions the tips of the cilia are in contact with the undersurface of the gel phase and coordinate their movement to push the mucus blanket upwards. Whilst it may only take 30–60 min for mucus to be cleared from

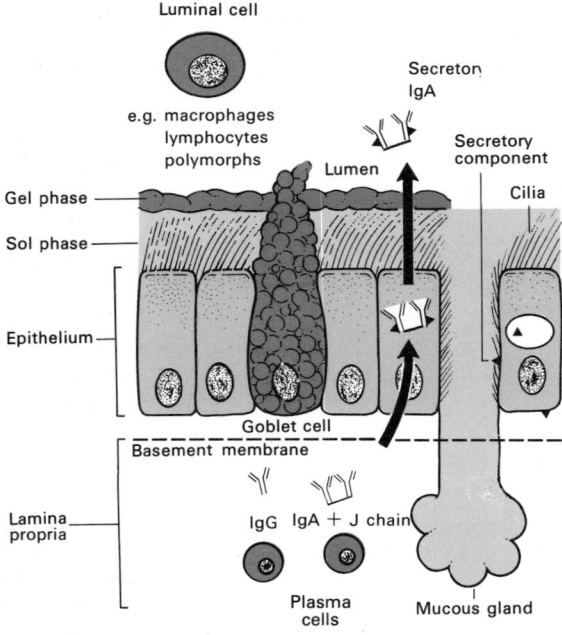

Fig. 12.10 Defence mechanisms present at the epithelial surface.

the large bronchi, there may be a delay of several days before clearance is achieved from respiratory bronchioles. One of the major long-term effects of cigarette smoking is a reduction in mucociliary transport. This contributes to recurrent infection and in the larger airways it prolongs contact with carcinogens.

Congenital defects in mucociliary transport occur. In the 'immotile cilia' syndrome there is an absence of the dynein arms in the cilia themselves, and in cystic fibrosis an abnormal mucus is associated with ciliary dyskinesia. Both diseases are characterized by recurrent infections and eventually with the development of bronchiectasis.

Humoral and cellular mechanisms

Non-specific soluble factors

- *Alpha-1-antitrypsin* is present in lung secretions. It inhibits chymotrypsin and trypsin and neutralizes proteases and elastase.
- *Lysozyme* is an enzyme found in granulocytes that has bacteriocidal properties.
- *Lactoferrin* is synthesized from epithelial cells and neutrophil granulocytes and has bacteriocidal properties.
- *Interferon* (see p. 137) is produced by most cells in response to viral infection. It is a potent suppressor of lymphocyte function and lowers the threshold for mast cell histamine release. It

renders other cells resistant to infection by any other virus.
- *Complement* is present in secretions. In association with antibodies, it plays an important cytotoxic role.

Alveolar macrophages
These are derived from precursors in the bone marrow and migrate to the lungs via the bloodstream. They phagocytose particles, including bacteria, and are removed by the mucociliary escalator, lymphatics and bloodstream. They are the dominant cell in the airways and comprise 90% of all cells obtained by bronchoalveolar lavage.

Macrophages (see p. 128) process antigens and play a part in both cellular and humoral immunity.

Lymphoid tissue (see p. 125)
The bronchus-associated lymphoid tissue consists of lymphocytes present either in aggregates (tonsils and adenoids) or scattered. It forms an important immunological defence mechanism. Lymphocytes become sensitized to antigens, resulting in local production of secretory IgA. IgG and IgE are also present in secretions derived from B lymphocytes in the lamina propria.

Respiratory symptoms

Runny, blocked nose and sneezing

Nasal symptoms are extremely common. The differentiation between the common cold or allergic rhinitis as a cause of 'runny nose' (rhinorrhoea), nasal blockage and attacks of sneezing is difficult. In allergic rhinitis, symptoms may be seasonal, following contact with grass pollen, or perennial, when the house-dust mite is the important allergen. Colds are frequent during the winter but, if more than three occur, the patient is probably suffering from perennial rhinitis rather than from infection due to a virus. Patients may be able to identify the cause of their symptoms if, for example, they sneeze whilst walking in the park in summer or after making beds.

Nasal secretions are usually thin and runny in rhinitis but thicker and yellow-green in the common cold. Nose bleeds and blood-stained nasal discharge are common occurrences and are not as serious as haemoptysis. Nevertheless, a blood-stained nasal discharge associated with nasal obstruction and pain may be the presenting feature of a nasal tumour. Total nasal blockage with loss of smell is often a feature of nasal polyps.

Cough

Cough is the commonest manifestation of lower respiratory tract disease. Smokers often have a morning cough with little sputum. Cough is the cardinal feature of chronic bronchitis, while sputum production and coughing, particularly at night, can be symptoms of asthma. Cough also occurs in asthmatics after mild exertion or following a forced expiration. A cough can also occur for psychological reasons.

A worsening cough is the commonest presenting symptom of a bronchial carcinoma and should not be overlooked. The explosive character of a normal cough is lost when laryngeal paralysis is present—a bovine cough—usually resulting from carcinoma of the bronchus infiltrating the left recurrent laryngeal nerve. Cough may be accompanied by stridor in whooping cough and in the presence of laryngeal or tracheal obstruction.

Despite the popularity of cough mixtures, the correct treatment of this symptom is to identify and treat the underlying cause. Cough may persist in some individuals for many weeks following a respiratory tract infection, perhaps as the result of persisting bronchial inflammation and increased airway responsiveness, a process that may settle with inhaled corticosteroid treatment.

Sputum

Approximately 100 ml of mucus is produced daily in a healthy, non-smoking individual. This flows at a regular pace up the airways, through the larynx, and is swallowed. Excess mucus is expectorated as sputum. The commonest cause of excess mucus production is cigarette smoking.

Mucoid sputum is clear and white but can contain black specks resulting from the inhalation of carbon. Yellow or green sputum is due to the presence of cellular material, including bronchial epithelial cells, or neutrophil or eosinophil granulocytes. Yellow sputum is not necessarily due to infection, as eosinophils in the sputum, as seen in asthma, can give the same appearance. The production of large quantities of yellow or green sputum is characteristic of bronchiectasis.

Blood-stained sputum (haemoptysis) varies from small streaks of blood to massive bleeding. It requires thorough investigation. The following should be borne in mind.

- The commonest cause of haemoptysis is acute infection but it should not be attributed to this without investigation.
- Other common causes are pulmonary infarction, bronchial carcinoma and tuberculosis.
- In lobar pneumonia, the sputum is rusty in appearance when blood is present.
- Pink, frothy sputum is seen in pulmonary oedema.
- In bronchiectasis, the blood is often mixed with purulent sputum.
- Large haemoptyses are usually due to bronchiectasis or tuberculosis.
- Uncommon causes of haemoptyses are idiopathic pulmonary haemosiderosis, Goodpasture's syndrome, trauma, blood disorders and benign tumours.

Haemoptysis should always be investigated. Often, the diagnosis can be made from a chest X-ray.

Firm plugs of sputum may be coughed up by patients suffering from an exacerbation of allergic bronchopulmonary aspergillosis; sometimes such sputum may appear as firm threads representing casts from inflamed bronchi.

Breathlessness

Breathlessness should be assessed in relation to the patient's life-style. For example, a moderate degree of breathlessness may be totally disabling if the patient has to climb many flights of stairs to reach home. A grading for breathlessness is given on p. 515.

The term *dyspnoea* should be used to describe a sense of awareness of increased respiratory effort that is unpleasant and that is recognized by the patient as being inappropriate. It is highly unlikely that a patient will use this term himself. Patients may complain of tightness in the chest; this must be differentiated from angina.

Orthopnoea (see p. 516) is breathlessness on lying down and is partly due to the weight of the abdominal contents pushing the diaphragm further into the thorax. Such patients are also made uncomfortable by bending over.

The terms *tachypnoea* and *hyperpnoea* refer, respectively, to an increased rate of breathing and an increased level of ventilation, which may be appropriate to the situation (e.g. during exercise). *Hyperventilation* is overbreathing and results in a lowering of the alveolar and arterial $P\text{CO}_2$.

Paroxysmal nocturnal dyspnoea is described on p. 516.

Respiratory diseases can cause breathlessness within minutes or hours or else more slowly over days, weeks or months. The typical causes of breathlessness over differing time periods are:

- *Sudden*
  Inhaled foreign body
  Pneumothorax
  Pulmonary embolism
- *Over a few hours*
  Asthma
  Pneumonia
  Pulmonary oedema
  Extrinsic allergic alveolitis
- *Intermittent*

Table 12.1 Physical signs of respiratory disease.

Pathological process	Chest wall movement	Mediastinal displacement	Percussion note	Breath sounds	Vocal resonance	Added sounds
Consolidation (i.e. lobar pneumonia)	Reduced on affected side	None	Dull	Bronchial	Increased	Fine crackles
Collapse						
Major bronchus	Reduced on affected side	Towards lesion	Dull	Diminished or absent	Reduced or absent	None
Peripheral bronchus	Reduced on affected side	Towards lesion	Dull	Bronchial	Increased	Coarse crackles
Fibrosis						
Localized	Reduced on affected side	Towards lesion	Dull	Bronchial	Increased	Coarse crackles
Generalized (e.g. cryptogenic fibrosing alveolitis)	Reduced on both sides	None	Normal	Vesicular	Increased	Coarse crackles
Pleural effusion (> 500 ml)	Reduced on affected side	Away from lesion (in massive effusion)	Stony dull	Vesicular reduced or absent	Reduced or absent	None
Large pneumothorax	Reduced on affected side	Away from lesion	Normal or hyperresonant	Reduced or absent	Reduced or absent	None
Asthma	Reduced on both sides	None	Normal	Vesicular Prolonged expiration	Normal	Expiratory polyphonic wheeze
Chronic bronchitis and emphysema	Reduced on both sides	None	Normal	Vesicular Prolonged expiration	Normal	Expiratory polyphonic wheeze and coarse crackles

Asthma
Pulmonary oedema
● *Over days*
Pleural effusions
Carcinoma of the bronchus/trachea
● *Over months or years*
Chronic bronchitis and emphysema
Cryptogenic fibrosing alveolitis
Occupational fibrotic lung disease
Non-respiratory causes—anaemia, hyperthyroidism

Wheezing

Wheezing is a common complaint and can be the result of airflow limitation due to any cause. The symptom of wheezing is *not* diagnostic of asthma; it may be absent in the early stages of this disease, and may also occur in patients with chronic bronchitis and emphysema.

Chest pain

The commonest type of chest pain encountered in respiratory disease is a localized sharp pain, often referred to as pleuritic. It is made worse by deep breathing or coughing and can be precisely localized by the patient. Localized anterior chest pain may be accompanied by tenderness of a costochondrial junction due to costochondritis. Pain in the shoulder tips suggests irritation of the diaphragmatic pleura, whereas central chest pain radiating to the neck and arms is typically of cardiac origin. Retrosternal soreness may occur in patients with tracheitis, and a constant, severe, dull pain may be the result of invasion of the thoracic wall by carcinoma.

Examination of the respiratory system

The nose

The anterior part of the nose can be examined using a nasal speculum and light source. In allergic rhinitis the mucosa lining the nasal septum and inferior turbinate appears swollen and a dark red or plum colour. Nasal polyps can also be identified, as can a frequent site of nasal haemorrhage (Little's area).

The chest (Table 12.1)

Radiology has become an essential part of examination of the chest. Diseases such as tuberculosis or lung cancer may not be detectable on clinical examination but are obvious on the chest X-ray. Conversely, the abnormal physical signs in asthma or chronic bronchitis may be associated with a normal chest X-ray.

Inspection

The patient should be observed carefully, paying particularly attention to mental alertness, cyanosis, breathlessness at rest, use of accessory muscles and any deformity or scars on the chest. A coarse tremor or flap of the outstretched hands indicates CO_2 intoxication. Prominent veins on the chest may imply obstruction of the superior vena cava. The jugular venous pressure should be assessed.

Central cyanosis (see p. 518) is assessed on the colour of the tongue and lips, and indicates a P_aO_2 below 6 kPa. Peripheral cyanosis is noted on the fingernails and skin of the extremities and in the absence of central cyanosis is due to a reduced peripheral circulation.

Finger clubbing is present when the normal angle between the base of the nail and the nail fold is lost. The base of the nail is fluctuant owing to increased vascularity, and there is an increased curvature of the nail in all directions, with expansion of the end of the digit. Some causes of clubbing are given in Table 12.2. Clubbing is not seen in chronic bronchitis.

Table 12.2 Some causes of finger clubbing.

Respiratory
Bronchial carcinoma, especially epidermoid
  (squamous cell) type—major cause
Chronic suppurative lung disease
  Bronchiectasis
  Lung abscess
  Empyema
Pulmonary fibrosis (e.g. cryptogenic fibrosing
  alveolitis)
Pleural and mediastinal tumours (e.g.
  mesothelioma)

Cardiovascular
Cyanotic heart disease
Subacute infective endocarditis

Miscellaneous
Congenital—no disease
Cirrhosis
Inflammatory bowel disease

Palpation

The position of the mediastinum should be ascertained by checking whether the trachea is central and whether the cardiac apex is in the fifth intercostal space. The supraclavicular fossa is examined for enlarged lymph nodes. The distance between the sternal notch and the cricoid cartilage (three to four finger breadths in full expiration) is reduced in patients with severe airflow limitation. Movement of the upper and lower parts of the chest should be assessed. Compression of the chest laterally and anteroposteriorly may produce a localized pain suggestive of a rib fracture.

Percussion

This should be performed symmetrically on both sides for comparison. Liver dullness is usually detected anteriorly at the level of the sixth rib. Liver and cardiac dullness are lost with over-inflated lungs. The percussion note is dull over consolidation and stony dull over a pleural effusion.

Auscultation

The diaphragm of the stethoscope should be used. The patient is asked to take deep breaths through the mouth. Inspiration sounds more prolonged than expiration. Healthy lungs filter off most of the high-frequency component, mainly due to turbulent flow in the larynx. Normal breath sounds are harsher anteriorly over the upper lobes (particularly on the right) and described as vesicular. Vesicular sounds may be loud in a thin healthy subject or soft in patients with emphysema. Breath sounds are reduced or absent in a pneumothorax, over a pleural effusion or when the bronchus to a lobe is obstructed by a carcinoma.

Bronchial breathing. These abnormal breath sounds are heard best over consolidated or collapsed lung and sometimes over areas of localized fibrosis or bronchiectasis. Such areas conduct the high-frequency hissing component of breath sounds well. Characteristically, the noise heard during inspiration and expiration is equally long but separated by a short silent phase. Bronchial breathing can be imitated by listening over the larynx, particularly if the subject breathes with the vocal cords in a position to sound a whispered 'eee'.

Whispering pectoriloquy (whispered, and therefore higher-pitched, sounds heards distinctly) invariably accompanies bronchial breathing.

Added sounds. Many terms are still used to describe additional sounds heard over the lung fields. The terms rhonchi, rales and crepitations are best discarded and replaced with the simple terms wheezes and crackles.

Wheeze is usually heard during expiration and

results from vibrations in the collapsible part of the airways when apposition occurs as a result of the flow-limiting mechanisms. Wheezes are heard in asthma and in chronic bronchitis and emphysema, but are not invariably present. In the most severe cases of asthma a wheeze may not be heard, as the air-flow may be insufficient to generate the sound. Wheezes may be monophonic (single large airway obstruction) or polyphonic (narrowing of many small airways).

Crackles. These brief crackling sounds are probably produced by opening of previously closed bronchioles, and their timing during breathing is of significance—early inspiratory crackles are associated with diffuse airflow limitation, whereas late inspiratory crackles are characteristically heard in pulmonary oedema, fibrosis of the lung and bronchiectasis. They may be described as fine or coarse but this is of no significance.

Pleural rub. This is a creaking or groaning sound that is usually well-localized. It is indicative of inflammation and roughening of the pleural surfaces, which normally glide silently over one another.

Vocal resonance and fremitus. Healthy lung attenuates high-frequency notes, leaving the booming low-pitched components of speech. Consolidated lung has the reverse effect, transmitting the high frequencies; the spoken word then takes on a bleating quality. Whispered speech can barely be heard over healthy lung, whereas consolidation allows its clear transmission. Sonorous sounds such as 'ninety-nine' are well transmitted across healthy lung to produce vibration that can be felt over the chest wall. Consolidated lung transmits these low-frequency noises less well, and pleural fluid severely dampens or obliterates the vibrations altogether.

Additional bedside tests

Since so many patients with respiratory disease have airflow limitation, air flow should be routinely measured at the bedside using a peak flow meter. This will provide a much more accurate assessment than any physical sign.

If signs and chest X-ray suggest pleural fluid, this can readily be confirmed by aspiration using a fine needle and a 20 ml syringe. The nature of the pleural fluid can be assessed (blood-stained, purulent or clear) and specimens should be sent immediately for bacterial culture and cytological examination for malignant cells (see below).

Investigation of respiratory disease

Routine haematological and biochemical tests

These should include tests for:

- Haemoglobin, to detect the presence of anaemia
- PCV (secondary polycythaemia occurs with chronic bronchitis and emphysema)
- Routine biochemistry

Other blood investigations sometimes required include α-1-antitrypsin levels, autoantibodies, and, in asthma, IgE to specific allergens (RAST; see p. 146) and *Aspergillus* antibodies.

Sputum

Sputum should be inspected for:

- *Colour*
  Yellow-green indicates inflammation (infection or allergy)
  Presence of blood suggests neoplasm or pulmonary infarct

Microbiological studies (Gram stain and culture) are not helpful in upper respiratory tract infections or in acute or chronic bronchitis. They are of value in:

- Pneumonia
- Diagnosis of tuberculosis (Ziehl–Nielsen stain)
- Unusual clinical problems
- *Aspergillus* lung disease

Cytology

This is extremely useful in the diagnosis of bronchial carcinoma. Advantages are:

- Quick result
- Cheap
- Non-invasive

However, its value depends on the presence of a reliable cytologist.

Transtracheal aspiration
This technique involves pushing a needle through the cricothyroid membrane, through which a catheter is threaded to a position just above the carina. This procedure induces coughing, and specimens are collected by aspiration or by the introduction and subsequent aspiration of sterile saline. It is an excellent technique (although not often required) for assessing infection in the lower respiratory tract because it obviates any possibility of contamination of the specimen with bacteria from the pharynx and mouth.

Table 12.3 Causes of collapse of the lung.

Tumours

Enlarged tracheobronchial lymph nodes due to:
 Malignant disease
 Tuberculosis

Inhaled foreign bodies (e.g. peanuts) in children,
 usually in the right main bronchus

Bronchial casts or plugs (e.g. allergic
 bronchopulmonry aspergillosis)

Retained secretions—postoperatively and in
 debilitated patients

Chest X-ray

The following must be taken into account when
viewing films:

- Centring of the film. The distance between each
  clavicular head and the spinal processes must be
  equal.
- Penetration.
- The view. Postero-anterior (PA) is the routine
  film. Antero-posterior (AP) films are only taken
  in very ill patients who are unable to stand up or
  be taken to the radiology department; the
  cardiac outline appears bigger and the scapulae
  cannot be moved out of the way.

The following should be noted:

- The shape and body structure of the chest wall
- Whether the trachea is central
- Whether the diaphragm is elevated or flat
- The shape, size and position of the heart
- The shape and size of the hilar shadows
- The vascular shadowing and the size and shape
  of any abnormalities of the lungs

X-ray abnormalities
Collapse and consolidation. The X-ray changes in
collapse of a whole lung are illustrated in Fig.
12.11. In collapse of the middle lobe, all that may
be detected is a loss of the clear outline of the right
atrium, which distinguishes it from collapse of the
right lower lobe. In consolidation, the segments or
lobes of the lung are opaque but the bronchi are
patent, producing an air bronchogram. Causes of
collapse are shown in Table 12.3.

Pleural effusion. Pleural effusions need to be more
than 500 ml to cause much more than blunting of
the costophrenic angle. On an erect film they
produce a characteristic shadow with a curved
upper edge rising into the axilla. If very large, the
whole of one side of the thorax may be opaque,
with shift of the mediastinum to the opposite side.

Fibrosis. Localized fibrosis causes streaky shadow-

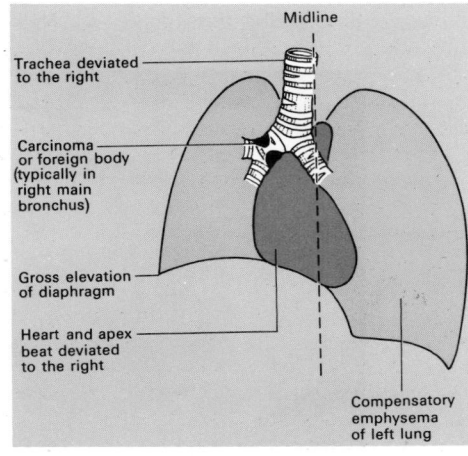

Fig. 12.11 Collapse of the right lung, showing a raised
right diaphragm and compensatory emphysema of the
left lung.

ing and the accompanying loss of lung volume
causes mediastinal structures to move to the same
side. More generalized fibrosis in the lung can lead
to a honeycomb appearance (see p. 690), seen as
diffuse shadows containing multiple circular trans-
lucences a few millimetres in diameter.

Round shadows. The causes of round shadows are
shown in Table 12.4.

Table 12.4 Causes of round shadows in the lung.

Carcinoma

Metastatic tumours (usually multiple shadows)

Tuberculoma (may be calcification within the lesion)

Lung abscess (usually with fluid level)

Encysted interlobar effusion (usually in horizontal
 fissure)

Hydatid cysts (rare and often with a fluid level)

Arteriovenous malformations (usually adjacent to a
 vascular shadow)

Aspergilloma

Rheumatoid nodules

Rare causes
 Bronchial carcinoid
 Cylindroma
 Chondroma
 Lipoma

Other shadows related to mediastinum
 Pericardium ⎫
 Oesophagus ⎬ Seen on lateral chest X-ray
 Spinal cord ⎭

(a)

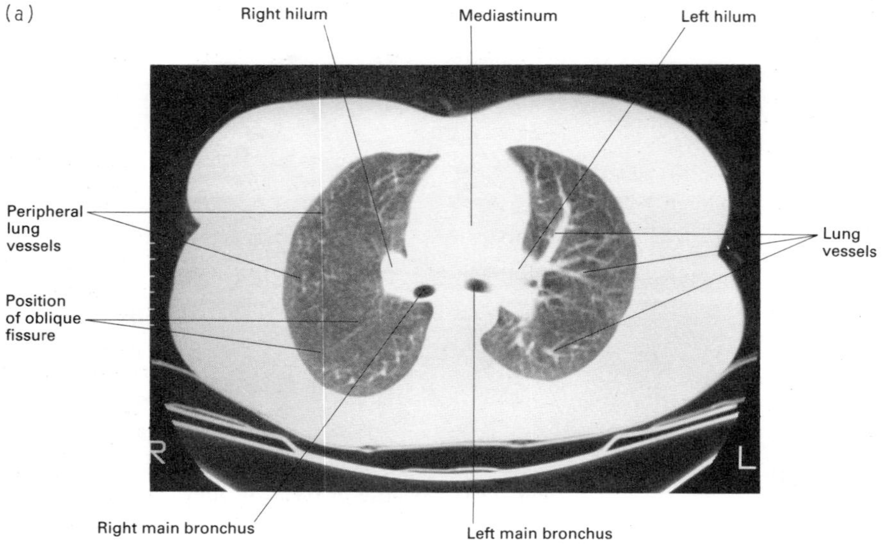

Right hilum

Mediastinum

Left hilum

Peripheral lung vessels

Position of oblique fissure

Lung vessels

R

L

Right main bronchus

Left main bronchus

(b)

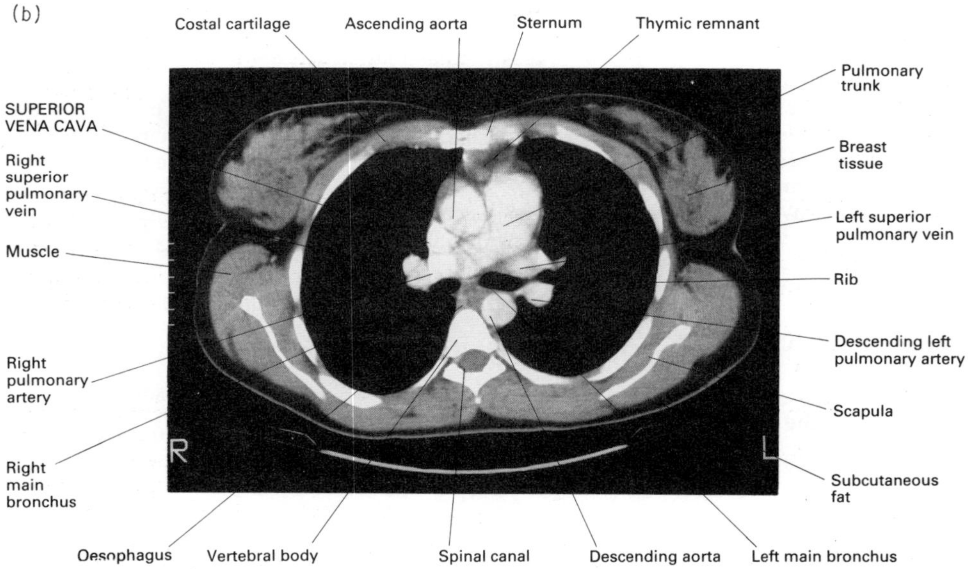

Costal cartilage

Ascending aorta

Sternum

Thymic remnant

Pulmonary trunk

SUPERIOR VENA CAVA

Right superior pulmonary vein

Breast tissue

Left superior pulmonary vein

Muscle

Rib

Descending left pulmonary artery

Right pulmonary artery

Scapula

Right main bronchus

R

L

Subcutaneous fat

Oesophagus

Vertebral body

Spinal canal

Descending aorta

Left main bronchus

(c)

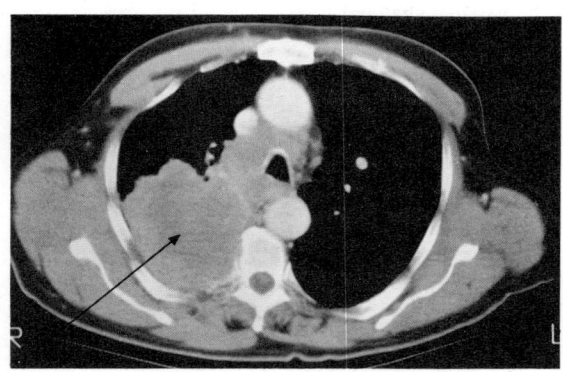

R

L

Fig. 12.12 CT scan of the lung. (a) Bone setting—showing normal mediastinal structures. (b) Soft-tissue setting—showing normal lung markings. (c) Scan showing a central carcinoma of the bronchus and enlarged lymph nodes.

Miliary mottling. This term describes numerous minute opacities, 1–3 mm in size, which are caused by many pathological processes. The commoner causes are miliary tuberculosis, pneumoconiosis, sarcoidosis, fibrosing alveolitis and pulmonary oedema, though the latter is usually perihilar and accompanied by larger, fluffy shadows. A rare but striking cause of miliary mottling is pulmonary microlithiasis.

Computed tomography

This technique is carried out by the rotation of an X-ray tube around the patient in a series of complete circles. The signals are detected by an array of scintillation crystals and are processed quantitatively by a computer to produce a two-dimensional image of high resolution for each axial scan or cut. CT gives a numerical indication of the relative densities of particular tissues, but only fat is different enough to be reliably diagnosed. Normal lung is of sufficiently low density (90% air, 10% soft tissue) to allow the trachea and main bronchus to show up on cuts, particularly when the latter are running at right angles or at the same plane rather than in an oblique direction. This is also true for the large pulmonary vessels and for other mediastinal structures to the extent that CT is the radiographic procedure of choice for investigating the mediastinum.

CT gives a much clearer indication of the extent of respiratory disease and is of particular value in:

- Assessing intrathoracic spread of carcinoma of the bronchus particularly into the mediastinal structures and bone
- Detecting pulmonary involvement in diseases such as sarcoid and lymphoma, not seen on chest radiographs
- Detecting pulmonary lesions in individuals exposed to industrial dust

CT is useful in staging of carcinoma of the bronchus and CT scanning should be extended to include the liver and adrenal glands. Although CT will identify enlarged mediastinal lymph nodes, it cannot reveal the aetiology. Histology needs to be obtained following mediastinoscopy and biopsy. Nevertheless, the absence of any lymph node enlargement on CT scanning is a useful indication favouring operability.

Magnetic resonance imaging (MRI)

This is being used particularly in bronchial carcinoma. It has no advantage over CT in most cases, but some mediastinal lymph node enlargement near major vessels is best detected by MRI. Pericardial involvement and secondaries are also detected clearly by MRI.

Radioisotope lung scanning

This technique has been widely used for the detection of pulmonary emboli.

Perfusion scan
Macro-aggregated human albumin labelled with technetium-99m is injected intravenously. The particles are of such a size that they impact in pulmonary capillaries, where they remain for a few hours. A gamma camera is then used to detect the position of the macro-aggregated human albumin. The resultant pattern indicates the distribution of pulmonary blood flow; cold areas occur where there is defective blood flow (e.g. in pulmonary emboli).

Disadvantages. Areas of lung with diminished perfusion caused by pulmonary emboli cannot be distinguished from those in which pulmonary blood flow has been closed down by poor ventilation of the adjacent lung. For example, mild asthma can cause a patchy appearance. (N.B. Peak flow should always be measured before a scan.)

In addition, in patients with an obvious radiological abnormality, a scan cannot differentiate pulmonary embolism from other causes of defective perfusion.

Value. Radioisotope scanning is particularly of value in patients whose chest X-ray is normal and in whom pulmonary embolism is suspected. Multiple cold areas on the scan with only a single abnormality on the X-ray support the diagnosis of pulmonary embolism.

Ventilation–perfusion scan
Xenon-133 gas is inhaled into the lung and its distribution is detected at the same time as a perfusion scan is carried out. Using the two scans, a pulmonary embolus causes a striking diminution of perfusion relative to ventilation. Other lung diseases (e.g. asthma or pneumonia) impair both ventilation and perfusion. Unfortunately, however, a pulmonary embolus often produces substantial changes in the lung substance (e.g. atelectasis) so that such a clear distinction is not always obvious. Nevertheless, this is a better technique than perfusion scan alone.

Disadvantages. Xenon-133 has only a short half-life and most laboratories do not have the necessary equipment for its measurement.

Respiratory function tests

In practice, airflow limitation can be assessed by use of relatively simple tests that have good intrasubject repeatability. Normal values are required for their interpretation since these tests vary

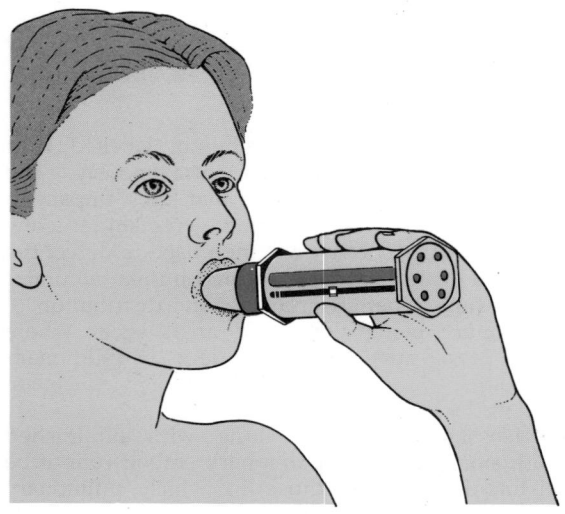

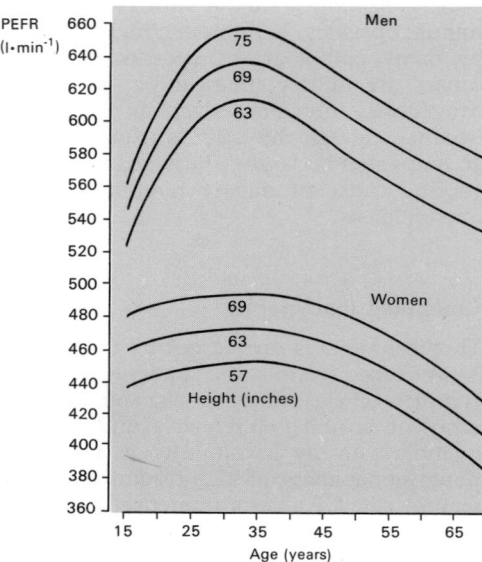

Fig. 12.13 Peak flow measurements. (a) Peak flow meter. The lips should be tight around the mouthpiece. (b) Graph of normal readings for men and women.

considerably, not only with sex, age and height, but also within individuals of the same age, sex and height. The standard deviation about the mean for a group of individuals is therefore very high; for example, the standard deviation for the peak expiratory flow rate is approximately $50 \text{ L} \cdot \text{min}^{-1}$ and for the forced expiratory volume in 1 s (FEV$_1$) it is approximately 0.4 L. Repeated measurements of lung function are required for assessing the progression of disease in an individual patient.

Tests of ventilatory function
These tests are mainly used to assess the degree of airflow limitation present during expiration.

Peak expiratory flow rate (PEFR). This is an extremely simple and cheap test. Subjects are asked to take a full inspiration to total lung capacity and then blow out forcefully into the mini-Wright peak flow meter (shown in Fig. 12.13), which is held horizontally; the lips must be placed tightly around the mouthpiece. The best of three tests is recorded.

This peak flow meter records the maximum expiratory flow rate within the first 2 ms of expiration. It is a reasonable measure of airflow limitation and the intrasubject repeatability is good. Regular measurements of peak flow rates on waking, during the afternoon, and before bed demonstrate the wide diurnal variations in airflow limitation that characterize asthma and allow an objective assessment of treatment to be made (see Fig. 12.14).

Spirometry. The Vitalograph spirometer measures the forced expiratory volume in 1 s (FEV$_1$) and the forced vital capacity (FVC). Both the FEV$_1$ and FVC

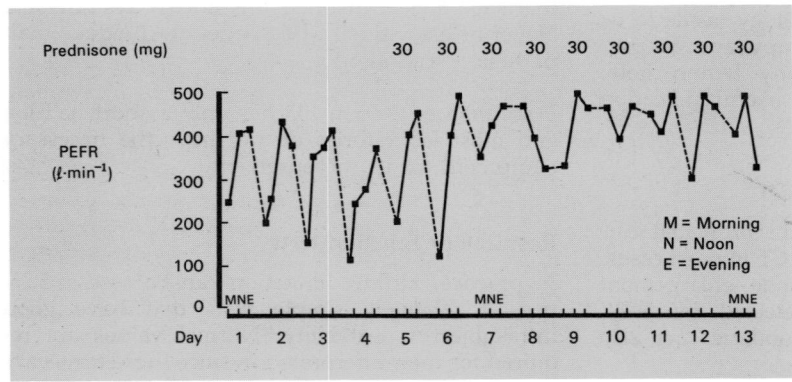

Fig. 12.14 Diurnal variability in airflow limitation, showing the effect of steroids.

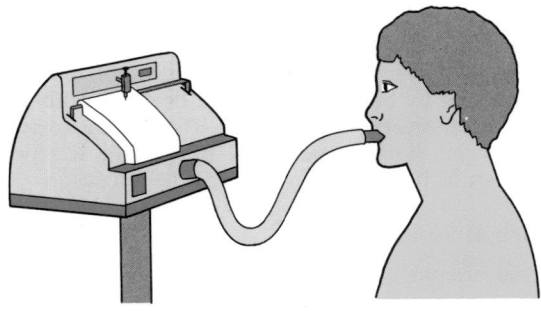

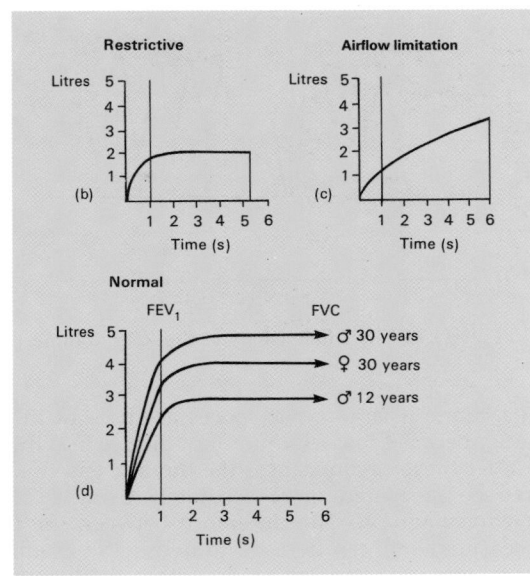

Fig. 12.15 Spirometry. (a) Diagram of a patient using a spirometer. (b) Graph showing restrictive pattern (FEV$_1$ and FVC reduced). (c) Graph showing airflow limitation (FEV$_1$ only reduced). (d) Graph showing normal patterns for age and sex.

are related to height, age and sex. The instrument used is shown in Fig. 12.15a. The technique involves a maximum inspiration followed by a forced expiration (for as long as possible) into the dry bellows spirometer. The act of expiration triggers the moving record chart, which measures volume against time. The record chart moves for a total of 5 s, but expiration should continue until all the air has been expelled from the lungs, as patients with severe airflow limitation may have a very prolonged forced expiratory time. This is demonstrated on the record chart in Fig. 12.15.

The FEV$_1$ expressed as a percentage of the FVC is an excellent measure of airflow limitation. In normal subjects it is around 75%. With increasing *airflow limitation* the FEV$_1$ falls proportionately more than the FVC, so that the FEV$_1$/FVC is reduced. With *restrictive lung disease* the FEV$_1$ and the FVC are reduced in the same proportion and the FEV$_1$/FVC remains normal or may even increase because of the enhanced elastic recoil.

It is important to realize that in chronic airflow limitation (particularly in emphysema and asthma) the total lung capacity is usually increased, yet there is nearly always some reduction in the FVC. This is the result of disease in the small airways causing obstruction to air flow before the normal residual volume is reached. This trapping of air within the lung (giving an increased residual volume) is a characteristic feature of these diseases.

Other tests. Tests such as the measurement of airways resistance in a body plethysmograph are more sensitive but the equipment is expensive and the necessary manoeuvres are too exhausting for many patients with chronic airflow limitation.

Flow volume loops. The ability to measure flow rates against volume (flow volume loops; see Fig. 12.8) enables a more sensitive analysis to be made of the site of airflow limitation within the lung. At the start of expiration from total lung capacity, the site of maximum resistance is the large airways, and this accounts for the flow reduction in the first 25% of the curve. As the lung volume reduces further, so the elastic pressures within the lung holding open the smaller airways reduce, and disease either of the lung parenchyma or the small airways themselves becomes readily apparent. For example, in diseases such as chronic bronchitis and emphysema, where the brunt of the disease falls upon the smaller airways, expiratory flow rates at 50% or 25% of the vital capacity may be disproportionately reduced when compared with flow rates at larger lung volumes.

Lung volume. The subdivisions of the lung volume are shown in Fig. 12.16. Tidal volume and vital capacity can be measured using a simple spirometer, but the total lung capacity (TLC) and the residual volume need to be measured by an alternative technique. TLC is measured by connecting the lungs to a reservoir containing a known amount of non-absorbable gas (helium) that can readily be measured. If the concentration of the gas in the reservoir is known at the start of the test and is measured after equilibration of the gas has occurred (when the patient has breathed in and out of the reservoir), the dilution of the gas will reflect the TLC. This technique is known as *helium dilution.* Residual volume can be calculated by subtracting the vital capacity from the TLC.

The TLC measured using this technique is

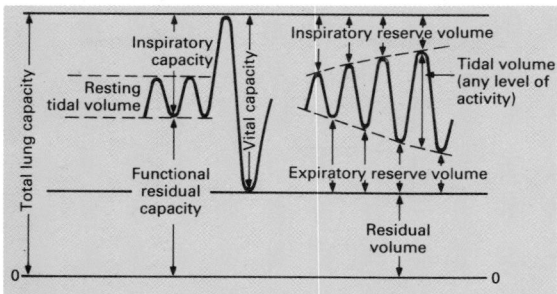

Fig. 12.16 The subdivisions of the lung volume.

inaccurate if large cystic spaces are present in the lung, because the helium cannot diffuse into them. Under these circumstances the thoracic gas volume can be measured more accurately using a body plethysmograph. The difference between the two measurements can be used to define the extent of non-communicating air space within the lungs.

Measurement of blood gases
This technique is described on p. 722.

The measurement of the partial pressure of both oxygen and carbon dioxide within arterial blood is an extremely useful test in diseases of the respiratory and circulatory systems. It is essential in the management of cases of respiratory failure and severe asthma, when repeated measurements are often the best guide to therapy.

Transfer factor. This measures the transfer of gas across the alveolar–capillary membrane and reflects the uptake of oxygen from the alveolus into the red cell. A low concentration of carbon monoxide is inhaled and is avidly taken up in a linear fashion by circulating haemoglobin, the amount of which must be known when the test is performed. In normal lungs the transfer factor is a true measure of the diffusing capacity of the lungs for oxygen and depends on the thickness of the alveolar–capillary membrane. In lung disease the diffusing capacity (D_{CO}) also depends on the $\dot{V}_A/Q$ relationship as well as on the area and thickness of the alveolar membrane. To control for differences in lung volume, the uptake of carbon monoxide is related to the lung volume; this is known as the transfer coefficient (K_{CO}).

Gas transfer is usually reduced in patients with severe degrees of emphysema and fibrosis. Overall gas transfer can be thought of as a relatively non-specific test of lung function but one that can be particularly used in the early detection and assessment of progress of diseases affecting the lung parenchyma (e.g. cryptogenic pulmonary fibrosis, sarcoidosis and asbestos).

Exercise tests

The predominant symptom in respiratory medicine is that of breathlessness. The degree of disability produced by breathlessness can be assessed before and after treatment by asking the patient to walk for 6 min along a measured track. This has been shown to be a reproducible and useful test.

Pleural aspiration

This should always be performed when fluid is present. An ordinary needle attached to a 20 ml syringe is used. The needle is inserted through an intercostal space over an area of dullness. Fluid is withdrawn and the presence of any blood is noted. Samples are sent for protein estimation, cytology and bacteriological examination, including culture and Ziehl–Nielsen stain for tuberculosis. Large amounts of fluid can be aspirated through a large needle to help relieve extreme breathlessness.

Pleural biopsy

Experienced operators obtain tissue in nearly all patients and, provided multiple specimens are taken, positive results may be expected in up to 80% of cases of tuberculosis and in 60% of cases of malignancy. The technique is illustrated in Fig. 12.17.

Mediastinoscopy and scalene node biopsy

This technique, which is seldom necessary, involves inspection of the mediastinal structures using a mediastinoscope inserted by blunt dissection downwards from behind the proximal end of the clavicle. Subsequent biopsy of tissue may be performed.

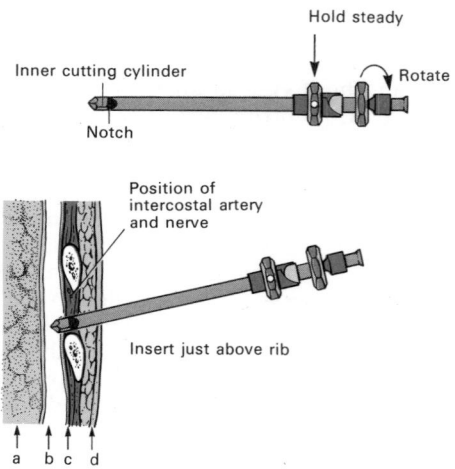

Fig. 12.17 Technique of pleural biopsy. The biopsy needle is shown penetrating the chest wall. a = lung parenchyma; b = pleural space; c = muscle; d = skin and subcutaneous tissue.

Pleural biopsy

- Pleural biopsy is usually performed at the end of the aspiration of fluid.
- A small skin incision is made, as the end of the Abrams' pleural biopsy needle is fairly blunt.
- Once in place through the pleura, the back part of the needle is rotated to open the notch; this is kept pointing forward.
- With lateral pressure the needle is withdrawn so that the notch will snag against the pleura.
- The needle is held firmly and the hexagonal grip is twisted clockwise to cut the biopsy. To avoid damage to the intercostal vessel or nerve, the notch should never be directed upwards when the biopsy is taken.
- Several biopsies should be taken at different angles by repeated insertion of the needle.
- Specimens should be put in sterile saline for culture for tuberculosis and into 10% formol saline for histological examination.

Fibreoptic bronchoscopy

The introduction of this technique has transformed the investigation of pulmonary disease. Central bronchial lesions can be biopsied readily. Washings can be taken from lobes containing more peripheral lesions for cytological examination for malignant cells, and appropriate staining and culture for bacteria including *Mycobacterium* and *Pneumocystis carinii*.

Diffuse parenchymal lung disease can be investigated using transbronchial biopsy. The biopsy forceps are pushed as far as possible to the periphery of the lung, the patient is asked to breathe in, and the jaws of the forceps are closed, removing a small piece of peripheral airway and surrounding lung parenchyma. Biplanar screening allows isolated peripheral lesions to be biopsied in the same way. A histological diagnosis can be made in 95% of central lung cancers but in only 50–75% of peripheral lesions biopsied during fibreoptic bronchoscopy.

Peripheral lesions are best biopsied percutaneously using a fine needle under direct X-ray or CT control.

Broncho-alveolar lavage

This technique can be used both in patients who have disease confined to one lobe and in those with more diffuse lung disease. The tip of the fibreoptic bronchoscope is lodged in the segmental orifice and 20 ml of 0.9% sterile saline is squirted down the suction port of the bronchoscope and immediately aspirated. This is repeated five times; about 40–60% of the total volume is recovered. Fluid is strained through two layers of surgical gauze and the volume is noted. The cells are then

Fibreoptic bronchoscopy

This enables the direct visualization of the bronchial tree as far as the subsegmental bronchi under a local anaesthetic.

Indications

- Lesions requiring biopsy seen on chest X-ray
- Haemoptysis
- Stridor
- Positive sputum cytology for malignant cells with no chest X-ray abnormality
- Collection of bronchial secretions for bacteriology, especially tuberculosis
- Recurrent laryngeal nerve paralysis of unknown aetiology
- Infiltrative lung disease (to obtain a transbronchial biopsy)
- Investigation of collapsed lobes or segments and aspiration of mucus plugs

Procedure

- The patient is starved overnight.
- Atropine 0.6 mg i.m. is given 30 min before the procedure.
- Topical anaesthesia (xylocaine 4% spray) is applied to the nose, nasopharynx and pharynx.
- Intravenous sedation (e.g. diazepam 10 mg) may be needed.
- The bronchoscope is passed through the nose, nasopharynx and pharynx under direct vision to minimize trauma.
- Xylocaine (2 ml of 4%) is dropped through the instrument onto the vocal cords.
- The bronchoscope is passed through the cords into the trachea.
- All segmental and subsegmental orifices should be identified.
- Biopsies and brushings should be taken of macroscopic abnormalities or occasionally from peripheral lesions under radiographic control.

spun down and resuspended at a concentration of 1×10^7 cells per millilitre for differential counting. The changes seen in different diseases of the lung are shown in Table 12.5. Since there is a considerable overlap in the distribution of cells seen in broncho-alveolar wash specimens in different diseases, this technique has no value in diagnosis. However, it can be used to monitor progression of disease, since improvement is characterized by a reduction in the number of cells and a return towards the normal proportions of different cell types.

Skin-prick tests (Fig. 12.18)

The tip of a fine needle is placed through a drop of allergen solution on the volar surface of the forearm into the epidermis, which is gently pricked with an upward lifting motion. A separate needle

Table 12.5 Broncho-alveolar lavage—changes in cell numbers and proportions in different diseases.

Disease	Number of cells (× 10⁶/ml)	Alveolar macrophages	Per cent Lymphocytes T	B	Null	Neutrophils	Granulocytes Eosinophils	Mast cells/basophils
None	14	90	5	1	2	< 1	< 1	< 1
Smokers	→	→	→	→	→	↑	→	→
Sarcoidosis	↑ ↑	↓ ↓	↑ ↑	↑	↑	→	→	→
Cryptogenic fibrosing alveolitis	↑ ↑	↓	→	→	→	↑ ↑	→	→
Extrinsic allergic bronchiolar alveolitis	↑ ↑	↓	↑	→	→	↑	↑	→

→ = no change from normal; ↑ = increased from normal; ↑ ↑ = greatly increased from normal; ↓ = decreased from normal; ↓ ↓ = greatly decreased from normal

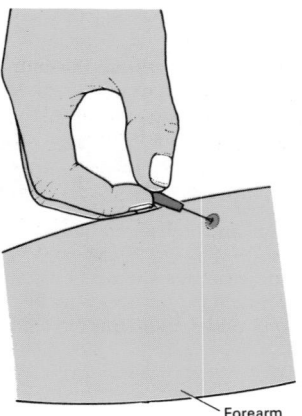

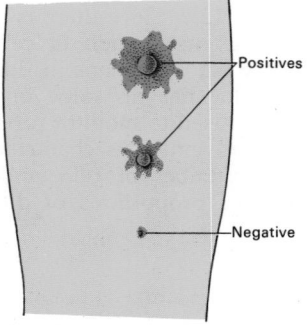

Fig. 12.18 The technique of skin-prick testing with allergen solutions, showing positive reactions with induration and surrounding erythema.

should be used for each allergen. Alternatively, a sterile allergen-coated lancet can be used in a similar way. A separate coated lancet is used for each allergen and has the advantage of speed and better preservation of the allergen and avoids contamination of test solutions over time. If the patient is sensitive to the allergen, a weal develops and the diameter of the induration (not the erythema) should be measured after 15 min. A weal of at least 2 mm diameter and greater than the reaction to the control solution is a positive test.

Skin tests can be inhibited by concurrent administration of antihistamines, so these should be stopped 48 h before testing. They are not inhibited by bronchodilators or corticosteroids.

With most allergens there is a good correlation between the diameter of the weal and levels of specific IgE antibody in the serum. The results should be interpreted in the light of the history (see p. 664).

A *late reaction* is the development of a larger, 1–5 cm, oedematous skin reaction 2–3 h after pricking. This occurs with allergens from *Aspergillus fumigatus*, but also follows large, immediate skin reactions induced by allergens from other common inhalant allergens.

Smoking

Epidemiology

General household surveys in the UK have shown a continuing decline in the prevalence of cigarette smoking in men but not women. In 1987, 44% of men and 34% of women aged 16 and over smoked tobacco in some form. Manufactured cigarettes were smoked by an equal proportion of both sexes (34%). Cigarette smoking is now commonest between the ages of 16 and 24 years (42% in both sexes). At the age of 15 more girls (27%) than boys (18%) smoke cigarettes. A greater proportion of professional workers than manual workers have given up smoking. In the USA the proportion of adult males who smoke is now only 36% and in women the prevalence is now 29%.

Dangers

Cigarette smoking is addictive. Smoking nearly always begins in adolescence for psychosocial reasons and, once it is a regular habit, the pharmacological properties of nicotine play an important part in persistence, conferring some advantage to the smoker's mood. Very few cigarette smokers (less than 2%) can limit themselves to occasional or intermittent smoking. The dangers are listed in Table 12.6.

There is a significant dose–response relationship between the smoking of 0–40 cigarettes daily and lung cancer mortality. Sputum production and airflow limitation increase with daily cigarette consumption, and effort tolerance decreases, partly due to high levels of carboxyhaemoglobin in bronchitis patients. Smoking and asbestos exposure are synergystic in producing bronchial carcinoma, increasing the risk in asbestos workers by up to 5–8 times that of non-smokers exposed to asbestos.

Cigarette smokers who change to other forms of tobacco are unlikely to reduce the risk, as they continue to inhale, and some of the highest levels of carboxyhaemoglobin have been found in cigar smokers.

Toxic effects

Cigarette smoke contains polycyclic aromatic hydrocarbons and nitrosamines, which are potent carcinogens and mutagens in animals. It causes release of enzymes from neutrophil granulocytes and macrophages that are capable of destroying elastin and leading to lung damage. Pulmonary epithelial permeability increases even in symptomless cigarette smokers, and correlates with the concentration of carboxyhaemoglobin in blood. This altered permeability possibly allows easier access to carcinogens.

Stopping smoking

If the entire population could be persuaded to stop smoking, the effect on health care in the Western World would be enormous. National campaigns run by central government linked to bans on advertisement and a substantial increase in the cost of cigarettes are the most certain ways of achieving this. Only 15% of general practitioners surveyed in 1982 actually encouraged their patients to give up smoking, yet simple advice and follow-up can motivate some 50% of their patients to stop. In smoking withdrawal clinics, success rates of 80% can be achieved in the first month, though only 15–20% of patients remain abstinent in the long term. Nicotine chewing gum has been advocated but is probably no better than verbal advice. Chest symptoms usually have to be severe to stop patients from smoking.

Table 12.6 The dangers of cigarette smoking.

Lung cancer
Chronic bronchitis and emphysema
Carcinoma of the oesophagus
Ischaemic heart disease
Peripheral vascular disease
Bladder cancer
An increase in abnormal spermatozoa
Memory problems

Maternal smoking
A decrease in birthweight of the infant
An increase in fetal and neonatal mortality

Passive smoking
Risk of pneumonia and bronchitis in infants of
   smoking parents
An increase in cough and breathlessness in smokers
   and non-smokers with chronic bronchitis,
   emphysema and asthma
Increased cancer risk

Diseases of the upper respiratory tract

The common cold (acute coryza)

This highly infectious illness comprises a mild systemic upset and prominent nasal symptoms. It is due to infection by rhinoviruses, the majority of which belong to the picornavirus group and exist in at least 100 different antigenic strains. Infectivity from close personal contact (nasal mucus on hands) or droplets is high in the early stages of the infection, and spread is facilitated by overcrowding and poor ventilation. On average, individuals suffer 2–3 colds per year but the incidence lessens with age, presumably as a result of accumulating immunity to the causative virus strains. The incubation is from 12 h to an upper limit of 5 days.

The clinical features are tiredness, slight pyrexia, malaise and a sore nose and pharynx. Profuse, watery nasal discharge, eventually becoming thick and mucopurulent, persists for up to a week. Sneezing is present in the early stage. Secondary bacterial infection occurs only in a minority.

Sinusitis

Sinusitis is an infection of the paranasal sinuses that often complicates upper respiratory tract infections, e.g. coryza or allergic rhinitis. Acute infections are usually caused by *Streptococcus pneumoniae* and *Haemophilus influenzae*. Symptoms include frontal headache and facial pain and tenderness, usually with nasal discharge, but are often difficult to differentiate from symptoms of the common cold.

Treatment is with antibiotics, e.g. amoxicillin. Rare complications include local and cerebral abscesses. Chronic sinusitis can be a cause of headaches, but often these headaches are due to tension.

Rhinitis

Rhinitis is present if sneezing attacks, nasal discharge or blockage occur for more than an hour on most days for:

● A limited period of the year (seasonal rhinitis)
● Throughout the whole year (perennial rhinitis)

Seasonal rhinitis
This is often called hay fever and is the most common of all allergic diseases. The term hay fever is inappropriate since fever rarely occurs and hay is not the cause. It is better described as seasonal allergic rhinitis. World-wide prevalence rates vary from 2% to 10%. Prevalence is maximum in the second decade, when up to 20% of young people suffer symptoms in June and July.

Nasal irritation, sneezing and watery rhinorrhoea are the most troublesome symptoms but many also suffer from itching of the eyes and soft palate and occasionally even itching of the ears due to the common innervation of the pharyngeal mucosa and the ear. In addition, approximately 20% suffer from attacks of asthma.

Symptoms in March, April or May are due to allergy to pollens from hazel, elder and birch trees (see Fig. 12.19). In London, UK, symptoms occur in:

● April and May owing to plane tree pollen.
● The first or second week of June owing to grass pollen, as pollen counts then exceed 50 grains per m³ of air. Symptoms continue till the end of July.
● August and September owing to moulds, particularly those from *Alternaria alternata*, which

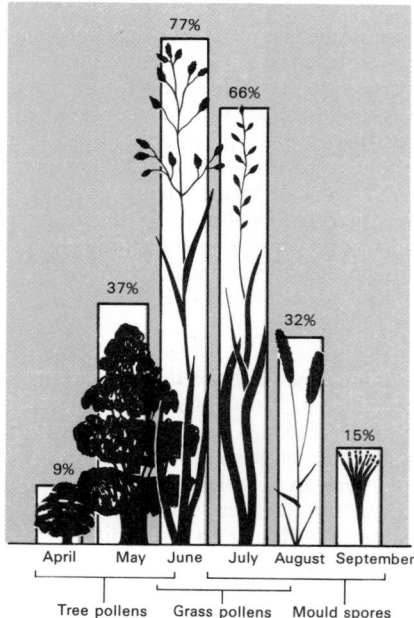

Fig. 12.19 Seasonal allergic rhinitis: giving the proportion of patients whose symptoms are worst in the month or months indicated. The causative agents are also shown.

grows on a variety of cultivated plants including wheat, and as 'early blight' on potatoes. *Cladosporium herbarum* grows around the roots of grass and its spores become airborne during lawn mowing. It causes allergic rhinitis throughout the summer months and may be identified in patients whose symptoms are not related to pollen counts.
● The autumn, when symptoms may develop from allergy to the spores of *Aspergillus fumigatus*, which readily grows on decaying plant material such as compost heaps and piles of leaves.

Figure 12.19 shows the proportion of patients with seasonal allergic rhinitis whose symptoms are worst in each month or months in relation to the common allergen.

Perennial rhinitis
Patients with perennial rhinitis rarely have symptoms that affect the eyes or throat. Half have symptoms predominantly of sneezing and watery rhinorrhoea, whilst the other half complain mostly of nasal blockage. The patient may lose the sense of smell and taste. A swollen mucosa can obstruct drainage from the sinuses, causing sinusitis in half of the patients. Perennial rhinitis is most frequent in the second and third decade, decreasing with age, and can be divided into three main types:

Perennial allergic rhinitis. The major cause of this is

an allergen called P1 contained in the faecal particles of the house-dust mite; these particles are approximately 20 μm in diameter (Fig. 12.20), not dissimilar in size to pollen grains. The house-dust mite itself is < 0.5 mm in size, invisible to the naked eye (Fig. 12.20), and is found in dust throughout the house, particularly in older, damp dwellings. They depend for nourishment upon desquamated human skin scales and are found in abundance (4000 mites per gram of surface dust) in human bedding.

The next most common allergens come from domestic pets and are proteins derived from urine or saliva spread over the surface of the animal as well as skin protein. Allergy to urinary protein from small mammals is a major cause of morbidity amongst laboratory workers.

Industrial dust, vapours and fumes are more likely to cause occupationally related perennial rhinitis than asthma.

The presence of perennial rhinitis makes the nose more reactive to non-specific stimuli such as cigarette smoke, washing powders, household detergents, strong perfumes and traffic fumes; these are *not* acting as allergens.

Perennial non-allergic rhinitis with eosinophilia. No extrinsic allergic cause can be identified in these patients, either from the history or on skin testing but, as in patients with perennial allergic rhinitis, eosinophilic granulocytes are present in nasal secretions.

Vasomotor rhinitis. These patients with perennial rhinitis have no demonstrable allergy or eosinophilia in nasal secretions. They may be suffering from non-specific nasal hyper-reactivity due to an imbalance of the autonomic nervous system innervating the erectile tissue (sinusoids) in the nasal mucosa.

Nasal polyps

These are round, smooth, soft, semitranslucent, pale or yellow, glistening structures attached to the nasal or sinus mucosa by a relatively narrow stalk or pedicle and occur in patients with both allergic and vasomotor rhinitis. They cause nasal obstruction, loss of smell and taste and mouth breathing, but rarely sneezing, since the mucosa of the polyp is largely denervated.

PATHOGENESIS

Sneezing, increased secretion and changes in mucosal blood flow are mediated both by efferent nerve fibres and by released mediators (see p. 668). Mucus production results largely from parasympathetic stimulation, whilst blood vessels are under both sympathetic and parasympathetic control.

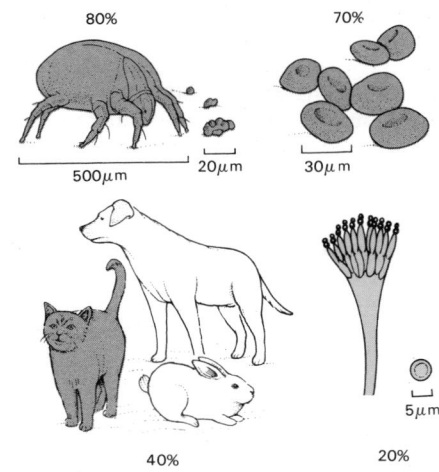

Fig. 12.20 Common allergens causing allergic rhinitis and asthma—the house-dust mite, faeces of house-dust mites, pollen grains, domestic pets, and moulds. Percentages are those of positive skin-prick tests to these allergens in patients with allergic rhinitis.

Sympathetic fibres maintain tonic contraction of blood vessels, keeping the sinusoids of the nose partially constricted with good nasal patency. Stimulation of the parasympathetic system dilates these blood vessels. This stimulation varies spontaneously in a cyclical fashion so that air intake alternates slowly over several hours from one nostril to the other. The erectile cavernous nasal sinusoids can be influenced by emotion, which, in turn, can affect nasal patency. It is thought that vasomotor rhinitis results from an imbalance in stimulation of the sympathetic and parasympathetic systems, with a preponderance of parasympathetic effects leading to nasal blockage.

Allergic rhinitis develops as a result of interaction between the inhaled allergen and adjacent molecules of IgE antibody. This is present on the surface of basophils and/or mast cells that are found in nasal secretions and within the nasal epithelium. Release of preformed mediators, in particular histamine, causes an increase in permeability of the epithelium, allowing allergen to reach IgE-primed mast cells in the lamina propria. Sneezing results from stimulation of afferent nerve endings and begins within minutes of the allergen entering the nose. This is followed by nasal secretion and eventually nasal blockage at a maximum of 15–20 min after contact with the allergen.

Although the mast cell contains or can generate many other potent vasomotor and chemotactic factors, the exact role for each of these has still to be evaluated (Fig. 12.32). It is likely that histamine plays a more important role in the development of allergic rhinitis than of asthma, since antihistamines are a useful and effective treatment for allergic rhinitis but are of little value in the everyday management of asthma. More mast cells are present in the nasal mucosa of individuals with rhinitis compared with those without rhinitis, and probably increase as allergen stimulation continues, accounting for the increasing responsiveness of the nose to lower amounts of grass pollen as the season continues. The mechanisms for recruitment of mast cells under these circumstances involves the release of interleukin-3 from T lymphocytes.

DIAGNOSIS AND INVESTIGATION

- A detailed history is mandatory for the diagnosis of allergic factors in rhinitis.
- Skin-prick testing (see Fig. 12.18) indicates that the mechanisms leading to allergic rhinitis (or asthma) are present in human skin. It does not necessarily mean that the particular allergen producing the weal causes the respiratory disease. However, if there is a positive clinical history for that allergen, a causative role is likely.
- Specific serum IgE antibody against the particular allergen provides the same information as the skin-prick test.
- The production of nasal secretions, sneezing and blockage can be compared after administration of allergen and saline. Such nasal provocation tests are rarely required to make the diagnosis.
- Stained smears of nasal secretion are of value in the following ways:
  (a) Eosinophilia (> 25% of total cells) indicates the presence of allergic rhinitis or non-allergic rhinitis with nasal eosinophilia, but is absent in vasomotor rhinitis.
  (b) Neutrophil granulocytes are seen in rhinovirus infection.

TREATMENT

Allergen avoidance
Removal of a household pet or total enclosure of industrial processes releasing sensitizing agents can lead to cure of rhinitis and, indeed, asthma.

Pollen avoidance is impossible. Contact may be diminished by wearing sunglasses, driving with the car windows shut, avoiding walks in the countryside (particularly in the late afternoon when the number of pollen grains is highest at ground level), and keeping the bedroom window shut at night. These measures are rarely sufficient in themselves to control symptoms. Exposure to pollen is generally lower at the seaside, where sea breezes keep pollen grains inland. Patients can be advised to avoid trouble by taking holidays in

Northern climates where pollen counts are lower or at times when the pollen season is over.

The house-dust mite infests most areas of the house, and is not confined to the bedroom. Mite counts are extremely low in hospitals where carpets are absent, floors are cleaned frequently and mattresses and pillows are covered in plastic sheeting that can be wiped down. Such conditions need to be reproduced in the home if mite counts are to be reduced to levels that can diminish symptoms. Antifungal agents (natamycin spray) have been used to kill fungi such as *Aspergillus* spp. (which help to break down human keratin for mite consumption), and acaricides, which directly kill mites, but these methods require long-term evaluation.

Antihistamines
Antihistamines remain the commonest therapy for rhinitis, and many can be purchased directly over the counter in the UK. They are particularly effective against sneezing, but are less effective against rhinorrhoea and have little influence on nasal blockage. Many antihistamines, e.g. chlorpheniramine (4 mg three times daily) or clemastine (1 mg twice daily), have sedative effects. Newer drugs such as astemizole (10 mg daily), cetirizine (10 mg once daily) and terfenadine (60 mg twice daily) are highly specific for H_1 receptors; they do not cross the blood–brain barrier and are therefore not associated with sedation. Although rarely sufficient for the treatment of rhinitis, antihistamines will control itching in the eyes and palate.

Decongestants
Drugs with sympathomimetic activity (alpha-adrenergic agents) are widely used for the treatment of nasal obstruction. They may be taken orally or more commonly as nasal drops or sprays (e.g. ephedrine nasal drops). Xylometazoline and oxymetazoline are widely used because they have a prolonged action and tachyphylaxis does not develop. Secondary nasal hyperaemia can occur some hours later as a rebound effect and rhinitis medicamentosa can develop if patients subsequently take increasing quantities of the local decongestant to overcome this phenomenon. Local decongestants may be the only effective treatment for vasomotor rhinitis, but patients must be warned about rebound nasal obstruction and must use the drug carefully. Usually, such preparations should only be prescribed for a limited period to open the nasal airways for administration of other therapy, particularly topical corticosteroids.

Anti-inflammatory drugs
These drugs, previously considered to act primarily by preventing release of mediators from mast cells and called therefore anti-allergic compounds, are

now known to influence a number of aspects of inflammation including mast and eosinophil activation and nerve function, and are best labelled anti-inflammatory drugs. Sodium cromoglycate applied topically in spray or powder form is of limited value in the treatment of allergic rhinitis, though is very effective in the management of allergic conjunctivitis. Ketotifen, an oral preparation considered to have potent antihistaminic and some anti-allergic activity, can be effective in both children and adults at a dose of 1 mg twice daily. Sedation is a problem initially in 20% of patients treated, though, as with other drugs with antihistaminic properties, many patients acclimatize to this and only 5% remain substantially sedated.

Corticosteroids
The most effective treatment for rhinitis is the use of small doses of topically administered corticosteroid preparations (e.g. beclomethasone spray twice daily). The amount used is insufficient to cause systemic effects and the effect is primarily anti-inflammatory. Preparations should be taken prior to the start of seasonal symptoms. The combination of a topical corticosteroid with a nonsedative antihistamine taken regularly is particularly effective.

Seasonal and perennial rhinitis respond readily to treatment with oral prednisolone 5–10 mg daily if other therapy has failed. Some patients with severe perennial rhinitis may require continuous small doses (2.5–5 mg) of daily prednisolone. Nasal polyps respond well to such oral doses of corticosteroids and their recurrence may be prevented by continuous application of topical corticosteroids.

Hyposensitization
The principle of hyposensitization is to inject gradually increasing amounts of the allergen that causes the patient's rhinitis to the point where symptoms begin to occur. This means that courses of hyposensitization must be tailored for each individual. Although its mode of action remains unknown, improvements in isolation of relevant allergens, better standardization and more stable preparations may make the technique more efficacious. In general, hyposensitization should be reserved for patients with allergic rhinitis caused by grass pollen or the house-dust mite, and it should be remembered that even in these cases symptomatic treatment is often more effective. Anaphylaxis can occur and suitable precautions should be taken (see p. 733).

Pharyngitis

Only about one-third of sore throats are due to infection with a haemolytic streptococcus and this proportion appears to be falling. The commonest viruses causing pharyngitis are those of the adenovirus group, which consists of about 32 serotypes. Endemic adenovirus infection causes the common sore throat, in which the oropharynx and soft palate are reddened and the tonsils are inflamed and swollen. Within one or two days the tonsillar lymph nodes enlarge. Occasionally, localized epidemics occur, particularly in schools in the summer-time, with episodes of fever, conjunctivitis, pharyngitis and lymphadenitis of the neck glands; these are due to adenovirus serotype 8. These diseases are self-limiting, and symptomatic treatment is all that is required.

Acute laryngotracheobronchitis

Acute laryngitis is an occasional but striking complication of upper respiratory tract infections, particularly those caused by viruses of the para-influenza group and the measles virus. Inflammatory oedema extends to the vocal cords and the epiglottis, causing considerable narrowing of the airway; in addition, there may be associated tracheitis or tracheobronchitis. Children under the age of 3 years are most severely affected. The voice becomes hoarse, the cough assumes a barking quality (croup) and there is audible laryngeal stridor. Progressive airways obstruction may occur, with recession of the soft tissue of the neck and abdomen during inspiration, and in severe cases central cyanosis may occur. Inhalation of steam may be helpful; in severe cases endotracheal intubation may be necessary. Oxygen and adequate fluids should be given. Rarely, a tracheostomy may be required.

Acute epiglottitis

Haemophilus influenzae type B can cause life-threatening infection of the epiglottis, a condition that is rare over the age of 5 years. The young child becomes extremely ill with a high fever, and severe airflow obstruction may rapidly occur. This is a life-threatening emergency and requires urgent endotracheal intubation and intravenous ceftazidime ($25–100 \ mg \cdot kg^{-1}$ in children). Chloramphenicol ($50–100 \ mg \cdot kg^{-1}$ in children) can also be used. The epiglottis, which is red and swollen, should not be inspected until facilities to maintain the airways are available.

Influenza (see p. 65)

The influenza virus belongs to the orthomyxovirus group and exists in two main forms—A and B. Influenza B is associated with localized outbreaks of milder nature, whereas influenza A is the cause of world-wide pandemics. Influenza A has a capacity to develop new antigenic variants at irregular intervals. Human immunity develops against the haemagglutinin (H) antigen and the neuraminidase (N) antigen on the viral surface. Major shifts in the antigenic make-up of influenza A viruses provide the necessary conditions for major pandemics, whereas minor antigenic drifts give rise to less severe epidemics because immunity in the population is less blunted.

The most serious pandemic of influenza occurred in 1918, and was associated with more than 20 million deaths world-wide. More recently, in 1957, a major shift in the antigenic make-up of the virus led to the appearance of influenza A2 type H2–N2, which caused a world-wide pandemic. A further pandemic occurred in 1968 owing to the emergence of Hong Kong influenza type H3–N2, and minor antigenic drifts have caused outbreaks around the world ever since.

CLINICAL FEATURES

The incubation period of influenza is usually 1–3 days. The illness starts abruptly with a fever, shivering and generalized aching in the limbs. This is associated with severe headache, soreness of the throat and a persistent dry cough that can last for several weeks. Influenza viruses can cause a prolonged period of debility and depression that may take weeks or months to clear; this is known as the post-viral syndrome.

COMPLICATIONS

Secondary bacterial infection, particularly with *Streptococcus pneumoniae* and *Haemophilus influenzae*, is common following influenza virus infection. Rarer, but more serious, is the development of pneumonia caused by *Staphylococcus aureus*, which has a mortality of up to 20%. Post-infectious encephalomyelitis rarely occurs after infection with influenza virus.

DIAGNOSIS

Laboratory diagnosis of all cases is not necessary. Definitive diagnosis can be established by demonstrating a fourfold increase in the complement-fixing antibody or the haemagglutinin antibody when measured before and after an interval of 1–2 weeks. Viral cultures are still a research procedure.

TREATMENT

Treatment is bed rest and aspirin, together with antibiotics for individuals with chronic bronchitis, or heart or renal disease.

PROPHYLAXIS

Protection by influenza vaccines is only effective in up to 70% of people and is of short duration, usually lasting for only a year. Influenza vaccine should not be given to individuals who are allergic to egg protein as some are manufactured in chick embryos. New vaccines have to be prepared to cover each change in viral antigenicity and are therefore in limited supply at the start of an epidemic. Routine vaccination is reserved for susceptible people with chronic heart, lung or kidney disease, and the elderly. In pandemics key hospital and health service personnel are also vaccinated.

Amantadine hydrochloride 100–200 mg daily may attenuate influenza A infection and should be reserved for individuals with chronic respiratory or cardiovascular disease who have not previously been immunized.

Inhalation of foreign bodies

Children inhale foreign bodies, frequently peanuts, more commonly than adults. In the adult, inhalation often occurs after an excess of alcohol or under general anaesthesia (loose dentures).

When the foreign body is large it may impact in the trachea. The person chokes and then becomes silent; death occurs unless the material is quickly removed.

Impaction usually occurs in the right main bronchus and produces:

- Choking
- Persistent monophonic wheeze
- Later, persistent suppurative pneumonia
- Lung abscess (common)

Treatment of inhaled foreign bodies

Emergency

The Heimlich manoeuvre is used to expel the obstructing object:

- Stand behind patient.
- Encircle your arms around the upper part of the abdomen just below the patient's rib cage.
- Give a sharp, forceful squeeze, forcing the diaphragm sharply into the thorax. This should expel sufficient air from the lungs to force the foreign body out of the trachea.

Non-emergency

Fibre optic bronchoscopy should be performed.

Diseases of the lower respiratory tract

Acute bronchitis

Acute bronchitis in previously healthy subjects is often viral. Bacterial infection with organisms such as *Streptococcus pneumoniae* and *Haemophilus influenzae* is a common sequel to viral infections, and is more likely to occur in individuals who are cigarette smokers and in those with chronic bronchitis and emphysema.

The illness begins with an irritating, unproductive cough, together with discomfort behind the sternum. This may be associated with tightness in the chest, wheezing and shortness of breath. The cough becomes productive, the sputum being yellow or green. There is a mild fever and a neutrophil leucocytosis; wheeze with occasional crackles can be heard on auscultation. In otherwise healthy adults the disease improves spontaneously in 4–8 days without the patient becoming seriously ill. Treatment with antibiotics may be given, e.g. amoxycillin 250 mg three times daily, though it is not known whether this hastens recovery in otherwise healthy individuals.

Chronic bronchitis and emphysema

Definitions
Chronic bronchitis is defined on the basis of the *history* as:

- Cough productive of sputum on most days for at least three months of the year for more than one year

Emphysema, on the other hand, is defined *pathologically* as:

- Dilatation and destruction of the lung tissue distal to the terminal bronchioles

Clinical observations led to the suggestion that there were two distinct types of patient:

- The *type A* fighter is *pink and puffing* in that, although he is very breathless, arterial tensions of oxygen and carbon dioxide are relatively normal and there is no cor pulmonale. These individuals were thought to be suffering predominantly from emphysema with little bronchitis.
- The *type B* non-fighter, on the other hand, is *blue and bloated*. He does not appear to be breathless, but has marked arterial hypoxaemia, carbon dioxide retention, secondary polycythaemia and cor pulmonale. These patients were thought to be suffering predominantly from chronic bronchitis.

Although this is an attractive concept and has some clinical usefulness, it is not supported by post-mortem studies that have shown no difference in the degree of mucous gland hyperplasia (i.e. bronchitis) or in the amount of emphysema in patients with type A compared with type B disease.

Autopsy studies have also shown that substantial numbers of centri-acinar emphysematous spaces are found in the lungs of 50% of British smokers over the age of 60 years and are unrelated to the diagnosis of significant respiratory disease before death.

Because of the difficulty of making a clear diagnosis between chronic bronchitis and emphysema during life, alternative terms such as chronic obstructive pulmonary disease (COPD), chronic obstructive lung disease (COLD) or chronic obstructive airways disease (COAD) were introduced to cover both of these conditions. These terms are unhelpful and should be replaced by the term 'chronic bronchitis and emphysema', as both these conditions coexist to a greater or lesser degree in each patient.

It is now recognized that the common tests for 'airway obstruction', the FEV_1 and PEFR, actually measure airflow limitation caused by both loss of elastic recoil and/or narrowing of airways. This has led to the introduction of the term 'chronic airflow limitation', which is the preferred terminology to describe the functional and physiological problem in chronic bronchitis and emphysema.

EPIDEMIOLOGY AND AETIOLOGY

Chronic bronchitis and emphysema (often referred to as the English disease) were always considered to be a particular problem in the UK, with a prevalence diagnosed on history of 17% in men and 8% in women in the age group 40–64 years. However, in the USA similar prevalence figures have been obtained and many developing countries are showing an increased prevalence.

There is no doubt that cigarette smoking is a major factor in the development of chronic bronchitis and emphysema. Not only are these diseases virtually confined to cigarette smokers, they are also related to the number of cigarettes smoked per day. The risk of death from chronic bronchitis and emphysema in patients smoking 30 cigarettes daily is 20 times that of a non-smoker. The bronchitis mortality amongst male doctors in relation to the number of cigarettes smoked is shown in Fig. 12.21.

Climate and air pollution are of less importance; nevertheless, there is a great increase in mortality from chronic bronchitis and emphysema during periods of heavy atmospheric pollution. The effect of urbanization, social class and occupation may also play a part in aetiology, but these effects are

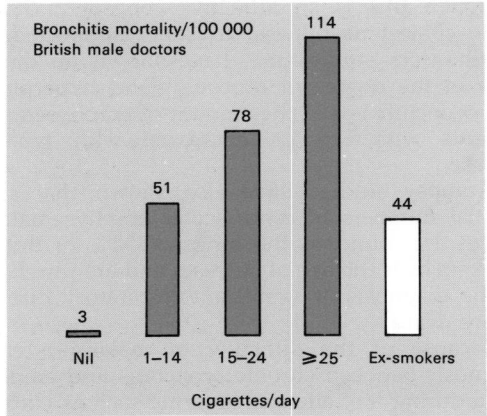

Fig. 12.21 Bronchitis death rates per 100 000 British male doctors according to their smoking habits. (From Doll R & Peto R (1976) *British Medical Journal* 2: 1525.)

difficult to separate from that of smoking.

The socioeconomic burden of chronic bronchitis and emphysema is considerable. Between 1976 and 1977 in the UK chronic bronchitis and emphysema were certified as causing 26 million lost working days for men and 2.6 million lost working days for women, accounting for some 10% of all days of sickness absence from work, much the highest of any defined disease entity. Nevertheless, the number of patients discharged from hospitals in the UK with this disease has been steadily falling; the death rate has also fallen in the last 20 years from 200 to 70 per 100 000.

PATHOPHYSIOLOGY

Chronic bronchitis

The most consistent pathological finding in chronic bronchitis is hypertrophy of the mucus-secreting glands of the bronchial tree. The hypertrophy of these mucous glands is evenly distributed throughout the lung, and is mainly seen in the larger bronchi. In addition, the number of mucus-secreting goblet cells increases. This leads to increased mucus production and the regular expectoration of sputum.

In more advanced cases the bronchi themselves are obviously inflamed and pus is seen in the lumen. Microscopically there is infiltration of the walls of the bronchi and bronchioles with acute and chronic inflammatory cells. The epithelial layer may become ulcerated and, when the ulcers heal, squamous epithelium may replace the columnar cells. The inflammation leads to widespread narrowing in the peripheral airways.

There is increasing evidence that the small airways are particularly affected early in the disease, initially without the development of any significant breathlessness. This initial inflammation of the small airways is reversible and accounts for the improvement in airway function if smoking is stopped in the early stages of the disease.

Further progression of the disease leads to progressive squamous cell metaplasia, and fibrosis of the bronchial walls. The physiological consequences of these changes is the development of airflow limitation. If the airway narrowing is combined with emphysema (causing loss of the elastic recoil of the lung) the resulting airflow limitation is even more severe.

Emphysema (Fig. 12.22)

Emphysema can be classified according to the site of damage:

- In *centri-acinar emphysema* distension and damage of lung tissue is concentrated around the respiratory bronchioles, whilst the more distal alveolar ducts and alveoli tend to be well-preserved. This form of emphysema is extremely common; when of modest extent, it is not necessarily associated with disability. Severe centri-acinar emphysema is associated with substantial airflow limitation.
- *Pan-acinar emphysema* is less common. Here, distension and destruction appear to involve the whole of the acinus, and in the extreme form, the lung becomes a mass of bullae. Severe airflow limitation and $\dot{V}_A/Q$ mismatch occur.
- In *irregular emphysema* there is scarring and damage affecting the lung parenchyma patchily without particular regard for acinar structure.

Emphysema can lead to expiratory airflow limita-

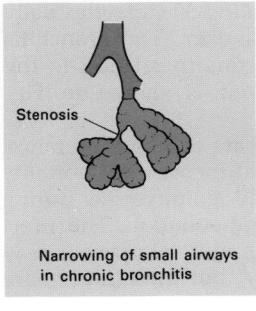

Narrowing of small airways in chronic bronchitis

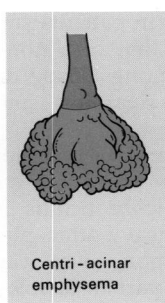

Centri-acinar emphysema

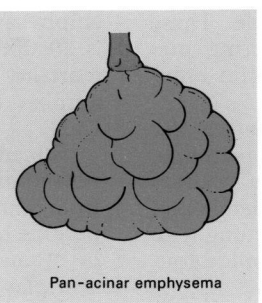

Pan-acinar emphysema

Fig. 12.22 The pathological features of chronic bronchitis and emphysema.

tion (see p. 632) and air trapping. The loss of lung elastic recoil results in an increase in total lung capacity while the loss of alveoli with emphysema results in decreased gas transfer.

$\dot{V}_A/\dot{Q}$ mismatch occurs partly because of damage and mucus plugging of smaller airways from chronic bronchitis and also because of the rapid expiratory closure of the smaller airways due to loss of elastic recoil from emphysema. This leads to a fall in P_aO_2 and a subsequent rise in P_aCO_2.

CO_2 is normally the major stimulant of the respiratory centre. In the face of a prolonged high P_aCO_2 this sensitivity is diminished and hypoxaemia becomes the chief drive to respiration. In this situation an attempt to abolish hypoxaemia by administration of oxygen can result in an increase in P_aCO_2 by decreasing the respiratory drive.

PATHOGENESIS

Cigarette smoking

Broncho-alveolar washes have shown that smokers have neutrophil granulocytes present within the lumen of the lung that are absent in non-smokers. Additionally, the small airways of smokers are infiltrated by granulocytes. These granulocytes are capable of releasing elastases and proteases, which possibly help to produce emphysema.

The hypertrophy of mucous glands in the larger airways is thought to be a direct response to persistent irritation resulting from the inhalation of cigarette smoke. The smoke has an adverse effect on surfactant, favouring overdistension of the lungs.

Infections

Infections are frequent and are often the precipitating cause of acute exacerbations of the disease. However, the role of infection in the development of the progressive airflow limitation that characterizes disabling chronic bronchitis and emphysema is far less clear. Nevertheless, release of enzymes from the excess neutrophil granulocytes found in infections probably adds to the lung damage.

Alpha-1-antitrypsin deficiency

This was first discovered in the 1960s in a family with early-onset emphysema. Many different phenotypes of alpha-1-antitrypsin deficiency have been recognized and these are also associated with liver disease (see p. 272). The three main types are MM (normal), MZ (heterozygous deficiency) and ZZ (homozygous deficiency) groups; these are defined by the serum level of antitrypsin. About 1 child in 5000 in Britain is born with the homozygous deficiency, but not all develop chest disease. Those who do develop breathlessness under the age of 40 years have radiographic evidence of basal emphysema and are usually, but not always, cigarette smokers. Purulent sputum

contains enzymes (elastases and proteases) that are normally inhibited by alpha-1-antitrypsin, and lack of this compound allows lung breakdown to proceed unchecked. This led to an attractive hypothesis for the mechanism of tissue damage in chronic bronchitis and emphysema, but no decrease in other forms of enzyme inhibition has been demonstrated.

CLINICAL FEATURES

Symptoms

The characteristic symptoms of chronic bronchitis and emphysema are cough with the production of sputum, wheeze and breathlessness following many years of a smoker's cough. Colds seem to 'go down to the chest' and frequent infective exacerbations occur, giving purulent sputum. Symptoms can be worsened by factors such as cold, foggy weather and atmospheric pollution. With advanced disease, breathlessness becomes severe even after mild exercise such as dressing.

Signs

In mild disease there are no signs apart from 'wheeze' throughout the chest. In severe disease, the patient is tachypnoeic, with prolonged expiration. The accessory muscles of respiration are used and there may be intercostal indrawing on inspiration and pursing of the lips on expiration (see Fig. 12.7). Chest expansion is poor, the lungs are hyperinflated, and there is loss of the normal cardiac and liver dullness.

The 'pink puffer' is always breathless and is not usually cyanosed. Rarely oedema or heart failure may be seen.

The 'blue bloater' is oedematous, deeply cyanosed, with hypoventilation and often little respiratory effort. These patients are likely to have hypercapnoea, which gives the following physical findings:

- Peripheral vasodilatation
- A bounding pulse
- Later, a coarse flapping tremor of the outstretched hands

More severe hypercapnoea leads to:

- Confusion
- Progressive drowsiness and coma with papilloedema

There is often considerable overlap between these two clinical patterns.

COMPLICATIONS

Respiratory failure

The latter stages of chronic bronchitis and emphysema are characterized by the development of respiratory failure. For practical purposes this is said to occur when there is either a P_aO_2 of less than 8 kPa (60 mm Hg) or a P_aCO_2 of more than 7 kPa (55 mm Hg) (see Chapter 13).

The persistence of chronic alveolar hypoxia and hypercapnia leads to constriction of the pulmonary arterioles and subsequent pulmonary arterial hypertension.

Cor pulmonale

Patients may develop cor pulmonale (see p. 608), which is defined as heart disease secondary to disease of the lung. It is characterized by pulmonary hypertension, right ventricular hypertrophy, and eventually right heart failure. On examination, the patient is centrally cyanosed (owing to the lung disease) and, when heart failure develops, breathlessness and ankle oedema occur. Initially a prominent parasternal heave may be felt due to right ventricular hypertrophy and a loud pulmonary second sound may be heard. In very severe pulmonary hypertension there is incompetence of the pulmonary valve. With right heart failure, tricuspid incompetence may develop with a greatly elevated JVP, ascites and upper abdominal pain due to swelling of the liver.

DIAGNOSIS

This is usually clinical. There is a history of breathlessness and sputum production in a lifetime smoker. It is unwise to make a diagnosis of chronic bronchitis and emphysema in the absence of cigarette smoking unless there is a family history of lung disease suggestive of a deficiency of alpha-1-antitrypsin.

In clinical practice, emphysema is often incorrectly diagnosed on signs of overinflation of the lungs (e.g. loss of liver dullness on percussion), since this may occur with other diseases such as asthma. Furthermore, centri-acinar emphysema may be present without signs of overinflation. Some elderly men develop a barrel-shaped chest due to osteoporosis of the spine and a consequent

decrease in height. This should not be attributed to emphysema.

In a number of patients the airflow limitation is reversible and the distinction between asthma and chronic bronchitis and emphysema can be difficult.

INVESTIGATION

- *Lung function tests* show evidence of airflow limitation (see Figs. 12.8 and 12.15). The ratio of the FEV_1 to the FVC is reduced and the PEFR is low. Lung volumes may be normal or increased, and the gas transfer coefficient of carbon monoxide is low when significant emphysema is present.
- On *chest X-ray* the diagnosis of chronic bronchitis and emphysema is not always possible, even when the disease is advanced. The classic features are the presence of bullae, severe overinflation of the lungs with low, flattened diagphragms, and a large retrosternal air space on the lateral film. There may also be a deficiency of blood vessels in the peripheral half of the lung fields compared with relatively easily visible proximal vessels.

  The chest X-ray can be normal even with advanced disease.
- The *haemoglobin level* and *PCV* may be elevated.
- *Blood gases* are often normal. In the advanced case there is evidence of hypoxaemia and hypercapnia.
- *Sputum examination* is unnecessary in the ordinary case as *Streptococcus pneumoniae* or *Haemophilus influenzae* are the only common organisms to produce acute exacerbations.
- *Electrocardiogram.* In cor pulmonale the P wave is taller (P pulmonale) and there may be right bundle branch block (rSR′ complex) and the changes of right ventricular hypertrophy.

TREATMENT

The single most important aspect in the manage-

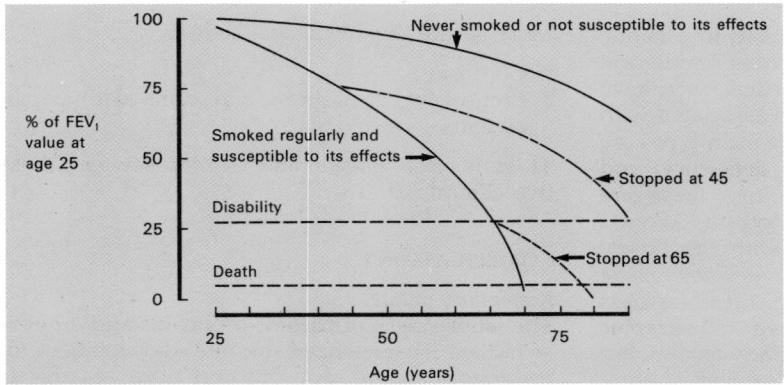

Fig. 12.23 Influence of smoking on airflow limitation. (From Fletcher CM & Peto R (1977) *British Medical Journal* **1**: 1645.)

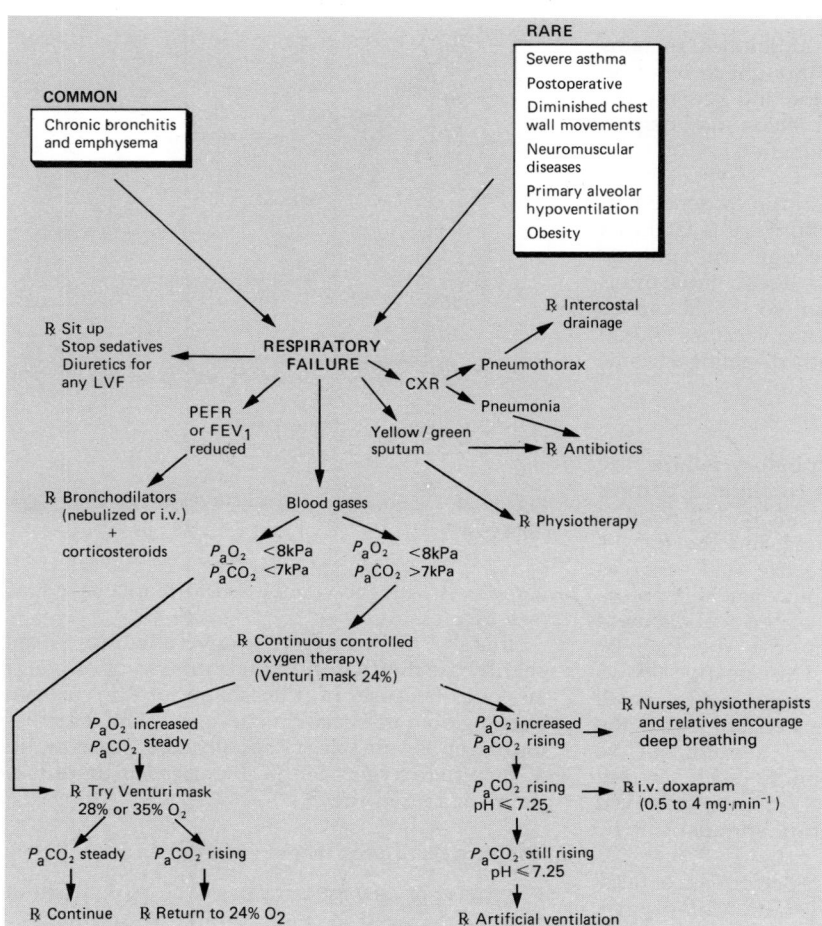

Fig. 12.24 Algorithm for the treatment of respiratory failure. LVF = left ventricular failure.

ment of chronic bronchitis and emphysema is to persuade the patient to stop smoking. Even at a late stage of the disease this may slow down the rate of deterioration and prolong the time before disability and death occur (Fig. 12.23). Accompanying heart failure should be treated (see p. 564).

Drug therapy

Drug therapy is used both for the short-term management of exacerbations and for the long-term relief of symptoms. In some cases the therapy is similar to that used in asthma (see p. 670).

Bronchodilators. Many patients feel less breathless following the inhalation of a beta-adrenoceptor agonist such as salbutamol (200 µg 4–6 hourly). Objective evidence of improvement in the peak flow or FEV_1 may be small, but with severe disability it may be of considerable help.

Corticosteroids. In symptomatic patients with chronic bronchitis and emphysema, a trial of corticosteroids is always indicated, since a propor-

tion of patients have a large, unsuspected, asthmatic element to their disease and airway function may improve considerably. Prednisolone 30 mg daily should be given for 2 weeks, with measurements of lung function before and after the treatment period. If there is objective evidence of a substantial degree of improvement in airflow limitation (> 15%), prednisolone should be gradually reduced and replaced by inhaled corticosteroids (beclomethasone 100–500 µg three times daily).

Antibiotics. Prompt antibiotic treatment shortens exacerbations and should always be given in acute episodes as they may prevent subsequent further lung damage. Patients can be given a supply of antibiotics to keep at home to start as soon as their sputum turns yellow or green. Treatment should be with amoxycillin 500 mg three times daily. Amoxycillin-resistant *Haemophilus influenzae* has become an increasing problem, occurring in up to 10% of isolates from sputum. Resistance to cefaclor is significantly less frequent and it may become the antibiotic of choice.

Long-term treatment with antibiotics remains controversial. They were once thought to be of no value, but eradication of infection and keeping the lower respiratory tract free of bacteria may help to prevent deterioration in lung function.

Mucolytics and vaccines. There is little evidence that mucolytics are of any benefit, though it is vital that patients are encouraged to cough up sputum. Symptomatic treatment with steam inhalations may help to liquefy the sputum so that it can be more easily coughed up. Influenza vaccines should be given yearly to patients with disabling chronic bronchitis and emphysema.

Treatment of respiratory failure

There are many causes of respiratory failure (see Fig. 12.24) but by far the most common is chronic bronchitis and emphysema. In this type II respiratory failure the P_aCO_2 is elevated and the P_aO_2 is reduced. It is important to realize that whereas hypercapnoea is intoxicating, hypoxaemia is potentially lethal. The primary aim of the management of respiratory failure is to improve the P_aO_2 by continuous oxygen therapy. This nearly always leads to a rise in the P_aCO_2 (see p. 63). Small increases in P_aCO_2 can be tolerated but not if the pH falls dramatically. The pH should not be allowed to fall below 7.25; under such circumstances, increased ventilation must be achieved either by the use of a respiratory stimulant or by artificial ventilation.

Figure 12.25 shows a fixed-performance mask (Venturi mask) for the administration of oxygen. This style of mask is used when only low concentrations of oxygen can be given. It should be

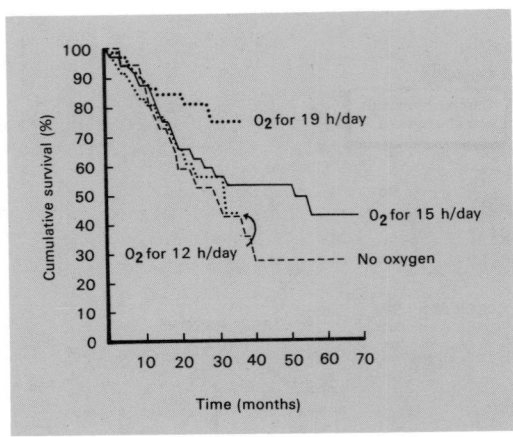

Fig. 12.26 Cumulative survival curves for patients receiving oxygen.

compared with the variable-performance face mask (see Fig. 13.16).

Initially, 24% oxygen is given, which is only slightly greater than the concentration of oxygen in air but, because of the shape of the oxygen–haemoglobin dissociation curve, this small increase in oxygen is valuable. Gradually, the concentration of inspired oxygen can be increased if there is no dramatic rise in the P_aCO_2.

Additional measures. These include:

- *Removal of retained secretions.* The patient should be encouraged to cough to remove secretions. If this fails, bronchoscopy and/or aspiration via an endotracheal tube may be necessary. A tracheostomy is only rarely required.
- *Respiratory stimulants.* Doxapram, 0.5–4 mg·min^{-1} by slow i.v. infusion, may help in the short term to arouse the patient and to stimulate coughing, with clearance of some secretions.
- *Assisted ventilation* (see p. 724). This is occasionally used for patients with chronic bronchitis and emphysema with severe respiratory failure when there is a definite precipitating factor and the overall prognosis is reasonable. This can be a difficult ethical problem.

Corticosteroids, antibiotics and bronchodilators should also be administered (see above).

Long-term oxygen therapy

Two controlled trials (chiefly in men) have indicated that the continuous administration of 2 litres of oxygen per minute via nasal prongs to achieve an oxygen saturation of greater than 90% for large proportions of the day can prolong life. Survival curves from these two studies are shown in Fig. 12.26. Only 30% of those not receiving long-term oxygen therapy survived for more than 5 years. A

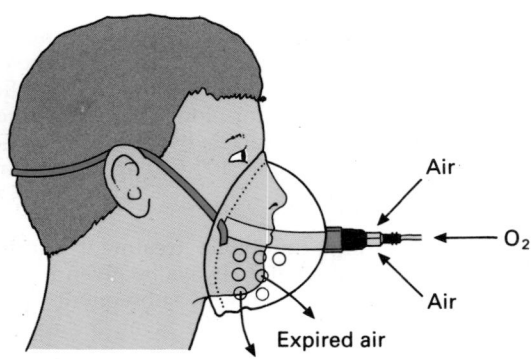

Fig. 12.25 'Fixed-performance' device for administration of oxygen to spontaneously breathing patients (Venturi mask). Oxygen is delivered through the injector of the Venturi mask at a given flow rate. A fixed amount of air is entrapped and the inspired oxygen can be accurately predicted. Masks are available to deliver 24%, 28% and 35% oxygen.

fall in pulmonary artery pressure was achieved if oxygen was given for 15 h daily, but substantial improvement in mortality was only achieved by the administration of oxygen for 19 h daily. These results suggest that long-term continuous domiciliary oxygen therapy will benefit patients who have:

- Chronic bronchitis and emphysema with an FEV_1 of less than 1.2 litres
- A P_aO_2 on air of less than 9 kPa (68 mm Hg)
- Carboxyhaemoglobin of less than 3%, i.e. patients who have stopped smoking

The provision of 19 h of oxygen daily at a flow rate of $1–3\ L\cdot min^{-1}$ to increase the arterial oxygen saturation to over 90% needs 20 oxygen cylinders per week. This is extremely expensive. Oxygen concentrators are cheaper and are now available through the health service in the UK.

Additional therapy

Pulmonary hypertension can be partially relieved by the use of oral beta-adrenoceptor stimulants such as salbutamol (4 mg three times daily), but whether this is useful in the long-term is unknown.

The sensation of breathlessness can be reduced by the use of either promethazine 125 mg daily or dihydrocodeine $1\ mg\cdot kg^{-1}$ by mouth. Reduced breathlessness and increased exercise tolerance also result from the combined administration of dihydrocodeine and oxygen delivered from a portable cylinder.

Exercise training

A modest increase in exercise capacity with diminution in the sense of breathlessness and improved general well-being can result from exercise training. Regular training periods can be instituted at home; climbing stairs or walking fixed distances combined with regular clinic visits for encouragement. Breathing exercises are probably of less value.

PROGNOSIS

In general, 50% of patients with severe breathlessness die within 5 years (Fig. 12.26), but even in the severe group stopping smoking helps the prognosis.

Nocturnal hypoxia

It has been shown that patients with chronic bronchitis and emphysema who show severe arterial hypoxaemia also suffer from profound nocturnal hypoxaemia with a P_aO_2 as low as 2.5 kPa (19 mm Hg), particularly during the rapid eye movement (REM) phase of sleep.

Because patients with chronic bronchitis and emphysema are already hypoxic, the fall in P_aO_2 produces a much larger fall in oxygen saturation (owing to the steepness of the oxyhaemoglobin dissociation curve) and desaturation of up to 50% occurs. The mechanism is alveolar hypoventilation due to:

- Inhibition of intercostal and accessory muscles in REM sleep
- Shallow breathing in REM sleep, which reduces ventilation, particularly in severe chronic airways disease
- An increase in upper airway resistance due to a reduction in muscle tone

These nocturnal hypoxaemic episodes are associated with a further rise in pulmonary arterial pressure, and the majority of deaths in patients with chronic bronchitis and emphysema occur during the night, possibly due to cardiac arrhythmias. These patients additionally show severe secondary polycythaemia, partly as a result of the severe nocturnal hypoxaemia.

Each episode of desaturation is usually terminated by arousal from sleep, so that normal sleep is reduced and the patient suffers from daytime sleepiness. Treatment is with nocturnal administration of oxygen.

Patients with arterial hypoxaemia should never be given sleeping tablets, which will further depress respiratory drive.

Obstructive sleep apnoea

This occurs during sleep, particularly rapid eye movement (REM) sleep, and is characterized by:

- Hypersomnolence
- Heavy snoring
- Restless sleep
- Poor concentration
- Morning headache
- Impotence

It is caused by the apposition of the tongue and palate to the posterior pharyngeal wall as illustrated in Fig. 12.27. In order to overcome the resulting asphyxia, the sufferer must partially or completely arouse, thus increasing the drive to the pharyngeal muscles, causing them to pull apart with a loud snort. The patient then goes back to sleep and the cycle is repeated at an interval of 30–120 s. Important contributory factors are obesity, a small pharyngeal lumen and chronic airflow limitation.

Correctable factors occur in about one-third of cases and include:

- Encroachment on pharynx: obesity, acromegaly, enlarged tonsils
- Nasal obstruction: nasal deformities, rhinitis, polyps, adenoids

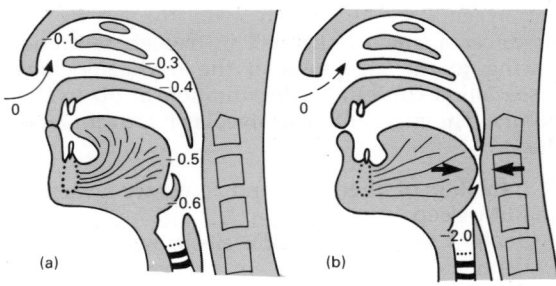

Fig. 12.27 Section through head, showing pressure changes (kPa) in (a) the normal situation and (b) obstructive sleep apnoea. There is a pressure drop during inspiration as air is sucked through the turbinates and in patients with obstructive sleep apnoea this is sufficient to collapse the pharynx, obstructing inspiration.

- Respiratory depressant drugs: alcohol, sedatives, strong analgesics

The diagnosis can usually be made by non-invasive ear or finger oximetry, best performed at home, accompanied by observation of the pattern of the snore–silence–snore cycle by the patient's family. Arterial oxygen saturation falls significantly in a cyclical manner.

Management consists of correction of treatable factors, e.g. tonsillectomy, together with, if necessary, continuous nasal positive airway pressure delivered by a nasal mask during sleep. Such systems raise the pressure in the pharynx by about 1 kPa, keeping the walls apart.

Bronchiectasis

Bronchiectasis may be defined simply as dilatation of the bronchi. Bronchial walls become inflamed, thickened and irreversibly damaged. The mucociliary transport mechanism is impaired and frequent bacterial infections ensue. Clinically, the disease is characterized by cough productive of large amounts of sputum.

EPIDEMIOLOGY

Prior to the discovery and clinical use of antibiotics, bronchiectasis was a frequent outcome of slowly resolving pneumonia. Most cases now arise in childhood and even the incidence in this age group has dropped. Both sexes can develop bronchiectasis, but an increased male preponderance over 45 years has been noted.

AETIOLOGY

The aetiology is uncertain but bronchial obstruction followed by infection plays a major role.

Bronchiectasis is a rare complication of whoop-

ing cough and measles in the Western World. Localized bronchiectasis also rarely results from tuberculous enlargement of lymph nodes at the hilum of the lung, particularly around the origin of the middle-lobe bronchus. Bronchial obstruction in children from other causes (e.g. inhaled peanuts) can give rise to gross suppurative lung disease and residual bronchiectasis.

Progressive bronchiectasis has been described in non-smoking patients of both sexes, with no other underlying cause. This syndrome is known as chronic bronchial sepsis.

Cystic fibrosis (p. 663) also leads to bronchiectasis, as over 75% of children with cystic fibrosis now survive to adult life. Bronchiectasis can also be associated with other congenital abnormalities— e.g. Kartagener's syndrome, which is characterized by sinusitis and transposition of viscera with bronchiectasis, associated with 'immotile cilia'.

CLINICAL FEATURES

Patients with mild bronchiectasis only produce yellow or green sputum after an infection, often viral. Localized areas of the lung may be particularly affected, when sputum production will depend on position. As the condition worsens, the patient suffers from persistent halitosis, recurrent febrile episodes with malaise, and episodes of pneumonia. Clubbing occurs, and coarse crackles can be heard over the infected areas, usually the bases of the lungs. When the condition is severe there is continuous production of foul-smelling, thick, khaki-coloured sputum. Haemoptysis, either as blood-stained sputum or as a massive haemorrhage, can occur. Breathlessness may result from airflow limitation.

INVESTIGATION

- The *chest X-ray* may be quite normal or may show dilated bronchi with thickened bronchial walls and sometimes multiple cysts containing fluid.
- CT scanning can show bronchial wall thickening (Fig. 12.28).
- *Bronchograms* This investigation is uncomfortable for the patient and is only required if the diagnosis is in doubt or where there is reason to believe that the disease may be localized and therefore amenable to surgical treatment. The left lower lobe and lingula are the commonest sites for localized disease.
- *Sputum examination* with culture and sensitivity of the organisms is essential for adequate treatment. The major pathogens are *Staphylococcus aureus*, *Pseudomonas aeruginosa*, *Haemophilus influenzae* and anaerobes. Other pathogens include *Streptococcus pneumoniae* and *Klebsiella pneumoniae*. *Aspergillus fumigatus* can be isolated

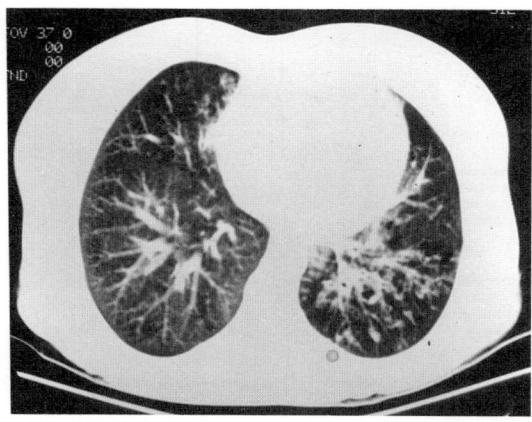

Fig. 12.28 CT scan showing bronchiectasis in the left lower lobe. Note dilated bronchi with thickened wall.

from 10% of sputum specimens in cystic fibrosis, but the role of this organism is uncertain.

TREATMENT

Postural drainage
Postural drainage is of vital importance and patients must be trained to tip themselves into appropriate positions at least three times daily for 10–20 min. Most patients find that lying over the side of the bed with head and thorax down is the most effective position.

Antibiotics
Experience from the treatment of cystic fibrosis suggests that bronchopulmonary infections should be eradicated if progression of the disease is to be halted. In mild cases, intermittent chemotherapy with amoxycillin 500 mg 8–hourly may be the only therapy needed. Flucloxacillin 500 mg 6-hourly is the best treatment if *Staphylococcus aureus* is isolated. Chloramphenicol is a useful drug in persistent infection.

If the sputum remains yellow or green despite regular physiotherapy and intermittent chemotherapy, or if lung function deteriorates despite treatment with bronchodilators, continuous oral chemotherapy should be considered.

A major problem is infection with *Pseudomonas aeruginosa*, for which only parenteral or aerosol chemotherapy is effective. Drug regimens involving tobramycin or gentamicin (80 mg i.v. bolus 8-hourly) together with carbenicillin or azlocillin (5 g i.v. over 20 min 8-hourly) are often required. High sputum levels of antibiotics can be achieved by inhalation. A treatment regimen of carbenicillin 1 g and gentamicin 80 mg given by a compressor-driven nebulizer twice daily has been found to be of benefit in young adult patients with chronic *Pseudomonas* infection. Ceftazidime intravenously

(2 g bolus 8-hourly) or by inhalation (1 g twice daily) has been shown to be equally effective.

Bronchodilators
Bronchodilators may be useful in patients with demonstrable airflow limitation.

Surgery
Unfortunately, bronchiectasis is rarely sufficiently localized for surgery to be of any value.

COMPLICATIONS

The incidence of complications has fallen with antibiotic therapy. Pneumonia, pneumothorax, empyema and metastatic cerebral abscess can occur. Severe, life-threatening haemoptysis can also occur, particularly in patients with cystic fibrosis.

Cystic fibrosis

Cystic fibrosis (CF) is due to a dysfunction of all exocrine glands resulting in abnormal mucus production. The classical form of the syndrome includes bronchopulmonary infection and pancreatic insufficiency, with a high sweat sodium and chloride concentration. It is a recessively inherited disorder with a carrier frequency in Caucasians of 1 in 2000 (see p. 117). There is a gene mutation on the long arm of chromosome 7 (7q 21.3 → 7q 22.1). A specific deletion in the coding region (the codon for phenylalanine at position 508 in the amino acid sequence [$\triangle$F 508] has been found resulting in a defect in a transmembrane regulator protein (see p. 293).

The frequency of $\triangle$F 508 mutation is 70% in the USA and UK, < 50% in southern Europe and 30% in Ashkenazic families. The identification of this transmembrane regulator protein will allow more accurate detection of carriers of the mutant gene.

CLINICAL FEATURES

Although the lungs of babies born with CF are structurally normal at birth, respiratory symptoms are usually the presenting feature. CF is now the commonest cause of recurrent bronchopulmonary infection in childhood, and is an important cause in early adult life. Finger clubbing is almost universal, haemoptysis is frequent and breathlessness occurs in the later stages as airflow limitation develops. Older children may also develop nasal polyps.

Puberty and skeletal maturity are delayed in most patients with the disease. Males are almost always infertile owing to failure of development of the vas deferens and epididymis. Females are able to conceive, but often develop secondary amenorrhoea as the disease progresses.

About 85% of patients have symptomatic steatorrhoea owing to pancreatic dysfunction (see p. 293). Children may be born with meconium ileus due to the viscoid consistency of meconium in CF and later in life develop the meconium ileus equivalent (MIE) syndrome, an important cause of small intestinal obstruction unique to CF.

Cholesterol gallstones appear to occur with increased frequency and cirrhosis develops in about 5% of older patients.

DIAGNOSIS

The diagnosis of CF in older children and adults may be difficult. It depends on the clinical history together with:

- A family history of the disease
- A high sweat sodium concentration over 60 mmol·L^{-1}. (Meticulous technique by laboratories performing regular sweat analysis is essential, but the test is still difficult to interpret in adults.)
- Absent vas deferens and epididymis.
- Immunoreactive trypsin (p. 293).

TREATMENT

Treatment for the respiratory disease is described under bronchiectasis on p. 663. The treatment of pancreatic insufficiency is described on p. 293. A few patients have now undergone successful heart–lung transplantation but their long-term survival following this procedure is not yet known.

PROGNOSIS AND COUNSELLING

The prognosis has consistently improved; most children now survive into their teens. The long-term outlook is uncertain, but progressive respiratory failure almost inevitably occurs. Genetic counselling for this disease is improving with the discovery of the gene abnormality; widespread screening programmes are being developed.

Asthma

Asthma is defined as partial obstruction to airflow in the intrathoracic airways that varies in severity over short periods of time, either spontaneously or as a result of treatment. The diagnosis of asthma depends upon showing these changes objectively using lung function tests.

PREVALENCE

Until recently it was considered that asthma affected approximately 5% of the population at some stage during their life. Increasing recognition of the disease (and possibly an increasing incidence) suggests that the prevalence, particularly in

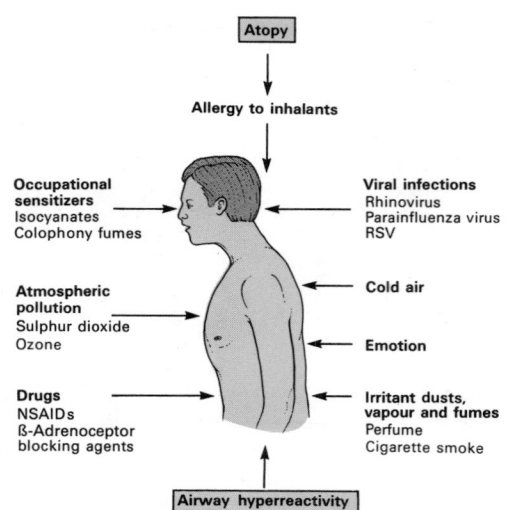

Fig. 12.29 Causes of asthma.

the second decade of life, may be as high as 10–15%. There is also a geographical variation, with asthma being common in, for example, New Zealand, but being much rarer in Far Eastern countries such as China and Malaysia. Long-term follow-up in developing countries suggests that the disease may become more frequent as individuals become more 'Westernized'. Studies of occupational asthma suggest that a high percentage of the work-force, perhaps up to 20%, may become asthmatic if exposed to potent sensitizers.

AETIOLOGY AND PATHOGENESIS

There are two major factors involved in the development of extrinsic asthma and many other stimuli that can precipitate attacks (Fig. 12.29).

Atopy and allergy

The term 'atopy' was used by clinicians at the beginning of the century to describe a group of disorders, including asthma and hay fever, that appeared:

- To run in families
- To have characteristic wealing skin reactions to common allergens in the environment
- To have circulating antibody in their serum that could be transferred to the skin of non-sensitized individuals.

The term is now best used to describe those individuals who readily develop antibodies of immunoglobulin E (IgE) class against common materials present in the environment. Such antibodies are present in 30–40% of the population, the proportion being greatest in the third and fourth decades of life and reducing with age. It now seems likely that IgE antibody production is controlled by a gene on chromosome 11.

The allergens involved are similar to those in rhinitis, though the particle size of pollens (> 20 μm) means that they are much more likely to cause conjunctivitis, rhinitis and pharyngitis than asthma. Allergens from the faecal particles of the house-dust mite are the most important extrinsic cause of asthma world-wide. The fungal spores from *Aspergillus fumigatus* give rise to a complex series of lung disease, including asthma (see p. 687).

Increased responsiveness of the airways of the lung (airway hyper-reactivity)
The definition of asthma used in North America incorporates a well-known feature of the disease—an increased responsiveness of the airways to non-specific stimuli (i.e. airway hyper-reactivity). Bronchial reactivity can be demonstrated by asking the patient to inhale, gradually increasing concentrations either of histamine or methacholine (*bronchial provocation tests*). This induces a transient episode of airflow limitation in susceptible individuals (approximately 20% of the population); the dose of the agonist (provocation dose) necessary to produce a 20% fall in FEV_1 is known as the $PD_{20}FEV_1$. Patients with clinical symptoms of asthma respond to very low doses of methacholine, i.e. they have a low $PD_{20}FEV_1$ (< 6 micromoles). In general, the greater the degree of hyper-reactivity, the more persistent the symptoms and the greater the need for treatment.

Some patients also react to methacoline but at higher doses and include those with:

- Attacks of asthma only on extreme exertion
- Wheezing or prolonged periods of coughing following a viral infection
- Problems with asthma only during the pollen season
- Allergic rhinitis, but not complaining of any lower respiratory symptoms until specifically questioned

Although the degree of hyper-reactivity can itself be influenced by allergic mechanisms (see. p. 667 and Fig. 12.32), its pathogenesis and mode of inheritance remain to be elucidated.

PATHOGENESIS AND PRECIPITATING FACTORS

Occupational sensitizers
Over 200 materials encountered at the work-place are known to give rise to occupational asthma. The seven most important causes are recognized occupational diseases in the UK and patients in insurable employment are therefore eligible for statutory compensation provided they apply within 10 years of leaving the occupation in which the

Table 12.7 Occupational asthma in the UK.

Cause	Source
Non-IgE related	
Isocyanates	Polyurethane varnishes Industrial coatings
Colophony fumes	Soldering Electronics industry
IgE related	
Allergens from animals and insects	Laboratories
Allergens from flour and grain	Farmers Millers Grain handlers
Proteolytic enzymes	Manufacture (but not use) of 'biological' washing powders
Complex salts of platinum	Metal refining
Acid anhydrides and polyamine hardening agents	Industrial coatings

asthma developed (Table 12.7). The development of asthma following exposure to some of these materials is linked to the development of specific IgE antibody in serum in some cases, whilst in others the cause has yet to be determined.

The proportion of employees developing occupational asthma depends primarily upon the level of exposure. Proper enclosure of industrial processes or appropriate ventilation can greatly reduce the risk. Atopic individuals develop occupational asthma more rapidly when exposed to agents causing the development of specific IgE antibody. Non-atopic individuals can also develop asthma when exposed to such agents, but usually after a longer period.

Non-specific factors
The characteristic feature of bronchial hyper-reactivity in asthmatics means that as well as reacting to specific antigens their airways will also respond to a wide variety of non-specific stimuli.

Cold air and exercise. Most asthmatics experience an attack of wheezing after prolonged and continuous exercise. Typically, the attack does not occur during the exercise period but at its conclusion. The inhalation of cold, dry air will also precipitate an attack. In both cases the wheezing is thought to be precipitated by the cooling and drying of the epithelial lining of the bronchi. Exercise and cold air provocation tests can be performed.

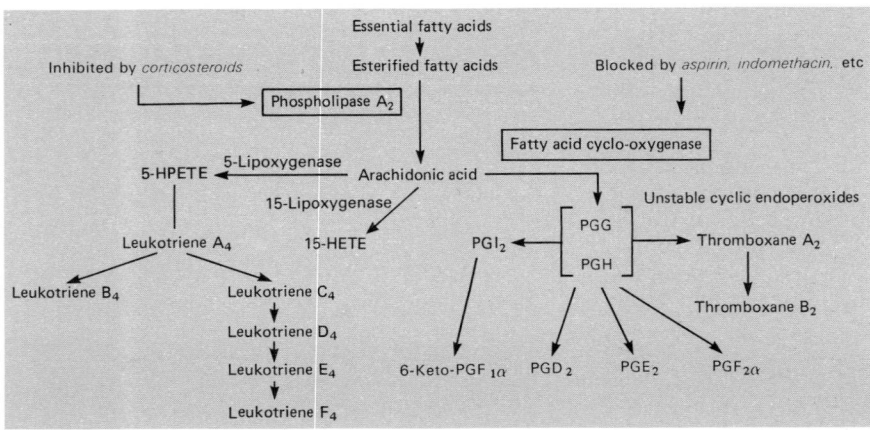

Fig. 12.30 Arachidonic acid metabolism and the effect of drugs.

Atmospheric pollution and irritant dusts, vapours and fumes. Many patients with asthma experience worsening of symptoms on contact with cigarette smoke, car exhaust fumes, strong perfumes or high concentrations of dust in the atmosphere. Further minor epidemics of the disease have occurred during periods of heavy atmospheric pollution in industrial areas, caused by the presence of high concentrations of sulphur dioxide and ozone in the air.

Emotion. It is well known that emotional factors may influence asthma, but there is no evidence that patients with the disease are any more psychologically disturbed than their non-asthmatic peers.

Drugs. Non-steroidal anti-inflammatory drugs (NSAIDs), particularly aspirin, have an important role in the development and precipitation of attacks in approximately 5% of patients with asthma. This effect is almost universal in those individuals who have both nasal polyps and asthma. The precise mechanism involved is unknown but it is thought that treatment with these drugs leads to an imbalance in the metabolism of arachidonic acid. NSAIDs inhibit arachidonic acid metabolism via the cyclo-oxygenase pathway, preventing the synthesis of prostaglandins. It is suggested that under these circumstances arachidonic acid is preferentially metabolized via the lipoxygenase pathway, resulting in the production of leukotrienes, previously known as the slow-reacting substances for anaphylaxis (see Fig. 12.30).

The airways of the lung have a direct parasympathetic innervation that tends to produce bronchoconstriction. There is no direct sympathetic innervation of the smooth muscle of the bronchi, and antagonism of parasympathetically induced bronchoconstriction is critically dependent upon circulating adrenaline acting through beta-2 receptors on the surface of smooth muscle cells.

Inhibition of this effect by beta-adrenoreceptor-blocking drugs such as propranolol leads to bronchoconstriction and airflow limitation, but only in asthmatic subjects. The so-called selective beta-1-adrenoceptor-blocking drugs such as atenolol may still induce attacks of asthma; their use in asthmatic patients for hypertension or angina should be questioned and calcium antagonists such as nifedipine should be used if appropriate.

Allergen-induced asthma
The experimental inhalation of allergen by atopic asthmatic individuals leads to the development of four types of reaction, as illustrated in Fig. 12.31.

The commonest reaction is *immediate asthma*, in which airflow limitation begins within minutes of contact with the allergen, reaches its maximum in 15–20 min and subsides by 1 h.

Many asthmatics subsequently develop a more prolonged and sustained attack of airflow limitation that responds poorly to inhalation of bronchodilator drugs such as salbutamol—the *late-phase reaction*.

The combination of an immediate reaction followed by a late reaction is known as a *dual asthmatic response*.

The inhalation of some materials, particularly occupational sensitizers such as the isocyanates, usually causes the development of an *isolated late reaction* with no preceding immediate response.

The development of the late-phase reaction is associated with an increase in the underlying level of airway hyper-reactivity such that individuals may show continuing episodes of asthma on subsequent days—*recurrent asthmatic reactions*.

The pathogenesis of asthma is complex and not fully understood. It involves a number of cells, mediators, nerves and vascular leakage that can be activated by several different mechanisms, of which exposure to allergens is the most important (Fig. 12.32).

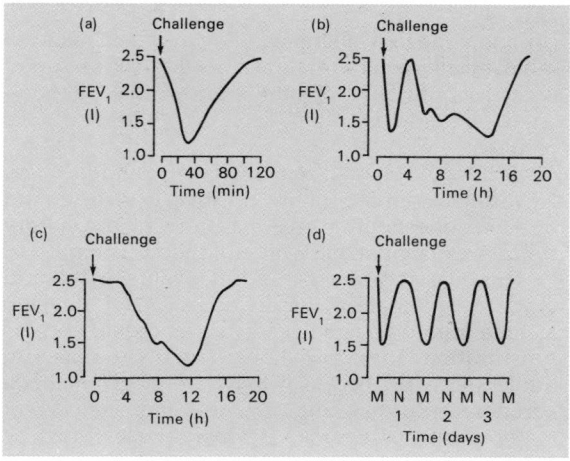

Fig. 12.31 Different types of asthmatic reactions following challenge with allergen. (a) Immediate asthma. (b) Dual asthmatic response. (c) Isolated late reaction. (d) Recurrent asthmatic reactions. M = midnight; N = noon.

● *Mast cells* (p. 128). These are increased in both the epithelium and surface secretions of asthmatics and can generate and release powerful smooth muscle and vasoactive mediators, such as histamine, prostaglandin D_2 (PGD_2) and leukotriene C_4 (LTC_4), which cause the immediate asthmatic reaction. Since potent beta-2-adrenoceptor agonists such as salbutamol have little effect on airway inflammation or hyper-reactivity but inhibit mast cell mediator release, many other factors are now considered important in the pathogenesis of late and recurrent asthmatic reactions leading to more severe asthma.

● *Epithelium.* Epithelial cells are shed during exacerbations of asthma (they can readily be identified in sputum), causing increased permeability to inhaled allergens, exposure of afferent

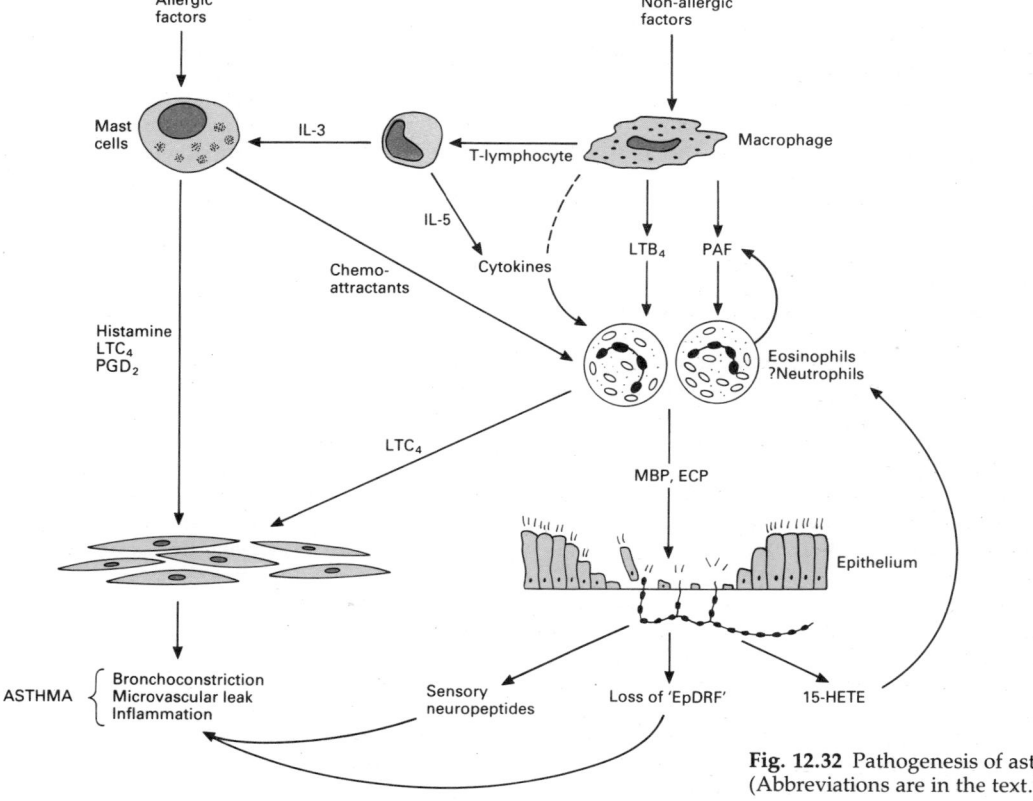

Fig. 12.32 Pathogenesis of asthma. (Abbreviations are in the text.)

nerve endings, loss of the putative epithelial-derived relaxant factor (EpDRF) and encephalinase capable of breaking down sensory neuropeptides, and generation of chemoattractant factors such as 15-hydroxyeicosatetranoic acid (15-HETE).

- *Basement membrane.* Recently biopsy studies have shown that the sub-basement membrane region, the lamina reticularis, is widened even in the mildest asthmatics owing to increased deposition of collagen Types III and V and fibronectin, indicating that inflammation occurs at the earliest stages of the disease.
- *Nerves.* Damage or loss of epithelial cells exposes C-fibre afferent nerve endings that can release the sensory neuropeptides substance P, neurokinin A and calcitonin gene-related peptide, contributing towards bronchoconstriction, microvascular leakage and mucus secretion.
- *Macrophages and lymphocytes.* These cells are abundant in the bronchial mucous membrane. Macrophages may play a particularly important role in the initial uptake and presentation of allergens to lymphocytes. They can release prostaglandins, thromboxanes, leukotriene B_4 (LTB_4) and platelet activating factor (PAF). Lymphocytes show evidence of activation and the release of lymphokines may play an important part in the migration and activation of mast cells (interleukin 3) and eosinophils (interleukin 5). The activity of both macrophages and lymphocytes is influenced by corticosteroids but not beta-2-adrenoceptor agonists.
- *Eosinophils.* These cells are found in large numbers in the bronchial secretions of asthmatics. When activated, they release LTC_4, PAF and basic proteins such as major basic protein (MBP) and eosinophil cationic protein (ECP) that are toxic to epithelial cells. Both the number and activation of eosinophils is rapidly decreased by corticosteroids.
- *Mediators.* The exact role of the many potent smooth muscle and vasoactive mediators, including LTC_4, LTD_4, thromboxanes and the sensory neuropeptides, as well as the chemoattractants LTB_4 and PAF, remains unknown and awaits the introduction of effective and specific antagonists. Studies with potent selective H_1 antagonists have shown that histamine plays only a small role in the pathogenesis of the persisting airflow limitation of asthma.

CLASSIFICATION

Traditionally, asthma has been divided into:

- Extrinsic—implying a definite external cause
- Intrinsic or cryptogenic—when no causative agent can be identified

Typically, *extrinsic asthma* occurs in atopic individuals who show positive skin-prick reactions to common inhaled allergens. Positive skin tests to inhalant allergens are shown in 90% of children, whereas only 50% of adults show this phenomenon. Eczema is often seen in childhood (see p. 1003).

Intrinsic asthma often starts in middle age. Nevertheless, many show positive skin tests and on close questioning give a history of respiratory symptoms compatible with childhood asthma.

This classification is of little value in clinical practice. Non-atopic individuals may develop asthma in middle age from extrinsic causes such as sensitization to occupational agents or aspirin intolerance, or because they were given beta-adrenoreceptor-blocking agents for concurrent hypertension or angina. Extrinsic causes must be considered in all cases of asthma and, where possible, avoided.

CLINICAL FEATURES

Patients suffering from asthma exhibit virtually indentical symptoms to those suffering from airflow limitation caused by chronic bronchitis and emphysema. Wheezing attacks and episodic shortness of breath are almost universal. Symptoms are usually worst during the night. Cough is a frequent symptom that sometimes predominates and is often misdiagnosed as being due to bronchitis. Nocturnal cough can be a presenting feature.

There is a tremendous variation in the frequency and duration of the attacks. Some patients may have only one or two attacks a year that last for a few hours, whilst others may have attacks lasting for weeks. Some patients can have chronic symptoms. Attacks may be precipitated by all the factors illustrated in Fig. 12.29; the signs of asthma are illustrated in Table 12.1.

INVESTIGATION

There is no single satisfactory diagnostic test for all asthmatic patients.

Lung function tests

Traditionally, the diagnosis of asthma is based on the demonstration of a greater than 15% improvement in FEV_1 or PEFR following the inhalation of a bronchodilator. However, this is often not present if the asthma is in remission or in very severe chronic disease, when little reversibility can be demonstrated.

Peak flow charts

Measurements of PEFR on waking, in the middle of the day, and before bed are particularly useful in demonstrating the variable airflow limitation that characterizes the disease. An example is shown in

Fig. 12.14. This technique is also of help in the longer-term assessment of the patient's disease and its response to treatment. Peak flows need to be measured over several days and preferably over a weekend or short holiday if the effect of work exposure is also being studied.

Exercise tests

These have been widely used in the diagnosis of asthma in children. Ideally, the child should run for 6 min on a treadmill at a work-load sufficient to increase the heart rate above 160 beats per min. A negative test does not rule out asthma.

Histamine or methacholine bronchial provocation tests (see p. 665)

This test indicates the presence of airway hyper-reactivity, a feature found in all asthmatics, and can be particularly useful in investigating those patients whose main symptom is cough. The test should not be performed on individuals who have poor lung function (FEV_1 < 1.5 litres).

Trial of corticosteroids

Prednisolone 30 mg orally should be given daily for 2 weeks to all patients who present with severe airflow limitation. A substantial improvement (> 15%) confirms the presence of an asthmatic element and that the administration of steroids will prove beneficial to the patient. The dose is slowly reduced over several weeks and is replaced by inhaled corticosteroids in those who will benefit.

Blood and sputum tests

Patients with asthma may have an increase in the number of eosinophils in peripheral blood (> 0.4 × 10^9/litre). This is rarely helpful in the diagnosis. The presence of large numbers of eosinophils, particularly when present in clumps in sputum, is helpful in the differential diagnosis of asthma from chronic bronchitis and emphysema.

Chest X-ray

There are no diagnostic features of asthma on the chest X-ray. A chest X-ray may be helpful in excluding a pneumothorax, which can occur as a complication, or in detecting the pulmonary shadows associated with allergic broncho-pulmonary aspergillosis.

Skin tests

Skin-prick tests should be performed in all cases of asthma to help identify extrinsic causes. Experimentally, the inhalation of an allergen that gives rise to a large weal on skin testing will almost always produce an attack of asthma in patients with the disease, but whether this occurs in everyday life depends on the concentrations encountered in the atmosphere.

Allergen provocation tests

These are seldom, if ever, required in the clinical investigation of patients. An exception is the investigation of food allergy causing asthma. This diagnosis is difficult; blind oral challenges with the food disguised in opaque gelatine capsules are necessary to confirm or refute a causative link (see p. 170).

MANAGEMENT

Asthma is an extremely common disease producing considerable morbidity. The aim of treatment must be to allow the asthmatic patient to lead as normal a life as possible. Sufficient therapy should be administered to enable the patient to keep fit and take part in sporting activities. Children should not be prevented from taking part in games because of their asthma. Since it is a chronic disease, patients must understand the purpose of each treatment and be able to take part in the management of their own disease. Many asthmatics belong to self-help groups whose aim is to further their understanding of the disease and to foster self-confidence and fitness.

Control of extrinsic factors

Avoidance of exposure to extrinsic agents remains difficult and is described in detail in the management of allergic rhinitis.

Avoidance of major allergens (e.g. the house-dust mite) can be helpful, but is difficult to achieve, short of living at high altitude where mites cannot survive, or in hospital where the environment is too hostile (see p. 652). The development of an effective acaricide harmless to man could prove valuable in the management of asthma.

Individuals intolerant to aspirin may benefit, though are rarely cured, by avoiding salicylates. Other agents, e.g. preservatives and colouring materials such as tartrazine, should be avoided if shown to be a causative factor. Fifty per cent of individuals sensitized to occupational agents may be cured if they are kept permanently away from exposure. The remaining 50% continue to have symptoms as severe as when exposed to materials at work. This is particularly so if they had been symptomatic for a long time before the diagnosis was made.

This underlines two points:

- The importance of the rapid identification of extrinsic cases of asthma and their removal wherever possible (e.g. the family pet)
- Once extrinsic asthma is initiated, it may become self-perpetuating

Hyposensitization

This form of treatment is not as effective for allergic asthma as for allergic rhinitis and is rarely advised for the management of asthma alone.

Drug treatment

The mainstay of asthma therapy is the use of therapeutic agents delivered as aerosols or powders direct into the lungs. The advantages of this method of administration are obvious. Drugs are delivered direct to the lung and the first-pass metabolism in the liver is avoided; both these factors mean that much lower doses are necessary and unwanted effects are slight.

Inhaled therapy

Use of an inhaler

- The canister is shaken.
- The patient exhales to functional residual capacity (not residual volume), i.e. normal expiration.
- The aerosol nozzle is placed to the open mouth.
- The patient simultaneously inhales rapidly and activates the aerosol.
- Inhalation is completed.
- The breath is held for 10 s if possible.
- Even with good technique only 15% of the contents is inhaled and 85% is deposited on the wall of the pharynx and ultimately swallowed.

Spacers

These are plastic conical spheres inserted between the patient's mouth and the inhaler. They are designed to reduce particle velocity so that less drug is deposited in the mouth. Spacers also diminish the need for coordination between aerosol activation and inhalation. They are useful in children and in the elderly.

The effective use of inhaled therapy depends upon careful instruction and training of the patient. At best only 15% of the aerosolized material will enter the respiratory tract. Many patients and doctors remain frightened to use aerosols because in the early 1960s there was a parallel between an increase in sudden deaths from asthma and sales of isoprenaline (a non-selective beta-adrenoceptor agonist) aerosols. In fact this was largely due to insufficient treatment of asthmatic patients with corticosteroids such that they took increasing doses of isoprenaline, but died of asthma.

Beta-2-adrenoceptor agonists. The newer bronchodilator preparations contain beta-adrenoceptor agonists that, unlike isoprenaline, are selective for the beta-2-adrenoceptors of the respiratory tract and do not stimulate the beta-1-adrenoceptors of the myocardium. These drugs are potent bronchodilators in that they cause relaxation of bronchial smooth muscle. Such treatment is very effective in relieving symptoms but does little for the underlying inflammatory nature of the disease. Inhalants such as salbutamol (100 µg per puff) or terbutaline (250 µg per puff) should be prescribed as two puffs four times daily. New highly selective and potent beta-2-adrenoceptor agonists are becoming available (salmeterol and formoterol) that importantly are effective by inhalation for up to 12 hours, reducing the need for administration to twice daily. Only the mildest asthmatics with intermittent attacks should rely upon this treatment alone. Some patients use nebulizers at home for self-administration of salbutamol or terbutaline. Such treatment is very effective owing to the high dose delivered, but patients must not rely on repeated home administration of nebulized beta-2-adrenoceptor agonists for worsening asthma, and must be encouraged to seek medical advice urgently if their condition does not improve. Tablets of beta-2-adrenoceptor agonists are less effective than when inhaled. To help those who cannot coordinate activation of the aerosol and inhalation, new devices that are breath-activated have been developed.

Anti-cholinergic bronchodilators. Muscarinic receptors are found in the respiratory tract; large airways contain mainly M3 receptors whereas the peripheral lung tissue contains M3 and M1 receptors. Non-selective muscarinic antagonists such as atropine were used for relief of bronchoconstriction whilst currently ipratropium bromide 20–40 µg three or four times daily by aerosol inhalation is used and is also additive to β adrenoreceptor stimulants.

Anti-inflammatory drugs. The exact mode of action of sodium cromoglycate (a mast cell stabilizer) remains unknown. This drug is particularly effective in patients with mild but frequent asthma. It must be taken regularly either in the form of a Spincap containing 20 mg or in aerosol form from a metered-dose inhaler delivering 5 mg per puff. The dose should be two puffs four times daily from an inhaler, or one Spincap three or four times daily.

Ketotifen is a potent antihistamine that is also considered to have mast-cell stabilizing properties. The indications for its use are identical to those for sodium cromoglycate. Its advantage is that it can be given as a single 1 mg tablet twice daily and therefore can be given to small children who find it difficult to use a Spinhaler or a metered-dose inhaler, and it may be effective against allergic disease affecting the eyes, nose and lungs.

Inhaled corticosteroids. All patients who have regular persisting symptoms in spite of treatment with a beta-2-adrenoceptor agonist and sodium cromoglycate or ketotifen need regular treatment with inhaled corticosteroids. Beclomethasone dipropionate is available in doses of 50 and 250 µg per puff, and budesonide is available in doses of 200 µg per metered inhalation. High-dose beclomethasone and budesonide should be reserved for patients who have not responded to beclomethasone 50 µg per puff. The unwanted effects of inhaled corticosteroids are oral candidiasis, which may develop in 5% of patients, and hoarseness due to the effect of corticosteroids on the laryngeal muscles. Inhaled corticosteroids have now been widely used for 15 years and no significant long-term unwanted effects have been detected.

Oral corticosteroids. Use of oral corticosteroids is necessary for those individuals not controlled on inhaled corticosteroids. The dose should be kept as low as possible to avoid side-effects. The effect of short-term treatment with prednisolone 30 mg daily is shown in Fig. 12.14. Some patients require continuing treatment with oral corticosteroids. Recent studies suggest that treatment with low doses of methotrexate (15 mg weekly) can significantly reduce the dose of prednisolone needed to control the disease.

Antibiotics. There is no evidence that antibiotics are helpful in the management of patients who suffer from properly diagnosed asthma. However, wheezing frequently occurs in exacerbations of chronic bronchitis and emphysema associated with infected sputum.

Yellow or green sputum containing eosinophils and bronchial epithelial cells may be coughed up in acute exacerbations of asthma. This is not due to bacterial infection and antibiotics are not required.

Management of severe asthma

Although this condition is often called 'status asthmaticus', it is better considered as severe asthma that has not been controlled by the patient's use of medication. Patients with severe asthma have:

- Tachycardia.
- Pulsus paradoxicus (> 10 mm Hg). In very severe asthma no paradoxicus is detected.
- Wheezing. Chest may be silent in severe asthma owing to insufficient airflow.

PEFR should be measured in all patients presenting with severe asthma, and if below 150 L·min^{-1} (in adults), the patient should be admitted to hospital.

Treatment is commenced with 5 mg of nebulized salbutamol or terbutaline and a chest X-ray is taken to exclude a pneumothorax. If no improvement occurs with nebulized therapy, salbutamol or terbutaline should be administered by intravenous infusion. Intravenous aminophylline is now not used for severe asthma because of its narrow therapeutic index. Hydrocortisone 200 mg i.v. should be administered 4-hourly for 24 h and 30 mg of predisolone should be given orally daily. Patients who do not respond to this regimen may require ventilation.

Treatment of severe asthma

At home

- The patient is assessed. Tachycardia with pulsus paradoxicus and cyanosis indicate a severe attack.
- If the PEFR is less than 150 L·min^{-1} (in adults), an ambulance should be called. All doctors should carry peak flow meters.
- Nebulized salbutamol or terbutaline 5 mg is administered.
- Hydrocortisone sodium succinate 200 mg i.v. is given.
- Oxygen is given if available.

In hospital

- The patient is reassessed.
- Oxygen is given via a variable-performance mask.
- The PEFR is measured using a low-reading peak flow meter, as an ordinary meter only measures from 60 L·min^{-1} upwards.
- Nebulized salbutamol or terbutaline 5 mg is given initially.
- Hydrocortisone 200 mg i.v. is given 4-hourly for 24 h, followed by prednisolone 30 mg orally daily for 2 weeks.
- Arterial blood gases are measured; if the $P_a CO_2$ is greater than 7 kPa, ventilation should be considered.
- A chest X-ray is performed to exclude pneumothorax.
- Nebulized salbutamol or terbutaline 5 mg is administered 4-hourly.
- One of the following intravenous infusions is given if no improvement is seen:
  Salbutamol 3–20 µg·min^{-1}, or
  Terbutaline 1.5 µg·min^{-1}

Patients should be kept in hospital for at least 5 days, since the majority of sudden deaths occur 2–5 days after admission. Oral corticosteroids should be gradually reduced on an outpatient basis until an appropriate maintenance dose or substitution by inhaled corticosteroid aerosols can be achieved.

If the patient's PEFR is greater than 150 L·min^{-1}, patients may improve dramatically on nebulized therapy and may not require hospital admission. Their regular treatment should be increased, probably to include treatment for 2 weeks with 15–30 mg of prednisolone followed by a gradual reduction in the oral dose and substitution by an inhaled corticosteroid preparation.

PROGNOSIS

Although asthma often improves in children as they reach their teens, it is now realized that the disease frequently returns in the second, third and fourth decades. Overall, in adults, there is a tendency for asthma to improve with age.

Diseases of the lung parenchyma

PNEUMONIAS

Pneumonia may be defined as an inflammation of the substance of the lungs. It is usually caused by bacteria. Clinically it presents as an acute illness characterized in the majority of cases by the presence of cough, purulent sputum and fever together with physical signs or radiological changes compatible with consolidation of the lung.

The advent of antibiotics might have been expected to decrease dramatically the mortality from pneumonia. However, mortality statistics obtained from death certificates show the reverse. This is because the dramatic decrease in deaths from pneumonia in children under 10 years has been counterbalanced by an increase in deaths from pneumonia in individuals over the age of 70 years.

CLASSIFICATION

Pneumonia can be classified both anatomically and on the basis of the aetiology.

Site

Pneumonias are either localized, e.g. affecting the whole of one lobe, or diffuse, when they primarily affect the lobules of the lung, often in association with the bronchi and bronchioles, a condition referred to as 'bronchopneumonia'.

Aetiology

An aetiological factor can be discovered in approximately 75% of patients. The term 'atypical pneumonias' was used to describe pneumonia caused by agents such as *Mycoplasma*, influenza A virus, *Chlamydia* and *Coxiella burnetii*. These types of pneumonia alone account for almost one-fifth of the cases of pneumonia (see Table 12.8) and the term 'atypical' should be dropped. Pneumonias may also result from:

- Chemical causes, e.g. aspiration of vomit (see p. 676)
- Radiotherapy (see p. 693)
- Allergic mechanisms (see p. 687)

Mycobacterium tuberculosis is an important cause of pneumonia; it is considered separately, since both its mode of presentation and its treatment are very different from the infective agents shown in Table 12.8.

Precipitating factors

- *Streptococcus pneumoniae*—often follows influenza or parainfluenza viral infection

- Hospitalized 'ill' patients—often infected with Gram-negative organisms
- Cigarette smoking
- Alcohol
- Bronchiectasis (e.g. in cystic fibrosis)
- Bronchial obstruction (e.g. carcinoma)—occasionally associated with infection with 'non-pathogenic' organisms
- Immunosuppression (e.g. AIDS or treatment with cytotoxic agents)—organisms include *Pneumocystis carinii*, *Mycobacterium avium*, cytomegalovirus
- Intravenous drug abuse—frequently associated with *Staphylococcus aureus* infection
- Inhalation from oesophageal obstruction—often associated with infection with anaerobes

CLINICAL PRESENTATION

The clinical presentation varies according to the immune state of the patient and the infecting agent. In the commonest type of pneumonia—caused by *Streptococcus pneumoniae*—there is often a preceding history of a viral infection. The patient rapidly becomes more ill with a high temperature (up to 39.5°C), pleuritic pain and a dry cough. A day or two later, rusty-coloured sputum is produced and at about the same time the patient may develop labial herpes simplex. The patient breathes rapidly and shallowly, the affected side of the chest moves less, and signs of consolidation may be present together with a pleural rub.

INVESTIGATION

Chest X-ray confirms the area of consolidation but radiological changes lag behind the clinical course so that X-ray changes may be minimal at the start of illness. Conversely, consolidation may remain on the chest X-ray for several weeks after the patient is clinically cured. The chest X-ray should always return to normal by 6 weeks, except in patients with severe airflow limitation. Persistent changes on the chest X-ray after this time suggest a bronchial abnormality, usually a carcinoma, with persisting secondary pneumonia. Chest X-rays should rarely be repeated more frequently than at weekly intervals during the acute illness and then at 6 weeks after discharge from hospital.

In *Streptococcus pneumoniae* pneumonia, there is often a white blood cell count that is greater than 15×10^9/litre (90% polymorphonuclear leucocytosis) and an ESR greater than 100 mm·h^{-1}.

The individual features of different pneumonias are given below. The overall investigation and management is shown in Fig. 12.33 and discussed on p. 677.

Mycoplasma pneumonia

This is a common cause of pneumonia. It often occurs in patients in their teens and twenties,

Table 12.8 The aetiology of pneumonia in the UK.

Infecting agent	Frequency as a cause of pneumonia (%)	Clinical circumstance
Streptococcus pneumoniae	50	Community pneumonia, patients usually previously fit
Mycoplasma pneumoniae	6	As above
Influenza A virus (usually with a bacterial component)	5	As above
Haemophilus influenzae	5	Pre-existing lung disease chronic bronchitis and emphysema
Chlamydia psittaci	3	Contact with birds (though not inevitable)
Staphylococcus aureus	2	Children, intravenous drug abusers, associated with influenza virus infections
Legionella pneumophila	2	Institutional outbreaks (hospitals and hotels), sporadic, endemic
Coxiella burnetii	1	Abattoir and animal-hide workers
Pseudomonas aeruginosa	< 1	Cystic fibrosis
Pneumocystis carinii *Actinomyces israelii* *Nocardia asteroides* Cytomegalovirus *Aspergillus fumigatus*	< 1	AIDS, lymphomas, leukaemias, use of cytotoxic drugs and corticosteroids
Anaerobic organisms	< 1	Inhalation pneumonia, alcohol abuse, postoperative
None isolated	25	—

frequently amongst those living in boarding institutions. Generalized features such as headaches and malaise often precede the chest symptoms by 1–5 days. Cough may not be obvious initially and physical signs in the chest may be scanty.

On chest X-ray, usually only one of the lower lobes is involved but sometimes there may be dramatic shadowing in both lower lobes. There is frequently no correlation between the X-ray appearances and the clinical state of the patient.

The white blood cell count is not raised. Cold agglutinins occur in half of the cases. The diagnosis is confirmed by a rising antibody titre. Treatment is with erythromycin 500 mg × 4 daily for 7–10 days. Tetracycline is effective.

Although most patients recover in 10–14 days,

the disease can be protracted, with cough and X-ray appearance lasting for weeks and relapses occurring. Lung abscesses and pleural effusions are rare.

Extrapulmonary complications can occur at any time during the illness and occasionally dominate the clinical picture. Most are rare but they include:

- Myocarditis and pericarditis
- Rashes and erythema multiforme
- Haemolytic anaemia and thrombocytopenia
- Myalgia and arthralgia
- Meningo-encephalitis and other neurological abnormalities
- Gastrointestinal symptoms (e.g. vomiting, diarrhoea)

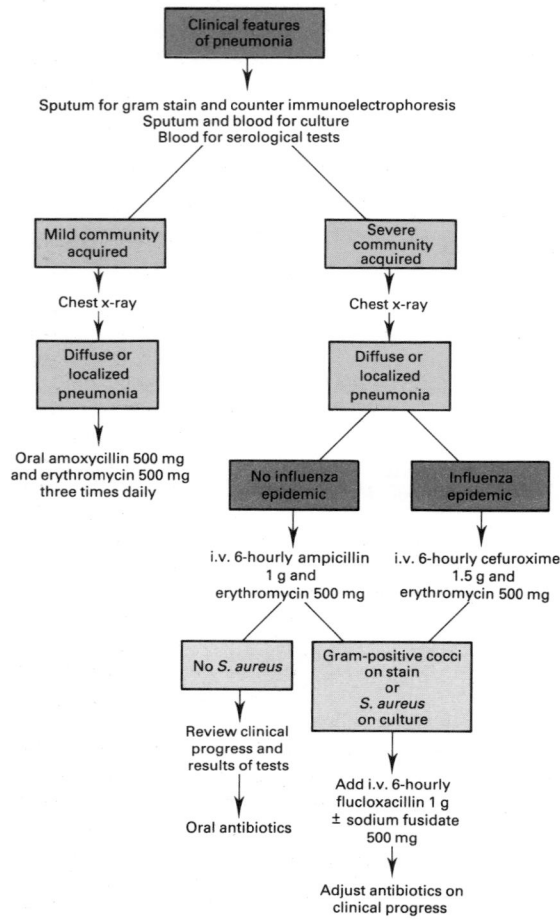

Fig. 12.33 Algorithm for the management of pneumonia (see also p. 677).

Viral pneumonia

Viral pneumonia is uncommon in adults, bacteria being the usual cause of the pneumonia *per se*. Influenza A virus or adenovirus infection can occasionally produce pneumonia.

Other pneumonias

Haemophilus influenzae

H. influenzae is frequently identified in the yellow-green sputum produced during exacerbation of chronic bronchitis. It is therefore not surprising that this organism may be the cause of pneumonia in people suffering from chronic bronchitis and emphysema. The pneumonia can be diffuse or confined to one lobe. There are no special features to separate it from other bacterial causes of pneumonia. It responds well to treatment with amoxycillin.

Chlamydia psittaci (see p. 55)

Typically the individual has been working with infected birds, especially parrots, but a history of contact is not always elicited. The incubation period is 1–2 weeks and the disease may pursue a very low-grade course over several months. Symptoms include malaise, high fever, cough and muscular pains. The liver and spleen are occasionally enlarged and scanty 'rose spots' may be seen on the abdomen. The chest X-ray shows segmental or a diffuse pneumonia. Occasionally the illness presents with a high, swinging fever and dramatic prostration with photophobia and neck stiffness that can be confused with meningitis. The diagnosis is confirmed by the demonstration of a rising titre of complement-fixing antibody. Tetracycline is the antibiotic of choice.

Staphylococci

Staphylococcus aureus normally only causes a pneumonia after a preceding influenzal viral illness. The infection starts in the bronchi, leading to patchy areas of consolidation in one or more lobes, which break down to form abscesses. These may appear as cysts on the chest X-ray.

Pneumothorax, effusion and empyemas are frequent. Septicaemia develops with metastatic abscesses in other organs.

Fulminating staphylococcal pneumonia occurring in influenza epidemics can lead to death in hours. All patients with this type of pneumonia are very ill; intravenous antibiotics must be administered promptly, but are not always effective.

Areas of pneumonia (septic infarcts) are also seen in staphylococcal septicaemia. This is frequently seen in intravenous drug abusers and also in patients with central catheters being used for parenteral nutrition. The infected puncture site is the source of the *Staphylococcus*. Pulmonary symptoms are often few but breathlessness and cough occur and the chest X-ray reveals areas of consolidation. Abscess formation is frequent.

Diagnosis and treatment are shown in Fig. 12.33.

Coxiella burnetti (Q-fever) (see p. 55)

The patient develops systemic symptoms of fever, malaise and headache, often associated with multiple lesions on the chest X-ray. The illness may run a chronic course and is occasionally associated with endocarditis. Diagnosis is made by an increase in the titre of complement-fixing antibody, and erythromycin or tetracycline is the usual treatment.

Legionella pneumophila (see p. 39)

Three epidemiological patterns of this disease are recognized:

● Outbreaks amongst previously fit individuals staying in hotels, institutions or hospitals where the shower facilities or cooling systems have been contaminated with the organism

- Sporadic cases occurring in many parts of the world where the source of the infection is unknown
- Outbreaks occurring in immunocompromised patients and in middle-aged and elderly male smokers

Legionella grows well in water over 25°C in temperature, and the infection is almost certainly spread by the aerosol route. Adequate chlorination and temperature control are important factors in the prevention of the disease.

The incubation period is 2–10 days. Males are affected twice as commonly as females. The infection may be mild, but the characteristic picture is of malaise, myalgia, headache and a fever with rigors and a pyrexia of up to 40°C. Half of the patients have gastrointestinal symptoms, with nausea, vomiting, diarrhoea and abdominal pain. Patients may be acutely ill, with mental confusion and other neurological signs. Haematuria occurs and occasionally renal failure.

The patient is tachypnoeic with initially a dry cough that later may become productive and purulent. The chest X-ray usually shows unilateral lobar and then multilobar shadowing, sometimes with a small pleural effusion. Cavitation is rare.

A strong presumptive diagnosis of *Legionella pneumophila* infection is possible in the majority of patients if they have three of the four following features:

- A prodromal virus-like illness
- A dry cough, confusion or diarrhoea
- Lymphopenia without marked leucocytosis
- Hyponatraemia

Hypoalbuminaemia and abnormal levels of liver enzymes are common in this disease. The diagnosis is confirmed by a change in antibody titre, but the quickest way is by the direct immunofluorescent staining of the organism in the pleural fluid, sputum or bronchial washings. A Gram stain does not detect the organism. Culture is possible but takes up to 3 weeks.

The organism is sensitive to erythromycin, which is the antibiotic of choice. Rifampicin is also being used. Mortality can be up to 30% in elderly patients but most patients recover spontaneously.

Gram-negative bacteria

These are the cause of many hospital-acquired pneumonias but they are occasionally responsible for cases in the community.

Klebsiella pneumoniae. Pneumonia due to *Klebsiella* usually occurs in the elderly with a history of heart or lung disease, diabetes, alcohol excess or malignancy. The onset is often sudden, with severe systemic upset. The sputum is purulent, gelatinous or blood-stained. The upper lobes are more commonly affected and the consolidation is often extensive. There is often swelling of the infected lobe so that on the lateral chest X-ray there is bulging of the fissures. The organism can be found in the sputum or in the blood. Treatment is dependent on the sensitivity of the organism, but a cephalosporin or chloramphenicol is usually required. The mortality is high, partly owing to the presence of an underlying condition.

Pseudomonas aeruginosa. Pneumonia due to this organism is of considerable significance in patients with cystic fibrosis, since it correlates with a worsening clinical condition and mortality. It is also seen in patients with neutropenia following cytotoxic chemotherapy. The isolation of *Pseudomonas aeruginosa* must be interpreted with care because the organism grows well on bacterial culture medium and may simply represent contamination from the upper airways. *Pseudomonas aeruginosa* infection requires combination treatment with tobramycin 3–5 mg·kg^{-1} i.v. or i.m. daily in 8-hourly doses together with carbenicillin 5 g i.v. 4–6 hourly. These antibiotics can be inhaled direct into the lung via nebulizers by patients with cystic fibrosis (see p. 663).

Pseudomonal infection should respond to the above regimen, but modifications may have to be made in the light of sensitivity testing. Tobramycin is nephrotoxic and produces vestibular damage, so that blood levels should be monitored. Two new antipseudomonal penicillins have been introduced—azlocillin and ticarcillin—both of which have greater activity than carbenicillin against these organisms. Pseudomonal and other Gram-negative infections also respond well to treatment with the 4-quinolone antibiotic ciprofloxacin (100–200 mg i.v. over 30–60 min twice daily) or ceftazidime (2 g bolus i.v. 8-hourly).

Branhamella catarrhalis. This organism, previously known as *Neisseria catarrhalis*, has been found to be associated with exacerbations of chronic bronchitis and occasionally with fatal pneumonia. An important point about this organism is that some strains produce a β-lactamase capable of destroying amoxycillin. The exact role of this organism in bronchopulmonary infection remains to be determined.

Anaerobic bacteria

Infections with these organisms usually occur in those with an underlying condition, e.g. diabetes, and are often associated with aspiration. Bacteroides is the commonest organism and is sensitive to metronidazole. The prognosis depends largely on the precipitating cause.

Pneumonias due to opportunistic infections
These are commonly becoming recognized in the immunocompromised patient.

Pneumocystis carinii. It is by far the commonest opportunistic infection, accounting for 80% of the cases of pneumonia in patients with acquired immunodeficiency syndrome (AIDS) (see p. 68). It is also seen in patients receiving immunosuppressive therapy. In the poorer parts of the world, however, *Pneumocystis* pneumonia is not infrequently found in malnourished children.

It is likely that infection with the organism occurs by inhalation, perhaps in childhood, and the organism may remain latent for many years, being reactivated when immunosuppression occurs. Clinically the pneumonia is associated with a high fever, breathlessness and dry cough. In patients with AIDS, however, the clinical features are different, with a much more insidious onset, though fever, dyspnoea, dry cough, weight loss and diarrhoea do occur. Marked hypoxaemia is characteristic.

The typical radiographic appearance is of diffuse bilateral alveolar and interstitial shadowing beginning in the perihilar regions and spreading out in a butterfly pattern.

Investigation includes fibreoptic bronchoscopy with transbronchial biopsies and bronchial washing and aspiration; the diagnosis can be made in 95% of cases by this method. Shadowing on the chest X-ray in AIDS patients, though most commonly due to *Pneumocystis carinii* can result from:

- Cytomegalovirus
- *Mycobacterium avium intracellulare*
- *Mycobacterium tuberculosis*
- *Legionella pneumophila*
- Pyogenic bacteria
- Kaposi's sarcoma
- Lymphoid interstitial pneumonia
- Non-specific interstitial pneumonitis

Treatment of *Pneumocystis carinii* is with high-dose co-trimoxazole (120 mg·kg^{-1} daily in divided doses) given initially intravenously for 2 weeks and continued for 1 week orally. Unwanted effects occur in up to 80% of cases and include nausea, skin rashes and agranulocytosis. Recently nebulized pentamidine 600 mg once daily for 21 days has been shown to be effective in milder cases. It is almost without unwanted effects, apart from cough during administration that can be reduced by previous nebulized salbutamol. Either low-dose co-trimoxazole (960 mg once daily) or once-monthly nebulized pentamidine have been shown to help prevent recurrence of *Pneumocystis carinii* pneumonia in AIDS patients.

The mortality partly depends on the underlying condition; with treatment it is approximately 25%.

Actinomyces israeli (see p. 40). The clinical picture is that of severe pneumonia, lung abscess or empyema.

Nocardia asteroides. This produces a similar picture to *Actinomyces*, though of greater severity. The chest X-ray often shows irregular opacities in one or both lungs, particularly in the mid-zones.

Cytomegalovirus (see p. 58). Bronchitis and pneumonia may occur but these are usually a more minor part of the generalized systemic illness.

Aspergillus fumigatus (see p. 687). This fungus gives rise to a widespread invasion of lung tissue in patients who are immunocompromised. It is a serious pneumonia that is usually rapidly fatal.

Rare infective causes of pneumonia

Pneumonia may be seen in the course of infection by *Bordetella pertussis*, typhoid and paratyphoid bacillus, brucellosis, leptospirosis and a number of viral infections including measles, chickenpox and glandular fever. It is not usually a major feature. Details of these infections are described in Chapter 1.

Aspiration pneumonia

The acute aspiration of gastric contents into the lungs can produce an extremely severe and sometimes fatal illness due to the intense destructiveness of gastric acid—the Mendelson syndrome. It can complicate anaesthesia, particularly during pregnancy.

In the absence of a tracheo-oesophageal fistula, aspiration only occurs during periods of impaired consciousness (e.g. during sleep), in reflux oesophagitis or oesophageal stricture, or in bulbar palsy. Because of the bronchial anatomy, the most usual site for spillage is the posterior segment of the right lower lobe. The persistent pneumonia is often due to anaerobes and it may progress to lung abscess or even bronchiectasis. It is vital to identify any underlying problem, since appropriate corrective measures can lead to resolution of the pulmonary problems.

Diffuse pneumonia (bronchopneumonia)

Diffuse pneumonia is very common. It is differentiated from severe bronchitis by signs of bronchial breathing or patchy shadows on the chest X-ray.

Widespread diffuse pneumonia is a common terminal event, largely resulting from an inability of patients dying from other conditions (e.g. cancer) to cough up retained secretions, allowing infection to develop throughout the lungs. Treatment in this situation is rarely appropriate.

Complications of pneumonia

Lung abscess

This term is used to describe severe localized suppuration in the lung associated with cavity formation on the chest X-ray, often with the presence of a fluid level, and not due to tuberculosis.

Causes of lung abscesses are many, but the commonest is aspiration, particularly amongst alcoholics following aspiration pneumonia. Lung abscesses also frequently follow the inhalation of a foreign body into a bronchus and occasionally occur when the bronchus is obstructed by a bronchial carcinoma.

Abscesses may develop during the course of specific pneumonias, particularly when the infecting agent is *Staphylococcus pyogenes* or *Klebsiella pneumoniae*. Septic emboli, usually staphylococci, result in multiple lung abscesses. Infarcted areas of lung may occasionally cavitate and rarely become infected. Amoebic abscesses may occasionally develop in the right lower lobe following transdiaphragmatic spread from an amoebic liver abscess.

The clinical features are those of persisting and worsening pneumonia associated with the production of large quantities of sputum, which is often foul-smelling owing to the growth of anaerobic organisms. There is usually a swinging fever. Chronic or subacute lung abscesses follow an inadequately treated pneumonia. Fever, malaise and weight loss occur. The chest signs may be few but clubbing often develops. The patient is often anaemic with a high ESR.

Empyema

Empyema means the presence of pus within the pleural cavity. This usually arises after the rupture of a lung abscess into the pleural space or from bacterial spread from a severe pneumonia. Typically an empyema cavity becomes infected with anaerobic organisms and the patient is severely ill with a high fever and a neutrophil granulocytosis.

Investigation

Bacteriological investigation of lung abscess and empyema is best conducted on specimens obtained by transtracheal aspiration, bronchoscopy or percutaneous transthoracic aspiration.

Treatment

Although anaerobic organisms are found in up to 70% of lung abscesses and empyemas, there is usually a mixed flora, often with aeorbes, particularly *Streptococcus milleri*. Anaerobic cocci, black-pigmented bacteroids and fusobacteria are the commonest anaerobes found.

Antibiotics should be given to cover both aerobic and anaerobic organisms; prolonged courses are often necessary. Treatment should be amoxycillin 1 g i.v. 6-hourly, erythromycin 500 mg i.v. 8-hourly and metronidazole 500 mg i.v. 8-hourly for 5 days, followed by oral amoxycillin and metronidazole for a prolonged period. Abscesses occasionally require surgery.

Empyemas should be treated by prompt tube drainage or rib resection and drainage of the empyema cavity followed by appropriate antibiotic treatment for up to 6 weeks.

Management of pneumonia

This is shown in the algorithm given in Fig. 12.33.

Sputum should always be sent for culture, but in mild cases treatment should be started immediately with oral amoxycillin and erythromycin.

More severe cases need to be admitted to hospital and a chest X-ray performed. Other investigations required are:

- Sputum—Gram stain and culture
- White blood-cell count is raised above 15×10^9/L (with a high neutrophil count) in more than 50% of patients with pneumococcal pneumonia but only in 10% of cases of *Legionella* or *Mycoplasma* pneumonia
- Blood culture

Treatment should be started immediately (without waiting for the result of these investigations). In more than 20% of cases, more than one organism is involved.

Further investigations may be necessary for the diagnosis of certain types of pneumonia:

- *Mycoplasma* antibodies (IgM and IgG)—in acute and convalescent samples. Cold agglutinins present in 50%.
- *Legionella* antibodies—immunofluorescent tests.
- Pneumococcal antigen—latex tests on sputum, urine and serum (three to four times more sensitive than sputum or blood cultures).

A high percentage of organisms causing pneumonia (e.g. *Mycoplasma pneumoniae*, *Haemophilus influenzae* and *Legionella pneumophila*) will not respond to penicillin. This drug should no longer be prescribed and should be replaced by a combination of bactericidal antibiotics that cover the commonest organisms. Treatment is commenced with ampicillin 1 g i.v. 6-hourly together with erythromycin 500 mg i.v. 6-hourly. The purpose of this programme is to treat pneumonia with sufficient doses of appropriate antibiotics at the earliest stage. The treatment can always be modified and reduced in the light of clinical progress and subsequent bacteriological and serological findings.

The chances of identifying a causative organism are greatly decreased in individuals who have received antibiotics in the week prior to their admission to hospital.

The overall mortality for pneumonia is currently 5% but for pneumonia due to *Staphyloccus aureus* it is in excess of 25%. Patients who die from pneumonia usually have not received the appropriate antibiotics in sufficient doses before or during the early stages of hospital admission.

Penicillin allergy

This often poses a difficult problem. Only about 1 in 10 individuals who claim to have developed an allergic response to penicillins actually show such a reaction on further exposure. Nevertheless, a history of penicillin allergy cannot be overlooked and a cephalosporin, e.g. oral cefaclor 250 mg 8-hourly or i.v. cefuroxime 1.5 g 6–8-hourly, should be given instead of amoxycillin despite a 10% cross-reactivity between the two groups. If the patient has a definite history of severe reaction, then erythromycin and chloramphenicol should be used, depending on the severity of the disease.

General measures

These include care of the mouth and skin. Fluids should be encouraged, to avoid dehydration. The patient is normally nursed sitting up or in the most comfortable position. Cough should normally be encouraged, but if it is unproductive and distressing, suppressants such as codeine linctus can be given.

Pleuritic pain may require analgesia, but powerful analgesia (e.g. opiates) should be used with care because they cause respiratory depression.

In severe hypoxia, oxygen therapy should be given; however, since the hypoxia is often due to a physiological shunt (see p. 634), it may make little difference to the hypoxaemia.

Severe hospital-acquired pneumonias

These should be treated in the same way as severe community-acquired pneumonias having taken appropriate samples for culture and sensitivities. However, as anaerobic organisms may be involved, the treatment should include metronidazole if the clinical state does not improve. Immunosuppressed patients may require very high-dose broad-spectrum antibiotics as well as antifungal and antiviral agents.

TUBERCULOSIS (see p. 40)

Tuberculosis is a disease of great antiquity and has even been found in Egyptian mummies. It remains a major disease of mankind on a world-wide basis. Indeed, until 50 years ago virtually everyone throughout the world was infected at some time in their lives. Fortunately, effective host defence mechanisms and the small number of infecting bacilli meant that most people overcame the primary infection, and it was only when host defences were poor or the infecting dose was large that clinical disease occurred. In Western countries, better nutrition and improved social conditions have meant that the disease is now rarely encountered in the indigenous population; however it may still be seen in conditions of social deprivation, where immunosuppressive drugs have altered the host defence mechanisms, or in acquired immunodeficiency syndrome (AIDS). Nevertheless, estimates suggest that, world-wide, ten million people develop clinical tuberculosis annually, with three million dying from the disease.

The risk of developing tuberculosis is between 20 and 50 times greater in the developing than in the Western World.

EPIDEMIOLOGY

In the UK the incidence of tuberculosis in immigrants from the Asian subcontinent and West Indies is 40 and four times as common, respectively, as in the native white population. This has led to great variation in the frequency of the disease in different areas of the UK.

Mortality from tuberculosis in the UK has fallen dramatically from 150 per 100 000 at the turn of the century to less than 5 per 100 000 in the 1980s. This steady decline was occurring long before the advent of antituberculous treatment, though this did cause an accelerated decrease in death rates. The fall in mortality is particularly marked in the younger age group and is less prominent in older people.

PATHOLOGY

The first infection with *Mycobacterium tuberculosis* is known as primary tuberculosis. It is usually subpleural, often in the mid to upper zones. Within an hour of reaching the lung, tubercle bacilli reach the draining lymph nodes at the hilum of the lung and a few escape into the bloodstream.

The initial reaction comprises exudation and infiltration with neutrophil granulocytes. These are rapidly replaced by macrophages that ingest the bacilli. These interact with T lymphocytes with the development of cellular immunity that can be demonstrated 3–8 weeks after the initial infection by the development of a positive reaction in the skin to an intradermal injection of protein from tubercle bacilli (tuberculin).

At this stage the classical pathology of tuberculosis can be seen. Granulomatous lesions consist of a central area of necrotic material of a cheesy nature, called caseation, surrounded by epithelioid cells and Langhans' giant cells with multiple nuclei, both cells being derived from the macro-

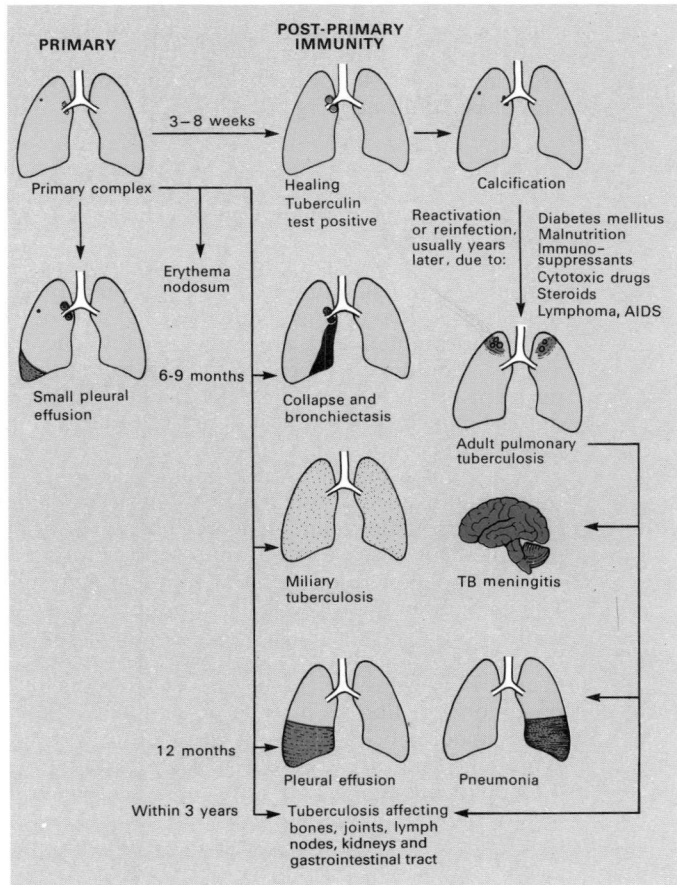

Fig. 12.34 The manifestations of primary and post-primary tuberculosis.

phage. Lymphocytes are present and there is a varying degree of fibrosis. Subsequently the caseated areas heal completely and many become calcified. It is now known that at least 20% of these calcified primary lesions contain tubercle bacilli, initially lying dormant but capable of being activated by depression of the host defence system. Reactivation leads to typical post-primary pulmonary tuberculosis with cavitation, usually in the apex or upper zone of the lung. 'Post-primary tuberculosis' refers to all forms of tuberculosis that occur after the first few weeks of the primary infection when immunity to the mycobacterium has developed.

CLINICAL FEATURES AND INVESTIGATION

Primary tuberculosis is symptomless in the great majority of individuals. Occasionally there may be a vague illness, sometimes associated with cough and wheeze. A small transient pleural effusion or erythema nodosum may occasionally occur, both representing allergic manifestations of the infective process.

Enlargement of lymph nodes compressing the bronchi can give rise to collapse of segments or lobes of the lung. Apart from cough and a monophonic wheeze, the individual remains remarkably well and the collapse disappears as the primary complex heals. Occasionally, persistent collapse can give rise to subsequent bronchiectasis, often in the middle lobe (Brock's syndrome).

The manifestations of primary and post-primary tuberculosis are shown in Fig. 12.34, together with the times when they usually occur. Extrapulmonary manifestations are summarized on p. 40. Miliary tuberculosis can occur within 3 years of the primary infection, or can occur much later as a manifestation of reactivation or, rarely, reinfection with tubercle bacillus.

Reactivation in the lung, or indeed in any extrapulmonary location, can occur as immunity wanes, usually with age and chronic ill-health (see Fig. 12.34).

Miliary tuberculosis

This disease is the result of acute diffuse dissemination of tubercle bacilli via the bloodstream. It can be a difficult diagnosis to make, particularly in older people, where it is particularly covert. This form of disseminated tuberculosis is universally fatal without treatment.

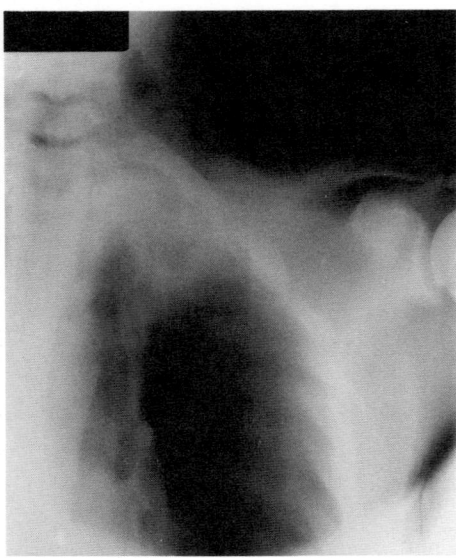

Fig. 12.35 Chest X-ray showing tuberculosis of left upper lobe with cavitation.

It may present in an entirely non-specific manner with the gradual onset of vague ill-health, loss of weight and then fever. Occasionally the disease presents as tuberculosis meningitis. Usually there are no abnormal physical signs in the early stages, although eventually the spleen and liver become enlarged. Choroidal tubercles are seen in the eyes. These lesions are about a quarter of the diameter of the optic disc and are yellowish and slightly shiny and raised in nature, later becoming white in the centre. There may be one or many in each eye.

The chest X-ray may be entirely normal in miliary tuberculosis as the tubercles are not visible until the miliary shadows are 1 or 2 mm in diameter; they have a hard outline. The lesions can increase in size up to 5–10 mm. Sarcoidosis and staphylococcal or mycoplasma pneumonia may mimic the chest X-ray appearance of miliary tuberculosis.

The Mantoux test is positive but may occasionally be negative in people with very severe disease. Transbronchial biopsies may frequently be positive before any abnormality is visible on the chest X-ray. CT scanning may reveal lung parenchymal abnormalities at an earlier stage.

Biopsy and culture of liver and bone marrow may be necessary in patients presenting with a pyrexia of unknown origin (PUO). In the past, a trial of antituberculous therapy was often used in individuals with a PUO. The fever should settle within 2 weeks of starting chemotherapy if it is due to tuberculosis. This approach is still occasionally used in susceptible individuals when a diagnosis cannot be confirmed.

Pulmonary tuberculosis
Typically there is gradual onset of symptoms over weeks or months. Tiredness, malaise, anorexia and loss of weight together with a fever and cough remain the outstanding features of pulmonary tuberculosis. Drenching night sweats are now rather uncommon and are more usually due to anxiety. Sputum in tuberculosis may be mucoid, purulent or blood-stained. Many patients suffer a dull ache in the chest and it is not uncommon for patients to complain of recurrent colds.

A pleural effusion or pneumonia can be the presenting feature of tuberculosis. Physical examination is of little value. Finger clubbing is only present if the disease is advanced and associated with considerable production of purulent sputum. There are often no physical signs in the chest even in the presence of extensive radiological changes, though occasionally persistent crackles may be heard. Physical signs of an associated effusion, pneumonia or fibrosis may be present.

An abnormal chest X-ray is often found with no symptoms, but the reverse is extremely rare—pulmonary tuberculosis is unlikely in the absence of any radiographic abnormality. The chest X-ray (Fig. 12.35) typically shows patchy or nodular shadows in the upper zones, loss of volume, and fibrosis with or without cavitation. Calcification may be present. The X-ray appearances alone may strongly suggest tuberculosis, but every effort must be made to obtain microbiological evidence. The X-rays do not give an indication of the activity of the disease. Very similar chest X-ray appearances occur in histoplasmosis and other fungal infections of the lung, including cryptococcosis, coccidioidomycosis and aspergillosis.

Lymph node tuberculosis manifestation
The patient presents with a tender lump, usually supraclavicular or in the anterior triangle of the neck. This form of tuberculosis is discussed on p. 41.

DIAGNOSIS

- Chest X-ray.
- The sputum is stained with Ziehl–Nielsen (ZN) stain for acid and alcohol-fast bacilli (AAFB).
- The sputum is cultured on Dover's or Lowenstein–Jensen medium for 4–8 weeks. Cultures to determine the sensitivity of the bacillus to

antibiotics take a further 3–4 weeks.

- Fibre optic bronchoscopy with washings from the affected lobes is useful if no sputum is available. This has replaced techniques such as gastric washings.
- Biopsies of the pleura, lymph nodes and solid lesions within the lung (tuberculomas) may be required to make the diagnosis.

PREVENTION

BCG vaccination

Vaccination with BCG (Bacille Calmette–Guérin) has been given to schoolchildren in the UK since 1954. BCG is a bovine strain of *Mycobacterium tuberculosis* that lost its virulence after growth in the laboratory for many years. Early trials showed that it decreases the risk of developing tuberculosis by about 70%. With the continuing decrease in the incidence of tuberculosis it is becoming less cost-effective to administer this vaccine, and the procedure is being stopped in certain areas of the UK. However, in other areas with a high immigrant population, the vaccine is being administered 6 weeks after birth rather than at the traditional age of 13 years. This is to prevent the disease from developing in young children, where it can progress extremely rapidly and in whom any delay in diagnosis can be fatal. BCG is only given to individuals who are tuberculin-negative; those with positive tests are further screened by a chest X-ray. BCG should be given at a dose of 0.1 ml intradermally to children and adults, but at a dose of 0.05 ml to infants. The practice of BCG vaccination in the UK, thereby producing cellular immunity and a positive tuberculin test, is an important reason why the Mantoux test is of little value in clinical practice for subsequent diagnosis of active disease.

Contact tracing

Tuberculosis is spread from person to person and effective tracing of close contacts has helped to limit spread of the disease as well as to identify diseased individuals at an early stage. Screening procedures involve screening all close family members or other individuals who share the same kitchen and bathroom facilities. Occasionally, close contacts at work or school may also be screened. Contacts who are ill should be thoroughly investigated for tuberculosis. If they are well, a chest X-ray is taken and a tuberculin test is performed.

In adults, provided the chest X-ray is negative and the tuberculin test is positive, nothing more need be done. In children, a positive tuberculin test is usually taken as evidence of infection, and treatment is instituted. If the tuberculin test is negative in children and young adults ($<$ 35 years)

Tuberculin testing

Mainly used for:

- Contact tracing
- BCG vaccination programmes

It is rarely of any value in the diagnosis of TB.

Patients are tested with:

- Purified protein derivative (PPD) of *Myobacterium tuberculosis* or
- Old tuberculin (OT)

The test is based on cell-mediated immunity with the development of induration and inflammation at the site of infection due to infiltration with mainly T lymphocytes.

The Mantoux test

This is used for individual patients.

- 0.1 ml of a 1 : 1000 strength PPD (equivalent to 10 tuberculin units) is injected intradermally.
- The induration is measured (not the erythema) after 72 h. The test is positive if the induration is 10 mm or more in diameter.

The Tine test

This is a simple test used for large-scale screening.

- Four pointed needles mounted on a plastic base are used.
- The tips of the needles are covered with OT and are pressed firmly into the skin once.
- The presence of papules that are confluent with each other after 72 h indicates a positive result.

it is repeated at 6 weeks, and if it remains negative then BCG is administered. If it has become positive (without BCG), this is again taken as an indication of active disease and the individual is treated.

Children under the age of 1 year who have a family member with tuberculosis are given chemoprophylaxis with a daily dose of isoniazid 5–10 $mg \cdot kg^{-1}$ for 6 months together with immunization with a strain of BCG that is resistant to isoniazid.

In general, much greater emphasis is placed on contact tracing and investigation of those under the age of 35 years and in some immigrant groups (Irish and Asian) in whom the disease is more virulent and prevalent.

TREATMENT

Bed rest does not affect the outcome of the disease. Some patients will require hospitalization for a brief period; these include ill patients, those in whom the diagnosis is uncertain and, most importantly, those individuals from whom it is essential to gain cooperation. The most important factor in the successful treatment of tuberculosis lies in the continual self-administration of drugs for 6 months; lack of patient compliance is a major reason why 5% of patients do not respond to treatment. *In vitro* resistance to one or more of the antituberculous drugs occurs in less than 1% of patients in the UK.

Long stay in hospital is now only required for persistently uncooperative patients, many of whom are homeless and abuse alcohol. With modern drugs the time required for treatment can be reduced.

Six-month regimen

This has now become standard practice for patients with pulmonary disease: daily administration of rifampicin 600 mg and isoniazid 300 mg. (For those whose body weight is below 55 kg, rifampicin is reduced to 450 mg daily.) These are given as combination tablets and are taken 30 min before breakfast, since the absorption of rifampicin is influenced by food. This is supplemented for the first 2 months by pyrazinamide at a dose of 1.5 g (body weight < 55 kg) or 2.0 g daily. Studies have indicated that pyrazinamide is of particular value in treating mycobacteria present within macrophages and for this reason it may have a very valuable effect on preventing subsequent relapse.

Longer regimens

Treatment of lymph node and/or bone tuberculosis should be continued for a total of 9 months and of tuberculous meningitis for 12 months. The drugs used are the same as for pulmonary tuberculosis with pyrazinamide prescribed for the first 2 months only.

Unwanted effects of drug treatment

Rifampicin. This drug induces liver enzymes, which may be transiently elevated in many patients. The drug should only be stopped if the serum bilirubin becomes elevated; which is extremely rare. Thrombocytopenia has been reported. Rifampicin stains body secretions pink and the patients should be warned of the change in colour of their urine, tears and sweat. Induction of liver enzymes means that concomitant drug treatment may be made less effective (see Chapter 14) and oral contraception should not be used.

Isoniazid. This gives rise to very few unwanted effects. At high doses it may produce a peripheral neuropathy but this is extremely rare when the normal dose of 200–300 mg is given daily. Nevertheless, it is customary to prescribe pyridoxine 10 mg daily to prevent this effect (see Fig. 3.6). Occasionally, isoniazid gives rise to allergic reac-

tions in the form of a skin rash and fever, and hepatitis occurs in less than 1%. The latter, however, may be fatal if the drug is continued.

Ethambutol. This drug can cause a dose-related retrobulbar neuritis that presents with colourblindness for green, reduction in visual acuity and a central scotoma. It usually reverses provided that the drug is stopped when symptoms develop; patients should therefore be warned of its effects. Because of this problem ethambutol is rarely used unless resistance of *M. tuberculosis* is present to one or more of the other drugs.

All patients should be seen by an ophthalmologist prior to treatment.

Pyrazinamide. The main unwanted effect of this drug is severe hepatic toxicity, though recent experience suggests that this is much rarer than initially thought using present dosage schedules. Gout due to hyperuricaemia may occur.

Streptomycin. The main unwanted effect of streptomycin is irreversible damage to the vestibular nerve. It is more likely to occur in the elderly and in those with renal impairment. Allergic reactions to streptomycin are more common than to rifampicin, isoniazid and pyrazinamide. This drug is only used if patients are very ill and not responding adequately to therapy.

Follow-up

Patients should be seen regularly for the duration of chemotherapy and once more after 3 months, since relapse, though very unlikely, usually occurs within this period of time.

Chemoprophylaxis

Patients who have any chest X-ray changes compatible with previous tuberculosis and who are about to undergo long-term treatment that has an immunosuppressive effect, such as renal dialysis or treatment with corticosteroids, should receive chemoprophylaxis with isoniazid 200–300 mg daily.

Non-tuberculous mycobacteria

Mycobacterium kansasii occurs in water and milk, though not in soil. Disease caused by this mycobacteria has mainly been described in Europe and the USA. It rarely causes a relatively benign type of human pulmonary disease, usually in middle-aged males. Men working in dusty jobs (e.g. miners) appear to be especially at risk, as are those who have underlying chronic bronchitis and emphysema. *Mycobacterium avium intracellulare* is an important cause of pulmonary infection in AIDS patients.

GRANULOMATOUS LUNG DISEASE

A granuloma is a mass or nodule composed of chronically inflamed tissue formed by the response of the mononuclear phagocyte system (macrophage/histiocyte) to a slowly soluble antigen or irritant. If the foreign substance is inert (e.g. an inhaled dust), the phagocytes turn over slowly; if the substance is toxic or reproducing, the cells turn over faster, producing a granuloma.

A granuloma is characterized by epithelioid multinucleate giant cells, as seen in tuberculosis. Granulomas may be caused by:

- Tuberculosis (see p. 40)
- Fungal and helminthic infections
- Hypersensitivity reactions
- Neoplasms

They are also found in disorders with no known cause, such as sarcoidosis.

Sarcoidosis

Sarcoidosis is a multisystem granulomatous disorder, commonly affecting young adults and usually presenting with bilateral hilar lymphadenopathy, pulmonary infiltration and skin or eye lesions. The diagnosis is confirmed on the histological evidence of widespread, non-caseating, epithelioid granulomas in more than one organ. Poisoning with beryllium can rarely produce a clinical and histological picture identical to sarcoidosis, though contact with this element is now strictly controlled.

EPIDEMIOLOGY AND AETIOLOGY

Sarcoidosis is a common disease that is often detected by mass X-ray studies. There is great geographical variation. The prevalence in Britain is approximately 19 in 100 000 of the population. It is common in the USA but is uncommon in Japan. The course of the disease is much more severe in American blacks than in whites. There is no relation with any histocompatibility antigen, but cases of sarcoidosis are seen within families, possibly suggesting an environmental factor. Other aetiological factors suggested are an atypical mycobacterium or fungus, the Epstein–Barr virus, pine pollen (because of the increased incidence of sarcoidosis in the south-eastern states of the USA) and occupational, genetic, social or other environmental factors (a higher incidence occurs in rural rather than in urban populations); none have been substantiated.

IMMUNOPATHOLOGY

- The typical sarcoid granuloma consists of focal accumulation of epithelioid cells, macrophages and lymphocytes, mainly T cells.
- There is a depressed cell-mediated reactivity to tuberculin and other antigens such as *Candida albicans*.
- There is an overall lymphopenia; circulating T lymphocytes are low but B cells are slightly increased.
- Broncho-alveolar lavage shows a great increase in the number of cells; lymphocytes (particularly CD4 helper cells) are greatly increased (see Table 12.5).
- The number of alveolar macrophages is increased but they represent a reduced percentage of the total number of cells.
- Transbronchial biopsies show infiltration of the alveolar walls and interstitial spaces with mononuclear cells, mainly T cells, prior to granuloma formation.

It now seems likely that the decrease in circulating T lymphocytes and changes in delayed hypersensitivity responses are the result of sequestration of lymphocytes within the lung. There is no evidence to suggest that patients with sarcoidosis suffer from an overall defect in cellular immunity, since the frequency of fungal, viral and bacterial infections is not increased and there is no substantiated evidence of a greater risk of developing malignant neoplasms.

CLINICAL FEATURES

The peak incidence is in the third and fourth decades, with a female preponderance. Sarcoidosis can affect many different organs of the body. The commonest presentation is with respiratory symptoms or abnormalities found on chest X-rays (50%). Fatigue or weight loss occurs in 5%, peripheral lymphadenopathy in 5% and a fever in 4%. A chest X-ray may be negative in up to 20% of non-respiratory cases, though lesions may be detected later.

Bilateral hilar lymphadenopathy is a characteristic feature of sarcoidosis. It is often symptomless and simply detected on a routine chest X-ray. Occasionally, the bilateral hilar lymphadenopathy is associated with a dull ache in the chest, malaise and a mild fever.

Although the chest X-ray may not show any evidence of infiltration in the lung fields, evidence from CT scanning, transbronchial biopsies and broncho-alveolar lavage indicate that the lung parenchyma is nearly always involved.

The differential diagnosis of the bilateral hilar lymphadenopathy includes:

- Lymphoma—though it is rare for this only to affect the hilar lymph nodes.
- Pulmonary tuberculosis—though it is rare for the hilar lymph nodes to be symmetrically enlarged.
- Carcinoma of the bronchus with malignant spread to the contralateral hilar lymph nodes—again it is rare for this to give rise to a typical symmetrical picture.

In the early stages it may be difficult to distinguish enlarged lymph nodes on the chest X-ray from the pulmonary arteries, and lymph node enlargement is not always symmetrical. It is for these reasons that, in the absence of additional erythema nodosum (see below), histological confirmation of the disease process is advisable.

Pulmonary infiltration

This type of sarcoidosis may be progressive and may lead to increasing effort dyspnoea and eventually cor pulmonale and death. The chest X-ray shows a mottling in the mid-zones proceeding to generalized fine nodular shadows. Eventually, widespread pulmonary line shadows develop, reflecting the underlying fibrosis. A honeycomb appearance can occasionally occur. Pulmonary function tests show a typical restrictive lung defect (see below).

It is possible to have a normal chest X-ray with abnormal lung function tests, and conversely, lung infiltration may be present on the X-ray with lung function tests in the normal range.

Extrapulmonary manifestations

Skin and ocular sarcoidosis are the commonest extrapulmonary presentations.

Skin sarcoidosis. This is seen in 10% of cases; apart from erythema nodosum, a chilblain-like lesion known as lupus pernio is seen, as are nodules (see p. 1034). Sarcoidosis is the commonest cause of erythema nodosum (see p. 1016). The association of bilateral symmetrical hilar lymphadenopathy with erythema nodosum only occurs in sarcoidosis.

Anterior uveitis. This is common and may present with misting of vision, pain and a red eye, but posterior uveitis may simply present as progressive loss of vision. Although ocular sarcoidosis accounts for about 5% of uveitis presenting to ophthalmologists, evidence of asymptomatic uveitis may be found in up to 25% of patients with sarcoidosis. Conjunctivitis may occur and retinal lesions have been recognized recently.

Keratoconjunctivitis sicca and lacrymal gland enlargement may also occur. Uveoparotid fever is a syndrome of bilateral uveitis and parotid gland enlargement together with occasional development of facial nerve palsy and is sometimes seen with sarcoidosis.

Metabolic manifestations. It is rare for sarcoidosis to present with problems of calcium metabolism, though hypercalcaemia is found in 10% of established cases. Hypercalcaemia and hypercalciuria are important complications since they can lead to the development of renal calculi and nephrocalcinosis. The cause of the hypercalcaemia has been shown to be the high circulating 1,25-dihydroxy vitamin D_3, 1α-hydroxylation occurring in sarcoid macrophages in the lung in addition to that taking place in the kidney.

The central nervous system. Involvement of the CNS is rare (2%) but can lead to severe neurological disease (see p. 936).

Bone involvement. Arthralgia without erythema nodosum is seen in 5% of cases. Bone cysts are found, particularly in the digits, with associated swelling. In the absence of swelling, routine X-rays of the hands are unnecessary.

Hepatosplenomegaly. Sarcoidosis is a cause of hepatosplenomegaly, though it is rarely of any clinical consequence.

Cardiac involvement. Cardiac involvement is rare (3%). Ventricular dysrhythmias, conduction defects and cardiomyopathy with congestive cardiac failure may be seen.

INVESTIGATION

Transbronchial biopsy is the most useful investigation. Positive results are seen in 90% of cases of pulmonary sarcoidosis with or without X-ray evidence of lung involvement. The test provides positive histological evidence of a granuloma in approximately one-half of patients with clinically extrapulmonary sarcoidosis in whom the chest X-ray is normal.

The Kveim test, which involved an intradermal injection of sarcoid tissue, was regularly used for confirmation of the diagnosis. It should not now be used because of the risk of transmission of infection. It is less sensitive than, less specific than and has been superseded by the transbronchial biopsy.

The tuberculin test is negative in 80% of patients with sarcoidosis; it is of no diagnostic value.

The serum level of angiotensin-converting enzyme (ACE) is two standard deviations above the normal mean value in over 75% of patients with untreated sarcoid. Raised (but lower) levels are also seen in patients with lymphoma, pulmonary tuberculosis, asbestosis and silicosis, rendering the test of no diagnostic value. However, it is a simple test and is of use in assessing the activity of the disease and therefore as a guide to treatment with corticosteroids. Reduction of serum ACE during treatment with corticosteroids has not, however, yet been proved to reflect resolution of the disease.

Lung function tests show a restrictive lung defect with pulmonary infiltration. There is:

- A decrease in total lung capacity
- A decrease in both FEV_1 and FVC
- A decrease in gas transfer

PROGNOSIS

It is now clear that sarcoidosis is a much more severe disease in certain racial groups, particularly American blacks, where death rates of up to 10% have been recorded. It is probable that the disease is fatal in less than 1 in 20 individuals in the UK, most often as a result of respiratory failure and cor pulmonale but, rarely, from myocardial sarcoidosis and renal damage.

The chest X-ray provides a guide to prognosis. The disease remits by 2 years in over two-thirds of patients with hilar lymphadenopathy alone, in approximately one-half with hilar lymphadenopathy plus chest X-ray evidence of pulmonary infiltration, but in only one-third of patients with X-ray evidence of infiltration without any demonstrable lymphadenopathy.

TREATMENT

Both the need to treat and the value of corticosteroid therapy are contested in many aspects of this disease.

Hilar lymphadenopathy on its own with no evidence of chest X-ray involvement of the lungs or decrease in lung function tests does not require treatment. Persisting infiltration on the chest X-ray or abnormal lung function tests are unlikely to improve without corticosteroid treatment. If the disease is not improving spontaneously 6 months after diagnosis, treatment should be started with prednisolone 30 mg for 6 weeks, reducing to alternate day treatment with prednisolone 15 mg for 6–12 months. Although there are no controlled trials that have proved the efficacy of such treatment, it is difficult to withhold corticosteroids when there is continuing deterioration of the disease.

Topical or systemic prednisolone should be given for patients suffering from involvement of the eyes or the presence of persistent hypercalcaemia. The erythema nodosum of sarcoidosis will respond rapidly to a short course of prednisolone 5–15 mg for 2 weeks.

Myocardial sarcoidosis and neurological manifestations are also treated with prednisolone, and uveoparotid fever responds rapidly to steroids.

Histiocytosis X

There are three variants of this disease, all characterized by the presence of granulomas consisting predominantly of characteristic histiocytes intermingled with eosinophilic and neutrophilic granulocytes, giant cells and lymphocytes. Electron microscopic studies have shown that the histiocytes contain granules characteristic of Langerhan cells. Fibrosis may occur early, with the development of multiple small cysts producing a honeycomb appearance.

Eosinophilic granuloma
This is the commonest variant in adults. It presents with increasing effort dyspnoea and cough. The chest X-ray shows diffuse bilateral mottling with translucencies with thick walls, and gas transfer is decreased. Recurrent pneumothorax occurs. The granulomas can also be found in bones.

Letterer–Siwe disease
This is usually a fatal disease of infancy that occurs under the age of 3 years. It is a widespread disease with skin lesions, lymphadenopathy, hepatosplenomegaly and bone lesions.

Hand–Schüller–Christian disease
This usually begins under the age of 5 years. It is characterized by defects in bone, exophthalmos and diabetes insipidus. Pulmonary lesions show diffuse nodular shadows with hilar lymphadenopathy simulating sarcoidosis.

Both Hand–Schüller–Christian disease and eosinophilic granuloma may recover spontaneously; survival for 20 years has been reported for both conditions.

Treatment is with corticosteroids and cyclophosphamide, though there is no evidence as yet that this treatment substantially alters the outcome.

Wegener's granulomatosis

This disease of unknown aetiology is characterized by lesions involving the upper respiratory tract, the lungs and the kidneys. Often the disease starts with severe rhinorrhoea with subsequent nasal mucosal ulceration followed by cough, haemoptysis and pleuritic pain. Occasionally there may be involvement of the skin and nervous system. A chest X-ray usually shows single or multiple nodular masses or pneumonic infiltrates with cavitation. The most remarkable radiographic feature is the migratory pattern, with large lesions clearing in one area and new lesions appearing in another.

The typical histological changes are usually best

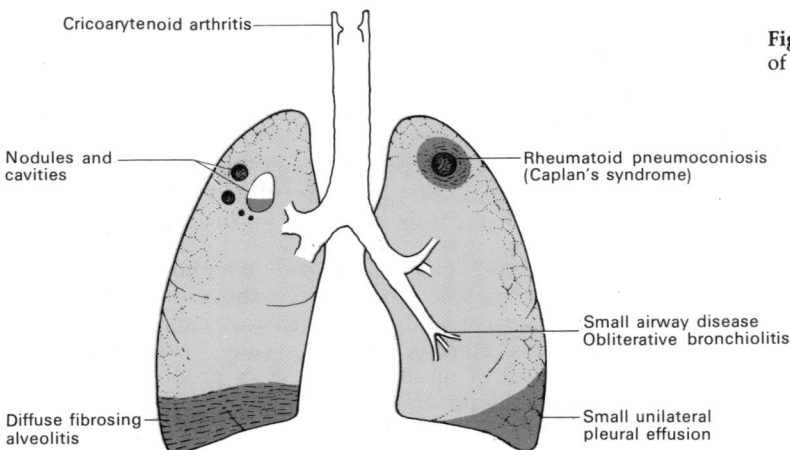

Fig. 12.36 The respiratory manifestations of rheumatoid disease.

Cricoarytenoid arthritis

Nodules and cavities

Rheumatoid pneumoconiosis (Caplan's syndrome)

Small airway disease
Obliterative bronchiolitis

Diffuse fibrosing alveolitis

Small unilateral pleural effusion

seen in the kidneys, where there is a necrotizing glomerulonephritis.

This disease was once invariably fatal but responds well to treatment with cyclophosphamide 150–200 mg daily. A variant of Wegener's granulomatosis called 'mid-line granuloma' particularly affects the nose and paranasal sinuses and is particularly mutilating; it has a poor prognosis.

RESPIRATORY MANIFESTATIONS OF SYSTEMIC CONNECTIVE-TISSUE DISEASE

Rheumatoid disease (see p. 384)

The features of respiratory involvement in rheumatoid disease are illustrated in Fig. 12.36.

Pleural adhesions, thickening and effusion are the commonest lesions. The effusion is often unilateral and tends to be chronic. It has a low glucose content but this can occur in any chronic pleural effusion.

Rheumatoid diffuse fibrosing alveolitis can be considered as a variant of the cryptogenic form of the disease (see p. 640). The clinical features and gross appearance are the same but the disease is often more chronic.

Rheumatoid nodules showing the typical histological appearances are rare in the lung. On the chest X-ray these appear as single or multiple nodules ranging in size from a few millimetres to a few centimetres. The nodules frequently cavitate. They usually produce no symptoms but can give rise to a pneumothorax or pleural effusion.

Obliterative disease of the small bronchioles is rare. It is characterized by progressive breathlessness and irreversible airflow limitation. Corticosteroids may prevent progression.

Involvement of the cricoarytenoid joints gives rise to dyspnoea, stridor, hoarseness and occasionally severe obstruction necessitating tracheostomy. Caplan's syndrome is due to a combination of dust

inhalation and the disturbed immunity of rheumatoid arthritis. It occurs particularly in coal-worker's pneumoconiosis but it can occur in individuals exposed to other dusts, such as silica and asbestos. Typically the lesions appear as rounded nodules 0.5–5 cm in diameter, though sometimes they become incorporated into large areas of fibrosis that are indistinguishable radiologically from progressive massive fibrosis. There may be little evidence of simple pneumoconiosis prior to the development of the nodule.

These lesions may precede the development of the arthritis. Rheumatoid factor is always present in the serum.

Systemic lupus erythematosus (see p. 391)

The commonest respiratory manifestation of this disease, occurring in up to two-thirds of cases, is the development of pleurisy, with or without an effusion. Effusions are usually small and bilateral. Basal pneumonitis is often present, perhaps as a result of poor movement of the diaphragm, or restriction of chest movements due to pleural pain. Pneumonia also occurs, either due to infection or to the disease process itself. Unlike rheumatoid arthritis, diffuse pulmonary fibrosis is rare.

Systemic sclerosis

Autopsy studies have indicated that there is almost always some evidence of diffuse fibrosis of alveolar walls and obliteration of capillaries and the alveolar space. Severe changes result in nodular then streaky shadowing on the chest X-ray, followed by cystic changes, ending up with a honeycomb lung. Function tests indicate a restrictive lesion and poor gas transfer.

Pneumonia may occur due to inhalation from the dilated oesophagus. Breathlessness may be worsened by restriction of chest wall movement

Table 12.9 Common types and characteristics of pulmonary infiltration with eosinophilia.

Disease	Symptoms	Blood eosinophils (%)	Multi-system involvement	Duration	Outcome
Simple pulmonary eosinophilia (Löeffler's syndrome)	Mild	10	None	< 1 month	Good
Prolonged pulmonary eosinophilia	Mild/moderate	> 20	None	> 1 month	Good
Asthmatic bronchopulmonary eosinophila	Moderate/severe	5–20	None	Years	Fair
Tropical pulmonary eosinophilia	Moderate/severe	> 20	None	Years	Fair
Hypereosinophilic syndrome	Severe	> 20	Always	Months/years	Poor
Polyarteritis nodosa	Severe	> 20	Always	Months/years	Poor/fair

due to thickening and contraction of the skin and trunk.

PULMONARY INFILTRATION WITH EOSINOPHILIA (PIE)

The common types and characteristics of these diseases are shown in Table 12.9. They range from very mild, simple, pulmonary eosinophilias to the usually fatal polyarteritis nodosa.

Simple and prolonged pulmonary eosinophilia

Simple pulmonary eosinophilia is a relatively mild illness with a slight fever and cough and usually lasting for less than 2 weeks. It is probably due to a transient allergic reaction in the alveolus. Many allergens have been implicated, including *Ascaris lumbricoides*, *Ankylostoma braziliense* and *Trichuris trichiura* as well as drugs such as para-amino-salicylic acid, aspirin, penicillin, nitrofurantoin and sulphonamides. Often, no allergen is identified. No treatment is required and the disease is self-limiting. Occasionally, however, the disease becomes more prolonged, with a high fever lasting for over a month. There is usually an eosinophilia in the blood and this condition is called *'prolonged pulmonary eosinophilia'*. Similar allergens are thought to be involved, with the addition of *Strongyloides stercoralis*. In both conditions the chest X-ray shows either localized or diffuse opacities. Corticosteroid therapy is indicated, with resolution of the disease over the ensuing weeks.

Asthmatic bronchopulmonary eosinophilia

This is characterized by the presence of asthma,

transient fleeting shadows on the chest X-ray, and blood or sputum eosinophilia. By far the commonest cause world-wide is allergy to *Aspergillus fumigatus* (see below), although *Candida albicans* may be an allergen in a small number of patients. In many, the appropriate allergen has still to be identified.

Diseases caused by *Aspergillus fumigatus*

The various types of lung disease caused by *Aspergillus fumigatus* are illustrated in Fig. 12.37.

The spores of *Aspergillus fumigatus* (5 μm in diameter) are readily inhaled and are present in the atmosphere throughout the year, though they are at their highest concentration in the late autumn. They can be grown from the sputum in up to 15% of patients with chronic lung disease in whom they do not produce disease. They are an important cause of extrinsic asthma in atopic individuals.

Allergic bronchopulmonary aspergillosis (Fig. 12.37)
In allergic bronchopulmonary aspergillosis the *Aspergillus* actually grows in the walls of the bronchi and eventually produces proximal bronchiectasis. There are episodes of eosinophilic pneumonia throughout the year, particularly in late autumn and winter. The episodes present with a wheeze, cough, fever and malaise. They are associated with expectoration of firm sputum plugs containing the fungal mycelium, which results in the clearing of the pulmonary infiltrates on the chest X-ray. Occasionally the large mucus plugs obliterate the bronchial lumen, causing collapse of the lung.

Repeated episodes of eosinophilic pneumonia left untreated can result in progressive pulmonary fibrosis that is often seen in the upper zones and

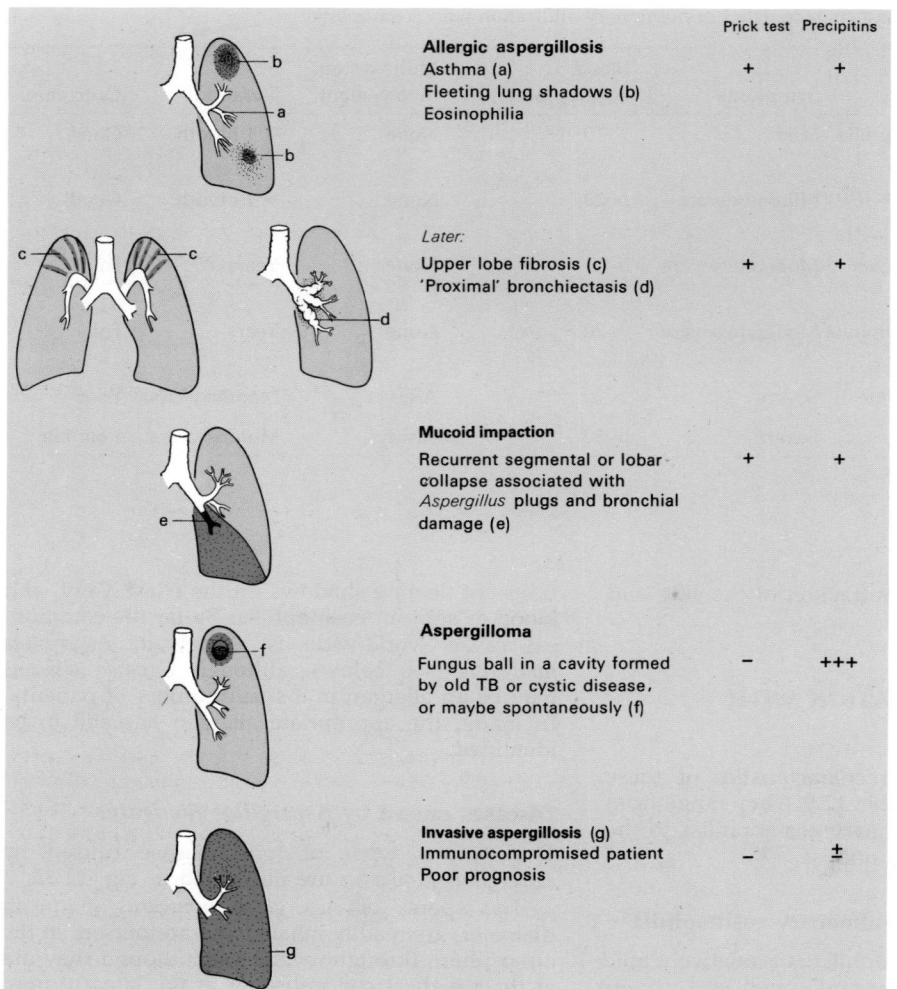

	Prick test	Precipitins
Allergic aspergillosis Asthma (a) Fleeting lung shadows (b) Eosinophilia	+	+
Later: Upper lobe fibrosis (c) 'Proximal' bronchiectasis (d)	+	+
Mucoid impaction Recurrent segmental or lobar collapse associated with *Aspergillus* plugs and bronchial damage (e)	+	+
Aspergilloma Fungus ball in a cavity formed by old TB or cystic disease, or maybe spontaneously (f)	−	+++
Invasive aspergillosis (g) Immunocompromised patient Poor prognosis	−	±

Fig. 12.37 Diseases caused by *Aspergillus fumigatus*.

can give rise to a similar chest X-ray appearance to that produced by tuberculosis.

The peripheral blood eosinophil count is usually raised, and total levels of IgE are extremely high (both that specific to *Aspergillus* and non-specific). Skin-prick testing with protein allergens from *Aspergillus fumigatus* gives rise to positive immediate skin tests. Sputum may show eosinophils and mycelia, and precipitating antibodies are usually found in the serum.

Lung function tests show a decrease in lung volumes and gas transfer in more chronic cases but in all cases evidence of reversible airflow limitation can be demonstrated.

Treatment for this allergic pneumonia is with prednisolone 30 mg daily, which readily causes clearing of the pulmonary infiltrates. Frequent episodes of the disease can be prevented by long-term treatment with prednisolone, but doses as high as 10–15 mg daily are usually required. Moderately severe asthma itself requires continu-

ous treatment with oral corticosteroids. Inhaled corticosteroids do not influence the occurrence of pulmonary infiltrates but are useful for the asthmatic element of the disease.

Aspergilloma (Fig. 12.37)

This is a totally separate disease from allergic bronchopulmonary aspergillosis. It simply represents the growth within previously damaged lung tissue of *Aspergillus fumigatus*, which forms a ball of mycelium within lung cavities. The typical appearance on the chest X-ray is of a round lesion with an air 'halo' above it. The continuing antigenic stimulation gives rise to large quantities of precipitating antibody in the serum. The aspergilloma itself causes little trouble, though occasionally massive haemoptysis may occur, requiring resection of the damaged area of lung containing the aspergilloma. Although treatment with antifungal agents, such as amphotericin (250 μg·kg⁻¹ i.v.), has been tested in both allergic bronchopulmonary aspergillosis and aspergilloma, this has had little success, though it remains the only treatment for invasive aspergillosis, when it is often combined with flucytosine (200 mg·kg^{-1} i.v. daily in four doses).

Tropical pulmonary eosinophilia

This condition presents with cough and wheeze together with fever, lassitude and weight loss. The typical appearance of the chest X-ray is of bilateral hazy mottling that is frequently uniformly distributed in both lung fields. The individual shadows may be as large as 5 mm or may become more confluent, giving the appearance of pneumonia. It is found in many tropical countries, but particularly in the Asian subcontinent, and it now seems fairly certain that the disease represents an allergic reaction to microfilaria, probably from *Wuchereria bancrofti*.

The disease is characterized by a very high eosinophil count in peripheral blood. The filarial complement fixation test is positive in almost every case. The treatment of choice is diethylcarbamazine at a dose of 5 mg·kg^{-1} body weight for 10–14 days; this usually produces a good response.

The hypereosinophilic syndrome

This disease is characterized by eosinophilic infiltration in various organs, sometimes associated with an eosinophilic arteritis. The heart muscle is particularly involved, but pulmonary involvement in the form of pleural effusion or interstitial lung disease occurs in about 40% of cases. Typical features are fever, weight loss, recurrent abdominal pain, persistent non-productive cough and congestive cardiac failure. Corticosteroid treatment may be of value in some cases.

Polyarteritis nodosa (see p. 397)

This is a rare disease characterized by foci of necrotizing arteritis that sooner or later affect many organs in the body. The lungs are rarely involved, except in the variant of polyarteritis nodosa known as the Churg–Strauss syndrome (see below).

The upper respiratory tract may be involved, with nasal obstruction and rhinorrhoea. The chest X-ray may show consolidation that is ill-defined and transgresses anatomical boundaries. These shadows may disappear and reappear over periods of 2–12 weeks, and some may represent intra-alveolar haemorrhage or pulmonary infarcts. The overall 5-year survival for polyarteritis nodosa is 80% with corticosteroids and immunosuppressive therapy.

Allergic granulomatosis (Churg–Strauss syndrome)
The pathology of this condition is dominated by an eosinophilic infiltration and it occurs in patients usually in their fourth decade who have a previous history of rhinitis and asthma. It may simply represent an unusual progression of allergic disease in a subset of predisposed individuals. It is characterized by a high blood eosinophil count, vasculitis of small arteries and veins, and extravascular granulomas. The lungs, peripheral nerves and skin are most often affected and renal failure is much less common than in generalized polyarteritis nodosa. Transient patchy pneumonia-like shadows may occur as in polyarteritis nodosa, but sometimes these can be massive and bilateral. Skin lesions include tender subcutaneous nodules as well as petechial or purpuric lesions. The disease responds well to corticosteroids.

GOODPASTURE'S SYNDROME AND IDIOPATHIC PULMONARY HAEMOSIDEROSIS

Goodpasture's syndrome (see also p. 441)

This disease, like polyarteritis nodosa, affects the lung and the kidneys. The disease often starts with an upper respiratory tract infection followed by cough and intermittent haemoptysis, tiredness and eventually anaemia, though massive bleeding may occur. The chest X-ray shows transient blotchy shadows due to intrapulmonary haemorrhage. These features usually precede the development of an acute glomerulonephritis by several weeks or months. The course of the disease is variable; some spontaneously improve while others proceed to renal failure. The disease usually occurs in individuals over 16 years of age. It is thought to be due to a type II cytotoxic hypersensitivity reaction, the hypothesis being that there may be a shared antigen between a virus and the basement membrane of both kidney and lung. Antiglomerular basement membrane antibodies are found in the serum. An association with influenza A2 virus has been reported. Treatment is with corticosteroids, but plasmapheresis to remove the antibodies has led to dramatic improvement in some cases.

Idiopathic pulmonary haemosiderosis

This is a similar disease to Goodpasture's syndrome, but the kidneys are less frequently involved. Most cases occur in children under 7 years of age. Characteristically, haemosiderin-containing macrophages are found in the sputum. The child develops a chronic cough and anaemia and the chest X-ray shows diffuse shadows due to intrapulmonary bleeding, and eventually miliary nodulation. There is an association with a sensitivity to cow's milk, and an appropriate diet is usually tried. The prognosis in general is poor and treatment with corticosteroids or azathioprine is usually given.

PULMONARY FIBROSIS AND HONEYCOMB LUNG

Pulmonary fibrosis is the end result of many diseases of the respiratory tract. It may be:

- Localized, e.g. following unresolved pneumonia
- Bilateral, e.g. in tuberculosis
- Widespread, e.g. in cryptogenic fibrosing alveolitis, due to drugs (busulphan, bleomycin and cyclophosphamide) or in industrial lung disease

Sometimes with widespread fibrosis a typical radiological appearance is seen that is known as honeycomb lung. This refers to the presence, often diffusely in both lungs, of cysts between 0.5 and 2 cm in diameter that are thick-walled and do not fill with opaque material on bronchography. The cystic air spaces probably represent dilated and thickened terminal and respiratory bronchioles. The main causes are shown in Table 12.10.

Cryptogenic fibrosing alveolitis (CFA)

This relatively rare disorder of unknown aetiology causes diffuse fibrosis throughout the lung fields, usually in late middle age. The cardinal features are progressive breathlessness and cyanosis, which eventually lead to respiratory failure, pulmonary hypertension and cor pulmonale. Gross clubbing occurs in two-thirds of cases and bilateral fine end-inspiratory crackles are heard on auscultation. Rarely, an acute form known as the Hamman–Rich syndrome occurs. The chest X-ray appearance initially is of ground-glass appearance, progressing to obvious small nodular shadows with streaky fibrosis and finally a honeycomb lung.

A number of autoimmune diseases are seen in association with this condition. For example, chronic active hepatitis occurs in 5–10% of cases.

Table 12.10 The main causes of honeycomb lung.

Localized
Systemic sclerosis
Sarcoidosis
Tuberculosis
Asbestosis
Berylliosis
Diffuse
Cryptogenic fibrosing alveolitis
Rheumatoid lung
Histiocytosis X
Tuberose sclerosis
Neurofibromatosis

Similar lung changes are also seen in rheumatoid arthritis, systemic sclerosis and Sjögren's syndrome, often associated with Raynaud's phenomenon.

CFA has also been reported in association with coeliac disease, ulcerative colitis and renal tubular acidosis.

PATHOGENESIS

Histologically there are two main features:

- Cellular infiltration and thickening and fibrosis of the alveolar walls
- Increased cells within the alveolar space (mainly shed type II pneumocytes and macrophages)

The pathogenesis of damage and fibrosis is complex and several factors are involved (see Fig. 12.38).

INVESTIGATION

- Respiratory function tests show a restrictive ventilatory defect—the lung volumes are reduced, the FEV_1 and FVC ratio is normal to high (with both values being reduced) and gas transfer is reduced.
- Blood gases show an arterial hypoxaemia with normal P_aCO_2
- The ESR is high.
- Broncho-alveolar lavage (Table 12.5) shows increased numbers of cells (particularly neutrophils)
- Antinuclear factor is positive in one-third of patients
- Rheumatoid factor is positive in 50% of patients
- In younger patients histological confirmation may be necessary, requiring a transbronchial lung biopsy or even an open lung biopsy to obtain a larger specimen.

DIFFERENTIAL DIAGNOSIS

The diagnosis of CFA can be made in an elderly person presenting with the above signs and laboratory test results. In younger people the differential diagnosis includes extrinsic allergic alveolitis, bronchiectasis, chronic left heart failure, sarcoidosis, industrial lung disease and lymphangitis carcinomatosa.

PROGNOSIS AND TREATMENT

The median survival time for patients with CFA is approximately 5 years. Treatment with large doses of prednisolone (30 mg daily) is usually prescribed for disabling disease, though its benefit has still to be proved by appropriate controlled trials. Azathioprine or cyclophosphamide may also be used. Supportive treatment includes oxygen therapy.

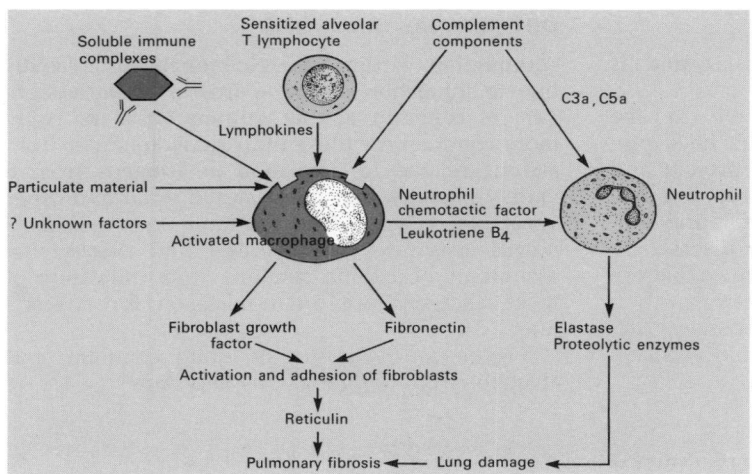

Fig. 12.38 Possible mechanisms involved in the activation of a macrophage and leading to the production of fibrosis.

Extrinsic allergic alveolitis

In this disease there is a widespread diffuse inflammatory reaction in both the small airways of the lung and alveoli. It is due to the inhalation of a number of different antigens, as illustrated in Table 12.11. By far the commonest of these diseases world-wide is farmer's lung, which affects up to 1 in 10 of the farming community in poor, wet areas around the world. In Western countries the incidence is almost certainly declining as more mechanized farming procedures are introduced.

PATHOGENESIS

Histologically there is an initial infiltration of the small airways and alveolar walls with neutrophils followed by lymphocytes and macrophages, leading to the development of non-caseating granulomas. These comprise multinucleated giant cells, occasionally containing the inhaled antigenic material. The major allergic response to the inhaled antigens is through cellular immunity, though there is evidence in some cases of an additional immediate hypersensitivity reaction involving specific IgE antibody and the deposition of immune complexes. All these mechanisms can attract and activate alveolar macrophages, so that continued antigenic exposure results in the development of pulmonary fibrosis.

CLINICAL FEATURES

The typical history is that of the onset of fever, malaise, cough and shortness of breath several hours after exposure to the causative antigen. For example, a farmer forking hay in the morning may only notice symptoms during the late afternoon and evening that resolve by the following morning. On examination the patient may have a fever, tachypnoea and coarse end-inspiratory crackles and wheezes throughout the chest. Cyanosis may be severe even at rest. Continuing exposure leads to a chronic illness characterized by severe weight loss, effort dyspnoea and cough, and the features of fibrosing alveolitis (see p. 690).

The chest X-ray shows fluffy nodular shadowing with the subsequent development of streaky shadows, particularly in the upper zones, and, in very advanced cases, honeycomb lung.

Table 12.11 Extrinsic allergic bronchiolar alveolitis.

Disease	Situation	Antigens
Farmer's lung	Forking mouldy hay or any other mouldy vegetable material	Thermophilic acinomycetes and *Micropolyspora faeni*
Bird fancier's lung	Handling pigeons, cleaning lofts or budgerigar cages	Proteins present in the 'bloom' on the feathers and in excreta
Maltworker's lung	Turning germinating barley	*Aspergillus clavatus*
Humidifier fever	Contaminated humidifying systems in air conditioners or humidifiers in factories (especially in printing works)	Possibly a variety of bacteria or amoebae (e.g. *Naegleria gruberi*)

INVESTIGATION

- The polymorphonuclear leucocyte count is raised in acute cases.
- Precipitating antibodies are present in the serum. A quarter of pigeon fanciers have precipitating antibody against pigeon protein and droppings in their serum but only a small proportion have lung disease. Precipitating antibodies are evidence of *exposure*, not disease.
- Lung function tests show a restrictive ventilatory defect with a decrease in gas transfer.
- Broncho-alveolar lavage (Table 12.5) shows increased cells (lymphocytes and granulocytes).

DIFFERENTIAL DIAGNOSIS

Although an extrinsic allergic bronchiolar alveolitis due to inhalation of the spores of *Micropolyspora faeni* is common among farmers, it is probably more common for these individuals to suffer from asthma related to inhalation of antigens from a variety of mites that infest stored grain and other vegetable material. The common ones are *Glyciphagus domesticus*, *G. destructor* and *Acarus siro*. Symptoms of asthma resulting from inhalation of these allergens are often mistaken for farmer's lung.

Pigeon fancier's lung is quite common, but alveolitis from budgerigars is very rare.

Table 12.12 Drug-induced respiratory disease.

Disease	Drugs
Asthma ± rhinitis	Penicillins Sulphonamides Cephalosporins Aspirin NSAIDs Tartrazine Iodine-containing contrast media Non-selective beta-adrenceptor- blocking drugs (e.g. propranolol) Suxamethonium Thiopentone
Diffuse lung injury infiltrate and/or fibrosis	Amiodarone Hexamethonium Nitrofurantoin Paraquat Continuous oxygen Cytotoxic agents—many, particularly busulphan, CCNU, bleomycin

Pulmonary eosinophilia	Antibiotics
	    Penicillin
	    Tetracycline
	    Sulphonamides
	NSAIDs
	Anti-epileptic
	    Phenytoin
	    Carbamazepine
	Others
	    Chlorpropamide

Opportunistic pulmonary infections	Corticosteroids Azathioprine Other cytotoxic drugs
Respiratory depression	Sedatives Opiates
SLE-like syndrome including pulmonary infiltrates, effusions and fibrosis	Hydralazine Procainamide Isoniazid Para-aminosalicylic acid

MANAGEMENT

Prevention is the aim. This can be achieved by change in work practice, with the use of silage for animal fodder and the drier storage of hay and grain. It is difficult to control pigeon fancier's lung, since individuals remain addicted to their hobby.

Prednisolone, initially in large doses of 30–60 mg daily, is necessary to cause regression of the early stages of the disease. Established fibrosis will not resolve and in some patients the disease may progress inexorably to respiratory failure in spite of intensive therapy. Farmer's lung is a recognized occupational disease in the UK and sufferers are entitled to compensation depending on their degree of disability.

Humidifier fever

Humidifier fever may present with the typical features of extrinsic allergic bronchiolar alveolitis without any radiographic changes. This disease has occurred in outbreaks in factories in the UK, particularly in printing works. In North America it is more commonly found in office blocks with contaminated air-conditioning systems. The cause remains unknown but probably involves several bacteria or even amoebae.

Humidifier fever can be prevented by sterilization of the recirculating water used in the very large humidifying plants in industry.

Drug-induced lung disease

Drugs may produce a wide variety of disorders of the respiratory tract. Pulmonary infiltrates with fibrosis may result from the use of a number of cytotoxic drugs used in the treatment of cancer. The commonest cause of these reactions is bleomycin. The pulmonary damage is dose-related, occurring when the total dosage is greater than 450 mg, but will regress in some cases if the drug is stopped. The most sensitive test is a decrease in gas transfer and therefore gas transfer should be measured repeatedly during treatment with the drug. The use of corticosteroids may help resolution.

Some of the most important drugs affecting the respiratory tract are shown in Table 12.12, together with the types of reaction they produce. The list is not exhaustive; for example, over 20 different drugs are known to produce a systemic lupus erythematosus-like syndrome, sometimes complicated by pulmonary infiltrates and fibrosis. Paraquat ingestion (see p. 750) can cause severe pulmonary oedema and death, and fibrosis develops in many of those who survive.

RADIATION DAMAGE

Irradiation of the lung during radiotherapy can cause a radiation pneumonitis. Patients complain of breathlessness and a dry cough. Radiation pneumonia results in a restrictive lung defect. Corticosteroids should be given in the acute stage.

Occupational lung disease

Exposure to dusts, gases, vapours and fumes at work can lead to the development of the following types of lung disease:

- Acute bronchitis and even pulmonary oedema from irritants such as sulphur dioxide, chlorine, ammonia or the oxides of nitrogen
- Pulmonary fibrosis due to mineral dust
- Occupational asthma (see Table 12.7)
- Extrinsic allergic bronchiolar alveolitis (see Table 12.11)
- Bronchial carcinoma due to industrial agents (e.g. asbestos, polycyclic hydrocarbons, radon in mines)

The degree of fibrosis that follows inhalation of mineral dust varies. While iron (siderosis), barium (baritosis) and tin (stannosis) lead to dramatic dense nodular shadowing on the chest X-ray, their effect on lung function and symptoms is minimal. Exposure to silica or asbestos, on the other hand, leads to extensive fibrosis and disability. Coal dust has an intermediate fibrogenic effect and accounts for 90% of all compensated industrial lung diseases. Lung fibrosis from exposure to asbestos has become an increasing problem. The term pneumoconiosis means the accumulation of dust in the lungs and the reaction of the tissue to its presence. The term is not wide enough to encompass all occupational lung disease and is now generally used in relation to coal dust and its effects on the lung.

Coal-worker's pneumoconiosis

Improved conditions in the coal industry have led to a considerable reduction in the number of cases of pneumoconiosis to about 2 per 1000 wage earners. The disease is caused by dust particles approximately 2–5 μm in diameter that are retained in the small airways and alveoli of the lung. The incidence of the disease is related to total dust exposure, which is highest at the coal face, particularly if ventilation and dust suppression are poor. Two very different syndromes result from the inhalation of coal.

Simple pneumoconiosis

This simply reflects the deposition of coal dust in the lung. It produces a fine micronodular shadow on the chest X-ray and is by far the commonest type of pneumoconiosis. It is graded on the chest X-ray appearance according to standards set by the International Labour Office (see below). Considerable dispute remains about the effects of simple pneumoconiosis on respiratory function and symptoms, many arguing that the development of the latter is largely due to chronic bronchitis and emphysema, commonly related to cigarette smoking.

Categories of simple pneumoconiosis are as follows:

1 Small round opacities are definitely present but are few in number.
2 Small round opacities are numerous but normal lung markings are still visible.
3 Small round opacities are very numerous and normal lung markings are partly or totally obscured.

The importance of simple pneumoconiosis is that it may lead to the development of progressive massive fibrosis (see below). This virtually never occurs on a background of category 1 simple pneumoconiosis but occurs in 30% of those with cateogry 3. Usually category 2 simple pneumoconiosis, which carries a 7% risk of developing PMF, must be present before benefit may be awarded for disability.

Progressive massive fibrosis (PMF)

The lesions in this disease are round fibrotic masses several centimetres in diameter, almost invariably in the upper lobes and sometimes having necrotic central cavities. The pathogenesis of PMF is still not understood, though it now seems clear that some fibrogenic promoting factor is present in individuals developing the disease.

Table 12.13 The effects of asbestos on the lung.

	Exposure	Chest X-ray	Lung function	Symptoms	Outcome
Asbestos bodies	Light	Normal	Normal	None	Evidence of asbestos exposure only
Pleural plaques	Light	Pleural thickening (parietal pleura) and calcification (also in diaphragmatic pleura)	Mild restriction	Rare, occasional mild effort dyspnoea	No other sequelae
Bilateral diffuse pleural thickening	Light/moderate	Bilateral diffuse thickening (of both parietal and visceral pleura) more than 5 mm thick and extending over more than one-quarter of the chest wall	Restrictive ventilatory defect	Effort dyspnoea	May progress in absence of further exposure
Mesothelioma	Light (20–40 year interval from light exposure to disease)	Pleural effusion, usually unilateral	Restrictive ventilatory defect	Pleuritic pain increasing dyspnoea	Median survival 2 years
Asbestosis	Heavy (5–20 year interval from exposure to disease)	Diffuse bilateral streaky shadows, honeycomb lung	Severe restrictive ventilatory defect and reduced gas transfer	Progressive dyspnoea	Poor, progression in some cases after exposure ceases
Asbestos exposure and carcinoma of the bronchus		The features of asbestosis, bilateral diffuse pleural thickening or bilateral pleural plaques plus those of bronchial carcinoma			Fatal

This was thought to be *Mycobacterium tuberculosis*, but is now thought to be immune complexes, analogous to the development of large fibrotic nodules in coal miners with rheumatoid arthritis (Caplan's syndrome). The development of both rheumatoid factor and antinuclear factor in the serum of patients with PMF is common, as it is in those suffering from asbestosis and silicosis. Pathologically there is apical destruction and disruption of the lung, resulting in emphysema and airway damage. Lung function tests show a mixed restrictive and obstructive ventilatory defect with loss of lung volume, irreversible airflow limitation and reduced gas transfer.

The patient with PMF suffers considerable effort dyspnoea, usually with a cough. The sputum can be black. The disease can progress (or even develop) after exposure to coal dust has ceased. Eventually respiratory failure may intervene.

Silicosis

This disease is now relatively uncommon though it may still be encountered in workers in foundries where sand used in moulds has to be removed from the metal casts (fettling), in sand blasting, and amongst stone-masons and pottery and ceramic workers.

Silicosis is caused by the inhalation of silica (silicon dioxide). This dust is highly fibrogenic. For example, a coal miner can remain healthy with 30 g of coal dust in his lungs but would be dead if he had inhaled 3 g of silica. Silica seems particularly toxic to alveolar macrophages and readily initiates the fibrogenic mechanism (see Fig. 12.38). The chest X-ray appearances and clinical features of the disease are similar to those of PMF. The chest X-ray appearance is distinctive: thin streaks of calcification are seen around the hilar lymph nodes ('eggshell' calcification).

Asbestosis (Table 12.13)

Asbestos is a mixture of silicates of iron, magnesium, nickel, cadmium and aluminium, and has the unique property of occurring naturally as a fibre. It possesses remarkably resistant properties to heat, acid and alkali, hence its widespread use. Asbestos is mined in southern Africa, Canada and the USSR. World production is still 5 million tons, of which 90% is chrysotile, 6% crocidolite and 4% amosite in type.

Chrysotile or white asbestos is the softest asbestos fibre. Each fibre is often as long as 2 cm but only a few micrometres thick. It is less fibrogenic than crocidolite.

Crocidolite (blue asbestos) is particularly resistant to chemical destruction. It exists in straight fibres up to 50 μm in length and 1–2 μm in width. It is now known that this type of asbestos is by far the most important in the development of all types of asbestosis and particularly of mesothelioma. This may be due to the fact that it is readily trapped in the lung. Its long, thin shape means that it can be inhaled, but subsequent rotation against the long axis of the smaller airways, particularly in turbulent airflow during expiration, causes the fibres to impact. Crocidolite is also particularly resistant to macrophage and neutrophil enzymic destruction. Exposure to asbestos occurred particularly in naval ship-building yards and in power stations but its ubiquitous use meant that light exposure was common. Up to 50% of urban dwellers had evidence of asbestos bodies (asbestos fibre covered in protein secretions) in their lungs at postmortem. New regulations in the UK prevent the use of crocidolite and severely restrict the use of chrysotile, and enforce careful dust control measures. These changes should eventually abolish the problem.

There is an important synergistic relationship between asbestosis and cigarette smoking and the development of bronchial carcinoma, usually adenocarcinoma; the risk is increased fivefold. There is also an increased risk in non-smokers and it is also present in workers exposed to asbestos who do not have clinically recognized asbestosis but who do have pleural plaques or thickening. It is important to remember that workers will continue to be exposed to blue asbestos in the course of demolition or in the replacement of insulation, and that there is a considerable time lag between exposure and development of the disease, particularly mesothelioma (20–40 years).

The diseases caused by asbestos are summarized in Table 12.13. Bilateral diffuse pleural thickening, asbestosis, mesothelioma and asbestos-related carcinoma of the bronchus are all eligible for compensation in the UK under the Social Security Act of 1975, but account for only one-quarter of the number of cases of compensation compared to coal-worker's pneumoconiosis. Asbestosis is the disease most frequently compensated (900 cases per year). This progressive disease is characterized by breathlessness and is accompanied by finger clubbing and bilateral basal end-inspiratory crackles. Fibrosis not detectable on chest X-ray may be revealed on CT scan. No treatment is known to alter the progress of the disease, though corticosteroids are often prescribed.

The number of cases of mesothelioma presenting for compensation has increased fivefold in the last decade to over 400 cases per year. Often open lung biopsy is needed to obtain sufficient tissue for diagnosis. No treatment influences the universally fatal outcome. Although pleural effusions are the commonest presentation of mesothelioma, occasionally they may have a benign origin and may regress spontaneously.

Byssinosis

This disease occurs world-wide but is declining rapidly in areas where the numbers of people employed in cotton mills are falling. In the UK the disease is confined to areas of Lancashire and Northern Ireland. The symptoms start on the first day back at work after a break (Monday sickness) with improvement as the week progresses. Tightness in the chest, cough and breathlessness occur within the first hour in dusty areas of the mill, particularly in the blowing and carding rooms where raw cotton is cleaned and the fibres are straightened.

The exact nature of the disease and its aetiology remain disputed. Two important features are that pure cotton does *not* cause the disease, and that cotton dust has some effect on airflow limitation in all those exposed. Individuals with asthma are particularly badly affected by exposure to cotton dust. The most likely aetiology is endotoxins from bacteria present in the raw cotton causing constriction of the airways of the lung. There are no changes on the chest X-ray and there is considerable dispute as to whether the progressive airflow limitation seen in some patients with the disease is due to the cotton dust or to other effects such as cigarette smoking or co-existent asthma.

Berylliosis

Beryllium–copper alloy has a high tensile strength and is resistant to metal fatigue, high temperature and corrosion. It is used in the aerospace industry, in atomic reactors and in many electrical devices.

Although beryllium is inhaled into the lungs, it causes a systemic poisoning that gives rise to a clinical picture similar to sarcoidosis. The major chronic problem is that of progressive dyspnoea with pulmonary fibrosis. However, strict control of levels in the working atmosphere have made the disease a rarity.

Tumours of the lung

Bronchial carcinoma accounts for 95% of all primary tumours of the lung. Alveolar cell carcinoma accounts for 2% of lung tumours and other less malignant or benign tumours account for the remaining 3%.

Benign tumours

Pulmonary hamartoma
This is the most common benign tumour of the lung and is usually seen as a very well-defined round lesion 1–2 cm in diameter in the periphery of the lung. Growth is extremely slow, but the tumour may reach several centimetres in diameter. Rarely it arises from a major bronchus and causes obstruction.

Bronchial carcinoid
This rare tumour resembles intestinal carcinoid tumour and is locally invasive, eventually spreading to mediastinal lymph nodes and finally to distant organs. It is a highly vascular tumour that projects into the lumen of a major bronchus causing recurrent haemoptysis. It grows slowly and eventually blocks the bronchus, leading to lobar collapse. Rarely, it gives rise to the carcinoid syndrome.

Cylindroma, chondroma and lipoma
These are extremely rare tumours that may grow in the bronchus or trachea, causing obstruction.

DIAGNOSIS AND TREATMENT

These tumours are diagnosed in the same way as bronchial carcinoma. Treatment is surgical and should not be delayed when collapse of a lobe is imminent or when obstruction is increasing.

Lung cysts

These may be congenital, bronchogenic cysts or may result from a sequestrated pulmonary segment. Hydatid disease causes fluid-filled cysts. Thin-walled cysts are due to lung abscesses, which are particularly found in staphyloccal pneumonia, tuberculous cavities, septic pulmonary infarction, primary bronchogenic carcinoma, cavitating metastatic neoplasm, or paragonimiasis caused by the lung fluke *Paragonimus westermani*.

Table 12.14 Death rates from lung cancer (age standardized per 100 000) according to tobacco consumption in male British doctors.

Non-smokers	10
Ex-smokers	43
Continuing smokers	
Any tobacco	104
Pipe/cigar	58
Cigarette	140
Number of cigarettes	
1–14 ⎫	78
15–24 ⎬ per day	127
25 or more ⎭	251

MALIGNANT TUMOURS

Bronchial carcinoma

This is the most common malignant tumour in the Western World and is now the third most common cause of death in the UK after heart disease and pneumonia. Mortality rates world-wide are highest in Scotland, closely followed by England and Wales. In the UK, 35 000 people die each year from bronchial carcinoma, with a male-to-female ratio of 3.5 : 1. Although the rising mortality from this disease has levelled off in men, it continues to rise in women, accounting for 1 in 8 of all deaths from malignant disease in women, second only to carcinoma of the breast.

The strength of the association between cigarette smoking and bronchial carcinoma overshadows any other aetiological factors (Table 12.14) but there is a higher incidence of bronchial carcinoma in urban compared with rural areas, even when allowance is made for cigarette smoking. Passive smoking (the inhalation of other people's smoke by non-smokers) increases the risk of bronchial carcinoma by a factor of 1.5. Occupational factors include exposure to asbestos, and an association is also claimed for workers in contact with arsenic, chromium, iron oxide, petroleum products and oils, coal tar, products of coal combustion, and radiation. Tumours associated with occupational factors are mostly adenocarcinomas and appear to be less related to cigarette smoking.

Cell types
Bronchial carcinoma is divided into small-cell carcinoma and non-small-cell carcinoma, a division based on the characteristics of the disease and its response to treatment. Studies of mean doubling times of carcinomas indicate that development from the initial malignant change to presentation takes many years; for adenocarcinoma it takes approximately 15 years, for squamous carcinoma 8 years and for small-cell carcinoma 3 years.

Non-small-cell carcinoma. The commonest carcinoma in this group is the *squamous* or *epidermoid carcinoma*, accounting for approximately 40% of all carcinomas. It occasionally cavitates, and widespread metastases occur relatively late.

Large-cell carcinoma represents a less well-differentiated tumour that metastasizes early. It accounts for 25% of all tumours.

Adenocarcinoma arises peripherally from mucous glands in the small bronchi and often produces a subpleural mass. Invasion of the pleura and the mediastinal lymph nodes is common, as are metastases in the brain and bones. Adenocarcinoma accounts for approximately 10% of all bronchial carcinomas and frequently arises in or around scar tissue. It is the commonest bronchial carcinoma associated with asbestos and is proportionally more common in non-smokers, in women, in the elderly, and in the Far East.

Alveolar cell carcinoma (bronchiolar carcinoma) accounts for only 1–2% of lung tumours and occurs either as a peripheral solitary nodule or as diffuse nodular lesions of multicentric origin. Occasionally this tumour is associated with expectoration of very large volumes of mucoid sputum.

Small-cell carcinoma. This tumour, often called oat-cell carcinoma, accounts for 20–30% of all lung cancers. It arises from endocrine cells (Kulchitsky cells). These cells are members of the APUD (amine precursors and uptake decarboxylation) system, which explains why many polypeptide hormones are secreted by these tumours. Small-cell carcinoma is now considered to be a systemic disease. Although the tumour is rapidly growing and highly malignant, it is the only one of the bronchial carcinomas that responds to chemotherapy.

CLINICAL FEATURES

The frequencies of the common symptoms of lung cancer on presentation are shown in Table 12.15. Chest pain and discomfort are often described as fullness and pressure in the chest. Sometimes the pain may be pleuritic owing to invasion of the pleura or ribs.

Commonly there are no abnormal physical signs. Enlarged supraclavicular lymph nodes are frequently found with small-cell carcinoma. There may be signs of a pleural effusion or of lobar collapse. Signs of an unresolved pneumonia or of associated underlying disease (e.g. diffuse pulmonary fibrosis in asbestosis) may be present.

Table 12.15 The frequency of the common presenting symptoms of bronchial carcinoma.

Symptom	Frequency
Cough	42%
Chest pain	22%
Cough and pain	15%
Coughing blood	7%
Chest infection Malaise Weight loss Shortness of breath Hoarseness Distant spread No symptoms	< 5% each

Table 12.16 Non-metastatic extrapulmonary manifestations of bronchial carcinoma (percentage of all cases).

Metabolic (universal at some stage)
Loss of weight
Lassitude
Anorexia

Endocrine (10%) (usually small-cell carcinoma)
Ectopic adrenocorticotrophin syndrome
Syndrome of inappropriate secretion of antidiuretic
    hormone (SIADH)
Hypercalcaemia (usually squamous cell carcinoma)
Rarer—hypoglycaemia, thyrotoxicosis,
    gynaecomastia

Neurological (2–16%)
Encephalopathies—including subacute cerebellar
    degeneration
Myelopathies—motor neurone disease
Neuropathies—peripheral sensorimotor
    neuropathy
Muscular disorders—polymyopathy, myasthenic
    syndrome (Eaton Lambert syndrome)

Vascular and haematological (rare)
Thrombophlebitis migrans
Non-bacterial thrombotic endocarditis
Microcytic and normocytic anaemia
Disseminated intravascular coagulopathy
Thrombotic thrombocytopenic purpura
Haemolytic anaemia

Skeletal
Clubbing (30%)
Hypertrophic osteoarthropathy (± gynaecomastia)
    (3%)

Cutaneous (rare)
Dermatomyositis
Acanthosis nigricans
Herpes zoster

Direct spread
The tumour may directly involve the pleura and ribs. Carcinoma in the apex of the lung can erode the ribs and involve the lower part of the brachial plexus (C8, T1 and T2), causing severe pain in the shoulder and down the inner surface of the arm (Pancoast's tumour). The sympathetic ganglion may also be involved, producing Horner's syndrome (see p. 886). Further extension may involve the recurrent laryngeal nerve as it passes down the aortic arch, causing unilateral vocal cord paresis with hoarseness and a bovine cough, and rarely the tumour may cause spinal cord compression.

Bronchial carcinoma can also directly invade the phrenic nerve, causing paralysis of the diaphragm.

It can involve the oesophagus, producing progressive dysphagia, and the pericardium, producing pericardial effusion and malignant dysrhythmias. It can also involve the superior vena cava, producing superior vena caval obstruction leading to early morning headache, facial congestion and oedema involving the upper limbs; the jugular veins are distended, as are the veins on the chest that form a collateral circulation with veins arising from the abdomen.

Metastatic complications
Bony metastases are common, giving rise to severe pain and pathological fractures. There is frequent involvement of the liver. Secondary deposits in the brain present as a change in personality, epilepsy or a focal neurological lesion. Carcinoma of the bronchus is a cause of secondary deposits in the adrenal gland.

Non-metastatic extrapulmonary manifestations
Although approximately 10% of small-cell tumours are thought to produce ectopic hormones at some stage, clinically important extrapulmonary manifestations are relatively rare apart from finger clubbing (Table 12.16).

Hypertrophic pulmonary osteoarthropathy (HPOA) (see also p. 408) occurs in approximately 3% of all bronchial carcinomas, particularly squamous-cell carcinomas and adenocarcinomas. Symptoms include joint stiffness and severe pain in the wrists and ankles, sometimes associated with gynaecomastia. X-rays show the characteristic proliferative periostitis at the distal ends of long bones, which have an onion-skin appearance. HPOA is invariably associated with clubbing of the fingers. It may regress after resection of the lung tumour or as a result of vagotomy at thoracotomy.

INVESTIGATION

Chest X-ray
This is the most valuable screening test for bronchial carcinoma. It is a relatively insensitive test, however, since the tumour mass needs to be between 1 and 2 cm in size to be recognized reliably. CT scanning can identify small tumour masses, but is at present too time-consuming and expensive to replace the chest X-ray.

About 70% of all bronchial carcinomas arise centrally, the rest peripherally (particularly adenocarcinomas). At the time of clinical presentation the chest X-ray will demonstrate over 90% of carcinomas. A small proportion arise within the main bronchus or trachea or else present with metastatic or non-metastatic complications but with no detectable mass on the chest X-ray.

Bronchial carcinoma can appear as round shadows on a chest X-ray (see p. 641). Characteristically the edge of the tumour has a fluffy or spiked appearance, though sometimes it may be entirely smooth with cavitation, particularly when the tumour is epidermoid in type. Carcinoma can also cause collapse of the lung.

Carcinoma causing partial obstruction of a bronchus interrupts the mucociliary escalator, and bacteria are retained within the affected lobe. This gives rise to the so-called secondary pneumonia that is commonly seen on a chest X-ray of a patient presenting with bronchial carcinoma.

The hilar lymph nodes on the side of the tumour are frequently involved in carcinoma of the lung. A large pleural effusion may also be present.

Carcinoma can spread through the lymphatic channels of the lung to give rise to lymphangitis carcinomatosa; this is usually unilateral and associated with striking dyspnoea. The chest X-ray shows streaky shadowing throughout the lung. This appearance may be seen in both lungs, particularly when it is due to metastatic spread, usually from tumours below the diaphragm (the stomach and colon) and from the breast.

Computed tomography

CT is particularly useful for identifying pathological changes in the mediastinum (e.g. enlarged lymph nodes (see Fig. 12.12), local spread of the tumour) and for identifying secondary spread of carcinoma to the opposite lung by detecting masses too small to be seen on the chest X-ray. Lymph nodes larger than 1.5 cm are considered pathological, although whether they are due to metastatic tumour, reactive hyperplasia or previous lung disease (i.e. TB) can only be determined by biopsy. A normal CT scan prior to surgery excludes the need for mediastinoscopy and node biopsy. CT scanning is of little help in assessing operability of peripheral cancer since these rarely metastasize to the mediastinum.

Magnetic resonance imaging may have some advantages over CT in mediastinal lesions when they are near to major vessels.

Fibreoptic bronchoscopy (see p. 647)

This technique is used to obtain cytological specimens from peripheral lesions as well as to obtain biopsy evidence of any tumours seen. If the carcinoma involves the first 2 cm of either main bronchus, the tumour is inoperable. Widening and loss of the sharp angle of the carina indicates the presence of enlarged mediastinal lymph nodes, either malignant or reactive. They can be biopsied by passage of a needle through the bronchial wall. Vocal cord paresis on the left indicates involvement of the recurrent laryngeal nerve and inoperability.

Transthoracic fine-needle aspiration biopsy

This involves the direct aspiration through the chest wall of peripheral lung lesions under appropriate X-ray or CT screening. Specimens can be obtained from 75% of peripheral lesions that could not be biopsied transbronchially. Pneumothorax occurs in 25% of patients, occasionally requiring drainage. Mild haemoptysis occurs in 5%. Implantation metastases do not occur.

TREATMENT

Unlike other cancers, there has been no improvement in survival from carcinoma of the bronchus. Only 20% of patients are alive one year after diagnosis and only 6–8% after 5 years (cf. 50% for breast or cervix).

Surgery

The only treatment of any value for non-small-cell cancer of the lung is surgery. Only 20% of all cases are suitable for resection and only 25–30% survive for 5 years. The mortality of thoracotomy in patients over 65 years with metastatic disease exceeds the expected 5-year survival rate and should therefore be avoided.

Pre-operative assessment. Radionuclide scanning for detection of metastatic disease in liver and bone is rarely positive in the absence of symptoms or abnormal enzyme tests (serum alkaline phosphatase) and is therefore unnecessary. A normal CT scan indicates no mediastinal spread of the tumour and favours curative resection.

Because of their common aetiology, chronic bronchitis and emphysema are frequently present. An FEV_1 of less than 1.5 litres is not compatible with an active life following pneumonectomy, although the surgery itself can be successfully accomplished. This also applies when the gas-transfer test is reduced by 50%.

Radiation therapy for cure

High-dose radiotherapy (6500 rad; 65 Gy) can produce results that are as good as those of surgery in patients who are fit and who have slowly growing squamous carcinoma. It is the treatment of choice if the tumour is inoperable for reasons such as poor lung function.

Radiation pneumonitis (defined as an acute infiltrate precisely confined to the radiation area and occurring within 3 months of radiotherapy) develops in 10–15%. Radiation fibrosis, a fibrotic change occurring within a year or so of radiotherapy and not precisely confined to the radiation area, occurs to some degree in all cases. These complications are usually of little importance.

Symptomatic radiation treatment

Bone pain, haemoptysis and the superior vena cava syndrome respond favourably to irradiation in the short term.

Chemotherapy
This is not effective for the treatment of non-small-cell cancer of the lung. The reverse is true for small-cell cancer, where single or combination chemotherapy has resulted in a fivefold increase in median survival from 2 to 10 months. A small number of patients enjoy several years of remission. The best results are achieved by simultaneous use of three or four of the following drugs: vincristine, cyclophosphamide, doxorubicin, lomustine, methotrexate and etoposide (see p. 373), although the unwanted effects are greater than with single-agent chemotherapy such as etoposide.

Laser therapy
This is a rapidly developing area. Good results have been achieved for reduction in tumour mass and relief of symptoms (breathlessness, stridor) in patients with tracheal tumours or obstruction to a main bronchus.

Terminal care (see p. 374)
Patients dying of cancer of the lung need attention to their overall well-being. They must not be ignored simply because they cannot be cured. A lot can be done to make the patient's remaining life symptom-free and as active as possible.

Daily treatment with prednisolone (up to 15 mg daily) may improve appetite. Morphine or diamorphine must be given regularly for pain, either in the form of a sustained-release morphine sulphate tablet twice daily or else as regular elixirs or injections. Many patients benefit from a continuous subcutaneous injection of opiates given by a pump. Candidiasis and other infections in the mouth are common and must be looked for and treated. Patients taking opiates are frequently constipated, so regular laxatives should be prescribed. Short courses of palliative radiotherapy for bone pain, severe cough or haemoptysis are helpful.

Both the patient and the relatives require counselling, a task that should be shared between nurses, social workers, hospital chaplains and doctors.

SCREENING FOR LUNG CANCER

Screening programmes (yearly chest X-ray, 4-monthly sputum cytology) have been tried in high-risk groups but the success rate is minimal, underlining the need for prevention.

Secondary tumours

Metastases in the lung are very common and usually present as round shadows 1.5–3 cm in diameter. They may be detected on chest X-ray in patients already diagnosed as having carcinoma.

The primary is usually in the

- Kidney
- Prostate
- Breast
- Bone
- Gastrointestinal tract
- Cervix or ovary

They nearly always develop in the parenchyma and are often relatively asymptomatic even when the chest X-ray shows extensive pulmonary metastases. It is rare for metastases to develop in the bronchi, when they may present with haemoptysis.

Carcinoma, particularly of the stomach, pancreas and breast, can involve mediastinal glands and spread along the lymphatics of both lungs (lymphangitis carcinomatosa), which can lead to progressive and severe breathlessness. On the chest X-ray, bilateral lymphadenopathy is seen together with streaky basal shadowing fanning out over both lung fields.

Occasionally a pulmonary metastasis may be detected as a *solitary round shadow* on chest X-ray in an asymptomatic patient. The commonest primary tumour to do this is a renal carcinoma. The differential diagnosis includes:

- Primary bronchial carcinoma
- Tuberculoma
- Benign tumour of the lung
- Hydatid cyst

Single pulmonary metastases can be removed surgically but, as CT scans usually show the presence of small metastases undetected on chest X-ray, surgery is seldom performed.

Disorders of the chest wall and pleura

Trauma

Trauma to the thoracic wall can be due to penetrating wounds and can lead to pneumo- or haemothoraces.

Rib fractures
Rib fractures can be caused by trauma or coughing (particularly in the elderly), and can occur in patients with osteoporosis. Pathological rib fractures may be due to metastatic spread from carcinoma of the bronchus, breast, kidney, prostate and thyroid. Ribs can also become involved by a mesothelioma. Fractures may not be readily visible on a postero-anterior chest X-ray, and lateral X-rays and oblique views may be necessary.

Pain may prevent adequate chest expansion and coughing and this can lead to pneumonia.

Treatment is with adequate analgesia using oral agents or by local infiltration or an intercostal nerve block.

More than one fracture in one rib can lead to a flail segment with paradoxical movement, i.e. part of the chest wall moves inwards during inspiration. This can produce inefficient ventilation and may require intermittent positive-pressure ventilation.

Rupture of the trachea or a major bronchus
Rupture of the trachea or even a major bronchus can occur during deceleration injuries, leading to pneumothorax, surgical emphysema, pneumomediastinum and haemoptysis. Surgical emphysema is caused by air leaking into the subcutaneous connective tissue; this can also occur after the insertion of an intercostal drainage tube. A pneumomediastinum occurs when air leaks from the lung inside the parietal pleura and extends along the bronchial walls.

Rupture of the oesophagus
Rupture of the oesophagus from external injury, endoscopic procedures, bougienage or necrotic carcinoma may lead to the serious complication of mediastinitis. This requires vigorous antibacterial chemotherapy.

Lung contusion
This causes widespread fluffy shadows on the chest X-ray due to intrapulmonary haemorrhage. This may give rise to adult respiratory distress syndrome or shock lung (see p. 729).

Kyphoscoliosis

Kyphoscoliosis may be congenital, idiopathic, due to disease of the vertebrae such as TB or osteomalacia, or due to neuromuscular disease such as Friedreich's ataxia or poliomyelitis. The respiratory effects of severe kyphoscoliosis are often more pronounced than might be expected and respiratory failure and death often occur in the fourth or fifth decade. The abnormality should be corrected at an early stage if possible.

Ankylosing spondylitis

Limitation of chest wall movement is often well compensated by diaphragmatic movement and the respiratory effects of this disease are relatively mild. It is associated with upper lobe fibrosis of unknown aetiology.

Pectus excavatum and carinatum

Pectus excavatum causes few problems other than embarrassment due to the deep vertical furrow in the chest, which can be corrected surgically. The heart is seen to lie well to the left on the chest X-ray. Pectus carinatum (pigeon chest) is often the result of rickets. No treatment is required.

Dry pleurisy

'Dry pleurisy' is the term used to describe pleurisy when there is inflammation but no appreciable effusion. The localized inflammation produces sharp localized pain, made worse on deep inspiration, coughing and occasionally on twisting and bending movements. Common causes are pneumonia, pulmonary infarct and carcinoma. Rarer causes are rheumatoid arthritis and systemic lupus erythematosus.

Epidemic myalgia (Bornholm disease) is due to infection by coxsackie B virus. This illness is common in young adults in the late summer and autumn and is characterized by an upper respiratory tract illness followed by pleuritic pain in the chest and upper abdomen with tender muscles. The chest X-ray remains normal and the illness clears within 1 week.

Pleural effusion

A pleural effusion is an excessive accumulation of fluid in the pleural space. It can be detected on X-ray when 300 ml or more of fluid is present and clinically when 500 ml or more is present. The chest X-ray appearances range from the obliteration of the costophrenic angle to dense homogenous shadows occupying part or all of the hemithorax. Fluid below the lung (a subpulmonary effusion) can simulate a raised hemidiaphragm. Fluid in the fissures may resemble an intrapulmonary mass. The physical signs are shown in Table 12.1.

Diagnosis is by pleural aspiration (see p. 646). The fluid that accumulates may be a transudate or an exudate.

Transudates. Effusions that are transudates can be bilateral. The protein content is less than 30 g·L^{-1} and the lactic dehydrogenase is less than 200 i.u.·L^{-1}. Causes include:

● Heart failure
● Hypoproteinaemia (e.g. nephrotic syndrome)
● Constrictive pericarditis
● Hypothyroidism
● Ovarian tumours producing right-sided pleural effusion—Meigs' syndrome

Exudates. The protein content of exudates is greater than 30 g·L^{-1} and the lactic dehydrogenase is greater than 200 i.u.·L^{-1}. Causes include:

● Bacterial pneumonia (common)

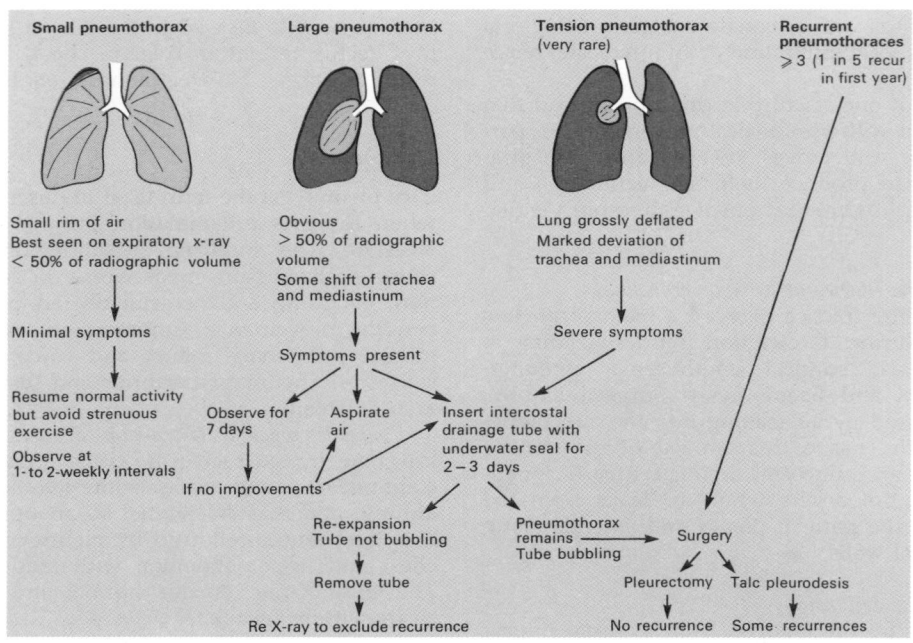

Fig. 12.39 Pneumothorax: an algorithm for management.

- Carcinoma of the bronchus (common) ⎫
- Pulmonary infarction (common) ⎬ Fluid may be blood-stained
- Tuberculosis ⎭
- Connective-tissue disease
- Post-myocardial infarction syndrome (rare)
- Acute pancreatitis (high amylase content) (rare)
- Mesothelioma (rare)
- Sarcoidosis (very rare)
- Yellow-nail syndrome (effusion due to lymph-oedema) (rare)
- Familial mediterranean fever (rare)

Pleural biopsy (see p. 646) may be necessary to diagnose the cause of the effusion. Treatment is of the underlying condition.

Malignant pleural effusions
Malignant pleural effusions that reaccumulate and are symptomatic can be aspirated to *dryness* followed by the instillation of a sclerosing agent such as tetracycline or bleomycin. Effusions should be drained slowly since rapid shift of the mediastinum causes severe pain and occasionally shock. This treatment produces only temporary relief.

Chylothorax

This is due to the accumulation of lymph in the pleural space, usually resulting from leakage from the thoracic duct due to trauma or to infiltration by carcinoma.

Empyema

This is the presence of pus in the pleural space and can be a complication of pneumonia (see p. 677).

Pneumothorax

'Pneumothorax' means air in the pleural space. It may occur due to trauma to the chest or may be spontaneous. Pneumothorax may be localized if the visceral pleura has previously undergone adhesion to the parietal pleura, or generalized if the whole hemithorax contains air. Normally the pressure in the pleural space is negative but this is lost once a communication is made with atmospheric pressure; the elastic recoil pressure of the lung then causes it to partially deflate. If the communication between the airways and the pleural space remains (an open pneumothorax), a bronchopleural fistula is created. Once the communication between the lung and the pleural space is obliterated, air will be reabsorbed at a rate of 1.25% of the total radiographic volume of the hemithorax per day. Thus, a 50% collapse of the lung will take 40 days to reabsorb completely once the pneumothorax is closed.

It has been postulated that a valvular mechanism may develop through which air can be sucked during inspiration but not expelled during expiration. The intrapleural pressure remains positive throughout breathing, the lung deflates further, the mediastinum shifts, and venous return to the heart decreases, with increasing respiratory and cardiac embarrassment. This tension pneumothorax is rare unless the patient is on positive ventilation.

Spontaneous pneumothorax
This usually occurs in young males, the male-to-female ratio being 6 : 1. It is caused by the rupture of a pleural bleb, usually apical, and is thought to be due to congenital defects in the connective tissue of the alveolar walls. Both lungs are affected with equal frequency. Often these patients are tall and thin.

In patients over 40 years of age, the usual cause is underlying chronic bronchitis and emphysema. Rarer causes include bronchial asthma, carcinoma, a lung abscess breaking down and leading to bronchopleural fistula, and severe pulmonary fibrosis with cyst formation.

The sudden onset of unilateral pleuritic pain or increasing breathlessness are the usual presenting features. If the pneumothorax enlarges or a tension pneumothorax develops, the patient becomes more breathless and may develop pallor and tachycardia. There may be few physical signs if the pneumothorax is small. The characteristic features and management are shown in Fig. 12.39. The main aim is to get the patient back to active life as soon as possible.

Disorders of the diaphragm

Diaphragmatic fatigue

The diaphragm can become fatigued if the force of contraction during inspiration exceeds 40% of the force it can develop in a maximal static effort. When this occurs acutely in patients with exacerbations of chronic airflow limitation or cystic fibrosis or in quadriplegics, positive-pressure ventilation is required followed by attempts to increase the strength and endurance of the diaphragm by breathing against a resistance for 30 min a day.

Unilateral diaphragmatic paralysis is common and symptomless. The affected diaphragm is usually elevated and moves paradoxically on inspiration. A sniff causes the paralysed diaphragm to rise, the unaffected diaphragm to descend. Causes include:

- Surgery
- Carcinoma of the bronchus with involvement of the phrenic nerve
- Neurological, including poliomyelitis, herpes zoster
- Trauma to cervical spine, birth injury, subclavian vein puncture
- Infection: tuberculosis, syphilis, pneumonia

Bilateral diaphragmatic weakness or paralysis causes breathlessness in the supine position and is a cause of sleep apnoea leading to daytime headaches and somnolence. Tidal volume is decreased and respiratory rate increased. Vital capacity is substantially reduced when lying down, and sniffing causes a paradoxical inward movement of the abdominal wall best seen in the supine position. Causes include viral infections, multiple sclerosis, motor neurone disease, poliomyelitis, Guillain–Barré syndrome, quadriplegia after trauma and rare muscle diseases. Treatment is either diaphragmatic pacing or night-time assisted ventilation.

Complete eventration of the diaphragm (invariably left-sided) is a congenital condition in which muscle is replaced by fibrous tissue. It presents as marked elevation of the left hemidiaphragm, sometimes associated with gastrointestinal symptoms. Partial eventration, usually on the right, causes a hump (often anteriorly) on the diaphragmatic shadow on X-ray.

Hernias occur through the diaphragm, the commonest being through the oesophageal hiatus, but occasionally anteriorly, through the foramen of Morgani, posterolaterally through the foramen of Bochdalek or at any site following traumatic tears.

Hiccups—see p. 173.

Mediastinal lesions

The mediastinum is defined as the region between the pleural sacs. It is additionally divided as shown in Fig. 12.40. Tumours affecting the mediastinum are rare.

Retrosternal or intrathoracic thyroid

The commonest mediastinal tumour is a retrosternal or intrathoracic thyroid, which is nearly always an extension of the thyroid present in the neck. Enlargement of the thyroid by a colloid goitre or malignant disease and, rarely, in thyrotoxicosis causes displacement of the trachea and oesophagus to the opposite side. Symptoms of compression develop insidiously before producing the cardinal feature of dyspnoea. Very occasionally an intrathoracic thyroid may be the cause of dysphagia and, rarely, of hoarseness of the voice and vocal-cord paralysis from stretching of the recurrent laryngeal nerve. The treatment is surgical removal.

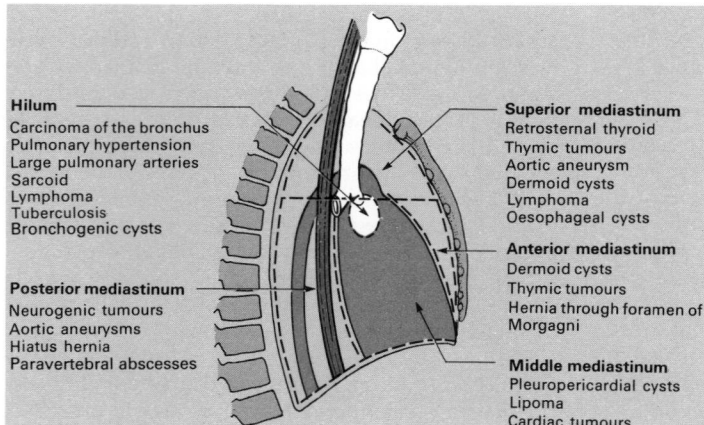

Fig. 12.40 Subdivisions of the mediastinum and mass lesions.

Hilum
Carcinoma of the bronchus
Pulmonary hypertension
Large pulmonary arteries
Sarcoid
Lymphoma
Tuberculosis
Bronchogenic cysts

Posterior mediastinum
Neurogenic tumours
Aortic aneurysms
Hiatus hernia
Paravertebral abscesses

Superior mediastinum
Retrosternal thyroid
Thymic tumours
Aortic aneurysm
Dermoid cysts
Lymphoma
Oesophageal cysts

Anterior mediastinum
Dermoid cysts
Thymic tumours
Hernia through foramen of Morgagni

Middle mediastinum
Pleuropericardial cysts
Lipoma
Cardiac tumours

Thymic tumours

The thymus is large in childhood and occupies the superior and anterior mediastinum. It involutes with age but may be enlarged both by cysts, which are rarely symptomatic, or tumours, which may cause the symptoms of myasthenia gravis or may lead to compression of the trachea or, rarely, the oesophagus. Surgery is the treatment of choice. Approximately half of the patients presenting with a thymic tumour have myasthenia gravis.

Pleuro-pericardial cysts

These cysts, which may be up to 10 cm in diameter, are filled with clear fluid and are usually situated anteriorly in the cardiophrenic angle on the right in 70% of cases. Infection only rarely occurs; malignant change does not occur. The diagnosis is usually made by needle aspiration. No treatment is required, but these patients should be followed up as an increase in cyst size suggests an alternative pathology; surgical excision is then advisable.

Further reading

Clark TJH & Godfrey S (eds) (1983) *Asthma*, 2nd edn. London: Chapman and Hall.

Davies RJ and Ollier S (1989) *Allergy the Facts*. Oxford University Press.

Seaton A, Seaton D, Leitch AG (1989) *Crofton and Douglas's Respiratory Diseases*, 4th edn. Oxford: Blackwell Scientific.

Mackay I (1989) *Rhinitis, Mechanisms and Management*. London: Royal Society of Medicine Services.

13

Intensive Care Medicine

Introduction

A glossary of terms and abbreviations used in this chapter is given in the Appendices.

Intensive care medicine (or 'critical care medicine') is concerned predominantly with the management of patients with acute life-threatening conditions ('the critically ill') in a specialized unit. It also encompasses the resuscitation and transport of those who become acutely ill, or are injured, either elsewhere in the hospital or in the community.

An intensive care unit is fully equipped with monitoring and technical facilities. Patients can receive intensive nursing care and the constant attention of appropriately trained medical staff. These conditions and facilities are not available on a general ward.

In all critically ill patients, the immediate objective is to preserve life and prevent, reverse or minimize damage to vital organs such as the brain and the kidneys. This is achieved by supporting cardiovascular and respiratory function in order to maximize delivery of oxygen to the tissues.

In this chapter only cardiovascular and respiratory problems are discussed. Many patients have failure of other organs such as the kidney and liver as well; treatment of these is dealt with in the appropriate chapters. Feeding the critically ill patient is discussed in Chapter 3.

Oxygen delivery

Oxygen delivery (oxygen flux) is defined as the total amount of oxygen delivered to the tissues per unit time. It is dependent on the volume of blood flowing through the microcirculation per minute (i.e. the total cardiac output—Q_t) and the amount of oxygen contained in that blood (i.e. the arterial oxygen content—C_aO_2). Oxygen is transported in combination with haemoglobin or dissolved in plasma. The amount combined with haemoglobin is determined by the oxygen capacity of the haemoglobin (usually taken as 1.34 ml O_2 per gram of haemoglobin) and its percentage saturation with oxygen (SO_2), while the volume dissolved in plasma depends on the partial pressure of oxygen (PO_2). Except when hyperbaric oxygen is administered, the amount of dissolved oxygen in plasma is sufficiently small to be ignored for most practical purposes.

The concept of oxygen flux (see text)

Oxygen flux = Cardiac output × Arterial oxygen content

Oxygen flux = Cardiac output × [(Hb × SO_2 × 1.34) + (P_aO_2 × 0.003)]

For representative values in a normal adult, and ignoring the small amount of dissolved oxygen:

$$1000 \text{ ml·min}^{-1} = 5000 \text{ ml} \times \tfrac{15}{100} \text{ g·ml}^{-1} \times \tfrac{99}{100} \times 1.34$$

Since oxygen consumption is normally approximately 250 ml·min^{-1}, there is an excess of supply over demand that provides a margin of safety if oxygen consumption increases or oxygen delivery falls.

Clinically, however, the concept of oxygen flux provides little information about the relative flow to individual organs. Furthermore, some organs have high oxygen requirements relative to their blood flow and may become hypoxic even if the overall oxygen flux is apparently adequate.

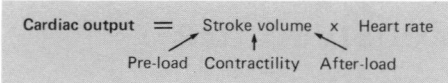

Fig. 13.1 The determinants of cardiac output.

CARDIAC OUPUT

Cardiac output is the product of heart rate and stroke volume, and is affected by changes in either (Fig. 13.1).

Heart rate

Extreme bradycardias and tachycardias can both cause reductions in cardiac output.

Increased heart rate
When heart rate increases, the duration of systole remains essentially unchanged, whereas diastole, and thus the time available for ventricular filling, becomes progressively shorter, and the stroke volume eventually falls. In the normal heart this occurs at rates greater than about 160 beats per minute, but in those with cardiac pathology, especially when this restricts ventricular filling (e.g. mitral stenosis), stroke volume may fall at much lower heart rates. Furthermore, tachycardias cause a marked increase in myocardial oxygen consumption and this may precipitate ischaemia in areas of the myocardium that have reduced coronary perfusion.

Decreased heart rate
When the heart rate falls, a point is reached at which the increase in stoke volume is insufficient to compensate for the bradycardia and again cardiac output falls.

Alterations in heart rate are often caused by disturbances of rhythm (e.g. atrial fibrillation, complete heart block or junctional arrhythmias), in which ventricular filling is not augmented by atrial contraction and stoke volume therefore falls.

Stroke volume

Three factors determine the stroke volume: pre-load, myocardial contractility and after-load (see p. 562).

Pre-load
This is defined as the tension of the myocardial fibres at the end of diastole, just before the onset of ventricular contraction, and is therefore related to the degree of stretch of the fibres (Fig. 13.2). The main factor influencing pre-load is the venous return. As the end-diastolic volume of the ventricle increases, stroke volume rises (Fig. 13.3).

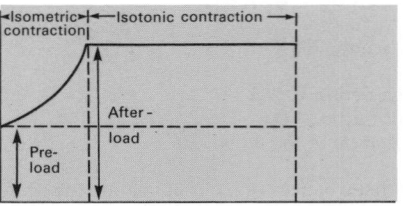

Fig. 13.2 The relationship between myocardial tension and contraction. 'Pre-load' is the tension of the myocardial fibres prior to the onset of systole and depends on the degree to which they are passively stretched. During isometric contraction the tension in the contractile elements increases. The tension required to open the aortic valve and eject blood from the ventricle is the 'after-load'.

Myocardial oxygen consumption ($\dot{V}_mO_2$) increases only slightly with an increase in pre-load and this is therefore the most efficient way of improving cardiac output.

Myocardial contractility
The state of myocardial contractility determines the response of the ventricles to changes in pre-load and after-load. Contractility is often reduced in intensive-care patients, either as a result of pre-existing myocardial damage, e.g. ischaemic heart disease, or the acute disease process itself. Changes in myocardial contractility alter the slope and position of the Starling curve; the resulting worsening ventricular performance is manifested as a depressed, flattened curve (Fig. 13.3).

After-load
This is defined as the myocardial wall tension developed during systolic ejection (Fig. 13.2). In the case of the left ventricle it is determined by the resistance imposed by the aortic valve, the peripheral vascular resistance and the elasticity of the major blood vessels.

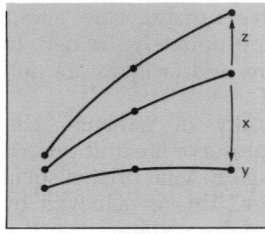

Fig. 13.3 Ventricular function (Starling) curve. As pre-load is increased, stroke volume rises. If the ventricle is overstretched, stroke volume will fall (x). In myocardial failure, the curve is depressed and flattened (y). Increasing contractility shifts the curve upwards and to the left (z).

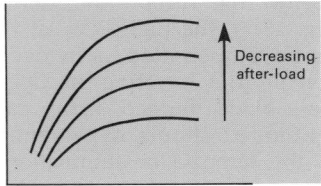

Fig. 13.4 The effect of changes in after-load on the ventricular function curve. At any given pre-load, decreasing after-load increases the stroke volume.

Decreasing the after-load can increase the stroke volume achieved at a given pre-load (Fig. 13.4), whilst also reducing the ventricular wall tension and the myocardial oxygen consumption. The reduction in wall tension may lead to an increase in coronary blood flow, thereby improving the myocardial oxygen supply–demand ratio.

An *increase* in after-load, on the other hand, can cause a fall in stroke volume and is a potent cause of increased $\dot{V}_mO_2$. Right ventricular after-load is normally negligible because the resistance of the pulmonary circulation is very low.

OXYGENATION OF THE BLOOD

Oxygen content (C_aO_2) is dependent on the amount of haemoglobin present per unit volume of blood, its oxygen capacity and its percentage saturation with oxygen. For this reason, maintenance of an 'adequate' haemoglobin concentration is essential in critically ill patients. However, tissue oxygenation is also dependent on blood flow. This is in turn determined not only by the cardiac output and its distribution, but also by the viscosity of the blood. The latter depends largely on the packed cell volume (PCV) and it is generally considered that the optimal balance between oxygen-carrying capacity and tissue flow is achieved at a PCV of approximately 30–35%.

Oxyhaemoglobin dissociation curve

The saturation of haemoglobin with oxygen is determined by the partial pressure of oxygen (PO_2) in the blood, the relationship between the two being described by the oxyhaemoglobin dissociation curve (Fig. 13.5). The sigmoid shape of this curve is important clinically for a number of reasons.

- Falls in P_aO_2 may be tolerated provided that the percentage saturation remains above 90%.
- Increasing the P_aO_2 to above normal has only a minimal effect on oxygen content unless hyperbaric oxygen is administered (when the amount

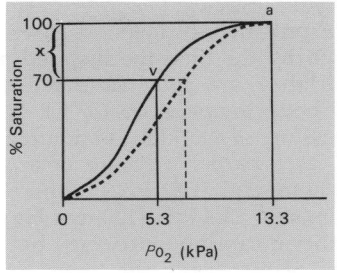

Fig. 13.5 The oxyhaemoglobin dissociation curve: a = arterial point; v = venous point; x = arteriovenous oxygen content difference.

The curve will move to the right (broken line) in the presence of acidosis (metabolic or respiratory), pyrexia or an increased red-cell 2,3-DPG concentration. For a given arteriovenous oxygen content difference, the mixed venous PO_2 will then be higher. Furthermore, if the mixed venous PO_2 is unchanged, the arteriovenous oxygen content difference increases and more oxygen is off-loaded to the tissues (see p. 296).

of oxygen in solution in plasma becomes significant).
- Once on the steep 'slippery slope' of the curve, a small decrease in P_aO_2 can cause large falls in oxygen content, while increasing P_aO_2 only slightly (e.g. by administering 28% oxygen to a patient with chronic bronchitis) can lead to useful increases in oxygen saturation.

The P_aO_2 is in turn influenced by the alveolar oxygen tension (P_AO_2), the efficiency of pulmonary gas exchange, and the partial pressure of oxygen in mixed venous blood ($P_{\bar{v}}O_2$).

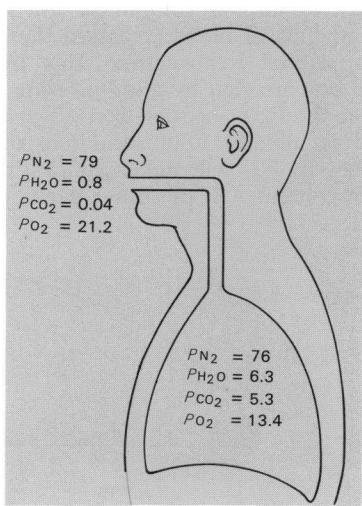

Fig. 13.6 The partial pressures of inspired and alveolar gas (values given in kilopascals).

Alveolar oxygen tension
The partial pressures of inspired gases are shown in Fig. 13.6. By the time the inspired gases reach the alveoli they are fully saturated with water vapour at body temperature (37°C), which has a partial pressure of 6.3 kPa (47 mm Hg) and contains CO_2 at a partial pressure of approximately 5.3 kPa (40 mm Hg). The P_AO_2 is thereby reduced to approximately 13.4 kPa (100 mm Hg).

The clinician can influence P_AO_2 by administering oxygen or increasing the barometric pressure (i.e. administering hyperbaric oxygen). Because of the reciprocal relationship between the partial pressures of oxygen and carbon dioxide in the alveoli, a small increase in P_AO_2 can be produced by lowering the P_ACO_2 (e.g. using intermittent positive pressure ventilation—IPPV).

Pulmonary gas exchange
In *normal* subjects there is a small alveolar–arterial oxygen difference ($P_{A-a}O_2$). This is due to:

- A small (0.133 kPa, 1 mm Hg) pressure gradient across the alveolar membrane
- A small amount of blood (2% of total cardiac output) bypassing the lungs via the bronchial and thebesian veins.

Pathologically there are three causes of a $P_{A-a}O_2$ difference:

- *Diffusion defect.* This is not an important cause of hypoxaemia even in conditions such as fibrosing alveolitis, in which the alveolar capillary membrane is considerably thickened. Certainly carbon dioxide is not affected, as it is much more soluble than oxygen.
- *Right-to-left shunts.* In certain congenital cardiac lesions, e.g. Fallot's tetralogy and when a segment of lung is completely unventilated, a large amount of blood bypasses the lungs and causes arterial hypoxaemia. This hypoxaemia cannot be corrected by administering oxygen to increase the P_AO_2, because blood leaving normal alveoli is already fully saturated and further increases in PO_2 will not significantly affect its oxygen content. On the other hand, because of

the shape of the carbon dioxide dissociation curve (Fig. 13.7), the high PCO_2 of the shunted blood can be compensated for by overventilating patent alveoli, thus lowering the CO_2 content of the effluent blood. Indeed, many patients with acute right-to-left shunts hyperventilate in response to the hypoxia or stimulation of stretch receptors in the lung, so that the P_aCO_2 is normal or low.

- *Ventilation/perfusion ($\dot{V}/\dot{Q}$) mismatch.* This is discussed in more detail in Chapter 12.

  Diseases of the lung parenchyma result in a $\dot{V}/\dot{Q}$ mismatch, producing an increase in alveolar dead space and hypoxaemia. The former can be compensated for by increasing overall ventilation. In contrast to the hypoxia resulting from a true right-to-left shunt (see above), that due to areas of low $\dot{V}/\dot{Q}$ can be partially corrected by administering oxygen and thereby increasing the P_AO_2 even in poorly ventilated areas of lung.

Mixed venous PO_2 ($P_{\bar{v}}O_2$)
This is the partial pressure of oxygen in pulmonary arterial blood that has been thoroughly mixed during its passage through the heart. If P_aO_2 remains constant, the $P_{\bar{v}}O_2$ will fall if more oxygen has to be extracted from each unit volume of blood arriving at the tissues. A fall in $P_{\bar{v}}O_2$ will occur if the cardiac output and thus oxygen delivery falls and/or tissue oxygen requirements increase. If $P_{\bar{v}}O_2$ falls, the effect of a given degree of pulmonary shunting on arterial oxygenation will be exacerbated. Thus, worsening arterial hypoxaemia does not necessarily indicate a deterioration in pulmonary function but may instead reflect a fall in cardiac output and/or a rise in oxygen consumption.

The $P_{\bar{v}}O_2$ is also influenced by the position of the oxyhaemoglobin dissociation curve (Fig. 13.5), a factor not incorporated in the concept of oxygen flux. Thus, if the arteriovenous oxygen content difference remains constant, a shift of the curve to the right, which occurs with acidosis, hypercarbia,

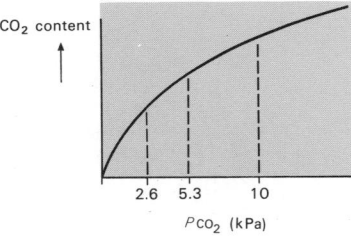

Fig. 13.7 The carbon dioxide dissociation curve. Note that in the physiological range the curve is essentially linear.

Table 13.1 Causes of shock.

Cardiogenic (e.g. ischaemic cardiac damage)

Mechanical
  Obstruction to outflow (e.g. pulmonary embolus)
  Restricted cardiac filling (e.g. cardiac tamponade)

Peripheral circulation
  Hypovolaemic:
    Exogenous losses (e.g. haemorrhage, burns)
    Endogenous losses (e.g. sepsis, anaphylaxis)
  Normovolaemic:
    Dilatation
    Sequestration   } (e.g. sepsis, anaphylaxis)
    Arteriovenous shunting

pyrexia and a rise in red-cell 2,3-diphosphogly-cerate (2,3-DPG) levels, may cause the $P_{\bar{v}}O_2$ to rise. If the $P_{\bar{v}}O_2$ remains unchanged, more oxygen will be unloaded at tissue level. A shift of the curve to the left, on the other hand, will cause a fall in the $P_{\bar{v}}O_2$. It might be argued, then, that under certain circumstances an acidosis may be beneficial in terms of tissue oxygenation, provided that it is not severe enough to interfere with cardiac function. It is probable though, that shifts of the dissociation curve are of little clinical significance.

Acute disturbances of haemodynamic function (shock)

Shock is difficult to define. The term is used to describe acute circulatory failure resulting in generalized cellular hypoxia due to inadequate or inappropriately distributed tissue perfusion.

CAUSES

The causes are shown in Table 13.1. Very often shock can result from a combination of these factors.

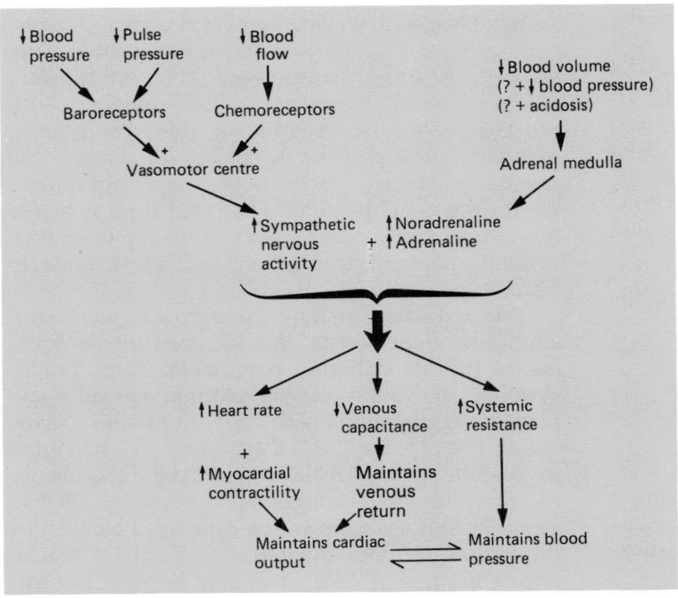

PATHOPHYSIOLOGY

Sympatho-adrenal response to shock (Fig. 13.8)

Hypotension stimulates the baroreceptors, and to a lesser extent the chemoreceptors, causing increased sympathetic nervous activity. Later this is augmented by the release of catecholamines from the adrenal medulla. The resulting vasoconstriction, together with increased myocardial contractility and heart rate helps to restore blood pressure and cardiac output. Opioid peptides containing the enkephalin sequence have been identified within the same chromaffin cells as catecholamines and are also released into the circulation in shock.

Reduction in perfusion of the renal cortex stimulates the juxtaglomerular apparatus to release renin. This converts angiotensinogen to angiotensin I, which is in turn converted in the lungs to the potent vasoconstrictor angiotensin II. Angiotensin II also stimulates secretion of aldosterone by the adrenal cortex, causing sodium and water retention. This helps to restore the circulating volume.

Neuroendocrine response to shock

- Release of pituitary hormones: adrenocorticotrophic hormone (ACTH), growth hormone (GH), vasopressin (antidiuretic hormone, ADH) and β-endorphin. (Endogenous opioid peptides such as β-endorphin, dynorphin and the enkephalins may be partly responsible for some of the cardiovascular changes.)
- Release of cortisol, which causes fluid retention and antagonizes insulin.
- Release of glucagon, which raises blood sugar.

Fig. 13.8 The sympatho-adrenal response to shock.

Release of mediators

The presence of severe infection (often with bacteraemia or endotoxaemia) or of large areas of devitalized tissue (e.g. following trauma or major surgery) can trigger a massive inflammatory response with systemic activation of leucocytes and release of a variety of potentially damaging 'mediators'. Although clearly beneficial when targeted against local areas of infection or necrotic tissue, dissemination of this response can produce widespread tissue damage.

Activation of complement cascade

One of the many functions of the complement system is to attract and activate leucocytes, which then marginate on to endothelium and release inflammatory mediators such as proteases and toxic oxygen radicals; these can produce local tissue damage. For example, the free radical superoxide (O_2^-) can participate in a number of chemical reactions, yielding hydrogen peroxide (H_2O_2) and hydroxyl radicals (OH^-), which can damage cell membranes, interfere with the function of a number of enzyme systems and increase capillary permeability.

Cytokines

Macrophage- and lymphocyte-derived cytokines such as the interleukins and tumour necrosis factor (TNF) are involved in the pathogenesis of shock. TNF release initiates many of the responses to endotoxin.

Platelet-activating factor

This vasoactive lipid is released from various cell populations, such as leucocytes and macrophages, in shock. Its effects, which are caused both directly and through the secondary release of other mediators, include hypotension, increased vascular permeability and platelet aggregation.

Products of arachidonic acid metabolism (see Fig. 12.30)

Arachidonic acid, derived from the increased breakdown of membrane phospholipid, is metabolized to form prostaglandins and leukotrienes, which are important inflammatory mediators. Prostaglandins currently thought to be of importance in shock include:

- Prostacyclin, which is a vasodilator and inhibits platelet aggregation
- Thomboxane A_2, which causes pulmonary vasoconstriction and activates platelets
- $PGF_2\alpha$, which may be responsible for the early phase of pulmonary hypertension commonly seen in experimental septic shock

Leukotrienes have a variety of effects including a reduction in cardiac output, vasoconstriction, increased vascular permeability and platelet activation.

Lysosomal enzymes

These are released in response to hypoxia, ischaemia, sepsis and acidosis. As well as being directly cytotoxic, they can cause myocardial depression and coronary vasoconstriction. Furthermore, lysosomal enzymes can convert inactive kininogens, which are usually combined with α-2-globulin, to vasoactive kinins such as bradykinin. These substances can cause vasodilatation and increased capillary permeability, as well as myocardial depression. They can also activate clotting mechanisms.

Microcirculatory changes

Since shock is a syndrome caused by inadequate tissue perfusion, the final common pathway for the pathophysiological changes is the microcirculation.

In the *early stages of septic shock* there is vasodilatation, arteriovenous shunting, increased capillary permeability and a defect of oxygen utilization by the tissues. Initially, before hypovolaemia supervenes, or when therapeutic replacement of circulating volume has been adequate, cardiac output is usually high and peripheral resistance low. Vasodilatation and increased capillary permeability also occur in anaphylactic shock.

In the initial stages of *other forms of shock*, and when hypovolaemia supervenes in sepsis and anaphylaxis, increased sympathetic activity causes constriction of both pre-capillary arterioles and, to a lesser extent, the post-capillary venules. This helps to maintain the systemic blood pressure. In addition, the hydrostatic pressure within the capillaries falls and fluid is mobilized from the extravascular space into the intravascular compartment. If shock persists, the accumulation of metabolites, such as lactic acid and carbon dioxide, combined with the release of vasoactive substances, causes relaxation of the pre-capillary sphincters, while the post-capillary venules, which are more sensitive to hypoxic damage, become relatively unresponsive to these substances and remain constricted. Blood is therefore sequestered within the dilated capillary bed and fluid is forced into the extravascular spaces, causing interstitial oedema, haemoconcentration, and an increase in viscosity.

This reduction in flow through the microcirculation, combined with the increase in viscosity, makes the blood highly coagulable. There is also systemic activation of the clotting cascade and platelet aggregation with clot formation occurs within the capillary bed. Plasminogen is converted to plasmin, which breaks down these clots, liberating fibrin/fibrinogen degradation products (FDPs). The cells that are supplied by capillaries blocked by this process of disseminated intravascular coagulation (DIC) (see p. 343) inevitably become hypoxic and eventually die. Tissue ischaemia is further exacerbated as capillaries are compressed by interstitial oedema. In this way vital organs may suffer serious damage. Finally, because clotting factors and platelets are consumed in DIC, they are unavailable for haemostasis elsewhere and a coagulation defect results—hence the alternative name for DIC of 'consumption coagulopathy'. This process occurs earlier and is more severe in septicaemic shock.

The capillary endothelium can be damaged by a number of factors, (particularly in septic shock), including DIC, microemboli, release of vasoactive compounds, complement, and activated leucocytes. Capillary permeability is thereby increased and fluid is lost into the extravascular space, causing further hypovolaemia, interstitial oedema and organ dysfunction.

Metabolic changes

Once the supply of oxygen to the cells is insufficient for continuation of the tricarboxylic acid (TCA) cycle, production of energy in the form of ATP becomes dependent on anaerobic metabolism. Under these circumstances, glucose is metabolized in the normal way to pyruvate but is then converted to lactate instead of entering the Krebs cycle. The H^+ ions released cause a metabolic acidosis. This pathway is relatively inefficient in terms of energy production. Despite the increased cellular permeability to glucose that is induced by hypoxia, shocked patients are often hyperglycaemic because of the elevated circulating levels of insulin antagonists such as cortisol, growth hormone and catecholamines, as well as catecholamine-induced glycogen breakdown. Blood levels of fatty acids and amino acids also rise. Eventually, because of the reduced availability of ATP, the sodium pump fails, cells swell due to accumulation of salt and water, and potassium losses increase. In the final stages, release of lysosomal enzymes may contribute to cell death.

Multiple organ failure (MOF)

Impaired tissue perfusion and microcirculatory abnormalities, often combined with the systemic release of 'mediators' (see above) can damage vital organs. The most severely ill patients may develop multiple organ failure, which is almost invariably associated with persistent sepsis. Following severe shock, damage to the mucosa of the gastrointestinal tract may allow bacteria or endotoxin within the gut lumen to gain access to the circulation, thereby perpetuating the generalized inflammatory response. In most cases the lung is the first organ to be affected with the development of the adult respiratory distress syndrome (ARDS) (see below). Secondary pulmonary infection is common in

ARDS, acting as a further stimulus to the inflammatory response. Later, liver and renal failure develop. Characteristically, these patients initially have a hyperdynamic circulation with vasodilatation and a high cardiac output. Eventually, however, cardio-vascular collapse supervenes and is the usual terminal event. The mortality of MOF is extremely high; factors affecting outcome include the number of organs that fail and the duration of organ failure.

CLINICAL SIGNS

Although many clinical features are common to all types of shock there are certain important respects in which they differ.

Hypovolaemic shock

- Inadequate tissue perfusion:
  (a) Skin—cold, pale, blue, slow capillary refill
  (b) Kidneys—oliguria, anuria
  (c) Brain—confusion and restlessness
- Increased sympathetic tone:
  (a) Tachycardia
  (b) Sweating
  (c) Blood pressure—may be maintained initially (despite up to a 25% reduction in circulating volume if the patient is young and fit), but later hypotension supervenes
- Metabolic acidosis and tachypnoea

Additional clinical features may occur in the following types of shock.

Cardiogenic shock

- Signs of myocardial failure—e.g. raised JVP, pulsus alternans, 'gallop' rhythm, basal crackles

Mechanical shock

- Elevated JVP
- Pulsus paradoxus in cardiac tamponade
- Kussmaul's sign (JVP rises on inspiration) in cardiac tamponade
- Signs of pulmonary embolism (if present)

Anaphylactic shock (see p. 733)

- Signs of profound vasodilatation:
  (a) Warm peripheries
  (b) Low blood pressure
- Urticaria
- Bronchospasm
- Oedema of the face, pharynx and larynx
- Hypovolaemia due to capillary leak

Septic shock

- Pyrexia and rigors

- Early signs (warm normotensive or warm hypotensive):
  - (a) Vasodilatation, warm peripheries
  - (b) Bounding pulse
  - (c) Rapid capillary refill
- Late signs (cold hypotensive):
  - (a) Hypotension and signs as for hypovolaemic shock (see above)
  - (b) Myocardial depression
- Other signs:
  - (a) Jaundice
  - (b) Coma (rare)
  - (c) Signs of DIC

The diagnosis of septicaemia is easily missed. In the elderly, the classical signs may not be present and, for example, mild confusion, tachycardia and tachypnoea may be the only clues, sometimes associated with unexplained hypotension or a reduction in urine output.

MONITORING

Invasive monitoring is unnecessary in straightforward cases, such as a fit young man with moderate traumatic haemorrhage, but will be required in the more seriously ill patients and in those who fail to respond to initial treatment (see later). Clinical assessment must never be neglected.

Clinical indices of tissue perfusion

Pale, cold skin, delayed capillary refill and the absence of visible veins in the hands and feet indicate poor perfusion. Skin-temperature measurements can help clinical evaluation as

---

Radial artery cannulation

Technique
- The arm is supported, with the wrist extended, by an assistant.
- The radial artery is palpated where it arches over the head of the radius.
- In conscious patients, local anaesthetic is injected to raise a weal over the artery, taking care not to puncture the vessel or obscure its pulsation.
- A small skin incision is made over the proposed puncture site.
- A small parallel-sided cannula (20 gauge for adults, 22 gauge for children) is used in order to allow blood to flow past the cannula. Teflon is less irritant.
- The cannula is inserted over the point of maximal pulsation and advanced in line with the direction of the vessel at an angle of approximately 30°.
- 'Flashback' of blood into the cannula indicates that the radial artery has been punctured.
- The cannula is threaded off the needle into the vessel and the needle withdrawn.
- The cannula is connected to a non-compliant manometer line filled with heparinized saline. This is then connected via a transducer and continuous flush device to an oscilloscope, which records the arterial pressure.

Complications
- Thrombosis
- Loss of arterial pulsation
- Distal ischaemia, e.g. digital necrosis (rare)
- Accidental injection of drugs—can produce vascular occlusion
- Disconnection—leading to hypovolaemia

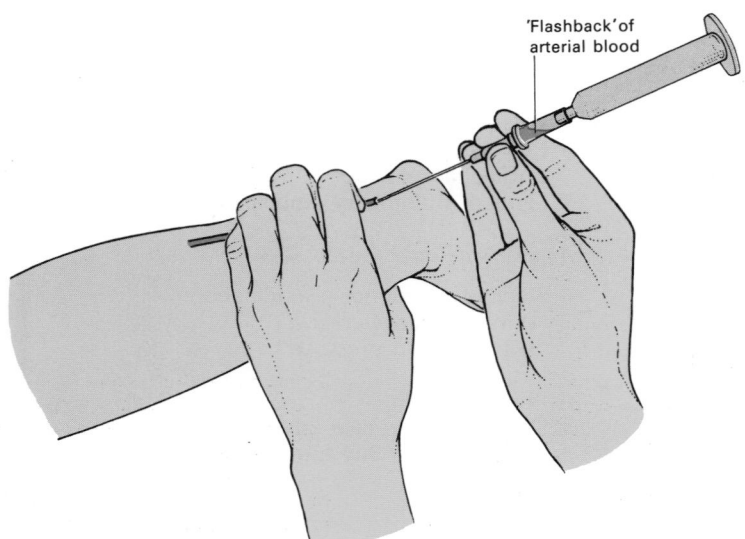

'Flashback' of arterial blood

Fig. 13.9 Percutaneous cannulation of the radial artery.

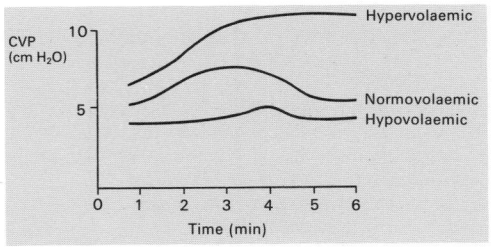

Fig. 13.10 The effects of rapid administration of a 'fluid challenge' to patients with a central venous pressure within the normal range. (From Sykes MK (1963) Venous pressure as a clinical indication of adequacy of transfusion. *Annals of the Royal College of Surgeons of England* **33**: 185–197. With permission.)

vasoconstriction is an early compensatory response.

Urinary flow is a sensitive indicator of renal perfusion and haemodynamic performance.

Blood pressure

This usually reflects the adequacy of the cardiac output. However, if there is vasoconstriction with a high peripheral resistance, the blood pressure may be normal, even when the cardiac output is reduced.

The asbolute level of blood pressure is also important, since hypotension may jeopardize perfusion of vital organs.

Blood pressure is traditionally measured with a sphygmomanometer, but automated instruments using a microphone to detect Korotkoff's sounds or continuous monitoring with an intra-arterial cannula, usually in the radial artery, can be used (Fig. 13.9).

Central venous pressure (CVP)

This provides a fairly simple method of assessing the adequacy of a patient's circulating volume and the contractile state of the myocardium. The absolute value of the CVP is not as important as its response to a fluid challenge (the infusion of 100–200 ml of fluid over 1–3 min) (Fig. 13.10). The hypovolaemic patient will initially respond to transfusion with little or no change in CVP, together with some improvement in cardiovascular function (falling heart rate, rising blood pressure and increased peripheral temperature). As the normovolaemic state is approached, the CVP usually rises slightly and stabilizes, while other cardiovascular values normalize. At this stage, volume replacement should be slowed, or even stopped, in order to avoid overtransfusion. Overtransfusion is indicated by an abrupt and sustained rise in CVP, often accompanied by some deterioration in the patient's condition. In cardiac failure the venous pressure is unusually high; the patient will not respond to volume replacement, which will cause a further, sometimes dramatic, rise in CVP.

The CVP may be read intermittently using a manometer system (Fig. 13.11) or continuously using a transducer connected to an oscilloscope, similar to that used for intra-arterial monitoring.

Common pitfalls in interpreting CVP results are:

- Blocked catheter. This results in a sustained high reading.
- Manometer or transducer wrongly positioned. Failure to level the CVP after changing the patient's position is a common cause of erroneous readings.
- Incorrect calibration. If an electronic transducer and oscilloscope are used, the system should be zeroed and calibrated prior to use.

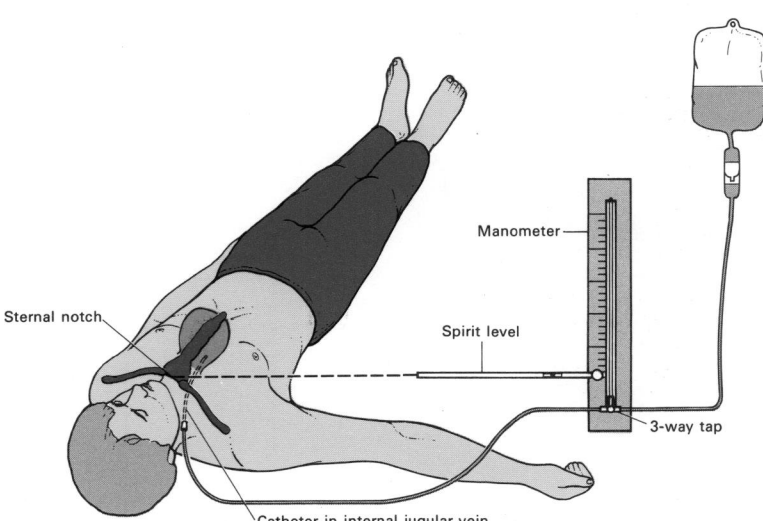

Fig. 13.11 Central venous pressure measurement using a manometer system. The reading must be referred to the level of the right atrium (indicated by the axillary fold or, provided the patient is supine, the sternal notch) using a spirit level.

- One or more infusions in progress through the CVP catheter. The CVP catheter may be used for other infusions and the pressure measured intermittently. A falsely high reading will result if these fluids continue to be administered by an infusion pump while the pressure is recorded.
- Catheter tip in right ventricle. If the catheter is advanced too far, an unexpectedly high pressure is recorded.

The catheter should be positioned in the superior vena cava. It is usually inserted via a percutaneous puncture of a subclavian or internal jugular vein (Fig. 13.12).

Left atrial pressure

Under most circumstances the CVP is an adequate guide to the filling pressures of both sides of the heart. However, in many critically ill patients this is not the case and there is a disparity in function between the two ventricles. Most commonly, left ventricular performance is worst, so that the left ventricular function curve is displaced downward and to the right (Fig. 13.13). This situation is encountered in some patients with clinically significant ischaemic heart disease and has also been reported in major trauma, sepsis, peritonitis, hepatic failure, valvular heart disease and after cardiac surgery. High right ventricular filling pressures, with normal or low left atrial pressures, are less common but may occur in right ventricular ischaemia and in situations where the pulmonary vascular resistance (i.e. right ventricular after-load) is raised, such as acute respiratory failure and pulmonary embolism.

These discrepancies between right and left ventricular performance can be exacerbated by the use of inotropic and vasoactive drugs. If there is a

PROCEDURE FOR CANNULATION OF THE INTERNAL JUGULAR VEIN

- The procedure is explained to the patient.
- The patient is placed head-down to distend the central veins (this facilitates cannulation and minimizes the risk of air embolism).
- The skin is cleaned. Sterile precautions are taken throughout the procedure.
- Local anaesthetic (1% plain lignocaine) is injected intradermally to raise a weal at the apex of a triangle formed by the two heads of sternomastoid with the clavicle at its base.
- A small incision is made through the weal.
- The cannula is inserted through the incision and directed laterally downwards and backwards until the vein is punctured just beneath the skin and deep to the lateral head of sternomastoid.
- It is checked that venous blood is easily aspirated using a syringe attached to the cannula.
- The cannula is threaded off the needle into the vein.
- The CVP manometer line is connected.
- If the catheter is in a large vein, venous blood will flow back when the giving-set tap is open and the infusion bottle is on the floor.
- The CVP is measured. The fluid level in the manometer should then fall rapidly and fluctuate with respiration.
- A chest X-ray should be taken to verify that the tip of the catheter is in the superior vena cava and to exclude pneumothorax.

Possible complications

- Accidental arterial puncture (carotid or subclavian)
- Damage to thoracic duct on left
- Air embolism
- Pneumothorax
- Thrombosis
- Catheter-related sepsis

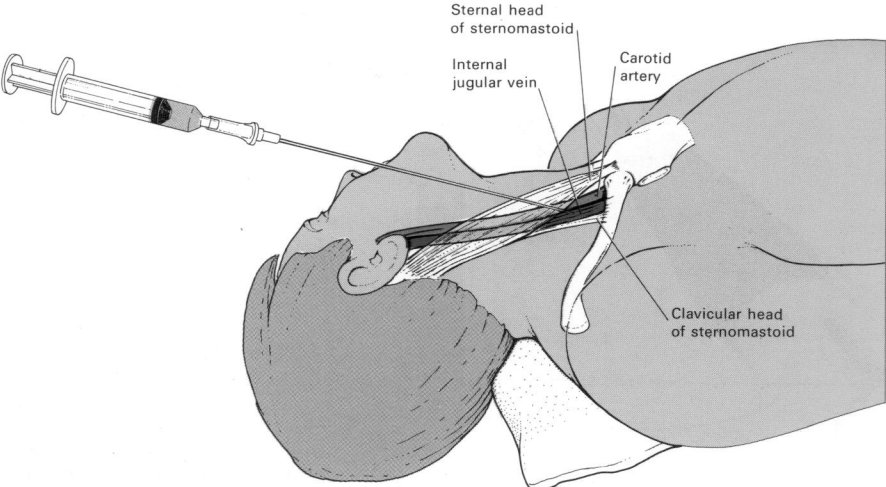

Fig. 13.12 Cannulation of the right internal jugular vein with a catheter-over-needle device.

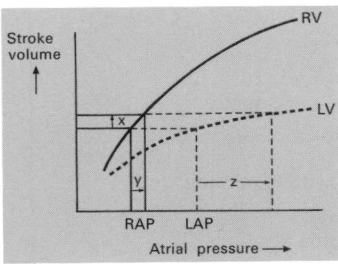

Fig. 13.13 Left ventricular (LV) and right ventricular (RV) function curves in a patient with left ventricular dysfunction. Since the stroke volume of the two ventricles must be the same (except perhaps for a few beats during a period of circulatory adjustment), left atrial pressure (LAP) must be higher than right atrial pressure (RAP). Moreover, an increase in stroke volume (x) produced by a small rise in RAP (y) will be associated with a marked increase in LAP (z).

disparity in ventricular function after cardiac surgery, then the left atrium can be cannulated directly. If the thorax is not open, however, some other means of determining left ventricular filling pressure must be devised.

Pulmonary artery pressure

A 'balloon flotation catheter' enables prompt and reliable catheterization of the pulmonary artery, without the need for screening, and minimizes the incidence of arrhythmias.

These 'Swan–Ganz' catheters can be inserted centrally through the femoral vein or via a vein in the antecubital fossa. Passage of the catheter from the major veins, through the chambers of the heart, into the pulmonary artery and into the wedge position is monitored and guided by the pressure waveforms recorded from the distal lumen (Fig. 13.14). A chest X-ray should always be obtained to check the final position of the catheter. Once in place, the balloon is deflated and the pulmonary artery mean systolic and end-diastolic pressures (PAEDP) can be recorded. The pulmonary capillary wedge pressure (PCWP) is measured by re-inflating the balloon, thereby propelling the catheter distally until it impacts in a medium-sized pulmonary artery. In this position there is a continuous column of fluid between the distal lumen of the catheter and the left atrium, so that PCWP is usually a reflection of left atrial pressure.

The technique is generally safe—the majority of complications are related to user inexperience. Pulmonary artery catheters should preferably be removed within 72 h, since the incidence of complications then increases progressively (Table 13.2).

Cardiac output

The only quantitatively accurate methods for measuring cardiac output are invasive. Of these, the thermodilution technique is most commonly

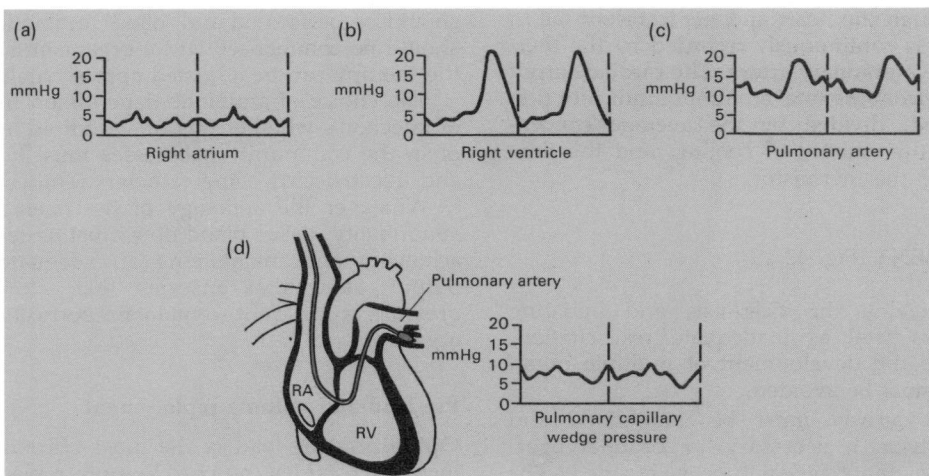

Fig. 13.14 Passage of a Swan–Ganz catheter through the chambers of the heart into the 'wedge' position. (a) Once in the thorax, marked respiratory oscillations are seen. The catheter should be advanced further towards the lower superior vena cava/right atrium, where oscillations become more pronounced. The balloon should then be inflated and the catheter advanced. (b) When the catheter is in the right ventricle there is no dicrotic notch and the diastolic pressure is close to zero. The patient should be returned to the horizontal, or slightly head-up, position before advancing the catheter further. (c) When the catheter reaches the pulmonary artery a dicrotic notch appears and there is elevation of the diastolic-presure. The catheter should be advanced further with the balloon inflated. (d) Reappearance of a venous waveform indicates that the catheter is 'wedged'. The catheter is not advanced further. The balloon is deflated to obtain the pulmonary artery pressure. The balloon is inflated intermittently to obtain the pulmonary capillary wedge pressure.

Table 13.2 Some complications of Swan–Ganz catheters.

Complication	Comments
Arrhythmias	May occur during passage of catheter through right ventricle Usually benign Can often be prevented with lignocaine
Sepsis	May occur at insertion site Septicaemia or endocarditis may develop
Knotting	May occur when catheter coils in right ventricle
Valve trauma	Occurs if catheter withdrawn with balloon inflated or due to valves repeatedly closing on catheter
Thrombosis/embolism	
Pulmonary infarction	May occur if catheter remains in 'wedge' position
Pulmonary artery rupture	Usually fatal May occur if balloon is inflated when catheter already 'wedged'
Balloon rupture/leak/embolism	Rare

used clinically. This uses a modified Swan–Ganz catheter with a lumen opening in the right atrium and a thermistor located a few centimetres from its tip. A known volume (usually 10 ml) of ice-cold 5% dextrose is injected as a bolus into the right atrium. This mixes with, and cools, the blood passing through the heart and the transient fall in temperature is continuously recorded by the thermistor in the pulmonary artery. The cardiac output is computed from the total amount of indicator (i.e. cold) injected, divided by the average concentration, i.e. the amount of cooling, and the time taken to pass the thermistor.

MANAGEMENT (Fig. 13.15)

Delay in making the diagnosis and initiating treatment, as well as inadequate resuscitation, contribute to the development of multiple organ failure and must be avoided.

A patent airway must be maintained and oxygen is given. If necessary, an oropharyngeal airway or an endotracheal tube is inserted. The latter has the advantage of preventing aspiration of gastric contents. *Very rarely* emergency tracheostomy is indicated (see below).

The underlying cause of shock should be corrected, e.g. haemorrhage should be controlled or infection eradicated. In patients with septic shock, every effort must be made to identify the source of infection and isolate the causative organism. As well as a thorough history and clinical examination, X-rays, ultrasonography and CT scanning may be required to locate the origin of the infection. Appropriate samples (urine, sputum, cerebrospinal fluid, pus drained from abscesses) should be sent to the laboratory for microscopy, culture and sensitivities. Several blood cultures should be performed and 'blind' antibiotic therapy should be commenced. If an organism is isolated, the therapy can be adjusted appropriately.

The choice of antibiotic depends on the source of infection—whether this was acquired in hospital or in the community. Abscesses must be drained and infected indwelling catheters removed.

Whatever the aetiology of the haemodynamic abnormality, tissue blood flow must be restored by achieving and maintaining an adequate cardiac output, as well as ensuring that arterial blood pressure is sufficient to maintain perfusion of vital organs.

Pre-load and volume replacement

Optimizing pre-load is the most efficient way of increasing cardiac output. Volume replacement is obviously essential in hypovolaemic shock but it is also required in anaphylactic and septic shock because of vasodilatation, sequestration of blood and loss of circulating volume due to capillary leak. Low-output, high-resistance septic shock is usually the result of hypovolaemia. Thus, patients with sepsis will often respond well to expansion of the circulating volume, and are thereby frequently converted to a high-output, low-resistance state.

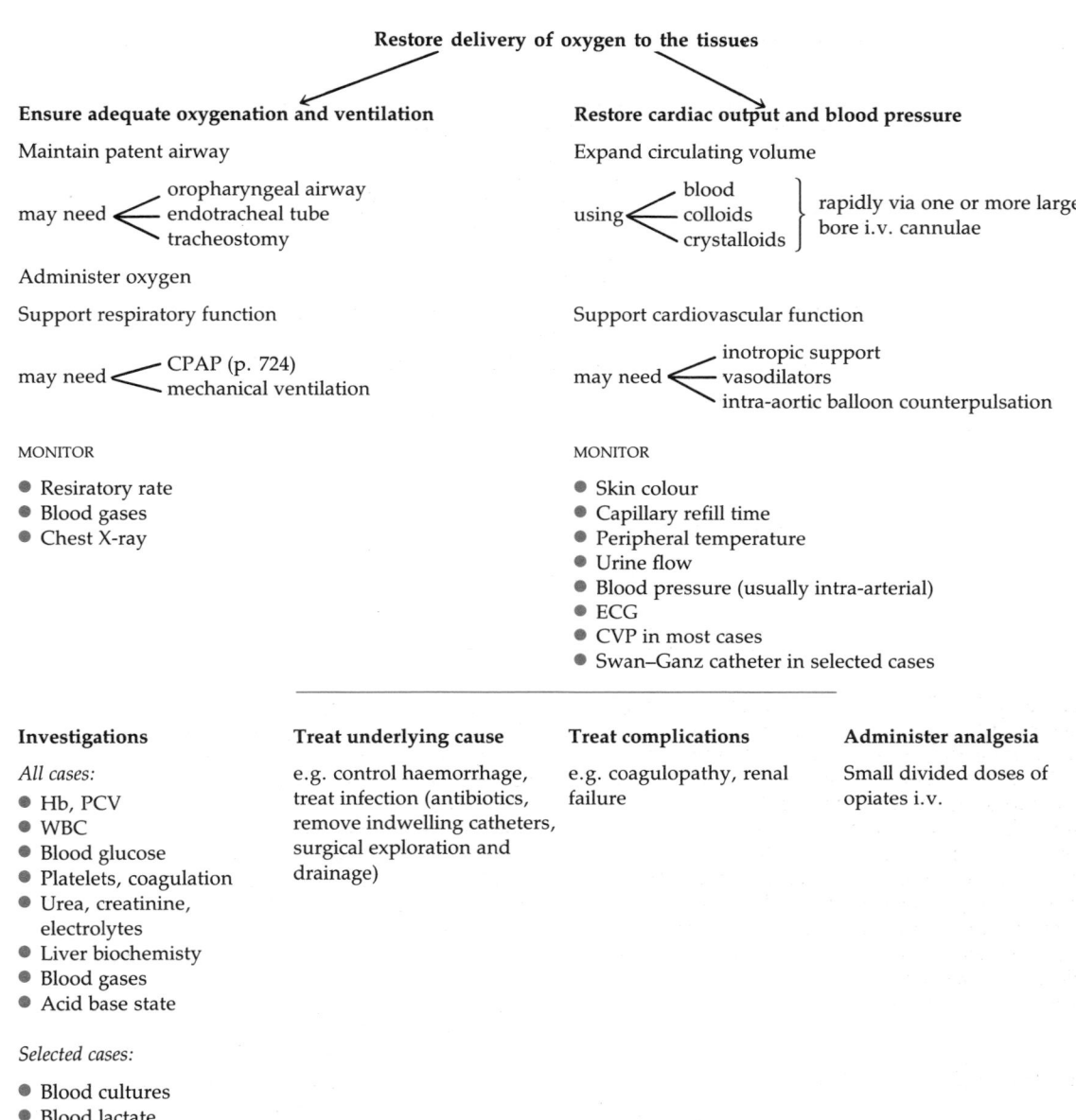

Restore delivery of oxygen to the tissues

Ensure adequate oxygenation and ventilation

Maintain patent airway

may need ← oropharyngeal airway
endotracheal tube
tracheostomy

Administer oxygen

Support respiratory function

may need ← CPAP (p. 724)
mechanical ventilation

MONITOR

- Resiratory rate
- Blood gases
- Chest X-ray

Restore cardiac output and blood pressure

Expand circulating volume

using ← blood
colloids
crystalloids } rapidly via one or more large bore i.v. cannulae

Support cardiovascular function

may need ← inotropic support
vasodilators
intra-aortic balloon counterpulsation

MONITOR

- Skin colour
- Capillary refill time
- Peripheral temperature
- Urine flow
- Blood pressure (usually intra-arterial)
- ECG
- CVP in most cases
- Swan–Ganz catheter in selected cases

Investigations

All cases:

- Hb, PCV
- WBC
- Blood glucose
- Platelets, coagulation
- Urea, creatinine, electrolytes
- Liver biochemisty
- Blood gases
- Acid base state

Selected cases:

- Blood cultures
- Blood lactate
- FDPs

Treat underlying cause

e.g. control haemorrhage, treat infection (antibiotics, remove indwelling catheters, surgical exploration and drainage)

Treat complications

e.g. coagulopathy, renal failure

Administer analgesia

Small divided doses of opiates i.v.

Fig. 13.15 Management of shock.

In mechanical shock, high filling pressures may be required to maintain an adequate stroke volume. Even in cardiogenic shock, careful volume expansion may, on occasions, lead to a useful increase in cardiac output. On the other hand, patients with severe cardiac failure, in whom ventricular filling pressures may be markedly elevated, often benefit from measures to reduce pre-load (and after-load) such as the administration of diuretics and vasodilators (see below).

The circulating volume must be replaced quickly (in minutes not hours) to reduce tissue damage and prevent acute renal failure. Fluid is administered via wide-bore intravenous cannulas to allow large volumes to be given quickly and the effect is continuously monitored.

Care must be taken to prevent volume overload, which leads to cardiac dilatation, a reduction in stroke volume, and a rise in left atrial pressure with a risk of pulmonary oedema. Pulmonary oedema is more likely in very ill patients because of a low colloid osmotic pressure (usually due to a low serum albumin) and disruption of the alveolar–capillary membrane (e.g. in adult respiratory distress syndrome). The development of pulmonary oedema can also be influenced by other unquantifiable factors, such as the hydrostatic and oncotic pressures within the interstitial spaces. Since the pulmonary lymphatics remove excess fluid, pulmonary oedema will only occur when this mechanism is overwhelmed or impaired. Left ventricular filling pressures should therefore not be allowed to rise to more than 15–18 mm Hg in the critically ill. In general, however, many more patients are undertransfused rather than overtransfused.

Choice of fluid for volume replacement

Blood. This is conventionally given for haemorrhagic shock as soon as it is available. In extreme emergencies, uncross-matched group 0 negative blood can be used, but an emergency cross-match can be performed in about 30 min and is as safe as the standard procedure. Donor blood is often separated into its various components for storage, necessitating the transfusion of packed red cells to maintain haemoglobin and plasma, or a plasma substitute for volume replacement.

Complications of blood transfusion are discussed on p. 329. Special problems arise when large volumes of stored blood are transfused rapidly. These include:

- *Temperature changes.* Bank blood is stored at 4°C and transfusion may result in hypothermia, peripheral venoconstriction, (which slows the rate of the infusion) and arrhythmias. Therefore, blood should be warmed if possible prior to the transfusion.
- *Coagulopathy.* Stored blood has essentially no effective platelets and is deficient in clotting factors. Large transfusions can therefore produce a coagulation defect. This may need to be treated by replacing clotting factors with fresh frozen plasma and the administration of platelet concentrates.
- *Metabolic acidosis/alkalosis.* Stored blood is now preserved in citrate/phosphate/dextrose (CPD) solution, which is less acidic than the acid/citrate/dextrose (ACD) solution used previously. Metabolic acidosis attributable solely to blood transfusion is rare. A metabolic alkalosis often develops 24–48 h after a large blood transfusion, probably mainly due to metabolism of the citrate; this will be exacerbated if the preceding acidosis has been corrected with intravenous sodium bicarbonate.
- *Hypocalcaemia.* Stored blood is anticoagulated with citrate, which binds calcium ions. This can reduce total body ionized calcium levels and cause myocardial depression. This is uncommon in practice, but if necessary can be corrected by administering 10 ml of 10% calcium chloride intravenously.
- *Increased oxygen affinity.* In stored blood, the red-cell 2,3-DPG content is reduced, so that the oxyhaemoglobin dissociation curve is shifted to the left. The oxygen affinity of haemoglobin is therefore increased and oxygen delivery is impaired. This effect is less marked with blood stored in CPD. Red-cell levels of 2,3-DPG are substantially restored within 12 h of transfusion.
- *Hyperkalaemia.* Potassium in the plasma rises progressively as blood is stored. However, hyperkalaemia is rarely a problem as prewarming of the blood increases red-cell metabolism—the sodium pump becomes active and potassium levels fall.
- *Microembolism.* Microaggregates in stored blood may be filtered out by the pulmonary capillaries. This process is thought by some to contribute to the adult respiratory distress syndrome.

Because of these problems, the use of crystalloid solutions, plasma, plasma substitutes and oxygen-carrying solutions for volume replacement is assuming greater importance.

Crystalloid solutions. Although crystalloid solutions, e.g. saline, are cheap, convenient to use and free of side-effects, the administration of large volumes of these fluids to critically ill patients should, in general, be avoided. They are rapidly lost from the circulation into the extravascular spaces and volumes of crystalloid 2–4 times that of colloid are required to achieve an equivalent haemodynamic response.

Colloidal solutions. These produce a greater, and more sustained increase in plasma volume, with associated improvements in cardiovascular function and oxygen transport. They also increase colloid osmotic pressure.

Plasma protein fraction (PPF), a natural colloid that is isotonic with plasma, is now widely available, although expensive. In normal subjects it will expand the circulating volume by an amount roughly equivalent to the volume infused. It has a half-life in the circulation of 15–17 days, although this is considerably reduced in those with increased capillary permeability. It has the same sodium content as plasma. Anaphylactoid reactions are rare (< 1% of cases). PPF should not generally be used for routine volume replacement, since other cheaper solutions are equally effective in the short term.

Dextrans are polymolecular polysaccharides in either 5% dextrose or normal saline. Low-molecular-weight dextran (dextran 40; mol. wt 40 000) has a powerful osmotic effect, so that fluid moves from the extravascular to the intravascular compartment, thereby expanding the circulating volume by approximately twice the volume infused. Although viscosity is reduced, this may be counterbalanced by a decrease in the flexibility of the red cells. The disadvantages of dextran 40 are that it is rapidly excreted by the kidneys, it forms a complex with fibrinogen, thereby inducing a coagulopathy, and it coats the red-cell membrane so that blood must be taken for cross-matching before administering dextran.

Dextran 70 (mol. wt 70 000) is also hyperoncotic, although less so than dextran 40, and also interferes with cross-matching. However, it has a longer half-life and is probably the most suitable dextran for routine use.

There is a small risk of allergic reactions (0.07–1.1% of cases). Normally a dose of 1.5 g dextran per kilogram of body weight should not be exceeded because of the risk of renal damage.

Gelatin solutions (haemaccel, gelofusin) have an average molecular weight of 35 000, which is isoosmotic with plasma. They are cheap. Large volumes can be administered, since coagulation defects do not occur and renal function is not impaired. However, because they readily cross the glomerular basement membrane, their half-life in the circulation is only 2–3 h and they can promote an osmotic diuresis. Allergic reactions occur in up to 10% of cases.

Hydroxyethyl starch (HES) has a mean molecular weight of approximately 450 000 and a half-life of about 6 h. Volume expansion is equivalent to, or slightly greater than, the volume infused. The incidence of allergic reactions is approximately 0.1%. Although more expensive than gelatins, HES is a valuable volume expander.

Oxygen-carrying blood substitutes. The ideal solution for volume replacement should have:

- An oncotic pressure similar to plasma
- A long half-life
- No adverse side-effects
- No requirement for cross-matching
- A long shelf-life at room temperature
- Oxygen-carrying properties

Some progress has been made towards attaining these objectives with the development of *fluorocarbon emulsions* (e.g. Fluosol-DA); these contain HES, electrolytes and an emulsifying agent. Although they are excellent volume expanders, the disadvantage is that they have a linear oxygen dissociation curve and they therefore only contribute significantly to oxygen delivery when alveolar oxygen tension is high. A number of serious adverse reactions to Fluosol-DA have been reported.

Haemoglobin solutions also have potential as oxygen-delivering resuscitation fluids, but their use is limited by their short intravascular retention time and their high affinity for oxygen.

Myocardial contractility and inotropic agents

Myocardial contractility can be impaired by hypoxaemia, severe acidosis and hypocalcaemia, as well as by some drugs (e.g. beta-blockers, antiarrhythmics and sedatives). Acidosis should only be corrected when it is severe (pH < 7.2) and is thought to be impairing cardiovascular performance. Sodium bicarbonate 8.4% should then be administered in small (50 ml) aliquots, guided by frequent acid–base measurements, until the pH is returned to a safe level. Sodium overload, marked alkalosis and a shift in the oxyhaemoglobin curve to the left are potential hazards.

When a patient remains hypotensive despite adequate volume replacement, and perfusion of vital organs is jeopardized, pressor agents may be administered to improve cardiac output and blood pressure. In some cases inotropic agents are given to redistribute blood flow (e.g. dopamine can be used to increase renal perfusion—see below). There is evidence that survival of patients with septic or traumatic shock (as well as following major surgery and in those with ARDS) is associated with supranormal values for cardiac output, oxygen delivery and oxygen consumption. Some now advocate that in the most severely ill patients, and in those who fail to respond to simple measures, treatment should be directed at increasing these variables until they equal or exceed the median values found in survivors.

It must be remembered, however, that all inotropes increase myocardial oxygen consumption, particularly if a tachycardia develops, and that this can lead to an imbalance between myocardial oxygen supply and demand, with the development or extension of ischaemic areas. For this reason such agents should be used with caution, particularly in cardiogenic shock following myocardial infarction.

All inotropic agents should be administered via a large central vein, and their effects carefully monitored.

Some of the currently available inotropes are considered here (see also p. 566).

Adrenaline

Adrenaline stimulates both alpha- and beta-adrenergic receptors, but at low doses beta effects seem to predominate. This produces a tachycardia, with an increase in cardiac index and a fall in peripheral resistance. At higher doses, alphamediated vasoconstriction develops. If this produces a useful increase in perfusion pressure, urine output may increase and renal failure may be avoided. However, as the dose is further increased, cardiac output may actually fall, accompanied by marked vasoconstriction, tachycardia and a metabolic acidosis. A reduction in renal blood flow then occurs, with oliguria and a risk of acute renal failure. Prolonged high-dose administration may eventually cause peripheral gangrene. For these reasons the minimum effective dose should be used for as short a time as possible. The addition of low-dose dopamine to the regimen may help to preserve renal function (see below). Despite its disadvantages, adrenaline remains a useful potent inotrope and is used when other agents have failed.

Noradrenaline
This is predominantly an alpha-adrenergic agonist. It may be of value in those with severe hypotension associated with a low systemic resistance, for example in septic shock. There is a risk of producing excessive vasoconstriction with impaired organ perfusion and increased after-load. Noradrenaline administration must therefore be accompanied by full haemodynamic monitoring, including determination of cardiac output (see above) and calculation of the peripheral resistance. Noradrenaline is not often used on its own.

Isoprenaline
This beta-adrenergic stimulant has both inotropic and chronotropic effects. It reduces peripheral resistance by dilating skin and muscle blood vessels and diverts flow away from vital organs such as the kidneys. The increase in cardiac output produced by isoprenaline is mainly due to the tachycardia, and this, together with the development of arrhythmias, seriously limits its value. There are now few indications for isoprenaline in the critically ill adult.

Dopamine
The actions of dopamine are complex but its main action is on β-adrenoreceptors. Compared with isoprenaline, this agent:

- Causes less tachycardia
- Is less arrhythmogenic
- Has a relatively greater effect on stroke volume.

When used in low doses, dopamine acts on specific dopaminergic receptors and the peripheral resistance falls, largely due to dilatation of the splanchnic and renal vasculature. Renal and hepatic blood flow increase, urine output and renal function are improved, and it is possible that failure of these organs is thereby prevented. At higher doses, however, dopamine causes the release of noradrenaline, and vasoconstriction occurs, causing an increased after-load and raising ventricular filling pressures. This is particularly dangerous in those with cardiac failure in whom left atrial pressure is already high.

Dopexamine
This analogue of dopamine is a vasodilator that does not stimulate alpha-receptors. It is a positive inotrope and increases renal blood flow.

Dobutamine
Dobutamine is closely related to dopamine:

- It has no specific effect on the renal vasculature although urine output often increases as cardiac output and blood pressure improve.
- It reduces systemic resistance and improves cardiac performance, thereby decreasing both after-load and ventricular filling pressures.
- It produces a greater improvement in cardiac output than dopamine for a given increase in myocardial oxygen consumption.

For these reasons, dobutamine is probably the agent of choice in patients with cardiogenic shock and cardiac failure.

Enoximone (see Fig. 11.51)
This recently introduced agent, active both orally and intravenously, has inotropic and vasodilator properties. Its mode of action has not been precisely defined but probably involves inhibition of phosphodiesterase. It may prove to be particularly useful in the management of cardiac failure.

Summary
Many still consider dopamine to be the inotrope of choice in most critically ill patients, largely because of its effects on splanchnic blood flow. Dobutamine is equally popular and is particularly indicated in patients in whom the vasoconstriction caused by dopamine could be dangerous (i.e. patients with cardiac disease and septic patients with fluid overload or myocardial failure). The combination of dobutamine and noradrenaline is currently popular for the management of patients who are shocked with a low systemic resistance. Dobutamine is given to achieve an optimal cardiac output, while noradrenaline is used to restore an adequate blood pressure by reducing vasodilatation.

Adrenaline, because of its potency, remains a useful agent in those patients unresponsive to other measures, particularly after cardiac surgery.

Diuretic therapy (see p. 565)

Diuretics increase salt and water excretion by the kidneys, thereby decreasing ventricular filling pressure (pre-load). This is the major form of therapy in sodium retention with fluid overload.

Vasodilator therapy (see also p. 565)

In selected cases, after-load reduction may be used to increase stroke volume and decrease myocardial oxygen requirements by reducing the systolic ventricular wall tension and increasing stroke volume. Vasodilatation also decreases heart size and the diastolic ventricular wall tension so that coronary blood flow is improved. The relative magnitude of the falls in pre-load and after-load depends on the pre-existing haemodynamic disturbance, concurrent volume replacement and the agent selected (see below).

Vasodilator therapy is most beneficial in patients with cardiac failure in whom the ventricular function curve is flat (see Fig. 13.4) and falls in pre-load have only a limited effect on stroke volume. This form of treatment may therefore sometimes be useful in cardiogenic shock and in the management of patients with pulmonary oedema associated with low cardiac output. Vasodilators may also be valuable in shocked patients who remain vasoconstricted and oliguric.

Such therapy is potentially dangerous and should be guided by continuous haemodynamic monitoring, including pulmonary artery catheterization or direct measurement of left atrial pressure. The circulating volume must be adequate before treatment is started. Falls in pre-load should be prevented, except in those with cardiac failure, in order to avoid serious reductions in cardiac output and blood pressure. If diastolic pressure is allowed to fall, coronary blood flow may be jeopardized and, particularly if a reflex tachycardia develops in response to the hypotension, myocardial ischaemia may be precipitated.

Alpha-adrenergic antagonists

These predominantly dilate arterioles and therefore mainly influence after-load.

Phenoxybenzamine is unsuitable for use in the critically ill because of its slow onset (1–2 h to maximum effect) and prolonged duration of action (2–3 days).

Phentolamine is very potent with a rapid onset and short duration of action (15–20 min). It can be used for short-term control of blood pressure in a hypertensive crisis, but can produce a marked tachycardia.

Vasodilators acting directly on the vessel wall

These agents are those most commonly used to achieve vasodilatation in the critically ill.

Hydralazine. This predominantly affects arterial resistance vessels. It therefore reduces after-load and blood pressure, while cardiac output and heart rate usually increase. Hydralazine is usually given as an intravenous bolus to control acute increases in blood pressure, particularly after cardiac surgery.

Sodium nitroprusside (SNP). This dilates arterioles and venous capacitance vessels, as well as the pulmonary vasculature. This agent therefore re-duces the after-load and pre-load of both ventricles and can improve cardiac output and the myocardial oxygen supply/demand ratio. It has been suggested that SNP can exacerbate myocardial ischaemia by producing a 'steal' phenomenon in the coronary circulation.

The effects of SNP are rapid in onset and spontaneously reversible within a few minutes of discontinuing the infusion.

A large overdose of SNP can cause cyanide poisoning, with intracellular hypoxia caused by inhibition of cytochrome oxidase, the terminal enzyme of the respiratory chain. This is manifested as a metabolic acidosis and a fall in the arterio-venous oxygen content difference.

Nitroglycerine (NTG) and isosorbide dinitrate (ISDN). These are both predominantly venodilators. They can therefore cause marked reductions in pre-load, which may be associated with falls in cardiac output and compensatory vasoconstriction. For the reasons discussed above, they are of most value in those with cardiac failure in whom pre-load reduction may reduce ventricular wall tension and improve coronary perfusion without adversely affecting cardiac performance. Furthermore, these agents may reverse myocardial ischaemia by increasing and redistributing coronary blood flow. They are therefore often used in preference to SNP in patients with cardiac failure and/or myocardial ischaemia. Both NTG and ISDN reduce pulmonary vascular resistance, an effect that can occasionally be exploited in patients with a low cardiac output secondary to pulmonary hypertension.

Mechanical support of the myocardium

Intra-aortic balloon counterpulsation (IABCP) is the most widely used technique for mechanical support of the failing myocardium. It is discussed on p. 545.

Adjunctive therapy in shock

Attempts have been made to identify agents that would prevent the release, or inhibit the effects, of the various mediators released in shock. For example, non-steroidal anti-inflammatory agents (which inhibit cyclo-oxygenase) have been used to limit prostaglandin production, naloxone has been used to block the effects of endogenous opioid peptides and recently monoclonal antibodies to TNF have been developed and investigated.

In animal studies very large doses of steroids have been shown to reduce mortality in septic shock, but clinical trials in man have shown that steroids are of no benefit and their administration to such patients is no longer recommended.

Respiratory failure

TYPES AND CAUSES

Respiratory failure occurs when pulmonary gas exchange is sufficiently impaired to cause hypoxaemia with or without hypercarbia. In practical terms respiratory failure is present when the P_aO_2 is < 8 kPa (60 mm Hg) or the P_aCO_2 is > 7 kPa (55 mm Hg). It can be divided into:

- Type I respiratory failure, in which the P_aO_2 is low and the P_aCO_2 is normal or low
- Type II respiratory failure, in which the P_aO_2 is low and the P_aCO_2 is high

Type I or 'acute hypoxaemic' respiratory failure occurs with diseases that damage lung tissue, with hypoxaemia due to right to left shunts or V/Q mismatch. Common causes include pulmonary oedema, pneumonia, adult respiratory distress syndrome and, in the chronic situation, pulmonary fibrosing alveolitis.

Type II or 'ventilatory failure' occurs when alveolar ventilation is insufficient to excrete the volume of carbon dioxide being produced by tissue metabolism. Inadequate alveolar ventilation is due to reduced ventilatory effort, inability to overcome an increased resistance to ventilation, failure to compensate for an increase in dead space and/or carbon dioxide production, or a combination of these factors. The most common cause is chronic bronchitis and emphysema. Other causes include chest-wall deformities, respiratory muscle weakness (e.g. Guillain–Barré syndrome) and depression of the respiratory centre.

MONITORING

A clinical assessment of respiratory distress should be made on the following criteria:

- The use of accessory muscles of respiration
- Tachypnoea
- Tachycardia
- Sweating
- Pulsus paradoxus
- Inability to speak
- Signs of carbon dioxide retention (see p. 657)

This can be supplemented by measuring tidal volume and vital capacity. Blood gas analysis should be performed to guide oxygen therapy and to provide an objective assessment of respiratory function.

The most sensitive clinical indicator of increasing respiratory difficulty is a rising respiratory rate. Tidal volume is a less sensitive indicator.

Minute ventilation rises initially in acute respiratory failure and falls precipitously only at a late stage when the patient is exhausted. Vital capacity is often a better guide to deterioration and is particularly useful in patients with respiratory inadequacy due to neuromuscular problems, e.g. the Guillain–Barré syndrome, in which the vital capacity decreases as weakness increases.

Blood gas analysis

Automation of measurements can give a false impression of reliability and accuracy and may lead to an uncritical acceptance of the results. Errors can result from malfunction of the analyser or incorrect sampling techniques. Care must be taken over the following.

- The sample should be analysed immediately or the syringe should be immersed in iced water (the end having first been sealed with a plastic cap) to prevent the continuing metabolism of white cells causing a reduction in PO_2 and a rise in PCO_2.
- The sample must be adequately anticoagulated to prevent clot formation within the analyser. However, excessive dilution of the blood with heparin, which is acidic, will significantly reduce its pH. Heparin (1000 i.u.·ml^{-1}) should just fill the dead space of the syringe, i.e. approximately 0.1 ml. This will adequately anticoagulate a 2 ml sample.
- Air almost inevitably enters the sample. The gas tensions within these air bubbles will equilibrate with those in the blood, thereby lowering the PCO_2, and, usually, raising the PO_2 of the sample. However, provided the bubbles are ejected immediately by inverting the syringe so that the needle is pointing upwards and expelling the air that rises to the top of the sample, their effect is insignificant.

It is unnecessary to use glass syringes, since diffusion of gases into the walls of plastic syringes is not a significant problem.

Normal values of blood-gas analysis are shown in Table 13.3.

The interpretation of the results of blood gas analysis can be considered in two separate parts:

Table 13.3 Normal values for measurements obtained when blood gas analysis is performed.

H^+	35–45 nmol·L^{-1}	(pH 7.35–7.45)
PO_2	10–13.3 kPa	(75–100 mm Hg)
PCO_2	4.8–6.1 kPa	(36–46 mm Hg)
Plasma HCO_3^-	22–26 mmol·L^{-1}	
O_2 saturation	95–100%	

- Disturbances of acid–base balance
- Alterations in oxygenation

Interpretation of results requires a knowledge of the history, the age of the patient, the inspired oxygen concentration and any other relevant treatment (e.g. the administration of sodium bicarbonate, and the ventilator settings for those on mechanical ventilation).

Disturbances of acid–base balance
The physiology of acid–base control is discussed on pp. 502–504. Acid–base disturbances can be described in relation to the diagram illustrated in Fig. 10.9, which shows P_aCO_2 plotted against arterial $[H^+]$.

Both acidosis and alkalosis can occur, each of which may be either metabolic (primarily affecting the bicarbonate component of the system) or respiratory (primarily affecting PCO_2). Compensatory changes may also be apparent. In clinical practice, arterial $[H^+]$ values *outside* the range 18–126 nmol·L^{-1} (pH 6.9–7.7) are very rarely encountered.

Respiratory acidosis. This is caused by retention of carbon dioxide. The P_aCO_2 and $[H^+]$ rise. A chronically raised P_aCO_2 is compensated by renal retention of bicarbonate and the $[H^+]$ returns towards normal. A constant arterial bicarbonate concentration is then usually established within 2–5 days. This represents a primary respiratory acidosis with a compensatory metabolic alkalosis (see p. 510). Common causes of respiratory acidosis include ventilatory failure and chronic bronchitis and emphysema (type II respiratory failure where there is a high P_aCO_2 and a low P_aO_2—see Chapter 12).

Respiratory alkalosis. In this case the reverse occurs and there is a fall in P_aCO_2 and $[H^+]$, often with a small reduction in bicarbonate concentration. If hypocarbia persists, some degree of renal compensation may occur, producing a metabolic acidosis, although in practice this is unusual. A respiratory alkalosis is often produced, intentionally or unintentionally, when patients are artificially ventilated; it may also be seen with hypoxaemic (type I) respiratory failure (see Chapter 12), hyperventilation and in those living at high altitudes.

Metabolic acidosis. This may be due to excessive acid production, most commonly lactic acid during an episode of shock or following cardiac arrest. A metabolic acidosis may also develop in chronic renal failure and following the loss of large amounts of alkali, e.g. from the gut or from the kidney in renal tubular acidosis.

Respiratory compensation for a metabolic acidosis is usually slightly delayed because the blood–brain barrier initially prevents the respiratory centre from sensing the increased blood $[H^+]$. Following this short delay, however, the patient hyperventilates and 'blows off' carbon dioxide to produce a compensatory respiratory alkalosis. There is a limit to this respiratory compensation, since values for P_aCO_2 less than about 1.4 kPa (11 mm Hg) are, in practice, never achieved. It should also be noted that respiratory compensation cannot occur if the patient's ventilation is controlled.

Metabolic alkalosis. This can be caused by loss of acid, e.g. from the stomach with nasogastric suction or in high intestinal obstruction, or excessive administration of absorbable alkali. Overzealous treatment with intravenous sodium bicarbonate is frequently implicated.

Respiratory compensation for a metabolic alkalosis is often slight and it is rare to encounter a $P_aCO_2 > 6.5$ kPa (50 mm Hg), even with severe alkalosis.

Alterations in oxygenation
When interpreting the P_aO_2 it is important to remember that it is the oxygen content of the arterial blood that matters and that this is determined by the percentage saturation of haemoglobin with oxygen. The relationship between the latter and the PO_2 is determined by the oxyhaemoglobin dissociation curve. In general, if the saturation is greater than 90%, oxygenation can be considered to be adequate. It must be remembered, however, that on the steep portion of the oxygen dissociation curve small falls in P_aO_2 will cause significant reductions in oxygen content. P_aO_2 is also influenced by factors other than pulmonary function, including alterations in $P_{\bar{v}}O_2$ caused by changes in the metabolic rate and/or cardiac output.

MANAGEMENT OF RESPIRATORY FAILURE

Conventional management of patients with respiratory failure includes the administration of supplemental oxygen, the control of secretions, the treatment of pulmonary infection, the control of bronchospasm and measures to limit pulmonary oedema.

Oxygen therapy

Methods of oxygen administration
Oxygen is initially given via a face mask. In the majority of patients (except patients with chronic bronchitis and chronically elevated P_aCO_2) the concentration of oxygen given is not important and oxygen can therefore be given by a simple face mask or nasal cannula (Fig. 13.16). With these

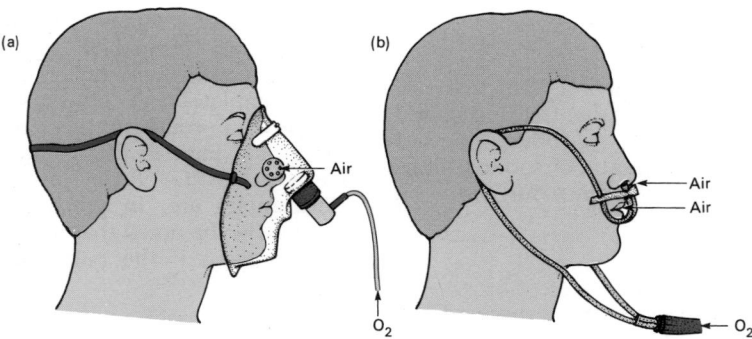

Fig. 13.16 Methods of administering supplemental oxygen to the unintubated patient. (a) Simple face mask. (b) Nasal cannulas.

devices the inspired oxygen concentration varies from about 35% to 55%, with oxygen flow rates of between 6 and 10 L·min^{-1}. Nasal cannulas are often preferred because they are less claustrophic and do not interfere with feeding or speaking, but they can cause ulceration of the nasal or pharyngeal mucosa. Figure 13.16 should be compared with the fixed performance mask shown in Fig. 12.25, with which the oxygen concentration can be controlled. It is vital to use this latter type of mask in patients with chronic bronchitis and emphysema with chronic type II failure.

Oxygen toxicity
Experimentally, mammalian lungs have been shown to be damaged by continuous exposure to high concentrations of oxygen; oxygen toxicity in humans is less well proven. Nevertheless, it is reasonable to assume that high concentrations of oxygen might damage the lungs and so the lowest inspired oxygen concentration compatible with adequate arterial oxygenation should be used. Long-term administration of 50% oxygen or less, or of 100% oxygen for less than 24 h, is probably safe. *Dangerous hypoxia should never be tolerated through a fear of oxygen toxicity.*

Respiratory support

If, despite the above measures, the patient continues to deteriorate or fails to improve, the institution of some form of respiratory support should be considered.

The various techniques of respiratory support currently available are shown in Table 13.4.

Negative-pressure ventilation
'Tank' ventilators were at one time widely used for the treatment of ventilatory failure complicating polio, and are still occasionally employed for long-term ventilation of patients with chronic respiratory failure due to neuromuscular disease or skeletal deformity. The patient's body is enclosed in an airtight 'tank' within which a negative pressure is created intermittently by a separate pump. Cuirass ventilators encase only the thorax.

Intermittent positive-pressure ventilation (IPPV)
IPPV has a number of important advantages over negative-pressure ventilation. In particular, the airway is secured and protected and secretions can be aspirated more easily. In addition, IPPV can be used more successfully in those with diseases

Table 13.4 Techniques for respiratory support.

Technique	Comments
Negative-pressure ventilation	Performed using a tank or cuirass ventilator (rarely used)
Intermittent positive-pressure ventilation (IPPV)	May be given with positive end-expiratory pressure (PEEP)
Continuous positive airway pressure (CPAP)	Given via an endotracheal tube or mask
Intermittent mandatory ventilation (IMV)	May be given with PEEP
High-frequency jet ventilation (HFJV)	

involving the lung parenchyma. Furthermore, access to and movement of the patient is relatively unrestricted.

In recent years a number of refinements and modifications of IPPV have been described, including intermittent mandatory ventilation (IMV), and IPPV with positive end-expiratory pressure (PEEP) (sometimes known as continuous positive-pressure ventilation; CPPV). These will be discussed later in this chapter.

The rational use of IPPV depends on a clear understanding of its potential beneficial effects, as well as its dangers.

Beneficial effects. These include:

- *Improved carbon dioxide elimination.* By adjusting the volume of ventilation, the P_aCO_2 can be returned to within normal limits.
- *Relief from exhaustion.* Artificial ventilation removes the work of breathing and relieves the extreme exhaustion that may be present in patients with respiratory failure. In some cases, if ventilation is not instituted, this exhaustion may culminate in respiratory arrest.
- *Effects on oxygenation.* In those with severe pulmonary parenchymal disease, the lungs may be very stiff and the work of breathing is therefore greatly increased. Under these circumstances the institution of IPPV may significantly reduce total body oxygen consumption; consequently $P_{\bar{v}}O_2$, and thus P_aO_2, may improve. Because ventilated patients are connected to a leak-free circuit it is possible to administer high concentrations of oxygen (up to 100%) accurately and to apply a positive end-expiratory pressure. In selected cases the latter may reduce shunting and increase P_aO_2 (see below).

Indications

- *Acute respiratory failure* with signs of severe respiratory distress, (e.g. respiratory rate > 40 min^{-1}, inability to speak, patient exhausted) persisting despite maximal therapy. Confusion, a decreased conscious level, a rising P_aCO_2 and extreme hypoxaemia are further indications. Care should be taken before ventilating patients with chronic lung disease as patients previously severely incapacitated will be difficult to wean off the ventilator and also relapse early. The most important criteria are the patient's previous exercise tolerance and ability to lead an independent existence.
- *Acute ventilatory failure* due, for example, to myasthenia gravis or Guillain–Barré syndrome. Artificial ventilation should be instituted when the vital capacity has fallen to < 10–15 ml·kg^{-1}. This will avoid complications such as atelectasis and infection as well as preventing unexpected respiratory arrest. The tidal volume and respiratory rate are relatively insensitive in the above conditions and change late in the course of the disease. A high P_aCO_2 (particularly if rising) is an indication for urgent artificial ventilation.

- *Other indications* include:
  Prophylactic post-operative ventilation in poor risk patients
  Head injury with acute brain oedema. Intracranial pressure is decreased by elective hyperventilation as this reduces cerebral blood flow
  Trauma—chest injury and lung contusion
  Severe left ventricular failure with pulmonary oedema (see p. 568)
  Coma with breathing difficulties, e.g. following drug overdose

Institution. IPPV requires endotracheal intubation. If the patient is conscious the procedure must be fully explained before anaesthesia is induced. Intubating patients in severe respiratory failure is an extremely hazardous undertaking and *should only be performed by experienced staff.* In extreme emergencies it may be preferable to ventilate the patient by hand using an oropharyngeal airway, a face mask and a self-inflating bag until experienced help arrives. The patient is usually hypoxic and hypercarbic, with increased sympathetic activity, and the stimulus of laryngoscopy and intubation can precipitate dangerous arrhythmias and even cardiac arrest. If possible, therefore, the ECG should be monitored, and the patient pre-oxygenated with 100% oxygen before intubation. In some deeply comatose patients, no sedation will be required, but in the majority of patients a short-acting intravenous anaesthetic agent followed by muscle relaxation will be necessary.

The complications of endotracheal intubation are given in Table 13.5.

Endotracheal tubes can now safely be left in place for several weeks and tracheostomy is therefore less often performed. Tracheostomy may be required for the long-term control of excessive bronchial secretions, particularly in those with a reduced conscious level, and/or to maintain an airway and protect the lungs in those with impaired pharyngeal and laryngeal reflexes.

The only indication for immediate tracheostomy is a life-threatening obstruction of the upper respiratory tract that cannot be bypassed with an endotracheal tube. However, tracheostomy performed under these circumstances can be extremely hazardous. Other indications are head and neck injuries, including burns to the face and upper airway.

Tracheostomy has a mortality rate of up to 3%. Complications of tracheostomy are shown in Table 13.6.

Dangers of IPPV. General dangers include:

Table 13.5 Complications of endotracheal intubation.

Complication	Comments
Immediate	
Tube in one or other bronchus (usually the right)	Avoid by checking both lungs are being inflated, i.e. both sides of the chest move and air entry is heard on auscultation. X-ray to check position of tube and to exclude lung collapse.
Tube in oesophagus	Gives rise to hypoxia and abdominal distension.
Early	
Migration of the tube out of trachea	
Leaks around the tube	
Obstruction of tube due to kinking or secretions	A dangerous complication. The patient becomes distressed, cyanosed and has poor chest expansion. The following should be performed immediately:
	• Manual inflation with 100% oxygen
	• Endotracheal suction
	• Check position of tube
	• Deflate cuff
	• Check tube for 'kinks'
	If no improvement, change the endotracheal tube.
Late	
Mucosal oedema and ulceration	
Damage to the cricoarytenoid cartilages	
Tracheal narrowing and fibrosis	

• Complications inherent in endotracheal intubation or tracheostomy.
• Disconnection or mechanical failure. These are unusual but dangerous. A method of manual ventilation, e.g. a self-inflating bag, must always be available by the bedside.
• Barotrauma. Overdistension of the lungs during IPPV can rupture alveoli and cause air to dissect centrally along the perivascular sheaths. This pulmonary interstitial air can sometimes be seen on chest X-ray as linear or circular perivascular collections or subpleural blebs. Other complications are pneumothorax, pneumomediastinum, pneumoperitoneum and subcutaneous emphysema. Intra-abdominal air originating from the alveoli is probably always associated with pneumomediastinum.

The incidence of barotrauma is greatest in those patients who require high inflation pressures, with or without a positive end-expiratory pressure, and the risk of pneumothorax is increased in those with destructive lung disease (e.g. staphylococcal pneumonia, emphysema), asthma or fractured ribs.

A tension pneumothorax can be rapidly fatal in ventilated patients with respiratory failure. Suggestive signs include the development or worsening of hypoxia, fighting the ventilator, an unexplained increase in inflation pressure, as well as hypotension and tachycardia, sometimes accompanied by a rising CVP. Examination may reveal unequal chest expansion, mediastinal shift (deviated trachea, displaced apex beat) and a hyperresonant hemithorax. Although, traditionally, breath sounds are diminished over the pneumo-

Table 13.6 Complications of tracheostomy.

As for endotracheal intubation (Table 13.5), plus:

Early

Surgical complications:
  Pneumothorax
  Haemorrhage
Tube misplaced in pretracheal subcutaneous tissues
Subcutaneous emphysema

Intermediate

Erosion of tracheal cartilages (may cause tracheo-
oesophageal fistula)
Erosion of innominate artery (may lead to fatal
haemorrhage)
Infection

Late

Tracheal stenosis at level of stoma, cuff or tube tip
Collapse of tracheal rings at level of stoma

thorax, this sign can be extremely misleading in ventilated patients. If there is time, the diagnosis can be confirmed by chest X-ray.

Other dangers of IPPV include:

- *Respiratory complications.* Patients ventilated with small tidal volumes become progressively more hypoxic. This is probably due to collapse of peripheral alveoli and can largely be prevented by using large tidal volumes (10–15 ml·kg^{-1}) and reducing the respiratory rate (usually to 10–12 per min) to avoid hypocarbia.
  Secondary pulmonary infection is a common and ominous complication of IPPV.
- *Cardiovascular complications.* The intermittent application of positive pressure to the lungs and thoracic wall impedes venous return and distends alveoli, thereby 'stretching' the pulmonary capillaries and causing a rise in pulmonary vascular resistance. Both these mechanisms can produce a fall in cardiac output. This may be exacerbated by a reduction in myocardial contractility caused by humoral or reflex mechanisms and possibly impaired coronary perfusion.
  In *normal subjects*, the fall in cardiac output is prevented by the constriction of capacitance vessels, which restores venous return. Hypovolaemia, pre-existing pulmonary hypertension, right ventricular failure and autonomic dysfunction (as may be present in those with Guillain–Barré syndrome, acute spinal cord injury or diabetes) will exacerbate the haemodynamic disturbance. Expansion of the circulating volume, on the other hand, can often restore cardiac output.
  In *patients with heart failure*, a paradoxical rise in blood pressure and cardiac output may occur in response to positive pressure ventilation. This may be due to reversal of hypoxia and a reduction in oxygen consumption, both of which will reduce the burden on a failing heart. A further possible benefit in those with cardiac failure is that a reduction in pre-load will reduce ventricular wall tension, allowing increased coronary blood flow and improved myocardial function. Moreover, when the ventricular function curve is flat, the fall in pre-load has little effect on stroke volume, whilst stiff lungs limit the transmission of high inflation pressures to the great veins and pulmonary capillaries. Therefore, IPPV should be used without hestitation in patients with cardiogenic pulmonary oedema who have severe respiratory distress and exhaustion.
- *Gastrointestinal complications.* Initially, many artificially ventilated patients will develop abdominal distension associated with an ileus. The cause is unknown, although the use of non-depolarizing neuromuscular blocking agents may in part be responsible.
- *Salt and water retention.* IPPV, particularly with positive end-expiratory pressure, causes increased ADH secretion and possibly a reduction in circulating levels of atrial naturetic peptide. Combined with a fall in cardiac output and a reduction in renal cortical blood flow, these can cause salt and water retention leading to interstitial oedema. This fluid retention is often paticularly noticeable in the lungs, possibly because IPPV interferes with pulmonary lymphatic drainage.

Selection of the pattern of ventilation. The aim is to achieve optimal gas exchange while minimizing adverse effects on the cardiovascular system.

The duration of the inspiratory phase must be sufficient to allow adequate gas distribution to all distal lung segments; inspiration should therefore last for between 1.5 and 2.0 s. In order to minimize the fall in cardiac output, expiration should take at least twice as long as inspiration and both inflation and deflation should be relatively rapid. The influence of the shape of the inspiratory wave-form on the efficiency of gas exchange is less certain.

Positive end-expiratory pressure (PEEP). A positive airway pressure can be maintained at a chosen level throughout expiration by attaching a threshold resistor valve to the expiratory limb of the circuit. PEEP should be considered if it proves impossible to achieve adequate oxygenation of arterial blood (more than 90% saturation) using conventional positive-pressure ventilation without raising the inspired oxygen concentration to potentially dangerous levels (conventionally > 50%). PEEP is not, however, a panacea for all patients who are hypoxic and, indeed, it may often be detrimental, not least because the use of levels of PEEP in excess of 5 cm H_2O is associated with an increased risk of barotrauma. Although some have used extremely high levels of PEEP (e.g. 60 cm H_2O) most recommend that pressures in excess of 15–20 cm H_2O should not be exceeded.

The primary effect of PEEP is to re-expand underventilated lung units. Provided that hypoxaemia is due to airway closure, this will reduce the shunt and increase the P_aO_2.

Unfortunately, the inevitable rise in mean intrathoracic pressure that follows the application of PEEP may further impede venous return, increase pulmonary vascular resistance and thus reduce cardiac output. This effect is probably least when the lungs are stiff. Moreover, the rise in pulmonary vascular resistance may be associated with dilatation of the right ventricle and distortion of the left ventricular cavity by the displaced interventricular septum. This is thought to restrict left ventricular filling and reduce stroke volume. The fall in cardiac output can be ameliorated by expanding the circulating volume, although in some cases inotropic support may be required. Thus, although arterial oxygenation is often improved by the application of PEEP, a simultaneous fall in cardiac output can lead to a reduction in total oxygen delivery.

The net effect of PEEP in an individual patient is therefore often unpredictable and is dependent on a balance of several factors. The most beneficial effects occur in those patients with large shunts due to alveolar collapse, stiff lungs, and good cardiovascular function, e.g. a young, fit patient with the adult respiratory distress syndrome. However, in patients with normal or high lung volumes, compliant lungs and only a modest degree of shunting, any improvement in P_aO_2 may be negated by the fall in cardiac output, particularly in those with poor cardiovascular function. Thus, PEEP should not be used in patients with emphysema or asthma and is usually of little benefit in those with fibrotic lung disease or bacterial pneumonia. Furthermore, in patients with only localized areas of diseased lung (e.g. unilateral aspiration pneumonia), PEEP may adversely affect oxygenation by overexpanding normal lung tissue and diverting blood to underventilated lung units.

Other techniques for respiratory support

Continuous positive airway pressure (CPAP). The application of CPAP achieves for the spontaneously breathing patient what PEEP does for the ventilated patient. Oxygen and air are delivered under pressure via an endotracheal tube or occasionally via a tightly fitted face mask. Not only can it improve oxgenation but the lungs become less stiff, breathing becomes easier and vital capacity improves.

Intermittent mandatory ventilation (IMV). This technique allows the patient to breathe spontaneously between the 'mandatory' tidal volumes delivered by the ventilator. Most modern ventilators will time these mandatory breaths to coincide with the patient's own inspiratory effort (synchronized IMV–SIMV). IMV can be used with or without PEEP or CPAP. It was originally introduced as a technique for weaning patients from artifical ventilation but is increasingly being used as an alternative to conventional IPPV.

High-frequency jet ventilation (HFJV). Adequate oxygenation and CO_2 elimination can be achieved by injecting gas into the trachea at rates of up to several thousand breaths per minute. In clinical practice rates of between 60 and 300 breaths per minute are usually employed.

Potential advantages of HFJV are largely related to the low peak airway pressures; thus cardiac output is maintained and the risk of barotrauma is negligible. Moreover, HFJV can be used to ventilate patients with large air leaks due, for example, to a bronchopleural fistula or lung lacerations. The place of HFJV in the management of patients with acute respiratory failure is less clear.

Weaning

It is important to discontinue artificial ventilation, and, if possible, to extubate the patient as soon as possible. On the other hand, premature attempts at weaning may be dangerous and can adversely affect the morale of conscious patients.

Because they perform no work during conventional mechanical ventilation, the respiratory muscles eventually become weak and uncoordinated. Moreover, there is usually some persisting abnormality of lung function. Thus, in patients who have been artificially ventilated for any length of time, spontaneous respiration usually has to be resumed gradually.

Criteria for weaning patients from artificial ventilation. Clinical assessment is of paramount importance when deciding whether a patient can be weaned from the ventilator. The patient's conscious level, psychological state, metabolic function, the effects of drugs, cardiovascular performance and mechanical factors must all be taken into account. Objective criteria are based on an assessment of pulmonary gas exchange (blood gas analysis), lung mechanics and muscular strength.

Techniques for weaning. Patients who have received artificial ventilation for less than 24 h, e.g. elective IPPV after major surgery, can usually resume spontaneous respiration immediately and no weaning process is required. This procedure can also be adopted for those who have been ventilated for longer periods but who clearly fulfil the objective criteria for weaning.

The *traditional* method of weaning in difficult cases is to allow the patient to breathe entirely spontaneously for a short time, following which IPPV is re-instituted. The periods of spontaneous breathing are gradually increased and the periods of IPPV are reduced. Initially it is usually advisable to ventilate the patient throughout the night. This method has several practical disadvantages: during the period of spontaneous respiration the patient may develop progressive hypoxia and/or hypercarbia as well as an increasing sympathetic drive, resulting in tachycardia and hypertension. After a predetermined period, or earlier if tachypnoea and exhaustion develop, the patient is reconnected to IPPV. At this time, respiratory drive is high, synchronization with the ventilator is difficult and heavy sedation may be required. It is then necessary to wait until the effects of these drugs have worn off before trying another period of spontaneous respiration. This method is stressful and tiring both for patients and staff. However, some patients do not tolerate IMV (see below) and this method of weaning may then be necessary.

The above disadvantages may be overcome by using IMV. This provides a smoother, more controlled method of weaning; it may also enable weaning to commence at an earlier stage than is possible using the conventional method. There is no evidence, however, that IMV enables patients who could not be weaned using conventional methods to resume spontaneous respiration, and in some cases the weaning process may be unnecessarily prolonged.

The application of CPAP can prevent the alveolar collapse, hypoxaemia and fall in compliance that might otherwise occur when patients start to breathe spontaneously. It is therefore often used during weaning with IMV and in spontaneously breathing patients prior to extubation, particularly when they were previously receiving IPPV with PEEP.

Extubation. This should not be considered until the patient can cough, swallow, protect his own airway and is sufficiently alert to be cooperative. Patients who fulfil these criteria can be extubated provided their respiratory function has improved sufficiently to sustain spontaneous ventilation indefinitely. This is often difficult to assess and is usually largely based on the patient's ability to breathe spontaneously via the endotracheal tube over a period of time. In those who have undergone prolonged artificial ventilation, this period may need to be 24–48 h, or even longer, while patients ventilated for less than 12–24 h can often be extubated within 10–15 min. During this 'trial of spontaneous respiration' the patient should be closely observed for any signs of respiratory distress.

ADULT RESPIRATORY DISTRESS SYNDROME (ARDS)

DEFINITION AND CAUSES

This syndrome was originally described in 1967 as acute respiratory distress in adults characterized by severe dyspnoea, tachypnoea, cyanosis refractory to oxygen therapy, loss of lung compliance and diffuse alveolar infiltrates seen on the chest X-ray. ARDS can therefore be defined as diffuse pulmonary infiltrates, refractory hypoxaemia and respiratory distress. A PCWP less than 16 mm Hg is often included in the definition in an attempt to exclude cardiogenic pulmonary oedema. ARDS can occur as a non-specific reaction of the lungs to a wide variety of insults, including shock (especially septic shock), fat embolism, trauma, burns, pancreatitis, cardiopulmonary bypass, lung contusion, inhalation of smoke or toxic gases, Goodpasture's syndrome, amniotic fluid embolism and aspiration pneumonia. Superadded infection is a common feature of ARDS, which now usually occurs in association with multiple organ failure and persistent sepsis.

PATHOPHYSIOLOGY

Non-cardiogenic pulmonary oedema
This is the main feature of ARDS and is associated with an increased pulmonary capillary permeability. This is due to damage to the alveolar–capillary membrane caused by the microcirulatory changes and release of inflammatory mediators as described previously (see p. 710).

Pulmonary hypertension
This is a common feature of ARDS. Initially, mechanical obstruction of the pulmonary circulation may occur as a result of vascular compression by interstitial oedema and subsequently oedema of the vessel wall itself. Later, constriction of the pulmonary vasculature may develop in response to increased autonomic nervous activity and circulating substances such as catecholamines, 5-HT, thromboxane, fibrin/fibrinogen degradation products, complement and activated leucocytes. Those vessels supplying alveoli with low oxygen tensions constrict (the 'hypoxic vasoconstrictor response'), diverting pulmonary blood flow to better oxygenated areas of lung, thus limiting the degree of shunt. In some patients with ARDS and pulmonary hypertension, angiography will reveal 'beading' of the arterioles and peripheral 'pruning' of the pulmonary vasculature. This suggests fibrin deposition and is associated with a marked increase in dead space and a poor prognosis, despite attempts to reverse the process using heparin and streptokinase. In this situation, subpleural lung segments are infarcted but continue to be ventilated and are therefore liable to rupture. In others,

angiography is normal, pulmonary hypertension is absent, and in these the 'wet lung' usually responds to dehydration and respiratory support.

Hyaline membranes
These are seen microscopically in the lungs of patients with ARDS and consist of necrotic type I pneumocytes and coagulated intralveolar proteins derived from the pulmonary exudate.

Fibrosis
Within seven days of the onset of ARDS, activated fibroblasts are seen in the interstitial spaces. Subsequently, interstitial fibrosis progresses, with loss of elastic tissue and obliteration of the lung vasculature. These changes are probably irreversible, although lung function often returns virtually to normal in patients who recover from ARDS, particularly in the young and non-smokers; residual X-ray changes are usually limited to a few linear scars.

CLINICAL PRESENTATION

The first sign of the development of ARDS is often an unexplained tachypnoea, followed by increasing hypoxaemia. Later, the chest X-ray shows bilateral, diffuse shadowing with an alveolar pattern and air bronchograms that may then progress to the picture of complete 'white-out'.

MANAGEMENT

This is based on treatment of the underlying condition (e.g. eradication of sepsis, excision of necrotic tissue) and supportive measures such as oxygen, CPAP, and IPPV/IMV with PEEP. Pulmonary oedema formation should be minimized by controlling left atrial pressure and, if possible, maintaining plasma proteins, particularly albumin, close to the normal range. However, once plasma enters the interstitial space, the transvascular oncotic gradient disappears and the main determinants of interstitial oedema formation become the microvascular hydrostatic pressure and lymphatic drainage. There is therefore some controversy concerning the relative merits of colloids or crystalloids for volume replacement in patients likely to develop ARDS, or in whom the condition is established. Cardiovascular support and the reduction of oxygen requirements are also important.

The administration of high-dose steroids to patients with established ARDS does not appear to improve outcome and current evidence suggests that prophylactic administration to those at risk of developing ARDS is of no value. Moreover, there is a suggestion that steroids may have an adverse effect on the prognosis of ARDS and their use is no longer recommended.

PROGNOSIS

Despite the treatment outlined, the mortality from established severe ARDS remains high at more than 50% overall. Approximately 40% of uncomplicated cases die, but the mortality rises with increasing age and failure of other organs. Many of those dying with ARDS now do so as a result of multiple organ failure and haemodynamic instability rather than impaired gas exchange.

Brain death

Brain death means 'the irreversible loss of the capacity for consciousness combined with the irreversible loss of the capacity to breathe'. Both these are essentially functions of the brain stem. Death, if thought of in this way, can arise either from causes outside the brain (i.e. respiratory and cardiac arrest) or from causes within the head. With the advent of artificial ventilation it became possible to support such a dead patient temporarily, although in all cases cardiovascular failure eventually supervenes and progresses to asystole.

Before considering a diagnosis of brain death it is essential that certain preconditions and exclusions are fulfilled.

Preconditions
- The patient must be in apnoeic coma (i.e. unresponsive and on a ventilator, with no spontaneous respiratory efforts).
- Irremediable structural brain damage due to a disorder that can cause brain stem death must have been diagnosed with certainty (e.g. head injury, intracranial haemorrhage).

Exclusions
- The possibility that unresponsive apnoea is the result of poisons, sedative drugs or neuromuscular blocking agents must be excluded.
- Hypothermia must be excluded as a cause of coma. The central body temperature should be more than 35°C.
- There must be no significant metabolic or endocrine disturbance that could produce or contribute to coma. There should be no profound abnormality of the plasma electrolytes, acid–base balance, or blood glucose levels.

Diagnostic tests for the confirmation of brain death

All brain stem reflexes are absent in brain death.

The following tests should not be performed in the presence of seizures or abnormal postures.

- The pupils should be fixed and unresponsive to bright light. Both direct and consensual light reflexes should be absent. The size of the pupils is irrelevant, although most often they will be dilated.
- Corneal reflexes should be absent.
- Oculocephalic reflexes should be absent, i.e. when the head is rotated from side to side, the eyes move with the head and therefore remain stationery relative to the orbit. In a comatose patient whose brain stem is intact, the eyes will rotate relative to the orbit (i.e. doll's eye movements will be present).
- There are no vestibulo-ocular reflexes on caloric testing (see p. 893).
- There should be no motor responses within the cranial nerve territory to painful stimuli applied centrally or peripherally. Spinal reflexes may be present.
- There must be no gag or cough reflex in response to pharyngeal, laryngeal or tracheal stimulation.
- Spontaneous respiration should be absent. The patient should be ventilated with 5% CO_2 in 95% O_2 for 10 min and then disconnected from the ventilator for a further 10 min. Oxygenation is maintained by insufflation with 100% oxygen at high flow rates via a catheter placed in the endotracheal tube. The patient is observed for any signs of spontaneous respiratory efforts. A blood gas sample should be obtained during this period to ensure that the P_aCO_2 is sufficiently high to stimulate spontaneous respiration (> 6.7 kPa [50 mm Hg]).

The examination should be performed (and repeated after a few hours) by two doctors of senior status a minimum of 6 h after the onset of coma or, if due to cardiac arrest, at least 24 h after restoration of an adequate circulation.

It is not necessary to perform confirmatory tests such as EEG and carotid angiography, as these may be misleading.

In suitable cases and provided the patient was carrying a donor card and/or the consent of relatives has been obtained, the organs of those in whom brain stem death has been established may be used for transplantation. In all cases in the UK the coroner's consent must be obtained.

Results, costs and patient selection for intensive care

For many critically ill patients, intensive care is undoubtedly life-saving and resumption of a normal life-style is to be expected.

In the most seriously ill patients, however, immediate mortality rates are high, a significant number die soon after discharge from the intensive care unit, and the quality of life for some of those who do survive may be poor. Moreover, intensive care is expensive, particularly for those with the worst prognosis.

Inappropriate use of intensive care facilities has other implications. The patient may experience unnecessary suffering and loss of dignity, while relatives may also have to endure considerable emotional pressures. In some cases treatment may simply prolong the process of dying, or sustain life of dubious quality, and in others the risks of interventions may outweigh the potential benefits.

Rational selection of those patients most likely to benefit from intensive care is therefore clearly desirable, both for a humane approach to the management of the critically ill and to ensure optimal use of relatively scarce resources.

Currently decisions to limit therapy, or not to resuscitate in the event of cardiorespiratory arrest, are made jointly by the medical staff of the unit, the primary physician or surgeon and the nurses, normally in consultation with the patient's family.

Scoring systems

A variety of scoring systems have been developed that can be used to evaluate the severity of a patient's illness. These have included an assessment of the severity of the acute disturbance of physiological function (acute physiology and chronic health evaluation—APACHE) and a measure of the therapeutic effort expended on a patient (therapeutic intervention scoring system—TISS). Other systems have been designed for particular categories of patient (e.g. the injury severity score for trauma victims). The APACHE score is widely applicable and has been extensively validated. It can accurately quantify the severity of illness and predict the overall mortality for large groups of critically ill patients, and is therefore useful when auditing a unit's clinical activity, for comparing results in different centres and as a means of characterizing groups of patients in clinical studies. No scoring system has yet been devised, however, that can predict with certainty the outcome in an individual patient and they must not, therefore, be used in isolation as a basis for limiting or discontinuing treatment.

Further reading

Hinds CJ (1987) *Intensive Care: A Concise Textbook*. London: Baillière Tindall.
Rippe JM, Irwin RS, Alpert JS & Dalen JE (eds) (1985) *Intensive Care Medicine*. Boston/Toronto: Little, Brown and Company.
Tinker J & Rapin M (eds) (1983) *Care of the Critically Ill Patient*. Berlin: Springer-Verlag.

14

Adverse Drug Reactions and Poisoning

Adverse drug reactions

The size of the problem

Any substance that possesses useful therapeutic effects may also produce unwanted, toxic or adverse effects. The incidence of adverse drug reactions in the population is not really known. A survey of 1160 patients given a variety of drugs showed that the incidence of adverse reactions increased with age from about 3% in patients 10–20 years of age to about 20% in patients 80–89 years of age. It has been estimated that about 0.5% of patients who die in hospital do so as a result of their treatment rather than the condition for which they were admitted.

Classification

Adverse drug reactions can be classified in several ways. They may be divided into reactions due to:

- Overdosage
- Intolerance
- Side-effects
- Secondary effects
- Idiosyncrasy
- Hypersensitivity

Another system of classification divides them into two types:

- Type A—the results of an exaggerated but otherwise normal pharmacological action of a drug
- Type B—totally aberrant effects not expected from the known pharmacological actions of a drug

In this chapter adverse drug reactions are divided into three types (see Table 14.1):

- Dose-dependent
- Dose-independent
- Pseudoallergic

The mechanisms underlying many drug reactions, however, are unclear and these reactions cannot at present be classified easily, e.g. hepatotoxicity and analgesic nephropathy.

Dose-dependent reactions

These occur in all patients given sufficiently large doses of any drug. The effects produced may be further subdivided into:

- Reactions that are predictable, being exaggerated therapeutic actions, e.g. depression of cardiac contractility by lignocaine or quinidine, or cen-

Table 14.1 Comparison between dose-dependent, dose-independent and pseudoallergic reactions.

	Dose-dependent	Dose-independent	Pseudoallergic
All patients	Yes	No	No
All drugs	Yes	No	No
Previous exposure necessary	No	Yes	No
Treatment	Reduce dose	Stop drug	Avoid drug or Reduce dose

tral nervous depression by barbiturates or narcotics

- Reactions that appear to be unrelated to their therapeutic effects, e.g. the ototoxicity produced by streptomycin

The first group, being predictable, can be anticipated and looked for without much difficulty. The second unpredictable group poses serious problems of recognition and quantification, particularly with a new drug.

Factors that influence the dose at which these dose-dependent effects appear are described on p. 734.

Dose-independent reactions

These occur in only a small proportion of patients and tend to be limited to certain well-defined manifestations. The possibility, however, of new syndromes occurring must never be overlooked. These reactions usually occur in patients who have previously been exposed and sensitized to the drug itself, to another drug of the same chemical class, or to one of another class of drugs that shares similar antigenic properties. For example, exposure to one form of penicillin usually produces a state of hypersensitivity to other penicillin derivatives, and, in a small proportion of patients, also to cephalosporin derivatives which share cross-antigenicity with the 6-amino-penicillanic acid nucleus.

Most drugs are of relatively low molecular weight and only become antigenic when they are combined covalently and irreversibly with other substances of high molecular weight, usually proteins. The drug is then said to be a *hapten*. Sometimes it is a metabolite of the drug or an impurity produced during manufacture that acts as the hapten. The most common of these dose-independent reactions are acute hypersensitivity reactions. These are due to the release of histamine and other mediators following the interaction of antigen with antibody (IgE) produced by B lymphocytes and bound to the cell membranes of mast cells or circulating basophils. The released substances cause rashes, oedema and the more serious effects of bronchospasm, peripheral vasodilatation and cardiovascular collapse—the anaphylactic reaction.

Circulating antigen–antibody complexes (immune complexes) cause the serum sickness syndrome. They are deposited in the basement membrane of the renal glomerulus and elsewhere.

Delayed hypersensitivity reactions, such as contact dermatitis, are due to the formation of sensitized T lymphocytes, which activate a cell-mediated immune response.

Other forms of dose-independent reactions include various blood dyscrasias. These may involve the production of antibodies to circulating blood elements, leading to:

- Thrombocytopenic purpura (e.g. with quinine)
- Haemolytic anaemia (e.g. with methyldopa)
- Depression of bone-marrow function, either selective (e.g. agranulocytosis) or total (aplastic anaemia). For example, chloramphenicol is a very effective antibiotic, but about one person in every 20 000 develops a fatal aplastic anaemia that is unrelated to the dose administered and which cannot at present be predicted by any pre-dose screening test. The exact mechanism of this aplasia is unknown.

Anaphylaxis

Anaphylaxis usually follows injections or occasionally insect bites.

Clinical features
Bronchospasm
Laryngeal spasm
Breathlessness
Cyanosis
Hypotension
Nausea, vomiting, diarrhoea

Treatment
Lay patient head down
Ensure airway free
Monitor blood pressure

Give:

Adrenaline i.m. 0.5–1.0 mg every 15 min
Intravenous infusion
Oxygen by variable concentration mask
Chlorpheniramine 10–20 mg slow i.v. infusion over 24 h
Hydrocortisone 100 mg i.v. every 4 h
In severe cases, continue prednisolone 20 mg every 6 h

Pseudoallergic reactions

In some susceptible patients, substances mimic the allergic reactions described under dose-independent reactions but without the same immunological mechanisms occurring. Unlike allergic reactions they occur on first contact with a drug rather than after previous sensitizing exposure. Susceptibility to such a reaction appears to be determined by genetic and environmental factors. These reactions are produced by compounds that are able to release histamine and other mediators directly from mast cells without involving an antigen–antibody reaction. Examples are:

- The itching, bronchospasm and vasodilatation due to histamine release by morphine
- The flushing, urticaria, angio-oedema, conjunctivitis, rhinitis, bronchial asthma, hypotension and even fatal shock produced by aspirin

It is probable that reactions to many other drugs

Table 14.2 Agents that are believed to be capable of producing pseudoallergic reactions through release of histamine and other mediators.

Aspirin and other non-steroidal anti-inflammatory drugs

Barbiturates

Anaesthetics (intravenous)

Neuromuscular blocking drugs

Morphine

Chlorpropamide/alcohol interaction (p. 840)

Sodium cromoglycate

Polypeptides, gamma-globulin

Dextrans and other colloids

Radiographic contrast media

Cremophor (solvent for some intravenous drugs)

Tartrazine

Intravenous compounds vitamins B and C (Parenterovite)

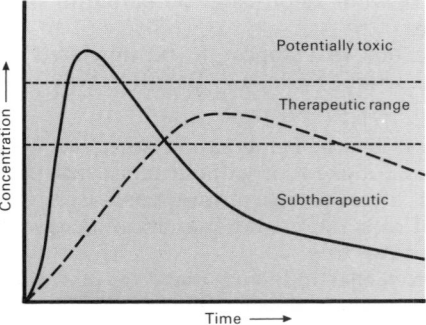

Fig. 14.1 Relationships between blood drug concentration and effect and time after oral administration.

are also due to this mechanism (see Table 14.2). An interesting example is the anaphylactic response produced by aspirin in one patient with urticaria pigmentosa and generalized mastocytosis.

If use of the particular drug to which the pseudoallergic reaction occurs cannot be avoided, its dose should be kept as low as possible, or, in the case of intravenous administration, it should be given by slow infusion rather than rapid injection. Sometimes it is possible to desensitize a patient by starting with a small dose of the drug and gradually increasing it under supervision.

Factors influencing dose-dependent adverse drug reactions

Formulation

The active agent represents only a small proportion of the total weight of a tablet or capsule. Similarly, drugs for injection require solubilization or suspension in a fluid vehicle of varying complexity. Other constituents of dosage forms, called *excipients*, are not necessarily inert, and may play an important part in facilitating or hindering the absorption of a drug. The proportion of an administered drug dose that reaches its site of action in the systemic circulation is known as its bioavailability. If the drug is given intravenously its bioavailability is 100%.

The dose-dependent adverse effects of many drugs are related to higher blood levels than those

necessary for their therapeutic action (see Fig. 14.1). A formulation that results in such high blood levels may, therefore, produce unacceptable effects. In the case of a poorly soluble drug, its physical form may be important in determining its dissolution rate and, therefore, its rate of absorption. For example, when the particle size of digoxin was reduced by a manufacturer, many patients experienced digitalis toxicity because the rate and extent of absorption was increased. Similarly, the influence of a change of the excipient on a drug's bioavailability was seen in Australia when a manufacturer of phenytoin capsules changed from using the relatively water-insoluble calcium sulphate to the much more soluble lactose. This led to an increase in the bioavailability of phenytoin, which was even more marked because of the 'saturation kinetics' that phenytoin exhibits.

Modification of the physical form of a drug, and changes in other constituents, permits the development of 'controlled release' formulations. These produce sustained levels within the therapeutic range and prevent early peak blood levels that enter the toxic range (see Fig. 14.1). This effect is particularly useful in drugs with a short half-life.

Route of administration

Parenteral administration of a drug may produce higher peak levels than are produced by oral administration, and may therefore produce more marked concentration-related adverse effects. For example, the intravenous administration of many drugs, particularly as bolus injections, may produce unwanted cardiac or central nervous effects. Intrathecal penicillin can produce encephalopathy and convulsions due to the toxic effects of high concentrations on the central nervous system; this route is nowadays seldom used.

Adverse reactions may occur owing to accidents during administration; for example, arterial rather than venous injection of thiopentone results in vascular spasm, arterial thrombosis and gangrene.

Pregnancy

Some drugs given in the first three months of pregnancy may cause congenital abnormalities and are said to be teratogenic. The best known example of a teratogenic drug is thalidomide, which resulted in bizarre and therefore easily recognizable abnormalities such as absent or grossly abnormal limbs (amelia, phocomelia). Stilboestrol administration during pregnancy produced adenosis and adenocarcinoma of the vagina in the female offspring when they reached their late teens or early twenties. This was recognized because of the normally relatively low incidence of this carcinoma in this age group. Low-grade teratogens that cause only minor deformities infrequently are likely to be unrecognized or demonstrated only with difficulty. Other drugs that are known or suspected to be teratogenic are given in Table 14.3.

Drugs given after the period of organogenesis may affect the growth or function of normally-formed fetal tissues or organs. The more important of these drugs are given in Table 14.4.

Age

Some drugs produce specific adverse effects at the extremes of life.

Neonates

In the neonatal period, drug-metabolizing enzymes may be deficient for at least a month after birth,

Table 14.3 Agents known or suspected to be teratogenic in man.

Definite or strongly suspected teratogens
Thalidomide
Anticonvulsants
Antineoplastic drugs
Folic acid antagonists
Alcohol
Warfarin
Lithium
Oestrogens
Stilboestrol
Androgenic steroids
Etretinate
Isotretinoin
Podophyllum resin
Organic mercury
Possible teratogens
Inhalational anaesthetics
Vitamin A
Progestogens
Live vaccines (some)
Radiographic dyes
Penicillamine
Progesterones (high-doses)

Table 14.4 Drugs that may have unwanted effects on the fetus during intrauterine life if given to the mother.

Drug	Effect
Antibacterial drugs	
Tetracyclines	Dental discoloration
Aminoglycosides	Eighth nerve damage
Novobiocin Sulphonamides	Jaundice, kernicterus
Antithyroid drugs	
Iodides Carbimazole Lithium Povidone-iodine	Neonatal hypothyroidism, goitre
Anticoagulants Warfarin	Fetal and neonatal haemorrhage
Hypoglycaemics Sulphonylureas	Fetal and neonatal hypoglycaemia
Cardiovascular drugs Beta-agonists	Fetal tachycardia, delayed labour
Beta-antagonists Reserpine	Fetal and neonatal bradycardia, impaired adrenergic responses
Central nervous system drugs	
Narcotics Alcohol Barbiturates Benzodiazepines	Central nervous depression, withdrawal syndromes
Corticosteroids and sex hormones	Fetal and neonatal adrenal suppression, virilization of female fetus
Non-steroidal anti-inflammatory drugs	
Aspirin Indomethacin	Premature closure of fetal ductus arteriosus, delayed labour, increased blood loss

particularly in the premature neonate. Neonates have problems in effectively metabolizing vitamin K analogues, suphonamides, barbiturates, morphine and curare. One of the most dramatic examples is the production of the 'grey baby' syndrome by chloramphenicol in premature infants. This consists of circulatory collapse and muscular hypotonia and is thought to be due to a combination of defective hepatic conjugation of chloramphenicol and accumulation of unconjugated drug because of immature renal excretion.

In addition to hepatic immaturity, newborn infants have a relatively lower glomerular filtration

Table 14.5 Adverse drug reactions associated with inherited enzyme deficiencies.

Deficient enzyme	Drugs involved	Adverse effects
Cholinesterase	Succinylcholine	Prolonged neuromuscular blockade, apnoea
N-Acetyltransferase	Isoniazid	Peripheral neuropathy
	Procainamide Phenelzine Hydralazine	Systemic lupus erythematosus
Glucose-6-phosphate dehydrogenase	Primaquine Sulphonamides Nitrofurantoin Quinine Chloramphenicol	Haemolysis
Glutathione peroxidase	Sulphonamides	Haemolysis
Methaemoglobin reductase	Sulphonamides Nitrites	Methaemoglobinaemia
Mixed function oxidase (cytochrome P450)	Debrisoquine	Hypotension
	Phenformin (withdrawn)	Lactic acidosis
	Metoprolol	Bradycardia, marked beta-blockade

rate and renal plasma flow than adults, which results in reduced excretion of drugs such as aminoglycosides and digoxin.

The elderly

Elderly patients are more susceptible than younger people to most dose-related adverse drug reactions.

Reduced hepatic drug extraction and metabolism occurs with increasing age. This contributes to the increased incidence of adverse effects in older patients following the administration of central depressant drugs such as sedatives, tranquillizers and hypnotics. Age-related changes in the sensitivity of the central nervous system to the effects of these compounds may also be involved.

Glomerular filtration rate falls with age, leading to the accumulation of drugs principally excreted unchanged by the kidney. In view of this, doses of digoxin, lithium and aminoglycosides have to be reduced in elderly patients.

Increasing age is also associated with changes in body composition, as well as with a general tendency to a decrease in body weight. Both of these may influence the distribution and tissue levels of administered drugs.

Differences in enzyme activity

Differences in enzyme activity between individuals may be either inherited or acquired.

Inherited

There are marked differences in the rates of drug metabolism between individuals. Some of these are known to be due to polymorphic genetic control of the metabolic pathways involved (see Table 14.5).

Other examples include the exacerbation of acute intermittent porphyria by barbiturates and the occurrence of a rare familial resistance to coumarin anticoagulants.

Acquired enzyme inhibition

Many adverse drug reactions occur due to the administration of drugs which cause inhibition of enzymes.

Monoamine oxidase. This is a widely distributed enzyme that is responsible for the intercellular degradation of, amongst other monoamines, adrenaline, noradrenaline, dopamine and 5-hydroxytryptamine (serotonin). Its inhibition by monoamine oxidase inhibitors (MAOIs) may, therefore, given rise to serious adverse effects from the following agents if taken concurrently (see Fig. 14.2):

- Indirectly acting sympathomimetic amines such as ephedrine and phenylpropanolamine, whose pressor and cardiac actions are due to the release of noradrenaline from adrenergic nerve terminals and are potentiated by MAO inhibition
- Foods that contain tyramine, such as cheeses, wines, meat and yeast products. Tyramine is an

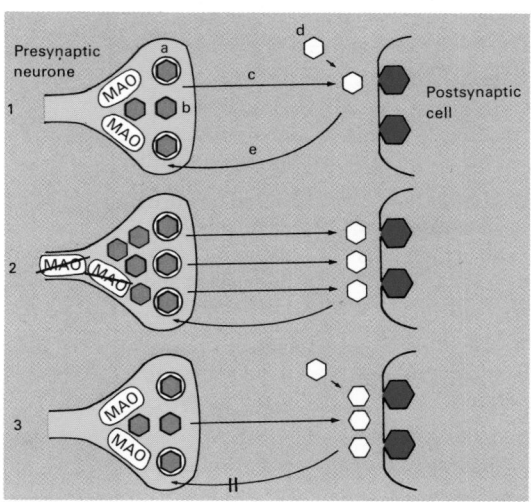

Fig. 14.2 Mechanisms by which monoamine oxidase inhibitors and monoamine reuptake inhibitors influence indirectly and directly acting sympathomimetic amines. a = granular stores of catecholamine; b = free cytoplasmic catecholamine; c = catecholamine released into synaptic cleft by nerve impulse or indirectly acting amine such as ephedrine or tyramine; d = exogenously administered directly acting amine such as noradrenaline; e = reuptake of catecholamine into the neurone, terminating its action. (1) Normal synapse; (2) Monoamine oxidase inhibition leads to increased catecholamine release by nerve impulse or sympathomimetic amine; (3) Monoamine reuptake inhibition e.g. tricyclics leads to increased effects of transmitter or administered amine.

indirectly acting amine with similar actions to phenylpropanolamine
- Monoamine-reuptake inhibiting (tricyclic) antidepressants, which can cause serious central nervous stimulation, convulsions and circulatory collapse if given together with an MAOI
- Antihypertensive drugs such as reserpine, guanethidine and bethanidine that release noradrenaline from its neuronal stores and so can produce serious hypertension
- Pethidine, which may produce severe narcotic effects with coma and hyperthermia in patients receiving MAOIs, possibly owing to raised levels of cerebral 5-hydroxytryptamine

Xanthine oxidase. Inhibition of xanthine oxidase by allopurinol can lead to reduced breakdown of purines such as 6-mercaptopurine and azathioprine, with an increased risk of their dose-dependent adverse effects, for example on the bone marrow.

Aldehyde dehydrogenase. This is inhibited by disulfiram, resulting in an accumulation of acetaldehyde after ingestion of alcohol, with the resulting 'antabuse' reaction of flushing, hypotension, head-ache, sweating, nausea, vomiting and even cardio-vascular collapse. This forms the basis of one approach to the management of alcohol dependence (see p. 993). A similar reaction may occur with the antimicrobial drug metronidazole.

Competition by drugs for hepatic drug-metabolizing pathways is not uncommon and is becoming increasingly recognized as a basis for adverse drug interactions. For example, cimetidine increases the anticoagulant effect of warfarin, the sedative effect of diazepam and the beta-adrenoreceptor blocking action of propranolol by inhibiting their hepatic metabolism. Sulphonamides decrease phenytoin metabolism so that toxic levels may be reached.

Acquired enzyme induction
The activity of hepatic drug-metabolizing enzymes may be increased by a large number of common substances, including insecticides, pesticides, polycyclic aromatic hydrocarbons, and some drugs such as barbiturates, phenytoin, carbamazepine and rifampicin. Such enzyme induction results in increased drug metabolism and breakdown, reducing the therapeutic activity of certain drugs. Examples include oral anticoagulants, corticosteroids and the contraceptive pill. The importance of enzyme induction lies in the exaggerated effects that can occur if the inducing drug is discontinued and the drug whose metabolism was being induced, e.g. warfarin, continues to be given in an increased dosage.

Protein binding

Many drugs are loosely bound to plasma and tissue proteins. The free unbound fraction is pharmacologically active. This fraction is increased in conditions in which hypoproteinaemia occurs (see Table 14.6). Competition between drugs for common binding sites can lead to a transient increase in free levels of one following its displacement by another, but the clinical importance of this is uncertain because increased clearance of the free fraction occurs, which tends to re-establish the original equilibrium between free and bound drug levels.

Route and kinetics of metabolism

Adverse reactions are particularly likely to occur where the relationship between drug dose and blood level is non-linear, so that relatively small increments in the dose given may lead to unexpectedly large increases in the blood level. Such a relationship is typical of saturation kinetics, in which hepatic metabolizing pathways become saturated or exhausted at a certain dose. Above this dose, proportionately more unchanged drug enters the systemic circulation. An important

Table 14.6 Influence of disease on drug toxicity through changes in pharmacokinetics.

Disease	Mechanism	Drugs involved	Effects
Liver disease; renal disease; cancer	Reduced serum albumin	Acidic drugs, e.g. aspirin	Increased free drug, risk of increased toxicity
Acute and chronic inflammation, myocardial infarction, surgery, trauma, cancer	Increased α-1-acid glycoprotein	Basic drugs, e.g. beta-antagonists, anti-arrhythmics	Reduced free drug, possibility of reduced therapeutic and toxic effects
Renal disease; cardiac failure	Reduced renal excretion	Digoxin, aminoglycosides, lithium	Increased therapeutic and toxic effects
Chronic liver disease; cardiac failure	Reduced hepatic uptake and clearance	Centrally acting drugs, steroids, warfarin, propranolol, tolbutamide, theophylline, lignocaine	Increased therapeutic and toxic effects
Cardiac failure	Reduced gastrointestinal perfusion and drug absorption	Digoxin	Possibility of reduced absorption and therapeutic effects, but importance uncertain

example of this phenomenon is seen with phenytoin (Fig. 14.3).

Some adverse effects are due not to the parent compound but to highly reactive metabolites. For example, when paracetamol is taken in overdose the capacity of hepatic conjugating mechanisms is exceeded and a hepatotoxic metabolite is formed and accumulates.

Excretion

Many drugs are excreted by the kidney, while others are reabsorbed. Changes in urinary pH affect elimination; for example, the excretion of the acidic drug aspirin is increased, whereas that of the basic drug mexiletine is reduced, by alkalinization of the urine. This may be important clinically in patients who have a persistently high urine pH from renal disease or a vegetarian diet. Competition for renal tubular excretion also occurs, e.g. penicillin competes with probenecid.

Local factors

The therapeutic action of some drugs is markedly dependent on the local physiological environment at its site of action. A good example is the effect of myocardial potassium concentration on the cardiac actions of digitalis glycosides, hypokalaemia leading to enhancement of their action, with the risk of toxicity. Another example is the influence of changes in sodium and potassium status on the response to lithium.

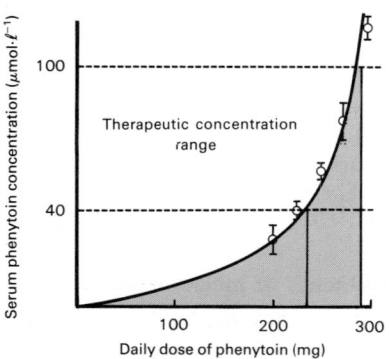

Fig. 14.3 Saturation kinetic as exhibited by phenytoin. The measurements were obtained from one patient on several maintenance doses of phenytoin and show a curvilinear relationship between dose and serum concentration. Note the relatively small dose range compatible with a therapeutic concentration. (Modified from Turner P & Richens A (1981) *Clinical Pharmacology*, 4th edn. Edinburgh: Churchill Livingstone. With permission.)

Table 14.7 Some clinically important drug interactions leading to adverse effects.

Drug A *may interact with*	Drug B	Potential results	Mechanism
Reduced hepatic excretion			
Carbamazepine Phenytoin Diazepam Propranolol Theophylline Coumarin anticoagulants	Cimetidine Sodium valproate Chloramphenicol Ciprofloxacin Sulphonamides Tolbutamide Indomethacin Clofibrate Tamoxifen	Potentiation of drug A	Inhibition of hepatic enzymes by drug B
Reduced renal excretion			
Penicillins Cephalosporins Dapsone	Probenecid	Increased plasma levels of drug A	Reduced tubular secretion of drug A
Mexiletine Amphetamine	Antacids (systemically absorbed)	Increased plasma levels of drug A	Reduced excretion of drug A in alkaline urine
Inhibition of neuronal uptake			
Monoamine reuptake inhibiting anti-depressants, e.g. imipramine, amitriptyline Fenfluramine	Noradrenaline Adrenaline Phenylephrine	Potentiation of pressor action of drug B	Inhibition by drug A of neuronal uptake of drug B (see Fig. 14.2)
Inhibition of monoamine oxidase			
MAOIs e.g. phenelzine	Amphetamine Ephedrine Phenylpropanolamine Pseudoephedrine Fenfluramine Levodopa Tyramine-containing food and wines	Acute hypertensive crisis	Release by drug B of monoamine stores increased by drug A (see Fig. 14.2)
	Pethidine and other narcotics Fluoxetine	Central nervous excitation, coma	Increased 5-HT activity
Summation of effects			
Barbiturates Benzodiazepines	Alcohol Other CNS depressants	Increased CNS depression	Summation of CNS depression
Monoamine reuptake inhibiting antidepressants, e.g. imipramine, amitriptyline	Anticholinergics Antihistamines Antiparkinsonian drugs	Excessive central and peripheral atropine-like effects	Summation of anti-cholinergic actions
	Monoamine oxidase inhibitors e.g. phenelzine	Central nervous excitation, coma	Increased central monoamine activity
Thiazide and loop diuretics	Corticosteroids Carbenoxolone	Hypokalaemia	Renal potassium loss

Table continued overleaf

Table 14.7 (*continued*)

Drug A *may interact with*	Drug B	Potential results	Mechanism
Angiotensin-converting enzyme inhibitors, e.g. captopril, enalapril	Potassium-sparing diuretics	Hyperkalaemia	Potassium retention
Anti-arrhythmic drugs	Beta-adrenoceptor blocking drugs, particulaly propranolol	Myocardial depression	Summation of myocardial depression
Antihypertensive drugs	Vasodilators Alcohol Fenfluramine Levodopa Bromocriptine	Hypotension	Summation of hypotensive effects
Loop diuretics	Aminoglycosides Cephaloridine Cephalothin	Increased nephrotoxicity and ototoxicity	Uncertain
Others			
Digoxin	Thiazide and loop diuretics	Toxicity of drug A	Hypokalaemia
	Quinidine Amiodarone Nifedipine Verapamil	Toxicity of drug A	Clearance of drug A reduced by drug B
Lithium	Haloperidol	Involuntary movements	Uncertain
Competitive neuromuscular blocking drugs, e.g. tubocurarine	Aminoglycosides Propranolol Lithium Quinidine	Potentiation of drug A	Uncertain
Metronidazole Chlorpropamide	Alcohol	Flushing, hypotension	Uncertain
Alcohol	Disulfiram	'Antabuse' reaction: flushing, hypotension, tachycardia, arrhythmias	Inhibition by drug B of metabolism of drug A, producing acetaldehyde accumulation
Azathioprine 6-Mercaptopurine	Allopurinol	Toxicity of drug A	Xanthine oxidase inhibition by drug B

Drug interactions

Drugs can interact within the body in many ways that may lead to adverse effects. Some important examples are given in Table 14.7.

Patient compliance

Patient compliance is also a factor in adverse reactions. Compliance is influenced by the drug formulation, frequency of dosage, number of drugs prescribed, and by the patient's age and ability to comprehend instructions.

Influence of disease on adverse drug reactions

Disease processes may increase the risk and severity of adverse drug reactions in several ways.

- Disease may lead to changes in the pharmacokinetics of a drug. A reduction in protein binding or reduced renal or hepatic clearance will potentiate the effects of certain drugs (Table 14.6).
- Changes in receptor density and function may occur. For example, there is evidence that the enhanced bronchoconstrictor effects of beta-adrenoceptor antagonists in asthmatics patients

Table 14.8 Some examples of enchanced drug toxicity associated with inherited diseases.

Inherited disease	Drug	Reaction
Haemophilia and von Willebrand's disease	Salicylates	Prolongs bleeding time
Hereditary myopathies, myotonia congenita	Halothane Caffeine Succinylcholine Potassium chloride	Malignant hyperthermia (malignant hyperpyrexia)
Osteogenesis imperfecta	Halothane Succinylcholine	Pyrexia
Periodic paralysis	Potassium chloride Insulin Adrenaline Ethanol Liquorice derivatives	Paralysis
Familial dysautonomia	Cholinergic and adrenergic agonists	Denervation supersensitivity

Table 14.9 Some examples of drug toxicity associated with disease states, the nature of which is not yet understood.

Disease	Drug	Reaction
Glandular fever (infectious mononucleosis)	Ampicillin Amoxycillin	Rash
Hypothyroidism Respiratory failure	CNS depressants	Enhanced CNS depression and respiratory failure
Burns Renal failure Polyneuropathy	Succinylcholine	Release of potassium-producing cardiac arrhythmias
Rheumatoid arthritis and other connective tissue diseases	Salicylates	Hepatotoxicity (rare)
Cystic fibrosis	Isoprenaline Theophylline	Bronchospasm
Renal failure	Clofibrate (withdrawn) Benzodiazepines Monoamine reuptake inhibiting antidepressants (tricyclic)	Severe myopathy Fatal dialysis dementia

may be due to a reduction ('down regulation') in beta receptor number produced by long-term treatment with beta-agonists such as salbutamol. The sensitivity of patients with myasthenia gravis to the neuromuscular blocking effects of streptomycin, neomycin or kanamycin may be due to drug-induced changes in cholinergic receptors.

● Some inherited diseases are associated with enhanced drug toxicity (see Table 14.8).

There are also several examples of disease-related enhanced drug toxicity the nature of which is not yet understood (Table 14.9).

Monitoring adverse drug reactions

Clinical trials of new drugs are conveniently classified into:

● Phase 1, in which the drug is given to a small number of normal volunteers in closely controlled and supervised conditions to study its kinetics and pharmacological effects
● Phase 2, in which the drug is given to a relatively small number of patients with the disease for which its use is proposed. The

therapeutic efficacy, correct dosage and pharma-cokinetics of the drug are determined by comparing the data with those for normal subjects to obtain some evidence of its safety

- Phase 3, in which the clinical evaluation of the drug is extended to large numbers of patients (perhaps hundreds). Trials include comparisons with placebos and with established treatments
- Phase 4 (post-marketing surveillance, PMS), in which long-term assessment of the safety and efficacy of the drug is made in thousands of patients, following the licensing of the drug for marketing

Experience has shown that careful observation of patients in phase 2 and phase 3 clinical trials is only likely to detect those adverse reactions that occur in 1% or more of patients exposed to a drug. Adverse reactions with an incidence of less than 1% require detection in phase 4 (PMS) studies.

Several countries have developed systems for collecting information about suspected adverse drug reactions. In the UK two systems are of particular interest.

Prescription event monitoring (PEM)

The PEM scheme involves identifying doctors and their patients as the prescriptions for a particular drug pass through the central Prescription Pricing Authority office. Relevant prescriptions are photo-copied and the copies are sent in confidence to the Drug Surveillance Research Unit in Southampton. Each 'test' drug under investigation is matched with a 'control' drug that is chemically or pharmacologically similar and already marketed for the same indications. Similar numbers of patients receiving each drug are selected and a simple questionnaire is sent to their general medical practitioners, requesting information on age, new diagnoses or events that have come to the doctor's attention, and reasons for any referral to a consultant or admission to hospital. PEM should be able to identify adverse drug reactions that have an incidence of 1 in 3000 or greater.

Yellow card system

The voluntary yellow card system has been the most productive to date in the UK for identifying important adverse drug reactions. Yellow reply-paid cards are supplied to doctors and dentists, who are encouraged to use them to report any suspected adverse drug reactions to the government's advisory Committee on Safety of Medicines. Although the rate of reporting is low, this system has drawn attention to the association of oral contraceptives and thromboembolism, hepatitis and methyldopa, jaundice and halothane, and extrapyramidal effects and metoclopramide. At present, only this system is potentially capable of detecting risk at all levels of incidence.

When suspicion has been aroused through the yellow card system, the existence or otherwise of a true association between a reported event and the implicated drug must be demonstrated epidemiologically by case control or cohort studies, and by clinical pharmacological and toxicological studies of the possible mechanisms involved.

The problems associated with long-term surveillance of many thousands of patients must not be underestimated. Such studies are costly in both time and money, and it is difficult to maintain the integrity of the study cohort, the interest and commitment of the doctors, and the compliance of the patients.

Reduction of adverse drug reactions

The incidence of adverse drug reactions can be reduced by:

- The development and marketing of safer drugs by the pharmaceutical industry
- Tighter control by drug-regulatory authorities within government on the licensing, promotion and marketing of drugs

Table 14.10 Drugs for which plasma concentration monitoring may be helpful.

Drug	Therapeutic plasma concentration range	Toxic levels	Optimum time for sampling after dose (h)
Carbamazepine	21–42 μmol$\cdot$L^{-1}	> 42 μmol$\cdot$L^{-1}	> 8
Digoxin	1.3–2.6 nmol$\cdot$L^{-1}	> 2.6 nmol$\cdot$L^{-1}	> 8
Gentamicin	Trough < 2 mg$\cdot$L^{-1}	> 2 mg$\cdot$L^{-1}	6–8
	Peak 4–8 mg$\cdot$L^{-1}	> 12 mg$\cdot$L^{-1}	1
Lithium	0.4–1.2 mmol$\cdot$L^{-1}	> 1.5 mmol$\cdot$L^{-1}	> 10
Phenytoin	40–80 μmol$\cdot$L^{-1}	> 80 μmol$\cdot$L^{-1}	> 10
Theophylline	55–110 μmol$\cdot$L^{-1}	> 110 μmol$\cdot$L^{-1}	> 4

In addition, the doctor must think carefully about every drug he or she prescribes.

The hazards of adverse drug reaction can be substantially reduced by:

- Understanding the mechanisms underlying the reactions
- Excluding a history of adverse reaction
- Individualizing drug dosage

Prescribing manuals and therapeutic textbooks give recommended ranges of drug doses. The choice of dose for an individual patient, however, depends on a large variety of factors, including genetic and environmental factors, most of which are still only poorly understood. The prescribing doctor must, therefore, determine the optimum drug dose for the patient from the advised range given by considering the factors already discussed and on the basis of his or her own experience. In some cases the dose can be decided by monitoring its therapeutic effect; for example, prothrombin time can be measured when using an oral anticoagulant drug, or blood sugar when using insulin or an oral hypoglycaemic drug. In addition, for drugs with a narrow therapeutic ratio (i.e. the ratio of the dose necessary to produce a therapeutic effect to that necessary to produce a toxic effect), or whose kinetics are not linear, titration of the dose to obtain a desirable blood level may be of value. Such control is called 'therapeutic drug monitoring', and is particularly helpful with digoxin, gentamicin, lithium and phenytoin, whose potentially toxic concentrations are relatively close to the therapeutic range (see Table 14.10).

Maintaining a low threshold of suspicion

Most important of all is that all prescribing doctors should be continually aware of the possibility that any clinical or life event (e.g. an accident) may be associated in some way with a patient's treatment. The lower the threshold of suspicion on the part of the doctor, the lower the risk of serious long-term adverse drug reactions in the patient.

Poisoning

In most hospitals in the Western World the commonest reason for acute admission to a medical ward is poisoning. Such poisoning is usually by self-administration of prescribed or over-the-counter medicines. Occasionally, however, toxic agents are accidentally ingested or inhaled at home or work or are administered with criminal intent.

Self-poisoning is often a cry for help, in which the patient takes whatever drug is easily available at home. Doctors should therefore always prescribe

---

Types of poisoning

Self-poisoning refers to the deliberate ingestion of an overdose of a drug or some other substance not meant for consumption.

Suicide is the term applied to all patients who die whether it was their intention to kill themselves or not.

Accidental poisoning occurs mostly in children below 5 years of age, but can occur in adults, e.g. from the accidental inhalation of a gas, ingestion of fluid from a wrongly labelled bottle, stings and bites, or eating poisonous foods (such as toadstools).

Non-accidental poisoning is the deliberate administration of a poison to a child.

Homicidal poisoning.

---

limited amounts of drugs, and it is advisable to keep only small amounts of tablets, preferably foil-wrapped, in the home. Patients should be advised about the potential danger of drugs that should be kept out of reach of children.

The majority of cases (80%) of self-poisoning do not require intensive medical management but all require a sympathetic and caring approach to their problems. Both the patient and the family may require psychiatric help (see p. 984) and the social services should be contacted to help with social and domestic problems.

In England there were 97 000 hospital admissions in 1982 for self-poisoning, the commonest being with psychotropics (29 000), and analgesics and antirheumatic drugs (26 000). In the same year in England and Wales there were 2208 deaths from poisoning, of which 237 were due to co-proxamol (paracetamol and dextropropoxyphene), 163 to paracetamol alone and 131 to amitriptyline. This pattern is reflected in many other countries where similar medicines are available.

Information from other continents is difficult to compare, but in Asia and Africa it seems that poisoning is a significant medical problem, with children a particularly vulnerable group. In Cairo, over half of the enquiries at the poisons reference centre involve the poisoning of children. The proportion of accidental poisoning in Asia and Africa is higher than in Europe and North America.

The number of admissions from self-poisoning is increasing. However, as a result of good supportive care and the reduced availability of coal gas and barbiturates, the mortality of patients is declining and is now well under 1%. Studies of the drugs involved reveal that:

- Acute overdoses usually involve more than one drug.
- Alcohol is the most commonly implicated second 'drug' in mixed self-poisonings; 60% of

men and 45% of women consume some alcohol at the same time as the drug.
- There is a poor correlation between the drug history and the toxicological findings. Therefore, patients' statements about the type and amount of drug ingested should not be relied on.
- The use of minor tranquillizers and antidepressants is increasing, but there is a decrease in the number of overdoses with barbiturates, which are virtually unavailable in the UK.

HISTORY

Eighty per cent of adults are conscious on arrival at hospital and the diagnosis of self-poisoning can usually be made easily from the history. In the unconscious patient a history from friends or relatives is helpful and the diagnosis can often be inferred from tablet bottles or a suicide note brought by the ambulance attendants.

It should be emphasized that in any patient with an altered conscious level, drug overdose must always be considered in the differential diagnosis.

EXAMINATION

On arrival at hospital the patient must be assessed urgently in the A and E Department. The following should be evaluated:

- Level of consciousness—a useful practical grading is:

I Drowsy but responds to commands
II Unconscious but responds to mild stimulation
III Unconscious but responds only to maximal painful stimuli (sternal rubbing)
IV Unconscious and no response
- Respiratory effort and cyanosis
- Blood pressure and pulse rate
- Pupil size and reaction to light (NB opiates constrict)
- Evidence of head injury or drug addiction

If the patient is unconscious the following should also be checked:

- Presence or absence of cough and gag reflex
- Temperature—measured with a low-reading rectal thermometer

The physical signs that may aid identification of the agents responsible for poisoning are shown in Fig. 14.4.

Principles of management

Most patients with self-poisoning require only general care and support of the vital systems. However, for a few drugs additional therapy is required.

Blood and urine samples should always be taken on admission for the determination of drug

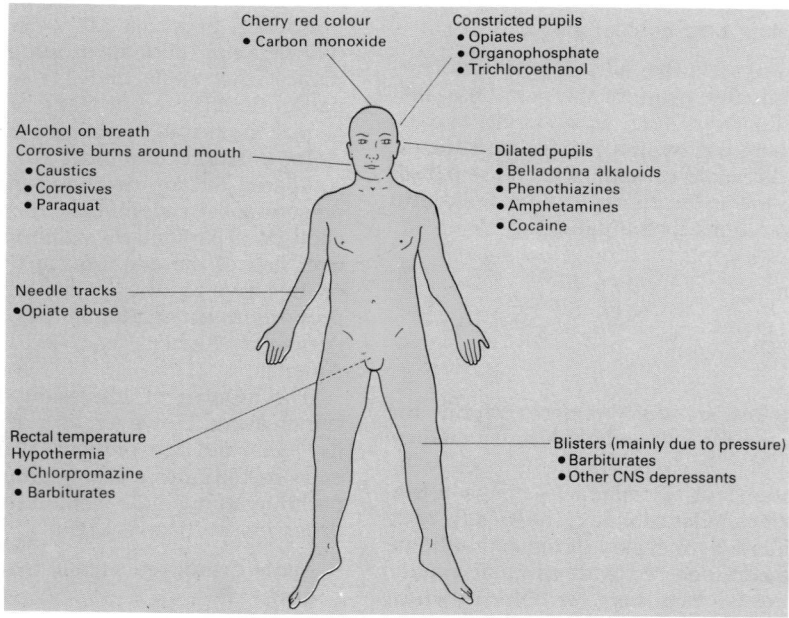

Fig. 14.4 Physical signs that may aid the identification of agents responsible for poisoning.

Table 14.11 Causes of hypotension after drug overdose.

An expanded venous bed due to venous vasodilatation

Hypovolaemia due to inadequate fluid intake in prolonged coma

Institution of IPPV in an already hypovolaemic patient

Myocardial depression due to the direct effect of the drug, exaggerated by hypoxia, acidosis and hypothermia

levels, as these are invaluable for the management of certain poisons and are helpful in legal problems. Drug screens of blood and urine are occasionally indicated in the seriously ill, unconscious patient in whom the cause of coma is unknown.

Routine haematological and biochemical investigations are of value, particularly in the differential diagnosis of coma.

Care of the unconscious patient (see also p. 907)

In all cases the patient should be nursed in the lateral position with the lower leg straight and the upper leg flexed; in this position the risk of aspiration is reduced. A clear passage for air should be encouraged by the removal of any obstructing object, vomit or dentures, and by backward elevation of the mandible. Nursing care of the mouth and pressure areas should be instituted. Catheterization of the bladder is usually unnecessary as bladders can be emptied by gentle suprapubic pressure. Insertion of venous cannulae and i.v. fluids are usually unnecessary unless the patient has been unconscious for more than 24 hours.

Respiratory support

If respiratory depression is minimal, oxygen (approximately 60%) should be administered via a mask. A naso- or oropharyngeal airway should be inserted and constant observation is mandatory to detect any further depression of ventilation.

Loss of the cough or gag reflex is the prime indication for intubation. The gag reflex is assessed by positioning the patients on their side and making them gag using a sucker. In most patients the reflexes are depressed sufficiently to allow intubation without the use of sedatives or relaxants. The complications of endotracheal tubes are discussed on p. 726.

If ventilation remains inadequate, intermittent positive-pressure ventilation (IPPV) should be instituted (see p. 724). Blood gas analysis is useful to confirm the need for IPPV. Hypoxaemia is common in the unconscious patient, particularly after the ingestion of opiates and barbiturates, and can easily go undetected without blood gas analysis.

Cardiovascular support

Hypotension is a common feature of drug overdose and is caused by the physiological effects listed in Table 14.11. The classic features of shock—tachycardia and pale cold skin—may be present, but vasodilatation may also be seen, e.g. with barbiturate overdose.

In the majority of cases, hypotension is mild and elevation of the feet is the only treatment required. In patients with more severe hypotension, volume expanders such as dextran should be used. In severely hypotensive patients, the measurement of central venous pressure (CVP) is helpful. Urine output (aiming for $0.5 \text{ ml·kg}^{-1}\text{·h}^{-1}$) is also an important longer-term guide to the adequacy of the circulation, as many vasodilated overdose patients are adequately perfused with a systolic blood pressure of as low as 90–100 mm Hg. Some hypotensive patients may need to be catheterized in order to monitor urine output.

If a patient fails to respond to the above measures, intensive therapy is required (see p. 716).

Arrhythmias are commonly seen with tricyclic antidepressants. Known arrhythmogenic factors such as hypoxia, acidosis and hypokalaemia should be corrected.

Special problems

Hypothermia. Defined as a rectal temperature of below 35°C, this is a common problem, especially in older patients or those poisoned with chlorpromazine or a similar neuroleptic. Hypothyroidism should always be excluded. Hypothermia is compounded by drug-induced vasodilatation and environmental exposure. The patient should be covered with a 'space blanket' and given intravenous and intragastric fluids at normal body temperature. Inspired gases should also be warmed to 37°C.

Rhabdomyolysis. Rhabdomyolysis can occur from pressure necrosis in drug-induced coma or it may complicate heroin abuse without coma. The risk of renal failure from myoglobinaemia is potentiated by dehydration and acidosis.

Convulsions. These may occur in serious tricyclic antidepressant poisoning, and in antihistamine, anticonvulsant or phenothiazine poisoning. Diazepam 10 mg i.v. is the standard treatment for fits of any cause. The patient should also receive a loading dose of phenytoin (1 g administered intravenously over 4 h via a central vein) and a maintenance dose of 100 mg 8-hourly if the fits are not immediately controlled. Persistent fits must be controlled rapidly, as they may otherwise result in severe hypoxia, brain damage and laryngeal trauma.

Stress bleeding. Measures to prevent stress ulceration of the stomach should be started on admission in all patients who are unconscious and require intensive care. Administration of antacid by intragastric tube is usually adequate although H_2 antagonists are often used.

SPECIFIC MANAGEMENT

Many techniques have been developed to decrease drug absorption and increase drug elimination, but most of these manoeuvres are only helpful with a few drugs. These, as well as antidotes to specific drugs, are described below.

Decreasing drug absorption

Vigorous attempts to empty the gastrointestinal tract are indicated when drugs that cause potentially fatal complications other than coma or respiratory depression have been ingested. Examples of such drugs are aspirin, paracetamol, colchicine, organophosphates, iron salts and tricyclic antidepressants. It is important to remember that the risk of aspiration into the lungs associated with the use of gastric lavage may well cause more problems than the effects of the drugs themselves.

Induced emesis. Induced emesis may be useful in small children as they are more difficult to lavage. It is rarely used in adults, as only small amounts of drug are recovered.

Paediatric ipecacuanha emetic mixture (*not* the undiluted fluid extract) is the emetic of choice. The dose is 10 ml for a child. Other emetics such as apomorphine, saline, copper sulphate and mustard are dangerous and should not be used.

Gastric lavage. This procedure is of use only when a large quantity of drug has been taken. The earlier gastric lavage is performed, the greater the amount of drug that is retrieved. It is of little value after 4 h except for the drugs shown in Table 14.12. Lavage is contraindicated for some poisons, e.g. corrosives, petrol or paraffin.

Absorbants. If administered promptly (within 1 h) and in sufficiently large amounts, activated charcoal (25–100 g) significantly reduces the gastrointestinal absorption of many drugs. Charcoal can

Table 14.12 Drugs for which gastric lavage is useful more than 4 h after ingestion.

Salicylates
Basic drugs such as quinidine or tricyclic antidepressants, where gastric emptying is delayed
Paracetamol

be administered by mouth, or more commonly by a nasogastric tube. The latter reduces the possibility of inhalation, which can cause severe pulmonary damage. However, because of this risk and questionable effectiveness, activated charcoal has been withdrawn in the UK.

Technique of gastric lavage

- Should be performed by an experienced nurse and doctor.
- The main danger is from pulmonary aspiration, and it is vital that the tracheobronchial tree is protected either by an intact cough reflex or by a cuffed endotracheal tube.
- The patient should be positioned lying on his left side, with his head over the end or side of the bed so that the mouth and throat are at a lower level than the larynx and trachea.
- A wide-bore tube (Jacques' gauge 30) is lubricated with glycerine or Vaseline and passed into the stomach. Aspiration is performed first, and then followed by lavage using 300 ml of water at body temperature for the first washing.
- This process should be repeated at least three or four times, using up to 500 ml of water on each occasion.
- An aliquot of the washing should be saved in case it is needed for drug analysis.

Increasing drug elimination

Forced alkaline diuresis. This potentially lethal technique is rarely necessary, as few drugs are excreted in their unchanged form. Its benefits have been shown to be outweighed by its serious complications. It is mainly used in salicylate poisoning, which is discussed on p. 747.

Peritoneal dialysis. The use of this technique is limited by its low efficacy but it may be indicated for patients severely poisoned by ethylene glycol.

Haemodialysis. This technique may be useful for patients with severe poisoning by lithium salts or methyl or ethyl alcohols. Rarely, patients with severe salicylate poisoning (blood salicylate level > 900 mg·L^{-1} or 6.5 mmol·L^{-1}) refractory to forced alkaline diuresis may be helped by haemodialysis.

Haemoperfusion. This is very rarely used. It involves the passage of blood through devices containing absorbent particles, such as activated charcoal or resins, to which drugs are adsorbed. Its use should be considered in patients severely posioned with certain drugs (e.g. theophylline) who fail to improve despite the use of adequate supportive measures.

Antagonizing the effects of poisons

These techniques will be considered under the individual drugs. Specific antidotes are available for a small number of drugs. Antidotes act in a number of ways:

- Interaction with poison to form an inert complex that is then excreted, e.g. desferrioxamine in iron overdose
- Acceleration or detoxification of a poison, e.g. *N*-acetylcysteine in paracetamol poisoning
- Prevention of the formation of a more toxic compound, e.g. ethanol used as a competitive substrate for the metabolizing enzyme to prevent formation of toxic metabolites in methanol poisoning
- Competition with the poison for essential receptors, e.g. naloxone in opiate poisoning
- Blockade of receptors through which the toxic effects are mediated, e.g. atropine used to block cholinergic receptors in organophosphate poisoning

Specific drug problems

In this section only specific treatment regimens will be discussed. The general principles of management of self-poisoning will always be required.

ANALGESICS

Analgesic poisoning is common in some areas, accounting for one-third of all cases of self-poisoning admitted to hospital. Salicylate poisoning has decreased over the past decade, while paracetamol poisoning has increased.

Combinations of aspirin or paracetamol and narcotic analgesics such as codeine or dextropropoxyphene are frequently taken. Co-proxamol, a combination of paracetamol and dextropropoxyphene can cause severe respiratory depression and is a major cause of death.

Accidental poisoning with analgesics has decreased since the introduction of child-resistant bottles.

Salicylates

Salicylates are well absorbed from the stomach and small intestine. They are metabolized to form salicyluric acid and salicyl phenolic glucuronides, a process that is saturated at therapeutic dosage. At high doses, renal excretion becomes important. Overdosage stimulates the respiratory centre, directly increasing the depth and rate of respiration and thereby producing a respiratory alkalosis. Compensatory mechanisms include renal excretion of bicarbonate and potassium, which results in a metabolic acidosis. Salicylates also interfere with carbohydrate, fat and protein metabolism, as well as with oxidative phosphorylation. This gives rise to increased lactate, pyruvate and ketone bodies, all of which contribute to the acidosis.

Symptoms and signs of salicylate poisoning include tinnitus, nausea and vomiting, overbreathing, hyperpyrexia and sweating with a tachycardia. Alternatively, the patient may appear completely well, even with high blood levels of salicylate. The ingestion of 10–20 g of aspirin by an adult (or one-tenth of this amount for a child) is likely to cause moderate or severe toxicity.

With severe intoxication (salicylate levels 800–1000 mg·L^{-1}; 5.6–7.2 mmol·L^{-1}), confusion, delirium, convulsions and coma result. It should be remembered that consciousness is not impaired unless the blood salicylate level is very high or, more commonly, another drug has been taken.

Cerebral and pulmonary oedema are serious complications, and may be exacerbated by forced diuresis.

TREATMENT

Aspirin delays gastric emptying and gastric lavage should be performed up to 12 h after the ingestion in all but the mildest cases.

Intravenous fluids may be necessary to correct dehydration and hypokalaemia. Occasionally intramuscular vitamin K is required to correct hypoprothrombinaemia. Making the urine alkaline is also effective in increasing urine salicylate excretion.

Forced alkaline diuresis is used if the blood level exceeds 500 mg·L^{-1} (3.6 mmol·L^{-1}). Increasing the pH of the urine from 7 to 8 increases the renal excretion of salicylic acid by about a factor of 10. In the first hour, 1500 ml of fluid should be given as 500 ml 5% dextrose, 500 ml 1.4% sodium bicarbonate and then 500 ml 5% dextrose again. Sufficient potassium should be mixed with each 500 ml bag to keep the serum potassium level above 3.5 mmol·L^{-1}. If less than 200 ml of urine is produced in the first hour, diuresis should be discontinued. The urine pH should be measured regularly—every 15 or 30 min—and kept at between 7.5 and 8.5. The plasma pH and arterial blood gases should be monitored at least 2-hourly to ensure that it does not rise above 7.6; the plasma electrolytes should also be measured. If facilities are not available for constant observation by medical and nursing staff, alkaline diuresis may be more dangerous than the salicylate poisoning itself and should not be used.

Paracetamol (see also p. 257)

Self-poisoning with paracetamol is common and the outcome can often be fatal. Paracetamol is converted to a toxic metabolite, N-acetyl-p-benzo-quinonimine, which is normally rapidly conjugated with reduced glutathione. After a large overdose, glutathione is depleted and the reactive intermediate binds covalently to liver-cell membranes causing necrosis. Marked liver necrosis can occur with as little as 10 g (20 tablets), and death with 15 g. The prothrombin time is the best guide to the severity of the damage.

The clinical features in the first 24 h include nausea and vomiting, but consciousness is preserved. Most patients recover within 48 h, but some develop liver failure, which usually becomes apparent in 72–96 h. Acute renal failure can occur sometimes in the absence of severe liver damage.

MANAGEMENT (Fig. 14.5)

Blood for paracetamol levels, liver biochemistry and prothrombin time should be taken immediately. Intravenous N-acetylcysteine is the treatment of

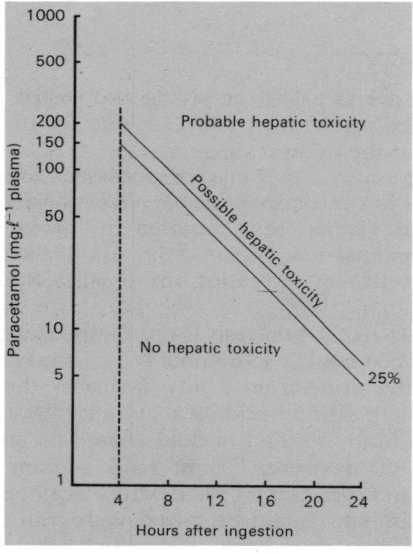

Fig. 14.5 Normogram for paracetamol.

Cautions for use of this chart:

- The units of measurement must be the same as used in this nomogram.
- Serum levels drawn before 4 h may not represent peak levels.
- The graph should be used only in relation to a single acute ingestion.
- The lower solid line 25% below the standard nomogram is included to allow for possible errors in paracetamol plasma assays and estimated time from ingestion of an overdose.

choice and provides sulphydryl groups that increase the availability of hepatic glutathione. Treatment should be started in all patients who have taken a large dose of paracetamol as soon as possible, even before the blood paracetamol level is known. The infusion can be stopped if the blood level is below the toxic range of 200 mg·L^{-1} (1.32 mmol·L^{-1}) at 4 h after ingestion, as liver damage is unlikely below this figure. For maximum protective action, treatment (300 mg·kg^{-1} over 20 h) should ideally be started within 8 h but it may be worthwhile up to 24 h, unless the prothrombin time is increased, when it is too late as the liver is already damaged. Oral therapy with N-acetylcysteine is used in some countries and oral methionine occasionally outside hospitals. Side-effects of N-acetylcysteine include convulsions and anaphylaxis in up to 5% of cases.

In addition to using specific antidotes, gastric lavage, a 5% dextrose drip to prevent hypoglycaemia, correction of any electrolyte imbalance and, if the prothrombin time is prolonged, the administration of vitamin K may be necessary.

Poisoning with paracetamol and dextropropoxyphene (co-proxamol) is complicated by respiratory depression. Since dextropropoxyphene is an opiate, naloxone should be given intravenously in an initial dose of 0.4–2.0 mg, and repeated at 2–3 min intervals up to a total of 10 mg if necessary. If this combination is taken with alcohol, death may occur rapidly from respiratory depression.

Patients should be transferred to a specialized liver unit if:

- Prothrombin time > 30 s at 48 h, or > 50 s at 72 h
- Serum creatinine > 200 mmol·L^{-1}
- There is metabolic acidosis (pH < 7.3)

Transfer should take place before hypotension and hepatic encephalopathy, as deterioration can be rapid. For prognosis of liver damage, see p. 257.

NSAIDs

Self-poisoning with NSAIDs has increased, particularly as ibuprofen is available without prescription. Overdoses will produce a variety of effects including nausea, vomiting, headache, tinnitus and gastrointestinal bleeding. Severe poisoning causes widespread metabolic abnormalities, hepatic and renal damage, and convulsions occur with mefenamic acid. Treatment is supportive.

Opiates

Opiates produce respiratory depression leading to coma. Pin-point pupils are seen. Naloxone 0.4–1.2 mg i.v. is a competitive antagonist but, as it is short-acting, repeated injections may be required.

Psychotrophic drugs

Benzodiazepines

Benzodiazepines are commonly taken in cases of self-poisoning, accounting for 40% of all drug overdosages in the UK. On their own they are remarkably safe but they potentiate the CNS-depressant effects of other drugs taken with them, such as barbiturates or ethanol. Benzodiazepines produce drowsiness, ataxia, dysarthria, nystagmus and sometimes coma. Mild hypotension and respiratory depression may occur. Most patients recover within 24 h. Deaths from benzodiazepines alone are rare. Flumazenil, a benzodiazepine antagonist, is only useful for severe respiratory depression but the patient should be carefully monitored.

Antidepressants

Monoamine oxidase inhibitors (MAOIs). Self-poisoning with MAOIs is uncommon and has a lower toxicity than with tricyclic antidepressants. Symptoms do not usually develop for at least 12 h after the overdose, when catecholamine levels in the tissues have risen. The clinical features include central nervous system overactivity, with agitation, hallucinations and muscle rigidity. Facial grimacing and writhing movements of the limbs and trunk may occur. There is usually dilatation of the pupils, tachycardia, a rising blood pressure and profuse sweating, although hypotension may occur. Muscle tone may be exaggerated and convulsions are common. Hyperpyrexia also occurs.

Gastric lavage is performed, see p. 746.

Tricyclic antidepressants. Most of the features of self-poisoning with these agents are due to the anticholinergic effects of the drugs. Clinical features include a decrease in the level of consciousness, but deep coma does not usually occur. Convulsions, increased muscle tone, hyper-reflexia and extensor plantar responses sometimes occur. The pupils are usually fixed and dilated and there may be ophthalmoplegia and gaze paralysis. Urinary retention may be present. Cardiovascular effects include hypotension and sinus tachycardia. More serious tachyarrhythmias and conduction defects are uncommon and are thought to be due to the quinidine-like action of these drugs. Ventricular arrhythmias are a cause of death in the first few hours following overdose.

If more than 15 tablets have been taken or if the patient is unconscious, gastric lavage should be performed within 4 h of admission to hospital. Cardiac arrhythmias may need treatment but often this is not necessary. Anti-arrhythmic therapy is often not effective; correction of any accompanying acidosis and hypoxia is more important.

Most patients recover consciousness within 24 h, while most cardiac abnormalities settle within 12 h.

Newer antidepressants such as mianserin produce only mild clinical effects, with drowsiness, hypotension and sinus tachycardia, which are much less severe than with the tricyclic antidepressants.

Lithium. Self-poisoning with this agent usually occurs in patients on long-term maintenance therapy. It is sometimes accidental owing to:

- Impairment of lithium elimination by the kidney, owing to the administration of a diuretic
- Other factors affecting water and electrolyte balance, such as nausea, vomiting, diarrhoea or exposure to high temperatures

In acute overdoses there is a delayed onset of symptoms of more than 12 h due to the slow entry of lithium into the tissues.

Clinical features include nausea, vomiting, diarrhoea, apathy and decreased consciousness. There may be restlessness and ataxia with increased muscle tone and rigidity. Electrolyte disturbances, such as hypokalaemia, occur with ECG changes. Acute renal failure is a rare complication. Coma is associated with a bad prognosis.

Serum lithium concentrations correlate poorly with the severity of acute lithium poisoning but, nevertheless, levels in excess of 20 $mmol\cdot L^{-1}$ are often serious.

Intravenous fluids are necessary to maintain a good urinary output. Forced diuresis should not be used but haemodialysis may be helpful in severe cases.

Phenothiazines. Clinical features include hypotension, hypothermia, CNS and respiratory depression, arrhythmias and dyskinesia. The latter can be treated with benztropine 2 mg i.v.

Cardiorespiratory drugs

These may be taken deliberately or sometimes accidentally by the elderly, often when one tablet is mistaken for another.

Beta-adrenoceptor blocking drugs

A small overdose of these drugs produces a bradycardia, but a large overdose can produce convulsions, coma, severe bradycardia and hypotension. Atropine 0.6–1.2 mg i.v. is given. Glucagon in a bolus dose of 10 mg i.v. followed by an infusion of 3 $mg\cdot h^{-1}$ should be used for severe hypotension. This agent activates adenyl cyclase, promoting formation of cAMP, which is a direct beta-stimulant of the heart.

Digoxin

Self-poisoning with this agent is uncommon but chronic poisoning in patients on digoxin is frequent. Clinical features include nausea, vomiting and cardiac arrhythmias, such as heart block and various tachyarrhythmias, including ventricular tachycardia.

Treatment is supportive. Cardiac abnormalities are treated, and hypokalaemia should be corrected.

Purified Fab fragments of digoxin antibody are available.

Theophylline

Overdosage causes vomiting, restlessness, agitation, tachycardia and dilated pupils. Convulsions, arrhythmias and hypokalaemia are seen in severe cases. Gastric lavage is performed.

Other

Self-poisoning by cardiorespiratory drugs is becoming more frequent. Overdosage results in an exaggerated pharmacological effect and treatment should be aimed at counteracting this, e.g. an overdose of salbutamol is treated with a beta-blocker.

Household and industrial poisons

Virtually all substances found in the home have been ingested either by adults because of poorly labelled bottles or accidentally by children. Occasionally household agents are deliberately taken. Many kitchen products contain bleaches (sodium hypochlorite or hydrogen peroxide), acids or alkalis and the main problem after poisoning with them is their corrosive action on the gut. There is an immediate burning pain in the lips, mouth, throat, retrosternal area and stomach, and ulceration may follow. Vomiting may occur, with blood in severe cases. The major long-term complication is oesophageal stricture. Poisoning with sodium hypochlorite should be treated with sufficient water or milk to dilute it. Gastric lavage is contraindicated unless very substantial quantities have been taken. Alkalis should not be neutralized.

Some household products contain solvents, e.g. acetone in nail varnish remover or toluene in paints, which may be sniffed accidentally or intentionally (see p. 755).

Paraquat

Over the last few years, accidental poisoning with paraquat has become less common and deliberate self-poisoning now accounts for most cases. Para-quat is found in commonly used brands of weedkiller as an aqueous 20% solution (Gramoxone) or 2.5% solution (Weedol). A dose of 1.5 g may be fatal. Clinical features include ulcers in the mouth and oesophagus, diarrhoea and vomiting, epistaxis, pulmonary oedema, and later pulmonary fibrosis, respiratory failure and renal failure. Treatment is with gastric lavage with Fuller's earth and purging with magnesium sulphate. Haemodialysis may be useful in removing the paraquat if the plasma level is high.

The outcome can be predicted by relating the plasma paraquat concentration to the number of hours that have elapsed since ingestion. It is doubtful whether any treatment affects the outcome.

CARBON MONOXIDE

Carbon monoxide poisoning is a worldwide problem. Domestic gas in the UK (except in Northern Ireland) does not contain carbon monoxide, but the combustion of any fuel gas in the absence of adequate oxygen and ventilation may lead to domestic carbon monoxide poisoning. The other common sources of carbon monoxide are the exhaust fumes of petrol engines and from certain gas appliances that use propane and butane gases.

Carbon monoxide combines readily with haemoglobin to form carboxyhaemoglobin, thus preventing the formation of oxyhaemoglobin. The clinical features of carbon monoxide poisoning include mental impairment, including coma in severe cases. Headache, nausea and vomiting, and the classic pink colour of the skin due to the carboxyhaemoglobin are seen. More severe toxicity produces widespread effects, including myocardial damage and respiratory distress. Treatment consists of removing the patient from the carbon monoxide source, and giving as high a concentration of oxygen as possible.

DISC BATTERIES

Batteries more than 20 mm in diameter can lodge in the oesophagus and a chest X-ray should always be performed. Batteries should be removed by endoscopy because they may break open liberating mercury and manganese, which have corrosive effects. Most batteries will pass through the gut in 48 h but, if they do not and are seen on X-ray to be disintegating, they should be surgically removed.

INSECTICIDES

Carbamates and organophosphate insecticides are used extensively in agriculture. They may be ingested accidentally, inhaled, or absorbed through the skin when protective clothing is not worn. These agents are potent inhibitors of cholinesterase and produce an accumulation of acetylcholine. Carbamate poisoning is generally less severe and of shorter duration.

The clinical features are due to the muscarinic and nicotinic effects of acetylcholine. They include nausea, vomiting, hypersalivation, muscle weakness, bronchospasm, and respiratory failure; convulsions may also occur. The plasma cholinesterase activity will be low.

Treatment involves washing any contaminated skin. Atropine 2 mg i.v. is given repeatedly to obtain full atropinization. Pralidoxime mesylate 1 g i.v, a cholinesterase reactivator, is used in severe cases.

CYANIDE

Cyanide is found in a wide range of industrial compounds, e.g. rodenticides and fertilizers. Hydrogen cyanide is also released from polyurethane foams.

Ingestion or inhalation of this agent produces rapid onset of dizziness and headache, followed by acute shortness of breath, shock and eventual coma. Cyanosis is not present and the skin colour is red. There may be an odour of bitter almonds. Cyanide inhibits cytochrome oxidase, preventing cellular respiration, which leads to hypoxia, metabolic acidosis and frequently death. Treatment is urgent; oxygen is given and an intravenous combination of sodium nitrite (300 mg over 3 min) and sodium thiosulphate (12.25 g over 10 min). This is followed by 600 mg of dicobalt edetate intravenously over 1 min and 300 mg given a minute later if no recovery occurs. 50% Dextrose 50 ml i.v. should also be given after the dicobalt edetate.

METHANOL, ETHANOL AND ETHYLENE GLYCOL

These agents are all chiefly metabolized by alcohol dehydrogenase in the liver. In poisoning, there is increased lactate formation, which increases the metabolic acidosis found after methanol (due to formate) or ethylene glycol ingestion (due to glycolate).

Minor poisoning with methanol causes headache, breathlessness and photophobia. In severe poisoning there is papilloedema and eventually optic atrophy and blindness. Poisoning with methanol is treated with gastric lavage and correction of acidosis with bicarbonate infusion. Ethanol infusion and haemodialysis are used to remove methanol in patients who have taken more than 30 g of methanol and who have a blood level of methanol greater than 500 mg·L^{-1} (15.6

mmol·L^{-1}). Intravenous folinic acid may prevent ocular toxicity.

Ethanol poisoning produces severe depression of consciousness and hypoglycaemia, particularly in children. Treatment usually only consists of gastric lavage with an endotracheal tube in position. The use of fructose is no longer advised and peritoneal dialysis or haemodialysis is only indicated for very severe cases. Chlormethiazole, used for alcohol withdrawal, is dangerous if the patient takes alcohol and should therefore be used as an inpatient therapy only.

Poisoning with ethylene glycol (antifreeze) causes gastrointestinal upset and neurological involvement, including coma, followed by cardiorespiratory collapse and acute renal failure. Treatment is by gastric lavage and correction of the acidosis with intravenous sodium bicarbonate and of the hypocalcaemia with intravenous calcium solutions. Ethanol is given orally or intravenously to maintain an ethanol blood level of 1000 mg·L^{-1} in severe cases to inhibit the metabolism of ethylene glycol. Haemodialysis is indicated in patients who have taken more than 50 g of ethylene glycol or who have plasma levels greater than 500 mg·L^{-1} (8.1 mmol·L^{-1}).

HEAVY METALS

Mercury

Chronic mercury poisoning causes tremor (hatters' shakes), excessive salivation, scanning speech, anxiety and depression. In the hatters' trade a rabbit fur was stirred in vats of hot mercuric nitrate to make felt, and inhalation of the vapour led to signs of chronic mercury poisoning.

Acute mercury poisoning is seen after the ingestion of mercuric salts (e.g. mercuric chloride), inhalation of mercuric vapours or the ingestion of mercury oxide in 'button' batteries. It is treated by induced emesis, lavage and injections of dimercaprol or penicillamine.

Lead

Acute lead poisoning is rare. Chronic lead poisoning, however, commonly occurs.

Occupational lead poisoning
This is a notifiable disease in the UK and work with lead is covered by strict regulations. Most lead poisoning occurs in scrap metal or smelting workers. Blood levels in these workers should be lower than 800 μg·L^{-1} (4 mmol·L^{-1}).

Domestic lead poisoning
This usually occurs in children owing to the ingestion of old lead-based paint around the home.

Most toys now have lead-free paint. Chronic ingestion of water from lead pipes and acute accidental ingestion of fluid from car batteries are other frequent causes of lead poisoning.

After absorption, lead interferes with haem and globin synthesis (see p. 302). It also binds to bone, and in patients suffering from chronic exposure small amounts of lead can be found in many tissues.

CLINICAL FEATURES

- Anorexia, nausea and vomiting
- A blue line on the gums
- Constipation and severe abdominal colic
- Dense metaphyseal bands at the growing end of long bones, particularly the wrist and knee in children (lead lines)
- Anaemia, with erythrocytes showing basophil stippling
- Peripheral nerve lesions giving wrist drop and foot drop, with muscle involvement
- Lead encephalopathy, with eventual seizures and impairment of consciousness

The diagnosis is made on the basis of the clinical features. The blood level of lead is very variable; levels above 800 $\mu g \cdot L^{-1}$ (4 mmol$\cdot L^{-1}$) are toxic.

TREATMENT

It is most important to remove the source of lead intoxication. Sodium calcium edetate (calcium EDTA), D-penicillamine and dimercaprol have all been used for treatment.

Iron

Poisoning with iron tablets is often accidental in children. Symptoms include nausea, vomiting, abdominal pain, diarrhoea and haematemesis due to a direct corrosive effect. In severe cases, hypotension, hepatic damage and coma can occur. Gastric lavage and intragastric desferrioxamine 5–10 g and 2 g i.m. 12-hourly or a slow i.v. infusion of 15 $mg \cdot kg^{-1} \cdot h^{-1}$ (maximum 80 $mg \cdot kg^{-1}$ in 24 h).

Arsenic

Acute poisoning with arsenic causes vomiting, abdominal pain and diarrhoea. It is treated with rehydration and dimercaprol. Chronic poisoning causes excess salivation, weakness, anorexia and polyneuritis. There is a 'raindrop' pigmentation of the skin. Arsenic accumulates in the hair and the nails.

Venomous animals

Snakes

The adder (*Vipera berus*) is the only poisonous snake native to the UK. However, a number of dangerous snakes are kept as pets, and worldwide venomous snakes still cause significant mortality. There are three types of venomous snake:

- Viperidae, which have long erectile fangs. They are subdivided into two types:
  - (a) *Viperidae* (true vipers, e.g. Russell's viper [dabora], European adder), which are found in all parts of the world except America and the Asian Pacific
  - (b) *Crotalidae* (pit-vipers, e.g. rattlesnakes, Malayan pit-viper), which are found in Asia and America. They have small heat-sensitive pits between the eyes and the nostrils

  The venom of both of these classes of snake is vasculotoxic.
- Elapidae (cobras, mambas, kraits, coral-snakes), which are found in all parts of the world except Europe. They have short, unmoving fangs and the venom produces neurotoxic features. Venom from the Asian cobra and the African spitting cobra also produces local tissue necrosis
- Hydrophidae (sea-snakes), which are found in Asian Pacific coastal waters. They have short fangs and flattened tails. The venom is myo-toxic.

CLINICAL FEATURES

Viperidae
Russell's viper is the most important cause of snakebite mortality in India, Pakistan and Burma. There is local swelling at the site of the bite, which may become massive. Local tissue necrosis may occur, particularly with cobra bites. Evidence of systemic involvement occurs within 30 min, including vomiting, evidence of shock and hypotension; haemorrhage due to incoaguable blood can be fatal.

Elapidae
There is not usually any swelling at the site of the bite. Vomiting and shock occur and are followed by muscle weakness, with paralysis of the respiratory muscles in severe cases. Cardiac muscles can also be involved.

Hydrophidae
Systemic features are muscle involvement, myalgia and myoglobinuria, which can lead to acute renal failure. Cardiac and respiratory paralysis may occur.

MANAGEMENT

A firm pressure bandage should be placed over the bite and the limb immobilized. This greatly delays the spread of the venom.

Arterial tourniquets should not be used and incision or excision of the bite area should not be performed. The type of snake should be identified if possible.

Often no venom has been injected by the snake bite and antivenoms are not generally indicated unless systemic effects are present. Antivenoms can cause severe allergic reactions and should not be given purely because a bite has occurred. Nevertheless, careful observation for 12–24 h is necessary and antivenom must always be given when indicated, as the mortality of snake bite is 10–15% with certain snakes.

General supportive measures should be given as necessary, as for all poisoning. These include diazepam for anxiety and intravenous fluids with volume expanders for hypotension. Treatment of acute respiratory, cardiac and renal failure is instituted as necessary.

Specific measures, i.e. antivenoms, can rapidly neutralize venom, but only if an amount in excess of the amount of venom is given. Antivenoms cannot reverse the effects of the venom so they must be given early. They do minimize some of the local effects and may prevent necrosis at the site of the bite. Antivenoms should be administered intravenously by slow infusion, the same dose being given to children and adults.

Allergic reactions are frequent, and adrenaline (1 in 1000 solution) should be available. Antivenoms are usually rapidly effective. In severe cases the antivenom infusion should be continued even with allergic reactions, with subcutaneous injections of adrenaline being given as necessary. Large quantities of antivenom may be required. Some forms of neurotoxicity, such as those induced by the death adder, respond to anticholinesterase therapy with neostigmine and atropine.

Local wounds often require little treatment. If necrosis is present, antibiotics should be given together with initially minimal surgical treatment. Skin grafting may be required later. Antitetanus prophylaxis must be given.

Antivenoms must be kept readily available in all snake-infested areas.

Scorpions

Scorpion stings are a serious problem in the tropics and cause 1000 deaths per year in Mexico. The poison glands are situated in the end of the tail.

Severe pain occurs immediately at the site of puncture, followed by swelling. This should be treated by a firm pressure bandage to avoid the spread of the neurotoxic venom. Signs of systemic involvement include vomiting, respiratory depression and haemorrhage. Treatment is supportive. Antivenom is available in certain countries.

Spiders

The black widow spider (*Latrodectus mactans*) is found in North America and the tropics and occasionally in Mediterranean countries. The bite quickly becomes painful and generalized muscle pain, sweating, headache and shock occur. No systemic treatment is required except in cases of severe systemic toxicity, when specific antivenom should be given where this is available.

Loxosceles causes many bites in Central and South America. *L. reclusa*, the brown recluse spider, is also found in the southern USA. Spiders are often found in bedrooms, so that patients are often bitten at night. There is a burning pain at the site of the bite, followed by a necrotic ulcer in some cases. Systemic effects, which include fever, vomiting and haemolysis, are rare. No treatment is indicated except in severe cases, when an antivenom should be given if available.

Phoneutria nigriventer, the banana spider, and *Atrax robustus*, the Sydney funnel-web spider, can both give nasty bites, which are occasionally fatal.

Insects

Insect stings, e.g. from wasps and bees, and bites, e.g. from ants, produce pain and swelling at the puncture site. Death occurs (12 per year in the UK) and is usually due to anaphylaxis, which requires urgent treatment (see p. 733). Patients who have severe local reactions to stings or a mild anaphylactic reaction should carry a Medi-jet syringe for self-administration of adrenaline should a further sting occur. Desensitization can be carried out, but the course is prolonged and often needs to be repeated.

Marine animals

There are many poisonous fish that can be dangerous. They are usually found in tropical waters but cases have been described worldwide. Stingrays and scorpion fish are two examples that sting by injecting venom through barbed spines. There is immediate severe local pain and swelling, which may be followed by tissue necrosis. Systemic effects include diarrhoea, vomiting, hypotension, cardiac arrhythmias and convulsions. Treatment is supportive. Care should always be taken in waters where these fish are known to be present.

Venomous Coelenterata include jellyfish, sea anemones and the Portuguese man-of-war. The tentacles contain toxin that, following a sting, produces painful wheals at the site of contact.

These wheals may become necrotic. Rarely there are systemic side-effects, including abdominal pain, diarrhoea and vomiting, hypotension and convulsions. Treatment consists of removing the tentacles, having first applied acetic acid (vinegar) to them. Alcohol compounds should not be used.

Molluscs

Only the octopus and cone-shells are venomous to man. The blue-ringed octopus, which is found in Australia, has toxic saliva, which flows into the wounds from the beak of the octopus and can cause serious systemic effects.

In cone-shells the venom is found in association with their radular teeth. A bite initially produces local numbness, which can then spread over the body and may eventually lead to paralysis.

Seafood poisoning

This can occur with fish and shellfish. In some cases it is attributable to toxins, but most poisonings occur as a result of pathogens such as *Salmonella* or hepatitis A virus. Ichthyosarcotoxic fish contain toxins in their blood, skin and muscle and are the commonest cause of poisoning.

Ciguatera. Poisoning occurs chiefly with the reef-dwelling fish from around the Pacific and Caribbean. The fish contain ciguatoxins from the plankton *Gambia discus*. Most cases of poisoning are due to the red snapper, grouper, barracuda and amberjack fish but many other species may be responsible. The poisonous fish cannot be distinguished from identical fish that do not contain the poison. The toxin is unaffected by cooking.

Symptoms occur from a few minutes to 30 h after ingestion of the fish. They include numbness and paraesthesia of the lips, abdominal pain, nausea, vomiting and diarrhoea. Visual blurring, photophobia, a metallic taste in the mouth, myalgia and eventual hypotension and shock can also occur.

Treatment is symptomatic, but symptoms can last for up to 2 weeks.

Scromboid fish. Fish such as tuna, mackerel and skipjack contain a high degree of histidine. This is decarboxylated by bacteria to histamine and, particularly if the fish are allowed to spoil, large amounts can accumulate in the fish, producing flushing, burning, pruritus, headache, urticaria, nausea, vomiting and bronchospasm 2–3 h after ingestion. Treatment is symptomatic; care should be taken only to eat fresh fish.

Tetrodotoxin-containing puffer-fish are found in both sea and freshwater areas of Asia, India and the Caribbean. Symptoms that follow ingestion are circumoral paraesthesia, malaise and hypotension, with more severe cases producing ataxia and neuromuscular paralysis. The mortality is 50–60%.

Shellfish. Bivalve molluscs, e.g. mussels, oysters, scallops and clams, can aquire the neurotoxin saxitoxin from the dinoflagellate *Gonoyaulax*. These protozoa colour the sea red and molluscs should never be taken from such areas. Symptoms are similar to those caused by tetrodotoxin, but are usually less severe. Treatment is symptomatic.

Plants

Many plants are known to be poisonous, but in practice it is unusual for severe poisoning to occur. Children are the usual victims. Only two people are known to have died from plant poisoning in the UK since the early 1970s. The commonest effects of nettles and poison ivy are dermatitis followed by vomiting. Poisonous plants commonly ingested include hemlock, labernum, deadly nightshade and green potatoes. Deadly nightshade (*Atropa belladonna*) contains hyoscyamine and hyoscine. When ingested these cause the anticholinergic effects of a dry mouth, nausea and vomiting, eventually leading to blurring of the vision, hallucinations, confusion and hyperpyrexia.

Mushrooms

There are many poisonous mushrooms that can be confused with edible fungi and be eaten by mistake. Nevertheless, apart from transient nausea, vomiting and diarrhoea, which can occur with many species, very severe reactions are rare.

Fatal mushroom poisoning is almost invariably due to *Amanita phalloides* (the death-cap mushroom). This fungus contains phallotoxins and amatoxins, both of which interfere with cell metabolism. Toxicity is increased if the mushrooms are eaten raw, as some toxins are inactivated by heat. In general, the sooner the symptoms occur, the less serious the poisoning, depending on the type of mushroom ingested. Within 2 h, nausea, vomiting, diarrhoea and sweating occur. After about 6 h, patients complain of headache and dizziness, and severe vomiting occurs at about 12 h. After 72 h, the more serious complications of hepatocellular and renal failure may occur, which have a high mortality.

The diagnosis is made by obtaining a careful history, with identification of the mushroom if possible. Amatoxins can be measured in the blood by radioimmunoassay.

Treatment should include gastric aspiration and lavage and general support. There is some evidence that haemodialysis may be of some value.

Other mushrooms that are poisonous include:

- *Amanita muscaria* (fly agaric), which contains a little muscarine and other hallucinogenic substances

- *Coprinus atramentarius* (ink cap), which contains a dehydrogenase inhibitor with a disulfiram-like effect, producing flushing, swelling, a rash on the face and hands, and cardiovascular effects, particularly after alcohol
- *Amanita pantherina* (false blusher), which produces similar features to deadly nightshade because of its atropine-like effects

Drug abuse (see p. 994)

Solvents

Solvent abuse has become a common problem, particularly in teenagers who inhale volatile organic solvents such as toluene in glues ('glue sniffing'). Many other solvents, such as aerosols (hair lacquer), antifreeze and petrol, can also be misused. Solvents are applied to a piece of cloth or put into a plastic bag and inhaled, often until consciousness is lost. The patient presents either in the acute intoxicated state or as a chronic abuser with excoriation and rashes over the face and a peripheral neuropathy. Death can occur and is probably due to cardiac arrhythmias. Stigmata of solvent abuse include sores or a rash round the nose and mouth and glue on the clothing.

Other drugs

Drug addicts frequently overdose themselves and are commonly admitted to hospital with the signs of opiate injection. Tell-tale injection sites and pinpoint pupils are important clues. Naloxone is given in the same dosage as for co-proxamol overdose (see p. 748).

Cannabis
Cannabis is usually smoked and often taken casually. Initially there is euphoria, followed by drowsiness and sleep. Redness of the conjunctivae and pupil dilatation are seen. No specific treatment is required.

Amphetamines
Amphetamines are taken for their stimulatory effect. In overdose there is confusion, delirium, hallucinations and violent behaviour. Cardiac arrhythmias can be a major problem. Treatment is with sedatives, such as diazepam. Forced acid diuresis may be used but is rarely required.

Cocaine
Cocaine can be taken by injection, inhalation or ingestion. It produces excitement, overalterness, euphoria and restlessness. This is followed by

delirium, tremor, convulsions and cardiac arrhythmias, which may cause cardiac failure. Respiratory failure may also occur.

Treatment is symptomatic and supportive. There is no specific antidote.

Poison information services

Information on poisoning can be obtained from the poisons information services at the following numbers:

National Poisons Information Service

Belfast	0232 240503
Cardiff	0222 569200
Dublin	0001 745588
Edinburgh	031 229 2477
	031 229 2441 (Viewdata)
London	071 407 7600 or 071 635 9191

Other centres

Birmingham	021 554 3801
Leeds	0532 430715 or 0532 432799
Newcastle	0632 325131

Laboratory analysis may help in the diagnosis and manangement of some cases. Information on the available services can be obtained from the National Poisons Information Service in London.

Further reading

Crome P (1982) Antidepressant overdosage. *Drugs* **23**: 431–461.

Davies DM (ed) (1986) *Textbook of Adverse Drug Reactions*, 3rd edn. Oxford: Oxford University Press.

Henry J & Volans G (1984) *ABC of Poisoning*. Part 1. *Drugs*. London: British Medical Association.

Kallos P & West GB (1983) Pseudo-allergic reactions in man. In Turner P & Shand DG (eds) *Recent Advances in Clinical Pharmacology*, Vol. 3, pp. 235–252. Edinburgh: Churchill Livingstone.

Prescott LF (1983) Paracetamol overdosage—pharmacological considerations and clinical management. *Drugs* **25**: 270–314.

Turner P, Richens A & Routledge P (1986) *Clinical Pharmacology*, 5th edn. Edinburgh: Churchill Livingstone.

Vale JA & Meredith TJ (1985) *Concise Guide to the Management of Poisoning*, 3rd edn. Edinburgh: Churchill Livingstone.

15

Environmental Medicine

Heat

In health, the core temperature of man is maintained by the thermoregulatory centre in the hypothalamus at a constant 37°C. Heat is produced by cellular metabolism, and is lost through the skin by vasodilatation and sweating and in air expired from the lungs. Sweating occurs when the ambient temperature is greater than 32.5°C and during exercise. The evaporation of sweat is an important mechanism in keeping the skin cool and the body temperature down.

Acclimatization
Acclimatization to a hotter climate takes 1–2 weeks. There is a gradual increase in sweating, and the sweat has a lower salt content. This process allows increased evaporation.

Heat cramps

These are painful cramps in the muscles (usually of the legs) after exercise. They often occur in fit young people who are well acclimatized when they take vigorous exercise in hot weather. The symptoms are thought to be the result of a low extracellular sodium caused by replenishment of water but not salt during prolonged sweating. The cramps respond to salt and water replacement and can be prevented by increasing dietary salt intake.

Heat exhaustion

This usually occurs in subjects who are not acclimatized and who undertake heavy exercise. It typically occurs in troops who are suddenly landed in a hot climate without prior acclimatization. Heat exhaustion is caused by water depletion, or salt and water depletion, due to sweating. Water loss can be as high as 5–6 litres per day, and up to 20 g of salt can be lost.

Common symptoms are giddiness, generalized fatigue, weakness and syncope. Many patients are not seriously affected, but they may go on to develop hypotension, a rise in body temperature of 38–40°C, and signs of volume depletion. Dehydration and delirium can eventually occur. Sweating usually continues until the late stages. The serum sodium can be high in water depletion, but is normal or low if both water and salt are depleted.

TREATMENT

The patient is removed from the heat and cooled using cold sponging and fans.

Oral rehydration with both salt and water may be all that is required; 25 g of sodium chloride and 5 litres of water in the first 24 h is given, with adequate replacements thereafter. In severe heat exhaustion, intravenous fluid is required. Isotonic saline is usually given, depending on the level of sodium in the serum. Careful monitoring is required and any subsequent potassium loss must be corrected.

Heat stroke

Heat stroke is an acute life-threatening situation when the body temperature is above 41°C. The patient suffers from headache, nausea, vomiting and weakness. The skin is hot. Sweating is often absent, but this is not invariable, even in severe heat stroke. Neurological involvement leads to confusion, delirium and eventually coma.

Heat stroke occurs in hot, humid climates with little cooling wind, even without exercise. Patients are usually unacclimatized; in some, sweating is limited owing to prickly heat (i.e. inflammation of the sweat glands after prolonged exposure to high temperatures). Old age, diabetes and alcohol are all further precipitating factors.

The diagnosis is clinical. The patient must be rapidly removed from the hot area, and then cooled with sponging and ice if available.

Unconscious patients need to be managed in intensive care (see p. 705) and rapid cooling with ice packs started. Fluids may be required, but these must be given with care as hypovolaemia is not present in many patients.

Prompt treatment is essential and can lead to a rapid and complete recovery; any delay may be fatal.

COMPLICATIONS

- Shock
- Cerebral oedema
- Renal and hepatic failure

Treatment of the complications is described in the appropriate chapters.

Malignant hyperpyrexia

This is discussed on p. 963.

Cold

Hypothermia is defined as a fall in the core (i.e. rectal) temperature to below 35°C. It is frequently lethal when the core temperature falls below 32°C.

Frostbite is local cold injury that occurs when tissue freezes.

Hypothermia

Hypothermia occurs in a variety of clinical settings:

- *In the home environment.* Hypothermia may occur in cold climates when there is poor heating, inadequate clothing and poor nutrition. Depressant drugs (e.g. hypnotics), alcohol, hypothyroidism or intercurrent illness may also contribute. Hypothermia is commonly seen in the poor and elderly, the latter having a diminished ability to feel cold and often a decrease in the insulating fat layer. Infants and neonates become hypothermic very rapidly at normal room temperature because of their relatively large surface area and lack of subcutaneous fat.
- *During exposure to extremes of temperature outside.* Hypothermia is a prominent cause of death in climbers, skiers, Arctic and Antarctic travellers and in wartime. Wet, cold conditions and wind-chill, physical exhaustion and inadequate clothing are common contributory factors.
- *Following immersion in cold water.* Dangerous hypothermia can develop after several hours immersion at temperatures of 15–20°C. Below 12°C the patient's limbs become anaesthetized and paralysed and take some hours to recover after the patient is rescued.

CLINICAL FEATURES

Mild hypothermia (32–35°C) causes shivering and initially a feeling of intense cold. The subject is alert and usually takes appropriate action to rewarm, e.g. huddling, extra clothing or exercise. As the core temperature falls, severe hypothermia (below 32°C) initially causes impairment of judgement (including awareness of the cold) and later leads to altered consciousness and coma. Death follows, usually from ventricular fibrillation.

DIAGNOSIS

If a thermometer is available (which must be low reading), the diagnosis is straightforward. If not, a rapid clinical assessment should be made. The hypothermic patients feels cold to the touch—the abdomen, groin and axillae are cold and clammy. If consciousness is impaired (i.e. if the patient is uncooperative, sleepy or in a coma) the core temperature is almost certainly below 32°C; this is a medical emergency.

SEQUELAE

The pulse rate and volume fall, and respiration becomes shallow and slow. Muscle stiffness develops and the tendon reflexes are depressed. The systemic blood pressure falls. As coma ensues, the pupillary and other brainstem reflexes are lost (the pupils are fixed and may be dilated in severe hypothermia).

Metabolic changes are variable, with either metabolic acidosis or alkalosis occurring. Arterial oxygen tension readings may appear normal since they are measured at room temperature, but these measurements are falsely high as the arterial PO_2 falls 7% per °C fall in temperature.

Ventricular arrhythmias (tachycardia and fibrillation) or asystole are the usual cause of death and may occur during treatment. 'J' waves—rounded waves above the isoelectric line immediately after the QRS complex—are pathognomic of hypothermia. Prolongation of the PR interval, QT interval and QRS complex also occur.

MANAGEMENT

The principles of management of this serious emergency are to rewarm the patient gradually while correcting metabolic abnormalities and treating cardiac arrhythmias. Hypothyroidism must always be looked for (see p. 802).

If the patient is awake, with a temperature above 32°C, rewarming can be achieved by placing the patient in a warm room, using 'space blankets', and giving warm fluids orally. Outdoors, the same result can be achieved by adding extra clothing, huddling with the subject, and using a warmed sleeping bag. Rewarming may take several hours. Alcohol should be avoided—it may add to confusion, boost confidence factitiously, cause peripheral vasodilatation (and further heat loss) or precipitate hypoglycaemia.

Severe hypothermia
In severe hypothermia, the patient may appear

dead. (Hypothermia should always be excluded before brain death is diagnosed.) Warming should take place gradually, aiming at an increase in temperature of 1°C per hour. The patient should be covered with a 'space blanket' and placed in a warm room. Direct surface heat from an electric blanket is also helpful. Any underlying condition should be treated promptly. Drug overdose should always be excluded.

Warmed intravenous fluids are given slowly and metabolic disturbances are corrected. Hypothyroidism, if present, should be treated with triiodothyronine 10 µg i.v. 8-hourly. Various methods of artificial rewarming have been suggested—warm humidified air by inhalation, gastric or peritoneal lavage, or haemodialysis—but in practice these are rarely used. The cardiac rhythm should be monitored and arrhythmias corrected.

Careful monitoring of all vital functions is required; appropriate treatment and intensive care are given as necessary.

PREVENTION

Prevention of hypothermia is particularly important in the elderly, who should be advised to try to improve general heating and insulation in the house. Heat should be provided in the bedrooms, and the use of safe electric blankets advised. Financial help will be needed by many patients. Constant supervision should be given during cold spells, when warm food and extra blankets must be provided.

Frostbite

The formation of ice crystals in the skin and superficial tissues begins when the temperature there falls to −3°C; ambient temperatures generally have to be below −6°C for this to occur.

RECOGNITION

Frostbitten tissue is pale, greyish and initially doughy to the touch. Later it freezes hard, when it looks (and feels) like meat taken from a deep freeze. This condition may occur when working or exercising in low temperatures and typically develops without the patient's knowledge. Hands and feet that have 'lost their feeling' are an important feature when the temperature is below −5°C, as frostbite may then develop insidiously.

MANAGEMENT

The frostbitten patient should, if possible, be transported (or walk, even on frostbitten feet) to a place of safety before treatment commences. Warming using the body heat of a companion or by immersion in water at 39 to 42°C should be

continued until obvious thawing occurs. This may be painful. Blisters will form within several days and, depending on the degree of frostbite, a blackened carapace or shell develops as the blisters regress or burst. Dry, non-adherent dressings and strict aseptic precautions are essential. Frostbitten tissues are anaesthetic and are at risk from infection and further trauma. Recovery takes place over many weeks. Surgery may be required, but should be avoided in the early stages, as it is difficult to predict the eventual amount of recovery.

High altitudes

The partial pressure of ambient (and hence alveolar and arterial) oxygen falls in a near-linear relationship to altitude (Fig. 15.1).

Below 3000 m there are few important clinical effects. Commercial aircraft are pressurized to 2750 m and the resulting hypoxia causes breathlessness only in those with severe cardiorespiratory disease. The incidence of thromboembolism is however, slightly greater than at sea level in sedentary travellers on long flights.

Above 3000–3500 m, hypoxia causes a spectrum of related clinical syndromes that affect visitors to high altitudes, principally climbers, trekkers, skiers and troops (Table 15.1). These conditions, which often coexist, occur largely during the acclimatization process. This may last some weeks, but enables man to live (permanently if necessary) at altitudes up to about 5600 m. At greater heights, although man can survive for days or weeks, deterioration due to chronic hypoxia is inevitable.

It has now been demonstrated on several

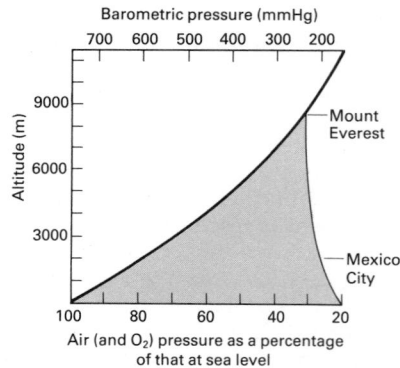

Fig. 15.1 Diagram to show the decrease in oxygen and barometric pressure with increasing altitude.

Table 15.1 Conditions caused by sustained hypoxia.

Condition	Incidence	Usual altitude
Acute mountain sickness	70%	3500–4000 m
Acute pulmonary oedema	2%	4000 m
Acute cerebral oedema	1%	4500 m
Retinal haemorrhages	50%	5000 m
Deterioration	100%	5600 m
Chronic mountain sickness	Rare	4500 m

occasions that ascent to the highest of the world's summits is possible without the use of supplementary oxygen. At the summit of Everest the barometric pressure is 34 kPa (253 mm Hg). This enables an acclimatized mountaineer to have an alveolar PO_2 of 4.0–4.7 kPa (30–35 mm Hg)—near the physiological limits of man.

Acute mountain sickness (AMS)

This term is used to describe the malaise, nausea, headache and lassitude that are common above 3500 m. Following arrival at this altitude there is usually a latent interval of 6–36 h before the onset of symptoms. Treatment is rest, with analgesics being given if necessary; recovery is almost invariable.

Prophylactic treatment with the carbonic anhydrase inhibitor acetazolamide is of value in reducing the symptoms of AMS, since these are partly due to the development of alkalosis.

In a minority of cases, the more serious sequelae of high-altitude pulmonary oedema (HAPO) and high-altitude cerebral oedema (HACO) occur.

High-altitude pulmonary oedema (HAPO)
Predisposing factors include youth, rapidity of ascent, heavy exertion and the presence of mountain sickness. Breathlessness, with frothy blood-stained sputum indicates established HAPO. Unless treated rapidly this leads to cardiorespiratory failure, collapse and death. Milder forms of HAPO are common, presenting with breathlessness that is not severe; it is important to recognize them.

High-altitude cerebral oedema (HACO)
Cerebral oedema is a poorly understood sequel of hypoxia. It is probably the result of the abrupt increase in cerebral blood flow that occurs even at modest altitudes of 3500–4000 m. Headache is usual, and is accompanied by varying disturbances of cerebral function; drowsiness, ataxia, nystagmus and papilloedema are common. Coma and death follow if the condition progresses.

Treatment
Any but the milder forms of AMS require urgent treatment. Oxygen should be given if it is available, and descent to a lower altitude should take place as quickly as possible. Dexamethasone or betamethasone are effective treatments in HAPO or HACO. Diuretics are of little value.

Retinal haemorrhages

Small 'flame' haemorrhages in the nerve fibre layer of the retina are common above 5000 m. They are usually symptomless unless they cover the macula, when there is painless loss of central vision. Recovery is usual.

Deterioration

Prolonged residence between 5600 and 7000 m leads to a syndrome of weight loss, anorexia and listlessness after several weeks. Above 7500 m deterioration develops more quickly, although it is possible to survive for a week or more at altitudes over 8000 m.

Chronic mountain sickness

This rare syndrome occurs in long-term residents of high altitudes after several decades. It has been described clearly only in the Andes, but may occur in Tibet and elsewhere in central Asia.

Polycythaemia, drowsiness, cyanosis, finger clubbing, congested cheeks and ear lobes, and right ventricular enlargement occur. The condition is gradually progressive.

By way of contrast, coronary artery disease and hypertension are rare in the native populations of high altitude.

Diving

The increases in ambient pressure to which a diver is exposed at various depths are summarized in Table 15.2.

Table 15.2 Pressure in relation to sea depth.

Sea depth (m)	Absolute pressure (atmospheres)	mm Hg
0	1	760
10	2	1520
50	6	4560
90	10	7600

Various methods are used to supply air to the diver. With the simplest, e.g. a snorkel, the limiting factor, which occurs below 0.5 m, is the respiratory effort required to suck air into the lungs. At greater depths this 'forced negative-pressure ventilation' ultimately results in pulmonary capillary damage and haemorrhagic pulmonary oedema. Scuba tanks, the method commonly used for sporting diving down to 50 m, carry compressed air at a pressure balanced with the water pressure.

Divers who work at great depths for commercial purposes or for underwater exploration breathe helium/oxygen or nitrogen/oxygen mixtures delivered by hose from the surface.

A wide variety of complex medical problems may affect divers at all depths. These are summarized below.

PROBLEMS DURING COMPRESSION
(i.e. descent)

Barotitis ('ear squeeze') and barosinusitis ('sinus squeeze')

Barotitis is the term used to describe acute vertigo occurring due to otitis media or the passage of water into the middle ear at depths of from 5 to 20 m. It is prevented by inflating the middle ear (by blowing or swallowing with an open glottis against closed lips and nostrils). Treatment of the serous otitis media is with nasal vasoconstrictor drops (phenylephrine). Rupture of the tympanic membrane may occur.

Barosinusitis is the term used to describe the sinus pain and the later damage to the walls of paranasal air sinuses that occurs during compression. It can be prevented by avoiding diving when the respiratory airways are blocked, e.g. owing to upper respiratory infection or allergic rhinitis.

Nitrogen narcosis

When compressed air is breathed below 30 m the narcotic effects of nitrogen cause impairment of cerebral function with changes of mood and performance that may be life-threatening. The condition reverses rapidly on ascent.

Nitrogen narcosis is avoided by replacing air with helium/oxygen mixtures, which can enable divers to descend to 700 m.

At these great depths neurological disturbances occur that are believed to be the result of the direct effects of pressure on neurones. Tremor, hemiparesis and psychological changes may occur.

Oxygen narcosis

Pure oxygen cannot be used for diving because oxygen becomes toxic to the lungs when the alveolar oxygen pressure exceeds 1.5 atmospheres absolute (5 m of water) and to the nervous system at around 10 m of water.

In the lungs, linear atelectasis appears and there is endothelial cell damage with exudation and pulmonary oedema. In the nervous system there is initially a feeling of apprehension, nausea and sweating, followed by muscle twitching and generalized convulsions, which may be fatal under water.

PROBLEMS DURING DECOMPRESSION

Decompression sickness ('the bends') occurs on returning to the surface and is caused by the release of inert gases, usually nitrogen or helium, which form bubbles in the tissues as the ambient pressure falls. It only occurs when the diver ascends too rapidly. Decompression tables are available for calculating the time needed to come to the surface safely from any given depth.

Decompression sickness

This can take a mild form (type 1 'non-neurological bends'), with skin irritation, mottling or limb pain only, or be more serious (type 2 'bends'), in which a variety of neurological features appear. Patients with type 2 'bends' may develop cortical blindness, hemiparesis, sensory disturbances or cord lesions. If nitrogen bubbles occur in the pulmonary vessels, divers experience retrosternal discomfort, dyspnoea and cough ('the chokes'). These symptoms develop within minutes or hours of a dive.

Treatment is with oxygen. In addition, all but the mildest forms of decompression sickness (i.e. skin mottling alone) require recompression, usually in a pressure chamber.

A long-term problem is aseptic necrosis caused by infarction due to nitrogen bubbles lodging in nutrient arteries supplying bone. It is seen in 5% of deep sea divers. Neurological damage may also persist.

Lung rupture, pneumothorax and surgical emphysema

These emergencies occur principally when divers 'breath-hold' while making emergency ascents after losing their gas supply. Following lung rupture the patient notes severe dyspnoea, cough and haemoptysis. Pneumothorax and emphysema usually respond to 100% oxygen. Air embolism may occur and should be treated with recompression.

Ionizing radiation

Ionizing radiation is either penetrating (X-rays, gamma rays or neutrons) or non-penetrating (alpha or beta particles). Penetrating radiation affects the whole body, while non-penetrating radiation only affects the skin. All radiation effects, however, depend on the type of radiation, the distribution of dose and the dose rate.

Absorption of doses greater than 100 rads of gamma radiation, e.g. following survival from a nuclear explosion or nuclear power plant accident, causes acute radiation syndromes of varying severity. Long-term effects also occur, sometimes decades after exposure, as radiation increases the rate of mutagenesis.

Radiation dosage is measured in joules per kilogram ($J \cdot kg^{-1}$); 1 $J \cdot kg^{-1}$ is also known as 1 gray (1 Gy). This is equivalent to 100 rads. Radioactivity is measured in becquerels (Bq); 1 Bq is equal to the amount of radioactive material in which there is one disintegration per second. 1 curie (Ci) is equal to 3.7×10^{10} Bq.

Radiation differs in the density of ionization it causes. Therefore a dose equivalent called a sievert (Sv) is used. This is the absorbed dose weighted for the damaging effect of the radiation. The annual background radiation is approximately 2.5 mSv.

Excessive exposure to ionizing radiation occurs following accidents in hospitals, industry, nuclear power plants and strategic nuclear explosions.

Mild acute radiation sickness

Nausea, vomiting and malaise follow doses of approximately 1 Gy (75–125 rad). Lymphopenia occurs within several days, followed 2–3 weeks later by a fall in all white cells and platelets. There is a late risk of leukaemia and solid tumours.

Severe acute radiation sickness

Many systems are affected; the extent of the damage depends on the dose of radiation received. The effects of radiation are summarized in Table 15.3.

Haemopoietic syndrome
Absorption of doses between 2–10 Gy (200 and 1000 rad) is followed by early and transient vomiting in some individuals, followed by a period of relative well-being. Lymphocytes are particularly sensitive to radiation damage and severe lymphopenia develops over several days. A decrease in granulocytes and platelets occurs 2–3 weeks later as no new cells are being formed by the damaged marrow. Thrombocytopenia with bleeding develops and frequent, overwhelming infections occur, with a very high mortality.

Gastrointestinal syndrome
Absorption of doses greater than 6 Gy (600 rad) causes vomiting several hours after exposure. This then stops, only to recur some 4 days later accompanied by severe diarrhoea. Owing to radiation inhibition of cell division, the villous lining of the intestine becomes denuded. Intractable bloody diarrhoea follows, with dehydration, secondary infection and death.

CNS syndrome
Exposures above 30 Gy (3000 rad) are followed rapidly by nausea, vomiting, disorientation and coma; death due to severe cerebral oedema follows in 36 h.

Radiation dermatitis
Skin erythema, purpura, blistering and secondary infection occur. Total loss of body hair is a bad prognostic sign and usually follows an exposure of at least 5 Gy (500 rad).

Late effects of radiation exposure
The survivors of the nuclear bombing of Hiroshima and Nagasaki have provided information on the long-term effects of radiation. The risk of developing acute myeloid leukaemia or cancer, particularly of the skin, thyroid and salivary glands, increases.

Infertility, teratogenesis and cataract are also late sequelae of radiation exposure.

TREATMENT

Acute radiation sickness is a medical emergency. Hospitals should be immediately informed of the type and length of exposure so that suitable arrangements can be made to receive the patient.

Table 15.3 The effects of radiation.

Acute effects
Haemopoietic syndrome
Gastrointestinal syndrome
CNS syndrome
Radiation dermatitis

Delayed effects
Infertility
Teratogenesis
Cataract
Neoplasia
   Acute myeloid leukaemia
   Thyroid
   Salivary glands
   Skin
   Others

The initial radiation dose absorbed can be reduced by removing clothing contaminated by radioactive materials.

Treatment of radiation sickness is largely supportive and consists of prevention and treatment of infection, haemorrhage and fluid loss. Storage of the patient's white cells and platelets for future use should be considered, if feasible.

Accidental ingestion or exposure to bone-seeking radioisotopes (e.g. strontium-90 and caesium-137) should be treated with chelating agents (e.g. EDTA) and massive doses of oral calcium. Radioiodine contamination should be treated immediately with potassium iodide 133 mg per day. This will block 90% of radioiodine absorption by the thyroid if given immediately before exposure.

Electric shock

Electric shock may produce clinical effects in three ways:

● *Pain and psychological sequelae.* The common 'electric shock' is usually a painful but harmless stimulus that is an unpleasant and frightening experience. It produces no lasting neurological damage or cutaneous evidence of damage.
● *Disruption of specific biological processes.* Ventricular fibrillation, muscular contraction and spinal cord damage follow a major shock. These are seen typically following a lightning strike.
● *Electrical burns.* These are either superficial burns (e.g. lightning may cause a fern-shaped burn), or necrosis of subcutaneous tissues due to the heat generated by the electricity.

Smoke

Smoke consists of particles of carbon in hot air and gases. These particles are mainly coated with organic acids and aldehydes. Use is widespread of synthetic materials (e.g. polyvinyl chloride) that release other substances, such as carbon monoxide and hydrochloric acid, on combustion. Respiratory symptoms may be immediate or delayed. Patients are dyspnoeic and tachypnoeic. Laryngeal stridor may require intubation. Hypoxia and pulmonary oedema can be fatal. Treatment is to remove the subject from the smoke and give O_2. Intensive care may be required.

Noise

The intensity of sound is expressed in terms of the square of the sound pressure. The bel is a ratio and is equivalent to a 10-fold increase in sound intensity; a decibel (dB) is one-tenth of a bel. Sound is made up of a number of frequencies ranging from 30 hertz (Hz) to 20 kHz, with most being between 1 and 4 kHz. When measuring sound, these different frequencies must be taken into account. In practice a scale known as A-weighted sound is used; sound levels are reported as dB(A). A hazardous sound source is defined as one with an overall sound pressure greater than 90 dB(A).

Repeated prolonged exposure to loud noise, particularly in the frequency range of 2–6 kHz, causes first temporary and later permanent hearing loss due to damage to the organ of Corti, with destruction of hair cells and, eventually, the auditory neurones. This is a common occupational problem, not only in industry and the armed forces, but also in the home (e.g. from electric drills and sanders), in sport (e.g. motor racing) and in entertainment (pop stars, their audiences and disc jockeys).

Serious noise-induced hearing loss is almost wholly preventable by personal protection (ear muffs, ear plugs); little treatment can be offered once deafness becomes established.

Drowning and near drowning

Drowning is a common cause of accidental death, accounting for over 100 000 deaths annually world-wide. Approximately 40% of drownings occur in children under 5 years of age. Exhaustion, alcohol, drugs and hypothermia all contribute to the overall problem.

'Dry' drowning
Ten to twenty per cent of drownings occur without aspiration of water into the lungs. Laryngeal spasm is thought to occur, which leads to asphyxia and cerebral anoxia from airway blockage. This can occur in both salt and fresh water.

'Wet' drowning
Following submersion in water, the subject panics and struggles, and this is followed by breath-holding with eventual swallowing and inhalation of water. This leads to asphyxia and death. The

difference between salt water and fresh water drowning has been overemphasized. In clinical practice there is no difference in serum electrolytes or blood volume in subjects who recover (near drowning).

EMERGENCY TREATMENT

It must be remembered that patients can survive up to 30 minutes under water without suffering brain damage and if the water is near 0°C this time can be much longer. The exact reasons for this are not clearly understood, but it is probably related to the protective role of the diving reflex. It has been shown experimentally that submersion in water causes a reflex slowing of the pulse and vasoconstriction. In addition, hypothermia decreases oxygen consumption of both the heart and brain.

Patients should be turned to one side and the mouth cleared of any debris. Mouth-to-mouth respiration should be immediately started together with cardiac resuscitation if this is appropriate (see p. 542).

Mouth-to-mouth resuscitation should always be attempted, even in the absence of a pulse and the presence of fixed dilated pupils, as patients can frequently make a dramatic recovery.

All patients should be subsequently admitted to hospital for intensive monitoring. Intensive care therapy may be required, and patients are liable to develop the adult respiratory distress syndrome (ARDS).

PROGNOSIS

The prognosis is good if the patient is fully conscious on admission to hospital but poor if the patient is still in a coma.

Motion sickness

This common problem, particularly in children, is caused by repetitive stimulation of the labyrinth of the ear. It occurs frequently at sea and in cars, but may occur on horseback or on less usual forms of transport such as camels or elephants. Nausea, sweating, dizziness, vertigo and profuse vomiting occur, accompanied by an irresistable desire to stop moving.

Prophylactic antihistamines or vestibular sedatives (hyoscine or cinnarizine) are of some value.

Further reading

Auerbach PS & Geehr EC (1983) *Management of Wilderness and Environmental Emergencies*. London: Macmillan.
Nelson RN, Rund DA & Keller MD (1985) *Environmental Emergencies*. Philadelphia: W.B. Saunders.

16

Endocrinology

Introduction

Hormones are chemical messengers produced by a variety of specialized secretory cells. They may be transported to a distant site of action (the classical 'endocrine' effect) or may act directly upon nearby cells ('paracrine' activity). Additionally, in the hypothalamus and elsewhere in the brain there are many such cells secreting hormones, some of which have true endocrine or paracrine activity, while others behave more like neurotransmitters.

Synthesis, storage and release of hormones

Under either neural or endocrine stimulation the cell increases production of its specific hormone product. This is often in the form of a precursor molecule that may itself be biologically inactive. The prohormone is often further processed before packaging into granules which are transported to the plasma membrane before release.

Plasma transport

Most hormones are secreted into the systemic circulation but, in the hypothalamus, they are released into the pituitary portal system. Much higher concentrations of the releasing factors thus reach the pituitary than occur in the systemic circulation.

Many hormones are bound to proteins within the circulation. Only the free (unbound) hormone is available to the tissues and thus biologically active. The binding serves to buffer against very rapid changes in plasma levels of the hormone. This principle is important in interpreting many tests of endocrine function, which often measure total rather than free hormone since binding proteins are frequently altered in disease states. Binding proteins frequently comprise both specific, high-affinity proteins of limited capacity, such as thyroxine-binding globulin (TBG) and other less-specific low-affinity ones, such as prealbumin and albumin. The most important and clinically relevant binding proteins are shown in Table 16.1.

Hormone action

Hormones act at the cell surface and/or within the cell. Many hormones bind to specific cell-surface receptors where they trigger internal messengers (Fig. 16.1a). These 'second messengers', for example, cyclic AMP for ACTH, LH and FSH and calcium for vasopressin and angiotensin II, then cause rapid alterations in cell-membrane ion transport or slower responses such as DNA, RNA and protein synthesis. Some hormones act by activation of the membrane-bound phosphoinositide pathways. Other hormones, especially steroids, enter most cells of the body where they act on intracellular protein receptors, often altering the activity of intracellular enzymes by phosphorylation or dephosphorylation. Steroid hormone receptor com-

Table 16.1 Plasma hormones with important binding proteins.

Hormone	Binding protein(s)
Thyroxine (T_4)	Thyroxine-binding globulin (TBG) Thyroxine-binding prealbumin (TBPA) Albumin
Triiodothyronine (T_3) (less bound than T_4)	Thyroxine-binding globulin (TBG) Albumin
Cortisol	Cortisol-binding globulin (CBG)
Testosterone Oestradiol	Sex hormone-binding globulin (SHBG)

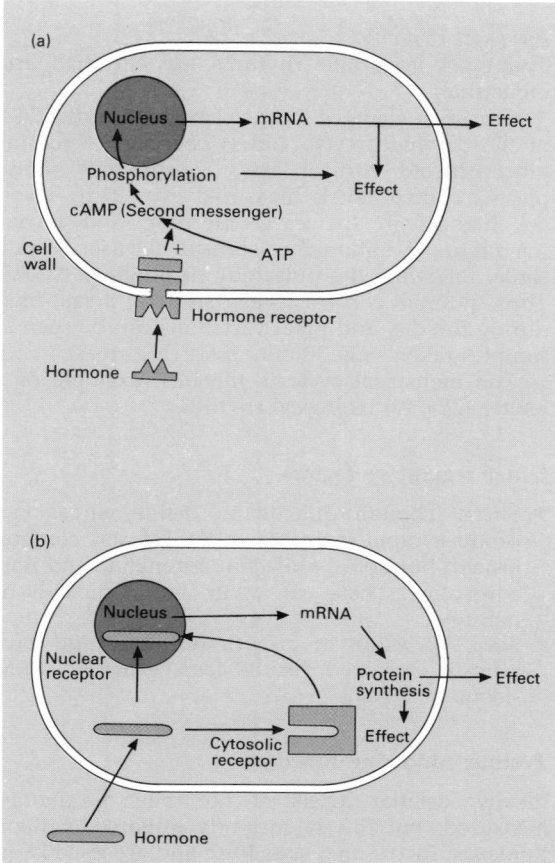

Fig. 16.1 (a) Binding of hormone to cellular surface receptor with subsequent release of a second messenger, here cAMP, which initiates intracellular mechanisms leading to mRNA production and the hormonal 'effect'. (b) Steroid and thyroid hormones enter the cell and bind to a cytosolic or core protein to initiate mRNA production and subsequent hormone 'effect'.

plexes are usually transported into the nucleus (Fig. 16.1b), where they interact with DNA to regulate gene transcription, and thus protein synthesis. The characteristics of different hormone systems are shown in Table 16.2.

The sensitivity and/or number of receptors for a hormone is often decreased after prolonged exposure to a high hormone concentration, the receptors thus becoming less sensitive ('down-regulation') (e.g. angiotensin II receptor, β-adrenoceptor). The reverse is true when stimulation is absent or minimal, the receptors showing increased numbers or sensitivity ('up-regulation').

Control and feedback

Most hormone systems are controlled by some form of feedback; an example is the hypothalamic–pituitary–thyroid axis (Fig. 16.2).

- Thyrotrophic-releasing hormone (TRH) is secreted in the hypothalamus and travels via the portal system to the pituitary where it stimulates the thyrotrophs to produce thyroid-stimulating hormone (TSH).
- TSH is secreted into the systemic circulation where it stimulates increased thyroidal iodine uptake and thyroxine and tri-iodothyronine synthesis and release.
- Serum levels of thyroxine (T_4) and tri-iodothyronine (T_3) are thus increased by TSH; in addition, the conversion of T_4 to T_3 (the more active hormone) in peripheral tissues is stimulated by TSH.
- T_4 and T_3 then enter cells where they bind to nuclear receptors and promote increased metabolic and cellular activity.
- Blood levels of T_3 and T_4 are sensed by receptors in the pituitary and possibly the hypothalamus. If they rise above the normal range TRH and TSH production is suppressed, leading to less T_4 and T_3 secretion.
- Peripheral T_3/T_4 levels thus fall to normal.
- If, however, T_3 and T_4 levels are low (e.g. post-thyroidectomy), increased amounts of TRH and thus TSH are secreted, stimulating the remaining thyroid to produce more T_3 and T_4; blood levels of T_4/T_3 *may* be restored to normal, although at the expense of increased TSH drive, reflected by a high TSH level ('compensated euthyroidism').

Table 16.2 Characteristics of different hormone systems.

	Peptides and catecholamines	Steroids and thyroid hormones
Protein binding:	No	Yes
Changes in plasma concentrations:	Rapid changes	Slow fluctuations
Plasma half-life:	Short (seconds to minutes)	Long (minutes to days)
Type of receptors:	Cell membrane	Intracellular
Mechanism:	Activate pre-formed enzymes	Stimulate protein synthesis
Speed of effect:	Rapid (seconds to minutes)	Slow (hours to days)

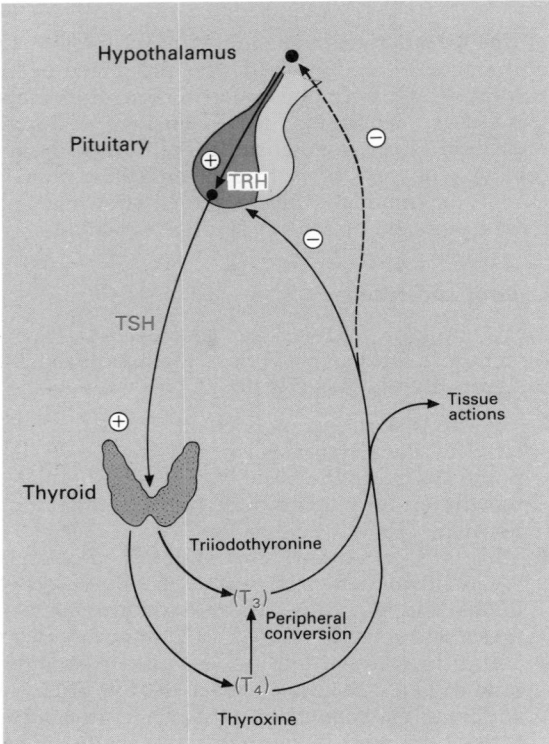

Fig. 16.2 The hypothalamic—pituitary—thyroid feedback system. The dotted line indicates *probable* negative feedback at hypothalamic level.

This is known as a 'negative feedback' system, referring to the effect of T_4 and T_3 on the pituitary and hypothalamus. There are also positive feedback systems, classically seen in the regulation of the normal menstrual cycle.

Patterns of secretion

Hormone secretion may be continuous or intermittent. The former is shown by the thyroid hormones, where T_4 has a half-life of 7–10 days and T_3 of about 6–10 h. Levels over the day, month and year show very little variation. In contrast, secretion of the gonadotrophins, luteinizing hormone and follicle-stimulating hormone (LH and FSH), is normally pulsatile, with major pulses released every 2 h or so. Continuous infusion of LH to produce a steady equivalent level does *not* produce the same result (e.g. ovulation in the female) as the intermittent pulsatility, and may indeed produce 'down-regulation' and amenorrhoea. This principle is employed therapeutically to produce very low androgen or oestrogen levels, both in carcinoma of the prostate in men and in infertility in women, using the long-acting superactive GnRH analogue buserelin.

Biological rhythms

The most important rhythms are circadian and menstrual.

Circadian changes means changes over the 24 h of the day/night cycle and is best shown for the glucocorticoid cortisol axis. Figure 16.3 shows plasma cortisol levels measured over 24 h—levels are highest in the early morning and lowest overnight. Additionally, cortisol release is pulsatile, following the pulsatility of pituitary ACTH. Thus 'normal' cortisol levels (stippled areas) vary during the day and great variations can be seen in samples taken only 30 min apart (Fig. 16.3).

The menstrual cycle is the best example of a longer (28-day) biological rhythm.

Other regulatory factors

- *Stress*. Though difficult to define, stress can produce rapid increases in ACTH and cortisol, growth hormone, prolactin, adrenaline and noradrenaline. These can occur within seconds or minutes.
- *Sleep*. Secretion of growth hormone and prolactin is increased during sleep, especially REM sleep.

Testing endocrine function

Ideally, cellular levels of hormones would be measured, but this is currently impossible. Body fluids are the normal substitute and are usually an excellent approximation but it must be remembered that they do not always reflect tissue action of the relevant hormone.

Blood levels

Assays for all important hormones are now available. Obviously the time, day and condition of

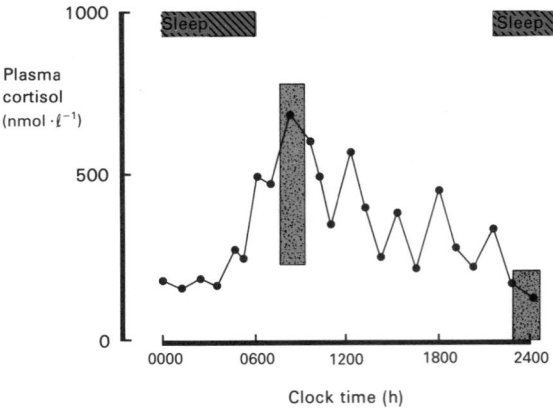

Fig. 16.3 Plasma cortisol levels during a 24-hour period. Note both the pulsatility and the shifting baseline. Normal ranges for 0900 and 2400 are shown hatched.

measurement may make great differences to hormone levels. The method and timing of samples will depend upon the characteristics of the endocrine system involved.

- Basal levels are especially useful for systems with long half-lives, e.g. T_4 and T_3. These vary little over the short term and random samples are therefore satisfactory.
- Basal samples may also be satisfactory if interpreted with respect to normal ranges for the time of day/month, diet, posture concerned. Examples are FSH, oestrogen and progesterone and aldosterone. All relevant details *must* be recorded or the data may prove uninterpretable.
- Stress-related hormones (e.g. catecholamines, prolactin, GH and cortisol) may require samples to be taken via an indwelling needle some time after venepuncture. Otherwise, high levels may be artefactual.

Urine collections

- 24-Hour collections have the advantage of providing an 'integrated mean' of a day's secretion but are often incomplete or wrongly timed. They also vary with sex and body size or age. Written instructions should be provided.

Saliva is sometimes used for steroid estimations, especially in children.

Stimulation and suppression tests
These are valuable in instances of hormone deficiency or excess:

- Where secretory capacity of a gland is damaged, maximal stimulation by the trophic hormone will give a diminished output. Thus, in the Synacthen (SYNthetic-ACTH-en) test for adrenal reserve (Fig. 16.4a), subject A shows a normal response (stippled area); subject B with primary hypoadrenalism (Addison's disease) demonstrates an impaired cortisol response to ACTH (Fig. 16.4).
- In contrast, a patient with a hormone-producing tumour usually fails to show normal negative feedback. A patient with Cushing's disease (excess pituitary ACTH) will thus fail to suppress ACTH and cortisol production when given a dose of synthetic steroid, as would normal subjects. Figure 16.4b shows the response of a normal subject (A) given dexamethasone at midnight; cortisol is suppressed the following morning. Subject B with Cushing's disease shows inadequate suppression.

The detailed protocol for each test must be followed exactly, since slight differences in technique will produce variations in results. Details of commoner tests are given in the Appendix.

Measurement of hormone concentrations
Circulating levels of most hormones are very low (10^{-9}–10^{-12} mol·L^{-1}) and cannot be measured by simple chemical techniques. The most widely used methods are radioimmunoassay and immunoradiometric assays. Radioimmunoassay is illustrated in Fig. 16.5.

- A known volume of sample is mixed with a known amount of radioactively labelled hormone.
- To this is added a known amount of specific antibody to the hormone. The antibody will attach to labelled and unlabelled hormone in proportion to their relative concentrations.
- Antibody-bound hormone and remaining free hormone can be separated and the bound or free radiolabelled part can be counted. In the instance shown, bound label is counted: the amount will vary depending on the hormone concentration in the sample.
- A set of 'standards' of known hormone level is included with the unknown samples; all are

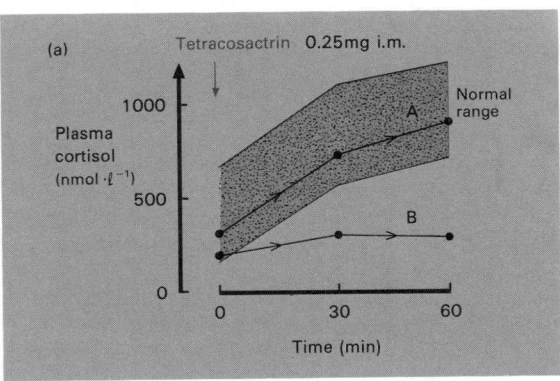

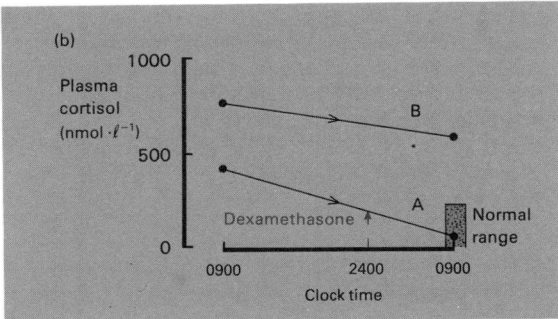

Fig. 16.4 (a) Short ACTH stimulation test showing a normal response in a healthy subject (A) and a decreased response in a patient with Addison's disease (B). (b) Dexamethasone suppression tests in a normal subject (A) and a patient with Cushing's disease (B), showing inadequate suppression.

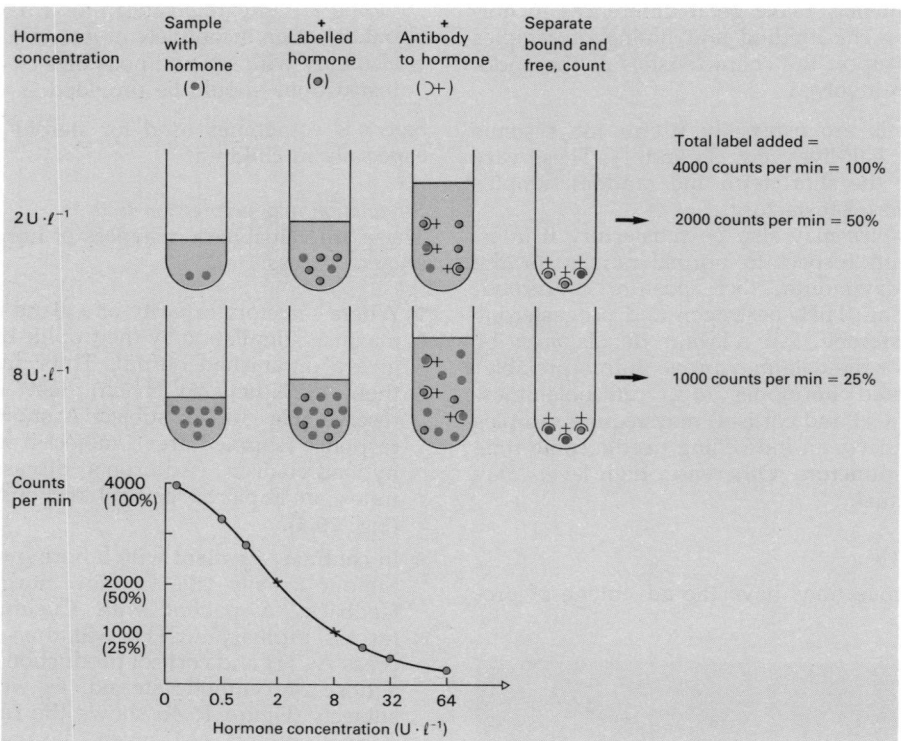

Fig. 16.5 The principles of radioimmunoassay. A known volume of sample is mixed with a known amount of radioactively labelled hormone. To this is added a known amount of specific antibody to the hormone. The antibody will attach to labelled and unlabelled hormone in proportion to their relative concentrations. Antibody-bound hormone and remaining free hormone can be separated and the bound or free radiolabelled part can be counted. In the instance shown, bound label is counted—the amount will vary depending on the hormone concentration in the sample.

A set of 'standards' of known hormone level is included with the unknown samples; all are treated in exactly the same way. From the standards a 'standard curve' is produced, showing the variation in counts per minute, or percentage total binding, with increasing concentrations of hormone. The 'unknown' samples will produce a number of counts; by reading off the graph the concentration of hormone originally present in the sample can be determined.

treated in exactly the same way.
- From the standards a 'standard curve' is produced (Fig. 16.5) showing the variation in counts·min^{-1}, or percentage total binding, with increasing concentrations of hormone.
- The 'unknown' samples will produce a number of counts; by reading off the graph the concentration of hormone originally present in the sample can be determined.

Radioimmunoassay has limitations; in particular the *immunological* activity of a hormone, as used in developing the antibody, may not necessarily correspond to *biological activity*. Nevertheless, reliable radioimmunoassays for most hormones are available, many at local hospitals and others at national level (in the UK by the Supraregional Assay Service).

It is, however, widely being replaced by immunoradiometric assays (IRMA). These rely on highly specific antibodies (usually monoclonal) that are themselves labelled rather than labelling the hormone concerned. Usually employing a solid-phase system, the principles are otherwise similar to those of RIA, requiring incubation and separation of bound and free fractions, except that the 'signal' is obviously proportional to the amount of substance present (i.e. this is a saturation analysis). It will also be immediately apparent that the label need not be a radioactive label but may be a fluorescent or coloured substance.

An introduction to endocrine disease

Most endocrine disease is extremely simple to understand—there is either too much of a hormone or too little! The underlying pathology, such as a tumour, may also cause local symptoms.

EPIDEMIOLOGY

The commonest endocrine disorders, excluding diabetes (Chapter 17), are:

Table 16.3 Common presenting complaints in endocrine disease.

Body size and shape
Short stature
Tall stature
Excessive weight or weight gain
Loss of weight

'Metabolic' effects
Tiredness
Weakness
Increased appetite
Decreased appetite
Polydipsia/thirst
Polyuria/nocturia
Tremor
Palpitation
Anxiety

Local effects
Swelling in the neck
Carpal tunnel syndrome
Bone or muscle pain
Protrusion of eyes
Visual loss (acuity and/or fields)
Headache

Reproduction/sex
Loss or absence of libido
Impotence
Oligomenorrhoea/amenorrhoea
Subfertility
Galactorrhoea
Gynaecomastia
Delayed puberty
Precocious puberty

Skin
Hirsuties
Hair thinning
Pigmentation
Dry skin
Excess sweating

- Thyroid disorders, affecting 4–8 new patients per primary care physician per year
- Children with short stature or delayed puberty
- Subfertility, affecting 5–10% of all couples, often with an endocrine component, and increasingly treatable
- Menstrual disorders and excessive hair growth in young women
- Primary hyperparathyroidism, affecting about 0.1% of the population
- Osteoporosis

While most other endocrine conditions are very uncommon, they often affect young people and are usually curable or completely controllable with appropriate therapy.

Hormones are also widely used therapeutically:

- Oral contraceptive pill use, the choice of perhaps 40% of women aged 18–35 using contraception
- Hormone replacement therapy (oestrogens + progestogens) for postmenopausal women
- Corticosteroid therapy is widely used in non-endocrine disease such as asthma

SYMPTOMS

Common endocrine presenting symptoms are shown in Table 16.3, which demonstrates the many effects that hormonal abnormalities can produce.

Hormones produce widespread effects upon the body; focal symptoms are less common than with other systems. Many endocrine symptoms are diffuse and vague, and the differential diagnosis is often wide.

In addition, there are close physiological, and sometimes anatomical, relationships between different glands. Thus excessive growth *may* be caused by excess pituitary growth hormone production, *possibly* from a tumour, which *might* affect control of gonadal, breast, thyroid and adrenal function. If the tumour is large it *could* cause visual

Table 16.4 Endocrine disease—past, family and social histories.

Past history
Necessary details may include:
Previous pregnancies (ease of conception, postpartum haemorrhage)
Relevant surgery (e.g. thyroidectomy, orchidopexy)
Radiation (e.g. to neck, gonads, thyroid)
Drug exposure (e.g. chemotherapy, sex hormones, oral contraceptives)
In childhood, developmental milestones and growth

Family history
Family history of:
Autoimmune disease
Endocrine disease
Essential hypertension
Diabetes

Family details of:
Height
Weight
Body habitus
Hair growth
Age of sexual development

Social history
Detailed records of alcohol intake (e.g. subfertility, obesity)
Drug abuse (e.g. cannabis and subfertility)
Full details of occupation, access to drugs, chemicals, etc.
Diet, e.g. salt, liquorice, iodine

field defects and even affect the hypothalamus, *perhaps* producing diabetes insipidus. Such possible connections and implications need to be recognized and investigated.

HISTORY AND EXAMINATION

Specific dates of onset of symptoms, how they were noticed and how they have progressed is vital. Not all questions are necessary or relevant for all patients; the skill is to ask the right ones!

Examination, too, must be selective and thoughtful, though general observation is vital. Conditions such as acromegaly and Cushing's syndrome are usually immediately apparent to the alert, though 'lateral thinking' is often necessary—for example, the need to check visual fields in these two examples.

Physical signs are listed under the relevant systems, and Table 16.4 describes the details that should be elicited in past, family and social

histories. A full drug history is mandatory as endocrine problems are quite often iatrogenic (Table 16.5).

Specific points about endocrine disease

As with other systems, endocrine diseases may be congenital or acquired and can be caused by a variety of pathologies. However, several forms of illness are commoner than in other systems.

Autoimmune disease
Organ-specific autoimmune diseases have now been shown for every major endocrine organ (Table 16.6). They are characterized by the presence of specific antibodies in the serum, often present years before clinical symptoms are evident. The conditions are usually commoner in women and have a strong genetic component, often with an identical-twin concordance rate of 50% and with HLA associations (see individual diseases).

Table 16.5 Drugs and endocrine disease.

Drug[a]	Effect
Drugs inducing endocrine disease	
Chlorpromazine Metoclopramide Oestrogens	Increase prolactin, causing galactorrhoea
Iodine Amiodarone	Hyperthyroidism
Lithium Amiodarone	Hypothyroidism
Chlorpropamide	Inappropriate ADH secretion
Drugs simulating endocrine disease	
Sympathomimetics Amphetamines	Mimic thyrotoxicosis or phaeochromocytoma
Liquorice Carbenoxolone	Mineralocorticoid activity; can simulate aldosteronism
Purgatives Diuretics	Hypokalaemia Secondary aldosteronism
Exogenous hormones or stimulating agents Use, abuse or misuse, by patient or doctor, of the following:	
Steroids	Cushing's disease Diabetes
Thyroxine	Thyrotoxicosis factitia
Vitamin D preparations Milk and alkali preparations	Hypercalcaemia
Insulin Sulphonylureas	Hypoglycaemia

[a] Drugs causing gynaecomastia are listed in Table 16.18.
Amiodarone may cause both hypo- and hyperthyroidism.

Table 16.6 Types of autoimmune disease.

Organ	Antibody	Clinical syndrome
Stimulating		
Thyroid	Thyroid-stimulating immunoglobulin (TSI, TSAb)	Graves' disease, neonatal thyrotoxicosis
	Thyroid growth immunoglobulin	Goitre
Destructive		
Thyroid	Thyroid microsomal antibody (peroxidase enzyme)	Primary hypothyroidism (myxoedema)
	Thyroglobulin	
Adrenal	Adrenal cortex	Primary hypoadrenalism (Addison's disease)
Pancreas	Islet cell	Type I (insulin-dependent) diabetes
Stomach	Gastric parietal cell	Pernicious anaemia
	Intrinsic factor	
Skin	Melanocyte	Vitiligo
Ovary	Ovary	Primary ovarian failure
Testis	Testis	Primary testicular failure
Parathyroid	Parathyroid chief cell	Primary hypoparathyroidism
Pituitary	Pituitary-specific cells	Selective hypopituitarism, e.g. GH deficiency, hyperprolactinaemia

N.B.: Other related diseases include myasthenia gravis and autoimmune liver disease.

Endocrine tumours

Hormone-secreting tumours occur in all endocrine organs, most commonly pituitary, thyroid and parathyroid. Fortunately, they are more commonly benign than malignant. While often considered to be 'autonomous', that is independent of the physiological control mechanisms, many do show evidence of feedback occurring at a higher 'set-point' than normal (e.g. ACTH secretion from a pituitary basophil adenoma).

Enzymatic defects

The biosynthesis of most hormones involve many stages. Deficient or abnormal enzymes can lead to absent or reduced production of the terminal hormone. In general, severe deficiencies present early in life with obvious signs; partial deficiencies usually present later with mild signs or are only evident under stress. An example of an enzyme deficiency is congenital adrenal hyperplasia.

Receptor abnormalities

Hormones work by activating cellular receptors. There are rare conditions in which hormone secretion and control are normal but the receptors are defective: thus, if androgen receptors are defective, normal levels of androgen will not produce masculinization (e.g. testicular feminization, p. 794). There are also a number of rare syndromes of diabetes and insulin resistance from receptor abnormalities (Chapter 17).

Central control of endocrine function

Anatomy

Many peripheral hormone systems are controlled by the hypothalamus and pituitary. The hypothalamus is sited at the base of the brain around the third ventricle and above the pituitary stalk, which leads down to the pituitary itself.

Figure 16.6 shows the important anatomical relationships of the hypothalamus and pituitary. The optic chiasm is just above the pituitary fossa; any expanding lesion from the pituitary or hypothalamus can produce visual field defects by pressure on the chiasm. The pituitary is itself encased in a bony box; any lateral, anterior or posterior expansion must cause bony erosion. Upward expansion of the gland through the diaphragma sellae is termed 'suprasellar extension'. The normal fossa is of very variable size but a true lateral X-ray should show a well-defined outline with a single floor. The commonest cause of apparent abnormality is a poorly aligned film.

Embryologically, the anterior pituitary is formed from Rathke's pouch ('endodermal') which meets an outpouching of the third ventricular floor to become the posterior pituitary.

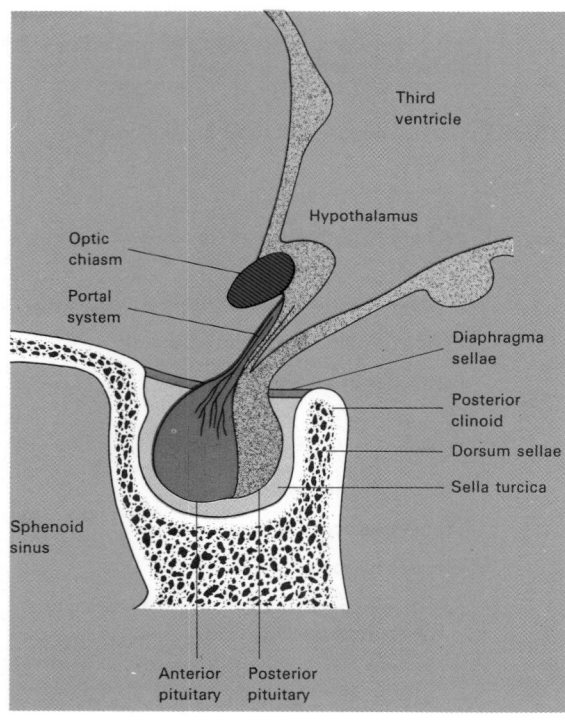

Fig. 16.6 A sagittal section of the pituitary fossa, showing the important anatomical relationships.

Physiology

The hypothalamus contains many vital centres for such functions as appetite, thirst, thermal regulation and sleep/waking. It acts as an integrator of many neural and endocrine inputs to control the release of releasing factors. Amongst other important influences it plays a role in the circadian rhythm, the menstrual cyclicity, stress, exercise and mood. From the hypothalamus a portal system runs down the stalk to the pituitary through which releasing factors are transported.

The release of most *anterior* pituitary hormones is controlled in the same way. Releasing or inhibitory hormones (Table 16.7) produced in the hypothalamus travel down the portal system and stimulate or inhibit specific cells within the pituitary. These cells then stimulate or inhibit the synthesis and release of trophic hormones, which stimulate the peripheral glands. This pattern is illustrated in Fig. 16.7. Many hormones are under dual control of stimulatory and inhibitory hypothalamic factors. Thus, growth hormone release is stimulated by GHRH but inhibited by somatostatin. TSH release is stimulated by TRH but partially inhibited by somatostatin. Some hormones have a dual stimulatory control, e.g. CRF and vasopressin are endogenous stimulators of ACTH release. Uniquely, prolactin is under inhibitory dopaminergic control and stimulatory TRH

Table 16.7 Nomenclature and biochemistry of hypothalamic, pituitary and peripheral hormones.

Hypothalamic hormones	Pituitary hormones	Peripheral hormones
Gonadotrophin-releasing hormone (LHRH, GnRH) (Decapeptide)	Luteinizing hormone (LH) Follicle-stimulating hormone (FSH) (Two-chain (α, β) peptides MW 32 000)	Oestrogens/androgens (Steroid ring)
Prolactin inhibiting factor (PIF) (Dopamine)	Prolactin (PRL) (Single peptide chain MW 23 000)	—
Growth hormone-releasing factor (GHRH) (40 amino acids) Somatostatin (GHRIH) (Cyclic peptide, 14 amino acids)	Growth hormone (GH) (Single chain peptide MW 23 000)	Somatomedin C (IGFI) and others (Small peptides MW 5000–9000)
Thyrotropin-releasing hormone (TRH) (Tripeptide)	Thyroid-stimulating hormone (TSH) (Two-chain (α, β) peptide MW 28 000)	Thyroxine, triiodothyronine (T_4, T_3) (Thyronines)
Corticotrophin-releasing factor (CRF) (41 amino acids)	Adrenocorticotrophic hormone (ACTH) (Single chain peptide, 39 amino acids MW 4500)	Cortisol (Steroid ring)
Vasopressin, anti-diuretic hormone (ADH) (Nonapeptide)	—	—
Oxytocin (Nonapeptide)	—	—

N.B.: The alpha chains of LH, FSH and TSH are identical.
IGF = insulin-like growth factor.
Biochemical structure shown in brackets.

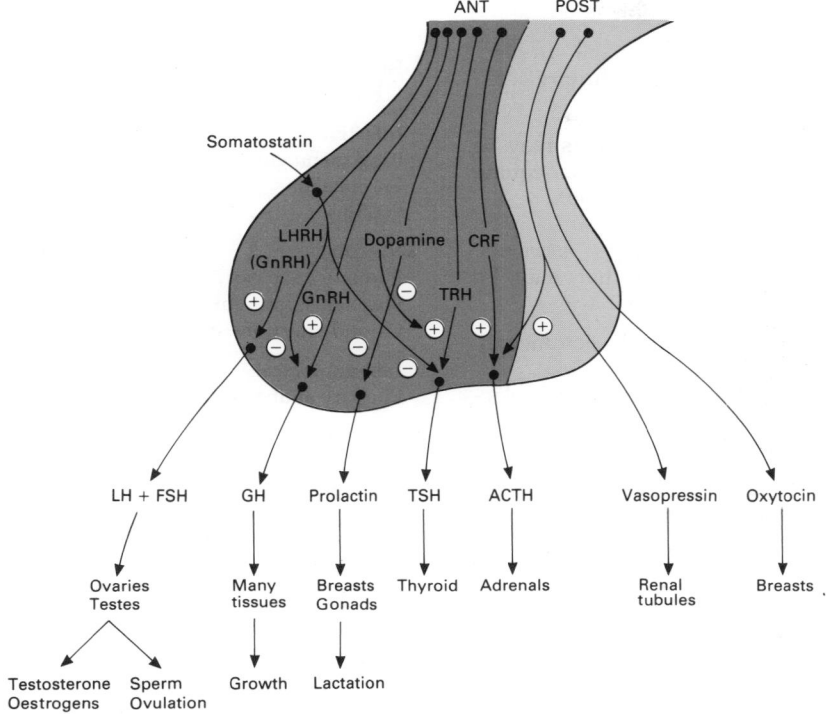

Fig. 16.7 Hypothalamic releasing hormones and the pituitary trophic hormones. + = stimulation; − = inhibition.

control (Fig. 16.7).

In contrast, the *posterior* pituitary acts merely as a storage organ. Antidiuretic hormone (ADH, vasopressin) and oxytocin, both non-peptides, are synthesized in the supraoptic and paraventricular nuclei in the anterior hypothalamus. They are then transported along a single axon and stored in the posterior pituitary. This means that damage to the stalk or pituitary does not prevent synthesis and release of ADH and oxytocin. ADH is discussed on p. 818; oxytocin produces milk ejection and uterine myometrial contraction.

Elucidation of the structures of the hypothalamic hormones, mainly by molecular biological techniques, has allowed their synthesis and the production of agonist and antagonist analogues. Thus, GnRH, CRF, GHRH and vasopressin are widely used both in testing function and therapeutically, while analogues of GnRH and vasopressin are employed therapeutically (see sections on Reproduction and Thirst).

Endorphins and the ACTH families of peptides
Recent discoveries include the endorphins (ENDogenous mORPHINe), some of which are derived from part of the ACTH precursor molecular (Fig. 16.8). This scheme demonstrates some of the complex processing of pituitary peptides including the role of a 'prohormone', from which the major hormone, ACTH, is split.

The endorphins have opioid activity and are thought to be mediators of stress-induced analgesia. They have also been found within the gut but their physiological role remains uncertain. The hypothalamus also contains large amounts of other neuropeptides such as natriuretic factor, bombesin

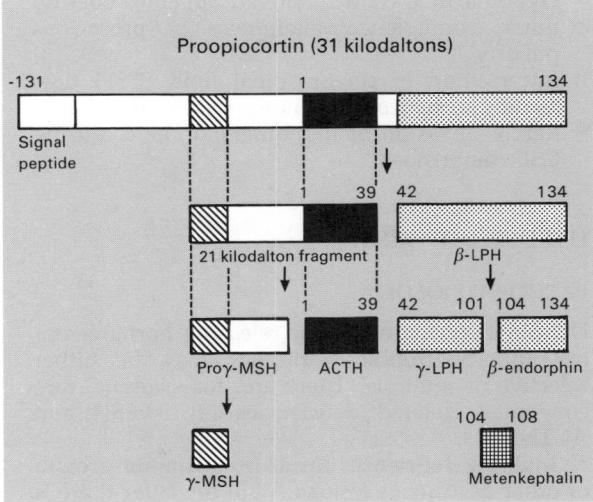

Fig. 16.8 Processing of the ACTH precursor molecule (proopiocortin) illustrating some of the products. MSH = melanocyte-stimulating hormone; LPH = lipotrophin.

and VIP (vasoactive intestinal peptide) that can also alter pituitary hormone secretion.

Presentations of hypothalamic and pituitary disease

As with most endocrine disease, problems may be caused by excess hormone secretion, inadequate production, or by local effects of a tumour.

Overproduction of hypothalamic–pituitary hormones. There are three major conditions that may be caused by tumour or hyperplasia:

- Growth hormone excess, leading to acromegaly or gigantism
- Prolactin excess (prolactinoma or hyperprolactinaemia)
- Cushing's disease (excess ACTH secretion)

Tumours producing LH, FSH or TSH are very rare. Some apparently 'non-functioning' tumours may produce the alpha subunit of LH, FSH and TSH (Table 16.7).

Underproduction of hormone. This may be due to disease at either hypothalamic or pituitary level producing hypopituitarism.

Local effects. Pituitary and hypothalamic lesions, hormonally active or not, can cause symptoms by infiltration of, or pressure on:

- The visual pathways, with field defects and visual loss
- The cavernous sinus, with III, IV and VI cranial nerve lesions
- Bony structures and the meninges surrounding the fossa, with headache
- Hypothalamic centres: altered appetite, obesity, thirst, somnolence/wakefulness or precocious puberty
- Interruption of cerebrospinal fluid (CSF) flow leading to hydrocephalus
- Rarely, invasion of the sphenoid sinus causing CSF rhinorrhoea

HYPOPITUITARISM

PATHOPHYSIOLOGY

Deficiency of hypothalamic releasing hormones or of pituitary trophic hormones may be either selective or multiple. There are, for example, rare congenital isolated deficiencies of LH/FSH and ACTH.

Multiple deficiences result from tumour growth or other destructive lesions. With the latter there is generally a progressive loss of anterior pituitary function in the order shown from left to right in Fig. 16.7. GH and gonadotrophins are usually first

Table 16.8 Causes of hypopituitarism.

Congential
Isolated deficiency of pituitary hormones (e.g. Kallmann's syndrome)

Infective
Basal meningitis (e.g. tuberculosis)
Encephalitis
Syphilis

Vascular
Pituitary apoplexy
Sheehan's syndrome (postpartum necrosis)
Carotid artery aneurysms

Immunological
Pituitary antibodies

Neoplastic
Pituitary or hypothalamic tumours
Craniopharyngioma
Meningiomas
Gliomas
Pinealoma
Secondary deposits, especially breast

Traumatic
Skull fracture
Surgery, especially transfrontal

Infiltrations
Sarcoidosis
Histiocytosis X
Haemochromatosis

Others
Radiation damage
Fibrosis
Chemotherapy
Empty sella syndrome

'Functional'
Anorexia nervosa
Starvation
Emotional deprivation

affected. Rather than prolactin deficiency, hyperprolactinaemia occurs relatively early because of loss of tonic inhibitory control by dopamine. TSH and ACTH are usually last to be affected. Panhypopituitarism refers to deficiency of all anterior pituitary hormones; it is most commonly caused by pituitary tumours.

Vasopressin and oxytocin secretion will only be significantly affected if the hypothalamus is involved.

CAUSES

Disorders causing hypopituitarism are listed in Table 16.8; pituitary and hypothalamic tumours are the commonest.

CLINICAL FEATURES

Symptoms and signs depend upon the extent of hypothalamic and/or pituitary deficiencies. Loss of libido, amenorrhoea and impotence are symptoms of gonadotrophin and the resultant gonadal deficiencies, while hyperprolactinaemia may cause galactorrhoea and hypogonadism. GH deficiency is 'silent' except in children. Secondary hypothyroidism and adrenal failure lead to tiredness, slowness of thought and action, and mild hypotension. Panhypopituitarism may give the classical picture of pallor with hairlessness ('alabaster skin').

Particular syndromes related to hypopituitarism include:

- *Kallmann's syndrome* (isolated gonadotrophin deficieny, which leads to hypogonadism); see p. 784.
- *Sheehan's syndrome.* This situation, now rare, is pituitary infarction following postpartum haemorrhage.
- *Pituitary apoplexy.* A pituitary tumour may infarct or haemorrhage into itself. This may produce severe headache sometimes followed by acute life-threatening hypopituitarism.
- *The empty sella syndrome.* This is sometimes due to a defect in the diaphragma and extension of the subarachnoid space ('cisternal herniation') or may follow spontaneous infarction of a tumour. All or most of the sella turcica may be devoid of apparent pituitary tissue, but, despite this, pituitary function is usually normal, the pituitary being eccentrically placed and flattened against the floor or roof of the pituitary fossa.

INVESTIGATION

Each axis of the hypothalamic–pituitary system may require separate investigation. The presence of normal gonadal function (ovulatory menstruation or normal libido/erections) suggests that multiple defects of anterior pituitary function are unlikely. Tests range from the simple basal levels, e.g. T_4 for the thyroid axis, to stimulatory tests for the pituitary, and tests of feedback for the hypothalamus (Table 16.9).

TREATMENT

Steroid and thyroid hormones are essential for life. Both may be given as oral replacement drugs, aiming to restore the patient to clinical and biochemical normality (Table 16.10). Growth hormone therapy may be given if necessary in the growing child and sex hormone production may be restored with androgens and oestrogens for symptomatic control; if necessary, human chorionic gonadotrophin (HCG) (mainly LH) and Pergonal or Metrodin (mainly FSH) can be given if fertility is desired. Pulsatile LHRH therapy has been used where there is residual pituitary function but is expensive and time-consuming.

Two warnings are necessary:

- Thyroid replacement should not commence until normal glucocorticoid function has been demonstrated or replacement steroid therapy initiated.
- Glucocorticoid deficiency may mask impaired urine concentrating ability, diabetes insipidus

Table 16.9 Tests for hypothalamic–pituitary (HP) function.

Axis	Tests for end-organ product	Feedback hormone	Tests for pituitary reserve	Tests for hypothalamic feedback
Anterior pituitary				
HP-ovarian	Plasma oestradiol Plasma progesterone Ultrasound (pelvic)	LH FSH	LHRH test	Clomiphene test
HP-testicular	Plasma testosterone Sperm count	LH FSH	LHRH test	Clomiphene test
Growth	Plasma GH/SmC	SmC	GRF test	Insulin tolerance test
Breast	Plasma prolactin	—	—	
Thyroid	Plasma T_4/T_3	TSH	TRH test	—
Adrenal	Plasma cortisol	ACTH	CRF test	Insulin tolerance test
Posterior pituitary				
Thirst	Plasma and urine osmolalities	Vasopressin response to small amounts of hypertonic saline (300 mmol·L^{-1})		

SmC = somatomedin C.

Table 16.10 Replacement therapy for hypopituitarism.

Axis	Usual replacement	Additional therapy
Gonadal	Males: testosterone 250–500 mg every 3–4 weeks Females: cyclical oestrogen/progestogen	HCG plus FSH (Pergonal) to produce testicular development, spermatogenesis or ovulation; used for infertility (Pulsatile LHRH used in both sexes)
Breast (prolactin)	Bromocriptine 3–15 mg daily as replacement inhibition	—
Growth	None usually needed in adult, though GH has effects on muscle mass	For growth, GH injections
Thyroid	Thyroxine 0.1–0.2 mg daily	—
Adrenal	Hydrocortisone 15–40 mg daily Prednisolone 5–10 mg daily (Normally no need for mineralocorticoid replacement)	ACTH (tetracosactrin) to prevent or reverse adrenal suppression
Thirst	Desmopressin 10–20 μg one to three times daily by nasal spray	Carbamazepine, thiazides or chlorpropamide are sometimes useful in mild diabetes insipidus

HCG = Human chorionic gonadotrophin (mainly LH).

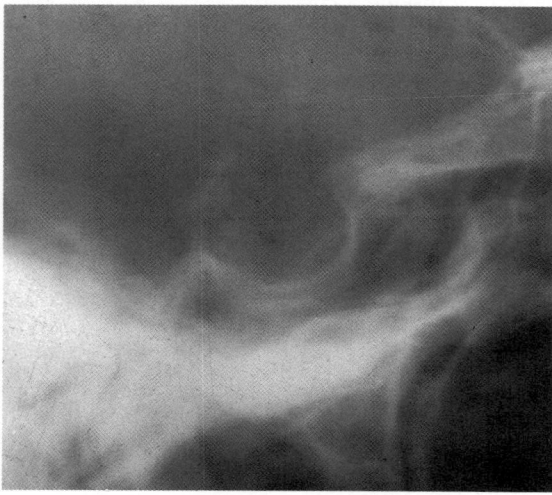

Fig. 16.9 Lateral skull X-ray showing double floor and enlargement of the pituitary fossa in a patient with acromegaly.

only becoming apparent *after* steroid replacement.

PITUITARY TUMOURS

Tumours are amongst the commonest causes of hypopituitarism. Investigation of a possible tumour follows three lines:

1 *Is there a hormonal excess?* The clinical features of acromegaly and Cushing's disease or hyperprolactinaemia are usually, but not always, obvious.

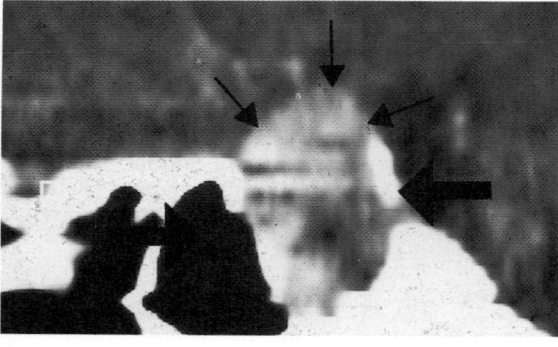

Fig. 16.10 CT scan (sagittal reconstruction) showing a pituitary tumour with suprasellar extension.

Hyperprolactinaemia may be clinically 'silent'.
2 *Are any hormones deficient?* Clinical examination may give clues; thus, short stature in a child with a pituitary tumour is likely to be due to GH deficiency. A slow, lethargic adult with pale skin is likely to be TSH and/or ACTH deficient. Milder deficiencies may not be obvious, and require specific testing (Table 16.9).
3 *Is there a tumour?* How big is it and what anatomical effects is it exerting? Investigations include:

● Lateral skull X-rays may show enlargement of the fossa. This is a common incidental finding and requires further investigation (Fig. 16.9).
● Visual fields. These should be plotted formally by Goldmann perimetry or by confrontation at

Table 16.11 Characteristics of pituitary tumours.

Tumour/condition	Usual size	Commonest clinical presentation
Prolactinoma	Most < 10 mm (microprolactinoma)	Galactorrhoea, amenorrhoea, hypogonadism, impotence
	Some > 10 mm (macroprolactinoma)	As above, plus headaches, visual field defects, hypopituitarism
Acromegaly	Medium-large (90% + of skull X-rays abnormal)	Change in appearance, visual field defects, chance observation, hypopituitarism
Cushing's disease	Most small, or hyperplasia rather than tumour	Central obesity, chance observation (local symptoms rare)
Nelson's syndrome	Often large	Post-adrenalectomy, pigmentation, sometimes local symptoms
Non-functioning tumours	Often large	Visual-field defects, headaches, hypopituitarism (small ones often found incidentally at post mortem)
Craniopharyngiomas	Often very large and cystic (skull X-ray abnormal in 50% +, calcification common)	Headaches, visual field defects, growth failure (50% below age 20, about 15% arise within sella)

the bedside using a small red pin as target. Common defects are upper temporal quadrantanopias and bitemporal hemianopias (see p. 884).
- High-resolution CT scanning with reconstruction is the investigation of choice (Fig. 16.10), though MRI is probably preferable when it is available (Fig. 16.11).

The common types of pituitary tumour (Table 16.11) are:

- Prolactinomas (histologically chromophobe adenomas)
- Non-functioning tumours, usually chromophobe adenomas
- Acidophil adenomas—acromegaly
- Basophil adenomas or hyperplasia—Cushing's disease and Nelson's syndrome

The differential diagnosis additionally includes craniopharyngioma, a usually cystic hypothalamic tumour arising from Rathke's pouch and often

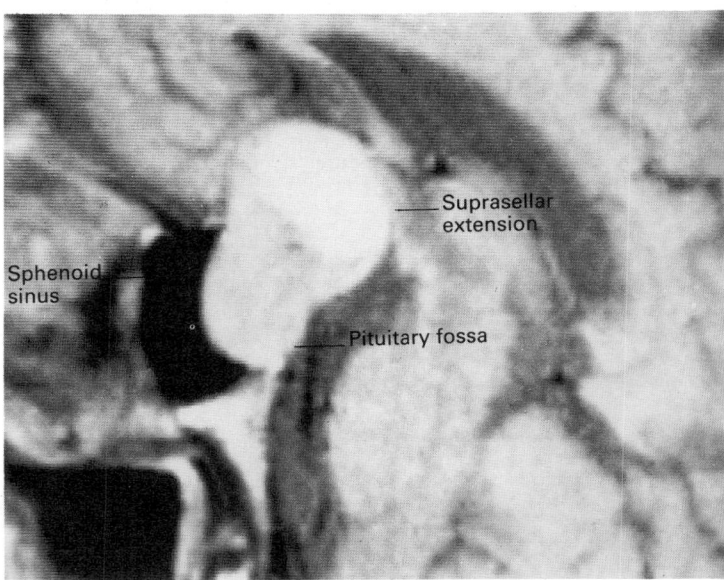

Fig. 16.11 MRI of pituitary fossa showing tumour with suprasellar extension.

mimicking an intrinsic pituitary lesion. Though presenting at any age, it is the commonest tumour in children and is ofen calcified. Less common are meningiomas, gliomas, chondromas, pinealomas and carotid artery aneurysms masquerading as tumours.

TREATMENT

Therapy has three aims:

1 *Removal/control of the tumour* (Table 16.12)

- Surgical removal is ideal and can be performed trans-sphenoidally or by the open transfrontal route. The former is suitable when the tumour is small, confined within or a little above the fossa and when there is no major suprasellar extension; it has become much more widely used of late. The transfrontal route is used for significant suprasellar extensions or when there is hypothalamic tumour. When surgical removal is incomplete, radiotherapy should be given to prevent recurrence—many believe radiotherapy should be given for most tumours except microadenomas or if the patient is elderly. Immunostaining of the removed material may allow confirmation of the tumour cell type and activity.

  Complications of trans-sphenoidal surgery include meningitis and CSF leaks, and naso-septal perforations.

- Radiotherapy can be given as either conventional external therapy using a three-beam technique (40–45 Gy, not exceeding 1.8 Gy per

fraction). An alternative is the trans-sphenoidal implantation of radioactive yttrium needles, which provide high-level local radio-activity to the tumour site. This requires great expertise and has best been used for Cushing's disease.

- Medical means may shrink or control a tumour, especially if it is considered inoperable, and sometimes for long-term therapy (especially for prolactinomas). Bromocriptine, mentioned below, is often used to obtain shrinkage of a large tumour before deciding on the possibility of subsequent trans-sphenoidal surgery or radiotherapy—the latter cannot be given when a tumour extends much above the sella as there is a danger of visual pathway and hypothalamic damage.

- With small tumours producing no pressure symptoms and without endocrine deficit, observation alone may be indicated with regular visual-field assessments.

2 *Reduction of excessive hormone secretion.* This may ultimately be achieved by eradication of the tumour as above, but medical control is often possible in the short-term and occasionally as long-term therapy:

- Prolactinomas usually respond to bromocriptine, a dopamine agonist agent, which often also produces significant tumour shrinkage as well as control of the galactorrhoea (see p. 791).

- Acromegaly also responds with some lowering of growth hormone levels on bromocriptine, though the response is often incomplete

Table 16.12 Comparisons of primary treatment for pituitary tumours.

	Advantages	Disadvantages
Surgical		
Transsphenoidal adenomectomy or hypophysectomy	Relatively minor procedure	Limited value if significant suprasellar extension
		Needs considerable expertise
		Risks of CSF leakage/meningitis
Transfrontal	Good access to suprasellar region	Major procedure
		Danger of frontal lobe damage
		High chance of subsequent hypopituitarism
Radiotherapy		
External (40–50 Gy)	Non-invasive	Slow action
	Prevents recurrence	May not be effective
Yttrium implantation	High local dose	Later hypopituitarism
		Great expertise needed
Medical		
Bromocriptine (for prolactinomas and acromega) Octreotide (for acromegaly)	Non-invasive Reversible	Not curative, long-term
		Significant side-effects in minority
		Expensive

and tumour shrinkage is less likely. Long-acting somatostatin analogues, e.g. octreotide, can also cause significant reduction of GH in acromegaly.

- ACTH secretion cannot usually be controlled medically, but the inhibition of cortisol synthesis and release can be achieved by the 11-hydroxylase blocker, metyrapone, or aminoglutethimide.

3 *Replacement of deficient hormone production.* See Table 16.10.

WEIGHT, EXERCISE AND STRESS

The importance of these factors in hypothalamic–pituitary function has only recently been fully realized. Anorexia nervosa, the 'slimming disease' commonly affecting young females, is associated with major functional hypopituitarism (see p. 995). This often presents as amenorrhoea, without which the diagnosis is extremely unlikely. Anorexia is an extreme example, but more marginal degrees of underweight are a cause of secondary amenorrhoea and oligomenorrhoea, and are often unrecognized as a cause of subfertility. Similar effects are seen in female athletes undergoing heavy training with menstrual irregularity that invariably reverts to normal when training stops.

Stress, though difficult to define, also affects endocrine function, especially menstruation. Emotional deprivation in childhood is an important cause of growth retardation and may be mediated by reduced GH secretion.

Reproduction and sex

Normal physiology of the female and male reproductive systems will first be considered, then their common disorders.

Embryology

Until 8 weeks the sexes share a common development, with a primitive genital tract including the Wolffian and Müllerian ducts. There are additionally a primitive perineum and primitive gonads. In the *presence* of a Y chromosome the potential testis develops while the ovary regresses. In the *absence* of a Y chromosome, the potential ovary develops and related ducts form a uterus and the upper vagina. Production of Müllerian inhibitory factor, from the early 'testis' produces atrophy of the Müllerian duct, while, under the influence of testosterone and dihydrotestosterone, the Wolffian duct differentiates into an epididymis, vas defer-

Table 16.13 Definitions in reproductive medicine.

Menarche	Age at first period
Primary amenorrhoea	Failure to begin spontaneous menstruation by age 16
Secondary amenorrhoea	Absence of menstruation for 3 months in a woman who has previously had cycles
Oligomenorrhoea	Irregular long cycles; often used for any length of cycle above 32 days
Dyspareunia	Pain or discomfort in the female during intercourse
Libido	Sexual interest or desire; often difficult to assess and is greatly affected by stress, tiredness and psychological factors
Menstruation	Onset of spontaneous (usually regular) uterine bleeding in the female
Impotence	Inability of the male to achieve or sustain an erection adequate for satisfactory intercourse
Azoospermia	Absence of sperm in the ejaculate
Oligospermia	Reduced numbers of sperm in the ejaculate; normal values are disputed
Virilization	Occurrence of male secondary sexual characteristics in the female

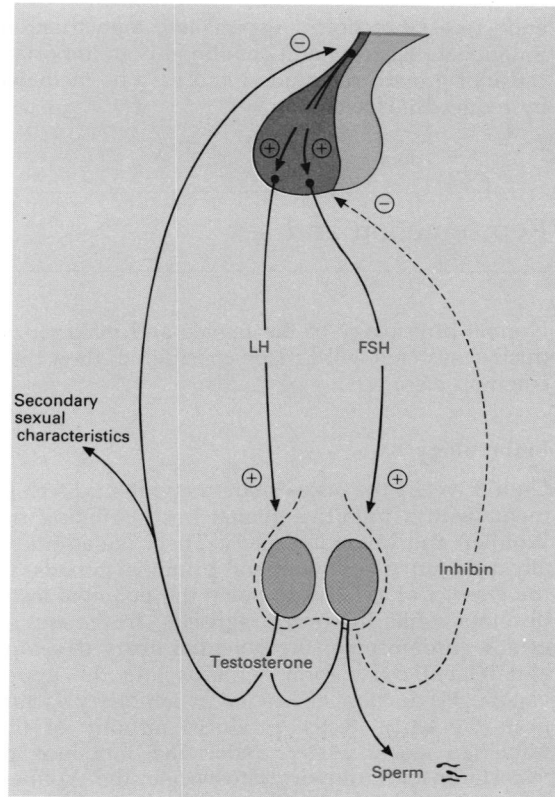

Fig. 16.12 The male hypothalamic—pituitary—gonadal axis.

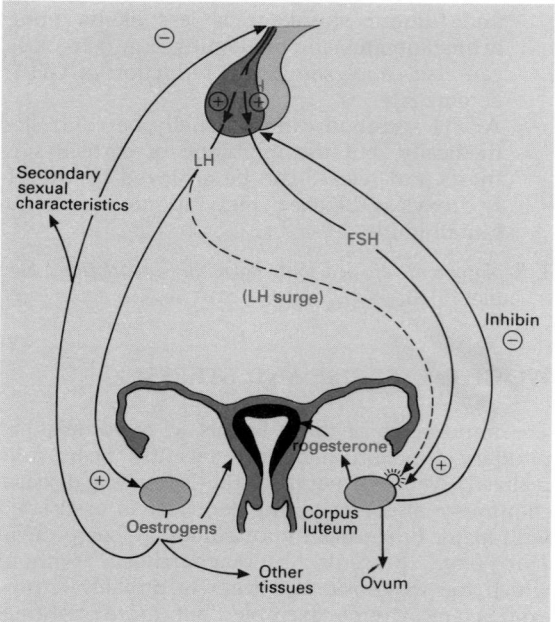

Fig. 16.13 The female hypothalamic—pituitary—gonadal axis.

ens, seminal vesicles and prostate. Androgens induce transformation of the perineum to include a penis, penile urethra and scrotum containing the testes, which descend in response to androgenic stimulation. At birth testicular volume is 0.5–1 ml.

Definitions

Relevant terminology is shown in Table 16.13.

Physiology

The male
An outline of the hypothalamic–pituitary–testicular axis is shown in Fig. 16.12.

- Pulses of LHRH (GnRH) are released from the hypothalamus and stimulate LH and FSH release from the pituitary.
- LH stimulates testosterone production from Leydig's cells of the testis.
- Testosterone acts systemically to produce male secondary sexual characteristics, anabolism and the maintenance of libido. It also acts locally within the testis to aid spermatogenesis.
- FSH stimulates the Sertoli's cells in the semini-

ferous tubules to produce mature sperm and the feedback hormone *inhibin*.
- Testosterone feeds back on the hypothalamus/ pituitary to inhibit LHRH secretion.
- Inhibin appears to feedback on the pituitary to decrease FSH secretion.

The secondary sexual characteristics of the male for which testosterone is necessary are the growth of pubic, axillary and facial hair, enlargement of the external genitalia, deepening of the voice, sebum secretion, muscle growth and frontal balding.

The female
The female situation is more complex (Figs. 16.13 and 16.14).

- In the adult female, higher brain centres impose a menstrual cycle of 28 days upon the activity of hypothalamic GnRH.
- Pulses of GnRH stimulate release of pituitary LH and FSH.
- LH stimulates ovarian androgen production.
- FSH stimulates follicular development and aromatase activity (an enzyme required to convert ovarian androgens to oestrogens). FSH also stimulates inhibin from ovarian stromal cells. Inhibin, in turn, inhibits FSH release.
- Although many follicles are 'recruited' for development in early folliculogenesis, by day 8–10 a 'leading' follicle is selected for development into a mature Graafian follicle.
- Oestrogens show a double feedback action on the pituitary, initially inhibiting gonadotrophin

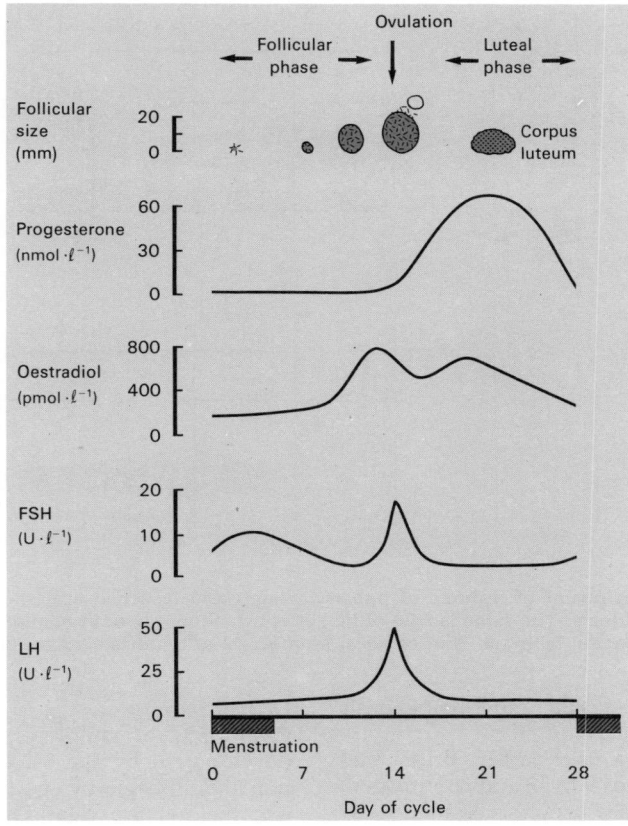

Fig. 16.14 Hormonal and follicular changes during the normal menstrual cycle.

secretion (negative feedback), but later high-level exposure results in increased GnRH secretion and increased LH sensitivity to GnRH (positive feedback).

● This leads to the mid-cycle LH surge, which induces ovulation (Fig. 16.14).

● The follicle then differentiates into a corpus luteum, which secretes both progesterone and oestradiol during the second half of the cycle (luteal phase).

● Oestrogen initially and then progesterone cause uterine endometrial proliferation in preparation for possible implantation; if implantation does not occur, the corpus luteum regresses and progesterone secretion falls and the endometrium is shed (menstruation).

● If a pregnancy ensues, HCG (human chorionic gonadotrophin) production from the corpus luteum will maintain corpus luteum function till 10–12 weeks, by which time the placenta will be making sufficient oestrogens and progesterone to support itself.

Oestrogens also induce secondary sexual character-istics, especially development of the breast and nipples, vaginal and vulval growth and pubic hair development. They also induce growth and maturation of the uterus and tubes. They do not, however, usually increase breast size in other circumstances.

Puberty

The mechanisms initiating puberty are poorly understood but are thought to result from withdrawal of central inhibition of GnRH release. LH and FSH are both low in the pre-pubertal child. In early puberty, FSH begins to rise first, initially in nocturnal pulses; this is followed by a rise in LH with a subsequent increase in testosterone/oestrogen levels. The milestones of puberty in the two sexes are shown in Fig. 16.15.

In boys, pubertal changes begin between 10 and 14 years and are complete between 15 and 17 years. The genitalia develop, testes enlarge and the area of pubic hair increases. Peak height velocity is reached between ages 12 and 17 during stage 4 of

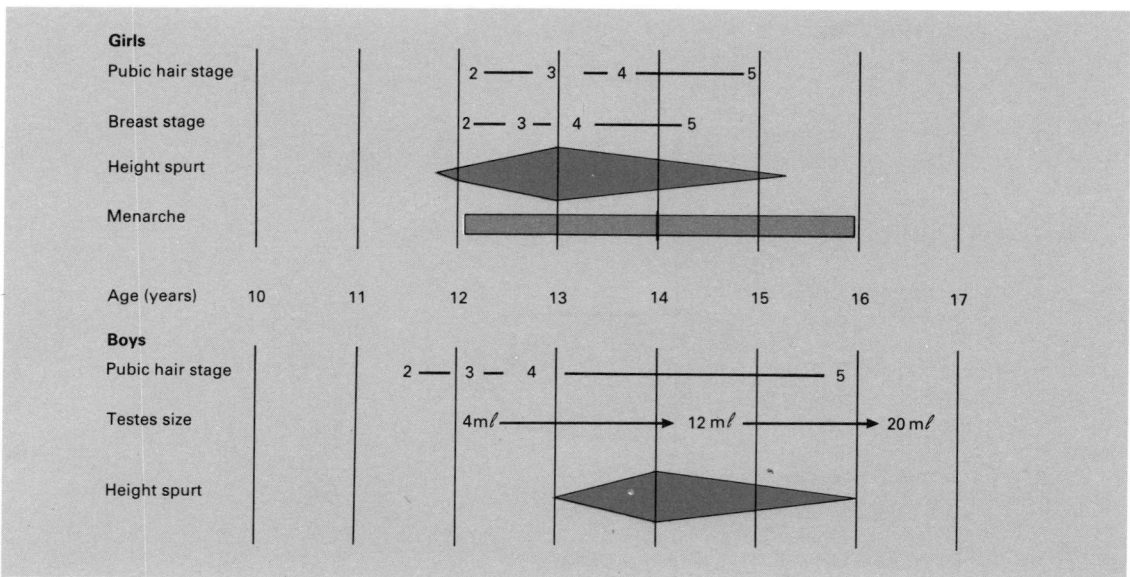

Fig. 16.15 The age of development of features of puberty. Stages and testicular size show mean ages and all vary considerably between individuals. The same is true of height spurt, shown here in relation to other data. The ages of menarche show approximate 5th, 50th and 95th centiles. Numbers 2 to 5 indicate stages of development.

testicular development. Full spermatogenesis occurs comparatively late.

In girls, events start a year earlier. Breast bud enlargement begins at ages 9 to 13 and continues to 12 to 18 years. Public hair growth commences at ages 9 to 14 and is completed at 12 to 16½ years. Menarche occurs relatively late (age 11 to 15) but peak height velocity is reached much earlier than in boys (age 10 to 13½ years).

Precocious puberty
Development of menarche (girls) or secondary sexual characteristics (boys) before the age of nine is premature, and may take the following forms:

- Idiopathic precocity (common in girls). This is a diagnosis of exclusion with no apparent cause for premature entry into puberty and an early growth spurt. Treatment is with cyproterone acetate, an anti-androgen with progestational activity, but LHRH analogues causing suppression of gonadotrophin release with reduced sex hormone production are likely to supersede this.
- Cerebral precocity. Many causes of hypothalamic disease, especially tumours, may present in this way. In boys this must be rigorously excluded.
- Forbes–Albright's syndrome, usually in girls, with precocity, polyostotic fibrous dysplasia and skin pigmentation.
- Premature thelarche is early breast development alone, usually transient between ages 2 and 4.
- Premature adrenarche is early development of pubic hair without significant other changes.

Delayed puberty
Over 95% of children show signs of pubertal development by age 14. In its absence, investigation should begin by age 15. Causes of hypogonadism (below) are clearly relevant but most cases represent constitutional delay.

- In constitutional delay, pubertal development, bone age and stature should be in parallel.
- In boys, testicular volume > 5 ml indicates the onset of puberty. A rising serum testosterone is an earlier clue.
- In girls, the breast bud is the first sign. Ultrasound allows assessment of ovarian and uterine development.
- Basal LH/FSH levels may identify the site of a defect, and LHRH tests can indicate the stage of early puberty.
- If any progression at all occurs clinically, observation is usually indicated.
- Low-dose sex hormone therapy to induce puberty is possible when delay is great and problems are serious (e.g. severe teasing at school).

The menopause

The menopause, or cessation of periods, occurs about the age of 50. During the late 40s, FSH initially, and then LH concentrations begin to rise, probably as follicle supply diminishes. Oestrogen levels fall and the cycle becomes disrupted. Most women notice irregular scanty periods coming on over a variable period, though in some, sudden amenorrhoea or menorrhagia occur. Eventually the menopausal pattern of low oestradiol levels with grossly elevated LH and FSH (usually > 50 and > 25 U·L^{-1}, respectively) is established.

Features of oestrogen deficiency are hot flushes, which occur in most women and can be disabling, vaginal dryness and atrophy of the breasts. There may also be vague symptoms of loss of libido, loss of self-esteem, non-specific aches and pains, irritability, depression, loss of concentration and weight gain. Women become very liable to osteoporosis and premenopausal protection from ischaemic heart disease disappears. When hormone replacement therapy (HRT) is given, the oestrogen should be given cyclically with a progestogen to prevent endometrial carcinoma from unopposed oestrogen action.

Some of the usual hazards of oestrogens apply (see below) but most physicians are now treating symptomatic patients much more widely and some recommend the widespread use of HRT, though still much less widely than in the USA. Current evidence suggests that when given *with* a progestogen, the benefits far outweigh the small risks, unless there are clear contraindications. The overall benefits may be summarized as follows:

● Symptomatic improvement in many, but not all, menopausal symptoms for the majority of women. Oestrogen-deficient symptoms respond well to oestrogen replacement, the vaguer symptoms generally, but not always, less well.
● Reduction in ischaemic heart disease and cerebrovascular disease mortality. Blood pressure falls in the majority.
● Protection against fractures of wrist, spine and hip, secondary to osteoporosis, at least where HRT is used before the age of 60. This is due to predominant protection of trabecular rather than cancellous bone.

Apart from individual risks from oestrogen therapy (e.g. migraine, thrombosis)—and even with these the effect of HRT may not parallel those of the 'pill'—the main concerns have been induction of cancer of the uterus or breast. Given with a progestogen, the risk of uterine cancer is not significantly increased, while the data on breast carcinoma are conflicting. There is of course the inconvenience of withdrawal bleeds, unless a hysterectomy has been performed. The preferred route of administration is oral, but implants and skin patches may become preferable in the future.

Premature menopause
The commonest cause of early menopause in the 20s and 30s is ovarian failure which is usually autoimmune in nature. HRT should be given.

The ageing male
In the male there is no sudden 'change of life'.

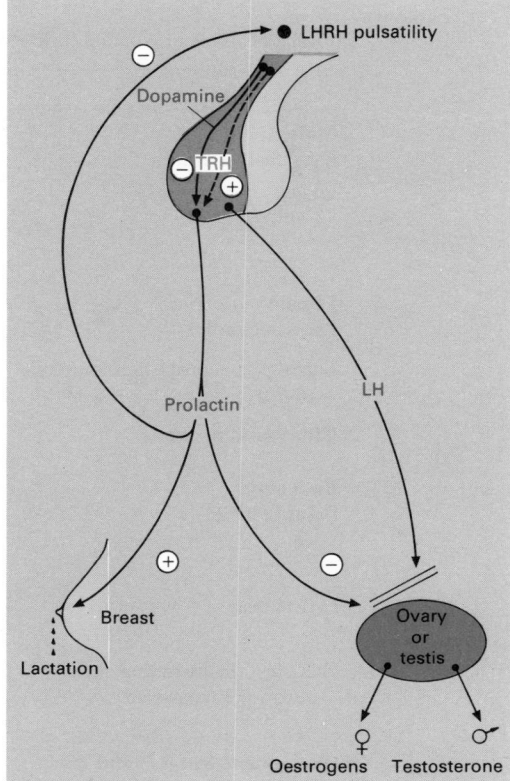

Fig. 16.16 The control of prolactin secretion.

Sexual and menstrual disorders

History
Libido
Potency
Frequency of intercourse
Menstruation—relation of symptoms to cycle
Breasts (? galactorrhoea)
Hirsuties

Physical signs
Evidence of systemic disease
Secondary sexual characteristics
Genital size (testes, ovaries, uterus)
Cliteromegaly
Breast development, gynaecomastia
Galactorrhoea
Extent/distribution of hair

However, there is a progressive loss in sexual function with reduction in morning erections and frequency of intercourse. The age of onset varies widely but overall testicular volume diminishes and gonadotrophin levels gradually rise.

Physiology of prolactin secretion

The hypothalamic–pituitary control of prolactin secretion is illustrated in Fig. 16.16. It is under

Table 16.14 Tests of gonadal function.

	Uses/comments
Male	
Basal testosterone	Normal levels exclude hypogonadism
Sperm count	Normal count excludes any deficiency Motility and abnormal sperms should be noted
Female	
Basal oestradiol	Normal levels exclude hypogonadism
Luteal phase progesterone (days 18–24)	If > 30 nmol·l^{-1}, suggests ovulation
Ultrasound of ovaries	To confirm ovulation
Both sexes	
Basal LH/FSH	Demonstrates state of feedback system for hormone production (LH) and germ cell production (FSH)
LHRH test	Shows adequacy (or otherwise) of LH and FSH stores in pituitary
HCG test (testosterone or oestradiol measured)	Response shows potential of ovary or testis; failure demonstrates primary gonadal problem
Clomiphene test (LH and FSH measured)	Tests hypothalamic negative feedback system
Post-coital test	Demonstrates state of sperm and sperm–mucus interaction

tonic dopamine inhibition and other factors known to increase prolactin secretion (e.g. TRH) are probably of less importance. Prolactin stimulates milk secretion but also reduces gonadal activity. It decreases LHRH pulsatility at hypothalamic level and, to a lesser extent, blocks the action of LH on the ovary or testis, producing hypogonadism. These actions may be clinically important.

DISORDERS OF SEX AND REPRODUCTION

CLINICAL FEATURES

A detailed history and examination of all systems is required.

Tests of gonadal function
The patient is his/her own best assay for gonadal endocrine function. A man having regular satisfactory intercourse or a woman with regular ovulatory periods is most unlikely to have significant *endocrine* disease. When symptoms are present, much can be deduced by basal measurements of the gonadotrophins, oestrogens/testosterone and prolactin:

● A low testosterone or oestradiol with high gonadotrophins indicates primary gonadal disease. Both testosterone and oestrogen circulate largely bound to sex hormone-binding globulin (see p. 764).

● In contrast, low levels of LH/FSH and testosterone/oestradiol imply hypothalamic and/or pituitary disease.

● Confirmation of normal female reproductive endocrinology requires the demonstration of ovulation; this is achieved by measurement of luteal phase serum progesterone and/or by ovarian ultrasound.

● Demonstration of normal male and female function requires a pregnancy; in the male, in the first instance there should be a healthy sperm count (20–200 $\times$ 10^4/ml): good motility ($> 60\%$ Grade I) and few abnormal forms ($< 20\%$).

● Hyperprolactinaemia can be confirmed or excluded by direct measurement of preferably 2–3 samples. Levels may increase with stress; ideally, a cannula should be inserted and samples taken through it 30 min later.

● The clomiphene test examines hypothalamic negative feedback. Clomiphene is a competitive oestrogen antagonist that binds to, but does not activate oestrogen receptors, thus inducing a rise

Table 16.15 Effects of androgens and consequences of androgen deficiency in the male.

Physiological effect	Consequences of deficiency
General	
Maintenance of libido	Loss of libido
Deepening of voice	High-pitched voice (if pre-pubertal)
Frontotemporal balding	Smooth skin
Facial, axillary and limb hair	Decreased hair
Pubic hair	
Maintenance of male pattern	Thinning and loss of pubic hair
Testes and scrotum	
Maintenance of testicular size/ consistency	Small soft testes
Rugosity of scrotum	Poorly developed penis/scrotum
Maintenance of erectile/ejaculatory function	Loss of erections/ejaculation
Stimulation of spermatogenesis	Subfertility
Skeletal	
Epiphyseal fusion	Eunuchoidism (if pre-pubertal)
Maintenance of muscle bulk	Decreased muscle bulk and power

in gonadotrophin secretion in the normal subject.

More detailed tests are indicated in Table 16.14.

DISORDERS IN THE MALE

Hypogonadism

CLINICAL FEATURES

Male hypogonadism may be a presenting complaint or an incidental finding, e.g. during investigation for infertility. The testes may be small and soft. Except with infertility, the complaints are usually of androgen deficiency (Table 16.15) rather than deficiency of sperm production. Sperm only makes up a very small proportion of seminal fluid volume.

Causes of male hypogonadism are shown in Table 16.16.

INVESTIGATION

Testicular disease may be initially apparent but basal levels of testosterone, LH and FSH should be measured. These will allow the distinction between primary gonadal (testicular) failure and hypothalamic–pituitary disease to be made. Biopsy of the testes may be indicated though rarely yields a treatable cause.

Skull radiology, pituitary CT scan, prolactin levels and other pituitary function tests may be needed. Depending on the causes, semen analysis,

Table 16.16 Causes of male hypogonadism.

Reduced gonadotrophins (hypothalamic–pituitary disease)
Hypopituitarism
Selective gonadotrophic deficiency (Kallmann's syndrome)
Hyperprolactinaemia
Primary gonadal disease (congenital)
Anorchia/Leydig cell agenesis
Chromosome abnormality (e.g. Klinefelter's syndrome)
Enzyme defects
5α-Reductase deficiency
Primary gonadal disease (acquired)
Testicular torsion
Castration
Local testicular disease
Chemotherapy/radiation toxicity
Renal failure
Cirrhosis/alcohol
Sickle cell disease
Androgen receptor deficiency

chromosomal analysis (e.g. to exclude Klinefelter's syndrome) and bone age estimation may be required.

TREATMENT

The cause can rarely be reversed. Replacement therapy should be commenced (Table 16.17).

Table 16.17 Androgen replacement therapy.

Preparation	Dose	Remarks
Testosterone mixed esters	250–500 mg i.m. every 3–6 weeks	Injection can be painful Usual maintenance therapy
Testosterone propionate	50–100 mg i.m. every 1–2 weeks	Frequent injections needed as half-life is short Good initial therapy
Testosterone undecanoate	80–240 mg daily, orally in divided doses	Variable dose, irregular absorption Very expensive

N.B.: Mesterolone and methyltestosterone are no longer advised; they are weakly active and can cause cholestasis.

Primary gonadal failure should be treated with androgens. Patients with hypothalamic–pituitary disease may be given LH and FSH (Pergonal) or pulsatile LHRH if fertility is required, otherwise they should receive androgen replacement.

Special instances of hypogonadism include:

- *Cryptorchidism.* By the age of 5 years both testes should be in the scrotum. After that age the germinal epithelium is increasingly at risk; lack of descent by puberty is associated with infertility. Surgical exploration and orchidopexy are usually undertaken but a short trial of HCG occasionally induces descent. Intra-abdominal testes have an increased risk of developing malignancy; if presentation is after puberty, orchidectomy is advised.
- *Klinefelter's syndrome ('seminiferous tubule dysgenesis').* This chromosomal disorder (47 XXY) involves loss of both Leydig cells and seminiferous tubular dysgenesis. Patients usually present with poor sexual development, small or undescended testes, gynaecomastia or infertility. They are sometimes mentally retarded. Clinical examination shows small pea-size but firm testes, usually gynaecomastia and often signs of androgen deficiency. Confirmation is by chromosomal analysis. Treatment is androgen replacement therapy, though if the patient is mentally subnormal this should be used carefully. No treatment is possible for the abnormal seminiferous tubules and infertility.
- *Isolated deficiency of LHRH or LH/FSH (Kallmann's syndrome).* Also known as hypogonadotrophic hypogonadism, this is often associated with decreased sense of smell (anosmia), and sometimes with other bony (cleft-palate), renal and cerebral abnormalities (e.g. colour blindness). It is often familial and is usually X-linked. Management is that of secondary hypogonadism; fertility is possible.
- *Oligospermia or azoospermia.* These may be secondary to androgen deficiency and corrected by replacement but more often they result from primary testicular diseases and are rarely treatable.
- *Azoospermia* with normal testicular size and low FSH levels suggests a vas deferens block.

Lack of libido and impotence

Many patients with impotence have no definable organic cause. A careful history of physical disease, related symptoms, stress and psychological factors, together with drug and alcohol abuse, must be taken. The presence of nocturnal emissions and frequent satisfactory morning erections largely excludes endocrine disease as a cause.

True erectile difficulty may be psychological, neurogenic, vascular, endocrine or related to drugs. Vascular disease may be more common than realized and is often associated with vascular problems elsewhere. The endocrine causes are those of hypogonadism (above) and can be excluded by normal testosterone, gonadotrophin and prolactin levels. Autonomic neuropathy, most commonly from diabetes mellitus, is the commonest identifiable cause on clinical examination. Many drugs can be responsible—cannabis, diuretics, metoclopramide, bethanidine/guanethidine, methyldopa and beta-blockers all produce impotence. Psychogenic impotence is frequently a diagnosis of exclusion, though complex tests of penile vasculature and function are now available in some centres.

Apart from cessation of the offending drug, methods of treatment include vacuum condoms, intracavernosal injections of papaverine and phentolamine, penile implants and vacuum expanders; specialist advice is essential. If no organic disease is found, or if there is clear evidence of psychological problems, the couple should receive psychosexual counselling.

Gynaecomastia

Gynaecomastia is development of breast tissue in the male. Causes are shown in Table 16.18.

Pubertal gynaecomastia occurs in perhaps 50% of normal boys, often asymmetrically. It usually resolves spontaneously within 6–18 months but after this duration may require surgical removal, as

Table 16.18 Causes of gynaecomastia.

Physiological
  Neonatal
  Pubertal
  Old age

Hyperthyroidism

Liver disease

Oestrogen-producing tumours (testis, adrenal)

HCG-producing tumours (testis, lung)

Starvation/refeeding

Carcinoma of breast

Drugs
  Oestrogenic
    Oestrogens
    Digitalis
    Cannabis
    Diamorphine
  Anti-androgens
    Spironolactone
    Cimetidine
    Cyproterone
  Others
    Gonadotrophins
    Cytotoxics

fibrous tissue will have been laid down. The cause is thought to be relative oestrogen excess.

In the older male, gynaecomastia requires a full assessment to exclude potentially serious underlying disease, such as bronchial carcinoma and testicular tumours (e.g. Leydig cell tumour). Drug effects are common (especially digoxin and spironolactone) and once these are excluded most cases have no definable cause.

DISORDERS IN THE FEMALE

Hypogonadism

Impaired ovarian function, whether primary or secondary, will lead both to oestrogen deficiency and abnormalities of the menstrual cycle. The latter is very sensitive to disruption, cycles becoming anovulatory and irregular before disappearing altogether. Symptoms will depend on the age at which the failure develops. Thus, before puberty, primary amenorrhoea possibly with delayed puberty will occur; if after puberty, secondary amenorrhoea and possibly hypogonadism will result.

Oestrogen deficiency
The physiological effects of oestrogens and symptoms/signs of deficiency are shown in Table 16.19.

Amenorrhoea

Absence of periods or markedly irregular infrequent periods (oligomenorrhoea) are a common presentation, often the earliest, of female gonadal disease. Important factors in clinical asessment of such patients are shown in Table 16.20.

Pregnancy. This must *always* be considered.

Table 16.19 Effects of oestrogens and consequences of oestrogen deficiency.

Physiological effect	Consequence of deficiency
Breast Development of connective and duct tissue Nipple enlargement and areolar pigmentation	} Small, atrophic breasts
Pubic hair Maintenance of female pattern	Thinning and loss of pubic hair
Vulva and vagina Vulval growth Vaginal glandular and epithelial proliferation Vaginal lubrication	Atrophic vulva Atrophic vagina Dry vagina and dyspareunia
Uterus and tubes Myometrial and tubal hypertrophy Endometrial proliferation	Small, atrophic uterus and tubes
Skeletal Epiphyseal fusion Maintenance of bone mass	Eunuchoidism (if pre-pubertal) Osteoporosis

Table 16.20 Clinical assessment of amenorrhoea.

History
? Pregnant
Age of onset
Age of menarche, if any
Sudden or gradual onset
General health
Weight, absolute and changes in recent past
Stress (job, lifestyle, exams, relationships)
Excessive exercise
Drugs
Hirsuties, acne, virilization
Headaches/visual symptoms
Sense of smell
Past history of pregnancies
Past history of gynaecological surgery

Examination
General health
Body shape and skeletal abnormalities
Weight and height
Hirsuties and acne
Evidence of virilization
Maturity of secondary sexual characteristics
Galactorrhoea
Normality of vagina, cervix and uterus

- Genital tract abnormalities, such as imperforate hymen, should be remembered, especially in primary amenorrhoea.
- Weight-related amenorrhoea. A minimum body weight is necessary for regular menstruation. This condition is common and may be seen at weights within the 'normal' range. Many of these subjects may have additional minor endocrine disease (e.g. polycystic disease) but restoration of body weight to above the 50th centile is often helpful. Similar problems occur with intensive physical training. Anorexia nervosa (see p. 995).
- Hypothalamic amenorrhoea. Some dispute the existence of this condition, linking all amenorrhoea to low weight or increased stress. A few patients, however, do appear to have defective cycling mechanisms without apparent explanation.
- Severe illness, even in the absence of weight loss.
- After stopping the contraceptive pill.

INVESTIGATION

Basal levels of FSH, LH oestrogen and prolactin allow initial distinction between primary gonadal and hypothalamic–pituitary causes (Table 16.21). Ovarian biopsy is necessary to confirm the diagnosis of primary ovarian failure. Subsequent investigations are also shown in Table 16.21.

TREATMENT

Treatment is that of the cause wherever possible (e.g. hypothyroidism, low weight, stress, excessive exercise).

Primary ovarian disease is rarely treatable except in the rare condition of 'resistant' ovary, where high-dose Pergonal can occasionally lead to folliculogenesis. Hyperprolactinaemia should be corrected (see below). Polycystic ovarian syndrome is discussed below.

Hirsuties

PATHOPHYSIOLOGY

The extent of hair growth varies between individuals, families and races, being more extensive in the Mediterranean and Asian populations. Soft vellous hair on the face and elsewhere is not sex-hormone dependent, nor is hair on the forearm or lower leg. Hair in the beard, moustache, breast, chest, axilla, abdominal midline, pubic and thigh areas is sex-hormone dependent. Any excess in the latter regions is thus usually a mark of increased ovarian or adrenal androgen production. Hair has a long growing cycle with spontaneous variations and clinical changes are therefore slow.

CLINICAL FEATURES

The complaint is common and often accompanied by severe anxiety and social stress. Important questions are:

- Age and speed of onset. Rapid progression and prepubertal or late onset suggest a more serious cause.
- Accompanying virilization (cliteromegaly, frontal balding, male phenotype, greasy skin, acne). This implies significant androgen excess.
- Menstruation. The greater the disruption the more likely a serious cause.

CAUSES AND INVESTIGATION

These are summarized in Table 16.22.

TREATMENT

The underlying cause should be removed in the rare instances where this is possible (e.g. drugs, adrenal or ovarian tumours). Other therapy is either local or systemic.

Local therapy
Plucking, bleaching, depilatory cream or wax and shaving may all help and are underused. Electrolysis is slow and expensive.

Systemic
Oestrogens (e.g. oral contraceptives) reduce free

Table 16.21 Differential diagnosis and investigation of amenorrhoea.

Diagnosis	Biochemical markers	Secondary tests
Ovarian failure		
Ovarian dysgenesis[a]	High FSH	Repeat FSH
Premature ovarian failure[a]	High LH	Karyotype (see p. 113)
Steroid biosynthetic defect[a]		Laparoscopy/biopsy of ovary
(Ovariectomy)		Serum oestradiol
(Chemotherapy)		HCG stimulation
Partial ovarian failure		
Resistant ovary syndrome	High LH	Serum oestradiol
Polycystic ovarian syndrome[a]	High FSH	Serum testosterone, androgens, SHBG
		Ultrasound of ovary
		Serum prolactin
		Laparoscopy and biopsy of ovary
Gonadotrophin failure		
Hypothalamic-pituitary disease[a]	Low LH	X-ray pituitary fossa
Kallmann's syndrome[a]	Low FSH	Serum oestradiol
Anorexia[a]		LHRH test
Weight loss[a]		Clomiphene test
General illness[a]		Serum thyroxine
Hypothyroidism[a]		Serum prolactin
Hyperprolactinaemia		
Prolactinoma[a]	High prolactin	Repeat prolactin (if > 2000 mU·L^{-1} then
Idiopathic hyperprolactinaemia		tumour probable)
Hypothyroidism[a]		Pituitary fossa X-ray
Polycystic ovarian disease[a]		CT scan of pituitary fossa
Drugs		Serum thyroxine
Others (Cycle defect? Other endocrine disease?)		
Hypothalamic cause[a]	Normal LH	Serum thyroxine
Weight gain/loss[a]	Normal FSH	Serum testosterone, SHBG
Mild polycystic disease	Normal prolactin	Laparoscopy and biopsy of ovary
Cushing's syndrome		
Thyrotoxicosis		
Post-pill amenorrhoea		
Androgen excess		
Gonadal tumour	High androgen	Androgen measurement (testosterone, androstenedione)
Uterine/vaginal abnormality		
Imperforate hymen[a]		Examination under anaesthesia plus
Absent uterus[a]		endometrial biopsy
Lack of endometrium		Progestogen challenge

[a] These conditions may present as primary amenorrhoea.

androgens by increasing SHBG levels when these are low. Prednisolone given in a reversed circadian manner (5 mg at night, 2.5 mg in the morning) may rarely improve hirsuties in polycystic ovarian syndrome when given alone.

Cyproterone acetate (50–200 mg/day) is an anti-androgen but is also teratogenic and a weak glucocorticoid and progestogen. Given continuously it produces amenorrhoea, and so is normally given for days 1–14 of each cycle. In women of childbearing age, contraception is essential.

Other agents of doubtful efficacy include spironolactone, bromocriptine and cimetidine.

Polycystic ovarian syndrome

PATHOPHYSIOLOGY

This very common condition, originally known in

Table 16.22 Conditions causing hirsuties.[a]

Condition	Clinical presentation	Menstruation	Investigations (results)
Hirsuties without virilization			
Familial/racial	Family history often present Long history, beginning after menarche	Normal	Normal
Idiopathic	Long history, beginning after menarche	Normal	Normal
Polycystic ovarian syndrome (mild)	Long history, beginning after menarche Sometimes acne or greasy skin	Normal to chaotic	Androgens($\uparrow$) SHBG ($\downarrow$) LH ($\uparrow$) Ultrasound of ovary
Late-onset congenital adrenal hyperplasia	Often before menarche Often short stature Sometimes acne or greasy skin	Variable	17-Hydroxyprogesterone ($\uparrow$)
Hirsuties with virilization			
Polycystic ovarian syndrome (severe)	Long history, beginning after menarche	Chaotic or amenorrhoea	Androgens ($\uparrow$) SHBG ($\downarrow$) LH ($\uparrow$) Ultrasound
Ovarian neoplasms	Short history, any adult age	Usually amenorrhoea	Ultrasound of ovary Laparoscopy and biopsy of ovary
Congenital adrenal hyperplasia	Infancy or childhood	—	17-Hydroxyprogesterone ($\uparrow$) Pregnanetriol ($\uparrow$) ACTH ($\uparrow$)
Adrenal tumours	Any age	Usually amenorrhoea	CT scan of adrenal

[a] Drugs causing hirsuties include androgens, phenytoin, diazoxide, minoxidil, cyclosporin and some progestogens.

its severe form as the Stein–Leventhal syndrome, is characterized by multiple ovarian cysts and by excess androgen production from the ovaries and adrenals, although whether the basic defect is in the ovary, adrenal or pituitary, remains unknown. The ovarian cysts represent arrested follicular development.

CLINICAL FEATURES

It is a common cause of amenorrhoea/oligomenorrhoea, hirsuties or acne, usually beginning shortly after menarche. It is sometimes associated with marked obesity. Mild virilization occurs in severe cases.

INVESTIGATION

The most accurate investigation is ovarian ultrasound, although a skilled observer is necessary and some apparently normal women show the abnormality. The typical ultrasonic features are those of a thickened capsule, multiple 3–5 mm cysts and a hyperechogenic stroma. Biochemically there are increased free androgens, though total testosterone may be normal. SHBG is low. The LH : FSH ratio is usually raised (> 2 : 1) but the FSH is normal or low. Mild hyperprolactinaemia is common but rarely exceeds 1500 mU·L^{-1}.

TREATMENT

This depends upon whether the aim is to produce fertility, regularize periods or reduce hirsuties.

- Reverse circadian rhythm prednisolone (2.5 mg in the morning, 5 mg on retiring) to suppress pituitary production of ACTH upon which adrenal androgens partly depend. Regular ovulatory cycles often ensue; hirsuties seldom respond to this treatment alone.
- Use of oestrogens/oral contraceptives for hirsuties (see above).

For fertility

- Clomiphene 50–200 mg/day from days 2–6 of cycle (or tamoxifen 10–40 mg/day) + HCG 5000 units i.m. on day 12/13. This can occasionally cause ovarian hyperstimulation and specialist supervision is necessary.
- Rarely, wedge resection or laser surgery of the ovary.

Hyperprolactinaemia

Increased prolactin levels (> 400–600 mU·L^{-1}) may be physiological, pathological or secondary to drug therapy (Table 16.23). Not all patients with galactorrhoea have hyperprolactinaemia, but the other causes are poorly understood ('normoprolactin-aemic galactorrhoea').

CLINICAL FEATURES

Hyperprolactinaemia *per se* usually presents with:

- Galactorrhoea, spontaneous or expressible (60% of cases)
- Oligo- or amenorrhoea
- Decreased libido in both sexes
- Decreased potency
- Subfertility
- Symptoms or signs of oestrogen or androgen deficiency. In the long-term osteoporosis may result
- In the peri-pubertal, as delayed or arrested puberty

Additionally, headaches and/or visual-field defects may be present if there is a pituitary tumour (more common in men).

INVESTIGATION

Once physiological and drug causes have been excluded:

Table 16.23 Causes of hyperprolactinaemia.

Physiological
Sleep (REM phase)
Pregnancy
Suckling
Nipple stimulation
Stress
Coitus

Pathological
Production by tumours
   Prolactinomas
   Occurs in some acromegalics
Interference with stalk
   Any hypothalamic/pituitary tumour
Idiopathic hyperprolactinaemia
Polycystic ovarian syndrome
Primary hypothyroidism
Chest wall injury
Renal failure
Liver failure

Drug-induced
Dopamine antagonists
   (e.g. metoclopramide and phenothiazines)
Oestrogens
Opiates
Cimetidine
Methyldopa
Reserpine

- At least three prolactin levels should be measured. Mean levels of $> 2000\text{--}3000 \text{ mU·L}^{-1}$ suggest a prolactinoma.
- A good quality skull X-ray should be obtained.
- Visual fields should be checked.
- Anterior pituitary function should be assessed if there is any clinical evidence of hypopituitarism or radiological evidence of tumour.
- A CT scan of the pituitary is necessary if there is an obvious tumour, and desirable if not. MRI may give additional detail.

Macroprolactinoma refers to tumours above 10 mm in diameter, microprolactinoma to smaller ones. The size of the prolactinoma may affect the choice of treatment.

TREATMENT

Treatment is dependent upon circumstances and facilities. Hyperprolactinaemia should be reduced with bromocriptine, a dopamine agonist. Initial doses should be small (e.g. 1.25 mg) and taken *during* food, beginning at bedtime. The dose should be gradually increased, usually to 2.5 mg three times daily, judged on clinical response and prolactin levels. Maintenance doses are 2.5–15 mg/day in divided doses. Side-effects include nausea and vomiting, dizziness and syncope, constipation and cold peripheries.

If a tumour is present this is likely to shrink with bromocriptine. Definitive therapy is controversial and will depend upon the size of the tumour, the patient's wish for fertility and local facilities.

- Trans-sphenoidal surgery often restores normo-prolactinaemia but there is a considerable late recurrence rate (50% at 5 years). Bromocriptine may produce hardening of the tumour and surgery should not be delayed beyond 2–3 months' treatment.
- Radiotherapy is only slowly effective and can sometimes cause hypopituitarism. It should, however, be used after surgery in larger tumours, especially where families are complete.
- Small tumours in asymptomatic patients may need only observation.
- Rarely, tumours enlarge during pregnancy to produce headaches and visual defects. Bromocriptine should be re-started.

ORAL CONTRACEPTION

The combined oestrogen–progestogen pill is widely used for contraception and has a low failure rate (< 1 per 100 woman-years). Current pills usually contain 20–30 µg of oestrogen, usually ethinyl-oestradiol, together with a variable amount of one of several progestogens.

The mechanisms of action is two-fold:

- Suppression by oestrogen of gonadotrophins, thus preventing follicular development, ovulation and luteinization
- Progestogen effects on cervical mucus, making it hostile to sperm

Side-effects of these preparations are shown in Table 16.24. Most of the serious side-effects are rare. While some problems require immediate cessation of the pill, the importance of other milder side-effects must be judged against the hazards of pregnancy occurring with inadequate contraception, especially if other effective methods are not practicable or acceptable. It is clear, however, that the hazards of the combined pill are much greater in women over 35, especially in smokers and those with other risk factors for cardiovascular disease (e.g. hypertension, hyperlipidaemias). The 'mini-pill' (progestogen only) is less effective but is often suitable where oestrogens are contraindicated (Table 16.24).

Table 16.24 Adverse effects and drug interactions of oral contraceptives (mixed oestrogen/progesterone combinations).

General
Weight gain
Loss of libido
Pigmentation (chloasma)
Breast tenderness
Increased growth rate of some malignancies

Cardiovascular
Increased blood pressure[a]
Deep vein thrombosis[a]
Myocardial infarction
Stroke

Gastrointestinal
Nausea and vomiting
Abnormal liver biochemistry[a]
Gallstones increased
Hepatic tumours

Nervous system
Headache
Migraine[a]
Depression[a]

Gynaecological
Amenorrhoea
'Spotting'
Cervical erosion

Haematological
Increased clotting tendency

Endocrine/metabolic
Impaired glucose tolerance
Worsened lipid profile

Drug interactions (reduced contraceptive effect due to enzyme induction)
Antibiotics
Barbiturates
Phenytoin
Carbamazepine
Rifampicin

[a] Common reasons for *stopping* oral contraceptives.

SUBFERTILITY

This term, kinder than infertility, is defined as the inability of a couple to conceive after 1 year of unprotected intercourse. Investigation requires the combined skills of gynaecologist, endocrinologist and, ideally, andrologist. Both partners must be considered and every aspect of the physiology critically examined.

CAUSES (Fig. 16.17)

- About 30% of couples have an identifiable male factor.
- Female tubal problems account for perhaps 20%; a similar proportion have ovulatory disorders.
- Inadequate intercourse, hostile cervical mucus and vaginal factors are uncommon (5%).
- 15% have no apparent explanation ('idiopathic').
- A significant proportion have both male and female problems.

CLINICAL ASSESSMENT

Both partners should be seen, *not* just the woman, and the following factors checked:

- *The man:* previous testicular damage (e.g. orchitis, trauma, undescended testes), urethral symptoms and venereal problems, local surgery and use of alcohol and drugs
- *The woman:* previous pelvic infection, regularity of periods, previous surgery, alcohol intake and smoking. Adequacy of body weight (p. 788)
- *Together:* frequency and adequacy of intercourse, use of lubricants

Examination should include an assessment of secondary sexual characteristics, body habitus and general health. In men, size and consistency of the testes are important, plus exclusion of a varicocele. In women, vaginal examination allows a check on the uterus and ovaries.

INVESTIGATION

Appropriate tests for particular defects are shown in Fig. 16.17.

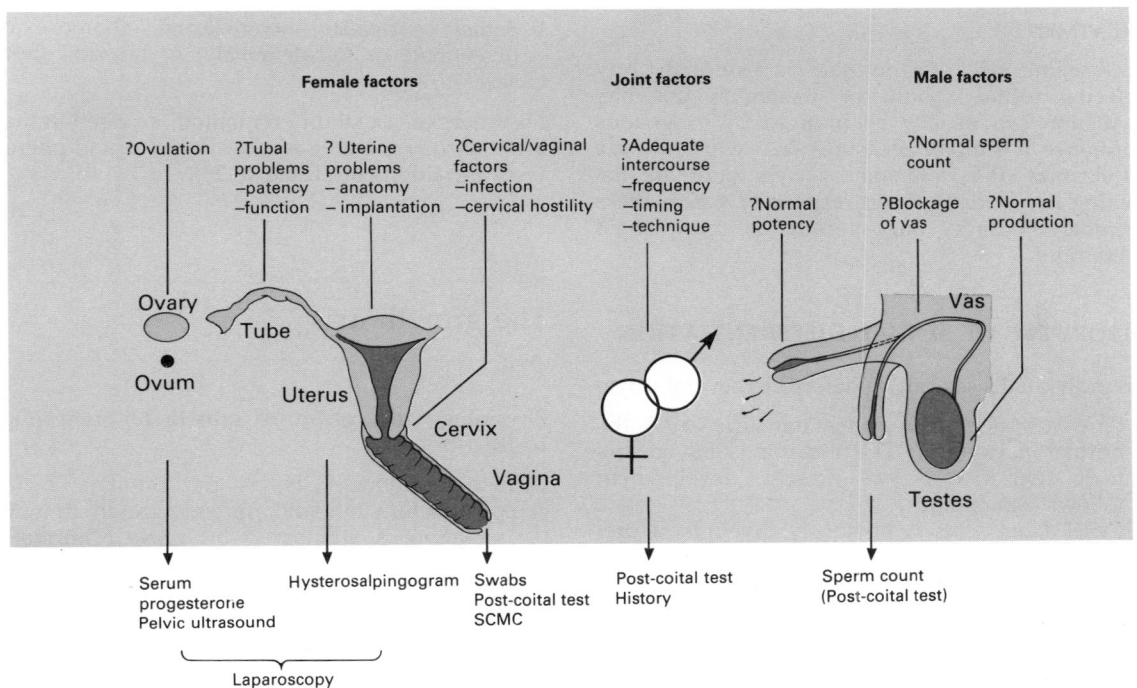

Fig. 16.17 The major factors involved in subfertility and their investigation. SCMC = sperm—cervical mucus contact test.

Table 16.25 Disorders of sexual differentiation.

Condition	Chromosomes	Gonads	Phenotype	Remarks
Turner's syndrome	45XO	Streak	Female	Often morphological features (short stature, web neck, coarctation of aorta)
Gonadal dysgenesis	46XY	Streak or minimal testes[a]	Immature female	
Congenital adrenal hyperplasia	46XX	Ovary	Female with variable virilization	Obvious androgen excess
Virilizing tumour	46XX	Ovary	Female with variable virilization	
True hermaphroditism	46XX/XY or mosaic	Testis and ovary	Male or ambiguous	
Klinefelter's syndrome	47XXY	Small testes	Male, often with gynaecomastia	Many are hypogonadal
Testicular feminization	46XY	Testes[a]	Ambiguous or infantile female	Androgen receptor defective
Testicular synthetic defects	46XY	Testes[a]	Cryptorchid, ambiguous	
5α-Reductase deficiency	46XY	Testes	Cryptorchid, ambiguous	Impaired conversion of testosterone to dihydrotesterone
Anorchia	46XY	Absent	Immature female	

[a] Gonadectomy advised because of high risk of malignancy.

TREATMENT

Counselling of both partners is essential. Any defect(s) found should be treated if possible. Ovulation can usually be induced by exogenous hormones if simpler measures fail, while *in vitro* fertilization (IVF) and similar techniques are becoming more widely used, especially where there is tubal blockage, oligospermia or unexplained subfertility.

DISORDERS OF SEXUAL DIFFERENTIATION

An individual's sex can be defined in several ways:

- *Chromosomal sex.* The normal female is 46 XX, the normal male 46 XY. The Y chromosome confers male sex; if it is not present, development follows female lines.
- *Gonadal sex.* This is obviously determined predominantly by chromosomal sex but requires normal embryological development.
- *Phenotypic sex*—the normal physical appearance and characteristics of male and female body shape. This in turn is a manifestation of gonadal sex and subsequent sex hormone production.
- *Social sex (gender)*—heavily dependent on phenotypic sex and normally assigned on appearance of the external genitalia at birth.

- *Sexual orientation*—heterosexual, homosexual (male/male or female/female) or bisexual (both sexes).

Disorders of sexual differentiation are rare but may affect chromosomal, gonadal endocrine and phenotypic development (Table 16.25).

The growth axis

Physiology and control of growth hormone (Fig. 16.18)

Growth hormone (GH) is the pituitary factor responsible for stimulation of body growth in man. Its secretion is stimulated by growth hormone releasing hormone (GHRH), released into the portal system from the hypothalamus; it is also under inhibitory control by growth hormone release inhibiting hormone (GHRIH, somatostatin). Growth hormone stimulates the hepatic production of an intermediate, somatomedin C—also known as insulin-like growth factor (IGF-1), that actually stimulates growth. Plasma levels of IGF-1, however, reflect local growth activity poorly. The metabolic actions of the system are:

- Increasing collagen and protein synthesis
- Promoting retention of calcium, phosphorus and nitrogen, necessary substrates for anabolism
- Opposing the action of insulin

Growth hormone release is intermittent and mainly nocturnal, especially during sleep. The frequency and size of GH pulses increase during the growth spurt of adolescence and decline thereafter. Acute stress and exercise both stimulate GH release while, in the normal subject, hyperglycaemia suppresses it.

Normal growth

Factors other than GH involved in linear growth in the human are:

- *Genetic.* Children of two short parents will probably be short
- *Nutritional.* Adequate nutrients must be available; impaired growth can result from inadequate dietary intake or small-bowel disease (e.g. coeliac disease)
- *General health.* Any serious systemic disease in childhood is likely to reduce growth (e.g. renal failure)
- *Emotional deprivation and psychological factors.* These can impair growth by complex, poorly understood mechanisms

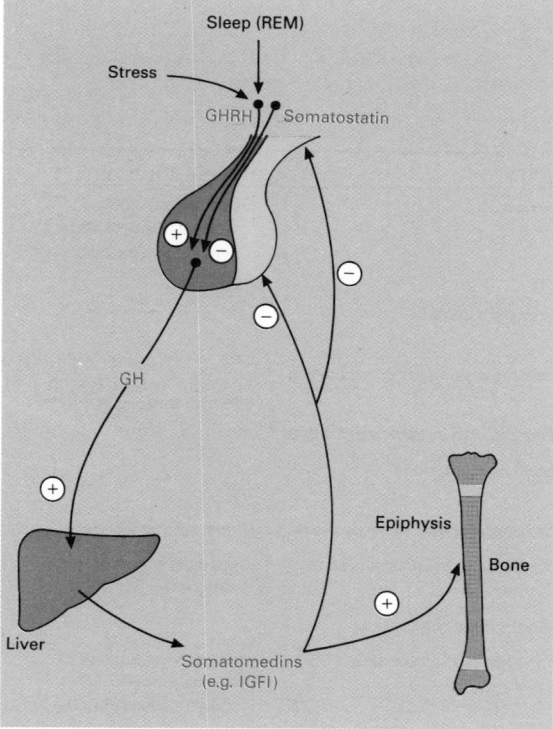

Fig. 16.18 The control of growth hormone and somatomedin secretion.

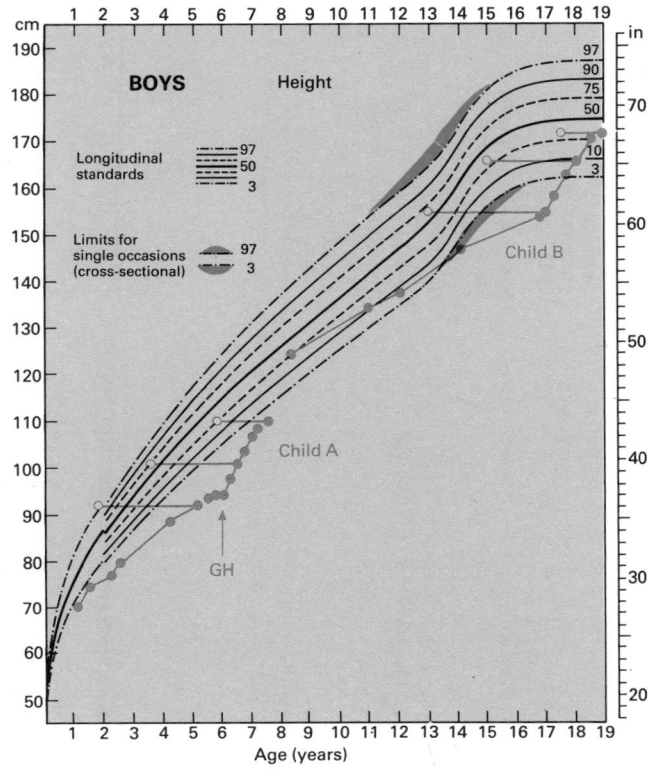

Fig. 16.19 A height chart for boys. Child A illustrates the course of a child with hypopituitarism, initially treated with cortisol and thyroxine, but showing growth only after growth hormone treatment. The open circles show the data corrected for bone age. (Based on a Tanner–Whitehouse chart, reference 1A, reproduced by permission of Castlemead Publications.)

Assessment of growth

Charts showing the range of height and weight with age for normal British children are available (Fig. 16.19). Height must be measured very carefully, ideally at the same time of day on the same instrument by the same observer.

In general, there are three overlapping phases of growth: infantile (0–2 years), which appears largely substrate (food) dependent; childhood (2–puberty), which is largely GH dependent; and the adolescent 'growth spurt', dependent on GH and sex hormones.

More important than current height is height velocity, which requires at least two measurements some months apart and, ideally, multiple serial measurements. This is a rate of *current* growth (cm/year), while attained height is largely dependent upon *previous* growth. Standard deviation scores (SDS) based on the degree of deviation from age–sex norms are widely used by experts—these and growth velocities are far more sensitive than simple charts in assessing growth.

The future height of a child can be predicted approximately from the parental heights ('midparental height'):

- *For a boy*, 13 cm (5 inches) is added to his mother's height and the mean parental height is then calculated.

- *For a girl*, 13 cm (5 inches) is subtracted from the father's height before taking the mean.

Thus, for a boy with a father of 5 ft 10 in and mother of 5 ft 1 in, the corrected heights are 5 ft 10 in and 5 ft 6 in—his predicted height is 5 ft 8 in. A daughter of the same parents would be expected to be 5 ft 3 in (mean of 5 ft 5 in and 5 ft 1 in).

GROWTH FAILURE—SHORT STATURE

When a child or his parents complain of short stature particular attention should focus on:

- Possible systemic disorder—especially small-bowel disease
- Evidence of skeletal or other congenital abnormalities
- Endocrine status—particularly primary hypothyroidism
- Dietary intake and use of drugs, especially steroids for asthma
- Emotional, psychological, family and school problems

School, clinic and home records of height and weight should be obtained if possible to allow growth-velocity calculation. If unavailable, such data must be obtained prospectively.

Table 16.26 Clinical features of common causes of short stature.

	Family history	Growth pattern	Clinical features	Time of puberty	Bone age	Remarks
Constitutional delay	Often present	Rather slow from birth	Immature but appropriate	Late but spontaneous	Moderate delay but maturing	Often difficult to differentiate from GH deficiency; growth velocity measurement vital
Familial short stature	Positive	Slow from birth	Normal	Normal	Normal	Need heights of all family members
GH insufficiency	Rare	Slow	Immature, often overweight	Delayed	Moderate to marked delay; not progressing	Early investigation and treatment vital; increased suspicion if child is plump
Primary hypothyroidism	Rare	Slow	Immature	Delayed	Markedly delayed	Measure TSH and T_4 in all cases of short stature; clear clinical signs often not present
Small-bowel disease	Sometimes	Slow	Immature, usually thin for height	Delayed	Delayed	Diarrhoea plus macrocytosis/anaemia; occasionally no gastrointestinal symptoms

---

Problems of growth and development

History
Rate of growth (home/school records, e.g. heights on kitchen door)
Change in appearance (old photos)
Change in shoe/glove/hat size
Age of appearance of pubic hair, breasts, menarche

Physical signs
Evidence of systemic disease
Body size, relative weight, proportions (span versus height)
Skin thickness, interdental separation
Facial features
Spade hands/feet
Grading of secondary sexual characteristics

A child with normal growth velocity is unlikely to have significant endocrine disease. However, low growth velocity without apparent systemic cause requires further investigation. Sudden cessation of growth suggests major physical disease; if no gastrointestinal, respiratory, renal or skeletal abnormality is apparent, then a cerebral tumour or hypothyroidism are likeliest. Slow-growing children require full endocrine assessment.

Features of the commoner causes of growth failure are given in Table 16.26.

INVESTIGATION

Systemic disease having been excluded, the following should be undertaken:

- *Thyroid function tests:* serum TSH and T_4 to exclude hypothyroidism
- *GH status:* basal levels are of little value. The GH response to bovril, exercise, clonidine, arginine and insulin are all used; a normal peak response is > 20 mU·L^{-1}. The most useful test is the insulin tolerance test (ITT). In early puberty the ITT is most usefully performed after stilboestrol priming, which enhances the GH response to hypoglycaemia.
- *Assessment of bone age:* left hand and wrist X-rays allow assessment of bone age; the knee, the state of epiphyseal closure.

TREATMENT

- Systemic illness should be treated.
- Primary hypothyroidism: replace with thyroxine 0.05–0.2 mg/day.
- GH insufficiency: human GH was previously used but was withdrawn as cases of Creutzfeld–Jacob disease were reported. It has been superseded by (very expensive) recombinant GH, which is given as nightly injection in doses of 10–20 units/m^2 of body surface area. GHRH has

been used experimentally. Treatment should be supervised in expert centres.

GROWTH HORMONE EXCESS—GIGANTISM AND ACROMEGALY

Growth hormone stimulates skeletal and soft-tissue growth. GH excess therefore produces gigantism in children (if acquired before epiphyseal fusion) but acromegaly in adults.

Tall stature

The commonest cause is hereditary (two tall parents!) or idiopathic (constitutional). It can occasionally be due to thyrotoxicosis. GH excess is a very rare cause and is usually clinically apparent.

Acromegaly

This is due to a pituitary tumour in almost all cases. Hyperplasia due to GHRH excess is rare.

CLINICAL FEATURES

Symptoms and signs of acromegaly are shown in Fig. 16.20. One-third of patients present with changes in appearance, one-quarter with visual-field defects or headaches; in the remainder the diagnosis is made by an alert observer in another clinic, e.g. diabetic, hypertension, dental, dermatology.

INVESTIGATIONS

- GH is normally undetectable in adults except during stress or as occasional spikes but, unless levels are always below 1 mU·L^{-1}, one cannot exclude the diagnosis. Only IRMA assays have this degree of sensitivity.
- The glucose tolerance test is diagnostic. Acromegalics fail to suppress GH below 1 mU·L^{-1}; about 25% of acromegalics have a diabetic glucose tolerance test.
- Lateral skull X-rays: abnormal in 90% as the tumours are relatively large.
- Visual fields: field defects are common.
- High-resolution CT scans are virtually never normal and MRI often gives even better definition of tumour extent.
- Pituitary function: partial or complete anterior hypopituitarism is common.
- Prolactin: hyperprolactinaemia occurs in 30% of patients.

MANAGEMENT AND TREATMENT

Untreated acromegaly results in markedly reduced survival with most deaths from heart failure, coronary artery disease and hypertension related

Symptoms of acromegaly

Change in appearance
Increased size of hands/feet
Headaches
Visual deterioration
Tiredness
Weight gain
Amenorrhoea/oligomenorrhoea
Galactorrhoea
Impotence or poor libido
Deep voice
Goitre
Breathlessness
Excessive sweating
Pain/tingling in hands
Polyuria/polydipsia
Muscular weakness
Joint pains

Old photographs are frequently useful.
Symptoms of hypopituitarism may be
  present as well.

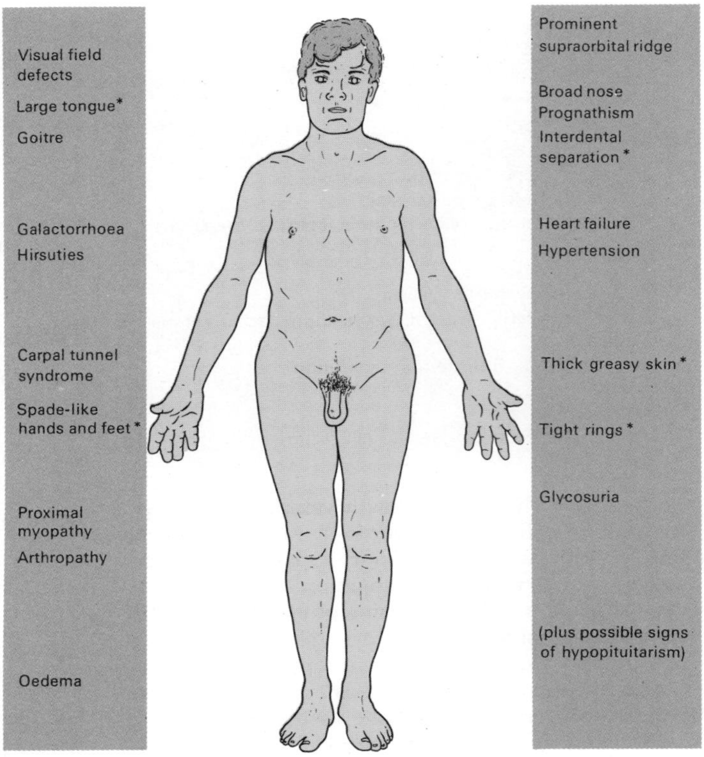

Visual field defects
Large tongue*
Goitre

Galactorrhoea
Hirsuties

Carpal tunnel syndrome
Spade-like hands and feet*

Proximal myopathy
Arthropathy

Oedema

Prominent supraorbital ridge

Broad nose
Prognathism
Interdental separation*

Heart failure
Hypertension

Thick greasy skin*

Tight rings*

Glycosuria

(plus possible signs of hypopituitarism)

(plus signs of hypopituitarism)

Fig. 16.20 The signs of acromegaly.
Asterisks indicate signs of greater discriminant
value.

causes. Treatment is therefore indicated in all
except the elderly or those with minimal abnormalities. The general pros and cons of surgery,
radiotherapy and medical treatment are discussed
above (p. 777).

Preferred treatment is controversial and complete cure is often slow, if possible at all. The
choice lies between:

- Trans-sphenoidal surgery with subsequent
  radiotherapy if excision is incomplete. Many
  authorities would give postoperative radiotherapy in nearly all cases, as the tumours
  frequently recur.
- Transfrontal surgery for big tumours with pressure effects. Postoperative radiotherapy is again
  usually given.
- External radiotherapy (takes 3–10 years to be
  effective) plus bromocriptime.
- A synthetic analogue of somatostatin (GHRIH—
  p. 772) called octreotide is now the treatment of
  choice. It has to be given by subcutaneous
  injection in doses of 50–200 µg 8-hourly but may
  be associated with mild steatorrhoea and an
  increased incidence of gallstones. It is extremely
  expensive.
- Bromocriptine alone, usually reserved for the
  elderly and frail. It can be given to shrink
  tumours prior to definitive therapy or to control
  symptoms and persisting GH secretion. It is
  probably only effective in mixed somatotroph

and mammotroph tumours. The dose is 10–60
mg/day (higher than for prolactinomas) but
should start slowly (see Hyperprolactinaemia). It
has largely been replaced by octreotide.

Hypopituitarism should be corrected and concurrent diabetes and/or hypertension should be treated conventionally; both usually improve with
treatment of the acromegaly.

The thyroid axis

The metabolic rate of many tissues is controlled by
the thyroid hormones, and overactivity and underactivity of the gland pose common clinical problems.

Anatomy

The gland consists of two lateral lobes connected
by an isthmus. It is closely attached to the thyroid
cartilages and to the upper end of the trachea, and
thus moves on swallowing. It is often palpable in
normal women.

Embryologically it originates from the base of
the tongue and descends to the middle of the neck.
Remnants of thyroid tissue can sometimes be

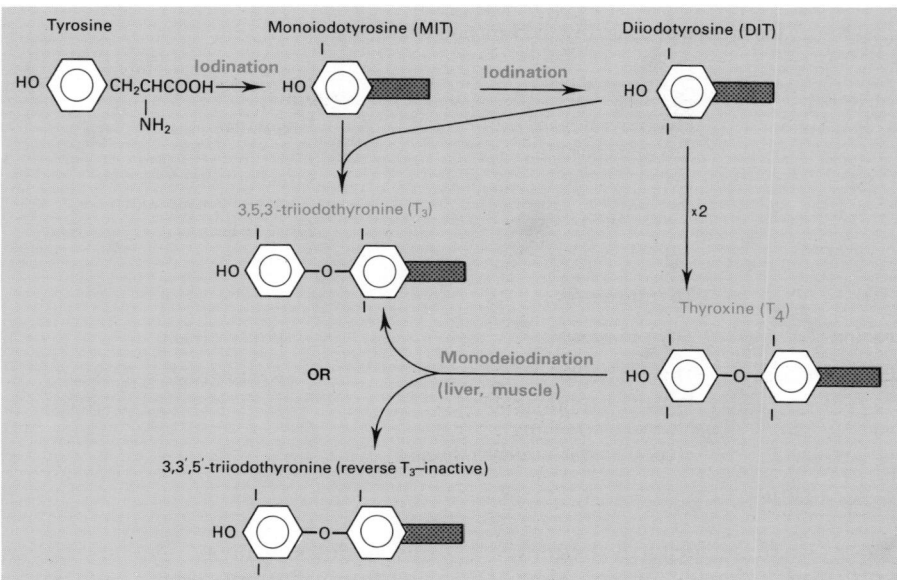

Fig. 16.21 The synthesis and metabolism of the thyroid hormones. The shaded areas denote the side-chain shown for tyrosine.

found at the base of the tongue (lingual thyroid) and along the line of descent. The gland has a rich blood supply from superior and inferior thyroid arteries.

The thyroid consists of follicles lined by cuboidal epithelioid cells. Inside is the colloid, which is an iodinated glycoprotein, thyroglobulin, synthesized by the follicular cells. Each follicle is surrounded by basement membrane, between which are parafollicular cells containing calcitonin-secreting C cells.

Table 16.27 Factors affecting thyroxine-binding globulin (TBG) levels.

Increased TBG
Hereditary
Pregnancy
Oestrogen therapy
Oral contraceptive use
Hypothyroidism
Phenothiazines
Acute viral hepatitis

Decreased TBG
Hereditary
Androgens
Corticosteroid excess
Thyrotoxicosis
Nephrotic syndrome
Major illness
Malnutrition
Chronic liver disease

Drugs causing altered binding
Non-steroidal anti-inflammatory drugs
Phenytoin

Biochemistry

The thyroid hormones, thyroxin (T_4) and triiodothyronine (T_3) are synthesized within the gland (Fig. 16.21).

More T_4 than T_3 is produced but T_4 is converted in some peripheral tissues (liver, kidney and muscle) to the more active T_3 by 5'-monodeiodination; an alternative 3'-monodeiodination yields the inactive reverse T_3 (rT_3).

In plasma, more than 99% of all T_4 and T_3 is bound to hormone-binding proteins (thyroxine-binding globulin, TBG; thyroid-binding pre-albumin, TBPA, and albumin). Only free hormone is available for tissue action, where T_3 binds to specific nuclear receptors within the cell. Factors affecting TBG are shown in Table 16.27.

Physiology of the hypothalamic–pituitary–thyroid axis (Fig. 16.2)

- Thyrotrophin-releasing hormone (TRH) is released in the hypothalamus and stimulates release of thyroid-stimulating hormone (TSH) from the pituitary.
- TSH stimulates the TSH receptor in the thyroid to increase synthesis of both T_4 and T_3 and also to release stored hormone, producing increased plasma levels of T_4 and T_3.
- T_4 and T_3 feed back on the pituitary and perhaps hypothalamus to reduce TRH and TSH secretion.

Thyroid function tests

Radioimmunoassays for total T_4, free T_4, Total T_3, free T_3 and IRMAs for TSH are widely available.

Table 16.28 Advantages and limitations of usual thyroid function tests.

Test	Most useful in	Not useful or possibly misleading in
Total thyroxine (T$_4$)	Hypothyroidism[a] Thyrotoxicosis[a]	Pregnancy Oestrogen therapy Oral contraceptive use 'Sick euthyroid syndrome' Drug therapy, e.g. NSAIDs Neonates
Free thyroxine (T$_4$)	Thyrotoxicosis	
Total triiodothyronine (T$_3$)	Thyrotoxicosis[a]	Hypothyroidism
TSH (immunoradiometric assay)	Thyrotoxicosis[a] Primary hypothyroidism[a] Neonatal screening[a] Hypothalamic-pituitary disease	'Sick euthyroid' syndrome Early in treatment of toxicosis

[a] Tests of first choice in this situation.

There are only minor significant circadian rhythms, and measurements may be made at any time. Particular uses of the tests are summarized in Table 16.28.

Tests include:

- *TSH measurement.* IRMAs for TSH now differentiate between normal and low levels and TSH levels now thus discriminate between hyperthyroidism, hypothyroidism and euthyroidism (Table 16.28). There are pitfalls, however. These are mainly with hypopituitarism, with the 'sick euthyroid' syndrome and with dysthyroid eye disease, all of which may give 'false' (i.e. misleading, not incorrect) low results implying hyperthyroidism. As a single test of thyroid function it is the most sensitive in most circumstances but most laboratories prefer to perform at least two tests—serum T$_3$ or free T$_3$ where hyperthyroidism is suspected, serum T$_4$ or free T$_4$ where hypothyroidism is likely.
- *Thyroid hormone uptake tests* (THUT) are now used much less. There are many forms of this measurement of free protein-binding sites, used to calculate the 'free thyroxine index' (FTI). Depending on the method of calculation, high values may imply hypothyroidism or hyperthyroidism; check with your laboratory. TBG is sometimes measured directly.
- *'Free' T$_4$ tests* attempt to measure only the unbound active hormone. They thus avoid the need for thyroid hormone uptake tests and calculation of the FTI. Though not perfect, many of them are adequate for clinical use.
- *TRH test.* This has been rendered almost obsolete except for investigation of hypothalamic–pituitary dysfunction. Primary hypothyroid patients show a high basal TSH level with an excessive rise; hyperthyroid subjects show suppression with a minimal increment of TSH. Flat responses are also seen with solitary autonomous nodules, Graves' eye disease and excessive thyroxine replacement, and in patients on steroids or with Cushing's syndrome.

Problems in interpretation of thyroid function tests
There are three major areas of difficulty.

Serious acute or chronic illness. Thyroid function is affected in several ways, with reduced concentra-

Table 16.29 Causes of hypothyroidism.

Primary
Congenital
  Agenesis
  Ectopic thyroid remnants

Defects of hormone synthesis
  Iodine deficiency
  Dyshormonogenesis
  Antithyroid drugs
  Other drugs, e.g. lithium, amiodarone

Autoimmune
  Atrophic thyroiditis
  Hashimoto's thyroiditis

Infective
  Post subacute thyroiditis

Post-surgery

Post-irradiation
  ^{131}I therapy
  External neck irradiation

Infiltration
  Tumour

Peripheral resistance to thyroid hormone

Secondary
Hypopituitarism
Isolated TSH deficiency

tion and affinity of binding proteins, decreased peripheral conversion of T_4 to T_3, with more rT_3 and reduced hypothalamic–pituitary TSH production. Systemically ill patients can therefore have an apparently low total and free T_4 and T_3 with a normal or low basal TSH (the 'sick euthyroid' syndrome). Levels are usually only mildly below normal and the tests should be repeated after resolution of the underlying illness.

Pregnancy and oral contraceptives. These lead to greatly increased TBG and thus to high or high–normal total T_4 and high THUT levels. The normal physiological changes during pregnancy are not fully understood but rarely cause clinical problems.

Drugs. Many drugs affect thyroid function tests by interfering with protein binding. The commonest are listed in Table 16.29. Basal TSH should be measured.

Thyroid autoimmunity

Antibodies to the thyroid are common and may be either destructive or stimulating; both occasionally coexist in the same patient.

Destructive antibodies may be directed against the microsomes or against thyroglobulin; the antigen for thyroid microsomal antibodies has now been identified as the peroxidase enzyme. They may be detected by haemagglutination techniques and affect up to 20% of the population, especially older women, but only 10–20% of these develop overt hypothyroidism.

A heterogenous group of stimulatory antibodies, termed thyroid-stimulating immunoglobulin/antibody (TSI, TSAb), also exist. These may stimulate the TSH receptor, producing Graves' disease and/or increase cell division and goitre formation.

Long-acting thyroid stimulator (LATS) and LATS-protector (LATS-P) have also been described but bear little correlation to clinical thyroid disease.

HYPOTHYROIDISM

PATHOPHYSIOLOGY

Underactivity of the thyroid may be *primary*, from disease of the thyroid or *secondary* to hypothalamic–pituitary disease (reduced TSH drive) (Table 16.29).

Causes of primary hypothyroidism
Atrophic (autoimmune) hypothyroidism. This is the commonest cause of hypothyroidism and is associated with microsomal autoantibodies leading to lymphoid infiltration of the gland and eventual atrophy and fibrosis. It is six times more common in females and the incidence increases with age. The condition is associated with other autoimmune disease such as pernicious anaemia.

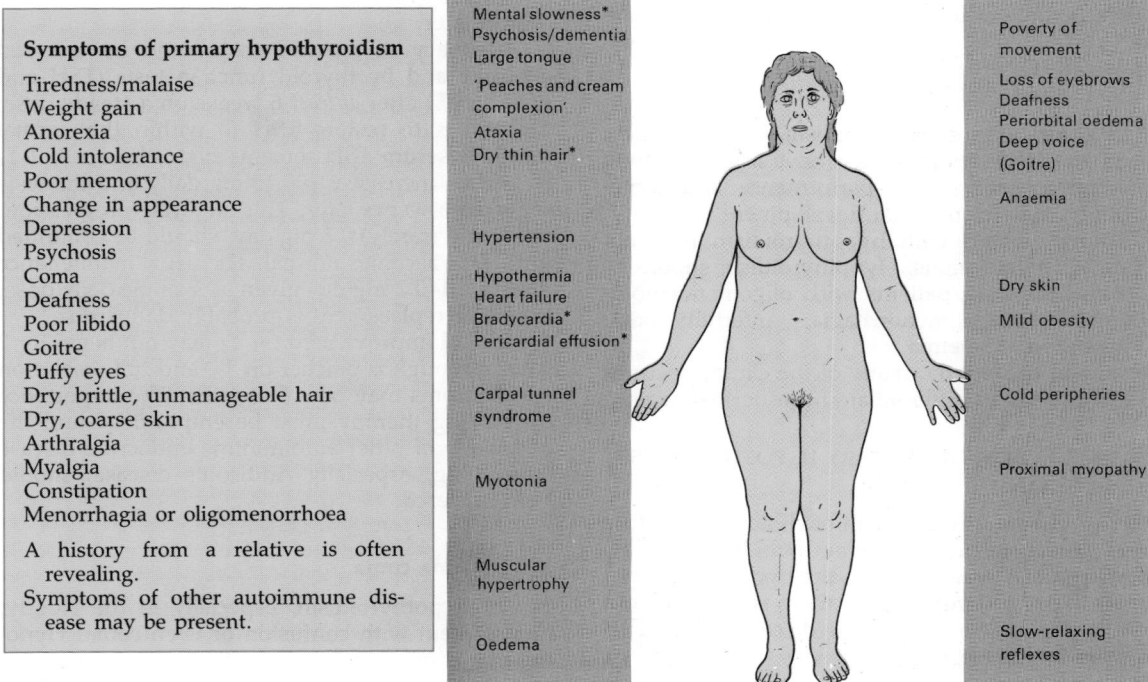

Symptoms of primary hypothyroidism
Tiredness/malaise
Weight gain
Anorexia
Cold intolerance
Poor memory
Change in appearance
Depression
Psychosis
Coma
Deafness
Poor libido
Goitre
Puffy eyes
Dry, brittle, unmanageable hair
Dry, coarse skin
Arthralgia
Myalgia
Constipation
Menorrhagia or oligomenorrhoea
A history from a relative is often revealing.
Symptoms of other autoimmune disease may be present.

Mental slowness*
Psychosis/dementia
Large tongue
'Peaches and cream complexion'
Ataxia
Dry thin hair*

Hypertension

Hypothermia
Heart failure
Bradycardia*
Pericardial effusion*

Carpal tunnel syndrome

Myotonia

Muscular hypertrophy

Oedema

Poverty of movement

Loss of eyebrows
Deafness
Periorbital oedema
Deep voice
(Goitre)

Anaemia

Dry skin

Mild obesity

Cold peripheries

Proximal myopathy

Slow-relaxing reflexes

Fig. 16.22 The signs of hypothyroidism. Asterisks indicate signs of greater discriminant value.

Hashimoto's thyroiditis. This form of autoimmune thyroiditis, again commoner in women and commonest in late middle age, produces atrophic changes with regeneration, leading to goitre formation. This is usually firm and rubbery but may range from soft to hard. Thyroid microsomal antibodies are again present, often in very high titres. Patients may be hypothyroid or euthyroid. Thyroxine therapy may shrink the goitre even when the patient is not hypothyroid, though this may take a long time.

Iodine deficiency. In mountainous areas (the Alps, Himalayas, South America, Central Africa) dietary iodine deficiency still exists. Goitre, occasionally massive, is common and was formerly seen in the UK as 'Derbyshire neck'. The patients may be euthyroid or hypothyroid depending on the severity of iodine deficiency.

Dyshormonogenesis. This rare condition is due to genetic defects in the synthesis of thyroid hormones; patients develop hypothyroidism with a goitre. One particular familial form is associated with sensorineural deafness (Pendred's syndrome).

CLINICAL FEATURES (Fig. 16.22)

Hypothyroidism may produce many symptoms. The classical picture of the slow, dry-haired, thick-skinned, deep-voiced patient with weight gain, cold intolerance, bradycardia and constipation makes the diagnosis easy; the term 'myxoedema' refers to the accumulation of mucopolysaccharide in subcutaneous tissues. Milder symptoms are, however, more common.

Special difficulties in diagnosis may arise:

- Children with hypothyroidism may not show classical features but often have a slow growth velocity, poor school performance and sometimes arrest of pubertal development.
- Young women with hypothyroidism may not show obvious signs. Hypothyroidism should be excluded in all patients with oligomenorrhoea/amenorrhoea, menorrhagia, infertility and hyperprolactinaemia.
- Among the elderly, many of the clinical features are difficult to differentiate from normal ageing.

INVESTIGATION OF PRIMARY HYPOTHYROIDISM (Table 16.28)

TSH is now the investigation of choice; a high TSH level confirms primary hypothyroidism. A low total or free T_4 level confirms the hypothyroid state and is especially important if there is any evidence of hypothalamic and pituitary disease, when TSH may be low or normal.

Thyroid and other organ-specific antibodies may be present. Other abnormalities include:

- Anaemia. This is usually normochromic and normocytic in type but it may be macrocytic (sometimes this is due to associated pernicious anaemia) or microcytic (in women, due to menorrhagia).
- Increased aspartate transferase levels, from muscle and/or liver.
- Increased creatine kinase levels.
- Hypercholesterolaemia.
- Hyponatraemia due to an increase in antidiuretic hormome (ADH) and impaired free water clearance.

TREATMENT

Replacement therapy with thyroxine (T_4) is given for life. The starting dose will depend upon the age and fitness of the patient, especially cardiac performance. In the young and fit, 0.1 mg/day is suitable, while 0.05 mg/day is more appropriate for the old or frail. T_3 offers no significant advantage over T_4.

Patients with ischaemic heart disease require even lower initial doses, especially if the hypothyroidism is severe and long-standing.

Most physicians would begin with 0.025 mg/day and perform serial ECGs, increasing the dose at 2–6 week intervals if angina does not occur or worsen and the ECG does not deteriorate. Some however, would use T_3 beginning with 2.5–5 µg 8-hourly, doubling the dose every 48 h up to 10 µg three times daily. If progress is satisfactory, T_4 (0.1 mg/day) is then started and T_3 is discontinued 5 days later.

Adequacy of replacement should be assessed clinically and by thyroid function tests (TSH and possibly T_4) after *at least* 6 weeks on a steady dose; the aim is to restore TSH to within the normal range. If serum TSH remains high, the dose of T_4 should be increased to 0.15 mg daily and the tests repeated 6 weeks later. This stepwise progression, to 0.2 and (rarely) 0.3 mg/day, should be continued until TSH becomes normal. The usual maintenance dose is 0.1–0.2 mg/day given as a single daily dose; excessive replacement is probably dangerous.

Clinical improvement on T_4 may not begin for 2 weeks, though is quicker on T_3, and full resolution of symptoms may take 6 months. The importance of life-long therapy must be emphasized and the possibility of other autoimmune endocrine disease developing, especially Addison's disease, should be considered.

Myxoedema coma

Severe hypothyroidism, especially in the elderly, may present with confusion or even coma. Hypothermia is often present and the patient may have severe cardiac failure, hypoventilation, hypoglycaemia and hyponatraemia.

The mortality was previously at least 50% and patients require full intensive care. Optimal treatment is controversial, physicians advising tri-iodothyronine (T_3) orally or i.v. in doses beginning as low as 2.5 µg every 8 hours; 2.5–5 µg 8-hourly is probably most suitable. Large i.v. doses should *not* be used.

Additional measures should include:

- Oxygen (by ventilation if necessary)
- Monitoring of cardiac output and pressures via Swan–Ganz catheter
- Gradual re-warming
- Hydrocortisone 100 mg i.v. 8-hourly
- Dextrose infusion to prevent hypoglycaemia

'Myxoedema madness'

Depression is common but occasionally with severe hypothyroidism in the elderly the patient may become frankly demented or psychotic, sometimes with striking delusions. This may occur shortly *after* starting thyroxine replacement.

Screening for hypothyroidism

The incidence of congenital hypothyroidism is approximately 1 : 3500 births. Untreated, severe hypothyroidism leads to permanent neurological and intellectual damage ('cretinism'). Routine screening of the newborn using a blood-spot, as in the Guthrie test, to detect a high TSH level as an indicator of primary hypothyroidism is efficient; cretinism is prevented if thyroxine is started within the first few months of life.

Screening of elderly patients is controversial but there is little doubt that the incidence of unsuspected thyroid disease in those over 65 years is 1–3%. With this and undiagnosed hyperthyroidism many physicians believe in screening of all elderly hospital attenders.

GOITRE (THYROID ENLARGEMENT)

Goitre is more common in women than in men and may be either physiological or pathological.

CLINICAL FEATURES

Most commonly a goitre is noticed as a cosmetic defect by the patient or by friends or relatives. The majority are painless but pain or discomfort can occur in acute varieties. Goitres can produce dysphagia and difficulty in breathing, implying oesophageal or tracheal compression.

Clinical examination should record the size, shape, consistency and mobility of the gland as well as whether its lower margin can be demarcated (thus implying the absence or retrosternal extension). A bruit may be present. Associated

Table 16.30 Causes of goitre.

Physiological
Puberty
Pregnancy

Autoimmune
Graves' disease
Hashimoto's disease

Thyroiditis
Acute (de Quervain's thyroiditis)
Chronic fibrotic (Reidel's thyroiditis)

Iodine deficiency (endemic goitre)

Dyshormonogenesis

Goitrogens (e.g. sulphonylureas)

Multinodular goitre

Diffuse goitre
Colloid
Simple

Cysts

Tumours
Adenomas
Carcinoma
Lymphoma

Miscellaneous
Sarcoidosis
Tuberculosis

lymph nodes should be sought and the tracheal position determined if possible. Examination should never omit an assessment of the patient's clinical thyroid status.

Specific enquiry should be made about any medication, especially iodine-containing preparations.

ASSESSMENT

Two facts are essential about any goitre: its pathological nature and the patient's thyroid status.

The nature can often be judged clinically. Goitres are usually separable into diffuse and nodular types, the causes of which differ (Table 16.30).

Particular points of note are:

- *Puberty and pregnancy* may produce a diffuse increase in size of the thyroid.
- *In Graves' disease* (autoimmune hyperthyroidism) the gland is again diffusely enlarged, often somewhat firm and frequently associated with a bruit.
- *Acute tenderness* in a diffuse swelling, sometimes severe pain, is suggestive of an acute viral thyroiditis (de Quervain's). This is usually asso-

ciated with a systemic viral illness and may produce transient clinical hyperthyroidism with an increase in serum T_4.

- *Pain* in a goitre may be caused by thyroiditis, bleeding into a cyst or (rarely) a thyroid tumour.
- *Simple goitre:* in this instance no clear cause is found for enlargement of the thyroid, which is usually smooth and soft. It may be associated with thyroid growth-stimulating antibodies.
- *Nodular goitres* may have multiple or solitary nodules. Commonest is the multinodular goitre, especially in older patients. The patient is usually euthyroid but may be hyperthyroid. Multinodular goitre is the commonest cause of tracheal and/or oesophageal compression and may cause laryngeal nerve palsy. It may also extend retrosternally.
- *Solitary nodules* present a difficult problem. A history of pain, rapid enlargement or associated lymph nodes in such a situation suggests the possibility of thyroid carcinoma. The majority of such nodules are, however, cystic or benign and, indeed, may simply be the largest solitary nodule of a multinodular goitre. Risk factors for malignancy include previous irradiation, long-standing iodine deficiency and occasional familial cases. Solitary toxic nodules (Plummers's syndrome) are quite uncommon and may be associated with T_3 production.
- *Fibrotic goitre* (Reidel's thyroiditis): this rare condition usually producing a 'woody' gland is associated with other midline fibrosis and is often difficult to distinguish from carcinoma, being irregular and hard.
- *Excessive doses of carbimazole* or propyl-thiouracil will induce goitre.
- *Iodine deficiency* and dyshormonogenesis (see above) can also cause goitre.
- Rarely the thyroid is the site of a *metastatic* deposit or the site of origin of a lymphoma.

INVESTIGATION

Clinical findings will dictate appropriate initial tests:

- *Thyroid function tests.* TSH plus T_4 or T_3 (Table 16.28).
- *Chest and thoracic inlet X-rays* to detect tracheal compression and large retrosternal extensions.
- *Thyroid scan (iodine or technetium).* This should be done whenever any doubt remains as to the nature of a lesion or when retrosternal extension is suspected. It demonstrates active thyroid tissue and is most useful for single toxic nodules (with suppression of the remaining gland uptake) and multinodular goitres. 'Cold' areas (without uptake) are likely to be cysts, fibrotic areas or tumours. The chance of a 'cold nodule' being malignant is about 10%. Iodine scans are particularly useful in demonstrating retrosternal

extension, ectopic thyroid tissue and biologically active thyroid carcinoma.
- *Ultrasound scan.* This technique, with improving resolution, can distinguish cystic from solid thyroid nodules; completely cystic lesions are very rarely malignant.
- *Fine-needle biopsy.* With fine needles and cytology in expert hands this technique is of increasing value. Local complications are rare. The risk of missing small areas of malignant change in cold nodules, theoretically high, has not proved to be so.

TREATMENT

During puberty and pregnancy a goitre associated with euthyroidism rarely requires intervention. If euthyroid, the patient should be reassured that spontaneous resolution is likely.

In other situations the patient should be rendered euthyroid.

Indications for surgical intervention are:

- *The possibility of malignancy.* A history of rapid growth, pain, cervical lymphadenopathy or previous irradiation to the neck warrant exploration. Until recently most physicians have advised removal of all 'cold nodules' because of the 10% risk of carcinoma. Needle biopsy/cytology render this unnecessary.
- *Pressure symptoms* on the trachea or, more rarely, oesophagus also warrant surgery. The possibility of retrosternal extension should be excluded.
- *Cosmetic reasons.* A large goitre is often a considerable anxiety to the patient even though functionally and anatomically benign.

THYROID CARCINOMA

The different types of thyroid carcinoma, their characteristics and treatment are listed in Table 16.31. The tumour is relatively uncommon, being responsible for 400 deaths annually in the UK.

Particular points are:

- *Papillary and follicular carcinomas* may take up iodine, shown by scanning. Such patients after total thyroidectomy may be given a therapeutic radioiodine dose, which will be taken up by remaining thyroid tissue or metastatic lesions. Replacement thyroxine will subsequently be needed and should suppress TSH, which may otherwise stimulate any residual differentiated carcinoma. Lungs and bone are the commonest sites of metastases, while local invasion is often a problem. The measurement of thyroglobulin in plasma has been used as a tumour marker for the presence of neoplastic tissue.
- *Anaplastic carcinomas* and lymphoma do not respond to radioactive iodine.

Table 16.31 Types of thyroid malignancy.

Cell type	Frequency	Behaviour	Spread	Prognosis
Papillary	70%	Occurs in young people, slow-growing	Local, sometimes lung/bone secondaries	Good, especially in young
Follicular	20%	Commoner in females	Metastases to lung/bone	Good if resected
Anaplastic	< 5%	Aggressive	Locally invasive	Very poor
Lymphoma	< 2%	Variable		Sometimes responsive to radiotherapy
Medullary cell	5%	Often familial	Local and metastases	Poor

● *Medullary carcinoma*, often associated with multiple endocrine neoplasia (see p. 830), is usually treated by total thyroidectomy. The patient's family should be screened for this and other endocrine neoplastic conditions.

HYPERTHYROIDISM

Hyperthyroidism is common, affecting perhaps 2–5% of all females at some time. Nearly all cases are caused by intrinsic thyroid disease; a pituitary cause is extremely rare (Table 16.32).

Graves' disease

This, the commonest cause, is an autoimmune process in which serum IgG antibodies bind to the thyroid TSH receptor and produce stimulation of thyroid hormone production, behaving like TSH. The antibodies, known as thyroid-stimulating immunoglobulins or antibodies (TSI or TSAb) may now be measured in serum.

Associated with the thyroid disease in many cases are eye changes (see below) and other signs such as vitiligo and pretibial myxoedema. Rarely lymphadenopathy and splenomegaly may occur. Graves' disease is also associated with other autoimmune disorders such as pernicious anaemia and myasthenia gravis.

The natural history is one of fluctuation, many patients showing a pattern of alternating relapse and remission; perhaps only 40% of subjects have a single episode.

Toxic solitary adenoma/nodule (Plummer's disease)

This is the cause of about 5% of cases of hyperthyroidism. It does not usually remit after a course of antithyroid drugs.

Toxic multinodular goitre

This commonly occurs in older women; again antithyroid drugs are rarely successful in inducing a remission.

CLINICAL FEATURES OF HYPERTHYROIDISM

The symptoms of hyperthyroidism affect many systems; they and relevant signs are shown in Fig. 16.23.

Symptomatology and signs vary with age and with the underlying aetiology. Important points are:

● The eye signs, pretibial myxoedema and thyroid acropachy only occur in Graves' disease. 'Pretibial myxoedema' is an infiltration on the shin, essentially only occurring with eye disease (see below). Thyroid acropachy is very rare and consists of clubbing, swollen fingers and periosteal new bone formation.
● In the elderly a frequent presentation is with atrial fibrillation, other tachycardias and/or heart failure, often with few other signs. Thyroid function tests are mandatory in any patient with unexplained atrial fibrillation.
● Children frequently present with excessive height or excessive growth rate, or with behavioural problems such as hyperactivity. They may also show weight gain rather than loss.
● Some elderly patients present with a clinical picture more like hypothyroidism; so-called 'apathetic thyrotoxicosis'.

Table 16.32 Causes of hyperthyroidism.

Graves' disease
Solitary toxic nodule/adenoma
Toxic multinodular goitre
Acute thyroidits
   Viral
   Autoimmune
   Post-irradiation
Thyrotoxicosis factitia (secret T_4 consumption)
Exogenous iodine
Drugs—amiodarone
Metastatic differentiated thyroid carcinoma
TSH-secreting tumours (e.g. pituitary)
HCG-producing tumours
Hyperfunctioning ovarian teratoma (struma ovarii)

Only the first three are common.

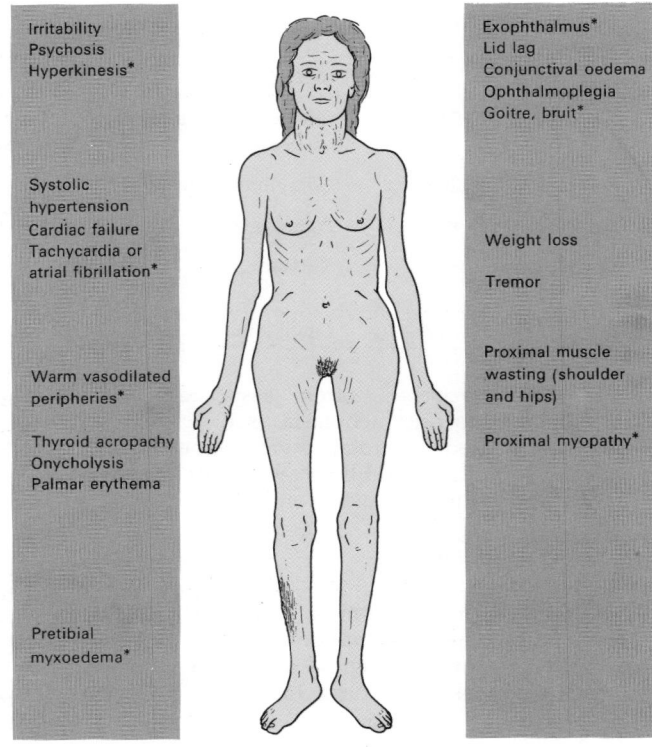

Symptoms of thyrotoxicosis

Weight loss
Increased appetite
Irritability/behaviour change
Restlessness
Malaise
Muscle weakness
Tremor
Choreoathetosis
Breathlessness
Palpitation
Heat intolerance
Vomiting
Diarrhoea
Eye complaints*
Goitre
Oligomenorrhoea
Loss of libido
Gynaecomastia
Onycholysis
Tall stature (in children)

* Only with Graves' disease.

Irritability
Psychosis
Hyperkinesis*

Systolic
hypertension
Cardiac failure
Tachycardia or
atrial fibrillation*

Warm vasodilated
peripheries*

Thyroid acropachy
Onycholysis
Palmar erythema

Pretibial
myxoedema*

Exophthalmus*
Lid lag
Conjunctival oedema
Ophthalmoplegia
Goitre, bruit*

Weight loss

Tremor

Proximal muscle
wasting (shoulder
and hips)

Proximal myopathy*

Fig. 16.23 The signs of hyperthyroidism. Asterisks indicate signs of greater discriminant value.

DIFFERENTIAL DIAGNOSIS

Thyrotoxicosis is often clinically obvious but treatment should never be instituted without biochemical confirmation.

Differentiation of the mild case from anxiety states may be difficult; useful positive clinical markers are eye signs, proximal myopathy and wasting. The hyperdynamic circulation with warm peripheries with thyrotoxicosis compared with the clammy hands of anxiety.

INVESTIGATION

TSH is suppressed though most physicians also like to confirm the diagnosis with a raised T_3 or T_4; the former is more sensitive as there are occasional cases of 'T_3 toxicosis'. TSI estimation is available in some centres.

The TRH test is now very rarely necessary. A normal TSH rise excludes the diagnosis; a flat response is characteristic but not diagnostic.

TREATMENT

Three possibilities are available: antithyroid drugs, surgery and radioiodine. Practices and beliefs differ widely within and between countries; it also depends on patient preference and local expertise. Some general guidelines are:

- Patients with large goitres, single or multiple nodular goitres are unlikely to remit after a course of antithyroid drugs.
- In the UK, radioiodine is rarely given to those under the age of 40.
- Patient preference, with informed discussion, must be given great weight.

Antithyroid drugs

Carbimazole is most often used in the UK. Occasionally propylthiouracil is also used. Methimazole, the active metabolite of carbimazole, is used in the USA. These drugs inhibit the formation of thyroid hormones and also have minor other actions; carbimazole/methimazole is also a mild immunosuppressive agent. Initial doses and side-effects are detailed in Table 16.33.

Though thyroid hormone synthesis is reduced very quickly, the long half-life of thyroxine (7 days) means that clinical benefit is not apparent for 10–20 days. As many of the manifestations of hyperthyroidism are mediated via the sympathetic system, beta-blockers are used to provide rapid partial symptomatic control; they also decrease peripheral conversion of T_4 to T_3. Drugs preferred are those

Table 16.33 Drugs used in the treatment of thyrotoxicosis.

Drug	Usual starting dose	Side-effects	Remarks
Anti-thyroid drugs			
Carbimazole	10–20 mg 8-hourly	Rash, nausea, vomiting, arthralgia, agranulocytosis (0.1%), jaundice	Active metabolite is methimazole Mild immunosuppressive activity
Propylthiouracil	100–200 mg 8–hourly	Rash, nausea, vomiting, agranulocytosis	Blocks conversion of T_4 to T_3
Beta-blockers for symptomatic control			
Propranolol	40–80 mg 6 to 8-hourly	Avoid in asthma; use with care in heart failure Usual beta-blocker side-effects	Use beta-blocking agents *without* intrinsic sympathomimetic activity May need higher doses in hyperthyroidism as metabolism is increased
Nadolol	40–240 mg daily		

without intrinsic sympathomimetic activity (Table 16.33). They should not be used alone for hyperthyroidism except when the condition is self-limiting, e.g. subacute thyroiditis.

Subsequent management is either by gradual dose reduction or a 'block and replace' regime.

Gradual dose titration

● Review after 4–6 weeks and reduce dose of carbimazole depending on clinical state and T_4/T_3 levels. TSH levels may remain suppressed for long periods.
● When euthyroid, stop beta-blockers.
● Review after 2–3 months and, if controlled, reduce carbimazole. Once-daily dosage is now possible.
● Gradually reduce dose to 5 mg/day over 12–18 months if thyrotoxicosis remains controlled.
● When euthyroid on 5 mg/day carbimazole, discontinue.
● About 50% of patients will relapse, mostly within the following 2 years. Long-term anti-thyroid therapy is then used or surgery is considered (see below).
● Propylthiouracil is used in similar fashion but doses required are tenfold higher (50–500 mg/day).

'Block and replace' regime. With this policy, full doses of antithyroid drugs, usually carbimazole 30–45 mg/day, are given to suppress the thyroid completely while replacing thyroid activity with T_4 0.1 mg/day. This is continued usually for 18 months, the claimed advantages being the avoidance of over- or undertreatment and the better use of the immunosuppressive action. Against this there is no 'feel' for whether the patient is likely to relapse as with the titration method.

Toxicity (Table 16.33). The major side-effect is agranulocytosis that occurs in approximately 1 in 1000 patients within 3 months of treatment. All patients must be warned to seek immediate medical attention if they develop unexplained fever or sore throat. If toxicity occurs on carbimazole, propylthiouracil may be used and vice versa; side-effects are rarely repeated on the other drug.

Surgery—subtotal thyroidectomy
Thyroidectomy should only be performed in patients who have previously been rendered euthyroid. Conventional practice is to stop the anti-thyroid drug 10–14 days before operation and to give potassium iodide (60 mg three times daily), which reduces the vascularity of the gland.

Particular indications for surgery are:

● Patient choice.
● A large goitre is unlikely to respond to anti-thyroid medication.

Indications for either surgery or radioiodine are:

● Persistent drug side-effects (also suitable for radioiodine)
● Poor compliance with drug therapy
● Recurrent hyperthyroidism after drugs

The operation should be performed by an experienced surgeon to reduce the chance of complications:

● Early postoperative bleeding causing tracheal compression and asphyxia is a rare emergency requiring immediate removal of all clips/sutures to allow escape of the blood/haematoma.
● Laryngeal nerve palsy (1%); vocal chord movement should be checked preoperatively. Mild hoarseness is more common.
● Transient hypocalcaemia in up to 10% but with

permanent hypoparathyroidism in less than 1%.
- Recurrent hyperthyroidism (less than 5%).
- Hypothyroidism—about 10% of patients are hypothyroid within one year and this percentage increases with time. It is likeliest if microsomal antibodies are positive. Automated computer thyroid registers with annual TSH screening is used in some regions.

Radioactive iodine

Iodine-131 in an empirical dose (usually 18–40 × 10^{10} Bq) accumulates in the thyroid and destroys the gland by local radiation. Early discomfort in the neck and immediate worsening of hyperthyroidism are sometimes seen; again patients must be rendered euthyroid before treatment though they have to stop antithyroid drugs about 5 days before radioiodine. If worsening occurs, the patient should not receive carbimazole for 2–3 days after radioiodine, as it will prevent radioiodine uptake by the gland. They should receive propranolol (Table 16.33) until carbimazole can be re-started.

Apart from the immediate problems above, a major complication is the progressive incidence in subsequent hypothyroidism affecting the majority of subjects over the following 20 years. Though 75% of patients are rendered euthyroid in the short-term, a small proportion remain hyperthyroid; increasing the radioiodine dose reduces recurrence but increases the rate of hypothyroidism. Again, long-term surveillance of thyroid function is necessary.

Special situations in hyperthyroidism

Thyroid crisis

This rare condition, with a mortality of 10%, is a rapid deterioration of thyrotoxicosis with hyperpyrexia, severe tachycardia and extreme restlessness. It is usually precipitated by stress, infection, surgery in an unprepared patient or radioiodine therapy. With careful management it should no longer occur.

Treatment is urgent. Propranolol in full doses is started immediately together with potassium iodide, antithyroid drugs, corticosteroids (which suppress many of the manifestations of hyperthyroidism) and full supportive measures.

Hyperthyroidism in pregnancy and neonatal life

Maternal hyperthyroidism during pregnancy is uncommon and usually mild. Diagnosis can be difficult because of misleading thyroid function tests, although TSH is largely reliable. The pathogenesis is almost always Graves' disease. TSI crosses the placenta to stimulate the fetal thyroid. Carbimazole also crosses the placenta, but thyroxine does so poorly. The smallest dose of carbimazole necessary is used and the fetus must be monitored (see below). The paediatrician should be informed and the infant checked immediately after birth—overtreatment with carbimazole can cause fetal goitre.

If necessary (high doses needed, poor patient compliance or drug side-effects), surgery can be performed, preferably in the second trimester. Radioactive iodine is absolutely contraindicated.

The fetus and maternal Graves' disease

Any mother with a history of Graves' disease may have circulating TSI. Even if she has been treated (e.g. by surgery), the immunoglobulin may still be present to stimulate the fetal thyroid, and the fetus can thus become hyperthyroid, while the mother remains euthyroid.

Any such patient should therefore be monitored during pregnancy. Fetal heart rate provides a direct biological assay of thyroid status, and monitoring should be performed at least monthly. Rates above 160/min are strongly suggestive of fetal hyperthyroidism and maternal treatment with carbimazole and/or propranolol may be used. To prevent the mother becoming hypothyroid, thyroxine may be given as this does not easily cross the placenta. Sympathomimetics, used to prevent premature labour, are contraindicated as they may provoke fatal tachycardias in the fetus.

Thyrotoxicosis may also develop in the neonatal period as TSI has a half-life of approximately 3 weeks. Manifestations in the newborn include irritability, failure to thrive and persisting weight loss, diarrhoea and eye signs. Thyroid function tests are difficult to interpret as neonatal normal ranges vary with age.

Untreated neonatal thyrotoxicosis is probably associated with hyperactivity in later childhood.

Thyroid eye disease

This is also known as dysthyroid eye disease or ophthalmic Graves' disease.

PATHOPHYSIOLOGY

The evidence suggests that the exophthalmos of Graves' disease is due to specific antibodies that cause retro-orbital inflammation and subsequent oedema. Histology shows the classical lymphocytic infiltration of autoimmune disease. It is not due to TSH, LATS or LATS-P. While often associated with Graves' hyperthyroidism, it need not be so and patients may be hyperthyroid, euthryoid or hypothyroid.

CLINICAL FEATURES

The clinical appearances are characteristic (Fig. 16.24). Proptosis and limitation of eye movements are direct effects of the inflammation, while conjunctival oedema, lid lag and corneal scarring are

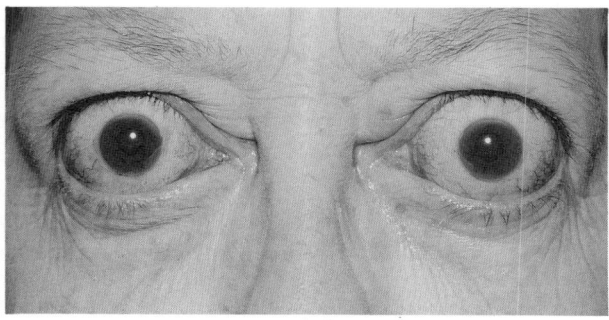

Fig. 16.24 The signs of thyroid eye disease.

Eye complaints

History
Difficulty in reading/distant vision
Double vision
Grittiness
Protrusion

Physical signs
Decreased acuity
Limitation of eye movements
Conjunctivitis/chemosis
Lid lag/lid retraction
Exophthalmos

---

secondary to the proptosis and lack of eye cover. The ability to close the eyes completely is important, as otherwise corneal damage may occur. Eye manifestations often do not parallel the clinical course of Graves' disease—in particular the degree of toxicosis.

INVESTIGATIONS

Few investigations are necessary if the appearances are characteristic and bilateral. TSH and T_3 or T_4 should be measured.

The exophthalmos should be measured to allow progress to be monitored. If appearances or measurements are markedly discrepant in the two eyes, other retro-orbital space-occupying lesions should be considered: CT scanning of the orbits will exclude other causes and show enlarged muscles and oedema.

TREATMENT

If abnormal, thyroid function should be normalized. Direct treatment may be either local or systemic:

- Methylcellulose eye drops are given to aid lubrication.

- Lateral tarsorrhaphy will aid closure if lids cannot be closed.
- If more severe, systemic steroids (prednisolone 30–120 mg/day) may reduce inflammation.
- Irradiation of the orbits is also used in severe instances.
- Surgical decompression of the orbit(s) is occasionally needed.
- Corrective eye muscle surgery may improve diplopia due to ocular palsies.

The glucocorticoid axis

Adrenal anatomy and function

The human adrenal comprises an outer cortex with three zones (reticularis, fasciculata and glomerulosa) producing steroids and an inner medulla that synthesizes, stores and secretes catecholamines. The adrenal steroids are grouped into three classes based on their predominant physiological effects:

- *Glucocorticoids.* These are named after their effects on carbohydrate metabolism; major actions are listed in Table 16.34.
- *Mineralocorticoids.* Their predominant effect is on the extracellular balance of sodium and potassium in the distal tubule of the kidney: aldosterone is the predominant mineralocorticoid in man (about 50%); corticosterone makes a small contribution. The weak mineralocorticoid activity of cortisol is also important since it is present in considerable excess. Aldosterone is produced solely in the zona glomerulosa.
- *Androgens.* Although they are secreted in considerable quantities, most have only relatively weak androgenic activity.

The relative potency of common steroids is shown in Table 16.35.

Table 16.34 The actions of glucocorticoids.

Increased or stimulated
Gluconeogenesis
Glycogen deposition
Protein catabolism
Fat deposition
Sodium retention
Potassium loss
Free water clearance
Uric acid production
Circulating neutrophils

Decreased or inhibited
Protein synthesis
Host response to infection
Lymphocyte transformation
Delayed hypersensitivity
Circulating lymphocytes
Circulating eosinophils

Biochemistry

All steroids have the same basic skeleton (Fig. 16.25a) and the chemical differences between them are slight. The major biosynthetic pathways are also shown in Fig. 16.25b.

Physiology

Glucocorticoid production by the adrenal is under hypothalamic/pituitary control (Fig. 16.26). Corticotrophin-releasing factor (CRF) is secreted in the hypothalamus in response to circadian rhythm, stress and other stimuli. It travels down the portal system to stimulate adrenocorticotrophic hormone (ACTH) release from the anterior pituitary corticotrophs. Circulating ACTH stimulates cortisol production in the adrenal. The cortisol (or any other synthetic corticosteroid) secreted feeds back on the hypothalamus and pituitary to inhibit further CRF/ACTH release. The set point of this system clearly varies through the day according to the circadian rhythm, and is usually overridden by severe stress.

Following adrenalectomy or Addison's disease, cortisol secretion will be absent or reduced; ACTH levels will therefore rise.

Mineralocorticoid secretion is mainly controlled by the renin–angiotensin system (see p. 827).

Investigation of glucocorticoid abnormalities

Basal levels
ACTH and cortisol are released episodically. The following precautions are therefore necessary when taking a blood sample:

- Sampling time should be accurately recorded.
- Stress should be minimized.
- Sampling should be delayed for 48 h after admission if Cushing's syndrome is suspected.
- Appropriate normal ranges (for time of day and method of assay) should be used.

Suppression and stimulation tests are used in instances of excess and deficient cortisol production respectively.

Dexamethasone suppression tests
Administration of synthetic glucocorticoid to a normal subject produces prompt feedback suppression of CRF and ACTH levels and thus of endogenous cortisol secretion (prednisolone and

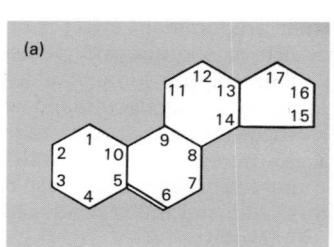

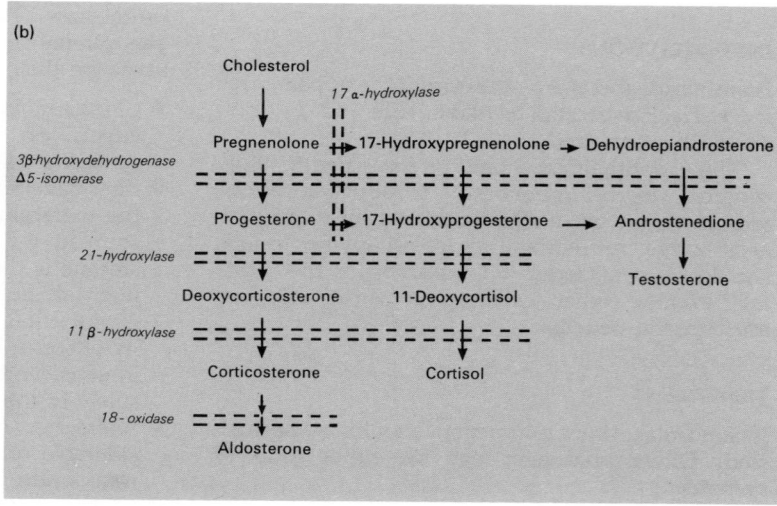

Fig. 16.25 (a) The steroid molecule. (b) The major steroid biosynthetic pathways.

Table 16.35 Glucocorticoid and mineralocorticoid potency of equal amounts of common steroids.

Steroid	Glucocorticoid effect[a]	Mineralocorticoid effect[a]
Cortisol (hydrocortisone)	1	1
Prednisolone	4	0.7
Dexamethasone	40	2
Aldosterone	0.1	400
Fludrocortisone	10	400

[a] Cortisol is arbitrarily defined as 1.

dexamethasone are not measured by most cortisol assays). Three forms of the test, used in the diagnosis and differential diagnosis of Cushing's syndrome, are available (Table 16.36).

ACTH stimulation tests
Synthetic ACTH (tetracosactrin, which consists of

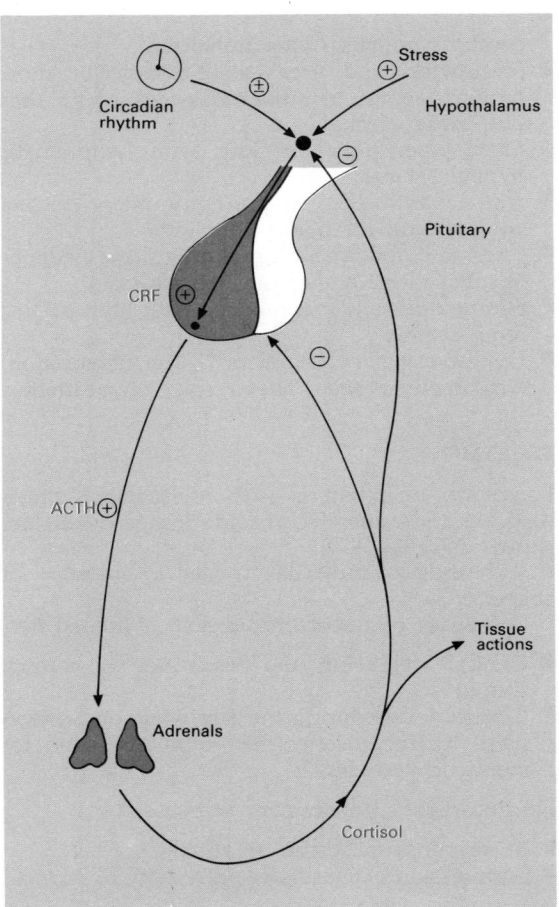

Fig. 16.26 Control of the hypothalamic–pituitary–adrenal axis. CRF = corticotrophin-releasing factor.

the first 24 amino acids of human ACTH) is given to stimulate adrenal cortisol production. Details are given in Table 16.36.

ADDISON'S DISEASE—PRIMARY HYPOADRENALISM

PATHOPHYSIOLOGY AND CAUSES

In this rare condition there is destruction of the entire adrenal cortex. Glucocorticoid, mineralocorticoid and sex steroid production are therefore all reduced. This differs from hypothalamic–pituitary disease, in which mineralocorticoid secretion remains largely intact, being predominantly stimulated by angiotensin II. Also, adrenal sex steroid production by the adrenals is largely independent of pituitary action. Reduced cortisol levels lead, through feedback, to increased ACTH production, which is responsible for the hyperpigmentation.

Primary hypoadrenalism shows a marked female preponderance and is now most often caused by autoimmune disease rather than TB (Table 16.37).

CLINICAL FEATURES

The clinical features of Addison's disease are shown in Fig. 16.27. The symptomatology of Addison's disease is often vague—weakness, tiredness, weight loss and anorexia predominate.

Important features are:

● Pigmentation (dull, slaty, grey-brown) in the mouth (opposite the molars), hand and all flexural regions is the predominant sign. It is particularly significant if it occurs in a recent scar.

● Postural hypotension, due to hypovolaemia and sodium loss, is usually present even if supine blood pressure is normal.

Table 16.36 Details of dexamethasone suppression and ACTH (Synacthen) tests.

Test	Protocol	Measure	Positive test	Use
Dexamethasone				
Overnight	Take 1–2 mg on going to bed on day −1	Plasma cortisol at 0900 h on day 0	Plasma cortisol < 180 nmol·L^{-1}	Outpatient screening test
'Low-dose'	0.5 mg 6-hourly × 8 doses from 0900 h on day 0	Plasma cortisol at 0900 h on days 0 and +2	Plasma cortisol < 180 nmol·L^{-1} on second sample	For diagnosis of Cushing's syndrome. May not suppress in obesity and depression
'High-dose'	2 mg 6-hourly × 8 doses from 0900 h on day 0	Plasma cortisol at 0900 h on days 0 and +2 (24 h urinary steroids on days −1 and +2)	Plasma cortisol on day +2 < 50% of that on day 0	Differential diagnosis of Cushing's syndrome; pituitary-dependent disease suppresses in about 90%
ACTH (Synacthen)				
Short	Tetracosactrin 0.25 mg i.m. at time 0	Plasma cortisol at time 0, +30 and +60 min	Cortisol at +30 min > 690 nmol·L^{-1}. Rise > 330 nmol·L^{-1}	To exclude primary adrenal failure
Long	Depot tetracosactrin 1 mg i.m. at time 0	Plasma cortisol at time 0, +1, +2, +3, +4, +5, +8 and +24 h	Maximum > 1000 nmol·L^{-1}	To demonstrate/exclude adrenal suppression

INVESTIGATION

Once Addison's disease is suspected, investigation is urgent. If the patient is seriously ill or very hypotensive, hydrocortisone 100 mg should be given i.m., ideally after a blood sample is taken for later measurement of plasma cortisol, or an ACTH stimulation test can be performed immediately. Full investigation should be delayed until emergency treatment has improved the patient's condition.

Otherwise, tests are as follows:

- Single cortisol measurements are virtually of no value.
- The short ACTH stimulation test should be performed (Table 16.36). An absent or impaired cortisol response is seen, confirmed if necessary by a long ACTH stimulation test to exclude adrenal suppression by steroids.
- A 0900 h plasma ACTH level; a high level (> 80 ng·L^{-1}) with low or low–normal cortisol

Table 16.37 Causes of primary hypoadrenalism.

Autoimmune disease
Tuberculosis
Surgical removal
Haemorrhage/infarction
  Meningococcal septicaemia
  Venography
Infiltration
  Malignant destruction
  Amyloid
Schilder's disease (adrenal leukodystrophy)

confirms primary hypoadrenalism.

- Electrolytes and urea: these classically show hyponatraemia, hyperkalaemia and a high urea but can be normal.
- Blood glucose may be low, with symptomatic hypoglycaemia.
- Adrenal antibodies are present in many cases of autoimmune adrenalitis.
- Chest and abdominal X-rays may show evidence of tuberculosis and/or calcified adrenals.
- Serum aldosterone is reduced with high plasma renin activity.
- Hypercalcaemia and anaemia (after rehydration) are sometimes seen. They resolve on treatment.

TREATMENT

Long-term treatment is with replacement glucocorticoid and mineralocorticoid; dosage details are shown in Table 16.38.

Tuberculosis must be treated if present or suspected.

Adequacy of glucocorticoid dose is judged by:

- Clinical well-being and restoration of normal weight
- Cortisol levels during the day while on replacement hydrocortisone (this cannot be used for synthetic steroids)

Fludrocortisone replacement is assessed by:

- BP response to posture (it should not fall)
- Suppression of plasma renin activity to normal

Patient advice
All patients requiring replacement steroids should:

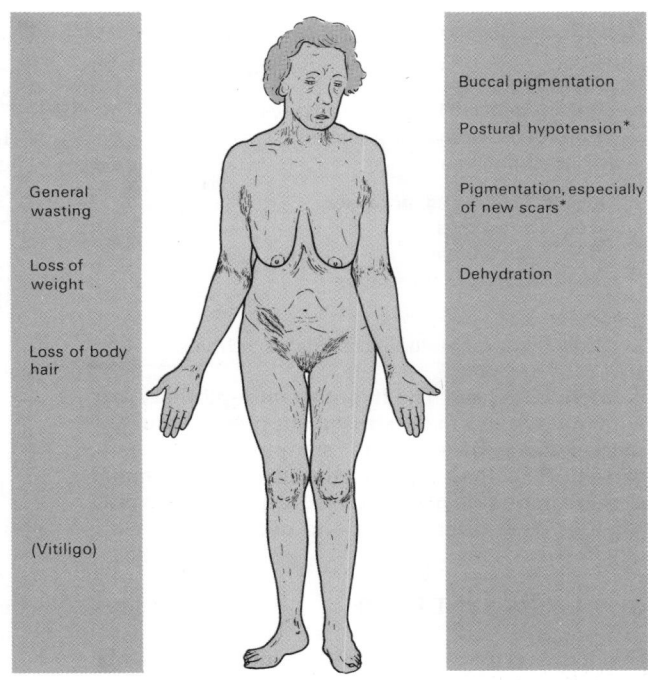

Symptoms of primary hypoadrenalism

Weight loss
Anorexia
Malaise
Weakness
Fever
Depression
Impotence/amenorrhoea
Nausea/vomiting
Diarrhoea
Confusion
Syncope from postural hypotension
Abdominal pain
Constipation
Myalgia
Joint or back pain

Features of other autoimmune disease
(e.g. vitiligo) are quite common.

General wasting

Loss of weight

Loss of body hair

(Vitiligo)

Buccal pigmentation

Postural hypotension*

Pigmentation, especially of new scars*

Dehydration

Fig. 16.27 The signs of primary hypoadrenalism (Addison's disease). Asterisks indicate signs of greater discriminant value.

- Carry a steroid card.
- Wear a Medic-Alert bracelet; this gives details of their condition so that emergency replacement therapy can be given if they are found unconscious.
- Keep an ampoule of hydrocortisone at home in case oral therapy is impossible, and the GP has to be called.

Acute hypoadrenalism
The major deficiencies are of salt, steroid and glucose.

Table 16.38 Average replacement steroid dosages for adults with primary hypoadrenalism.

Drug	Dose
Glucocorticoid	
Cortisol	30 mg daily—20 mg on waking, 10 mg at 1800 h
or Prednisolone	7.5 mg daily—5 mg on waking, 2.5 mg at 1800 h
or Dexamethasone	0.75 mg daily—0.5 mg on waking, 0.25 mg at 1800 h
Mineralocorticoid	
Fludrocortisone	0.05–0.4 mg daily

- Assuming normal cardiovascular function, 1 litre of normal saline should be given over 30–60 min with 100 mg of intravenous hydrocortisone.
- Dextrose should be infused if hypoglycaemia is present.
- Subsequent saline requirements may be for several litres within 24 h (assessing with CVP line if necessary) plus hydrocortisone, 100 mg i.m. 6-hourly, until the patient is clinically stable.
- Oral replacement medication is then started, initially hydrocortisone about 20 mg 8-hourly or equivalent, reducing to 20 mg + 10 mg or equivalent over a few days.
- Fludrocortisone is unnecessary acutely as the high cortisol doses provide sufficient mineralocorticoid activity—it should be introduced later.

SECONDARY HYPOADRENALISM

This may arise from hypothalamic–pituitary disease or from long-term steroid therapy leading to hypothalamic–pituitary–adrenal suppression.

Most patients with the former have panhypopituitarism (p. 774) and need thyroxine replacement as well as cortisol; in this case hydrocortisone *must* be started before thyroxine.

The commonest cause of hypoadrenalism is long-term corticosteroid medication for non-

Table 16.39 Causes of Cushing's syndrome.

ACTH-dependent disease
Pituitary-dependent (Cushing's disease)
Ectopic ACTH-producing tumours
ACTH administration

Non-ACTH-dependent causes
Adrenal adenomas
Adrenal carcinomas
Glucocorticoid administration

Others
Alcohol-induced pseudo-Cushing's syndrome

---

endocrine disease. The hypothalamic–pituitary axis and the adrenal may both be suppressed and the patient may have vague symptoms of feeling unwell. The long ACTH stimulation test should demonstrate a delayed cortisol response. Weaning off steroids is often a long and difficult business.

CUSHING'S SYNDROME

Cushing's syndrome is the term used to describe the clinical state of increased free circulating glucocorticoid. It occurs most often following the therapeutic administration of synthetic steroids (see below); all the spontaneous forms of the syndrome are rare.

PATHOPHYSIOLOGY AND CAUSES

The causes of Cushing's syndrome are usually subdivided into two groups (Table 16.39):

● Increased circulating ACTH, from the pituitary, ectopic tumour or medical administration, with consequential glucocorticoid excess, known as Cushing's disease
● A primary excess of endogenous or exogenous glucocorticoid hormone alone, with subsequent (physiological) suppression of ACTH

CLINICAL FEATURES

The predominant clinical features of Cushing's syndrome are those of glucocorticoid excess and are illustrated in Fig. 16.28.
 Particular points include:

● Pigmentation only occurs with ACTH-dependent causes.
● A Cushingoid appearance can be caused by excess alcohol consumption (pseudo-Cushing's syndrome)—the pathophysiology is poorly understood, though cortisol levels are certainly increased.
● Impaired glucose tolerance or frank diabetes are common, especially in the ectopic ACTH syndrome.
● Hypokalaemia due to the mineralocorticoid

Symptoms of Cushing's syndrome

Weight gain (central)
Change in appearance
Depression
Psychosis
Insomnia
Amenorrhoea/oligomenorrhoea
Poor libido
Thin skin/easy bruising
Hair growth/acne
Muscular weakness
Growth arrest in children
Back pain
Polyuria/polydipsia

Old photographs may be useful.
Symptoms of hypopituitarism are
 rare.

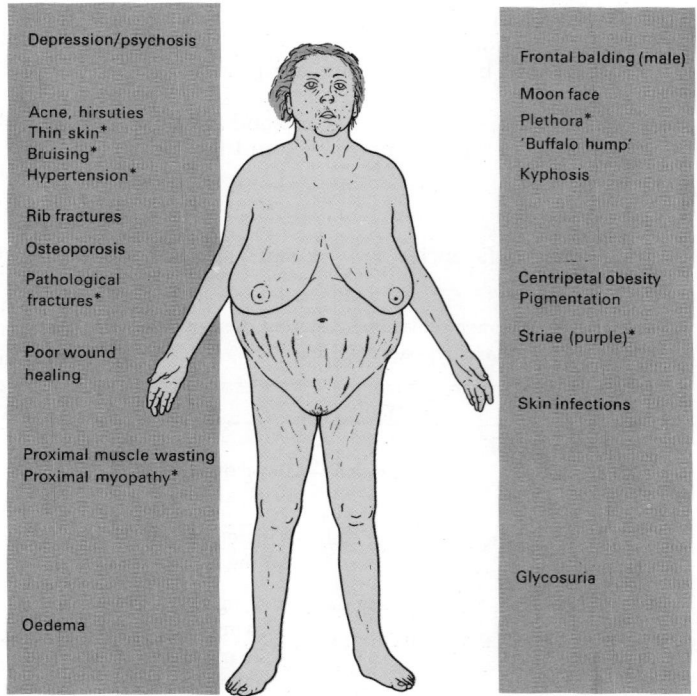

Depression/psychosis

Acne, hirsuties
Thin skin*
Bruising*
Hypertension*

Rib fractures

Osteoporosis

Pathological fractures*

Poor wound healing

Proximal muscle wasting
Proximal myopathy*

Oedema

Frontal balding (male)

Moon face
Plethora*
'Buffalo hump'
Kyphosis

Centripetal obesity
Pigmentation

Striae (purple)*

Skin infections

Glycosuria

Fig. 16.28 The signs of Cushing's syndrome. Asterisks indicate signs of most value in discriminating Cushing's syndrome from simple obesity and hirsuties.

activity of cortisol is common with ectopic ACTH secretion.

DIAGNOSIS

There are two phases to the investigation:

- Confirmation of the presence or absence of Cushing's syndrome
- Differential diagnosis of its cause

Confirmation rests on demonstrating inappropriate cortisol secretion, not suppressed by exogenous glucocorticoids: difficulties occur with obesity and depression where cortisol dynamics are often abnormal. Random cortisol measurements are of no value.

Out-patient screening methods include:

- 24 h urinary free cortisol measurements. Repeatedly normal values (corrected for body mass) render the diagnosis most unlikely.
- The overnight dexamethasone suppression test (Table 16.36). Normal suppression reliably excludes the diagnosis but failure to suppress is not diagnostic and needs further investigation.

In-patient tests involve:

- Circadian rhythm. After 48 h in hospital, cortisol samples are taken at 0900 h and 2400 h (without warning the patient). Normal subjects show a pronounced circadian variation (Fig. 16.3); those with Cushing's syndrome have high evening cortisol levels, though the 0900 h value may be normal.
- Low-dose dexamethasone test (Table 16.36). Patients with Cushing's syndrome fail to suppress plasma or urinary cortisol levels.
- Insulin tolerance test. This is useful in depression or obesity, when abnormal circadian and suppression responses are seen. The normal rise of cortisol with hypoglycaemia does not occur in patients with Cushing's syndrome.

Differential diagnosis of the cause
This can be extremely difficult. The classical ectopic ACTH syndrome is distinguished by a short history, pigmentation and weight loss, unprovoked hypokalaemia, clinical or chemical diabetes and plasma ACTH levels above 200 ng·L^{-1}. Severe hirsuties/virilization suggests an adrenal tumour.

Biochemical and radiological procedures for diagnosis include:

- Adrenal CT scan. Adrenal adenomas and carcinomas causing Cushing's syndrome are relatively large and always detectable by CT scan. Carcinomas are distinguished by large size, irregular outline and signs of infiltration or metastases.
- Pituitary CT or MRI. Of less value than the

adrenal scan; only a minority of tumours of significant size are detected with confidence, and indeed over 80% of skull X-rays are normal.
- Plasma potassium levels. All diuretics must be stopped. Hypokalaemia is common with ectopic ACTH secretion.
- High-dose dexamethasone test (Table 16.36). Failure of urinary or plasma cortisol suppression suggests an ectopic source of ACTH or an adrenal tumour. The metyrapone test has been shown to be of little value.
- Plasma ACTH levels. Low or undetectable ACTH levels (< 10 ng·L^{-1}) on two or more occasions are a reliable indicator of non-ACTH dependent disease.
- Corticotrophin-releasing hormone test. Exaggerated ACTH responses to exogenous CRF suggest pituitary-dependent Cushing's disease.
- Chest X-ray is mandatory to demonstrate a carcinoma of the bronchus or a bronchial carcinoid. Lesions may be very small; if ectopic ACTH is suspected, whole-lung and mediastinal CT scan should be performed.

Further investigations may involve selective catherization of jugular veins and inferior petrosal sinus for pituitary lesions, or throughout the body in a search for ectopic sources. Bronchoscopy, cytology and regional arteriograms are sometimes necessary.

TREATMENT

Untreated Cushing's syndrome has a very bad prognosis, with death from hypertension, myocardial infarction, infection and heart failure. Whatever the underlying cause, cortisol hypersecretion should be controlled prior to surgery or radiotherapy. Considerable morbidity and mortality is otherwise associated with operating on unprepared patients. The usual drug is metyrapone, an 11-hydroxylase blocker, which is given in doses of 750 mg to 4 g daily in 3–4 divided doses. Plasma cortisol should be monitored, aiming to reduce the mean level during the day to 300–400 nmol·L^{-1}, equivalent to normal production rates. Aminoglutethimide is sometimes used, but trilostane has been abandoned.

Choice of treatment depends upon the cause.

Cushing's disease (pituitary-dependent hyperadrenalism)
Treatment options are surgery, radiotherapy and medical control; the choice remains controversial.

Trans-sphenoidal removal of the tumour, by an experienced surgeon, is probably the treatment of choice. Selective surery nearly always leaves the patient ACTH-deficient immediately postoperatively and this is considered a good prognostic sign. Transfrontal surgery is very rarely necessary because most tumours are small, though they are occasionally locally invasive.

Yttrium implantation of radioactive needles in the fossa produces good results in some centres but it is not generally available.

External irradiation alone is slow, only effective in 20–50% and of little value except in those unfit for, or unwilling, to have surgery. Children, however, respond much better to radiotherapy, 80% being cured.

Medical therapy to reduce ACTH (e.g. bromocriptine, cyproheptadine) is rarely effective and bilateral adrenalectomy is now very little used.

Other causes
Adrenal adenomas should be resected after preparation with metyrapone. Contralateral adrenal suppression may last for years.

Carcinomas are highly aggressive and the prognosis is poor. In general, if there are no widespread metastases, tumour bulk should be reduced surgically and the adrenolytic drug *op*′DDD given; new preparations have reduced the side-effects of nausea/vomiting and ataxia. Some would also give radiotherapy to the tumour bed after surgery.

Ectopic tumour sources should be removed if possible. Otherwise chemotherapy/radiotherapy should be used, depending on the tumour. Control of the Cushing's syndrome with metyrapone is beneficial for symptoms.

If the source is not clear, cortisol hypersecretion should be controlled with medical therapy until a diagnosis can be made.

Nelson's syndrome

This rare syndrome is of increased pigmentation associated with an enlarging pituitary tumour occurring afer bilateral adrenalectomy. The tumour may be locally invasive but most physicians believe it can be prevented by pituitary radiotherapy soon after adrenalectomy, though the latter is now rarely used.

CONGENITAL ADRENAL HYPERPLASIA (CAH)

PATHOPHYSIOLOGY

This condition results from a deficiency of an enzyme in the steroid synthetic pathways, most commonly 21-hydroxylase. As a result, cortisol secretion is reduced and feedback leads to increased ACTH secretion to maintain adequate cortisol—this in turn leads to diversion of the steroid precursors into the androgenic steroid pathways (Fig. 16.29). Thus, 17-hydroxy progesterone, androstenedione and testosterone levels are increased, leading to virilization. Rarely, aldosterone synthesis is impaired with resultant salt wasting. The 21-hydroxylase deficiency has been shown to be due to defects on chromosome 6 near the HLA-region.

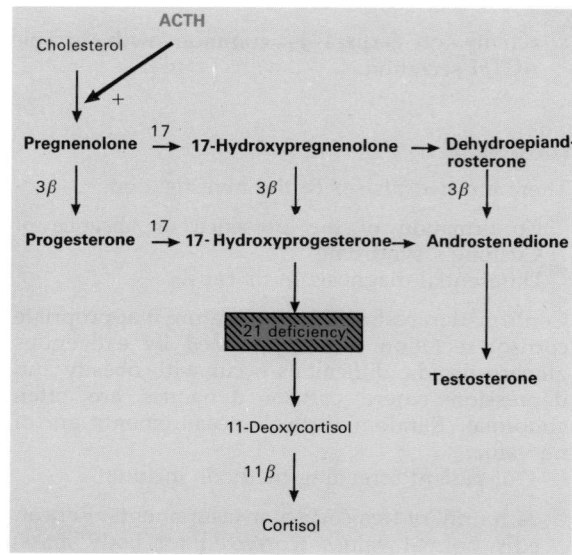

Fig. 16.29 Effects of congenital adrenal hyperplasia (21-hydroxylase deficiency) on steroid biosynthesis. Precursors and products present in excess appear in bold type. Those present in normal or reduced quantity appear in lighter type.

CLINICAL FEATURES

If severe, this presents at birth with sexual ambiguity or adrenal failure. In the female, clitoral hypertrophy, urogenital abnormalities and labioscrotal fusion are common, but the syndrome may be unrecognized in the male. Precocious puberty with hirsuties is a later presentation, while some milder cases only present in adult life, usually accompanied by primary amenorrhoea. Hirsutism developing before menarche is suggestive of CAH.

INVESTIGATION

- 17-Hydroxyprogesterone levels are increased (Fig. 16.29).
- Urinary pregnanetriol excretion is increased.
- Basal ACTH levels are raised.

TREATMENT

Replacement of glucocorticoid activity and mineralocorticoid activity if deficient is as for primary hypoadrenalism (see above). Correct dosage is often difficult to establish in the child but should ensure normal 17-hydroxyprogesterone and ACTH levels while allowing normal growth; excessive replacement leads to stunting of growth.

USES AND PROBLEMS OF THERAPEUTIC STEROID THERAPY

Apart from their use as therapeutic replacement for endocrine deficiency states, synthetic glucocorti-

Table 16.40 Common therapeutic uses of glucocorticoids.

Respiratory disease
Asthma
Chronic bronchitis and emphysema
Sarcoidosis
Hay fever (usually topical)

Cardiac disease
Post-myocardial infarction syndrome

Renal disease
Some nephrotic syndromes

Gastrointestinal disease
Ulcerative colitis
Crohn's disease
Chronic active hepatitis

Obstetrics
Prevention/treatment of ARDS (p. 729)

Rheumatological disease
Systemic lupus erythematosus
Polymyalgia rheumatica

Neurological disease
Cerebral oedema

Skin disease

Tumours
Hodgkin's lymphoma
Other lymphomas

Transplantation
Immunosuppression

Table 16.41 Adverse effects of corticosteroid therapy.

PHYSIOLOGICAL

Adrenal and/or pituitary suppression

PATHOLOGICAL

Cardiovascular
Increased blood pressure

Gastrointestinal
Peptic ulceration exacerbation (possibly)
Pancreatitis

Renal
Polyuria
Nocturia

Central nervous
Depression
Euphoria
Psychosis
Insomnia

Endocrine
Weight gain
Glycosuria/hyperglycaemia/diabetes
Impaired growth
Amenorrhoea

Bone and muscle
Osteoporosis
Proximal myopathy and wasting
Aseptic necrosis of the hip
Pathological fractures

Skin
Thinning
Easy bruising

Eyes
Cataracts

Increased susceptibility to infection
(signs and fever are frequently masked)
Septicaemia
TB
Skin, e.g. fungi

---

coids are widely used for many non-endocrine conditions (Table 16.40).

Short-term use (e.g. for acute asthma) carries little risk of significant side-effects except for the simultaneous suppression of immune responses. The danger lies in their continuance, often through medical oversight or patient default.

Long-term therapy with synthetic or natural steroids will, in most respects, mimic endogenous Cushing's syndrome. Exceptions are the relative absence of hirsuties, acne, hypertension and severe sodium retention, as the synthetic steroids have low androgenic and mineralocorticoid activity.

Excessive doses of steroids may also be absorbed from skin when strong dermatological preparations are used but inhaled steroids very rarely cause Cushing's syndrome, although they may cause adrenal suppression.

The major hazards are detailed in Table 16.41; in the long-term many are of such severity that the clinical need for *high*-dose steroids should be continually and critically assessed.

Supervision of steroid therapy

All patients receiving steroids should carry a steroid card and know that:

- Long-term steroid therapy must never be stopped suddenly. Doses should be reduced very gradually, with most being given in the morning at the time of withdrawal—this minimizes adrenal suppression.
- Doses need to be increased in times of serious intercurrent illness (defined as presence of a fever), accident and stress. Double doses should be taken during these times.
- Other physicians, anaesthetists and dentists must be told about their steroid therapy.

Table 16.42 Steroid cover for operative procedures.

Procedure	Premedication	Intra- and postoperative	Resumption of normal maintenance
Simple procedures (e.g. gastroscopy, simple dental extractions)	Hydrocortisone 100 mg i.m.	—	Immediately if no complications
Minor surgery (e.g. varicose veins, hernias)	Hydrocortisone 100 mg i.m.	Hydrocortisone 100 mg i.m. every 6 h for 24 h	After 24 h if no complications
Major surgery (e.g. hip replacement, vascular surgery)	Hydrocortisone 100 mg i.m.	Hydrocortisone 100 mg i.m. every 6 h for 72 h	After 72 h if normal progress and no complications; perhaps double normal dose for next 2–3 days
GI tract surgery or major thoracic surgery (not eating or ventilated)	Hydrocortisone 100 mg i.m.	Hydrocortisone 100 mg i.m. every 6 h for 72 h or longer if still unwell	When patient eating normally again; until then higher doses (50 mg 6-hourly) may be needed

Steroids and surgery

Any patient receiving steroids or who has recently received them and may still be suppressed requires careful control of steroid medication around the time of surgery. Details are shown in Table 16.42.

The thirst axis

Thirst and water regulation is largely controlled by antidiuretic hormone (ADH, vasopressin). This is synthesized in the hypothalamus and migrates in neurosecretory granules along axonal pathways to the posterior pituitary.

Changes in plasma osmolality are sensed by osmoreceptors in the anterior hypothalamus. Vasopressin secretion is suppressed at levels below 280 mosmol·kg^{-1}, thus allowing maximal water diuresis. Above this level, plasma vasopressin increases in direct proportion to plasma osmolality. At the upper limit of normal (295 mosmol·kg^{-1}) maximum antidiuresis is achieved and thirst is experienced at about 298 mosmol·kg^{-1}.

Other factors affecting vasopressin release are shown in Table 16.43.

At normal concentrations the kidney is the predominant site of action. Via a cyclic AMP mechanism it allows the collecting tubule to become permeable to water, thus permitting re-absorption of hypotonic luminal fluid. At high concentrations vasopressin also causes vasoconstriction.

Disorders of vasopressin secretion or activity include:

- Inappropriate excess of the hormone (SIADH)
- Deficiency as a result of hypothalamic disease (diabetes insipidus)
- 'Nephrogenic diabetes insipidus'—a condition in which the renal tubules are insensitive to vasopressin, an example of a receptor abnormality

While all these are uncommon, they need to be distinguished from the occasional patient with 'hysterical water drinking' and those whose renal tubular function has been impaired by electrolyte abnormalities, such as hypokalaemia or hypercalcaemia.

Syndrome of inappropriate antidiuretic hormone (SIADH)

CLINICAL FEATURES

The presentation is usually vague, with confusion, nausea, irritability and, later, fits and coma. There is no oedema. Mild symptoms usually occur with plasma sodium levels below 125 mmol·L^{-1} and serious manifestations are likely below 115 mmol·L^{-1}.

The syndrome must be distinguished from those causing similar dilutional hyponatraemia from excess dextrose infusion or diuretic administration (thiazides or amiloride—see p. 496).

Table 16.43 Factors affecting vasopressin release.

Increased by:	Decreased by:
Increased osmolality	Decreased osmolality
Hypovolaemia	Hypervolaemia
Hypotension	Hypertension
Nausea	Ethanol
Hypothyroidism	Alpha-adrenergic
Angiotensin II	stimulation
Adrenaline	
Cortisol	
Nicotine	
Antidepressants	

BIOCHEMISTRY

The usual features are:

- Dilutional hyponatraemia due to excessive water retention
- Low plasma osmolality with higher 'inappropriate' urine osmolality
- Continued urinary sodium excretion
- Absence of hypertension or hypokalaemia
- Normal renal and adrenal function

The causes are listed in Table 16.44.

Table 16.44 Causes of the syndrome of inappropriate ADH (SIADH).

Tumours	**Metabolic causes**
Small cell carcinoma of lung	Alcohol withdrawal
Prostate	Porphyria
Thymus	**Drugs**
Pancreas	Chlorpropamide
Lymphomas	Carbamazepine
	Cyclophosphamide
Pulmonary lesions	Vincristine
Pneumonia	
Tuberculosis	
Lung abscess	
CNS causes	
Meningitis	
Tumours	
Head injury	
Subdural	
Cerebral abscess	
SLE vasculitis	

TREATMENT

The underlying cause should be corrected where possible. For symptomatic relief:

- Fluid intake should be restricted to 500–1000 ml/day.
- Plasma osmolality and sodium and body weight should be measured frequently.
- If water restriction is poorly tolerated or ineffective, demethylchlortetracycline (600–1200 mg/day) may be given; this inhibits the action of vasopressin on the kidney causing a reversible form of nephrogenic diabetes insipidus. It may, however, cause photosensitive rashes.
- When very severe, hypertonic saline (300 mmol·L^{-1} slowly i.v.) is rarely given and frusemide may be used. These should be used with extreme caution.

Diabetes insipidus (DI)

CLINICAL FEATURES

Deficiency of vasopressin leads to polyuria, noc-

Table 16.45 Causes of diabetes insipidus.

Cranial diabetes insipidus
Congenital

Idiopathic

Tumours
  Craniopharyngioma
  Pituitary with suprasellar extension
  Hypothalamic tumour, e.g. glioma
  Metastases, especially breast
  Lymphoma/leukaemia

Infections
  Tuberculosis
  Meningitis
  Cerebral abscess

Infiltrations
  Sarcoidosis
  Histiocytosis X

Post-surgical
  Transfrontal
  Transsphenoidal

Post-radiotherapy

Vascular
  Haemorrhage/thrombosis
  Sheehan's syndrome

Nephrogenic diabetes insipidus
Idiopathic

Renal tubular acidosis

Hypokalaemia

Hypercalcaemia

Drugs, e.g.
  Lithium
  Demethylchlortetracycline (demeclocycline)
  Glibenclamide

turia and compensatory polydipsia. Urine output may reach as much as 10–15 L/day, leading to dehydration that may be very severe if the thirst mechanisms are impaired or the patient is denied fluid.

Causes of DI are listed in Table 16.45. The commonest is hypothalamic–pituitary surgery, following which transient DI is common, frequently remitting after a few days or weeks. Primary overdrinking (polydipsia) is a common differential diagnosis (Table 16.45).

DI may be masked by simultaneous cortisol deficiency—cortisol replacement allows a water diuresis and DI then becomes apparent.

DIDMOAD syndrome (Wolfram syndrome) is a rare recessive disorder comprising diabetes insipidus, diabetes mellitus, optic atrophy and deafness.

BIOCHEMISTRY

- High or high-normal plasma osmolality with low urine osmolality (in primary polydipsia plasma osmolality tends to be low)
- Resultant high or high-normal plasma sodium
- Failure of urinary concentration with fluid deprivation
- Restoration of urinary concentration with vasopressin or an analogue

The latter two points may be studied with a formal water-deprivation test (see Appendix). In normal subjects, plasma osmolality remains normal while urine osmolality rises above 700 mosmol·kg^{-1}. In DI, plasma osmolality rises while the urine remains dilute, only concentrating after exogenous vasopressin is given.

TREATMENT

Synthetic vasopressin (desmopressin, DDAVP) is the treatment of choice. It is given intranasally, 10–20 µg once to three times daily or intramuscularly 2–4 µg daily. Response is variable and must be monitored carefully with fluid input/output charts and plasma osmolality measurements.

Alternative agents in mild DI, probably working by sensitizing the tubules to endogenous vasopressin, include thiazide diuretics, carbamazepine 200–400 mg/day or chlorpropamide (200–350 mg/day). These are now rarely used, especially with the risk of hypoglycaemia from chlorpropamide.

Nephrogenic diabetes insipidus

In this condition, renal tubules are resistant to normal or high levels of plasma vasopressin. It may be inherited as a sex-linked recessive or can be acquired as a result of renal disease, drug ingestion, hypocalcaemia or hypokalaemia. Wherever possible the cause should be reversed.

Other causes of polyuria and polydipsia

Diabetes mellitus, hypokalaemia and hypercalcaemia are diagnoses to be considered. In the case of diabetes mellitus the cause is an osmotic diuresis secondary to glycosuria and this leads to dehydration and an increased perception of thirst due to hypertonicity of the extracellular fluid. Both hypokalaemia and hypercalcaemia lead to 'nephrogenic diabetes insipidus' whereby the kidney becomes relatively insensitive to the actions of vasopressin.

Primary, or hysterical polydipsia is a relatively common cause of thirst and polyuria. It is a psychiatric disturbance characterized by the excessive intake of water. Plasma sodium and osmolality fall as a result and the urine produced is *appropriately* dilute. Vasopressin levels become virtually undetectable. Prolonged primary polydipsia may lead to the phenomenon of renal 'medullary washout', with a fall in the concentrating ability of the kidney.

Characteristically the diagnosis is made by a water-deprivation test; a low plasma osmolality is usual at the start of the test, and since vasopressin secretion and action can be stimulated, the patient is able to concentrate his/her urine (albeit his 'maximum' concentrating ability may be impaired), the initially low urine osmolality gradually increasing with the duration of the water deprivation.

Skeletal endocrinology

Bone forms 25% of a normal adult's weight; its major mineral constituents are calcium, phosphate and, to a much lesser extent, magnesium. In the adult there is a continuous process of bone remodelling and resorption, and not a static framework. While exchange of calcium between bone and plasma is only 10–15 mmol/day, over a year 20% of total bone calcium is exchanged.

Physiology, structure and function of bone

Bone is a collagen-based matrix with mineral laid down upon it. Its structural strength depends upon both components, but uncalcified bone is soft (e.g. in osteomalacia) and defective collagen leads to brittle bones (e.g. osteogenesis imperfecta).

Bone deposition is carried out by osteoblasts, whereas resorption depends on osteoclasts. The local factors controlling the relative activity of these processes is poorly understood but it is certainly dependent on hormonal factors. Procollagen is synthesized in osteoblasts and modified to yield collagen, which is a semi-rigid rod-like molecule of general formula 333 × (glycine–proline–amino acid) that polymerizes in a staggered linear fashion and is joined by cross-linkages. After formation, calcium hydroxyapatite crystallization occurs between and around the collagen fibrils.

Osteoclasts stimulated by parathyroid hormone (PTH), appear on the surface of bone, and cause bone resorption.

Bone metabolism and mineralization is thus dependent on:

- Collagen synthesis
- Absorption and availability of calcium, affected by vitamin D
- Bone resorption and deposition, largely under hormonal control

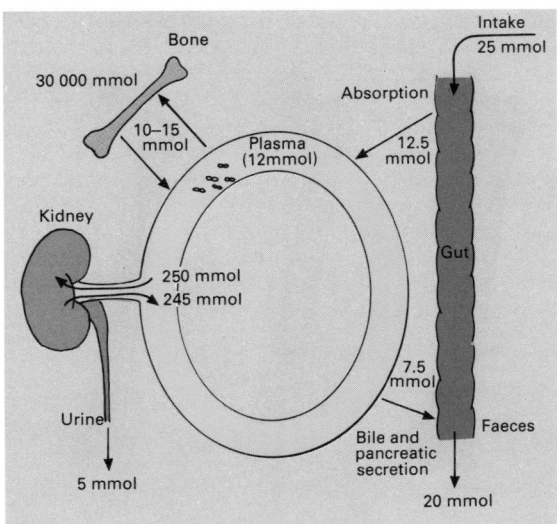

Fig. 16.30 Calcium exchange in the normal human. The fluxes shown are per day.

Calcium absorption and distribution

Normal Western adult calcium consumption is approximately 800–1000 mg daily (20–25 mmol of Ca^{2+}), though it is much lower in some less-affluent countries. Calcium deficiency does not appear to be a significant cause of bone disease, probably because calcium absorption increases in states of dietary calcium deficiency. Absorption is, however, sometimes reduced by generalized malabsorption.

Calcium fluxes between gut, plasma, bone and kidney are shown in Fig. 16.30. The circulating pool of calcium (about 12 mmol in total) is tiny compared with the bony reservoir and small compared with the daily fluxes.

Vitamin D metabolism (see p. 158)

Vitamin D metabolism is illustrated in Fig. 3.4. The predominant active metabolite is 1,25-dihydroxy-cholecalciferol.

Cholecaliferol (vitamin D_3) from the diet and a precursor synthesized in the skin from cholesterol under ultraviolet light stimulation (usually sunlight) are hydroxylated within the liver to form the principal circulating metabolite 25-hydroxychole-calciferol (25-OHCC). This is further hydroxylated within the kidney to either 1,25-dihydroxychole-calciferol (1,25-DHCC)—the active metabolite—or to a similar but physiologically inactive product, 24,25-dihydroxycholecalciferol (24,25-DHCC). The relative amount of 1,25-DHCC compared with 24,25-DHCC produced increases with low plasma calcium, partially under parathyroid hormone control.

Regulation of plasma calcium: the parathyroids

Parathyroid hormone (PTH) levels rise as plasma calcium falls. The effects of PTH, secreted by the four parathyroid glands, are several, all serving to raise plasma calcium:

> Increased tubular reabsorption of calcium
> Increased excretion of phosphate
> Increased osteoclastic resorption of bone
> Increased intestinal absorption of calcium
> Increased synthesis of 1,25-DHCC

The effects are mediated at membrane receptors on the target cells, with resultant increased adenyl cyclase activity (see Fig. 3.5).

While the parathyroids are usually situated posterior to the upper and lower lobes of the thyroid, additional local ones are sometimes seen and they may also occasionally be found elsewhere in the neck or in the mediastinum.

Other calcium regulatory factors
Calcitonin. This hormone is produced by thyroid C-cells. Its physiological importance in man as a hypocalcaemic hormone remains uncertain. Plasma levels rise with increasing plasma calcium, and it is known to inhibit osteoclastic bone resorption and increase renal excretion of calcium and phosphate. However, total thyroidectomy (absent calcitonin) and medullary carcinoma (excess calcitonin) have few skeletal effects. It is, however, used in the treatment of Paget's disease (p. 421) and, rarely, in hypercalcaemia.

Glucocorticoids. Steroids have complex actions on bone, essentially leading to excessive bone resorption and osteoporosis.

Sex hormones. Androgens and/or oestrogens have several effects on the skeleton:

- In puberty they induce the growth spurt and subsequent epiphyseal closure.
- Both influence skeletal calcium content, especially post-menopausal oestrogen deficiency, which leads to progressive bone loss.

Growth hormone. Acting via the somatomedins (IGF 1, p. 749) GH stimulates growth of cartilage.

Thyroid hormones. Excess T_4 and T_3 cause increased bone turnover, while hypothyroidism leads to growth delay.

The role of magnesium

Total body magnesium is about 25 g. Plasma magnesium ranges between 0.7 and 1.1 mmol·L^{-1}, and generally follows plasma calcium. Magnesium deficiency prevents the release of PTH; the level should be measured when there are signs or symptoms of hypocalcaemia unresponsive to calcium administration.

The role of phosphate

Phosphate forms an essential part of most biochemical systems from nucleic acids downwards. About 80% of all body phosphorus is within bone, plasma phosphate normally ranging from 0.80–1.40 $mmol \cdot L^{-1}$. Phosphate reabsorption from the kidney is decreased by PTH, thus hyperparathyroidism is associated with low plasma levels. High levels are found in hypoparathyroidism and in renal failure when normal excretion does not occur.

Measurement of plasma calcium, phosphate and PTH

Total plasma calcium is normally 2.2–2.6 $mmol \cdot L^{-1}$. Usually only 40% of total plasma calcium is ionized and physiologically relevant; the remainder is protein-bound or complexed and thus unavailable to the tissues. Ionized calcium is difficult to measure but very dependent upon protein—in particular albumin—concentration. An approximate correction for plasma calcium is to add or subtract 0.02 $mmol \cdot L^{-1}$ for every gram per litre by which the simultaneous albumin lies below or above a standard figure (normally 40 or 47 $g \cdot L^{-1}$). Thus, a total calcium of 2.22 $mmol \cdot L^{-1}$ with an albumin of 35 $g \cdot L^{-1}$ will become 2.32 $mmol \cdot L^{-1}$ (corrected to 40 $g \cdot L^{-1}$).

For critical measurements, samples should be taken in the fasting state without use of a cuff, as this affects protein concentration.

Parathyroid hormone assays are available in special centres, now improved with two-site immunoradiometrics that only measure the intact molecule and not fragments; interpretation requires simultaneous plasma calcium and phosphate measurements.

METABOLIC BONE DISEASE

Osteomalacia

PATHOPHYSIOLOGY

This results from inadequate mineralization of the osteoid framework, leading to soft bones. It is thus usually caused by a defect in vitamin D availability or metabolism. The effect on bone is shown in Fig. 16.31.

CAUSES

- Deficiency of vitamin D: dietary plus inadequate sunlight exposure (see above) often seen in Asian immigrant females in the UK
- Malabsorption: patients after gastric surgery,

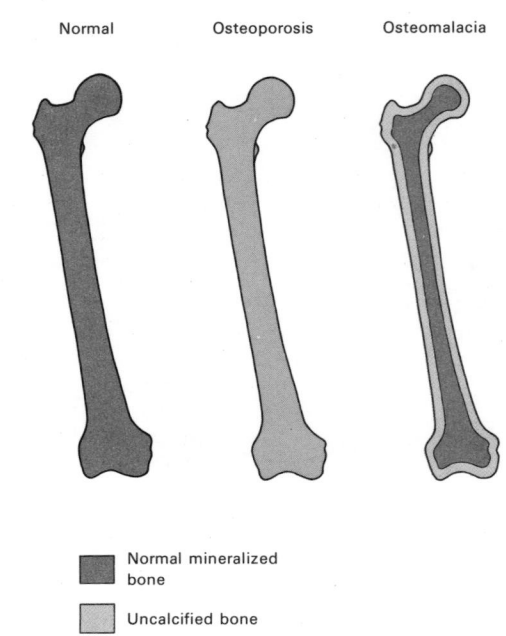

Fig. 16.31 Diagrammatic representation of the effects of osteoporosis and osteomalacia on the density and calcification of bone.

those with coeliac disease and those with deficient bile salt production
- Renal disease leading to inadequate conversion of 25-OHCC to 1,25-DHCC (see p. 477)

Less common are hepatic failure (reduced 25-OHCC) and phenytoin or barbiturate therapy (which induce the mixed function oxidase system and affect vitamin D metabolism). Vitamin D-resistant rickets (familial hypophosphataemia) is an X-linked disorder with hypophosphataemia, phosphaturia and rickets.

CLINICAL FEATURES

Childhood rickets usually presents with bony deformity or failure of adequate growth. In the adult, osteomalacia may produce bone and muscle pain and tenderness, often due to subclinical fractures. There is often a marked proximal myopathy, with a characteristic 'waddling' gait.

DIAGNOSIS

Certain diagnosis can only be made by bone biopsy with demonstration of increased unmineralized bone; undecalcified bone must be used. The procedure is uncomfortable and clinically rarely necessary.

The following biochemical and radiological findings are characteristic:

- Low serum phosphate.

- Increased serum alkaline phosphatase.
- Low or low-normal plasma calcium, corrected for albumin (see above).
- A low phosphate-calcium product is a useful screening test but use your local laboratory normal.
- X-rays show defective mineralization, especially in the pelvis, long bones and ribs, often with Looser's zones (linear areas of low density).

TREATMENT

Vitamin D replacement is given, usually as calciferol (500–5000 units/day) or the newer active metabolite (1-cholecalciferol (alfacalcidol) 1 μg/day). Plasma calcium must be checked regularly, as hypercalcaemia can be produced. Calcium supplements should not be given long-term unless there is a dietary deficiency.

Higher doses are needed when renal disease or resistance is present.

Osteoporosis

PATHOPHYSIOLOGY

Osteoporosis is reduced bone mass per unit bone volume (Fig. 16.31). This leads to reduced strength and increased risk of fracture, often with even minor trauma. Measurement of bone mass by densitometry and similar techniques is difficult and not generally available—plain radiography gives only very crude clues to the presence of osteoporosis.

The following factors are relevant:

- Bone mass decreases with increasing age.
- Osteoporosis is commonest in post-menopausal

Table 16.46 Causes of osteoporosis.

Old age
Post-menopausal
Endocrine causes Cushing's syndrome Diabetes mellitus Thyrotoxicosis Hypogonadism Acromegaly
Rheumatoid arthritis (localized only)
Immobilization Long-term bed rest
Weightlessness
Chronic renal failure
Drugs Glucocorticoids Heparin (long term)
Alcohol

women, as oestrogens prevent bone resorption. This group has a high prevalence of osteoporosis and fractures, most commonly Colles', femoral neck and vertebral sites.

- Inadequate dietary calcium intake is thought to be a further factor, with the average adult intake in patients with osteoporosis being 500–700 mg/day (12.5–17.5 mmol/day of Ca^{2+}) being only half that required to maintain balance.
- Physical activity, especially during growth, may promote increased bone mass. Excessive exercise in women, however, may produce hypogonadism (p. 778).

Other conditions causing osteoporosis are listed in Table 16.46.

CLINICAL FEATURES

The commonest presentation is of acute bone pain secondary to a suspected or actual fracture.

INVESTIGATION

- Plain radiology is of limited value—the reduction in density must be extreme before it can be detected with certainty. Crush fractures and complete vertebral collapse are common. There tends to be vertebral biconcavity.
- Fresh fractures may be highlighted by bone scanning (technetium-99).
- Plasma calcium, phosphate and alkaline phosphatase are all normal except following a recent fracture, when the latter may be raised. The disorder is one of bone mass not of calcium metabolism *per se*.
- Secondary deposits or multiple myeloma may need exclusion.
- The possibilities of thyrotoxicosis, Cushing's syndrome and diabetes mellitus may require the usual tests.
- Histological examination by transiliac biopsy is sometimes used to confirm the diagnosis. Coincident osteomalacia is sometimes present.
- Bone mass measurement (densitometry) is not widely available and CT scanning is little used. MRI may prove of greater value.

TREATMENT

Treatment of the established disease is unsatisfactory because bone mass has already been lost. Prophylaxis for high-risk individuals is therefore preferable.

Fractures should be treated by conventional orthopaedic means. Fresh fractures of the spine require short-term bed rest with adequate analgesia and, if necessary, muscle relaxants.

Treatment of the underlying osteoporosis is the same as that for prophylaxis.

PROPHYLAXIS

This area is controversial and the scientific evidence is conflicting. The following measures have been suggested but, apart from the first, are not widely accepted.

- Oestrogen therapy is of proven value and is being increasingly used as evidence accumulates that the potential side-effects (thrombosis, endometrial carcinoma, hypertension) are less than the benefits. Those with premature menopause or ovariectomy, those with high-risk factors, e.g. nullipara, the hypogonadal, those with family history of osteoporosis, should certainly be treated and many believe hormone replacement therapy (HRT) should be given to most women (see p. 782).
- Dietary calcium may be increased to above 1.5 g/day (40 mmol of Ca^{2+}), especially for postmenopausal women.
- Moderate exercises against gravity, e.g. walking, running and competitive sports, may also retard bone loss. This is often painful or impossible in those with established disease.

Fluoride, calcitonin and diphosphonates are being investigated but their use cannot be advised at present.

Paget's disease

See page 421.

HYPOCALCAEMIA AND HYPOPARATHYROIDISM

PATHOPHYSIOLOGY

Hypocalcaemia may be due to deficiencies of calcium homeostatic mechanisms, secondary to high phosphate levels or other causes of hypocalcaemia (Table 16.47). Hypoparathyroidism is uncommon.

CAUSES

- Renal failure is the commonest cause of hypocalcaemia.
- In postoperative thyroidectomy and parathyroidectomy, hypocalcaemia is usually transient.
- Idiopathic hypoparathyroidism is one of the rarer autoimmune disorders. Vitiligo, cutaneous moniliasis and other autoimmune diseases are often seen.
- DiGeorge syndrome is familial and associated with intellectual impairment, cataracts, calcified basal ganglia and occasionally with organ-specific autoimmune disease.
- Pseudohypoparathyroidism is a syndrome of end-organ resistance to parathyroid hormone. It

Table 16.47 Causes of hypocalcaemia.

Increased phosphate
Chronic renal failure
Phosphate therapy

Drugs
Calcitonin
Diphosphonates

Miscellaneous
Acute pancreatitis
Citrated blood in massive transfusion

Hypoparathyroidism
Congenital deficiency (DiGeorge's syndrome)
Idiopathic hypoparathyroidism (autoimmune)
After neck operations
Severe hypomagnesaemia

Resistance to PTH
Pseudohypoparathyroidism

Vitamin D
Deficiency
Resistance to vitamin D

is associated with short stature, short metacarpals and intellectual impairment. Pseudopseudohypoparathyroidism is the situation of the phenotypic defects without the calcium abnormalities.

CLINICAL FEATURES

The symptoms are those of neuromuscular irritability and neuropsychiatric manifestations. Parasthesiae, circumoral numbness, cramps, anxiety and tetany are followed by convulsions, laryngeal stridor, dystonia and psychosis.

Two important signs of hypocalcaemia are Chvostek's sign—gentle tapping over the facial nerve causes twitching of the facial muscles—and Trousseau's signs, where inflation of sphygmomanometer cuff above diastolic BP for 3 min induces tetanic spasm of the fingers and wrist. Severe hypocalcaemia may cause papilloedema and a prolonged Q–T interval on the ECG.

INVESTIGATION

The clinical picture is usually diagnostic and is confirmed by a low serum calcium. Additional tests include:

- Blood urea, creatinine
- High phosphate levels
- Absent or low PTH levels
- Parathyroid antibodies (not widely available)
- Vitamin D metabolite levels
- X-rays of metacarpals showing short fourth metacarpals, which occur in pseudohypoparathyroidism.

TREATMENT

Urgency of treatment depends upon severity of symptoms and degree of hypocalcaemia. If severe (e.g. tetany), intravenous calcium (10 ml initially, then 10–40 ml of 10% calcium gluconate in a litre of saline over 4–8 h) is given. Oral calcium supplements (2–10 g/day, 40–200 mmol of Ca^{2+}) are rarely sufficient alone.

1α-hydroxylated derivatives of Vitamin D are now preferred for their shorter half-life. Usual maintenance doses per day are 1 µg for 1α-OHD (alfacalcidol) and 1,25 OHD (calcitriol) and 0.25 mg for dihydrotachysterol. During treatment, plasma calcium must be monitored frequently to prevent hypercalcaemia.

HYPERPARATHYROIDISM AND HYPERCALCAEMIA

Hypercalcaemia is much commoner than hypocalcaemia, and is frequently detected incidentally with multichannel chemical analysers. Mild, asymptomatic hypercalcaemia occurs in about 1 in 1000 of the population and is usually due to primary hyperparathyroidism.

True hypercalcaemia should always be confirmed on a carefully collected specimen (see above).

PATHOPHYSIOLOGY AND CAUSES

Major causes of hypercalcaemia are listed in Table 16.48; primary hyperparathyroidism and malignant disease are the commonest.

Hyperparathyroidism may be primary, secondary or tertiary.

- Primary hyperparathyroidism is caused by single (80+%) or multiple (5%) parathyroid adenomas or by hyperplasia (10%). Parathyroid carcinoma is rare (2%) though usually with severe hypercalcaemia.
- Secondary hyperparathyroidism is physiological compensatory hypertrophy of all four parathyroids due to hypocalcaemia (e.g. in renal failure or vitamin D deficiency). PTH levels are raised but calcium levels are low or normal; PTH levels fall to normal after correction of the cause of hypocalcaemia.
- Tertiary hyperparathyroidism is the development of apparently autonomous parathyroid hyperplasia after long-standing secondary hyperparathyroidism, most often in renal failure. Plasma calcium and PTH are both raised, the latter often grossly so. Parathyroidectomy is necessary at this stage.

CLINICAL FEATURES

The symptoms and signs of hypercalcaemia are

Table 16.48 Causes of hypercalcaemia.

Excess PTH
Primary hyperparathyroidism
Tertiary hyperparathyroidism
Ectopic PTH secretion (very rare indeed)

Excess action of vitamin D
Iatrogenic or self-administered excess
Sarcoidosis

Excess calcium intake
'Milk alkali' syndrome

Drugs
Thiazides

Malignant disease
Secondary deposits
Production of osteoclastic factors by tumours
Myeloma

Other endocrine disease
Thyrotoxicosis
Addison's disease

Miscellaneous
Long-term immobility
Familial hypocalcuric hypercalcaemia

now more often mild and general rather than the severe renal and bone problems seen years ago:

- General—malaise, depression.
- Renal—renal colic from stones, polyuria/nocturia, haematuria and hypertension. The polyuria results from the effect of hypercalcaemia on the renal tubules reducing concentrating ability, a form of nephrogenic diabetes insipidus.
- Bones—bone pain.
- Abdominal—abdominal pain, sometimes peptic ulceration.

Particular points of note are:

- Malignant disease is usually advanced by the time hypercalcaemia occurs as a result of bony metastases. The common tumours are bronchus, breast, myeloma, oesophagus, thyroid, prostate, lymphoma and renal cell carcinoma. 'Ectopic PTH secretion' is very rare. Recent studies have produced evidence of a PTH-related protein, a 141-amino-acid polypeptide, the sequence of which shows an initial approximate homology with PTH. The biological action appears to lie in the first 34 amino acids. Local bone-resorbing cytokines and prostaglandins may be important locally where there are metastatic skeletal lesions leading to local mobilization of calcium by osteolysis with subsequent hypercalcaemia. They probably rarely cause hypercalcaemia by a generalized 'hormonal' action.

- Severe hypercalcaemia (> 3 mmol$\cdot$L^{-1}) is usually associated with malignant disease, hyperparathyroidism, renal dialysis or vitamin D therapy.
- Corneal calcification is a marker of long-standing hypercalcaemia.
- In primary hyperparathyroidism only 5–10% have definite bony lesions and 20–40% renal involvement.

INVESTIGATION AND DIFFERENTIAL DIAGNOSIS

- Several fasting calcium and phosphate samples should be taken. Hypophosphataemia is common in primary hyperparathyroidism.
- PTH levels should be measured. Detectable levels during hypercalcaemia are inappropriate and imply hyperparathyroidism.
- Abdominal X-rays may show renal calculi or nephrocalcinosis. Renal function must be measured.
- High-definition hand X-rays may show subperiosteal erosions in the middle or terminal phalanges.
- A hydrocortisone suppression test is often helpful; plasma calcium in hyperparathyroidism is resistant to suppression by steroids (10 days of hydrocortisone 40 mg three times daily); this also occurs with some malignancies. In sarcoidosis, vitamin D-mediated hypercalcaemia and some malignancies, suppression to normal or near-normal levels is seen.
- Protein electrophoresis for myeloma, TSH, T$_3$ for thyrotoxicosis, biopsy for sarcoidosis.
- PTH reduces renal tubular reabsorption of bicarbonate, thus slightly reducing the plasma level. As a consequence, the plasma chloride is elevated in primary hyperparathyroidism.

If primary hyperparathyroidism is confirmed, the following may be helpful in localization, though adenomas are usually small:

- Ultrasound, though insensitive to small tumours, is simple and safe.
- CT scan, though very high resolution is needed. MRI may prove more sensitive.
- Radioisotope 'subtraction' scans: a picture of the parathyroid tissue is derived from the difference in uptake between thallium-201 (taken up by thyroid and parathyroid) and technetium-99m (thyroid only). Reports on its efficacy are conflicting.
- Barium swallow may show indentation of the oesophagus by an adenoma.
- PTH venous catheterization is usually reserved for previous operative failures.

TREATMENT OF PRIMARY HYPERPARATHYROIDISM

Indications for surgery in hyperparathyroidism remain controversial. All agree that with renal disease or bone involvement surgery is indicated, there being no long-term medical treatment. The situation in which the plasma calcium is mildly raised (2.65–3.0 mmol$\cdot$L^{-1}) is disputed; most physicians feel that probable symptoms of hypercalcaemia, which may be mild and non-specific, should lead to parathyroidectomy. Those who are asymptomatic should receive careful follow-up; development of renal, bone or other symptoms then warrants surgery.

Surgery
Parathyroid surgery should only be performed by experienced surgeons. Ninety per cent of these patients have adenomas rather than hyperplasia but the minute glands may be very difficult to define. It is also very difficult to distinguish between an adenoma and normal parathyroid.

If initial exploration is unsuccessful, venous catheterization for PTH levels may be helpful if CT or MRI is not; a few parathyroids lie in ectopic sites elsewhere in the neck and upper mediastinum.

Postoperative care
The main danger postoperatively is hypocalcaemia (see above):

- Chvostek and Trousseau signs should be sought regularly.
- Daily plasma calcium measurements are needed for 2–5 days.
- Mild transient hypoparathyroidism often occurs for 1–2 weeks, possibly owing to suppression of the other parathyroids. Depending on severity, oral or intravenous calcium should be given temporarily.
- A few patients develop long-standing surgical hypoparathyroidism.

TREATMENT OF SECONDARY HYPERPARATHYROIDISM

Treatment depends upon the primary pathology, although steroids are often useful. Emergency treatment is discussed below.

TREATMENT OF ACUTE HYPERCALCAEMIA

This is an emergency, leading to nausea and vomiting, nocturia and polyuria, drowsiness and altered consciousness. The serum calcium is greater than 3 mmol$\cdot$L^{-1}, sometimes as high as 5 mmol$\cdot$L^{-1}.

While investigations of the cause (if unknown) is underway, immediate treatment is mandatory if the patient is seriously ill or plasma calcium is very high (> 3.5 mmol$\cdot$L^{-1}):

- Adequate rehydration (3–4 litres/day of saline for 2–3 days) is essential in all cases.
- Prednisolone (30–60 mg/day) is effective in a few

states, especially myeloma, sarcoidosis and vitamin D excess. In others it has little or no value.

- Intravenous diphosphonates (e.g. etidronate disodium and aminohydroxypropylidene biphosphonate (APD) are new, but probably the treatment of choice for hypercalcaemia of malignancy. The intravenous dose is 7.5 mg·kg^{-1} per day for 3 successive days for etidronate. A new biphosphate, pamidronate disodium, has just been introduced—the dosage is 15–90 mg as an infusion in normal saline or 5% dextrose over 2–8 h, or in smaller doses over 2–4 days.
- Mithramycin (plicamycin) (25 μg·kg^{-1} i.v. over 4–6 h) is often effective for 48 h.
- Calcitonin (200 units 6-hourly i.v.) has an acute but very short-lived hypocalcaemic action; it is now little used.
- Oral phosphate (sodium cellulose phosphate 5 g three times daily) produces diarrhoea; intravenous phosphate rapidly lowers calcium levels but is dangerous.

Once the calcium is reduced to levels where the patient is no longer acutely ill, routine investigation can proceed.

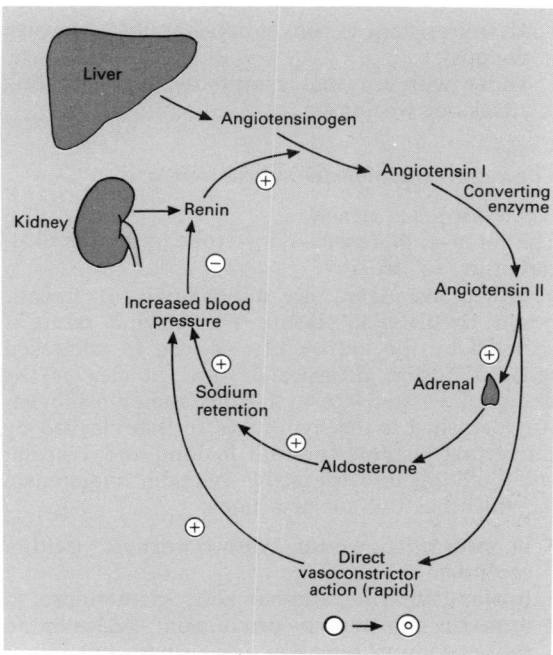

Fig. 16.32 The renin–angiotensin–aldosterone system.

Endocrinology of blood pressure control

The control of blood pressure (BP) is complex involving neural, cardiac, hormonal and many other mechanisms.

BP is dependent upon cardiac output and peripheral resistance. Although cardiac output can be increased in endocrine disease (e.g. thyrotoxicosis) the main role of hormonal mechanisms is control of peripheral resistance and of circulating blood volume. The oral contraceptive pill is a common endocrine cause of hypertension.

When to investigate for secondary hypertension?

Endocrine causes account for less than 5% of all hypertension (Table 16.49). It is impracticable and unnecessary to screen all hypertensive patients for secondary causes. The highest chances of detecting such causes are in:

- Subjects under 35 years old, especially those without a family history of hypertension
- Those with accelerated (malignant) hypertension
- Those with indications of renal disease (proteinuria, unequal renal sizes)
- Those with hypokalaemia before diuretic therapy

Table 16.49 Endocrine causes of hypertension.

Excessive renin, and thus angiotensin II, production
Renal artery stenosis
Other local renal disease
Renin-secreting tumours

Excessive production of catecholamines
Phaeochromocytoma

Excessive GH production
Acromegaly

Excessive aldosterone production
Adrenal adenoma (Conn's syndrome)
Idiopathic adrenal hyperplasia
Dexamethasone-suppressible hyperaldosteronism

Excessive production of other mineralocorticoids
Cushing's syndrome (massive excess of cortisol, a weak mineralocorticoid)
Congenital adrenal hyperplasia (in some cases)
Tumours producing other mineralocorticoids, e.g. corticosterone

Exogenous 'mineralocorticoids'
Liquorice ingestion
Abuse of mineralocorticoid preparations

- Those resistant to conventional antihypertensive therapy
- Those with unusual symptoms (e.g. sweating attacks or weakness)

The renin–angiotensin–aldosterone axis

Biochemistry and actions
The renin–angiotensin–aldosterone system is illustrated in Fig. 16.32.

Angiotensinogen, an α-2-globulin of hepatic origin, circulates in plasma. The enzyme, renin, is secreted by the kidney in response to decreased renal perfusion pressure or flow; it cleaves the decapeptide angiotensin I from angiotensinogen. Angiotensin I is inactive but is further cleaved by converting enzyme (present in lung and vascular endothelium) into the active peptide, angiotensin II, which has two major actions:

- It causes powerful vasocontriction (within seconds).
- It stimulates the adrenal zona glomerulosa to increase aldosterone production. Aldosterone causes sodium retention and urinary potassium loss (hours to days).

The vasoconstrictor action of angiotensin II is short-term, while the sodium retention induced by aldosterone increases total body sodium and BP in the longer term.

As BP increases and sodium is retained, the stimuli to renin secretion are reduced. Dietary sodium excess will tend to suppress renin secretion, whereas sodium deprivation or urinary sodium loss will increase it.

Atrial natriuretic factor/peptide (ANP)

These peptides are secreted from atrial granules. They produce marked effects on the kidney, increasing sodium and water excretion and glomerular filtration rate and lowering BP, plasma renin activity and plasma aldosterone. They appear to play a significant role in cardiovascular and fluid homeostasis but there is no evidence of primary defects in their secretion causing disease.

Analogues that as well as inhibiting the aminopeptidases that break down ANP are under development and might prove of value in producing a sodium diuresis.

RENIN (AND ANGIOTENSIN) DEPENDENT HYPERTENSION

Many forms of unilateral and bilateral renal diseases are associated with hypertension. The classic example is renal artery stenosis: the major hypertensive effects of this and other situations such as renin-secreting tumours are directly or indirectly due to angiotensin II.

Renin inhibitors have been produced, though none are yet available for clinical use. They appear to hold promise as antihypertensive agents.

Renal artery stenosis

This is discussed on p. 454.

DISORDERS OF ALDOSTERONE

Primary hyperaldosteronism
PATHOPHYSIOLOGY

This rare condition (< 1% of all hypertension) is caused by excess aldosterone production leading to sodium retention, potassium loss and the combination of hypokalaemia and hypertension.

CAUSES (Table 16.49)

Adrenal adenomas (Conn's syndrome) account for 60% of cases; 30% are due to bilateral adrenal hyperplasia, which may be secondary to excess of a pituitary aldosterone stimulating factor that is as yet unidentified.

CLINICAL FEATURES

The usual presentation is with hypertension and hypokalaemia (< 3.5 mmol·L^{-1}), although 20% of patients have initial potassium levels of 3.5–4.2 mmol–L^{-1}. The few symptoms are non-specific; muscle weakness, nocturia and tetany are rarely seen. The hypertension may be severe and associated with renal and retinal damage.

Adenomas, often very small, are commoner in young females, while bilateral hyperplasia rarely occurs before age 40 and is commoner in males.

INVESTIGATION

The characteristic features are:

- Hypokalaemia. A high-salt diet should be given for several days before testing and diuretics must be stopped 3 weeks before investigation; plasma samples must be separated quickly. Bethanidine or prazosin may be used for temporary control of blood pressure because they do not alter renin or aldosterone secretion.
- Urinary potassium loss. Levels over 30 mmol/day *during* hypokalaemia are inappropriate.
- Elevated plasma aldosterone levels that are not suppressed with saline infusion (300 mmol over 4 h) or fludrocortisone administration.
- Suppressed plasma renin activity. Beta-blockers and other drugs may interfere with renin activity.

Once a diagnosis of aldosteroinism is established, differentiation of adenoma from hyperplasia involves adrenal CT or MRI (not infallible as tumours may be very small), complex biochemical testing, adrenal scintillation scanning (now rarely needed) and venous catheterization.

TREATMENT

An adenoma should be surgically removed; BP falls in 70%. Those with hyperplasia should be treated with the aldosterone antagonist spironolactone (100–400 mg/day); side-effects include nausea, rashes and gynaecomastia. Amiloride (10–40 mg/day) is an alternative, especially as spironolactone has been linked with tumour development in animals. Calcium channel blockers are also effective.

Secondary hyperaldosteronism

This situation arises when there is excess renin (and hence angiotensin II) stimulation of the zona glomerulosa. Common causes are accelerated hypertension and renal artery stenosis, when the patient will be hypertensive. Causes associated with normotension include congestive cardiac failure and cirrhosis, where excess aldosterone production contributes to sodium retention.

Spironolactone is of value in both situations. Angiotensin-converting enzyme inhibitors e.g. captopril, enalapril or lisinopril, are effective in heart failure.

Hypoaldosteronism

Except as part of primary hypoadrenalism (Addison's disease—p. 811), this is very uncommon.

THE ADRENAL MEDULLA

The major catecholamines, noradrenaline and adrenaline, are produced in the adrenal medulla (Fig. 16.33) although most noradrenaline is derived from sympathetic neuronal release. While noradrenaline and adrenaline undoubtedly produce hypertension when infused, they probably play little part in BP regulation in normal man.

Phaeochromocytoma

Phaeochromocytomas, tumours of the sympathetic nervous system, are very rare (less than 1 in 1000 cases of hypertension). Ninety per cent arise in the adrenal, 25% are multiple and 10% are malignant. Some are associated with multiple endocrine neoplasia syndromes (p. 831).

PRESENTATION

The clinical features are those of catecholamine excess and are frequently, but not necessarily, intermittent (Table 16.50).

DIAGNOSIS

The possibility needs to be considered quite frequently in patients with hypertension. Specific tests are:

- Measurement of urinary metabolites (vanillylmandelic acid (VMA) and metanephrines—Fig. 16.33) is a useful screening test; normal levels on three 24-hour collections virtually exclude the diagnosis. Many drugs and dietary vanilla interfere with these tests.
- If high VMAs are found, plasma catecholamines may be estimated.

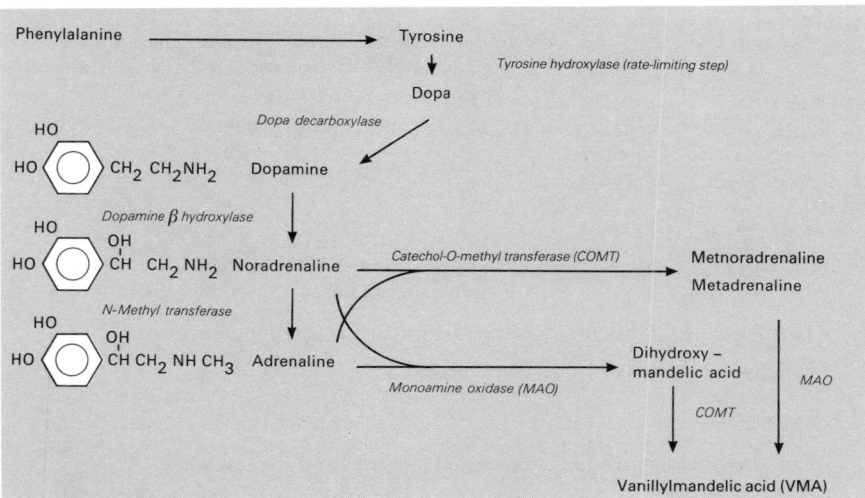

Fig. 16.33 The synthesis and metabolism of catecholamines.

- CT scans, initially of the abdomen, are usually helpful as the tumours are often large.

Table 16.50 Symptoms and signs of phaeochromocytoma.

Symptoms
Anxiety or panic attacks
Palpitations
Tremor
Sweating
Headache
Flushing
Nausea and/or vomiting
Weight loss
Constipation or diarrhoea
Raynaud's phenomenon
Chest pain
Polyuria/nocturia

Signs
Hypertension—intermittent or constant
Tachycardia plus arrhythmias
Bradycardia
Orthostatic hypotension
Pallor or flushing
Glycosuria
Fever
(Signs of hypertensive damage)

- Scanning with [^{131}I]-metaiodobenzylguanidine produces specific uptake in sites of sympathetic activity.

TREATMENT

Tumours should be removed if this is possible. Medical pre- and perioperative treatment is vital and includes complete alpha- and beta-blockade with phenoxybenzamine (20–40 mg/day initially), then propranolol (120–140 mg/day), plus transfusion of whole blood to re-expand the contracted plasma volume. Labetolol is not recommended. Surgery in the unprepared patient is fraught with dangers of both hyper- and hypotension; expert anaesthetic help is vital and sodium nitroprusside should be available in case sudden severe hypertension develops.

When operation is not possible, combined alpha- and beta-blockade can be used long-term.

Other endocrinological disorders

Diseases of many glands

Multiple gland failure
This is caused by autoimmune disease (see Table 16.6).

Table 16.51 Multiple endocrine neoplasia (MEN) syndrome.

Organ	Frequency	Tumours/manifestations
TYPE 1		
Parathyroid	95%	Adenomas/hyperplasia
Pituitary	70%	Adenomas—prolactinoma, ACTH or growth hormone secreting (acromegaly)
Pancreas	50%	Islet cell tumours (secreting insulin, glucagon, somatostatin, VIP, pancreatic polypeptide) Zollinger–Ellison syndrome
Adrenal	40%	Non-functional adenoma
Thyroid	20%	Adenomas—multiple or single
TYPE 2a		
Adrenal	Most	Phaeochromocytoma (70% bilateral) Cushing's syndrome
Thyroid	Most	Medullary carcinoma (calcitonin producing)
Parathyroid	60%	Hyperplasia
TYPE 2b		

Type 2a with Marfanoid phenotype and intestinal and visceral ganglioneuromas.
Neuromas also present around lips and tongue.

Multiple endocrine neoplasia (MEN)

This is the name given to the simultaneous or metachronous recurrence of tumours involving a number of endocrine glands (see Table 16.51). They are inherited in an autosomal dominant manner and are thought to arise from the expression of a recessive oncogenic mutation.

An affected person may pass on the mutation to his offspring in the germ cell, but for the disease to become evident a somatic mutation must also occur, e.g. deletion or loss of a normal homologous chromosome. The defect in MEN 1 is on the long arm of chromosome 11 near an area containing a number of oncogenes that encode for proteins with fibroblastic growth factor activity. The gene for MEN 2a is on chromosome 10 close to the retinol-binding gene.

MANAGEMENT

Management is surgical.

- *Type 1.* All four parathyroid tumours are removed (as all may be involved) followed by vitamin D (1,25-dihydrocalciferol) replacement therapy. Pancreatic tumours are often multiple and recurrence after partial pancreatectomy is invariable. Other tumours are treated surgically if necessary.
- *Type 2.* Tumours may also be recurrent or bilateral and a careful follow-up is necessary.

Screening of relatives. A careful family history should first be taken. If negative, it does not exclude involvement and it may need repeating at regular (1–5 year) intervals.

- *Type 1.* Fasting calcium estimation. (If elevated, look for other manifestations of MEN 1).
- *Type 2.* (a) Medullary carcinoma of thyroid (MCT). Pentagastrin and calcium infusion test with measurement of calcitonin to pick up 'C' cell hyperplasia (> doubling of the calcitonin level is abnormal.
    (b) Phaeochromocytoma. VMA and metanephrine estimations.

Both first- and second-degree relatives should be screened biochemically. Genetic markers can be used to predict presymptomatic relatives. For example, in Type 2a, polymorphic variants of the retinol-binding protein (*RBP*) gene can be used.

Ectopic hormone secretion

This terminology refers to hormone secretion from a non-endocrine cell, most usually seen in tumours that have some degree of embryological resemblance to specialist endocrine cells. The clinical effects may be those of the hormone produced, with or without manifestations of systemic malignancy.

The commonest situations seen are:

- Hypercalcaemia of malignant disease, often from squamous cell tumours or lung and breast, often with bone metastases. It is mediated by various factors, but very rarely by PTH itself (see p. 825).
- Syndrome of inappropriate ADH section (p. 818). Again, this is commonest from a primary lung tumour.
- The ectopic ACTH syndrome (p. 816). Small-cell carcinoma of the lung, carcinoid tumours and medullary thyroid carcinomas are the commonest causes.
- Production of insulin-like activity may result in hypoglycaemia (p. 859).

Further reading

Baillière's Clinics in Endocrinology and Metabolism—a series of up-to-date reviews of specific topics. London: Baillière Tindall.

Besser GM & Cudworth AG (1987) *Clinical Endocrinology—An Illustrated Text.* London: Gower.

DeGroot LJ, Reed Larsen P, Refetoff S & Stanbury JB (1984) *The Thyroid and Its Disorders*, 5th edn. New York: Wiley.

Greenspan FS & Forsham PH (eds) (1986) *Basic and Clinical Endocrinology*, 2nd edn. Los Altos: Lange Medical Publishers.

Hall R, Anderson J, Smart GA & Besser GM (eds) (1990) *Fundamentals of Clincial Endocrinology*, 4th edn. London: Pitman Medical.

Martin CR (1985) *Endocrine Physiology*. Oxford: Oxford University Press.

Wilson JB & Foster DW (eds) (1985) *Textbook of Endocrinology*, 7th edn. Brighton: Holt-Saunders.

17

Diabetes Mellitus and Other Disorders of Metabolism

Diabetes mellitus

Introduction

Diabetes means excessive urination. Earlier generations of physicians, obliged to taste the urine, distinguished the honey flavour of diabetes mellitus from the tasteless urine of diabetes insipidus. Diabetes mellitus is a group of metabolic disorders characterized by chronic hyperglycaemia. The metabolic disturbance involves the metabolism of fat and protein as well as that of carbohydrates, reflecting a state of insulin deprivation. This in turn may be due to deficient insulin secretion, to factors opposing the tissue effects of insulin, or to both. Untreated diabetes results in characteristic clinical symptoms; these vary in intensity, and may culminate in the hyperglycaemic emergencies of diabetic ketoacidosis or non-ketotic hyperosmolar coma. Diabetes is usually irreversible and while it allows the patient to have a reasonably normal lifestyle, its late complications result in a consider-

ably reduced life expectancy. These complications include accelerated arterial disease and a characteristic microangiopathy. Macrovascular disease leads to an increased prevalence of coronary artery disease and peripheral vascular disease, while microvascular damage contributes to diabetic retinopathy and diabetic nephropathy.

Diabetes is common, affecting some 30 million people world-wide. Its causes are incompletely understood, but it is clear that the disease is often multifactorial and that both genetic and environmental factors are involved. Primary diabetes mellitus has two main forms: insulin-dependent (IDDM) and non-insulin-dependent (NIDDM), which are also referred to as type I and type II diabetes.

Insulin secretion

Insulin is the key hormone involved in the storage and controlled release within the body of the chemical energy available from food. It is synthesized in the beta cells of the pancreatic islets in the form of proinsulin, which is stored in secretory

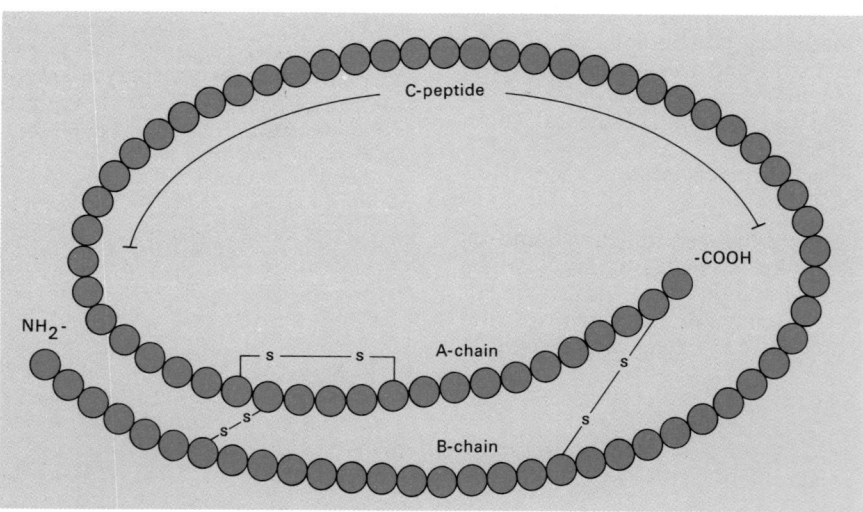

Fig. 17.1 The proinsulin molecule. During the process of insulin secretion, C-peptide (connecting peptide) breaks off and insulin is released as two peptide chains linked by disulphide bridges.

granules close to the cell membrane. A biochemically inert peptide fragment known as connecting (C) peptide breaks off from proinsulin (Fig. 17.1) in the secretory process, so that equimolar quantities of insulin and C-peptide are released into the circulation. Insulin enters the portal circulation, and is carried to the liver, its prime target organ. About 50% of secreted insulin is extracted and degraded in the liver; the residue is broken down by the kidney. C-peptide is only partially extracted by the liver (and hence provides a useful index of the rate of insulin secretion), but is mainly degraded by the kidney.

The insulin receptor is a glycoprotein of approximate molecular weight 400 kD present on many target cells (Fig. 17.2). Insulin molecules bind to these receptors, forming a complex that promotes glucose uptake.

An outline of glucose metabolism

Blood glucose levels are closely regulated in health and rarely stray outside the range of 3.5–8.0 $mmol \cdot L^{-1}$, despite the varying demands of food, fasting and exercise. The principal organ of glucose homeostasis is the liver, which absorbs and stores glucose (as glycogen) in the post-absorptive state and releases it into the circulation between meals to match the rate of glucose utilization by peripheral tissues.

Glucose production. About 200 g of glucose is produced and utilized each day. More than 90% is derived from the liver, three-quarters from glyco-

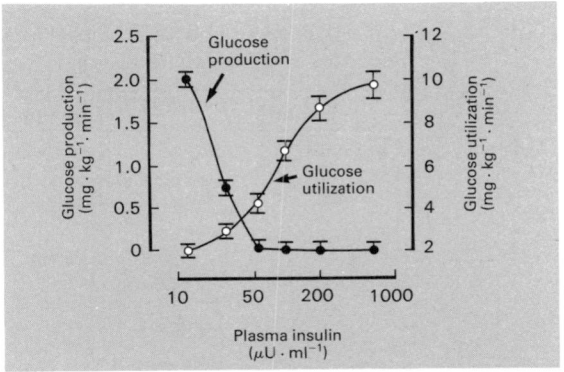

Fig. 17.3 The effect of different insulin levels on glucose production and glucose utilization. Hepatic glucose production rises as insulin levels fall. Conversely, peripheral uptake of glucose is promoted at high insulin levels.

gen and one-quarter from gluconeogenesis. The remaining 5–10% derives from renal gluconeogenesis.

Glucose utilization. The brain is the major consumer of glucose. Its requirement is $1 \ mg \cdot kg^{-1}$ body weight per minute, or 100 g daily in a 70 kg man. Glucose uptake by the brain is obligatory and is not dependent on insulin, and the glucose used is oxidized to carbon dioxide and water.

Other tissues, such as muscle and fat, are facultative glucose consumers. The effect of insulin peaks associated with meals is to lower the threshold for glucose entry into cells; at other times, energy requirements are largely met by fatty-acid oxidation. Glucose taken up by muscle is stored as glycogen or broken down to lactate, which re-enters the circulation and becomes an important substrate for hepatic gluconeogensis. Glucose is used by fat tissue as a source of energy and as a substrate for triglyceride synthesis; lipolysis releases fatty acids from triglyceride together with glycerol, another substrate for hepatic gluconeogenesis.

Hormonal regulation. Insulin is the major regulator of intermediary metabolism, although its actions are modified in important respects by other hormones. Dose–response curves for the production and utilization of glucose are shown in Fig. 17.3.

At low insulin levels, glucose production is maximal and utilization is minimal; at high levels the situation is reversed. At intermediate plasma insulin levels of 40–50 $mU \cdot L^{-1}$, glucose production is largely suppressed but utilization remains low. This observation forms the theoretical basis for the low-dose insulin regimen used to treat diabetic ketoacidosis (see below).

The effect of counter-regulatory hormones (gluc-

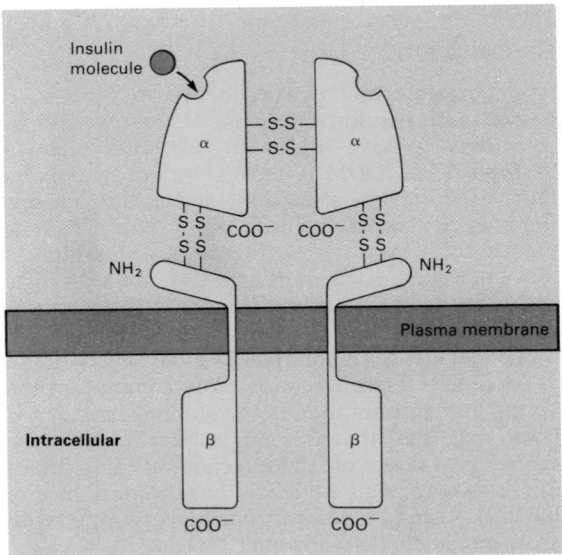

Fig. 17.2 The insulin receptor consists of α and β subunits linked by disulphide bridges. The β subunits straddle the cell membrane and initiate some of the intracellular actions of insulin.

Table 17.1 Opposing actions of insulin and two of its antagonists—glucagon and adrenaline.

Insulin	Action	Glucagon and adrenaline
	Glucose production by liver:	
↓	Glycogenolysis	↑
↓	Gluconeogenesis	↑
	Glucose utilization by:	
↑	Fat and muscle	↓
↓	Lipolysis	↑
↓	Ketogenesis	↑

agon, adrenaline, cortisol and growth hormone) is to shift the dose–response curves to the right, resulting in greater production of glucose and less utilization for a given level of insulin.

The opposing actions of insulin and two of its antagonists are summarized in Table 17.1.

Detailed understanding of the actions of insulin at a molecular level remains tantalizingly incomplete but very rapid progress has been made in recent years. Isolation and characterization of the insulin receptor has been an important advance. The receptor is a glycoprotein that straddles the cell membrane and consists of a dimer with two α subunits, which include the binding sites for insulin, and two β subunits, which traverse the cell membrane and initiate at least some of the intracellular actions of insulin. The DNA sequence coding for the receptor has been isolated and sequenced and is located on the short arm of chromosome 19.

After binding, the insulin–receptor complex is internalized by the cell with subsequent degradation of insulin and recycling of the receptor to the cell surface.

TYPES OF DIABETES

Diabetes may be primary or secondary (see Table 17.2). Although IDDM (type I diabetes) and NIDDM (type II diabetes) represent two distinct diseases from the epidemiological point of view, clinical distinction may sometimes be difficult. The two disease processes should, in clinical terms, be visualized as opposite ends of a continuous spectrum (Table 17.3).

Insulin-dependent diabetes mellitus (IDDM; type I diabetes)

EPIDEMIOLOGY

Approximately one person in 300 in the UK is treated with insulin, but some of these would be considered to have NIDDM by the criteria shown in Table 17.3. IDDM is most common in populations of European extraction, and within Europe there is a marked increase in incidence as one moves north from the Mediterranean—the highest incidence occurs in northern Scandinavia. The frequency of IDDM in various countries is shown in Fig. 17.4.

The incidence in childhood is maximal at 10–13 years of age. Presentation is more common in the spring and autumn than in the summer, and it has been suggested that this might be related to the greater prevalence of viral infections at these times. There is now good evidence that the incidence of IDDM is rising, at least in northern Europe, with an approximate doubling over the past 20–30 years.

AETIOLOGY

Genetic susceptibility
IDDM is not genetically predestined, but an

Table 17.2 Causes of secondary diabetes.

Liver disease
Cirrhosis

Pancreatic disease
Cystic fibrosis
Chronic pancreatitis
Tropical diabetes
Pancreatectomy
Haemochromatosis
Carcinoma of the pancreas

Endocrine disease
Cushing's syndrome
Acromegaly
Thyrotoxicosis
Phaeochromocytoma

Drug-induced disease
Thiazide diuretics
Steroid therapy

Insulin-receptor abnormalities
Congenital lipodystrophy
Acanthosis nigricans

Genetic syndromes, e.g. Friedrich's ataxia

Table 17.3 The spectrum of diabetes: a comparison of insulin-dependent diabetes mellitus (IDDM) and non-insulin-dependent diabetes mellitus (NIDDM).

	IDDM (type I)	NIDDM (type II)

Epidemiology	Patients are:
	  Younger
	  Usually lean
	  European extraction
	    (most commonly)
	
	Seasonal incidence
	
	? Viral aetiology
		Patients are:
		  Older
		  Often overweight
		  All racial groups
		    (increasing incidence in
		    affluent immigrants)

Heredity	HLA-DR3 or DR4 in 95%
	
	30–50% concordance in
	  identical twins
		No HLA links
		
		90% concordance in identical
		  twins

Pathogenesis	Autoimmunity:
	  Islet cell antibody
	  Insulin autoantibodies
	  Insulitis
	  Associations with other
	    organ-specific
	    autoimmune diseases
		No evidence of immune
		  disturbance

Clinical	Insulin deficiency
	
	May develop ketoacidosis
	
	Always need insulin
		Partial insulin deficiency,
		  insulin resistance
		
		May develop non-ketotic
		  hyperosmolar state
		
		Sometimes need insulin

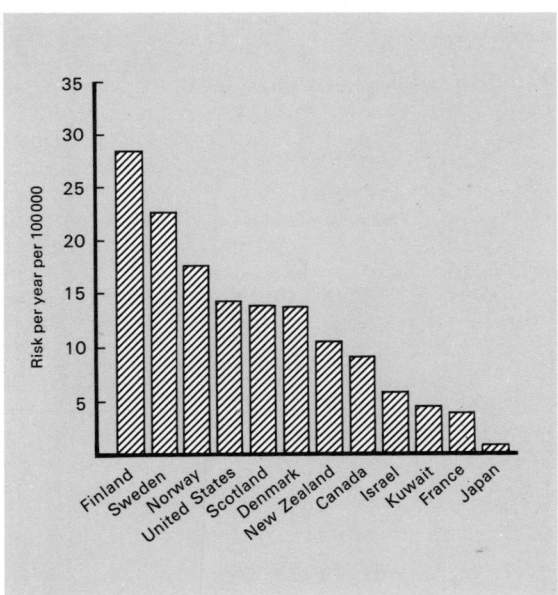

Fig. 17.4 The incidence of insulin-dependent diabetes mellitus (type I diabetes) in different countries.

increased susceptibility to the disease may be inherited.

Idential twins
The identical twin of a patient with IDDM has a 30–50% chance of developing the disease. This implies that non-genetic factors must also be involved.

Inheritance
The child of an insulin-dependent diabetic patient has an increased chance of developing IDDM. This risk, curiously, is greater with a diabetic father (between 1 in 20 and 1 in 40) than with a diabetic mother (1 in 40–80). The overall risk for a second sibling is 1 in 20, rising to 1 in 6 for an HLA-identical sibling.

HLA system. Ninety-five per cent of IDDM patients carry HLA-DR3, HLA-DR4 or both. Other reported HLA associations in the A and B regions are secondary to linkage disequilibrium (Fig. 17.5). Even stronger associations are being reported with the DQ region.

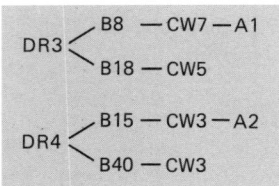

Fig. 17.5 HLA axes of susceptibility for diabetes.

DR3 and DR4 are common antigens present in 50% of the UK population. The relative risk conferred by DR3 is estimated at 7 times, that of DR4 at 9 times, and that of both DR3 and DR4 at 14 times normal. Since this risk is additive, a model based on two susceptibility genes (one associated with DR3 and one with DR4) has been proposed.

In contrast, individuals with HLA-DR2 have a considerably reduced risk (0.12 times normal) of developing diabetes. The reasons for this protective effect are unclear.

The insulin gene. Associations between IDDM and other chromosomes (apart from chromosome 6) have been described. A polymorphous DNA region close to the insulin gene on chromosome 11 has been studied, and short, intermediate and long insertions (see p. 107) have been reported. Homozygosity of the short (class I) allele is found in some 80% of patients with IDDM as against 40% of controls.

Immunological aspects
Several pieces of evidence suggest that autoimmune processes are involved in the pathogenesis of IDDM.

Association with other autoimmune disease. Autoimmune thyroid disease, Addison's disease and pernicious anaemia are more common in patients and their relatives.

Immunogenetic associations. The association between DR3, DR4 and diabetes, and the protective effect of DR2 might represent idiosyncracies in the immune process that result in increased (or reduced) susceptibility.

The insulitis process. Autopsies of patients who died soon after diagnosis are characterized by infiltration of the pancreatic islets by mononuclear cells. A similar pattern occurs in other autoimmune diseases, e.g. thyroiditis.

Immune abnormalities at diagnosis. About 70% of newly presenting patients have islet-cell antibodies. These react with human islets and can be detected by immunofluorescence. They usually become undetectable within a few years of diagnosis. In such patients increased numbers of activated T lymphocytes may also be present in the circulation at diagnosis.

Environmental factors
A viral aetiology has been suspected for many years. This is based on the seasonal incidence of the condition, anecdotal associations, and analysis of viral antibody titres at diagnosis. IgM antibodies to Coxsackie B4 have been reported in 20–30% of new cases. However, in view of the long prodromal period (see below), it seems likely that viruses precipitate rather than initiate the onset of diabetes.

The diabetes prodrome
Prospective study of first-degree relatives of children with diabetes has revealed that islet-cell antibodies may appear in the circulation months or even years before diagnosis. Insulin antibodies have also been reported in this period, and abnormalities of insulin secretion in response to intravenous glucose may develop.

The sequence of events leading to diagnosis may be as shown in Fig. 17.6. Better understanding of this sequence may in time permit strategies of prevention to be tested.

Non-insulin-dependent diabetes mellitus (NDDM; type II diabetes)

EPIDEMIOLOGY

Unlike IDDM this is relatively common in all populations enjoying an affluent lifestyle. Large

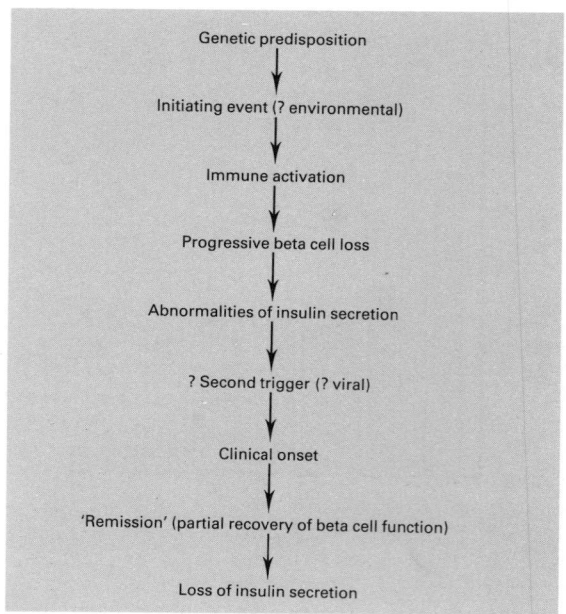

Fig. 17.6 The possible sequence of events leading to the development of IDDM.

Table 17.4 Frequency of non-insulin-dependent diabetes mellitus in various populations (WHO criteria).

Group	Age (years)	Rate (%)
USA	20–74	6.9
USA—Mexican immigrants	25–65	17.0
USA—Pima Indians	25+	25.5
Malta	15+	7.7
Indonesia	15+	1.7
New Guinea (highlands)	20+	0.0

differences in prevalence have been reported. The disease may be present in a subclinical form for years before diagnosis, and the incidence increases markedly with age and degree of obesity. The onset may be accelerated by the stress of pregnancy, drug treatment or intercurrent illness. Estimates of prevalence using the WHO criteria would suggest an overall prevalence of around 2% in the UK; the rate is about fivefold higher in Asian immigrants.

The rates shown in Table 17.4 have been reported in various populations.

Epidemiological surveys have shown that indolent well-fed populations are 2–20 times as likely to develop NIDDM as lean populations of the same race.

AETIOLOGY

Genetics
Identical twins of a patient with NIDDM have an almost 100% chance of developing diabetes. About 25% of patients have a first-degree relative with NIDDM. Certain families exist in which diabetes appears to travel as an autosomal dominant characteristic, but study has been limited by the lack of a useful genetic marker for the condition.

Immunology
There is no evidence of immune involvement in its pathogenesis.

Insulin secretion and action
Patients with NIDDM, unlike those with IDDM, retain about 50% of their beta-cell mass at autopsy.

Abnormalities of insulin secretion develop early in the course of the disease. Normal subjects have a biphasic insulin response to intravenous glucose. In NIDDM the first-phase insulin response to intravenous glucose is lost, and insulin secretion in response to oral glucose is delayed and exaggerated. The majority of patients manifest reduced insulin secretion relative to the prevailing glucose concentration, and there is progressive beta-cell loss occuring in many patients, although not to the extent seen in IDDM. It is not known whether this is due to 'exhaustion' of surviving beta cells or to some independent process of damage. Islet amyloid deposits are commonly seen in NIDDM, destroying the cells and interfering with glucose and hormone transport. The amyloid deposits are derived from islet amyloid polypeptide (IAPP), which may oppose the action of insulin, possibly explaining the insulin resistance that is also present. Obesity is present in 80% of such patients, but insulin resistance may also be marked in lean patients.

Impaired glucose tolerance

If an oral glucose tolerance test is administered at random to a large population, 1–2% will be found to have unsuspected diabetes. A much larger group—5% or more (depending on the age, race and nutritional state of the population)—fall into an intermediate category now referred to as impaired glucose tolerance (IGT). The criteria for this category are given below. Follow-up of patients in this case shows that some (2–4% yearly) go on to develop diabetes, but that the abnormality does not progress in the majority. Classification is complicated by the poor reproducibility of the oral glucose tolerance test and the group is certainly heterogeneous. Some are obese, some have liver disease, and others are on medication that impairs glucose tolerance; individuals in this category are at increased risk of arterial disease but do not develop the specific microvascular complications of diabetes.

Tropical diabetes

A distinct variety of diabetes has been described. This is found only in developing countries on or near the equator. The following features have been described.

- Onset is before the age of 30.
- There is a history of severe malnutrition.
- There is insulin dependence, sometimes with severe but fluctuating insulin resistance.
- Ketoacidosis does not develop when insulin is withdrawn.

There are two main variants:

- *Fibrocalculous pancreatic diabetes.* This is associated with exocrine pancreatic deficiency, pancreatic fibrosis (often leading to calcification) and the presence of stones in the pancreatic duct. There may be a history of recurrent abdominal pain, and in 75% of cases there is evidence of pancreatic calcification on plain abdominal X-ray. Most populations in which this condition arises are subject to malnutrition and have a diet based on cassava. Cyanates are present in the cassava root and may be a factor in the pancreatic damage.

- *Protein-deficient pancreatic diabetes.* This form appears to be a direct consequence of malnutrition. The main differences from the fibrocalculous variant are that exocrine pancreatic function is unimpaired and there is no evidence of pancreatic fibrosis or calcification. Abdominal pain is not a feature.

In both forms of tropical diabetes, insulin secretion is preserved, although impaired; this is the likely explanation for the observed resistance to ketosis.

The oral glucose tolerance test

After an overnight fast, 75 g of glucose is taken in 250–350 ml of water. Blood samples are taken in the fasting state and 2 h after the glucose has been given.

A specific enzymatic glucose assay must be used. Plasma glucose levels are 10% higher than whole blood.

Diabetes
This is present when the fasting *blood* glucose is over 6.7 mmol·L^{-1} and/or when the 2-hour value is over 10 mmol·L^{-1}. Corresponding values for *plasma* glucose are 7.8 mmol·L^{-1} and 11.1 mmol·L^{-1}.

Impaired glucose tolerance
This is present when the fasting blood glucose is below 6.7 mmol·L^{-1} and when the 2-hour value is between 6.7 and 10 mmol·L^{-1}. Corresponding values for *plasma* glucose are 7.8 and 11.1 mmol·L^{-1}. Impaired glucose tolerance can only be diagnosed using the oral glucose tolerance test.

Intermediate sampling times (e.g. 30 min and 60 min) are not needed for the diagnosis of diabetes by WHO criteria. However, simultaneous blood and urine glucose measurements can be used to define a low renal threshold for glucose.

Diabetes can usually be diagnosed on the basis of fasting or random blood glucose measurements (see text). *The glucose tolerance test should be reserved for borderline cases only.*

CLINICAL PRESENTATION OF DIABETES

Acute presentation
Young people often present with a brief 2–4 week history and report the classic triad of symptoms:

- *Polyuria*, due to the osmotic diuresis that results when blood glucose levels exceed the renal threshold
- *Thirst*, due to the resulting loss of fluid and electrolytes
- *Weight loss*, due to fluid depletion and the accelerated breakdown of fat and muscle secondary to insulin deficiency

Ketoacidosis may be the presenting feature if these early symptoms are not recognized and treated.

Subacute presentation
The clinical onset may be over several months, particularly in older patients. Thirst, polyuria and weight loss are usual features but medical attention is sought for such symptoms as lack of energy, visual blurring due to refractive errors, or pruritus vulvae or balanitis due to *Candida* infection.

Complications
Complications may be the presenting feature. These include:

- Staphylococcal skin infections
- Retinopathy noted during a visit to the optician
- A polyneuropathy causing tingling and numbness in the feet
- Impotence
- Arterial disease, resulting in myocardial infarction or peripheral gangrene

Asymptomatic diabetes
Glycosuria or a raised blood glucose may be detected on routine examination (e.g. for insurance purposes) in individuals who deny any symptoms of ill health.

Physical examination

This is often unrewarding but evidence of weight loss and dehydration may be present, and the breath may smell of ketones. Older patients may present with established complications, and the presence of the characteristic retinopathy is diagnostic of diabetes.

INVESTIGATION OF DIABETES

The diagnosis is usually simple. Blood glucose levels are so closely controlled by the body that even small deviations become important.

- In *symptomatic* patients, a single elevated blood glucose, measured by a reliable method, indicates diabetes.
- In *asymptomatic* or *mildly symptomatic* patients, the diagnosis is made on:
  - (a) One, preferably two, fasting venous *blood* glucose levels above 6.7 mmol·L^{-1} (120 mg·dl^{-1}); the equivalent venous *plasma* level is 7.8 mmol·L^{-1} (140 mg·dl^{-1})
  - (b) One, preferably two, random values above 10 mmol·L^{-1} (180 mg·dl^{-1-1}) in venous whole blood or 11.1 mmol·L^{-1} (200 mg·dl^{-1}) in venous plasma
- A glucose tolerance test (GTT) is unnecessary when the criteria above are satisfied, and should be reserved for true borderline cases.

- Glycosuria is measured using sensitive glucose-specific dipstick methods. Glycosuria is not diagnostic of diabetes but indicates the need for further investigation. About 1% of the population have renal glycosuria. This is an inherited low renal threshold for glucose, transmitted either as a Mendelian dominant or recessive trait.

Other investigations

No further tests are needed to diagnose diabetes. Other routine investigations including screening the urine for proteinuria, a full blood count, urea and electrolytes, and a fasting blood sample for cholesterol and triglycerides. The latter test is useful to exclude an associated hyperlipidaemia but should only be performed after blood glucose levels have been brought under control.

It is important to remember that diabetes may be *secondary* to other conditions (see Table 17.2), may be *precipitated* by underlying illness and be *associated* with autoimmune disease or hyperlipidaemia.

TREATMENT OF DIABETES

Guidelines to therapy

All patients with diabetes require diet therapy. Good glycaemic control is unlikely to be achieved with insulin or oral therapy when diet is neglected, especially when the patient is also overweight.

Insulin is always indicated in a patient who has been in ketoacidosis, and is usually indicated in patients who present under the age of 40. Insulin is also indicated in older patients following primary or secondary failure of oral therapy (see below). Tablets should be avoided in younger patients and are contraindicated in pregnancy.

In older patients the approach to therapy is empirical. Diet alone should be tried in the first instance, and dietary knowledge and compliance should always be reassessed with care before proceeding to the next step. This is of particular importance in the obese patient who fails to lose weight.

When diet fails to achieve satisfactory control, thin patients are usually treated with a sulphonylurea drug, and obese patients with a biguanide. Primary failure of treatment occurs when these agents (alone or in combination) never achieve the desired level of control. Other patients may show a good initial response followed by progressive loss of control over the succeeding months or years; this is referred to as secondary failure of treatment.

Since this approach is largely empirical, it is not surprising that practice differs from one country to another. For example, metformin (the only biguanide in common use) is very widely employed in France, tends to be used less in the UK, and is not licensed in the USA. Criteria of control also vary, so that what is classed as primary failure at one centre may be seen as a success in another. The most widespread error in management is procrastination; the patient whose control is inadequate on tablets should start insulin without undue delay.

Recent evidence suggests that the progression of vascular complications including retinopathy can be reduced by regular low dose aspirin therapy.

Diet

The diet for a diabetic patient is no different from the diet considered healthy for the population as a whole.

Carbohydrate

This should consist of unrefined carbohydrate rather than simple sugars such as sucrose. Carbohydrate is absorbed relatively slowly from fibre-rich foods, preventing the rapid swings in circulating glucose seen when refined sugars are ingested. For example, the glucose peak seen after eating an apple is much flatter than that seen after drinking the same amount of carbohydrate as apple juice.

The total amount of carbohydrate in the diet should provide 50–55% of the total calories.

Fat

The traditional diabetic diet was low in carbohydrates and therefore high in fat (Table 17.5). Not only was this high fat content inappropriate for patients already predisposed to arterial disease, but glucose tolerance actually deteriorates rather than improves on a low-carbohydrate diet.

Table 17.5 Comparison of the composition of the traditional and modern diabetic diets.

	Percentage of calories	
	Traditional diet	Modern diet
Protein	12	15
Fat	66	35
Carbohydrate	22	50

Calories

This should be tailored to the needs of the patient.

- The overweight diabetic patient is started on a reducing diet of approximately 1000–1600 kcal per day (4000–6000 kJ).
- The lean patient is put on an isocaloric diet.
- Patients who are underweight because of untreated diabetes require energy supplementation.

Table 17.6 Drugs used in non-insulin-dependent diabetes mellitus.

	Duration of action	Excretion	Dose per 24 h
Sulphonylureas			
Tolbutamide	6–8 h	Hepatic	1–2 g in divided doses
Chlorpropamide	36–48 h	Hepatic and renal	100–500 mg
Glibenclamide	12–20 h	Hepatic and renal	2.5–20 mg
Gliclazide	10–12 h	Hepatic and renal	40–320 mg
Biguanides			
Metformin	12–20 h	Unchanged in urine	1–2 g in 2–3 doses

Prescribing a diet
Most people find it extremely difficult to modify their eating habits, and repeated advice and encouragement are needed if this is to be achieved. A diet history is taken, and the diet prescribed should involve the least possible interference with the lifestyle of the patient. It is important to stress that patients on insulin or oral agents should eat the same amount at the same time each day. Patients on insulin require snacks between meals and at bedtime to buffer the effect of injected insulin. Alcohol is not forbidden but its calorific content should be taken into account. Patients on insulin should be warned to avoid alcoholic binges since these may precipitate severe hypoglycaemia.

The role of patient education
The care of diabetes is based on self-management by the patient, who is helped and advised by those with specialized knowledge. The quest for improved glycaemic control has made it clear that whatever the technical expertise applied, the outcome depends on willing cooperation by the patient. This in turn depends on an understanding of the risks of diabetes and the potential benefits of glycaemic control and other measures such as maintaining a lean weight, stopping smoking and taking care of the feet.

If accurate information is not supplied, misinformation from friends and other patients will take its place. For this reason, many patients have exaggerated fears of, for example, blindness (about 1 patient in 20 is blind after 30 years of diabetes), death during hypoglycaemia (extremely rare), or the risk of passing diabetes on to their children (2–5% of offspring develop IDDM).

Organized training programmes involving nurse specialists, dietitians and chiropodists as well as physicians are now a recognized part of good modern diabetes care.

Tablet treatment (see Table 17.6)

Sulphonylureas
These have two main actions:

- They increase basal and stimulated insulin secretion.
- They reduce peripheral resistance to insulin action.

The effects upon insulin secretion are most marked in the early stages of treatment, but the peripheral effects are more important for maintenance therapy. The sulphonylureas should be avoided in young ketotic patients, who require early insulin therapy, and are contraindicated in pregnancy. Insulin should be substituted during major surgery or severe intercurrent illness.

These drugs have similar actions and potency. All should be used with care in patients with liver disease, and only those primarily excreted by the liver should be given to patients with renal impairment. Tolbutamide is the safest drug in the very elderly because of its short duration of action. Chlorpropamide has the disadvantages of a long duration of action and a wider range of side-effects, and is now less widely used.

Drug interactions (see p. 739). All sulphonylureas bind to circulating albumin and may be displaced by other drugs, such as sulphonamides, that compete for their binding sites. Their clinical effect may be reduced by thiazide diuretics or steroid therapy.

Side-effects. Hypoglycaemia is the most common side-effect and may be severe and prolonged. Skin rashes and other sensitivity reactions may occur.

Chlorpropamide use is often associated with a facial flush when alcohol is taken. It may also cause a cholestatic jaundice and (at high doses) a dilutional hyponatraemia.

Biguanides
Metformin acts by reducing glucose absorption from the gut and by increasing insulin sensitivity. Unlike the sulphonylureas it does not induce hypoglycaemia in normal volunteers. It is usually reserved for patients in middle or old age,

Table 17.7 Human insulin preparations.

Manufacturer		Eli Lilly[a]	Nordisk[a]	Novo[a]
Soluble		Humulin S	Human Velosulin	Human Actrapid
Zinc		Humulin Zn	—	Human Semitard (amorphous zinc)
				Human Ultratard (crystalline zinc)
				Human Monotard (amorphous 30%, crystalline 70%)
Protamine (Isophane)		Humulin I	Human Insulatard	Human Protaphane
Soluble: Protamine mixtures		(*% soluble*)		
	10%	Humulin M1	—	—
	20%	Humulin M2	—	—
	30%	Humulin M3	Human Mixtard	Human Actraphane
	40%	Humulin M4	—	—
	50%	—	Human Initard	—

[a] Produced by recombinant DNA technology.

particularly for the overweight. It may be given in combination with sulphonylureas when a single agent has proved to be ineffective.

Its side-effects include anorexia, epigastric discomfort and diarrhoea. Lactic acidosis has occurred in patients with severe hepatic or renal disease, and metformin is contraindicated when these are present.

Insulin treatment

Injections

Most people have a fear of injecting themselves, and insulin therapy should begin with a lesson in injection technique. A disposable 10–16 mm needle (depending on adiposity) should be used to its full depth at 90° to the skin. The thighs and abdomen are the most convenient areas, and the injection site used should be changed regularly to prevent areas of lipohypertrophy. The rate of insulin absorption depends on local subcutaneous blood flow, and is accelerated by exercise, local massage or a warm environment. Absorption is more rapid from the arm than from the abdomen, and is slowest from the thigh. All these factors can influence the shape of the insulin profile.

All patients need careful training for a life with insulin, but routine hospital admission is unnecessary where facilities for community support exist.

Choice of insulin

Species. Insulin is found in every creature with a backbone, and the central part of the molecule is constant. (For example, fish insulin produces hypoglycaemia in man.) Differences in the amino acid sequence after the antigenicity of the molecule. Beef insulin has three amino acids that are different from human insulin, and pork insulin has only one; the latter is therefore less antigenic.

Human insulin is produced by:

- Chemical substitution of an amino acid in position 30 of the beta-chain of pork insulin.
- DNA coding of *Escherichia coli* to produce proinsulin, with enzymatic cleavage to insulin (bioengineering).

All forms of injected insulin, even human, may result in antibody formation, but insulin antibodies usually have little clinical importance. Human insulin has largely replaced the other varieties.

Purity. Earlier preparations of insulin contained glucagon and other impurities. Modern insulins are now of high purity, having only a single sharp peak on electrophoresis.

Formulation (see Table 17.7). There are two main types of insulin:

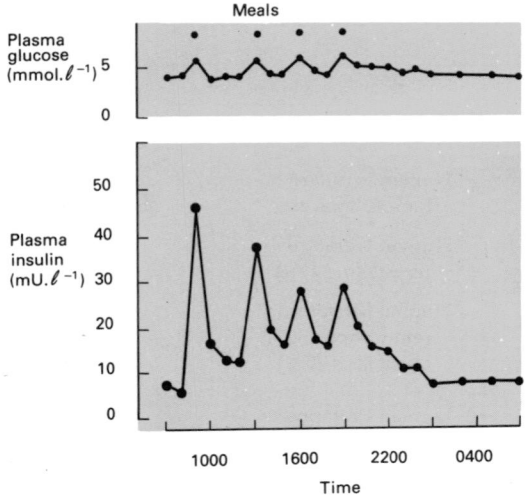

Fig. 17.7 Glucose and insulin profiles in normal subjects.

- Insulin prepared in a clear solution (soluble or crystalline). These insulins are short-acting and are the only insulins to be used in emergencies such as ketoacidosis or for surgical operations.
- Insulins pre-mixed with retarding agents (either protamine or zinc) that precipitate crystals of varying size according to the conditions employed. These insulins are intermediate- or long-acting.

All insulins are available in solutions containing 40, 80 and 100 units per millilitre, but in the UK the standard insulin available is 100 units per millilitre.

Clinical use
In normal subjects a sharp rise in insulin occurs after meals; this is superimposed on a constant background of insulin secretion (Fig. 17.7). Insulin therapy attempts to reproduce this pattern. In order to achieve this, a common strategy is to give intermediate-acting insulin to control the afternoon and night blood sugar level, and short-acting insulins morning and evening to match meal times (Fig. 17.8a).

Ideal control is often hard to achieve for the following reasons.

- The insulin is given into the systemic circulation rather than the portal circulation.
- Subcutaneous soluble insulin takes 60–90 min to achieve peak plasma levels—the onset and off-set of action are too slow.
- The absorption of subcutaneous insulin into the circulation is variable; the longer-acting the preparation, the more erratic the absorption.
- Basal insulin levels are constant in the normal state, but injected insulin invariably peaks and declines, with resulting swings in metabolic control.

Individuals vary and therapy must be tailored accordingly. One approach to therapy is outlined here.

- Young patients are started on two injections daily of an intermediate insulin at a dose of 8–10 u twice daily. Some recovery of endogenous insulin secretion may occur over the first few months ('the honeymoon period') and the insulin dose may need to be reduced. Requirements rise thereafter and soluble insulin is added to the regimen. As a rule of thumb, two-thirds of the daily dose is given in the morning, and two-thirds of each injection is given as intermediate insulin.
- A multiple injection regimen is flexible and highly acceptable for most young patients with established IDDM.
- Twice-daily injections of pre-mixed soluble and isophane insulins, e.g. Mixtard, are effective in the majority of patients with NIDDM.
- Older patients may sometimes manage adequately on a single daily injection.

If glycaemic control is inadequate with the standard approach, the alternatives are multiple insulin injections or continuous subcutaneous insulin infusion (CSII). Both methods require a planned approach to life, with special attention to diet and exercise and frequent blood-glucose testing.

Multiple injections. The introduction of 'pen injection' devices has made this approach much more acceptable in patients. Three variants are shown diagrammatically in Fig. 17.8b–d.

Infusion devices. CSII is delivered by a small pump strapped around the waist that infuses a constant trickle of insulin under the skin. Meal-time doses are delivered when the patient touches a button on the side of the pump.

This approach has the advantage of smoothing blood glucose levels to prevent swings to hyper- and hypoglycaemia, and is particularly useful in the overnight period. It also has the advantage of flexibility concerning meal times, which is of great value to patients in busy jobs who cannot always live by the clock. Disadvantages include the nuisance of being attached to a gadget, skin infections, and the risk of ketoacidosis if the flow of insulin is broken (since these patients have nö protective reservoir of depot insulin). Infusion pumps should only be used by specialized centres able to offer a round-the-clock service to their patients.

Social implications
Patients starting on insulin need to inform the driving licence authorities and their insurance companies. They are also wise to inform their employers. Certain types of work are unsuitable

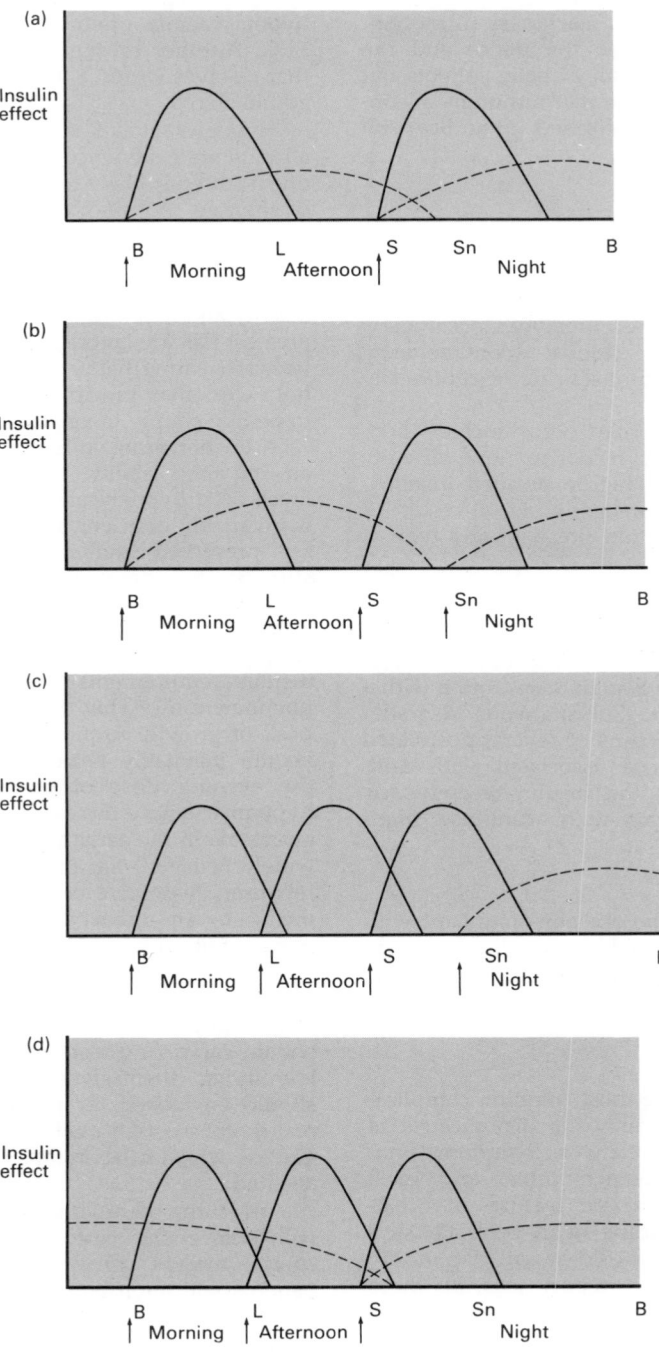

Fig. 17.8 Insulin regimens. Profiles of soluble insulins are shown as solid lines and intermediate- or long-acting as broken lines. The arrows indicate when the injections are given. (a) Twice daily soluble and intermediate. (b) Splitting the evening injection. (c) Three times daily soluble with long-acting insulin given before supper. B = breakfast; L = lunch; S = supper; Sn = snack (bedtime).

for insulin-treated patients, including driving a heavy goods vehicle, working at heights, or working close to dangerous machinery in motion. Certain professions such as the police and the armed forces are barred to all diabetic patients but there are few other limitations, although a considerable amount of ill-informed prejudice still exists.

Complications

At the injection site. Shallow injections result in intradermal insulin delivery and scarring. Injection site abscesses occur but are rare.

Local allergic responses sometimes occur early in therapy but usually resolve spontaneously. Generalized allergic responses are exceptionally rare.

Lipodystrophies that may occur include lipoatrophy, a local allergic response now virtually abolished by the use of highly purified insulins, and lipohypertrophy, occurring as a result of overuse of a single injection site with any type of insulin.

Insulin resistance. The most common cause of mild insulin resistance is obesity. Occasional unstable patients require massive insulin doses, often with a fluctuating requirement. Subcutaneous degradation of injected insulin is one of several postulated causes. Insulin resistance associated with antibodies directed against the insulin receptor has been reported in patients with acanthosis nigricans.

Weight gain. Patients who are non-compliant with their diet and predisposed to weight gain may show progressive weight gain on treatment, especially if the insulin dose is increased inappropriately, making them feel hungry.

Hypoglycaemia. This is the most common complication of insulin therapy and is a major cause of anxiety for patients and relatives. Symptoms typically develop over a few minutes, and most patients experience 'adrenergic' features of sweating, tremor and a pounding heart beat. Physical signs include pallor and a cold sweat. A minority of long-standing patients report loss of these warning symptoms and may in consequence drift into severe hypoglycaemia. Such patients appear pale, drowsy or detached, signs that their relatives quickly learn to recognize. Behaviour is clumsy or inappropriate, and some become irritable or even aggressive. Others slip rapidly into hypoglycaemic coma.

Occasionally, patients develop convulsions during hypoglycaemic coma, especially at night. It is important not to confuse this with idiopathic epilepsy, especially since patients with frequent hypoglycaemia often have abnormalities on the EEG. Another presentation is with a hemiparesis that resolves within a few minutes when glucose is administered.

Hypoglycaemia is a common problem. Virtually all patients experience intermittent symptoms and one in three is likely to go into coma at some stage of therapy. A minority suffer attacks that are so frequent and severe as to be virtually disabling.

Hypoglycaemia results from an imbalance between injected insulin and a patient's normal diet, activity and basal insulin requirement. The times of greatest risk are before meals and during the night. Irregular eating habits, unusual exertion and alcohol excess may precipitate episodes; others appear to be due simply to variation in insulin absorption.

A further problem is that diabetic patients have an impaired ability to counter-regulate glucose levels after hypoglycaemia. The glucagon response is invariably deficient, even though the alpha cells are preserved and respond normally to other stimuli. The adrenaline response may also fail in patients with a long duration of diabetes.

Noctural hypoglycaemia is commonly caused by attempts to compensate for the slight increase in insulin requirements from 4 a.m. (the 'dawn phenomenon'). This is related to the nocturnal peak of growth hormone secretion. Since injected insulin inevitably peaks and declines, increasing the evening dose of insulin to combat fasting hyperglycaemia increases the risk of hypoglycaemia in the early hours of the morning. It was widely believed that this hypoglycaemia caused a rebound hyperglycaemia (the 'Somogyi effect') owing to an unbalanced counter-regulatory response, but in practice fasting hyperglycaemia is usually due to insulin deficiency.

The diagnosis of hypoglycaemia is simple and can usually be made on clinical grounds. Patients should carry a card or wear a bracelet or necklace identifying themselves as diabetic, and these should be looked for in unconscious patients. If real doubt exists, it will do no harm to administer glucose whilst a laboratory blood glucose result is awaited.

Any form of rapidly assimilated carbohydrate will relieve the early symptoms, and patients should always carry sugar or sweets. Drowsy patients will often be able to take carbohydrate in liquid form, e.g. proprietary glucose drinks. Unconscious patients should be given intravenous glucose (50 ml of 50% dextrose solution) or intramuscular glucagon (1 mg). Glucagon acts by mobilizing hepatic glycogen, and works almost as rapidly as glucose. It is simple to administer and can be given at home by relatives. Glucose reserves should be replenished with oral glucose once the patient revives.

Measuring control

The 'artificial pancreas' is a system of blood glucose control that works by continuous blood glucose analysis. This is fed into a computer, which delivers an appropriate amount of insulin into the circulation. Patients on insulin need to devise their own simplified form of this feedback loop.

Urine tests

Urine tests are simple to perform, and it can usually be assumed that a patient with consistently negative tests and no symptoms of hypoglycaemia is well controlled. Even so, the correlation between urine tests and simultaneous blood glucose is poor. This is because:

- Changes in urine glucose lag behind changes in blood glucose.
- The mean renal threshold is around 10 $mmol \cdot L^{-1}$ but the range is wide (7–13 $mmol \cdot L^{-1}$). The threshold also rises with age.
- Urine tests can give no guidance concerning blood glucose levels below the renal threshold.

Dipstick tests based on specific enzymatic reactions for glucose have now superseded the older tablet method for testing the urine.

Urinary ketones may also be measured by a dipstick test. This is rarely helpful in routine outpatient management, but can be useful in special situations such as intercurrent infections. Heavy ketonuria can inhibit some dipstick tests for glucose, and a combined stick (measuring both glucose and ketones) may be of value.

Blood glucose levels

Blood glucose levels provide the best assessment of day-to-day control. A fasting glucose level is a useful guide to therapy in NIDDM since it correlates well with other measures of control, but this is not the case in IDDM.

A random blood glucose test (e.g. in the clinic) is of limited value, but patients may easily be taught to provide their own profiles by testing finger-prick blood samples with reagent strips and reading these with the aid of a visual scale or reflectance meter. It has been amply demonstrated that most patients are willing and able to provide reasonably accurate results provided they have been properly taught how to do so.

Blood is taken from the side of a finger tip (*not* from the tip, which is densely innervated) using a special lancet such as a Monolet, which can be fitted to a spring-loaded device. The standard flat steel lancets provided in many hospitals are unsuitable for this technique. Patients are asked to take regular profiles (e.g. four daily samples on 2 days each week) and to note these in a diary or record book. They are encouraged to adjust their

insulin dose as appropriate and should ideally be able to obtain advice over the telephone when needed.

Glycosylated haemoglobin (HbA_{1c})

Glycosylation of haemoglobin occurs as a two-step reaction, resulting in the formation of a covalent bond between the glucose molecule and the terminal valine of the β-chain of the haemoglobin molecule. The rate at which this reaction occurs is related to the prevailing glucose concentration. Glycosylated haemoglobin can be distinguished by techniques such as electrophoresis, and is expressed as a percentage of the normal haemoglobin. The usefulness of this test is that it condenses all the changes in blood glucose levels over several weeks into a single value that is related to the mean blood glucose over the same period. The figure will, however, be misleading if the life-span of the red cell is reduced. HbA_{1c} provides a rapid assessment of the level of glycaemic control in a given patient, but blood glucose testing is needed before the clinician can know what to do about it.

Glycosylated plasma proteins ('fructosamine') may also be measured as an index of control. Glycosylated albumin is the major component and fructosamine measurement relates to glycaemic control over the preceding 1–3 weeks. The technique is cheaper and quicker than HbA_{1c} measurement and lends itself to automization, but correlation between the two analyses is surprisingly weak. The clinical value of fructosamine estimation is still rather uncertain.

Does good glycaemic control matter?

The answer to this question involves a number of separate issues.

1 Is poor control associated with an increased risk of microvascular complications?

Retrospective studies have repeatedly shown that those with the worst control have the highest rate of complications.

2 Is this increased risk reversible?

There are many difficulties in answering this question:

- The gestation of diabetic complications is lengthy, often 10–20 years.
- Control was difficult to quantify before HbA_{1c} tests were introduced.
- Good control is difficult to achieve, so comparisons have usually been between 'poor and worse' control rather than between 'good and bad'.
- Some patients are easier to bring into good control than others, so the groups selected as 'well' or 'poorly' controlled in previous studies were not strictly comparable.

Prospective randomized studies are therefore

Table 17.8 Terms used in uncontrolled diabetes.

Ketonuria	Detectable ketone levels in the urine; it should be appreciated that ketonuria occurs in fasting non-diabetics and may be found in relatively well-controlled patients with IDDM
Ketosis	Elevated plasma ketone levels in the absence of acidosis
Diabetic ketoacidosis	A metabolic emergency in which hyperglycaemia is associated with a metabolic acidosis due to greatly raised (> 5 mmol·L^{-1}) ketone levels
Non-ketotic hyperosmolar coma	A metabolic emergency in which uncontrolled hyperglycaemia induces a hyperosmolar state in the absence of significant ketosis
Lactic acidosis	A metabolic emergency in which elevated lactate levels induce a metabolic acidosis; in diabetic patients this is rare and associated with biguanide therapy

needed. Studies in experimental animals strongly suggest that improved control is protective. Studies in man are now under way but face considerable technical problems.

3 Can established complications be halted or reversed by intensive insulin therapy?

Insulin infusion devices have made near-normal blood glucose control possible for closely supervised groups of patients. Studies in patients with established retinopathy or nephropathy have shown that early retinopathy benefits from 2–3 years of intensive therapy, but that patients with more advanced retinal changes or proteinuria do not. Retinopathy may show a transient deterioration in the most strictly controlled group. These observations suggest that microvascular lesions may be self-perpetuating once a threshold level of damage has been reached.

4 Is macrovascular disease influenced by control?

Patients with impaired glucose tolerance have an increased rate of large vessel disease but rarely develop microvascular lesions. This might be because large arteries are more sensitive to elevated glucose levels, but it has also been suggested that hyperinsulinaemia (present in many patients with NIDDM and a common consequence of insulin treatment) is a cause of accelerated atherogenesis. At present there is little evidence that good glycaemic control protects against arterial disease.

DIABETIC METABOLIC EMERGENCIES

The main terms used are defined in Table 17.8.

Diabetic ketoacidosis

CAUSES

Diabetic ketoacidosis is the hallmark of IDDM. Its main causes can be grouped as follows:

- Previously undiagnosed diabetes
- Interruption of insulin therapy
- The stress of intercurrent illness

It is important to note that the majority of cases reaching hospital could have been *prevented* by earlier diagnosis, better communication between patient and doctor, and better patient education.

The most common error of management is for a patient to reduce or omit insulin because he feels unable to eat owing to nausea or vomiting. This is a factor in at least 25% of all hospital admissions. Insulin should never be stopped.

PATHOGENESIS

Ketoacidosis is a state of uncontrolled catabolism associated with insulin deficiency. Insulin deficiency is a necessary precondition since only a modest elevation in insulin levels is sufficient to inhibit hepatic ketogenesis. Even so, stable patients

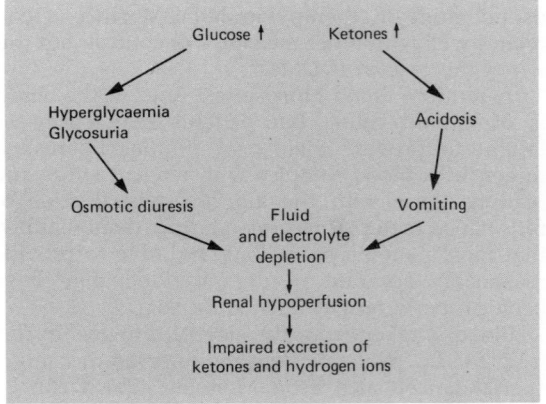

Fig. 17.9 Dehydration occurs during ketoacidosis as a consequence of two parallel processes. Hyperglycaemia results in osmotic diuresis, and hyperketonaemia results in acidosis and vomiting. Renal hypoperfusion then occurs and a vicious circle is established as the kidney becomes less able to compensate for the acidosis.

do not readily develop ketoacidosis when insulin is withdrawn. Other factors include counter-regulatory hormone excess and fluid depletion. The combination of insulin deficiency with excess of its hormonal antagonists leads to the parallel processes shown in Fig. 17.9.

In the absence of insulin, hepatic glucose production accelerates and peripheral uptake by tissues such as muscle is reduced. Rising glucose levels lead to an osmotic diuresis, loss of fluid and electrolytes, and dehydration. Plasma osmolality rises and renal perfusion falls.

In parallel, rapid lipolysis occurs, leading to elevated circulating free fatty-acid levels. The free fatty acids are broken down to fatty acyl-CoA within the liver cells, and this in turn is converted to acetoacetate (ketone bodies) within the mitochondria (Fig. 17.10).

Accumulation of ketone bodies produces a metabolic acidosis. This is typically associated with nausea and vomiting, leading to further loss of fluid and electrolytes. The excess ketones are excreted in the urine but also appear in the breath, producing a distinctive smell similar to that of acetone. Respiratory compensation for the acidosis leads to hyperventilation, graphically described as 'air hunger'. Progressive dehydration impairs renal excretion of hydrogen ions and ketones, aggravating the acidosis. As the pH falls below 7.0 [(H$^+$) > 100 nmol·L^{-1}), pH-dependent enzyme systems in many cells function less effectively. Untreated, severe ketoacidosis is invariably fatal.

CLINICAL FEATURES

The features of ketoacidosis are those of uncontrolled diabetes with acidosis, and include prostration, hyperventilation (Kussmaul respiration), nausea, vomiting and, occasionally, abdominal pain. The latter is sometimes so severe as to cause confusion with a surgical acute abdomen.

Some patients are mentally alert at presentation, but confusion and stupor are common. About 5%

present in coma. Evidence of marked dehydration is present and the eyeball is lax to pressure in severe cases. Hyperventilation is present but becomes less marked in very severe acidosis owing to respiratory depression. The smell of ketones on the breath allows an instant diagnosis to be made by those able to detect the odour. The skin is dry and the body temperature is often subnormal, even in the presence of infection; in such cases, pyrexia may develop later.

DIAGNOSIS

This is confirmed by demonstrating hyperglycaemia with ketonaemia or heavy ketonuria, and acidosis. No time should be lost and treatment is started as soon as the first blood sample has been taken.

Hyperglycaemia is demonstrated by Stix testing, while a blood sample is sent to the laboratory for confirmation. Ketonaemia is confirmed by centrifuging a blood sample and testing the plasma with Ketostix or Acetest tablets. An arterial blood sample is taken for blood gas analysis.

Further investigations are detailed below.

MANAGEMENT

The principles of management are as follows.

- *Replace the fluid losses.*
- *Replace the electrolyte losses.* Potassium levels need to be monitored with great care to avoid the cardiac complications of hypo- or hyperkalaemia.
- *Restore the acid–base balance.* A patient with healthy kidneys will rapidly compensate for the metabolic acidosis once the circulating volume is restored. Bicarbonate is seldom necessary, although it is usual for this to be given at a pH below 7.0 ([H$^+$] > 100 nmol·L^{-1}).
- *Replace the deficient insulin.* Traditionally, soluble insulin was given as a bolus with half the dose

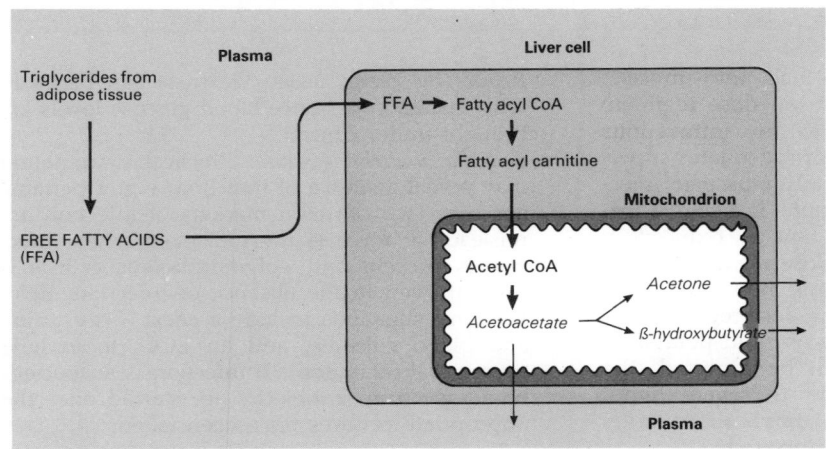

Fig. 17.10 Ketogenesis. During insulin deficiency, lipolysis accelerates and free fatty acids taken up by liver cells form the substrate for ketone formation (acetoacetate, acetone and β-hydroxybutyrate) within the mitochondrion.

GUIDELINES FOR THE DIAGNOSIS AND MANAGEMENT OF DIABETIC KETOACIDOSIS

Diagnosis

- Hyperglycaemia—measure blood glucose
- Ketonaemia—test plasma with Ketostix/Acetest
- Acidosis—measure blood gases

Investigations

- Blood glucose
- Urea and electrolytes
- Osmolality
- Full blood count
- Blood gases
- Blood and urine culture
- Chest X-ray
- ECG

Management

Insulin   i.v. 6 units stat, then 6 units hourly by infusion OR
                       i.m. 20 units stat, then 6 units hourly by i.m. injection

Fluid replacement   Normal saline 0.9% (150 mmol each of Na^+ and Cl^- per litre) 4 litres in 4 h, then 1 litre 4-hourly. Add KCl 20 mmol to each litre

IF:

- Blood pressure is below 80 systolic, give 2 units whole blood or plasma.
- pH below 7.0 ([H^+] > 100 $nmol \cdot L^{-1}$), give sodium bicarbonate 1.26% (150 mmol each of Na^+ and HCO_3 per litre) 500 ml over 1 h. Add KCl 20 mmol; rate should not exceed 20 $mmol \cdot L^{-1}$ over 1 h.
- Plasma Na^+ over 150 $mmol \cdot L^{-1}$, give up to 1 litre of ½-normal (0.45%) saline but continue with normal saline thereafter.

Special measures

- Broad-spectrum antibiotics if infection is likely
- Bladder catheter if no urine is passed after 4 h
- Nasogastric tube if in coma
- CVP line in elderly or shocked patients
- Consider subcutaneous Heparin in the comatose, elderly or obese

Subsequent management

- Monitor glucose hourly ⎫ for 8 h.
  Monitor electrolytes 2-hourly ⎭
- Adjust K^+ replacement according to results. (Use ECG monitor as additional check.)
- When blood glucose falls to 10–12 $mmol \cdot L^{-1}$, change infusion fluid to 10% dextrose plus 20 mmol KCl, 500 ml 4-hourly. Continue insulin 3 units hourly by infusion or 6 units 2-hourly by i.m. injection

injected into a vein and half into muscle. Modern treatment is with a low-dose regimen; soluble insulin is given as an intravenous infusion where facilities for adequate supervision exist, or as hourly intramuscular injections. The subcutaneous route is avoided because subcutaneous blood flow is reduced in shocked patients. The low-dose regimen lowers blood glucose by suppressing hepatic glucose production, whereas the high-dose regimen also promotes rapid entry of glucose and potassium into muscle cells. As might be expected, the high-dose regimen can lead to severe hypoglycaemia or hypokalaemia, complications largely avoided by the low-dose approach.

- *Replace the energy losses.* Dextrose can be given with insulin cover once blood glucose levels are brought under control.
- *Seek the underlying cause.* Physical examination may reveal a source of infection, e.g. a perianal abscess. Two common markers of infection are misleading: fever is unusual even when infection is present and polymorpholeucocytosis is present even in the absence of infection. Relevant investigations include a chest X-ray, urine and blood cultures, and an ECG (to exclude myocardial infarction). If infection is suspected, broad-spectrum antibiotics are started once the appropriate cultures have been taken.

ELECTROLYTE CHANGES IN DIABETIC KETOACIDOSIS AND NON-KETOTIC HYPEROSMOLAR COMA

Examples of blood values

	Severe ketoacidosis	Non-ketotic hyperosmolar coma
Na^+ ($mmol \cdot L^{-1}$)	140	155
K^+ ($mmol \cdot L^{-1}$)	5	5
Cl^- ($mmol \cdot L^{-1}$)	100	110
HCO_3^- ($mmol \cdot L^{-1}$)	5	30
Urea ($mmol \cdot L^{-1}$)	8	15
Glucose ($mmol \cdot L^{-1}$)	30	50
Arterial pH	7.0	7.35

The *osmolality* can be measured directly, or can be calculated approximately from the formula:

$$Osmolality = 2(Na^+ + K^+) + glucose + urea$$

The normal range is 285–300 $mmol \cdot L^{-1}$

For example, in the example of severe ketoacidosis given above:

$$Osmolality = 2(140 + 5) + 30 + 8 = 328 \ mmol \cdot L^{-1}$$

and in the example of non-ketotic hyperosmolar coma:

$$Osmolality = 2(155 + 5) + 50 + 15 = 385 \ mmol \cdot L^{-1}$$

The *anion gap* is calculated as $(Na^+ + K^+) - (Cl^- + HCO_3)$ (see p. 505). The normal anion gap is less than 17.

In the example of ketoacidosis the anion gap is 40, and in the example of non-ketotic hyperosmolar coma the anion gap is 20. Mild hyperchloraemic acidosis may develop in the course of therapy. This will be shown by a rising plasma chloride and persistence of a low bicarbonate even though the anion gap has returned to normal.

Problems of managment

- *Hypotension.* This may lead to renal shutdown. Plasma expanders (or whole blood) are therefore given if the systolic blood pressure is below 80 mm Hg. A central venous pressure line is useful in this situation. A bladder catheter is inserted if no urine is produced within 4 h, but routine catheterization is unnecessary.
- *Coma.* The usual principles apply (see p. 905). It is essential to pass a nasogastric tube to prevent aspiration and the rare but fatal complication of acute gastric dilatation.
- *Cerebral oedema.* This rare but feared complication has mostly been reported in children or young adults. The mortality is high.
- *Hypothermia.* Severe hypothermia with a core temperature below 33°C may occur and may be overlooked unless a rectal temperature is taken with a low-reading thermometer.
- *Late complications.* These include stasis pneumonia and deep-vein thrombosis, and occur especially in the comatose or elderly patient.
- *Complications of therapy.* These include hypoglycaemia and hypokalaemia. Overenthusiastic fluid replacement may precipitate pulmonary oedema in older patients. Hyperchloraemic acidosis, usually mild, may develop in the course of fluid therapy. The nature of a persistent acidosis may be overlooked if the plasma chloride level has not been estimated.

Subsequent management

Intravenous fluids are stopped once the metabolic condition is under control and the patient is able to take the necessary fluids by mouth. Insulin is given as three or four soluble subcutaneous doses per day until a maintenance regimen can be restarted.

Sliding-scale regimens are often unnecessary and may even delay the establishment of stable blood glucose levels.

The treatment of diabetic ketoacidosis is incomplete without a careful enquiry into the causes of the episode and advice as to how to avoid its recurrence.

Non-ketotic hyperosmolar coma

This condition, in which severe hyperglycaemia develops without significant ketosis, is the metabolic emergency characteristic of uncontrolled NIDDM. Patients present in middle or later life, often with previously undiagnosed diabetes. Common precipitating factors include consumption of glucose-rich fluids (e.g. Lucozade), concurrent medication such as thiazide diuretics or steroids, and intercurrent illness.

Non-ketotic coma and ketoacidosis represent two ends of a spectrum rather than two distinct disorders. The biochemical differences may partly be explained as follows:

- The extreme dehydration characteristic of non-

ketotic coma may be related to age. Old people experience thirst less acutely, and more readily become dehydrated. In addition, the mild renal impairment associated with age results in increased urinary losses of fluid and electrolytes.
- The degree of insulin deficiency is less severe in non-ketotic coma. Endogenous insulin levels are sufficient to inhibit hepatic ketogenesis, whereas glucose production is unrestrained.

CLINICAL PRESENTATION

The characteristic clinical features are dehydration and stupor or coma. Impairment of consciousness is directly related to the degree of hyperosmolality. Evidence of underlying illness such as pneumonia or pyelonephritis may be present, and the hyperosmolar state may predispose to stroke, myocardial infarction or arterial insufficiency in the lower limbs.

INVESTIGATION AND TREATMENT

These are according to the guidelines for keto-acidosis, but care must be taken with the amount of fluid and insulin given. Plasma osmolality is monitored and half-normal saline (i.e. 0.45%) is used for initial rehydration in severe cases. Normal saline (0.9%) remains the standard fluid for rehydration.

PROGNOSIS

The reported mortality is around 20–30%, mainly because of the advanced age of the patients and the frequency of intercurrent illness. Unlike keto-acidosis, non-ketotic coma is not an absolute indication for subsequent insulin therapy, and survivors may do well on diet and oral agents.

Lactic acidosis

Lactic acidosis may occur in diabetic patients on biguanide therapy. Phenformin, the agent responsible in the great majority of reported cases, has now been withdrawn. The risk in patients taking metformin is extremely low provided that the therapeutic dose is not exceeded and the drug is withheld in patients with advanced hepatic or renal dysfunction.

Patients present with a severe metabolic acidosis, usually without significant hyperglycaemia or ketosis, and treatment is by rehydration and infusion of bicarbonate. The mortality is in excess of 50%.

COMPLICATIONS OF DIABETES

When insulin was introduced it was assumed that it would provide complete and adequate replacement therapy, just as thyroxine does in hypothyroidism.

Time proved that insulin-treated patients still have a considerably reduced life expectancy. Those diagnosed before the age of 20 have only a 50–60% chance of living past the age of 45, although there are recent indications of improved survival. The excess deaths are mainly due to diabetic nephropathy, but there is also a considerable excess cardiovascular mortality. Heart disease, peripheral vascular disease and stroke are the major causes of death in patients over the age of 50.

Large-vessel disease
Diabetes is a risk factor in the development of atherosclerosis. This risk is related to that of the background population. For example, Japanese diabetics are much less likely to develop atherosclerosis than patients in Europe but are much more likely to develop it than non-diabetic Japanese. The excess risk to diabetics compared with the general population increases as one moves down the body:

- Stroke is twice as likely
- Myocardial infarction is 3–5 times as likely and women with diabetes lose their pre-menopausal protection from coronary artery disease
- Amputation of a foot for gangrene is 50 times as likely

Diabetes is additive with other risk factors for large-vessel disease. In other words, the diabetic who smokes or is obese, hypertensive or hyperlipidaemic adds the risks conferred by these conditions to that of diabetes itself.

Microvascular complications
In contrast to macrovascular disease, which is prevalent in Western populations as a whole, microvascular disease is specific to diabetes. Small blood vessels throughout the body are affected but the disease process is of particular danger in three sites:

- The retina
- The renal glomerulus
- The nerve sheath

Diabetic retinopathy, nephropathy and neuropathy tend to manifest 10–20 years after diagnosis in young patients. They present earlier in older patients, probably because these have had unrecognized diabetes for months or even years prior to diagnosis.

Diabetic eye disease

Diabetes can affect the eyes in a number of ways. The most common and characteristic form of involvement is diabetic retinopathy. About one in three young patients is likely to develop visual

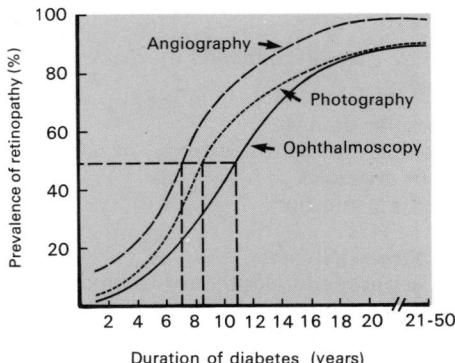

Fig. 17.11 Almost all patients show some evidence of retinopathy within 20 years of diagnosis; angiography and retinal photography are more sensitive than ophthalmoscopy.

problems, and in the UK 5% have become blind after 30 years of diabetes; diabetes is the commonest cause of blindness in the population as a whole up to the age of 60.

Other forms of eye disease may also occur:

- The lens may be affected by reversible osmotic changes in patients with acute hyperglycaemia, causing blurred vision, or by cataracts.
- Rubeosis iridis (new vessel formation in the iris) may develop as a late complication of diabetic retinopathy and can cause glaucoma.
- External ocular palsies, especially of the sixth nerve, can occur.

The natural history of retinopathy (Fig. 17.11)
Diabetes causes increased thickness of the basement membrane and increased permeability of the retinal capillaries. Aneurysmal dilatation may occur in some vessels while others become occluded. These changes are first detectable by fluorescein angiography, a technique in which a fluorescent dye is injected into an arm vein and photographed in transit through the retinal vessels.

Background retinopathy. The first abnormality visible through the ophthalmoscope is the appearance of dot 'haemorrhages', which are actually due to capillary microaneurysms. Leakage of blood into the deeper layers of the retina produces the characteristic 'blot' haemorrhage, while exudates of fluid rich in lipids and protein give rise to hard exudates. These have a bright yellow-white colour and a sharply defined margin.

These changes rarely develop in young patients with a duration of diabetes under 10 years, but by 20 years virtually all eyes will show changes on fluorescein angiography, and most will at least manifest the occasional dot haemorrhage on careful ophthalmoscopy. In contrast, retinopathy may be

present at diagnosis or shortly thereafter in older patients.

Background retinopathy does not in itself constitute a threat to vision but may progress to two other distinct forms of retinopathy: maculopathy or proliferative retinopathy.

Diabetic maculopathy. This may lead to blindness in the absence of proliferation in the older patient with NIDDM. It is characterized by strings of hard exudates arranged in horseshoe or circular fashion around the central and lateral part of the macula. These may cause loss of visual acuity by occluding the central part of the retina and regular testing of visual acuity is essential in screening for this condition. Oedema and ischaemia of the macula may also occur. Maculopathy can usually be diagnosed by measurement of visual acuity and use of the ophthalmoscope, but more elaborate techniques are needed to diagnose macular oedema and ischaemia.

Proliferative retinopathy. This dangerous form of retinopathy appears to develop on a basis of retinal ischaemia. The earliest sign is the appearance of 'cotton-wool spots', representing patches of retinal oedema. Unlike hard exudates they may also occur in severe hypertensive retinopathy. The term 'soft exudate' is often used synonymously but is best avoided. Cotton-wool spots are greyish-white, have indistinct margins and a dull matt surface, unlike the glossy appearance of hard exudates. Venous beading and/or venous loops are other recognized pre-proliferative changes.

Hypoxia is thought to be the signal for formation of new vessels. These lie superficially or grow forward into the vitreous, resembling fronds of seaweed. They branch repeatedly, are fragile, bleed easily (because they lack the normal supportive tissue) and may give rise to a fibrous-tissue reaction.

Haemorrhages can be pre-retinal or into the vitreous. A vitreous haemorrhage presents as a loss of vision in one eye, sometimes noticed on waking, or as a floating shadow affecting the field of vision. Ophthalmoscopy gives the appearance of a featureless, grey haze. Partial recovery of vision is the rule, as the blood is reabsorbed, but repeated bleeds may occur.

Loss of vision may also result from fibrous proliferation associated with new vessel formation. This may give rise to traction bands that contract with the course of time, producing retinal detachment.

Cataracts
Senile cataracts develop some 10–15 years earlier in diabetic patients than in the remainder of the population.

Juvenile or 'snowflake' cataracts are much less

common. These are diffuse, rapidly progressive cataracts associated with very poorly controlled diabetes. They should be distinguished from temporary lens changes that occasionally appear during hyperosmolar coma and resolve when the coma is brought under control.

Examination of the eye

Careful systematic examination of the eye is essential. Visual fields, acuity and eye movements are tested, and the pupils are dilated with a quick-acting mydriatic such as tropicamide 0.5%. Dilating drugs should not be used in patients with a history of glaucoma or cataract surgery, except with the advice of an ophthalmologist.

The examination begins at arm's length. At this distance, cataracts are silhouetted against the red reflex of the retina. The ophthalmoscope is advanced until the retina is in focus. The examination begins at the optic disc, moves through each quadrant in turn, and ends with the macula (since this is least comfortable for the patient). The ophthalmoscope is then adjusted to the +10 dioptre lens for examination of the cornea, anterior chamber and lens. The location of abnormalities should always be sketched in the notes for future reference.

Management of diabetic eye disease

There is no specific medical treatment for background retinopathy, but patients are advised not to smoke and hypertension should be treated. Rapid progression may occur in pregnant patients and in those with nephropathy, and these groups need frequent monitoring. All patients with retinopathy should be examined regularly in the clinic and, if possible, also supervised by an ophthalmologist. Referral to an ophthalmologist is particularly important in the following circumstances:

- Deteriorating visual acuity
- Extensive hard exudates
- Pre-proliferative changes (cotton-wool spots or venous beading)
- New vessel formation

The ophthalmologist may perform fluorescein angiography to define the extent of the problem. Maculopathy and proliferative retinopathy are treatable by retinal photocoagulation with lasers; in the latter condition early effective therapy reduces the risk of visual loss by about 50%. The value of photocoagulation is particularly marked in those with disc (as against peripheral) new vessels. In one trial only 15% of treated, as against 50% of untreated, eyes with disc new vessels progressed to legal blindness. Treatment in this case is by panretinal photocoagulation with 2000–5000 laser burns to each eye.

The diabetic kidney

The kidney may be damaged by diabetes in three main ways:

- Glomerular damage
- Ischaemia due to hypertropy of afferent and efferent arterioles
- Ascending infection

Diabetic glomerulosclerosis

Clinical nephropathy secondary to glomerular disease usually manifests 15–25 years after diagnosis and affects 30–40% of patients diagnosed under the age of 30. It is the leading cause of premature death in young diabetic patients. Older patients may also develop nephropathy, but the proportion affected is much smaller.

The earliest functional abnormality in the diabetic kidney is renal hypertrophy associated with a raised glomerular filtration rate; this appears soon after diagnosis and is related to poor glycaemic control.

The initial structural lesion in the glomerulus is thickening of the basement membrane. Associated changes may result in disruption of the protein cross-linkages that make the membrane an effective filter. In consequence, a progressive leak of protein into the urine occurs. The earliest evidence of this is 'microalbuminuria' (i.e. amounts of urinary albumin so small as to be undetectable by dipsticks (see p. 430)), which in turn progresses to frank proteinuria. Light-microscopic changes of glomerulosclerosis become manifest; both diffuse

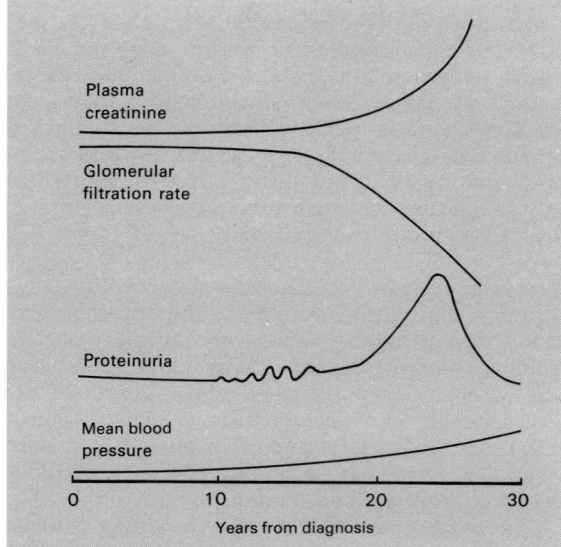

Fig. 17.12 Schematic representation of the natural history of nephropathy. The typical onset is 15 years after diagnosis. Intermittent proteinuria leads to persistent proteinuria. In time, the plasma creatinine rises as the glomerular filtration rate falls.

and nodular glomerulosclerosis can occur. The latter is sometimes known as the Kimmelstiel–Wilson lesion. At a later stage still, the glomerulus is replaced by hyaline material.

Microalbuminuria is followed by intermittent Albustix-positive proteinuria, and then persistent proteinuria. At this stage the plasma creatinine is normal but the average patient is only some 8–10 years from end-stage renal failure. The proteinuria may become so heavy as to induce a transient nephrotic syndrome, with peripheral oedema and hypoalbuminaemia.

Patients with nephropathy typically show a normochromic normocytic anaemia and a raised ESR. Hypertension is a common development and may itself damage the kidney still further. A rise in plasma creatinine is a late feature that progresses inevitably to renal failure, although the rate of progression may vary widely between individuals.

The natural history of this process is shown in Fig. 17.12. A curious feature is that almost all patients with long-established diabetes have abnormalities on renal biopsy but only a proportion develop the features of a progressive renal disease.

Ischaemic lesions
Arteriolar lesions, with hypertrophy and hyalinization of the vessels, affect both afferent and efferent arterioles. The appearances are similar to those of hypertensive disease but are not necessarily related to the blood pressure in patients with diabetes.

Infective lesions
Urinary tract infections are more common in women but not men with diabetes. Ascending infection may occur because of bladder stasis due to autonomic neuropathy, and infections more easily become established in damaged renal tissue. Autopsy material frequently reveals interstitial changes suggestive of infection, but ischaemia may produce similar changes and the true frequency of pyelonephritis in diabetes remains uncertain.

Untreated infections in diabetics can result in renal papillary necrosis, in which renal papillae are shed in the urine, but this complication is rare.

Diagnosis and management of diabetic nephropathy
The earliest clinical feature is proteinuria. Unfortunately, this is a sign of established and progressive disease. Poor glycaemic control is undoubtedly a risk factor in the development of nephropathy, but the established disease does not respond to improved control. For this reason it is now common for patients to be screened for microalbuminuria and there are indications that the process may still be reversible at this early stage before stick detection is possible. In patients with diabetes, frank proteinuria usually, but not invariably, implies diabetic nephropathy. It is important to consider and exclude other possible causes of renal disease. Clinical suspicion may be provoked by an atypical history, the absence of diabetic retinopathy (usually but not invariably present with diabetic nephropathy) and the presence of haematuria. Renal biopsy should be considered in such cases, but in practice is rarely necessary or helpful. The risk of intravenous urography is increased in diabetes, especially if patients are allowed to become dehydrated prior to the procedure, and a renal ultrasound is preferable. Other investigations include repeated microscopy and culture of the urine, 24 h urine collections to quantify protein loss and to measure creatinine clearance, and regular measurement of the plasma creatinine level.

Management of diabetic nephropathy is similar to that of other causes of renal failure, with the following provisos:

- Oral hypoglycaemic agents partially excreted via the kidney (e.g. chlorpropamide) must be avoided.
- Insulin sensitivity increases and drastic reductions in dosage may be needed.
- Meticulous control of hypertension helps to postpone renal failure.
- Diabetic retinopathy tends to progress rapidly and frequent ophthalmic supervision is essential.

Management of end-stage disease is complicated by the fact that patients often have other complications of diabetes such as blindness, autonomic neuropathy or peripheral vascular disease. Vascular shunts tend to calcify rapidly and hence chronic ambulatory peritoneal dialysis may be preferable to haemodialysis, and the failure rate of renal transplants is somewhat higher than in non-diabetic patients. A recent trend is to perform a segmental pancreatic graft at the same time as a renal graft. Although pancreatic grafts have a limited viability, owing to progressive fibrosis within the graft, they may give the patient a year or so of freedom from insulin injections.

Recent evidence suggests that diabetic nephropathy is becoming less common as diabetes care improves.

Diabetic neuropathy

Diabetes can damage peripheral nervous tissue in a number of ways. The vascular hypothesis postulates occlusion of the vasa nervorum as the prime cause. This seems likely in isolated mononeuropathies but the diffuse symmetrical nature of the common forms of neuropathy implies a metabolic cause. Since hyperglycaemia leads to increased formation of sorbitol and fructose in Schwann cells, accumulation of these sugars may disrupt function and structure.

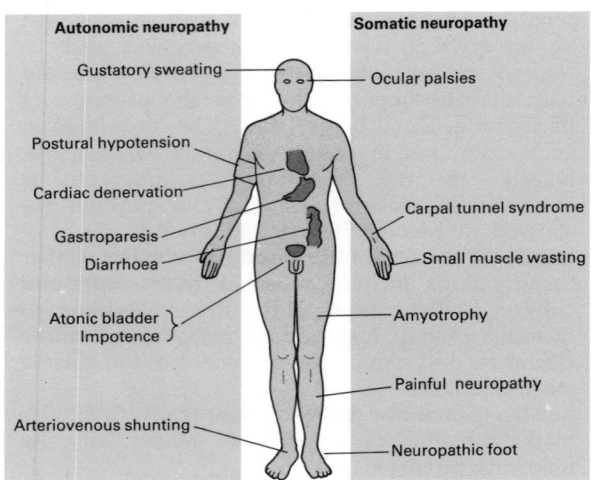

Fig. 17.13 The neuropathic man.

The earliest functional change in diabetic nerves is delayed nerve conduction velocity; the earliest histological change is segmental demyelination, due to damage to Schwann cells. In the early stages axons are preserved, implying prospects of recovery, but at a later stage irreversible axonal degeneration develops.

The following varieties of neuropathy may occur (Fig. 17.13):

● Symmetrical sensory polyneuropathy (distal)
● Mononeuropathy and multiple mononeuropathy:
  (a) Cranial nerve lesions
  (b) Isolated peripheral nerve lesions
  (c) Diabetic amyotrophy
● Autonomic neuropathy

Symmetrical sensory polyneuropathy
This is often unrecognized by the patient in its early stages. Early clinical signs are loss of vibration sense, pain sensation (deep before superficial) and temperature sensation in the feet. At later stages patients may complain of a feeling of 'walking on cotton wool' and can lose their balance when washing the face or walking in the dark owing to impaired proprioception. Involvement of the hands leads to the familiar 'stocking and glove' distribution. Complications include unrecognized trauma, beginning as blistering due to an ill-fitting shoe or a hot water bottle, and leading to ulceration.

A diffuse, painful neuropathy is a rare but unpleasant complication. The patient describes burning or crawling pains in the feet, shins and anterior thighs. These symptoms are typically worse at night, and pressure from bedclothes may be intolerable. Acute painful neuropathy is an occasional presenting feature, which usually responds to improved glycaemic control. A more chronic form, developing later in the course of the disease, is sometimes resistant to almost all forms of therapy. Neurological assessment is difficult because of the hyperaesthesia experienced by the patient, but muscle wasting is not a feature and objective signs can be minimal.

Involvement of motor nerves to the small muscles of the feet gives rise to interosseous wasting. Unbalanced traction by the long flexor muscles leads to a characteristic shape of the foot, with a high arch and clawing of the toes, which in turn leads to abnormal distribution of pressure on walking, resulting in callus formation under the first metatarsal head or on the tips of the toes and perforating neuropathic ulceration.

Neuropathic arthropathy (Charcot's joints) may sometimes develop in the ankle. The hands show small-muscle wasting as well as sensory changes but it is important to differentiate these signs and symptoms from those of the carpal tunnel syndrome, which occurs with increased frequency in diabetes and may be amenable to surgery.

Mononeuropathy and multiple mononeuropathy
Cranial nerve lesions. Isolated or multiple palsies of nerves to the external eye muscles, especially the third and sixth nerves, are more common in diabetes. A characteristic feature of diabetic third nerve lesions is that pupillary reflexes are retained owing to sparing of pupillomotor fibres. Full recovery is the rule.

Isolated peripheral nerve lesions. Manifestations may be sensory, motor, or mixed, and multiple nerves may be involved ('mononeuritis multiplex'). The onset is usually abrupt and sometimes painful; recovery is typically slow and incomplete. Lesions are more likely to occur at common sites for external pressure palsies or nerve entrapment, e.g. the median nerve in the carpal tunnel.

Diabetic amyotrophy. This condition is usually seen in older men with diabetes. Presentation is with painful wasting, usually asymmetrical, of the quadriceps muscles. Features include extreme wasting with loss of the knee jerks, and extreme tenderness of the affected area. An extensor plantar response sometimes develops and CSF protein content is elevated. Diabetic amyotrophy is usually associated with periods of poor glycaemic control and may be present at diagnosis; unlike other forms of diabetic neuropathy, amyotrophy often resolves in time with careful control of the blood glucose.

Autonomic neuropathy
Patients with evidence of somatic neuropathy will also have damage of the sympathetic and para-

sympathetic nervous systems. In the early stages these autonomic lesions are asymptomatic and can only be detected with special tests, but they may later give rise to disabling symptoms.

The cardiovascular system. Vagal neuropathy results in tachycardia at rest and loss of sinus arrhythmia. At a later stage the heart may become denervated (resembling a transplanted heart). Cardiovascular reflexes such as the Valsalva manoeuvre are impaired.

Postural hypotension occurs owing to loss of sympathetic tone to peripheral arterioles. A warm foot with a bounding pulse is sometimes seen in a polyneuropathy as a result of peripheral vasodilatation.

Gastrointestinal tract. Vagal damage can lead to gastroparesis, often asymptomatic, but sometimes leading to intractable vomiting. Diarrhoea often occurs at night accompanied by urgency and incontinence. Diarrhoea and steatorrhoea may occur owing to bacterial overgrowth and treatment is with antibiotics.

Bladder involvement. Loss of tone, incomplete emptying, and stasis (predisposing to infection) can occur, and may ultimately result in an atonic, painless, distended bladder.

Impotence. This is common. The first manifestation is incomplete erection which may in time progress to total impotence; retrograde ejaculation also occurs. However, impotence in diabetes is not always due to autonomic neuropathy. Other causes include anxiety, depression, alcohol excess, drugs, primary or secondary gonadal failure and (rarely) disease of the iliac vessels. Treatment is difficult and depends largely on sympathetic counselling of both partners, although some patients may benefit from intracavernous injection of paparaverine (see p. 787).

The diabetic foot

Many amputations in diabetes could be delayed or prevented by more effective patient education and medical supervision. Ischaemia, infection and neuropathy combine to produce tissue necrosis. Although these factors may coexist, it is important to distinguish between the ischaemic and the neuropathic foot (Table 17.9).

Management of the diabetic foot
Many diabetic foot problems are avoidable, so patients need to learn the principles of foot care and should be advised concerning appropriate footwear and the risks of smoking. Older patients should visit a chiropodist regularly and should not cut their own toe-nails.

Table 17.9 Distinguishing features between ischaemia and neuropathy in the diabetic foot.

	Ischaemia	Neuropathy
Symptoms:	Claudication Rest pain	Usually painless Sometimes painful neuropathy
Inspection:	Dependent rubor Trophic changes	High arch Clawing of toes No trophic changes
Palpation:	Cold Pulseless	Warm Bounding pulses
Ulceration:	Painful Heels and toes	Painless Plantar

Once tissue damage has occurred in the form of ulceration or gangrene, the aim is preservation of viable tissue. The two main threats are:

- *Infection.* This rapidly takes hold in a diabetic foot, and early effective antibiotic treatment is essential. Collections of pus are drained and excision of infected bone is needed if osteomyelitis develops. Regular X-rays of the foot are needed to check on progress.
- *Ischaemia.* The blood flow to the feet is assessed clinically or with the Doppler ultrasound stethoscope. Femoral arteriography may be performed, since localized areas of occlusion may be amenable to bypass surgery.

Foot problems are the major cause of hospital bed occupancy by diabetic patients. Good liaison between surgeon and physician is essential if this period in hospital is to be used efficiently. When irreversible arterial insufficiency is present, it is often quicker and kinder to opt for an early major amputation rather than subject the patient to a debilitating sequence of conservative procedures.

Infections

There is no evidence that diabetic patients with good glycaemic control are more prone to infection than normal subjects. However, poorly controlled diabetes entails increased susceptibility to the following infections:

- *Skin*
  (a) Staphylococcal infections (boils, abscesses, carbuncles)
  (b) Mucocutaneous candidiasis
- *Urinary tract*
  (a) Urinary tract infections (in women)
  (b) Pyelonephritis
  (c) Perinephric abscess
- *Lungs*
  (a) Staphylococcal and pneumococcal pneumonia

(b) Gram-negative bacterial pneumonia
(c) Tuberculosis

One reason why poor control lends to infection is that chemotaxis and phagocytosis by polymorphonuclear leucocytes is impaired at high blood glucose levels.

Conversely, infections may lead to loss of glycaemic control, and are a common cause of ketoacidosis. Insulin-treated patients need to increase their dose by up to 25% in the face of infection, and non-insulin-treated patients may need insulin cover while the infection lasts. Patients should be told never to omit their insulin dose, even if they are nauseated and unable to eat; instead they should seek urgent medical advice.

Skin and joints (see p. 1035 and p. 409)

Joint contractures in the hands are a common consequence of childhood diabetes. The sign may be demonstrated by asking the patient to join his hands as if in prayer; the metacarpophalangeal and interphalangeal joints cannot be apposed. Thickened, waxy skin can be noted on the backs of the fingers. These features may be due to glycosylation of collagen and are not progressive. The condition is sometimes referred to as diabetic cheiroarthropathy.

Osteopenia in the extremities is also described in IDDM but rarely leads to clinical consequences.

SPECIAL SITUATIONS

Surgery

Smooth control of diabetes minimizes the risk of infection and balances the catabolic response to anaesthesia and surgery. The procedure for insulin-treated patients is simple:

- Soluble insulin only is given for 2–3 days before surgery.
- Whenever possible, diabetic patients should be first on the morning theatre list.
- An infusion of glucose, insulin and potassium is given during surgery. The insulin can be injected into the glucose solution or administered by syringe pump. A standard combination is 16 units of soluble insulin with 10 mmol KCl in 500 ml of 10% dextrose, infused at 100 ml·h^{-1}.
- Postoperatively, the infusion is maintained until the patient is able to eat. Glucose levels are checked 2–4-hourly and potassium levels are monitored.

The same approach is used in the emergency situation, with the exception that an insulin infusion or subcutaneous injections of 4–6 units of soluble insulin hourly may be needed to bring the blood glucose under control prior to surgery.

Non-insulin-treated patients should stop medication 2 days before the operation. Patients with mild hyperglycaemia (fasting blood glucose below 8 mmol·L^{-1}) can be treated as non-diabetic. Those with higher levels are treated with soluble insulin prior to surgery, and with glucose, insulin and potassium during and after the procedure, as for insulin-treated patients.

Pregnancy and diabetes

Modern management has transformed the outcome of pregnancy in women with diabetes. Thirty years ago one pregnancy in three ended with the death of the fetus or neonate. Today, the results in specialized centres approach those of non-diabetic pregnancy. This improvement is due to meticulous glycaemic control and careful medical and obstetric management.

Glycaemic control in pregnancy
The patient should perform daily home blood glucose profiles; the renal threshold falls in pregnancy and urine tests are therefore of little or no value. Insulin requirements rise, and intensified insulin regimens may become necessary. The aim is to maintain blood glucose and HbA$_{1c}$ levels within the normal range.

When the pregnancy is planned, good control is sought prior to conception.

General management
The patient is seen at intervals of 2 weeks or less at a clinic managed jointly by obstetrician and physician. Routine admission at 32 weeks is no longer necessary, and, circumstances permitting, the aim should be outpatient management with a spontaneous vaginal delivery at term.

Obstetric problems associated with diabetes
Poorly controlled diabetes is associated with macrosomia, hydramnios, pre-eclampsia and intrauterine death. Ketoacidosis in pregnancy carries a 50% fetal mortality, but maternal hypoglycaemia is relatively well tolerated.

Neonatal problems
Maternal diabetes, especially when poorly controlled, is associated with fetal macrosomia. The infant of a diabetic mother is more susceptible to hyaline membrane disease than non-diabetic infants of similar maturity. In addition, neonatal hypoglycaemia may occur. The mechanism is as follows: maternal glucose crosses the placenta, but insulin does not; the fetal islets hypersecrete to combat maternal hyperglycaemia, and a rebound to hypoglycaemic levels occurs when the umbilical cord is severed.

These complications are due to hyperglycaemia in the third trimester. Poor glycaemic control in the first trimester carries an increased risk of congenital malformations, particularly of the cardiovascular and central nervous systems. For this reason, women with diabetes should be advised to achieve optimum glycaemic control before conception.

Gestational diabetes
This term refers to diabetes that develops in the course of pregnancy and remits following delivery.

The diabetes is typically asymptomatic and is demonstrated biochemically on the basis of random testing or an oral glucose tolerance test. Since the renal threshold for glucose falls during normal pregnancy and glucose tolerance deteriorates, the condition may easily be misdiagnosed. Current practice in many centres is to screen for this condition using glucose levels in blood samples taken at antenatal clinics. A value above 6.4 mmol·L^{-1} within 2 h of a meal, or above 5.8 mmol·L^{-1} therafter, represents a deviation above the ninety-ninth percentile and indicates the need for an oral glucose tolerance test.

Treatment is with diet in the first instance, but most patients require insulin cover during the pregnancy. Oral agents are avoided because of the potential risk to the fetus.

Gestational diabetes has been associated with a higher frequency of obstetric problems, fetal macrosomia and neonatal hypoglycaemia. It is likely to recur in subsequent pregnancies, and non-insulin-dependent diabetes may develop later in life.

Not all diabetes presenting in pregnancy is gestational. True IDDM may develop, and swift diagnosis is essential to prevent the development of ketoacidosis. Hospital admission is required if the patient is symptomatic, or has ketonuria or a markedly elevated blood glucose level.

Brittle diabetes

There is no precise definition for this term, which is used to describe patients with recurrent keto-acidosis and/or recurrent hypoglycaemic coma. Of these, the largest group is made up of those who experience recurrent severe hypoglycaemia.

Recurrent severe hypoglycaemia
This affects 1–3% of insulin-dependent patients. Most are adults who have had diabetes for more than 10 years. By this stage endogenous insulin secretion is negligible in the great majority of patients. Pancreatic alpha cells are still present in undiminished numbers, but the glucagon response to hypoglycaemia is virtually absent. Long-term patients are thus subject to fluctuating hyper-insulinaemia due to erratic absorption of insulin from injection sites, and lack a major component of the hormonal defence against hypoglycaemia. In this situation adrenaline secretion becomes vital,

but this too may become impaired in the course of diabetes. Loss of adrenaline secretion has been attributed to autonomic neuropathy, but this is unlikely to be the sole cause; central adaptation to recurrent hypoglycaemia may also be a factor.

The following factors may also predispose to recurrent hypoglycaemia:

- *An unrecognized low renal threshold for glucose.* Attempts to render the urine sugar-free will inevitably produce hypoglycaemia.
- *Excessive insulin doses.* A common error is to increase the *dose* when a patient needs more frequent injections to overcome a problem of *timing*.
- *Endocrine causes.* These include pituitary insufficiency, adrenal insufficiency and premenstrual insulin sensitivity.
- *Alimentary causes.* These include exocrine pancreatic failure and diabetic gastroparesis.
- *Renal failure.* This is associated with falling insulin requirements and unstable control.
- *Patient causes.* The patient may be unintelligent, feckless or may manipulate their therapy.

Recurrent ketoacidosis
This usually occurs in adolescents or young adults, and the most severe form is more common in girls. Although metabolic decompensation may develop very rapidly, it is often impossible to pin-point an underlying abnormality. Many theories exist concerning the causes of this condition, but all agree that it is heterogenous. The following categories have been suggested:

- *Iatrogenic.* Inappropriate insulin combinations may be a cause of swinging glycaemic control. For example, a once-daily regimen may cause hypoglycaemia during the afternoon or evening and pre-breakfast hyperglycaemia due to insulin deficiency.
- *Intercurrent illness.* Unsuspected infections, including urinary tract infections and tuberculosis, may be present. Thyrotoxicosis can also manifest as unstable glycaemic control.
- *Psychosocial causes.* These certainly form the largest category. It has been suggested that neuroendocrine mechanisms such as catecholamine secretion might mediate the metabolic disturbance. Other patients undoubtedly manipulate their illness, whether consciously or unconsciously.
- *Unknown aetiology.* The most 'brittle' patients of all are usually female, aged 15–25 and often overweight, and typically suffer from amenorrhoea. The insulin requirement is variable but is often high. Sophisticated 'cheating' has been detected in some of these patients, but this should never be assumed without convincing proof.

Hypoglycaemia

Hypoglycaemia develops when hepatic glucose output falls below the rate of glucose uptake by peripheral tissues. Hepatic glucose output may be reduced by:

- The inhibition of hepatic glycogenolysis and gluconeogenesis by insulin
- The depletion of hepatic glycogen reserves by malnutrition, fasting, exercise or advanced liver disease
- Impaired gluconeogenesis (e.g. following alcohol ingestion)

In the first of these categories, insulin levels are raised and the liver contains adequate glycogen stores, and the hypoglycaemia can be reversed by injection of glucagon. In the other two situations, insulin levels are low and glucagon is ineffective.

Peripheral glucose uptake is accelerated by high insulin levels and by exercise, but these conditions are normally balanced by increased glucose output. Insulin or sulphonylurea therapy for diabetes accounts for the vast majority of cases of severe hypoglycaemia encountered in an A and E department.

The commonest symptoms and signs of hypoglycaemia are neurological. The brain consumes about 50% of the total glucose produced by the liver. This high energy requirement is needed to generate ATP used to maintain the potential difference across axonal membranes.

Insulinomas

Insulinomas are pancreatic islet cell tumours that secrete insulin. Most are sporadic but some patients have multiple tumours arising from neural-crest tissue (multiple endocrine adenomatosis). Some 95% of these tumours are benign. The classic presentation is with fasting hypoglycaemia, but early symptoms may also develop in the late morning or afternoon. Recurrent hypoglycaemia is often present for months or years before the diagnosis is made, and the symptoms may be atypical or even bizarre; the presenting features in one series are given in Table 17.10. Common

Table 17.10 Presenting features of insulinoma.

Diplopia
Sweating, palpitations, weakness
Confusion or abnormal behaviour
Loss of consciousness
Grand mal seizures

misdiagnoses include psychiatric disorders, epilepsy and cerebrovascular disease.

DIAGNOSIS

Whipple's triad remains the basis of clinical diagnosis. This is satisfied when:

- Symptoms are associated with fasting or exercise
- Hypoglycaemia is confirmed during these episodes
- Glucose relieves the symptoms

A fourth criterion—demonstration of inappropriately high insulin levels during hypoglycaemia—may usefully be added to these.

In practice, the diagnosis is confirmed by the demonstration of hypoglycaemia in association with inappropriate and excessive insulin secretion. Hypoglycaemia is demonstrated by:

- Measurement of overnight fasting (16 h) glucose and insulin levels on three occasions. About 90% of patients with insulinomas will have low glucose and non-suppressed (normal or elevated) insulin levels.
- Performing a prolonged supervised fast. Whipple's triad can be demonstrated in about 95% of patients in the course of a 48-hour fast.

Autonomous insulin secretion is demonstrated by lack of the normal feedback suppression during hypoglycaemia. This may be shown by:

- Measuring insulin, C-peptide or proinsulin levels during a spontaneous episode of hypoglycaemia
- Inducing hypoglycaemia. Since pharmaceutical insulin does not contain C-peptide, an insulin tolerance test is performed and C-peptide is assayed as an index of endogenous insulin secretion. An alternative is to infuse fish insulin, which does not interfere with the assay for human insulin, and to measure circulating insulin levels. These tests are potentially hazardous, and should be resorted to only when real doubt exists concerning the diagnosis.

Many patients also have an abnormal (diabetic) glucose tolerance test, but this has no diagnostic value.

TREATMENT

The most effective therapy is surgical excision of the tumour. It is usual to perform pancreatic angiography preoperatively in an attempt to localize the tumour, but the majority of insulinomas can be palpated by a skilled surgeon. Localization is also possible using a rapid insulin assay on blood sampled at different levels from the pancreatic vein.

Medical treatment with diazoxide is useful when the insulinoma is malignant, in patients in whom a tumour cannot be located, and in elderly patients with mild symptoms.

Hypoglycaemia with other tumours

Hypoglycaemia may develop in the course of advanced cachectic disease, and has been described in association with many tumour types. Certain massive tumours, especially sarcomas, are associated with hypoglycaemia, possibly because the tumour is consuming large amounts of glucose. Other tumour types appear to secrete substances with insulin-like action, but true ectopic insulin secretion is extremely rare.

Post-prandial hypoglycaemia

If frequent *venous* blood glucose samples are taken following a prolonged glucose tolerance test, about one in four subjects will have at least one value below 3 mmol·L^{-1}. The arteriovenous glucose difference is quite marked during this phase, so that very few are truly hypoglycaemic in terms of arterial (or capillary) blood glucose content. Failure to appreciate this simple fact led some authorities to believe that post-prandial (or reactive) hypoglycaemia was a potential 'organic' explanation for a variety of complaints that might otherwise have been considered psychosomatic. An epidemic of false 'hypoglycaemia' followed, particularly in the USA. Later work showed a poor correlation between symptoms and biochemical hypoglycaemia. Even so, a number of otherwise normal people occasionally become pale, weak and sweaty at times when meals are due, and report benefit from advice to take regular snacks between meals.

True post-prandial hypoglycaemia may develop in the presence of alcohol, which 'primes' the beta cells to produce an exaggerated insulin response to carbohydrate. The person who substitutes alcoholic beverages for lunch is particularly at risk. Post-prandial hypoglycaemia sometimes occurs after gastric surgery, owing to rapid gastric emptying and mismatching of food and insulin. This is referred to as 'dumping' but it is rarely a clinical problem (see p. 193).

Hepatic and renal causes of hypoglycaemia

The liver can maintain a normal glucose output despite extensive damage, and hepatic hypoglycaemia is uncommon. It is particularly a problem with fulminant hepatic failure following poisoning with, for example, paracetamol.

The kidney has a subsidiary role in glucose production (via gluconeogenesis in the renal cor-

tex), and hypoglycaemia is sometimes a problem in terminal renal failure.

Hereditary fructose intolerance occurs in 1 in 20 000 live births and can cause hypoglycaemia (p. 862).

Endocrine causes of hypoglycaemia

Endocrine disorders resulting in deficiencies of hormones antagonistic to insulin are rare but well-recognized causes of hypoglycaemia. These include hypopituitarism, isolated ACTH deficiency and Addison's disease.

Drug-induced hypoglycaemia

Many drugs have been reported to produce isolated cases of hypoglycaemia, but usually only when other predisposing factors are present. The following are among the more important:

- *Sulphonylureas* may be used in the treatment of diabetes or may be taken by non-diabetics in suicide attempts.
- *Quinine* may produce severe hypoglycaemia in the course of treatment for falciparum malaria.
- *Salicylates* may cause hypoglycaemia following accidental ingestion by children, but this complication is very rare in adults.
- *Propranolol* has been reported to induce hypoglycaemia in the presence of strenuous exercise or starvation.

Alcohol-induced hypoglycaemia

Alcohol-induced hypoglycaemia was first described in poorly-nourished chronic alcoholics but may also present in binge drinkers and in children who have taken relatively small amounts of alcohol. Alcohol inhibits gluconeogenesis and is most likely to induce hypoglycaemia when taken by fasting or malnourished individuals or children, who have no hepatic glycogen reserve. The clinical presentation is with coma and hypothermia.

Factitious hypoglycaemia

This is a relatively common variant of self-induced disease. Hypoglycaemia is produced by surreptitious self-administration of insulin or sulphonylureas. Many patients in this category have been extensively investigated for an insulinoma. Measurement of C-peptide levels during hypoglycaemia should identify patients who are injecting insulin; sulphonylureas may be picked up by chromatography of plasma or urine.

Table 17.11 Composition of major lipoprotein classes.

	Protein	Triglyceride	Cholesterol	Phospholipid	Major apoproteins
Chylomicrons	2%	85%	4%	9%	B, CI, CII, CIII
VLDL	10%	50%	15%	18%	B, CI, CII, CIII, E
LDL	23%	10%	45%	20%	B
HDL	55%	4%	17%	24%	A-I, A-II

Disorders of lipid metabolism

Cholesterol and triglycerides are insoluble and are transported between the intestine, liver and periphery in the form of soluble complexes known as lipoproteins. These circulate as spherical particles with an envelope of phospholipid and apoproteins and at non-polar lipid core. They can be divided by density, configuration and electrophoretic mobility into chylomicrons, very low-density lipoproteins (VLDLs), intermediate-density lipoproteins (IDLs), low-density lipoproteins (LDLs) and high-density lipoproteins (HDLs) (Table 17.11).

Chylomicrons are large particles composed mainly of triglyceride. They are synthesized in the small-intestinal mucosa and provide the main form of transport for dietary fat. They also contain phospholipid, a small amount of cholesterol, apoprotein B-48 (apo B-48) and apo A-I, A-II, and acquire apo C-II and apo E, transferred from HDLs (Fig. 17.14). Chylomicrons give the post-prandial plasma a lactescent appearance that normally clears within a few hours. The chylomicrons are catabolized to form chylomicron remnants by lipoprotein lipase

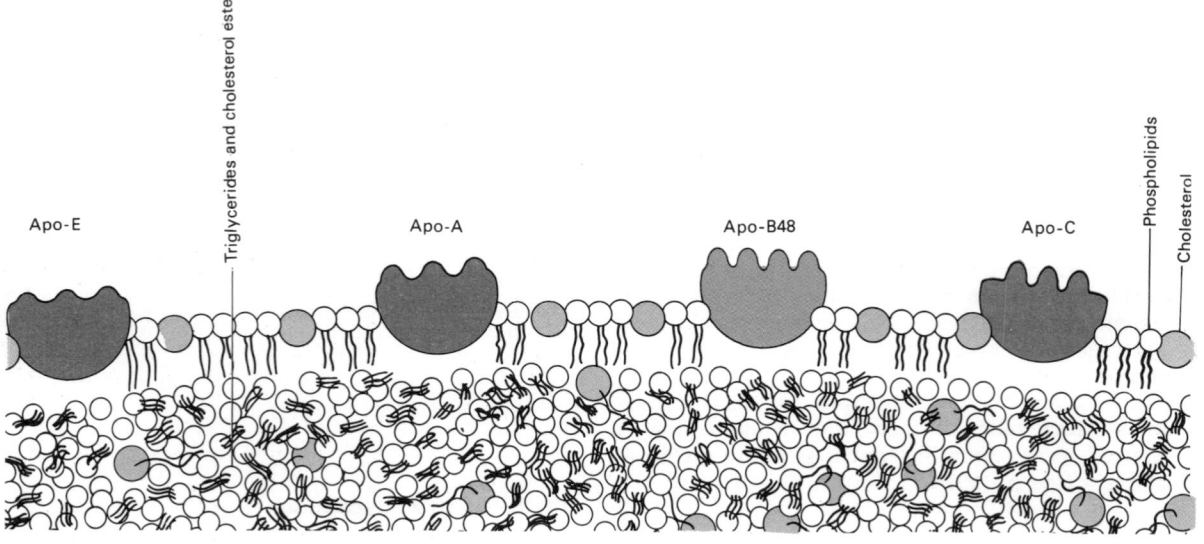

Fig. 17.14 Schematic diagram of the surface of a chylomicron particle (2000–5000 Å) showing the apoproteins lying in the membrane.

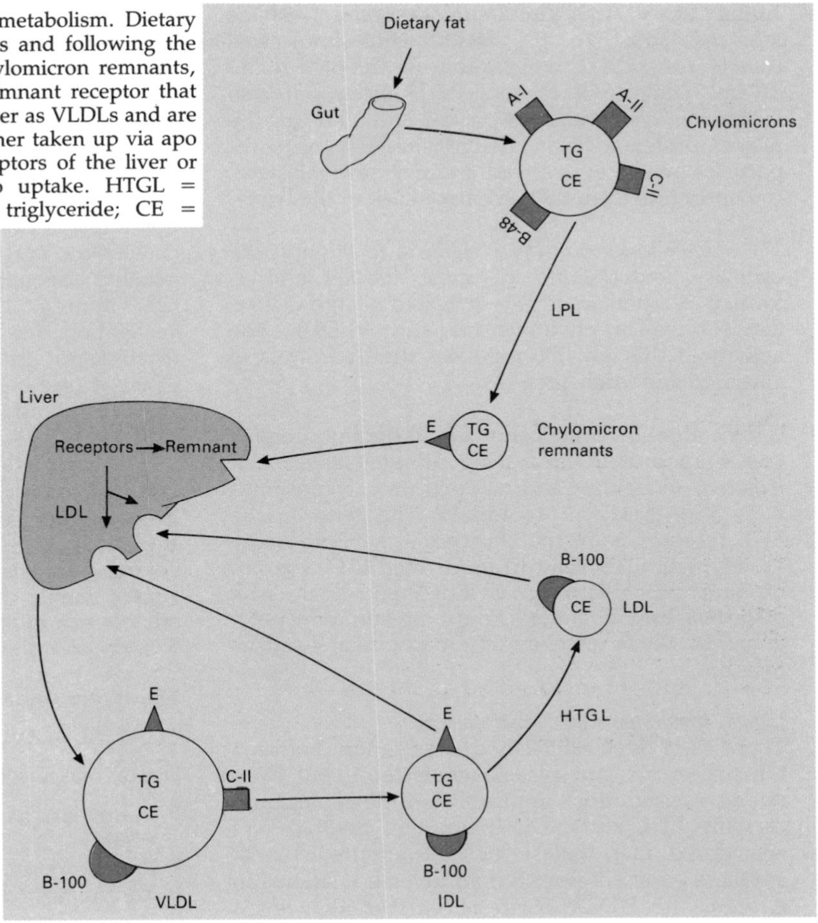

Fig. 17.15 Pathways of lipoprotein metabolism. Dietary fat is incorporated into chylomicrons and following the hydrolysis of triglycerides forms chylomicron remnants, which are taken up by a hepatic remnant receptor that recognizes apo E. Lipids leave the liver as VLDLs and are hydrolysed into LDLs. These are either taken up via apo E recognition sites by the LDL receptors of the liver or further processed to LDL prior to uptake. HTGL = hepatic triglyceride lipase; TG = triglyceride; CE = cholesterol ester.

(activated by apo C-II) in peripheral tissues as well as by hepatic lipase (Fig. 17.15). Triglyceride is progressively removed by lipolysis to remove free fatty acids. Some apo A-I, A-II and apo C are transferred to HDLs. Chylomicron remnants are eventually taken up by specific apo B and apo E receptors in the liver.

VLDLs are synthesized mainly in the liver and represent endogenous triglyceride synthesis. They contain apo B-100 and apo E. VLDLs are also catabolized by lipoprotein lipase in the peripheral tissues. The breakdown of VLDLs and transfer of some apoproteins to HDLs give rise to smaller, denser remnant particles, some of which can be identified as IDLs.

IDLs are taken up by the hepatocyte LDL receptors by binding to the apo E on the IDL surface. Alternatively, IDLs are converted by further hydrolysis of triglycerides (probably by hepatic lipase) to LDLs.

LDLs are the major cholesterol-carrying lipoprotein in normal plasma, their main protein being (as for VLDLs) apo B-100. The majority of LDLs enter the liver cells after binding to high-affinity receptors found in the coated pit region that recognize apo B-100. After binding, the LDL is internalized and metabolized, releasing free cholesterol that partly contributes to endogenous cholesterol (Fig. 2.9, p. 124).

A 'scavenger pathway' is also available to clear LDLs. An acetyl-LDL receptor is available in many tissues including macrophages and sinosoidal endothelial cells in the liver. These specifically take up LDLs that have been modified by oxidation. It is this mechanism that seems to convert macrophages to foam cells found in the fatty streak—the earliest lesion in atherosclerosis.

HDLs are produced in the liver and intestine and

contain 20–50% of circulating cholesterol. HDLs are the substrate for lecithin:cholesterol acyl transferase (LCAT), which catalyses the conversion of free cholesterol to cholesterol ester and also lecithin to lysolecithin. Apo A-I and A-II are the major proteins. This heterogeneous group of particles may be involved in reverse cholesterol transport (i.e. from the periphery back to the liver).

The enzyme lipoprotein lipase (LPL) is situated in the capillary endothelium of most tissues and is formed as a precursor. It is activated by apo C-II on the surface of chylomicrons and VLDLs. The activity of this enzyme regulates the hydrolysis of all triglyceride-rich proteins.

Genetic control. So far genes for 10 apolipoproteins and 4 lipoprotein processing proteins have been isolated, sequenced and mapped on chromosomes 1, 2, 3, 6, 8, 11, 15, 16 and 19. The gene for the LDL receptor is on the short arm of chromosome 19. Hyperlipidaemias can be divided into a group of rare but relatively well-defined single-gene disorders and a larger group, presumably polygenic, in which genetic and environmental factors overlap.

Lipids, lipoproteins and atherosclerosis
There is a well-established association between atherosclerosis and plasma cholesterol, but even stronger associations appear when the cholesterol-carrying LDL and HDL lipoprotein fractions are considered. LDL-cholesterol levels are predictive of coronary heart disease, but an inverse relationship is seen with HDL-cholesterol, so that high levels appear to be protective.

Cholesterol deposited in atheromatous lesions is derived from LDL and enters the lesion at a rate dependent upon the plasma concentrations. The protective role of HDL may be in mediating hepatic cholesterol excretion by reverse transport of cholesterol from the periphery.

The atherogenicity of triglyceride-rich lipoproteins is less clear but there are strong epidemiological associations with ischaemic heart disease and peripheral vascular disease. Marked hypertriglyceridaemia (> 10 mmol·L^{-1}) carries a risk of pancreatitis and is another indication for treatment.

In males the incidence of coronary heart disease is least in those with cholesterol values below 5.2 mmol·L^{-1}, rises linearly to a level of 6.5 mmol·L^{-1}, and rises even more steeply above this point. Since the population mean lies around 5.6 mmol·L^{-1}, the inference is that most people in Western societies might benefit from having a lower cholesterol, especially since there is now evidence that lowering cholesterol does indeed reduce the incidence of coronary heart disease. These observations have profound social implications, while incidentally generating an enormously profitable market for the pharmaceutical industry.

Whilst many of us might derive some benefit from dietary modification and attention to other potential coronary risk factors, there is at present little evidence to support routine screening for cholesterol in the healthy population, although this has its advocates.

Modification of diet reduces cholesterol by 15–25% and triglyceride by 20–40%. Diet modification alone is therefore appropriate for those in the cholesterol range from 5.2–6.4 mmol·L^{-1}, and is usually adequate for those in the range from 6.5–8 mmol·L^{-1}. Above 8 mmol·L^{-1}, further investigation for underlying disease (e.g. hypothyroidism) and to characterize the lipoprotein disorder (see below) is called for. Diet remains the basis of therapy and lipid-lowering agents are an adjunct. Advice should be geared to the individual patient rather than to the biochemistry report. For example, obesity and other coronary risk factors need to be taken into account, and a more aggressive approach is called for if the patient is young, has established arterial disease, or has a strong family history of this. Conversely, the relative risk of hypercholesterolaemia is reduced in women and diminishes with increasing age.

The hyperlipidaemias

CLINICAL FEATURES

Features associated with hyperlipidaemia include:

- Xanthelasmas (cholesterol deposits on the eyelid)
- Premature arcus in the cornea
- Xanthomas (cholesterol deposits in the skin)
- Rarely, lipaemia retinalis (turbid blood in the retinal vessels)

Evidence of possible underlying disorders (Table 17.12) such as hypothyroidism should be sought.

INVESTIGATION

Initial investigation involves measurement of the fasting cholesterol and triglyceride levels. The

Table 17.12 Secondary causes of raised cholesterol and triglyceride.

Raised cholesterol
Diet
Hypothyroidism
Liver disease
Nephrotic syndrome
Porphyria

Raised triglyceride
Obesity
Poorly controlled diabetes
Alcohol excess
High-carbohydrate diet
Renal failure
Oestrogen therapy

Table 17.13 Lipid-lowering agents.

Type	Dose	Comments
Ion-exchange resins		
Cholestyramine	12-24 g daily	Gastrointestinal side-effects, e.g. constipation, indigestion, nausea Increases VLDL. Unsuitable for hypertriglyceridaemia
Fibrates		
Bezafibrate	200 mg three times daily (with food)	Well-tolerated
Gemfibrizil	600 mg twice daily	
Nicotinic acid derivatives		
Nicotinic Acid	100–200 mg initially 1–2 g three times daily maximum	Flushing and GI upset limit tolerance
Probucol	500 mg twice daily (with food)	
HMG CoA reductase inhibition		
Simvastatin	10–40 mg taken in the evening	Not fully evaluated. Resistant cases only. Caution with liver disease

patient follows his normal diet for the preceding 2 weeks, and drugs that may affect lipid metabolism are withdrawn. The result may be influenced by acute illness, but the test may be performed soon after myocardial infarction and any high levels confirmed before treatment is started.

Values should be assessed according to the age of the patient. Results over the ninety-fifth percentile should be investigated further, including measurement of HDL–cholesterol and lipoprotein electrophoresis.

Examination of stored serum provides useful information: a diffuse milky appearance usually means raised VLDL, whereas a creamy upper layer with clear plasma beneath indicates chylomicronaemia. Family members should be investigated when a primary hyperlipidaemia is suspected.

GENERAL MANAGEMENT OF HYPERLIPIDAEMIAS

General principles are:

- The maintenance of a lean body weight
- A low-fat diet
- Avoidance of alcohol
- Avoidance of oestrogens and thiazides
- Avoidance of smoking
- The treatment of diabetes and hypertension when present
- Moderate exercise

Lipid-lowering agents (Table 17.13)
These may be effective in one of three ways:

- Reduced synthesis of VLDLs and LDLs (e.g. nicotinic acid).
- Enhanced VLDL clearance (e.g. bezafibrate).
- Enhanced LDL catabolism (e.g. cholestyramine, which is a non-absorbable anion exchange resin that binds bile acids in the gut lumen, thus reducing the enterohepatic circulation and enhancing cholesterol conversion to bile acids).
- HMG-Co-A reductase inhibition. Drugs such as simvastatin inhibit this rate-limiting enzyme in cholesterol synthesis and consequently there is an increase in LDL receptor expression.

Cholestyramine reduced the incidence and progression of coronary disease in a large cohort of American men with raised cholesterol levels. Until wider clinical experience has been obtained, simvastatin should be reserved for resistant hypercholesterolaemia (> 7.8 mmol$\cdot$L^{-1}).

Table 17.14 Classification of hyperlipidaemias.

Disease	WHO type	Cholesterol	Triglyceride	Possible protein abnormality	Physiological abnormality
Familial hypercholesterolaemia	IIa IIb	↑	N (↑)	LDL receptor (Apo B-100)	↑ LDL
Polygenic hypercholesterolaemia (common)	II	↑	N	(LDL receptor)	↑ LDL
Familial dysbetalipoproteinaemia (broad β disease, remnant hyperlipoproteinaemia)	III	↑	↑	Apo E LDL receptor	↑ IDL ↑ CM[a] remnants
Familial hypertriglyceridaemia	IV	N	↑	Apo B LPL Apo C-II	↑ VLDL ↑ CM
Familial combined hyperlipidaemia	IIa IIb IV	↑	↑	Apo B	↑ VLDL ↑ LDL
Lipoprotein lipase deficiency, Apo C-II deficiency	I V	N	↑	LPL defect Apo C-II	↑ CM ↑ VLDL

[a] CM = chylomicrons.

CLASSIFICATION OF HEREDITARY HYPERLIPIDAEMIAS (Table 17.14)

This is complex and many find it confusing. This is because the standard Fredrickson/WHO classification is based on patterns found during laboratory analysis rather than on disease entities. These patterns may result from a variety of disease processes and sometimes overlap.

Familial hypercholesterolaemia is characterized by hypercholesterolaemia due to raised LDL levels. There can be mild elevation in triglycerides and VLDLs. It is autosomal dominant in inheritance with an incidence of 1 : 500 heterozygotes in the population. The metabolic defect is related to binding and internalization of LDL to its receptor protein. A familial apo B-100 defect giving raised LDLs has recently been described.

Heterozygotes often develop coronary artery disease between the third and fourth decade of life and account for 5% of survivors of myocardial infarction under the age of 60. Premature arcus and xanthomas may be present and cholesterol levels are markedly elevated. Homozygotes have grossly elevated cholesterol (usually > 16 mmol·L^{-1}) and marked xanthomatosis and develop coronary artery disease whilst in their teens.

Treatment is with a low-cholesterol diet, cholestyramine and nicotinic acid, and can be very effective if this regimen is followed conscientiously. In refractory cases, simvastatin should be used.

Familial dysbetalipoproteinaemia. This is characterized by raised cholesterol and triglyceride levels due to raised IDLs and chylomicron remnants. The defect is due to an abnormal form of apoprotein E—Apo E-2, which fails to bind to specific receptors, so that lipoproteins are not cleared. The disease develops in adult life, and is often associated with obesity, glucose intolerance and hyperuricaemia. Palmar xanthomas may be present and are diagnostic. The risk of coronary artery and peripheral vascular disease is increased.

Treatment is by weight reduction and reduced dietary cholesterol and fat. Nicotinic acid may also be necessary.

Familial hypertriglyceridaemia is an autosomal dominant disorder associated with raised VLDLs. The exact mechanism is unclear. There is an association with diabetes. It is exacerbated by a number of environmental factors including obesity, alcohol, diuretics (thiazides), oral contraceptive pill and glucocorticoids. Eruptive xanthomas are present; pancreatitis occurs. Treatment is with weight reduction, low-fat diet, alcohol avoidance, careful control of diabetes and oral gemfibrozil for patients with very high triglyceride levels. The risk of coronary disease is small.

Familial combined hyperlipidaemia. This common disorder has raised cholesterol and triglyceride levels and has an increased risk of coronary artery disease. The precise mechanism is unclear but it is probably related to dysfunction of apo B.

Lipoprotein lipase or Apo C-II deficiency is a rare autosomal recessive condition and is characterized by the presence of chylomicrons in fasting plasma. Chylomicrons cannot be metabolized due to deficiency of extra-hepatic LPL or its co-factor Apo C-II.

Patients present in childhood with hepatosplenomegaly, eruptive xanthomas and lipaemia retinalis; some experience recurrent pancreatitis. Despite the raised triglyceride levels there is little evidence of premature vascular disease. Treatment is with a strict low-fat diet (10–25% of dietary energy). Fish oils, containing polyunsaturated omega-3 fatty acids, are also used.

Hypolipidaemia

Low lipid levels can be found in severe protein–energy malnutrition. They are also seen occasionally with severe malabsorption and in intestinal lymphangiectasia.

Abetalipoproteinaemia

This is described on p. 210.

Familial alpha-lipoprotein deficiency (Tangier disease)

One of the two HDL apoproteins, apo A-I, is deficient in homozygotes with this very rare disease, so that there is little HDL in plasma. Tangier disease is inherited as an autosomal recessive. The serum cholesterol is low, but serum triglycerides are normal or high. Cholesterol accumulates in reticulo-endothelial tissue, although the mechanism is uncertain, producing enlarged and orange-coloured tonsils and hepatosplenomegaly. There are also corneal opacities and a polyneuropathy.

Inborn errors of carbohydrate metabolism

Glycogen storage disease

All mammalian cells can manufacture glycogen, but the main sites of its production are the liver and muscle. Glycogen is a high-molecular-weight glucose polymer. In glycogen storage disease there is either an abnormality in the molecular structure or an increase in glycogen concentration owing to a specific enzyme defect. Almost all these conditions are autosomal recessive in inheritance and present in infancy, except for McArdle's disease, which presents in adults.

Table 17.15 shows the classification and clinical features of some of these diseases. New specific enzyme defects, e.g. liver phosphorylase, phosphorylase kinase, are being recognized.

Galactosaemia

Galactose is normally converted to glucose. However, a deficiency of the enzyme galactose-1-phosphate uridyl transferase results in accumulation of galactose-1-phosphate in the blood. This deficiency, inherited as an autosomal recessive, results in hypoglycaemia and acidosis in the neonate. Progressive hepatosplenomegaly, catar-

Table 17.15 Some glycogen storage diseases.

Type	Affected tissue	Enzyme defect	Clinical features	Tissue needed for diagnosis[a]	Outcome
I (Von Gierke)	Liver, intestine, kidney	Glucose-6-phosphatase	Hepatomegaly, hypoglycaemia, stunted growth, obesity, hypotonia	Liver	If patients survive initial hypoglycaemia, prognosis is good; hyperuricaemia is a late complication
II (Pompé)	Liver, muscle, heart	Lysosomal α-glucosidase	Heart failure, cardiomyopathy	Leucocytes, liver, muscle	Death in first 6 months; juvenile and adult variants seen
III (Forbes)	Liver, muscle (abnormal glycogen structure)	Amylo-1,6-glucosidase	Like type I	Leucocytes, liver, muscle	Good prognosis
IV (Anderson)	Liver (abnormal glycogen structure)	1,4-α-glucan branching enzyme	Failure to thrive, hepatomegaly, cirrhosis and its complications	Leucocytes, liver, muscle	Death in first 3 years
V (McArdle)	Muscle only	Phosphorylase	Muscle cramps and myoglobinuria after exercise (in adults)	Muscle	Normal life span; exercise must be avoided

[a] Tissue obtained is used for the biochemical assay of the enzyme.

acts, renal tubular defects and mental retardation occur.

Treatment is with a galactose-free diet, which, if started early, results in normal development. Untreated patients die within a few days. Prenatal diagnosis and diagnosis of the carrier state are possible by measurement of the level of galactose-1-phosphate in the blood.

Galactokinase deficiency also results in galactosaemia and early cataract formation.

Defects of fructose metabolism

Absorbed fructose is chiefly metabolized in the liver to lactic acid or glucose. Three defects of metabolism occur; all are inherited as autosomal recessive traits:

- *Fructosuria* is due to fructokinase deficiency. It is a benign condition.
- *Fructose intolerance* is due to fructose-1-phosphate aldolase deficiency. Fructose-1-phosphate accumulates after fructose ingestion, resulting in symptoms of hypoglycaemia. Hepatomegaly and renal tubular defects occur but are reversible on a fructose-free diet. Intelligence is normal.
- *Fructose-1,6-diphosphate deficiency* leads to a failure of gluconeogenesis, and to hepatomegaly.

Pentosuria

Pentosuria is due to L-xylulose reductase deficiency. It has no clinical significance.

Inborn errors of amino-acid metabolism

Inborn errors of amino-acid metabolism are chiefly inherited as autosomal recessive conditions. The major ones are shown in Table 17.16.

AMINO-ACID TRANSPORT DEFECTS

Amino acids are filtered by the glomerulus but 95% of the filtered load is reabsorbed in the proximal convoluted tubule by an active transport mechanism.

Aminoaciduria results from:

- Abnormally high plasma amino-acid levels (e.g. phenylketonuria)
- Any inherited disorder that damages the tubules secondarily (e.g. galactosaemia)
- Tubular reabsorptive defects, either generalized (e.g. Fanconi syndrome) or specific (e.g. cystinuria)

Amino-acid transport defects can be congenital or acquired.

Generalized aminoacidurias

Fanconi syndrome
This occurs in a juvenile form (De Toni–Fanconi–Debré syndrome) or in adult life. There is defective tubular reabsorption of:

- Most amino acids
- Glucose
- Phosphate, resulting in hypophosphataemic rickets
- Bicarbonate, with failure to transport hydrogen ions, causing a renal tubular acidosis that then produces a hyperchloraemic acidosis

Other abnormalities include:

- Hypouricaemia
- Potassium depletion, primary or secondary to the acidosis
- Polyuria
- Increased excretion of immunoglobulins and other low-molecular-weight proteins

Various combinations of the above abnormalities have been described.

The juvenile form begins at the age of 6–9 months, with failure to thrive, vomiting and thirst. There is also acidosis, dehydration and vitamin D-resistant rickets.

In the adult, the disease is similar to the juvenile form, but osteomalacia is a major feature.

Treatment is with large doses of vitamin D (e.g. 1–2 µg of 1-α-hydroxycholecalciferol with regular blood calcium monitoring).

Lowe's syndrome (oculocerebrorenal dystrophy)
In this syndrome there is generalized aminoaciduria combined with mental retardation, hypotonia, congenital cataracts and an abnormal skull shape.

Specific aminoacidurias

Cystinuria
There is defective tubular reabsorption and jejunal absorption of cystine and the dibasic amino acids lysine, ornithine and arginine. Inheritance is either completely or incompletely recessive, so that heterozygotes who have increased excretion of lysine and cystine only can occur. Cystine absorption from the jejunum is impaired but, nevertheless, cystine in peptide form can be absorbed. Cystinuria leads to urinary stones and is responsible for approximately 1–2% of all urinary calculi. The disease often starts in childhood, although most cases present in adult life.

Table 17.16 The major inborn errors of amino-acid metabolism.

Disease	Enzyme defect	Incidence	Biochemical and clinical features	Treatment	Prognosis
Albinism	Tyrosinase	1 in 13 000	Amelanosis—whitish hair, pink-white skin, grey-blue eyes Nystagmus, photophobia, strabismus	Symptomatic	—
Alkaptonuria	Homogentisic acid oxidase	1 in 100 000	Homogentisic acid polymerizes to produce a black-brown product that is deposited in cartilage and other tissue (ochronosis) Urine darkens on standing Sweat stains clothing Arthritis	None	Good
Homocystinuria			Homocystine is excreted in urine		
Type I	Cystathionine synthetase		Mental handicap Marfan-like syndrome Thrombotic episodes	—	—
Type II	Methylene tetrahydrofolate reductase		Survivors have mental retardation	—	Mainly die as neonates
Phenylketonuria	Phenylalanine-4-hydroxylase	1 in 20 000	Brain damage with mental retardation and epilepsy Phenylpyruvate and its derivatives excreted in urine	Diet low in phenylalanine in first few months of life prevents damage	—
Histidinaemia	Histidine deaminase	Very rare	Mental retardation	—	—
'Maple syrup' disease	Branched-chain ketoacid decarboxylase	Very rare	Failure to thrive Fits, neonatal acidosis and severe cerebral degeneration Valine, isoleucine, leucine and their derivatives are excreted in urine A milder form is seen	—	Early death
Oxalosis (hyperoxaluria)	Glyoxylic acid dehydrogenase	Very rare	Nephrocalcinosis, renal stones, renal failure due to deposition of calcium oxalate	—	Death occurs in first two decades

There are many other enzyme defects producing, for example, alaninaemia, ammonaemia, argininaemia, citrullinaemia, isovaleric acidaemia, lysinaemia, ornithinaemia or tyrosinaemia.

Treatment is with a high fluid intake in order to keep the urinary cystine concentration low. Patients are encouraged to drink up to 3 litres over 24 h and to drink even at night. Penicillamine should be used for patients who cannot keep the cystine concentration of their urine low.

The condition cystinosis (see p. 869) must not be confused with cystinuria.

Hartnup's disease
There is defective tubular reabsorption and jejunal absorption of most neutral amino acids but not their peptides. The resulting tryptophan malabsorption produces nicotinamide deficiency (see p. 162). Patients can be asymptomatic, but others develop evidence of pellagra, with cerebellar ataxia, psychiatric disorders and skin lesions. Treatment is with nicotinamide and often brings about considerable improvement.

Tryptophan malabsorption syndrome (blue diaper syndrome)
This is due to an isolated transport defect for tryptophan; the tryptophan excreted oxidizes to a blue colour on the baby's diaper.

Familial iminoglycinuria
This occurs when there is defective tubular reabsorption of glycine, proline and hydroxyproline. It seems to have few clinical effects.

Methionine malabsorption syndrome
This is due to failure to absorb and excrete methionine, and results in diarrhoea, vomiting and mental retardation. Patients characteristically have an oast-house smell.

Mucopolysaccharide disorders

Mucopolysaccharide disorders are inherited clinical syndromes due to the failure of the normal breakdown of complex carbohydrates. Partially degraded glycosaminoglycans accumulate in the skeleton, connective tissues and central nervous system.

Hurler's syndrome

This is inherited as a recessive disorder. Affected infants deteriorate after the first few months of life, both mentally and physically. Patients are short and have a characteristic facial appearance (gargoylism) with a flattened nose bridge and an open mouth with a large tongue. Death occurs in late childhood, usually from pneumonia.

Hunter's syndrome

This is similar to Hurler's syndrome but it is inherited in an X-linked recessive manner.

Morquio syndrome

In this syndrome the child becomes progressively more deformed and dwarfed. Intelligence is normal.

Lysosomal storage diseases (sphingolipidoses)

Lysosomal storage diseases are due to inborn errors of metabolism which are mainly inherited in an autosomal recessive manner.

Sphingolipids are degraded by a series of lysosomal enzymes, and accumulate when there is a deficiency of these enzymes.

Gaucher's disease
In Gaucher's disease there is an accumulation of glucocerebroside in the reticuloendothelial system, particularly the liver, bone marrow and spleen. There are three clinical types, the commonest presenting in adult life with an insidious onset of hepatosplenomegaly. There is a high incidence in Ashkenazi Jews (1 in 3000 births), and patients have a characteristic pigmentation on exposed parts, particularly the forehead and hands. Typical Gaucher cells are found in the bone marrow, which are glucocerebroside-containing reticuloendothelial histiocytes. Patients develop anaemia, evidence of hypersplenism and pathological fractures due to bone involvement. Nevertheless, many have a normal life-span.

Acute Gaucher's disease presents in infancy or childhood with rapid onset of hepatosplenomegaly with neurological involvement due to Gaucher cells in the brain. The outlook is poor.

Niemann–Pick disease
This is due to the accumulation of sphingomyelin in reticuloendothelial macrophages in many organs, particularly the liver, spleen, bone marrow and lymph nodes. The disease usually presents within the first 6 months of life with mental retardation and hepatosplenomegaly. Typical foam cells are found in the marrow, lymph nodes, liver and spleen.

Tay–Sachs disease (familial amaurotic idiocy)
In this conditioin there is accumulation of GM2 gangliosides in the central nervous system and

peripheral nerves. It is particularly common (1 : 2000) in Ashkenazi Jews. There is a progressive degeneration of all cerebral function, with fits, epilepsy, dementia and blindness and death usually occurs before 2 years of age. The macula has a characteristic cherry spot appearance.

Fabry's disease
This X-linked recessive condition is due to a deficiency of alpha-galactosidase, causing an accumulation of alpha-galactosyl-lactosyl-ceramide in various tissues including the liver, kidney, blood vessels and the ganglion cells of the nervous system. The patients present with peripheral nerve involvement, but eventually most patients develop renal problems in adult life.

DIAGNOSIS

Many of the sphingolipidoses can be diagnosed by demonstrating the enzyme deficiency in the appropriate tissue.
Prenatal diagnosis is becoming possible in a number of the conditions by obtaining specimens of amniotic cells (see p. 119). Carrier states can also be identified, so that sensible genetic counselling can be given.

Cystinosis

In cystinosis, cystine accumulates in the reticuloendothelial cells. It is inherited in an autosomal recessive manner. The exact defect is unknown but it is thought to be a defect of cystine transport across the lysosomal membrane. Three forms are recognized: the infantile form is usually fatal in the first year owing to renal failure; the intermediate form presents in early/young adult life with fever and renal problems; and the adult form is benign. The generalized aminoaciduria seen in these patients often causes confusion with the Fanconi syndrome. Corneal deposits of cystine are seen.

Amyloidosis

This is a disorder of protein metabolism in which there is extracellular deposition of insoluble fibrillar protein, either localized or widely distributed throughout the body.
Characteristically the amyloid protein consists of β-pleated sheets that are responsible for the insolubility and resistance to proteolysis. A smaller part of the protein is the amyloid P component (AP), which is derived from normal circulatory glycoprotein and is related to the acute-phase reactant (CRP).
Amyloid in tissues appears as an amorphous, homogenous substance that stains pink with haematoxylin and eosin and stains red with Congo red, which also shows a green fluorescence in polarized light.

Hereditary systemic amyloidosis

In the Portuguese type I neuropathic amyloidosis, fibrils composed of prealbumin formed into β sheets are found, producing a polyneuropathy.
In *familial Mediterranean fever*, renal amyloidosis is a common serious complication. Deposition of AA fibrils occurs.

Local amyloidosis

Deposits of amyloid fibrils of various types can be localized to various organs or tissues, e.g. skin, heart and brain. A new amyloid syndrome due to β2 microglobulin deposition as amyloid fibrils has been seen in patients on chronic dialysis.

Senile amyloid

Amyloid deposits are frequently found in the elderly. In particular, cerebral deposits of the A4 protein are found, and this protein is also seen in the brains of patients with Down's syndrome and Alzheimer's disease (see p. 949).

Immunocyte-related amyloidosis

In this variety, the deposits consist of amyloid light (AL) chain fragments. The molecular weights of these fragments range from 5000 to 25 000. The amyloidosis is usually associated with lymphoproliferative diseases of the B-cell lineage, e.g. myeloma, Waldenstrom's macroglobulinaemia or non-Hodgkin's lymphoma.

CLINICAL FEATURES

The clinical features are related to the organs involved, patients presenting with heart failure, nephrotic syndrome, purpura or bleeding, peripheral neuropathy or weight loss. Weakness and paraesthesia of the hand may occur due to the carpal tunnel syndrome. On examination, a characteristic feature is macroglossia, which only occurs in this form of amyloidosis. Hepatomegaly and occasionally splenomegaly are seen.

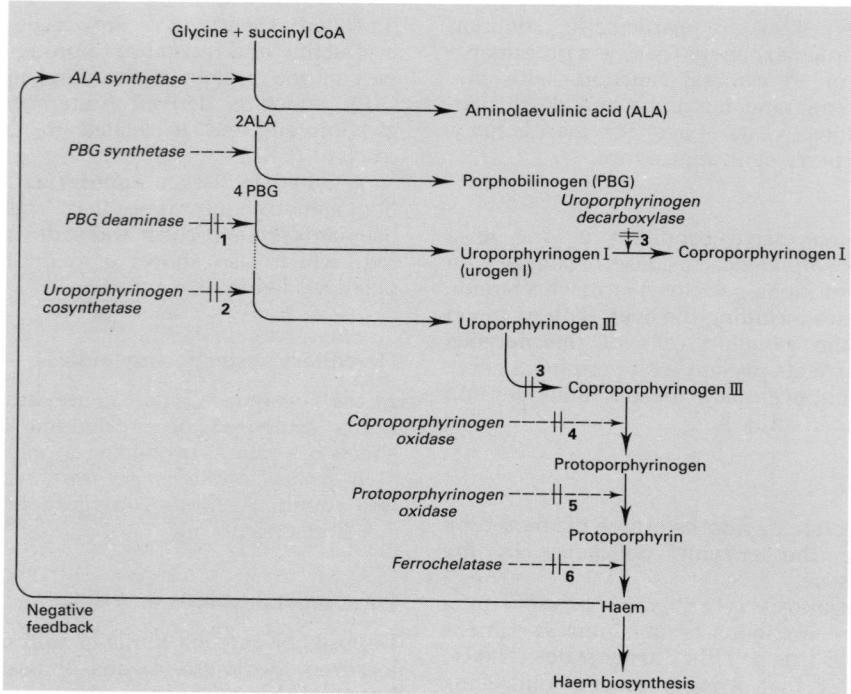

Fig. 17.16 Porphyrin metabolism. The numbers indicate the blocks occurring in forms of porphyria. 1 = acute intermittent porphyria; 2 = congenital (erythropoietic) porphyria; 3 = porphyria cutanea tarda; 4 = hereditary coproporphyria; 5 = variegate porphyria; 6 = erythropoietic protoporphyria.

Table 17.17 The classification of porphyrias.

	Hepatic	Erythropoietic
Acute:	Acute intermittent porphyria Variegate porphyria Hereditary coproporphyria	
Non-acute:	Porphyria cutanea tarda	Congenital porphyria Erythropoietic 　protoporphyria

INVESTIGATION

The diagnosis is made on the presence of the characteristic histological features mentioned above in a biopsy of the rectum or gums. The bone marrow may show plasma cells in primary amyloidosis or a lymphoproliferative disorder. A paraproteinaemia and light chains in the urine may be seen as a result of associated conditions.

TREATMENT

Treatment is symptomatic or of the associated cause.

Reactive systemic amyloidosis

In reactive systemic amyloidosis, the amyloid (AA) is composed of protein A (molecular weight 8500), which is a precursor of the normal serum component serum amyloid A (SAA), an acute-phase reactant. Overproduction of SAA as well as its degradation to AA determines whether amyloidosis occurs. This type of amyloidosis, which used to be known as secondary amyloidosis, involves the spleen, liver, kidney and adrenal glands. It is associated with long-standing chronic infections (e.g. tuberculosis), inflammation (e.g. rheumatoid arthritis), malignancy (e.g. Hodgkin's disease), and also occurs in familial Mediterranean fever (FMF).

Clinically there is hepatosplenomegaly. Hepatic failure and renal failure with renal-vein thrombosis or the nephrotic syndrome may develop.

The porphyrias

This heterogeneous group of rare inborn errors of metabolism is caused by abnormalities of enzymes involved in the biosynthesis of haem, resulting in overproduction of the intermediate compounds called porphyrins (Fig. 17.16).

Structurally, porphyrins consist of four pyrrole rings. These pyrrole rings are formed from the precursors glycine and succinyl-CoA, which are converted to δ-aminolaevulinic acid (δ-ALA) in a reaction catalysed by the enzyme δ-ALA synthetase. Two molecules of δ-ALA condense to form a pyrrole ring.

Porphyrins can be divided into uro-, copro- or protoporphyrins depending on the structure of the side-chain. They are termed type I if the structure is symmetrical and type III if it is asymmetrical. Both uro- and coproporphyrins can be excreted in the urine.

The sequence of enzymatic changes in the production of haem is shown in Fig. 17.16. The chief rate-limiting step is the enzyme δ-ALA synthetase, as an increase in this enzyme results in an overproduction of porphyrins. Haem provides a negative feedback mechanism on this enzyme.

In porphyria the excess production of porphyrins occurs either in the liver (hepatic porphyrias) or in the bone marrow (erythropoietic porphyria), but porphyrias can also be classified in terms of clinical presentation as acute or non-acute. Acute porphyrias usually produce neuropsychiatric problems and are associated with excess production and urinary excretion of δ-ALA and porphobilinogen; these metabolites are not increased in non-acute porphyrias. The second control mechanism is therefore uroporphyrinogen-I-synthetase (see Fig. 17.16); this is depressed or normal in the acute porphyrias and raised in non-acute cases.

A classification of porphyrias is given in Table 17.17.

Acute intermittent porphyria

This is an autosomal dominant disorder. Presentation is in early adult life, usually around the age of 30, and women are affected more than men. It may be precipitated by alcohol and drugs such as barbiturates and oral contraceptives, but a wide range of lipid-soluble drugs have also been incriminated. The abnormality lies at the level of porphobilinogen synthetase in the haem biosynthetic pathway (see Fig. 17.16).

Presentation is with:

● Abdominal pain, vomiting and constipation (90%)
● Peripheral polyneuropathy (sensory and motor) (70%)
● Hypertension and tachycardia (70%)
● Neuropsychiatric disorders (such as depression, anxiety, and frank psychosis) (50%)

The diagnosis should be considered whenever there is a combination of these cardinal features or:

● A family history of porphyria.
● The urine turns red-brown or red on standing. A classic bedside test for excess porphobilinogen may be performed by adding one volume of urine to one volume of Ehrlich's aldehyde, which produces a pink colour. If excess porphobilinogen is present, the pink colour persists when two volumes of chloroform are added.

Other investigations

● Normal blood count; occasional neutrophil leucocytosis
● Abnormal liver biochemical tests—elevated bilirubin and transferases
● Blood urea often raised

Screening. Urinalysis is not adequate and measurement of erythrocyte PBG deaminase and ALA synthetase is extremely sensitive.

MANAGEMENT

Managment of the acute episodes is largely supportive. A high carbohydrate intake is maintained (this has an indirect effect on porphyrin overproduction), and a narcotic may be given for pain. Intravenous haematin infusion also appears to be of benefit.

Management in the remission period is by avoidance of possible precipitating factors.

Other acute porphyrias

Variegate porphyria
This combines many of the features of acute intermittent porphyria with those of a cutaneous porphyria. A bullous eruption develops on exposure to sunlight owing to the activation of porphyrias deposited in the skin. There is an increased production of protoporphyrinogens owing to an abnormality of protoporphyrinogen oxidase in the haem biosynthetic pathway (see Fig. 17.16).

Hereditary coproporphyria

This is extremely rare and broadly similar in presentation to variegate porphyria. The distinction is based on biochemical analysis.

Porphyria cutanea tarda (cutaneous hepatic porphyria) (see p. 1036)

This condition, which has a genetic predisposition, presents with a bullous eruption on exposure to sunlight; the eruption heals with scarring. Alcohol is the most common aetiological agent. There is an abnormality in hepatic uroporphyrinogen decarboxylase. Evidence of biochemical or clinical liver disease may also be present. Polychlorinated hydrocarbons have been implicated and porphyria cutanea tarda has been seen in association with benign or malignant tumours of the liver.

The diagnosis depends on demonstration of increased levels of urinary uroporphyrin. Histology of the skin shows subepidermal blisters with perivascular deposition of PAS-staining material. The serum iron and transferrin saturation are often raised. The liver biopsy shows mild iron overload as well as features of alcoholic liver disease.

Remission can be induced by venesection; this should be repeated if the urinary uroporphyrin rises in the remission phase. Chloroquine may also have a useful role in promoting urinary excretion of uroporphyrins.

Erythropoietic porphyrias

Congenital porphyria

This is extremely rare and is transmitted as an autosomal recessive trait. Its victims show extreme sensitivity to sunlight and develop disfiguring scars. Dystrophy of the nails, blindness due to lenticular scarring, and brownish discoloration of the teeth also occur.

Erythropoietic protoporphyria

This is commoner than congenital porphyria and is inherited as an autosomal dominant trait. It presents with irritation and burning pain in the skin on exposure to sunlight. Hepatic involvement may also occur. Diagnosis is made by fluorescence of the peripheral red blood cells and by increased protoporphyrin in the red cells and stools. Oral β-carotene provides effective protection against solar sensitivity; the reason for this is not known.

Further reading

Besser GM, Bodansky HJ and Cudworth AG (1988) *Clinical Diabetes*. London: Gower.

Bliss M (1983) *The Discovery of Insulin*. Edinburgh: Paul Harris.

Bloom A & Ireland J (1980) *A Colour Atlas of Diabetes*. London: Wolfe Medical.

Galton DJ (1985) *Molecular Genetics of Common Metabolic Disease*. London: Edward Arnold.

Havel JR (ed.) (1982) *Lipid Disorders*. Medical Clinics of North America, vol. 66, No. 2. Philadelphia: WB Saunders.

Keen H & Jarrett J (eds) (1982) *Complications of Diabetes*, 2nd edn. London: Edward Arnold.

McColl KEL, Moore MR & Goldberg A (1982) Porphyrin metabolism—the porphyrias. In Hardisty RN & Weatherall DJ (eds) *Blood and its Disorders*. 2nd edn. Oxford: Blackwell Scientific.

Stanbury JB, Wyngaarden JB, Fredrickson DS, Goldstein JL & Brown MS (eds) (1982) *The Metabolic Basis of Inherited Disease*, 5th edn. New York: McGraw-Hill.

World Health Organization (1985) *Diabetes Mellitus. Report of a WHO study group*. WHO Technical Report series 727, Geneva.

18

Neurological Disease and Diseases of Voluntary Muscle

neurological conditions of the Indian subcontinent, South-East Asia and Africa include:

- Leprosy
- Tuberculosis (meningitis, tuberculoma)
- Meningococcal meningitis
- Tetanus
- Rabies
- Cerebral malaria
- Multiple vitamin deficiencies
- Cysticercosis
- Neurological complications of AIDS (Africa and S-E Asia)

Table 18.1 Neurological diseases: annual incidence rates per 100 000 population in the UK.

Disorder	Rate
Herpes zoster	440
Back pain and sciatica	300
Stroke	150
Epilepsy and single seizures	50
Dementia	50
Polyneuropathy	40
Transient ischaemic attacks	30
Bell's palsy	25
Parkinson's disease	20
Alcoholism (neurological complications)	20
Meningitis	15
Encephalitis	15
Subarachnoid haemorrhage	15
Metastatic brain tumour	15
Benign brain tumour	10
Primary malignant brain tumour	5
Metastatic cord tumour	5
Trigeminal neuralgia	4
Multiple sclerosis	3
Motor neurone disease	2
All primary muscle disease	1.5
Intracranial abscess	1
Benign spinal cord tumour	1
Huntington's disease	0.4
Myasthenia gravis	0.4

Introduction

The spectrum of diseases seen in neurological practice over the last four decades has been dramatically changed by prevention and treatment, e.g. poliomyelitis and Parkinson's disease. In current practice the majority of patients attending neurologists do not have sinister conditions. Tension headaches, migraine, dizziness and malaise are common presenting symptoms and frequently cause difficulty. 'Neurological' symptoms may be the presenting features of common psychological illness (e.g. depression or anxiety) that require sympathy, interpretation and treatment.

The neurological diseases seen commonly in the UK and some important rarer conditions are summarized in Table 18.1.

Neurology in developing countries

Low standards of nutrition, hygiene and education, with widespread economic hardship, contribute to different patterns of disease. Common

Of these, only TB and meningococcal infection are seen commonly in Europe. AIDS, however, is increasing.

Prevalence rates often differ widely from annual incidence rates; these will be mentioned under the individual diseases.

Symptoms

There are two essential questions in any neurological diagnosis:

1 What is/are the site(s) of the lesion(s)?
2 What is the likely pathology?

Most of the diagnoses in neurology are made on a detailed history alone. The method of recording the details is beyond the scope of this chapter, but an important point is that the history should read chronologically and portray the *story* of the disease. A summary should conclude the history.

HEADACHE

Headache at some time is an almost universal experience. It varies from an infrequent and trivial nuisance to a symptom of serious disease.

Mechanism of headache

Pain receptors are found in the vessels at the base of the brain (both arterial and venous) and in the meninges. These receptors are also present in extracranial vessels, the muscles of the scalp, neck and face, the paranasal sinuses, the eyes and the teeth. The brain substance itself is almost devoid of pain receptors.

The pain of headache is mediated by mechanical and chemical (e.g. 5-hydroxytryptamine, histamine) stimulation of receptors: nerve impulses are carried centrally via the fifth and ninth cranial nerves and via the upper cervical sensory roots.

Pressure headaches

Intracranial mass lesions displace the meninges and the basal vessels. When these structures are physically moved by changes in cerebrospinal fluid pressure (e.g. coughing), pain is exacerbated. Cerebral oedema, which accumulates around mass lesions, causes further shift. Headache is typically worse after lying down for some hours (as cerebral oedema develops).

Any headache, however mild, that is present on waking and which is made worse by coughing, straining or sneezing may well be due to displacement or dilatation of the intracranial vessels and *may* be due to a mass lesion. These are often called 'the headaches of raised intracranial pressure'. Vomiting often accompanies them.

Headache of subacute onset

The onset and progression of a headache over days or weeks with or without the features of 'pressure headaches' should always raise the suspicion of an intracranial mass lesion or serious intracranial disease.

Encephalitis (see p. 932) and viral meningitis (see p. 931) should be considered. Giant-cell arteritis causes headache, with scalp tenderness, particularly over the age of 60.

A single episode of severe headache

This common emergency is caused principally by:

- Subarachnoid haemorrhage
- Migraine

and occasionally

- Meningitis

Particular attention should be paid to the suddenness of onset (suggestive of subarachnoid), neck stiffness and vomiting (meningeal irritation) and rashes and fever (meningitis).

Recurrent headaches

Migraine (p. 941) and tension headache (p. 940) are the commonest causes of recurrent pain. Sinusitis, glaucoma and migrainous neuralgia should also be considered. Hangover headache is usually obvious! Malignant hypertension occasionally causes a patient to seek medical advice because of headache. Headaches are not caused by essential hypertension.

Intermittent hydrocephalus due to an intraventricular tumour is a rare cause of recurrent prostrating headache with weakness of the lower limbs.

'Eyestrain' from refractive error is an unusual cause of headache.

Headache following head injury

Subdural haematoma (p. 915) should be considered, whether or not the headaches are suggestive of a mass lesion. The vast majority of post-traumatic headaches (p. 944), which last days, weeks or months are not, however, associated with any serious intracranial cause.

Table 18.2 Common neurological causes of difficulty in walking.

Spasticity
Parkinson's disease
Cerebellar ataxia
Sensory loss (joint position)
Distal weakness
Proximal weakness
Apraxia of gait

Chronic headaches

Almost all recurring headaches with a history going back for several years or more are due to muscle tension and/or migraine (see p. 940). Depression usually accompanies them.

Dizziness and vertigo

'Dizziness' is a word patients use for a wide variety of complaints ranging from a vague feeling of unsteadiness to severe, acute vertigo. It is also frequently used to describe the light-headedness that is felt in anxiety and 'panic attacks', during palpitations, and in syncope or chronic ill health. Therefore, the *site* of this symptom must be determined, i.e. whether it is perceived in the limbs, the chest or the head.

Vertigo (an illusion of movement) is a more definite symptom. It is usually a sensation of rotation in which the patient feels that their surroundings are spinning or moving. Vertigo indicates disease of the labyrinth, vestibular pathways or their central connections.

Blackouts

Like dizziness, 'blackouts' is a vague, descriptive term implying either altered consciousness, visual disturbance or falling. Epilepsy, syncope, hypoglycaemia and other conditioins must be considered (see p. 920). A careful history, particularly from an eye-witness, is essential.

DIFFICULTY IN WALKING

This is a common presenting complaint in neurological disease; the main causes are given in Table 18.2. Arthritis and muscle pain also alter the gait, making it stiff and slow. The recognition of an abnormal gait is important in diagnosis.

Spasticity

Spasticity (see p. 896) with or without pyramidal weakness causes stiffness and jerkiness of gait, which is maintained on a narrow base. The toes catch level ground, causing wearing down and scuffing of the toes of the shoes. The pace shortens. Clonus may be noticed as involuntary extensor jerking of the legs.

When the problem is predominantly unilateral and weakness is marked (in a hemiparesis), the weaker leg drags stiffly and is circumducted.

Parkinson's disease (see p. 922)

Here there is muscular rigidity in both the extensors and the flexors of the limbs. Power remains normal. The gait slows; the pace shortens to a shuffle. The base remains narrow. Falls occur. A stoop is apparent and swinging of the arms is diminished. The gait is 'festinant', i.e. hurried, as small rapid steps are taken. There is particular difficulty in initiating movement and in turning quickly. Sometimes when the patient stops or is halted, a few rapid, small and unsteady backward steps are taken; this is known as retropulsion.

Cerebellar ataxia

In disease of the lateral lobes of the cerebellum the stance becomes broad-based, unstable and tremulous. The gait tends to veer towards the side of the more affected cerebellar lobe (see p. 898).

In disease of the cerebellar vermis (a midline structure), the trunk becomes unsteady and there is a tendency to fall backwards (truncal ataxia).

Sensory ataxia

The ataxia of peripheral sensory lesions (e.g. polyneuropathy, p. 953) is due to diminution of the sense of proprioception (joint position). The patient cannot perceive accurately the position of the legs. The gait becomes broad-based and high-stepping or 'stamping'.

The ataxia is made worse by removal of additional sensory input, e.g. in the dark or when the eyes are closed. This is the basis of a positive Romberg's test, which was first described in the sensory ataxia of tabes dorsalis (see p. 933).

Weakness of the lower limbs

With distal weakness the affected leg is lifted over obstacles. When the dorsiflexors of the foot are weak, such as in a common peroneal nerve palsy (see p. 953), the foot, having been lifted, returns to the ground with a visible and audible 'slap'.

Weakness of proximal lower limb muscles (e.g. polymyositis, muscular dystrophy) leads to difficulty in rising from the sitting position. Once upright, the patient walks with a waddling gait, the pelvis being ill-supported by each lower limb as it carries the full weight of the body.

Apraxia of gait

In frontal-lobe disease (e.g. tumours, hydro-cephalus, infarction) the central organization of walking is disturbed. The patient is able to move the legs normally while sitting or lying but cannot walk in an organized way. This is known as 'apraxia of gait'—a failure of the skilled movement of walking. Urinary incontinence and a degree of dementia are often present.

Neurological examination

The following headings summarize the essential elements of the clinical examination:

- State of consciousness, arousal
- Appearance, attitude, insight
- Mental state (see p. 966)
- Orientation in time and place
- Recall of recent and distant events/memory
- Level of intellect
- Language and speech/cerebral dominance
- Disorders of higher function (e.g. apraxia)
- Gait
- Romberg's test
- The skull—shape, circumference, bruits
- The neck—stiffness, palpation and auscultation of carotid arteries
- *The cranial nerves*—see discussion of individual nerves
- *The motor system*
  (a) Upper limbs:
      Wasting and fasciculation
      Posture of the outstretched arms—drift, re-bound, tremor
      Tone—if increased, is it spasticity or 'extra-pyramidal' rigidity?
      Power—weakness may be graded roughly into 'slight', 'moderate' or 'severe' or numerically (0–5) (Table 18.3)
      Tendon reflexes: + or ++ = normal; +++ = increased; 0 = absent even with reinforcement
  (b) Thorax and abdomen:
      Respiration
      Abdominal reflexes and muscles
  (c) The lower limbs:
      Wasting and fasciculation
      Tone, power and tendon reflexes
      Plantar responses
- Co-ordination and fine movements
- *The sensory system.* First, the patient is asked whether or not the feeling in the limbs, face and trunk is entirely normal.
  (a) Posterior columns:
      Light touch

Table 18.3 Grades of muscle weakness (Medical Research Council).

Grade	Definition
0	No contraction
1	Flicker of contraction
2	Active movement with gravity eliminated
3	Active movement against gravity
4	Active movement against gravity and resistance
5	Normal power

      Vibration (using a 128 Hz tuning fork)
      Joint position
      Two-point discrimination (normal: 0.5 cm on fingertips, 2 cm on soles)
  (b) Spinothalamic tracts:
      Pain (pin prick)—using a clean pin
      Temperature
  Chart of areas of abnormal sensation

Short neurological examination

A detailed neurological examination is time-consuming and is not necessary in all patients, particularly those without symptoms suggestive of neurological disease. A short examination will detect the majority of defects.

Short neurological examination

Look at the patient

- General demeanour
- Speech
- Gait
- Arm swinging

Examine head

- Fundi
- Pupils
- Eye movements
- Facial movements
- Tongue

Examine upper limbs

- Posture of outstretched arms
- Wasting, fasciculation
- Power, tone
- Co-ordination
- Reflexes

Examine lower limbs

- Power (hip flexion, ankle dorsiflexion), tone
- Reflexes
- Plantar responses

Assess sensation

- Ask the patient

Investigation

The history and examination remain most valuable 'tests' in neurology but computed tomography (CT) and other non-invasive tests have revolutionized the management of patients.

PRELIMINARY INVESTIGATION

Examples of helpful routine investigations are given in Table 18.4.

SPECIALIZED TESTS

Skull X-rays

Plain X-rays should not be done unnecessarily. Examples of diagnostically important changes are:

- Fractures and lesions of the vault (e.g. osteolytic lesions)
- Enlargement or destruction of the sella turcica (e.g. intrasellar tumour, raised intracranial pressure)
- Intracranial calcification (e.g. tuberculoma, oligodendroglioma, wall of an aneurysm, cysticercosis)
- Pineal calcification (to show midline shift)

Spinal X-rays

These show fractures and degenerative, destructive and congenital bone lesions.

Table 18.4 The value of some investigations in neurological disease.

Test	Yield
Urinalysis	Glycosuria (polyneuropathy), ketones (coma), Bence Jones proteins (cord compression)
Blood picture	Macrocytosis (B_{12} deficiency), high ESR (giant cell arteritis)
Serum electrolytes	Hyponatraemia, hypokalaemia (weakness)
Blood glucose	Hypoglycaemia (coma), diabetes mellitus (coma)
Serum calcium	Hypocalcaemia, tetany
Chest X-ray	Bronchial carcinoma, spinal or rib lesions, thymoma

Computed tomography (CT)

Method. This technique uses a collimated X-ray beam moving synchronously with detectors across a slice of brain between 2 mm and 13 mm thick. The transmitted X-irradiation from an element, or pixel of that slice (< 1 mm^2) is processed by computer and a numerical value (the Hounsfield number) is assigned to its density (air $= -1000$ units; water $= 0$; bone $= +1000$ units).

The difference in X-ray attenuation between bone, brain and CSF makes it possible to distinguish normal and infarcted tissue, tumour, extravasated blood and oedema. Examples of normal CT scans are shown in Fig. 18.1.

The image can be enhanced with intravenous contrast media to show areas of increased blood supply and oedema more clearly. Additional information about the subarachnoid space and the cerebral ventricles is obtained by scanning after the intrathecal injection of water-soluble contrast media (e.g. metrizamide) or air. In general, lesions greater than 1 cm in diameter can be visualized on CT scans.

The method is safe (apart from occasional systemic reactions to contrast); the irradiation involved is small.

Uses. CT scanning is used for the diagnosis of:

- Cerebral tumours
- Intracerebral haemorrhage and infarction
- Subdural and extradural haematoma
- Subarachnoid haemorrhage
- Lateral shift of midline structures and displacement of the ventricular system
- Cerebral atrophy
- Pituitary lesions
- Spinal lesions (with CT myelography)

The CT scan can also be used to show that a brain is anatomically normal with a high degree of accuracy.

Limitations

- Lesions under 1 cm in diameter may be missed.
- Lesions with attenuation close to that of bone may be missed if they are near the skull.
- Lesions with attenuation similar to that of brain may be difficult to diagnose (e.g. 'isodense' subdural haematoma).
- The results are poor when the patient cannot cooperate; a general anaesthetic may occasionally be necessary.

Magnetic resonance imaging (MRI)

This technique makes use of the properties of protons aligned in a strong magnetic field. The protons are bombarded with radiofrequency waves at right angles to generate images. The equipment

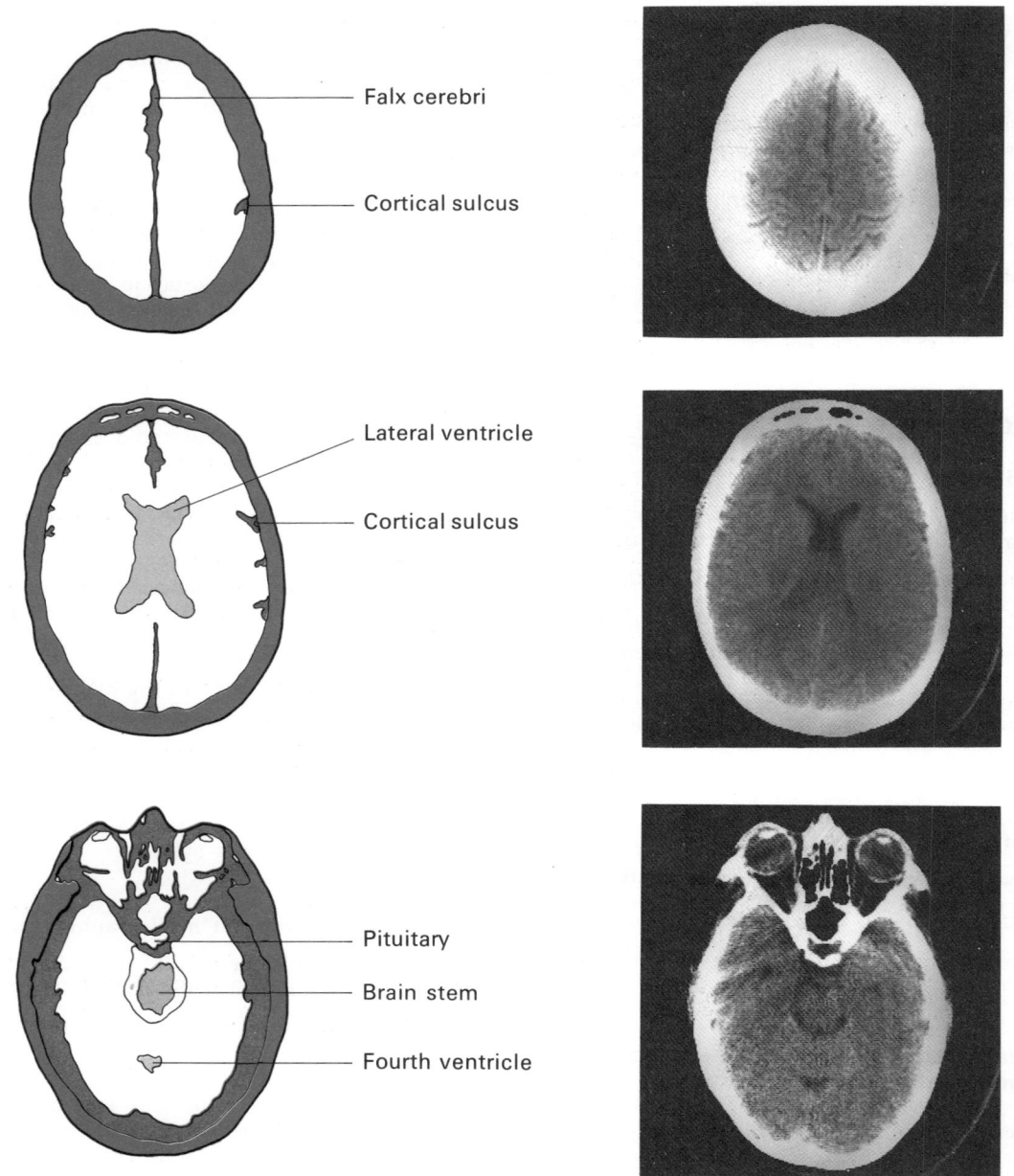

Fig. 18.1 Normal CT head scan: transverse sections at three levels.

is expensive and still restricted to specialized units.

The particular value of MRI scanning is its ability to distinguish between white matter and grey matter (Fig. 18.2) in the brain. Brain tumours, syringomyelia, the lesions of multiple sclerosis and lesions in the posterior fossa and at the foramen magnum are demonstrated well. In the spinal cord the technique can visualize tumours, cord compression and vascular malformations.

Cerebral angiography and digital imaging

This demonstrates the cerebral arterial and venous systems. Contrast is injected intra-arterially or intravenously.

Carotid and vertebral arteriography is used for the demonstration of aneurysms, arteriovenous malformations and venous occlusion. Films of the aortic arch and the carotid and vertebral arteries demonstrate occlusion, stenoses and atheromatous

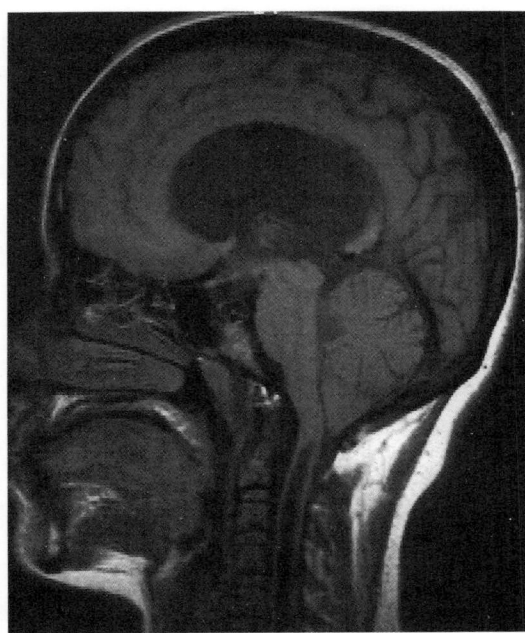

Fig. 18.2 MRI scan showing lesions of multiple sclerosis. (Courtesy of MRI Ltd, London.)

plaques. Spinal angiography is used to investigate arteriovenous malformations of the cord.

Conventional arteriography is invasive and requires a general anaesthetic; it should rarely be performed outside a specialist centre. It carries a mortality of around 1% and a 1% risk of stroke.

Digital subtraction angiography (DSA), using a computerized subtraction technique is superseding traditional angiography. Contrast is injected intravenously or intra-arterially. No anaesthetic is necessary.

Myelography

A water-soluble radiopaque dye is injected into the lumbar (or rarely cervical) subarachnoid space and viewed by conventional X-rays or CT. This is used in the diagnosis of tumours of the spinal cord and other causes of cord compression.

Radiculography is an examination confined to the lumbar region to show the anatomy of nerve roots.

Isotope brain and bone scanning

A radioisotope, usually [^{99m}Tc]pertechnate is injected intravenously to detect:

- Vascular tumours
- Arteriovenous malformations
- Cerebral infarcts
- Subdural haematoma

Isotope brain scanning is safe, non-invasive and

cheap but has largely been overtaken by CT scanning because of the high incidence of false-negative isotope scans.

Isotope bone scanning is useful for detecting vertebral lesions (e.g. metastases).

Electroencephalography

The electroencephalogram (EEG) is recorded from scalp electrodes on 16 channels simultaneously for 10–30 min. The main value of the EEG is in the diagnosis of epilepsy and diffuse brain diseases.

Epilepsy (see p. 916). Spikes, or spike and wave abnormalities occur, but it should be emphasized that patients with epilepsy may have a normal EEG between fits.

Diffuse brain disorders. Slow-wave EEG abnormalities are seen in encephalitis, dementia and metabolic states (e.g. hypoglycaemia and hepatic coma).

Brain death (see p. 730). The EEG is isoelectric (i.e. flat). An EEG is no longer necessary to confirm the diagnosis of brain death in the UK.

Electromyography and nerve conduction studies

Electromyography. A concentric needle electrode is inserted into voluntary muscle. The amplified recording is viewed on an oscilloscope and heard through a speaker. The following can be demonstrated:

- Normal interference pattern
- Denervation and re-innervation
- Myopathic, myotonic or myasthenic changes (see p. 959)

Peripheral nerve conduction. Four measurements are of principal value in the diagnosis of neuropathies and nerve entrapment:

- Mean conduction velocity (motor and sensory) (see Fig. 18.3)
- Distal motor latency
- Sensory action potentials
- Muscle action potentials

Cerebral-evoked potentials

Visual-evoked potentials record the time taken for the response to a retinal stimulus to travel to the occipital cortex. Their value is chiefly in documenting previous retrobulbar neuritis (see p. 885), which causes a permanent delay in the latency despite clinical recovery of vision.

Similar techniques exist for the measurement of auditory and somatosensory potentials (from an arm or leg).

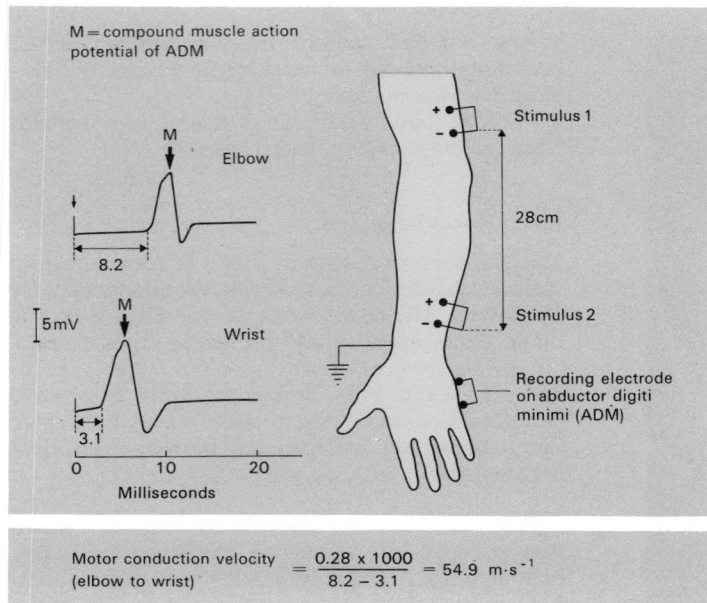

M = compound muscle action potential of ADM

M   Elbow

8.2

5 mV   M   Wrist

3.1

0   10   20
Milliseconds

Stimulus 1

28 cm

Stimulus 2

Recording electrode on abductor digiti minimi (ADM)

$$\text{Motor conduction velocity (elbow to wrist)} = \frac{0.28 \times 1000}{8.2 - 3.1} = 54.9 \text{ m·s}^{-1}$$

Fig. 18.3 Measurement of motor conduction velocity of the ulnar nerve. A recording electrode on the abductor digiti minimi records the muscle action potential (M) from the ulnar nerve at the elbow (stimulus 1) and at the wrist (stimulus 2). From these values the motor conduction velocity can be calculated.

LUMBAR PUNCTURE

Examination of the CSF

Indications for lumbar puncture

- Diagnosis of meningitis and encephalitis
- Diagnosis of multiple sclerosis and neurosyphilis
- Intrathecal injection of contrast media and drugs
- Diagnosis of suspected subarachnoid haemorrhage (sometimes)
- Measurement of CSF pressure (e.g. in benign intracranial hypertension, p. 940)
- Removal of CSF therapeutically (e.g. in benign intracranial hypertension)
- The diagnosis of miscellaneous conditions (e.g. certain polyneuropathies, sarcoidosis, intrathecal neoplastic involvement)

Contraindications for lumbar puncture

- Suspicion of a mass lesion in the brain or spinal cord. Caudal herniation of the cerebellar tonsils ('coning') may occur if an intracranial mass is present and the pressure below is reduced by removal of CSF. This is extremely dangerous (p. 939).
- Any cause of raised intracranial pressure.
- Local infection near the site of puncture.
- Congenital lesions in the lumbosacral region (e.g. meningomyelocele).
- Platelet count below 40×10^9/L and other clotting abnormalities, including anticoagulant drugs.
- Unconscious patients and those with papilloedema must have a CT scan before lumbar puncture.

LUMBAR PUNCTURE

Lumbar puncture should not be performed in the presence of raised intracranial pressure or when an intracranial mass lesion is a possibility.

Technique

- The patient is placed on the edge of the bed in the left lateral position with the knees and chin as close together as possible.
- The third and fourth lumbar spines are marked. The fourth lumbar spine usually lies on a line joining the iliac crests.
- Using sterile precautions, 2% lignocaine is injected into the dermis by raising a bleb in either the third or fourth lumbar interspace.
- The special lumbar puncture needle is pushed through the skin in the midline. It is pressed steadily forwards and slightly towards the head.
- When the needle is felt to penetrate the dura mater, the stylet is withdrawn and a few drops of CSF are allowed to escape.
- The CSF pressure can now be measured by connecting a manometer to the needle. The patient's head must be on the same level as the sacrum. Normal CSF pressure is 60–150 mm H_2O. It rises and falls with respiration and the heart beat.
- Specimens of CSF are collected in three sterilized test tubes and sent to the laboratory. An additional sample in which the sugar level can be measured, together with a simultaneous blood sample for blood sugar measurement, should be taken when relevant (e.g. in meningitis).
- Patients are usually asked to lie flat after the procedure to avoid a headache that may develop but this is probably of little value. Analgesics may be required.

Table 18.5 The normal CSF.

Appearance	Crystal clear Colourless
Pressure	60–150 mm of CSF with patient recumbent
Cell count	< 5 per mm^3 No polymorphs Mononuclear cells only
Protein	0.2–0.4 g·L^{-1}
Glucose	⅔ to ½ of blood glucose
IgG	< 15% of total CSF protein
Oligoclonal bands	Absent

These contraindications are relative, i.e. there are circumstances when LP is carried out in spite of them.

The composition of the normal CSF is shown in Table 18.5. Changes of diagnostic importance are mentioned under the sections on individual diseases.

Biopsy

Muscle. Biopsy is useful in the diagnosis of inflammatory and dystrophic disorders of muscle (see p. 960).

Peripheral nerve. Biopsy, usually of the sural nerve, is carried out to aid diagnosis in certain polyneuropathies, e.g. vasculitides.

Brain. Brain biopsy (e.g. of a non-dominant frontal lobe) is undertaken to diagnose inflammatory and degenerative brain diseases.

   CT-guided stereotactic biopsy of intracranial mass lesions is being used increasingly. It is less traumatic and more accurate than conventional biopsy through a skull burr hole or craniotomy.

Psychometric assessment

Formal psychometric testing is used to assess intellectual function. Preservation of the verbal IQ (a measure of past attainments) in the presence of deterioration of the performance IQ (a measure of present abilities) is a useful indicator of dementia. Low subtest scores (e.g. for block design, speech or constructional skills) indicate impaired function of specific regions of the brain. The main limitation of these techniques is that depression and lack of concentration can also impair scores.

Miscellaneous tests

Certain specialized tests are employed in the diagnosis of individual (and often rare) neurological diseases. Examples are:

- Serum enzymes liberated from muscle—greatly raised in many primary muscle diseases (see p. 959). Creatine phosphokinase is the enzyme usually assayed in most laboratories.
- Serum copper and caeruloplasmin in Wilson's disease (see p. 271).
- Antibodies to acetylcholine receptor protein in myasthenia gravis (see p. 961).

Functional anatomy

The functional unit of the nervous system is the neurone, with its cell body and axon, which terminates at a synapse. The specificity, size and type of each group of neurones varies greatly. For example an alpha motor neurone of the anterior horn cell of the lumbar spinal cord has an axonal length of over a metre and innervates several hundred to 2000 muscle fibres—to form the motor unit. By contrast, a spinal or intracerebral internuncial neurone may have an axon under 100 μm in length and terminate solely on one or other neuronal cell body.

   It is now generally agreed that transmission at most if not all synapses is mediated by chemical neurotransmitters. These transmitters are released by action potentials passing down the axon. They then react with the receptors on the postsynaptic cell body, increasing its ionic permeability and propagating a further action potential within it.

   This combination of electrical activity in the axon and chemical release at the synapse is the basis of all neurological function.

   Important neurotransmitter substances are:

- Acetylcholine
- Noradrenaline
- Adrenaline
- 5-hydroxytryptamine
- γ Aminobutyric acid
- Opioid peptides
- Prostaglandins
- Histamine

The exact role of these neurotransmitters in pathogenesis is being evaluated.

The cerebral cortex

CEREBRAL LOCALIZATION

This subject causes everyone considerable difficulty. The following paragraphs summarize the areas of principal clinical importance in general medicine.

The dominant hemisphere

The concept of cerebral dominance arose with the observation that right-handed stroke (and other) patients with acquired language disorders, had destructive lesions within the left hemisphere. Almost all right-handed people have language function in the left hemisphere; so do over 70% of those who are apparently left-handed.

Destructive lesions within the left fronto-temporo-parietal region cause disorders of:

● Spoken language—known as aphasia or dysphasia
● Writing—known as agraphia
● Reading—known as alexia

The non-dominant hemisphere

Disorders in right-handed patients with *right* hemisphere lesions are more difficult to define but comprise abnormalities of perception of internal and external space. Examples of this are losing the way in familiar surroundings, failing to put on clothing correctly ('dressing apraxia') or failure to draw simple shapes ('constructional apraxia').

APHASIA AND DYSARTHRIA

Aphasia (or dysphasia) is a loss or defect in language and is caused by left fronto-temporo-parietal lesions.

Dysarthria is simply disordered articulation. Any lesion that produces paralysis, slowing or incoordination of the muscles of articulation or local discomfort will cause dysarthria. Examples are upper and lower motor lesions of the lower cranial nerves, cerebellar lesions, Parkinson's disease and local lesions of the mouth, larynx, pharynx and tongue. Many aphasic patients are also somewhat dysarthric.

Some varieties of aphasia

Broca's aphasia (expressive aphasia, anterior aphasia)
A lesion in the left frontal lobe causes reduced fluency of speech with comprehension relatively preserved.

The patient is mute and makes great efforts to initiate speech. Language is reduced to a few disjointed words and there is failure to construct sentences.

Patients who recover from this form of aphasia say that they knew what they wanted to say but 'could not get the words out'.

Wernicke's aphasia (receptive aphasia, posterior aphasia)
A left temporo-parietal lesion leaves language that is fluent but the words themselves are incorrect. This varies from the insertion of a few incorrect or non-existent words into fluent speech (when it may be difficult to recognize aphasia) to a profuse outpouring of jargon, i.e. rubbish with wholly non-

Table 18.6 Principal disorders seen with a destructive lesion of the cortex in a right-handed individual.

Site of lesion	Disorder
Either frontal region	Intellectual impairment Personality change Urinary incontinence Mono- or hemiparesis
Left frontal region	Broca's aphasia
Left temporoparietal region	Acalculia Alexia Agraphia Wernicke's aphasia Right–left disorientation Homonymous field defects
Right temporal region	Confusional states Failure to recognize faces Homonymous field defects
Either parietal region	Contralateral sensory loss or neglect Constructional apraxia[a] Agraphaesthesia[b] Failure to recognize surroundings Limb apraxia Homonymous field defects
Right parietal region	Dressing apraxia Failure to recognize faces Neglect of left limbs
Occipital lobes and occipitoparietal region	Visual field defects (see p. 884) Visuospatial defects Disturbances of visual recognition

[a] Inability to draw or construct shapes and patterns.
[b] Inability to recognize shapes drawn on the palm.

existent words. This may be so bizarre as to be confused with psychotic behaviour.

Patients who have recovered from Wernicke's aphasia say that when aphasic they found the speech of others like a wholly unintelligible foreign language, and though they knew they were speaking could neither stop themselves nor understand what they said.

Nominal aphasia (anomic aphasia or amnestic aphasia)
This describes difficulty naming familiar objects. When it occurs in a severe and isolated form it is caused by a left posterior temporal/inferior parietal lesion. Naming difficulty is, however, an early sign in all types of aphasia.

Global aphasia (central aphasia)
This is the expressive disturbance characteristic of Broca's aphasia and the loss of comprehension of Wernicke's. It is due to widespread damage to the areas concerned with speech and is the commonest form of aphasia after a severe left hemisphere infarct. Writing and reading are also affected.

CLINICAL FEATURES OF FOCAL CEREBRAL LESIONS

Focal lesions of the cerebral cortex cause symptoms and signs by three processes:

- Destruction or suppression of function of cortical neurones and surrounding structures (see Table 18.6)
- Synchronous discharge of neurones by irritative lesions which cause partial (focal) seizures that may become generalized seizures (see Table 18.7)
- Displacement of the intracranial contents (see p. 938) and surrounding cerebral oedema

Table 18.7 Effects of an irritative lesion of the cortex.

Site of lesion	Effects
Frontal region	Partial seizures—focal motor seizures of contralateral limbs Conjugate deviation of head and eyes away from the lesion
Temporal region	Formed visual hallucinations Complex partial seizures Memory disturbances (e.g. déjà vu)
Parietal region	Partial seizures—focal sensory seizures of contralateral limbs Crude visual hallucinations, (e.g. shapes in one part of the field)
Occipital region	Visual disturbances (e.g. flashes)

MEMORY AND ITS DISORDERS (p. 974)

Disorders of memory follow damage to the medial surface of the temporal lobe and its brain-stem connections, including the hippocampi, fornices and mammillary bodies. Bilateral lesions are usually necessary to cause amnesia.

It is characteristic of all organic disorders of memory that more recent events are recalled poorly in contrast to the relative preservation of distant memories.

Memory loss is a part of dementia of any cause and occurs in a wide variety of clinical situations (Table 18.8).

Table 18.8 Causes of amnestic syndrome.

Alcohol (Wernicke–Korsakoff syndrome)
Head injury (severe)
Anoxia
Posterior cerebral artery occlusion (bilateral)
Herpes simplex encephalitis
Chronic sedative abuse
Bilateral invasive tumours
Arsenic poisoning
Following hypoglycaemia

The cranial nerves

THE OLFACTORY NERVE (FIRST CRANIAL NERVE)

This sensory nerve arises from olfactory (smell) receptors in the nasal mucosa. Branches pierce the cribriform plate and synapse in the olfactory bulb. The olfactory tract then passes to the olfactory cortex in the anteromedial surface of the temporal lobe.

Loss of the sense of smell (anosmia) occurs with head injury and tumours of the olfactory groove (e.g. meningioma, frontal glioma).

The sense of smell is often lost, sometimes permanently, after upper respiratory viral infections. It is diminished in nasal obstruction.

THE OPTIC NERVE (SECOND CRANIAL NERVE) AND THE VISUAL SYSTEM

The optic nerve carries axons from the ganglion cells of the retina to the lateral geniculate bodies. The visual pathway is shown in Fig. 18.4. It should be noted that the lens causes the image on the retina to be inverted. Thus, an object in the lower

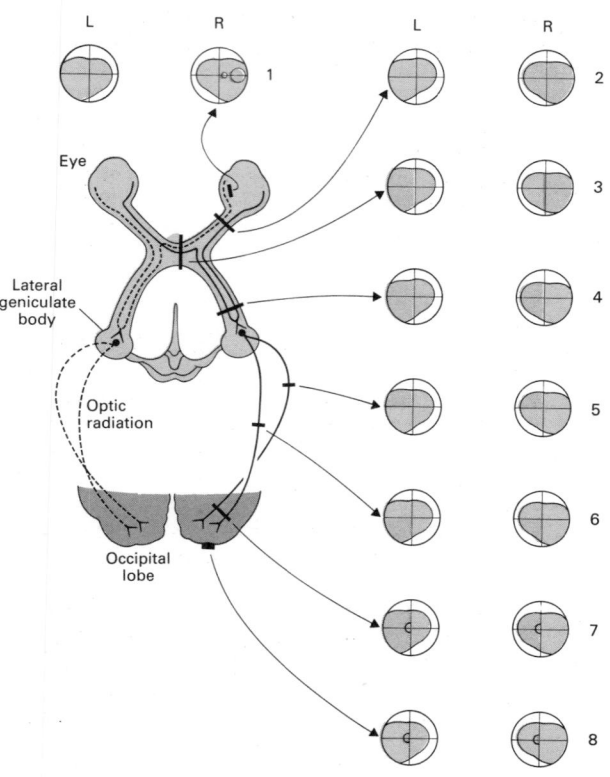

Fig. 18.4 The visual pathway (see text).

part of the visual field is projected to the upper retina and an object in the temporal half of the visual field is projected to the nasal half of the retina.

At the optic chiasm, fibres travelling in the nasal portions of the optic nerves cross to the opposite sides, where they join uncrossed temporal fibres from the lateral portion of each optic nerve. One optic tract thus carries fibres from the temporal side of the ipsilateral retina and the nasal side of the contralateral retina.

From the lateral geniculate body, fibres pass in the optic radiation to the visual cortex of the occipital lobe.

The visual field projected to each optic tract, radiation and cortex is called 'homonymous', to indicate the different (i.e. bilateral) origins of each pathway. (A homonym is the same word used to denote different things.)

Field defects are 'hemianopic' when half the field is affected, and 'quadrantanopic' when a quadrant is affected. 'Congruous' denotes symmetry and 'incongruous' lack of symmetry.

Visual acuity

This should be tested with a Snellen test chart and corrected for refractive errors with lenses or a pinhole. The corrected visual acuity should be recorded. The normal acuity should be 6/6 to 6/9 in both eyes.

Visual field defects

These should be charted by confrontation with white and red headed pins and, if abnormal or in doubt, recorded in detail with a Goldman (or similar) screen. The common defects are shown in Fig. 18.4.

Retinal and local eye lesions (Fig. 18.4, site 1)
Lesions of the retina produce either scotomata (small area of visual loss) or peripheral visual loss (tunnel vision). Common causes are diabetic retinal vascular disease, glaucoma and retinitis pigmentosa.

Local lesions of the eye (e.g. cataract) can also cause visual loss.

Optic nerve lesions (Fig. 18.4, site 2)
Unilateral visual loss, commencing as a central or paracentral scotoma, is characteristic of optic nerve lesions. Complete lesions of the optic nerve produce total unilateral visual loss with loss of pupillary light reflex (direct and consensual) when the blind eye is illuminated.

The causes of optic nerve lesions are given in Table 18.9. The principal pathological appearances of the visible part of the nerve, the disc, are:

- Disc swelling (papilloedema)
- Pallor (optic atrophy)

Papilloedema (Table 18.10). This means swelling of the papilla—the optic disc. The earliest ophthalmoscopic signs are redness of the disc followed by blurring and heaping up of its margins (the nasal margin first). There is loss of the normal, visible, spontaneous pulsation of the retinal veins. The

Table 18.9 Principal causes of an optic nerve lesion.

Optic and retrobulbar neuritis

Optic nerve compression (e.g. tumour or aneurysm)

Toxic optic neuropathy (e.g. tobacco, ethambutol, methyl alcohol, quinine)

Syphilis

Ischaemic optic neuropathy (e.g. in giant cell arteritis)

Papilloedema of any cause

Hereditary optic neuropathies

Severe anaemia

Vitamin B_{12} deficiency

Trauma

Infective—spread of paranasal sinus infection or orbital cellulitis

Table 18.10 Causes of papilloedema.

Intracranial mass lesions
Brain oedema, e.g. encephalitis, trauma
Subarachnoid haemorrhage
Benign intracranial hypertension
Metabolic causes, e.g. CO_2 retention, chronic anoxia, hypocalcaemia
Accelerated hypertension
Optic neuritis
Disc infiltration, e.g. leukaemia
Ischaemic optic neuropathy
Retinal venous obstruction (thrombosis, orbital lesions)

physiological cup becomes obliterated and the disc engorged, with dilatation of its vessels and the retinal veins. Small haemorrhages surround the disc.

True disc oedema should be distinguished from various conditions that simulate it. Marked hypermetropic (long-sighted) refractive errors make the disc appear pink, distant and ill-defined. Opaque (myelinated) nerve fibres near the disc and hyaline bodies (drusen) can be mistaken for disc swelling.

In difficult cases fluorescein angiography is diagnostic. In papilloedema, fluorescein injected intravenously leaks from the disc capillaries and may be seen and photographed.

Early papilloedema from causes other than optic neuritis (see below) often produces few visual symptoms, the patient's complaints being those of the underlying disease.

As disc oedema develops there is enlargement of the blind spot and blurring of the vision. As the disc becomes engorged its arterial blood flow is reduced and, in severe papilloedema, infarction of the nerve occurs, often suddenly, with resulting blindness.

Optic neuritis. Optic neuritis is swelling of the optic disc due to inflammation of the optic nerve. The commonest cause is demyelination (e.g. multiple sclerosis). Disc swelling due to optic neuritis is distinguished from other causes of disc oedema by the occurrence of early and severe visual loss.

The term retrobulbar neuritis implies that the inflammatory process is 'behind the bulb' (i.e. the eye), so that no abnormality may be seen with the ophthalmoscope in spite of visual impairment.

Optic atrophy. Disc pallor (optic atrophy) may follow a variety of pathological processes, including infarction of the nerve, demyelinating optic neuritis (in multiple sclerosis), optic nerve compression, syphilis, B_{12} deficiency and toxins (e.g. quinine and methyl alcohol).

Optic atrophy is described as consecutive or secondary when it follows papilloedema. The degree of visual loss depends upon the underlying pathology.

Defects of the optic chiasm (Fig. 18.4, site 3)
Bi-temporal hemianoptia defects occur when a lesion compresses the central part of the chiasm. Common causes are:

- Pituitary neoplasm
- Craniopharyngioma
- Secondary neoplasm

Defects of the optic tract and optic radiation (Fig. 18.4, sites 4, 5 and 6)
Homonymous hemianopia or quadrantanopia are the typical field defects caused by unilateral compression or infarction of these structures. Optic tract lesions are rare.

Temporal lobe lesions (due to tumour or infarction) cause upper quadrantanopic defects; parietal lobe lesions cause lower quadrantanopic defects.

Defects of the occipital cortex (Fig. 18.4, sites 7 and 8)
Homonymous hemianopic defects are caused by unilateral posterior cerebral artery infarction. The macular region (at the occipital pole) is spared because it has a separate blood supply from the middle cerebral artery.

Damage to one occipital pole causes a small, congruous, scotomatous, homonymous hemianopia (site 8).

Widespread bilateral occipital lobe damage by tumour, trauma or infarction causes the syndrome of 'cortical blindness' (Anton's syndrome). The patient is blind but characteristically lacks insight into the degree of visual loss and may deny it. The pupillary responses are normal (see also p. 911).

The pupils

Sympathetic impulses from fibres in the nasociliary nerve stimulate the dilator muscle of the pupil (dilator pupillae) and cause the pupil to dilate.

Sympathetic fibres to the eye (and face) originate in the hypothalamus, pass uncrossed through the midbrain and lateral medulla and emerge from the spinal cord at T1 (close to the lung apex). Postganglionic fibres begin in the superior cervical ganglion. These pass to the pupil in the nasociliary nerve from a plexus surrounding the internal carotid artery. Those fibres to the face (sweating and pilo-erection) form a plexus surrounding the external carotid artery. This arrangement is of clinical importance in Horner's syndrome (see p. 886).

Parasympathetic impulses that pass from the ciliary ganglion in the short ciliary nerves to the sphincter muscle of the pupil (sphincter pupillae) cause the pupil to constrict.

An outline of the arrangement of parasympa-

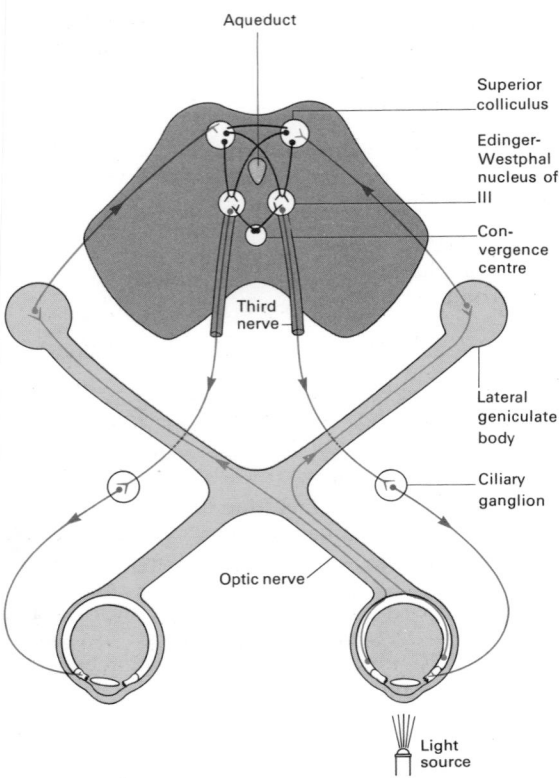

Labels in figure:
Aqueduct
Superior colliculus
Edinger-Westphal nucleus of III
Convergence centre
Third nerve
Lateral geniculate body
Ciliary ganglion
Optic nerve
Light source

Fig. 18.5 The pupils: afferent and parasympathetic efferent pathways. Fibres concerned with the pupillary light reflex bypass the lateral geniculate body and go to the pretectale muscles.

thetic fibres to the pupils and the mechanism of the light reflex is shown in Fig. 18.5.

The light reflex. Afferent fibres in each optic nerve (some crossing in the chiasm, see Fig. 18.5) pass to both lateral geniculate bodies and relay to the Edinger–Westphal nuclei.

Efferent (parasympathetic) fibres from each Edinger–Westphal nucleus pass via the third nerve to the ciliary ganglion and thence to the pupil.

Light constricts the pupil of the eye being tested (direct reflex) and the contralateral pupil (consensual reflex).

The convergence reflex. Fixation on a near object requires convergence of the ocular axes and is accompanied by pupillary constriction.

The afferent fibres in each optic nerve, which pass through both lateral geniculate bodies, also relay to the convergence centre. This centre receives 1a spindle afferent fibres from the extraocular muscles—principally the medial recti, which are innervated by the third nerve. The efferent route is from the convergence centre to the Edinger–Westphal nucleus, ciliary ganglion and

pupils. Voluntary or reflex fixation on a near object is thus accompanied by appropriate convergence and pupillary constriction.

Clinical abnormalities of the pupils
Degenerative changes in old age. The pupil tends to become small (3–3.5 mm) in old age (senile miosis) and may be irregular; a bright light is necessary to demonstrate constriction and the convergence reflex is sluggish. A slight difference between the size of the pupils is common (physiological anisocoria) but the changes may cause confusion with the Argyll Robertson pupil.

The Argyll Robertson pupil. This is a small, irregular (3 mm or less) pupil that is fixed to light but constricts on convergence. The lesion is believed to be in the area surrounding the aqueduct.

The Argyll Robertson pupil is (almost) diagnostic of neurosyphilis. Similar changes are occasionally seen in diabetes mellitus.

The myotonic pupil (Holmes–Adie pupil). This is a dilated pupil seen most commonly in young women. It is usually unilateral. There is no reaction (or a very slow reaction) to a bright light and also an incomplete constriction to convergence. The condition is due to denervation in the ciliary ganglion.

The myotonic pupil is of no pathological significance but is often associated with diminished or absent tendon reflexes.

Table 18.11 Causes of Horner's syndrome.

Hemisphere and brain stem lesions
Massive cerebral infarction
Pontine glioma
Lateral medullary syndrome
'Coning' of the temporal lobe
Cervical cord lesions
Syringomyelia
Cord tumours
T1 root lesions
Bronchial neoplasm (apical)
Apical TB
Cervical rib
Brachial plexus trauma
Sympathetic chain in the neck
Following thyroid/laryngeal surgery
Carotid artery occlusion
Neoplastic infiltration
Cervical sympathectomy
Miscellaneous
Congenital
Migrainous neuralgia (usually transient)

Horner's syndrome. This syndrome is due to interruption of sympathetic fibres to one eye. It presents as unilateral pupillary constriction with slight ptosis and enophthalmos. The conjunctival vessels may be injected. There is loss of sweating of the same side of the face or body; the extent depends upon the level of the lesion. The syndrome indicates a lesion of the sympathetic pathway on the same side. Causes of Horner's syndrome are given in Table 18.11.

The level of the lesion is indicated by the distribution of the loss of sweating:

● Central lesions affect sweating over the entire half of the head, arm and upper trunk.
● Lesions of the neck proximal to the superior cervical ganglion cause diminished sweating on the face.
● Lesions distal to the superior cervical ganglion do not affect sweating at all.

Pharmacological tests may indicate the level of the lesion. For example, a lesion distal to the superior cervical ganglion causes denervation hypersensitivity of the pupil, which dilates when 1 : 1000 adrenaline is instilled. This dose has little effect on the normal pupil or a proximal lesion. In clinical practice the test is of limited value.

Other abnormalities of the pupils seen in coma are discussed on p. 906.

THE OCULAR MOVEMENTS AND THIRD, FOURTH AND SIXTH CRANIAL NERVES

The control of eye movement can be divided into:

● The central upper motor neurone mechanisms, which drive the normal yoked parallel movements of the eyes (conjugate gaze)
● The oculomotor, abducens and trochlear nerves and the muscles they supply

Conjugate gaze
Fast voluntary and reflex eye movements originate in each frontal lobe. Fibres pass in the anterior limb of the internal capsule and cross in the pons to end in the parapontine reticular formation (PPRF; Fig. 18.6a); the PPRF was previously known as 'the centre for lateral gaze'.

The PPRF is close to each sixth nerve nucleus. It also receives fibres from:

● The ipsilateral occipital cortex. These pathways are concerned with movements to track or pursue objects within the visual fields.
● Both vestibular nuclei. These pathways are concerned with the relationship between eye movements and the position of the head and neck (doll's head reflexes, see p. 731).

The PPRF co-ordinates lateral eye movements through the medial longitudinal fasciculus (MLF)

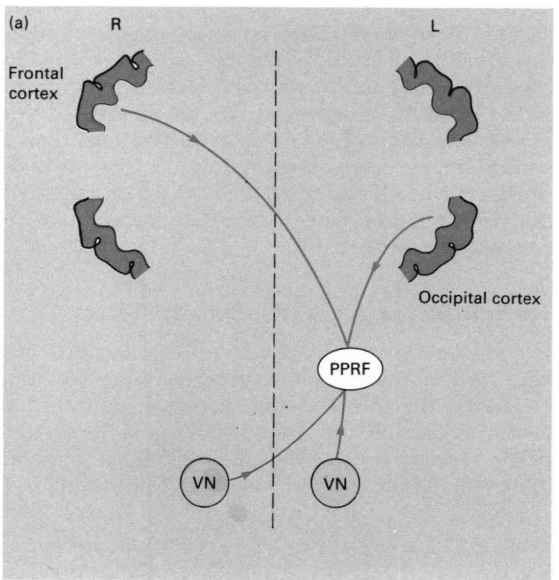

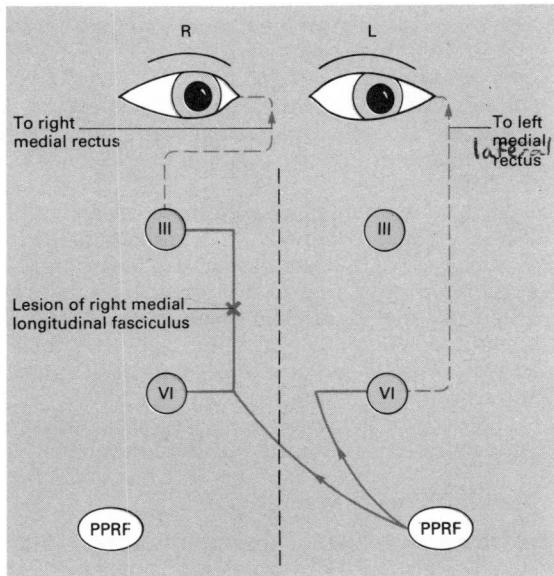

Fig. 18.6 (a) Conjugate lateral gaze: principal input to parapontine reticular formation (PPRF). VN = vestibular nucleus. Impulses from the *right* frontal cortex drive *left* PPRF, which also receives fibres from the vestibular nuclei and occipital cortex. (b) Conjugate lateral gaze: principal output from PPRF (see text for explanation). Impulses thus generated within the *left* PPRF pass to both the ipsilateral VI nerve nucleus (lateral rectus muscle, abduction) and via the medial longitudinal fasciculus to neurones in the *left* third nerve nucleus (medial rectus muscle, adduction). Thus voluntary gaze to the *left* is initiated in the *right* frontal cortex. (From Bannister R (1985) *Brain's Clinical Neurology*, 6th edn. Oxford: Oxford University Press.)

(Fig. 18.6b). Fibres from the PPRF pass to both the ipsilateral sixth nerve nucleus and, having crossed the midline, the opposite third nerve nucleus via the MLF. Each sixth nerve nucleus (supplying the lateral rectus) and the opposite third nerve nucleus (supplying the medial rectus and others) are thus linked. The eyes move with parallel axes and at the same velocity.

Abnormalities of conjugate lateral gaze

It is important to understand that a destructive lesion of one side of the brain allows the eyes to be driven laterally by the intact opposite pathway.

A destructive frontal-lobe lesion (e.g. an infarct) causes failure of conjugate lateral gaze to the side opposite to the lesion (Fig. 18.6a). In an acute lesion the eyes are often deviated past the midline to the side of the lesion and therefore look *towards the normal limbs*. There is usually a contralateral hemiparesis.

An irritative frontal-lobe lesion (e.g. an epileptic focus), by stimulating the opposite PPRF, drives the eyes away from the side of the lesion.

A unilateral destructive brain stem lesion involving the PPRF causes failure of horizontal conjugate gaze towards the side of the lesion. There is usually a hemiparesis and the eyes are deviated *towards the paralysed limbs*.

Doll's head reflexes and skew deviation
These are of diagnostic value in coma (p. 731).

Internuclear ophthalmoplegia
Internuclear ophthalmoplegia (INO) is one of the commoner complex brain-stem signs that involve the oculomotor system. It is due to a lesion within the MLF.

It is a common sign in multiple sclerosis (MS). When present bilaterally it is almost pathognomonic of MS. Unilateral lesions are also caused by small brain stem infarcts. In a right INO there is a lesion of the right MLF (see Fig. 18.6b). On attempted left lateral gaze the right eye fails to adduct. The left eye develops coarse nystagmus in abduction.

The side of the lesion is on the side of impaired adduction, not on the side of the nystagmus.

Abnormalities of vertical gaze

A failure of up gaze is caused by an upper brain-stem lesion, such as a supratentorial mass pressing from above, or a tumour of the brain stem (e.g. a pinealoma). When the pupillary convergence reflex fails, this combination is called Parinaud's syndrome.

Defective up gaze also occurs in certain degenerative disorders (e.g. progressive supranuclear palsy, see p. 925).

Impairment of up gaze also occurs as part of normal ageing.

Weakness of the extraocular muscles (diplopia)

Diplopia (double vision) implies that there is weakness of one or more of the extraocular muscles.

The cause is usually a lesion of the third, fourth or sixth cranial nerves (or a combination of these) or their nuclei, or disease of the neuromuscular junction (myasthenia gravis) or the ocular muscles.

Squint (strabismus)
This is the appearance of the eyes when the visual axes fail to meet at the fixation point.

Paralytic squint. Paralytic or 'incomitant' squint occurs when there is an acquired defect of the movement of an eye. There is a squint (and hence diplopia) maximal in the direction of action of the weak muscle.

Non-paralytic squint. Non-paralytic or 'concomitant' squint describes a squint beginning in childhood in which the angle between the visual axes does *not* vary when the eyes are moved, i.e. the squint remains the same in all directions of gaze. Diplopia is almost never a symptom. The deviating eye (the one that does not fixate) usually has defective vision; this is called 'amblyopia ex anopsia'.

Non-paralytic squint may be latent, i.e. only visible at certain times, such as when the patient is tired.

The *cover test* is used to assess squint and to recognize latent squint. The patient is asked to fix on an object. The eye that is apparently fixing the object centrally is covered. If the uncovered eye makes any movement to take up fixation, then a squint must have been present. The test is repeated with the opposite eye—the fixing eye will not move when the other, squinting, eye is covered or uncovered.

The oculomotor nerve (third cranial nerve)

The nucleus of the third nerve lies ventral to the aqueduct in the midbrain. Efferent fibres to four external ocular muscles (the superior, inferior and medial recti, and the inferior oblique), the levator palpebrae superioris and the sphincter pupillae (parasympathetic) enter the orbit through the

Table 18.12 Common causes of an oculomotor nerve lesion.

Aneurysm of the posterior communicating artery
'Coning' of the temporal lobe (p. 938)
Infarction of the nerve
In diabetes mellitus
Atheroma
Midbrain infarction
Midbrain tumour

superior orbital fissure.

The common causes of an oculomotor nerve lesion are given in Table 18.12. Signs of such a lesion are:

- Unilateral complete ptosis
- The eye facing 'down and out'
- Fixed and dilated pupil

'Sparing of the pupil' means that the parasympathetic fibres which run in a discrete bundle on the superior surface of the nerve are undamaged by the lesion and the pupil reacts normally.

In diabetes, infarction of the nerve usually spares the pupil.

In a third nerve palsy the eye can still abduct (sixth nerve) and 'intort' (fourth nerve). When a patient with a right third nerve lesion attempts to converge and look downwards, the conjunctival vessels of the right eye can be seen to twist clockwise; this is 'intortion' and indicates that the trochlear nerve is intact.

The trochlear nerve (fourth cranial nerve)

The trochlear nerve supplies the superior oblique muscle.

An isolated fourth nerve lesion is a rarity. The head is tilted away from the side of the lesion. The patient complains of diplopia when attempting to look down and away from the affected side.

The abducens nerve (sixth cranial nerve)

The abducens nerve supplies the lateral rectus muscle.

In a sixth nerve lesion there is a convergent squint with diplopia maximal on looking to the side of the lesion. The eye cannot be abducted beyond the midline.

There are many causes of a sixth nerve lesion. The nerve may be involved in the brain stem, e.g. in multiple sclerosis. In raised intracranial pressure it is compressed against the tip of the petrous temporal bone. The nerve sheath may be infiltrated by tumours, particularly nasopharyngeal carcinoma. An isolated sixth nerve palsy due to infarction may occur in diabetes mellitus. A sixth nerve lesion is a common sequel of head injury.

THE TRIGEMINAL NERVE (FIFTH CRANIAL NERVE)

The trigeminal nerve is mainly sensory but contains some motor fibres.

Sensory fibres (see Figs. 18.7 and 18.11) from the three divisions—ophthalmic (V_1), maxillary (V_2) and mandibular (V_3)—pass to the trigeminal ganglion at the apex of the petrous temporal bone. From here central fibres enter the brain stem. Ascending fibres transmitting the sensation of light touch enter the nucleus in the pons. Descending fibres carrying pain and temperature sensation form the spinal tract of the fifth nerve and end in the spinal nucleus in the medulla and upper cervical cord.

Motor fibres arise in the upper pons and join the mandibular branch to supply the muscles of mastication.

Signs of a trigeminal nerve lesion
Diminution of the corneal reflex is often the first sign of a fifth nerve lesion.

A complete fifth nerve lesion causes unilateral sensory loss on the face, tongue and buccal mucosa. The jaw deviates to the side of the lesion when the mouth is opened.

Central (brain-stem) lesions of the lower trigeminal nuclei (e.g. in syringobulbia, see p. 946) produce a characteristic circumoral sensory loss.

When the spinal tract (or spinal nucleus) alone is involved, the sensory loss is restricted to pain and temperature sensation, i.e. 'dissociated' (see p. 902).

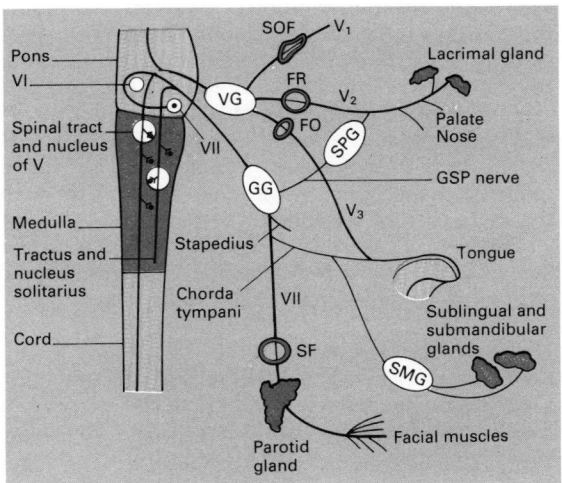

Fig. 18.7 Fifth and seventh cranial nerves and their relationships. SOF = superior orbital fissure; FR = foramen rotundum; FO = foramen ovale; SF = stylomastoid foramen; SPG = sphenopalatine ganglion; GG = geniculate ganglion; VG = gasserian ganglion; SMG = submandibular ganglion; GSP = greater superficial petrosal.

Causes of trigeminal nerve lesions
Brain stem. Lesions at this site involve the nuclei and central connections, and include:

● Brain stem glioma
● Multiple sclerosis
● Infarction
● Syringobulbia

Cerebello-pontine angle. Here the nerve is compressed by:

● Acoustic neuroma
● Meningioma
● Secondary neoplasm

Apex of the petrous temporal bone. Infection from chronic middle-ear disease involves the nerve at this site. The combination of this sign with pain and a sixth nerve lesion is called Gradenigo's syndrome.

Cavernous sinus. Here the trigeminal ganglion is compressed by:

● Aneurysm of internal carotid artery
● Extension of a pituitary neoplasm
● Cavernous sinus thrombosis
● Secondary neoplasm

The trigeminal ganglion is infected in ophthalmic herpes zoster (see p. 933), the commonest lesion of the ganglion.

Peripheral branches of the trigeminal nerve. These are affected by neoplastic infiltration of the skull base.

Trigeminal neuralgia

Trigeminal neuralgia ('tic douloureux') is a condition of unknown cause, seen most commonly in old age. It is almost always unilateral.

SYMPTOMS

Severe paroxysms of knife-like or electric-shock-like pain, lasting seconds, occur with the distribution of the fifth nerve. The pain tends to commence in the mandibular division (V_3) and spreads to the maxillary (V_2) and (rarely) to the ophthalmic division (V_1). It occurs many times a day.

Each paroxysm is stereotyped, brought on by stimulation of a specific 'trigger zone' in the face. Washing, shaving, a cold wind or eating are examples of the trivial stimuli that may provoke the pain. The face may be screwed up in agony (hence 'tic'—an involuntary movement).

The pain characteristically does not occur at night. Spontaneous remissions last for months or years before recurrence.

SIGNS

There are no signs of trigeminal nerve dysfunction. The corneal reflex is preserved. Diagnosis is on clinical grounds alone.

TREATMENT

The anticonvulsant carbamazepine 600–1200 mg daily suppresses attacks in the majority of patients. Phenytoin and clonazepam are also used, but are less effective.

If drug therapy fails, surgical procedures (radio-frequency extirpation of the ganglion, nerve decompression or sectioning of the sensory root) are useful in difficult cases. Alcohol injection into the trigeminal ganglion or peripheral fifth nerve branches can also be carried out.

'Secondary' trigeminal neuralgia

Trigeminal neuralgia also occurs in multiple sclerosis (see p. 928), with lesions of the cerebellopontine angle (see below) and with tumours of the fifth nerve (e.g. neuroma). These lesions are usually accompanied by physical signs (e.g. a depressed corneal reflex).

Idiopathic trigeminal neuropathy

A chronic and isolated fifth nerve lesion may sometimes develop without any apparent cause. When sensory loss is severe, trophic changes (facial scarring and corneal ulceration) occur.

Post-herpetic neuralgia (see p. 933)

This may occur in the distribution of one division of the trigeminal nerve, commonly the first.

THE FACIAL NERVE (SEVENTH CRANIAL NERVE)

This nerve is largely motor in function, supplying the muscles of facial expression. The nerve carries sensory taste fibres from the anterior two-thirds of the tongue via the chorda tympani. The complex arrangement of the nerves to the face, their nuclei and connections is shown in Fig. 18.7.

The facial nerve arises from the seventh nerve nucleus in the pons and leaves the skull through the stylomastoid foramen.

Part of each facial nucleus supplying the upper face (principally the frontalis muscle) receives some supranuclear fibres from each hemisphere.

Unilateral facial weakness
Lower motor neurone (LMN) lesions. A unilateral LMN lesion causes weakness of *all* the muscles of facial expression on the same side. The face,

especially the angle of the mouth, falls, and dribbling occurs from the corner of the mouth. There is weakness of frontalis and of eye closure since the upper facial muscles are weak. Corneal ulceration may occur if the cornea is exposed during sleep. The platysma muscle is also weak.

Upper motor neurone (UMN) lesions. UMN lesions cause weakness of the lower part of the face on the side opposite the lesion. The frontalis muscle is spared; the normal furrowing of the brow is preserved, and eye closure and blinking are not affected.

In UMN lesions there is relative preservation of spontaneous 'emotional' movement (e.g. smiling) compared with voluntary movement.

Causes of facial weakness

The commonest cause of facial weakness is a supranuclear lesion, e.g. cerebral infarction, leading to UMN facial weakness and hemiparesis.

Lesions at four other levels may be recognized by the associated signs.

Pons. The sixth nerve nucleus is encircled by the seventh nerve fibres and is therefore often involved in pontine lesions of the seventh nerve, causing a lateral rectus palsy.

If there is accompanying damage to the neighbouring PPRF (see p. 887) and corticospinal tract, there is the combination of:

- LMN facial weakness
- Failure of conjugate lateral gaze (towards the lesion)
- Contralateral hemiparesis

Causes include pontine tumours (e.g. glioma), demyelination and vascular lesions.

The facial nucleus is affected in poliomyelitis (see p. 59) and in motor neurone disease (see p. 947); the latter usually causes bilateral weakness.

Cerebellopontine angle. The fifth, sixth and eighth nerves are affected with the seventh nerve in lesions in the cerebellopontine angle. Causes are acoustic neuroma and meningioma.

Within the petrous temporal bone. The geniculate ganglion (a sensory ganglion for taste) lies at the genu of the facial nerve (see Fig. 18.7). Fibres join the facial nerve in the chorda tympani and carry taste from the anterior two-thirds of the tongue. The (motor) nerve to the stapedius muscle leaves the facial nerve distal to the genu.

Lesions within the petrous temporal bone cause:

- Loss of taste on the anterior two-thirds of the tongue
- Hyperacusis (an unpleasantly loud distortion of noise) due to paralysis of the stapedius muscle

Causes include:

- Bell's palsy
- Trauma
- Infection of the middle ear
- Herpes zoster (Ramsay Hunt syndrome)
- Tumours (e.g. glomus tumour)

Within the face. Branches of the facial nerve pierce the parotid gland and supply the muscles of facial expression. The nerve can be damaged here by parotid gland tumours, mumps (epidemic parotitis), sarcoidosis (see p. 683) and trauma.

The nerve is also affected in polyneuritis (e.g. Guillain–Barré syndrome, see p. 954), usually bilaterally.

Weakness of the muscles of the face also occurs in primary muscle disease and disease of the neuromuscular junction. Weakness is usually bilateral. Causes include:

- Dystrophia myotonica (p. 962)
- Facio-scapulo-humeral dystrophy (p. 963)
- Myasthenia gravis (p. 961)

Bell's palsy

This is a common, acute, isolated facial nerve palsy believed to be due to a viral infection that causes swelling of the nerve within the petrous temporal bone.

SYMPTOMS

The patient notices marked unilateral facial weakness, sometimes with loss of taste on the anterior two-thirds of the tongue. Pain behind the ear is common at onset. The diagnosis is made on clinical grounds. *No* other cranial nerves are involved.

MANAGEMENT AND COURSE

Spontaneous improvement usually occurs towards the end of the second week. Thereafter, continuing recovery occurs but this may take 12 months to become complete. About 15% of patients are left with a severe, unsightly, residual weakness.

Electrophysiological tests are of some help in predicting the outcome. After the third week, the absence of an evoked potential from muscle (the nerve is stimulated over the parotid gland) indicates that recovery is unlikely.

Steroids (e.g. prednisolone 60 mg daily, reducing to nil over 10 days) or ACTH reduce the proportion of patients left with a severe deficit, provided the drugs are given at the onset.

A tarsorrhaphy (suturing of the upper to the lower lid) may be necessary if there is prolonged corneal exposure. Adhesive tape is a useful measure.

Cosmetic surgery and/or re-innervation (e.g. anastomosis of the lingual nerve to the facial nerve) are sometimes indicated after a year has elapsed from the initial attack if there is severe residual paralysis.

The condition occasionally recurs and is very rarely bilateral.

Ramsay Hunt syndrome

This is herpes zoster (shingles) of the geniculate ganglion.

There is a facial palsy (identical to Bell's palsy) with herpetic vesicles in the external auditory meatus (which receives a sensory twig from the facial nerve) and sometimes in the soft palate. Deafness may occur.

Treatment for shingles should be given (see p. 1025).

Hemifacial spasm

This is an irregular clonic spasm of the facial muscles, usually occurring in middle-aged women. It varies in severity from a mild inconvenience to a severe and disabling condition when it affects all the facial musculature of one side.

The causes are:

- Idiopathic
- Acoustic neuroma
- Paget's disease of the skull
- Following Bell's palsy
- Pressure from aberrant vessels in the cerebellopontine angle

SIGNS

There are clonic spasms of the facial muscles on one side. A mild LMN facial weakness is common.

MANAGEMENT

Mild cases require no treatment. In severe cases various destructive or decompressive procedures on the facial nerve in the cerebellopontine angle are helpful. Local injection of botulinum toxin reduces the movements for some months. Drugs are of no value.

Myokymia

Facial myokymia is a rare, continuous, fine, sinuous movement of the lower face that is seen in brain stem lesions (e.g. multiple sclerosis, brain stem glioma).

The term myokymia is also used to describe the innocent twitching around the eye that commonly occurs in fatigue.

THE VESTIBULOCOCHLEAR NERVE (EIGHTH CRANIAL NERVE)

This nerve has two parts—cochlear and vestibular.

Cochlear nerve

Auditory fibres from the spiral organ (of Corti) in the cochlea pass to the cochlear nuclei in the pons. Fibres from these nuclei cross the midline and pass upwards through the medial lemnisci to the medial geniculate bodies and the temporal gyri.

The symptoms of a cochlear nerve lesion are deafness and tinnitus. The signs are of hearing loss, with bone conduction decreased as well as air conduction. This is called sensorineural or perceptive deafness.

Vestibular nerve

Vestibular fibres from the three semicircular canals, the saccule and the utricle pass to the vestibular nuclei in the pons. Vestibular nerve fibres also pass directly to the cerebellum.

The vestibular nuclei are connected to the spinal cord, the cerebellum, the nuclei of the ocular muscles and the parapontine reticular formation (PPRF), the spinal muscles and the temporal lobe.

The maintenance of balance and posture depends in part upon impulses passing between the neck and spinal muscles and the vestibular system.

The main symptom of a vestibular lesion is vertigo. Vomiting frequently accompanies acute vertigo of any cause. Nystagmus is the principal physical sign, often with loss of balance.

Vertigo

Vertigo, the definite illusion of movement of the subject or surroundings, indicates a disturbance of vestibular, brain stem or, rarely, cortical function. The principal causes are given in Table 18.13.

Deafness and tinnitus accompanying vertigo indicate that its origin is from the ear or the eighth cranial nerve.

Nystagmus

Nystagmus is a rhythmic oscillation of the eyes. It is a sign of disease of either the ocular or the vestibular system and its connections. Nystagmus

Table 18.13 Principal causes of vertigo.

Ménière's disease
Drugs (e.g. gentamicin, anticonvulsant intoxication)
Toxins (e.g. ethyl alcohol)
'Vestibular neuronitis'
Multiple sclerosis
Migraine
Acute cerebellar lesions
Cerebellopontine angle lesions
Partial seizures (temporal lobe focus)
Brain stem ischaemia or infarction
Benign positional vertigo

is described as either 'pendular' or 'jerk'.

For true nystagmus to be present it must be sustained and demonstrable within binocular gaze.

Pendular nystagmus. Pendular movement means movements to and fro which are similar both in velocity and amplitude. Pendular nystagmus is almost always binocular, horizontal and present in all directions of gaze.

It is seen when there is poor visual fixation (e.g. long-standing, severe visual impairment) or as a congenital lesion, when it is sometimes associated with head-nodding. It very rarely occurs in 'neurological' diseases.

Jerk nystagmus. Jerk nystagmus (the usual nystagmus of neurological disease) has a fast and a slow component to the rhythmic movement. It is seen in vestibular, brain stem, cerebellar and (very rarely) cortical lesions.

The direction of the nystagmus is named after the *fast* component, which can be thought of as a reflex attempt to correct the slower component.

Considerable difficulties exist when attempts are made to use the direction of jerk nystagmus alone as a localizing sign, although it is both a common and valuable indication of abnormality. The following are useful starting points:

- Horizontal or rotary nystagmus may be either of peripheral (middle ear) or central (brain stem and its connections) origin. In peripheral lesions it is usually transient (minutes or hours): in central lesions it is long-lasting (weeks, months or more).
- Vertical nystagmus is caused only by central lesions.
- Down-beat nystagmus, a rarity, is caused by lesions around the foramen magnum.

Investigation of vestibulocochlear nerve lesions

Audiometry is of value in distinguishing sensorineural deafness from conductive deafness.

Caloric tests are used to assess function of the labyrinth. These record the evoked nystagmus when first cold, then warm, water is run into the external meatus. Decreased or absent nystagmus indicates ipsilateral labyrinth, eighth nerve or brain stem involvement. In the normal caloric test:

- *Cold* water in the *left* ear causes nystagmus to the *right*
- *Warm* water in the *left* ear causes nystagmus to the *left*

The right ear would give opposite responses.

Auditory evoked potentials record the response from a repetitive 'click' stimulus. The level of the lesion may be detected by abnormalities in the response.

Lesions of the eighth nerve and its connections

Lesions at five levels can be recognized by the associated signs.

Cortex. Vertigo sometimes occurs as an aura in a partial seizure of temporal lobe origin.

Deafness is very rare in cortical lesions.

Pons. Vertigo is common with demyelinating or vascular lesions of the brain stem that involve the vestibular nuclei and their connections. A sixth or seventh nerve lesion, internuclear ophthalmoplegia or contralateral hemiparesis help localization. Nystagmus is frequently present.

Deafness is very rare in pontine lesions.

Cerebellopontine angle. Perceptive deafness occurs. Sixth, seventh and fifth nerve lesions develop, followed by cerebellar signs (ipsilateral) and later 'pyramidal' signs (contralateral). Nystagmus is usually present.

Causes include acoustic neuroma, meningioma and secondary neoplasm.

Petrous temporal bone. A seventh nerve lesion may be present. Causes include trauma, middle ear infection and Paget's disease of bone.

End-organ disease. The main causes are:

- Ménière's disease
- Drugs (e.g. gentamicin)
- Noise
- Middle-ear infection
- Intrauterine rubella
- Congenital syphilis
- Mumps
- 'Vestibular neuronitis'

Ménière's disease

This condition is characterized by recurrent attacks of the three symptoms—vertigo, tinnitus and deafness. It is associated with a dilatation of the endolymph system of unknown cause.

SYMPTOMS

The sudden, unprovoked attacks of vertigo with vomiting and loss of balance last from minutes to hours. Tinnitus and deafness accompany an attack but may be overshadowed by the degree of vertigo. The attacks are recurrent over months or years. Ultimately deafness develops and the vertigo ceases.

SIGNS

Nystagmus often accompanies an attack. Sensorineural deafness may be found.

MANAGEMENT

Medical treatment with vestibular sedatives (e.g. cinnarazine or prochlorperazine) is unsatisfactory. Each attack is, however, self-limiting. Betahistine 8 mg three times daily is sometimes helpful.

Recurrent severe attacks may require surgery (e.g. ultrasound destruction of the labyrinth or vestibular nerve section).

Vestibular neuronitis

This common but poorly understood syndrome describes an acute attack of severe vertigo with nystagmus, often with vomiting, but without loss of hearing. It is believed to follow or accompany viral infections that affect the labyrinth.

The disturbance lasts for several days or weeks but is self-limiting and rarely recurs. Treatment is with vestibular sedatives. The condition is sometimes followed by benign positional vertigo. Very similar symptoms may be caused by demyelination or vascular lesions within the brain stem.

Benign positional vertigo and positional nystagmus

Positional vertigo is vertigo precipitated by head movements, usually into a particular position. It may occur when turning in bed or on sitting up. The vertigo is transient, lasting seconds or minutes.

Vertigo can be produced by moving the patient's head suddenly (Hallpike's test). There is a latent interval of a few seconds, followed by nystagmus.

The syndrome of benign positional vertigo sometimes follows 'vestibular neuronitis', head injury or ear infection. It usually lasts for some months. There are no sequelae, although the condition sometimes recurs. Treatment is with vestibular sedatives.

Positional nystagmus (and vertigo) that is without a latent interval and does not fatigue is occasionally seen with neoplasms of the posterior fossa.

THE GLOSSOPHARYNGEAL AND VAGUS NERVES (NINTH AND TENTH CRANIAL NERVES)

The glossopharyngeal nerve

This mixed nerve arises in the medulla and leaves the skull through the jugular foramen with the vagus and accessory nerves.

Its sensory fibres supply all sensation to the tonsillar fossa and pharynx (the afferent pathway of the gag reflex), and taste to the posterior third of the tongue.

Motor fibres supply the stylopharyngeus muscle, autonomic fibres supply the parotid gland, and a sensory branch supplies the carotid sinus.

Isolated lesions are most unusual, since lesions at the jugular foramen also affect the vagus and sometimes the accessory nerves.

Glossopharyngeal neuralgia
This is a rare, severe, paroxysmal neuralgia. Pain involves the pharynx and is triggered by swallowing.

The vagus nerve

This mixed nerve supplies the striated muscle of the pharynx (efferent pathway of the gag reflex), the larynx (including the vocal cords via the recurrent laryngeal nerves) and the upper oesophagus.

There are some sensory fibres from the larynx.

Parasympathetic fibres supply the heart and abdominal viscera.

Ninth and tenth nerve lesions

A unilateral lesion of the ninth nerve causes diminished sensation on one side of the pharynx. A unilateral tenth nerve lesion causes unilateral failure of voluntary and reflex elevation of the soft palate, which is drawn to the side opposite the lesion. Individual lesions of these nerves are unusual.

Bilateral combined lesions of the ninth and tenth nerves cause weakness of elevation of the palate, depression of palatal sensation and loss of the gag reflex. The cough is depressed and the vocal cords are paralysed. The patient complains of difficulty in swallowing, choking (particularly with fluids) and hoarseness.

The causes of ninth and tenth nerve lesions are given in Table 18.14.

Table 18.14 Principal causes of lesions of the ninth, tenth and eleventh cranial nerves.

Site	Pathology
Brain stem	Infarction
	Syringobulbia
	Motor neurone disease (motor fibres)
	Poliomyelitis (motor fibres)
Jugular foramen	Carcinoma of nasopharynx
	Glomus tumour
	Internal jugular vein thrombosis
Neck and nasopharynx	Carcinoma of nasopharynx
	Metastases
	Polyneuropathy

Lesions of the recurrent laryngeal nerves
Unilateral paralysis of this important branch of each vagus causes hoarseness (dysphonia) and depression of the forceful, explosive part of the cough reflex. Bilateral acute lesions, e.g. postoperatively, are a serious emergency and cause respiratory obstruction.

The left recurrent laryngeal nerve (which loops beneath the aorta) is more commonly affected than the right.

Causes of recurrent laryngeal nerve lesions include:

● Mediastinal tumours
● Aneurysm of the aorta
● Trauma or surgery to the neck

THE ACCESSORY NERVE (ELEVENTH CRANIAL NERVE)

This motor nerve to the trapezius and sternomastoid muscles arises in the medulla and leaves the skull through the jugular foramen with the ninth and tenth nerves.

A lesion of the eleventh nerve causes weakness of the sternomastoid (rotation of the head and neck to the opposite side) and the trapezius (shoulder shrugging). The principal causes are shown in Table 18.14.

THE HYPOGLOSSAL NERVE (TWELFTH CRANIAL NERVE)

The motor nerve to the tongue arises in the medulla and leaves the skull through the anterior condylar foramen.

Twelfth nerve lesions

A lower motor neurone lesion of the twelfth nerve leads to unilateral weakness, wasting and fasciculation of the tongue. When protruded the tongue deviates towards the weaker side.

Some causes of a hypoglossal nerve (or nucleus) lesion are:

● *In the brain stem:*
   Motor neurone disease
   Syringobulbia
   Poliomyelitis
● *At the skull base:*
   Trauma
   Tumours
      Nasopharyngeal carcinoma
      Glomus tumour
● *In the neck:*
   Trauma
   Tumours

Bilateral supranuclear (upper motor neurone) lesions cause the tongue movements to be slow; in addition the tongue cannot be protruded very far. There is no fasciculation.

BULBAR AND PSEUDOBULBAR PALSY

A *bulbar palsy* describes weakness of lower motor neurone type of the muscles supplied by the lower cranial nerves whose nuclei lie in the medulla (the 'bulb'). The weakness is caused by lesions of the lower cranial nerve nuclei, the (ninth to twelfth) cranial nerves themselves or the muscles they supply.

The symptoms, signs and causes of a bulbar palsy are mentioned under the sections on the ninth to twelfth cranial nerves. Isolated lesions of these nerves are rare.

In *pseudobulbar* palsy, bilateral supranuclear (upper motor neurone) lesions of the lower cranial nerves cause weakness and poverty of movement of the tongue and the pharyngeal musculature. Signs of a pseudobulbar palsy are a stiff, slow, spastic tongue (which is not wasted) and dysarthria with a 'gravelly' spastic voice that is slow and sounds 'dry'. The gag reflex and palatal reflex are preserved. The jaw jerk is exaggerated. Emotional lability (inappropriate laughing or crying) often accompanies pseudobulbar palsy. The principal causes are:

● Motor neurone disease, in which there are often both upper and lower motor neurone lesions
● Multiple sclerosis, in which it occurs mainly as a late event
● Cerebrovascular disease, in which it may occur with multi-infarct dementia

Severe difficulty with swallowing, dysarthria and a slow-moving tongue also occur in the late stages of Parkinson's disease and this should be distinguished from both pseudobulbar and bulbar palsy.

The motor system

THE CORTICOSPINAL TRACTS

The corticospinal tracts originate from the neurones of the fifth layer of the cortex and terminate on the motor nuclei of the cranial nerves and anterior horn cells of the spinal cord. The pathways of importance (see Fig. 18.8) in clinical diagnosis decussate in the medulla and pass to the contralateral halves of the cord as the crossed lateral corticospinal tracts. This is the 'pyramidal'

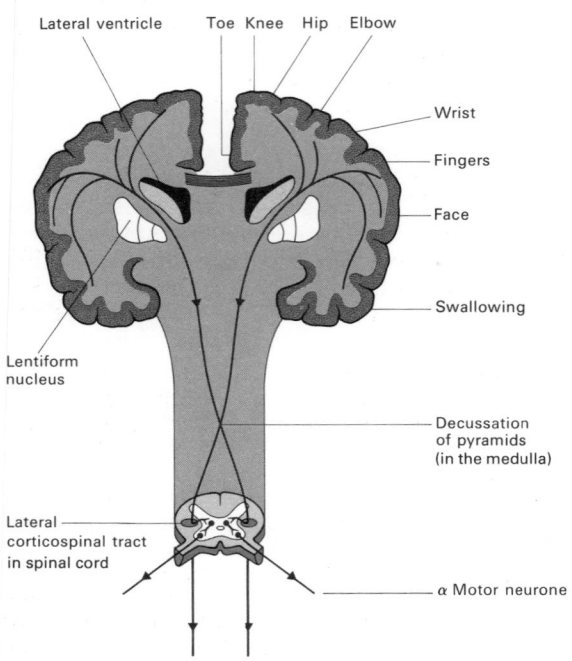

Fig. 18.8 The crossed corticospinal ('pyramidal') tracts.

system, disease of which causes upper motor neurone (UMN) lesions.

A small proportion of the corticospinal outflow remains uncrossed (the anterior corticospinal tracts).

Characteristics of UMN lesions (Table 18.15)

Drift of the upper limb
In the normal individual the outstretched upper limbs are held symmetrically, even when the eyes are closed. In a 'pyramidal' lesion, the affected upper limb drifts downwards, medially and tends to pronate and flex slightly. This important sign may occur early, before weakness is evident.

Weakness
A UMN ('pyramidal') lesion above the decussation causes weakness of the contralateral limbs, i.e. a hemiparesis. In an acute, severe lesion such as an infarct of the internal capsule, this weakness will be dense, but in partial lesions there is a characteristic *pattern* of weakness in the limbs: in the upper limb the flexors are stronger than the extensors, and in the lower limb the extensors are stronger than the flexors. In the upper limb the weaker movements are thus shoulder abduction and elbow extension; in the forearm and hand, the wrist and finger extensors and abductors are weaker than their antagonists. In the lower limb the weaker movements are flexion and abduction of the hip,

flexion of the knee, and dorsiflexion and eversion of the ankle.

When the UMN lesion is below the decussation, the hemiparesis is on the same side as the lesion.

Increase in tone (spasticity)
An acute lesion of one pyramidal tract causes a flaccid paralysis (and areflexia). An increase in tone follows within several days owing to loss of the inhibitory effect of the corticospinal pathway and an increase in spinal reflex activity. This increase in tone affects all muscle groups on the affected side but is most easily detected in the stronger muscles. It is characterized by changing resistance to passive movement; the change may be sudden—the 'clasp-knife' effect. The tendon reflexes are exaggerated and clonus can commonly be demonstrated.

Changes in superficial reflexes
The plantar response becomes extensor. In a severe lesion (e.g. an infarct of the internal capsule causing hemiplegia) this response can be elicited from a wide area of the affected limb. As recovery occurs the area that is sensitive becomes smaller until only the posterior third of the lateral aspect of the sole is receptive. The stimulus may have to be unpleasant (an orange stick is the correct instrument to use). For the response to be certainly extensor, the dorsiflexion of the great toe should be accompanied by fanning of the toes.

The abdominal (and cremasteric reflexes) are abolished on the affected side.

The signs of a pyramidal lesion may be minimal. Weakness, spasticity or changes in superficial reflexes may predominate. The absence of one group of signs does not exclude a UMN lesion.

Clinical patterns of upper motor neurone disorders

Two main patterns of clinical features occur in UMN (pyramidal) disorders: hemiparesis and paraparesis.

Hemiparesis means weakness of the limbs of one side; it is usually (but by no means always) caused by a lesion within the brain. Paraparesis means weakness of both lower limbs and is

Table 18.15 Signs of an upper motor neurone lesion.

Drift of upper limb
Weakness with a characteristic distribution
Increase in tone of the spastic type
Exaggerated tendon reflexes
An extensor plantar response
Loss of abdominal reflexes
No muscle wasting
Normal electrical excitability of muscle

Table 18.16 Causes of a spastic paraparesis.

Spinal lesions
Spinal cord compression (see Table 18.47)
Multiple sclerosis, myelitis (e.g. VZV)
Motor neurone disease
Subacute combined degeneration of the cord
Syringomyelia
Syphilis
Familial or sporadic paraparesis
Vascular disease of the cord
Non-metastatic manifestation of malignancy
Tropical spastic paraparesis (HTLV-1)

Cerebral lesions[a]
Parasagittal cortical lesions
  Meningioma
  Venous sinus thrombosis
Hydrocephalus
Multiple cerebral infarction

---

[a] All are rare causes of a paraparesis.

characteristically diagnostic of a spinal cord lesion.

The terms hemiplegia and paraplegia strictly indicate total paralysis but the terms are often used loosely to describe severe weakness.

Hemiparesis
The level of a unilateral lesion of the corticospinal tracts may be determined by the accompanying features.

Motor cortex. Weakness localized to one contralateral limb (monoplegia) or part of a limb is characteristic of an isolated lesion of the motor cortex. There may be a defect in higher cortical function (e.g. aphasia). Focal epilepsy may occur.

Internal capsule. Since the corticospinal fibres are tightly packed in the internal capsule, occupying about 1 cm^2, a small lesion causes a large deficit. For example, an infarct of a small branch of the middle cerebral artery (see p. 910) causes a sudden, dense, contralateral hemiplegia that includes the face.

Pons. A pontine lesion is rarely confined to the corticospinal tract alone. Adjacent structures such as cranial nerve nuclei (e.g. of the sixth or seventh nerve) are involved, causing ipsilateral cranial nerve lesions with contralateral hemiparesis.

Spinal cord. A lesion of one lateral corticospinal tract in the cord causes an ipsilateral UMN lesion and is indicated by a reflex level in the upper limbs (e.g. absent biceps jerk) or the presence of a Brown–Séquard syndrome (see p. 902). A spinal cord cause of a hemiparesis is unusual.

Paraparesis. Paraparesis (or tetraparesis, when the four limbs are involved) indicates bilateral damage to the corticospinal tracts. Spinal cord disease is the usual cause, but bilateral cerebral lesions can cause a similar picture (see Table 18.16).

THE EXTRAPYRAMIDAL SYSTEM AND THE CONTROL OF MOVEMENT

The extrapyramidal system is a general term for the basal ganglia. In disorders of this system, the commonest of which is Parkinson's disease, there is a combination of:

- Reduction in movement, i.e. bradykinesia (slow movement) or akinesia (no movement)
- Involuntary movements (tremor, chorea, dystonia or athetosis)
- Rigidity

Anatomy and physiology

Structure
The corpus striatum, consisting of the caudate nucleus, globus pallidus and putamen (the latter two forming the lentiform nucleus) lies close to the substantia nigra, thalami and subthalamic nuclei. There are interconnections between these structures and the cerebral cortex, the cerebellum and the reticular formation, the cranial nerve nuclei (particularly the vestibular nerve) and the spinal cord.

The overall function of this complex system is the initiation and modulation of movement. The system modulates cortical motor activity by a series of hypothetical servo loops.

It is now clear that in many basal ganglia disorders there are substantial and specific changes in neurotransmitter profile rather than discrete anatomical lesions.

In Parkinson's disease there is *reduction of*:

- Dopamine (to 10% of normal) in the putamen and substantia nigra
- Noradrenaline and 5-hydroxytryptamine (to 40% of normal) in the putamen
- Glutamic acid decarboxylase (GAD) in substantia nigra and cerebral cortex. GAD is the enzyme responsible for synthesizing γ-amino-butyric acid (GABA)

Cholinergic activity is relatively well-preserved in Parkinson's disease.

Changes in the neurotransmitter profile are associated with characteristic clinical patterns. For example:

- In Parkinson's disease an increase in dopamine activity (due to levodopa therapy) relieves rigidity. In excess (in both normal people and those with Parkinson's disease), levodopa therapy causes chorea.

- In Huntington's disease (chorea) there is a marked reduction in acetycholine and GABA activity in the striatum. Dopamine activity is normal.
- In normal people an increase in acetylcholine activity or a decrease in dopamine activity causes rigidity and bradykinesia (parkinsonism). For example, reserpine (which depletes neurones of dopamine) and phenothiazines or butyrophenones (which block dopaminergic neurones) cause or exacerbate parkinsonism.

Clinically, extrapyramidal disorders are classified broadly into the akinetic-rigid syndromes (see p. 922), in which poverty of movement predominates, and the dyskinesias, in which there are a variety of involuntary movements.

THE CEREBELLUM

The cerebellum receives afferent fibres from:

- Proprioceptive organs in joints and muscles
- The vestibular nuclei
- The basal ganglia
- The corticospinal system

Efferent fibres pass from the cerebellum to:

- Each red nucleus
- The vestibular nuclei
- The basal ganglia
- The anterior horn cells

Each lateral lobe of the cerebellum coordinates movement of the ipsilateral limb. The vermis (a midline structure) is concerned with maintenance of axial (midline) posture and balance.

Cerebellar lesions

Expanding mass lesions within the cerebellum produce hydrocephalus, causing severe headaches, vomiting and papilloedema. 'Coning' of the cerebellar tonsils through the foramen magnum and respiratory arrest occur, often within hours. Very rarely 'tonic seizures' of the limbs occur with cerebellar masses.

Lateral cerebellar lobes
A lesion within one cerebellar lobe (e.g. a tumour or infarction) causes disruption of the normal sequence of movements (dyssynergia) on the side of the lesion.

Posture and gait. The outstretched arm is held still in the early stages of a cerebellar lesion but there is rebound overshoot when the limb is pressed downwards by the examiner and released. Gait is ataxic with a broad base; the patient falters towards the side of the lesion.

Tremor and ataxia. Movement is imprecise in direction, in force and in distance (dysmetria).

Rapid alternating movements (tapping, clapping or rotary movements of the hand) are clumsy and disorganized (dysdiadochokinesis).

'Intention tremor' (action tremor, with past-pointing) is seen when the 'finger–nose–finger' and 'heel–shin' tests are performed.

Nystagmus (see p. 892). Coarse horizontal nystagmus appears with cerebellar lobar lesions. Its direction is towards the side of the lesion.

Dysarthria. Speech is affected (usually with bilateral lesions). A halting, jerking dysarthria results—the 'scanning speech' of cerebellar lesions.

Other signs. Titubation—rhythmic tremor of the head in either to and fro ('yes–yes') movements or rotary ('no–no') movements—also occurs, mainly when cerebellar connections are involved (e.g. in

Table 18.17 Principal causes of cerebellar syndromes.

Tumours	Haemangioblastoma
	Medulloblastoma
	Secondary neoplasm
	Compression by acoustic neuroma
Vascular lesions	Haemorrhage
	Infarction
	Arteriovenous malformation
Infection	Abscess
	AIDS
	Kuru
Developmental	Arnold–Chiari malformation
	Basilar invagination
	Cerebral palsy
Toxic and metabolic	Anticonvulsant drugs
	Chronic alcohol abuse
	Following carbon monoxide poisoning
	Lead poisoning
Inherited	Friedreich's ataxia
	Ataxia telangiectasia
	Essential tremor
Miscellaneous	Multiple sclerosis
	Hydrocephalus
	Post-infective cerebellar syndrome of childhood
	Hypothyroidism
	Non-metastatic manifestation of malignancy
	Cerebral oedema of chronic hypoxia

essential tremor and multiple sclerosis).

Hypotonia and depression of reflexes are also sometimes seen with cerebellar disease but are usually of little value as localizing signs. 'Pendular', i.e. slow, reflexes also occur.

Midline cerebellar lesions

Lesions of the cerebellar vermis have a dramatic effect on the equilibrium of the trunk and axial musculature. Truncal ataxia causes difficulty in standing and sitting unsupported, with a rolling, broad, ataxic gait.

Lesions of the flocculonodular region cause vertigo, vomiting and ataxia of gait if they extend to the roof of the fourth ventricle.

Table 18.17 summarizes the main causes of cerebellar disease.

TREMOR

Tremor is an oscillation, regular and sinusoidal, of a part or parts of the body. Different varieties are outlined below.

Postural tremor

Everyone has a physiological tremor of the outstretched hands at 8–12 Hz. This is increased with anxiety, hyperthyroidism and certain drugs (lithium, sodium valproate and sympathomimetics) or in mercury poisoning. A coarse, postural tremor is seen in chronic alcoholism and in benign essential tremor (usually at 5–8 Hz). Postural tremor does not worsen on movement.

Intention tremor

Tremor that is exacerbated by action, with past-pointing and accompanying slowness and incoordination of rapid alternating movement (dysdiadochokinesis), occurs in cerebellar lobe disease and with lesions of cerebellar connections. Titubation (tremor of the head) and nystagmus may be present.

Rest tremor

This is present at rest, is between 4–7 Hz and is not made worse by action. It occurs primarily in Parkinson's disease and is sometimes described as 'pill-rolling' between the thumb and index finger.

Other tremors

Tremor is seen following lesions of the red nucleus (e.g. infarction, demyelination) and rarely with frontal-lobe lesions.

LOWER MOTOR NEURONE LESIONS

The lower motor neurone (LMN) is the motor pathway from the anterior horn cell (or cranial

Table 18.18 Signs of a lower motor neurone lesion.

Weakness
Wasting
Hypotonia
Reflex loss
Fasciculation
Fibrillation potentials (detected electromyographically—see p. 880)
Contractures of muscle
'Trophic' changes in skin and nails

nerve nucleus) via a peripheral nerve to the motor end plate.

The motor unit consists of a single anterior horn cell, the single fast-conducting alpha motor nerve fibre that leaves the spinal cord via the anterior root, and the group of muscle fibres (100–2000) being supplied via the mixed peripheral nerve. Anterior horn cell activity is modulated by the impulses from:

- The corticospinal tracts
- The extrapyramidal system (basal ganglia and cerebellum)
- Afferent fibres from the posterior roots

Signs of an LMN lesion

Voluntary muscle depends upon the motor unit for all movement and also for its metabolic integrity. Signs follow rapidly if the LMN is interrupted at any point in its course (Table 18.18). Wasting appears within 3 weeks of the development of an LMN lesion. Fasciculation occurs and is due to visible contractions of single motor units.

Causes of an LMN lesion

Examples of LMN lesions at various levels are:

- Anterior horn cell—poliomyelitis, motor neurone disease
- Spinal root—cervical and lumbar root lesions, neuralgic amyotrophy
- Peripheral (or cranial) nerve—nerve trauma or compression, polyneuropathy

THE SPINAL REFLEX ARC

The components of the spinal reflex arc are illustrated in Fig. 18.9. The stretch reflex is the physiological basis for the tendon reflexes. For example, in the knee jerk, a tap on the patellar tendon activates stretch receptors in the quadriceps. Impulses in first-order sensory neurones pass directly to lower motor neurones (L3 and L4), which activate the quadriceps, causing a contraction.

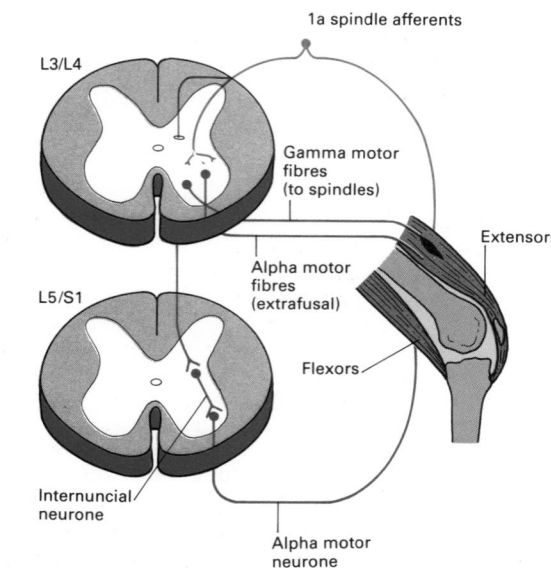

Fig. 18.9 The knee jerk: an example of a spinal reflex arc.

Loss of a tendon reflex is caused by a lesion anywhere along the spinal reflex path. The reflex lost indicates the level of the lesion (Table 18.19).

Reinforcement
Distraction of the patient's attention, clenching the teeth or pulling of the interlocked fingers increases the activity of the stretch reflex. Such 'reinforcement' manoeuvres should be carried out before a reflex is recorded as absent.

The sensory system

Peripheral nerves and spinal roots

Peripheral nerves carry all modalities of sensation from either free or specialized nerve endings to the dorsal root ganglia and thus to the cord.

The sensory distribution of the spinal roots (dermatomes) is shown in Fig. 18.10.

Table 18.19 Spinal levels of tendon reflexes.

Spinal level	Reflex
C5–6	Supinator
C5–6	Biceps
C7	Triceps
L3–4	Knee
S1	Ankle

The spinal cord (Fig. 18.11)

Posterior columns
For clinical purposes, the sensory modalities of vibration sense, joint position, light touch and two-point discrimination travel uncrossed in the posterior columns to the gracile and cuneate nuclei in the medulla. Axons from second-order neurones cross the midline in the brain stem to form the medial lemniscus and pass to the thalamus.

Spinothalamic tracts
Fibres carrying pain and temperature sensation synapse in the dorsal horn of the cord, cross the cord and pass as the spinothalamic tracts to the thalamus and reticular formation.

The sensory cortex

The projection of fibres from the thalamus to the sensory cortex of the parietal region is shown in Fig. 18.11. Connections also exist between the thalamus and the motor cortex.

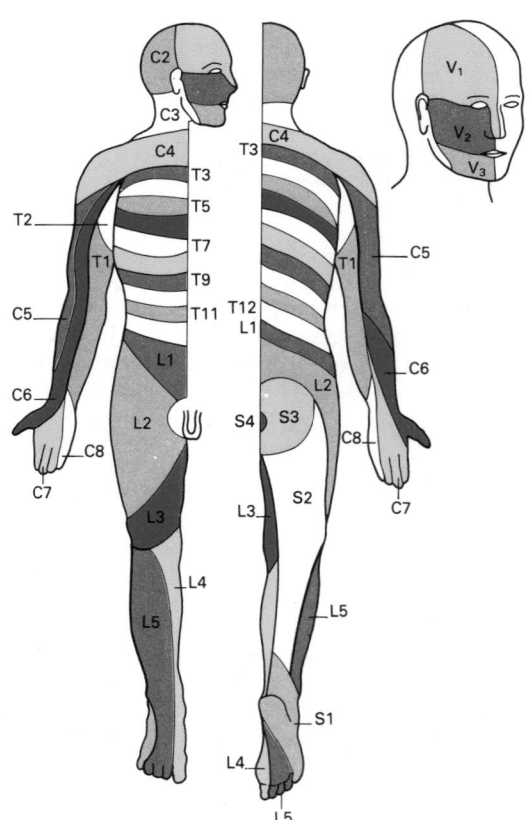

Fig. 18.10 The dermatomes.

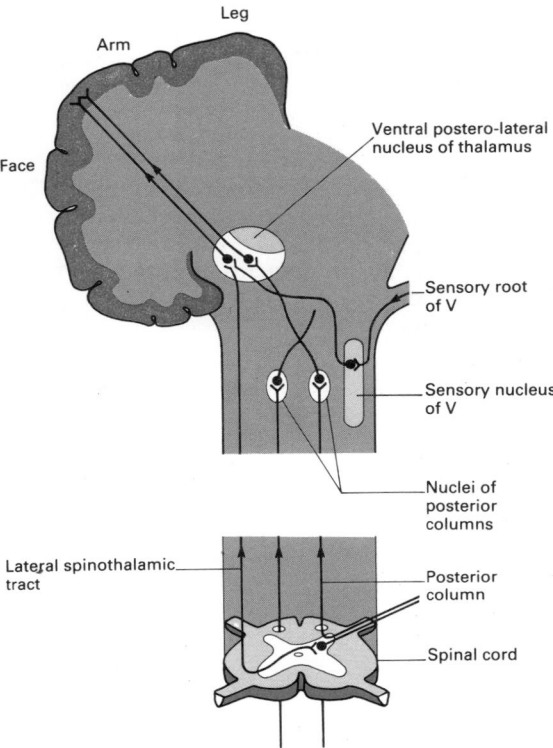

Fig. 18.11 The principal sensory pathways. The posterior columns remain uncrossed until the medulla. The spinothalamic tracts cross close to their entry into the spinal cord.

LESIONS OF THE SENSORY PATHWAYS

Paraesthesiae, numbness and pain are the principal symptoms of lesions of the sensory pathways below the level of the thalamus. The quality and distribution of the symptoms may suggest the site of the lesion.

Peripheral nerve lesions

The symptoms are felt in the distribution of the affected peripheral nerve (see p. 952).

Section of a nerve is followed by complete sensory loss. Nerve entrapment (see p. 952) causes numbness, pain and tingling. Tapping the site of compression sometimes causes a sharp, electric-shock-like pain in the distribution of the nerve (Tinel's sign).

Neuralgia
Neuralgia refers to local pain of great severity in the distribution of a damaged nerve. Examples are:

- Trigeminal neuralgia (p. 890)
- Post-herpetic neuralgia (p. 933)
- Causalgia

Spinal root lesions

Root pain
The pain of root compression is referred to the myotome supplied by that root and there is also a tingling discomfort in the dermatome. The pain is made worse by manoeuvres that either stretch the nerve root (as in straight leg raising) or increase the pressure in the spinal subarachnoid space (as in coughing and straining).

Cervical and lumbar disc protrusions (see p. 957) are common causes of root lesions.

Dorsal root lesions
Section of a dorsal root causes loss of all modalities of sensation in the appropriate dermatome. However, the overlap with adjacent dermatomes may make it difficult to detect anaesthesia if only a single root is affected.

Lightning pains. Tabes dorsalis (now a rarity) is a form of neurosyphilis that causes a low-grade inflammation of the dorsal roots and root entry zone of the cord. Its presentation includes irregular, sharp, momentary stabbing pains that involve one or two spots, typically in a calf, thigh or ankle.

Spinal cord lesions

Posterior column lesions. Posterior column lesions cause:

- Tingling of a limb
- Electric-shock-like sensations
- Clumsiness
- Numbness
- Band-like sensations

These symptoms are often felt vaguely without a clear sensory level on the side of the lesion.

Position sense, vibration sense, light touch and two-point discrimination are lost below the level of the lesion. Loss of position sense produces sensory ataxia (see p. 875).

Lhermitte's phenomenon
This is an electric-shock-like sensation radiating down the trunk and limbs that is produced by neck flexion. It indicates a cervical cord lesion. Lhermitte's sign is common in acute exacerbations of multiple sclerosis (see p. 927). It also occurs in cervical spondylotic myelopathy (see p. 957), subacute combined degeneration of the cord (see p. 956) and radiation myelopathy (p. 945).

Spinothalamic tract lesions
Pure spinothalamic lesions cause isolated contra-

lateral loss of pain and temperature sensation below the level of the lesion. This is called 'dissociated sensory loss', i.e. pain and temperature are 'dissociated' from light touch, which is preserved.

The spinal level is modified by the lamination of fibres within the spinothalamic tracts. Fibres from the lower spinal roots lie superficially and are therefore damaged first by compressive lesions from outside the cord. As an external compressive lesion (e.g. a midthoracic extradural meningioma; see Fig. 18.12) enlarges, the spinal sensory level ascends as deeper fibres become involved. Conversely, a central lesion of the cord (e.g. a syrinx, see p. 946) affects the deeper fibres first.

Symptoms of spinothalamic tract lesions are the absence of pain (resulting in painless burns and minor injuries) or the loss of temperature sensation. Perforating ulcers and neuropathic joints may follow.

Spinal cord compression

This important syndrome causes a progressive spastic paraparesis (or tetraparesis) with sensory loss below the level of the lesion. Sphincter disturbance is common.

Root pain is frequent but not invariable. It is felt characteristically at the site of compression. With a lesion of the thoracic cord (e.g. an extradural meningioma), pain radiates in a band around the chest and is made worse by coughing, straining and jarring, as the meningeal sheath of the nerve is stretched.

Involvement of one spinothalamic tract (contralateral loss of pain and temperature) together with one corticospinal tract (ipsilateral 'pyramidal' signs) is known as the 'Brown–Séquard syndrome' of hemisection of the cord.

Paraparesis and spinal cord disease are discussed further on pp. 897 and 944.

Pontine lesions

Pontine lesions lie above the decussation of the posterior columns. Since the medial lemniscus and spinothalamic tracts are close together, there is loss of all forms of sensation on the side opposite the lesion. The upper cranial nerve nuclei are often also involved.

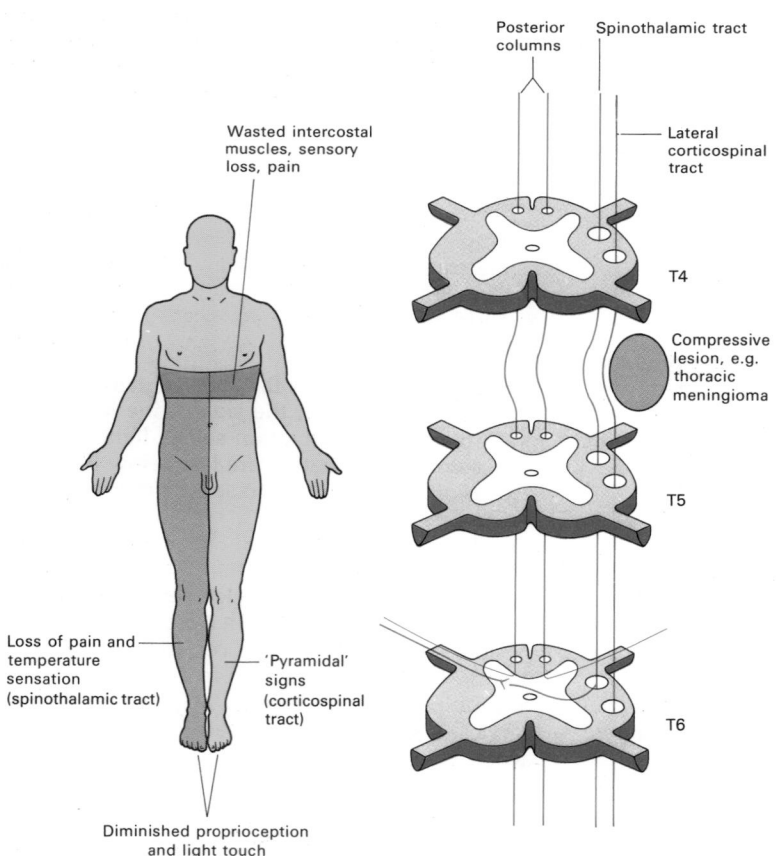

Fig. 18.12 The clinical features of spinal cord compression and their production.

Thalamic lesions

Thalamic lesions may produce loss of sensation to all modalities of sensation on the opposite side of the body; this is an unusual clinical picture.

Spontaneous pain may also occur. Thalamic pain, sometimes called the 'thalamic syndrome', is usually caused by a small thalamic infarct. The patient develops a hemiparesis that recovers partially. There remains a constant deep-seated pain that affects the paretic limbs. It is often very severe. Movement does not change the pain, which continues night and day. Extreme anguish is usual and the secondary depression that follows may lead to suicide.

Cortical lesions

Pain is not a feature of destructive cortical lesions.

Irritative phenomena (e.g. partial seizures) in the parietal cortex cause tingling sensations in the affected part.

Sensory loss, neglect of one side and subtle disorders of sensation may occur with lesions of the parietal cortex.

PAIN AND DISTURBANCE OF SENSATION

Pain fibres

Primary afferent axons (2–5 μm, thinly myelinated fibres and smaller, unmyelinated C fibres) pass in the peripheral nerves to the dorsal horn of the spinal cord. Some axons synapse in the substantia gelatinosa of the dorsal horn (an area richly supplied with opioids). Others pass to the contralateral spinothalamic tracts (see Fig. 18.11).

The gate theory of pain

This suggests that pain sensation is altered by other afferent impulses (e.g. touch, pressure, vibration) that enter the spinal cord and have a 'gating' or inhibitory effect on impulse transmission. Thus, pain sensation may be modulated by other sensory modalities. For example, local heat and transcutaneous electrical stimulation are sometimes useful in the management of chronic pain.

Opioid peptides
Naturally occurring opioid peptides act as neurotransmitters and are widely distributed within the central nervous system. They are found mainly within the substantia gelatinosa of the dorsal horn, in the periaqueductal grey matter and in the midline raphe nuclei of the brain stem. Three classes of peptide and receptor have now been recognized (Table 18.20). β-Endorphin is the most potent known endorphin and has a powerful

Table 18.20 Opioid peptides.

Peptide	Receptor
Enkephalins	delta receptors
Dynorphins	kappa receptors
Endorphins	mu receptors

analgesic action. Morphine and other opiates act at the μ receptors.

Psychological aspects of pain

Pain is difficult to quantify and its interpretation depends not only on the patient's description but also on the experience, personality and mood of the doctor. Depression is an almost invariable companion of chronic pain.

CONTROL OF PAIN

Chronic and recurrent pain is disabling and distressing to the patient and has important secondary effects upon a family and household members. Multidisciplinary Pain Relief Clinics are sometimes helpful in providing specific and skilled supportive therapy, but the management of pain should be part of the skills of all doctors. Treatments available include:

Oral therapy with:

- Analgesics ranging from simple pain-killing drugs (such as aspirin, paracetamol, co-proxamol) to opiates (e.g. morphine or diamorphine). Sufficient analgesia can only be gauged by frequent assessment of the patient.
- Psychotropic drugs, e.g. phenothiazines, tricyclic antidepressants.
- Specific drugs for defined conditions, e.g. carbamazepine for trigeminal neuralgia.

Parenteral therapy

- Analgesics given i.m. or i.v.
- Analgesics (e.g. opiates) by continuous subcutaneous infusion (portable pump) in terminal care. These are sometimes valuable in the management of patients at home.

Epidural drugs

- Local anaesthetics, e.g. lignocaine or the long-acting bupivacaine.
- Phenol or alcohol injection to destroy nerve roots (e.g. when infiltrated with secondary neoplasms).
- Opiates administered by epidural catheter and syringe pump.

Local injection

- Corticosteroids and lignocaine injected directly into a painful area.

Sympathetic block

- Long-acting local anaesthetics are injected into the sympathetic chain under X-ray screening control.

Transcutaneous electrical nerve stimulation (TENS)

- A portable stimulator is used (e.g. in post-herpetic neuralgia).

Neurosurgery

- Tractotomy—section or radiofrequency lesion in the spinothalamic tract of the cord.
- Electrical stimulation by implanted electrodes in the thalamus or posterior columns of the cord.

Miscellaneous

- Acupuncture
- Alternative medicine

Control of the bladder and sexual function

Afferent fibres (T12–S4) record changes in pressure within the bladder and tactile sensation in the genitalia.

Disorders of micturition

Bilateral upper motor neurone lesions cause frequency of micturition and incontinence. The bladder is small and unusually sensitive to small changes in intravesical pressure.

Lower motor neurone lesions (which must be bilateral to cause urinary symptoms) cause a flaccid, atonic bladder, which overflows without warning.

Frontal-lobe lesions (e.g. dementia, hydrocephalus) cause a disturbance of awareness of micturition, resulting in incontinence.

Impotence

Failure of erection of the penis (or clitoris) and ejaculation is caused by bilateral upper or lower motor lesions. Depression is also a common cause of impotence. Endocrine aspects of impotence are discussed on p. 786.

Unconsciousness and coma

The central reticular formation, which extends from the brain stem to the thalamus, influences the state of arousal. This complex process involves interactions between the reticular formation, the cortex and brain stem, and all sensory pathways.

Disturbed consciousness

Definitions

- *Consciousness* means awareness of oneself and the surroundings in a state of wakefulness.
- *Clouding of consciousness* is reduced wakefulness or awareness.
- *Sleep* is a state of mental and physical inactivity from which the subject can be roused.
- *Stupor* is an abnormal, sleepy state from which the patient can be aroused by stimuli that may need to be repeated or vigorously applied.
- *Confusion* is the state of altered consciousness in which patients are bewildered and misinterpret the world around them.
- *Delirium* is a state of high arousal (seen typically in delirium tremens, see p. 992) in which there is confusion and often hallucinations.
- *Coma* is a state of unrousable unresponsiveness. A grading system for coma used particularly in patients with head injury is shown in Table 18.22. An alternative grading system is given on p. 744.

Causes of coma

Altered consciousness is produced by three types of process affecting the brain stem, reticular formation and the cerebral cortex.

Table 18.21 Efferent nerve supply of the bladder and genitalia.

Type of nerve supply	Source	Structure/function supplied
Parasympathetic	S2–S4	Detrusor muscle contraction
		Genitalia (penile erection, engorgement of clitoris)
Somatic	Pudendal nerves	External sphincter
Sympathetic	T12–L2	Trigone
		Ejaculation, orgasm

Table 18.22 Glasgow Coma Scale.

	Score
Eye opening (E)	
Spontaneous	4
To speech	3
To pain	2
Nil	1
Motor response (M)	
Obeys	6
Localizes	5
Withdraws	4
Abnormal flexion	3
Extensor response	2
Nil	1
Verbal response (V)	
Orientated	5
Confused conversation	4
Inappropriate words	3
Incomprehensible sounds	2
Nil	1

Coma score = E + M + V (minimum = 3; maximum = 15)

- *Diffuse brain dysfunction*. Generalized metabolic (e.g. uraemia) or toxic (e.g. septicaemia) disorders can depress brain function.
- *Direct effect on the brain stem*. Lesions of the brain stem itself damage the reticular activating system.
- *Indirect effect on the brain stem*. Mass lesions above the tentorium cerebelli compress or damage the ascending reticular activating system in the brain stem.

It is important to understand that single focal brain lesions of the cerebral hemispheres do not produce coma unless they compress the brain stem. Oedema frequently surrounds hemisphere lesions, contributing greatly to their effects.

Other coma-like states include 'the locked-in syndrome', a state of unresponsiveness due to massive brain stem infarction. The patient is unable to communicate or move (except sometimes the eyes) but has a functioning cerebral cortex. The 'chronic vegetative state', a sequel of head injury, for example, implies loss of sentient behaviour, i.e. the patient perceives little or nothing but lies awake, breathing spontaneously: widespread cerebral damage is present.

Unresponsiveness of psychological origin may cause difficulty in the differential diagnosis of apparent coma.

The principal causes of coma and stupor are shown in Table 18.23. A common cause of coma is self-poisoning (see p. 743).

THE UNCONSCIOUS PATIENT

Immediate assessment

Immediate action, which takes only seconds, is essential (Table 18.24).

A history should then be obtained from accompanying relatives, friends, ambulance drivers or the police. Many patients with diabetes mellitus, epilepsy or hypoadrenalism, and those who take corticosteroids, wear or carry identifying discs or cards; these should be looked for.

Further examination

- The depth of coma should be recorded (Table 18.22).
- A full general and neurological examination should then be carried out.

GENERAL EXAMINATION

Temperature
This is raised in infection and hyperpyrexia and low in hypothermia.

Table 18.23 Principal causes of coma and stupor.

Diffuse brain dysfunction
Drug overdose, alcohol
CO poisoning, anaesthetic gases
Hypoglycaemia, hyperglycaemia
Hypoxic/ischaemic brain injury
Hypertensive encephalopathy
Renal failure
Hepatic failure
Respiratory failure with CO_2 retention
Hypercalcaemia, hypocalcaemia
Hypoadrenalism, hypopituitarism and
    hypothyroidism
Hyponatraemia, hypernatraemia
Metabolic acidosis
Hypothermia, hyperpyrexia
Trauma—following closed head injury
Epilepsy—following a generalized seizure
Encephalitis, cerebral malaria
Subarachnoid haemorrhage
Metabolic rarities e.g. porphyria

Direct effect on brain stem
Brain stem haemorrhage or infarction
Brain stem neoplasm
Brain stem demyelination
Wernicke–Korsakoff syndrome
Trauma

Indirect effect on brain stem
Hemisphere tumour, infarction, abscess,
    haematoma, encephalitis or trauma
Cerebellar lesions

Table 18.24 Immediate action in patients with coma (see also p. 744).

Examine	Action
Airway	Clear, and intubate if necessary
Pulse (? absent) Pulses (? fixed, dilated)	Perform cardiopulmonary resuscitation if appropriate
For presence of trauma	If head injury present, anticipate deterioration

Skin
The following should be noted:

- Colour (cyanosis, jaundice, purpura, rashes, pigmentation)
- Texture (coarse and dry in hypothyroidism)
- Presence of injection sites (diabetics, drug addicts)

Breath
Alcohol or ketones may be smelt. In hepatic failure and uraemia a distinct fetor is present.

Respiration
Depressed but regular respiration occurs in most states of stupor and coma. The presence of particular types of respiration may point to the diagnosis:

- *Cheyne–Stokes respiration* (periodic respiration) is alternating hyperpnoea and apnoea. In neurological disease it implies bilateral cerebral dysfunction, usually deep in the hemispheres or in the upper brain stem, and may be a sign of incipient 'coning'. It may occur in metabolic comas, particularly if there is CO_2 retention from pulmonary disease.
- *Kussmaul (acidotic) respiration* is deep-sighing hyperventilation that occurs principally in diabetic ketoacidosis and uraemia.
- *Central neurogenic (pontine) hyperventilation* describes the sustained, rapid, deep breathing seen in patients with pontine lesions.
- *Ataxic respiration* is the shallow, halting respiration that occurs when the medullary respiratory centre is damaged. It is frequently a pre-terminal event.
- *Vomiting, hiccup and excessive yawning* may indicate a lesion in the lower brain stem in a stuporose patient.

NEUROLOGICAL EXAMINATION

Head and neck
The patient should be examined for evidence of trauma and neck stiffness.

Pupils
The size of the pupils and their reaction to light should be recorded. The following patterns may be seen:

- Dilatation of one pupil, which becomes fixed to light, indicates herniation of the uncus of the temporal lobe ('coning') and compression of the third nerve. This is a potential neurosurgical emergency.
- 'Pinpoint' light-fixed pupils occur with pontine lesions (e.g. a pontine haemorrhage) that interrupt the sympathetic pathways.
- Mid-position or slightly dilated pupils (4–6 mm) fixed to light and sometimes irregular are seen when damage to the midbrain interrupts the pupillary light reflex.
- Horner's syndrome (ipsilateral pupillary constriction and ptosis, see p. 886) occurs with lesions of the hypothalamus and also in 'coning'.
- Fixed, dilated pupils are a cardinal sign of brain death. They also occur in deep coma of any cause, but particularly coma due to barbiturate intoxication or hypothermia.
- Mid-point pupils that react to light are characteristic in coma of metabolic origin and coma due to most CNS-depressant drugs.

Other pupillary changes due to drugs are described on p. 744.
N.B.— No mydriatic drugs should be given to the unconscious patient.

Fundi
Papilloedema or retinal haemorrhage should be recorded.

Ocular movements
In most cases of coma the eyes are slightly divergent. Slow, roving eye movements, usually horizontal, are seen in light coma.

Vestibulo-ocular reflexes
Passive head rotation causes conjugate ocular deviation in the direction opposite to the induced head movement (doll's head reflex). This reflex is lost in very deep coma and is absent in brain stem lesions. It is absent in brain death.

Conjugate ocular deviation is seen towards the irrigated ear when ice-cold water is run into the external auditory meatus; this is known as the caloric or vestibulo-ocular reflex and indicates that the brain stem is intact. In coma, this test is used mainly in the diagnosis of brain death (see p. 731).

Abnormalities of conjugate gaze (see p. 888). Sustained conjugate lateral gaze occurs towards the side of a destructive hemisphere lesion ('the eyes look *towards the normal limbs*') because damage to supranuclear pathways prevents contralateral gaze.

In a pontine brain-stem lesion, sustained conjugate lateral gaze occurs away from the side of the lesion, *'towards the paralysed limbs'*.

Rarely, an irritative lesion in the frontal region (e.g. an epileptic focus) may drive the eyes away from the affected hemisphere, i.e. conjugate deviation may occur away from the side of the lesion.

Skew deviation (where one eye is deviated upwards and the other down) is a rare sign. It indicates a brain-stem lesion.

Spontaneous eye movements. Spontaneous eye movements (other than roving eye movements) are distinctly unusual in coma of any cause.

The sudden, brisk, downward-'diving' eye movement seen in pontine (or cerebellar) haemorrhage is known as ocular 'bobbing'.

Motor responses
Impairment of consciousness makes it difficult to recognize focal neurological signs. The following should be looked for:

- The response to visual threat in a stuporose patient—asymmetry indicates hemianopia.
- Tone—the only evidence of a hemiparesis may be abnormal flaccidity on the affected side.
- The response to painful stimuli—this may be asymmetrical.
- The facial appearance—drooping of one side of the face, unilateral dribbling, or blowing in and out of the paralysed cheek may occur.
- Asymmetry of the tendon reflexes.
- Asymmetry of the plantar responses. Both are, however, frequently extensor in coma of any cause.
- Asymmetry of decerebrate and decorticate posturing.

INVESTIGATION

In many instances the cause of coma will be evident from the history and examination (e.g. head injury, cerebral haemorrhage, self-poisoning), and appropriate investigations should be carried out.

If the cause is still unclear, further investigations will be necessary.

Blood and urine

- Drugs screen, e.g. salicylates, diazepam
- Routine biochemistry, e.g. urea, electrolytes, glucose, calcium, liver biochemistry
- Metabolic and endocrine studies, e.g. thyroid function tests, serum cortisol
- Blood cultures

Rarities such as cerebral malaria or porphyria should also be considered.

CT head scan
This may indicate an otherwise unsuspected mass lesion or intracranial haemorrhage.

CSF examination
Lumbar puncture should only be performed in coma after careful assessment of the case. It is contraindicated if an intracranial mass lesion is a possibility. A CT scan is often necessary to exclude this. CSF examination is likely to alter therapy only if undiagnosed meningo-encephalitis is present.

MANAGEMENT

The unconscious patient needs careful nursing, meticulous attention to the airway and frequent observation to detect any change in vital function. Longer-term management requirements are:

- Skin: turning, skin care, avoidance of pressure sores, removal of rings
- Oral hygiene: mouth washes, suction
- Eye care: taping of lids, prevention of corneal damage, irrigation
- Fluids: intragastric or i.v. fluids
- Calories—liquid diet through a fine intragastric tube, 3000 kcal (1255 kJ) daily
- Sphincters: catheterization only if necessary (Paul's tubing if possible); avoidance of constipation (evacuate rectum manually if necessary)

Brain death

This is described on p. 730.

Cerebrovascular disease

Stroke is a principal cause of death and chronic disability in all developed countries. Strokes cause about 10 deaths per 100 000 population per annum in Europe and USA in those aged 40 years, rising to 1000 per 100 000 per annum at 75 years. Arterial thromboembolism is the commonest cause of stroke. The incidence of stroke is decreasing, probably owing to the treatment of hypertension.

Cerebrovascular disease comprises:

- Thromboembolic infarction
- Primary intracranial haemorrhage
- Subarachnoid haemorrhage
- Subdural and extradural haemorrhage and haematoma
- Cortical venous and dural venous sinus thrombosis

Definitions

Stroke. This is a focal neurological deficit due to a vascular lesion. It is usually of rapid onset and, by definition, lasts longer than 24 h if the patient survives. Hemiplegia due to middle cerebral arterial thromboembolism is a common example.

A stroke is said to be 'completed' when the deficit has reached its maximum, usually within 6 h of onset. It is 'in-evolution' when it is becoming worse, usually within 24 h of onset.

These definitions, although valuable, are arbitrary. The clinical picture of 'stroke' may also be caused by tumour, abscess, subdural haematoma or, rarely, by demyelination.

Transient ischaemic attack (TIA). This is a focal deficit lasting less than 24 h. There is complete clinical recovery. The attack is usually of sudden onset. TIAs have a tendency to recur.

Pathophysiology

Difficulties occur in the diagnosis of cerebrovascular disease because similar clinical events can be caused by different pathological processes.

Completed stroke. A completed stroke is caused by:

- Embolism from a distant site and subsequent brain infarction
- Thrombosis of a cerebral vessel and subsequent brain infarction
- Haemorrhage into the brain

Table 18.25 Risk factors and predisposing causes in cerebrovascular disease.

Risk factors
Hypertension
Diabetes mellitus
Obesity
Family history
Cigarette smoking
Hyperlipidaemia
Oral contraceptives
Alcohol

Predisposing causes
Extracranial atheroma
Intracranial atheroma
Heart disease, e.g. mitral stenosis
Low cerebral perfusion, e.g. hypotension
Berry aneurysms
Arteriovenous malformation
Miscellaneous:
Hyperviscosity, e.g. polycythaemia
Arteritis e.g. SLE
Trauma
Bleeding disorders
Metabolic diseases, e.g. homocystinuria (very rare)

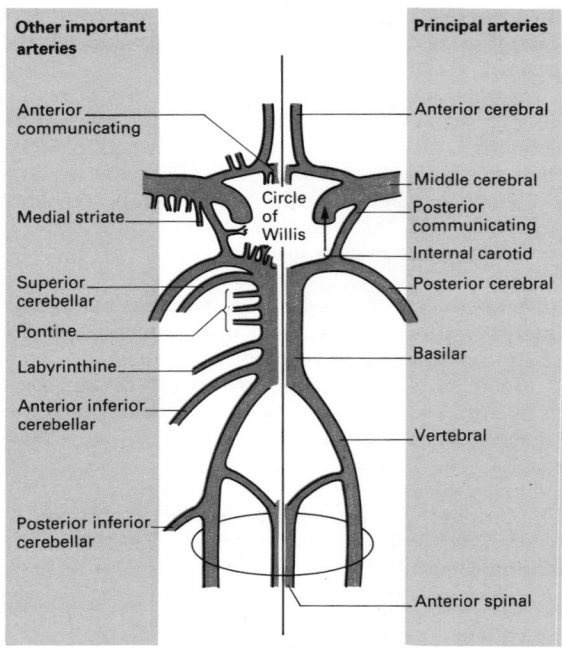

Fig. 18.13 The arteries supplying the brain.

TIAs. TIAs are caused either by the passage of microemboli or, less commonly, by a fall in cerebral perfusion (e.g. due to a cardiac dysrhythmia, postural hypotension or decreased flow through atheromatous vertebral arteries). Small areas of brain infarction or even haemorrhage may less commonly also cause a clinical TIA.

The underlying risk factors and predisposing pathology are shown in Table 18.25.

Thromboembolism from vascular disease outside the brain is the cause of about 70% of strokes and 90% of TIAs.

The principal sources of emboli are atheromatous plaques within the great vessels, the carotid and vertebral systems, or the heart (from mitral or aortic valves, or from mural thrombi formed on diseased heart muscle).

Vascular anatomy

An understanding of normal arterial anatomy and the likely sites of atheromatous plaques and stenotic lesions is important.

The circle of Willis (Fig. 18.13) is supplied by the two internal carotid arteries and by the basilar artery, which is formed by the union of the two vertebral arteries. Proximal to the circle, atheromatous plaques and stenoses are common at the following sites (see Fig. 18.15, p. 910):

- The origins of the common carotid arteries

- The origins of the internal carotid arteries
- Within the carotid syphon (in the cavernous sinus)
- Within the subclavian vessels
- The origins of vertebral arteries.

The distribution of the anterior, middle and posterior cerebral arteries, which supply the cerebrum, is shown in Fig. 18.14.

Autoregulation. The smooth muscle of small intracerebral arteries responds directly to changes in pressure gradient across the vessel wall. In the normal situation, constant cerebral blood flow (CBF) can be maintained with systolic blood pressures between 80 and 170 mm Hg (i.e. the CBF is independent of perfusion pressure).

In disease states, CBF autoregulation may fail. The contributory causes are:

- Severe hypotension (systolic BP < 75 mm Hg)
- Severe hypertension (systolic BP > 180 mm Hg)
- Increase in blood viscosity (polycythaemia, hyperviscosity syndromes)
- Raised intracranial pressure
- Changes in arterial PO_2 and PCO_2

TRANSIENT ISCHAEMIC ATTACKS (TIAs)

Symptoms. TIAs cause sudden loss of function in one region of the brain. Symptoms usually reach their peak in seconds and last for minutes or hours (but by definition < 24 h).

The general site of the cerebral lesion is often suggested by the clinical pattern of the attack.

Signs. The diagnosis of a TIA is often based upon the description of a past event. During an attack the loss of function can be demonstrated. Consciousness is usually preserved.

There may be clinical evidence of a source of embolus, such as:

- Valvular heart disease or endocarditis
- Recent myocardial infarction
- Atrial fibrillation (or other dysrhythmia)
- Carotid artery stenosis (arterial bruit)
- Difference between right and left brachial blood pressure (subclavian stenosis)

There may be other clinical evidence of associated disease, such as:

- Atheroma
- Hypertension
- Postural hypotension
- Bradycardia or low cardiac output
- Diabetes mellitus
- Arteritis (rare)
- Polycythaemia (rare)

Specific types of TIA
The clinical features of many of the forms of TIA are given in Table 18.26. Hemiparesis, vertigo or aphasia are the commonest complaints.

Table 18.26 Features of transient ischaemic attacks.

Anterior circulation (carotid system)	Posterior circulation (vertebrobasilar system)
Amaurosis fugax	Diplopia, vertigo, vomiting
Aphasia	Choking and dysarthria
Hemiparesis	Ataxia
Hemisensory loss	Hemisensory loss
Hemianopic visual loss	Hemianopic visual loss
	Transient global amnesia
	Tetraparesis
	Loss of consciousness (rare)

Two examples are mentioned briefly here.

Amaurosis fugax. This is a sudden transient loss of vision in one eye due to the passage of emboli through the retinal arteries. The emboli are sometimes visible through an ophthalmoscope. Amaurosis fugax is suggestive of a TIA in the anterior circulation and is often the first clinical evidence of carotid stenosis. It may also herald a hemiparesis.

Transient global amnesia. Episodes of amnesia with

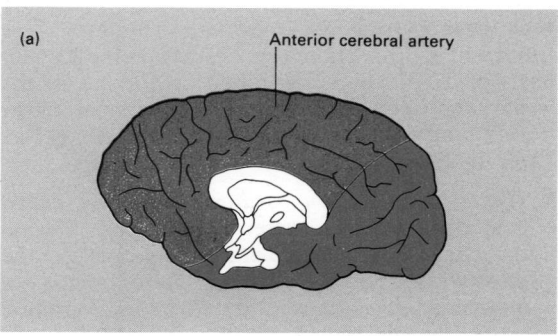

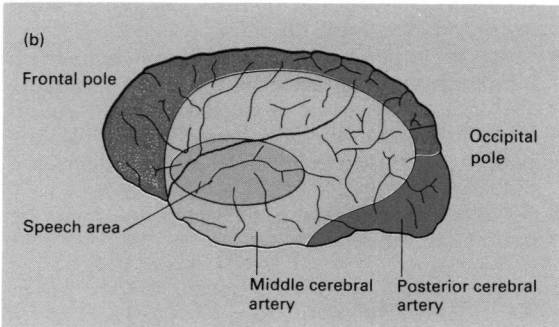

Fig. 18.14 The distribution of the three major cerebral arteries. (a) Medial view. (b) Lateral view.

confusion lasting for several hours are probably caused by ischaemia in the posterior circulation.

Differential diagnosis
TIAs must be distinguished (usually on wholly clinical grounds) from other causes of transient loss of function.

Focal epilepsy is usually accompanied by 'irritative phenomena' (e.g. jerking of the limbs) and characteristically there is a 'march' of events, with some progression. In a TIA the maximum deficit is usually apparent immediately.

Migraine, with a focal prodrome, sometimes causes diagnostic confusion. Headache is distinctly unusual in a TIA and there are usually no visual disturbances suggestive of migraine.

Prognosis
A TIA is an important prognostic event. Prospective studies have shown that five years after the TIA:

- One out of six patients will have suffered a stroke
- One out of four patients will have died (usually from heart disease or stroke)

A TIA in the anterior circulation is generally of more serious prognostic significance than a TIA in the posterior circulation.

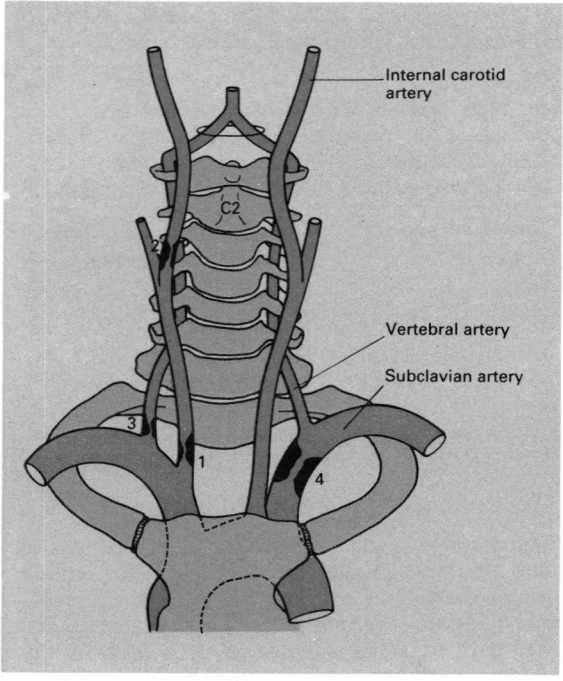

Fig. 18.15 The principal sites of atheroma in extracerebral vessels: (1) common carotid artery; (2) internal carotid artery; (3) vertebral artery; (4) subclavian artery.

CEREBRAL INFARCTION

Main cerebral infarction from thromboembolism typically produces a stroke, but small infarcts may present as TIAs or may even be symptomless. The clinical picture is very variable and depends on the site and extent of the infarct. It is no longer usual to attempt to subdivide the site into the precise distribution of a single branch vessel. Nevertheless, the site of cerebral infarction may be inferred from the pattern of the physical signs (e.g. cortex, internal capsule, brain stem).

SYMPTOMS AND SIGNS

The commonest stroke is the hemiplegia caused by infarction of the internal capsule following thromboembolism of a branch of the middle cerebral artery. A similar picture is caused by internal carotid occlusion (Fig. 18.15).

The signs are those of an acute upper motor neurone lesion of one side, including the face. Aphasia is usual when the dominant hemisphere is affected. The limbs are at first flaccid and areflexic. Headache is unusual and consciousness is not lost.

After a variable period the reflexes recover and become exaggerated and an extensor plantar response appears. Weakness is maximal at first, and recovers gradually over the course of days, weeks or months.

Brain-stem infarction
Infarction in the brain stem causes complex patterns of dysfunction depending on the site of the lesion and its relationship to the cranial nerve nuclei, long tracts and brain-stem connections (see Table 18.27).

- *The lateral medullary syndrome,* formerly called posterior inferior cerebellar artery (PICA) thrombosis, or Wallenberg's syndrome, is the most widely recognized syndrome of brain-stem infarction. It is caused by PICA or vertebral artery thromboembolism (Fig. 18.16). There is sudden vertigo, vomiting and ipsilateral ataxia, with contralateral loss of pain and temperature sensation (see Table 18.28).
- *Coma* may be caused by bilateral brain-stem infarction that damages the reticular formation.
- *The 'locked in syndrome'* is caused by upper brain-stem infarction; despite being conscious, the patient cannot speak, swallow or move the limbs.
- *Pseudobulbar palsy* (see p. 895) may be caused by brain-stem infarction.

Other types of infarction
Lacunar infarction. Lacunes are small (< 1.5 cm^3) areas of infarction seen at postmortem in patients with hypertension. Pure motor stroke, pure sen-

Table 18.27 Features of brain stem infarction.

Clinical feature	Structure involved
Hemiparesis or tetraparesis	Corticospinal tracts
Sensory loss	Medial lemniscus and spinothalamic tracts
Diplopia	Oculomotor system
Facial numbness	Fifth nerve nuclei
Facial weakness (LMN)	Seventh nerve nucleus
Nystagmus, vertigo	Vestibular connections
Dysphagia, dysarthria	Ninth and tenth nerve nuclei
Dysarthria, ataxia, hiccups, vomiting	Brain stem and cerebellar connections
Horner's syndrome	Sympathetic fibres
Altered consciousness	Reticular formation

Table 18.28 Features of the lateral medullary syndrome.

Ipsilateral	Contralateral
Facial numbness (V)	Spinothalamic sensory loss
Diplopia (VI)	Hemiparesis (mild, unusual)
Nystagmus	
Ataxia	
Horner's syndrome	
IX and Xth nerve lesions	

sory stroke, sudden unilateral ataxia and sudden dysarthria with a clumsy hand are typically caused by single lacunar infarcts. Lacunar infarction may be symptomless.

Multi-infarct dementia. Multiple lacunes or larger infarcts cause the picture of generalized intellectual loss that is sometimes seen in patients with cerebrovascular disease. The condition tends to occur with a stepwise progression with each subsequent infarct. The final picture is of dementia, pseudobulbar palsy and a shuffling gait with small steps. There may be confusion clinically with Parkinson's disease, and this syndrome has been called 'atherosclerotic parkinsonism' in the past.

Hemianopic visual loss or cortical blindness (Anton's syndrome, see p. 885). This may follow infarction of the posterior cerebral arteries.

Weber's syndrome. This consists of an ipsilateral third nerve paralysis with a contralateral hemiplegia due to a lesion in one half of the midbrain. Paralysis of upward gaze, due to a lesion localized in the region of the red nucleus, may also occur.

Watershed infarction. This describes the multiple cortical infarcts that occur during prolonged episodes of very low cerebral perfusion (e.g. following massive myocardial infarction or hypotensive therapy). The border zones between the areas supplied by the anterior, middle and posterior cerebral arteries are damaged. A syndrome of cortical visual loss and memory and intellectual impairment is typical.

IMMEDIATE MANAGEMENT

The initial decision whether to admit a stroke patient to hospital depends upon the clinical state and facilities available at home. Often the practical

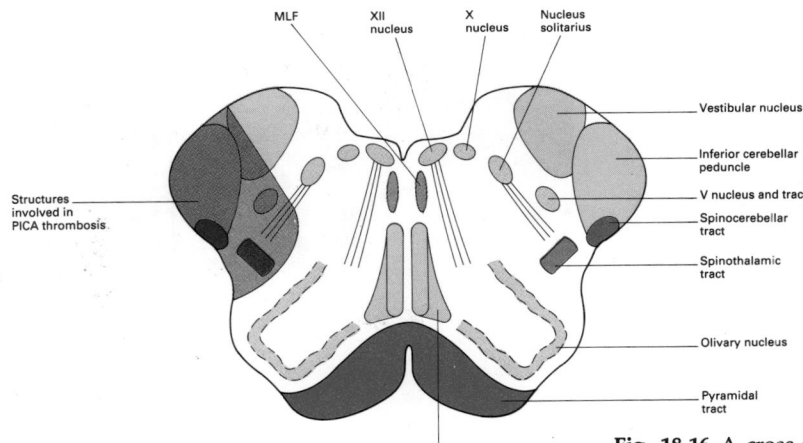

Fig. 18.16 A cross-section of medulla showing posterior inferior cerebellar artery (PICA) thrombosis. MLF = medial longitudinal fasciculus. (Modified from Ross Russell RW & Wiles CM (1986) *Neurology* (Integrated Science Series). London: Heinemann.)

Table 18.29 Preliminary investigation in stroke.

Test	Yield
Urinalysis, blood sugar	Diabetes mellitus
Haemoglobin	Polycythaemia
White cell count	Infection
ESR, CRP	Inflammation
Serology for syphilis	Possible neurosyphilis
Chest X-ray	Neoplasms
ECG	Recent infarct, dysrhythmia

difficulties of caring for the disabled for what may be a prolonged period determine these immediate decisions. In practice, many TIAs and mild strokes can be managed at home and specialist advice sought when necessary.

The management of the unconscious patient is described on p. 907.

EXAMINATION

In the examination, particular care should be taken to find a possible source of embolus (e.g. carotid bruit, atrial fibrillation, valve lesion or evidence of endocarditis) and to determine whether hypertension or postural hypotension is or has been present. There may be evidence of other emboli or a history of previous TIAs.

The brachial blood pressure should be measured in each arm; a difference of more than 20 mm Hg is suggestive of stenosis of a subclavian artery.

INVESTIGATION

The usual investigations in thromboembolic stroke and their potential yields are listed in Table 18.29.

Blood cultures should be taken if there is any possibility of endocarditis.

Autoantibody studies should be considered in young patients (e.g. presentation of systemic lupus erythematosus, p. 391).

Specialist investigation of thromboembolic stroke
Lumbar puncture is no longer a routine investigation in stroke. It is indicated only in special circumstances (e.g. when blood syphilitic serology is positive).

Investigation such as CT scanning and angiography are expensive and the information gained rarely changes the management in the elderly patients in whom stroke and TIA are most common. These studies are not often indicated in patients over 65 years unless there is doubt about the aetiology of the stroke.

All young stroke and TIA patients (below 60 years) should, however, be considered for both CT scanning and angiography. A specialist opinion may be necessary to decide the timing and indications.

CT scanning. CT scanning will usually site a lesion and distinguish between a haemorrhage and infarction. It will also rule out (or show unexpected) mass lesions, e.g. subdural haematoma, tumour or abscess.

Carotid doppler and duplex scanning. These ultrasound studies are of value in screening for carotid artery disease: in skilled hands they are highly effective in demonstrating internal carotid artery stenosis, the principal surgical target in stroke patients.

Angiography. Angiography (conventional carotid arteriography or DSA) is valuable in anterior circulation TIAs to diagnose surgically accessible arterial stenoses (mainly internal carotid artery stenosis).

There is a high probability of finding a carotid stenosis when there is a loud localized carotid bruit in the neck.

The majority of normotensive young patients (below 60 years) with TIA or stroke in the anterior circulation who recover well should be considered for angiography, though the yield in terms of internal carotid (and other accessible) arterial stenoses is under 5%. In more elderly patients, the risks of the procedure and the relatively poor results of vascular surgery in preventing further stroke usually make further investigation unwise.

Vertebral and arch angiography are rarely performed following posterior circulation TIAs and strokes unless there is a clinical suggestion of subclavian artery disease.

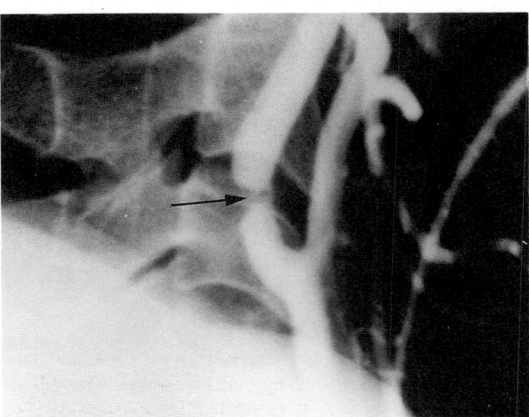

Fig. 18.17 Carotid arteriogram showing a tight stenosis of internal carotid artery (arrow).

TREATMENT

Surgical approaches

Internal carotid endarterectomy. This is considered in patients who are shown to have internal carotid artery stenosis (Fig. 18.17) that narrows the arterial lumen by more than 70%. The results of surgery are still being evaluated. The procedure has a mortality around 5%.

Extracranial–intracranial bypass. Anastomosis of the superficial temporal artery (external carotid) through a burr hole to a cortical branch of the middle cerebral artery (internal carotid) was widely advocated in the decade 1975–85 when there had been internal carotid occlusion. The indications for the procedure are still being assessed but a recent trial suggests no overall benefit.

Medical therapy

All risk factors (see Table 18.25) should be identified and, if possible, treated.

Hypertension. The control of high blood pressure is the single most important factor in the prevention of stroke. The annual incidence of stroke is falling in countries where active treatment of hypertension is undertaken.

Other measures. Anticoagulants are used when there is atrial fibrillation, other paroxysmal dysrhythmias or when there are certain cardiac valve lesions (uninfected) or cardiomyopathies. They can also be used in 'stroke in evolution'. Anticoagulants are potentially dangerous in the 2 weeks following cerebral infarction because of the risk of provoking cerebral haemorrhage. There are wide differences in clinical practice regarding their use. Aspirin (see p. 345) may offer some protection against further episodes of TIA or cerebral infarction.

Ticlopidine (see p. 345) 250 mg twice daily has been shown to reduce the rate of subsequent stroke or myocardial infarction in men and women who have had a recent thromboembolic stroke, but further studies are necessary.

Polycythaemia should be treated (p. 325).

Baclofen (a GABA antagonist) is sometimes helpful in the management of severe spasticity following stroke (p. 946).

REHABILITATION

Physiotherapy and speech therapy

Skilled physiotherapy is of particular value in the first few months following the stroke. It is helpful in relieving spasticity, preventing contractures and teaching stroke patients to use walking aids. The effect of physiotherapy on the longer-term outcome is inadequately researched.

Speech therapy is frequently recommended in aphasia. It is possible that the spontaneous return of speech is hastened as much by normal conversation with a relative as by a therapist, though the trained therapist has a vital understanding of the problems and frustration of the aphasic patient.

Both physiotherapy and speech therapy have an undoubted psychological role. Stroke is frequently a devastating event and, particularly when it occurs during working life, radically alters the pattern of the patient's remaining years. Many patients become unemployable and cannot lead independent lives. The financial consequences to the sufferer are usually considerable. The loss of self-esteem makes secondary depression common.

Following recovery from stroke, various aids and modifications may be necessary at home, for example stair rails, portable lavatories, bath rails, hoists, sliding boards, wheelchairs, tripods, modification of doorways and sleep arrangements, stair lifts and kitchen modifications. A visit to the patient's home with the occupational therapist and their primary care physician to discuss these problems is valuable.

PROGNOSIS

Between one-third and one-half of patients will die in the first month following a stroke. This early mortality is lower for thromboembolic infarction (under a quarter) than for intracerebral haemorrhage (around three-quarters). A poor outcome is likely when there is coma, a defect in conjugate gaze and a severe hemiplegia. Recurrent strokes are common (10% in the first year) and, in addition, many patients die subsequently of a myocardial infarction. Of initial survivors 30–40% are alive after 3 years.

Gradual improvement usually follows stroke, although the patient may be left with a severe residual deficit. Of those who survive a stroke, about one-third return to independent mobility and one-third have severe disability requiring permanent institutional care.

If, in general, there is sufficient language to be intelligible at 3 weeks, the outlook for recovery of fluent speech is good. Many stroke patients are, however, left with word-finding difficulties.

PRIMARY INTRACRANIAL HAEMORRHAGE

Intracerebral haemorrhage

AETIOLOGY

Rupture of microaneurysms (Charcot–Bouchard aneurysms, 0.8–1.0 mm in diameter) is the principal cause of primary intracerebral haemorrhage. This occurs typically in patients with hypertension and occurs at well-defined sites—basal ganglia, pons, cerebellum and subcortical white matter.

Saccular ('berry') aneurysms and arteriovenous malformations also bleed into the brain.

RECOGNITION

Although CT scanning is of great help in establishing the diagnosis, there is no entirely reliable way of distinguishing between haemorrhage and infarction, as both produce a focal deficit. Cerebral haemorrhage, however, tends to be accompanied by a severe headache and to cause a more severe general deficit (e.g. coma) than a thromboembolic stroke.

MANAGEMENT

The general management of cerebral haemorrhage is as for cerebral infarction, although the immediate prognosis is not as good. Only when an intracerebral haematoma behaves as an expanding mass lesion causing deepening coma and coning should urgent surgical removal be considered. Anticoagulant drugs are of course contraindicated.

Cerebellar haemorrhage

It is important to recognize cerebellar haemorrhage because it causes an acute hydrocephalus. There is headache and rapid reduction of consciousness with signs of brain-stem origin (e.g. nystagmus, ocular palsies). The gaze deviates to the side of the lesion. Emergency surgery may be necessary to remove a cerebellar haematoma.

SUBARACHNOID HAEMORRHAGE

The term subarachnoid haemorrhage (SAH) describes spontaneous rather than traumatic arterial bleeding into the subarachnoid space.

INCIDENCE

SAH accounts for 10% of cerebrovascular disease and has an annual incidence of 15 per 100 000.

CAUSES

The causes of SAH are shown in Table 18.30. It is unusual to find any contributing disease.

Saccular ('berry') aneuryms (Fig. 18.18)
Saccular aneurysms form on the circle of Willis and its adjacent branches. The common sites of aneurysms are:

- Junction of the posterior communicating and the internal carotid artery—posterior communicating artery aneurysm
- Junction of the anterior communicating artery and the anterior cerebral artery—anterior communicating artery aneurysm

Table 18.30 Causes of subarachnoid haemorrhage.

Saccular ('berry') aneurysms	70%
Arteriovenous malformation	10%
No lesion found	20%

Rare associations
Bleeding disorders
Mycotic aneurysms (endocarditis, see p. 598)
Acute bacterial meningitis
Brain tumours (e.g. metastatic melanoma)
Arteritis (e.g. systemic lupus erythematosus)
Spinal SAH from a spinal arteriovenous
  malformation
Co-arctation of the aorta
Marfan's syndrome, Ehlers–Danlos syndrome
Polycystic kidneys

- Bifurcation of the middle cerebral artery—middle cerebral artery aneurysm

Other sites are on the basilar artery, the posterior inferior cerebellar artery, the intracavernous internal carotid artery and the ophthalmic artery. Saccular aneurysms are an incidental finding in 1% of autopsies and may be multiple.

Aneurysms cause symptoms either by spontaneous rupture (when there is usually no preceding history) or by pressure effects on surrounding

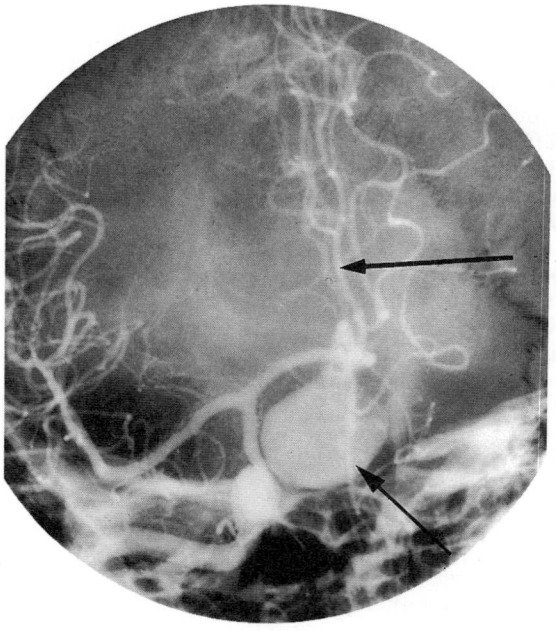

Fig. 18.18 Carotid arteriogram showing a large aneurysm of the anterior communicating artery (bottom arrow). The top arrow indicates the anterior cerebral arteries.

structures, e.g. a posterior communicating aneurysm may cause a painful third nerve palsy (see p. 888).

Arteriovenous malformation (AVM)

This is a lesion of developmental origin, usually within the hemisphere. An AVM may cause epilepsy, which is often focal. Once an AVM has ruptured to cause an SAH there is a tendency to re-bleed at a rate of 10% per year.

CLINICAL FEATURES OF SAH

The onset is sudden with a devastating headache, often occipital. This is usually followed by vomiting and often by loss of consciousness. The patient remains comatose or drowsy for several hours to several days. Less-severe headaches may cause diagnostic difficulties.

On examination, there is neck stiffness and a positive Kernig's sign. Papilloedema is sometimes present and may be accompanied by retinal haemorrhages and subhyaloid haemorrhage (massive retinal haemorrhage tracking beneath the hyaloid membrane).

INVESTIGATION

CT scanning shows subarachnoid or intraventricular blood. The CSF is yellow (xanthochromic) several hours after SAH. Lumbar puncture is not necessary if the diagnosis is made by CT.

Carotid and vertebral angiography is usually performed in all patients who are potentially fit for surgery (i.e. those who are young—below 55–60 years—and not in coma) to establish the site of the bleeding.

DIFFERENTIAL DIAGNOSIS

SAH must be differentiated from severe migraine. This is sometimes difficult. Acute meningitis may also cause a very abrupt headache.

COMPLICATIONS

Blood clot in the subarachnoid space can lead to obstruction of CSF flow and hydrocephalus. This can be asymptomatic but can be a cause of deteriorating conscious level a few days or weeks after the initial event. Diagnosis is by CT and a drainage procedure may be required.

MANAGEMENT

Nearly half the cases of SAH are either dead or moribund before they reach hospital. Of the remainder, a further 10–20% die in the early weeks in hospital from further bleeding.

Patients who are comatose or who have severe

neurological deficits have a poor prognosis. In others, where angiography demonstrates aneurysm, a direct neurosurgical approach to clip the neck of the aneurysm is carried out. In selected cases the results of surgery are excellent.

The immediate treatment of patients with SAH is bed rest and supportive measures. Hypertension should be controlled. Dexamethasone and anti-fibrinolytic agents are often prescribed, but their place in therapy is dubious. Nimodipine, a calcium-channel blocking agent, has been shown to reduce the mortality.

Severe spasm of the intracranial arteries sometimes complicates SAH and is a poor prognostic sign. Hydrocephalus may also follow a bleed.

It is usual to refer all cases of SAH to a specialist centre for a decision about angiography and possible surgery.

SUBDURAL AND EXTRADURAL HAEMORRHAGE AND HAEMATOMA

These conditions are of great neurosurgical importance as both may cause death unless treated promptly.

Subdural haematoma (SDH) (see Fig. 18.20b, p. 936)

SDM occurs when blood accumulates in the subdural space following rupture of a vein. It is almost always due to head injury, which may be minor, but the latent interval between injury and symptoms may be weeks or months. Chronic SDH is common in the elderly and in patients with alcohol abuse.

Headache, drowsiness and confusion are common; the symptoms are indolent and often fluctuate. Focal deficits such as hemiparesis or sensory loss may develop and epilepsy may occur. Stupor and coma gradually ensue.

Extradural haemorrhage (see Fig. 18.20a)

This follows a tear of a branch of a middle meningeal artery, usually underlying a linear skull fracture. Blood accumulates rapidly over minutes or hours in the extradural space. The most characteristic picture is of a head injury with a brief duration of unconsciousness followed by a 'lucid interval' of recovery. The patient then develops a progressive hemiparesis and stupor, and rapid transtentorial 'coning', with first an ipsilateral dilated pupil, followed by bilateral fixed dilated pupils, tetraplegia and death.

An acute subdural haemorrhage presents in a similar way.

MANAGEMENT

The diagnosis of extradural or subdural haemorrhage or haematoma is confirmed by CT scan and/or arteriography. MRI scanning is also used.

Surgical drainage is carried out. If it is performed early, the outlook is excellent. When far from specialist help (e.g. in wartime or at sea), drainage should be carried out when the diagnosis is suspected on clinical grounds alone; this procedure has been life-saving.

In the elderly, some SDHs resolve spontaneously and can be monitored with serial CT scans.

CORTICAL VENOUS AND DURAL VENOUS SINUS THROMBOSIS

These are unusual complications of skull and paranasal (air) sinus infection, dehydration or severe intercurrent illness. There is also an association with pregnancy and the contraceptive pill.

Cortical venous thrombosis
The venous infarct caused by the thrombosis leads to focal signs (e.g. hemiparesis) and epilepsy. There is often a fever.

Dural venous sinus thromboses
Cavernous sinus thrombosis. This causes ocular pain, proptosis and chemosis. An external and internal ophthalmoplegia with papilloedema develop.

Lateral and sagittal sinus thrombosis. This causes raised intracranial pressure with headache, papilloedema and often epilepsy.

MANAGEMENT

Treatment and investigation is directed at the underlying cause of the thrombosis. Anticonvulsants are used in epilepsy and antibiotics in infection. Anticoagulants are sometimes used.

Epilepsy and other causes of recurrent loss of consciousness

EPILEPSY

An epileptic seizure is a convulsion or transient abnormal event experienced by the subject due to a paroxysmal discharge of cerebral neurones. Epilepsy, by definition, is the continuing tendency to have such seizures, even if a long interval separates attacks.

INCIDENCE

Epilepsy is a common condition. Some 3% of the

Table 18.31 Classification of epilepsy.

Generalized seizures
1 Absence seizures[a]
Typical absences with 3-Hz spike-and-wave discharge (petit mal)
Atypical absences with other EEG changes
2 Myoclonic seizures
3 Tonic–clonic seizures (grand mal, major convulsions)[a]
4 Tonic seizures
5 Akinetic seizures
Partial seizures
These start by activation of a group of neurones in one part of one hemisphere. They are also called focal seizures.
1 Simple partial seizures (no impairment of consciousness),[a] e.g. Jacksonian seizures
2 Complex partial seizures (with impairment of consciousness)[a]
3 Partial seizures evolving to tonic–clonic seizures[a]
4 Apparent generalized tonic–clonic seizures, with EEG but not clinical evidence of focal onset[a]

[a] Common varieties of epilepsy.

population have two or more seizures during their lives. In Britain approximately 65 people suffer from their first seizure each day. Around a quarter of a million people in Britain take anticonvulsants. In Asia the prevalence is similar to that in Western nations; the condition is said to be over twice as common in Africa.

PATHOPHYSIOLOGY

The spread of electrical activity between cortical neurones is normally restricted. Synchronous discharge of neurones in normal brain takes place in small groups only; these limited discharges are responsible for the normal rhythms of the electroencephalogram (EEG).

During a seizure, large groups of neurones are activated repetitively and 'hypersynchronously'. There is a failure of inhibitory synaptic contact between neurones. This causes high-voltage spike-and-wave activity on the EEG.

Epileptic activity confined to one area of the cortex is associated with specific symptoms and signs (partial seizures). This activity may remain focal or may spread to cause paroxysmal activity in both hemispheres and a generalized convulsion. This spread is called secondary generalization of a partial seizure.

Seizure threshold
Each individual has a threshold for seizure activity. Experimentally some chemicals (e.g. pentylene-

tetrazol, a gas) induce seizures in all subjects. Individuals who are more likely than others in the population to have seizures in response to various stimuli, for example, flashing lights, are said to have a 'low seizure threshold', although this is a concept, not an actual measurement.

CLASSIFICATION

Epilepsy is classified according to the clinical type of seizure (Table 18.31).

Generalized seizures
Tonic–clonic seizures (grand mal seizures, generalized convulsions). Following a vague warning, the body enters a rigid tonic phase that lasts for up to a minute. The subject may utter a cry and fall, sometimes injuring himself. The tongue may be bitten and there may be incontinence of urine or faeces.

This is followed by a convulsion (the clonic phase) in which the muscles jerk rhythmically. This lasts a few seconds to a few minutes. Seizures are usually self-limiting, leaving the patient drowsy or in coma for several hours.

Typical absences (petit mal). This type of generalized epilepsy is almost invariably a disorder of childhood, and by definition an attack is accompanied by 3-Hz spike-and-wave in the EEG. The child ceases activity, stares and pales slightly. The eyelids may twitch. The attack lasts for a few seconds only. A few jerks may occur.

After an attack, the child carries on as if nothing had happened. Typical absence attacks are never due to identifiable local lesions. Children with typical absence attacks may in adult life develop generalized seizures.

The term *petit mal* should not be used to describe the absence attacks of partial seizures (see below).

Partial seizures (focal seizures)
The hallmark of a partial seizure is a discharge from a focal group of neurones. The seizure frequently has clinical features that provide evidence on its site of origin.

When these features precede a grand mal fit, the warning they give to the patient or relatives is called the 'aura' and the seizure is said to become secondarily generalized.

Jacksonian (motor seizures). These simple partial seizures originate in the motor cortex. Jerking movements typically begin at the angle of the mouth or in the thumb and index finger, spreading to involve the limbs on the side opposite the epileptic focus. The clinical evidence of this spread of activity is called 'the march' of the seizure. Conjugate gaze (see p. 888) may deviate away from a frontal lobe focus (an 'adversive seizure').

Paralysis of the affected limbs may follow for several hours (Todd's paralysis).

Temporal lobe seizures. These complex partial seizures are associated with strange disturbances of smell or feelings of unreality ('jamais vu') or undue familiarity ('déja vu') with the surroundings. Visual hallucinations (visions or faces) may be seen. Absence attacks or vertigo may occur.

Many other types of partial seizure are known, e.g. autonomic disturbances with piloerection or flushing, sensory disturbances (parietal cortex), crude visual shapes (occipital cortex) or strange sounds (auditory cortex).

AETIOLOGICAL AND PRECIPITATING FACTORS
(Table 18.32)

A cause for epilepsy is found in under one quarter of patients. A number of secondary factors may trigger seizures in those with a low seizure threshold.

Family history. About 30% of patients with epilepsy have a history of seizures in first-degree relatives. Usually the mode of inheritance is uncertain; a low seizure threshold appears to run in some families. Generalized typical absence seizures (petit mal) are sometimes inherited as an autosomal dominant trait with variable penetrance.

Trauma and surgery. Perinatal trauma (causing cerebral contusion and haemorrhage) and fetal anoxia are common causes of seizures in childhood. Hypoxic damage to the medial temporal lobes (medial temporal sclerosis) is an important cause.

Head injury is sometimes followed by epilepsy within the first week ('early' epilepsy) or many

Table 18.32 Aetiological and precipitating factors in epilepsy.

Family history
Trauma and surgery
Pyrexia
Intracranial mass lesions
Cerebral infarction
Drugs, alcohol and drug withdrawal
Encephalitis
Metabolic abnormalities
Degenerative brain disorders
Photosensitivity and auditory stimuli

months or years later ('late' epilepsy). To cause epilepsy, the injury must (almost always) be sufficient to cause coma. The presence of early epilepsy, a depressed skull fracture, cerebral contusion, a dural tear or intracranial haematoma increases the incidence of late post-traumatic epilepsy.

Surgery to the cerebral hemispheres is followed by seizures in about 10% of patients.

Pyrexia. High fevers in children under 5 years are sometimes associated with generalized seizures ('febrile convulsions'). In the majority there is no tendency for the seizures to recur in adult life.

Intracranial mass lesions. All mass lesions affecting the cerebral cortex may cause epilepsy—either partial or secondary generalized seizures. If the onset of seizures is in adult life, the chance of an unsuspected mass lesion being present is around 3%.

Hydrocephalus, of any cause, may be associated with seizures.

Cerebral infarction. Seizures may follow cerebral infarction, especially in the elderly.

Drugs, alcohol and drug withdrawal. Phenothiazines, monoamine oxidase inhibitors, tricyclic antidepressants, amphetamines, lignocaine and nalidixic acid may occasionally provoke fits either in overdose or in therapeutic doses in individuals with a low seizure threshold.

Chronic alcohol abuse is a common cause of seizures. These occur either while drinking or during periods of abstention. Alcohol-induced hypoglycaemia can also provide attacks.

Withdrawal of anticonvulsant drugs (especially phenobarbitone) and withdrawal of benzodiazepines may provoke seizures.

Encephalitis and other inflammatory conditions of the brain. Seizures are frequently the presenting feature of encephalitis, chronic meningitis (e.g. TB), cerebral abscess, cortical venous thrombosis and neurosyphilis.

Metabolic abnormalities. Seizures may occur with the following metabolic abnormalities:

- Hypocalcaemia
- Hypoglycaemia
- Hyponatraemia
- Acute hypoxia
- Porphyria
- Uraemia
- Hepatic failure

Degenerative brain disorders. Seizures can occur in Alzheimer's disease and in many rarer degenerative diseases. Epilepsy is three times more common in patients with multiple sclerosis than in the general population.

Photosensitive and other types of reflex epilepsy. Seizures are sometimes precipitated by flashing lights or a flickering television screen. This photosensitivity can be seen on the occipital recording of the EEG. Very rarely other stimuli provoke attacks.

INVESTIGATION

The diagnosis of epilepsy is established from evidence witnessed during an attack. It is preferable to interview a witness personally, if this is possible. Investigation of epilepsy of adult onset, although once always advocated, is not recommended, as the yield of treatable lesions is extremely low. The electroencephalogram (EEG) is the single most useful investigation in the study of a seizure, though it has distinct limitations.

The electroencephalogram in epilepsy

- During a seizure the EEG is almost invariably abnormal, because epileptic activity reaches the surface of the brain.
- EEG evidence of seizure activity is shown typically by a cortical spike focus (e.g. in a temporal lobe) or by generalized spike-and-wave activity.
- In petit mal, 3-Hz spike-and-wave activity is seen. It is always present during an attack and is frequently seen in the inter-ictal intervals (i.e. between attacks).
- A normal EEG between attacks does *not* exclude epilepsy. Many people suffering from epilepsy have normal inter-ictal EEG activity. In addition, an abnormal inter-ictal EEG does not prove that an attack was epileptic.
- EEG telemetry, with video recordings of attacks has greatly added to the value of this investigation in the study of attacks of disturbed consciousness whose nature is uncertain.

Other investigations

Routine investigations (blood picture, serum biochemistry, chest X-ray) may indicate an underlying

Table 18.33 Suggested scheme for the use of anticonvulsant drugs.

Type of seizure	Drug
Generalized tonic–clonic seizures	Phenytoin
Generalized absence (petit mal) seizures	Sodium valproate
Partial seizures	Carbamazepine Sodium valproate

Table 18.34 Therapeutic levels of anticonvulsant drugs.

Drug	Adult daily dose	Therapeutic level
Phenytoin	300 mg	40–80 μmol·L^{-1}
Carbamazepine	200 mg × 3	20–50 μmol·L^{-1*}
Sodium valproate	200 mg × 3	200–700 μmol·L^{-1*}

* Poorly defined.

metabolic or structural cause. Such tests are normal in idiopathic epilepsy.

CT scanning is always indicated in adults who have seizures of recent onset with physical signs, but in general the diagnostic yield of scanning after single or recurrent seizures is low. Investigation of first attacks is unrewarding.

TREATMENT

Emergency measures
The emergency treatment of a seizure is simply to ensure that the patient harms himself as little as possible and that the airway is patent in a prolonged seizure and in post-ictal coma. Wooden mouth gags, tongue forceps and physical restraint frequently cause injury rather than prevent it.

If there is any suspicion of hypoglycaemia, blood should be taken for the measurement of glucose, and intravenous glucose should be given.

Long-term anticonvulsant drugs
Anticonvulsant drugs are indicated in recurrent seizures. Phenytoin, carbamazepine and sodium valproate are the most effective drugs prescribed. Phenobarbitone, primidone and the benzodiazepine clonazepam are also used. There are differences in opinion about the most appropriate drugs for each particular variety of seizure: one suggested scheme is given in Table 18.33.

Phenytoin has the advantage of being cheap and effective. Its therapeutic level in serum is well

Table 18.35 Idiosyncratic unwanted effects of anticonvulsant drugs.

Drug	Side-effects
Phenytoin	Rashes Blood dyscrasias Lymphadenopathy Systemic lupus erythematosus
Carbamazepine	Rashes Blood dyscrasias, particularly severe leucopenia
Sodium valproate	Anorexia Hair loss Liver damage

defined and the serum level of phenytoin should be monitored in the majority of patients (Table 18.34). The therapeutic serum levels of other anticonvulsants are less clearly defined and routine estimations are not usually performed.

It is preferable to try to use one drug alone in the treatment of epilepsy, although a second (or third) drug may be needed in resistant cases.

Unwanted effects. Intoxication with all anticonvulsants causes a syndrome of ataxia, nystagmus and dysarthria.

Chronic administration of phenytoin can cause gum hypertrophy, hypertrichosis, osteomalacia, folate deficiency, polyneuropathy and encephalopathy. The more common idiosyncratic (i.e. non-dose-related) side-effects are summarized in Table 18.35.

The question of withdrawal of drug therapy is often raised by the patients. Unfortunately, withdrawal can be socially disastrous for the patient in preventing him from driving. Careful discussion with an experienced physician is important: withdrawal should not be considered until the patient has been free of all fits for at least 2 years.

Status epilepticus
This is when seizures follow each other without recovery of consciousness. It is a medical emergency with a mortality of 10–15%. When grand mal seizures follow one another there is a serious risk of death from cardiorespiratory failure. Several treatment regimes are available. Immediate i.v. injection of diazepam 10 mg followed by i.v. infusion of 200 mg·L^{-1} over 24 h is the first line of treatment. Chlormethiazole 0.8% should be given by intravenous infusion if status epilepticus continues or returns. Phenytoin i.v., phenobarbitone i.v., clonazepam i.v. are also used.

'Status' can also occur in absence seizures and in focal epilepsy. Ventilatory support must be available when status is treated. 'Epilepsy partialis continua' is a continuous seizure of a small part of the body, e.g. a finger, without loss of consciousness. It is often due to a cortical neoplasm.

Neurosurgical treatment
Several surgical approaches have been used in epilepsy. The most important is amputation of the anterior temporal lobe (usually of the non-dominant side) in those with partial seizures or partial seizures that are secondarily generalized. Indications include poor control on drug therapy and a clearly defined focus of abnormal electrical activity.

The social consequences of epilepsy

The great majority of patients with epilepsy can be managed by a general practitioner or as an outpatient, and have infrequent seizures that alter the pattern of their lives relatively little. In the small minority who have exceedingly frequent seizures, treatment in hospital or residential care is necessary.

There remains, however, a considerable social stigma attached to the diagnosis, an important fact to be considered when the nature of attacks of disturbed consciousness is uncertain. Employers are reluctant to take on patients who have seizures.

Present trends are to encourage both adults and children with epilepsy to lead lives as unrestricted as possible, though with simple, sensible provisos such as avoiding swimming alone and dangerous sports such as rock-climbing or solo canoeing. It is also wise to advise on simple domestic matters, e.g. that the bathroom door should remain unlocked.

Driving and epilepsy

Those who have suffered from more than one seizure are unable to hold a driving licence in Britain unless they satisfy the following criteria:

- They shall have been free from *any* form of epileptic attack whilst awake for a period of 2 years prior to the issue of a licence.
- In the cases of attacks whilst asleep, the attacks must have occurred *only* whilst asleep and the patient must not have had an attack for 3 years prior to the issue of a licence.

The rules for those holding Public Service Vehicle and Heavy Goods Vehicle licences (PSV & HGV) are stricter: any attack after the age of 3 years automatically bars an applicant indefinitely from holding such a licence.

It is the duty of a doctor to inform patients of these regulations: the patient should then write to the licensing authorities. Similar strict regulations exist for potential aircraft pilots, sea captains and other similar activities. The correct diagnosis of an attack at any age has therefore become of major social and legal importance.

OTHER CAUSES OF RECURRENT ATTACKS OF DISTURBED CONSCIOUSNESS AND FALLS
(Table 18.36)

Episodes of transient disturbance of consciousness and falls are common clinical problems. It is usually possible to distinguish between a 'fit' (a seizure), a 'faint' (syncope) and other types of attack from the history given by the patient and the account of an eye witness.

Syncope ('fainting', vasovagal attacks) and related disorders

Sudden reflex bradycardia and peripheral and splanchnic vasodilatation leading to loss of consciousness occurs commonly in response to prolonged standing, fear, venesection or pain. It almost never occurs in the recumbent posture. The subject falls to the ground and is unconscious for less than 2 min. Recovery is rapid. A few jerking movements are uncommon but do occur. Incontinence of urine is exceptional.

This is the 'simple faint' from which the majority of the population suffer at some time, particularly in childhood, in youth or in pregnancy.

Other forms of syncope

Syncope may occur after micturition in men (particularly at night) and when the venous return to the heart is obstructed by breath-holding and severe coughing.

The syndrome of carotid sinus syncope is believed to be due to excessive sensitivity of the sinus to external pressure. It may occur in elderly patients who lose consciousness on touching of the neck.

Postural hypotension occurs in patients with impaired autonomic reflexes, e.g. in the elderly, in autonomic neuropathy, or with ganglion-blocking drugs used in hypertension, with phenothiazines, levodopa or tricyclic antidepressants.

Transient cerebral ischaemia in the posterior cerebral circulation may cause episodes of loss of consciousness.

Cardiac arrhythmias (cardiac syncope, Stokes–Adams attacks—see p. 550) are important causes of recurrent episodes of loss of consciousness, particularly in the elderly. There is sometimes a preceding warning of palpitations (either fast or slow). The loss of consciousness is sudden and accompanied by pallor. Exceptionally, there are convulsive movements ('anoxic convulsions'). Flushing may occur when the patient recovers. The usual cardiac arrhythmias that cause loss of

Table 18.36 Causes of attacks of disturbed consciousness and falling.

Epilepsy	Drop attacks
	Night terrors in
Syncope	children
Micturition syncope	Psychogenic attacks
Cough syncope	Panic attacks
Breath holding (children)	Hyperventilation
Postural hypotension	
Carotid sinus syncope	Hypoglycaemia
TIA	Hypoglycaemia
Cardiac arrhythmias	
Effort syncope	Vertigo
	Hydrocephalus
Narcolepsy and cataplexy	Choking

consciousness are paroxysmal bradycardias (e.g. in complete heart block) or tachycardias (e.g. ventricular tachycardias, ventricular fibrillation). Supraventricular tachycardias are unusual causes of loss of consciousness.

Effort syncope (syncope on exertion) is of cardiac origin (e.g. aortic stenosis, hypertrophic obstructive cardiomyopathy).

INVESTIGATION

Syncope and related conditions where cerebral blood flow is impaired can usually be distinguished from epilepsy on the clinical history alone.

Cardiac monitoring may sometimes be necessary to detect an arrhythmia.

MANAGEMENT

The immediate management of syncope, or impending syncope, is to lie the patient down, to elevate the lower limbs and to record the pulse. In the rare circumstances, where cerebral blood flow cannot be restored, e.g. in a dentist's chair, syncope may be followed by cerebral infarction.

Drop attacks

These sudden episodes of weakness of the lower limbs with falling but without loss of consciousness occur in middle-aged women. They are believed to be due to sudden changes in tone in the lower limbs, presumably of brain-stem origin. Previously they have been regarded as forms of TIA, from which they are distinct.

Panic attacks, night terrors and psychogenic attacks

Panic attacks are usually associated with an autonomic disturbance, e.g. tachycardia, sweating and piloerection. Consciousness is usually preserved. Hyperventilation (see below) is common.

Night terrors are sudden episodes seen in children who awake as if from a dream in a state of terror.

Psychogenic attacks cause considerable difficulty in diagnosis. Attacks resembling grand mal fits may occur but more usually there are bizarre and irregular limb movements.

Hypoglycaemia (see also p. 858)

Hypoglycaemia causes attacks in which the patient either feels unwell or may lose consciousness, sometimes with a convulsion. There is often some warning, with hunger, shaking and sweating. There is prompt relief with i.v. (or oral) glucose.

Hypoglycaemic attacks unrelated to diabetes are rare. Most patients who feel unwell after fasting or in the early morning have no serious organic disease.

Hypocalcaemia and hyperventilation

A grand mal fit may accompany hypocalcaemia (see p. 824).

The alkalosis accompanying hyperventilation leads to a feeling of light-headedness, which may be accompanied by circumoral and peripheral tingling and tetany (e.g. carpopedal spasm) (see p. 824).

Vertigo

Acute episodes of vertigo may cause prostration: consciousness is sometimes lost for a few seconds.

Choking

Sudden prostration sometimes follows choking, particularly when a large bolus of meat obstructs the larynx. The patient goes blue, is speechless and may die in the attack if the obstruction is not relieved.

Treatment involves immediately grasping the patient around the abdomen and squeezing hard in an effort to eject the food (see p. 654, Heimlich manoeuvre).

SLEEP AND ITS DISTURBANCES

Sleep is required on a regular basis. The reason for this is unclear; it is postulated that the laying down of memory is one important component. Complex pathways between the cortex and reticular formation are involved in the production and maintenance of sleep. During a normal night's sleep there are periods of deep sleep associated with rapid eye movement (REM). Dreaming occurs during REM sleep.

In *insomnia* sleep is fitful. Less time than usual is spent in REM sleep.

In *sleep apnoea* the normal short periods of apnoea seen during REM sleep are prolonged. This occurs with brain stem lesions and with upper airways obstruction, when it is accompanied by snoring. The latter is particularly important in patients with chronic bronchitis and emphysema, who may become severely hypoxic (see p. 661).

Narcolepsy and cataplexy

Narcoleptic attacks are periods of irresistible sleep in inappropriate circumstances. They may occur when there is little distraction, after meals, while travelling in a vehicle, or without obvious cause. Genetically, narcolepsy is strongly associated with HLA-DR2.

Cataplexy is a sudden loss of tone in the lower limbs with preservation of consciousness. Attacks are set off by sudden surprise or emotion.

The two conditions are related and may be accompanied by hypnagogic hallucinations (terrifying hallucinations on falling asleep), hypnopompic hallucinations (on waking) and sleep paralysis (a frightening inability to move whilst drowsy). The EEG is normal in these attacks.

Treatment is with methyl phenidate, other amphetamine-like drugs, or small doses of tricyclic antidepressants.

Parkinson's disease and other movement disorders

Disorders of movement can be classified broadly into akinetic-rigid syndromes, where there is loss of movement with increase in muscle tone, and dyskinesias, where there are added movements outside voluntary control. Both are due to disorders of the extrapyramidal system.

Parkinson's disease is much the commonest of these conditions. A classification of movement disorders is given in Table 18.37.

AKINETIC-RIGID SYNDROMES

PARKINSON'S DISEASE

In 1817, James Parkinson, a physician in Hoxton, London, described the clinical appearance of patients with the 'shaking palsy'. The disease is common and world-wide, with prevalence increasing sharply with age to about 1 in 200 in those over

Table 18.37 A classification of movement disorders.

Akinetic-rigid syndromes
Parkinson's disease
Drug-induced parkinsonism, e.g. phenothiazines
MPTP-induced parkinsonism
Post-encephalitic parkinsonism
'Parkinsonism plus'
Childhood akinetic-rigid syndromes

Dyskinesias
Essential tremor
Chorea
Hemiballismus
Myoclonus
Tick or 'habit spasms'
Torsion dystonias

70 years. The condition is clinically distinct from other 'parkinsonian' syndromes.

There are few clues as to its cause:

- Patients who develop the disease have smoked less and die less frequently from lung cancer than the normal population.
- Minute doses of a pyridine compound (see p. 924) cause a severe parkinsonian syndrome. The significance of this to idiopathic Parkinson's disease is not clear.
- Survivors of encephalitis lethargica, which is presumed to be a viral disease, develop parkinsonism. However, it is not thought that the idiopathic disease is related to this or to another infective agent.
- The condition is not inherited.

PATHOLOGY

In the pars compacta of the substantia nigra there is progressive cell degeneration and the appearance of eosinophilic inclusion bodies (Lewy bodies). Degeneration also occurs in other brainstem nuclei. Biochemically there is loss of dopamine (and melanin) in the striatum that correlates well with the areas of cell loss and also with the degree of akinesia. The underlying cause of these biochemical changes remains obscure (see p. 897).

CLINICAL FEATURES

There is a combination of tremor, rigidity and akinesia, together with important changes in posture.

Symptoms
The commonest symptoms are tremor and slowness of movement. Patients also complain that the limbs feel stiff and ache and that fine movements are difficult. The slowness of movement causes the characteristic symptoms of difficulty in rising from a chair or getting into or out of bed. Writing becomes small (micrographia) and spidery, with a tendency to tail off at the end of a line. Other evidence of the disease often comes from relatives who have noted slowness and an impassive facial expression.

Signs
Tremor. This is a characteristic 4–7 Hz rest tremor that is usually decreased by action and increased by emotion. 'Pill-rolling' movements of the fingers and thumbs may be seen. The shaking is sometimes unilateral or more prominent on one side.

Rigidity. Stiffness of the limbs develops that can be felt throughout the range of movement and equally in opposing groups of muscles (in contrast to the selective increase in tone found in spasticity). This 'lead-pipe' rigidity is often more marked on one side and is present in the neck and axial muscles (where it is difficult to examine).

The rigidity is usually more easily felt when a joint is moved slowly and gently. Simultaneous active movement of the opposite limb increases the tone of the side under examination. When combined with tremor, the smooth plasticity of the increase in tone is broken up into a jerky resistance to passive movement, a phenomenon known as 'cogwheeling'.

Akinesia. The poverty and slowing of movement (bradykinesia) is an additional handicap, distinct from rigidity. There is difficulty in initiating movement. Rapid finger movements (such as piano-playing movements) become indistinct, slow and tremulous. The immobility of the face gives a mask-like facies with the appearance of depression. The frequency of spontaneous blinking is reduced, causing a 'serpentine stare'.

Postural changes. A stoop is characteristic and the gait is shuffling, festinant and with poor arm swinging. The posture is sometimes called 'simian' to describe the forward flexion, immobility of the arms and lack of facial expression. The patient sits with the trunk bent forward and motionless, without gesture or animation, but the limbs are tremulous. Balance is impaired, but despite this the gait remains on a narrow base. Falls are common as the usual corrective righting reflexes fail, the sufferer falling stiffly 'like a telegraph pole'.

Speech. Speech is altered to a monotonous slurring dysarthria, due to the combination of akinesia, tremor and rigidity. Dribbling is frequent, and dysphagia occurs as the disease progresses.

Other findings. Constipation is usual and urinary difficulties are common, especially in men. The skin is greasy and sweating is excessive.

Power remains normal until advanced akinesia makes its assessment difficult. There is no sensory loss, although patients often complain of discomfort in the limbs. The reflexes are normal (though they may be asymmetrical, following an asymmetrical increase in tone). The plantar responses are flexor.

Cognitive function is preserved, at least in the early stages. Dementia sometimes occurs in the late stages.

Natural history

Parkinson's disease progresses over a period of years, beginning as a mild inconvenience but slowly overtaking the patient. Remissions are unknown except for rare and remarkable short-lived periods of release. These tend to occur at times of great emotion, fear or excitement, when the sufferer is released for seconds or minutes and able to move quickly.

The rate of progression is very variable, with a benign form running over several decades. Usually the course is over 10–15 years, with death resulting from bronchopneumonia.

DIFFERENTIAL DIAGNOSIS

There is no laboratory test for the disease. The diagnosis is made on clinical grounds alone. The condition must be distinguished from other akinetic-rigid syndromes. Hypothyroidism and depression also cause slowing of movement.

Certain diffuse or multifocal brain diseases cause some features of 'parkinsonism' (i.e. the slowing, rigidity and tremor). Alzheimer's disease, multi-infarct dementia, and the sequelae of repeated head injury (e.g. in boxers) or hypoxia are the commoner examples.

TREATMENT

Older treatments with anticholinergic drugs altered the disease little, and frequently caused mental confusion. Benzhexol is still used in mild cases and as an adjunct to other therapy. Amantadine, originally introduced as an antiviral agent, is also sometimes helpful.

Levodopa

The introduction of levodopa in the late 1960s was a revolutionary therapeutic approach, apparently replacing the lost neurotransmitter dopamine. Today levodopa is usually combined with a peripheral decarboxylase inhibitor—benserazide (as Madopar) or carbidopa (as Sinemet). This combined therapy reduces the peripheral side-effects, principally nausea, of levodopa and its metabolites.

Treatment is commenced gradually (Madopar 125 mg or Sinemet '110' one tablet three times daily) and increased until either an adequate improvement has taken place or side-effects limit further increase in dose.

The great majority of patients with Parkinson's disease (but not other parkinsonian syndromes) improve initially with levodopa. The response in severe, previously untreated disease may be dramatic.

Unwanted effects of levodopa therapy. Nausea and vomiting within an hour of treatment are the commonest symptoms of the dose being too large. Confusion and visual hallucinations also occur. Chorea occurs in acute overdose.

As there are considerable problems with long-term treatment, levodopa therapy should not be started until necessary. Sometimes the drug appears to become ineffective, even with increasing doses. The disease progresses and the patient suffers from severe episodes of 'freezing' and falls. Fluctuation in the response to levodopa may also occur. The duration of action of the drug contracts, and the patient begins to suffer from a 'chronic levodopa syndrome', fluctuating between dopa-induced dyskinesias (chorea and dystonic movements) and severe and sometimes sudden immobility (on–off syndrome).

These are major and often insoluble problems in management. Approaches to treatment of the complications include the following:

- The interval between levodopa doses can be shortened and the individual doses reduced.
- Selegiline—a type B monoamine oxidase inhibitor—inhibits the catabolism of dopamine in the brain. This sometimes has the effect of smoothing out the response to levodopa.
- Bromocriptine—a directly acting dopaminergic agonist is sometimes used.
- 'Drug holidays'—periods of drug withdrawal—are sometimes helpful. They require close supervision since severe rigidity and akinesia follow the withdrawal of levodopa.

Psychiatric aspects

Depression is common in Parkinson's disease as the symptoms become worse and unresponsive to treatment. It is particularly difficult to treat, since type A monoamine oxidase inhibitor antidepressants (e.g. phenelzine) are absolutely contraindicated with levodopa, and tricyclic antidepressants (e.g. amitriptyline) have extrapyramidal side-effects.

All anti-parkinsonian drugs, particularly in high doses, may cause confusion with visual hallucinations, which may exacerbate an associated dementia.

Neurosurgery

Stereotactic placement of small lesions in the ventrolateral nucleus of the thalamus was commonly used in the two decades preceding the development of levodopa. The procedure was effective in reducing tremor but poor for relieving akinesia; it is now rarely performed.

Recent attempts to transplant fetal or autologous dopamine-containing tissue (adrenal medulla) to the cerebral ventricles or basal ganglia, though technically feasible, have not produced any major clinical improvement in patients with Parkinson's disease.

Physiotherapy and physical aids

Skilled and determined physiotherapy can improve the gait and help the patient to overcome particular problems.

Sensible guidance should be given about:

- Clothing—avoiding zips, fiddly buttons and

lace-up shoes.
- Cutlery—using built-up handles.
- Chairs—high, upright chairs are easier to rise from than deep, comfortable armchairs.
- Rails—should be fitted near the lavatory and bath.
- Shoes—should be easy to put on and have smooth soles.
- Flooring—patients' feet sometimes 'stick' to carpets and rugs and they prefer to walk on vinyl or linoleum.
- Walking aids are often a hindrance in the early stages but later a frame or a tripod may be helpful.

Drug-induced movement disorders

Reserpine, phenothiazines and butyrophenones induce a parkinsonian syndrome, with slowness and rigidity but usually little tremor. Methyldopa and tricyclic antidepressants also cause some slowing of movement. These syndromes tend not to progress. They respond poorly to levodopa. They disappear when the drug is stopped.

MPTP-induced parkinsonism. MPTP (1-methyl-4-phenyl-1,2,3,6-tetrahydropyridine) is an impurity produced inadvertently when opiate analgesics are synthesized illicitly. A few cases of a severe and largely irreversible parkinsonian syndrome have followed ingestion of minute quantities of MPTP. The relevance of this to idiopathic Parkinson's disease is not clear.

Other movement disorders due to neuroleptic drugs
Neuroleptic drugs (i.e. phenothiazines and butyrophenones) also produce other varieties of movement disorder. Three are described here.

Akathisia. This is a restless, repetitive and irresistible need to move.

Acute dystonic reactions. These sometimes follow, unpredictably, single doses of these drugs, even those used as antiemetics or vestibular sedatives (such as prochlorperazine and metoclopramide). Spasmodic torticollis, trismus and oculogyric crises (i.e. episodes of sustained upward gaze) may occur. These acute dystonias respond promptly to the intravenous injection of an anticholinergic drug (e.g. benztropine 1–2 mg).

Chronic tardive dyskinesias. These disabling disorders consist of mouthing and smacking of the lips, grimaces and contortion of the face and neck. They tend to occur some 6 months after commencing neuroleptic therapy and may be made temporarily worse when the offending drug is stopped. Only about half of the cases eventually recover.

Post-encephalitic parkinsonism

An epidemic of an encephalitic illness (encephalitis lethargica) occurred in 1918–1930 that left in its wake a severe extrapyramidal syndrome of parkinsonism with added dystonic movement disorders. Many of the survivors were permanently disabled. Occasionally, sporadic cases of the disease have been recorded recently in the UK; a recent epidemic may have occurred in Bulgaria.

'Parkinsonism plus'

This describes rare disorders in which there is parkinsonism and evidence of a separate pathology.

Progressive supranuclear palsy is the commonest disorder and consists of axial rigidity, dementia and signs of parkinsonism together with a striking inability to move the eyes vertically or laterally.

Other examples of 'parkinsonism plus' are the rare multiple system atrophies, e.g. olivo-ponto-cerebellar degeneration and primary autonomic failure (Shy–Drager syndrome).

Akinetic-rigid syndromes in children

A group of extremely rare disorders cause an akinetic-rigid syndrome in those under 20 years of age. The most important are Wilson's disease and athetoid cerebral palsy.

Wilson's disease
This is a rare and treatable disorder of copper metabolism that is inherited as an autosomal recessive disease. There is deposition of copper in the brain (particularly in the basal ganglia), in the cornea and in the liver (see p. 271). It is most important that all young patients with cirrhosis are screened for this condition, as the neurological damage is irreversible unless early treatment is instituted.

Children with the disease have an akinetic-rigid syndrome and/or dyskinesias followed by progressive intellectual impairment.

Diagnosis and treatment—see p. 272.

Athetoid cerebral palsy
Writhing movements of the limbs, sometimes with an increase in tone, are seen in cerebral palsy following kernicterus. This is now much less common following the prophylactic treatment of rhesus haemolytic disease.

DYSKINESIAS

Benign essential tremor

This common condition, often inherited as an autosomal dominant trait, causes tremor at 5–8 Hz that is usually worse in the upper limbs. The head is often tremulous (titubation) and also the trunk. Pathologically there is patchy neuronal loss in the cerebellum and cerebellar connections. Tremor is seen when the hands adopt a posture, such as holding a glass or a spoon. Oscillations are not usually present at rest nor do they worsen on movement.

Essential tremor may be seen at any age but occurs most frequently in the elderly. It is slowly progressive but rarely produces a severe disability. Writing is shaky and untidy but there is no micrographia. Anxiety exacerbates the tremor, sometimes dramatically.

Treatment is often unnecessary. Many of those affected are reassured to find they do not have Parkinson's disease, with which the condition is often confused.

Small doses of alcohol and beta-adrenergic blockers such as propranolol often reduce the tremor. The anticonvulsant primidone also helps some patients. Sympathomimetics (e.g. salbutamol) make the tremor worse.

Chorea

Chorea consists of jerky, quasi-purposive and sometimes explosive movements, following each other but flitting from one part of the body to another. The causes of chorea are listed in Table 18.38; the commoner conditions are outlined below.

Huntington's disease
Relentlessly progressive chorea and dementia in middle life are the hallmarks of this inherited disease.

The prevalence of the disease is about 1 in 20 000. It occurs world-wide. Inheritance is as an autosomal dominant trait with full penetrance; the children of an affected parent have a 50% chance of inheriting the disease as it rarely, if ever, jumps

Table 18.38 Causes of chorea.

Huntington's disease
Sydenham's chorea
Benign hereditary chorea
Abetalipoproteinaemia (see p. 210) and chorea
Chorea associated with:
Drugs—phenytoin, levodopa, alcohol
Thyrotoxicosis
Systemic lupus erythematosus
Polycythaemia vera
Encephalitis lethargica
Stroke
Trauma (subdural haematoma)
Tumour

a generation. The family history of the disease in previous generations is often concealed, either by design or default. Recent advances in gene mapping and linkage association suggest a gene defect, possibly at the G8 locus of chromosome 4.

Pathology. There is cerebral atrophy with marked loss of small neurones in the caudate nucleus and putamen. Important changes in neurotransmitters occur:

- There is reduction in the enzymes synthesizing acetylcholine and GABA in the striatum.
- There is depletion of GABA, angiotensin-converting enzyme and met-enkephalin in the substantia nigra.
- Somatostatin levels are high in the corpus striatum.

These changes may be secondary to the cell damage. In contrast to Parkinson's disease, dopamine and tyrosine hydroxylase activity are normal.

Management and course. There is steady progression, of both the dementia and chorea. No treatment arrests the disease, although phenothiazines may reduce the chorea by causing drug-induced parkinsonism. Tetrabenazine or sulpiride may help to control the chorea. Death usually occurs between 10 and 20 years after the onset.

There are at present no predictive tests for Huntington's chorea and some families choose to be sterilized in an effort to eradicate the gene. The discovery of a DNA marker makes prenatal diagnosis possible, but the exact inheritance is still being evaluated. Counselling in this tragic disease is vital.

Sydenham's chorea (St Vitus' dance)
Thomas Sydenham described this transient chorea of adolescence and childhood in 1686. Fewer than half of the cases follow within 3 months of rheumatic fever (see p. 583). It may recur, or appear, in adult life during pregnancy (chorea gravidarum) or in those taking oral contraceptives. In each case there is a diffuse mild encephalitis.

The onset of the chorea is usually gradual. Irritability, insolence and inattentiveness herald the onset of fidgety movements, which are sometimes predominantly unilateral. A minority of patients are confused. Although rheumatic heart disease is sometimes found, the child usually does not have a fever or other features of rheumatic fever. The antistreptolysin-O (ASO) titre and ESR are rarely raised.

Recovery occurs spontaneously within weeks or months.

Hemiballismus

Hemiballismus (also called hemiballism) describes violent swinging movements of one side of the body caused usually by infarction or haemorrhage in the contralateral subthalamic nucleus.

Myoclonus

Myoclonus is the sudden, involuntary jerking of a single muscle or a group of muscles. It occurs in a wide range of disorders and is sometimes provoked by a sudden stimulus such as a loud noise.

Benign essential myoclonus
Nocturnal myoclonus, i.e. sudden jerking of a limb or the body on falling asleep, is extremely common and not pathological.

'Paramyoclonus multiplex' is widespread, random muscle jerking usually occurring in adolescence. Fits do not occur.

Myoclonic epilepsy
Muscle jerking is a feature of many different forms of epilepsy.

Progressive myoclonic epilepsy
These very rare conditions include various familial and metabolic disorders where myoclonus accompanies a progressive encephalopathy.

An example is Lafora body disease, a syndrome of myoclonus, epilepsy and dementia, with mucopolysaccharide inclusion bodies in neurones, liver cells and intestinal mucosa.

Static myoclonic encephalopathy
Myoclonus may follow a severe brain insult such as severe cerebral anoxia following cardiac arrest.

Tics

Repetitive twitching movements of the face, neck or hand are part of our normal motor gestures. Patients or their relatives seek advice about them when they become too frequent or irritating. Simple transient tics, e.g. sniffing or a particular facial grimace, are common in childhood, but may persist into adult life.

The rare Gilles de la Tourette syndrome is the occurrence of multiple tics accompanied by sudden explosive barking and grunting with the utterance of sexually related obscenities. The condition develops in childhood or adolescence, in either sex, and is usually life-long. This is thought to be due to an organic disorder of the basal ganglia. Treatment with haloperidol is sometimes helpful.

Torsion dystonias

Dystonia implies a movement caused by a prolonged muscular contraction when a part of the body is thrown into spasm. A classification of these unusual conditions is given in Table 18.39.

Table 18.39 A classification of dystonias.

Generalized dystonia
Dystonia musculorum deformans
Drug-induced dystonia (e.g. metoclopramide)
Symptomatic dystonia (e.g. after encephalitis
  lethargica or in Wilson's disease)
Paroxysmal dystonia (very rare, familial, with
  marked fluctuation)

Focal dystonia
Spasmodic torticollis
Writer's cramp
Oromandibular dystonia
Blepharospasm
Hemiplegic dystonia (e.g. following stroke)

Dystonia musculorum deformans
This rare disease is frequently inherited (there are various modes of transmission) and commences in childhood as dystonic spasms of the limbs that affect gait and posture. It is gradually progressive, spreading to all parts of the body over one or two decades. Intellect is not impaired. Spontaneous remissions occasionally occur.

Spasmodic torticollis
Dystonic spasms gradually develop around the neck, usually in the third to fifth decade. They cause the head to turn (torticollis) or to be drawn backwards (retrocollis) or forwards.

Minor dystonic movements can also affect the trunk or limbs. A curious feature is that some patients have a 'trigger area', often on the jaw. Gentle pressure at this site relieves the involuntary movement.

Various psychiatric explanations have been advanced for this and other movement disorders, but it is now felt that they are organic conditions. Torticollis may remit but many cases remain for life.

Writer's cramp
This is a specific inability to perform a previously highly developed skilled movement, especially writing, due to a curious dystonic posturing. It occurs particularly in those who spend many hours each day writing, and is thus seen less frequently now than in former years. Other skilled functions of the hand are normal and there are no other neurological signs. Prolonged rest sometimes seems to help the condition but it may become a major disability.

Blepharospasm and oromandibular dystonia
These related conditions consist of spasms of forced blinking or involuntary movement of the mouth and tongue, e.g. lip-smacking and protrusion of the tongue and jaw. Speech may be affected.

TREATMENT
All dystonic movement disorders are particularly difficult to treat. Butyrophenones (e.g. haloperidol and sulpiride) are sometimes helpful. Blepharospasm can be helped by minute injections of botulinum toxin into the orbicularis oculi muscle.

Multiple sclerosis

Multiple sclerosis (MS) is a common disease of unknown cause in which there are multiple areas of demyelination within the brain and spinal cord. These are 'disseminated in time and place' (hence the old name 'disseminated sclerosis'). An acquired defect in the oligodendroglial cells that produce myelin is responsible.

The commonest age of onset is between 20 and 35 years. In the UK MS causes disability of varying degree in over 50 000 people.

PREVALENCE

The disease occurs world-wide, but the prevalence varies widely, being directly proportional to the distance from the equator. At 50–65°N (roughly Land's End to Iceland) the prevalence is 60–100 per 100 000 people; at latitudes less than 30°N the prevalence is less than 10 per 100 000; and at the equator it is a rarity. In the southern hemisphere the variation is similar, with progressive increase in prevalence away from the equator.

AETIOLOGY

The cause of the disease is unknown.

Familial incidence and HLA linkage
First-degree relatives of a patient have an increased chance of developing MS, although there is no clear-cut pattern of inheritance.

In Caucasians in northern Europe and the USA, there is a positive association between MS and antigens HLA-A3, B7 and DR2.

Infection
Although efforts to transmit MS experimentally have been uniformly unsuccessful, there is an abnormal immune response in MS patients, with an increase in the titres of serum and CSF antibodies to many common viruses, particularly measles.

Certain epidemic transmissible zoonoses, such as scrapie, a demyelinating disease in sheep, are pathologically similar to MS. HTLV-1 infection in man (tropical spastic paraparesis) is an example of a viral demyelinating disease.

Diet

It has been suggested that MS is related to the consumption of large quantities of animal fats. Surveys in Norway have shown that MS is distinctly uncommon in coastal fishing communities compared with agricultural areas. However, the role of diet is particularly difficult to evaluate.

PATHOLOGY

The essential features are plaques of demyelination, initially 2–10 mm in size (see Figure 18.19). These lesions are perivenular and have a predeliction for the following sites within the brain and spinal cord:

- Optic nerves
- Brain stem and its cerebellar connections
- Cervical cord
- Periventricular region

Plaques rarely destroy large groups of neighbouring anterior horn cells (so that muscle wasting is unusual) and never occur in the myelin sheaths of peripheral nerves. Re-myelination seldom occurs and the mechanism of the remission of symptoms is unclear.

CLINICAL FEATURES

No single group of signs or symptoms is diagnostic of MS. Despite this, the disease is often recognizable on clinical grounds. There are two patterns:

- Relapsing and remitting MS with lesions occurring in different parts of the CNS at different times
- Chronic progressive MS

Common presentations of MS are described below.

Optic neuropathy (ON)

Symptoms. The patient complains of blurring of vision in one eye. Mild ocular pain is usual. The symptoms progress, usually over days, to produce severe visual loss. Recovery occurs, typically within a month. Bilateral ON occasionally occurs.

Signs. The signs of ON depend upon the site of the plaque. When the lesion is in the optic nerve head there is disc swelling (optic neuritis). If the lesion is several millimetres proximal to the disc there are often no ophthalmoscopic features ('the doctor sees nothing and the patient sees nothing'); this is known as retrobulbar neuritis.

Optic neuritis is easily distinguished from papilloedema of other causes by the presence of early visual loss.

A relative afferent pupillary defect is often

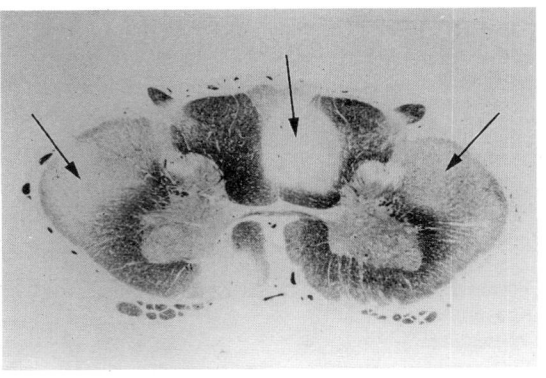

Fig. 18.19 Multiple sclerosis. Cross-section of the spinal cord showing demyelination (arrows) in the posterior column and lateral corticospinal tracts. (Courtesy of Professor W.I. Macdonald.)

present in the early stages. This persists after recovery.

Sequelae. There are usually no residual symptoms, but small scotomata and defects in colour vision can be demonstrated. Following the attack, disc pallor appears (optic atrophy), first in the temporal region and then spreading to affect the whole disc.

Brain-stem demyelination

An acute episode affecting the brain stem causes diplopia, vertigo, facial numbness or dysphagia. 'Pyramidal' signs in the limbs occur when the corticospinal tracts are involved.

A typical picture is sudden diplopia and vertigo with nystagmus, but without tinnitus or deafness. This lasts for some weeks before recovery. Diplopia may be caused by many different lesions—a sixth nerve lesion and an internuclear ophthalmoplegia are two examples.

Cord lesion

A spastic paraparesis is caused by demyelination in the cord. There is difficulty in walking and sensory disturbance. Urinary symptoms are common.

In the initial episode it may be impossible to decide, even with specialized tests, whether or not a lesion is due to demyelination. The appearance of subsequent lesions confirms the diagnosis. Remissions may last for many years; their length is unpredictable.

Unusual presentations

Epilepsy occurs more commonly in MS patients than in the general population. So, too, does trigeminal neuralgia (p. 890). Tonic spasms, brief spasms of a limb, are another unusual symptom of this disease.

The later stages of the disease are characterized by progressive disability with a spastic tetraparesis, ataxia, brain-stem signs, pseudobulbar palsy and incontinence of urine. Dementia is common. Death follows from uraemia and/or bronchopneumonia.

DIFFERENTIAL DIAGNOSIS

Few other neurological diseases of young people follow a similar relapsing and remitting course. Thromboembolism causes symptoms that are characteristically more sudden in onset. Other degenerative conditions such as Friedreich's ataxia are gradually progressive, without remissions.

Initially individual plaques (e.g. in the optic nerve, brain stem or cord) may cause diagnostic difficulty; they must be distinguished from compressive, inflammatory, mass or vascular lesions.

CNS sarcoidosis, systemic lupus erythematosus and Behçet's syndrome may mimic the relapsing pattern of MS.

INVESTIGATION

There is no single diagnostic test for MS. Examination of the peripheral blood and urine is unhelpful and there are no features on plain X-rays.

Examination of the CSF has long been used to support the diagnosis. Table 18.40 summarizes the investigations that are usually performed. The appearance and pressure of the fluid and the level of glucose are normal, and serological tests for syphilis are negative. The presence of oligoclonal bands of IgG indicate the production of immunoglobulin (to unknown antigens) within the central nervous system.

Electrophysiological tests

Delay in the visual-evoked response (VER) follows optic neuropathy. As some attacks are subclinical, a delayed VER may provide evidence of a second lesion within the central nervous system in, for example, an undiagnosed cord lesion.

Brain stem and somatosensory evoked potentials are also sometimes measured.

Peripheral nerve studies are normal. EEG recordings are unhelpful.

CT and MRI

Plaques of demyelination are sometimes seen as low-attenuation lesions on CT scans, although this is unusual. With chronic disease cerebral atrophy is seen.

MRI identifies plaques readily in MS and may be valuable in cases where there is doubt about the diagnosis (see Fig. 18.2).

MANAGEMENT AND PROGNOSIS

Once diagnosed, practical decisions need to be taken about employment, home and plans for the future in the face of a potentially disabling disease for which there is no curative treatment. It is now usual practice to inform patients of the diagnosis.

There is no method of predicting the course of MS but there is wide variation in its severity. Many MS patients live self-sufficient, productive lives while others are gravely disabled.

Wise counsel and honesty, tempered with reassurance of the benign course of many cases of MS, is important.

Many forms of therapy have been suggested for MS, including cryotherapy, pyrotherapy, vaccines, purified protein derivative (PPD), transfer factor, electrical stimulation, gluten-free diets, sunflower seed oil, arsenicals and hyperbaric oxygen. None of these has been shown to benefit patients.

Short courses of ACTH and corticosteroids are used widely in exacerbations and do sometimes appear to reduce temporarily the effect of a relapse. They do not influence the outlook in the long term. Immunosuppressants (azathioprine, cyclophosphamide) are also used, but there is no agreement about their value.

In any chronic neurological disease, treatment of intercurrent infections is important. Urinary infection frequently exacerbates the symptoms.

Muscle relaxants (e.g. baclofen, benzodiazepines and dantrolene) reduce the pain and discomfort of spasticity, particularly when there are flexor spasms of the lower limbs.

Table 18.40 The CSF in multiple sclerosis (MS).

Constituent	Normal	MS	Comments
Cell count	< 5 per mm^3	5–60 per mm^3	Rarely up to 100 per mm^3, typically mononuclear cells
Total protein	0.2–0.4 g·L^{-1}	0.4–1.0 g·L^{-1}	Normal in 40% of cases
IgG	< 15% of total protein	> 15% of total protein	Normal in 60% of cases
Oligoclonal IgG	Negative	Positive	Bands present in 80% of cases

Other measures

There is much that should be done for a patient with any chronic neurological disease. Practical advice at work, on walking aids, wheelchairs, car conversions, alterations to houses and gardens can be given. Support in a wide range of areas from fear and reactive depression to the sexual difficulties of the disabled is also helpful. Liaison between family practitioner, physiotherapist, occupational therapist and social worker is important.

Infective and inflammatory disease

MENINGITIS

Meningitis (inflammation of the meninges) may be caused by:

- Bacteria
- Viruses
- Fungi
- Other organisms
- Malignant cells
- Drugs and contrast media
- Blood (following subarachnoid haemorrhage)

The term is usually restricted to inflammation due to infective agents (see Table 18.41). Micro-

Table 18.41 Infective causes of meningitis in the UK.

BACTERIA
Neisseria meningitidis*
Haemophilus influenzae*
Streptococcus pneumoniae*
Mycobacterium tuberculosis
Treponema pallidum
VIRUSES
Echo
Coxsackie
Mumps
Epstein–Barr virus
Polio
Herpes simplex
HIV
FUNGI
Cryptococcus neoformans
(*Coccidioides immitis, Histoplasma capsulatum, Blastomyces dermatitidis* in USA)

* These organisms account for 70% of acute bacterial meningitis outside the neonatal period. A wide variety of bacteria are responsible for the remaining 30% of cases.

organisms reach the meninges either by direct extension from the ears, nasopharynx, a cranial injury or congenital meningeal defect, or by spread via the bloodsteam.

Immunocompromised patients (AIDS patients and those receiving cytotoxic drugs) are at an increased risk of meningitis, which may be caused by unusual organisms.

PATHOLOGY

In acute bacterial meningitis the pia-arachnoid is congested with polymorphs. A layer of pus forms that may organize to form adhesions, causing cranial nerve palsies and hydrocephalus. In tuberculous infection the brain is covered in a viscous grey-green exudate; numerous tubercles are found on the meninges. Cerebral oedema is common in bacterial meningitis.

In viral meningitis there is a predominantly lymphocytic inflammatory reaction in the CSF without the formation of pus or adhesions. There is no cerebral oedema unless viral encephalitis develops.

CLINICAL FEATURES (Table 18.42)

Meningitic syndrome

There is intense malaise, fever, rigors, severe headache, photophobia and vomiting. The patient is irritable and often prefers to lie still.

Neck stiffness and a positive Kernig's sign appear within a few hours. In milder cases (and

Table 18.42 Clinical clues in meningitis.

Clinical feature	Probable cause
Petechial rash	Meningococcal infection
Skull fracture Ear disease Congenital CNS lesion	Pneumococcal infection
Previous antibiotics	Partially treated bacterial infection
Immunocompromised patients	HIV infection Unusual organisms
Rash or pleurodynia	Enterovirus infection
International travel	Poliomyelitis Malaria
Occupational history (working with drains, canals, polluted river water; also swimming), prostration myalgia, conjunctivitis and jaundice	Leptospirosis

Table 18.43 Typical changes in the CSF in meningitis.

	Normal	Viral	Pyogenic	Tuberculosis
Appearance	Crystal clear	Clear/turbid	Turbid/purulent	Turbid/viscous
Mononuclear cells	< 5 per mm^3	10–100 per mm^3	< 50 per mm^3	100–300 per mm^3
Polymorph cells	Nil	Nil^a	200–3000 per mm^3	0–200 per mm^3
Protein	0.2–0.4 g·L^{-1}	0.4–0.8 g·L^{-1}	0.5–2.0 g·L^{-1}	0.5–3.0 g·L^{-1}
Glucose	> ½ blood glucose	> ½ blood glucose	< ⅓ blood glucose	< ⅓ blood glucose

^{a} Some polymorph cells may be seen in the early stages of viral meningitis.

many viral meningitides) there are few other signs, but it is most unreliable to rely on the clinical impression alone when assessing the severity of the infection.

In uncomplicated meningitis, consciousness is not impaired, although the patient may be delirious with a high fever. Papilloedema may occur. The appearance of drowsiness, lateralizing signs and cranial nerve lesions indicate a complication such as a venous sinus thrombosis (see p. 916), severe cerebral oedema or hydrocephalus, or an alternative diagnosis such as a cerebral abscess (see p. 936) or encephalitis (see p. 932).

Specific varieties of meningitis
Particular attention should be paid to rashes and associated clinical features (see Table 18.42), and a search should be made for infected foci.

Acute bacterial meningitis. The onset is sudden, with rigors and a high fever. A petechial rash, often sparse, is strong evidence of meningococcal meningitis. Septicaemia may present with acute septicaemic shock.

Viral meningitis. This is almost always a benign, self-limiting condition lasting 4–10 days. Headache may follow for some weeks but there are no serious sequelae.

Tuberculous meningitis. TB causes a chronic meningitis commencing with vague headache, lassitude, anorexia and vomiting. Meningitic signs may appear only after some weeks. Drowsiness, focal signs and seizures may occur. A similar picture occurs in cryptococcal meningitis, the commonest fungal meningitis in Europe.

Malignant meningitis. Malignant cells sometimes cause a subacute or chronic meningitic process. Meningitis, cranial nerve palsies, paraparesis and root lesions are seen, often in complex patterns. The CSF shows increased cells and protein and often a low glucose. Treatment is with intrathecal cytotoxic agents. The prognosis is poor.

DIFFERENTIAL DIAGNOSIS

Acute meningitis may resemble subarachnoid haemorrhage, severe migraine and other causes of a sudden severe headache. Meningitis should be considered in all patients who have headache and fever.

MANAGEMENT

Meningitis is an emergency that has a high mortality even in countries with highly developed systems of health care. Although viral meningitis is a self-limiting condition, untreated bacterial meningitis is lethal; in most series the death rate is around 15% even with treatment.

If meningococcal (or other acute bacterial) meningitis is diagnosed clinically, particularly in children, *immediate* treatment with i.v. benzylpenicillin should be started with subsequent urgent investigations. In this acute illness, minutes count.

If there is no suggestion of an intracranial mass lesion (when CT scanning should be performed), immediate lumbar puncture should be carried out. Typical changes in the CSF are shown in Table 18.43. CSF pressure is characteristically elevated. Blood should be taken for culture and glucose as well as for routine tests. Chest and skull films should be taken if possible.

Gram-staining of the CSF may demonstrate organisms (e.g. Gram-positive intracellular diplococci—pneumococcus; Gram-negative cocci—meningococcus). Ziehl-Nielsen stain demonstrates acid-fast bacilli (TB), though these organisms are rarely numerous. Indian ink stains fungi.

Many serological tests are now available for CSF. Syphilitic serology should always be carried out.

The clinical picture and CSF examination should allow at least a presumptive diagnosis of the cause of the meningitis to be made within several hours of presentation. Patients with impaired consciousness should be nursed as described on p. 907. General management includes diazepam for convulsions and analgesics for headache.

Treatment of bacterial meningitis

It is often possible to distinguish between viral, pyogenic, tuberculosis and other organisms from the clinical setting and immediate examination of the CSF. If bacterial meningitis is suspected, high doses of antibiotics are started. There should be close liaison with a microbiologist.

In an undiagnosed pyogenic infection in an adult, intravenous benzylpenicillin 2 g two-hourly and intravenous chloramphenicol 75 mg·kg^{-1} is given. If the diagnosis of pneumococcal or meningococcal infection has been made, penicillin alone is used. Chloramphenicol alone or third generation cephalosporins should be used in *Haemophilus* infections.

Tuberculous meningitis is treated for at least 9 months with antituberculous drugs; rifampicin, isoniazid and pyrazinamide is the usual combination (see p. 682).

It is no longer necessary to use intrathecal antibiotics.

Local infection (e.g. an infected paranasal sinus) should also be treated, surgically if necessary. Surgical repair of depressed skull fracture or meningeal tear may be necessary.

Polyvalent vaccines are available against recurrent pneumococcal meningitis (e.g. when there is a CSF leak following skull fracture) and against some strains of meningococci (p. 25).

Differential diagnosis of CSF pleocytosis

Difficulties occur in meningitis when a raised, often mixed (lymphocyte and polymorph) picture is found but no infecting organism. This is sometimes called 'aseptic meningitis'. The conditions listed in Table 18.44 should be considered.

Table 18.44 Causes of CSF pleocytosis.

Partially treated bacterial meningitis
Viral meningitis
TB or fungi
Neoplastic meningitis
Parameningeal foci (e.g. paranasal sinus)
Syphilis
Intracranial abscess
Cerebral venous or arterial infection
Following subarachnoid haemorrhage
Encephalitis, including AIDS
Rare causes (e.g. cerebral malaria, sarcoidosis, Behçet's syndrome, Lyme disease)

ENCEPHALITIS

Encephalitis is inflammation of brain parenchyma. It is caused by a wide variety of viruses and may also occur in bacterial and other infections.

Acute viral encephalitis

In many cases a viral aetiology is presumed but not confirmed serologically or by culture. The usual organisms cultured from cases of viral encephalitis in adults in Britain are echo, coxsackie, mumps and herpes simplex viruses.

Adenovirus, varicella zoster, influenza, measles and other viruses are rarer causes.

CLINICAL FEATURES

Many of these infections cause a mild self-limiting illness with headache and drowsiness. In a minority there is a more serious illness accompanied by focal signs, seizures and coma. Herpes simplex virus (HSV I) accounts for many of these severe infections in Britain and has a mortality of around 20% even with treatment. In the Far East the Japanese B arbovirus is a more usual, and epidemic, cause of severe encephalitis, with a high mortality.

DIFFERENTIAL DIAGNOSIS

This includes:

- Bacterial meningitis complicated by cerebral oedema and/or cerebral venous thrombosis
- Cerebral abscess
- Acute disseminated encephalomyelitis
- Toxic confusional states in febrile illnesses and in septicaemia

INVESTIGATION

Investigation in severe cases includes CT scanning (which characteristically shows areas of oedema). EEG (which shows slow-wave changes and/or 'periodic complexes') and viral serology of blood and CSF.

Brain biopsy is now seldom performed in the UK.

TREATMENT

Suspected herpes simplex encephalitis is immediately treated with intravenous acyclovir, the active form of which inhibits DNA synthesis. Phosphorylation of this drug is dependent upon the presence of viral thymidine kinase; thus the drug is specific for herpes virus infections. If the patient is in coma the outlook is poor whether or not drugs are given.

Supportive measures are required for comatose

patients. Seizures are treated with anticonvulsants. Prophylactic immunization is possible against Japanese B encephalitis and sometimes advised particularly for travellers to the Far East in endemic areas.

Acute disseminated encephalomyelitis (ADE)

This follows many common viral infections (e.g. measles, varicella zoster, mumps and rubella) and immunization against rabies, smallpox, influenza or pertussis. The clinical syndrome is often similar to acute viral encephalitis, with added focal brain stem and/or spiral cord lesions due to demyelination, but in which viral particles are not usually present. The prognosis is variable. Mild cases recover completely but in severe cases (those in coma) mortality is around 25% and the survivors often have permanent brain damage. Treatment is supportive, with steroids and anticonvulsants.

MYELITIS

Myelitis means inflammation of the spinal cord causing paraparesis or tetraparesis. It occurs with varicella zoster or as part of a post-infective encephalomyelitis. Poliomyelitis is a specific enterovirus infection of anterior horn cells (see p. 59).

Transverse myelitis is described on p. 945.

HERPES ZOSTER (SHINGLES)

This is a recrudescence of infection with varicella zoster virus within the dorsal root ganglia (of certain cranial nerves), the original infection having been acquired in an attack of chickenpox many years previously. The viruses causing chickenpox and shingles are identical.

CLINICAL FEATURES

The skin changes are described on p. 1025.

In the cranial nerves, herpes zoster has a predeliction for the fifth and seventh nerve. 'Ophthalmic herpes' is infection of the first division of the fifth nerve and may lead to corneal scarring and secondary panophthalmitis. 'Geniculate herpes' (the Ramsay–Hunt syndrome, see p. 892) leads to facial palsy accompanied by vesicles on the pinna, external auditory meatus and fauces.

The local complications of shingles are secondary bacterial infection, very rarely purpura and necrosis in the affected segment ('purpura fulminans'), generalized herpes zoster, and post-herpetic neuralgia.

A myelitis, meningoencephalitis or motor radiculopathy may be caused by varicella zoster.

Post-herpetic neuralgia

Post-herpetic neuralgia is pain in the zone of the previous eruption; it occurs in some 10% of patients. It is a burning, continuous pain responding poorly to all analgesics. Depression is almost universal. Treatment is unsatisfactory but there is a trend towards gradual recovery over 2 years.

NEUROSYPHILIS

Syphilis is described on p. 46.

Before penicillin therapy, some 10% of patients infected at sexual contact by the spirochaete *Treponema pallidum* developed tertiary neurological disease, often 10–25 years after the primary infection. A wide variety of syndromes were described, all of which are now clinical rarities. Neurosyphilis does, however, still occur, particularly in those who may have had many sexual partners.

For practical purposes, negative serological tests for syphilis in blood exclude the disease.

The main syphilitic syndromes are described below.

Asymptomatic neurosyphilis

This is the term used to describe positive CSF serology without signs.

Meningovascular syphilis

This presents as:

- A subacute meningitis often with cranial nerve palsies and papilloedema
- A focal form in which a gumma, an expanding intracranial mass, causes epilepsy, raised pressure and focal deficits, e.g. hemiplegia
- A paraparesis caused by a spinal meningovasculitis

Tabes dorsalis

This is a complex syndrome in which demyelination occurs in the dorsal roots. Many of the features are due to 'de-afferentation'. The elements of the syndrome are:

- Lightning pains (see p. 901)
- Ataxia, loss of reflexes, widespread sensory loss and some muscle wasting
- Neuropathic joints (Charcot's joints)
- Argyll Robertson pupils
- Ptosis and optic atrophy

General paralysis of the insane (GPI)

The grandiose title indicates that this is a syndrome of madness and weakness. The dementia is often similar to that associated with Alzheimer's disease (see p. 949). Progressive dementia, brisk reflexes, extensor plantar reflexes and tremor occur. Death follows within 3 years of the onset.

Argyll Robertson pupils are usually present. Seizures may occur.

Other forms

Mixtures of the syndromes described above occur.

In congenital neurosyphilis (acquired in utero), there are features of both tabes dorsalis and GPI in childhood; this is known as taboparesis.

In secondary syphilis, a self-limiting meningeal reaction occurs that may be symptomless or may cause a subacute meningitis.

TREATMENT

Benzylpenicillin 1 g daily by injection for 10 days in primary infection eliminates the risk of future tertiary syphilis. Established neurological disease can be arrested but not usually reversed with penicillin. Parenteral penicillin for 2–3 weeks is given for all forms of neurosyphilis. Allergic reactions (Jarisch–Herxhemier reactions) may occur; high-dose steroid cover is usually given with penicillin to reduce their severity.

AIDS AND THE NERVOUS SYSTEM

Individuals with HIV infection frequently present with or develop neurological disease. In addition, HIV-infected patients have a high rate of cerebrovascular disease. There is a variety of clinical neurological pictures, which may be confusing.

Meningitis

Acute aseptic meningitis. This is believed to be a primary HIV meningitis. Spontaneous recovery is usual.

Chronic meningitis. This may occur with HIV itself, fungi (e.g. *Cryptococcus neoformans*, or *Aspergillus*), TB, *Listeria monocytogenes*, *E. coli* or other organisms. Treatment is typically difficult and unsuccessful.

Diffuse encephalopathies

AIDS-dementia complex. This is a diffuse, progressive, usually fatal HIV-related dementia, sometimes associated with a cerebellar syndrome, thought to be due to a primary cerebral HIV infection.

Encephalitis. Cytomegalovirus, herpes simplex, *Toxoplasma* and other organisms cause a severe and often fatal encephalitis.

CNS lymphoma and progressive multifocal leucoencephalopathy (p. 935). These are progressive late complications of HIV infection. They are usually fatal.

Paraparesis

This occurs in AIDS in the following patterns:

Acute HIV transverse myelitis. This is believed to be a primary HIV myelitis. Spontaneous recovery is usual.

Myelopathy due to infection, e.g. with herpes simplex or zoster, cytomegalovirus.

CNS lymphoma. Lymphomatous masses that cause cord compression or malignant meningitis.

AIDS-related neuropathy

Three patterns occur:

- Mononeuropathy e.g. a common peroneal nerve lesion
- Mononeuritis multiplex (see p. 953)
- Polyneuropathy (see p. 953)

Management of AIDS. See p. 72.

OTHER INFECTIONS

The nervous system is involved in many infective diseases.

Rabies (see p. 67)
Rabies is transmitted to man from infected animals via penetrating wounds. The rabies virus multiplies in the wound and migrates via the peripheral nerves and dorsal root ganglia to the central nervous system. A fatal encephalitis follows in which, at autopsy, characteristic neuronal inclusion bodies (Negri bodies) are observed.

Tetanus (see p. 27)
Tetanus may follow even a trivial wound. There is liberation of a powerful toxin that travels within motor nerves to reach the central nervous system, where it binds irreversibly with certain sialic acid-containing gangliosides. The toxin blocks inhibition of spinal reflexes, resulting in spasms.

Botulism (see p. 28)
The paralytic symptoms of botulism are caused by a presynaptic block in neuromuscular transmission.

Lyme disease (see p. 52)
This produces a chronic radiculopathy. A paraparesis can occur.

Leprosy (see p. 41)
In tuberculoid leprosy a mononeuritis multiplex is seen. The infected nerves become large and palpable as hard cords. The peripheral nerves are also affected in lepromatous leprosy.

Table 18.45 Miscellaneous CNS infections.

Organism	Disease	CNS manifestation
Rickettsia	Typhus Scrub typhus Rocky mountain spotted fever	Meningo-encephalitis
Plasmodium falciparum	Malaria	Meningo-encephalitis
Toxoplasma gondii	Toxoplasmosis	Meningo-encephalitis (e.g. in AIDS)
Naegleria fowleri (a freshwater amoeba)		Meningo-encephalitis
Entamoeba histolytica	Amoebiasis	Brain abscess
Trypanosoma rhodesiense *Trypanosoma gambiense*	Trypanosomiasis	Subacute encephalitis
Echinococcus granulosus	Hydatid disease	Intracranial cysts
Taenia solium	Cysticercosis	Multiple intracranial cysts
Schistosoma mansoni	Schistosomiasis	Encephalopathy Cord lesions
Strongyloides stercoralis	Strongyloidiasis	Meningo-encephalitis

Poliomyelitis (see p. 59)
In this condition there is invasion of the anterior horn cells by the pathogenic virus. Many infections are subclinical but in a minority there is serious paralytic disease involving the respiratory muscles and sometimes causing a bulbar palsy.

Other examples of infection involving the central nervous system are summarized in Table 18.45.

MISCELLANEOUS CONDITIONS

Progressive rubella encephalitis
Some 10 years after the primary infection there is rarely a progressive syndrome of mental impairment, fits, optic atrophy, cerebellar and pyramidal signs. There is evidence of local antibody production against rubella viral antigen within the CNS.

Subacute sclerosing pan-encephalitis (SSPE)
The persistence of measles antigen in the CNS is believed to be the cause of this rare late sequel to measles infection. Progressive mental deterioration, fits, myoclonus and pyramidal signs occur, usually in a child. Diagnosis is confirmed by demonstrating a high titre of measles antibody in the blood and CSF.

Creutzfeldt–Jakob disease (CJD)
This is a slowly progressive dementia characterized pathologically by 'spongiform encephalopathy'. It

occurs world-wide and is transmitted by an agent resistant to many of the usual sterilization processes. The name given to such agents is 'slow' virus. Infection has been transmitted from post-mortem and surgical specimens and corneal grafts, and to the recipients of human growth hormone (which was obtained from human pituitary glands removed at autopsy). The pathology of CJD is very similar to bovine spongiform encephalopathy of cattle.

The condition has a long incubation period, sometimes up to several years. Death is almost invariable within 2 years from the onset of symptoms.

Kuru
This is a dementia and cerebellar ataxia occurring in the highlands of New Guinea. It is believed to have been spread by ritual cannibalism. Spongiform change occurs in the brain (very similar to that in Creutzfeldt–Jakob disease). This obscure condition is also believed to be transmitted by a slow virus.

Progressive multifocal leuco-encephalopathy
This is an opportunistic infection with the papovaviruses JC and SV-40 (and others) in patients who are immunocompromised. Multifocal demyelinating hemisphere lesions develop that contain virus particles. Death is usual after several years.

Reye's syndrome (see also p. 278)
This is a severe encephalitic illness, usually of

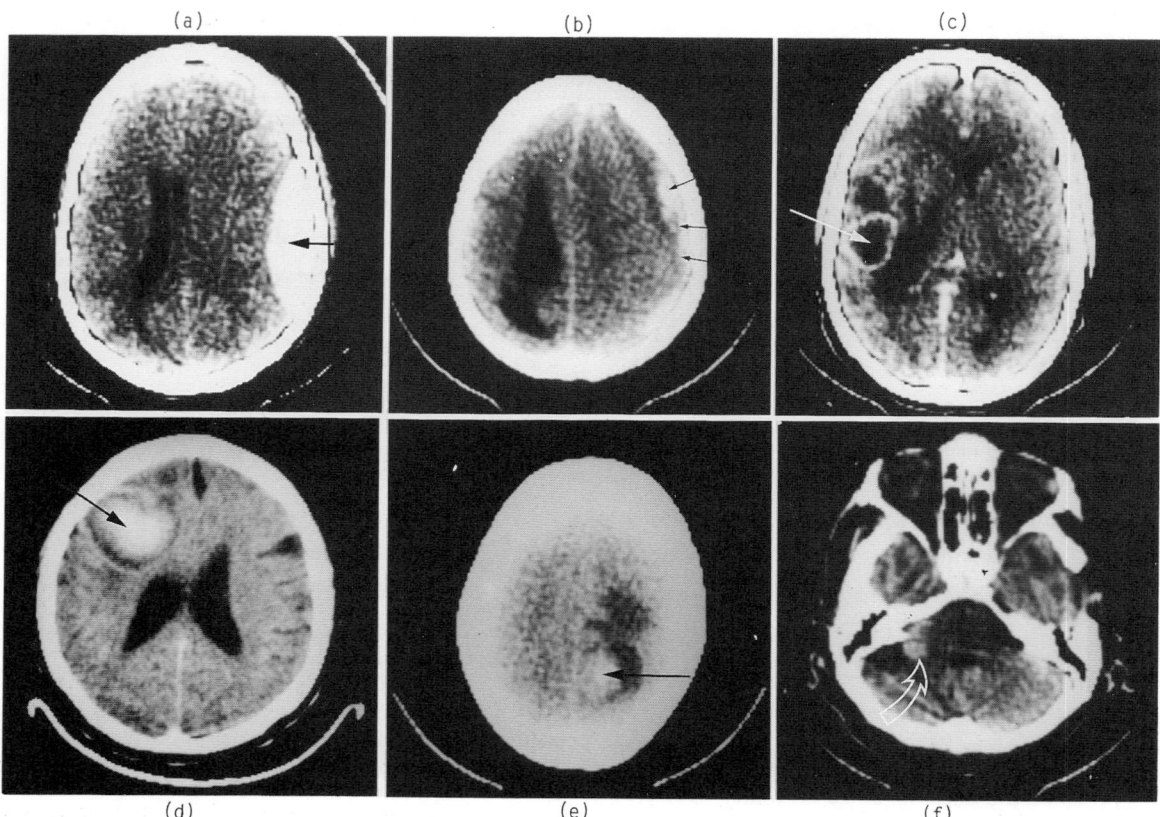

Fig. 18.20 CT scan appearances of various conditions. (a) Extradural haemorrhage. (b) Subdural haemorrhage. (c) Abscess. (d) Meningioma. (e) Secondary neoplasm. (f) Acoustic neuroma.

children, accompanied by fatty infiltration of the liver and hypoglycaemia. A viral cause has been postulated but other factors, including aspirin therapy, have also been implicated.

Mollaret's meningitis

This term is used to describe recurrent episodes of 'aseptic meningitis' over many years. A viral cause is postulated. Some of these patients are helped by treatment with the mitotic poison colchicine.

Vogt–Koyanagi–Harada syndrome

This is a recurrent inflammatory disease of cells of neural crest origin, causing uveitis, meningo-encephalitis, vitiligo, deafness and alopecia.

ME: Myalgic encephalomyelitis (epidemic neuromyasthenia) (see p. 972)

Headache, fever, lassitude, torpor, myalgia and depression sometimes follow viral infection (e.g. hepatitis, infectious mononucleosis, coxsackie infections). It is particularly difficult to distinguish between organic and psychological elements in these cases.

Sarcoidosis (see p. 683)

This condition may cause a chronic meningo-encephalitis with sarcoid lesions within the brain and spinal cord, a peripheral neuropathy, cranial nerve palsies (particularly bilateral seventh nerve palsies) or, rarely, a myopathy.

Behçet's syndrome (see p. 409)

The three principal features are recurrent oral and genital ulceration, inflammatory ocular disease and neurological syndromes. Brain-stem and cord lesions, aseptic meningitis, encephalitis and cerebral venous thrombosis also occur.

ABSCESSES WITHIN THE NERVOUS SYSTEM

Brain abscess (see Fig. 18.20c)

A focal area of infection within the cerebrum or cerebellum presents as an expanding mass lesion (see p. 938). The usual organisms are streptococci (aerobic, anaerobic and microaerophilic species), *Bacteroides* spp., staphylococci and enterobacteria. Mixed infections are common. Fungi can also cause brain abscesses. Multiple abscesses may develop. A parameningeal (e.g. ear, nose, paranasal sinus, skull fracture) or distant (e.g. lung, heart, abdomen) focus of infection may be present. Frequently no cause is found.

Tuberculoma

Tubercle bacilli cause chronic caseating intracranial granulomas—tuberculomas—which are the commonest single intracranial masses in areas such as India where TB is common. Tuberculomas either present as mass lesions or occur in the course of tuberculous meningitis. They may also be symptomless and appear on skull X-rays as areas of intracranial calcification.

CLINICAL FEATURES

Headache, focal signs (e.g. hemiparesis, aphasia, hemianopia), epilepsy and raised intracranial pressure occur. Fever, leucocytosis and a raised ESR are usual in cerebral abscess but are not always present. The presentation may thus be remarkably similar to many cerebral neoplasms. The symptoms may be indolent, developing over weeks, particularly in the cerebral hemispheres. Cerebellar abscesses tend to develop more acutely.

MANAGEMENT

Urgent CT scanning is essential. The search for a focus of infection should include a detailed examination of the skull, ears and paranasal sinuses.

Lumbar puncture is contraindicated in suspected brain abscess.

Treatment should be carried out with liaison between neurosurgeon and microbiologist. Surgical decompression may be necessary if antibiotics are unsuccessful. Despite treatment, the mortality of abscess remains high, at around 25%, and epilepsy is common in survivors.

Subdural empyema

This is usually secondary to local infection. The features are similar to those of a cerebral abscess.

Intracranial epidural abscess

Rarely, a collection of pus tracks along the intracranial epidural space, causing sequential cranial nerve lesions, typically without evidence of raised pressure. There is usually evidence of local infection. Drainage is necessary.

Spinal epidural abscess

Staphylococcus aureus is the usual organism responsible. It reaches the spine via the bloodstream, e.g. from a boil. There is fever and usually back pain followed by paraparesis or root lesions. Emergency myelography, decompression and antibiotics are indicated.

Intracranial tumours

Primary intracranial tumours account for approximately 10% of all neoplasms. The commoner varieties of tumours are outlined in Table 18.46; around one-quarter are metastases (Fig. 18.20e).

Differences between overall annual incidence rates (Table 18.1) and presentation as clinical problems (Table 18.46) are accounted for by the fact that small meningiomas and cerebral metastases are commonly found unexpectedly at postmortem.

Gliomas

These are malignant, intrinsic tumours that originate in neuroglia, usually within the cerebral hemispheres. Their cause is unknown. They are occasionally associated with neurofibromatosis.

Primary intracranial malignant tumours virtually never metastasize outside the CNS and spread only by direct extension.

Astrocytomas. These gliomas arise from astrocytes. They are classified into grades I–IV, depending on malignancy. Grade I astrocytomas grow slowly over many years while grade IV tumours cause death within several months.

Cystic astrocytomas occur in childhood, usually within the cerebellum. They are relatively benign.

Oligodendrogliomas. These arise from oligodendroglia and grow slowly, usually over several decades. Calcification is common.

Table 18.46 Relative frequency of common intracranial tumours on the basis of clinical presentation.

Tumour	Relative frequency
Primary malignant (glioma)	40%
Astrocytoma	
Oligodendroglioma	
Benign	30%
Meningioma	
Neurofibroma	
Metastases	25%
Bronchus	
Breast	
Stomach	
Prostate	
Thyroid	
Kidney	

Meningiomas (Fig. 18.20d)

These benign tumours arise from the arachnoid membrane and may grow to a large size, usually over years. When close to the skull they erode bone. They often occur along the intracranial venous sinuses, which they may invade. They are rare below the tentorium.

Neurofibromas

These arise from Schwann cells and occur principally in the cerebellopontine angle, where they arise from the eighth nerve sheath (see p. 893).

Other less common neoplasms include:

- Cerebellar haemangioblastoma
- Ependymoma of the fourth ventricle
- Colloid cyst of the third ventricle
- Pinealoma
- Chordoma of the skull base
- Glomus tumour—a vascular neoplasm of the jugular bulb
- Medulloblastoma—a cerebellar tumour of childhood
- Craniopharyngioma (see p. 778)

Pituitary tumours

These are discussed on p. 776.

CLINICAL FEATURES

Mass lesions within the cranium produce symptoms and signs in three co-existing ways:

- By the direct effects of the mass on surrounding structures, which are either destroyed or suffer impairment of function from infiltration, pressure or cerebral oedema
- By the effects of raised intracranial pressure and the shift of intracranial contents
- By provoking either generalized or partial seizures

Although neoplasms, either secondary or primary, are the commonest lesions to cause these effects, cerebral abscess, tuberculoma, subdural haematoma and intracranial haematoma may also produce symptoms and signs that may be clinically indistinguishable.

Direct effects of mass lesions
These will depend upon the site of the mass and its speed of growth. The hallmark of a mass lesion is a progressive deterioration of function.

Three examples of possible effects are given below:

- A left frontal meningioma (see Fig. 18.20d) will cause a vague disturbance of personality, apathy and impairment of intellectual function over several months. When the frontal speech area becomes affected, an expressive aphasia will develop. As the corticospinal pathways become involved, a right hemiparesis will follow.
- A right parietal glioma involving the fibres of the optic radiation will cause a left homonymous field defect. Cortical sensory loss and a left hemiparesis may follow. Partial seizures causing episodes of numbness of the left limbs may develop.
- A left eighth nerve sheath neurofibroma (an 'acoustic neuroma') (see Fig. 18.20f) growing in the cerebellopontine angle will cause progressive perceptive deafness (VIII), vertigo (VIII), numbness of the left side of the face (V) and facial weakness (VII), followed by cerebellar ataxia as the cerebellar connections are compressed.

The direct effects are commonly those that first bring the patient to seek medical attention. The rate of progression will vary greatly from a few days or weeks to several years in the case of a slowly enlarging mass. Since cerebral oedema surrounds many mass lesions it is often difficult on clinical grounds to distinguish its effect from that of the mass itself.

Raised intracranial pressure
The triad of headache, vomiting and papilloedema is an important, though relatively unusual, presentation of a mass lesion. These symptoms usually imply that obstruction to CSF pathways has occurred. Typically this picture is produced early by masses within the posterior fossa and as a later event with lesions above the tentorium.

Shift of the intracranial contents produces symptoms and signs that co-exist with the direct effects of an expanding mass:

- Distortion of the upper brain stem, as midline structures are displaced either caudally or laterally by a hemisphere mass (see Fig. 18.20), leads to impairment of consciousness (drowsiness progressing to stupor and coma).
- Compression of the medulla by herniation of the cerebellar tonsils caudally through the foramen magnum (an example of 'coning') causes impairment of consciousness, respiratory depression, bradycardia, decerebrate posturing and death.
- False localizing signs ('false' only because they are not related directly to the site of the mass) appear.

Three examples of false localizing signs are:

- A sixth nerve lesion, first on the side of a mass and later bilaterally, is caused as the nerve is compressed during its long intracranial course.
- A third nerve lesion develops as the uncus of the temporal lobe herniates caudally, compressing the third nerve against the petroclinoid

ligament and stretching it by downward displacement of the posterior communicating artery. The first sign of this is dilatation of the pupil as the parasympathetic fibres in the nerve are compressed.

- Hemiparesis on the *same* side (i.e. 'the one you don't expect') as a hemisphere tumour is caused by compression of the brain stem (the contralateral cerebral peduncle) on the free edge of the tentorium.

These false localizing signs are of importance in clinical neurology because their development indicates that a shift of the brain is taking place. Urgent surgical intervention may be necessary.

Seizures
Partial seizures, simple or complex, which may evolve to generalized tonic–clonic seizures are characteristic features of many hemisphere masses, whether malignant or benign. The site of origin of a partial seizure is frequently of localizing value (see p. 917). Generalized tonic–clonic seizures with EEG (but not clinical) evidence of a focal onset also occur.

INVESTIGATION

CT scan is the investigation of choice when the diagnosis of a tumour is suspected.

CT scan
It is important to emphasize that CT indicates only the site of a mass and not its nature. Cerebral abscess, cerebral infarction, benign and malignant tumours have characteristic, but not entirely diagnostic, appearances. Contrast enhancement adds to the discriminating ability of CT and should be used when a mass is suspected.

MRI
MRI is often more discriminating than other non-invasive tests, particularly for posterior fossa tumours.

EEG
The EEG may show electrical abnormalities in the region of a mass (but it may be normal): it is rarely of major value in management. The main exception is with cerebral abscess, where the EEG shows characteristic marked slow wave changes.

Technetium brain scan
This is sometimes useful to confirm the site of a lesion shown on CT, but the test discriminates poorly and misses many tumours. *Very* occasionally this test shows a lesion that has been missed by CT.

Skull films
Plain X-rays of the skull are discussed on p. 877. In pituitary and parasellar lesions they do give important information about changes in the dorsum sellae and clinoid processes. In hemisphere lesions, plain films are frequently abnormal but the test has little value as a screening process.

'Routine' tests
Since the proportion of cerebral tumours that prove to be metastases is high, 'routine' tests such as a chest X-ray are of great importance.

Specialized neuroradiology
Angiography, ventriculography and other contrast studies may sometimes be necessary to define the site or the blood supply of a mass.

Lumbar puncture
Lumbar puncture is contraindicated when the differential diagnosis includes any mass lesion.
Examination of CSF rarely yields diagnostically useful information in this situation, and the procedure may be followed by immediate herniation of the cerebellar tonsils. If there are pressing reasons for the procedure it should be carried out after careful assessment of the consequences and after a CT scan has been performed.

TREATMENT

Surgical exploration and either biopsy or removal of the mass is usually carried out to ascertain its nature. Some benign tumours can be removed in their entirety.

Radiotherapy is usually recommended for gliomas and for radiosensitive metastases. Chemotherapy is of little value in the majority of primary brain tumours.

Cerebral oedema surrounding a tumour is rapidly reduced by corticosteroids; dexamethasone or betamethasone are used by injection in an emergency. Intravenous mannitol may also be used as an osmotic diuretic.

Epilepsy is treated with anticonvulsants.

With all malignant brain tumours the overall outlook is poor, with less than 50% survival at 1 year. Meningiomas are, however, often removed in their entirety and thus cured.

Hydrocephalus

Hydrocephalus means that there is an excessive amount of CSF within the cranium. Although this also occurs in cerebral atrophy, in practice the term hydrocephalus is used to describe different syndromes in which there is, or has been, obstruction to CSF outflow with consequent high pressure and dilatation of the cerebral ventricles. Exceptionally an increase in CSF production occurs.

Infantile hydrocephalus

Enlargement of the head in infancy is diagnosed in about 1 in 2000 live births. There are several causes:

- *The Arnold–Chiari malformation.* There is elongation of the medulla and abnormal cerebellar tissue (the tonsils) in the cervical canal. Associated spina bifida is common. Syringomyelia may develop.
- *The Dandy–Walker syndrome.* There is cerebellar hypoplasia and obstruction to the outflow foramina of the fourth ventricle.
- *Stenosis of the aqueduct of Sylvius* (Fig. 18.21). This may be either congenital or acquired following neonatal meningitis or haemorrhage.

Hydrocephalus in adult life

Infantile hydrocephalus not infrequently becomes symptomatic only in adult life. The features are of headache, vomiting, papilloedema, ataxia and bilateral pyramidal signs.

Hydrocephalus in adults also occurs with:

- *Tumours of the posterior fossa and brain stem.* These obstruct the aqueduct or fourth ventricular outflow.
- *Subarachnoid haemorrhage, head injury or meningitis (particularly tuberculous).* The hydrocephalus is

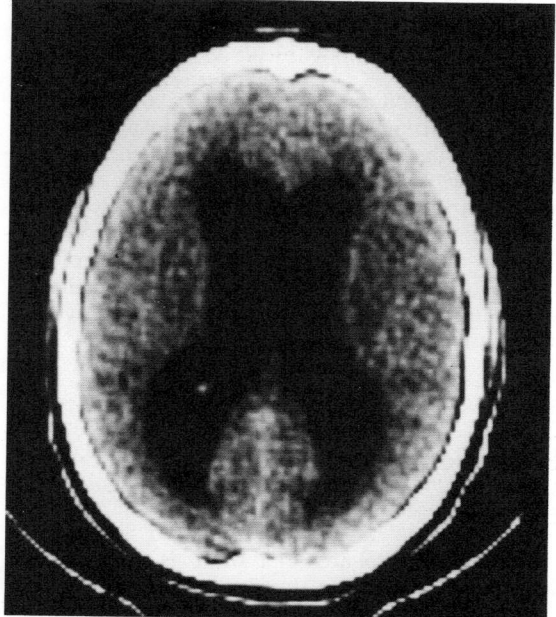

Fig. 18.21 Hydrocephalus on CT scan. Stenosis of the aqueduct of Sylvius causing gross ventricular dilatation.

often a transient phenomenon.

- *Tumours of the third ventricle.* A colloid cyst of the third ventricle causes enlargement of the lateral ventricles, headache and papilloedema.
- *Normal-pressure hydrocephalus.* In this syndrome enlarged cerebral ventricles occur without cortical atrophy. It presents with dementia, urinary incontinence and apraxia, usually in the elderly. The CSF pressure is characteristically normal. It is currently thought that this syndrome is the late result of previous episodes of high pressure, though usually of unknown cause.
- *Papilloma of the choroid plexus.* This is an extremely rare neoplasm that secretes CSF.

Ventriculoatrial or ventriculoperitoneal shunting may be necessary when hydrocephalus is diagnosed.

Benign intracranial hypertension (pseudotumour cerebri)

This syndrome consists of marked papilloedema without other signs in patients who are subsequently shown to have neither a mass lesion nor an increase in ventricular size. It occurs mainly in obese young women with vague menstrual irregularities. Steroid therapy is sometimes thought to be a cause and many other drugs have been occasionally implicated. Other causes of papilloedema should be excluded.

The condition is benign only in that it is not fatal. Infarction of the optic nerve occurs (with consequent blindness) when the papilloedema is severe and longstanding. Surgical decompression or shunting may be necessary. Thiazide diuretics appear to reduce the intracranial pressure in this condition. Weight reduction is important.

Headache, migraine and facial pain

'TENSION HEADACHE'

The vast majority of chronic and recurrent headaches are believed, on no good evidence, to be due to 'tension' within the scalp muscles. What is certain is that they are, in terms of pathology, innocent. 'Tight band' sensations, pressure behind the eyes, and throbbing and bursting sensations are common.

There may be obvious precipitating factors such as worry, noise, concentrated visual effort or fumes. Depression is also a frequent underlying cause. Tension headaches are often attributed to cervical spondylosis, refractive errors or high blood pressure; the evidence for these is poor. Similar headaches also follow head injuries, which may be minor.

There are no abnormal physical signs other than tenderness and tension in the nuchal and scalp muscles.

MANAGEMENT

This involves:

- Firm reassurance
- Avoiding the causes
- Analgesics
- Physical treatments—massage, relaxation
- Antidepressants—when indicated

Investigation may be needed to confirm the benign nature of the problem.

MIGRAINE

Migraine means recurrent headaches associated with visual and gastrointestinal disturbance; despite the origin of the word, it does not invariably mean unilateral headache.

INCIDENCE

About 10% of any population sampled admit to these symptoms.

MECHANISMS

The cause of migraine is unknown. The headache, often throbbing, is believed to be due to vasodilatation or oedema of blood vessels, with stimulation of nerve endings near affected extracranial and meningeal arteries. The release of vasoactive substances is thought to play a role; for example, the serum level of 5-hydroxytryptamine rises at the onset of the prodromal symptoms and falls during the headache.

Cerebral symptoms and signs (e.g. tingling of limbs, aphasia, weakness) are caused by ischaemia and/or depression of cortical function.

Definite precipitating factors are unusual. Some patients complain of symptoms at times of relaxation (e.g. weekend migraine). Others find that chocolate (high in phenylethylamine) and cheese (high in tyramine) precipitate attacks. Migraine is common around puberty, at the menopause and premenstrually, and sometimes increases in severity or frequency with the contraceptive pill or the development of hypertension.

There is no reason to suppose that migraine is associated with any major intracranial lesion. However, since migraine is such a common symptom complex, an intracranial mass lesion and migraine sometimes both occur in the same patient by coincidence.

Rarely, migraine follows head injuries.

CLINICAL PATTERNS

There are several types of migraine, the attacks varying from intermittent headaches barely distinguishable from tension headaches to discrete episodes that mimic thromboembolic cerebral ischaemia. The distinction between the variants is somewhat artificial.

The attack itself may be divided into:

- Prodromal symptoms
- Headache and associated symptoms

Prior to the attack some patients experience a feeling of well-being.

Classical migraine

Prodromal symptoms are usually visual and are related to ischaemia in the distribution of the intracranial arteries. There are unilateral patchy scotomata (when the retinal vessels are involved), unilateral blindness (involvement of the ophthalmic artery) and sometimes hemianopic field loss (involvement of the posterior cerebral artery). Teichopsia (flashes) and fortification spectra (jagged lines resembling battlements) are common.

Transient aphasia sometimes occurs, together with tingling, numbness or vague weakness of one side. The patient feels nauseated.

The prodrome lasts for 15 min to 1 h or more. Headache follows. This is occasionally hemicranial ('splitting the head') but often begins locally and becomes generalized. Nausea increases and vomiting follows. The patient is irritable and prefers to be in a darkened room. The superficial temporal artery (either or both) is engorged and pulsating.

After several hours the attack ceases. There is sometimes a diuresis towards the end of an attack. Sleep often follows.

Common migraine

This is the usual variety of migraine. Prodromal visual symptoms are vague. There is recurrent headache accompanied by nausea and malaise. Distinction from tension headache may be impossible.

Basilar migraine

The prodromal symptoms are due to ischaemia in the posterior cerebral circulation. Circumoral tingling, numbness of the tongue, vertigo, diplopia, transient blindness, syncope, dysarthria and ataxia occur.

Hemiplegic migraine

This is a rarity in which classical migraine is accompanied by hemiparesis. Recovery occurs within 24 h. Exceptionally, cerebral infarction follows.

Ophthalmoplegic migraine

This is a third (or exceptionally a sixth) nerve palsy occurring in a migraine attack. The condition is rare and is difficult to distinguish from other causes of a third nerve palsy (see p. 888) without investigation.

Facioplegic migraine

This rarity is unilateral facial weakness occurring during a migraine attack.

DIFFERENTIAL DIAGNOSIS

The sudden onset of headache may be similar to meningitis or subarachnoid haemorrhage.

The hemiplegic, visual and hemisensory symptoms must be distinguished from thromboembolic TIAs (see p. 909). In TIAs the maximum deficit is present immediately and headache is unusual.

Unilateral tingling or numbness should be distinguished from sensory epilepsy (partial seizures). In the latter a distinct 'march' of symptoms is usual.

MANAGEMENT

General measures
These include:

- Reassurance and relief of anxiety
- Avoidance of precipitating dietary factors (rarely helpful)
- Patients on oral contraceptives, a change in brand or stopping of the drug may help. Severe hemiplegic symptoms are an indication for stopping these drugs.

During the attack
Paracetamol or other simple analgesics should be given, with anti-emetics (e.g. metoclopramide) if necessary.

Ergotamine tartrate (1–2 mg orally or rectally, 360 μg by aerosol or 0.25–0.5 mg by injection) is sometimes, though not often, helpful if given early in attack. Ergotamine should not be used in patients with a history of vascular disease.

Prophylaxis
It is particularly difficult to discern the true (as opposed to placebo) effects of prophylactic drugs in migraine. When drugs are necessary, the following are used:

- Pizotifen (a 5-HT antagonist) 0.5 mg at night for several days, increasing to 1.5 mg at night. Common side-effects are slight weight gain and drowsiness
- Propranolol 10 mg three times daily, increasing to 40–80 mg three times daily
- Clonidine 0.025 mg three times daily, increasing to 0.075 mg three times daily

- Methysergide (a 5-HT antagonist) 2–6 mg daily. An occasional side-effect is retroperitoneal fibrosis, which precludes its use for longer than 6 months.

FACIAL PAIN

The face is richly supplied with pain-sensitive structures—the teeth, gums, sinuses, temporomandibular joints, jaw and eyes—disease of which causes facial pain. Facial pain is also caused by some specific neurological conditions; these are mentioned below.

Trigeminal neuralgia. This is described on p. 890.

Trigeminal nerve lesions. These are described on p. 889.

Post-herpetic neuralgia. This is described on p. 933.

Migrainous neuralgia
This condition, which is distinct from migraine despite its name, causes recurrent bouts of excruciating pain that wake the patient at night and are centred around one eye. It affects adults in the third and fourth decades and is more common in men. Alcohol sometimes precipitates an attack.

The pain lasts for several hours. Vomiting occurs. The face and nostril feel congested. A transient ipsilateral Horner's syndrome is common during the attack.

Despite the pain there are no serious sequelae. Treatment of the attack with analgesics is unhelpful. Prophylactic drugs for migraine are of little value. Lithium carbonate sometimes has a dramatic effect in preventing attacks: the drug level should be monitored carefully.

Atypical facial pain
Facial pain for which no cause can be found is seen in the elderly, mainly in women. It is believed to be a somatic equivalent of depression. Tricyclic antidepressants are sometimes helpful.

Other causes
Facial pain occurs in usual variants of migraine and in giant-cell arteritis (see below).

GIANT-CELL ARTERITIS (CRANIAL ARTERITIS, TEMPORAL ARTERITIS) (p. 398)

This important syndrome is a granulomatous arteritis of unknown aetiology occurring chiefly in those over the age of 60 and affecting in particular the extradural arteries. Other forms of arteritis, e.g. systemic lupus erythematosus (see p. 391) and polyarteritis nodosa (see p. 397) can present with similar features but with a more generalized arteritis affecting intracranial arteries and vasa nervorum of the cranial nerves. Giant cell arteritis is closely related to polymyalgia and these can occur in the same patient.

CLINICAL FEATURES

Headache
Headache is almost invariable. It is felt over the inflamed superficial, temporal or occipital arteries. Touching the skin over the inflamed vessel (e.g. combing the hair) causes pain. The arterial pulsation is soon lost and the artery becomes hard, tortuous and thickened. The skin over the vessels may be red. Rarely, gangrenous patches appear in the scalp.

Facial pain
Pain in the face, jaw and mouth occurs and is caused by inflammation of the facial, maxillary and lingual branches of the external carotid artery. Pain is characteristically worse on eating (jaw claudication). Opening the mouth and protruding the tongue is difficult. A painful, ischaemic tongue occasionally occurs.

Visual problems
Visual loss due to inflammation and occlusion of the ciliary and/or central retinal artery occurs in 25% of untreated cases. The patient complains of sudden uniocular visual loss, either partial or complete, which is painless. Amaurosis fugax (see p. 909) may precede total visual loss, which is usually permanent.

When the ciliary vessels are affected, the optic disc becomes swollen and pale (see p. 885). The retinal branch vessels are usually normal. If the central retinal artery is occluded, there is sudden unilateral blindness, pallor of the disc and retinal ischaemia.

Systemic features
Generalized limb pains, proximal limb girdle pain and tenderness, without joint effusion, i.e. polymyalgia rheumatica (see p. 398), occurs in half the cases. Weight loss, sweating and malaise also occur.

Rare complications
Brain-stem ischaemia, cortical blindness, ischaemic neuropathy of peripheral nerves, cranial nerve lesions, and involvement of the aorta, coronary, renal and mesenteric arteries are sometimes seen.

INVESTIGATION

The ESR is greatly elevated, 60–100 mm·h^{-1} being common, although very rarely the ESR is normal. Plasma α-2-globulins are raised and the albumin is occasionally reduced. Normochromic, normocytic anaemia occurs.

The diagnosis is usually confirmed by biopsy of a superficial temporal artery. A 1 cm (or greater) segment should be excised because the characteristic granulomatous changes within the walls (lymphocytes, plasma cells, multinucleate giant cells, destruction of the internal elastic lamina) may be patchy.

TREATMENT

The diagnosis should be established without delay because of the risk of blindness. High doses of steroids (prednisolone, initially 60–100 mg daily) should be started immediately in a patient with typical features even before the biopsy. The dose is reduced as the ESR falls. A characteristic of the condition is that the headache subsides within hours of the first large dose of steroid.

It is usually possible to stop steroid treatment after some months to several years.

Head injury

Over 100 000 patients with head injury are admitted to hospital in Britain annually. Around 400 of these patients have disturbance of consciousness for longer than a month. Road traffic accidents and alcohol abuse are the principal aetiological factors in this major cause of death and morbidity.

Skull fractures
Linear skull fracture of the vault or base is an indication of the severity of injury but is not necessarily associated with any neurological sequelae. Healing takes place and surgical intervention is usually unnecessary.

Depressed skull fracture of the vault is followed by a high incidence of post-traumatic epilepsy (see p. 917). Surgical elevation and debridement are usually necessary.

The principal local complications of skull fracture are:

- Rupture of a meningeal artery, causing an extradural haematoma (see p. 915).
- Tearing of dural veins, causing subdural haematoma (see p. 915) or CSF rhinorrhoea and otorrhoea with its risk of meningitis.

Brain damage
Older classifications attempted to separate 'concussion', in which transient coma was followed by complete recovery, from brain contusion after which there were prolonged coma and focal signs. There is little pathological support for this. The

mechanisms of brain damage following trauma are complex and interrelated. They involve:

- Direct axonal and neuronal damage
- Raised intracranial pressure
- Brain oedema
- Brain ischaemia
- Brain hypoxia

CLINICAL COURSE

In a mild injury a patient is first stunned or dazed for a few seconds or minutes. Loss of consciousness is transient and, following this the patient is alert, and there is no amnesia. The period of loss of consciousness indicates severity; over several *hours* is regarded as indicating severe brain injury. The Glasgow Coma Scale (p. 905) can be used to assess the degree of coma and brain damage as well as indicating prognosis; a low score implies a severe injury and 50% of such patients die or remain in a vegetative state.

Recovery may take a long period of time, depending on the severity of the injury. During early recovery patients are often restless and lethargic and they may have mild focal neurological deficits. Gradually patients become more alert to their surroundings.

LATE SEQUELAE

These are common causes of morbidity and have important social and medicolegal consequences. They include the following:

- Many patients with severe head injuries have prolonged and incomplete recoveries, and are left with impairment of higher cerebral function, hemiparesis and other deficits.
- Post-traumatic epilepsy may occur (see p. 917).
- 'Chronic traumatic encephalopathy' follows repeated (and often minor) injuries. This 'punch drunk' syndrome is dementia and presents with extrapyramidal and pyramidal signs. It is seen mainly in professional boxers.
- The 'post-traumatic syndrome' describes the vague complaints of headache, dizziness and malaise that follow even minor head injuries. Depression is prominent. Symptoms may be prolonged.
- 'Benign positional vertigo' (see p. 894) is a transient sequel of head injury.
- Chronic subdural haematoma (see p. 915).
- Hydrocephalus (see p. 939).

MANAGEMENT

Patients with head injury require skilled prolonged and energetic supportive therapy.

Acute management of the unconscious patient is described on p. 907.

REHABILITATION

Patients left with *severe* neurological deficits will require rehabilitation in specialized units. Recovery requires not only intensive physiotherapy but also the overall care of their mental state. Many patients are depressed and have behavioural problems and they and their families need long-term support and counselling.

Diseases of the spinal cord

The cord extends from C1 (its junction with the medulla) to the vertebral body of L1 (the conus medullaris).

The blood supply is via the anterior spinal artery and a plexus on the posterior cord. This network is supplied by the vertebral arteries, the thyrocervical trunk and several branches from the lumbar and intercostal vessels.

SPINAL CORD COMPRESSION

The clinical features are discussed on p. 897.

Acute cord compression is unmistakable. There is paralysis and sensory loss below the level of the lesion.

Chronic compression of the cord causes progressive difficulty in walking (see p. 875) over

Table 18.47 Causes of spinal cord compression.

Spinal cord neoplasms (see Table 18.48)

Disc and vertebral lesions
   Trauma
   Chronic degenerative

Inflammatory
   Epidural abscess
   Tuberculosis
   Granuloma

Vertebral neoplasms
   Metastases
   Myeloma

Epidural haemorrhage

Rarities
   Paget's disease
   Epithelial, endothelial and parasitic cysts
   Aneurysmal bone cyst
   Vertebral angioma
   Haematomyelia, arachnoiditis
   Osteoporosis

Table 18.48 Principal spinal cord neoplasms.

Extradural
Metastases:
  Bronchus
  Breast
  Prostate
  Lymphoma
  Thyroid
  Melanoma

Extramedullary
Meningioma
Neurofibroma
Ependymoma
Arteriovenous malformation

Intramedullary
Glioma
Ependymoma
Haemangioblastoma
Lipoma
Arteriovenous malformation
Teratoma

weeks, months or years. Spastic paraparesis with sensory loss is found. Sphincter disturbance is common.

It is frequently difficult to distinguish chronic cord compression from other causes of paraparesis and tetraparesis on clinical grounds alone (Tables 18.16 and 18.47).

Spinal cord neoplasms (Table 18.48)
Extramedullary tumours (extradural and intradural) cause cord compression gradually over weeks to months, with local or referred root pain and a sensory level (see p. 902).

Intramedullary tumours (e.g. glioma) typically have a very slowly progressive course over several years. Sensory disturbances similar to syringomyelia (see p. 946) may appear.

Disc and vertebral lesions
Central cervical disc protrusion and lumbar disc protrusion are considered on pp. 957 and 414, respectively.

Epidural abscess
This is described on p. 937.

Epidural haemorrhage and haematoma
These are rare sequelae of anticoagulant therapy, bleeding disorders and trauma. A rapidly progressive cord lesion develops.

Tuberculosis
Spinal TB is a frequent cause of cord compression in countries where TB is common (e.g. India, Pakistan, Bangladesh and Africa). There is destruc-

tion of vertebral bodies and disc spares, with spread of infection along the extradural space. Cord compression and paraparesis follow (Pott's paraplegia).

MANAGEMENT

Early recognition of the syndrome is vital. Surgical exploration is frequently necessary and, if this is not performed sufficiently early, irreversible paraplegia may follow.

Plain spinal films show degenerative bone disease and destruction of vertebrae by infection or neoplasm. Routine tests may indicate a primary neoplasm or infection.

Myelography, sometimes with CT scanning, is necessary. It should, if possible, be done promptly in a centre equipped to carry out neurosurgical exploration. The signs of cord compression may increase after lumbar puncture. MRI is also valuable.

The results following the early removal of benign tumours are excellent.

TRANSVERSE MYELITIS

This broad term is used to describe acute inflammation of the cord and paraplegia occurring with viral infection, MS and other inflammatory and vascular disorders (e.g. syphilis, radiation myelopathy, anterior spinal artery occlusion). Myelography is usually required to exclude a compressive lesion.

ANTERIOR SPINAL ARTERY OCCLUSION

Cord infarction, causing an acute paraparesis or tetraparesis (or tetraplegia) may occur in any thrombotic or embolic vascular disease (e.g. endocarditis, shock, atheroma, diabetes mellitus, syphilis, polyarteritis nodosa). It sometimes occurs during surgery to the posterior mediastinum, and follows dissection of the aorta and trauma. It occasionally occurs as an isolated event.

RADIATION MYELOPATHY

A mild paraparesis and sensory loss sometimes develops within several weeks to a year of radiotherapy if the cord has been damaged. Particular care is usually taken to shield the cord during radiotherapy.

METABOLIC AND TOXIC CORD DISEASE

Subacute combined degeneration of the cord due to vitamin B_{12} deficiency (see pp. 305 and 956) is the most important example of metabolic disease causing spinal cord damage.

Cord lesions may also be seen in severe malnutrition, when they are probably due to multiple B-vitamin deficiencies.

Lathyrism

This is an endemic, spastic paraparesis of central India caused by the toxin B-(N)-oxalylaminoalanine. It occurs when excessive quantities of a drought-resistant pulse, *Lathyrus sativus*, are consumed.

SYRINGOMYELIA AND SYRINGOBULBIA

Fluid-filled cavities within the spinal cord (myelia) and brain stem (bulbia) are the essential features of these conditions.

AETIOLOGY

A history of birth injury may be obtained and bony anomalies at the foramen magnum, spina bifida (see p. 950), Arnold–Chiari malformation (see p. 950) or hydrocephalus (see p. 939) are often seen.

It is believed that in the presence of an anatomical abnormality at the foramen magnum, the normal pulsatile CSF pressure waves are transmitted to the delicate tissues of the cervical cord and brain stem, with secondary cavity formation. The cavity, or syrinx, is in continuity with the central canal of the cord.

PATHOLOGICAL ANATOMY

The expanding cavity gradually destroys:

- The second-order spinothalamic neurones in the cervical cord
- The anterior horn cells
- The lateral corticospinal tracts

The vestibular system, trigeminal nuclei, sympathetic system and twelfth nerve nuclei may also be affected.

CLINICAL FEATURES

Patients usually present in the third to fourth decade.

Pain in the upper limbs is common. This may be exacerbated by exertion or coughing. Spinothalamic (pain and temperature) sensory loss in the upper limbs leads to painless burns. Difficulty in walking may occur.

The signs of a cavity in the cervical region are:

- Areas of dissociated sensory loss. These may extend in a bizarre distribution over the trunk and upper limbs.

- Loss of upper limbs reflexes.
- Wasting of the small muscles of the hand.
- Spastic paraparesis. This may initially be mild and symptomless.

Neuropathic joints, trophic skin changes and ulcers may follow.

When the cavity extends through the foramen magnum into the brain stem (syringobulbia), there is atrophy and fasciculation of the tongue, nystagmus, Horner's syndrome, hearing loss and impairment of facial sensation.

MANAGEMENT AND COURSE

The condition is intermittently progressive over several decades.

Investigation shows widening of the cervical canal on plain films, and frequently ventricular enlargement on CT scan. An MRI scan (the investigation of choice) demonstrates the intrinsic cavity. Myelography (which is sometimes followed by deterioration) shows widening of the cord and herniation of the cerebellar tonsils through the foramen magnum.

There is no curative treatment. Decompression of the foramen magnum sometimes reduces the rate of deterioration.

PARAPLEGIA (see p. 896)

MANAGEMENT

The patient who becomes paraplegic from any cause demands skilled and prolonged nursing care. Particular problems are discussed below.

Bladder. Intermittent (or continuous) catheterization is usually necessary initially. A reflex emptying bladder develops in permanent paraplegia, avoiding the need for catheterization and some of the risks of urinary stasis, infection, and renal and bladder calculi.

Bowel. Constipation and faecal impaction must be avoided. Manual evacuation is necessary following acute paraplegia, but reflex emptying later develops.

Skin care. The risk of pressure sores is great. Meticulous attention must be paid to cleanliness and to turning the patient every 2 h. The sacrum, iliac crests, greater trochanters, heels and malleoli should be inspected frequently. Ripple mattresses and water beds are useful.

If pressure sores develop, plastic surgical repair should be considered.

The lower limbs. Passive physiotherapy is helpful in avoiding contractures. Severe spasticity (with spasms either in flexion or extension) may be helped by dantrolene sodium, baclofen or diazepam.

General considerations

The general health and morale of the patient should be considered carefully and regularly. Any intercurrent infection (urinary or respiratory) is potentially hazardous and should be recognized and treated early, as chronic renal failure is the single most common cause of death in paraplegia.

Rehabilitation

Many patients with traumatic paraplegia or tetraplegia return to partial self-sufficiency and a wheelchair existence. Specialist advice from a skilled rehabilitation unit is necessary. Lightweight, specially adapted wheelchairs are often recommended. The patients have demanding practical, psychological and social needs but with guidance and help can often return to an active role in society.

Other causes of cord lesions

- Multiple sclerosis
- Motor neurone disease
- Familial or sporadic paraparesis
- Non-metastatic manifestation of malignancy (see p. 958)
- Neurosyphilis

Rarities, e.g. sarcoidosis (see p. 683), Behçet's syndrome (see p. 409)

Degenerative diseases

The term 'degenerative' underlines a present lack of understanding of the aetiology of this group of progressive diseases of the nervous system.

MOTOR NEURONE DISEASE (MND)

In this disease there is progressive degeneration of motor neurones in the spinal cord, in the somatic motor nuclei of the cranial nerves and within the cortex. The condition is sporadic and of entirely unknown cause. The prevalence is about 6 in 100 000, with an equal sex incidence. The onset is in middle life. The sensory system is not involved.

CLINICAL FEATURES

There are three patterns:

- Progressive muscular atrophy

- Amyotrophic lateral sclerosis
- Progressive bulbar palsy

Although useful as a means of understanding the disease, these are not distinct aetiological or pathological variants; the three merge later in the course of the condition.

Progressive muscular atrophy

Wasting often begins in the small muscles of one hand and spreads inexorably throughout the arm. Although it may begin unilaterally, wasting soon follows on the opposite side.

Fasciculation is common. It is due to the spontaneous firing of abnormally large motor units formed by the branching fibres of surviving axons that are striving to innervate muscle fibres that have lost their nerve supply. Cramps may occur but pain does not.

The physical signs are of wasting and weakness, with fasciculation that is often widespread. Tendon reflexes are lost when the reflex arc is interrupted (by anterior horn cell loss) but are often preserved or exaggerated because of the loss of motor neurones in the corticospinal tracts.

Amyotrophic lateral sclerosis (ALS)

'Lateral sclerosis' means disease of the lateral corticospinal tracts (i.e. a spastic paraparesis). 'Amyotrophy' means atrophy of muscle (which would be unusual in most other forms of spastic tetraparesis or paraparesis). The clinical picture is thus of a progressive spastic tetraparesis or paraparesis with added *lower* motor neurone signs and fasciculation. 'ALS' is the term usually given to MND in the USA.

Progressive bulbar palsy

Here the brunt of the onset of the disease falls upon the lower cranial nerve nuclei and their supranuclear connections. Dysarthria, dysphagia, nasal regurgitation of fluids and choking are common symptoms. For reasons unknown, this form of the disease is more common in women than in men. The characteristic features are of a bulbar and pseudobulbar palsy i.e. a mixture of upper and lower motor neurone signs in the lower cranial nerves, e.g. a wasted fibrillating tongue with a spastic weak palate.

COURSE

Remission is unknown. The disease progresses, spreading gradually and causes death, often from bronchopneumonia. Survival for more than 3 years is most unusual though there are rare 'benign' forms of the condition in which survival is prolonged.

The ocular movements are not affected. There are never cerebellar or extrapyramidal signs.

Table 18.49 Principal causes of dementia in adults and the features on which the diagnosis is made or excluded.

Condition	Diagnostic features
Alzheimer's disease	Clinical history, CT scan
Hypothyroidism	TSH levels and serum T4
Subacute combined degeneration of cord	MCV, blood picture, vitamin B_{12} assay
Pellagra	Dietary history
Hypoparathyroidism	Serum calcium level
Multiple cerebral infarction	CT scan
Alcohol/Wernicke–Korsakoff syndrome	Clinical history
Intracranial mass, hydrocephalus (including subdural haematoma)	Clinical features, CT scan
Chronic traumatic encephalopathy	Clinical history, CT scan
Huntington's disease	Family history, chorea
Multiple sclerosis	Clinical features, evoked potentials, CSF, MRI scan
Spongiform encephalopathy	EEG, ?cerebral biopsy
Progressive supranuclear palsy	Clinical features
General paralysis of the insane	Syphilitic serology
Poisoning by: Drugs (chronic barbiturate intoxication) Carbon monoxide Heavy metals (organic mercurials, manganese)	Drug levels and clinical history
Following prolonged anoxia or hypoglycaemia	Clinical findings
Chronic hepatic encephalopathy	Clinical features, liver biochemistry
AIDS encephalopathy	HIV serology
Uraemia, dialysis	Raised blood urea
Rare metabolic disorders, e.g. Wilson's disease	Serum copper level, caeruloplasmin level

N.B.: Depression may produce a clinical picture that is indistinguishable from dementia (see p. 979).

Awareness is preserved and dementia is unusual. Sphincter disturbance occurs late, if at all.

MANAGEMENT

There are no specific diagnostic tests and the diagnosis can often be made on clinical grounds alone. Cervical radiculopathy and myelopathy and the rare (almost extinct) syphilitic cervical pachymeningitis may sometimes cause diagnostic difficulty. Bulbar myasthenia gravis may sometimes appear similar in the early stages.

Denervation may be confirmed by electromyography, which characteristically shows chronic partial denervation with preserved motor conduction velocity. The CSF is usually normal (the protein may be slightly raised).

No treatment has been shown to influence the course of this disease. Management of these patients, who are often well-informed and aware of the outlook, is particularly difficult.

Spinal muscular atrophies

These are a group of rare genetically determined disorders of the motor neurone that give rise to slowly progressive, usually symmetrical, muscle wasting and weakness. An acute infantile type (Werdnig–Hoffman disease), a chronic childhood type (Kugelberg–Welander disease) and adult forms are recognized. Clinically these conditions may be confused with muscular dystrophies (see p. 962), hereditary neuropathies or motor neurone disease.

DEMENTIA (see p. 973)

The principal causes of progressive generalized failure of higher cerebral functions are shown in Table 18.49.

Alzheimer's disease

This term is now used for both senile and presenile dementia. Pathologically there is severe cortical neuronal loss, and the presence of 'neurofibrillary tangles' in degenerating neurones. Neither is specific for the disease.

Extracellular amyloid fibrils consisting of a 4-kD peptide called β-amyloid protein (A4 protein) accumulate in cerebral and meningeal microvessels and in the cores of the mature senile plaques seen in the cerebral cortex (see p. 869). The gene for the precursor protein of A4 (Pro A4) is localized close to the defect on chromosome 21 causing familial Alzheimer's disease. The significance of these findings is still unclear. A relationship between the ingestion, or accumulation of aluminium ions has been suggested, but is not proven.

CLINICAL FEATURES

The condition is seldom seen below the age of 50. A familial tendency is unusual. Memory failure, progressive intellectual decline and apathy, and on occasion, features of focal cortical disturbance such as aphasia occur. Severe depression may be present in the early stages. The disease is gradually progressive. 'Pyramidal' signs (e.g. extensor plantar reflexes) are sometimes found together with a stoop and expressionless face suggestive of Parkinson's disease. Epilepsy may occur.

INVESTIGATION

There are no characteristic changes in the peripheral blood, in the CSF or on EEG. Cortical atrophy is seen on a CT scan. Psychometric testing may be valuable in the early stages of the condition.

The purpose of investigation in dementia is to establish the diagnosis and to distinguish those causes for which some treatment may be available (Table 18.49).

TREATMENT

No treatment exists for Alzheimer's disease. Patients can remain at home if family support is adequate but hospital care often becomes necessary. The few treatable causes of dementia (e.g. hypothyroidism) require urgent therapy.

Pick's disease

Pick's disease is dementia in which the cortical atrophy is initially restricted to the frontotemporal region. The cause is unknown.

Congenital and inherited diseases

CEREBRAL PALSY

This term describes disorders apparent at birth or in childhood due to brain damage in the neonatal period leading to non-progressive deficits.

Mental retardation, varying from severe intellectual impairment to mild learning disorders, is common in all forms of cerebral palsy, but severe physical disability is not necessarily associated with a severe defect in higher cerebral function.

CAUSES

The precise cause of brain damage in an individual child may be difficult to determine. The following may be responsible:

- Hypoxia in utero and/or during parturition
- Trauma, during parturition or in the neonatal period
- Prolonged convulsions or coma (e.g. febrile convulsions, hypoglycaemia) in infancy
- Kernicterus
- Cerebral haemorrhage and infarction

CLINICAL FEATURES

Failure to achieve normal developmental milestones is often the earliest feature. More specific motor syndromes become apparent later in childhood or rarely, in adult life.

Spastic diplegia. This is spasticity (predominantly of the lower limbs) with 'scissoring' of the gait.

Athetoid cerebral palsy. This is described on p. 925.

Infantile hemiparesis. Hemiparesis may be noted at

birth or during childhood. Hemiatrophy of the limbs (and atrophy of contralateral hemisphere) is usual. Seizures are common.

Congenital ataxia. This is incoordination and hypotonia of the trunk and limbs.

DYSRAPHISM

Failure of normal fusion of the fetal neural tube leads to this group of congenital anomalies.

Anencephaly
Anencephaly is absence of the brain and cranial vault, and is incompatible with life.

Meningoencephalocele
This is an extrusion of brain and meninges through a midline skull defect that varies from a minor protrusion to a massive defect.

Spina bifida
In spina bifida there is failure of fusion of the neural tube, usually in the lumbosacral region. Several varieties occur.

Spina bifida occulta. This is failure of fusion of the vertebral arch only. There are rarely neurological abnormalities and a bony anomaly is seen on X-ray. It occurs in 3% of the population. A dimple or a tuft of hair may overlie the lesion.

Meningomyelocele and meningocele with spina bifida. Meningomyelocele consists of elements of the cord and lumbosacral roots contained within a meningeal sac that herniates through a defect in the vertebrae. In severe cases the lower limbs and sphincters are paralysed. The defect is visible at birth.
　　Meningocele is a meningeal defect alone.
　　Hydrocephalus is commonly associated with these abnormalities. Meningitis may follow if a sinus connects the spinal canal with the overlying skin.

BASILAR IMPRESSION OF THE SKULL (PLATYBASIA)

This is usually a congenital anomaly in which there is invagination of the foramen magnum and skull base upwards. The lower cranial nerves, medulla, upper cervical cord and roots are affected. It is often complicated by the Arnold–Chiari malformation, in which aberrant cerebellar tissue extends through the foramen magnum.
　　The condition also occurs in Paget's disease and rarely in osteomalacia.

NEUROECTODERMAL SYNDROMES

These are disorders in which organs derived from ectoderm show a tendency to form tumours and hamartomas, with lesions in the skin, eye and nervous system.

Neurofibromatosis (von Recklinghausen's disease)

This is characterized by multiple skin neurofibromas and pigmentation. The neurofibromas arise from the neurilemmal sheath. One new case occurs in every 3000 live births. The mode of inheritance is autosomal dominant.

CLINICAL FEATURES (see p. 1037)

Clinically neurofibromatosis can be divided into type 1 (or peripheral) and type 2 (bilateral acoustic or central). The predisposing gene for type 1 has been localized to chromosome 17 and for type 2 to the long arm of chromosome 22. The main application for these genetic markers will be for antenatal diagnosis and genetic counselling, although the severity of the disease itself will not be predictable.

Skin tumours
Subcutaneous, soft, sometimes pedunculated, tumours appear. They may be multiple.

Skin pigmentation
Multiple café-au-lait patches—pale brown macules 1–20 cm in diameter are found. These are common in the normal population but more than five patches is abnormal.

Neural tumours
Many neural tumours occur more frequently in von Recklinghausen's disease than in the general population, including:

- Cutaneous neurofibroma
- Eighth nerve sheath neurofibroma
- Spinal cord and nerve root neurofibroma
- Meningioma
- Glioma (including optic nerve glioma)
- Plexiform neuroma (massive cutaneous overgrowth)

Rarely, the benign tumours undergo sarcomatous change.

Associated abnormalities. These include:

- Scoliosis
- Orbital haemangioma
- Local gigantism of a limb
- Phaeochromocytoma and ganglioneuroma
- Renal artery stenosis
- Pulmonary fibrosis
- Obstructive cardiomyopathy
- Fibrous dysplasia of bone

TREATMENT

Surgery may be necessary for cosmetic reasons. Tumours causing pressure within the nervous system require excision, if this is feasible.

Tuberose sclerosis (epiloia)

This is a rare autosomal dominant condition whose principal features are adenoma sebaceum, epilepsy and mental retardation (often severe).

Adenoma sebaceum
These are reddish nodules (angiofibromas) that develop on the cheeks in childhood.

Other lesions
Other lesions include shagreen patches, amelanotic naevi, retinal phakomas (glial masses), renal tumours, glial overgrowth in brain and gliomas. Cardiac rhabdomyomas, hamartomas of lung and kidney, and polycystic kidneys may also occur.

Sturge–Weber syndrome (encephalofacial angiomatosis)

There is an extensive port-wine naevus on one side of the face (usually in the distribution of a division of the fifth nerve) and a leptomeningeal angioma.
Epilepsy is common. Familial occurrence is exceptional.

Von Hippel–Lindau syndrome (retinocerebellar angiomatosis)

This is the occurrence in families (dominant inheritance with variable penetrance) of retinal and cerebellar haemangioblastomas or, less commonly, haemangioblastomas of the cord and cerebrum. Renal, adrenal and pancreatic cysts (and haemangioblastomas) may also be found. Polycythaemia sometimes occurs.
There are numerous other disorders related to these conditions, for example, ataxia telangiectasia (see p. 139) and Osler–Weber–Rendu syndrome (see p. 337).

SPINOCEREBELLAR DEGENERATIONS

The classification of this large group of rare inherited disorders is complex. Three conditions will be mentioned here.

Friedreich's ataxia

This is a progressive degeneration of dorsal root ganglia, spinocerebellar tracts, corticospinal tracts and Purkinje cells of the cerebellum. Difficulty in walking occurs around the age of 12 and is progressive. The clinical findings are:

- Ataxia of gait and trunk
- Nystagmus (in 25%)
- Dysarthria
- Absent joint position and vibration sense in lower limbs
- Absent reflexes in lower limbs
- Optic atrophy (in 30%)
- Pes cavus
- Cardiomyopathy with T-wave inversion and left ventricular hypertrophy, arrhythmias.

Death is usual before the age of 40.

Hereditary spastic paraparesis

Isolated progressive paraparesis runs in some families. The inheritance is variable. Additional features including cerebellar signs, pes cavus, wasted hands and optic atrophy are sometimes seen. The conditions are usually mild and progress slowly over many years.

Ataxia telangiectasia (see p. 139)

This is a rare, autosomal recessive condition that produces a progressive ataxic syndrome in childhood and early adult life.
There is striking telangiectasia of the conjunctiva, nose, ears and skin creases. There are also defects in cell-mediated immunity and antibody production. A defect in DNA repair has been demonstrated. Death is usual by the third decade, either from infection or from the development of lymphoreticular malignancy.

PERONEAL MUSCULAR ATROPHY AND OTHER INHERITED NEUROPATHIES

These disorders are classified within a large and complex group—the hereditary motor and sensory neuropathies (HMSN).

Peroneal muscular atrophy

Peroneal muscular atrophy (Charcot–Marie–Tooth disease) is a common clinical syndrome in which there is distal limb wasting and weakness that slowly progresses over many years, mostly in the legs, with variable loss of sensation and reflexes. In advanced cases the distal wasting below the knees is so marked that the legs resemble 'inverted champagne bottles'. Mild cases have only pes cavus and clawing of the toes and may pass unnoticed.
Three forms are recognized:

- HMSN type I—a demyelinating neuropathy
- HMSN type II—an axonal neuropathy
- Distal spinal muscular atrophy

Both autosomal dominant and recessive inherit-

Table 18.50 Fibre types in peripheral nerves.

Type	Fibre diameter (μm)	Conduction velocity (m·s^{-1})	Function
A	10–18	90	Primary spindle afferents Alpha motor neurones
A	6–12	50	Touch and pressure afferents
A	4–8	30	Gamma afferents
B	2–6	10	Autonomic preganglionic
C	0.2–0.3	2	Pain and temperature afferents Autonomic postganglionic

ance is seen in different families. In HMSN type I with dominant inheritance (the commonest form), linkage has been demonstrated for the locus on the long arm of chromosome 1.

Optic atrophy, deafness, retinitis pigmentosa and spastic paraparesis are sometimes seen in variants of these conditions.

HMSN type III

This was formerly known as 'the hypertrophic neuropathy of Déjérine–Sottas'. It is an autosomal recessive demyelinating sensory neuropathy of childhood leading to severe incapacity during adolescence. It is notable because the CSF protein may be greatly elevated to 10 g·l^{-1} or more, and the CSF pathways are obstructed by greatly hypertrophied nerve roots.

Diseases of the peripheral nerves

The different nerve fibre types within a peripheral nerve are shown in Table 18.50. All are myelinated except the C fibres, which carry impulses from painful stimuli.

Two pathological processes affect peripheral nerves—axonal (or wallerian) degeneration and demyelination. Neuropathies are classified according to which process predominates.

Axonal degeneration

Axonal degeneration occurs after a nerve has been sectioned or its axon severely damaged. Within 7–10 days the axon and the myelin sheath distal to the injury degenerate and are inexcitable electric-

ally. When a motor nerve is damaged there is atrophy of the muscle fibres in the motor units it supplies. Denervation may be detected by recording fibrillation potentials on EMG.

Regeneration occurs by axonal growth down the nerve sheath and axonal sprouting from the stump. Growth takes place at a rate of up to 1 mm per day. In a chronic neuropathic process (e.g. motor neurone disease or polyneuropathy), sprouts from the terminal axons of *normal* motor axons reinnervate the denervated muscle fibres; giant polyphasic units are then seen on EMG.

Demyelination

Here damage to the myelin sheath (the axon itself is initially preserved) causes conduction block or marked slowing of conduction; this can be used to distinguish demyelination from axonal degeneration. Local demyelination is caused by pressure (compression and entrapment neuropathies) or by inflammation (e.g. Guillain–Barré syndrome).

Definitions

Neuropathy means a pathological process affecting a peripheral nerve or nerves.

Mononeuropathy is a process affecting a single nerve, and multiple mononeuropathy (or mononeuritis multiplex) is a process affecting several or multiple nerves.

Polyneuropathy is a diffuse, symmetrical disease process, usually progressing proximally. It is either acute, subacute or chronic. Its course may be progressive, relapsing or towards recovery. Polyneuropathy may be motor, sensory, sensorimotor (mixed) or autonomic.

Radiculopathy means a disease process affecting the nerve roots.

MONONEUROPATHIES

Peripheral nerve compression and entrapment
(Table 18.51)

Damage to a nerve by compression is either acute (e.g. due to a tourniquet or other sustained pressure) or chronic (entrapment neuropathy). In both, demyelination predominates, but some axonal degeneration occurs.

Acute compression usually affects nerves which are exposed anatomically (e.g. the common peroneal nerve at the head of the fibula).

Entrapment occurs where a nerve passes through relatively tight anatomical passages (e.g. the carpal tunnel).

These conditions are diagnosed largely from the clinical features. Diagnosis is confirmed by nerve

Table 18.51 Nerve compression and entrapment.

Nerve	Site of entrapment or compression
Median	Carpal tunnel
Ulnar	Cubital tunnel
Radial	Spiral groove of humerus
Posterior interosseous	Supinator muscle
Lateral cutaneous of thigh ('meralgia paraesthetica')	Inguinal ligament
Common peroneal	Neck of fibula
Posterior tibial	Flexor retinaculum (tarsal tunnel)

conduction studies and EMG. The commoner conditions are mentioned below.

Median nerve compression at the wrist (carpal tunnel syndrome)

This common syndrome is sometimes seen in:

- Hypothyroidism
- Diabetes mellitus
- Pregnancy
- Rheumatoid arthritis
- Acromegaly

The condition is, however, usually idiopathic. It causes nocturnal tingling and pain in the hand (and sometimes forearm) followed by weakness of the thenar muscles. Wasting of abductor pollicis brevis develops, with sensory loss of the palm and radial three-and-a-half fingers. Tinel's sign may be positive, i.e. tapping on the carpal tunnel will reproduce the pain.

Treatment with a splint at night or a local steroid injection in the wrist gives temporary relief. When the condition occurs in pregnancy (due to fluid retention) it is often self-limiting. Surgical decompression of the carpel tunnel is a simple and definitive treatment.

Ulnar nerve compression

This typically occurs at the elbow, where the nerve is compressed in the cubital tunnel. It follows fracture of the ulna or prolonged or recurrent pressure on the nerve at this site.

Wasting of the ulnar innervated muscles develops (hypothenar muscles and interossei) together with sensory loss in the ulnar one-and-a-half fingers.

Decompression and transposition of the nerve at the elbow may be necessary.

The deep (solely motor) branch of the ulnar nerve may be damaged in the palm by recurrent pressure from tools (e.g. screwdrivers), crutches or cycle handlebars.

Radial nerve compression

The radial nerve is compressed acutely against the humerus, e.g. when the arm is draped over a hard chair for several hours ('Saturday night palsy'). Wrist drop and weakness of finger extension and of the brachioradalis muscle follow. Recovery is usual within 1–3 months.

Meralgia paraesthetica

Burning, tingling and numbness on the antero-lateral aspect of the thigh is caused by entrapment of the lateral cutaneous nerve of the thigh beneath the inguinal ligament.

Many of the patients are obese; weight reduction helps to relieve the symptoms. Division of the inguinal ligament is not usually effective.

Common peroneal nerve palsy

When the common peroneal nerve is compressed against the head of the fibula (owing to prolonged squatting, wearing plaster casts, prolonged bed rest or coma) there is foot drop and weakness of eversion. A patch of numbness on the anterolateral border of the shin or dorsum of the foot may be found. Recovery is usual (but not invariable) within several months.

Multiple mononeuropathy (mononeuritis multiplex)

Multiple mononeuropathy occurs in:

- Diabetes mellitus
- Leprosy
- Connective tissue disease (polyarteritis nodosa, SLE, giant cell arteritis, rheumatoid arthritis)
- Sarcoidosis
- Malignancy
- Amyloidosis
- Neurofibromatosis
- AIDS

Diagnosis is largely clinical, supported by electrical studies. Treatment is that of the underlying disease.

POLYNEUROPATHIES

Although many toxins and disease processes are known to be associated with polyneuropathy (see below), the cause of the majority of cases remains undetermined. The commonest presentation is a chronic or subacute sensorimotor neuropathy. A classification of polyneuropathy is given in Table 18.52.

Table 18.52 Classification of polyneuropathy.

Idiopathic chronic sensorimotor neuropathies
Post-infective neuropathy (Guillain–Barré syndrome)
Drugs/toxic, metabolic and vitamin deficiency neuropathies
Neoplastic neuropathies
Neuropathies in connective tissue diseases
Autonomic neuropathies
Hereditary sensorimotor neuropathies

Idiopathic chronic sensorimotor neuropathies

The patient complains of a progressive symmetrical numbness and tingling in the hands and feet, which spreads proximally in a 'glove and stocking' distribution. There is distal weakness, which also ascends. Rarely the cranial nerves may be affected. Tendon reflexes involving affected nerves are lost. The symptoms may progress over many months, remain static or remit at any stage. Autonomic features are sometimes seen.

Investigation (nerve conduction studies, EMG) of the neuropathy shows either axonal degeneration or demyelination, or features of both of these processes. Some cases of demyelinating (not axonal) chronic sensorimotor neuropathy respond to steroid or immunosuppressive therapy.

Post-infective polyneuropathy (Guillain–Barré syndrome, acute inflammatory neuropathy)

CLINICAL FEATURES

This demyelinating neuropathy, which has an autoallergic basis, follows 1–3 weeks after a viral infection that is often trivial in nature. The patient complains of weakness of distal limb muscles or distal numbness. This ascends over several days or weeks. In mild cases there is little disability, but in some 20% of causes the respiratory and facial muscles are affected and the patient may become paralysed.

Weakness, areflexia and sensory loss are found.

Autonomic features (see below) are sometimes seen. There is a rare proximal form of the condition that initially affects the ocular muscles and in which ataxia is found (Miller Fisher syndrome).

DIAGNOSIS

This is established on clinical grounds and is confirmed by nerve conduction studies, which show the slowing of conduction or conduction block seen in demyelinating neuropathies. The CSF contains a normal cell count and sugar level but the protein is frequently raised to $1-3$ $g \cdot L^{-1}$.

The differential diagnosis includes other paralytic illnesses such as poliomyelitis, botulism or primary muscle disease.

TREATMENT AND COURSE

Treatment is essentially supportive, with particular attention to compensating for weakness of the respiratory and bulbar muscles. Ventilation may be necessary.

Corticosteroids are sometimes used to treat the Guillain–Barré syndrome but are not of proven value. Plasmapheresis has been shown to be of proven benefit in shortening the period of disability.

Recovery, though gradual over many months, is usual but may be incomplete.

Diphtheria

Demyelinating neuropathy is sometimes caused by the exotoxin of *Corynebacterium diphtheriae*. Palatal weakness followed by pupillary paralysis and a sensorimotor neuropathy occur several weeks after faucial infection. The condition is now rare in countries where immunization against diphtheria is practised.

Metabolic, toxic and vitamin-deficiency neuropathies

The commoner of these neuropathies are shown in Table 18.53. All are due to impairment of normal metabolism of the axon, myelin or both.

METABOLIC NEUROPATHIES

Diabetes mellitus
Several varieties of neuropathy occur in diabetes mellitus:

- Symmetrical sensory polyneuropathy
- Mononeuropathy and multiple mononeuropathy
  (a) Cranial nerve lesions

Table 18.53 Toxic, metabolic and vitamin deficiency neuropathies.

Metabolic	*Toxic*
Diabetes mellitus	Drugs
Uraemia	Alcohol
Hepatic disease	Industrial toxins
Thyroid disease	
Porphyria	*Vitamin deficiency*
Amyloid disease	B_1 (thiamine)
Malignancy	B_6 (pyridoxine)
Refsum's disease	Nicotinic acid
	B_{12}

(b) Isolated peripheral nerve lesions, e.g. median
(c) Diabetic amyotrophy
● Autonomic neuropathy

These are discussed in more detail on p. 853.

Uraemia
Progressive sensorimotor neuropathy occurs in chronic uraemia. The response to dialysis is variable but the neuropathy usually improves after renal transplantation.

Thyroid disease
A mild chronic sensorimotor neuropathy is sometimes seen in both hyper- and hypothyroidism.

Porphyria
Acute intermittent porphyria is a rare metabolic disorder (see p. 871) in which there are episodes of a severe, mainly proximal, neuropathy, sometimes associated with abdominal pain, confusion and later coma. Alcohol and barbiturates may precipitate attacks.

Amyloidosis
This is described on p. 869.

Refsum's disease
This is a rare condition inherited as an autosomal recessive trait. There is a sensorimotor polyneuropathy with ataxia, retinal damage and deafness. It is due to a defect in the metabolism of phytanic acid.

Table 18.54 Drug-associated neuropathies.

Drug	Neuropathy	Mode/site of action
Phenytoin Chloramphenicol Procarbazine	Sensory	Axon
Isoniazid	Sensory	Pyridoxine metabolism
Dapsone Gold Amphotericin	Motor	Axon
Nitrofurantoin Vincristine Chlorambucil Disulfiram Cisplatin	Sensorimotor	Axon
Perhexiline (not available in UK)	Sensorimotor	Myelin

TOXIC NEUROPATHIES

Alcohol
A polyneuropathy, mainly in the lower limbs, occurs in chronic alcoholics. Calf pain is common. The response to abstention is variable. Thiamine should be given.

Drugs
Many drugs have been reported to be associated with a polyneuropathy. The more important ones are shown in Table 18.54.

Industrial toxins
A wide variety of industrial toxins have been shown to cause polyneuropathy:

● Lead poisoning causes a motor neuropathy.
● Acrylamide (plastics industry), trichlorethylene (a solvent), hexane and other fat-soluble hydrocarbons (e.g. those inhaled in glue-sniffing, p. 994) cause a progressive polyneuropathy.
● Arsenic and thallium cause a polyneuropathy.

VITAMIN DEFICIENCY NEUROPATHIES

Vitamin deficiencies are an important cause of disease of the nervous system because they are potentially reversible if treated early (and progressive if not). They occur in malnutrition, when they are commonly multiple.

Thiamine (vitamin B₁)
Deficiency causes the clinical syndrome of beri-beri (see p. 160). The principal features are polyneuropathy, Wernicke's encephalopathy, an amnesic syndrome (Wernicke–Korsakoff psychosis) and cardiac failure. Alcohol abuse is the commonest cause in Western countries. Other neurological consequences of alcohol are summarized in Table 18.55.

Wernicke–Korsakoff syndrome. This important syndrome is an acute or gradual encephalopathy associated with alcohol abuse and other causes of thiamine deficiency. The typical triad comprises ocular signs, ataxia and a confusional state, but the condition occurs in partial forms. It is due to ischaemic damage to the brain stem and its connections. Clinical features include:

● *Ocular signs.* Nystagmus, bilateral lateral rectus palsies, conjugate gaze palsies, fixed pupils and, rarely, papilloedema are found.
● *Ataxia.* There is a broad-based gait, cerebellar signs in the limbs and vestibular paralysis (absent response to caloric stimulation).
● *Confusion.* Apathy, decreased awareness or restlessness, amnesia, stupor and coma occur.

Hypothermia and hypotension due to hypothalamic damage are rare findings.

Table 18.55 Effects of ethyl alcohol on the nervous system (see also Table 3.15 and p. 172).

Acute intoxication
Disturbance of balance, gait and speech
Coma
Head injury and its sequelae

Alcohol withdrawal
'Morning shakes'
Tremor of arms and legs
Delirium tremens

Thiamine deficiency
Polyneuropathy
Wernicke–Korsakoff syndrome

Epilepsy
Acute intoxication
Alcohol withdrawal
Hypoglycaemia

Cerebellar degeneration

Cerebral infarction

Cerebral atrophy
Dementia

Central pontine myelinolysis

Marchiafava–Bignami syndrome (a rare degeneration of the corpus callosum)

The condition is under-diagnosed. Erythrocyte transketolase activity is reduced but is of limited practical value because the measurement is rarely available.

Thiamine (i.m. or i.v.) should be given immediately if the diagnosis is in question. It is harmless; the condition is not. Untreated Wernicke–Korsakoff syndrome commonly leads to a severe irreversible amnesic syndrome and residual brainstem signs.

Pyridoxine (vitamin B_6)
Deficiency causes a mainly sensory neuropathy (p. 162). It may be precipitated during isoniazid therapy for TB in those who acetylate the drug slowly.

Vitamin B_{12}
Deficiency causes disease of the brain, spinal cord and peripheral nerves.

Subacute combined degeneration of the cord. This important syndrome of the spinal cord is a sequel of Addisonian pernicious anaemia and rarely other causes of vitamin B_{12} deficiency (see p. 305). It is frequently associated with a polyneuropathy.

The patient complains initially of numbness and tingling of the extremities. The signs are of distal sensory loss (particularly posterior column) with absent ankle jerks (due to the neuropathy) com-

bined with evidence of cord disease (exaggerated knee-jerk reflexes, extensor plantar responses). Optic atrophy and retinal haemorrhage may occur. In the later stages sphincter disturbance, weakness and dementia are seen.

Macrocytosis and megaloblastic changes in the bone marrow are invariable in subacute combined degeneration of the cord. The cause of the B_{12} deficiency should be established (see p. 305). Treatment with parenteral B_{12} reverses the peripheral nerve damage but has little effect on the CNS (cord and brain) signs.

Neoplastic neuropathy

Polyneuropathy is sometimes seen as a non-metastatic manifestation of malignancy (see p. 958).

In myeloma and other dysproteinaemic states, polyneuropathy occurs, probably owing to impaired perfusion of nerve trunks or to demyelination associated with allergic reactions within peripheral nerves.

Neuropathies associated with connective tissue diseases

Neuropathy occurs in systemic lupus erythematosus, polyarteritis nodosa, rheumatoid disease and giant-cell arteritis owing to microinfarction of peripheral nerves. This presents either as a multiple mononeuropathy or a symmetrical sensorimotor neuropathy.

Autonomic neuropathy

Autonomic neuropathy causes postural hypotension, retention of urine, impotence, diarrhoea (or occasionally constipation), diminished sweating, impaired pupillary responses and cardiac arrhythmia.

Many varieties of neuropathy affect autonomic function to a mild, and often subclinical, degree. Occasionally, when there is damage to small myelinated and non-myelinated B and C fibres, the clinical features of the autonomic neuropathy predominate. This situation may occur in diabetes mellitus, in amyloidosis and in the Guillain–Barré syndrome.

Hereditary sensorimotor neuropathies

These are described on p. 959.

PLEXUS LESIONS AND RADICULOPATHY

The common conditions that cause nerve root or lumbar or brachial plexus lesions are summarized in Table 18.56.

Table 18.56 Principal causes of plexus and nerve root lesions.

Plexus
Trauma
Malignant infiltration
Cervical rib
Neuralgic amyotrophy

Nerve root
Trauma
Herpes zoster
Meningeal inflammation (e.g. syphilis)
Tumours (neurofibroma, metastases)
Cervical and lumbar spondylosis

Cervical rib (thoracic outlet syndrome)

A fibrous band or cervical rib extending from the tip of the transverse process of C7 to the first rib stretches the lower roots of the brachial plexus (C8 and T1). There is pain along the ulnar border of the forearm, and sensory loss initially in the distribution of T1 with wasting of the thenar muscles, principally the abductor pollicis brevis muscle. Horner's syndrome may occur. The rib or band can be excised.

In other patients the rib or band causes subclavian artery or venous occlusion. The neurological and vascular problems rarely occur together.

Neuralgic amyotrophy

This is a condition in which severe pain in the muscles of the shoulder is followed by wasting, usually of the infraspinatus, supraspinatus, deltoid and serratus anterior muscles (a 'branchial plexus neuropathy'). The cause is unknown but, since the condition follows viral infection or immunization in some cases, an allergic basis is postulated.

Recovery of the wasted muscles occurs over some months.

Malignant infiltration

Metastatic disease of nerve roots of the brachial or lumbosacral plexus causes a painful radiculopathy.

A common example is an apical bronchial neoplasm (Pancoast's tumour) that causes a T1 lesion and involves the sympathetic outflow. There is wasting of the small muscles of the hand, pain and sensory loss in areas supplied by T1, and ipsilateral Horner's syndrome. This condition also occasionally occurs in apical TB.

Cervical and lumbar spondylosis (see Table 8.21)

Spondylosis describes the degenerative changes within vertebrae and intervertebral discs that occur during ageing or secondarily to trauma or rheumatoid disease. The changes are common in the lower cervical and lower lumbar region.

Several, often related, factors are important in producing signs and symptoms, including:

- Osteophytes—local overgrowth of bone
- Congential narrowing of the spinal canal
- Disc degeneration with posterior or lateral disc protrusion
- Ischaemic changes in the cord and nerve roots

The commoner clinical syndromes will be described.

Lateral cervical disc protrustion (Fig. 18.22)
The patient complains of pain in the upper limb. A C7 protrusion is the commonest lesion. There is root pain (see p. 901), which radiates into the affected myotome (scapula, triceps and forearm extensors in a C7 lesion) and a sensory disturbance (tingling, numbness) in the affected dermatome. There is weakness and, later, wasting of muscles innervated by the affected root (triceps and finger extensors in a C7 lesion) and reflexes using this root will be lost (the triceps jerk in a C7 lesion).

Although the initial pain is often severe, most cases recover with rest and analgesics. It is usual to immobilize the neck in a collar. Plain X-rays of the cervical spine (oblique views) show encroachment into the exit foraminae by osteophytes. In cases where recovery is delayed, root compression may be demonstrated at myelography and surgical root decompression performed.

Central cervical disc protrusion (cervical myelopathy)
Posterior disc protrusion (Fig. 18.22), which is common at C4/5, C5/6 and C6/7 levels, causes spinal cord compression (see p. 902). Congenital narrowing of the canal, osteophytic bars and ischaemia are contributory factors.

The patient complains of difficulty in walking. Frequently there are no symptoms in the neck. A

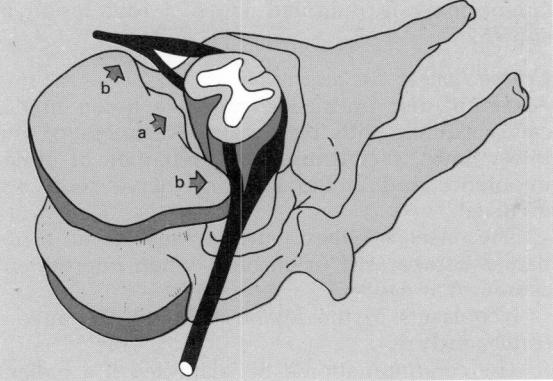

Fig. 18.22 Cervical spondylosis: (a) central and (b) lateral disc protrusion.

spastic paraparesis (or tetraparesis) is found, with variable sensory loss. A reflex level in the upper limbs and evidence of lateral disc protrusion may coexist.

Plain films may show narrowing of the sagittal diameter of the spinal canal and osteophytes but the changes correlate poorly with signs and symptoms. Myelography is necessary to demonstrate the level and extent of cord compression. MRI is increasingly being used.

Cervical laminectomy or anterior fusion of the vertebral bodies with removal of the disc may be necessary when the cord compression is severe or progressive. The results of surgery are often disappointing. Recovery of the 'pyramidal' signs is unusual, although progression may be halted.

A collar should be fitted. Manipulation of the neck should be avoided.

Thoracic disc protrusion

Central protrusion of a thoracic disc is a rare cause of paraparesis.

Lateral lumbar disc protrusion

The L5 and S1 roots are commonly compressed by lateral prolapse of the L4/5 and L5/S1 discs, respectively. There is low back pain and 'sciatica' (pain radiating down the buttock and lower limb). The onset may be acute and follow lifting a heavy weight, or may be subacute and apparently unrelated to exercise.

Straight leg raising is limited. There may be loss of reflexes (ankle jerk in an S1 root lesion or knee jerk in an L4/5 lesion) and weakness of plantar flexion (S1) or extension of the great toe (L5). Sensory loss may be found in the affected dermatome.

Plain films of the lumbar spine show narrowing of the disc space, osteophytes or a narrow canal. Unsuspected malignancy or infection may be demonstrated.

Most cases resolve with rest and analgesics. In the minority, myelography is necessary and laminectomy is indicated when a root lesion is shown.

Central lumbar disc protrusion

A central disc protrusion causes a lesion of the cauda equina with back pain, weakness of the lower limbs, sacral numbness, retention of urine, impotence and areflexia. Many nerve roots are involved.

The onset is either acute (a cause of an acute flaccid paraparesis) or chronic, when intermittent claudication occurs.

Neoplasms in the lumbosacral region cause a similar picture.

The condition should be suspected if a patient with back pain develops retention of urine. Urgent myelography and decompression is indicated.

Spinal stenosis

Narrowing of the lumbar spinal canal produces back pain (see p. 416) and is an important cause of buttock claudication. Congenital narrowing of the cervical canal predisposes to cervical myelopathy from minor disc protrusion.

Non-metastatic manifestations of malignancy

Many neurological syndromes may accompany malignancy. Clinical pictures include:

- Sensorimotor neuropathy
- Cerebellar syndrome
- Dementia and encephalopathy
- Myasthenic–myopathic syndrome (Eaton–Lambert syndrome)
- Progressive multifocal leucoencephalopathy
- Mononeuritis multiplex
- Cranial polyneuropathy
- Motor neurone disease variants
- Spastic paraparesis

The cause of most of these remains obscure. The clinical importance is that the neurological syndrome sometimes precedes clinical recognition of the neoplasm, which is often a small-cell carcinoma of the bronchus or a lymphoma. The neurological signs may recede if the tumour is resected or treated.

Diseases of voluntary muscle

Weakness is the predominant feature of a myopathy. Its distribution and pattern is of diagnostic importance. A classification of muscle disease is given in Table 18.57. Only the more common conditions are mentioned below.

PATHOPHYSIOLOGY

Muscle fibres are affected by:

- Acute inflammation and fibre necrosis (e.g. polymyositis)
- Chronic degeneration of muscle fibres (e.g. Duchenne muscular dystrophy)
- Regeneration and fibre hypertrophy
- Complex immune and metabolic disorders. For example:

Table 18.57 Classification of muscle disease.

ACQUIRED MYOPATHIES

Inflammatory myopathy
Polymyositis
  Alone
  With skin lesions (dermatomyositis)
  With collagen disease
  With malignancy
Viral, bacterial and parasitic infection
Sarcoidosis

Metabolic and endocrine myopathy, due to:
Corticosteroids/Cushing's syndrome
Thyroid disease
Calcium metabolism disorders
Hypokalaemia
Ethanol
Drugs

Myasthenic disorders
Myasthenia gravis
Myasthenic–myopathic (Eaton–Lambert) syndrome

GENETICALLY DETERMINED MYOPATHIES

Muscular dystrophies
Duchenne muscular dystrophy
Facio-scapulo-humeral dystrophy
Limb girdle dystrophy

Myotonias
Dystrophia myotonica
Myotonia congenita

Periodic paralyses
Hypokalaemic
Hyperkalaemic
Normokalaemic

Specific metabolic myopathies, e.g.
Myophosphorylase deficiency
Other defects of glycogen, fatty acid and
  mitochondrial metabolism
Malignant hyperpyrexia

(a) In myasthenia gravis, there is a reduction in the number of available acetylcholine receptors at the neuromuscular junction due to antibodies to the receptor protein.
(b) In myotonias, defective chloride ion membrane conductance is associated with delayed muscle relaxation.
(c) Enzyme defects in the glycolytic pathway (e.g. myophosphorylase deficiency) result in impaired force generation.

INVESTIGATION

Diagnosis is possible on clinical grounds alone in some myopathies. The distribution of weakness and the consistency of the muscles should be noted.

Serum muscle enzymes
Serum creatine phosphokinase (and aldolase) is greatly elevated in many dystrophies (e.g. Duchenne muscular dystrophy) and in inflammatory disorders of muscle (e.g. polymyositis). These enzymes are normal in myasthenia, and are usually normal in myotonias and chronic partial denervation.

Electromyography
When a muscle is weak the normal interference pattern is reduced. An EMG is useful to distinguish between primary muscle disease and denervation (e.g. motor neurone disease). The principal abnormalities are:

- *Myopathy.* Short duration 'spiky' polyphasic muscle action potentials are seen. Spontaneous fibrillation is occasionally recorded.
- *Denervation.* Fibrillation potentials of about 1 ms in duration and 50–200 µV in amplitude are seen, and are evidence of re-innervation.

Other changes. Myotonic discharges (in myotonias) consist of high-frequency activity that varies repeatedly to cause a characteristic sound on the loudspeaker.

In myasthenia gravis a characteristic decrement in the evoked muscle action potential follows stimulation of the motor nerve. The reverse is seen (an increment in repetitive response) in the rare myasthenic–myopathic syndrome (Eaton–Lambert syndrome), which may accompany carcinoma of the bronchus.

Muscle biopsy
Information about muscle fibre types (type 1 = slow; type 2 = fast), denervation, inflammation, dystrophic changes and muscle histochemistry is obtained by muscle biopsy. Electron microscopy is sometimes necessary.

In chronic partial denervation, 'fibre type grouping', i.e. groups of atrophic fibres of the same fibre type, is seen. Hypertrophic fibres also occur. In acute denervation, small angulated fibres are seen scattered randomly between normal fibres. In dystrophies and myositis, the muscle fibres are diffusely abnormal, the nuclei become central, and invasion by inflammatory cells and/or necrosis occurs.

Considerable experience is required to assess these changes accurately.

INFLAMMATORY MYOPATHIES

Polymyositis

This group of disorders is characterized by non-suppurative inflammation of skeletal muscle. The muscles are weak and usually painful. In many cases there are skin changes (dermatomyositis, see p. 1033) or other connective tissue diseases (see p. 1031).

CLINICAL FEATURES

'Polymyositis alone' is a rare disease, most common in the fourth and fifth decades. Symptoms are of difficulty in rising from a chair, climbing stairs or lifting. Weakness is typically proximal. The weak muscles ache and are sometimes tender and indurated.

As the disease progresses there may be widespread weakness and wasting, with dysphagia, respiratory muscle weakness and cardiac involvement.

INVESTIGATION

Preliminary investigations show a raised ESR and a mild normochromic normocytic anaemia. Antinuclear factor is sometimes positive. The serum creatine phosphokinase is usually (but not always) elevated.

The EMG shows myopathic changes. Occasionally fibrillation potentials occur and may cause diagnostic difficulty.

Muscle biopsy shows inflammatory changes with infiltration of the muscle by mononuclear cells.

DIFFERENTIAL DIAGNOSIS

Muscular dystrophies rarely progress as rapidly as polymyositis and there is no muscle pain. Pseudohypertrophy does not occur in polymyositis and there is no family history.

Motor neurone disease is always eventually accompanied by upper motor neurone signs, and prominent fasciculation is common.

TREATMENT

Corticosteroids and/or azathioprine or cyclophosphamide reduce the symptoms in about 75% of cases. Only rarely does the disease progress to cause grave disability or death from respiratory failure or cardiac involvement.

Other inflammatory myopathies

Muscle pain and weakness occur in trichinosis due to the ingestion of pork infected with *Trichinella spiralis*.

Acute myositis also occurs with coxsackie virus infections (see p. 61).

Tropical pyomyositis of central Africa is suppurative inflammation of muscle caused by staphylococci and other organisms.

An inflammatory myopathy may occur in sarcoidosis.

METABOLIC AND ENDOCRINE MYOPATHIES

Corticosteroids and Cushing's syndrome
Proximal muscle weakness occurs with prolonged high-dose steroid therapy (particularly with 9-α-fluorinated steroids such as dexamethasone and triamcinolone) and in Cushing's syndrome. Selective type-2 fibre atrophy is seen on muscle biopsy.

Thyroid disease (p. 798)
Several muscle diseases may occur:

- Thyrotoxicosis is sometimes accompanied by a severe proximal myopathy.
- In ophthalmic Graves' disease there is swelling and lymphocytic infiltration of the extraocular muscles (see p. 808).
- Hypothyroidism is sometimes associated with muscle pain and stiffness, resembling myotonia. A true proximal myopathy also occurs.
- There is also an association between thyrotoxicosis and myasthenia gravis, and between thyrotoxicosis and hypokalaemic periodic paralysis. Both associations are seen more frequently in South-East Asia.

Disorders of calcium metabolism
Proximal myopathy may occur in osteomalacia of any cause (see p. 822).

Hypokalaemia
Acute hypokalaemia (e.g. in diuretic therapy) causes a severe flaccid paralysis (periodic paralysis, see p. 963) that is reversed by correcting the electrolyte disturbance.

Chronic mild hypokalaemia (also commonly caused by diuretics) gives rise to a mild, mainly proximal, weakness.

Alcohol
Severe myopathy with muscle pain, necrosis and

Table 18.58 Drug-induced muscle disorders.

Disorder	Drugs responsible
Subacute proximal myopathy	Diamorphine Clofibrate Chloroquine Lithium Quinine
Myasthenic syndromes	D-Penicillamine Lithium Propranolol
Malignant hyperpyrexia	Psychotropic drugs General anaesthetics

myoglobinuria occurs in acute alcoholic excess. (A similar syndrome occurs in diamorphine and amphetamine addicts.) A subacute proximal myopathy occurs with chronic alcohol abuse.

Drugs

Many drug-induced muscle disorders have been described (see Table 18.58). Most respond to drug withdrawal.

DISORDERS OF THE NEUROMUSCULAR JUNCTION

Myasthenia gravis

This acquired condition is characterized by weakness and fatiguability of proximal limb, ocular and bulbar muscles. The heart is not affected.

The cause is unknown. IgG antibodies to acetylcholine receptor protein are found. Immune complexes (IgG and complement) are deposited at the post-synaptic membranes causing interference with and later destruction of the acetylcholine receptor.

Thymic hyperplasia is found in 70% of myasthenic patients below the age of 40. In 10% of patients a thymic tumour is found, the incidence increasing with age; antibodies to striated muscle can be demonstrated in these patients. Young patients without a thymoma have an increased association with certain HLA antigens B8, DR3.

There is an association between myasthenia gravis and thyroid disease, rheumatoid disease, pernicious anaemia and systemic lupus erythematosus. Myasthenia gravis is sometimes caused by D-penicillamine treatment in rheumatoid disease.

The prevalence is about 4 in 100 000. It is twice as common in women as in men, with a peak incidence around the age of 30 years.

CLINICAL FEATURES

Fatiguability is the single most important feature. The proximal limb muscles, the extraocular muscles, and the muscles of mastication, speech, and facial expression are those commonly affected in the early stages. Respiratory difficulties may occur.

Complex extraocular palsies, ptosis and a typical fluctuating proximal weakness are found. The reflexes are initially preserved but may be fatiguable. Muscle wasting is sometimes seen late in the disease.

INVESTIGATION

The clinical picture of fluctuating weakness may be diagnostic but many cases are initially diagnosed as 'hysterical'.

Tensilon (edrophonium) test

Edrophonium (an anticholinesterase) 10 mg i.v. is injected as a bolus after a test dose of 1–2 mg. Improvement in weakness occurs within seconds and lasts for 2–3 minutes when the test is positive. To be certain it is wise to have an observer present and to perform a control test using an injection of saline.

Occasionally the test itself causes bronchial constriction and syncope. It should not therefore be carried out where there are no facilities for resuscitation.

Serum acetylcholine receptor antibodies

These are present in 90% of cases of generalized myasthenia gravis. The antibodies are found in no other condition.

Nerve stimulation

There is a characteristic decrement in the evoked muscle action potential following stimulation of the motor nerve.

Other tests

Preliminary tests may show a mediastinal mass on chest X-ray that can be confirmed by mediastinal CT scanning.

Routine peripheral blood studies are normal (the ESR is not raised). Autoantibodies to striated muscle, intrinsic factor or thyroid may be found. Rheumatoid factor and antinuclear antibody tests may be positive.

Muscle biopsy is usually not performed but ultrastructural abnormalities can be seen.

COURSE AND MANAGEMENT

The severity of myasthenia gravis fluctuates but most cases have a protracted course. It is important to recognize respiratory impairment, dysphagia and nasal regurgitation; emergency assisted ventilation may be required in myasthenic crises.

Exacerbations are usually unpredictable but may be brought on by infections, by aminoglycosides or other drugs. Enemas (magnesium sulphate) may provoke severe weakness.

Oral anticholinesterases

Pyridostigmine (60 mg tablet) is the most widely used drug. Its duration of action is 3–4 h. The dose (usually 4–16 tablets daily) is determined by the patient's response.

Overdose of anticholinesterase causes severe weakness (cholinergic crisis).

Colic and diarrhoea may occur with anticholinesterases. Oral atropine 0.5 mg with each dose may reduce this.

Although anticholinesterases are of value in treating the weakness, they do not alter the natural history of the disease.

Thymectomy

Thymectomy offers long-term benefit, though the reason is uncertain. It improves the prognosis, particularly in patients below 40 years and in those who have had the disease for less than 10 years.

Following thymectomy, some 60% of non-thymoma cases improve. If a thymoma is present, surgery is necessary to remove a potentially malignant tumour, but it is unusual for the myasthenia to improve.

Immunosuppressant drugs

Corticosteroids are used when there is an incomplete response to anticholinesterases. There is improvement in 70% of cases, although this may be preceded by an initial relapse.

Azathioprine (and sometimes plasmapheresis) is combined with prednisolone in steroid-resistant cases.

Myasthenic–myopathic syndrome (Eaton–Lambert syndrome)

This is a rare non-metastatic manifestation of small-cell carcinoma of the bronchus. There is defective acetylcholine release at the neuromuscular junction. Proximal muscle weakness, sometimes involving the ocular and bulbar muscles, is found, with absent reflexes. Weakness tends to improve after muscular contraction (unlike myasthenia gravis).

Other myasthenic syndromes

Other rare myasthenic syndromes occur, for example, congenital myasthenia.

MUSCULAR DYSTROPHIES

These are progressive, genetically determined disorders of skeletal and sometimes cardiac muscle.

Duchenne muscular dystrophy (DMD)

This is inherited as an X-linked recessive disorder, but one-third of cases arise by spontaneous mutation. It occurs in 1 in 3000 male infants. Recently the DMD locus has been localized to the Xp21 region of the X chromosome and the disease is characterized by the absence of the gene product—the protein dystrophin, which is a rod-shaped cytoskeletal protein found in muscle. DMD is usually obvious by the fourth year, and causes death by the age of 20.

CLINICAL FEATURES

The boy has difficulty in running and in rising to an erect position, when he has to 'climb up his legs with his hands' (Gowers' sign).

There is initially a proximal limb weakness with pseudohypertrophy of the calves. The myocardium is affected. The boy becomes severely disabled by 10 years.

INVESTIGATION

The diagnosis is often made on clinical grounds alone.

The creatine phosphokinase is grossly elevated (100–200 times the normal level). Muscle biopsy shows characteristic variation in fibre size, fibre necrosis, regeneration and replacement by fat, and on immunochemical staining an absence of dystrophin. The EMG shows a myopathic pattern.

MANAGEMENT

There is no curative treatment. Passive physiotherapy helps to prevent contractures in the later stages of the disease. A recent trial of prednisolone therapy has shown a short-term improvement in muscle strength and function.

Carrier detection

A female with an affected brother has a 50% chance of carrying the gene. In carrier females, 70% have a raised creatine phosphokinase level and the remainder usually have EMG abnormalities or changes on biopsy. Accurate carrier and prenatal diagnosis can be made using cDNA probes that are co-inherited with the DMD locus.

Genetic advice explaining the inheritance of the condition and counselling about abortion should be given. Determination of the fetal sex by amniocentesis and selective abortion of a male fetus is sometimes carried out. Many proven carrier females choose not to have offspring.

Limb girdle and facio-scapulo-humeral dystrophy

These milder dystrophies are summarized in Table 18.59. There are many other varieties of muscular dystrophy.

MYOTONIAS

These conditions are characterized by myotonia, i.e. continued muscle contraction after the cessation of voluntary effort. The EMG is characteristic (see p. 879). The myotonias are important because patients tolerate general anaesthetics poorly. The commonest two of these rare conditions are mentioned below.

Dystrophia myotonica

This autosomal dominant condition causes progressive distal muscle weakness, with ptosis,

Table 18.59 Limb girdle and facio-scapulo-humeral dystrophies.

	Limb girdle	Facio-scapulo-humeral
Inheritance:	Autosomal recessive	Autosomal dominant
Onset:	10–20 years	10–40 years
Muscles affected:	Shoulder and pelvic girdle	Face, shoulder and pelvic girdle
Progress:	Severe disability within 20–25 years	Normal life expectancy, slow progression
Pseudohypertrophy:	Rare	Very rare
Serum creatine phosphokinase:	Raised (slightly)	Raised (slightly) or normal

weakness and thinning of the face and sternomastoids. Myotonia is usually present. The muscle disease is part of a larger syndrome comprising:

- Cataracts
- Frontal baldness
- Intellectual impairment (mild)
- Cardiomyopathy and conduction defects
- Small pituitary fossa and hypogonadism
- Glucose intolerance
- Low serum IgG

The onset of obvious clinical disease is usually between 20 and 50 years. The condition is gradually progressive. Phenytoin or procainamide sometimes helps the myotonia.

Myotonia congenita (Thomsen's disease)
This is an autosomal dominant disorder. An isolated myotonia, usually mild, occurs in childhood and persists throughout life. The myotonia is accentuated by rest and by cold. Diffuse muscle hypertrophy occurs and the patient appears to have well-developed muscles.

PERIODIC PARALYSES

These are rare membrane disorders characterized by intermittent flaccid muscle weakness and alterations in serum potassium.

Hypokalaemic periodic paralysis
This condition, usually inherited as an autosomal dominant trait, is characterized by generalized weakness (including the speech and bulbar muscles) that often starts after a heavy carbohydrate meal or after a period of rest after exertion. Attacks last for several hours. It is often first noted in the teenage years and tends to remit after the age of 35. The serum potassium is usually below 3.0 mmol·L^{-1} in an attack. The weakness responds to the administration of potassium chloride.

Similar weakness also occurs in hypokalaemia due to diuretics, and may occur during thyrotoxicosis.

Hyperkalaemic periodic paralysis
This condition, usually inherited as an autosomal dominant trait, is characterized by sudden attacks of weakness that are sometimes precipitated by exercise. Attacks start in childhood and tend to remit after the age of 20 years. They last from 30 min to 2 h. Myotonia may occur. The serum potassium is raised.

The attacks are terminated by intravenous calcium gluconate or chloride.

A very rare normokalaemic, sodium-responsive periodic paralysis also occurs.

SPECIFIC METABOLIC MYOPATHIES

This is a large group of rare, genetically determined muscle diseases. Two of these diseases will be mentioned here.

Myophosphorylase deficiency (McArdle's syndrome)
This is an autosomal recessive disorder in which there is a lack of skeletal muscle myophosphorylase. The disorder causes easy fatiguability and severe cramp on exercise, with myoglobinuria.

There is no rise in venous lactate during ischaemic exercise; this forms the basis of a test for the condition.

Malignant hyperpyrexia
Widespread skeletal muscle rigidity and hyperpyrexia developing as a sequel to general anaesthesia is due to an unknown muscle membrane defect. Sudden death during or after anaesthesia may occur in this rare condition, which is sometimes inherited as an autosomal dominant trait. Dantrolene is useful in controlling the rigidity.

Further reading

Aids to the Examination of the Peripheral Nervous System, 3rd edn. (1986) London: Baillière Tindall.

Bannister R (1985) *Brain's Clinical Neurology*, 6th edn. Oxford: Oxford University Press.

Patten J (1977) *Neurological Differential Diagnosis*. London: Harold Starke.

Ross Russell RW & Wiles CM (1986) *Neurology* (Integrated Clinical Science Series). London: Heinemann.

19
Psychological Medicine

related to alcohol and other forms of drug use and abuse.

In Britain, as in the rest of the Western World, there has ben a shift away from the long-stay mental hospital as the focus of psychiatric treatment and towards acute units in district general hospitals.

About 25% of all those referred to psychiatric departments are aged 65 years and over; this includes patients with disorders such as depression and confusional states, which may be reversible, and dementias, which usually are not. It has been estimated that in England about half a million people over 65 years suffer from moderate or severe dementia, and about one-quarter of these are aged 85 years or more.

THE PSYCHIATRIC INTERVIEW

The interview is of prime importance in making a psychiatric diagnosis:

- It is a technique for obtaining information.
- It serves as a standard situation in which to assess the patient's emotions and attitudes.
- The first interview serves to establish an understanding with the patient that will be the basis of any subsequent therapeutic relationship.

The psychiatric history

The history records data from several sources. It is concerned with the patient's complaints, his recent and remote past, and the patient's present life situation up to the time of referral or admission.

The history consists of:

- *Reason for referral*—a brief statement of why and how the patient came to the attention of the doctor
- *Complaints*—reported by the patient in his own words
- *Present illness*—a detailed account of the illness from the earliest time at which a change was noted until the patient came to the attention of the doctor
- *Family history*—this should focus on the family atmosphere in the patient's childhood, early stresses (including death or separation), and the occurrence of mental illness in family members
- *Personal history*—a short biography that covers childhood and school, jobs held and lost, marriage and divorce, children, and the present

Introduction

Psychiatry is the branch of medicine that is concerned with the study and treatment of disorders of mental function. A substantial proportion of patients seen by a doctor suffer from psychiatric illness rather than organic disease. Some of these psychiatric problems occur as a consequence of individual social circumstances that may be difficult to alter. Physical and psychiatric disorder often coincide because:

- Patients with psychiatric problems can present with physical manifestations (e.g. the irritable bowel syndrome).
- Chronic or severe physical ill-health can result in psychiatric disorder (e.g. depression in the setting of a chronic painful disorder).
- Psychiatric symptoms can be part of a physical disease complex (e.g. depression in hypothyroidism).
- Patients with established psychiatric disorders can also develop physical disease.

For these reasons, the psychological aspects of disease cannot be the exclusive preserve of psychiatrists but must be the concern of all doctors.

Approximately 15% of attenders at general practices in the UK suffer from psychiatric ill-health. Most of the illnesses are minor mood disorders, taking the form of various combinations of depression and anxiety, and about two-thirds are short-lived in nature and clear within 6 months. However, about 5% of general practice consultations involve patients suffering from major depression requiring energetic treatment. The major psychoses—schizophrenia and manic-depressive illness—are much less common in this setting. The general hospital physician and surgeon will tend to see psychiatric disorders that are associated with physical disease or caused by certain physical treatments as well as disorders

housing, social and financial situation
- *Personality*—this consists of a person's attitudes and beliefs, moral values and standards, leisure activities and interests, and usual reaction to stress and setback
- *Medical history*—this includes health during childhood, menstrual history, previous mental health and the use and abuse of alcohol, tobacco and drugs

Supplementary information should be obtained from a close relative or friend who can provide corroboration and additional details.

The mental state examination

Appearance and general behaviour
The patient's clothes, posture, facial expression, general grooming, and demeanour are noted. Posture and movement may also reflect mood. Any inappropriate activity or gross physical signs should also be noted. In the case of the mute or non-cooperative patient, this aspect of the examination should be quite detailed.

Speech
The form of the patient's speech (its rate and quantity) is assessed. Disorders of flow (e.g. whether there are interruptions, rapid shifts or sudden blocks) are relevant. Particularly unusual disturbances can be illustrated by recording typical excerpts.

Mood
This is the least objective part of the examination. Obvious misery, elation or anxiety should be noted. The patient's general feelings are explored (e.g. 'How do you feel in yourself?' 'How is your mood?'). Suicidal feelings are enquired about at this stage if a depressive mood is suspected (e.g. 'How desperate do you feel?' 'Have you ever felt like ending your life?' 'Have you found that you have been thinking of ways to do it?' 'Have you made an attempt?'). Likewise, where an expansive mood is noted, questions concerning elation, including the presence of excessive self-confidence, inflated self-assessment and extravagant plans, are raised. The constancy of mood during the interview, its appropriateness and its impact on the interviewer should be noted.

Enquiries should also be made concerning sleep, appetite, libido, fatigue and irritability.

Thought content
The patient's answers to questions such as 'What do you see as your main worries?' should be summarized. Questions should be asked concerning anxieties or preoccupations with the present life situation, with the future, with the past, and with the safety of themselves or others, and whether the worries interfere with concentration or sleep. Information should also be sought concerning the presence of phobias, obsessional ruminations, compulsions or rituals.

Abnormal beliefs and interpretations of events
The content, mode of onset and degree of fixity are noted of any abnormal beliefs:

- In relation to the environment (e.g. ideas of reference, misinterpretations or delusions). The patient is asked about beliefs that he is being persecuted, being treated in a special way or is the subject of an experiment.
- In relation to the body (e.g. ideas or delusions of bodily change).
- In relation to the self (e.g. delusions of passivity, influence, thought-reading or intrusion).

Abnormal experiences referred to the environment, body or self
The patient should be directly asked whether

Table 19.1 Assessment of cognitive functions.

Function	Questions
Orientation	What is the time/day/month/year? Where are you? What is this place? Whom do you recognize?
Concentration	Repeat months of the year backwards Take 7 serially from 100 (serial 7s) Repeat a span of digits (e.g. 5-figure: 43701; 6-figure: 732156)
Memory: Short-term	Recall test name and address after 2 and 5 min
Medium/long-term	Current affairs (e.g. name of the prime minister, occupant of the throne, events in the news) Dates of World War II
Intelligence	Simple arithmetic sums Meanings of words Meanings of proverbs Ability to read and write
Higher cortical function	Spatial awareness—drawing 3D objects Naming of objects Right–left discrimination ('Touch your left ear with your right hand')

he/she has experienced unusual, odd or abnormal experiences related to:

- The environment (e.g. hallucinations and illusions, which may be auditory, visual, tactile, olfactory or gustatory; feelings of familiarity or unfamiliarity; derealization; déjà-vu)
- The body (e.g. feelings of deadness, pain or other alterations of bodily sensation)
- The self (e.g. depersonalization; awareness of disturbance in the mechanism of thinking, or blocking, retardation or autochthonous ideas)

Cognitive state

This should be briefly assessed in every patient and related to his general intelligence. It may be impaired in organic mental illness. However, the patient who can give a clear and accurate history is unlikely to have cognitive impairment. Aspects to be tested are shown in Table 19.1.

Insight

The degree to which a patient recognizes that he is ill should be assessed at the end of the mental state examination.

Summary

The psychiatric history, present state and mental state examination can now be summarized in order to provide a differential diagnosis. In psychiatry, the term 'the formulation' is used to describe a concise assessment of the case, which includes a discussion of alternative ideas about diagnosis, aetiology, treatment and prognosis and the arguments for and against each alternative.

SIGNS AND SYMPTOMS OF PSYCHIATRIC DISORDER

Appearance and general behaviour

Facial appearance, posture and movement provide information about a patient's mood. Patients with retarded depression sit with shoulders hunched, immobile, and with the gaze directed at the floor. Agitated depressives are often tremulous and restless, adjusting their clothing and pacing up and down, while manic patients are often overactive and disinhibited.

Certain uncommon disorders of behaviour are encountered, mainly in schizophrenia. These include:

- *Stereotypy*, which is repetition of movements that do not appear to have a purpose; the movement may be repeated in a regular sequence (e.g. rocking backwards and forwards)
- *Mannerisms*, which are repeated movements that appear to have some functional significance (e.g. saluting)

- *Negativism*, when patients do the opposite of what is asked and actively resist efforts to persuade them to comply
- *Echopraxia*, when patients automatically imitate the interviewer's movements despite being asked not to do this

Speech

Disorders of thinking are usually recognized from the patient's speech.

Disorders of the stream of thought
There are abnormalities in the amount and speed of the thoughts experienced. At one extreme, there is *pressure of thought*, in which ideas arise in remarkable abundance and variety and pass rapidly through the mind. *Poverty of thought* is the opposite experience, when there appears to be a lack or absence of any thoughts whatsoever and the patient reports his mind to be blank or starved of ideas. Pressure of thought characteristically occurs in mania, and poverty of thought in depression; either may be experienced in schizophrenia. The stream of thought can also be suddenly interrupted. Minor degrees of this phenomenon are not uncommon, especially in normal people who are tired or tense. Severe *thought blocking*, in which there is a particularly abrupt and complete interruption of the stream of thought, strongly suggests schizophrenia. The patient often describes the experience as a sudden and complete emptying of his mind and may interpret the experience in an unusual way (e.g. as having had his thoughts removed by some alien person, presence or machine).

Disorders of the form of thought
These include flight of ideas, perseveration, and loosening of associations.

Flight of ideas. The patient's thoughts and speech move quickly from one topic to another, such that one train of thought is not completed before another appears. It is often accompanied by *clang associations* (the tendency to use two or more words with a similar sound), *punning* (the use of one word with two or more different meanings), rhyming, and responding to distracting cues in the immediate surroundings. Flight of ideas is characteristic of mania.

Perseveration. This is the persistent and inappropriate repetitions of the same thoughts or actions. It is often associated with dementia but can occur in other conditions.

Loosening of associations. This is manifested by a loss of the normal structure of thinking. The most striking impression is an extreme lack of clarity.

There are several forms. *Knight's move* or *derailment* denotes transition from one topic to another, either between sentences or within a sentence, with no logical relationship between the two topics and no evidence of flight of ideas as described above. When this abnormality is extreme and disrupts not merely the connections between sentences but also the finer grammatical structure of speech, it is termed *word salad* or *verbigeration*. One effect of loosened associations is sometimes termed 'talking past the point'; the patient always seems to get near to talking about the matter in hand but never quite gets there.

Mood

In psychiatric disorders, mood may be altered in three ways:

- Its nature may be changed.
- It may fluctuate more than usual.
- It may be inconsistent either with the patient's thoughts and actions or with occurrences in the patient's immediate environment.

Changes in the nature of mood

Changes in the nature of mood may be towards depression, elation or anxiety. *Depression* may mean the symptom of feeling sad, melancholic or low in spirits, or it may mean the syndrome of depression as characterized by low mood, lack of enjoyment, reduced energy and changes in appetite, sleep and libido. *Elation* refers to a subjective feeling of high spirits, vitality and even ecstasy, which may or may not be accompanied by exuberant behaviour, increased energy and overactivity. *Anxiety* is a common symptom of worry or apprehension that is often accompanied by physical symptoms such as palpitations, trembling, 'butterflies in the stomach' and hyperventilation.

Anxiety and depression can occur separately or together and may be associated with an obvious cause or may appear to arise without reason.

A *phobia* is an intense fear of a specific object, activity or situation coupled with a wish to avoid it. The fear is irrational in that it is out of all proportion to the real danger. The patient recognizes that it is an exaggerated fear but finds it difficult to control. Objects that provoke such fear include insects, spiders and other animals (e.g. dogs, cats, horses) or natural phenomena such as lightning or the dark. Situations that provoke phobic reactions include open spaces (agoraphobia), closed spaces such as lifts and underground trains (claustrophobia), high places, and crowds.

Changes in the fluctuation of mood

These may result in a total loss of emotion or an inability to experience pleasure. The former is termed *apathy*. When the normal variation of mood is reduced rather than lost, the mood is described as *blunted*. Emotions that are changeable in a rapid, abrupt and excessive way are termed *labile* emotions.

Inconsistent or inappropriate mood

This occurs when the normal emotional expression of the person fails to match his thoughts and actions. For example, a patient may laugh when describing the death of a close and loved relative. Such incongruity needs to be distinguished from laughter that indicates that someone is ill at ease when talking about a distressing subject.

Changes of mood are found in a variety of psychiatric disorders, including depression, mania, anxiety, organic psychoses and schizophrenia.

Thought content

As discussed earlier, thought content refers to the worries and preoccupations manifested by the patient and elicited on interview. Abnormal beliefs and experiences are, of course, part of the thought content, but are regarded as sufficiently important to be discussed separately (see below).

An important disorder of thought content is an *obsession*, which is a recurrent, persistent thought, impulse or image that enters the mind despite the individual's effort to resist it. The individual recognizes that the obsession is his own and is not implanted by anyone or arising from elsewhere.

A *compulsion* is a repetitive and seemingly purposeful action performed in a stereotyped way, referred to as a *compulsive ritual*. Compulsions are accompanied by a subjective sense that they must be carried out and by an urge to resist. Common obsessions concern dirt, contamination, orderliness and dread of illness, while corresponding compulsions would be repeated hand-washings and checkings.

Abnormal beliefs and interpretations of events

The main form of abnormal belief is the *delusion*.
Delusions can be:

- *Primary* or *autochthonous*, i.e. they appear suddenly and with full conviction but without any preceding or related mental events. For example, a patient on being offered a cup of tea suddenly believes that this indicates that the Russians have landed at Dover.
- *Secondary*, i.e. derived from some preceding morbid experience, such as a depressed mood or an auditory hallucination.

Delusions are classified according to their content, and include persecutory delusions (also called paranoid delusions), delusions of reference, guilt, worthlessness or nihilism, religious delusions, and delusions of grandeur, jealousy or control. These are further defined when discussed in relation to specific conditions.

Particular delusions concerning thought control can occur. Patients who have delusions of *thought insertion* believe that some of their thoughts are not their own but have been implanted by some outside force or agency. The same or other patients may believe that thoughts are taken out of their minds by external forces or agencies (*thought withdrawal*), while in delusions of *thought broadcasting* the patient believes that his unspoken thoughts are known to other people through radio, television, telepathy or in some other way. Feelings and actions may also be interpreted by the individual as being under the influence or control of some external, usually alien, power. Such *passivity* experiences, occurring in the absence of clear-cut brain diseases, are regarded as diagnostic of schizophrenia. The patient may merely assert that his behaviour is controlled from without and may be unable to give any further explanation. This is usually described as an *experience of passivity*. The patient may develop secondary delusions that explain this alien control as a result of witchcraft, hypnosis, radio waves, television—so-called *delusions of passivity*. The disturbances of thought control discussed above are examples of passivity experiences involving the thought processes.

Delusion

This is defined as an abnormal belief arising from distorted judgements and that is:

● Held with absolute conviction
● Not amenable to reason or modifiable by experience
● Not shared by those of a common cultural or social background
● Experienced as a self-evident truth of great personal significance
● False

Delusions should be distinguished from *overvalued ideas*, i.e. deeply held personal convictions that are understandable when the individual's background is known. *Ideas of reference* that fall short of delusions are held by people who are particularly self-conscious. Such individuals cannot help feeling that people take particular notice of them in public places, pass comment about them and/or observe things about them that they would prefer were ignored. Such feelings are not delusional in that the individual who experiences them realizes that they originate within him and that he is no more noticeable or noteworthy than anyone else, but nevertheless he cannot dismiss the feelings.

Abnormal experiences referred to the environment, body or self

Illusions are misperceptions of external stimuli and are most likely to occur when the general level of sensory stimulation is reduced.

Hallucinations are perceptions that are experienced in the absence of any external stimulus to the sense organs in the outside world (and are not within one's mind as in imagery). Normal people occasionally experience hallucinations, mainly auditory in type, particularly when tired and during the transition between sleeping and waking.

Hallucination

This is defined as a thorough conviction of a sensation when no external object to excite or provoke such a sensation is present. It is:

● A false perception and not a distortion
● Perceived as inhabiting objective space
● Perceived as having qualities of normal perceptions
● Perceived alongside normal perceptions
● Independent of the individual's will

Hallucinations can be *elementary* (e.g. bangs, whistles) or *complex* (e.g. faces, voices, music), and may be auditory, visual, tactile, gustatory, olfactory or of deep sensation.

A change in self-awareness such that the person concerned feels unreal is termed *depersonalization*. In this state the person feels detached or remote from his/her own experience and unable to feel emotion. The individual is aware of the subjective nature of this alteration. The feeling that the external environment has become unreal and/or remote is termed *derealization*. Both these phenomena occur in healthy people when they are tired, after sensory deprivation and during the use of hallucinogenic drugs, and also occur in certain conditions such as anxiety, depression, schizophrenia and temporal lobe epilepsy.

Cognitive state

There are four processes involved in normal memory:

● Registration—the ability to add new material to the existing memory stores
● Retention—the ability to retain the memory
● Recall—the ability to bring it back into awareness
● Recognition—the feeling of familiarity indicating that a particular person, event or object has been encountered before

Some patients describe the recognition of a situation, person or event as having been encountered before when it is in fact novel—the so-called *déjà vu* experience, whereas others report the reverse experience (*jamais vu*) when there is failure to recognize a situation, person or event that has been encountered before. Déjà vu experiences occur in healthy people as well as in anxiety states. Both types of experience can occur in epilepsy (see p. 917).

Patients with Wernicke–Korsakoff syndrome, who have extreme difficulty in remembering recent and past events, sometimes report remembering past events that have not actually taken place; this is known as *confabulation*. Failure of memory is termed *amnesia*.

Consciousness can be defined as the awareness of the self and the environment. Attention, concentration and memory are impaired and orientation is disturbed in any condition in which a disturbance of consciousness occurs. This subject is considered on p. 904.

Defence mechanisms

These are a series of subconscious mental processes. The individual is unaware that he is employing them although he may become aware of such motives through self-analysis or by having them pointed out to him. The defence mechanisms described below are amongst the commonest used and are useful in understanding many aspects of behaviour.

Repression is the exclusion from awareness of memories, emotions and/or impulses that would cause anxiety and distress if allowed to enter consciousness.

Denial, a related concept, is believed to be employed when a patient behaves as though unaware of something that he might reasonably be expected to know. One example would be a patient who, despite being told that a close relative has died, continues to behave as though he/she were still alive.

Regression is the unconscious adoption of patterns of behaviour appropriate to an earlier stage of development. It is often seen in ill people who become child-like and highly dependent in relation to their doctor and nursing care.

Projection involves the unconscious attribution to another person of thoughts or feelings that are in fact one's own.

Reaction formation refers to the unconscious adoption of behaviour opposite to that which reflect the individual's true feelings and intentions.

Displacement involves the transferring of emotion from a situation or object with which it is properly associated to another that gives less distress.

Rationalization refers to the unconscious process whereby a false but acceptable explanation is provided for behaviour that in fact has other, much less acceptable, origins.

Sublimation refers to the unconscious diversion of unacceptable outlets into acceptable outlets.

Identification refers to the unconscious process of taking on some of the characteristics or behaviours of another person, often to reduce the pain of separation or loss.

CAUSES OF PSYCHIATRIC DISORDER

A single psychiatric disorder may result from several causes.

Predisposing factors

These are factors, often operating from early life, that determine a person's vulnerability to psychological distress. Such causes include:

- Genetic endowment
- Environment *in utero*
- Personality
- Childhood trauma

There is evidence for a strong genetic factor in the psychoses, and a weaker genetic factor in the neurotic disorders. Intrauterine disturbances may result in minor organic damage to the brain and central nervous system, which in turn may render the individual liable to develop a serious mental disorder in later life in response to particular kinds of stress.

Personality results from the interaction of genetic endowment, uterine development, early childhood experience and various physical, psychological and social influences manifesting themselves up to and including adolescence. Certain personalities are believed to be particularly prone to develop certain disorders. For example, individuals who manifest certain obsessional traits as part of their personality have an increased risk of developing depressive and obsessional illnesses, while anxious, apprehensive individuals are prone to develop a variety of neurotic disorders. When taking the history, particular care should be taken to assess whether the individual's personality was well developed and mature *prior* to the development of the illness, as this will be a major factor in determining the outcome of treatment and the prognosis.

Table 19.2 Psychiatric symptoms commonly associated with physical diseases.

Symptom	Examples of physical disease
Depression	Carcinoma
	Infection
	Thyroid disorders
	Adrenal disorders
	Diabetes mellitus
Anxiety	Hyperthyroidism
	Phaeochromocytoma
	Hypoglycaemia
	Partial seizures
	Alcohol/drug withdrawal
Irritability	Head injury
	Premenstrual tension
	Early dementia
	Hypoglycaemia
Fatigue	Anaemia
	Sleep disorders
	Infections
	Carcinoma
Behavioural disturbance	Epilepsy
	Toxic confusional states
	Dementia
	Porphyria
	Hypoglycaemia

Precipitating factors

These are factors that occur shortly before the onset of a disorder and that appear to have caused it. They may be physical, psychological or social in nature. Whether they produce a disorder depends partly on their severity and partly on the presence of predisposing factors.

Physical precipitating factors include physical diseases (e.g. hypothyroidism, tumours, metabolic disorders) or drugs (e.g. steroids, hypotensives, alcohol). Psychological factors include loss of self-esteem due to a setback or misfortune such as marital infidelity or financial disaster. Social factors include moving house, job difficulties and family disturbances.

Occasionally, the same factor can act in more than one way. A head injury can induce psychological disturbances either through physical changes in the central nervous system or through the stress it provokes in the individual, while marital breakdown may lead to overindulgence in alcohol with secondary impairment of mental processes and psychiatric illness.

Perpetuating factors

These are factors that prolong the course of a disorder after it has occurred. For example, some psychiatric disorders lead to secondary demoralization. A medical student who suffers a depressive illness may well find it difficult to accept the diagnosis, may regard himself as weak and flawed, and may withdraw from social activities. Such a response could prolong the original disorder.

PSYCHIATRIC ASPECTS OF PHYSICAL DISEASE

Psychological and physical symptoms commonly occur together; surveys have shown that they tend to 'cluster' in some people, while others remain relatively free from illnesses. The commonest presentation of psychiatric ill-health in physically ill patients is as affective disorders or acute organic brain syndromes. The relationship between psychological and physical symptoms may be understood in one of three ways:

- Psychological distress and disorder can provoke and precipitate physical disease.
- Physical distress and disease can cause psychological ill-health (see Table 19.2), as can the medication given for the disease.
- Physical and psychological symptoms and disorders coexist because both are common, particularly in the elderly.

Physically ill patients often respond to their illness by feeling depressed, anxious, angry and/or unable to cope. Such reactions are very often transient and require little in the way of management other than recognition, reassurance and support. Sometimes however, they persist after the acute stage of the physical illness has passed. Certain factors also

Table 19.3 Factors increasing the risk of psychiatric illness in physically ill patients.

Patient
Previous history of psychiatric illness
History of difficulty in coping with stress
Disturbed personal, family or social circumstances

Setting
Intensive care units
Coronary care units
Renal dialysis units

Physical illness
Carcinoma
Endocrine disorders
Infections
Metabolic disorders
Head injury
Mutilating surgery

Physical treatment
Drugs (e.g. steroids)
Radiotherapy

increase the risk of a psychiatric disorder occurring in the setting of physical disease (Table 19.3). Treatment is the same as for physically healthy, psychiatrically ill patients, but care must be taken when prescribing psychotropic drugs to avoid drug interactions.

One symptom that can be thought of as both a physical and a psychological symptom is *pain*. It is the commonest medical symptom, can cause considerable psychological distress and can arise from psychological disturbance. The main sites of psychologically determined pain are the head, the neck, the lower back, the abdomen and the genitalia.

Psychologically determined pain is often continuous for lengthy periods and responds poorly to analgesics. It is often described by the patient as waxing and waning in response to emotional stress and, despite its severity, does not necessarily wake the patient from sleep. A particularly dramatic form of chronic, atypical pain is facial pain; antidepressant therapy has been found to be effective in up to 50% of such patients. Another common painful condition in which depression is often present but is 'masked' by the physical symptoms is the irritable bowel syndrome.

There has been much speculation about the existence of a chronic fatigue syndrome that might follow various infections, often viral. The cardinal symptom is fatigue, which, together with the associated symptoms of poor concentration and memory, irritability and alterations in sleep, resembles the older diagnosis of neurasthenia. Controversy currently exists concerning the precise status of myalgic encephalomyelitis (ME) consisting of aching muscles, 'inflamed' brain and spinal cord and fatigue, and attributed by some to infection with Epstein–Barr and/or other viruses. However, there is no good evidence for any infective cause of this condition at present.

CLASSIFICATION OF MENTAL ILLNESS

The concept of mental illness is complicated. The diagnosis is only made when:

- There is a recognizable disturbance in one or more psychological functions, e.g. perception, emotion, thought.
- The disturbance is not under the comprehensive control of the individual concerned.
- The disturbance usually (though not invariably) causes distress to the affected individual.
- The disturbance usually (though not invariably) requires expert, professional assessment and treatment for recovery.

Particular problems in psychiatry are posed by such conditions as sexual disorders, drug and

Table 19.4 A classification of psychiatric disorders.

Organic disorders (ICD 290–294)[a]
Functional psychosis 　Schizophrenia (ICD 295) 　Manic-depressive disorder (ICD 296)
Neurotic disorders 　Anxiety neurosis (ICD 300) 　Phobic neurosis (ICD 300.2) 　Obsessional neurosis (ICD 300.3) 　Hysteria (ICD 300.1) 　Hypochondriasis (ICD 300.7)
Personality disorders (ICD 301)
Sexual deviations and disorders (ICD 302)
Alcohol and drug dependence (ICD 303–305)
Other disorders e.g. anorexia nervosa (ICD 307.1)

[a] Three-digit numbers refer to the numbers of the diagnostic categories in the *Glossary of Mental Disorders*, part of the 9th revision of the International Classification of Diseases produced by the World Health Organization.

alcohol dependence and personality disorders.

The most widely used and inclusive classification of mental disorders is the World Health Organization's *Glossary of Mental Disorders*, which is part of the 9th revision of the International Classification of Diseases. In 1980, the third edition of the *Diagnostic and Statistical Manual* of the American Psychiatric Association (DSM III) was published. This scheme has five axes. The two main axes are:

- Psychiatric syndromes
- Personality disorders

The others are:

- Physical disorders
- Severity of psychological stressors
- Highest level of adaptive functioning

A simple classification of psychiatric disorders is shown in Table 19.4. The term *psychosis* is usually applied to a psychiatric disorder that significantly impairs insight, involves a substantial break with reality, exercises a major impact on the individual's personality and functioning, and usually requires specialized, inpatient treatment. Certain symptoms that by definition involve an impairment of reality, such as delusions, hallucinations and formal thought disorder, are often termed psychotic symptoms. In contrast, the term *neurosis* is applied to psychiatric disorders in which psychotic symptoms and features are absent, the patient's personality is relatively undamaged, and contact with reality is unimpaired. Neuroses can be thought of as exaggerated forms of the normal reactions to stressful events. Anxiety, depression, irritability and physical symptoms lacking an organic cause are experienced by many people in response to stressful circumstances and events. In the neuroses these symptoms become so intense as to be highly unpleasant and distressing and out of proportion to the severity of the stress.

Organic psychiatric disorders

Organic brain diseases result from structural pathology, as in senile dementia, or from disturbed central nervous system function, as in fever-induced delirium. A classification of organic brain syndromes, derived from the American classification, DSM III, is shown in Table 19.5.

Table 19.5 Classification of organic brain syndromes.

Delirium
Dementia
Amnestic syndrome
Organic delusional syndrome
Organic affective syndrome
Intoxication and withdrawal syndromes

Delirium

Delirium, also termed 'toxic confusional state', is an acute or subacute condition in which impairment of consciousness is accompanied by abnormalities of perception and mood. The impairment of consciousness can range from mild befuddlement to serious disorientation and confusion. The degree of impairment classically fluctuates, so that there are intermittent lucid periods. Confusion is usually worse at night. During the acute phase, thought and speech are incoherent, memory is impaired and misperceptions occur. Transient hallucinations, usually visual, and delusions may occur and, as a consequence, the patient may be frightened, suspicious, restless and uncooperative. A large number of diseases may be accompanied by delirium; this is particularly so in elderly patients. Some causes of delirium are listed in Table 19.6. Delirium usually clears within a few days as the underlying illness resolves. If the delirium runs a subacute course, more permanent disorders of cognition, memory or personality may occur.

Investigation and treatment of the underlying physical disease should be undertaken. The patient should be carefully nursed and rehydrated. Pain relief should be adequate and sedation provided if necessary. If a high fever is present, the temperature should be reduced with fans, ice-packs and

Table 19.6 Some causes of delirium.

Systemic infection
    Any infection, particularly with high fever (e.g. malaria, septicaemia)

Metabolic disturbance
    Hepatic failure
    Renal failure
    Disorders of electrolyte balance
    Hypoxia

Vitamin deficiency
    Thiamine (Wernicke–Korsakoff syndrome, beriberi)
    Nicotinic acid (pellagra)
    Vitamin B_{12}

Endocrine disease
    Hypoglycaemia

Brain damage
    Trauma
    Tumour
    Abscess
    Subarachnoid haemorrhage

Drug intoxication
    Anticonvulsant
    Anticholinergic
    Anxiolytic/hypnotic
    Opiates
    Industrial poisons, e.g. DDT, trichloroethylene

Drug/alcohol withdrawal

antipyretic drugs. All current drug therapy should be reviewed and, where possible, stopped. Benzodiazepines are the drugs of choice in the management of minor restlessness, but in severe delirium haloperidol is probably a more effective choice, the daily dose usually ranging between 10 and 60 mg. If necessary, the first dose of 2–10 mg can be administered intramuscularly.

Management of the disturbed or violent patient
Psychotic, organically impaired and intoxicated patients may be frightened, aggressive, confused and difficult to manage. It is important that those involved in their acute management refrain from threatening behaviour, appear in control (even if they do not feel it!) and avoid being drawn into a confrontation.

When evaluating a disturbed patient in the emergency department, a crucial question is: 'Could this behaviour be the result of an organic disturbance?' Organic psychiatric disorders, particularly those associated with drugs and alcohol, are important causes of behavioural and thought disturbances in emergency clinic attenders. Some organic disorders initially showing signs and

Table 19.7 Clinical features of delirium, dementia and acute functional psychosis.[a]

Feature	Delirium	Dementia	Acute functional psychosis
Onset	Sudden	Insidious	Sudden
24-h course	Fluctuating	Stable	Stable
Consciousness	Reduced	Clear	Clear
Attention	Globally impaired	Globally impaired	Variably affected
Cognition	Globally impaired	Globally impaired	May be selectively impaired
Hallucinations	Usually visual	Often absent	Mainly auditory
Delusions	Fleeting, poorly systematized	Often absent	Sustained, systematized
Orientation	Usually impaired	Often impaired	May be impaired
Psychomotor activity	Increased, reduced or shifting	Often normal	Varies from retardation to hyperactivity
Speech	Often slow, rapid or incoherent	Difficulty finding words, perseveration	Normal, slow or rapid
Involuntary movements	Often asterixis or coarse tremor	Often absent	Usually absent
Physical illness or drug toxicity	One or both are present	Often absent	Usually absent

[a] After Lipowski (1989) *New England Journal of Medicine* **320** (No. 9): 578–581 (with permission).

symptoms of psychosis, such as poisoning, meningitis and hypoxia, may be life-threatening. Treatment is with chlorpromazine in doses of 25–50 mg orally; i.m. haloperidol causes less hypotension and is an alternative.

Dementia

Dementia is defined as an acquired global impairment of intellect, memory and personality without impairment of consciousness. Usually, its onset is gradual, although a sudden change of environment, such as admission to hospital or an intercurrent illness, may bring it to light.

The symptoms and signs of dementia include:

- Memory impairment
- A decline in intellectual ability
- Coarsening of the personality
- A deterioration in social skills
- Disinhibition of behaviour
- Mood changes
- Paranoid delusions and hallucinations

Memory impairment, which affects short-term rather than long-term memories, is usually an early symptom. The intellectual decline is often gradual and alterations in personality follow. Depression, anxiety and irritability often accompany the intel-

lectual and behavioural deterioration, while in the later stages paranoid delusions, which may be accompanied by auditory and visual hallucinations, appear. Table 19.7 shows the features of dementia compared with delirium and an acute functional psychosis.

About 25% of the elderly population suffer from a psychiatric disability, mainly anxiety and depression. However, dementia affects about 10% of those aged over 65 years and 20% of those over 80 years of age—a total of 650 000 people in England and Wales. The causes are many and are, for the most part, irreversible. Among elderly patients, degenerative and vascular causes predominate.

The main causes of dementia are given in Table 18.49, p. 948.

Amnestic syndrome (see p. 883)

The amnestic syndrome is characterized by a marked impairment of memory occurring in clear consciousness and not as part of a delirium or dementia. Long-term memory is affected but the typical feature is impairment of short-term memory. Often the patient is blandly unconcerned and commonly displays confabulation. One of the commonest causes is severe thiamine deficiency secondary to chronic alcohol abuse but other, less common causes are shown in Table 18.8.

Organic delusional syndrome

The organic delusional syndrome is characterized by a mental state dominated by delusions that are often accompanied by a persistent and distressing misperception of the environment, sometimes referred to as 'delusional tone'. The delusions are very often persecutory but may also be hypochondriacal, pathologically jealous, grandiose or erotic.

Organic affective syndrome

The organic affective syndrome consists of marked mood changes that result from organic brain damage. There are depressive and manic phases, often occurring suddenly, or there may be a persistently dysphoric state. There is no significant intellectual loss, delusions or hallucinations, and a family history of affective disorder is uncommon.

Intoxication and withdrawal syndromes

These are discussed on p. 992.

Schizophrenia

The term 'schizophrenia' was coined by the Swiss psychiatrist Eugen Bleuler in 1908 as a 'rending (disconnection) or splitting of the psychic functions'. The normal integration of emotional and cognitive functions is ruptured in schizophrenia.

Table 19.8 Possible biological causes of schizophrenia.

Genetic
40% risk for children of 2 affected parents
50% risk for monozygotic twin of affected individual
Possible locus on chromosome 5

Dopamine
Dopamine agonists (e.g. amphetamine) exacerbate the condition
The therapeutic potency of neuroleptics is directly related to their ability to block dopamine receptors in the brain
Withdrawal of dopamine antagonists causes rebound of symptoms in some patients
Post-mortem studies show increased dopamine-binding sites in the brains of affected patients

Brain damage (e.g. in utero from long-acting virus)
Enlargement of lateral ventricles and widening of cerebral fissures and sulci on CT scans of a subgroup of patients

Other
Disturbance in transmethylation
Abnormalities in monoamine oxidase function

The annual prevalence of the condition ranges between 2 and 4 per 1000. The lifetime risk of contracting schizophrenia is 1%, but for first-degree relatives of sufferers it is 12%. High rates have been reported in north-west Yugoslavia and among the Tamils of south India.

CAUSES

No one cause has been identified to date. A number of possible causes have been implicated and are currently the subject of research. Biological causes are indicated in Table 19.8. Psychological theories suggest that schizophrenics have an impaired ability to handle the amount and speed of incoming perceptual stimuli and/or that some schizophrenics have a left hemisphere limbic dysfunction. A popular social theory suggests that disturbances in family relationships or communication are the cause, but the evidence is poor. Studies of so-called 'expressed emotion' suggest that schizophrenic patients are particularly vulnerable to highly expressed emotions, and such family atmospheres increase the chances of relapse in treated patients as do intensive psychotherapy and social demands.

CLINICAL FEATURES

The illness can begin at any age but is rare before puberty; the peak age of onset is in late adolescence and the early twenties. The overall sex incidence is about equal. Schizophrenia is probably not a specific condition but rather a number of clinical syndromes. The symptoms that have been considered as diagnostic of the condition have been termed 'first-rank' symptoms and were described by the German psychiatrist Kurt Schneider. They consist of:

● Auditory hallucinations—the patient hears his own thoughts spoken aloud and/or he hears one or several voices referring to himself in the third person or referring to him by name, and/or he hears voices commenting on his behaviour
● Thought withdrawal, insertion and interruption
● Thought broadcasting
● Delusional perceptions
● External control of emotions
● Somatic passivity and feelings—the patient believing that thoughts or acts are due to the influence of others

The World Health Organization's *International Pilot Study of Schizophrenia* has shown that the presence of any one of these symptoms, in the absence of physical disease, is highly discriminating for the diagnosis in a variety of countries and cultures. Other symptoms of acute schizophrenia include behavioural disturbances, thought disorder, hallucinations, delusions and mood abnormalities.

Chronic schizophrenia is characterized by thought

Table 19.9 Drugs causing psychosis.

Glucocorticoids
Anticholinergic agents
Sympathomimetic central stimulants
Phenytoin
Carbamazepine
Disulfiram
Metronidazole
Cardiac glycosides
Hallucinogens, e.g. LSD, mescaline
Amantadine

disorder and the so-called 'negative' symptoms of underactivity, lack of drive, social withdrawal and emotional emptiness. Motor disturbances can occur but they are extremely rare. Such disorders are often described as catatonic and include stupor, excitement, mannerisms, stereotypies and automatic obedience. Delusions in chronic schizophrenia are often held with little emotional response (the so-called 'systematized' delusions) and may be 'encapsulated' from the rest of the patient's beliefs and behaviour.

DIFFERENTIAL DIAGNOSIS

Schizophrenia must be distinguished from

- Organic psychiatric disorders
- Affective disorders
- Personality disorders

The most important organic disorders, particularly in young patients, are drug-induced psychoses and temporal-lobe epilepsy. Some of the drugs that can produce psychosis are listed in Table 19.9.

In older patients, any acute brain syndrome as well as dementia can present in a schizophrenia-like manner. A helpful diagnostic point is that clouding of consciousness and disturbances of memory do not occur in schizophrenia and visual hallucinations are unusual.

Affective disorders present with a more sustained disturbance of mood and any delusions and hallucinations that are detected are usually understandable in terms of the mood disturbance. 'First-rank' symptoms are not normally a feature of affective disorders. Differentiating insidiously arising schizophrenia from a personality disorder in a young person can be exceptionally difficult and the passage of time may be needed for the condition to be clarified.

COURSE AND PROGNOSIS (Table 19.10)

The prognosis of schizophrenia is highly variable. The patient's psychosocial environment appears important in that in an understimulating environment negative symptoms worsen, whereas in an excessively stimulating environment positive symptoms may emerge or worsen. Some patients only suffer acute episodes that leave them relatively unimpaired; others insidiously develop chiefly negative symptoms. The most common presentation and course is an initial acute episode of floridly positive symptoms followed by the emergence and persistence of negative symptoms.

A recent review of treatment studies suggests that between 15 and 25% of schizophrenics recover completely, another two-thirds will have relapses and may develop mild to moderate negative symptoms, while about 1 in 10 will become seriously disabled.

Table 19.10 Prognostic factors in schizophrenia.

	Good factors	Bad factors
Premorbid state	No family history of schizophrenia	Family history of schizophrenia
	Stable personality	Withdrawn, solitary, eccentric personality
	Warm personal relationships	Poor work record; poverty of relationships
	Stable home relationships	Stormy domestic situation
Features of illness	Identifiable precipitating factor or 'life event'	No obvious triggering factor or 'life event'
	Acute onset	Insidious onset
	Few first rank symptoms	Many first rank symptoms
	Disturbance of mood	No mood disturbance
	Initiative, interest and motivation maintained	Blunting of emotional responses; initiative, motivation and interest impaired
	Prompt treatment	Treatment delayed

Table 19.11 Unwanted effects of neuroleptic drugs.

COMMON EFFECTS

Extrapyramidal
Acute dystonia
Parkinsonism
Akathisia
Tardive dyskinesia

Autonomic
Hypotension
Failure of ejaculation

Anticholinergic
Dry mouth
Urinary retention
Constipation
Blurred vision

Metabolic
Weight gain

RARE EFFECTS

Hypersensitivity
Cholestatic jaundice
Leucopenia
Skin reactions

Other
Precipitation of glaucoma
Galactorrhoea
Amenorrhoea
Cardiac arrhythmias
Seizures
Retinal degeneration (with thioridazine in high
    doses)

TREATMENT

The best results are obtained by combining drug and social treatments.

Antipsychotic (neuroleptic) drugs
These reduce psychomotor excitement and control many of the symptoms of schizophrenia without causing disinhibition, confusion or sleep. Such drugs are most effective against acutely occurring, positive symptoms and least effective in the management of chronic, negative symptoms. Complete control of positive symptoms can take up to 3 months and premature discontinuation of treatment can result in prompt release.

The phenothiazines are the most extensively used group of neuroleptics. Chlorpromazine (100–1000 mg daily) is the drug of choice when a more sedating drug is required. Trifluoperazine is used when sedation is undesirable. Fluphenazine decanoate is used as a long-term prophylactic to prevent relapse (25–100 mg i.m. every 1–4 weeks). Promazine or thioridazine is useful in the elderly when it is desirable to reduce the risk of extra-pyramidal and anticholinergic side-effects.

Antipsychotic drugs block dopamine receptors. Their action on the basal ganglion may produce extrapyramidal side-effects. This limits their use in the maintenance therapy of many patients. They also block adrenergic and cholinergic receptors and thereby cause a number of unwanted effects (Table 19.11).

In patients manifesting good prognostic features and responding well to drugs, treatment may be discontinued under supervision after several months. Poor prognosis schizophrenia, on the other hand, usually requires regular maintenance therapy for many months or even years.

Social treatment
Social treatment involves attention being paid to the patient's environment and social functioning. Patients with any degree of residual impairment and negative symptoms usually require rehabilitation in a structured work and social environment. Parents and relatives need advice concerning the optimum amount of emotional and social stimulation to be provided for the patient. Some patients can manage a normal job, whereas others require a sheltered workshop. A very small number of severely disabled patients require long-term residential medical and nursing care.

Psychological treatment
This consists of reassurance, support and a good doctor–patient relationship. Psychotherapy of an intensive or exploratory kind is contraindicated.

Manic-depressive disorder

The central feature of this disorder is an abnormality of mood, either depression or elation or both. Mood is best considered in terms of a continuum ranging from severe depression at one extreme to severe mania at the other, with normal, stable mood at the centre (Fig. 19.1).

Manic-depressive disorders are divided into bipolar manic-depression, in which patients suffer attacks of both depression and mania, and unipolar disorders, in which there is either mania alone or, more commonly, depression alone. First-degree relatives of patients suffering from bipolar illness have an increased risk of manic-depressive illness but not those of patients with unipolar illness.

Depression is classically divided into endogenous depression and reactive depression, although the validity of this distinction is doubtful. The criteria of endogenous depression include:

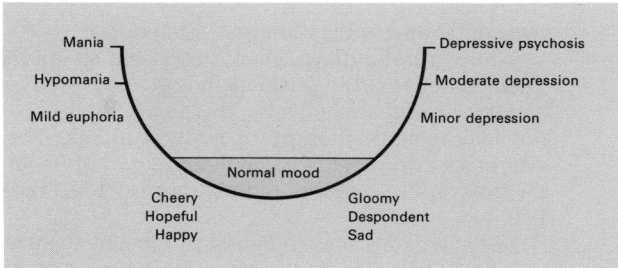

Fig. 19.1 Continuum of normal and abnormal mood.

- Pervasive and unresponsive depression
- Early morning waking
- Diurnal variation of mood (worse in the morning)
- Profoundly depressive ideas (e.g. guilt, suicidal feelings)
- The lack of an obvious precipitating cause
- A stable premorbid personality

The criteria of reactive depression include:

- A fluctuating depression responsive to environmental change
- Self-pity rather than self-blame
- A clear precipitating cause
- A vulnerable or predisposed personality
- Absence of the criteria of endogenous depression

A mixture of both types is a commoner presentation than a pure form of either.

CLINICAL FEATURES

The clinical features of *mania* reflect a marked elevation of mood (Table 19.12). The term *hypo-*

mania refers to a mild form of mania characterized by euphoria, overactivity and disinhibition. It can be difficult to distinguish this from simple exuberance, enthusiasm and good humour.

At the opposite pole of the affective continuum, *major depressive illness* is also characterized by disturbances of mood, talk, energy and ideation (Table 19.13). The mood may be described by the patient in physical terms, e.g. like a weight in the head, a tightness of the chest, or a feeling of almost physical pain. Depressed patients describe the world as grey, themselves as lacking a zest for living, and their bodies as devoid of pleasure and feeling. Anxiety is common, obsessional symptoms may emerge and, in the severer forms, delusions of guilt, persecution and of bodily disease are not uncommon. In severe depression apparent organic impairment, detectable on cognitive testing, can result in disorientation.

Table 19.12 Clinical features of mania.

Mood	Elevated, infectious, labile
Talk	Fast, pressurized, flight of ideas, punning, rhyming
Energy	Excessive, restless, distractible
Ideation	Grandiose, self-confident, delusions of wealth, power, influence or of religious significance, persecutory delusions
Cognition	Formal testing difficult, disturbance of retrieval of memories
Physical	Insomnia, mild to moderate weight loss
Behaviour	Disinhibition, increased sexual interest, excessive drinking or spending
Hallucinations	Fleeting auditory or, more rarely, visual

Table 19.13 Clinical features of depression.

Mood	Depressed, miserable, unhappy
Talk	Impoverished, slow, monotonous, incomplete
Energy	Lacking, retarded (in some cases agitation), apathetic
Ideation	Feelings of futility, guilt, self-reproach, unworthiness, hypochondriacal preoccupations, worrying, suicidal thoughts, delusions of guilt, nihilism, persecution
Cognition	Verbal memory impaired, 'pseudodementia' in elderly patients
Physical	Early waking, appetite and weight loss, constipation, loss of libido, impotence, fatigue, bodily aches and pains
Behaviour	Retardation or agitation, poverty of movement and expression
Hallucinations	Auditory—often abusive, hostile, critical

Table 19.14 Features that help distinguish major from minor depression.

	Minor	Major
Mood	Transiently low Responsive to environment	Persistently low Unresponsive to environment
Behaviour	Capable of being lifted out of gloom and sadness	Persistently agitated and/or retarded
Suicidal feelings	Fleeting	Persistent
Delusions	Absent	Often present
Physical symptoms	Vague aches and pains, some appetite and sleep loss	Persistent bowel changes, appetite and weight loss, sleep disturbance and early waking
Hallucinations	Absent	Occasionally present

Depression is a common experience. It occurs in the setting of physical disease, social stress, personal problems and life crises. It is important to distinguish the more severe and potentially life-threatening *major* form, requiring energetic treatment, from the less severe *minor* form, which, with simple support, sympathy and reassurance, usually lifts (see Table 19.14).

The aetiological factors in manic-depressive disorders are listed in Table 19.15.

DIFFERENTIAL DIAGNOSIS

This is shown in Table 19.16.

Occasionally, doctors are called upon to distinguish between 'normal' grief following a separation or bereavement, and depressive illness. A number of symptoms that commonly occur in depressive illness also follow bereavement, most notably sleep disturbance, appetite and weight loss, and tearfulness. However, a number of distinguishing features can usually be identified (see Table 19.17).

Two conditions presenting in women and characterized by disturbance of mood may well be related to manic-depressive disorders. These are the premenstrual syndrome and puerperal affective disorders.

The premenstrual syndrome

Symptoms consist of irritability, depression and tension during the 7- to 10-day premenstrual period. These symptoms are often accompanied by breast tenderness, a subjective feeling of weight gain and bloatedness, and headache, and are usually dramatically relieved with the onset of the period. Women who suffer from affective disorders may be more prone to experience premenstrual symptoms and to have exacerbations of their psychiatric disorder during the premenstrual phase.

The cause or causes of the premenstrual syndrome remain unclear and the various treatments proposed, which include the use of vitamin B_6, diuretics, progesterone, oral contraceptives, oil of evening primrose and oestrogen implants, remain empirical.

Puerperal affective disorders

In postpartum women, affective disorders also occur. Such disturbances are divided into 'maternity blues', postpartum ('puerperal') psychosis and chronic depression. Maternity blues is used to describe the brief episodes of emotional lability, irritability and tearfulness that occur in 65–90% of women 2–3 days postpartum and that resolve spontaneously in a few days. Postpartum psychosis occurs once in every 500–1000 births. Over 80% of cases are affective in type and the onset is usually within the first 2 weeks following delivery. In addition to the classical features of an affective psychosis, disorientation and confusion are often noted. Severely depressed patients may have delusional ideas that the child is deformed, evil or otherwise affected in some way, and such false ideas may lead to attempts to kill the child and to suicide. The response to speedy treatment is generally good. The recurrence rate for a depressive illness in a subsequent puerperium is 15–20%.

Less severe depressive disorders occur during the first postpartum year in 10–20% of mothers. Most patients recover after a few months. Social and psychological factors are important but the underlying aetiological factor is unknown.

TREATMENT

The treatment of affective disorders involves physical, psychological and social therapies. Hospitalization is usually required in the case of severely depressed, potentially suicidal patients and in mania. In general, neither severe depression nor mania respond to psychotherapy, and both require energetic physical treatment. Simple support, reassurance, sympathy and the opportunity to express

Table 19.15 Possible aetiological factors involved in manic-depressive disorders.

BIOLOGICAL

Genetic
10–15% of first degree relatives have an affective
  disorder (risk in community is 1–2%)
68% of monozygotic twins reared together or apart
  are concordant for manic-depressive disorder
23% of dizygotic twins are concordant
Possible links with genetic markers

Biochemical
Imbalance in neurotransmitters (e.g. monoamine
  neurotransmitters are depleted in depression, but
  increased in mania)
Loss of diurnal rhythm of plasma cortisol in
  depression
Hormonal factors (e.g. depression is more common
  after childbirth, in premenstrual phase, with use
  of oral contraceptives, and around the
  menopause)
Electrolytes—intracellular sodium is high in affective
  disorders

PSYCHOLOGICAL

Maternal deprivation
Psychoanalysis initially suggested that loss of
  maternal affection in early life predisposes
  individuals to affective disorder in later life. This
  association has more recently broadened to
  include any significant loss in early childhood

Learned helplessness
Experimental animals put in a position where they
  cannot escape or control punishing stimuli
  develop a behavioural syndrome that resembles
  depression in humans. It has led to the suggestion
  that a similar mechanism is at work in humans

SOCIAL

Stressful events
An excess of life events is found in the months
  before the onset of depression. Life events include
  bereavement, loss of a job, moving house,
  marriage and going on vacation

Vulnerability factors
In women, it has been claimed that certain factors
  render them vulnerable to become depressed.
  These include lack of a job outside the home, the
  presence of three or more young children in the
  family, and lack of a confiding, intimate
  relationship

Table 19.16 Differential diagnosis of manic-depressive disorders.

Condition	Comments
MANIA	
Drug-induced psychosis	Screen for suspected drugs (most notably amphetamines, cannabis)
Acute schizophrenia	Other classical (i.e. 'first rank') schizophrenic symptoms usually present or eventually emerge
Dementia	Global cognitive impairment may present with euphoria and irritability; in mania, any cognitive impairment improves with treatment
Hyperthyroidism	

DEPRESSION

Systemic physical disease
  Malignancy
  Hypothyroidism
  Hyperparathyroidism
  Cushing's syndrome
  Vitamin and mineral disorders
  Post-infection
  Multiple sclerosis
  Collagen disorders
  Cerebral ischaemia
  Congestive heart failure
  Porphyria

Drug-induced depression
  Corticosteroids
  Hormones
    Oestrogen
    Progesterone
  Hypotensive agents
    Reserpine
    Methyldopa
    Clonidine
  Antiparkinsonian drugs
    Levodopa
    Amantadine hydrochloride
  Anticancer drugs
    Vincristine
    Vinblastine

Psychiatric disorders
  Schizophrenia
  Alcohol abuse
  Drug abuse
  Anxiety neurosis
  Dementia (see Table 18.49)

Table 19.17 Bereavement reaction versus depressive illness following bereavement ('morbid grief reaction').

	Normal bereavement	Depressive illness
Onset	Immediately follows loss	Delay for weeks or months
Duration	Lasts weeks rather than months	Persists for weeks/months/years
Pattern	Person slowly accepts loss and adjusts accordingly	Patient denies loss and refuses to accept implications
Grief	Expressed openly	Difficulty in expressing grief
Guilt	Mild regret in early stages	Marked guilt often present

distress and negative feelings are often sufficient to bring about relief of minor depressive episodes.

Physical treatment of depression

The most frequently used drugs are the tricyclic and related antidepressants. Imipramine and amitriptyline are the two most commonly used. Many related compounds have been introduced, some having fewer autonomic and cardiotoxic effects. Imipramine and amitriptyline are given by mouth in initial doses of 25–75 mg daily, building up over a week to 150–250 mg daily. The full therapeutic impact takes up to 2 weeks to occur. These drugs potentiate the action of monoamines, noradrenaline and serotonin by inhibiting their reuptake into nerve terminals. Other tricyclics in common use include nortriptyline, doxepin, mianserin, clomipramine, lofepramine and trazodone. Tricyclic antidepressants have a number of side-effects (see Table 19.18); in patients with established cardiac disease mianserin, dothiepin or trazodone are preferred over the more cardiotoxic compounds.

A second group of antidepressants, the monoamine oxidase inhibitors (MAOIs), act by inhibiting the intracellular enzyme monoamine oxidase, leading to an increase of noradrenaline, dopamine and 5-hydroxytryptamine in the brain. There are two types:

- Hydrazine derivatives, e.g. isocarboxazid, phenelzine (potentially hepatotoxic)
- Amphetamine-related, e.g. tranylcypromine (potentially addictive)

The most widely used is phenelzine, which is given orally in doses of 30–60 mg daily. The onset of action of MAOIs is within 24–48 h. Unwanted effects include increased appetite and weight gain and difficulty in sleeping. MAOIs also produce hypertensive reactions with foods containing tyramine or dopamine and therefore a restricted diet is prescribed. These amines are normally broken down by monoamine oxidase in the gut mucosa and the liver. Tyramine is present in cheese, pickled herrings, yeast extract, certain red wines and any food, such as game, that has undergone partial decomposition. Dopa is present in broad beans. This 'tyramine reaction' is treated with intravenous phenotolamine. MAOIs interact with drugs such as pethidine (see p. 739) and cause liver damage. Particular caution should be taken when changing from a MAOI to a tricyclic or vice versa; it is safest to allow a 2-week drug-free interval between the two types of drug.

MAOIs are used in depressions that present with marked anxiety and obsessional or hypochondriacal features, and that lack marked biological symptoms characteristic of severe depression.

ECT (electroconvulsive therapy) is the most rapidly acting of the available physical treatments of depression. It can be the treatment of first choice in those cases where:

- The patient is dangerously suicidal
- A delay in treatment represents a serious risk to health
- The patient is refusing food and drink
- The patient is in a depressive stupor

The treatment involves the passage of an electric current, usually 80 V for a duration of 0.1–0.3 s, across two electrodes applied to the anterior temporal areas of the scalp. Before the treatment is given, the patient is anaesthetized (usually by means of thiopental 125–150 mg) and receives a muscle relaxant (usually suxamethonium 30–50 mg). A modified convulsion is produced. A course of six to eight treatments over 3 weeks has been shown to be superior to placebo treatment in severe depression characterized by retardation and delusions.

Table 19.18 Unwanted effects of tricyclic antidepressants.

Anticholinergic effects	*Convulsant activity*
Dry mouth	Lowered seizure
Constipation	threshold
Tremor	
Blurred vision	*Other effects*
Urinary retention	Weight gain
Postural hypotension	Sedation
	Mania
Cardiac effects	Agranulocytosis
ECG changes	(mianserin)
Arrhythmias	

ECT is sometimes used in the management of acute schizophrenia, but the evidence of its effectiveness in this condition is less clear.

ECT is a controversial treatment, yet it is remarkably safe and free of serious side-effects. Serious complications are rare. However, post-ictal, short-term retrograde amnesia and a temporary defect in new learning can occur but these are short-lived effects. The mode of action of ECT in depressive illness is unclear.

Physical treatment of mania

The main physical treatment in mania is the use of neuroleptic drugs such as chlorpromazine, haloperidol and pimozide. Doses similar to those used in schizophrenia are used. Excitement and overactivity are usually reduced within days, but elation, gradiosity and associated delusions often take longer to respond. If improvement does not occur rapidly, larger doses of haloperidol (up to 120 mg daily) may be required. First attacks of mania usually require treatment for up to 3 months. Subsequent attacks, especially if they occur rapidly on cessation of treatment, may need drugs for at least a year after hypomanic features have disappeared.

Lithium carbonate is used but it can take up to 10 days to take effect. Lithium is more commonly used as a prophylactic agent in patients who have a history of repeated episodes of mania and/or depression. In the body it substitutes for sodium and potassium ions and thus can exercise profound effects on a number of metabolic processes. Toxic symptoms begin to occur when the serum concentration exceeds 1.5 mmol·L^{-1} and regular serum estimations are required. Persistent vomiting or diarrhoea with fluid and electrolyte imbalance or diuretic therapy can precipitate toxic levels of lithium. The therapeutic range of lithium prophylaxis is between 0.4 and 1.2 mmol·L^{-1} although adequate prophylaxis can be obtained with plasma levels as low as 0.4–0.6 mmol·L^{-1}.

Lithium is rapidly absorbed from the gastrointestinal tract and more than 95% is excreted by the kidney, small amounts being found in the saliva and sweat. Renal clearance of lithium correlates with renal creatinine clearance. Its mode of action is unknown. Unwanted effects include:

- Gastrointestinal symptoms
- A fine tremor
- Polyuria and polydipsia
- Weight gain

At higher concentrations, toxic effects include drowsiness, blurred vision, a coarse tremor, ataxia and dysarthria. Such symptoms progress to delirium and convulsions, and coma and death can occur. Long-term effects include non-toxic goitre, hypothyroidism and nephrogenic diabetes insipidus.

Recently, carbamazepine has been found effective in the treatment of manic states and in prophylaxis. Some patients who do not respond to lithium may respond to carbamazepine. For antimanic treatment, dosage in the initial stage of treatment will be 200 mg once a day for 2 days, followed by 200 mg twice daily for 2 days, then 200 mg three times daily. Rarely dosage may have to be increased to a maximum of 1200 mg daily. The usual prophylactic dosage is 600 mg daily. The combination of lithium and carbamazepine is occasionally more effective than either drug alone.

Social treatment

Many patients with depression, particularly of the milder form, have associated social problems. Assistance with such social problems can make a significant contribution to clinical recovery. Other social interventions include the provision of group support, social clubs, occupational therapy and training to cope with particularly stressful situations.

Psychological treatment

The psychological treatments in affective disorders can be divided into:

- *Supportive:* Sympathy, reassurance and information should be part of every patient's treatment.
- *Dynamic psychotherapy* (see p. 989). This form of psychotherapy has a limited value in the treatment of affective disorders. In general, its use is restricted to the less severe cases.
- *Cognitive therapy.* This is a behavioural form of therapy that combines behavioural tasks with questioning and arguments designed to alter some of the ideas that are common among depressed patients and that appear to prolong their depression. Among these are negative interpretations of events and maladaptive assumptions (e.g. assuming that because a friend does not telephone it means he no longer cares about the patient). In treatment, the patient is required to record such ideas and examine the evidence for and against them. Patients are also encouraged to undertake some of the pleasurable activities they gave up when they became depressed. There is some evidence that the effects of cognitive therapy are about the same as those of antidepressant drugs in the treatment of mild to moderate depression.

COURSE AND PROGNOSIS

Between two-thirds and three-quarters of patients admitted with a major depressive illness will suffer at least one relapse requiring hospital admission. The number of less severe relapses is even higher. It has been estimated that between 15 and 20% of depressives never fully recover. It may take those who do recover between four and 18 months before they can expect to regain full social functioning.

Virtually all manic patients recover and the main problem is the prevention of relapse. Estimates of the proportion of patients who have only a single episode of mania vary widely between 1% and 50%! Subsequent depressive disorder is common in manic patients who relapse. Between 5% and 10% of manic-depressive sufferers develop a chronic disability that may follow the first episode. Between 5% and 10% become long-term hospital inpatients and an additional 25% have persistent affective symptoms that are disabling to some degree. The continuation of antidepressant therapy for up to 6 months after recovery from a depressive episode does reduce the probability of recurrence, while the use of lithium carbonate and carbamazepine as prophylactic therapy to prevent recurrence of bipolar manic-depressive swings is widely recommended.

Suicide and attempted suicide (deliberate self-harm) (see also p. 743)

Between 11% and 17% of people who have suffered a severe depressive disorder at any time will eventually commit suicide. About 1% of deaths in England and Wales each year are due to suicide, yielding a rate of 8 per 100 000. The rate increases with age, peaking for women in their sixties and for men in their seventies. The highest rates of suicide have been reported in Hungary (40 per 100 000) and East Germany (36 per 100 000), while the lowest are those of Spain (3.9 per 100 000) and Greece (2.8 per 100 000), but such

Table 19.19 Factors that increase the risk of suicide.

Living alone

Immigrant status

Recent bereavement, separation or divorce

Recent loss of a job or retirement

Living in a socially disorganized area

Male sex

Older age

Family history of affective disorder, suicide or alcohol abuse

Previous history of affective disorder, alcohol or drug abuse

Previous suicide attempt

Addiction to alcohol or drugs

Severe depression or early dementia

Incapacitating, painful physical illness

variations may reflect differences in reporting as much as genuine differences in frequency of suicide.

Factors that increase the risk of suicide are indicated in Table 19.19.

A distinction must be drawn between those who attempt suicide ('parasuicides') and those who are determined and eventually succeed (suicides). The following points should be considered:

- Suicide is commoner in men, while parasuicide is commoner in women.
- The majority of parasuicides occur in people under 35.
- The majority of suicides occur in people over 60.
- Approximately 90% of parasuicides involve self-poisoning.
- A formal psychiatric disorder is unusual in parasuicide.

There is, however, overlap between the two groups and between 1% and 2% of people who attempt suicide will kill themselves in the year following their original attempt. In Britain, over 100 000 suicide attempts are made each year, and the overwhelming majority of these are seen and treated within accident and emergency departments.

The guidelines given on p. 984 for the assessment of such patients will help to ensure that the important 'risk' factors relating to suicide are covered.

In general, it is worth trying to interview a family member or other close associate and check these points with him or her. Requests for immediate represcription or discharge should be denied, except in cases of essential medication (e.g. epileptics). In such cases, however, only 3 days' supply of medication should be given and the patient should be instructed to report to their general practitioner or to their psychiatric out-patient clinic for further supplies.

Neuroses and personality disorders

These disorders constitute the largest portion of psychiatric disorders, accounting for 50% of admissions to psychiatric hospitals, 75% of patients seen in psychiatric outpatient clinics, and over 90% of the psychiatric disorders seen and managed by general practitioners. There is an overlap between neuroses and personality disorders, although in general they can be distinguished.

Neurosis is defined below. Personality disorders are deeply ingrained maladaptive patterns of behaviour generally recognizable by the time of adolescence and often becoming less obvious in

Guidelines for possible psychiatric referral in deliberate self harm

Identification of the precipitant

- Was there a clear precipitant?
- What was the patient's state of mind at the time?
- Was the act premeditated or impulsive?
- Did the patient leave a suicide note?
- Had the patient taken pains not to be discovered?
- Did he make the attempt in familiar or strange surroundings (i.e. at home or away from home)?
- What are the patient's feelings about the attempt now?
- Was the patient under the influence of alcohol or drugs?

Present state examination

- Has the precipitant or crisis resolved?
- Is there continuing suicidal intent?
- Does the patient have any psychiatric symptoms?
- What is the patient's social support system?
- Has the patient harmed himself before?
- Has anyone in the family ever taken their life?
- Does the patient have a physical illness?

Indications for referral to a psychiatrist

Absolute indications include:

- Clinical depression
- Psychotic illness of any kind
- Clearly pre-planned suicidal attempts which were not intended to be discovered
- Persistent suicidal intent (the more detailed the plans, the more serious the risk)
- A violent method used

Other common indications include:

- Alcoholics and drug abusers
- Older patients over 45, especially if male
- Those with a family history of suicide
- Those with serious (especially incurable) physical disease
- Those living alone or otherwise unsupported
- Those in whom there is a major unresolved crisis
- Persistent suicide attemptors

middle or old age. The personality is abnormal either in the balance of its components, its quality or expression, or in its total aspect, and this deviation has an adverse effect upon the individual or on society.

The psychopath is a person who, as described by the Mental Health Amendment Act (1982) manifests 'a persistent disorder or disability of mind (whether or not including significant impairment of intelligence) which results in abnormally aggressive or seriously irresponsible conduct'. The individual tends to be emotionally cold and callous, shows little remorse or ability to learn from previous mistakes, tolerates frustration poorly, is impulsive and has considerable difficulty sustain-

ing roles requiring persistence and consistency, such as jobs, personal relationships and financial obligations.

Anxiety neurosis

An anxiety neurosis is a condition in which anxiety dominates the clinical symptoms.

CLINICAL FEATURES

The patient looks worried, has a tense posture, restless behaviour, a pale skin, and sweaty hands, feet and axillae. The physical and psychological symptoms (Table 19.20) result from either over-

Table 19.20 Physical and psychological symptoms of anxiety.

PHYSICAL

Gastrointestinal
Dry mouth
Difficulty in swallowing
Epigastric discomfort
Flatulence
Diarrhoea (usually frequency)

Respiratory
Feeling of chest constriction
Difficulty in inhaling
Overbreathing

Cardiovascular
Palpitations
Awareness of missed beats
Feeling of pain over heart

Genitourinary
Increased frequency
Failure of erection
Lack of libido

CNS
Tinnitus
Blurred vision
Dizziness

Other
Headache
Sleep disturbances

PSYCHOLOGICAL

Apprehension and fear
Irritability
Difficulty in concentrating
Distractability
Restlessness
Sensitivity to noise
Depression
Depersonalization
Obsessional symptoms

activity of the sympathetic nervous system or increased tension in the skeletal muscles. Sleep is disturbed: the patient has difficulty in getting to sleep because of worry and restlessness, and when he does sleep he wakes intermittently and may have unpleasant dreams. Another feature is the *hyperventilation syndrome*.

Sometimes the anxious patient has the conviction that he suffers from heart disease. The conviction is accompanied by palpitations, fatigue, breathlessness and inframammary pain. The terms 'cardiac neurosis', 'effort syndrome' and 'neurocirculatory asthenia' used to be applied to the disorder. Beta-blockers are sometimes useful in controlling these symptoms.

The hyperventilation syndrome

Features

Panic attacks—fear, terror and impending doom—accompanied by some or all of the following:

- Dyspnoea
- Palpitations
- Chest pain or discomfort
- Choking sensation
- Dizziness
- Paraesthesiae
- Sweating
- Carpopedal spasms

Cause

Overbreathing leading to a decrease in P_aCO_2 and an increase in arterial pH.

Diagnosis

A provocation test—voluntary overbreathing for 2–3 min—provokes similar symptoms; rebreathing from a paper bag relieves them.

Management

- Explanation and reassurance is given.
- The patient is trained in relaxation techniques and slow breathing.
- The patient is asked to breathe into a closed paper bag.

Types of anxiety
Anxiety may be divided into the following categories:

- A more or less continuous *state of anxiety* that fluctuates to some extent in response to environmental circumstances
- Sudden and unpredictable attacks of anxiety that are usually accompanied by severe physical symptoms—the so-called *panic attacks*
- *Phobic anxiety*, which is anxiety triggered by a single stimulus or set of stimuli that are predictable and that normally cause no particular concern to others

Table 19.21 The differential diagnosis of anxiety neurosis.

Psychiatric disorder	Physical disorder
Depressive illness	Hyperthyroidism
Schizophrenia	Hypoglycaemia
Presenile dementia	Phaeochromocytoma
Alcohol dependence	
Drug dependence	
Benzodiazepine withdrawal	

- An *anxious personality*—an individual who has a lifelong tendency to experience tension and anxiety, and to have a worrisome attitude towards life and a constant anticipation of setback and stress

DIFFERENTIAL DIAGNOSIS

This is given in Table 19.21.

AETIOLOGY

Genetic factors
Anxiety neurosis occurs in 15% of relatives of affected patients compared with 3% of the general population. (The genetic role is less important in phobic anxiety.)

Psychodynamic theory
This is a theoretical explanation that suggests that anxiety neurosis reflects overwhelming stress, anxiety and difficulties in the child–parent relationship in early childhood or even at birth. Psychoanalysts also interpret phobic neurosis as an unconscious avoidance of unacknowledged feelings of temptation (usually sexual), the phobia representing a displacement of the real fear (e.g. the agoraphobic patient is really afraid of the feelings of temptation aroused when meeting people in the street).

Learning theory
Anxiety is regarded as a fear response that has been attached to another stimulus through conditioning.

TREATMENT

Psychological treatment
For many brief episodes of anxiety neurosis, a discussion with a doctor involving explanation and reassurance concerning the nature of physical symptoms of anxiety is usually sufficient. Relaxation training can be as effective as drugs in relieving mild or moderate anxiety. Such an approach uses an elaborate system of exercises designed to bring about relaxation of individual groups of skeletal muscles and to regulate breath-

ing. A further development is anxiety management training, which involves two stages. In the first stage, verbal cues and mental imagery are used to arouse anxiety. In the second stage, the patient is trained to reduce this anxiety by relaxation, distraction and reassuring self-statements. Both of these approaches are forms of behaviour therapy.

The term behaviour therapy is applied to psychological treatments derived from experimental psychology and intended to change symptoms and behaviour. A behavioural therapy used in the treatment of phobias is desensitization. Patients are required to imagine the fear-provoking situations or objects, starting with those that evoke little fear, and progressing through carefully planned steps or a hierarchy to the most severe phobic stimulus. At each stage, anxiety is neutralized, usually by relaxation. Improvement in phobias is greater after this approach than after group or individual psychotherapy.

Flooding treatment is based on the finding that conditioned fear responses dissipate when experimental animals are prevented from running away from fear-provoking situations; if the animals are kept in the situation, the fear dies away. In flooding treatment, patients are required either to imagine or to enter feared situations in a way that maximizes anxiety. They continue to do this until the fear exhausts itself. In a variation on this approach, anxiety is increased still further by requiring the patient to imagine exaggerated scenes or situations; for example, a patient fearful of spiders might be required to imagine having hundreds of them crawling over his naked body. This procedure is termed implosion. There is little evidence that it is superior to the more straightforward desensitization.

The treatment of choice for agoraphobia is programmed practice. This combines exposure to real rather than imagined anxiety-provoking situations, with measures to control any anxiety experienced in these situations. The therapist teaches the patient how best to return to the feared situation and how to cope with the anxiety that results. This is carried out for at least one hour each day using situations chosen that give rise to moderate anxiety. Emphasis is placed on providing the patient with the knowledge required to plan his own treatment.

Non-behavioural treatments include individual and group-based psychotherapies. In general, however, behavioural therapy has replaced such approaches in the treatment of anxiety and phobias.

Physical treatment
Drugs used in the treatment of anxiety can be divided into two groups: those that act primarily on the central nervous system and those that block peripheral autonomic receptors. The main group of centrally acting anxiolytic drugs are the benzodiazepines. They appear to bind to specific receptors on neuronal cell membranes, producing a facilitation of the effects of the inhibitory transmitter γ-aminobutyric acid (GABA). Diazepam (5 mg twice daily to 10 mg three times daily in severe cases) and nitrazepam have relatively long half-lives (20–40 h) and are more suitable as antianxiety drugs than as hypnotic drugs, whereas oxazepam, temazepam and lorazepam have shorter half-lives and may be used as hypnotics.

Adverse effects include overdosage, which may be accidental or deliberate, and produces drowsiness, sleep, confusion, incoordination, ataxia, diplopia and dysarthria. Physical as well as psychological dependence has been described, and convulsions have occurred on withdrawal of such drugs after long-term administration. The withdrawal syndrome (Table 19.22) is particularly severe when high doses have been given, e.g. 30 mg of diazepam daily or more. Tolerance can occur with repeated doses and can lead to an escalation of dosage. Thus, if a benzodiazepine drug is prescribed for anxiety, it should be given in as low a dose and for as short a time as possible (i.e. for not more than 3–4 weeks).

Table 19.22 Withdrawal syndrome with benzodiazepines.

Insomnia
Anxiety
Tremulousness
Muscle twitchings
Perceptual distortions
Frank convulsions

Many of the symptoms of anxiety are due to an increased release of adrenaline and noradrenaline from the adrenal medulla and the sympathetic nerves. Thus, adrenergic blocking drugs such as propranolol (20–40 mg two or three times daily) are effective in reducing symptoms such as palpitations, tremor and tachycardia.

Obsessional neurosis and personality

Obsessional neuroses are characterized by obsessional thinking and compulsive behaviour (see p. 966) together with varying degrees of anxiety, depression and depersonalization. They account for some 2% of referrals to psychiatrists and have a prevalence in the general population of about 1 in 1000.

CLINICAL FEATURES

The obsessions and compulsions are so persistent and intrusive that they greatly impede the patient's functioning and cause considerable distress. There is a constant need to check that things have been done correctly and no amount of reassurance can remove the small amount of doubt that persists— the so-called 'folie de doute'. Some rituals are derived from superstitions, such as repetitive actions done a required number of times, with the need to start again at the very beginning if interrupted. When severe, obsessional neuroses last for many years and are very resistant to treatment. However, obsessional symptoms commonly appear in the setting of other disorders, most notably anxiety neurosis, depression, schizophrenia and organic cerebral disorders, and disappear rapidly with the resolution of such disorders.

Minor variants of morbid obsessional symptoms can be noted fairly frequently in people who are not regarded as ill or in need of treatment. The mildest grade is that of obsessional personality traits such as over-conscientiousness, tidiness, punctuality and other attitudes and behaviours indicating a strong tendency towards rigidity, conformity and inflexibility. Such individuals are perfectionists, have a poor tolerance of shortcomings in others and take pride in their high standards. When such traits are so marked that they override and dominate other aspects of the personality, in the absence of clear-cut obsessional thinking and compulsive rituals, the picture becomes that of an obsessional personality disorder.

AETIOLOGY

Genetic factors
Obsessional neuroses are found in 5–7% of the parents of obsessional patients. Such a finding may of course reflect environmental as well as genetic causes.

Organic factors
Symptoms have been seen following encephalitis lethargica and it has been suggested that organic factors may be involved. In most cases, however, there is no evidence of disease of the CNS.

Psychodynamic factors
Freud suggested that symptoms result from repressed impulses of an aggressive or sexual nature. He also suggested that they occur as a result of regression to the anal stage of development—an idea consistent with the obsessional patient's frequent concern over excretory functions and dirt.

Learning theory
This suggests that obsessional rituals are the equivalent of avoidance responses. However, anxiety actually increases rather than falls after some rituals, which is against such a theory.

TREATMENT

Psychological treatment
A form of behaviour therapy that is particularly effective in the treatment of obsessional rituals is response prevention. Patients are instructed not to carry out their rituals; initially there is a rise in distress but with persistence both the rituals and the distress diminish. Patients are encouraged to practise keeping them under control while returning to situations that normally make them worse.

Another approach known as 'modelling' involves demonstrating to the patient what is required and encouraging the patient to follow this example. In the case of hand-washing rituals, this might involve holding an allegedly 'contaminated' object and carrying out other activities without washing, the patient being encouraged to follow suit. When obsessional thoughts accompany rituals, thought stopping is advocated. In this procedure the patient is taught to arrest the obsessional thought by arranging a sudden intrusion (e.g. snapping an elastic band, clicking the fingers).

Physical treatment
Anxiolytic drugs provide short-term symptomatic relief. Any coexisting depression should be treated with an antidepressant. One tricyclic antidepressant believed to have a specific action against obsessional symptoms is clomipramine, but studies suggest that the drug effects are modest and only occur in patients with definitive depressive symptoms.

Psychosurgery is sometimes recommended in cases of severe obsessional neurosis. The development of stereotactic techniques has led to the replacement of the earlier, crude leucotomies with more precise surgical interventions such as subcaudate tractotomy and limbic leucotomy, with lesions placed in the cingulate area and the ventromedial quadrant of the frontal lobe. These are undertaken to relieve patients of obsessional symptoms unresponsive to other treatments. Psychosurgery is now only performed in specialist centres, and formal and detailed consent requirements are laid down in England and Wales in the Mental Health Act 1983.

PROGNOSIS

Two-thirds of cases improve within a year. The remainder run a fluctuating course. The prognosis is worse when the personality is obsessional and the symptoms are severe.

Hysterical neurosis and personality

Hysterical neurosis or hysteria is a condition in which there are symptoms and signs of disease with three characteristics:

- They occur in the absence of physical pathology.
- They are produced unconsciously.
- They are not caused by overactivity of the sympathetic nervous system.

The lifetime prevalence has been estimated at 3–6 per 1000 in women, with a lower incidence in men. Most cases begin before the age of 35 and it occurs rarely after 40 years. However, hysterical symptoms commonly occur after this age as part of some other disorder.

CLINICAL FEATURES

The various symptoms are usually divided into dissociative and conversion categories (Table 19.23). The term 'dissociative' indicates the seeming dissociation between different mental activities, and covers such phenomena as amnesia, fugues, somnambulism and multiple personality. The term 'conversion' derives from Freud's theory that mental energy can be converted into certain physical symptoms. Such symptoms include paralysis, fits, sensory loss, aphonia, blindness, deafness, disorders of gait and abdominal pain.

The main characteristics of hysterical symptoms include the following:

- They are not produced willfully or deliberately.
- They often reflect a patient's ideas about illness.
- They may imitate symptoms of a relative/friend who has been ill.
- There are obvious discrepancies between hysterical signs and symptoms and those of organic disease.
- The symptoms usually confer some advantage on the patient (so-called secondary gain).
- They are often accompanied by less than the expected amount of emotional distress ('belle indifference').

Hysterical amnesia commences suddenly. Patients are unable to recall long periods of their lives and may even deny any knowledge of their previous life or personal identity. A proportion who present thus have concurrent physical disease, especially epilepsy, multiple sclerosis or the effects of head injury. In a hysterical fugue, the patient not only loses his memory but wanders away from his usual surroundings, and when found, denies all memory of his whereabouts during his wandering. Apart from hysteria, fugue states are associated with epilepsy, depression and alcohol abuse.

Hysterical pseudodementia involves a memory loss and behaviour that initially suggest severe and generalized intellectual deterioration. Simple tests are answered wrongly but in such a way as to suggest that the correct answer is in the patient's mind. The Ganser syndrome is a rare condition composed of four features:

- The giving of 'approximate answers' (i.e. almost correct)

- Physical or mental symptoms of hysteria
- Hallucinations
- Clouding of consciousness

The relation of somnambulism, or sleepwalking, to other forms of hysteria is unclear, but its similarity to the condition arising through hypnosis suggests that it may be a form of dissociation.

In multiple personality, there are rapid alterations between two patterns of behaviour, each of which is forgotten by the patient when the other is present. Each 'personality' appears to be a complex and integrated set of emotional responses. The condition is rare.

A variation of hysteria is the epidemic or mass hysteria, seen mainly in institutions for girls or young women in which the combined effects of suggestion and shared anxiety produce explosive outbreaks of sickness or other disturbed behaviour. Another variant is Briquet's syndrome, which is said only to occur in women, follows an intractable course, runs in families and involves multiple somatic symptoms occurring in several different bodily systems for which no organic cause is found.

Patients with a hysterical personality are those who exhibit a particular set or cluster of personality traits that include a remarkable egocentricity, a manipulative skill and an ability to attract attention to themselves by dramatic initiatives, often of a sexually provocative or emotionally exaggerated fashion. Their emotions are described as shallow and labile and there is an 'acting' quality attached to much of what they do and say. Their personal relationships are often transient yet full of dramatic intensity. Such individuals, when they do develop genuine physical illness, may be dubbed 'hysterical' because they describe their symptoms and complaints in such an exaggerated manner.

DIFFERENTIAL DIAGNOSIS

The diagnosis of hysteria may be erroneously made because:

- The symptoms may be those of an as yet

Table 19.23 Common hysterical symptoms.

Dissociative (mental)	Conversion (physical)
Amnesia	Paralysis
Fugue	Disorders of gait
Pseudodementia	Tremor
Ganser syndrome	Aphonia
Somnabulism	Mutism
Multiple personality	Sensory symptoms
Psychosis	Repeated vomiting
	Globus hystericus
	Hysterical fits
	Dermatitis artifacta

undetected physical disease. For example, 'globus hystericus' (see p. 181) may actually be difficulty in swallowing secondary to an oesophageal cancer.

- Undetected brain disease (e.g. a tumour in the frontal lobe or early dementia) may in some way 'produce' hysterical symptoms.
- Physical disease may provide a non-specific stimulus to hysterical elaboration or an exaggeration of symptoms by a somewhat dramatic or histrionic patient.

Physical disease must be excluded. The distinction between hysteria and malingering (i.e. the conscious pretence of illness) should be considered but is difficult to make.

AETIOLOGY

Genetic factors
Studies have been inconclusive but reported rates in relatives of affected patients do appear higher than in the general population.

Psychodynamic factors
Central to the theory of psychoanalysis is the view that hysteria is the result of emotionally charged ideas lodged in the unconscious at some point in the past. Symptoms are explained as the combined effects of repression and the 'conversion' of psychic energy into physical channels.

Organic disease
Hysteria is sometimes associated with physical disease. However, it also quite clearly occurs in the absence of such pathology.

TREATMENT

Psychological treatment
Psychotherapy of a psychodynamic kind often uncovers striking memories of early childhood sexual experiences and other problems relevant to the patient's presenting condition. Psychodynamic psychotherapy is derived from psychoanalysis and is based on a number of key analytical concepts. These include Freud's ideas about psychosexual development, mechanisms of defence (including repression, projection and denial), free association as the method of recall, and the therapeutic techniques of interpretation including that of transference, defences and dreams. Such therapy usually involves once-weekly 50-minute sessions, the length of treatment varying between 3 months and 2 years. The long-term aim of such therapy is two-fold: symptom relief and personality change. Psychodynamic psychotherapy is classically indicated in the treatment of the neuroses and personality disorders, but to date there is a lack of convincing evidence concerning its superiority over other forms of treatment.

Simpler forms of psychotherapy involving more straightforward reassurance and explanation, greater involvement of the therapist in the actual sessions, and the elimination of factors that appear to reinforce symptoms, are as effective and probably more so than the more complex and time-consuming forms. Group psychotherapy involving six to eight patients, which facilitates the development of confidence, the recollection of painful experiences and the growth of social and interpersonal skills, is also useful in a number of neurotic and personality disorders, although its usefulness in hysterical neuroses is doubtful.

Abreaction brought about by hypnosis or by intravenous injections of small amounts of amylobarbitone with or without amphetamine may produce a dramatic, if short-lived, recovery. In the abreactive state, the patient is encouraged to relive the stressful events that provoked the hysteria and to express the accompanying emotions, i.e. to abreact. Such an approach has been useful in the treatment of acute hysterical neuroses in war time, but appear to be of much less value in civilian life.

Physical treatment
Drug treatments have no part to play in hysteria unless the symptoms are secondary to a depressive illness or anxiety neurosis requiring treatment.

PROGNOSIS

Most cases of recent onset recover quickly. Those that last longer than a year are likely to persist for a very long time.

Hypochondriacal neurosis

This is a neurotic disorder in which the conspicuous features are an excessive concern with one's health in general, in the integrity and functioning of some part of one's body or, less frequently, one's mind. Hypochondriasis may coexist with actual physical disease; the important point is that the patient's concern is out of all proportion and is unjustified. The symptoms of hypochondriasis occur in a variety of psychiatric disorders, particularly in depression and anxiety. When hypochondriacal tendencies are lifelong, the condition is more usually termed 'hypochondriacal personality'.

Alcohol abuse and dependence

There are a number of different types of alcohol abuse, and a wide range of physical, social and psychological problems are associated with excessive drinking. Until recently, much attention was devoted to the syndrome of alcohol dependence. In fact, doctors should be concerned with the health problems caused by alcohol abuse whether or not such abuse is related to actual physiological dependence on alcohol. The term 'alcoholism' is a confusing one with off-putting connotations of vagrancy, 'meths' drinking and social disintegration. It has recently been replaced by the term 'alcohol dependence syndrome', which has seven essential elements:

- A compulsive need to drink.
- A stereotyped pattern of drinking. Whereas the ordinary drinker varies his daily pattern, the addicted drinker drinks at regular intervals to avoid or relieve withdrawal symptoms.
- Drinking takes primacy over other activities.
- Tolerance to alcohol is altered. The dependent drinker is ordinarily unaffected by blood alcohol levels that would incapacitate a normal drinker. Increasing tolerance is an important sign of increasing dependence. In the later stages of dependence, tolerance falls.
- Repeated withdrawal symptoms. These occur some 8–12 h after cessation of drinking or after a sharp fall in blood alcohol in people who have been drinking heavily for many years. They characteristically appear on waking as a result of the fall in the blood alcohol level during sleep.
- Relief drinking. Many dependent drinkers take a drink early in the morning to stave off withdrawal symptoms. In most cultures, early morning drinking is diagnostic of alcohol dependence.
- Reinstatement after abstinence. A severely dependent drinker who drinks again after a period of abstinence is likely to relapse quickly and return to his old addictive pattern.

The 'problem drinker' is one who causes or experiences physical, psychological and/or social harm as a consequence of drinking alcohol. Many problem drinkers, while heavy drinkers, are not physiologically addicted to alcohol. Heavy drinkers are those who drink significantly more in terms of quantity and/or frequency than the average drinker. Binge drinkers are those who drink excessively in short bouts, usually 24–48 h long, separated by often quite lengthy periods of abstinence. Their overall monthly or weekly alcohol intake may be relatively modest. The interrelationship between these types of drinking is shown in Fig. 19.2.

Extent of the problem

A conservative estimate is that there are at least 300 000 people in Britain with alcohol-related problems. A survey on drinking in England and Wales found that 5% of men and 2% of women reported alcohol-related problems. People with serious drinking problems have an increased risk of dying that is between two and three times greater than that of members of the general population at the same age and sex. Approximately one in five male admissions to acute medical wards are directly or indirectly due to alcohol. Between 33% and 40% of A and E attenders have blood alcohol concentrations above the present legal limit for driving. Up to one in five seemingly healthy men attending health screening programmes are found to have biochemical evidence of heavy alcohol consumption, though they are a selected population coming mainly from the upper social classes. Of the 2000 patients on the practice list of the average general practitioner, about 100 will be heavy drinkers, 40 will be problem drinkers and 10 will be physically dependent on alcohol.

Over the past 30 years, the average British adult has almost doubled his alcohol consumption (from 5.2 litres of absolute alcohol per year in 1950 to 9.9 litres in 1983). Over that same time period, admissions to psychiatric hospitals for treatment of alcohol problems have increased more than 25-fold, cirrhosis rates have doubled, and drunkenness offences have risen from 60 000 to over 100 000 per year.

Detection

Many doctors still fail to recognize the heavy drinker and even the problem drinker. Greater

Table 19.24 Common alcohol-related psychological and social problems.

Psychological	Social
Depression	Marital and sexual difficulties
Anxiety and phobias	
Memory disturbances	Family problems
Personality disturbances	Child abuse
Delirium tremens	Employment problems
Attempted suicide	Financial difficulties
Pathological jealousy	Accidents at home, on the roads, at work
	Delinquency and crime
	Homelessness

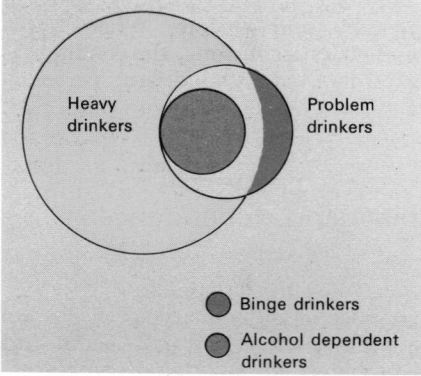

Fig. 19.2 The terminology of drinking.

Table 19.25 The CAGE questionnaire.[a]

1 Have you ever felt you ought to CUT down on your drinking?

2 Have people ANNOYED you by criticizing your drinking?

3 Have you ever felt bad or GUILTY about your drinking?

4 Have you ever had a drink first thing in the morning (an 'EYE-OPENER') to get rid of a hangover?

[a] From Mayfield D, McLeod G & Hall P (1974) *American Journal of Psychiatry* **131**: 1121–1123. With permission.

awareness is urgently needed to allow intervention at a stage when something can still be achieved, and to provide better statistics.

Alcohol abuse should be suspected in any patient presenting one or more physical problems commonly associated with excessive drinking (see Chapter 3, p. 171). Alcohol abuse may also be associated with a number of psychological symptoms and social problems (see Table 19.24). Certain features in the history should also raise suspicion, most notably:

- Absenteeism from work
- Frequent attendances for unexplained dyspepsia or gastrointestinal bleeds
- Hospital admissions for accidents of all kinds
- 'Fits', 'turns' or 'falls'

Certain signs may be helpful, if present, in detecting alcohol abuse in patients. These include:

- Plethoric face with/without telangiectases
- Bloodshot conjunctivae
- Smell of stale alcohol
- Facial appearance resembling Cushing's syndrome
- Marked tremor
- Signs of alcohol-related diseases

The patient's frequency of drinking and quantity drunk on typical occasions should be established. Patients can assess their alcohol consumption on the basis of units of alcohol. One standard unit of alcohol is equivalent to 8 g of absolute alcohol. This amount is found in:

- Half a pint of average-strength beer
- One standard UK measure of spirits
- One glass of sherry
- One glass of table wine

The following are useful guidelines:

- Drinking up to 20 units of alcohol a week for men and 13 units for women carries no long-term health risk.
- There is unlikely to be any long-term health damage between 21 and 36 units (men) and 14

and 24 units (women) provided that the drinking is spread throughout the week.
- Beyond 36 units a week in men and 24 units a week in women, damage to health becomes increasingly likely.
- Drinking above 50 units a week in men (35 units in women) is currently regarded as a definitive health hazard.

A number of questionnaires, such as the CAGE questionnaire (see Table 19.25), have been developed to help identify patients with alcohol-related problems. Two or more positive replies to the CAGE questionnaire are said to identify problem drinkers.

It is important to remember that there are a number of key 'at-risk' factors involved, which include:

- *Marital difficulties.* These may conceal heavy drinking or may be used to justify it.
- *Work problems.* Alcohol abusers have 2½ times as many days off work as more sober colleagues.
- *An affected relative.* Twenty-five per cent of the male relatives of alcohol abusers have similar problems.
- *High-risk occupations.* Examples of these include company directors, salesmen, doctors, journalists, publicans and seamen.
- Associated physical and mental conditions.

A number of laboratory tests are helpful in the identification of excess chronic alcohol consumption:

- *Blood alcohol.* This is useful in anyone suspected of but who denies drinking; most people have no detectable alcohol in their blood in the middle of the day.
- *Urinary alcohol.* A value exceeding 120 mg·dl^{-1} is suggestive of chronic alcohol abuse, and a value over 200 mg·dl^{-1} (44 mmol·L^{-1}) is said to be diagnostic.
- *Gamma glutamyl transpeptidase.* Elevated serum γ-GT activity is observed in about 75% of hospitalized alcoholics; in outpatients and heavy drinkers, the prevalence reaches 90%. Acute alcohol consumption does not lead to abnormal levels but regular, moderate drinkers often have a slight elevation of the γ-GT. Levels return to normal with abstention from alcohol.
- *Mean corpuscular volume.* An MCV of more than 96 fl is found in about 60% of alcohol abusers. The response to abstinence is a return to normal over a period of about 2 months.

Alcohol dependence syndrome

The alcohol dependence syndrome is usually very much easier to identify than problem-related drinking. Figure 19.3 outlines the main characteristics of the syndrome but these do not necessarily present

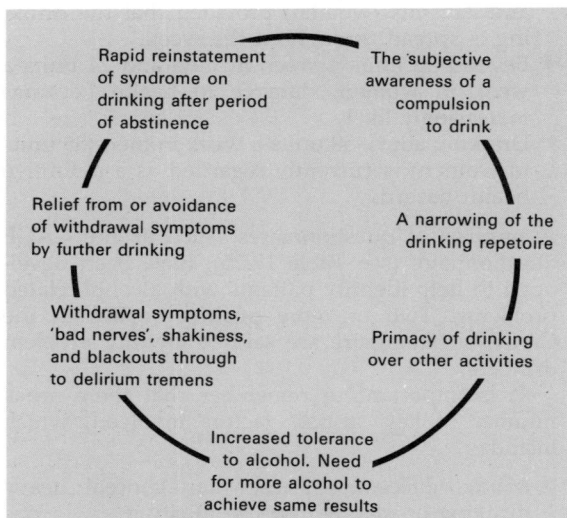

Fig. 19.3 Elements of the alcohol dependency syndrome.

Table 19.26 Symptoms of alcohol dependence.

Unable to keep to a drink limit

Difficulty in avoiding getting drunk

Spending a considerable time drinking

Missing meals

Memory lapses, 'blackouts'

Restless without drink

Organizing day around drink

Trembling after drinking the day before

Morning retching and vomiting

Sweating excessively at night

Withdrawal fits

Morning drinking

Decreased tolerance

Hallucinations, frank delirium tremens

in any particular order. Symptoms of alcohol dependence in a typical order of occurrence are shown in Table 19.26.

COURSE

The course of the alcohol dependence syndrome comprises three linked stages. The first stage is 'heavy' social drinking, i.e. the ingestion of three to five standard drinks (units) of alcohol a day for several years. This stage can continue asymptomatically for a lifetime or, because of a change of circumstances or peer group, it can revert to a more moderate pattern of drinking or can progress to the second stage of alcohol abuse. This stage is usually associated with frequent ingestion of more than eight drinks a day and there are associated

medical, legal, social and/or occupational complications. About half of such abusers either return to asymptomatic (controlled) drinking or achieve stable abstinence. In a small number of cases, such alcohol abuse can persist intermittently for decades with minor morbidity and become milder with time. About 25% of all cases of alcohol abuse will lead to chronic alcohol dependence, withdrawal symptoms and the eventual need for detoxification. This last stage most commonly ends in social incapacity and death or abstinence.

Evidence suggests that alcohol-dependent drinkers do not develop their dependence after a few drinks but that the disorder requires up to 10 years of heavy drinking to evolve (3–4 years in women). In some individuals who use alcohol to alter consciousness, obliterate conscience and defy social canons, dependence and apparent loss of control may appear in only a few months to a few years.

Withdrawal symptoms

Mild tremor, headache, nausea and general malaise are characteristic of the 'hangover'. Patients who are chronically alcohol-dependent often do not have these symptoms, partly because they are tolerant to alcohol and tend to continue to consume alcohol on the next day. Withdrawal from alcohol causes:

- Prominent tremor
- Insomnia
- Agitation
- Fits
- Delirium tremens (DTs)

Delirium tremens is the most serious withdrawal state and occurs 1–5 days after alcohol (or barbiturate) withdrawal. Patients are disorientated, agitated, and have a marked tremor and visual hallucinations (e.g. 'pink elephants').

Signs include sweating, tachycardia, tachypnoea and pyrexia. Additional signs include dehydration, infection, hepatic disease or the Wernicke–Korsakoff syndrome. If delirium tremens is not treated promptly, death can occur.

CAUSES

Genetic factors

Sons of alcoholics adopted away from home are four times more likely to develop drinking problems than the adopted away sons of non-alcoholics.

Environmental factors

A Boston follow-up study showed that 1 in 10 of boys who grew up in a household where neither parent abused alcohol subsequently became alcohol dependent compared with 1 in 4 of those reared by alcohol-abusing fathers and 1 in 3 of those reared by alcohol-abusing mothers.

Biochemical factors
Several factors have been suggested, including abnormalities in alcohol dehydrogenase, neurotransmitter substances and brain amino acids, such as γ-aminobutyric acid (GABA) but, to date, there is no conclusive evidence that these or other biochemical factors play a causal role.

Personality
Follow-up studies have failed to identify any trait or tendency that significantly distinguishes those who subsequently abuse alcohol from those who do not.

Psychiatric illness
This is not a common cause of addictive drinking but it is a treatable one. Some depressed patients drink excessively in the hope of raising their mood. Patients with anxiety states or phobias are also at risk.

Excess consumption in society
Recently, the idea has grown that rates of alcohol dependence and alcohol-related problems are related to the general level of alcohol consumption in society and, in turn, to factors that may control overall consumption, including price, licensing laws, the number and nature of sales outlets, and the customs and moral beliefs of society concerning the use and abuse of alcohol.

TREATMENT

Psychological treatment
Successful identification at an early stage constitutes an important treatment in its own right. It should lead to:

- The provision of information concerning safe drinking levels
- A recommendation to cut down where indicated
- Simple support and advice concerning associated problems

Table 19.27 Management of delirium tremens.

The patient should be hospitalized.
Chlormethiazole* 9–12 capsules (each capsule contains 192 mg) for 24 h, then reduced over 5 days, or diazepam 4–100 mg for 2 days then reduced.
Any dehydration should be corrected.
Any electrolyte imbalance should be corrected.
Any systemic infection should be treated.
B vitamins should be given parenterally.

* i.v. should be avoided.

Such an approach has been found to be as effective as more expensive and specialized forms of psychotherapy in the treatment of moderate to heavy non-addictive drinking. With addictive drinking, the most favoured psychological treatment is group therapy, which involves identification, confession, emotional arousal, the implantation of new ideas, and the long-term support by fellow-members of the group. Family and marital therapy involving both alcoholic and spouse may also be important.

Behaviour therapies involving teaching patients how to drink in a more controlled way are currently the subject of much study.

Physical treatment
Addicted drinkers often experience considerable difficulty when they attempt to reduce or stop their drinking. Withdrawal symptoms are a particular problem and delirium tremens needs urgent treatment (Table 19.27). Drugs that show cross-tolerance for alcohol, such as diazepam or chlormethiazole, may be used in a regimen that involves a steady reduction over 5–7 days. A useful chlormethiazole regimen is 9–12 capsules daily for 2 days, 6–8 daily for 3 days and 4–6 daily for a final 2 days. However, long-term treatment with drugs should not be prescribed in those patients who continue to abuse alcohol. Many alcohol abusers add dependence on diazepam or chlormethiazole to their problems.

Drugs such as disulfiram (Antabuse) react with alcohol to cause very unpleasant acetaldehyde intoxication and histamine release. A daily maintenance dose of such a drug means that an alcohol-dependent drinker must wait until the disulfiram is eliminated from the body before he can drink safely. Such drugs, therefore, can provide a 'chemical fence' around the drinker for at least 24 h. Disulfiram implants have been developed that have a treatment life of 6 months. As yet there is doubt as to whether their benefit is psychological rather than pharmacological.

OUTCOME

Whereas in the case of non-dependent heavy drinkers the goal of normal drinking within safe limits can be a very reasonable one, the alcohol-dependent drinker must be persuaded to abstain. Abstention, particularly after many years drinking, is a difficult goal and not surprisingly many fail in the attempt. Research suggests that between 40% and 50% of alcohol-dependent drinkers are abstinent or drinking very much less up to 2 years following intervention. Specialized treatment units, psychiatric treatment, group therapy and attendance at meetings of Alcoholics Anonymous—the self-help organization that provides members with a social structure to fill the gap previously occupied by drinking—are all potential elements in the attempt to keep the alcohol-dependent individual abstinent and healthy. To date, however, there is little convincing evidence that highly expensive, time-consuming and specialized modes of treatment are superior in their efficacy to straightforward advice, support, encouragement and monitoring.

Drug dependence

In addition to alcohol and nicotine, there are a number of psychotropic substances that are used for their effects on mood and other mental functions (Table 19.28).

Solvents

Adolescents engage in glue-sniffing for the intoxicating effects produced by the solvents inhaled. The glue is sniffed directly from tubes, plastic bags or smears on pieces of cloth. Tolerance develops over weeks or months. Intoxication is characterized by:

- Euphoria
- Excitement
- A floating sensation
- Dizziness
- Slurred speech
- Ataxia

Acute intoxication can cause amnesia and visual hallucinations. The habit is dangerous because:

- There is a risk of tissue damage, including damage to bone marrow, brain, liver and kidneys. Death can occur.
- Acute intoxication can also result in aggressive and impulsive behaviour.

Amphetamines and related substances

These have temporary stimulant and euphoriant effects that are followed by depression, anxiety and irritability. Psychological rather than true physical dependence is the rule. In addition to restlessness, overtalkativeness and overactivity, amphetamines can produce a paranoid psychosis indistinguishable from acute paranoid schizophrenia.

Cocaine

Cocaine is a CNS stimulant (with similar effects to amphetamines) derived from Erthroxylon coca trees grown in the Andes. In purified form it may be taken by mouth, sniffed or injected. If cocaine hydrochloride is converted to its base (crack) it can

Table 19.28 Commonly used drugs of dependence.

Stimulants	*Narcotics*
Methylphenidate	Morphine
Phenmetrazine	Heroin
Phencyclidine ('angel	Codeine
dust')	Pethidine
Cocaine	Methadone
Amphetamine derivatives	*Hypnotics*
Hallucinogens	Barbiturates
Cannabis preparations	Benzodiazepines
Solvents	
LSD	
Mescaline	

be smoked. This is an effective way of obtaining an intense stimulating effect and 'free-basing' has become common. Compulsive use and dependence are thought to occur more frequently amongst users who are free-basing. Dependent users take large doses and alternate between the withdrawal phenomena of depression, tremor and muscle pains, and the hyperarousal produced by increasing doses. Prolonged use of high doses produces irritability, restlessness, paranoid ideation and occasionally convulsions. Persistent sniffing of the drug can cause perforation of the nasal septum.

Hallucinogenic drugs

Hallucinogenic drugs such as lysergic acid diethylamide (LSD), cannabis and mescaline produce distortions and intensifications of sensory perceptions as well as frank hallucinations.

Cannabis
A widely used drug in some subcultures is cannabis, derived from the plant Cannabis sativa. It is not thought to cause physical dependence. The drug, when smoked, seems to exaggerate the preexisting mood, be it depression, euphoria or anxiety. There is no definite withdrawal syndrome or tolerance. There is disagreement over whether it can produce a psychosis.

Hypnotics

Other drugs of dependence include barbiturates and benzodiazepines. Discontinuing treatment with benzodiazepines may cause withdrawal symptoms such as anxiety, restlessness, tachycardia and sensory disturbances (see Table 19.22); for this reason, withdrawal should be supervised and gradual.

Narcotics

Physical dependence occurs with morphine, heroin and codeine as well as with synthetic and semisynthetic narcotic analgesics such as methadone and pethidine. These substances display cross-tolerance—the withdrawal effects of one are reduced by administration of one of the others. The psychological effect of such substances is of a calm, slightly euphoric mood associated with freedom from physical discomfort and a flattening of emotional response. This is believed to be due to the attachment of morphine and its analogues to receptor sites in the CNS normally occupied by endorphins. Tolerance to this group of drugs is rapidly developed and marked. Following abstinence it is rapidly lost. The abstinence syndrome consists of a constellation of signs and symptoms (see Table 19.29) that reach peak intensity on the second or third day after the last dose of the opiate. These rapidly subside over the next 7 days. Withdrawal is dangerous in patients with heart disease, tuberculosis or other chronic debilitating conditions.

Narcotic addicts are reported to have a high mortality rate due to acute illness associated with drug abuse. Heart disease (including infective endocarditis), tuberculosis and glomerulonephritis are common causes of death, while tetanus, malaria and acute viral hepatitis B are also causally related to addiction.

TREATMENT

The treatment of a narcotic drug overdose requires immediate action. If opioid overdose is suspected, naloxone given intravenously (see p. 748) can be life-saving and diagnostic. There should be an immediate recovery of consciousness or a lightening of the comatose state if the offending agent is an opioid. Care must be taken, however, as opiate

Table 19.29 Narcotic abstinence syndrome.

Yawning Rhinorrhoea Lacrimation Pupillary dilatation Sweating Piloerection Restlessness	12–16 h after last dose of opiate
Muscular twitches Aches and pains Abdominal cramps Vomiting Diarrhoea Hypertension Insomnia Anorexia Agitation Profuse sweating Weight loss	24–72 h after last dose of opiate

antagonists can precipitate violent abstinence symptoms. A constant infusion of naloxone hydrochloride may be required in methadone overdoses.

The treatment of chronic dependence is usually directed towards helping the addict to live without drugs. Some who cannot manage such a regimen may be maintained on oral methadone. In the UK, only specially licensed doctors may legally prescribe heroin and cocaine to an addict for maintenance treatment of addiction.

Causes of drug dependence

There is no single cause of drug dependence. Three factors appear important:

● Availability of drugs
● A vulnerable personality
● Social, particularly peer, pressures

Once regular drug taking is established, pharmocological factors are particularly important in determining dependence.

Eating disorders

Obesity (see p. 164)

The majority of cases of obesity are caused by a combination of constitutional and social factors that encourage overeating. It is relatively infrequent for psychological causes to be involved. However, even when obesity is not due to definite psychological causes, it may itself produce a psychological reaction of depression and tension, particularly if attempts by the patient to lose weight are repeatedly ineffective.

TREATMENT

Behavioural methods of treatment that make use of positive rewards for weight loss or for behaviour likely to lead to a reduction of weight have been attempted, but their efficacy is doubtful.

Anorexia nervosa

The main clinical criteria for diagnosis are:

● A body weight more than 25% below the standard weight
● An intense wish to be thin
● A morbid fear of fatness
● Amenorrhoea in women

Clinical features may include:

● Onset usually in adolescence

- A previous history of chubbiness or fatness
- A relentless pursuit of low body weight
- Usually a distorted image of her own body size
- The patient generally eating little
- Particular avoidance of carbohydrates
- Vomiting, excessive exercise and purging
- Amenorrhoea—an early symptom; in 20% it precedes weight loss
- Binge eating
- Usually a marked lack of sexual interest
- Lanugo

The physical consequences of anorexia include sensitivity to cold, constipation, hypotension and bradycardia. In most cases, amenorrhoea is secondary to the weight loss. Vomiting and abuse of purgatives may lead to hypokalaemia and alkalosis.

PREVALENCE

Case register data suggests a rate ranging from 1–10 per 100 000 females aged between 15 and 34 years. Surveys have suggested a prevalence rate of 1–2% among schoolgirls and university students. However, many more young women have amenorrhoea accompanied by less weight loss than the 25% required for the diagnosis. The condition is much less common among men. The onset in women is usually between 16 and 17 years of age and it seldom occurs after 30 years.

AETIOLOGY

Biological factors
Genetic. Six to ten per cent of siblings of affected girls suffer from anorexia nervosa. No study of monozygotic twins has been made so this increase could be due to environmental as much as genetic factors.

Hormonal. There could be a disturbance of hypothalamic function in that:

- Amenorrhoea precedes weight loss in 20% of sufferers.
- Hormonal disturbances include low luteinizing hormone levels with impaired response to luteinizing hormone releasing hormone and to clomiphene. However, such findings could be due to the effect of prolonged fasting.

Psychological factors
Individual. Patients usually have:

- A disturbance in body image
- Dietary problems in early life

Anorexia is seen as an escape from the emotional problems of adolescence and a regression into childhood.

Family. The specific pattern of relationships described is characterized by:

- Overprotectiveness
- Rigidity
- Lack of conflict resolution

Anorexia serves to prevent dissension in families. However, evidence in favour of such patterns is conflicting.

Social factors
There is a higher prevalence in higher social classes, and a high rate in certain occupational groups (e.g. ballet students and nurses) and in societies where cultural value is placed on thinness.

COURSE AND PROGNOSIS

The condition runs a fluctuating course, with exacerbations and partial remissions. Long-term follow-up suggests that about two-thirds of patients maintain normal weight and that the remaining third are split between those who are moderately underweight and those who are seriously underweight. Indicators of a poor outcome include:

- A long initial illness
- Severe weight loss
- Bulimia, vomiting or purging
- Difficulties in relationships

Suicide has been reported in 2–5% of patients with chronic anorexia nervosa. More than one-third have recurrent affective illness, and various family, genetic and endocrine studies have found associations between eating disorders and depression.

TREATMENT

Treatment can be conducted on an outpatient basis, but if the weight loss is severe it is accompanied by marked physical symptoms of lassitude, dizziness and weakness and/or electrolyte and vitamin disturbances; hospital admission may then be unavoidable. Rarely, the patient's weight loss may be so severe as to be life-threatening. If the patient cannot be persuaded to enter hospital, compulsory admission may have to be used.

Treatment goals include:

- Establishing a good relationship with the patient
- Restoring the weight to a level between the ideal body weight and the patient's idea of what her weight should be
- The provision of a balanced diet of at least 3000 calories in three to four meals per day
- The elimination of purgative and/or laxative use and vomiting

Treatment can be conducted on behavioural or

dynamic psychotherapeutic lines or on a combination of both. The usual behavioural approach is to remove privileges on the patient's admission and to restore them gradually as rewards for weight gain. Intense psychoanalytically-derived psychotherapy is not helpful. Family therapy involving the exploration of problems in family relationships and their modification through counselling has recently been explored; however, evidence that it is superior to simple supportive psychotherapy is lacking.

Bulimia nervosa

This refers to episodes of uncontrolled excessive eating, which are also termed binges. There is a preoccupation with food and a habitual adoption of certain behaviours that can be understood as the patient's attempts to avoid the fattening effects of periodic binges. These behaviours include:

- Self-induced vomiting
- Laxative abuse
- Misuse of drugs—diuretics, thyroid extract or anorectics

Additional clinical features include:

- Physical complications of vomiting:
  Cardiac arrhythmias ⎤
  Renal impairment   ⎬ Consequences of low K⁺
  Muscular paralysis   ⎦
  Tetany—from hypokalaemic alkalosis
  Swollen salivary glands ⎤ From vomiting
  Eroded dental enamel   ⎦
- Associated psychiatric disorders:
  Depression in reaction to vomiting
  Alcohol dependence
- Fluctuations in body weight
- Menstrual function—periods irregular but amenorrhoea rare
- Personality—neurotic traits present premorbidly

The prevalence of bulimia in community studies is high; it affects between 5 and 30% of girls attending high schools, colleges or universities in the US. Bulimia is often associated with anorexia nervosa. The prognosis is uncertain.

TREATMENT

As the condition has only recently been recognized, it is not yet clear what is the most effective form of treatment. Admission to hospital with careful control over eating has been advocated, while a behavioural approach involving careful diary-keeping regarding eating and making patients responsible for control is under extensive study. In this approach, patients attempt to identify and avoid any environmental stimuli or emotional changes that regularly precede the desire to binge. Preliminary results of this approach are promising.

Psychosexual disorders

Sexual disorders can be divided into sexual dysfunctions, sexual deviations and gender role disorders (see Table 19.30).

Sexual dysfunctions

Sexual dysfunction in men refers to repeated inability to achieve normal sexual intercourse, whereas in women it refers to a repeatedly unsatisfactory quality of sexual satisfaction. Problems of sexual dysfunction can usefully be classified into those affecting sexual desire, those affecting sexual arousal and those affecting orgasm. Among men presenting for treatment of sexual dysfunction, impotence is the most frequent complaint. The prevalence of premature ejaculation is low, while ejaculatory failure is rare.

Sexual drive is affected by constitutional factors, ignorance of sexual technique, anxiety about sexual performance, medical conditions and certain drugs (see Tables 19.31 and 19.32).

Table 19.30 Classification of sexual disorders.

Sexual dysfunction

Affecting sexual desire:
  Low libido

Impaired sexual arousal:
  Erectile impotence
  Failure of arousal in women

Affecting orgasm:
  Premature ejaculation
  Retarded ejaculation
  Orgasmic dysfunction in women

Sexual deviations

Variations of the sexual 'object'
  Fetishism
  Transvestism
  Paedophilia
  Bestiality
  Necrophilia

Variations of the sexual act:
  Exhibitionism
  Voyeurism
  Sadism
  Masochism
  Frotteurism

Disorders of the gender role

Transsexualism

Table 19.31 Medical conditions affecting sexual performance.

Endocrine	Renal
Diabetes mellitus	Renal failure
Hyperthyroidism	
Hypothyroidism	Neurological
	Neuropathy
Cardiovascular	Spinal cord lesions
Angina pectoris	
Previous myocardial	Musculoskeletal
infarction	Arthritis
	Respiratory
Hepatic	Asthma
Cirrhosis, particularly	Chronic bronchitis and
alcoholic	emphysema

The treatment of sexual dysfunction involves careful assessment, the participation where appropriate of the patient's partner, and specific therapeutic techniques, including relaxation, behavioural training and supportive counselling.

Sexual deviations

Nowadays, sexual deviations are more likely to be regarded as unusual forms of behaviour than as illnesses and doctors are only likely to be involved when the behaviour involves breaking the law (e.g. paedophilia or bestiality) and when there is a question of an associated mental or physical disorder. Homosexuality was formerly classified as an illness but today it is increasingly accepted as an alternative sexual lifestyle.

Transvestism is a form of sexual deviation in which individuals, usually men, dress in clothes of the opposite sex. The cross-dressing may either be a symptom of some other sexual deviation or may be employed as a means of fetishistic sexual excitement. It usually begins about puberty and the transvestite experiences sexual excitement and may masturbate when indulging in this behaviour. The overwhelming majority of cross-dressers believe that they are of the correct gender, in contrast to transsexuals (see below).

Table 19.32 Drugs adversely affecting sexual arousal.

Male arousal	Female arousal
Alcohol[a]	Alcohol[a]
Benzodiazepines	CNS depressants
Neuroleptics	Oral combined
Cimetidine	contraceptives
Narcotic analgesics	Methyldopa
Methyldopa	Clonidine
Clonidine	
Spironolactone	
Antihistamines	

[a] Alcohol 'increases the desire but diminishes the performance'.

Gender role disorders

Transsexualism involves a disturbance in sexual identity. The criteria for establishing sexual identity are described on p. 793.

In transsexualism, there is no evidence as yet of abnormality in the chromosomal or phenotypic sex and social sex conforms to biological sex. There is, however, a severe disturbance in psychosexual differentiation. A person's gender identity refers to the individual's sense of masculinity or femininity as distinct from sex. It is thought to arise from a biological component (prenatal endocrine influences), psychological imprinting and social conditioning. Disturbances in these three areas have variously been blamed for the cause of transsexualism. The four key features of transsexualism are:

- A sense of belonging to the opposite sex and of having been born into the wrong sex
- A sense of estrangement from one's own body; all manifestations of anatomical sexual identification are regarded as repugnant
- A strong desire to resemble physically the opposite sex and seek treatment, including surgery, towards this end
- A wish to be accepted in the community as belonging to the opposite sex

For males, treatment includes hormonal administration (oestrogen is used to produce some breast enlargement and fat deposition around hips and thighs) and, if surgery is to be recommended, a period of living as a woman as a trial beforehand. In the case of female transsexuals treatment involves surgery and the use of methyl testosterone.

Psychiatry and the law

At the heart of the relationship between psychiatry and the law is the issue of responsibility. Mental disorder, by virtue of its severity and/or quality, may impair the individual's responsibility for his thinking and actions. The law in most Western countries provides for the compulsory admission and/or treatment of the mentally disordered person for his own protection and/or the protection of others and for mitigation in the case of the mentally disordered individual who commits a criminal offence.

In England and Wales the law relating to the care and control of the mentally ill has evolved out of common law. The Act of Parliament that is crucially involved is the Mental Health Act of 1983. This Act is concerned not merely with provisions governing the compulsory admission and treat-

Table 19.33 Important sections of the Mental Health Act 1983.

Section	Duration	Signatures required	Purpose
2	28 days	Two doctors (one approved) plus nearest relative or social worker	Assessment and treatment
3	6 months	Two doctors (one approved) plus nearest relative or social worker	Treatment
4	72 h	One doctor plus relative or social worker	Emergency admission
5(2)	72 h	Doctor in charge of patient's care	Emergency detention of patient already in hospital
5(4)	6 h	Nurse (RMN)	Emergency detention of a patient already in hospital
136	72 h	Police officer	Psychiatric assessment of those in public places thought by police to be mentally ill and in need of a place of safety

ment of mentally disordered persons, but also with patients' rights, appeals tribunals and the overall supervision of the use of compulsory powers. The Act is divided into a number of sections, each of which deals with a different aspect of the process. The Mental Health (Scotland) Act 1984 and the Mental Health (Northern Ireland) Order 1986 contain clauses broadly similar to those in England and Wales.

Apart from one provision of the National Assistance Act 1948, the Mental Health Act 1983 is the only method whereby individuals can legally be deprived of their liberty without having committed a crime or being suspected of committing a crime. It is, therefore, very important that doctors understand the seriousness of their responsibility and the details of the legislation.

There are three conditions that need to be met before an appropriate compulsory section form is signed. The patient must:

- Be suffering from a defined mental disorder
- Be at risk to his/her and/or other people's health or safety
- Be unwilling to accept hospitalization voluntarily

The reasons why there is no alternative approach to the treatment suggested for the patient should be outlined.

Sexual deviance or alcohol or drug dependence are *not* mental disorders, but otherwise the definition of mental disorder is broad and includes:

- Mental illness
- Mental impairment
- Severe mental impairment
- Psychopathy

Any registered medical practitioner may sign a 'medical recommendation' under the Act, but the added signature of a specialist psychiatrist ap-

proved under Section 12 is needed for compulsory orders lasting for more than 72 h. Unless the patient is already in hospital, the nearest relative or an approved mental health social worker is also required to sign the application form. Important sections of the Act are detailed in Table 19.33.

Sections 4, 5(2), 5(4) and 136 cannot be extended by repetition. They must be converted to a Section 2 or 3 if prolonged detention is necessary. Likewise, Section 2 should be converted to a Section 3 if required. Patients on the longer orders (2 and 3) can appeal to a Mental Health Review Tribunal. The Act also deals with consent to treatment, guardianship, mentally abnormal offenders and hazardous treatments. A Mental Health Act Commission supervises the Act, provides second opinions and regularly visits hospitals. Although much of the process of detention against one's will is formalized, there is no liability for a doctor who acts in good faith with a patient's best interests at heart. Clearly written medical notes, accepted forms of treatment and common sense remain the basis of good practice.

Further reading

Clare AW (1980) *Psychiatry in Dissent*, 2nd edn. London: Tavistock Publications.

Gelder M, Gath D & Mayou R (1989) *Oxford Textbook of Psychiatry*, 2nd edn. Oxford: Oxford University Press.

Goldberg D & Huxley P (1980) *Mental Illness in the Community*. London: Tavistock Publications.

Silverstone T & Turner P (1982) *Drug Treatment in Psychiatry*, 3rd edn. London: Routledge & Kegan Paul.

20

Dermatology

Introduction

Skin diseases are extremely common but their exact prevalence is unknown. There are over 1000 different entities described but two-thirds of all cases are due to fewer than 10 conditions. These common conditions include acne, warts, eczema, infections due to bacteria, viruses and fungi, and psoriasis.

Some conditions, e.g. acne, may be part of normal development while others may be inherited, e.g. the Ehlers–Danlos syndrome. Skin disease may present as part of a systemic disease, e.g. the rash associated with systemic lupus erythematosus, or alternatively, a severe skin disease may cause systemic symptoms, e.g. pemphigus. Geographical factors are also important; in particular, skin conditions due to certain fungi and bacteria are more prevalent in the tropics.

Structure of the skin (Fig. 20.1)

The skin is divided into three layers:

- The epidermis
- The dermis
- The subcutaneous layer

The epidermis
The epidermis consists of stratified epithelium and is divided into two layers. The inner malpighian layer contains the germinal basal layer (stratum germinativum), above which lies the stratum spinosum or prickle cell layer; above this is the stratum granulosum. The outer layer consists of anucleate cornified cells (stratum corneum). The stratum lucidum lies between the granular and the cornified layers. The cells in the germinal basal

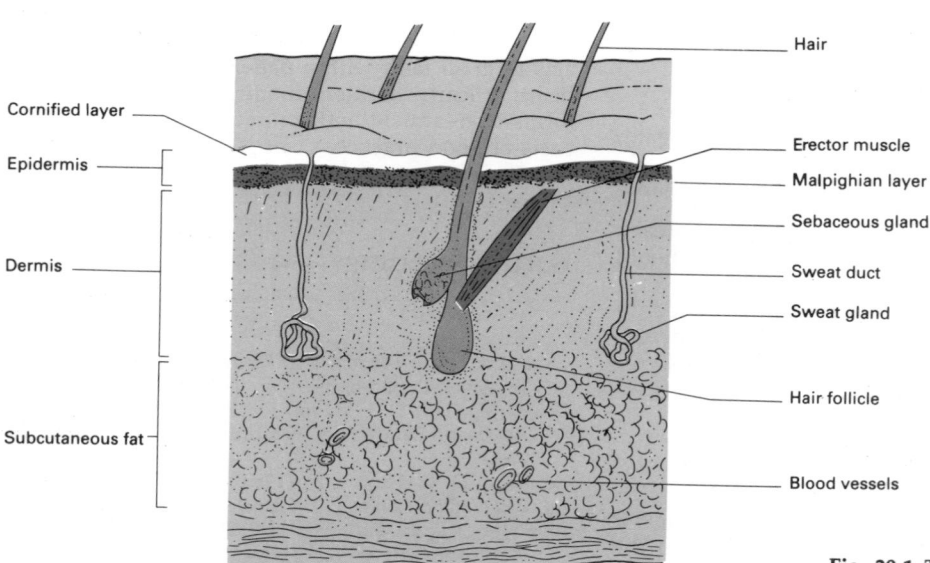

Fig. 20.1 The structure of the skin.

Cornified layer
Epidermis
Dermis
Subcutaneous fat

Hair
Erector muscle
Malpighian layer
Sebaceous gland
Sweat duct
Sweat gland
Hair follicle
Blood vessels

layer give rise to successive layers of cells that lose their nuclei and die as they reach the surface.

The cells in the epidermis consist of keratinocytes that move peripherally from the basal layer where they are continually formed by mitosis. Three other cell types are also seen:

- *Melanocytes* are dendritic cells that arise from the neural crest. They synthesize melanin and transfer it as pigment granules to the epidermal keratinocytes.
- *Langerhans' cells.* These are also dendritic cells that originate in bone marrow. They are in the suprabasal layers of the epidermis and their surfaces express HLA-DR and the antigens CD1 and CD4. They also have surface receptors for C_3 and the Fc fragment of IgG and can secrete interleukin 1. They therefore function as antigen-presenting and antigen-trapping cells and also cooperate with lymphocytes in eliciting an immune response.
- *Merkel cells* migrate from the neural crest and are most numerous on digital pads, lips, the oral cavity and hair follicles where they are involved in sensation. They act as mechanoreceptors and contain neurotransmitter materials.

Epidermodermal junction
The structure is shown in Fig. 20.8. Anchoring fibrils extend from the lamina densa into the dermis. This junctional area is highly antigenic and is the site of a number of disorders.

The dermis
The dermis contains connective tissue fibres, amorphous ground substance, blood vessels, nerves, lymphatics and muscles. The connective tissue fibres consist mainly of collagen (75%) but some are elastic or reticulin fibres. These are embedded in a mucopolysaccharide ground substance. Fibroblasts lie between the collagen bundles and elastic fibres run parallel and enclose the bundles. This gives the skin its elasticity. The cells within the dermis include leucocytes, histiocytes, fibroblasts and mast cells.

The sweat glands
The sweat glands are of two varieties:

- The *eccrine glands* are present all over the skin, particularly the palms, but not in mucous membranes. The glands are situated in the dermis and secrete a watery fluid containing chloride, lactic acid, fatty acids, urea, glycoproteins and mucopolysaccharides.
- The *apocrine glands* are large sweat glands whose ducts open into the hair follicles. They are found in the axillae, anogenital areas, nipples, areolae and scalp. They do not function until puberty. Modified glands produce wax in the ears, and also occur on the eyelids. They produce a white secretion containing proteins and complex carbohydrates.

The sebaceous glands
Sebaceous glands occur all over the skin (except on the palms and soles) but are most numerous on the scalp and face. They have no lumen and their secretion is due to decomposition of the cells. The secretion, called sebum, consists mainly of fatty acids and cholesterol and is discharged into the pilosebaceous follicle.

Hair
Each hair consists of a shaft of keratinized cells that is produced by the hair bulbs deep in the dermis and projects through the skin from the hair follicle. The hair follicle is richly supplied by nerves and blood vessels and contains melanin. There are three types of hair:

- Terminal—medullated coarse hair, e.g. scalp, mole, beard, eyebrows, pubic
- Vellus—non-medullated short, fine, downy hair, e.g. on the face of women and prepubertal boys
- Lanugo—hair covering the fetus

Every hair follicle has a phase of involution (catagen phase), a shedding phase (telogen phase) and a growth phase (anagen phase) which may last up to 3 years in scalp hair. The length to which hair can grow depends on the rate of growth and the length of the anagen phase, and it is cyclical. The anagen phase can vary depending on the site of the hair, e.g. 3–5 years on the scalp. Shed telogen or anagen hair can be distinguished as the 'club' of the telogen hair is depigmented.

Nails
Nails are hard, translucent plates of keratin that grow from beneath the nail fold. A fingernail takes up to 6 months to replace itself and its growth is affected by disease and malnutrition.

The subcutaneous layer
This contains fat, sweat glands and blood vessels.

Functions of the skin

The skin acts as a protective covering to the body. Its functions are as follows:

- It forms a physical barrier to antigens or bacteria.
- It prevents excessive absorption or loss of water.
- Its pigmentation prevents injury from ultaviolet light.
- Vitamin D is synthesized by sunlight in the epidermis.
- It is involved in temperature regulation.
- Sensations of pain, touch and temperature can be distinguished.
- It is involved in immunological reactions.

Table 20.1 Terminology used in skin diseases.

Annular lesions	Lesions occurring in rings
Atrophy	Thinning of skin
Bulla	A large vesicle
Crust	Dried exudate on the skin
Ecchymoses	Bruises more than 3 mm in diameter
Erythema	Redness
Erythroderma	Widespread redness of the skin with scaling
Excoriation	Linear marks due to scratching
Macule	A flat circumscribed area of discoloration
Maculopapule	A raised and discoloured circumscribed lesion
Nodule	A circumscribed large palpable mass > 1 cm in diameter
Papule	A circumscribed, raised, palpable area
Petechiae	Bruises less than 3 mm in diameter
Plaque	A disc-shaped lesion; can result from coalescence of papules
Purpura	Extravasation of blood into the skin; does not blanch on pressure
Pustule	A pus-filled blister
Scales	Dried flakes of dead skin from horny layer (keratin)
Telangiectasis	A visible small dilated vessel on the skin
Vesicle	A small, visible, fluid-filled blister
Weal	A transiently raised, reddened area associated with scratching

Terminology

The terms used to describe skin diseases are shown in Table 20.1.

History

The history should include questions on the patient's general health, past medical history, family history, occupation and any drugs being taken. A description of the skin lesion should be obtained, including its site of origin, spread, length of time it has been present, whether it is itchy or painful, whether it forms blisters or whether any ointment or medicines have helped.

Examination

A careful examination of the whole skin should be made, as clues to the diagnosis may be apparent in distant sites. If the nature of the skin disease is not obvious, a full general examination should be performed, as the skin disease may be a manifestation of a systemic disorder.

Pruritus

This is an itch occurring in many skin conditions, including:

- Scabies
- Atopic eczema
- Candidiasis
- Urticaria
- Insect bites (e.g. flea, bed-bug)

It also occurs with systemic conditions, often without obvious skin involvement. These include:

- Metabolic disease—hyperthyroidism, carcinoid syndrome
- Malignant disease—chronic lymphatic leukaemia, lymphoma, some carcinomas
- Haematological disease—polycythaemia vera
- Renal disease—chronic renal failure with uraemia
- Liver disease—cholestasis, particularly primary biliary cirrhosis
- Miscellaneous—senile pruritus, psychogenic, drugs, e.g. opiates

---

Investigation

- *Skin scrapings for fungi.* Scrapings from areas of involved skin are placed on a slide with 20% potassium hydroxide to clear extraneous material. Fungal mycelia, as well as parasites and lice, may be seen under the microscope.
- *Skin biopsy.* Skin should be removed in the shape of an ellipse along lines of stretch (Langer's lines). Biopsies should either be fixed in formalin or frozen immediately for immunofluorescence.
- *Wood's light.* This is an ultraviolet light that is shone on the skin. Normal hair and skin fluoresce bluish-white. Certain types of ringworm (*Microsporum audouini* and *M. canis*) fluoresce a greenish colour; erythrasma due to *Corynebacterium minutissemum* fluoresces pink/red.
- *Patch tests.* These are used to confirm allergic contact dermatitis.
- *Laboratory tests* for the exclusion of bacterial and fungal infections. Tests for SLE or thrombocytopenic purpura, for example, should be performed as appropriate.
- *Hair*—microscopy and root analysis.

- *Routine tests* such as blood counts and ESR and also urine testing, e.g. for glucose in diabetes, should be performed.

Dermatitis and eczema

Dermatitis implies inflammation of the skin and can be due to many causes. It is usual to prefix the term with the causal agent, e.g. solar dermatitis.

The characteristic features of dermatitis are:

- *A red and hot skin.* Dermatitis affects the epidermis and superficial dermis.
- *Oedema in acute stages.* This separates the keratinocytes (spongiosis) and produces intradermal vesicles.
- *Weeping and oozing* of fluid on to surface. Crusting is seen in acute phases and scaling and fissuring in chronic stages.
- *Excoriation* produced by intense itching. Chronic scratching leads to secondary thickening or lichenification of skin (Fig. 20.2).
- *Secondary infection.*
- *Impaired thermoregulation* and an increased blood flow leading to cardiac failure in very severe cases.

Acute and chronic stages can be seen in the same individual and the acute can resolve completely, leaving no skin abnormalities.

The meaning of the word 'eczema' is 'flowing over', which describes some of the above inflammatory changes. The words eczema and dermatitis are used somewhat interchangeably because in both conditions similar inflammatory changes occur in the skin. Use of the term eczema avoids the word 'dermatitis', which often conjures up ideas in the patient's mind of external irritants such as cause contact dermatitis.

Eczema occurs following a variety of stimuli.

ENDOGENOUS ECZEMA OR ATOPIC DERMATITIS

PATHOGENESIS

The word 'atopy' implies a capacity to hyper-react to common environmental factors. It can be demonstrated by multiple positive skin-prick tests (see p. 647). A positive test to a specific antigen does not necessarily indicate that this antigen is involved in causation of the skin disease, and removal of the antigen, e.g. from the diet, often does not improve the skin condition.

Serum levels of the IgE antibody are elevated in atopic eczema as in all atopic diseases; higher values are seen when eczema is combined with asthma. The significance of these raised levels in the pathogenesis of the eczema is unclear.

Diet
A few patients may be able to correlate the onset of itching and exacerbation of eczema with dietary factors such as eggs and milk and the removal of the food item will often improve the skin condition. Dietary changes may need to be assessed over a prolonged period and care taken over reintroduction of any offending food. Serious attempts at dietary restriction should be supervised by trained personnel.

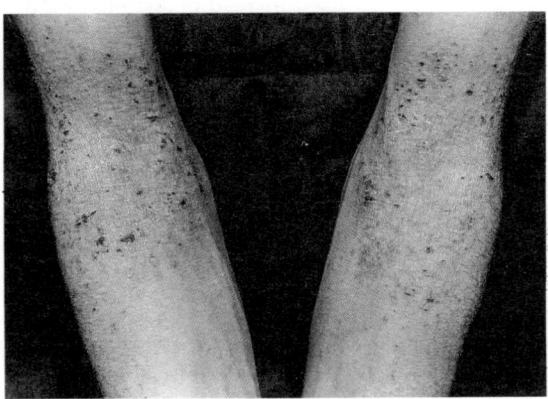

Fig. 20.2 Lichenification seen with chronic flexural eczema.

Genetic factors
There is a hereditary predisposition; when both parents have the disease, the risk of their offspring developing eczema is approximately 60%.

Exacerbating factors
Non-specific stimuli such as heat, humidity, drying of the skin and contact with woollen clothing may cause a flare-up of disease, and patients should be advised to avoid these trigger factors. Irritation may occur following contact urticaria when, for example, foods or animal saliva touch the skin of a sensitized individual.

In atopic patients *Staphylococcus aureus* is found more frequently on the normal skin or nasal mucosa than expected. It is present on the eczematous lesions in 90% of atopics and exacerbates the condition.

PATTERNS OF DISEASE

Infantile eczema
Erythema, weeping or scaling usually appear first on the facial skin after several months. Other body sites are less commonly affected.

Irritation produces restlessness and the child may rub his face or scalp on a pillow or the cotside. With time there is a gradual spread of the dermatitis to the flexures.

Flexural or childhood dermatitis
In toddlers and older children the skin folds are typically involved. Facial involvement may persist, partly owing to climatic factors, e.g. sunlight and low humidity.

Adult dermatitis
In those whose disease continues into adult life, the flexures at the neck, elbow, wrist, ankle or knee and the limbs are often involved. Chronic eczematous changes are common on the face, although any body site may be involved.

PROGNOSIS

With a typical pattern of involvement and an early onset, the prognosis is good. Some children will lose their disease in infancy, whilst others improve gradually so that by the early teens more than 90% will be clear of disease. Localized recurrence may occur in adult life if the skin is unduly stressed, e.g. the hands of nurses or hairdressers. An unusual pattern of eczema over extensor surfaces (reversed pattern) coming on later in childhood may represent more recalcitrant disease and the prognosis should be guarded.

TREATMENT

About a third of atopic children have a dry skin in

Table 20.2 Topical steroids.

Actions
Anti-inflammatory
Immunosuppressive
Decrease rate of epidermal turnover

Types
Many. Available in cream, ointment or lotion form. Vary in potency:

Mild, e.g. hydrocortisone 1%
Moderate, e.g. clobetasone butyrate 0.05%
Potent, e.g. betamethasone 0.1% (as valerate), hydrocortisone butyrate, fluocinolone acetonide 0.2%
Very potent, e.g. clobetasol propionate 0.05%

Compound preparations with, for example antibacterials, are available.

Uses
In general, the least potent effective preparation should be used. The use of potent preparations on the face should be avoided.

Side-effects
Thinning of skin
Spread of local infection
Telangiectasia and striae
Hair growth
Acne
Adrenal suppression with long-term use of potent preparations

Side-effects are chiefly associated with the more potent forms.

addition to eczema, so that the regular use of emollients such as aqueous cream or emulsifying ointment applied to a damp skin after bathing or used instead of soap is fundamental to a treatment regimen. The use of perfumed soaps and 'bubble baths' should be avoided. Non-perfumed cleansers and gels should be used for washing, with the use of soap limited. Sunny holidays at the sea will often stabilize the skin condition and a course of ultraviolet light treatment may bring a similar benefit.

For widespread regular use over months or years, a mild topical corticosteroid (Table 20.2), e.g. 1% hydrocortisone, is suitable; the cream base is the form best tolerated. Localized disease may require short courses of more potent topical corticosteroids on some occasions, especially when the skin is markedly thickened. The addition of tar as an alcoholic solution or as crude coal tar may also improve lichenified skin.

Bacterial infection seen with gross excoriation or with fissuring of the skin is treated with a steroid/antibiotic combination and systemic anti-

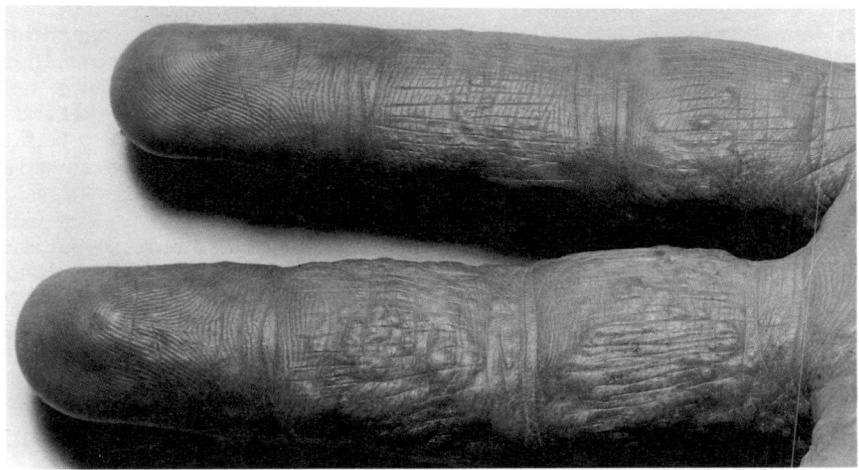

Fig. 20.3 Pompholyx.

biotics may be required.

The treatment of associated atopic disease, e.g. asthma, may in turn improve the state of the skin, the child's well-being and sleep pattern. Sedative antihistamines, such as promethazine hydrochloride elixir at night, will also help to prevent restless sleep and ceaseless scratching.

POMPHOLYX (Fig. 20.3)

This pattern of eczema commonly affects the sides of the fingers, palms, the toes or soles of the feet. Irritant vesicles are the initial feature, though with more serious attacks bullae may be seen.

The patients are usually in their twenties or thirties when they develop the disease. A previous history of atopy is not elicited in the majority of patients.

Some normal individuals develop irritant vesicles on the sides of the fingers in warm weather but there is no clear-cut relationship to sweating. Endogenous factors that trigger this type of eczema are not known. The role of dietary nickel provoking the disease in nickel-sensitive patients is controversial. Attacks may occur frequently and at regular intervals or merge.

TREATMENT

Drying and bacteriostatic solutions such as potassium permanganate 0.01% are used daily until weeping is controlled. Potent topical corticosteroids containing antibiotics or antiseptics may be necessary to control severe attacks, e.g. betamethasone 0.1% cream with neomycin or fluocinolone acetonide 0.025% cream with clioquinol.

Systemic treatment with steroids, e.g. i.m. tetracosactrin, given at regular intervals over weeks or even months, or prednisolone by mouth in doses of between 10 and 15 mg daily, may be necessary to break the frequency of attacks and heal the skin.

DISCOID OR NUMMULAR ECZEMA

The majority of individuals with this type of disease are middle-aged or elderly and have no previous history of skin disease. Papules and coin-shaped raised lesions associated with extreme itching occur on the limbs, most commonly on the lower leg; they may merge to form plaques. Annular patches may appear in association with other patterns of eczema during early life. The cause is unknown but bacterial antigens have been implicated. Eczematous lesions on the legs are sometimes due to venous incompetence (see p. 1038).

TREATMENT

Occlusive bandages containing zinc paste or ichthammol may help to alleviate itching and prevent incessant scratching. Impregnated steroid tape containing flurandrenolone 0.0125% may produce the same effect; intralesional triamcinolone or local potent topical corticosteroids improve the condition of the skin and give relief from itching. The disease often improves when the patient retires from work.

EXOGENOUS ECZEMA

Exogenous eczema can be divided into primary irritant dermatitis and true contact dermatitis associated with a cell-mediated immune response.

Primary irritant dermatitis

This is essentially a degreasing of the skin with a subsequent water loss followed by dryness, fissuring and cracking. It can occur both at work and in the home. Industrial solvents that remove greasy coatings covering metal components in industry can with equal efficiency remove surface lipids from the skin if they are not handled with care.

Housewives are also at risk; the changes in the skin occur in parallel with the extent of immersion of the hands in water, e.g. for washing of kitchen utensils, personal garments or napkins. Initially the skin beneath a ring is often involved, as neat detergent or soap powder tends to lodge there and erode the skin, which becomes eczematous. This spreads to the thin skin on the sides of the fingers, the webs and the backs of the hands; the palms are only affected in more severe and chronic disease. A similar type of disease may be seen in other occupations that involve wet work and the use of cleaning and detergent solutions, such as bar work and hairdressing.

Asteatotic eczema or eczema cracquele

This is a condition often seen in long-stay elderly hospital patients. Dryness of the skin is more evident with ageing. The condition is made worse by washing with soap. The eczema can result in a 'crocodile skin' appearance that is most noticeable on the lower limbs.

This condition may also be seen in hypothyroidism.

Although the skin may appear inflamed, the use of emollients and creams or soap substitutes has the greatest beneficial effect and topical corticosteroids are often unnecessary.

Allergic contact dermatitis

This is a good example of cell-mediated immune disease of type IV reaction. T lymphocytes are sensitized to the antigen, some time after the first contact.

Small-molecular-weight substances passing through the skin need to be linked to skin proteins (haptens) in order to sensitize. Langerhans' cells in the dermis present the antigen to lymphocytes. The sensitivity lasts for life.

CLINICAL FEATURES AND INVESTIGATION

An unusual pattern of rash with clear-cut demarcation or odd-shaped areas of erythema and scaling should arouse suspicion and in combination with a careful history indicate a cause. All areas of the skin may be involved, so that the back can be used as a convenient site for testing. The suspected allergen is then placed in contact with the skin as a patch test. If the causative agent cannot be clearly defined, e.g. in hand eczema, then a range of known everyday antigens can be tested, including materials such as rubber, nickel and medicaments. Positive readings will need to be interpreted with caution and may not have an obvious relevance when considering the patient's history or occupation.

If the major distribution of an eruption appears to involve exposed skin, then photo-patch testing may be required. Two identical sets of likely allegens are placed on the back; one set is exposed to long-wave ultraviolet light, with the second non-exposed set acting as a control.

Patch testing

The original skin disease should be in a quiescent phase before patch testing is done.

Systemic steroid therapy may alter the cutaneous response to an allergen.

- The back is a convenient site for testing.
- Sites for application of the antigen are clearly labelled and a map of their whereabouts is made.
- Materials are diluted in order to prevent irritant reactions and suspended in white soft paraffin.
- White soft paraffin should be used alone in some sites as a control.
- Each substance is then placed within an aluminium disc and kept in place next to the skin by adhesive strapping.
- The patches are taken off and an initial reading is made after 48 h.
- A positive reaction is indicated by an area of eczema.
- Further readings are taken at 96 h.
- Blistering may indicate a non-specific irritant effect but it can occur with soap or detergent materials.

TREATMENT

Treatment is to remove the known irritant or allergen if this is possible. Steroid creams are helpful for short periods when the disease is severe. Antipruritic agents may be necessary for symptomatic relief of itching.

MISCELLANEOUS

Exfoliative dermatitis (erythroderma)

In this condition the entire skin is erythematous, oedematous and scaly. The disease is rare and can be idiopathic (without a preceding skin condition) or can follow dermatitis, psoriasis or other skin disease. It can also be a reaction to many drugs e.g. sulphonamides, sulphonylureas, gold. It is also an occasional feature of systemic disorders, particularly the lymphomas.

MANAGEMENT

Body fluid loss can be considerable and the patient needs intensive medical care; systemic steroid therapy is often necessary.

Erythemato-squamous eruptions

PSORIASIS

This chronic skin disease is seen most commonly as erythematous well-demarcated silvery scaled plaques over extensor surfaces such as the elbows and knees, and in the scalp. In this common pattern the onset of the disease is unusual before 15 years of age, and the initial presentation may occur in old age. Psoriasis occurs throughout the world; in the temperate zones 2% of the population are affected. It is less common in some races with pigmented skins.

Genetic factors are important in the aetiology of the disease, and certain triggers initiate or exacerbate the condition. Characteristically there are periods of activity and remission that are often impossible to predict.

Arthropathy occurs in association with the skin disease in about 8–10% of individuals. Pathogenetic factors that link the two conditions are not clear, though abnormal vascular changes are seen in both.

AETIOLOGY

Genetic factors
The mode of inheritance of the disease is not known but certain HLA markers are recognized. HLA-B13, B16 and B17 are associated with an increased relative risk and HLA-CW6 has a risk increased up to 15 times that of the general population. The B loci occupy an area adjacent to the gene that expresses CW6. HLA-B27 is seen in up to 90% of individuals with ankylosing spondylitis and in 70% of individuals who develop a similar spinal arthropathy with psoriasis.

Infection
The role of infection as an exacerbating factor is suggested by the following observations:

- In children, superficial small patterned lesions of *guttate psoriasis* may appear over the trunk and limbs 10–14 days following a throat infection with beta-haemolytic streptococci, and up to 75% of these individuals have the HLA-CW6 marker.
- Patients with Reiter's syndrome (see p. 403) may develop skin lesions that are identical to those seen in psoriasis. Reiter's disease can occur after dysentery or after venereal contact, again suggesting an infective aetiology that might induce psoriasis.

Emotional trauma
It is a commonly expressed layman's view that many skin diseases are 'nervous' in origin. The role of emotional trauma in triggering psoriasis in a particular individual is best assessed over a long interval. For example, a child followed through to adolescence may be seen to have an exacerbation of the disease with the stress of school examinations. Patients can also develop a reactive psychological state owing to the severity of their skin disease. However, most patients appear as well-balanced individuals.

Mechanical trauma
Repeated trauma to the skin over the elbows and knees as part of everyday activity may explain the common involvement of these sites with psoriasis. In sedentary occupations, e.g. in chauffeurs, there may be intractable disease over the lumbosacral region. Scratching the skin when the disease is in an active phase may induce lesions along the line of trauma—the isomorphic response or Koebner phenomenon. Irritant types of psoriasis such as that affecting the scalp may be made worse by scratching.

Drugs
It is well recognized that lithium carbonate may induce intractable psoriasis. This agent inhibits adenylate cyclase activity, which may alter epidermal cell kinetics. Beta-receptor antagonists such as propranolol may exacerbate psoriasis through similar mechanisms.

PATHOGENESIS

The pathogenesis is unclear but a number of factors play a role.

Epidermal cell proliferation is seen in both the lesions and the uninvolved skin of psoriatics. There is a shortening of the epidermal cell cycle time and an increase in the number of proliferative cells in the growth fraction of the epidermis. Division is normally limited to the basal layer in normal skin but may extend over several layers within psoriatic plaques. Polyamines are known to be important in regulating cellular proliferation, and the levels of these substances and of their rate-limiting enzyme, ornithine decarboxylase, are elevated in psoriasis.

Arachidonic acid levels are greatly elevated in both uninvolved and lesional skin. Many stimuli that affect the cell membrane may cause a release of phospholipase and arachidonic acid and a number of inflammatory mediators are formed from arachidonic acid via the lipoxygenase pathway (see Fig. 12.30). The major initial metabolite in the lipoxygenase pathway is 5-hydroperoxyeicosatetraenoic acid (5-HPETE). This is the precursor of a family of peptido-HETEs, including the leukotrienes, that can alter enzyme pathways that control cell kinetics. Leukotrienes also have marked chemo-attractant properties.

Leukotriene B_4 (LT B_4) levels are elevated in lesional skin and the injection of this substance causes an increase in polymorphonuclear infiltration. Polymorphonuclear cell infiltration of the epidermis and the formation of Munro microabscesses are an important pathological feature in this disease. A variety of immune factors may also attract polymorphonuclear leucocytes; these include immune complexes and complement fragments.

Both humoral and cellular abnormalities have been demonstrated in psoriasis, including elevated IgA and alteration of T cell function. The relative lack of sensitization to the common sensitizer dinitrochlorobenzene (DNCB) in patients with psoriasis supports the concept of an altered cell-mediated immune response in this disease.

CLINICAL FEATURES

Plaque psoriasis
Lesions are well-demarcated, salmon pink in colour and are surmounted by silvery scaling that may be exaggerated by lightly traumatizing the skin with the edge of a fingernail.

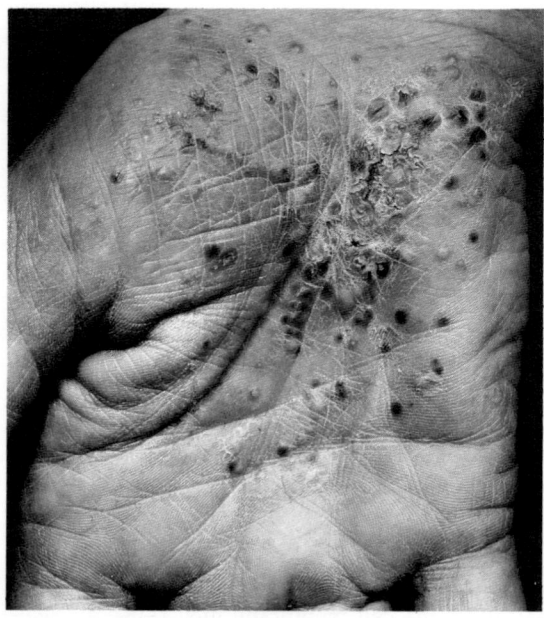

Fig. 20.4 Pustular psoriasis of the palm.

The majority of patients with a plaque type of psoriasis show involvement of the skin over the extensor surfaces of the limbs such as the elbows and knees, with scattered smaller lesions on the limbs and trunk that increase with exacerbation of the disease. Involvement of the scalp with thickened hyperkeratotic scale is common. This is most clearly seen at the hair margin or over the occiput.

The *arthropathy* associated with psoriasis is described on p. 408.

Flexural psoriasis
This is a less common type of psoriasis that may be seen together with plaques or may occur alone. Lesions have a pinkish glazed appearance, are clearly demarcated and non-scaly. The groin, perianal and genital skin are principally involved. Other sites include inframammary folds and the umbilicus. The condition may prove intractable in situations such as the inframammary fold of elderly women with large and pendulous breasts, or when associated with incontinence.

Pustular psoriasis
This may occur in various patterns and in children it is often an isolated finding involving a single digit. The nail dystrophy most commonly seen is yellow discoloration and thickening. Scaling may be pronounced over the digit and, in association with erythema, may spread over the finger.

In its most common form, pustular psoriasis affects the palms or soles with areas of well-demarcated scaling and erythema (Fig. 20.4). The pustules, which are sterile, may appear white, yellow or greenish in colour and when dried are deep brown. Pustulation may not always be evident and it is often associated with increased disease activity. When the condition is grossly hyperkeratotic and occurs in a conical or papular form it is termed '*rupioid*'; identical lesions are seen as one of the cutaneous features of Reiter's syndrome (keratoderma blennorrhagica).

The trunk and limbs may be involved by an almost universal scaling as *exfoliative or erythrodermic psoriasis*. When this condition is seen in association with superficial pustule formation it is termed 'generalized pustular psoriasis'. This is a serious and life-threatening condition with all the problems that are inherent in managing a patient with widespread burns. Such a disease may occur spontaneously but it is seen more frequently after the use of potent corticosteroid therapy given orally or by topical application.

Nail involvement
This can occur in isolation with no evidence of psoriasis elsewhere. The changes most commonly seen include pitting and onycholysis, when separation of the distal edge of the nail from the underlying vascular bed produces a whitish

appearance. A red/brown, salmon-pink or 'oil-stain' coloration may be seen over the nail proximal to the onycholysis. Less commonly the nails are ridged or furrowed. Hyperkeratosis beneath the nail is a pattern of the disease most often seen on the toe-nails, especially in association with pustular variants of psoriasis. When only one or two toe-nails are affected it may be difficult to distinguish from a fungal infection.

MANAGEMENT

The majority of patients can cope with the chronic nature of the disease but the physician must take an active role in treating exacerbations. Tolerance and understanding are required in helping patients to overcome the social stigma that may be associated with their disease.

Active treatment can be divided into regimens suitable for hospital in-patient or day-care centres and treatment that can be prescribed for use in the home. It is unreasonable to expect patients to go through lengthy rituals involving the application of messy topical agents routinely or for any length of time at home. The discoloration of personal garments and bed linen may cause further social or domestic upset and so medicaments containing tar or dithranol, which stain, should be confined to hospital use where possible.

In-patient regimens
Dithranol in concentrations of between 0.05% and 0.5% in zinc and salicylic acid paste (Lassar's paste) is applied to the lesional skin and is protected by wearing a tubular stockingette suit for 12–24 h. Repeated treatments are necessary. The application of this paste is preceded by a tar bath and minimal erythema doses of UVB (ultraviolet light of short wavelength). The intensity of the ultraviolet irradiation is gradually increased throughout the treatment period. Coal tar and salicylic acid ointment containing dithranol in concentrations of between 0.05% and 0.1% is applied overnight to the scalp and removed in the morning with a tar-containing shampoo. Coal tar is often used as an alternative to dithranol in the USA.

Out-patient treatments
- Dithranol is applied at increasing concentrations of between 1% and 3% mixed with 5% salicylic acid in white soft paraffin for up to 20 minutes' therapy and is then washed off. This type of short application enables these messy preparations to be confined to the bathroom of the patient's home. Regular use is quite often prevented by the degree of irritancy experienced and by the marked staining of the skin that is seen with the increasing dithranol concentration.

- Combined preparations of corticosteroids with dithranol or an alcoholic solution of coal tar are especially valuable at low concentrations in the treatment of flexural psoriasis, or for patients with widespread lesions who experience irritation with dithranol applied in a paste form. They are cosmetically aceptable for use in the home.
- Topical steroids can be used but long-term usage of potent steroids should be avoided.
- Low-dose tetracycline in prolonged courses may be helpful in unremitting pustular psoriasis on the palms and soles. This treatment tends to limit the accumulation of polymorphonuclear leucocytes, a prominent feature in the pathology of the disease.
- The retinoic acid derivative etretinate, taken by mouth (1 mg·kg^{-1} daily), is helpful in managing the above pattern of disease and other forms of psoriasis. However, long-term treatment may be required and this can cause loss of hair, hepatic disturbance, hyperlipidaemia and hyperostoses. As it is teratogenic it should not be given to pregnant women.
- PUVA therapy may improve or clear most patterns of psoriasis. Photosensitizing agents, e.g. psoralens, are taken orally 2 h before or applied topically 30 min before exposure to the long-wave ultraviolet light (UVA). Exposure for 2–15 min on two to three occasions each week usually results in clearance of the psoriasis in 10–12 weeks. Maintenance treatment is required every 2–3 weeks in most patients to keep the skin clear.
- NSAIDs. Troublesome joint disease may respond to these drugs.
- Cytotoxic drugs may help alleviate widespread intractable cutaneous disease and painful joints in older patients. Patients with severe chronic psoriasis may experience complete and long-term remission with methotrexate in doses of up to 30 mg once a week. Apart from bone-marrow suppression, cumulative dosage of this drug can lead to hepatic fibrosis. Liver biopsies are required before starting the drug and at yearly intervals, as routine blood tests cannot detect the liver fibrosis. The fibrotic changes tend to be non-progressive, if the drug is stopped. Hydroxyurea can be used and is not hepatotoxic. Azathioprine is more effective on the arthropathy.

SEBORRHOEIC DERMATITIS

Seborrhoeic dermatitis affects those areas of the skin where there is a high density of sebaceous glands. The cause is unknown and no consistent alteration in the function of the sebaceous glands has been demonstrated. For many years observers have attempted to link the disease to lipophilic yeasts that are present on the normal skin as saprophytes—e.g. *Pityrosporum orbiculare* and *P. ovale*, which occur on the trunk and scalp respectively. Bacterial infection has also been considered in the pathogenesis but infection is probably secondary to the skin maceration. Neurogenic factors play a role in that patients with Parkinson's disease may develop similar clinical features over their facial skin and continuing mental stress often exacerbates the disease. Patients are often fair-skinned types of Celtic origin and so genetic factors may also be relevant.

The prevalence of this condition in AIDS is approximately 80% and is correlated with a poor prognosis.

CLINICAL FEATURES

The scalp is principally involved and shows diffuse scaling and erythema. Papules and pustules may accompany these changes or present as the only manifestation of the disease. The spread locally is to the eyebrows, nasolabial folds, the ears and neck. Blepharitis and otitis externa can occur as single features, or they may accompany more widespread disease. Other skin sites affected include the sternal region, the thoracic spine and the paraspinal skin, the axillae, the groin folds and the perianal region. Greasy scales, weeping and maceration are seen with more severe or acute disease. On the back a folliculitis may be the predominant feature.

On occasions the condition may be seen together with more typical eczematous changes elsewhere on the skin; the term 'seborrhoeic eczema' is often used to describe this pattern.

TREATMENT

Shampoos that contain substances with a cytostatic action, e.g. selenium sulphide, zinc pyrithione or econazole, can give initial benefit to patients with a scaly and greasy scalp. With time the beneficial effect may be lost and it is a good principle to change the shampoo after 6–8 weeks. These shampoos tend to aggravate the scalp if there are marked inflammatory lesions and antiseptic preparations such as cetrimide or povidone-iodine in shampoo forms can be added.

A course of tetracycline in a dose of 250 mg twice daily before meals given for 2–3 months may lower the intensity of the inflammatory patterns of the disease.

Lotions, creams or antiseptic powders may help to diminish maceration of the skin involving body folds. Steroid creams should be those of relatively low potency, and preferably they should be combined with an antibiotic or antiseptic such as tetracycline or clioquinol.

Candidiasis may accompany chronic disease and imidazole/hydrocortisone combination creams often help this and other features of the disease.

LICHEN PLANUS

Lichen planus describes a condition in which the lesions are:

- Purplish in colour
- Polygonal in outline
- Planar or flat-topped papules

The cause is unknown but some gross forms of lichen planus may occur in association with diseases in which there is a profound immunological abnormality such as myasthenia gravis with thymoma, and with graft-versus-host disease. Lichen planus-like reactions occur with certain drugs such as sulphonamides (most commonly taken as sulphasalazine), sulphonylureas, methyldopa and thiazide diuretics. Patients with rheumatoid arthritis treated by agents that alter immune function, such as antimalarials, gold, levamisole or penicillamine, may also develop lichen planus-like lesions or lichenoid rashes.

PATHOLOGY

This is characteristic, with the epidermis showing hyperkeratosis, and a marked chronic lymphocytic infiltrate is seen at the epidermodermal junction. This infiltration consists principally of T cells and suggests an immunological reaction to an epidermal antigen.

CLINICAL FEATURES

The distribution of the lesions is peripheral, involving the wrists and ankles, usually symmetrically. The genitalia, scalp or nails are less frequently involved; with chronic disease the scarring that may occur can permanently damage the growth of hair or nails. Scarring may also accompany the less frequent annular patterns of the disease. Linear lesions may follow trauma or scratching (Koebner phenomenon) or may occur in children in a naevoid fashion along a limb. Trauma to the mucosa overlying the bite margin in the mouth commonly induces involvement at this site, producing distinctive pale white linear markings or patterns. Erosive changes may also be seen on the buccal mucosa or tongue or female genitalia.

The presence of Wickham's striae—fine white lacy patterning coursing over the papule—helps to distinguish this disease. Post-inflammatory hyperpigmentation is also a useful diagnostic sign if the disease is beginning to fade at the time of first presentation.

TREATMENT

Untreated, common patterns of the disease may last for 12–18 months. Hypertrophic lesions on the legs or annular patterns may be rather more persistent; recurrence may occur in about one-fifth of cases.

Widespread acute disease is often associated with intractable itching and this may require oral prednisolone for control, given over several months. Less acute disease may be managed with the topical application of potent corticosteroids together with a sedative antihistamine given at night to control the itching.

PITYRIASIS ROSEA

This is a self-limiting non-recurrent scaling maculopapular eruption occurring principally in children and young adults. It has a characteristic distribution, with lesions being predominant on the trunk and the proximal aspect of the limbs. The disease is less common in the summer, and current epidemiological evidence suggests an infective cause, most probably viral. Drugs, e.g. penicillamine, gold, may induce identical clinical features. Males and females are equally affected.

CLINICAL FEATURES

Commonly, a larger and more conspicuous lesion, 2–6 cm in diameter, will precede the more widespread rash by up to 10 days (the herald patch). Individual lesions are reddish-brown in colour, macular, scaled and discrete. They often course over the chest wall following the line of the ribs in a linear fashion. The proximal limb girdle is also affected but the face and scalp are rarely involved. Individual lesions especially over the neck, may show a collarette i.e. a border composed of a rim of scales that point towards the centre. Florid inflammatory papules may occasionally be seen, and individual lesions may be rather more hyperkeratotic on black or Asian skins. The eruption is only mildly pruritic and usually clears in 6–8 weeks without treatment.

Constitutional upset may be noticed prior to the onset of the rash or within the first few days of its appearance. This should help to distinguish the condition from secondary syphilis which it may closely resemble but in which systemic features are usually more severe.

Acne vulgaris

This chronic condition is associated with the blockage of the pilosebaceous duct and appears on areas of the skin, such as the face, chest and back, where sebaceous glands are most numerous and active.

Superficial blocking of the pilosebaceous orifice at the surface of the skin is manifest commonly as a comedo or 'blackhead'; this may be associated with or followed by a variety of inflammatory changes.

INCIDENCE

The incidence of acne vulgaris appears to be the same for both sexes; lesions are evident at a younger age in girls and occur with their earlier sexual maturation. The disease is usually more extensive and serious in males. The majority of patients are clear of acne lesions by their early twenties but about 6% of patients will have disease continuing between the ages of 25 and 40 years.

PATHOGENESIS

There is at the present time no unifying concept with which to explain the pathogenesis of the most common patterns of this disease.

Alteration of the sebaceous glands
The principal age of onset is at puberty when, under the influence of androgenic hormones, sebaceous glands hypertrophy and increase the production of sebum. A greasy skin and scalp usually accompany the polymorphic lesions, which are distributed on the face, chest and back. The secretion of sebum may, however, remain the same or even be increased in the twenties when the acne has cleared.

Microbiology
Propionibacterium acnes, an anaerobic diphtheroid, is present within the pilosebaceous duct, and has lipolytic enzymes capable of altering the local lipid constituents. The products of this organism's enzyme activity, principally fatty acids, have been obtained from within the duct; however, they have little inflammatory property when applied to the skin in the majority of acne subjects.

P. acnes has been shown to alter the cell-mediated immune response and to stimulate the classical and alternative complement pathways. The local accumulation of complement found in and around the duct may thus be due to the presence of *P. acnes*. Pro-inflammatory mediators, also induced by the organism, are chemo-attractant and are capable of producing some of the clinical features seen with active disease.

The sebaceous gland becomes decreased in size and activity when isotretinoin (13-*cis*-retinoic acid) is used in the treatment of acne, and the numbers of *P. acnes* diminish in parallel.

There is no convincing evidence, however, that the numbers of this organism are altered effectively by any of the oral antibiotics that are used in the treatment of the disease.

Keratinization

The superficial portion of the follicular duct undergoes keratinization and an early finding in acne is an increase in the amount of keratin material at this site. It is probable that one of the several effects of isotretinoin, which can so dramatically improve serious acne, is that it alters this abnormal production of keratin.

Androgens

The effect of androgens on the disease is clearly seen in a number of young women in whom the disease continues beyond the teens. Up to 50% of such patients may show evidence of increased circulatory androgen levels, with raised total and free testosterone and/or lowered sex hormone-binding globulin. The alteration of these abnormal findings with treatment may lead to the clinical improvement of seemingly intractable disease.

CLINICAL FEATURES

The 'blackhead' or comedo is the common first-stage lesion, the pigmentation being provided by melanin from the hair. In the absence of such lesions, the diagnosis of acne vulgaris is less likely. Closed comedones or 'whiteheads' are flesh-coloured lesions that are most commonly seen on the cheeks or chin, especially with incidental light or when the skin is slightly stretched. Such lesions represent very firmly obstructed follicles and are often the forerunners of more actively inflamed papules and pustules. Alteration of the water content of the keratin plugs may occur with hormonal changes during the menstrual cycle or with the application of moisturizing creams, e.g. in 'pomade acne', when whitehead lesions become predominant.

The development of inflammatory papules and pustules will follow the release into the skin of the contents of a blocked follicle and the diffusion of chemo-attractant materials across the wall. The pustules are sterile and produce no growth of organism with routine culture. More marked inflammatory changes may lead to large cysts, scarring and keloid formation.

Increased local trauma may cause exacerbation of the disease; this may occur with head-gear, the pressure of strapping across the shoulders or trunk, or on special sites, e.g. beneath the chin in professional violin players ('fiddler's neck').

When unusual sites are involved, such as the forearms and thighs, with eruptions that resemble acne on superficial inspection, on closer examination it will be seen that there is essentially a folliculitis and this can be produced by substances such as cutting oils in industry.

TREATMENT

Diet

Scientific studies show no relationship between food and acne. If, however, any individual experiences a worsening of their disease, after eating chocolate, for example, this should be removed from their diet.

Local applications

- A variety of abrasives, astringents or exfoliatives are useful particularly in comedonal disease. Most of these agents contain benzoyl peroxide in concentrations of between 2.5% and 10%, presented as lotions, creams or gels, alone or in combination with sulphur. Treatment should initially be with low concentrations (usually applied at night), with the concentration being increased with time and as tolerance develops. Erythema, dryness and scaling or peeling of the skin are often seen in the first weeks of treatment and diminish with time.
- Washing with povidone-iodine surgical scrub, which contains a surfactant, may 'freshen' the skin and give short-term relief from greasiness.
- Sunshine or ultraviolet light from artificial sources also helps this comedonal stage of the disease.
- Topical antibiotics available for use are clindamycin phosphate, tetracycline hydrochloride and erythromycin 2% in alcoholic solution.
- Topical retinoic acid (tretinoin) in concentrations of 0.01–0.025% in a lotion or a gel or 0.025–0.05% as a cream is helpful for the comedonal stage.

Systemic therapy

- *Antibiotics.* Pustular and inflammatory disease will respond to oral antibiotics such as tetracycline, oxytetracycline, erythromycin and co-trimoxazole. Treatment with tetracycline 250 mg two or three times daily is often not effective until the drug has been taken for 2 weeks and courses should extend over months. Iron and calcium will markedly diminish the absorption of oxytetracycline or tetracycline, which should therefore be given at least 30 min before food. The absorption of minocycline (100 mg daily) is less affected by food but the drug is more expensive. Topical antibiotics are a useful adjunct to treatment.
- *Hormones.* The alteration of abnormal hormone levels in women may often improve acne. The

Table 20.3 An aetiological classification of urticaria.

Idiopathic

Immunological mechanisms
IgE mediated:
  Atopy
  Physical, e.g. cold, dermographism
  Antigen sensitivity, e.g. pollens, foods, drugs,
    helminths
Complement mediated:
  Hereditary angio-oedema
  Serum sickness
  Blood transfusion reactions
  Necrotizing vasculitis

Non-immunological mechanisms
Mast cell-releasing agents:
  Opiates
  Radiological contrast media
  Antibiotics
Prostaglandin inhibitors:
  Aspirin
  Non-steroidal anti-inflammatory drugs
  Azo dyes
  Benzoates

use of a suitable oral contraceptive pill in which the progestogen component does not produce androgenic effects in the skin may help over the course of 6–8 months or more. Cyproterone acetate, an anti-androgen, has been combined at a low dosage (2 mg) with ethinyloestradiol (35 μg) to produce an oral contraceptive; this needs to be prescribed for periods of up to a year in order to gain full benefit for the skin.

- 13-cis *retinoic acid (vitamin A analogue)*. Severe cystic acne that is unresponsive to the treatments outlined above is the current indication for the use of isotretinoin. Four months of therapy in doses of 1.0 mg·kg^{-1} per day by mouth will produce a remission of the disease in more than 90% of patients for periods of up to 8 years. The side-effects are described on p. 1009.

Erythematous lesions

URTICARIA

The term 'urticaria' implies intermittent transient swelling of the skin with a loss of fluid from vessels into the extravascular space. Dermal swelling is associated with weals, whilst subcutaneous fluid collection is associated with brawny lesions around the lips and orbit (angio-oedema) or the genitalia. Attacks may be associated with pruritus.

The skin appears completely normal afterwards (within minutes or hours).

The passage of fluid out of the vessel may accompany the dilatation caused by mediators such as histamine released from neighbouring mast cells or by other vasoactive compounds such as kinins or prostaglandins. More severe vessel damage, e.g. the vasculitis associated with diseases such as systemic lupus erythematosus or allergic vasculitis, may produce weals in association with purpura and necrosis. On occasions, rather ordinary-looking weals may be accompanied by quite marked vessel damage and an inflammatory cell infiltrate seen on histological examination. Biopsies should therefore be obtained:

- When weals last longer than 2 days
- When weals are accompanied by purpuric staining
- When antibiotics and circulating immune complexes are present in the sera
- When attacks are accompanied by systemic features such as fever or arthralgia

An aetiological classification of urticaria is given in Table 20.3.

Chronic urticaria

This is arbitrarily defined as disease lasting for more than 6 weeks. Weals that irritate are seen on the trunk or limbs and usually last for several hours, or up to 12–24 h (Fig. 20.5). There may be accompanying angio-oedema and this feature may predominate in some patients with swelling of eyes or lips; swelling of the genitalia is less common.

PATHOGENESIS

Many trigger factors have been implicated, including salicylates, indomethacin, tartrazine dyes in food substances or benzoates used as preservatives. Such substances may exacerbate the disease when it is in the active phase in up to 40% of patients. Cross-reactivity between substances, e.g. tartrazine and salicylates is seen, but a search for a food 'allergen' is often unrewarding. A direct pharmacological effect on vessel reactivity is probable, and both aspirin and indomethacin are known to affect prostaglandin metabolism. Agents that can liberate histamine directly include morphine and codeine.

Type I hypersensitivity is more commonly seen with acute disease, or in atopic individuals, and may be triggered by, for example, penicillin in milk. Even when no obvious trigger factor is found there is a tendency towards resolution of the attacks over weeks or months in the majority of patients. In the recalcitrant case an exclusion diet may be used as a last resort, but this is often unhelpful.

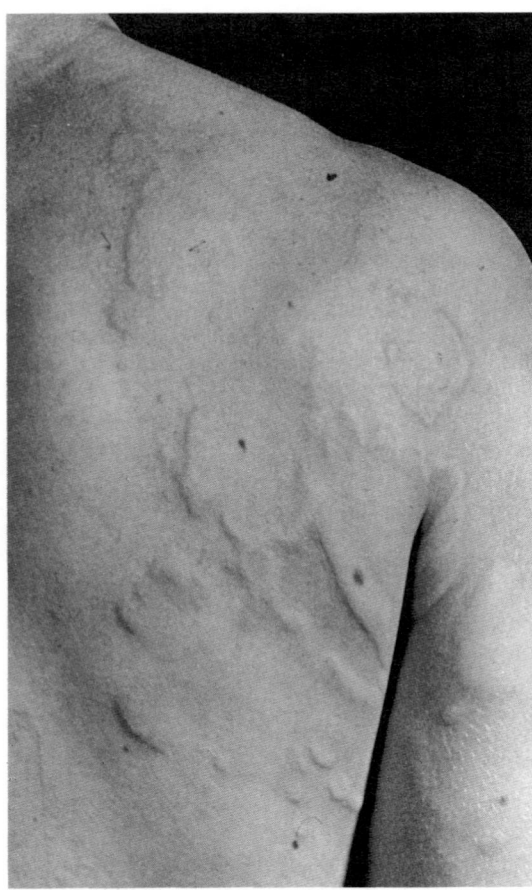

Fig. 20.5 Urticaria.

TREATMENT

Many patients can be managed as follows:

- A sedative H_1 antihistamine is given at night, such as long-acting chlorpheniramine maleate 8–12 mg, or brompheniramine (long-acting) 12–24 mg, or hydroxyzine hydrochloride 10–50 mg.
- Non-sedative H_1 antihistamines such as terfenadine 60 mg twice daily or astemizole 10 mg daily, cetirizine 10 mg daily are useful for daytime use.
- Angio-oedema will often respond better to agents with a wider spectrum of action such as hydroxyzine hydrochloride or cyproheptadine hydrochloride than to routine H_1-receptor-blocking agents.
- The combination of an H_1-receptor antagonist with an H_2-blocker such as cimetidine or ranitidine may stop attacks when other treatments fail.

Acute urticaria accompanied by anaphylaxis (see p. 733), for example from bee stings, snake bites or, less frequently, from food ingestion or drugs,

will require the use of adrenaline. Intravenous hydrocortisone or antihistamines may be given to limit the swelling when the crisis is over, for their effect is not seen for up to 20 min.

Physical urticarias

These may be produced by e.g. pressure, sweating, touch, heat, cold, ultraviolet light or water. These patterns of urticaria are less common and are most likely to be misdiagnosed. This is particularly true of conditions that are not easily reproduced in the clinic, e.g. pressure urticaria.

Cholinergic urticaria
This is not an uncommon pattern of disease and is seen in young adults. The weals are usually small, are often associated with erythema, and last 5–20 min. Attacks are triggered by exercise, hot baths, showers or emotional upset. Such factors may also cause itching but no obvious weals (especially in Blacks) and induce stress and panic reactions. Large quantities of histamine may be liberated during attacks and cause difficulty with breathing.

Patients should be advised to avoid histamine liberators such as codeine or aspirin. If attacks can be anticipated, pre-dosing with hydroxyzine, cyproheptadine or a non-sedative antihistamine such as terfenadine during the day may abort a reaction.

Dermographism (factitious urticaria)
This reaction represents an exaggeration of the third component of Lewis's triple response. A livid weal is produced in response to scratching in about 5% of the population; it is usually asymptomatic. Symptomatic disease occurs when symptoms of itching or discomfort occur after trauma to the skin. Patients may experience marked erythema and wealing when, for example, towelling dry after a bath. Complaints of generalized pruritus with, on occasions, nothing to see may prompt doctors to label the patient as neurotic.

Cold urticaria
This may be triggered by wind over the surface of the skin, e.g. when cycling, or by cold objects in contact with the skin, e.g. taking articles from a freezer. The weals may be reproduced in many patients by the application of an ice cube to the flexor aspect of the forearm. Anaphylaxis may accompany submersion of the body in cold water and patients need to be warned against bathing unaccompanied.

Solar urticaria
Ultraviolet light-induced weals may be seen on sites that are not normally exposed such as the upper arm, especially during the early summer; the

weals appear within minutes of sun exposure. The action spectra is variable between patients and it may need to be assessed in order to provide adequate sunscreens.

Aquagenic urticaria

Contact of the skin with water may induce itching with or without weals. Symptoms may be reproduced by touching the skin with wet gauze. This condition is often a presenting feature of polycythaemia vera.

HEREDITARY ANGIO-OEDEMA

This is a familial disease inherited in an autosomal dominant manner and many patients can give an account of crises occurring in relatives.

AETIOLOGY

The disease is associated with C1 esterase inhibitor deficiency (see p. 139), which may be qualitative or quantitative. This protein modulates the intravascular activation of complement and its deficiency leads to angio-oedema. Clinical features may not appear until adult life. Another form of disease, which is not familial, has recently been described in association with lymphoproliferative disorders.

CLINICAL FEATURES

Severe airways obstruction that is unresponsive to antihistamines may lead to death, and visceral oedema may produce attacks of abdominal pain. Attacks may be preceded by a prodromal rash evident as mild erythema or erythema marginatum. Trauma to the skin, e.g. knocking an arm on a doorpost, may trigger an attack, for C1 esterase inhibitor activity is evoked in the fibrinolytic cascade as well as in complement pathways. The disease must be differentiated from non-hereditary angio-oedema. Swellings may last for up to 72 h and are painful rather than irritant. Purpuric staining may occur, but pitting oedema is not seen.

An analysis of complement levels will demonstrate a low level of C1 esterase inhibitor or its deficient functional activity on laboratory testing; C2 and C4 levels are also reduced. The disease can be differentiated from that associated with lymphoma, when C1 levels are also low and there is no family history.

TREATMENT

Inhibitors of plasmin such as ε-aminocaproic acid or stanozolol (2.5–5 mg daily) and danazol (100–200 mg daily) (attenuated androgens) may be used for long-term treatment. Long-term usage in females may cause menstrual irregularity, fluid retention and androgenicity. Acute attacks may also require the use of fresh frozen plasma.

MASTOCYTOSIS

Mast cells are normally distributed in the connective tissue of the skin and other organs. These cells (see p. 128) release many substances, including histamines, from their granules. An increase in the number of mast cells is referred to as mastocytosis. It may be confined to the skin or, less frequently, may be widespread through all tissues including the viscera (systemic mastocytosis).

Cutaneous mastocytosis

Cutaneous disease is seen principally in children, whereas associated systemic disease is more common in adults. There is a positive correlation between a late onset in adult life, extent of skin involvement and systemic disease.

Clinical forms of the disease that affect principally the skin are varied. Cells may be concentrated into a tumour, often a solitary nodule of yellow/brown colour (mastocytoma). This occurs on the trunk or limbs in the first few years of life and regresses after an interval of 3–4 years.

In urticaria pigmentosa, macular or papular pigmented red/brown lesions are widely distributed on the trunk and are more sparse on the limbs. These lesions urticate on scratching. Trauma to the non-lesional skin may produce dermographism in many patients. Attacks of flushing or irritation of the skin may follow emotional upset or change of temperature or be precipitated by drugs that release histamine, such as codeine or aspirin. The majority of cases occur in children and the lesions fade in late childhood, but those patients with an onset in adult life tend not to lose their disease.

Children may be born with or develop in early infancy diffuse cutaneous mastocytosis, and blistering may be the first indication of the disease. Later in childhood the skin may be thickened and leathery, when markings and folds are exaggerated. Individual lesions are not seen and very rarely erythrodermic forms occur. Hepatomegaly and splenomegaly may occur with diffuse disease.

In adults an uncommon variant of urticaria pigmentosa occurs in which the predominant skin change is widespread telangiectasia. Pigmented lesions are small and macular and are associated with erythema.

In *systemic disease* the bone marrow and skeletal system are commonly involved but any organ can be affected, giving rise to symptoms such as headache and bronchospasm due to histamine release. The treatment is symptomatic and the prognosis is good in the majority.

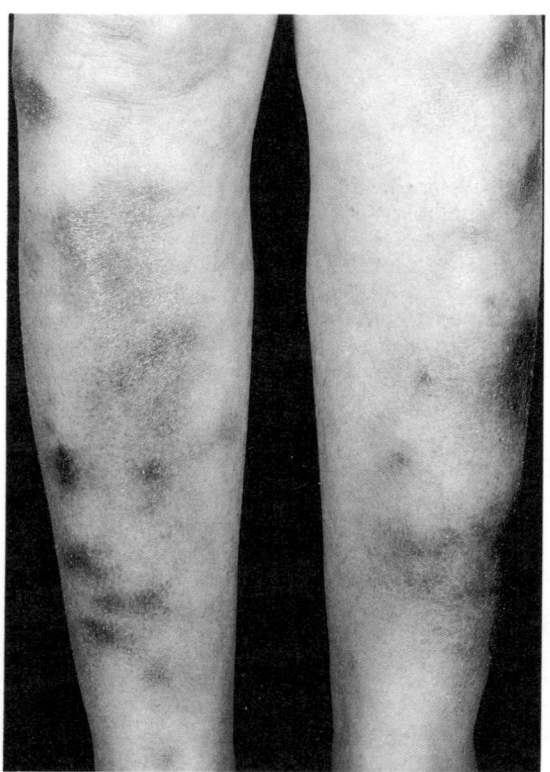

Fig. 20.6 Erythema nodosum on the shins.

ERYTHEMA NODOSUM

This is an acute and sometimes recurrent panniculitis that produces painful nodules or plaques on the shins (Fig. 20.6), with occasional spread to the thighs or arms. Adult females are principally affected.

Histological features suggest that this is an immunological reaction. Immune complex deposition within dermal vessels is an important component in the production of the symptom complex.

A wide range of antigenic stimuli may produce this lesion. Infectious conditions in which erythema nodosum may be seen include streptococcal infections, tuberculosis, leprosy (papules rather than nodules, which are disseminated widely over the skin), yersiniosis, tularaemia, blastomycosis, coccidioidomycosis, histoplasmosis, lymphogranuloma venereum, psittacosis and cat-scratch disease. Sarcoidosis is the commonest association in the UK. Erythema nodosum also occurs in 5–10% of cases of inflammatory bowel disease. Drugs that may produce this reaction include sulphonamides and possibly oral contraceptives. In half the cases no cause is found.

CLINICAL FEATURES

Painful nodules or plaques up to 5 cm in diameter appear in crops over 2 weeks and slowly fade to leave bruising and staining of the skin. Systemic upset is common, with malaise, fever and arthralgia; the condition is especially debilitating when it is recurrent.

INVESTIGATION

Investigations should attempt to exclude streptococcal disease, sarcoidosis and viral causes. The association with sarcoidosis is discussed on p. 683.

TREATMENT

Bed rest helps when systemic features and arthralgia are present. Non-steroidal, anti-inflammatory drugs such as indomethacin should be given to lessen the pain associated with the cutaneous and joint symptoms. Recovery may take weeks and recurrent attacks can occur.

ERYTHEMA MULTIFORME

This is an acute self-limiting and often recurrent condition affecting the skin and mucosal surfaces. There is evidence suggesting that circulating immune complexes are important in triggering the reaction in the skin, which occurs from 7–14 days following, for example, recurrent herpes simplex infection.

AETIOLOGY

Children, adolescents or young adults are principally affected. It is associated with:

- Herpes simplex infection (usually Type 1) in about one-third of cases. The virus is a common trigger factor for recurrent attacks.
- *Mycoplasma pneumoniae.*
- Drugs, e.g. sulphonamides, sulphonylurea derivatives (chlorpropamide) and, less commonly now, barbiturates.
- Other infections, including vaccinia or orf, streptococci, yersiniosis, tuberculosis and histoplasmosis.
- Connective-tissue diseases or neoplasia (rare precipitating factors).
- Topical applications triggering allergic reactions over the areas of skin on which they are placed—erythema multiforme lesions occur at the peripheries.

In half of the cases no cause can be found.

CLINICAL FEATURES

Symmetrically distributed erythematous papules evolve into concentric rings of varying colour. These are commonly seen on the back of the hands, palms and forearms, but may also be seen on the feet or toes. The lesions may show central pallor associated with oedema, bullae formation and peripheral erythema. Alternatively, pallor may be accompanied by central erythema or purpura. Frank bullae represent epidermal necrosis and the separation of this layer. Lesions often spread proximally along the limbs or affect dependent parts in prostrated patients.

The Stevens–Johnson syndrome describes a severe erythema multiforme with a widespread bullous disease associated with oral and genital ulceration and marked constitutional symptoms. Severe mucosal disease is seen with e.g. *Mycoplasma pneumoniae* infection and peripheral lesions may be few in number and difficult to discern, so that erythema multiforme may not easily be diagnosed.

Eye changes include conjunctivitis, ulceration of the cornea, uveitis or panophthalmitis, so that the opinion of an ophthalmologist should be sought in the early stages of disease. These latter features are often the most serious of the complications associated with erythema multiforme.

TREATMENT

The disease is usually self-limiting but death can occur with the Stevens–Johnson syndrome. The withdrawal of offending drugs and the prompt treatment of associated disease is important. It is unlikely that systemic steroid therapy alters the outcome, and such treatment has been shown to be disadvantageous in children. Care of the eye and mucosal ulceration are important, and in severe cases intravenous fluids and feeding may be required.

PYODERMA GANGRENOSUM (Fig. 20.7)

This is a characteristic non-infective, necrotizing ulceration of the skin that occurs in association with underlying systemic disease or blood dyscrasia in 50% of patients.

AETIOLOGY

Associated diseases are described in Table 20.4; these are diverse and give no obvious clue to a common pathogenesis. No constant abnormality of humoral or cell-mediated immunity has been demonstrated.

The pathological features include a massive polymorphonuclear cellular infiltrate with marked necrosis.

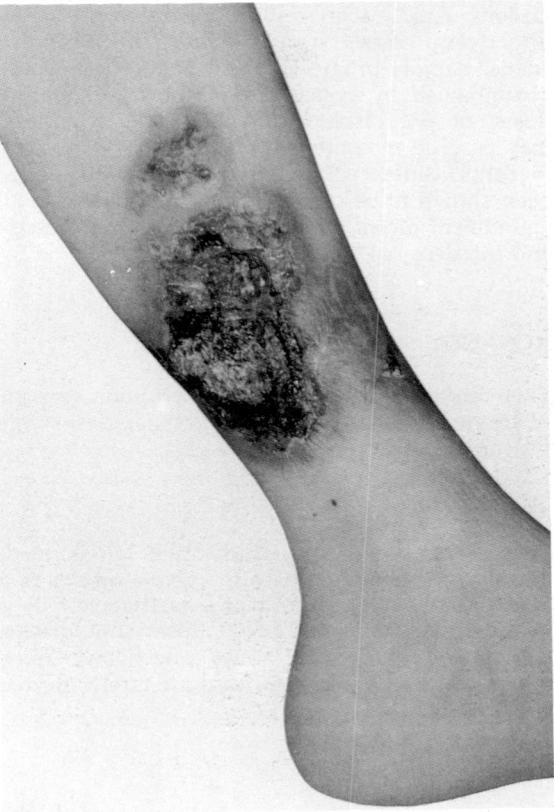

Fig. 20.7 Pyoderma gangrenosum.

CLINICAL FEATURES

Lesions most commonly arise as inflammatory pustules or papules that appear on the trunk and limbs. They may rapidly enlarge over several days to produce large necrotic ulcers with a crescentic or polycyclic outline and sloughy base, which undermines a raised purplish prominent rim. Other patients may have a more slowly progressive indolent ulcer.

Less frequently, but especially in association with acute myelogenous leukaemia, ulceration may be superficial and arise as necrotic bullae.

Table 20.4 Conditions associated with pyoderma gangrenosum.

Multiple myeloma
Other paraproteinaemias, especially IgA
Sero-negative and sero-positive arthropathy
Inflammatory bowel disease
Acute leukaemia
Polycythaemia vera
N.B.: No cause is found in 50% of cases.

TREATMENT

Lesions usually regress with the treatment of the underlying cause, e.g. colectomy in ulcerative colitis. Rapidly progressive and painful lesions are accompanied by systemic symptoms and require doses of prednisolone 80–100 mg. Azathioprine may be used in combination or alone.

Tetracyclines, colchicine and clofazimine have been shown to be of benefit in a few patients.

Indolent ulcers may respond to topical therapy and intralesional steroid injections.

ROSACEA

This chronic inflammatory facial eruption consists of erythema, often accompanied by papules, sterile pustules and telangiectasia.

AETIOLOGY

Those most commonly affected are fair-skinned, middle-aged females who often give a history of a ready flushing tendency which is triggered by a warm atmosphere, emotional upset, hot drinks, spicy food or alcohol. Males often have more severe disease but black Africans are rarely affected with rosacea.

PATHOGENESIS

There is no cohesive view that can explain the combination of clinical findings and pathological changes. Gastritis and other gastrointestinal diseases were once thought to play a role but recent observations have not confirmed this.

Histological sections frequently show changes that are interpreted as folliculitis, but a more constant feature is hyperplasia of the connective tissue around dilated blood vessels of the superficial dermis. This suggests that actinic (i.e. sunlight-induced) damage to the skin is an important component of the disease. The possibility that affected persons might be unduly sensitive to the effect of vasoactive mediators, such as sympathomimetic amines, histamine and acetylcholine has not been substantiated, though endogenous opiates may play a role.

CLINICAL FEATURES

Patients demonstrating the most florid aspects of the disease will have an intense erythema of the skin overlying the flush areas of the face, i.e. the cheeks, nose and chin. The presence of papules and pustules distinguishes rosacea from the facial eruptions of systemic lupus erythematosus. The lesions are intermittent initially, but with chronic disease the erythema is persistent and marked

telangiectasia appears. Other less-common features include lymphoedema of the cheeks or lower eyelids and rhinophyma. In the latter condition there is irregular thickening of the skin of the nose and the follicular orifices are enlarged. The skin of the nose is bright or purplish red. In severe cases there is marked thickening of the skin on the surrounding cheeks. Rhinophyma can occasionally be the only manifestation of rosacea.

Approximately one-half of the patients with rosacea have a variety of ocular lesions. Blepharitis and conjunctivitis are the most common findings, but episcleritis, iritis and keratitis also occur, the latter being a potentially serious complication.

TREATMENT

- Factors that provoke facial flushing should be avoided.
- Tetracycline in doses of 250 mg two or three times daily for periods of at least 12 weeks will improve the inflammatory aspect of the eruption in most patients.
- Metronidazole may be of help when tetracycline is not effective, but care must be taken with the use of this drug over prolonged periods. Two months' treatment at doses of 200 mg three times daily is often adequate.
- Hydrocortisone combined with 0.5–1% sulphur as a cream may bring some relief of facial discomfort.
- Isotretinoin (13-*cis*-retinoic acid) at doses of 0.5–1 mg·kg^{-1} for a period of 4 months has been shown to help resistant disease.

Rhinophyma is improved by shaving hypertrophic tissues from the nose, although re-growth of tissue freqently occurs.

Bullous diseases

In these rare disorders, bullae form the primary lesions and these result from cleavage at various levels at or near the epidermodermal junction. There is a significant mortality associated with the diseases and the treatments. Immunopathological findings are important in the confirmation of diagnosis, in monitoring disease activity, and for understanding the pathogenesis.

PEMPHIGUS

Pemphigus is a rare disease in which antibody, usually of the IgG class, reacts with an antigen at the surface of the epidermal cell that forms part of the intercellular cement substance. The interaction causes proteases and plasmin to be released and the cells lose their adhesion and become rounded (acantholysis). Such cells may be seen when blister fluid obtained from skin lesions is spread on to a slide (Tzanck smear) and examined under the microscope.

The zone of separation within the epidermis may vary; in pemphigus vulgaris it appears just above the basal layer; in superficial forms of pemphigus, clefts occur adjacent to the granular layer. Nikolsky's sign consists of extension of the zone of separation by light pressure or rubbing the skin.

Pemphigus vulgaris

Patients are usually between the ages of 40 and 60 years and are often Jewish. It is also common in India. Antigen–antibody complexes have been shown, on immunofluorescence, to localize within the intercellular substance of the epidermis, adjacent to clefts. Animal and human keratinocytes lose adhesion when cultured in the presence of sera from patients with pemphigus vulgaris.

CLINICAL FEATURES

There are several forms of pemphigus. In the most common form lesions may be confined to the mucosal surfaces in the early stages of the disease and in the mouth may present as bright red, sore and denuded mucosa. In a few patients this may be the only site involved; more commonly, however, thin-walled blisters appear over normal-looking skin elsewhere on the body. Such lesions soon rupture to leave moist eroded areas and secondary bacterial infection is common. When large areas of the skin are denuded, fluid loss and catabolic changes may produce severe metabolic disturbance. These metabolic changes may be compounded in the early stages of systemic steroid treatment.

Blisters may never be evident clinically in the more superficial patterns of pemphigus. A pemphigus-like eruption has been seen with drugs such as penicillamine, captopril and rifampicin.

INVESTIGATION

The diagnosis is confirmed by the cytological examination of blister fluid and by direct immuno-fluorescent staining of a skin sample obtained from the edge of a fresh blister. Fluorescent anti-human IgG and anti-human C3 outline the intercellular substance between the epidermal cells and the edges of the cleft in the skin that forms the blister.

Indirect immunofluorescence demonstrates the presence of circulating antibodies; the titres may reflect disease activity.

TREATMENT

Treatment includes general measures of controlling bacterial infection and fluid loss. Air beds are useful for nursing such patients. Prednisolone in doses of 60–100 mg daily or more may be needed to prevent new blisters forming, and drugs such as azathioprine or methotrexate may be required to enable the dose of steroid to be lowered at the earliest opportunity.

Bullous pemphigoid

Bullous pemphigoid tends to affect older people; most are more than 60 years old at the time of presentation. Direct immunofluorescence demonstrates staining of IgG and C3 at the basement membrane zones. On electron microscopy blister formation is seen at the level of the lamina lucida (Fig. 20.8). Circulating antibodies can be detected in the sera in 70% of patients.

CLINICAL FEATURES

The disease may begin with irritation and erythema of the skin occurring for weeks or months before blistering appears. Bullae then develop, often on an erythematous background but also on normal skin. These tense bullae, which are often secondarily infected, may be localized to one area of the skin (often the legs) or may be more widespread. Involvement of mucosae is rare.

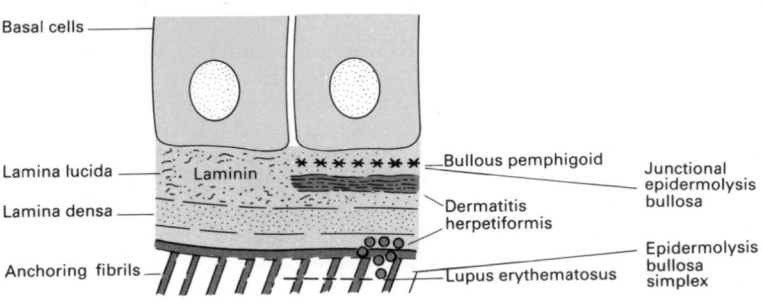

Fig. 20.8 Section of skin to show sites of damage or immune deposition in lupus erythematosus and some bullous diseases.

INVESTIGATION

The diagnosis may be confirmed by the immuno-fluorescent staining of the basement membrane with IgG.

TREATMENT

Smaller doses of prednisolone than those required for pemphigus (40–50 mg daily) are needed to control this disease. Steroid-sparing or substitution may again be achieved with azathioprine or methotrexate and in some patients with dapsone 50–100 mg per day.

It is possible to stop all medication in many patients after 2–3 years of treatment.

EPIDERMOLYSIS BULLOSA

This is the name given to a group of rare and largely genetically determined diseases that vary from localized disease on the soles of the feet in one form, to infants born with a loss of skin from large areas of their body surface at the other extreme.

PATHOGENESIS

In epidermolysis bullosa simplex, blistering arises within the basal cells of the epidermis, while in junctional epidermolysis bullosa the area of cleavage is within the lamina lucida. In the dystrophic form of the disease, separation occurs beneath the lamina densa within the superficial dermis.

CLINICAL FEATURES

Epidermolysis bullosa simplex
This presents within the first year of life, when blisters appear over contact areas of the skin such as the palms and knees; the soles often become affected when walking commences. Scarring is unusual.

Epidermolysis bullosa dystrophica
There are two forms of this disease:

- In the autosomal dominant form, bullae occur on the limbs in infancy.
- In the recessive form, bullae occur at birth and large areas of the skin are denuded with subsequent scarring; contracture and fusion of the skin between the fingers and toes leads to syndactyly. Ulceration of mucosal surfaces, e.g. tongue, oesophagus and the anal margin may be seen.

Epidermolysis letalis (junctional epidermolysis bullosa)
Epidermolysis letalis presents at birth with both mucosal disease and widespread erosions of the skin that often fails to heal. The child dies in infancy.

TREATMENT

There is a tendency for non-lethal forms of the disease gradually to improve through childhood. Protection of the skin and the prompt care of newly eroded skin may lessen scarring. Attention to nutrition, anaemia, eyes and mucosal surfaces is essential but at this time there is no good evidence that drugs will alter the extent of blistering.

DERMATITIS HERPETIFORMIS

Dermatitis herpetiformis produces an extremely itchy polymorphic rash that is symmetrically distributed over the extensor surfaces of the body. The unusual feature of this condition is that most patients also have a gluten-sensitive enteropathy, which is usually asymptomatic.

PATHOLOGY

The dermal papillae are infiltrated with neutrophils, eosinophils and fibrin. Later subepidermal vesicles develop. The major diagnostic pointer is IgA deposits in the normal skin, which can be seen on immunofluorescence. These deposits are usually granular and subepidermal but in 10–20% of patients they may be linear, with the deposits lying within the basal lamina. Linear deposits may also be seen in some other subepidermal blistering conditions. The small-bowel lesion is similar to that seen in coeliac disease (see p. 205) except that it is less severe and varying degrees of villous atrophy are seen; small-bowel lesions are associated with the granular IgA skin deposits.

Immunogenetic findings
The HLA markers and changes in humoral and cellular immunology are similar to those found in coeliac disease.

CLINICAL FEATURES

DH can occur at any age but is seen chiefly in the second, third and fourth decades. Erythematous plaques, excoriations, urticarial papules, crusts or vesicles appear on elbows, knees, shoulders, buttocks and scalp; the mucous membranes are occasionally affected. The lesions are extremely itchy and the vesicles have usually been burst by scratching, leaving encrusted lesions. The course of the disease is one of remissions and exacerbations. Patients can often predict an eruption 8–12 h before its onset because of localized itching. Gastrointestinal symptoms are rare, even with small intestinal lesions and steatorrhoea is seen in less than 5% of patients.

INVESTIGATION

The diagnosis is made on the clinical and histological appearance of the skin, by finding IgA deposits in normal skin, and by the response to dapsone.

TREATMENT

Dapsone 50–200 mg daily will usually control the rash within hours and on stopping the drug the symptoms promptly recur. Occasionally, higher doses of dapsone are required. Maintenance doses vary but patients can adjust their own medication to the minimal dose required to control the rash. Complications of dapsone therapy include haemolytic anaemia and methaemoglobulinaemia.

A gluten-free diet improves the intestinal lesions and also helps the skin lesions, leading to a reduction or cessation of dapsone.

Other conditions that produce blistering include porphyria and drug eruptions; these are discussed on pp. 1036 and 1039.

Infections

Some of the bacterial, viral and fungal infections that affect the skin are considered in this section. Many skin infections are considered under the individual causative organisms in Chapter 1.

BACTERIAL INFECTIONS

An important role of the intact skin is to prevent the entry of infective organisms. This is achieved by the following:

- The cornified surface on many body sites is difficult to breach and has a dessicating effect on some microorganisms.
- Surface long-chain fatty acids inhibit the growth of staphylococci.
- The resident flora on the skin surface can limit the growth of potential pathogens by the production of antimicrobial substances. This is especially useful on continually moist surfaces such as the flexures, where the opportunity for invasion is increased.

AETIOLOGY

- Trauma, or abrasion of the skin removes the stratum corneum and allows infection to occur much more readily; *Staphylococcus aureus* or *Streptococcus pyogenes* are the usual invaders. A cleft in the skin can often be seen at the site of entry of streptococci, e.g. below the ear-lobe when erysipelas ensues, causing cellulitis affecting the face.
- Viral disease or primary dermatoses may allow secondary bacterial infection, e.g. impetigo can follow a 'cold sore' or eczema.
- Other organisms that breach the skin include fleas and lice, and with subsequent itching and excoriation bacterial infection may spread. In patients with continuing bacterial infection (particularly children) an underlying disease such as infestation should always be sought.
- *Staphylococcus aureus* may form part of the flora of the nose in 20% of individuals. It can also be carried on perianal skin, especially in males. In the majority of infections, invasion of the skin remains localized to, for example, a hair follicle as a furuncle or boil. Toxins produced by staphylococci, e.g. exfoliatin are released by certain phage types and will cause separation of epidermal cells to produce *toxic epidermal necrolysis*. Toxic shock syndrome is associated with staphylococcal infection, serious systemic disease, wide-spread erythema and subsequent peeling of the skin. Erythrogenic staphylococcal toxins may produce a disease that resembles scarlet fever, which is induced by streptococci.

Staphylococcal infection (see p. 21)

Boils
Boils or furuncles are painful, erythematous, tender, papular lesions that are related to infection of the hair follicle and can occur on any part of the hair-bearing skin. They are most commonly seen on the neck, axillae, buttocks and thighs. Spread to involve several follicles will produce a carbuncle. Superficial infection of the follicle causes pin-point pustules over the face or legs, especially in children.

Follicular impetigo. Papular lesions may occur when the whole follicle is inflamed to produce sycosis. Sycosis barbae occurs when the beard area is involved. Less commonly, crusted, necrotic or scarred lesions occur on the scalp or face. Staphylococci can sometimes be isolated from these but the pathogenesis of such lesions is not clear.

Treatment of boils. Acute lesions should only be treated with systemic antibiotics if there is marked surrounding erythema or there are associated constitutional symptoms. When the lesion is beginning to 'point' then the overlying skin may be broken with a sterile needle and the area gently swabbed with an antiseptic, such as chlorhexidine or povidone-iodine.

Recurrent boils will require the long-term use of

an antiseptic regimen over several months, including bathing with povidone-iodine added to the bath or washing water. Affected sites and areas of carriage such as the nose or perianal skin will require the application of an antiseptic cream (containing chlorhexidine or neomycin) or dusting powder. With resistant staphylococci (MRSA, see p. 23) mupirocin in ointment form is applied to the nose or topically. Family members may also require treatment if, despite the above measures, chronic sepsis continues. Similar treatment may be required for staphylococcal infection associated with sycosis barbae.

Impetigo

This crusted eruption commonly seen on the face of children may be caused by staphylococci, streptococci or a combination of the two organisms. Staphylococcal infection induces superficial bullae, which are seldom evident because they quickly rupture to leave a moist yellow crusted surface with surrounding inflammation. Tyically the facial skin is involved and children are frequently affected. Bullous lesions are less commonly seen and are associated with the same phage type of staphyloccus that produces toxic epidermal necrolysis. The reason why the disease remains limited in some children whereas it becomes disseminated in others is not clear.

Treatment. Care should be taken to prevent or limit spread of the disease in families or institutions. Areas should be gently bathed with an antiseptic solution such as hexachlorophone or povidone-iodine. Similar preparations in a paint or powder form should be applied to the skin after cleansing. Systemic antibiotics are prescribed if infection is widespread. Rarely, nephrotoxic strains of streptococci are associated with impetigo; the sensitivity of staphylococci should be determined. Erythromycin or cephalosporins both give adequate levels in the skin when given by mouth.

Streptococcal infection

Erysipelas

This is most commonly seen in the skin as widespread erythema and cellulitis. The organisms gain entry through fissures in the skin, e.g. in a toe-cleft, and the skin becomes red, swollen and tender. Constitutional symptoms of fever, malaise and hallucinations often accompany the cutaneous features. With recurrent disease the area affected, e.g. the foot and lower leg, may become lymphoedematous.

Treatment. It is important to treat any underlying skin disease that may be associated with maceration or fissuring of the skin. Local antiseptics applied as paints or dusting powder should be used on areas of chronic fissuring. Foot soaks that are bacteriostatic and astringent, e.g. potassium permanganate 0.01% solution, might be prescribed when maceration of the toe-clefts is associated with excessive sweating. Recurrent erysipelas may require long-term prophylaxis with oral penicillin or erythromycin.

Ecthyma

This disease is not common nowadays in the UK except in drug addicts or patients with HIV infection. Chronic ulceration is produced by infection of the dermis and both *Streptococcus pyogenes* and *Staphylococcus aureus* may be isolated from the same wound.

Debilitation, poor hygiene or nutrition are important contributing factors. Often prolonged and intensive local antiseptic treatment combined with systemic antibiotics will be needed to heal the skin.

Erysipeloid

Erysipeloid is an acute infective disease of the skin. It is most often localized to areas that have been traumatized by contact with carcasses and bones of pigs, chickens or fish. The condition is therefore seen in butchers, meat porters, fishermen or, rarely, housewives. The causative organism is *Erysipelothrix insidiosa*, which also causes swine erysipelas, a serious and systemic disease of pigs. In humans, well-demarcated blue/red discoloration is noticed on the hands, fingers or arms. This follows several days after laceration or abrasion and clears without sequelae. Rarely, fever and malaise accompany the common cutaneous presentation and cases of systemic and cutaneous disease resembling swine erysipelas have been recorded.

The disease is self-limiting and lasts about 7–10 days. If treatment is required, then penicillin given for a week is effective.

Gram-negative infection

This type of infection may occur in moist wounds such as leg ulcers treated with occlusive bandages or dressings. *Pseudomonas aeruginosa* is the most frequent contaminant of such wounds. Astringent solutions such as acetic acid (1–2% solution) will often dry the skin sufficiently to discourage the growth of Gram-negative organisms. Potassium permanganate 0.01% can be used as an alternative for bathing the limb or may be applied as a compress.

Debilitated or immunocompromised patients may rarely develop necrotic skin lesions (from which *Pseudomonas* may be isolated) when local vasculitis follows *Pseudomonas aeruginosa* septicaemia (ecthyma gangrenosum).

Erythrasma

Chronic localized pigmented scaled lesions of the skin occur over skin flexures such as the axillae, groin, toe-webs and beneath the breasts.

The organism isolated from such sites is often a normal commensal of the skin, *Corynebacterium minutissimum*. It is not clear therefore why some adults are especially prone to the disease. Excessive sweating and poor hygiene are frequent accompanying features. Examination by Wood's light causes the organism to fluoresce, producing a pink-red colour.

Treatment. Oral erythromycin will eradicate extensive disease, and the drying of macerated skin with imidazole powders or topical fucidic acid cream will clear more limited infection.

Mycobacterial infection

Cutaneous disease can be due to *Mycobacterium tuberculosis* or *M. leprae*; both of which are uncommon in the Western hemisphere. It is also associated with atypical mycobacteria, including *M. ulcerans*, which causes tropical Buruli ulcer, and *M. marinum*, which causes fish tank or swimming pool granuloma.

Lupus vulgaris

This condition is the most common form of skin disease associated with tuberculosis. Two forms are recognized:

- Haematogenous spread from a reactivated primary lesion
- More rarely, following scrofuloderma, which occurs when the skin is ulcerated by the spread

of infection from an adjacent infected lymph gland or bone

Histologically, the cutaneous lesions show granulomas with central caseation. It is usual to be able to demonstrate the organism from the skin lesions.

Sites of involvement are usually on cooler areas of the skin, with the face being most frequently involved. Erythema, scaling and scarring plaques are seen (Fig. 20.9). In severe intractable disease subcutaneous tissues appear 'gnawed' and hence the term 'lupus' (meaning 'wolf').

Tuberculosis verrucosa cutis

Primary inoculation of the skin with *M. tuberculosis* may give rise to warty lesions on the skin of young children who come into contact with infected sputum or on the fingers of surgeons or pathologists who handle infected tissue.

Secondary inoculation of the skin occurs from endogenous sources, e.g. at the side of the mouth from infected sputum (tuberculosis orificalis cutis); it appears as a plaque or papule.

Tuberculides

Tuberculides form a group of poorly defined eruptions and our knowledge of their pathogeneses is incomplete. It is probable that they represent a reaction in the skin to the haematogenous spread of *M. tuberculosis*. They have declined in parallel with pulmonary tuberculosis. Included under this general heading are papulonecrotic tuberculide, lichen scrofulosorum and erythema induratum or Bazin's disease.

Treatment

Lupus vulgaris and other forms of tuberculosis of the skin should be treated with standard chemotherapy for 6–9 months (see p. 682). Tuberculides such as erythema induratum will clear on the same regimen.

Atypical mycobacterial infections

Skin granulomas develop where the skin is traumatized against the rough surface of the lining or surround of a swimming pool, or over a digit, hand or forearm abraded against the side of an aquarium during cleaning. The latter is the more common nowadays, when the patient presents with a chronic papular lesion on the finger, usually with scaling and less frequently with atrophic changes. On occasions more than one lesion may be seen following spread along cutaneous lymphatics. The organism causing this infection is *M. marinum*.

Lesions may clear over the course of months and routine antituberculous treatment is ineffective. Minocycline in doses of up to 100 mg twice daily for 6–8 weeks may hasten resolution of the lesions.

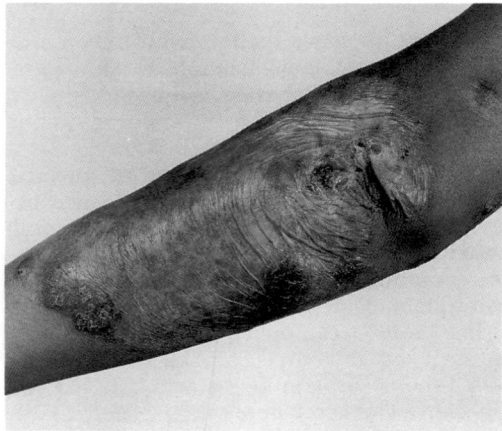

Fig. 20.9 Lupus vulgaris with active granuloma formation at the margins.

Leprosy (see p. 41)

M. lepra infection of the skin gives rise to leprosy. However, in order to lessen the stigma associated with the disease, the term Hansen's disease is preferred.

Tuberculoid leprosy. The organism may be confined to the primary site of involvement in neural tissue and from there there is a spread to the skin. Lesions are few and typically there are plaques with an elevated rim, dusky red in colour and with some central pallor. The surface of the skin is often dry over the lesion, hairless and insensitive. Local peripheral nerves may be enlarged.

Biopsy shows tuberculoid granulomas but no bacilli.

Lepromatous leprosy. Evidence of nerve involvement in the skin is often lacking and presenting signs may be in the respiratory system with nasal congestion. The plaques, nodules, macules and papules that occur are usually erythematous and multiple and have no appreciable loss of sensation. With untreated disease, the facial skin may become thickened and the remainder of the integument is often scaly and dry. Increasing nerve damage leads to loss of sensation, ulceration of limbs, loss of digits and muscle wasting.

Diagnosis and treatment are discussed on p. 44.

VIRAL INFECTIONS

Herpes simplex (see p. 56)

There are two types of herpes simplex virus (HSV) infection—HSV types I and II.

CLINICAL FEATURES

Primary herpes gingivostomatitis (HSV I) may be asymptomatic in children, but others can experience severe stomatitis associated with buccal ulceration, marked local lymph node enlargement and systemic features. Trauma to the skin may introduce the virus, as in gladiatoral or 'scrumpox'. Damage to the skin over a finger may produce a herpetic whitlow especially in nursing personnel.

Type II genital infection may not cause symptoms in females if it is intravaginal. Vulvovaginitis causes burning irritation, dysuria and lymph node enlargement. Extragenital infection on the thigh or buttock can cause myalgia, and dysaesthesiae of the affected overlying skin.

Recurrent disease may induce systemic upset with fever, headaches and meningeal irritation associated with the spread of the virus into the central nervous system. There is local dysaes-thesiae followed by vesiculation, weeping and crusting; less commonly local erythema and papule formation occur but no blistering. Depending on the degree of secondary bacterial infection, attacks clear, with separation of the crust, in 10–14 days.

COMPLICATIONS

Ocular complications. More serious and chronic disease can occur when the eye is the site of primary herpes infection or of recurrent attacks. Ulceration may give rise to marked local pain and oedema and produce keratitis, scarring and visual impairment.

Cutaneous complications. Recurrent herpes simplex type I infection is probably the most common cause of erythema multiforme, which occurs 10–14 days following vesiculation over the lips, face or mucous membranes.

Typical target or iris lesions appear usually over acral skin on the fingers, toes, palms or soles.

Eczema herpeticum. Atopic individuals can develop widespread disseminated viral infection at any time. This does not only occur when their eczema is in an active phase, nor does it occur on every occasion of contact. Nurses and parents with active cold sores should avoid nursing children with atopic eczema.

DIAGNOSIS

This is usually clinical. Rarely the virus may need to be cultured from the vesicles and differentiated immunologically from varicella zoster virus.

TREATMENT AND MANAGEMENT

Local drying agents such as ether or surgical spirit will promote crusting and diminish pain and discomfort.

Povidone-iodine has a mild antiviral action and is available in an alcoholic solution or paint form (10% w/v). The astringent effect is a useful adjunct to treatment and secondary infection may not occur so readily following its use.

Specific measures include the use of idoxuridine, acyclovir or adenosine arabinoside. Infection of the eye is improved by the use of local application of eye drops containing 0.1% idoxuridine or an ointment containing 0.5% idoxuridine. Adenosine arabinoside is available as 3% ointment. Idoxuridine 5–20% is applied to the skin in a vehicle such as dimethyl sulphoxide (DMSO), which aids the absorption of the active ingredient into the skin. The local applications need to be made at the onset of discomfort and for the ensuing few days.

Acyclovir, a thymidine analogue, is activated in

the presence of HSV thymidine kinase. Toxicity to normal tissues is therefore reduced and treatment with this agent in severe local infection or disseminated disease in neonates, atopic individuals or those with immune deficiency may greatly reduce morbidity and mortality. The compound is available for local use as a 5% cream. In tablet form, acyclovir 200 mg five times daily for 5 days is a normal dosage for type I infection. This may need to be increased or doubled when treating type II disease. Parenteral forms of the drug are also available for severely ill patients and for disseminated disease.

Women with genital herpes should undergo cervical screening as there may be a link with carcinoma of the cervix. This should always be performed if their sexual partners have recurrent disease.

Varicella (chickenpox)

This is a common infectious disease of childhood occurring in the winter and spring and caused by the varicella zoster virus (VZV) (see p. 57).

Herpes zoster (shingles)

This infection usually represents the re-emergence of the varicella zoster virus from posterior nerve roots in the spinal cord or cranial nerves into the skin (see p. 933).

AETIOLOGY

This disease affects patients in their middle years or old age. Factors that cause the re-emergence of the virus are often unknown and probably represent changes in the immune state of the host. The induction of an attack by local spinal disease or an occult concomitant malignancy is unusual.

CLINICAL FEATURES

The prodromal symptoms of pain, tingling and dysaesthesia may precede by days the re-emergence of the virus into the skin. It then produces characteristic vesicles, papules or bullous lesions throughout the dermatome. Unusual sites of involvement such as sacral nerve disease may give rise to visceral changes and lead to, for example, bladder dysfunction.

COMPLICATIONS

Secondary infection increases discomfort, and in an elderly person intractable post-herpetic neuralgia may follow an attack of shingles. Trophic ulcers are sometimes seen over the face in association with cranial nerve involvement. Trigeminal nerve disease (ophthalmic division) can lead to infection of the eye. Signs that include swelling of the eyelid, conjunctivitis or blistering at the side of the nose require an ophthalmic opinion.

TREATMENT

- Drying solutions such as calamine cream or lotion are soothing.
- Antiseptic powders containing povidone-iodine or hexachlorophane may help to limit secondary infection.
- Idoxuridine 20–40% in dimethyl sulphoxide (DMSO) may be applied where practical to the affected dermatome on dressings that are kept moist with the compound for the first 3–4 days of infection. This treatment should be limited to immunocompromised or elderly patients with severe disease.
- Acyclovir 800 mg orally five times daily for 7 days is now becoming the treatment of choice. Acyclovir cream 5% may be applied for less severe attacks.
- Prednisolone in doses of 40–60 mg decreasing over 3 weeks can prevent post-herpetic neuralgia in those over 60 years of age. Dissemination of disease is not seen with systemic steroids.
- Management of post-herpetic neuralgia is discussed on p. 933.

Orf

This disease is due to a pox virus infection that commonly affects young sheep, producing a pustular dermatitis. Vesiculopustular lesions appear around the mouth or feet of lambs, and persons coming into contact with the fluid from these may develop papular lesions on traumatized skin. Veterinary surgeons, farmers or their families and butchers are among those principally at risk.

Milker's nodes are produced by a pox virus that is morphologically identical to that of orf. Lesions are seen in farm workers handling the mouths or teats of cattle, and the organism may be carried by domestic cats.

CLINICAL FEATURES

Hands are usually affected. The lesions consist of red/blue papules, 1–2 cm in diameter, with a grey edge and surrounding erythema. Misguided incision of such a swelling may release antigen and produce erythema multiforme. Lesions settle in 6–8 weeks and immunity appears to be life-long.

Molluscum contagiosum

AETIOLOGY

This infection is usually grouped with other diseases caused by the pox viruses, but the virus is antigenically different. Atopic individuals appear to be especially prone to infection and in such persons lesions may be more numerous and difficult to eradicate.

CLINICAL FEATURES

Flesh-coloured, umbilicated papules are seen. They are usually not more than 5 mm in diameter, but the size may vary. Children are most commonly infected and flexural surfaces are the areas of skin most frequently involved. In adults, spread often occurs with sexual contact. Irritation over the surrounding skin may induce scratching and further spread. Single lesions may occur and become quite large and inflammatory and then the diagnosis may not be easy.

TREATMENT

The papules need only to be opened and the contents expressed; this often occurs with scratching although a sterile needle can be used. Silver nitrate or phenol may be applied or electrocautery or a hyfrecator (which seals blood vessels using a small charge of electricity but without heat) may be used. Associated changes in the skin, such as eczema, need to be treated in order to prevent scratching and further spread of lesions.

Warts

AETIOLOGY

The human papillomavirus (HPV) is within the genus papovavirus, which includes other species-specific viruses that infect domestic animals such as the dog, rabbit, horses or cattle. It has long been recognized that tumours induced in animals by this group of viruses may undergo malignant transformation, and the oncogenic potential for man is of increasing concern.

Types of virus
DNA hybridization techniques have demonstrated more than 50 different virus types, and immunocytochemical methods have identified virus particles in human tumours.

Previously warts have been classified according to the clinical appearance or anatomical site that they infect. It is now recognized that one or several viral types can be found in each of the clinically different lesions, e.g. plantar warts are caused by HPV-1 and HPV-4. The genus is divided into types according to the homology of the DNA pattern.

PATHOGENESIS

Viral DNA can be isolated from the basal cells of the epidermis, but the fully infective virion is only evident in more superficial epidermal cells. Cytology or histology shows gross disruption of the cells of the granular layer or below, which have intranuclear and cytoplasmic eosinophilic inclusions. Gross hyperkeratosis and parakeratosis are also associated with viral infection.

CLINICAL FEATURES

Common warts
Common warts are individual papular lesions with a coarse or roughened surface that are seen on the palmar aspect of the fingers and on the knees; other sites are less commonly affected. Children between the ages of 11–16 years are principally affected. Spread is associated with trauma. Many periungal warts are seen in nail biters, who may also have warts on or around their lips.

Plantar warts (verrucae)
These lesions are often solitary and are distributed over contact areas of the foot. When they overlie a bony prominence and are associated with marked hyperkeratosis, pain and tenderness when pressure is applied may be severe. Squeezing a plantar wart or verruca may more readily induce pain than pressing on the lesion and this is a useful test in differentiating a verruca from a callosity. Paring down the skin over a verruca will demonstrate a pit in the skin at which the surface markings come to an abrupt halt; they are, however, continuous over a callus. Maceration of the skin associated with sweating may induce many superficial lesions that form a mosaic wart.

Single filiform warts
These lesions occur on the face and at the nasal vestibule or around the mouth; they may also be seen over the face or neck of older patients.

Plane warts
Plane warts are flat-topped and slightly rough on the surface, which is often pigmented. They are usually 2–3 mm in diameter and may require incidental lighting to discern their outline. The face, around the mouth and chin are the sites most commonly involved, and the hyperpigmentation may give children an unwashed appearance. Young women are also affected and lesions may persist for years. The dorsa of the hands and knees are sometimes involved and trauma may demonstrate the Koebner phenomenon at these sites.

Gential warts
Genital warts often have a fleshy consistency. Maceration of the overlying keratin mass may produce whitish vegetations. There is evidence for venereal transmission and for malignant transformation in both sexes.

In the female the vulva is most frequently

involved at the introitus and over the labia; the perineum and perianal skin are less commonly involved. A thorough vaginal inspection should be undertaken in women with persistent genital infection or in those whose consorts have genital warts. There is increasing evidence to link HPV-6, -11, -16 and -18 with cervical dysplasia or frank malignant change.

Male infection involves the glans penis, prepuce, frenulum and coronal sulcus; the shaft and scrotum may bear sessile or flat-topped, papular warts.

TREATMENT

Spontaneous resolution is common and this makes it difficult to assess the value of therapy.

Keratolytics containing salicylic or lactic acid may lessen the unsightly appearance of common warts, which is peculiarly loathsome to so many patients.

Drying preparations may speed resolution if maceration of the skin over the hands and feet is associated with excessive sweating. Glutaraldehyde 10% w/v may be applied twice daily with a brush to individual lesions or wiped over the surface of mosaic warts. Soaks include formaldehyde as a formalin solution at concentrations of between 2% and 5%, or potassium permanganate 0.01%. Too strong solutions or too frequent applications may induce cracking or fissuring over areas of the skin such as the toe-clefts.

Destructive methods may hasten resolution by producing local inflammatory changes and enhancing immune reactions. These include chemical cautery, electrocautery and crysosurgery.

On some occasions curettage may prompt the resolution of painful verrucae but any scarring that accompanies such procedures may give rise to chronic pain, particularly when situated over pressure points.

FUNGAL INFECTIONS

Fungal infections of the skin can be divided into those associated with ·yeasts such as *Candida albicans* and others caused by dermatophytes or ringworm fungi.

Candidiasis

AETIOLOGY

Use of drugs such as corticosteroids, cytotoxics, antibiotics and oral contraceptives can predispose to candidiasis. It is now a major problem in patients with AIDS.

Local factors in the skin, such as maceration, may predispose to secondary invasion at sites such

as the groin or breast fold, particularly if obesity is present.

CLINICAL FEATURES

Oral candidiasis. This is discussed on p. 179.

Cutaneous candidiasis
Maceration of the skin in body folds, especially in the obese, induces erosion and intertrigo (Fig. 20.10). In a similar fashion, the wet napkins of infants may encourage opportunistic infection with *C. albicans*.

Pruritus vulvae
Candidiasis is a common cause of a vaginal discharge and leads to pruritus vulvae. It can be a presenting feature of diabetes mellitus. Other causes are:

- Vaginal discharge due to *Trichomonas*, *Gardenella* or other causes
- Scabies and pediculosis
- Contact dermatitis
- Senile atrophy
- Leukoplakia
- Psychogenic

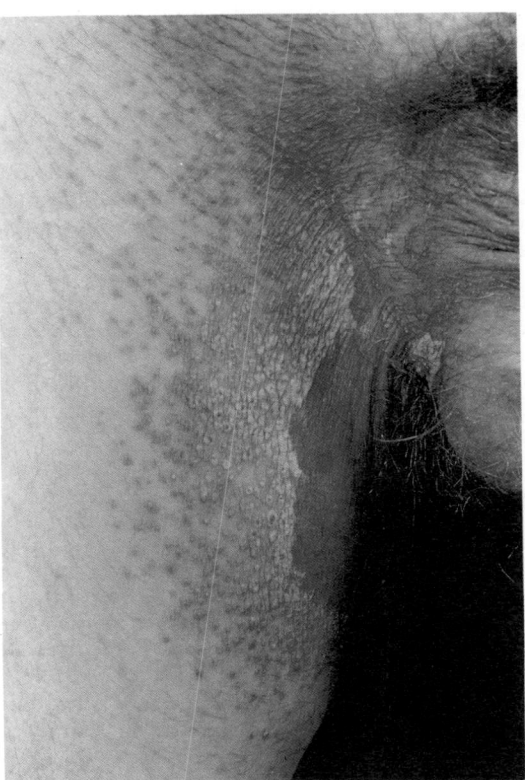

Fig. 20.10 Intertrigo with the typical satellite pustules seen with secondary candidiasis.

Aggravating factors include poor hygiene, obesity, tight clothing and excess washing with soap. Treatment depends on the cause.

Paronychia

Chronic maceration of the skin is important in the development of paronychial infection. Commonly the seal or eponychium at the proximal nail fold is lost by continual immersion of the hands in water or by manicure. A space is opened up beneath the nail fold and the continuing moist environment suits the growth of *C. albicans*.

Disease is manifest by a swelling or bolstering of the nail fold, erythema, pain and deformity of the nail plate. Greenish black discoloration of the nail plate often indicates concomitant infection with organisms such as *Pseudomonas aeruginosa*, which thrives in the same moist environment.

TREATMENT

An attempt to dry areas of contiguous skin, e.g. beneath the breasts by interposing an absorbent material between the two skin surfaces, is important. The routine use of a fine powder containing antifungal agents such as miconazole or clotrimazole as a talc after washing is helpful.

Specific antifungal agents used are nystatin, which has only topical activity, and an imidazole (e.g. clotrimazole or miconazole) cream, lotion, spray or powder. Fluconazole and itraconazole are new oral trizoles and are used particularly for vaginal candidiasis.

In severe intertrigo it is important to incorporate a low-potency steroid together with the antifungal agent in order to allay the inflammatory changes, itching and excoriation.

More serious and widespread disease in infants or those who are immunocompromised by disease or therapy may be effectively treated with oral ketoconazole 200–400 mg daily. The unusual but potentially serious hepatotoxic effects of this drug require that it should be reserved for very intractable or life-threatening disease.

Infection with dermatophytes or ringworm fungi

Dermatophytes or ringworm fungi are able to invade the keratinized tissue of the skin, nails or hair and include *Epidermophyton*, *Microsporum* or *Trichophyton*. The term 'tinea' means 'moth-eaten' and may be used to denote the pattern of involvement, e.g. tinea capitis.

The source of the fungus may be zoophilic (animal to man), anthrophilic (human to human) or geophilic (soil to man).

Scrapings taken from the skin and dissolved in 20% potassium hydroxide should reveal the presence of hyphae. A second sample is plated on a culture medium and incubated. Samples from nail clippings and hairs may be analysed in the same way.

Tinea capitis

This is now an uncommon disease in the UK. The organism most commonly involved is *Microsporum canis*, which is transmitted from the coats of dogs and cats.

CLINICAL FEATURES

Areas of scaling and hair loss are evident in children infected by *M. canis*, but at puberty changes within the hair itself limit infection. On occasions more marked inflammatory changes are seen with a boggy swelling in the scalp, surmounted by crusting and loss of or matting of the hair; this is called kerion. Scarring of the scalp that may follow such infection can lead to permanent hair loss.

Trichophyton species, *T. tonsurans* and *T. violaceum*, invade the hair shaft (endothrix) and often cause the hair to break off at the level of the scalp, producing a black dot appearance. More widespread and severe hair loss associated with a characteristic pattern of scaling in which yellowed keratin scale passes upwards along the hair shaft forming a scutulum or 'shield' shape is seen with the infection favus, which is caused by *T. schoenleini*. This infection is seen in the Middle East, southern Africa, Greenland and, less frequently, in Pakistan.

DIAGNOSIS

Examination by Wood's light produces a greenish fluorescence of the scalp when it is infected with *M. canis* and other species that invade the surface of the hair (ectothrix).

TREATMENT

It is important to treat the animal source of infection. Spread from human to human is unusual with infection produced by *M. canis*. Griseofulvin is given by mouth and treatment may need to be prolonged for up to 3 months. Itraconazole is now also being used. Antibacterial treatment may be required for suppurative disease (kerion), either topically or by mouth, in order to lessen the risk of scarring.

Tinea pedis

This refers to infection that involves principally the toe webs or the soles of the feet.

AETIOLOGY

The infecting organism is most commonly *Trichophyton rubrum* (colonies produce red coloration on culture). *Epidermophyton floccosum* and *T. mentagro-*

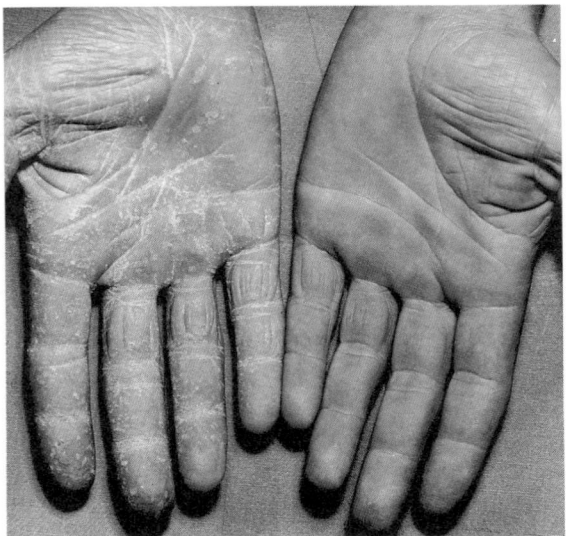

Fig. 20.11 Trichophyton rubrum infection of the right palm.

phytes are less commonly seen.

Occupations that produce maceration of the skin and communal spread include coal mining and working on submarines, where warm decks and rubber-soled shoes encourage infection. Athletic pursuits (athlete's foot infection), the wearing of occlusive footwear and swimming also encourage spread of these infections.

The disease is often intractable and *T. rubrum* infection may be especially difficult to eradicate, with the organism showing resistance to both topical and systemic fungicides.

CLINICAL FEATURES

Infection is mostly seen as:

- Scaling, maceration and erythema of the lateral toe webs
- Blistering lesions, often few in number on the plantar surface of the toes or foot
- Confluent erythema and scaling on the soles

Spread may occur to the palms (Fig. 20.11) or to the medial aspect of the thigh and perianal skin of males.

TREATMENT

Traditional foot powders often contain antifungal agents of low potency but their drying effect is useful when they are applied regularly. Drying foot soaks such as potassium permanganate 0.01% solution may discourage infection by preventing maceration.

Specific measures include oral griseofulvin. This may need to be given for periods of up to 3 months for disease associated with *T. rubrum* in doses of 500 mg twice daily. Imidazoles (clotrimazole or miconazole) can be applied overnight as a cream and used as a talc in powder form by day.

Tinea unguium

This most commonly affects the great-toe nails but several nails may be affected. It causes discoloration, chalky deposits, subungual hyperkeratosis and fragmentation of the nail plate. Infected fingernails show similar changes (Fig. 20.12) but are less frequently involved.

Unusual trauma associated with occupations and hobbies, congenital changes or malalignment may also produce misshapen great-toe nails. When several toe-nails are involved the differential diagnosis includes psoriasis.

DIAGNOSIS

Clippings taken from the free edge of the nail should be sent for culture. Usually the same organisms that cause tinea pedis are found.

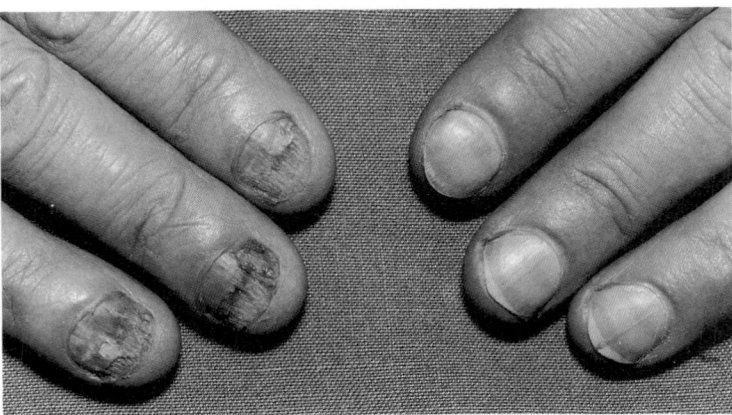

Fig. 20.12 Dystrophy of the fingernails associated with dermatophyte infection (tinea unguium).

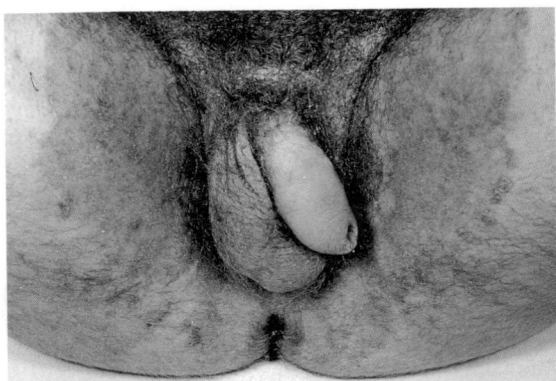

Fig. 20.13 Tinea cruris extending to perianal skin and buttocks.

TREATMENT

Nail-plate infection will require systemic treatment for up to 9 months for finger-nails and 2 years for toe-nails. Griseofulvin 0.5–1 g daily given for such a length of time is seldom associated with serious side-effects but it may fail to eradicate the infection even though the cosmetic appearance is improved. The combination of tioconazole lotion, which penetrates the nail, with griseofulvin can speed and increase the chances of clearing. Itraconazole is also used.

Tinea corporis

Infection of the skin of the groin (*tinea cruris*) is not infrequently seen in males with chronic infection of the feet, so that both areas should be examined at the same time. An area of erythema and scaling is surrounded by a well-defined edge and is often studded with pustules or papules. Infection may extend over the perianal skin (Fig. 20.13).

Tinea corporis may be evident in older members of the family, while children are infected on the scalp. Annular, erythematous and scaled lesions are then seen on the trunk or limbs. More inflammatory, pustular and indurated plaques affect the neck or shoulders of farm workers who come into contact with cattle infected with *Trichophyton verrucosum*.

Diagnosis is by direct microscopy and culture of skin scrapings.

Treatment is with griseofulvin and local antifungal cream.

INFESTATIONS

Scabies (the itch)

Scabies is a highly irritant condition occurring on the skin of an individual sensitized to the female mite of *Sarcoptes scabiei* or its products.

Mode of transmission

Transmission is by skin-to-skin contact with an affected individual and usually occurs in bed. Holding hands is a less common mode of spread from infested children. Warmth is necessary for the mite or acarus to remain mobile and thereby pass from one person to another.

Most individuals will only harbour about a dozen mature female acari. However, many thousands of mites may be associated with crusted or Norwegian scabies, and the affected individuals seem unable to mount the same sensitizing responses. This condition is more common in mentally subnormal individuals and immunocompromised individuals, who may have large numbers of mites, and this imposes a hazard for those who come into casual contact with them while they are in-patients in hospital.

CLINICAL FEATURES

Sites of predeliction for burrows include the finger webs, wrists, elbows, ankles, breasts and genitalia. Linear or curved tracts may be seen with a tiny vesicle at one end that contains the mite. The mite can be removed on the end of a needle, or the burrow scraped to reveal eggs, mite fragments or faeces as firm evidence of infestation.

Sensitivity to the mites' products occurs after 4–6 weeks, when individuals develop most commonly a widespread, highly irritant, excoriated and often secondary infected folliculopapular eruption. Secondary eczematous changes may be evident, or the patient (especially a child) may present with impetigo.

The diagnosis should be suspected if symptoms of itching are severe, when papules appear over genitalia and the history indicates that bed fellows, family or friends are also complaining of irritation. Infants develop papules on the palms, soles or the axillary folds and some adults suffer post-scabetic papules for up to several months after sensitization. Mites from dogs or birds may produce vesicular lesions, crusting or urticaria but infestation from these sources is not associated with burrows.

TREATMENT

All infested individuals and their close contacts should be treated. A lotion containing gamma-benzene hexachloride (lindane 0.1–1%) must be applied to all parts of the skin surface save the face and kept in contact with the skin for a full 24 h, so that hand-washing must be followed by re-application. The process is then repeated 24 h later and all personal garments, night attire and bed-linen should then be laundered in a washing machine. Neurotoxic effects from the absorption of lindane in young children occasionally occur and, alternatively, malathion should be used.

Pediculosis capitis (head lice)

This condition is prevalent in schoolchildren in the UK, with infestation also occurring (though less commonly) in those who have close contact with the children, e.g. mothers. The head louse itself is difficult to find within a thick head of hair but evidence of its presence is seen in the many eggs or 'nits' laid along the hair shafts. The initial lesions occur close to the scalp, especially over the occipital region and the nape of the neck. In children, infestation should be suspected when excoriation is seen and impetigo is evident around the hair margin. Infestation occurs from the close touching of heads and is often widespread within a class of schoolchildren.

TREATMENT

The mite is now resistant in many cases to gamma-benzene hexachloride so that more certain cure follows the application of malathion 0.5%. This is left on for 12 h overnight and removed with malathion shampoo. Cutting the hair facilitates the use of local applications. Thereafter a second application may be necessary at an interval of 7 days. Eggs are killed by this treatment and it is not necessary to continually attempt to remove them.

Pediculosis corporis (body lice)

This condition is usually found only in those with a gross lack of hygiene, such as vagrants. The skin of affected individuals is often thickened, pigmented and excoriated; lice, often few in number, may be evident on the seams of clothing worn next to the skin. The clothes should be autoclaved.

Pediculosis pubis (pubic lice)

Infestation is evident over the pubic hair, with occasional spread in hairy individuals on to the body or even the eyebrows. Contracting the disease is often related to promiscuity. Irritation is the initial symptom and patients are able to detect movement of the louse on skin covered by relatively sparse hairs. Treatment of the infestation is the same as that for head lice.

Arthropod-borne diseases

Development of these diseases depends on contact with the animals or birds that form the primary host for the causative organisms. These include *Cheyletielliae*, most commonly *C. yasgouri* or *C. parasitovorax*, from dogs, cats, rabbits and other pets. On close inspection of their coats such animals will often have evidence of scaling and thickening of the skin, on which mites are sometimes evident by their movement. Brushings are taken on to dark paper, which is then scanned for evidence of mites, fleas or their products. Bites should be suspected in those who have close contact with animals; the area of skin affected shows grouped vesiculopapular lesions.

TREATMENT

This must first begin with the elimination of the arthropod at its source. All other manoeuvres that attempt to produce symptomatic relief of itching associated with bites, such as repellants, calamine lotion, cream or antihistamines, give only temporary relief.

Cutaneous manifestations of systemic diseases

The skin is frequently involved in systemic diseases. In this section, only conditions with major cutaneous manifestations that are not dealt with elsewhere are considered.

CONNECTIVE-TISSUE DISEASES (see p. 391)

These systemic diseases often have cutaneous manifestations, which are described here.

Systemic lupus erythematosus (SLE)

Photosensitivity is a presenting feature in about one-fifth of patients and may occur with a greater frequency as the disease progresses.

The nose, cheeks (butterfly distribution) forehead, ears and the backs of the hands are affected by the non-specific changes of diffuse erythema or maculopapular lesions; blistering may accompany more acute disease.

More chronic changes on the backs of the hands or fingers include blue/red discoloration of the skin, reticulate patterning or poikiloderma (i.e. scarring, atrophic changes and vessel prominence combined with erythema). Nail-fold capillary dilatation and ragged cuticles with haemorrhages are seen in this disease, as well as in dermatomyositis and systemic sclerosis. Loss of tissue over finger pads associated with Raynaud's phenomenon (see p. 624) is seen, although this is a more prominent feature in systemic sclerosis or mixed connective-tissue disease.

Purpura and urticaria may be presenting features of SLE or they may accompany a more widespread vasculitis.

Alopecia occurs with either broken hairs, most noticeable over the frontal region, or diffuse hair loss associated with more severe generalized disease.

TREATMENT (see p. 393)

Protection against the sun is important.

Cutaneous (discoid) lupus erythematosus

This condition represents disease that is almost totally confined to the skin. There are two different patterns:

- Discoid lesions involving principally facial skin
- Widespread cutaneous disease, when the hands, feet, limbs and trunk may also be affected

Patients with widespread cutaneous disease may develop SLE, whilst patients with SLE may develop chronic discoid lesions.

Arthropathy, Raynaud's phenomenon, haematological abnormalities, a raised ESR and abnormal serological findings are sometimes seen with disease, which is seemingly limited to the skin. It may be difficult, therefore, to decide whether a patient has just cutaneous disease or a systemic illness. Obvious ill health, high levels of DNA binding and hypocomplementaemia, a positive lupus band test (typical immunofluorescent changes seen on a biopsy, suitably stained and taken from normal uninvolved skin) are important findings in SLE and these may help to differentiate the two conditions.

CLINICAL FEATURES

Women are twice as frequently affected as men, in contrast to SLE where the female-to-male ratio is 9 : 1. The peak incidence is later than SLE—between 40 and 50 years. In discoid LE the face, neck and, less commonly, the scalp are the principal sites of involvement. Erythematous scaled plaques, oval or round or contoured in outline may be seen (Fig. 20.14). Follicular plugging is characteristically seen; this may be demonstrated as spikes of keratin seen on the undersurface of a removed scale. Atrophy and scarring are common features and when these occur on the scalp, permanent hair loss follows. Although sunlight is an exacerbating factor in most patients, other forms of trauma to the skin, such as cold injury, may trigger the onset of new lesions or reactivate areas of previously involved skin.

Widespread, cutaneous disease may demonstrate similar morphological features, although scaling is not so pronounced. Reticulate patterning or smooth, shiny red/blue atrophic skin is seen, especially on the fingers or plantar aspect of the toes. Chilblain-like lesions may be seen at the same sites and on the heels or earlobes.

TREATMENT

Suitable protection from strong sun or cold should be worn. High-protection-factor sunscreens need to be applied regularly.

Hydroxychloroquine in doses of 200–400 mg daily during spring and summer gives extra protection from sunlight and settles inflammatory changes. Prolonged treatment at high dosage can produce permanent retinal damage so that an ophthalmic opinion should be sought prior to starting treatment and at regular intervals thereafter. Oral prednisolone is given for more florid cutaneous disease.

Potent topical corticosteroids may improve cutaneous lupus erythematosus; this disease is one indication for their application to facial skin. Treatment may need to be intensified when acute inflammatory changes affect the scalp so that scarring and permanent hair loss are prevented.

Other agents that have been used for recalcitrant patterns of disease include thalidomide, vitamin E and retinoids.

Systemic sclerosis and morphoea (scleroderma)

The term scleroderma means a thickening or hardening of the skin associated with an increase in its collagen content. Thickening of the skin also occurs in association with other conditions, such as

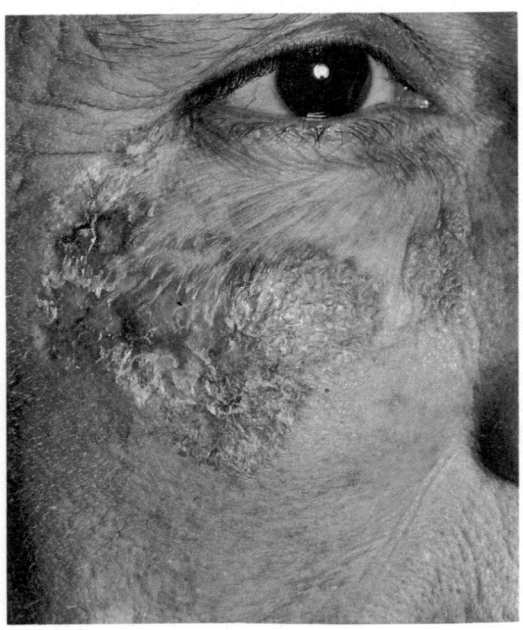

Fig. 20.14 Discoid lupus erythematosus.

porphyria or the carcinoid syndrome. In these conditions the lesion is called pseudoscleroderma. The generic term 'scleroderma' should therefore not be used, as systemic sclerosis and morphoea are distinct entities. Systemic sclerosis has both cutaneous and systemic features, whilst morphoea is confined to the skin.

Morphoea

Females are more frequently affected in a ratio of 3 : 1. It most commonly presents in young patients as a plaque of thickened red or blue skin, sometimes showing central pallor; the skin over the trunk and limbs is most frequently involved. A more superficial and widespread pattern of disease affects the trunk in middle-aged females. Children are affected by linear lesions seen on the skull and over the face and tissues underlying the skin may also be involved, producing facial hemiatrophy.

Plaques evolve to produce waxy, thickened skin that cannot be easily separated from the underlying tissue. Individual plaques may enlarge or new lesions appear over an interval and resolution is associated with hyperpigmentation that may never totally fade. Involvement of the limb may be associated with widespread and severe induration of the skin, muscle pain and joint stiffness.

Generalized cutaneous disease is rare.

TREATMENT

The early inflammatory changes, if severe and associated with oedema and induration may be limited by systemic steroids and azathioprine. It is difficult to treat well-established disease.

Systemic sclerosis (see p. 394)

In two-thirds of patients, Raynaud's phenomenon may be present for years or even decades prior to the development of other clinical features. Severe ischaemia associated with this disease may lead to severe ulceration, gangrene and a loss of digits.

Typically the skin in systemic sclerosis is bound down to underlying structures and the fingers taper (known as sclerodactly or acrosclerosis). Fibrotic changes around the joints may produce flexion deformities and prevent fine movements. A binding down of facial skin may produce beaking of the nose, a fixed facial expression, radial furrowing of the lips and limitation of mouth opening. Mat-like telangiectases on the face or hands and some proximal spread of skin thickening complete the usual picture. Calcium deposits are sometimes extruded from the skin over digits (CR(E)ST syndrome, see p. 395). Thickening of the skin and pigmentary changes are often seen at the base of the neck or over the cervical spine and shoulders.

The disease may sometimes present as puffiness or oedema of the hands or feet, with preceding or accompanying attacks of Raynaud's phenomenon, though circulatory impairment may not be evident. A more explosive onset with widespread or universal skin thickening and more extensive visceral disease is less common.

TREATMENT

Severe Raynaud's phenomenon may be helped by charcoal, chemical or preheated thermal glove warmers or electrically heated gloves. Nifedipine may limit the attacks. Severe ulceration or imminent gangrene may be prevented by the intravenous infusion of prostaglandin E_1 or prostacyclin. Dryness of the skin associated with hair loss, damage to sweat glands and sebaceous glands may respond to emollients and soap substitutes.

Dermatomyositis and polymyositis (see p. 396)

These uncommon diseases affect blood vessels, muscle and skin in a varying fashion.

Dermatomyositis when seen in childhood often has a marked vascular component. Disease in adults aged 40–60 years affects the skin and muscle tissue together. Proximal myopathy, often associated with malignant disease *per se*, and non-specific skin changes have sometimes been mislabelled as dermatomyositis. This misdiagnosis has probably given a falsely high incidence of associated malignant disease (10–25%) that can be seen in adults with dermatomyositis. Recently Coxsackie B virus has been isolated from muscle tissue.

CLINICAL FEATURES

The rash is often very distinctive and may display features of photosensitivity. Fingers show ragged cuticles and haemorrhages with dilated and altered nail-fold capillary changes (Fig. 20.15). Erythematous, blue plaques are evident over the dorsal aspect of the fingers, more especially over the small joints, with a similar but streaked appearance over the metacarpophalangeal joints. Mild scaling may accompany these findings.

Scaling and erythema are seen at the elbow, and on occasions blue/red discoloration and reticulate patterning of the skin over the wrists, knees, feet, arms or thighs are seen.

Facial changes may include a marked erythema resembling sunburn, but inflammation of the eyelids or heliotrope coloration suggest the true diagnosis. Other exposed skin, e.g. the 'V' of the neck or the upper arms, may show erythema and sunburn-like changes that may also cause confusion. Marked cutaneous changes may occur in the absence of muscle disease. Typically, however, patients experience a proximal muscle weakness, noticeable when getting off a lavatory or combing

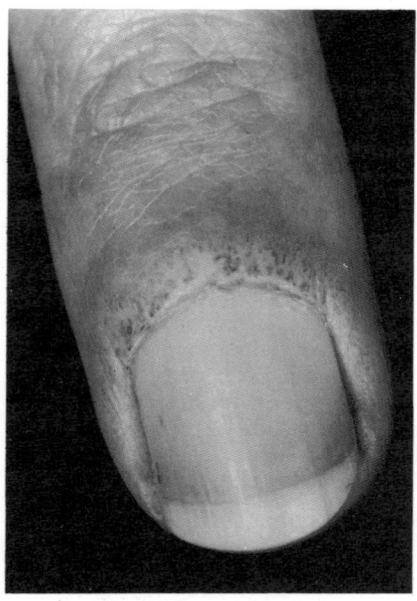

Fig. 20.15 Ragged cuticle and nail fold capillary dilatation associated with dermatomyositis.

the hair; dysphagia and respiratory muscle involvement are more rare.

INVESTIGATION

An underlying malignancy should be looked for. The malignancy may precede, accompany or follow the rash. Measurement of muscle enzyme levels and electromyogram (EMG) studies or muscle biopsy are helpful in the diagnosis and in following disease progress (see p. 959).

TREATMENT

The prevention of joint contractures is very important in the childhood pattern of disease and soft-tissue calcification may regress with time. In adults, prednisolone with or without azathioprine or methotrexate is given for muscle disease (see p. 396). Sun screening and topical corticosteroid therapy may help to limit changes in the skin in those patients with predominantly cutaneous disease.

SARCOIDOSIS

About one-quarter of patients with systemic sarcoidosis have skin lesions. There are many variants:

- Erythema nodosum (p. 1016), a non-specific reaction.
- Nodules, papules and plaques, red/blue or brown are seen particularly on the face, nose, ears and neck in chronic sarcoid. This is the most common specific form seen in Caucasians.
- Annular, macular lesions with central depigmentation are less common.
- Micropapular lesions are common in Afro-Caribbeans and are usually the same colour as the skin. They occur around the nasal alae within the vestibules, on the lips or cheeks or over the peri-orbital skin (Fig. 20.16).
- Lupus pernio, an uncommon variant, affects the nose with a diffuse bluish plaque with small papules within the swelling.
- Widespread cutaneous sarcoidosis is often papular or nodular. Occasionally, subcutaneous nodules are found. Sarcoidosis may appear in old scars.

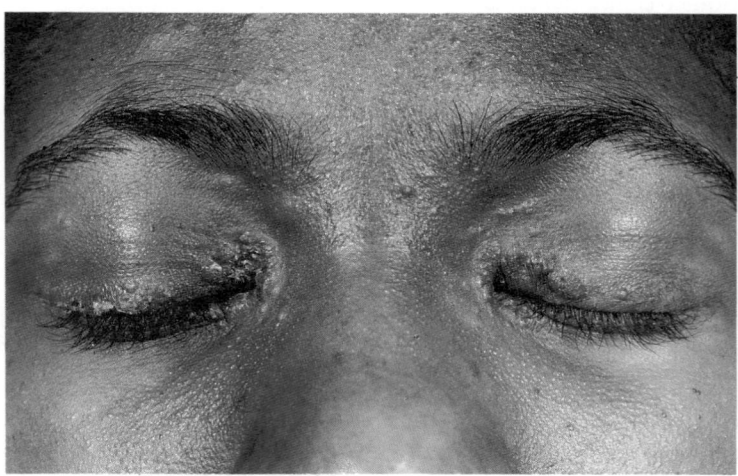

Fig. 20.16 Micropapular sarcoidosis affecting the eyelids.

Differential diagnosis of facial lesions includes leprosy and tuberculosis. Blue nodular lesions should be differentiated from lymphomas.

TREATMENT

Most cutaneous forms of sarcoidosis will improve with increasing doses of systemic steroids. Drugs such as methotrexate or chloroquine may help in reducing the dose of steroid required. Intralesional steroids can aid resolution on occasions. Lesions may often recur on withdrawal of drugs.

METABOLIC DISEASE

Diabetes mellitus (see p. 856)

Cutaneous abnormalities occur in more than 25% of patients with diabetes mellitus. They may be non-specific, such as infection with candidiasis, or so distinctive that the dermatologist may be able to predict the diagnosis of diabetes mellitus.

Secondary causes of diabetes (see p. 834), e.g. haemochromatosis and liver disease, may in themselves have cutaneous manifestations and these features are described under the appropriate disease heading.

Necrobiosis lipoidica (diabeticorum)
The association of this condition with diabetes is unpredictable; 50% of such cutaneous changes occur in non-diabetic patients. Necrobiosis lipoidica is an unusual complication of diabetes and is not necessarily related to other vascular complications. Nevertheless, small-vessel damage is thought to be a central feature of the pathogenesis. There is partial necrosis of dermal collagen and connective tissue and a histiocytic cellular response. It is more common in females, and presents in young adults or early middle life.

The skin over the shins is the site principally involved and pigmentary changes may cause the casual observer to associate the eruption with venous incompetence. On close examination the features are characteristic; erythematous plaques are seen that gradually develop a brown waxy discoloration that is more evident when stretching the skin. The skin's blood vessels are prominent because of the associated atrophic changes in the dermis. Fibrosis and scarring from previous ulceration may also be seen (Fig. 20.17).

Treatment is with support bandaging. The use of an antiseptic powder or spray such as povidone-iodine is useful when the skin is broken. Non-adhesive dressings should be used. Low dose aspirin may help to improve the healing of such lesions.

Diabetic dermopathy
This is also a common finding on the shins of

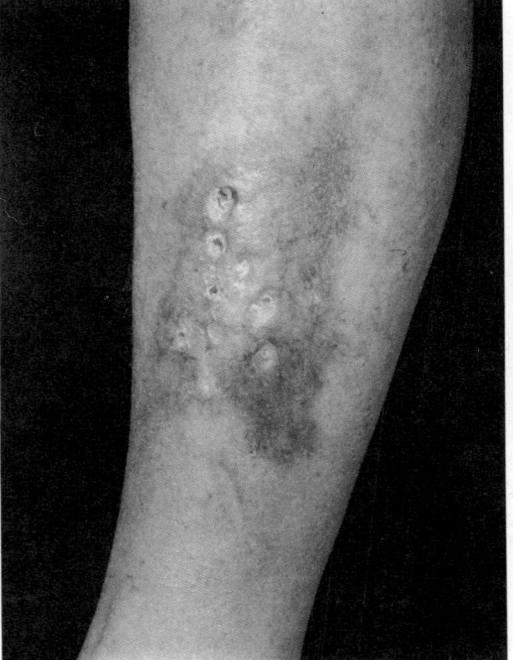

Fig. 20.17 Necrobiosis lipoidica.

diabetics. Initially the lesions are erythematous and papular but tend with time to become flat, hyperpigmented and atrophic. The changes are often seen in association with microangiopathy elsewhere. The pathogenesis of these lesions, which are not specific to diabetes mellitus, is unclear, although intimal thickening of small blood vessels has been demonstrated.

Diabetic stiff hands
This condition was first described in patients with juvenile-onset diabetes, but similar changes have been seen in middle-aged diabetics.

Tight, waxy skin principally affects the dorsum of the fingers and is associated with joint stiffness that can limit extensor movements of the small joints (cheiroarthropathy). Histological sections demonstrate thickening of dermal collagen.

Scleroedema
This condition is seen as a spreading erythema and induration of the skin that starts on the upper trunk of middle-aged diabetics. These changes are often heralded by a respiratory illness or by streptococcal infection. The lesion may become generalized over the trunk, limbs, hands and feet, although the genitalia tend to be spared. There is a spontaneous resolution with time.

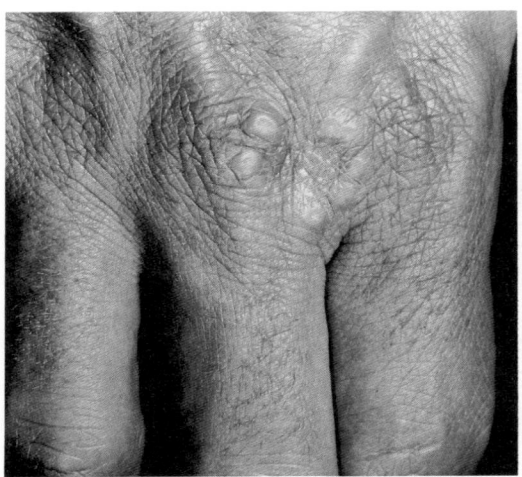

Fig. 20.18 Granuloma annulare.

Diabetic bullae

This is an unusual complication in which blisters develop on the feet and occasionally the hands. They are of an acute onset and occur without any obvious preceding trauma. The disease is sometimes associated with an extensive polyneuropathy. Histological section shows a cleft in the region of the lamina lucida but the cause is not known. Blisters clear in 2–5 weeks.

Granuloma annulare

This presents as flesh-coloured papules in annular or crescentic configurations, principally over the extensor surface of the joints of the fingers (Fig. 20.18). The feet, ankles, hands and wrists may be similarly affected. A disseminated pattern is probably triggered by sunlight but often involves covered areas of skin.

The association of such lesions with diabetes mellitus remains controversial; a few cases do not have overt diabetes but only impaired glucose tolerance. The pathology is similar to necrobiosis lipoidica and the two conditions may occur together.

Eruptive xanthomas

These may appear suddenly as crops of yellow papules on the knees, elbows, back and the buttocks. They are associated with hyperlipidaemia (see p. 862) and are particularly common in diabetics. They resolve with the control of the diabetes and hyperlipidaemia.

Other skin disorders

Infections and lipodystrophies are often seen in diabetes mellitus; they are discussed in Chapter 17.

Porphyria cutanea tarda (see p. 872)

Only the changes seen in porphyria cutanea tarda

are considered here. Similar changes in the skin may be seen with variegate porphyria and hereditary coproporphyria.

Cutaneous lesions occur on exposure to sunlight. These consist of increased fragility of the skin over the dorsum of the hands, fingers and face and are associated with erythema, blistering and scarring (Fig. 20.19). Hypertrichosis on the sides of the face and between the eyebrows and hair margin is common and may be associated with facial skin thickening and loss of hair (pseudoscleroderma). Hyperpigmentation or loss of pigment may also be seen on the facial skin. Itching may be troublesome.

The diagnosis and treatment are discussed on p. 871.

Cutaneous amyloidosis

Amyloidosis is discussed on p. 869.

Cutaneous forms of the disease may be widespread on the skin and mucosal surfaces or localized to particular areas. The skin is involved in about 40% of patients who have systemic amyloidosis in association with diseases such as myelomatosis.

The gums may appear nodular and waxy and bleed easily on trauma. Pale yellow-brown papules may appear over the basal conjunctivae and at other mucosal sites and purpura is seen following mild trauma.

Sites of predilection elsewhere on the skin include the eyelids, the nasolabial folds, the sides of the neck, and the flexural surfaces. Thickened indurated plaques may rarely affect the chest, abdomen or hands. Cutaneous changes are rare in the hereditofamilial patterns of disease.

Cutaneous disease where there is no evidence of systemic spread is seen in two forms: macular and lichen amyloidosis.

Macular amyloidosis

Macular amyloidosis is quite commonly seen on the shoulders, neck or upper back of patients of Asian origin. The hyperpigmented macular changes have a rippled appearance likened to the changes seen on a sandy beach at low tide. Patients are only concerned about the appearance of the lesions, which are dark grey/black in colour. The amyloid material is difficult to demonstrate on histology using routine methods.

Lichen amyloidosis

Lichen amyloidosis is an uncommon papular eruption that is often pruritic and occurs on the lower limbs. There is no explanation for the appearance of the amyloid material at this site. Other pruritic diseases on the lower legs are often hypertrophic, especially in patients of African or Asian origin. Diseases such as hypertrophic lichen

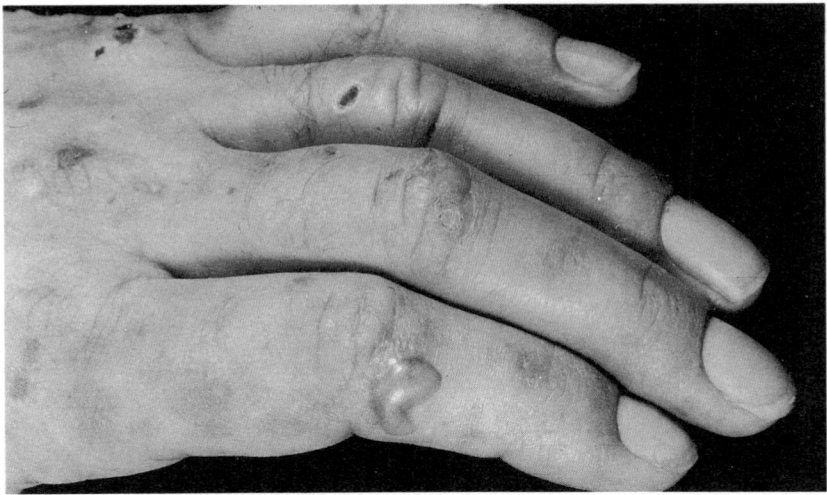

Fig. 20.19 Scarring and blister formation seen with porphyria cutanea tarda.

planus and lichen simplex may resemble the disease on superficial inspection. Close examination should, however, distinguish these diseases. The shiny warty close-set papules of lichen amyloidosis are characteristic of the disease.

CNS-RELATED DISEASES

The number of dermatoses that have been associated with diseases of the nervous system is large but most are extremely rare.

Neurofibromatosis (see p. 950)

The characteristic cutaneous features are hyperpigmentation (café-au-lait spots) and flesh-coloured smooth polypoid swellings, i.e. neurofibromas. Molluscum fibrosum (skin tags) are sessile pink-coloured tumours that are often numerous over the trunk. Plexiform neuromas are uncommon and tend to follow the course of a nerve, usually on the face or neck. In some areas there is overgrowth of skin and subcutaneous tissue in addition and this may give rise to gross disfigurement (elephantiasis neuromatosa). Oral lesions occur in up to 10% of patients.

Café-au-lait spots may suggest the diagnosis in children but there should be more than five in number to support it. The pigmentary changes must be differentiated from those seen in Albright's syndrome (see p. 781). In neurofibromatosis the café-au-lait spots show histologically the presence of giant melanosomes; these are rare in Albright's disease.

Tuberous sclerosis (epiloia) (see p. 951)

The cutaneous lesions in tuberous sclerosis are derived from connective tissue and are of several different types.

Adenoma sebaceum are erythematous papules or nodules on the cheeks or within the folds at the sides of the mouth or nose. The tumours are vascular and fibrous in origin. Periungual fibromas occur as pink, firm, claw-like tumours arising from and around the nail folds.

Shagreen patches are flesh-coloured tumours that are firm and plaque-like. They often have a wrinkled surface and are most frequently seen over the lumbosacral region.

Areas of macular hypopigmentation occur in ovoid or leaf-like shapes. They may be seen over the trunk or back and are most easily detected by examination by Wood's light. They appear early in childhood, associated in many cases with mental retardation.

Small erythematous papules on the face and cheeks may be treated with an electrical Hyfrecator or cautery.

Other CNS-related diseases

Naevoid lesions may be seen in conjunction with neurological disease; for example, in the epidermal naevus syndrome, pigmented naevi occur in a linear fashion on the limb or trunk and may be associated with epilepsy or mental retardation.

Gross ichthyotic changes may occur on the skin of patients with spastic diplegia and mental retardation in the Sjögren–Larsson syndrome.

MALIGNANT DISEASES

The skin can be involved by both primary and secondary tumours. Table 20.5 shows some cutaneous markers of malignant disease.

Table 20.5 Some cutaneous markers of malignant disease.

Acanthosis nigricans (p. 1047)

Erythema guratum repens
   concentric erythematous rings over whole body
   often carcinoma of the bronchus

Necrolytic migratory erythema—associated with a glucagonoma (p. 236)
Thrombophlebitis migrans—carcinoma of the pancreas
Dermatomyositis (p. 1033)
Peutz–Jegher syndrome (p. 233)
Gardner's syndrome (p. 234)
Erythroderma associated with T-cell lymphoma
Generalized pigmentation, e.g. Hodgkin's disease
Acquired icthyosis, e.g. lymphoma

Table 20.6 Causes of leg ulceration.

Venous insufficiency
Arterial insufficiency
Neuropathies, e.g. diabetic, leprosy, syphilis
Blood disorders, e.g. sickle cell disease, spherocytosis
Chronic infection, e.g. post-cellulitis
Pyoderma gangrenosum
Trauma or artefact

Vascular and lymphatic disorders

Cutaneous abnormalities are seen in many diseases of the arteries, veins and lymphatics. This section discusses skin ulceration and lymphoedema.

Venous ulcers

These are confined to the lower limbs and many are post-thrombotic. The increased hydrostatic pressure in the veins resulting from incompetent valves is reflected by increased capillary blood pressure. Leakage of plasma under pressure gives rise to perivascular fibrin deposition, impairing gaseous exchange across the vessel wall. Nutrition of the skin is then affected and leads to ischaemia and eventual ulceration. Ulcers around the ankle are often accompanied by:

- Hyperpigmentation following extravasation of red cells and haemosiderin deposition
- Dermatitis and excoriation due to pruritus
- White atrophy ('atrophie blanche') caused by hyalinization of skin vessels producing scars in the overlying skin
- Secondary infection with possible cellulitis or thrombophlebitis

The differential diagnosis of leg ulcers is shown in Table 20.6.

Arterial ulcers

Ulcers occurring in skin away from the ankle region are more commonly associated with arterial disease. This may accompany venous hypertension in the legs, especially in the elderly. Cold, atrophic skin with loss of hair, impalpable peripheral pulses with a history of claudication may suggest the diagnosis. The ulcers usually have a punched out appearance and are often very painful.

MANAGEMENT

- *General* management consists of reducing leg venous hypertension. This can be helped by wearing support bandages when standing or by elevation of the limbs when sitting or lying. Exercise should be encouraged and, if the patient is obese, weight reduction recommended.
- *Dermatitis* should be treated with bland non-steroidal applications such as zinc and salicylic acid paste. Impregnated bandages containing zinc and applied moist can dry out and stiffen to provide occlusion and support.
- *Ulcers* should be cleaned with normal saline or a weak potassium permanganate solution. A non-adhesive absorbent dressing should be applied with an elasticated bandage up to the knees. These dressings may be viscous materials, alginates, semipermeable films, hydrogels or hydrocolloids. These are expensive but covering the wound with a permeable membrane will diminish pain and encourage re-epithelialization. Clean granulating ulcers should have non-adherent dressings applied and left undisturbed for increasing periods as the ulcer heals. A debriding agent (e.g. hydrophilic polysaccharide beads) or surgery may be necessary to remove dead tissue. Pinch grafting may also be necessary. The grafts are removed from the thigh and dotted over the ulcers and left undisturbed for 10 days.
- *Infection.* Local antibiotics should be avoided if possible. Pseudomonas aeruginosa infection accompanies non-permeable occlusive bandages. Systemic antibiotics may be required for cellulitis.
- *Follow-up* care and preventative measures are

most important and elastic stockings may always be necessary.

- *Varicose veins.* Treatment may be necessary.

Pressure sores (decubitus ulcers)

These occur in elderly, immobile, unconscious or paralysed patients. They are due to skin ischaemia from sustained pressure over a bony point. Normal individuals feel the pain of continued pressure and even during sleep movement takes place to change position continually. General medical conditions such as protein–energy malnutrition and anaemia predispose to ulceration. The management consists of:

- Prevention with care of pressure areas.
- Treatment of general condition.
- Special mattresses and beds to relieve pressure areas.
- Topical treatment—keep ulcer clean and moist. (Many topical therapies are harmful.)
- Plastic surgery.

Lymphoedema

This is oedema due to lymphatic obstruction. The affected area is swollen and initially there is pitting. In chronic lymphoedema the skin becomes thickened and the oedema is permanent. Localized lymphoedema occurs transiently with any skin infection. The causes of chronic lymphoedema in the Western hemisphere include recurrent cellulitis, malignant disease due to infiltration or following treatment with surgery or radiotherapy, or recurrent cellulitis, or it can be familial with abnormal lymphatics. In the tropics, filariasis is a common cause. There are a number of rare congenital causes with abnormalities of the lymphatic vessels, such as the yellow-nail syndrome (see p. 1051).

Drug eruptions

Cutaneous eruptions account for one-third of all side-effects of drugs. It is sometimes difficult to differentiate an eruption due to a drug from one produced by the underlying illness. On occasions the effects of both are relevant to the onset of the rash, for example patients prescribed ampicillin for infectious mononucleosis will almost always develop a widespread morbilliform rash.

Patients often take many drugs together and it may be difficult to incriminate one agent in the production of the rash. *In vitro* testing of drugs in these situations is inadequate in establishing or predicting the likelihood of the drug causing the cutaneous side-effect.

The drugs mentioned below are only examples. If there is doubt about an eruption, the most likely drug to produce this should be stopped.

Urticaria (see p. 1013)

Urticaria may be associated with a type I IgE reaction and anaphylaxis in patients who are hypersensitive, for example, to penicillin. Urticaria can also occur in the serum sickness syndrome, IgG immune complex-mediated reactions occuring 1–2 weeks after drugs or serum, or lastly, by direct release of histamine. The latter include:

- Codeine, opiates and tubocurarine.
- Radiological contrast media.
- Aspirin and non-steroidal anti-inflammatory drugs, e.g. indomethacin may trigger blood vessel hyper-reactivity by affecting the production of arachidonic acid metabolites.

Allergic vasculitis and purpura

Drugs that produce vasculitis may activate the alternative pathway of complement or produce cryoglobulins and immune complexes in the serum. Antibody, principally IgA, may be deposited around damaged vessels in the kidney and skin. Purpuric lesions appear most frequently on the extremities and may be accompanied by urticaria, blisters, necrosis of the skin and ulceration.

Drugs that have been associated with this disease include allopurinol, sulphonamides, gold, hydrallazine, quinidine and methyldopa.

Purpura may be seen following drug-induced thrombocytopenia (p. 339). Drugs may combine with the platelets to form an antigen; antibody formation follows, leading to platelet destruction.

Erythema nodosum and erythema multiforme

Erythema nodosum and erythema multiforme may be induced by drugs; these are considered on p. 1016.

Erythematous morbilliform eruptions

These maculopapular erythematous reactions are the commonest type of drug eruption. They usually occur a week after starting the medication and are widespread on the trunk and over pressure sites such as the thighs, knees and elbows. Diffuse erythema may be accompanied by pruritus and followed by desquamation. An accompanying fever may cause confusion with viral illnesses. Paired sera for viral antibodies may help to establish the correct diagnosis in retrospect.

All penicillins, sulphonamides, gold and gentamicin are agents most likely to induce this type of reaction.

Lichen planus-like or lichenoid eruptions. These are discussed on p. 1010.

Photosensitizing agents. These are discussed on p. 1048.

Toxic epidermal necrolysis

This is the most serious type of drug-induced disease. It can be distinguished on histological grounds from the condition seen in children, which produces a similar clinical picture and is induced by staphylococci (see p. 22). There is superficial peeling of all the skin. The agents most likely to cause such disease are sulphonamides, allopurinol and barbiturates.

Fixed drug eruption

The pathogenesis of this type of reaction is unknown. The face, hands and genitalia are most commonly affected. Bright red, sometimes purpuric or even blistered plaques or annular lesions are seen. An accompanying burning discomfort is present. The lesions are fixed in site and appear within hours of the offending drug's administration. They will occur at exactly the same sites if the drug is given again at another time. Post-inflammatory hyperpigmentation is a striking feature.

Phenolphthalein in laxatives or as a colouring in sweets is a common cause. Other agents include tetracycline, sulphonamides, phenacetin, salicylates, the oral contraceptive pill and chlordiazepoxide.

Pigmentation

Pigmentation that occurs with oral agents is considered below (see p. 1045).

Exacerbation of pre-existing skin diseases

Pre-existing skin diseases may be exacerbated by drugs. Examples include lithium carbonate and β-receptor antagonists, which will exacerbate psoriasis.

Lupus erythematosus-like rash

This can be produced by drugs such as hydralazine, procainamide, phenytoin, penicillamine and isoniazid. The lesions are often reversed on stopping the drug.

Acneiform eruptions

These are papulopustular eruptions but usually without comedones. The major drugs are corticosteroids, oral contraceptives, androgens, iodides, anticonvulsants, isoniazid.

Eczematous reactions can be caused by e.g. sulphonamides, sulphonylureas. Sensitization can be by topical application.

Nails and hair. See p. 1049.

Naevi and tumours

The skin is a prime target for aberrant growth and tumour formation. It may be in direct contact with ionizing radiation and many chemical substances or micro-organisms that may act as inducers of abnormal cellular activity. There are also a large number of different cell types represented within the skin.

Many skin tumours are rare and in practice are confined to a few types.

Melanocytic naevus (naevocytic naevus)

This is a tumour produced by cells of neural crest origin, mainly melanocytes. Schwann cells may also contribute to the dermal aspect of these lesions. This is the most common type of skin tumour. It is pigmented and is referred to as a 'mole' in lay terms.

These tumours originate as a proliferation of melanocytes at the epidermodermal junction, so that clinically little growth above the skin surface is seen at this stage (*junctional naevus*).

With time, cells migrate downwards into the dermis and their bulk increases so that tumours become elevated above the skin surface. Both an epidermal and dermal component are now seen (*compound naevus*). Gradually the epidermal component becomes less obvious and the tumour becomes a cellular naevus; fibrotic changes and a loss of pigment may then cause a lesion to become less evident or disappear.

Such lesions may be present in childhood but they appear more obvious and increase their numbers with puberty. Sun-sensitive individuals tend to produce greater numbers, particularly on exposed areas of skin. There is therefore a greater number over the lateral aspect of the arm compared with the medial side. Pregnancy will also increase the numbers of naevi and the degree of hyperpigmentation.

The average count of melanocytic naevi on a Caucasian from the Western hemisphere is more than a dozen by the third decade. Junctional naevi and malignant melanomas should be differentiated by size, the even degree of pigmentation, the smoothness of the overlying epidermis and lack of symptoms in the former.

Congenital melanocytic naevi are often bigger and may cover large areas of the skin e.g. as a bathing trunk naevus. These have an irregular surface and an uneven degree of pigmentation. There is an increased potential for malignant change with larger lesions.

Juvenile melanoma (Spitz naevus)
These naevi are solitary pink or reddish-brown lesions on the face or limbs of children. A history of rapid growth is given and for this reason they are often removed.

Dermal melanocytes
A proliferation of naevus cells in the dermis may give rise to blue discoloration of the skin. The *mongolian spot* in children represents a more diffuse spread of such cells. When these are localized to form a slightly elevated papule, especially in adults, they are called a *'blue naevus'*.

Basal cell papilloma (seborrhoeic wart)

This is a benign proliferation of basal cells that produces a raised lesion with a varying degree of pigmentation. The number of these tumours increases with age. The consistency is often greasy and this aspect has led to the misnomer 'seborrhoeic wart'—the lesions are *not* related to sebaceous tissue growth. 'Senile wart' is another unacceptable term because the lesions may be seen in young adults.

The face and trunk are the sites most commonly affected. Marked hyperpigmentation may cause confusion with malignant melanoma. Maceration of these tumours from sweating may, in summertime, lead to irritation. The numbers present on the trunk may prohibit their removal in some patients, but readily traumatized or irritant lesions can be removed with a curette and the base cauterized, or they may be frozen with liquid nitrogen.

Keratoacanthoma

This rapidly growing tumour of the epidermis arises most commonly on the skin of the hand and face. The aetiology is unknown; it is possible that trauma initiates the event and viral DNA has been shown in these tumours. There is often evidence of chronic actinic damage of the surrounding skin (Fig. 20.20).

The lesions are often pale or flesh-coloured, well-demarcated papules and on occasions appear inflammatory. Usually 0.5–1 cm in diameter, they may reach 3–4 cm across in giant lesions. The increase in size is rapid and often alarming to the patient. The greatest diameter is attained in 4–8 weeks; involution then occurs and the centre becomes a keratinous crater. Regression may then become complete over several months but, since a ragged scar may be left, it is often better to remove the tumour by curettage. Histological sections may reveal changes that are difficult to differentiate from a squamous carcinoma.

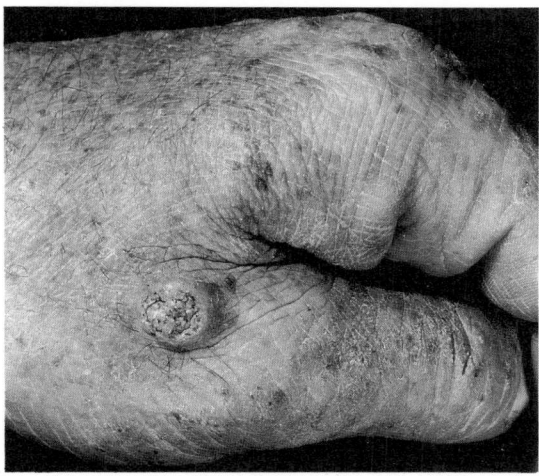

Fig. 20.20 Keratoacanthoma occurring on chronically sun-damaged skin.

Haemangiomas

Capillary naevus (naevus flammeus)
This is associated with a proliferation of capillaries in the superficial dermal capillary plexus. The salmon-coloured patch may be seen on the face or more commonly on the nape of the neck in up to 40% of infants. They may not fade from the latter site and are often covered by hair. Facial lesions occur on the glabella, forehead and eyelids and tend to fade away in the first year of life.

Port-wine stain
This is a tumour present at birth that consists of dilated capillary vessels with endothelial cell lining. The face and neck are most commonly affected and there is no natural regression with age. Those patients who experience such growths around the orbit may have in addition a proliferation of vessels on the meninges (Sturge–Weber syndrome) and neurological defects.

Camouflage is the only practical method of managing such lesions. Laser therapy is time-consuming, is only available at a few centres, and the best results appear to follow the treatment of such naevi in adults.

Cavernous haemangioma (strawberry naevus)
This tumour is not present at birth, but usually appears in the first month of life. Lesions are often well-circumscribed, round and lobulated and are usually seen on the face, neck or trunk. Growth continues in the first year in many patients; this is followed by slow involution, which is complete in the majority by 4–5 years, so that reassurance is often all that is required. Gross lesions warrant attempts at treatment when, for example, they obstruct the eye and threaten the development of

binocular vision. The bulk of such tumours may be reduced by systemic steroids or sclerosants. Some naevi show features of both capillary and cavernous tissue within a single tumour.

Cherry angioma (Campbell de Morgan's spot)
Campbell de Morgan's spots are angiokeratomas that appear as pinpoint lesions or naevi of several millimetres in diameter on the trunk or limbs with an increasing frequency throughout middle-age. Treatment is only required for cosmetic reasons; cautery or diathermy is effective.

Granuloma telangiectaticum

This tumour is a proliferation of dermal vasculature, so that the previous term pyogenic granuloma is a misnomer. Often trauma will initiate this growth on the finger or elsewhere on the skin. In children the trunk is a common site of involvement and there is a tendency for recurrence here from a deep-feeding vascular channel. Bleeding after trauma is a troublesome and worrying feature for some patients and older lesions may become fibrotic. Treatment is by curettage and cautery.

Epidermal naevus

This may appear as a single lesion unassociated with any other developmental abnormality or may occur together with, for example, neurological defects as part of a syndrome. Histologically, there is a proliferation of epidermal structures that are often mixed, so that verrucous, sebaceous, apocrine, eccrine or follicular changes may all occur. The predominant component will determine the clinical appearances. Some types of naevi may undergo malignant transformation, though this is not common.

Sebaceous naevi appear most frequently on the scalp as flesh-coloured, leaf-shaped tumours, which may with time undergo malignant transformation to form basal-cell carcinomata.

Histiocytoma (dermatofibroma)

This tumour is composed of blood vessels, histiocytes or dense fibrous tissue, according to the age of the tumour. It usually arises from trauma such as insect bites and is a common tumour on the legs or buttocks of adults, especially females. A firm tender papule develops, forming a button-like tumour on the surface of which the overlying skin can be wrinkled. The brown pigment or rapid growth may cause alarm and confusion with melanoma.

MALIGNANT TUMOURS

There is public concern about the increased numbers of malignant tumours of the skin and their association with sun exposure. The malignant transformation of pre-existing naevi or chronic inflammatory lesions on the skin are less common events.

Basal-cell carcinoma (rodent ulcer)

This is the most common cancer of the skin and is frequently seen on the face of middle-aged or elderly people in the UK, especially those with fair hair and blue eyes who are sun-sensitive and often of Celtic origin. Such tumours are seen at a younger age in those living nearer to the equator, but the reasons why tumours appear with such frequency on sites such as the periorbital skin, which is to some degree protected from sunlight, is not clear.

Other types of ionizing radiation such as X-rays, for example given to young adults for ankylosing spondylitis, have in the past produced sufficient stimulus for the development of basal-cell carcinomata at the irradiated site after a prolonged interval of 10–20 years. Arsenicals have only recently been abandoned as oral medication and may also cause cutaneous malignancy after a similar induction time.

CLINICAL FEATURES

Lesions are most commonly seen at the sides of the nose and around the orbit as flesh-coloured translucent papules or plaques with superficial dilated blood vessels coursing over the surface; central necrosis with ulceration or crusting is frequent (Fig. 20.21). Scarring or cystic or pigmented lesions are less common. There is a tendency for basal-cell

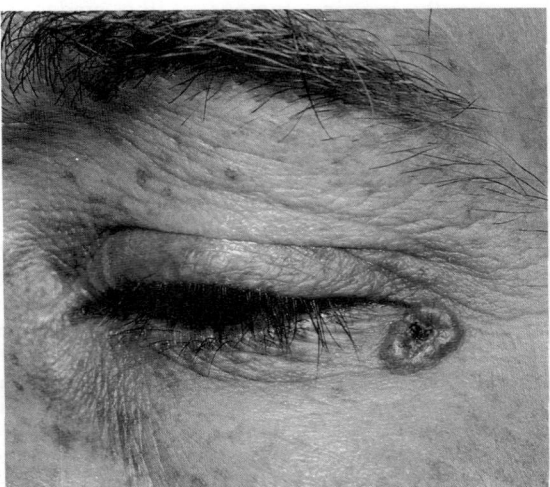

Fig. 20.21 Basal-cell carcinoma.

carcinomas to be locally invasive but metastasis is extremely rare.

Basal cell carcinomata and lesions appearing as small brown pigmented papules, which are often numerous, are seen in the basal cell naevus syndrome.

Superficial scarring or morphoeic basal cell carcinomas are more difficult to discern at their margins from normal skin; although uncommon they are important as they tend to follow tissue planes and invade an orifice such as the orbit. Treatment with X-rays is less effective for such tumours.

TREATMENT

Tumours are normally removed surgically or treated with cryotherapy or radiotherapy. However, lesions that become invasive or are less accessible to normal treatments may be removed by chemosurgery. In Mohs' method the tissue is fixed *in situ* and excised in a systematic fashion and examined immediately under a microscope to determine the presence or absence of tumour.

Squamous carcinoma

This invasive tumour with the ability to metastasize arises from the epidermis (keratinocytes) or skin appendages. It is most commonly seen on previously damaged or chronically irritated skin. It has also been associated with certain occupations (e.g. chemical carcinogens inducing cancer of the scrotum) or with certain social customs (e.g. tumours on the legs from radiant heat from fires). Albinism and xeroderma pigmentosum may produce severe actinic damage to the skin and frank malignancy at an early age. Viral disease may predispose to squamous carcinoma and the human papilloma virus may be isolated from the skin of patients with epidermodysplasia verruciformis.

CLINICAL FEATURES

Tumours are hyperkeratotic and crusted and are usually seen over sun-damaged skin, e.g. on the pinna. Induration of the tissue provides a further clue to the diagnosis. Ulceration may occur if the lesion is on sites such as the lips or genitalia. Papilliferous and more friable tumours may appear on relatively normal skin.

TREATMENT

Treatment is usually by excision. Tumours on the head and neck may also be treated by radiotherapy. Superficial lesions may be treated with cryosurgery.

Malignant melanoma

This tumour, formed by epidermal melanocytes, is rising in incidence throughout the world. This increase has been seen particularly in light-skinned people. The latitude and length of residence of these people in places such as Australia suggest that ultraviolet light exposure is important. An increase in tumours on skin that has not until recent years been commonly exposed, such as the legs of females, also indicates that chronic sun exposure is a significant factor.

Inheritance is also important in the dysplastic naevus syndrome, when large multiple and atypical naevi on the trunk show a familial trait and patients may develop multiple primary melanomas.

Malignant change is recognized in pre-existing naevi, especially pigmented naevi, that cover a large surface of the skin, e.g. bathing trunk naevi, and in lentigo maligna.

Lentigo maligna

Lentigo maligna represents an increased number of melanocytes at the epidermodermal junction. It begins as a flat freckle-like lesion, which in time changes colour and pattern as it grows. It occurs on the facial or sun-exposed skin of patients in their fifties or older. It is a precursor of malignant melanoma.

Malignant change in a mole should be suspected with a change in size, outline, colour, surface or elevation. Symptoms that include itching, bleeding after minor trauma or an increasing awareness of the tumour should also arouse suspicion.

The prognosis is directly related to the thickness of the tumour assessed at histological examination; patients with a tumour less than 1 mm thick have a 5-year survival rate of more than 90% but for tumours greater than 3.5 mm thick the 5-year survival rate is less than 50%.

The prognosis is also related to site; patients with a tumour on the trunk fair better than those with facial lesions, but melanomas on the trunk have a worse prognosis than those on the limbs. The depth of invasion of skin and local cellular reactions on histological section also indicate the prognosis.

TREATMENT

Excision is performed according to the depth of invasion with a wide excision of deeper invasive lesions followed by skin grafting. Deeply invasive lesions on a limb may be further treated by isolation and arterial perfusion with cytotoxic agents such as mustine hydrochloride. Radiotherapy, chemotherapy and immunotherapy have not yet been shown to materially alter the outlook for those with disseminated disease.

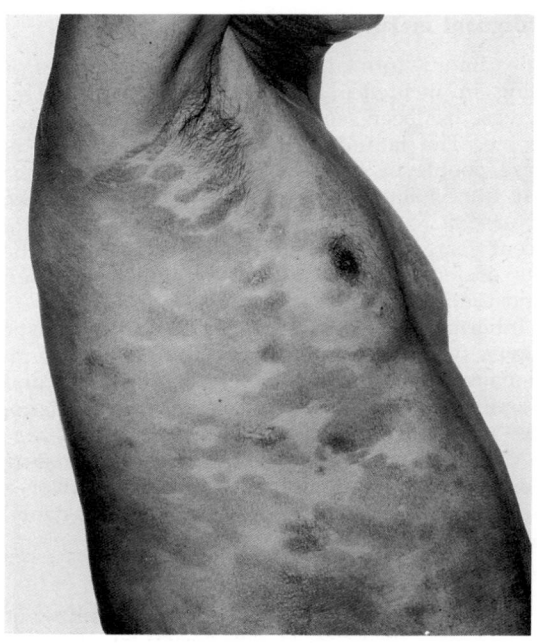

Fig. 20.22 Figurate erythema and plaque formation seen with mycosis fungoides.

Mycosis fungoides

This is a lymphomatous invasion of the skin by T lymphocytes (see p. 369) that may eventually form cutaneous tumours. In the final stages of the disease there is spread to lymph nodes and other organs. The name implies mushroom-like growths on the skin but these are a rare and often a terminal event.

In the Sézary syndrome the area of skin infiltration is greater. Both of these conditions are classified as a T-cell lymphoma.

CLINICAL FEATURES

The most common presentation of patients seen in the UK is with a pattern of scaling and erythema that may remain confined over areas such as on the buttocks, thighs or trunk as rather fixed patches for many years. Tumours may then develop initially as plaques (Fig. 20.22) and then as ulcerating nodules or masses; dissemination follows with visceral spread and death. With an onset in middle life or old age, patients will often die from other causes. Presentation with advanced disease and spread to local lymph nodes is uncommon in the UK but has been described more frequently in the USA.

TREATMENT

Topical mustine hydrochloride or PUVA (psoralens and ultraviolet A) or electron beam therapy may control widespread disease and plaque forms of the disease. The combination of prednisolone and chlorambucil may limit the spread of more advanced disease, but dissemination to the viscera is associated with the terminal phase of the disease. Multiple chemotherapeutic regimens are disappointing in their effect.

Metastases to any part of the skin can occur from many primary carcinoma sites including breast, stomach, lung and kidney.

Kaposi's sarcoma

Kaposi's sarcoma is a vascular, multifocal, malignant tumour. It is seen in:

- Patients with AIDS. The incidence is higher in homosexuals than in haemophiliacs.
- Immunosuppressed patients secondarily to chemotherapy.
- Elderly males of Jewish or Mediterranean origin (classic form).
- Africans: several forms are seen, viz. classical, locally aggressive or lymphadenopathic.

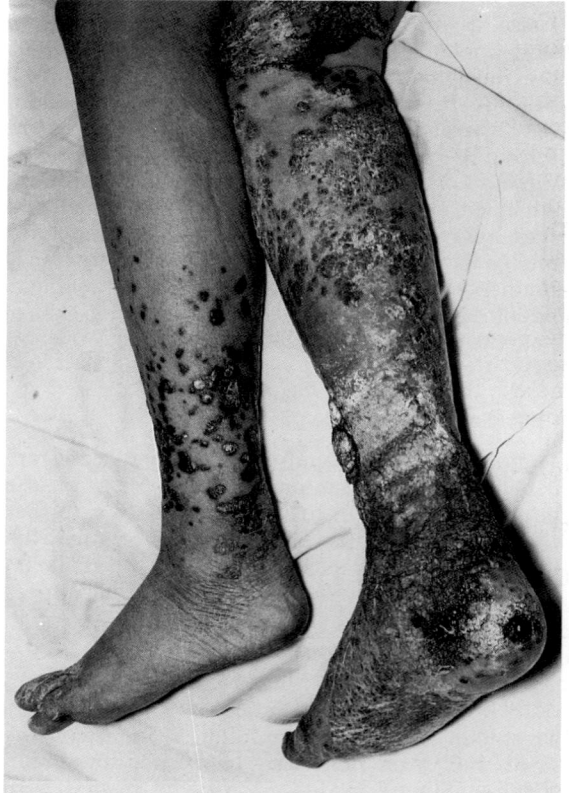

Fig. 20.23 Kaposi's sarcoma.

CLINICAL FEATURES

The initial lesion appears as a bruise that gradually darkens and becomes raised as a firm nodule (Fig. 20.23). Lesions are not usually painful or itchy initially and can develop at several sites all over the body.

Gastrointestinal lesions (approximately 40% of cases) are usually asymptomatic but later liver and lymph node involvement occur.

PROGNOSIS AND TREATMENT

The classic and African endemic varieties run an indolent course and are much less aggressive than that associated with AIDS. Lesions may progress rapidly, enlarge slowly over years or even regress. Treatment is with radiotherapy or chemotherapy. In AIDS a third of the patients may show a response but relapse later; prognosis is poor. The prognosis is good in the other forms and in those on immunosuppressive drugs the lesions may regress on stopping therapy.

Disorders of pigmentation

There are many factors that alter the hue of a normal skin. The principal pigments are melanin and haemoglobin or its breakdown products. Carotene, if taken in large amounts in the diet, is concentrated in subcutaneous fat and in keratin, giving a yellow coloration to the skin. The skin can also change its colour by deposition of abnormal substances or by alteration of melanogenesis. These substances include drugs, bilirubin, haemosiderin, heavy metals and the deposition of metal salts, dyes and inks in tattooing. In practice, patients are most concerned with alterations in the degree of melanin pigmentation. This is especially so in those races who have a greater deposition of melanin in their skin as a normal characteristic. Alteration in the degree of pigmentation in those with pigmented skins may be striking and give rise to much personal and social stress.

HYPOPIGMENTATION

Generalized hypopigmentation (albinism)

Albinism is inherited as an autosomal recessive disorder of melanin synthesis. This disorder produces a milky white skin, white hair, blue eyes and photophobia. There are different types, but in the commoner types there is a defect or inhibition of tyrosinase biosynthesis. In phenylketonuria (see p. 867) there is a failure to convert phenylalanine to tyrosine and hypopigmentation of the skin, hair and eyes occurs.

Localized hypopigmentation

Localized absence of melanocytes is seen in vitiligo. In post-inflammatory hypopigmentation some melanocytes are seen but these have reduced activity. In pityriasis versicolor the lipophilic yeast *Pityrosporon orbiculare* produces substances that have an inhibiting effect on melanocytes. This condition can be treated with itraconazole.

Industrial processes may expose the skin and melanocytes to substances, such as phenols, that are also toxic to the pigment-producing cells.

Vitiligo

This is a common skin disease affecting approximately 1% of the population. It has a familial incidence. Melanocytes are lost from affected areas of skin. The reason is unclear but hypotheses include the following:

- There may be autodestruction of melanocytes by the products of melanin synthesis.
- There may be autoimmune damage to melanocytes. Antigens have been detected on the surface of melanocytes and antimelanocyte antibodies have been detected in the sera of some patients. There is also an association of vitiligo with other diseases that demonstrate organ-specific antibody production, such as diabetes mellitus, thyroiditis and pernicious anaemia.
- Neurogenic dysfunction has been invoked as an important factor in the production of rare naevoid patterns of the disease that tends to affect the limbs.

CLINICAL FEATURES

More than half the patients notice a loss of pigment before the age of 20 years. Areas of pigment loss are usually symmetrical and often annular in outline, though other shapes and patterns may be evident. These areas tend to enlarge peripherally and present a convex edge to the normal pigmented skin. The initial areas of involvement often include the fingers, hands, face and genitalia. These regularly traumatized areas of skin may show evidence of the Koebner phenomenon (see p. 1007) when the disease is in an active phase.

TREATMENT

This is unsatisfactory. Traditional therapy in places such as the Middle East includes the use of psoralens obtained from plant sources and applied topically or taken in tablet form. These substances enter into the skin and are then activated by sunlight. PUVA therapy used in the treatment of psoriasis is derived from these observations. Many treatments with PUVA therapy are required for vitiligo and there is concern over the long-term effects of the continuing use of high-intensity ultraviolet light for long periods, especially in younger patients. Potent topical corticosteroids, probably through their action as anti-inflammatory agents, may induce repigmentation when applied to new lesions of vitiligo and a trial over a limited area of skin for a period of 6–8 weeks is warranted. There may be spontaneous recovery, especially in children.

Post-inflammatory hypopigmentation

This may follow trauma to the skin from chemicals or physical agents or following inflammatory skin diseases. It is a noticeable feature in some patients with eczema. Mild hypopigmentation on the cheeks of children may be associated with scaling and erythema. Inflammatory changes are usually more evident in winter-time and are associated with conditions of low humidity and drying winds.

The tanning of surrounding skin in summer will often make the eruption appear more striking, especially in dark-skinned children (pityriasis alba). Pityriasis versicolor may also tend to present in the summer for similar reasons.

TREATMENT

The intensity of local inflammatory changes will be reduced with topical corticosteroids. Soap substitutes and emollients should be used when dryness of the skin is evident.

HYPERPIGMENTATION

Hyperpigmentation is most commonly seen following sun exposure but may also follow inflammatory changes in the skin. It is often much more evident in those races whose skins are already heavily pigmented.

Epidermal naevi may contain an increased number of melanocytes and be pigmented. Melanin deposited in the dermis will often produce a blue discoloration of the skin, which is seen in the following:

- Mongolian blue spot on the backs of children, more especially those of Asian origin
- Naevus of Ito (on the neck)
- Naevus of Ota (on the face)
- Blue naevus

Brown-coloured naevoid lesions

In *neurofibromatosis*, café-au-lait patches and axillary freckling are seen.

Albright's syndrome (see p. 781) produces extensive light brown discoloration of the skin over the trunk, buttocks and thighs that is often asymmetrical and affects children of pre-school age.

Xeroderma pigmentosum is associated with a freckling type of hyperpigmentation on the face or other sun-exposed sites. In those patients with severe disease it is associated with solar damage and cutaneous malignancy, which may be evident early in childhood.

Freckling on the skin of fair-skinned and otherwise normal persons increases with the length of sun exposure. Histological sections appropriately stained demonstrate an increase in the size and shape of melanosomes within the melanocyte.

Lentigines

These are circumscribed dark brown macules that are less than 0.5 cm in diameter. There is a localized increase in the number of melanocytes seen on light microscopy and the degree of pigmentation is often much more intense clinically than that seen with freckles. A generalized distribution of lentigines may be seen as part of a syndrome that includes cardiac defects (*Leopard* or *Moynahan's syndrome*). In the *Peutz–Jegher syndrome* (orofacial lentiginosis) (see p. 233) lesions are localized to the face and hands and there is an association with intestinal polyposis.

Generalized hypermelanosis

Liver disease
In haemochromatosis there is a grey/black component to the hyperpigmentation that is more evident in sun-exposed areas of skin. Hypermelanosis may also be pronounced in patients with primary biliary cirrhosis.

Endocrine disease
In *Addison's disease* pigmentation may be diffuse but it is often much more pronounced on sun-exposed or traumatized skin, e.g. beneath bra straps or over the buccal mucosa in the mouth. Both ACTH and melanocyte-stimulating hormone (MSH) are increased but it is uncertain which plays the dominant role in producing the pigmentation. *Hyperthyroidism* may rarely produce a similar pattern of hyperpigmentation.

Acromegaly, Cushing's syndrome and ACTH therapy may also be associated with pigmentation that may be particularly pronounced in patients with sella turcica enlargement following adrenalectomy (Nelson's syndrome), when multiple lentigines and oral hyperpigmentation are also seen.

Pregnancy and the oral contraceptive pill may both produce an increase in pigmentation on the neck,

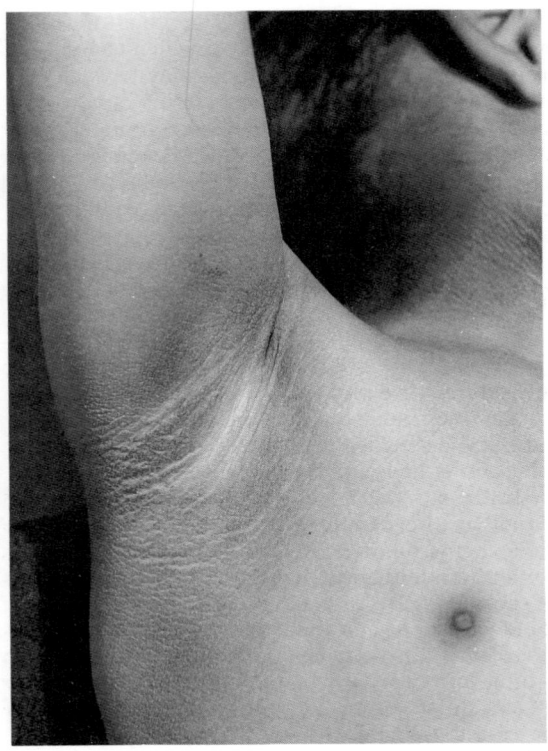

Fig. 20.24 Acanthosis nigricans.

the areolae of the breasts, over the abdominal skin and genitalia. Involvement of the face (melasma) may cause the patient to seek medical advice.

Neoplastic disease and cachexia can produce a general darkening of the skin colour; more marked changes occur with ectopic ACTH production.

Other diseases
Acanthosis nigricans is most commonly seen as localized hyperpigmentation of the neck, axillae (Fig. 20.24), groins or facial skin, but the changes may be generalized and profound. Velvety overgrowth of the skin at the flexures may be accompanied by filiform growths around the face, mouth or over the tongue, and by a curious roughness of the palmar or plantar skin (tripe palms). These changes are seen in middle-aged patients with visceral malignancies such as carcinoma of the stomach, but other types of neoplasia such as lymphomas have also been reported in association with these typical cutaneous features. Acanthosis nigricans can, however, occur without an underlying malignancy, with obesity in juveniles and together with endocrine diseases.

Renal failure is associated with hypermelanosis and an increase in MSH-like reactive hormone produc-

tion is seen in some patients. A yellow/brown, widespread coloration of the skin often occurs; scaling and irritation may also be seen. The relief of itching is difficult to achieve in such patients.

Systemic sclerosis may produce localized pigmentary changes in sites such as the nape of the neck or over the shoulder girdle, but hyperpigmentation may be profound and generalized in some patients. Thickening of the skin is usually present and should offer a clue as to the primary diagnosis.

Chemical deposition in the skin may occur as an occupational hazard, e.g. in those who process silver (argyria).

Mercurials may produce hypermelanosis, and gold when injected or taken by mouth may cause blue/black pigmentation, most evident on sun-exposed sites (chrysiasis).

The iron-containing pigment *haemosiderin* may also stimulate localized melanin production. This occurs on sites such as the legs of patients with varicose eczema following the loss of red cells into the skin. Mucocutaneous discoloration may also be seen with chronic lead poisoning.

Drugs
Mepacrine imparts a yellow colour to the skin but the sclera are spared. Chloroquine and chlorpromazine may produce bluish/grey coloration of the skin, especially in areas exposed to the sun. Arsenicals ingested over a long interval cause macular hyperpigmentation together with areas of hypopigmentation (rain-drop appearance).

Sunlight and the skin

The effects of ultraviolet light on the skin may be beneficial or damaging. The formation of vitamin D from sterol precursors in the skin is dependent on sunlight, and ultraviolet light exposure may be used with benefit in the treatment of chronic skin conditions such as acne, eczema and psoriasis.

Damaging effects, however, occur with chronic irradiation, giving rise to changes in connective tissues that produce ageing, wrinkling, altered texture, dryness and changes in skin pigmentation. Epidermal changes include hyperkeratosis, dysplasia and malignancy.

PHOTODERMATOSES

These can be divided into:

- Eruptions in which sunlight has a primary role
- Diseases in which sunlight is a trigger or an exacerbating factor

Primary photosensitivity

Polymorphic light eruption
The term 'polymorphic' refers to the difference in the morphology of the eruption between one patient and another. The lesions tend, however, to be monomorphic in any one individual.

Lesions are usually papulovesicular. Eczema, urticarial plaques or purpuric changes are less common. The rash is seen after a few hours of sun exposure and is most common on the chest and arms, the backs of the hands or lower legs. The eruption usually occurs in spring and early summer and improves as summer progresses and the skin 'hardens'. Fair-skinned individuals are most commonly affected by intense sunlight but those who have previously tanned easily and are of a darker complexion can also be affected. The papules may be associated with weeping and intense pruritus lasting for 5–10 days. The reaction can most readily be produced in the clinic or laboratory using high-intensity ultraviolet light at a wavelength of 320–420 nm.

Pre-treatment during spring-time with 12–18 treatments of PUVA may prevent the disease. Hydroxychloroquine given in doses of 400 mg daily for 2–3 weeks before and during sun exposure may prevent attacks. Topical corticosteroids such as betamethasone and high-factor sun-blocking creams (factors 15–18) also help to minimize the disease.

Hutchinson's summer prurigo
This rare disease usually has its onset before puberty. It affects both exposed and unexposed skin and may last throughout the year. Lesions are often excoriated and the necrotic papules may be quite disfiguring. The wavelengths responsible are usually in the sunburn range (290–320 nm). Sunscreen creams should be used but these do not offer sufficient protection in most cases. β-Carotene given by mouth may help a few patients.

Actinic reticuloid (chronic actinic dermatitis)
This is a rare condition affecting older men in which the gross thickening, coloration and texture of exposed skin may resemble lymphomatous infiltration, both clinically and on microscopy. Many patients have had eczema previously and a significant proportion of these patients also have a positive patch test to materials such as rubber or plants.

Clinical features include eczematous and purpuric lesions on non-exposed skin such as the legs, arms and trunk. Light sensitivity may be such that during active phases of the disease the only respite for patients is found in a darkened room. Protective clothing, sun-barrier creams, systemic steroid therapy, azathioprine, cytotoxic drugs and hydroxychloroquine may be required in combination to produce improvement.

Secondary photosensitivity

Topical agents
The application of perfumes (e.g. those containing bergaptine), sulphonamides and antimicrobial agents (e.g. halogenated salicylanilide) may produce photosensitive reactions. The latter group of compounds have largely been withdrawn.

Plant extracts such as psoralens commonly found in the family Umbelliferae are used in photochemotherapy (PUVA therapy). However, phytophotodermatitis may occur when the leaves of such plants (e.g. giant hogweed, wild parsley) abrade the skin surface. Psoralen compounds are absorbed into the skin and then activated by natural long-wavelength ultraviolet radiation. The linear configuration of the lesions should provide the clue to diagnosis.

Systemic agents
Systemic agents associated with photosensitivity include tetracyclines (chiefly chlortetracycline), thiazides, frusemide, phenothiazines and retinoids.

Disease states
Sunlight can exacerbate systemic lupus erythematosus. Antibodies produced against DNA denatured by ultraviolet light form immune complexes in the skin and other organs.

In porphyria, porphyrins deposited in the skin are activated by ultraviolet light.

Diseases of collagen and elastic tissue

The skin contains collagen types I, III and V within the dermis, type IV in the basement membrane, type VII in the anchoring fibrils and type VIII in the endothelium. Abnormalities of these can give rise to various skin disorders.

Ehlers–Danlos syndrome

This is a heterogeneous group of diseases in which at least nine different varieties have been described. Hyperextensibility, fragility and bruising of the skin occurs to a varying degree with each of the diseases and it is accompanied by the hypermobility of joints. Fragility of blood vessels occurs, and rarely aortic rupture.

The patterns of inheritance are varied and can be autosomal recessive, autosomal dominant or X-linked recessive.

The skin is velvety to the touch and hyperextensible but recoils normally on stretching. Trauma or laceration of the skin can lead to tissue-paper scars and poor wound healing. Pseudo-tumours may occur over the elbows and knees; they consist principally of fat, but may show signs of calcification.

Solar elastosis

Degradation of elastic fibrils in the skin normally occurs with ageing. This usually begins in early adult life but changes are more noticeable in the sixties and seventies. The clinical features are characterized by yellowish papules or plaques and wrinkling and are usually associated with pigmentation and keratoses on exposed skin.

Cutis laxa (generalized elastolysis)

This is a rare disease in which there are a number of variants. These are inherited as autosomal recessive, X-linked recessive or dominant traits. A defect in the cross-linking of elastin is suggested, but other abnormalities, including copper deficiency, have been reported. The subsequent changes in the skin, sometimes gross, may be evident at birth or arise at the time of puberty. The disfiguring changes may be severe with extreme laxity of the facial skin and massive folds over the trunk that have no recoil on stretching. Joint hypermobility is not a common feature.

Pseudoxanthoma elasticum

This is a generalized disorder of elastic tissue. The pathogenesis is unknown, and both autosomal dominant and recessive modes of transmission are seen. The skin, eyes and vascular structures are involved.

Cutaneous features are seen in childhood and are most evident over flexural surfaces and at the sides of the neck. Initially there is an accentuation of skin lines or folds and this is followed by thickening around yellowish diamond-shaped papules, producing a peau d'orange or plucked-chicken appearance. The skin may be lax and hang in folds. The skin demonstrates very little elastic recoil on stretching. The mucous membranes may also be affected. Long-term and high-dose treatment with D-penicillamine produces similar cutaneous features.

Widespread vascular changes are associated with fibrous proliferation and the deposition of calcium in the media of the arteries. Intermittent claudication and angina pectoris occur at an early age as a result. Gastrointestinal bleeding may be a troublesome feature. Splits in Bruch's membrane, which contains both elastin and collagen and separates the choroid from the retina, are demonstrated as angioid streaks on ophthalmoscopy.

Marfan's syndrome

A biochemical defect for this disease has not been identified, and some features of the condition may be seen in association with the Ehlers–Danlos syndrome or with homocystinuria. Inheritance is usually in an autosomal dominant manner.

Striae distensae are the only common dermatological sign, and the most impressive changes affect the skeleton. The facial appearance of affected patients may be distinctive, with elongation and asymmetry. A high-arched palate, although frequently described, is not a common feature. A tall stature, long thin digits and alteration in the body proportions are seen; the distance from the soles to the pubis (lower segment) is greater than the distance from the pubis to the vertex (upper segment). The arm span, measured from the extended fingers, often exceeds the height of the patient.

Joints. A laxity of ligaments may give rise to dislocation of joints such as the jaw or patellae. Steinberg's sign occurs when the thumbs are adducted over the palm and their tips are seen to cross the ulnar border of the hand. Inguinal or femoral hernias are often seen.

Respiratory system. Pulmonary changes include hernia of the diaphragm, emphysema and spontaneous pneumothorax.

Cardiovascular system. Cardiovascular symptoms follow the degeneration in the media of vessel walls. The aortic valve ring may dilate and produce an incompetent valve, and less commonly the mitral valve is similarly involved, producing the 'billowy valve syndrome' (see p. 590). Aneurysm formation may occur, usually in the ascending aorta, and may be followed by dissection and/or rupture.

Eyes. Weakness of the suspensory ligament of the lens may cause dislocation; this is a common clinical feature of the disease.

Diseases of the hair and nails

Both hair and nails are composed of keratin and are derived principally from the epidermal layer (see p. 1001). Each may be affected by the same type of disease process, e.g. lichen planus, or altered by conditions that affect primarily the epidermis.

DISORDERS OF HAIR GROWTH

The extent and distribution of body hair is largely determined genetically. At the time of puberty, terminal hair growth occurs in males on the beard area, over the upper lip, chest, abdomen and thighs. Androgens determine the extent of secondary sexual patterns of hair growth during adolescence in both sexes. In females any marked alteration in the extent of hair growth or hair loss at times other than at puberty or the menopause may reflect serious endocrine disturbance.

Hirsuties (see p. 788)

Hirsuties is defined as an excessive growth in females of hair of male type and distribution. In many parts of the world an excess of body hair is accepted as a racial characteristic or may, in addition, be seen as a family trait. In the Western World, excess body hair in females is considered less acceptable and women may become self-conscious about the extent of their hair growth.

Most hirsute females do not have recognizable clinical or biochemical evidence of endocrine disease, though this must be excluded by a careful history, examination and hormone profile where appropriate.

Some drugs alter the texture and extent of hair growth; these include cortisone, minoxidil, diazoxide, hydantoins and cyclosporin A. Here the hair growth is non-androgenic in pattern and the term *hypertrichosis* is used.

The problem should not be dismissed lightly as most women who are affected are not prepared to accept these cutaneous manifestations of androgenicity.

Methods of hair removal include removal by abrasion with mittens that have a roughened surface, shaving and plucking, but these give short-term relief. Depilatory creams and waxing should not be used frequently on facial hair but may be used elsewhere, such as on the legs.

Bleaching facial hair with peroxides will produce an acceptable appearance for fine hair. Coarse hairs are best dealt with by electrolysis but this needs to be performed by skilled personnel and may produce scarring, especially if acne is a concurrent problem on the chin. With severe hirsutism, anti-androgens (e.g. cyproterone acetate) or prednisolone (5 mg at night and 2.5 mg in the morning) may be used to produce a slowing of hair growth so that mechanical removal need not be so frequent or vigorous.

Hair loss

Hair loss that occurs to the extent that scalp skin becomes abnormally visible is termed alopecia. It may be permanent, when the hair follicles are damaged by scarring (e.g. in lichen planus or discoid lupus erythematosus), or may recover if the follicles are left intact (e.g. in some endocrine diseases or alopecia areata).

Diffuse hair loss
Hairs are lost in the telogen phase. Normally about 100 hairs are shed each day. In severe illness or following pregnancy there is an increase in the number of hairs entering the telogen phase (telogen effluvium). Hair loss is seen 3–4 months after the event when the new anagen hair pushes out the old telogen hair. Nail growth may be affected in the same way.

Other causes of diffuse hair loss include endocrine disease such as hyperthyroidism or hypothyroidism and androgen overactivity in both males and females. Iron deficiency, rapid weight loss associated with dieting, and drugs such as lithium or vitamin A and its derivatives also produce diffuse and treatable hair loss.

Alopecia areata
This occurs in both sexes and all races and is usually seen in young adults or children as a well-defined path of hair loss. Only 25% of cases are seen over the age of 40 years and 25% of patients give a family history of the condition.

AETIOLOGY

There is often a personal or family history of atopy. Alopecia areata occurs in association with autoimmune diseases such as thyrotoxicosis, Addison's disease, pernicious anaemia and chronic active hepatitis.

The association of alopecia areata with such diseases suggests that immune changes are important in the pathogenesis. It is also seen in association with Down's syndrome, vitiligo and hypogammaglobulinaemia.

CLINICAL FEATURES

Patients are often dark-skinned and patches of hair loss can occur over any part of the body, e.g. the beard area or eyebrows, but the scalp is most frequently affected. Asymptomatic loss may first be noticed by a relative or hairdresser. Patches tend to re-grow over the course of several months within the scalp margin in adults. An extension into the actual hair margin (ophiasis) is often less quick to recover. Children with an atopic background may lose all their scalp hair (alopecia totalis) and the prognosis in such patients should be guarded; alopecia totalis is seen less frequently in adults. Loss of hair from all body sites (alopecia universalis) may occur by extension from other sites but can also occur acutely.

The extension of hair loss occurs in a peripheral fashion; at the advancing edge, broken hairs (exclamation mark hairs) provide evidence of disease activity. Diffuse loss of hairs in alopecia areata is an infrequent occurrence and may be difficult to differentiate from other causes of hair loss.

Re-growing hair appears as a fine, depigmented downy growth. Areas of alopecia principally affect pigmented hair and premature greying is seen after diffuse hair loss.

TREATMENT

Large doses of corticosteroids will produce a regrowth of hair, but relapse occurs after treatment is stopped. Topical corticosteroids may also help to speed the rate of regrowth of hair. Other treatment modalities, effective in small numbers of patients, include PUVA therapy and topical minoxidil. This is available as a 2% solution. It will induce hair growth in about one-third of individuals but this tends to fall out on cessation of treatment.

Premature male-pattern baldness
Recession of the hair margin is an ageing characteristic of primates. This may appear early in males but such a pattern of loss in young females may indicate serious androgenicity. Vertical thinning is seen in association with margin recession in both sexes. In young women there is often evidence of androgen excess, which may be treated by anti-androgen therapy over an interval of a year with some recovery. The primary defect is atrophy of the hair follicle. It is due to a number of factors other than excess androgen activity, for antiandrogen therapy is not always effective in stimulating strong terminal hair growth in females.

Abnormalities of the hair shaft
The hair shaft may become twisted, beaded or broken, leading to hair loss. Short, unruly or broken hair is then the primary complaint. Similar patterns of loss will be seen with drying of the hair or the effect of weathering, cosmetics, bleaching agents or grooming.

Traction
Traction associated with fashion, traditional or ethnic practices, such as hot combing, braiding or plaiting, may also cause a localized hair fall, especially over the temporal region. Straightening or relaxing the hair, undertaken by those with naturally curly hair may, in addition, produce permanent root damage.

DISEASES OF THE NAILS

The nail plate grows continuously, although the rate varies with age, slowing with advancing years, and with some generalized diseases. Growth of fingernails is normally at a rate of about 1 cm every 3 months, so that renewal of a fingernail may take 6 months, and toe-nails, which grow more slowly, may take from 18 months to 2 years. An increase in the rate of growth of the nail plate occurs in psoriasis and other skin diseases.

The nail plate arises from the matrix and lies on the nail bed that also contributes to its growth. The hard outer layer is formed from the proximal matrix and the bulk of the nail, composed of soft keratin, is produced by the distal matrix.

The nail matrix lies within a fold of epidermis, so that dermatoses or infections that involve the posterior nail fold may also cause abnormalities of the nail plate; these include chronic paronychia, fungal disease, eczema and psoriasis. These nail changes have been discussed in the appropriate sections.

Congenital defects of the nail occur in conjunction with abnormalities of the epidermis, teeth or skeleton.

Nail disorders in generalized diseases

Clubbing. This is discussed on p. 639.

Connective tissue diseases
Short and brittle nails occur in severe circulatory disorders, e.g. Raynaud's phenomenon (see p. 624), especially in association with systemic sclerosis. Pterygium formation also occurs when a thin skin-fold merges with the cuticle, widening it by several millimetres. Chronic paronychia may persist despite all therapeutic manoeuvres in patients with severe digital ischaemia. Nail fold capillary dilatation and distortion or the absence of capillaries, usually with severe Raynaud's phenomenon, is seen in systemic sclerosis. Ragged cuticles containing haemorrhages are often most pronounced in patients with dermatomyositis.

Yellow nail syndrome
The nail plate is thickened, yellow in colour, smooth and with an increased lateral curvature. The rate of growth of the nail is reduced. Such nails are seen in association with chronic oedema of the hands, feet, ankles or face, congenital

lymphoedema, pleural effusions, chronic sinus infection and thyroid disease.

White bands
Distal white bands that are parallel to the lunula and separated from this and each other by a normal pink-coloured portion are seen in patients with hypoalbuminaemia. The nails return to normal when the level of protein is restored.

Half-and-half nails
This is the name given to nails in which the proximal nail is pale or white and the distal portion is red or brown in colour; these nails occur in renal failure.

Brown streaks
Longitudinal brown streaks are commonly seen in black patients when pigment cells are incorporated into the nail matrix. Alteration of pigment beneath the nails that is localized and not related to obvious trauma in white-skinned patients may require a biopsy of the nail to exclude subungual melanoma.

Onycholysis
Onycholysis or separation of the distal edge of the nail from the vascular nail bed will cause whiteness of the free edge and this most commonly follows trauma or faulty or excessive manicure. Psoriasis is another common cause and similar changes may be seen in thyrotoxicosis or following photo-onycholysis produced by photoactive drugs such as tetracycline or psoralens, as well as in porphyria.

Splinter haemorrhages
These are most frequently caused by trauma to the nail; subacute infective endocarditis, systemic lupus erythematosus and psoriasis are less common causes.

Koilonychia
Spoon-shaped nails or koilonychia is seen in association with iron deficiency anaemia but it may also follow trauma, e.g. in garage mechanics who regularly fit tyres.

Chronic paronychia
This is due to chronic infection from *Candida albicans*. It is rarely a manifestation of an under-lying systemic disease such as hypoparathyroidism, multiple endocrine disease or chronic iron deficiency.

Transverse lines
Transverse lines (Beau's lines) related to acute physical or psychiatric illness or the use of cytotoxic drugs represent a temporary arrest of growth. They may be associated with an arrest of hair growth and subsequent fall (telogen effluvium).

Blue discoloration of the nail
This may be seen in hepatolenticular degeneration (Wilson's disease) as blue lanulae.

Effects of drugs

A number of drugs, including antimalarials such as chloroquine may cause a blue/black discoloration of the nail plate. Mepacrine may stain the nail plate blue and fluoresces green on examination by Wood's light. Argyria occurring as an occupational disease or following, for example, the use of silver-containing nose drops will stain the nails a grey/blue colour. Phenothiazine produces a blue/black coloration that is often accentuated in summer-time.

Cytotoxic drugs
Diffuse, longitudinal or horizontal melanonychia affecting the nail base or nail plate may occur in association with pigmentary changes of the surrounding skin with doxorubicin, busulphan, cyclophosphamide and daunorubicin therapy.

Further reading

Baker H (ed) (1989) *Clinical dermatology*, 4th ed. London: Baillière Tindall.

Fitzpatrick TB (ed) (1987) *Dermatology in General Medicine*, 3rd ed. New York: McGraw–Hill.

Kirby J (1986) *Roxburgh's Common Skin Diseases*. London: Lewis.

Mackie R (ed) (1984) *Current Perspectives in Immunodermatology*. Edinburgh: Churchill Livingstone.

Appendices

Diets

These diets were compiled by Jasmine Challis, Senior Dietitian, and Eileen McKay, District Dietitian, St Bartholomew's Hospital, London.

DIABETIC DIET

The basic principles of the diabetic diet are given below.

- Sugar and foods with a high sugar content, e.g. sweets, chocolate, honey, preserves, sweet biscuits, cakes, ordinary fruit squashes and fizzy drinks, and sweet alcoholic drinks, generally should be avoided. (For some diabetics, these can be included if taken in conjunction with complex carbohydrates.)
- Fats should be used sparingly.
- Fibre intake should be increased by the use of wholemeal bread and high-fibre cereals, pulses and fruit.
- Salt should be used sparingly.
- Protein intake should be normal.
- Most vegetables, herbs, spices, condiments (except salt), tea, coffee, sugar-free squashes and fizzy drinks, and soda water are allowed freely.
- Carbohydrate foods with a low sugar content should provide a high proportion of the energy intake. Carbohydrate intake should be spread throughout the day to include between-meal and bedtime snacks.
- Alcohol can be taken in moderation.

Patients who are overweight are given an appropriate reducing diet until they achieve ideal weight.

To provide variety in the diet, a system of carbohydrate exchanges is used, some of which are listed below. Each of the following contains approximately 10 g of carbohydrate (CHO) and is equal to one 'exchange':

- 1 small slice bread
- 2 crackers or plain biscuits
- 1 digestive biscuit
- 1 portion of a breakfast cereal
- 1 small potato ('egg-sized')
- 1 heaped tablespoon boiled rice
- ⅓ pint (175 ml) milk
- 1 small carton plain yoghurt
- 2 tablespoons dried beans
- 1 apple, orange, pear or peach
- 1 small banana
- 1 small glass orange juice (100 ml)

SAMPLE MEAL PLAN

For a lean patient maintaining weight on 2000 kcal (8400 kJ) and 260 g of CHO (i.e. 50% of total energy as CHO).

	CHO (g)
Daily	
175 ml semi-skimmed milk for tea or coffee	10
20 g polyunsaturated margarine	
Breakfast (60 g CHO)	
2 portions of a breakfast cereal	20
175 ml semi-skimmed milk	10
2 slices wholemeal bread	20
Margarine from allowance	
100 ml orange juice	10
Mid-morning (20 g CH0)	
Large banana	20
Lunch (60 g CHO)	
4 slices wholemeal bread for sandwiches—	
with lean meat, and salad vegetables	40
Low-fat plain yoghurt	10
Pear	10
Mid-afternoon (20 g CHO)	
2 digestive biscuits	20
Evening meal (60 g CHO)	
Beef and butterbean casserole	10
Jacket potato	30
Vegetables	
Baked apple with dates	20
Bedtime (30 g CHO)	
Wholemeal fruit bun	30
	Total 260 g CHO

It should be remembered that patients will have to be instructed how to maintain their carbohydrate intake during illness, cope with their diet while travelling, and adjust their intake prior to exercise.

GLUTEN-FREE DIET

This is used for the treatment of coeliac disease and dermatitis herpetiformis.

The diet involves the exclusion of wheat, rye, barley and oats. *Any* food containing gluten— either as an obvious constituent (e.g. flour, bread) or as a 'hidden' ingredient (e.g. stock cubes, dessert mixes)—must be avoided.

Foods allowed

- Gluten-free (GF) bread*, CF crispbread*, GF pasta*
- GF flour*, soya flour, potato flour, pea flour, rice flour
- Soya bran, rice bran
- GF biscuits, GF cakes
- Breakfast cereals
- Rice, tapioca, sago, arrowroot, buckwheat, millet, maize
- Fresh or frozen meat, poultry, offal
- Plain fresh or frozen fish, fish canned in oil
- Eggs, plain cheeses
- Milk, cream, butter, margarine, oils
- Plain fresh, frozen or tinned vegetables and potatoes
- Tinned fruit in syrup or natural juice, fresh or frozen fruit
- Nuts
- Tea, coffee, fruit juice, fruit squash, fizzy drinks
- Sugar, glucose, boiled sweets, syrup, honey, jam, marmalade, jelly, gelatine
- Herbs, spices, mustard, vinegar, salt, pepper
- Monosodium glutamate
- Wine, beer, spirits, liqueurs

*Products prescribable on the National Health Service in the UK for coeliac disease and dermatitis herpetiformis.

In addition, any home-made items, e.g. soups or sauces, made with GF ingredients are obviously suitable.

Foods forbidden

- Ordinary bread, crispbreads, pasta
- Ordinary flour, rye flour, barley flour
- Wheat bran
- Ordinary biscuits and cakes
- Breakfast cereals made with wheat or oats
- Barley, oatmeal, semolina
- Meat pies, most beefburgers, most sausages, most tinned meats
- Fish with breadcrumbs or batter, fish cakes, fish in sauce
- Potato croquettes
- Fruit pies
- Some night-time drinks, barley water
- Most stock cubes and gravy mixes

The lists above are *not* comprehensive and it is not always possible to tell from a 'label' whether or not a manufactured product is gluten-free. In the UK The Coeliac Society produces a comprehensive list of manufactured foods which are gluten-free and patients prescribed such a diet are advised to join:

The Coeliac Society
PO Box 220
High Wycombe
Bucks HP11 2HY

DIETS IN RENAL DISEASE

Restricted-protein diet

This is used in the treatment of patients with symptomatic uraemia or in patients with asymptomatic moderate renal failure (creatinine clearance < 40 ml·min^{-1}) in the hope of slowing the rate of deterioration in renal function otherwise destined to occur.

Protein	0.6 g·kg^{-1} ideal body weight per day
Energy	35 kcal·kg (150 kJ·kg^{-1}) ideal body weight per day
Sodium	~ 50 mmol per day (unless salt waster)
Potassium	Restricted to ~ 50 mmol if the patient becomes hyperkalaemic

SAMPLE MENU PLAN

For 70 kg person, moderately active, not overweight:

Protein = 42 g; energy = 2500 kcal (10 500 kJ), sodium ~ 50 mmol; potassium ~ 50 mmol.

Breakfast
1 egg
2 slices white/wholemeal bread with unsalted polyunsaturated margarine or unsalted butter
Jam, marmalade or honey

Lunch
25 g meat or 40 g fish
2 slices white/wholemeal bread with unsalted polyunsaturated margarine or unsalted butter
1 portion vegetable
1 portion fruit and double cream

Evening meal
50 g meat or 75 g fish
150 g potatoes
1 portion vegetable
1 portion fruit and double cream

Daily
175 ml milk, 1 bottle Hycal or equivalent, 50 g unsalted butter or unsalted polyunsaturated margarine, 75 ml double cream

Suitable drinks
Tea, lemonade, cola drinks, bitter lemon—as part of fluid allowance

Allowed freely
Sugar, jam, honey, marmalade, boiled sweets, low-protein products.

A small amount of salt may be used in cooking but none added at table. See 'no-added-salt' diet for further restrictions. Salt intake may need to be increased, for example, in salt wasters.

Nephrotic syndrome

This diet contains 70–80 g of protein and 60–100 mmol sodium.

SAMPLE MEAL PLAN

Breakfast
Cereal with milk
2 slices toast with polyunsaturated margarine or butter

Main meal
100 g meat or 150 g fish
Potatoes or rice
Vegetables
Milk pudding, pudding with custard or fruit and ice cream

Snack meal
50 g meat or 75 g fish
Bread or potatoes
Vegetables or salad
Fruit

Daily
~ 1 pint of milk

Usually a small amount of salt may be used in cooking but none added at table. See 'no-added-salt' diet for further restriction.

Low-calcium, low-oxalate diet

This is required in hypercalciuric or hyperoxaluric stone formers, in combination with a high fluid intake (> 2 litres daily).

SAMPLE MEAL PLAN

Breakfast
1 egg
1 slice white bread with butter
Cereal

Main meal
Average helping of meat or fish
Potatoes or rice
Vegetables
Fruit or jelly

Snack meal
Average helping of meat or fish
2 slices white bread with butter

Daily
150 ml milk

Avoid
Foods rich in calcium, e.g. cheese, ice-cream, yoghurt, extra milk
Foods rich in oxalate, e.g. rhubarb, spinach, beetroot, beans

Tea intake is restricted to 4 cups daily.

DIET IN LIVER DISEASE

40 g protein, no-added-salt diet

This is used in the treatment of liver disease. See 'no-added-salt' diet for additional instructions.

SAMPLE MEAL PLAN

Daily
150 ml milk

Breakfast
Fruit juice
1 egg
1 slice bread or toast with butter and jam or marmalade
Tea or coffee with milk from allowance

Mid-morning
Fruit juice
Tea or coffee with milk from allowance

Lunch
25 g meat or 40 g fish or 1 egg or 1 small yoghurt or 3 tablespoons pulses
1 slice bread or equivalent
Vegetables or salad
Fruit

Mid-afternoon
1 slice bread with butter and jam or honey
Tea or coffee with milk from allowance

Evening meal
25 g meat or 40 g fish or 1 egg or 1 small yoghurt
    or 3 tablespoons pulses
1 slice bread or equivalent
Vegetables or salad
Fruit

Bedtime
1 slice bread or equivalent
Tea or coffee with remainder of milk allowance

Fat and fatty foods must be restricted if poorly tolerated. Alcohol must be avoided.

1 slice of bread may be exchanged for any of the following:

3 plain biscuits
2 crispbreads
1 small bowl breakfast cereal or porridge
2 tablespoons cooked rice or cooked pasta
2 small potatoes
1 small slice cake
1 tablespoon flour
1 tablespoon ice-cream

Extras
Sugar
Glucose
Boiled sweets
Mints
Fruit squash
Fizzy drinks
Fruit
Fruit juice

These are 'encouraged' in order to increase energy intake.

SALT-RESTRICTION DIETS

No-added-salt diet

This restricts sodium intake to between 60 and 100 mmol daily depending on energy intake. A small amount of salt may be used in cooking, but none must be used at table.

The following foods contain considerable amounts of sodium and *must be avoided*:

Bacon, ham, sausages, pâté
Cheese
Tinned fish and meat
Smoked fish and meat
Fish and meat pastes
Tinned vegetables
Tinned and packet soups
Sauce mixes
Bottled sauces and chutneys
Meat and vegetable extracts, stock cubes
Salted nuts and crisps
Soya sauce
Monosodium glutamate

40 mmol sodium diet

This is used in the treatment of ascites or severe oedema associated with salt and water retention. It is often used in conjunction with fluid restriction and/or diuretics.

In addition to avoiding the foods listed under 'no-added-salt' diet, the following restrictions apply:

● No salt to be used in cooking or at table
● Salt-free butter must be used
● Milk should be restricted to 300 ml daily
● Only 4 slices ordinary bread are permitted daily—extra bread must be salt-free
● Choose breakfast cereals that are free from added salt

22 mmol sodium diet

As above but replace ordinary bread with salt-free bread.

LOW-FAT DIET

If the body's ability to digest and/or absorb fat is impaired, a diet low in fat is indicated. In this case *all* fats, i.e. both animal and vegetable in origin, must be restricted.

Where fat tolerance is low it is better to distribute the fat intake throughout the day.

Care should be taken to check the fat content of manufactured foods.

SAMPLE MEAL PLAN

Daily
Low-fat milk as required
10 g butter or margarine or oil or 20 g 'low-fat' spread

Breakfast
Fruit or fruit juice
Breakfast cereal or porridge
Bread or toast with butter or margarine from allowance
Jam, marmalade or honey

Snack meal
Lean meat, chicken, low-fat cheese, egg, fish or baked beans
Bread, toast or crispbread
Vegetables or salad
Fruit or low-fat yoghurt

Main meal
Clear soup, fruit juice, melon or grapefruit
Lean meat, chicken or fish cooked without fat, beans or pulses
Potato, rice or pasta cooked without fat

Vegetables or salad
Fruit, jelly or pudding made with low-fat milk

Beverages
Tea, coffee, fruit juice, fruit squash or fizzy drinks

Extras
Boiled sweets, mints, fruit gums, meringues, water ice, ice lollies
Plain or semi-sweet biscuits
Herbs, spices, mustard, vinegar, pickles, oil-free salad dressings

REDUCING DIET

This diet is suitable for obese diabetics, although distribution of carbohydrate-containing foods may need modification for those on oral hypoglycaemic agents or insulin. Energy restriction is achieved by reducing *fat*, *sugar* and *alcohol*, while maintaining a modest intake of fibre-containing carbohydrate foods.

SAMPLE MEAL PLAN

Breakfast
Small cupful of breakfast cereal or porridge with low-fat milk, no sugar
1 slice wholemeal bread or toast with a little butter or margarine*

Snack meal
Average helping of lean meat, poultry, fish, eggs, cheese or small tin baked beans
Salad vegetables
2 slices wholemeal bread or 4 crispbread or 2 small potatoes
Fresh fruit or sugar-free, low-fat yoghurt

Main meal
Average helping of lean meat, poultry, fish, eggs, cheese or pulses
Cooked vegetable and/or side salad
1 small potato or 1 tablespoon boiled rice or 1 slice wholemeal bread
Fruit, fresh or tinned in natural juice

Low-fat milk (skimmed or semi-skimmed) should be used in tea and coffee. Artificial sweeteners may be used if necessary. Other suitable drinks include sugar-free squashes and fizzy drinks, soda water, and mineral water.

* Not more than 100 g of butter or margarine is allowed per week.

Avoid:
Sweets, chocolate, honey, preserves, sweet biscuits, cakes, tinned fruit in syrup, puddings

Ordinary fruit squash and fizzy drinks
Malted milk drinks and drinking chocolate
Fried foods, cream, mayonnaise, salad dressing, crisps, cream cheese, pastry, dumplings, avocado pear, nuts
Alcohol

CHOLESTEROL-LOWERING DIET

The diet involves reducing total fat intake (particularly saturated fat) and restricting foods high in cholesterol. Foods high in fibre are encouraged.
Overweight patients would normally be given a suitably modified reducing diet.

SAMPLE MEAL PLAN

Breakfast
Fruit or fruit juice
Cereal (preferably wholegrain) or porridge with low-fat milk
Bread (preferably wholemeal) with polyunsaturated margarine
Jam, marmalade or honey

Snack meal
Sandwich or salad with *lean* meat, fish or low-fat cheese
Bread or crispbread with polyunsaturated margarine *or* baked beans on toast
Fresh fruit or low-fat yoghurt

Main meal
Clear soup, fruit juice, melon or grapefruit
Lean meat or fish or low-fat cheese
Vegetables
Potatoes—jacket (with polyunsaturated margarine or low-fat yoghurt), boiled, mashed or fried in polyunsaturated oil, or pasta or rice
Fruit, jelly or pudding made with low-fat milk

Avoid:
Butter, lard, suet, cooking fats, other margarines, 'vegetable oils', coconut oil, salad cream, mayonnaise, egg yolk, whole milk, dried milk with added vegetable fat, cream, yoghurt made with whole milk
Duck, goose, offal, sausages, pâté, luncheon meat, salami-type sausages
Fish roe, prawns, shrimps
Avocado pear, nuts, crisps
Ice-cream, tinned and packet desserts, chocolate spread, lemon curd, chocolate, toffee, butterscotch, cocoa, drinking chocolate, malted milk drinks
All biscuits (except crispbreads, water biscuits, plain and semi-sweet biscuits), cakes, pastries, pies (unless made with suitable ingredients)

CHOLESTEROL- AND TRIGLYCERIDE-LOWERING DIET

In addition to the restrictions listed under the cholesterol-lowering diet, sugar and foods with a high sugar content must be avoided. Carbohydrate foods with a high fibre content are encouraged. Alcohol intake should be restricted.

For overweight patients a modified reducing diet is advised.

DIETS FOR SPECIFIC URINE COLLECTIONS

Diet for 5HIAA collections (Carcinoid)

The following items may need to be avoided prior to 5-hydroxyindole acetic acid (5HIAA) urine collections:

- Tomatoes and tomato products
- Broad beans
- Bananas
- Plums
- Pineapple
- Avocado pears
- Aubergines
- Plantain
- Papaw, passion fruit
- Nuts

Diet for VMA collections (Phaeo)

The following foods may need to be avoided prior to vanillylmandelic acid (VMA) urine collections:

- Vanilla essence
- Vanilla-containing foods
  Ice-cream
  Cakes
  Biscuits
  Puddings
  Desserts and dessert mixes
  Custard

- Bananas
- Nuts
- Chocolate and bedtime beverages
- Coffee
- Cola-flavoured drinks and foods

Standard total parenteral regiment for a 24-hour period

This regimen provides:

- 35–45 kcal·kg^{-1} (150–190 kJ·kg^{-1}) daily
- 35% of the non-protein energy as fat
- 65% of the non-protein energy as carbohydrate
- 14–20 g of nitrogen

The following are mixed in a 3-litre bag under laminar-flow conditions in the pharmacy:

1 L Synthamin 14 with electrolytes	348 kcal
0.5 L 20% Intralipid	900 kcal
1.5 L 20% dextrose	1200 kcal
	2448 kcal

+ 10 ml Vitlipid Adult (fat-soluble vitamins)
+ 10 ml Addamel (minerals)
+ 1 vial Solivito (water-soluble vitamins)
+ 15 units soluble insulin

Careful biochemical monitoring is essential.

Standard enteric diet

This is given in Table 3.13 (p. 167).

Normal values

These normal values were compiled by Ruth Halliday, SRN, and modified by Katherine Woodward , RGN, St Bartholomew's Hospital. Values vary from one laboratory to another. Please check with your own laboratory.

HAEMATOLOGY

Haemoglobin
    Male   14.0–17.7 g·dl^{-1}
    Female   12.2–15.2 g·dl^{-1}

Mean corpuscular haemoglobin (MCH)	27–33 pg
Mean corpuscular haemoglobin concentration (MCHC)	32–35 g·dl^{-1}
Mean corpuscular volume (MCV)	80–96 fl.
Packed cell volume (PCV)	
Male	0.42–0.53 L·L^{-1}
Female	0.36–0.45 L·L^{-1}
White cell count (WCC)	4–11 × 10^9/L
Basophil granulocytes	< 0.01–0.1 × 10^9/L
Eosinophil granulocytes	0.04–0.4 × 10^9/L
Lymphocytes	1.5–4.0 × 10^9/L
Monocytes	0.2–0.8 × 10^9/L
Neutrophil granulocytes	3.5–7.5 × 10^9/L
Total blood volume	60–80 ml·kg^{-1}
Plasma volume	40–50 ml·kg^{-1}
Platelet count	150–400 × 10^9/L
Serum B$_{12}$	160–925 ng·L^{-1} (150–675 pmol·L^{-1})
Serum folate	4–18 μg·L^{-1} (5–63 nmol·L^{-1})
Red cell folate	160–640 μg·L^{-1}
Red cell mass	
Male	25–35 ml·kg^{-1}
Female	20–30 ml·kg^{-1}
Reticulocyte count	0.2–2.0% of red cells (10–100 × 10^9/L)
Erythrocyte sedimentation rate (ESR)	< 20 mm in 1 h

Coagulation

Bleeding time	3–10 min
Partial thromboblastin time (PTTK)	30–50 s
Prothrombin time	16–18 s
International Normalised Ratio (INR)	1

BIOCHEMISTRY

Acid phosphatase	1–5 U·L^{-1}
Alanine aminotransferase (ALT)	5–30 U·L^{-1}
Albumin	34–48 g·L^{-1}
Alkaline phosphatase	25–115 U·L^{-1}
Alpha-1-antitrypsin	2–4 g·L^{-1}
Alpha-fetoprotein	< 10 kU·L^{-1}
Amylase	< 220 U·L^{-1}
Angiotensin-converting enzyme	204–358 U·L^{-1}
Aspartate aminotransferase (AST)	10–40 U·L^{-1}
Bicarbonate	22–30 mmol·L^{-1}
Bilirubin	< 17 μmol·L^{-1} (0.3–1.5 mg·dl^{-1})

Caeruloplasmin	$0.20–0.45$ g·L^{-1}
Calcium	$2.20–2.67$ mmol·L^{-1} ($8.5–10.5$ mg·dl^{-1})
Chloride	$100–106$ mmol·L^{-1}
Cholinesterase	$2.25–7.0$ U·L^{-1}
Copper	$12–25$ μmol·L^{-1} ($100–200$ mg·dl^{-1})
C-reactive protein	< 10 mg·L^{-1}
Creatinine	$60–120$ μmol·L^{-1} ($0.6–1.5$ mg·dl^{-1})

Creatinine kinase (CPK)
   Female $24–170$ U·L^{-1}
   Male $24–195$ U·L^{-1}

C_3	$0.55–1.20$ g·L^{-1}
C_4	$0.20–0.50$ g·L^{-1}
Ferritin	$5.8–120$ nmol·L^{-1} ($15–250$ μg·L^{-1})

Gamma-glutamyl transpeptidase (γ-GT)
   Male $11–50$ U·L^{-1}
   Female $7–32$ U·L^{-1}

Glucose	$4.5–5.6$ mmol·L^{-1} ($70–110$ mg·dl^{-1})
Glycosylated haemoglobin (HbA$_{1c}$)	$3.8–6.4\%$
Hydroxybutyric dehydrogenase (HBD)	$40–150$ U·L^{-1}

Immunoglobulins (11 years and over)
   IgA $0.8–4$ g·L^{-1}
   IgG $7.0–18.0$ g·L^{-1}
   IgM $0.4–2.5$ g·L^{-1}

Iron	$13–32$ μmol·L^{-1} ($50–150$ μg·dl^{-1})
Iron binding capacity (total) TIBC	$42–80$ μmol·L^{-1} ($250–410$ μg·dl^{-1})
Lactate dehydrogenase	$240–525$ U·L^{-1}
Lead	< 1.2 μmol·L^{-1}
Magnesium	$0.7–1.1$ mmol·L^{-1}
Osmolality	$280–296$ mosmol·kg^{-1}
Phosphate	$0.8–1.5$ mmol·L^{-1}
Potassium	$3.5–5.0$ mmol·L^{-1}
Protein (total)	$62–80$ g·L^{-1}
Sodium	$135–146$ mmol·L^{-1}
Urate	$180–420$ μmol·L^{-1} ($3.0–7.0$ mg·dl^{-1})
Urea	$2.5–6.7$ mmol·L^{-1} ($8–25$ mg·dl^{-1})
Vitamin A	$0.5–2.01$ μmol·L^{-1}

Vitamin D
   25-hydroxy $37–200$ nmol·L^{-1} ($0.15–0.80$ ng·L^{-1})
   1,25-dihydroxy $60–108$ pmol·L^{-1} ($0.24–0.45$ pg·L^{-1})

Zinc	$7–18$ μmol·L^{-1}

Lipids and lipoproteins

Cholesterol	$3.5–6.5$ mmol·L^{-1} (ideal < 5.2 mmol·L^{-1})

HDL cholesterol
 Male   0.9–1.4 mmol·L^{-1}
 Female   1.2–1.7 mmol·L^{-1}

Lipids (total)   4.0–10.0 g·L^{-1}

Lipoproteins
 VLDL   0.128–0.645 mmol·L^{-1}
 LDL   1.55–4.4 mmol·L^{-1}
 HDL Male   0.70–2.1 mmol·L^{-1}
   Female   0.50–1.70 mmol·L^{-1}

Non-esterified fatty acids
 Male   0.19–0.78 mmol·L^{-1}
 Female   0.06–0.9 mmol·L^{-1}

Phospholipid   2.9–5.2 mmol·L^{-1}

Triglycerides
 Male   0.70–2.1 mmol·L^{-1}
 Female   0.50–1.70 mmol·L^{-1}

Blood gases

Arterial P_{CO_2} 4.8–6.1 kPa (36–46 mm Hg)

Arterial P_{O_2} 10–13.3 kPa (75–100 mm Hg)

Arterial [H$^+$]   35–45 nmol·L^{-1}

Arterial pH   7.35–7.45

Urine values

Calcium   7.5 mmol daily or less (< 300 mg daily)

Copper   0.2–1.0 µmol daily

Creatinine   0.13–0.22 mmol·kg^{-1} body weight, daily

5-Hydroxyindole acetic acid   5–75 µmol daily; amounts lower in females than
                                          males

Protein (quantitative)   < 0.15 g per 24 h

Tests in endocrinology

These tests were compiled by Dr Paul Drury, Consultant Physician, King's College Hospital, London.

General

Different laboratories will have different normal ranges for many of these tests, and slightly different protocols—*always* consult the laboratory before performing or interpreting these tests. Also check whether plasma or serum is required, and whether any special handling is needed.

Time, date, stage of test and date of last menstrual period when appropriate should always be noted on the request form as they are critical for interpretation.

GONADAL AXIS

Basal levels

Basal levels are often sufficient to indicate the site of the problem; they may also indicate the stage of the menstrual cycle.

Male adult

Testosterone	10–35 nmol·L^{-1}
Luteinizing hormone (LH)	1–10 u·L^{-1}
Follicle-stimulating hormone (FSH)	1–7 u·L^{-1}

Female adult

	Follicular	Mid-cycle	Luteal	Postmenopausal
LH (u·L^{-1})	2.5–21	25–70	1–10	> 50
FSH (u·L^{-1})	1–10	6–25	0.3–21	> 25
Oestradiol (pmol·L^{-1})	< 110	500–1100	300–750	< 150
Progesterone (nmol·L^{-1})	< 12	—	> 30	< 3
Testosterone (nmol·L^{-1})	0.5–3.0			

LHRH test

100 μg of luteinizing hormone releasing hormone (LHRH) is given intravenously into an indwelling catheter at time 0; samples are taken at time 0, +20 and +60 min for LH and FSH. Normal responses are:

	20 min	60 min
Female (follicular phase)		
LH (u·L^{-1})	15–42	12–35
FSH (u·L^{-1})	1–11	1–25
Male		
LH (u·L^{-1})	13–58	11–48
FSH (u·L^{-1})	1–7	1–5

Sperm counts

Volume	0.1–11 ml
Density	1.5–375 × 10^6 ml
Motility	5–95%

Prolactin

Stress can affect prolactin levels. To establish a definite abnormality several samples should be taken, ideally through an indwelling venous catheter.

Normal levels are < 400 mu·L^{-1} in most laboratories. The significance of minor increases (400–600 mu·L^{-1}) is disputed. Levels above 2000–3000 mu·L^{-1} *suggest* the presence of a prolactinoma.

GROWTH AXIS

Basal levels

Growth hormone (GH) release is episodic; however, an undetectable or very low level (< 1 mu·L^{-1}) on a random sample excludes acromegaly.

Acromegaly

In normal subjects, GH levels are suppressed to below 1–2 mu·L^{-1} during an oral glucose tolerance test (for details see Chapter 17).

GH deficiency

In children, exercise and arginine are often used to stimulate GH secretion; a level above 20 mu·L^{-1} is a normal response. The insulin tolerance test is, however, the optimal test for adults and children.

Insulin tolerance test for GH reserve

After an overnight fast, a rapid-acting human insulin is administered at 0900 via an indwelling intravenous catheter. The dose is usually 0.15 u·kg^{-1} body weight but should be 0.1 u·kg^{-1} for hypopituitarism and 0.2–0.3 u·kg^{-1} in cases of insulin resistance (e.g. acromegaly, Cushing's syndrome). Clinical hypoglycaemia and a blood glucose < 2.2 mmol·L^{-1} should be produced; if not, repeat the dose at 45 min. Samples are collected at 0, +30, +45, +60, +90 and +120 min. A normal response for GH is > 20 mu·L^{-1}. A large breakfast should be given afterwards.

The test should not be used in patients with epilepsy, heart disease or profound hypopituitarism—a normal ECG and a cortisol result > 150 nmol·L^{-1} should be seen before the test. Syringes loaded with 50% dextrose and hydrocortisone must always be available during the test.

This test is also used to measure ACTH reserve (see below).

THYROID AXIS

Basal levels

Levels of the thyroid hormones vary very little by hour or day unless patients are acutely ill; basal levels thus usually suffice.

Total serum thyroxine (T_4)	60–160 nmol·L^{-1}
Total serum triiodothyronine (T_3)	1.2–3.1 nmol·L^{-1}
Free serum thyroxine (T_4)	13–30 pmol·L^{-1}
Thyroid-stimulating hormone (TSH)	0.5–5.0 mu·L^{-1}

TRH test—now much less used

200 µg of thyrotropin-releasing hormone (TRH) is given via an indwelling intravenous catheter at time 0 after a basal sample is collected; subsequent samples are taken at +20 and +60 min. Normal responses are:

0 min	0.5–5.0 mu·l^{-1}
20 min	3.4–20 mu·l^{-1}
60 min	< 20 min level
Increment	> 2.0 mu·l^{-1}

An excessive response indicates hypothyroidism; an inadequate one indicates either primary hyperthroidism or pituitary disease.

ADRENAL AXIS

Basal levels

Adrenocorticotrophic hormone (ACTH) and cortisol levels vary episodically and with a circadian rhythm; single untimed samples are of *very* little value. Normal values are as follows for circadian studies:

	0900	2400 (must be asleep)
ACTH	10–80 ng·L^{-1}	< 10 ng·L^{-1}
Cortisol	150–700 nmol·L^{-1}	< 150 nmol·L^{-1}

Short ACTH stimulation test

This test is used to exclude Addison's disease. After taking a first sample for cortisol, 0.25 mg of tetracosactrin is given at time 0. Further samples are taken at +30 and +60 min. Normal values are:

30 min	550–1160 nmol·L^{-1}
60 min	690–1290 nmol·L^{-1}
Increment	330–850 nmol·L^{-1}

Dexamethasone suppression tests

These are used to exclude Cushing's syndrome. They are described on p. 767.

Insulin tolerance test—for ACTH reserve

This can be used to measure ACTH reserve; details are given above. It should only be performed if the 0900 cortisol is > 180 nmol·L^{-1}.

A normal response to hypoglycaemia is a cortisol level ⩾ 550 nmol·L^{-1}; most authorities also demand an increment of > 180 nmol·L^{-1}.

ENDOCRINOLOGY OF BONE

Calcium levels only change abruptly after surgery or other therapy. They are, however, dependent on protein concentration and should be measured in incuffed samples. The values given below are for albumin levels of 47 g·L^{-1}; to correct, add or subtract 0.02 mmol·L^{-1} for each g·L^{-1} of albumin below or above 47 g·L^{-1}.

Serum calcium	2.20–2.67 mmol·L^{-1}
Serum phosphate	0.80–1.50 mmol·L^{-1}
Alkaline phosphatase	25–115 U·L^{-1}
Serum parathormone (PTH)	Very variable between assays
Vitamin D 25-hydroxy	37–200 nmol·L^{-1}

ENDOCRINOLOGY OF BLOOD PRESSURE AND THIRST

Blood pressure

Plasma renin activity (PRA) varies very widely according to method—your own laboratory should be consulted.

Aldosterone (and PRA) should be measured after at least 30 min recumbency and, possibly, after 4 h ambulation. Normal values are:

| Lying | 100–500 pmol·L^{-1} |
| Standing | 200–1000 pmol·L^{-1} |

Thirst

As a screening test, early morning plasma and urine osmolalities are measured. Normal values are:

Plasma 275–290 mosmol·kg^{-1}	Plasma and urine osmolalities must be interpreted together. Further study requires a water deprivation test.
Urine Above 600 mosmol·kg^{-1} suggests good concentration	

WEIGHT AND HEIGHT CHARTS

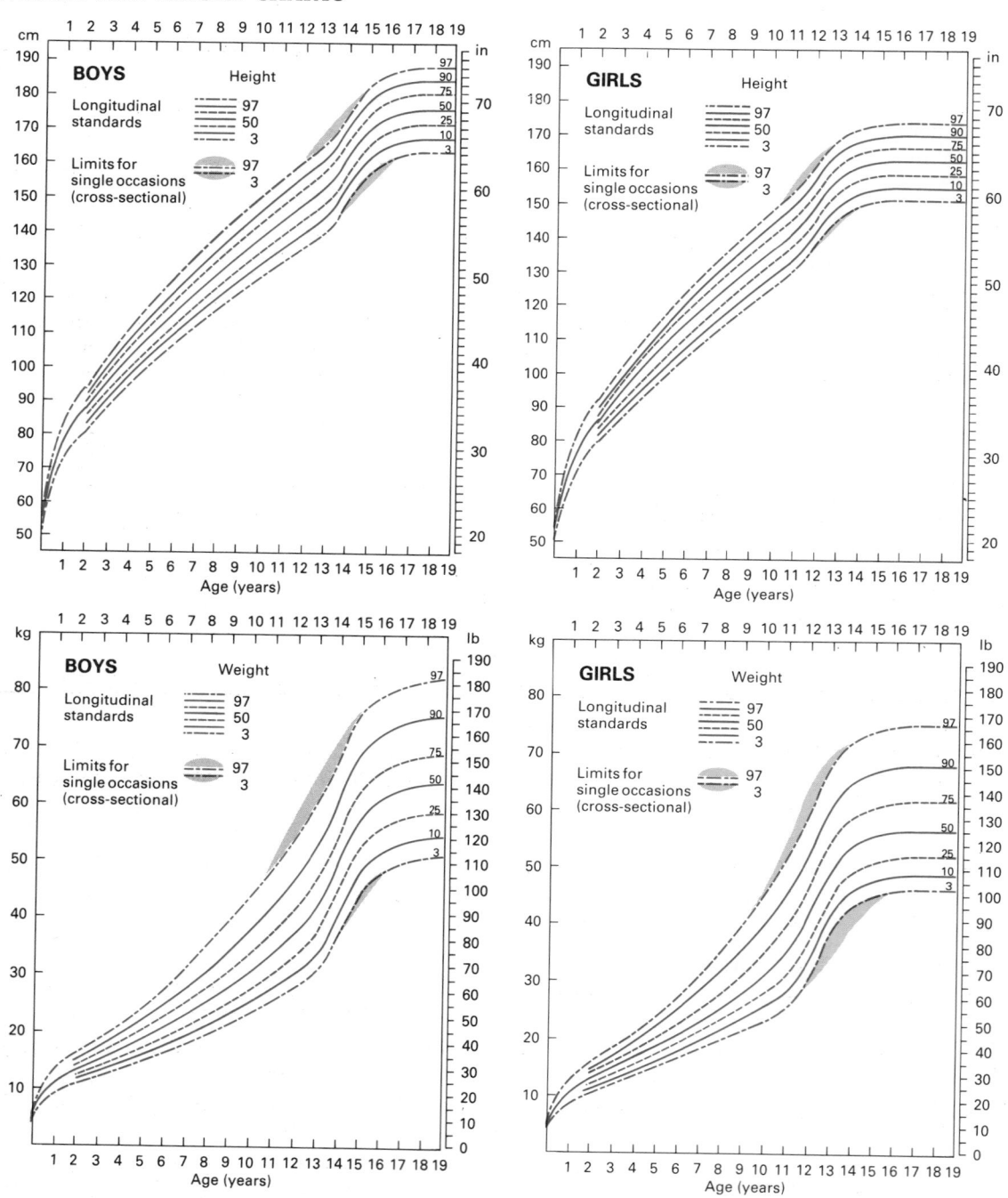

Based on Tanner–Whitehouse charts, reference 11A and 12A, reproduced by permission of Castlemead Publications.

Guidelines for body weight

Values given are weights without clothes.

Height (m)	Men (kg)			Women (kg)		
	Acceptable average	Acceptable weight range	Obese*	Acceptable average	Acceptable weight range	Obese*
1.45				46.0	42–53	64
1.48				46.5	42–54	65
1.50				47.0	43–55	66
1.52				48.5	44–57	68
1.54				49.5	44–58	70
1.56				50.4	45–58	70
1.58	55.8	51–64	77	51.3	46–59	71
1.60	57.6	52–65	78	52.6	48–61	73
1.62	58.6	53–66	79	54.0	49–62	74
1.64	59.6	54–67	80	55.4	50–64	77
1.66	60.6	55–69	83	56.8	51–65	78
1.68	61.7	56–71	85	58.1	52–66	79
1.70	63.5	58–73	88	60.0	53–67	80
1.72	65.0	59–74	89	61.3	55–69	83
1.74	66.5	60–75	90	62.6	56–70	84
1.76	68.0	62–77	92	64.0	58–72	86
1.78	69.4	64–79	95	65.3	59–74	89
1.80	71.0	65–80	96			
1.82	72.6	66–82	98			
1.84	74.2	67–84	101			
1.86	75.8	69–86	103			
1.88	77.6	71–88	106			
1.90	79.3	73–90	108			
1.92	81.0	75–93	112			
Body mass index†	22.0	20.1–25.0	30.0	20.8	18.7–23.8	28.6

* Value and above for all entries.
† Body mass index = weight (kg)/height^2 (M).

From Bray GA (ed) (1979) *Obesity in America*. Proceedings of the 2nd Fogarty International Centre Conference on Obesity, No. 79. Washington: US DHEW.

Abbreviations and symbols used in respiratory medicine

A–a	Difference of a gas pressure between alveolus (A) and pulmonary artery (a)
ARDS	Adult respiratory distress syndrome
C_aO_2	Arterial oxygen content
C_L	Lung compliance
FEV_1	Forced expiratory volume in 1 s
FRC	Functional residual capacity
FVC	Vital capacity during forced full expiration
IPPV	Intermittent positive pressure ventilation
LAP	Left atrial pressure
P_ACO_2	Partial pressure of carbon dioxide in alveolar gas
P_aCO_2	Partial pressure of carbon dioxide in arterial blood
PAEDP	Pulmonary artery end diastolic pressure
P_AO_2	Partial pressure of oxygen in alveolar gas

P_aO_2	Partial pressure of oxygen in arterial blood	$P_{\bar{v}}O_2$	Partial pressure of mixed venous oxygen
PAP	Pulmonary artery pressure	Q_t	Total cardiac output
$PD_{20\text{-}FEV1}$	Provocation dose producing a 20% reduction in FEV_1	RV	Residual volume
PCO_2	Partial pressure of carbon dioxide	SO_2	Percentage saturation of haemoglobin with oxygen
PCWP	Pulmonary capillary wedge pressure	TLC	Total lung capacity
PEFR	Peak expiratory flow rate; measured in litres per minute	$\dot{V}_{max}$	Maximal rate of air flow during forced expiration
P_ICO_2	Partial pressure of carbon dioxide in inspired air	V_A	Volume of alveolar gas
P_IO_2	Partial pressure of inspired oxygen	VC	Vital capacity
PEEP	Positive end-expiratory pressure	VT	Tidal volume
PO_2	Partial pressure of oxygen	$\dot{V}/\dot{Q}$	Ventilation : perfusion ratio

Index